W9-BQX-787

INFECTIOUS DISEASES OF THE DOG AND CAT

INFECTIOUS DISEASES OF THE DOG AND CAT

Second Edition

CRAIG E. GREENE,
D.V.M., M.S., Diplomate A.C.V.I.M.
(Internal Medicine and Neurology)
Gunst Professor, Department of Small Animal Medicine
College of Veterinary Medicine
The University of Georgia
Athens, Georgia

W.B. SAUNDERS COMPANY
A Division of Harcourt Brace & Company
Philadelphia London Toronto Montreal Sydney Tokyo

W.B. SAUNDERS COMPANY
A Division of Harcourt Brace & Company

The Curtis Center
Independence Square West
Philadelphia, Pennsylvania 19106

Library of Congress Cataloging-in-Publication Data

Infectious diseases of the dog and cat / [edited by] Craig E. Greene—2nd ed.
p. cm.

ISBN 0–7216–2737–4

1. Dogs—Infections. 2. Cats—Infections. I. Greene, Craig E.
SF 991.I54 1998 636.7′089′69—dc21

DNLM/DLC 97-30657

INFECTIOUS DISEASES OF THE DOG AND CAT ISBN 0–7216–2737–4

Printed in the United States of America.

Last digit is the print number: 9 8 7 6 5 4 3 2 1

To my wife, Jeanne, and son, Casey, for their understanding and personal sacrifice

To the contributors and the researchers in the field who have advanced our knowledge

And to the memory of Joanne Moyer, whose balanced attitude toward animal welfare and research should be admired by us all.

Contributors

Diane D. Addie, Ph.D., B.V.M.S.
University of Glasgow, Glasgow, Scotland, United Kingdom
Feline Coronavirus Infection

Max J. G. Appel, D.V.M., Ph.D.
Professor of Virology, James A. Baker Institute for Animal Health, College of Veterinary Medicine, Cornell University, Ithaca, New York
Canine Distemper, Lyme Borreliosis

Charles A. Baldwin, D.V.M., Ph.D.
Virologist, Veterinary Diagnostic Laboratory, and Associate Professor, Department of Medical Microbiology, College of Veterinary Medicine, The University of Georgia, Athens, Georgia
Arboviral Infections

Stephen C. Barr, B.V.Sc, M.V.S., Ph.D.
Associate Professor of Medicine, Department of Clinical Sciences, College of Veterinary Medicine, Cornell University, Ithaca, New York
Trypanosomiasis, Enteric Protozoal Infections, Cryptosporidiosis and Cyclosporiasis

Jeanne A. Barsanti, D.V.M., M.S., Diplomate A.C.V.I.M.
Professor and Chief, Small Animal Medicine Section, College of Veterinary Medicine; Internist, University of Georgia Veterinary Teaching Hospital, The University of Georgia, Athens, Georgia
Botulism, Genitourinary Infections

Derrick Baxby, B.Sc., Ph.D., F.R.C.Path.
Senior Lecturer, Department of Medical Microbiology, University of Liverpool, Liverpool, United Kingdom
Feline Poxvirus Infection

Malcolm Bennett, B.V.Sc., Ph.D., M.R.C.V.S.
Senior Lecturer, Department of Veterinary Pathology, University of Liverpool, Liverpool, United Kingdom
Feline Poxvirus Infection

Ernst L. Biberstein, D.V.M., Ph.D., Diplomate A.C.V.M.
Professor Emeritus, University of California, Davis, Davis, California
Laboratory Diagnosis of Fungal and Algal Infections

Edward B. Breitschwerdt, D.V.M.
Professor of Medicine and Infectious Diseases, College of Veterinary Medicine, North Carolina State University, Raleigh; Adjunct Assistant Professor of Medicine, Duke University Medical Center, Durham, North Carolina
Rocky Mountain Spotted Fever, Q Fever, and Typhus; Bartonellosis; Rhinosporidiosis

Cathy A. Brown, V.M.D., Ph.D., Diplomate A.C.V.P.
Assistant Professor, Veterinary Diagnostic Laboratory, College of Veterinary Medicine, The University of Georgia, Athens, Georgia
Leptospirosis

Steven C. Budsberg, D.V.M., M.S.
Professor, Department of Small Animal Medicine, College of Veterinary Medicine, The University of Georgia, Athens, Georgia
Musculoskeletal Infections

Janet P. Calpin, B.S., L.A.T.G.
Animal Resources, College of Veterinary Medicine, The University of Georgia, Athens, Georgia
Laboratory Diagnosis of Protozoal Infections, Infectious Disease Rule-Outs for Medical Problems

Clay A. Calvert, D.V.M.
Professor, Department of Small Animal Medicine and Surgery, College of Veterinary Medicine, The University of Georgia, Athens, Georgia
Canine Viral Papillomatosis, Cardiovascular Infections

Leland E. Carmichael, D.V.M., Ph.D., Dhc
The John M. Olin Professor of Virology, James A. Baker Institute for Animal Health, College of Veterinary Medicine, Cornell University, Ithaca, New York
Canine Herpesvirus Infection, Canine Brucellosis

M. Cecilia Castellano, D.V.M.
Assistant Professor, Small Animal Clinics, Facultad de Ciencias Veterinarias, Universidad Nacional de la Plata, La Plata, Republica Argentina
Rhinosporidiosis

Sharon A. Center, D.V.M., Diplomate A.C.V.I.M.
Professor, Internal Medicine, College of Veterinary Medicine, Cornell University, Ithaca, New York
Hepatobiliary Infections

Francis W. Chandler, D.V.M., Ph.D.
Professor of Pathology and Director, Barton Immunopathology Laboratory, Department of Pathology, Medical College of Georgia, Augusta, Georgia
Candidiasis, Torulopsosis, and Rhodotorulosis; Trichosporonosis; Pneumocystosis

Susan M. Cotter, DV.M., Diplomate A.C.V.I.M. (Internal Medicine and Oncology)
Professor of Medicine, School of Veterinary Medicine, Tufts University, North Grafton, Massachusetts
Feline Viral Neoplasia

Hollis Utah Cox, D.V.M., Ph.D., Diplomate A.C.V.M.
Professor of Veterinary Bacteriology, Department of Veterinary Microbiology and Parasitology, School of Veterinary Medicine; Chief of Microbiology Services, Louisiana Veterinary Medical Diagnostic Laboratory, Veterinary Teaching Hospital and Clinics, School of Veterinary Medicine, Louisiana State University, Baton Rouge, Louisiana
Staphylococcal Infections

Thomas M. Craig, D.V.M., Ph.D.
Professor, Department of Veterinary Pathobiology, College of Veterinary Medicine, Texas A&M University, College Station, Texas
Hepatozoonosis

Susan Dawson, B.V.M.S., Ph.D., M.R.C.V.S.
Research Assistant, Department of Veterinary Pathology, University of Liverpool, Liverpool, United Kingdom
Feline Respiratory Disease

Michael J. Day, B.V.M.S. (Hons), Ph.D., F.A.S.M., Diplomate E.C.V.P., M.R.C. Path., and F.R.C.V.S.
Senior Lecturer in Veterinary Pathology, Department of Pathology and Microbiology, University of Bristol, Bristol, United Kingdom
Aspergillosis and Penicilliosis

Elizabeth S. Didier, Ph.D.
Tulane Regional Primate Research Center, Tulane University, Covington, Louisiana
Encephalitozoonosis

Peter J. Didier, D.V.M., Ph.D.
Veterinary Pathologist, Tulane Regional Primate Research Center, Tulane University, Covington, Louisiana
Encephalitozoonosis

David W. Dreesen, D.V.M., M.P.V.M.
Professor of Medical Microbiology, College of Veterinary Medicine, The University of Georgia, Athens, Georgia
Rabies

J. P. Dubey, M.V.Sc., Ph.D.
Senior Scientist, Parasite Biology and Epidemiology Laboratory, United States Department of Agriculture, Beltsville, Maryland
Toxoplasmosis and Neosporosis, Enteric Coccidiosis

John K. Dunn, M.A., M. Vet. Sc., B.V.M.S, D.S.A.M., Diplomate E.C.V.I.M., M.R.C.V.S. and N.I.A.
University Lecturer in Small Animal Medicine and Clinical Pathology, Department of Clinical Veterinary Medicine, University of Cambridge, Madingley Road, Cambridge, United Kingdom
Fever

Robert W. Dunstan, D.V.M., M.S., Diplomate A.C.V.P.
Professor of Pathology, Department of Pathology, College of Veterinary Medicine, Michigan State University, East Lansing, Michigan
Sporotrichosis

David F. Edwards, D.V.M., Diplomate A.C.V.I.M. and A.C.V.P.
Professor, College of Veterinary Medicine, University of Tennessee, Knoxville, Tennessee
Actinomycosis and Nocardiosis

Herman F. Egberink, D.V.M., Ph.D.
Associate Professor, Department of Infectious Diseases and Immunology, Virology Unit, Veterinary Faculty, Utrecht University, Utrecht, The Netherlands
Feline Viral Papillomatosis

James F. Evermann, M.S.D., Ph.D.
Department of Veterinary Clinical Sciences and Washington Animal Disease Diagnostic Laboratory, College of Veterinary Medicine, Washington State University, Pullman, Washington
Laboratory Diagnosis of Viral and Rickettsial Infections

William R. Fenner, D.V.M.
Associate Professor, College of Veterinary Medicine, Ohio State University, Columbus, Ohio
Central Nervous System Infections

Luis Ferrer, D.V.M., Ph.D.
Professor, Faculty of Veterinary Science, Universitat Autònoma de Barcelona, Barcelona, Spain
Leishmaniasis

Carol S. Foil, M.S., D.V.M., Diplomate A.C.V.D.
Professor, Department of Veterinary Clinical Sciences, School of Veterinary Medicine, Louisiana State University, Baton Rouge, Louisiana
Miscellaneous Fungal Infections, Dermatophytosis

Richard B. Ford, D.V.M., M.S., Diplomate A.C.V.I.M.
Professor of Medicine, College of Veterinary Medicine, North Carolina State University, Raleigh, North Carolina
Canine Infectious Tracheobronchitis

William J. Foreyt, Ph.D.
Professor, College of Veterinary Medicine, Washington State University, Pullman, Washington
Salmon Poisoning Disease

James G. Fox, M.S., D.V.M.
Professor and Director, Division of Comparative Medicine, Massachusetts Institute of Technology, Cambridge; Adjunct Professor of Comparative Medicine, Tufts School of Veterinary Medicine, Grafton, Massachusetts; Adjunct Professor of Comparative Medicine, University of Pennsylvania School of Veterinary Medicine, Philadelphia, Pennsylvania
Campylobacter *Infections, Gastric Helicobacters, Intestinal and Hepatic Helicobacters*

Rosalind Gaskell, B.V.Sc., Ph.D., M.R.C.V.S.
Reader, Department of Veterinary Pathology, University of Liverpool, Liverpool, United Kingdom
Feline Respiratory Disease, Feline Poxvirus Infection

Urs Giger, P.D., Dr. Med. Vet., M.S., Diplomate A.C.V.I.M. and E.C.V.I.M.
Charlotte Newton Sheppard Professor of Medicine and Chief, Section of Medical Genetics, School of Medicine, University of Pennsylvania; Professor of Veterinary Medicine, School of Veterinary Medicine, University of Pennsylvania, Philadelphia, Pennsylvania; Professor of Internal Medicine, University of Zürich, Zürich, Switzerland
Immunodeficiencies and Infectious Diseases

Ellie J.C. Goldstein, M.D.
Clinical Professor of Medicine, School of Medicine, University of California, Los Angeles; Director, R.M. Alden Research Laboratory, Santa Monica-University of California, Los Angeles Medical Center, Santa Monica, California
Bite Wound Infections

John R. Gorham, D.V.M., Ph.D.
Professor, Department of Veterinary Microbiology and Pathology, College of Veterinary Medicine, Washington State University, Pullman, Washington
Salmon Poisoning Disease

Craig E. Greene, D.V.M., M.S., Diplomate A.C.V.I.M.
Gunst Professor, Department of Small Animal Medicine, College of Veterinary Medicine, The University of Georgia, Athens, Georgia
Antiviral Drugs; Canine Distemper; Infectious Canine Hepatitis and Canine Acidophil Cell Hepatitis; Canine Herpesvirus Infection; Nonrespiratory Parainfluenza Virus Infection of Dogs; Feline Panleukopenia; Feline Syncytium-Forming Virus Infection; Feline Paramyxovirus Infections; Hantavirus Infection; Rabies; Enterovirus Infections; Mumps and Influenza Virus Infections; Arthropod-Borne Encephalomyelitis; Borna Disease–Like Meningoencephalitis; Rocky Mountain Spotted Fever, Q Fever, and Typhus; Chlamydial Infections; Mycoplasmal, Ureaplasmal, and L-Form Infections; Antibacterial Chemotherapy; Streptococcal and Other Gram-Positive Bacterial Infections; Salmonellosis; Shigellosis; Yersiniosis; Tyzzer's Disease; Clostridium perfringens *Infection; Canine Brucellosis; Tetanus; Leptospirosis; Lyme Borreliosis; Melioidosis; Glanders; Tuberculous Mycobacterial Infections; Dermatophilosis; Feline Abscesses; Bite Wound Infections; Bartonellosis; Surgical and Traumatic Wound Infections; Antifungal Chemotherapy; Candidiasis, Torulopsosis, and Rhodotorulosis; Trichosporonosis; Protothecosis; Antiprotozoal Chemotherapy; African Trypanosomiasis; Cytauxzoonosis; Acanthamebiasis; Enteric Coccidiosis; Pneumocystosis;* Malassezia *Dermatitis; Otitis Externa; Respiratory Infections; Gastrointestinal and Intra-Abdominal Infections; Environmental Factors in Infectious Disease; Immunodeficiencies and Infectious Diseases; Fever; Immunocompromised People and Pets; Immunoprophylaxis and Immunotherapy; Canine Immunization Recommendations; Feline Immunization Recommendations; Canine and Feline Biologics Manufacturers and Products Available Worldwide; Laboratory Testing for Infectious Diseases of Dogs and Cats; Manufacturers of Diagnostic Test Kits and Their Products; Infectious Disease Rule-Outs for Medical Problems; Antimicrobial Drug Formulary*

Russell T. Greene, D.V.M., Ph.D., Diplomate A.C.V.I.M., A.C.V.M.
Owner, Phoenix Veterinary Internal Medicine Services, Phoenix, Arizona
Miscellaneous Bacterial Infections, Coccidioidomycosis

Danielle Gunn-Moore, B.V.M.S., M.R.C.V.S.
Lecturer in Veterinary Pathology, University of Bristol Veterinary School, Bristol, United Kingdom
Mycobacterial Infections

Gerryll Gae Hall, D.V.M.
Technical Services Veterinarian, Schering-Plough Animal Health, Companion Animal Business Unit, Union, New Jersey
Canine and Feline Biologics Manufacturers and Products Available Worldwide

David A. Harbour, B.Sc., Ph.D.
Senior Lecturer in Veterinary Virology, Department of Clinical Veterinary Science, Division of Molecular and Cellular Biology, University of Bristol, Langford, Bristol, United Kingdom
Feline Enteric Viral Infections

John W. Harvey, D.V.M., Ph.D.
Professor and Chair, Department of Physiological Sciences, College of Veterinary Medicine, University of Florida, Gainesville, Florida
Ehrlichiosis, Haemobartonellosis

Dwight C. Hirsh, D.V.M., Ph.D.
Professor of Microbiology, School of Veterinary Medicine; Chief, Microbiology Service, Veterinary Medical Teaching Hospital, School of Veterinary Medicine, University of California, Davis, Davis, California
Anaerobic Infections

Marian C. Horzinek, D.V.M., Ph.D.
Professor, Department of Infectious Diseases and Immunology, Virology Unit, Veterinary Faculty, Utrecht University, Utrecht, The Netherlands
Feline Viral Papillomatosis

Johnny D. Hoskins, D.V.M., Ph.D., Diplomate A.C.V.I.M.
Professor Emeritus, Department of Veterinary Clinical Sciences, School of Veterinary Medicine, Louisiana State University, Baton Rouge, Louisiana
Canine Viral Enteritis

Peter J. Ihrke, V.M.D.
Professor of Dermatology, Department of Medicine and Epidemiology, School of Veterinary Medicine, University of California, Davis; Adjunct Associate Professor of Dermatology, Stanford University, School of Medicine, Stanford; Chief, Dermatology Service, Veterinary Medical Teaching Hospital, School of Veterinary Medicine, University of California, Davis, Davis, California
Integumentary Infections

Gilbert J. Jacobs, D.V.M., Diplomate A.C.V.I.M.
Professor of Medicine, College of Veterinary Medicine, The University of Georgia, Athens, Georgia
Cryptococcosis

Spencer S. Jang, B.A.
Clinical Laboratory Technologist, Supervisor, Microbiology Service, Veterinary Medical Teaching Hospital, School of Veterinary Medicine, University of California, Davis, Davis, California
Anaerobic Infections, Laboratory Diagnosis of Fungal and Algal Infections

Oswald Jarrett, B.V.M.S., Ph.D.
Professor of Comparative Virology, Department of Veterinary Pathology, University of Glasgow, Glasgow, Scotland, United Kingdom
Feline Coronavirus Infection

Boyd R. Jones, B.V.Sc., F.A.C.V.Sc., M.R.C.V.S.
Professor, Small Animal Clinical Studies, University College Dublin, Dublin, Ireland
Enteric Bacterial Infections

Robert L. Jones, D.V.M., Ph.D.
Professor, Department of Microbiology, and Clinical Microbiologist, Diagnostic Laboratories, College of Veterinary Medicine and Biomedical Sciences, Colorado State University, Fort Collins, Colorado
Laboratory Diagnosis of Bacterial Infections

Arnold F. Kaufmann, D.V.M., M.S.
Retired, Formerly Chief, Emerging Diseases Branch, Division of Bacterial and Mycotic Diseases, National Center for Infectious Diseases, Centers for Disease Control and Prevention, Atlanta, Georgia
Tularemia

Frances A. Kennedy, D.V.M., M.S.
Pathologist, Animal Health Diagnostic Laboratory, College of Veterinary Medicine, Michigan State University, East Lansing, Michigan
Feline Adenovirus Infection

Ann B. Kier, D.V.M., Ph.D., A.C.L.A.M.
Professor, Department of Veterinary Pathobiology, College of Veterinary Medicine, Texas A&M University, College Station, Texas
Cytauxzoonosis

Stephen A. Kruth, D.V.M., Diplomate A.C.V.I.M.
Professor, Department of Clinical Studies, Ontario Veterinary College, University of Guelph, Guelph, Ontario
Gram-Negative Bacterial Infections, Endotoxemia

Gail A. Kunkle, D.V.M., Diplomate A.C.V.D.
Professor, College of Veterinary Medicine; Dermatology Service Chief, Veterinary Medical Teaching Hospital, University of Florida, Gainesville, Florida
Mycobacterial Infections

Michael R. Lappin, D.V.M., Ph.D.
Department of Clinical Sciences, College of Veterinary Medicine and Biomedical Sciences, Colorado State University, Fort Collins, Colorado
Ehrlichiosis, Laboratory Diagnosis of Protozoal Infections, Toxoplasmosis and Neosporosis

Dennis F. Lawler, D.V.M.
Veterinary Services Manager, Ralston Purina Co., St. Louis, Missouri
Prevention and Management of Infection in Catteries, Prevention and Management of Infection in Kennels

Alfred M. Legendre, D.V.M., M.S.
Department of Small Animal Clinical Sciences, College of Veterinary Medicine, University of Tennessee, Knoxville, Tennessee
Blastomycosis

Diane T. Lewis, D.V.M., Diplomate A.C.V.D.
Clinical Assistant Professor, College of Veterinary Medicine, University of Florida, Gainesville, Florida
Mycobacterial Infections

Hans Lutz, Dr. Med. Vet. habie.
Professor, School of Veterinary Medicine; Head, Clinical Laboratory, Department of Internal Veterinary Medicine, University of Zürich, Zürich, Switzerland
Feline Paramyxovirus Infections

Dennis W. Macy, D.V.M., M.S.
Professor of Internal Medicine and Oncology, College of Veterinary Medicine and Biomedical Sciences, Colorado State University, Fort Collins, Colorado
Plague

Charles L. Martin, D.V.M., M.S., Diplomate A.C.V.O.
Professor, Department of Small Animal Medicine, College of Veterinary Medicine, The University of Georgia, Athens, Georgia
Ocular Infections

Linda Medleau, D.V.M., M.S., Diplomate A.C.V.D.
Professor of Dermatology, College of Veterinary Medicine, The University of Georgia, Athens, Georgia
Cryptococcosis

Meri A. Miller, D.V.M., Diplomate A.C.V.I.M.
North Atlanta Veterinary Specialists, Alpharetta, Georgia
Leptospirosis

T. Mark Neer, D.V.M.
Professor of Medicine, Department of Clinical Sciences; Section Chief, Small Animal Medicine, Veterinary Teaching Hospital and Clinics, College of Veterinary Medicine, Louisiana State University, Baton Rouge, Louisiana
Ehrlichiosis

John F. Prescott, Vet. M.B., Ph.D.
Professor, Department of Pathobiology, Ontario Veterinary College, University of Guelph, Guelph, Ontario
Streptococcal and Other Gram-Positive Bacterial Infections

Hugh W. Reid, B.V.M.S., D.T.V.M., Ph.D., M.R.C.V.S.
Head, Immunobiology Division, Moredun Research Institute, Edinburgh, Scotland, United Kingdom
Arboviral Infections

Edmund J. Rosser, Jr., D.V.M., Diplomate, A.C.V.D.
Professor of Dermatology, Department of Small Animal Clinical Sciences, College of Veterinary Medicine, Michigan State University, East Lansing, Michigan
Sporotrichosis

Rance K. Sellon, D.V.M., Ph.D.
Assistant Professor of Medicine, Department of Veterinary Clinical Sciences, College of Veterinary Medicine, Washington State University, Pullman, Washington
Feline Immunodeficiency Virus Infection

John A. Shadduck, D.V.M., Ph.D.
Executive Vice President, Operations, Heska Corp., Fort Collins, Colorado
Encephalitozoonosis

Nick J.H. Sharp, B.Vet.Med., Ph.D.
Assistant Professor, College of Veterinary Medicine, North Carolina State University, Raleigh, North Carolina
Aspergillosis and Penicilliosis

Deborah C. Silverstein, D.V.M.
Resident, Emergency and Critical Care, Veterinary Medical Teaching Hospital, School of Veterinary Medicine, University of California, Davis, Davis, California
Laboratory Testing for Infectious Diseases of Dogs and Cats, Manufacturers of Diagnostic Test Kits and Their Products

Robbert J. Slappendel, D.V.M., Ph.D.
Associate Professor (Internal Medicine of Companion Animals), Faculty of Veterinary Medicine, Department of Clinical Sciences of Companion Animals, Utrecht University, Utrecht, The Netherlands
Leishmaniasis

Karen Snowden, D.V.M., Ph.D.
Assistant Professor, Department of Veterinary Pathobiology, College of Veterinary Medicine, Texas A&M University, College Station, Texas
Encephalitozoonosis

Jean Stiles, D.V.M., M.S., Diplomate A.C.V.O.
Associate Professor, Ophthalmology, College of Veterinary Medicine, The University of Georgia, Athens, Georgia
Ocular Infections

Reinhard K. Straubinger, Dr. Med. Vet., Ph.D.
Research Assistant II, New York State College of Veterinary Medicine, Cornell University, Ithaca, New York
Lyme Borreliosis

Joseph Taboada, D.V.M., Diplomate A.C.V.I.M.
Associate Professor of Medicine, Director of Professional Instruction and Curriculum, School of Veterinary Medicine, Louisiana State University, Baton Rouge, Louisiana
Babesiosis

Shelly L. Vaden, D.V.M., Ph.D.
Associate Professor of Internal Medicine, College of Veterinary Medicine, North Carolina State University, Raleigh, North Carolina
Canine Infectious Tracheobronchitis

Marc Vandevelde, Dr. Med. Vet.
Professor and Head, Animal Neurology, University of Bern, Bern, Switzerland
Pseudorabies, Neurologic Diseases of Suspected Infectious Origin

A.D.J. Watson, B.V.Sc., Ph.D., F.R.C.V.S.
Associate Professor in Veterinary Medicine, Department of Veterinary Clinical Sciences, The University of Sydney, New South Wales, Australia
Antiviral Drugs, Antibacterial Chemotherapy, Antifungal Chemotherapy, Antiprotozoal Chemotherapy, Antimicrobial Drug Formulary

Alice M. Wolf, D.V.M., Diplomate A.C.V.I.M. and A.B.V.P.
Professor, Department of Small Animal Medicine, College of Veterinary Medicine, Texas A&M University, College Station, Texas
Histoplasmosis

John C. Wright, Ph.D.
Professor of Psychology, Mercer University; Certified Applied Animal Behaviorist, Macon, Georgia
Bite Wound Infections

Preface

The first edition of this book published in 1990 was a sequel to the text *Clinical Microbiology and Infectious Diseases of the Dog and Cat,* which I edited in 1984. There are many changes and updates in this second edition compared with the preceding texts. The subject of infectious diseases has been rapidly advancing. In the last 8 years, many new infections of dogs and cats have been recognized. The use of molecular genetic techniques has had a dramatic impact on furthering our knowledge of infectious diseases of all species. Genetic methods have been used in the research laboratory to discover new organisms causing disease; re-examine genetic relatedness between pathogens and reclassify them; detect specific infectious agents from a diagnostic standpoint and detect carrier states; study the pathogenesis of infectious diseases; and determine if treatment has been efficacious in eliminating persistent pathogens. Although genetic amplification has revealed many new insights into infectious agents and the diseases they cause, the use of these tests in routine diagnostics is in its infancy. The proprietary nature of the reaction, its extreme sensitivity and need for continual monitoring, makes it a test confined to the reference laboratory. False-negative results can occur from interfering substances in biologic specimens, and false-positive results can occur from inadvertent contamination of reagents or the environment. Perhaps the future will see more routine use of these tools in the form of standard tests or possibly in-office kits.

Diseases caused by newly discovered agents in dogs and cats that are novel to this edition are feline adenovirus infection (Chapter 15), feline viral papillomatosis (Chapter 21), feline and canine ehrlichiosis (Chapter 28), typhus in cats (Chapter 29), various *Helicobacter* infections (Chapter 39), *Chryseomonas* infection (Chapter 46), mycobacterial infections (Chapter 50), *Bartonella* infections (Chapter 54), amoebiasis caused by *Willaertia* (Chapter 78), *Toxoplasma*-like infection of cats (Chapter 80), and transmissible myocarditis/diaphragmitis of cats (Chapter 87).

Previously established infections of other hosts that have now been recognized to occur in dogs or cats include canine parvovirus infection in cats (Chapter 8), bordetellosis in cats (Chapter 16), equine morbillivirus infection in cats (Chapter 18), hantavirus infection in cats (Chapter 20), Borna disease–like meningoencephalitis (Chapter 26), ehrlichial infections (Chapter 28), toxigenic streptococcal infections (Chapter 35), *Helicobacter* infections (Chapter 39), *Clostridium perfringens* type D infection in dogs (Chapter 39), rhodotorulosis (Chapter 66), and feline spongiform encephalopathy (Chapter 84).

A number of diseases or clinical problems given brief mention in previous editions have been given expanded coverage under individual section headings or their own chapters. These include gram negative bacterial infections (Chapter 37), surgical and traumatic infections (Chapter 55), African trypanosomiasis (Chapter 72), cyclosporiasis (Chapter 82), encephalitis in pug and Maltese dogs (Chapter 84), encephalitis in Yorkshire terriers (Chapter 84), steroid-responsive meningitis-arteritis (Chapter 84), immunodeficiencies and infectious diseases (Chapter 95), prevention and management of infection in catteries and kennels (Chapters 97 and 98, respectively), and immunocompromised people and pets (Chapter 99).

The emphasis of this book is on diagnosis and treatment of canine and feline infections. Each of the first four sections includes current information on diseases caused by viruses, rickettsiae, chlamydias, and mycoplasmas; bacteria; fungi and algae; and protozoa and unknown agents. Each of these major sections is introduced by a chapter that discusses routine diagnostic testing for the type of microorganisms in that section. The aim of these diagnostic chapters is to help the clinician determine the indications and methods for sample collection and laboratory submission, interpretation of results, and when applicable, performance of in-office diagnostic procedures. The therapy chapter following the diagnostic chapter includes the indications and pharmacologic considerations of antimicrobials used to treat various infections discussed in the respective section.

Section V involves the principles of diagnosis and therapy of infections in various body organ systems and the clinical problems related to infectious diseases, such as environmental control of infections, immunodeficiency disorders, prevention of infection in communal environments, immunocompromised people and pets, and immunization.

Modifications have been made to improve the readability and clinical usefulness of the book. Drug dosage tables have been furnished to give complete and consistent prescribing information in each chapter. The references from previous editions have generally been omitted from the text in chapters that have been updated. Those references cited are predominantly from 1990 to the present. These decisions were made by a mutual agreement between the editor and publisher to keep the size, and as a result, the cost of the book for the reader, within a reasonable limit.

A comprehensive drug formulary (Appendix 8) is referred to extensively throughout the book. The references cited in the formulary appear in the respective antimicrobial therapy chapters and elsewhere in the text.

All listed references have been reviewed in the preparation of the book but are not necessarily cited in each chapter. The reader is referred to the previous edition's chapter by citation in the text to obtain information on original references. Those interested in a complete historical bibliographic listing for each disease should consult the texts of 1984 and 1990 along with the present edition. Together, bibliographic information in these texts should provide the reader with a relatively extensive listing of veterinary literature on a given subject.

The number of appendices has been reduced from previous editions but the volume of material has expanded. Because of space limitations, the appendices on staining and microscopic techniques and environmental survival of infectious agents have been omitted. The reader should consult the first edition for such information, which has undergone minimal change. The appendix on interstate and international travel requirements was not included because the most current information can be obtained by contacting respective state offices or consulates. Much of this information is also available on the worldwide web.

A number of the appendices have been updated and expanded. These include those concerning immunization guidelines (Appendices 1 and 2) and the availability of biologics worldwide (Appendix 3). Laboratories performing diagnostic tests for each disease are listed in Appendix 5. Commercial test kits are listed in Appendix 6. A new addition to this text is an extensive worldwide formulary of drug manufacturers and antimicrobial drugs (Appendix 8). This formulary is cross referenced in each chapter. It refers to tabulated dosage information throughout the book. It took countless hours to compile this information from thousands of literature sources. Extensive information on drugs used to treat microbial infections is thus consolidated. I have found this formulary to be an invaluable tool during my clinical duties. I hope that you too may find it of similar benefit.

CRAIG E. GREENE

Acknowledgments

One person can ultimately be held responsible for coordinating and editing a textbook, but the work cannot be completed without the assistance of many others. My contributors were unselfish in their commitment to add yet another task to their already busy schedules. I certainly could not have done the work or provided the needed expertise without their assistance.

I must first thank my loyal and dedicated editorial assistant, Janet Calpin, a technician in Animal Resources at the University of Georgia. As in the previous texts, she was involved in all phases of this book through its inception and completion. This book would not have been possible without her commitment. Anyone who uses this reference has her to thank for its existence. Mamie Watson was intricately involved in all the typing of the manuscript for submission to the publisher. She is meticulous and accurate in her keyboard skills and medical vocabulary, which helped us in viewing and submitting the manuscript and tabular material in a format that mimicked the final published work. Library assistance of Elizabeth Bloemer, Linda Tumlin, JoAnne Giel, and Lucy M. Rowland was of great benefit in obtaining many of the needed publications. Lynn Reece was adept at producing many of the maps and pathogenesis algorithms by computer to give these entries accuracy and consistency. The secretaries of the Department of Small Animal Medicine, Diane Embrick, Mamie Watson, and Fran Cantrell, helped me with all my obligations so that I could retain my sanity and meet all my other obligations. Many people in the Educational Resource Center, headed by Dr. Lari Cowgill, assisted me at some point in compiling illustrative material. For this edition, Susan Brinkley was the administrative secretary who kept projects on track. Vivian Freeman and Ladonna Allen helped with duplicating. Photographic needs were managed by Jeanne Ann Davidson and Joey Rodgers. The artwork of medical illustrator Kip Carter and the illustrations of Dan Beisel were used again. In addition, Kip did two additional life cycle drawings that were used in the chapters on borreliosis and coccidioidomycosis. Thel Melton helped with reproduction of some maps for bartonellosis. Some of the original graphics by Harsh Jain were published again in this edition. I greatly appreciate the lending of photographic material by many persons. They are acknowledged at the respective figures. Members of the Clinical Pharmacy Staff, including Dr. Doug Kemp, Dr. Heather Fitzsimons, Dr. Jim Evans, and Tony Hughey, were helpful in assisting me in obtaining literature and information for compiling the drug formulary.

Many people helped me with their expertise in reviewing particular sections of the book. Janet Foley and Niels Pedersen, University of California, Davis, reviewed the section on feline coronavirus infection. Marc Vandevelde, University of Bern, Switzerland, reviewed the section on borna disease–like meningoencephalitis. Jackie Dawson of the Centers for Disease Control and Prevention, Atlanta, Georgia, and Yasuko Rikihisa of The Ohio State University, Columbus, Ohio, reviewed the tabular information on serologic cross-reactivity among ehrlichial species. Susan Little of the Department of Microbiology and Parasitology, The University of Georgia, reviewed the species information of *Ehrlichia.* Steve Barthold, of the University of California, Davis, reviewed the section on Lyme borreliosis. Jeff Watts of Pharmacia & Upjohn Animal Health reviewed the tabular information on oral microflora isolated from dogs and cats and from bite wound infections.

Private practitioners have also contributed to this book by their many questions and their determination in finding new therapies for unresponsive infectious diseases. Drs. Brad and Barry Fly of Nashville, Tennessee, found that imidocarb is effective in the treatment of cytauxzoonosis (Chapter 76); Dr. Stuart Bleck, of Lexington, Massachusetts, with the permission of his client, Judy Boyer, determined that her dog's *Mycobacterium avium-intracellulare* complex infection was kept in remission with combination chemotherapy (Chapter 50). Dr. Tom Chamberlain of Williamsburg, Virginia, determined that *Pentatrichomonas* infection in cats would respond to paromomycin (Chapter 78).

I am appreciative of the manufacturers listed in Appendix 3 for providing us with the information needed to compile the detailed international information on available canine and feline biologics. Laboratories listed in Appendices 5 and 6 were very helpful in providing the information on their testing services and kits, respectively.

I am indebted to those who have provided me with research and clinical support on infectious diseases over the years. My most recent graduate students, Andre Jaggy, Perry Jameson, and Michelle McDermott, have worked on various infectious disease problems in my research. In the last year, Macon Miles has been my dedicated student research assistant who, along with Michelle Kaplan and Elise Knappenberger, have helped me sustain my research efforts on bartonellosis during this long process. Dr. Donald Dawe, Pat Schroeder, Leigh Rheny, Lisa Johnson, and Amanda Bearss of the Clinical Immunology and Infectious Disease Laboratory have helped in the development and implementation of diagnostic testing and monitoring of clinical and research animals. Richard and Joanne Moyer, formerly of Crozet, Virginia, have provided financial support through the memorial fund of Edward Gunst, Richmond, Virginia, and established the Gunst Professorship at The University of Georgia, College of Veterinary Medicine. I am fortunate to be awarded this position at this time. Joanne passed away unexpectedly while suffering from a terminal illness on April 11, 1997. She was a client, a mentor, and a respected person in her continual quest for animal welfare. At the same time, she had a responsible attitude concerning the need for medical research on animals and its benefits for animal and human well being. I am grateful for the impact that she had on me and my career.

I would also like to thank Dr. Keith Prasse, Dean of the College of Veterinary Medicine; Dr. Clarence Rawlings, Head of the Department of Small Animal Medicine; and the faculty, staff, and students of The University of Georgia, College of

Veterinary Medicine, for making it a respected veterinary institution as well as an enjoyable place to work.

The people at W.B. Saunders Company have done an exceptional job in their efforts with this book. Ray Kersey has been my editor and allowed me the creative freedom to bring you this book in its best possible form for the lowest cost to the reader. He placed me in the very competent hands of Dave Kilmer, developmental editor, who answered all my questions and put me in touch with all the other specialists I needed, including Cass Stamato in editorial, Al Beringer in typesetting, Jeff Gunning in production, Doug Yeager in art and design, and Mary Anne Folcher in copy editorial. The copy editor of the submitted manuscript was Mary McCoy, whose editing and medical knowledge, along with all the others at Saunders, gave the book a consistent format. This book will be current at the time it is published because it is set from electronic copy. The galleys have been updated to the current literature during the editing process. Only 6 months have elapsed from the time the final version of the chapters was delivered until publication.

Comments on the text, ideas for future editions, correction of errors, citation of omissions, or information and facts that will benefit the advancement of our knowledge of infectious diseases are appreciated.

CRAIG E. GREENE

Contents

Section II
Bacterial Diseases

Section V
Clinical Problems

Appendices

NOTICE

Section

I

VIRAL, RICKETTSIAL, CHLAMYDIAL, AND MYCOPLASMAL DISEASES

Chapter

1

Laboratory Diagnosis of Viral and Rickettsial Infections

James F. Evermann

Accurate diagnosis of viral and rickettsial diseases requires a concerted effort between the veterinarian and the diagnostic laboratory. A definitive determination relies on analysis of clinical signs and results of laboratory analyses of antemortem or postmortem specimens.[5, 28, 31] The trends in laboratory detection of viruses and rickettsiae have taken a dual pathway. The first pathway is the development of more sensitive assays for the early recognition of disease and initiation of therapy for the affected animal and the implementation of prevention measures for susceptible contacts. Pursuit of a laboratory diagnosis is important when an animal has clinical manifestations that may be caused by any one of a number of infectious agents, such as those causing feline upper respiratory disease and canine enteritis. A laboratory diagnosis can also assist in predicting the impact of the infectious disease on the affected animal and other animals with which it has contact. This is especially true of diseases for which there are no current vaccines, such as FIV and CHV infections.[2, 4]

The second pathway involves the detection of viruses and rickettsiae in subclinically affected animals that are in the incubatory phases or are recovered carriers. The reasons for this approach have been increased client concern for their pets with life-threatening diseases such as FIP and increased recognition of zoonotic infections.[8, 11] Of greater concern to veterinarians and physicians is the potential zoonotic transmission of disease from pet animals maintained within convalescent centers and home care facilities for immunocompromised people.[1] Rabies and the tick-borne rickettsial infections are examples of potential zoonoses.[15, 27]

The interest of the clinician submitting specimens directly influences the type of diagnostic assay that should be selected (Table 1–1). The identification of the critical points for testing during the infectious process allows for early intervention and minimizes the loss associated with the disease outcome (Fig. 1–1).[24] The *first* of five critical points (CPs) is at the initial interaction between the infectious agent and the pet animal. Certain infections may be acquired by in utero transmission such as CHV, by cat bite such as FIV, or by tick vectors such as RMSF. The *second* CP follows shortly after the onset of infection. Very sensitive assays such as the FeLV-ELISA for antigen may detect transiently viremic cats

Table 1–1. Interpretation of Laboratory Analysis in a Case in Which Canine Parvoviral Enteritis Was Suspected or Being Monitored for on the Basis of Clinical Signs or At-Risk Category[a]

CLINICAL INQUIRY	TEST(S)	LEVEL OF INTERPRETATION
1. Is the dog infected with CPV?	ELISA for antigen	Yes/no
2. When was the dog exposed?	IgM serology	7–10 days
3. Is the CPV a new strain or variant?	Virus isolation, neutralization with monoclonal antibody	Strains 2, 2a, or 2b
4. Are other infectious agents present?	EM-virus isolation	Rotavirus, coronavirus, calicivirus
	ELISA for antigen	Rotavirus
	Bacteriology	*Salmonella* sp., *Campylobacter* sp., *E. coli*
	Parasitology	*Giardia* sp.
5. Is the dog protected or at risk?	IgG serology, HI serology	≥ 1:100 (IgG); or ≥ 1:80 (HI)
6. Is the dog shedding low levels of virus subclinically?	Nucleic acid–based (PCR) assays	Yes/no

[a]Interpretation is dependent on the level of clinical inquiry and the types of laboratory tests used.

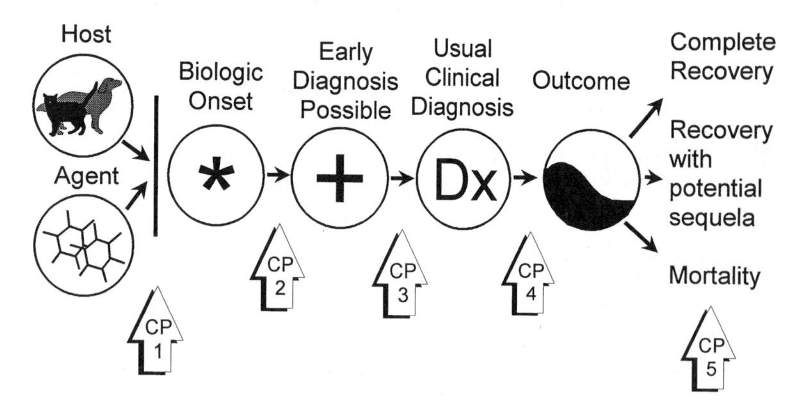

Figure 1–1. Scheme depicting the infection-disease spectrum with critical points (CP) identified to assist the clinician in monitoring preclinical infections, usual clinical symptoms, and the outcome of the disease. Modified from Sackett et al: *In* Sackett DL, Haynes RB, Guyatt GH, et al (eds): Clinical Epidemiology. A Basic Science for Clinical Medicine. Little, Brown, 1991, p 156, with permission.

within 2 weeks after initial infection. The *third* CP is at the time of presentation of the animal with clinical illness. This point is exemplified by a dog with diarrhea that is shedding large quantities of CPV in the feces. At the *fourth* CP, the diagnosis of an infectious disease process may alter the outcome of the disease by prompt therapy and supportive care such as with severe upper respiratory disease with FCV and FHV. The *fifth* and final CP may be overlooked but is the aftermath of disease in which complete or partial recovery with sequelae may occur, such as with CDV. Testing at this time may help to limit the spread of infection from the diseased animal to other animals in the household. Diagnostic assays to determine shedding patterns, animals at risk, and prognoses for recovering animals are very important after the outcome period.[28, 31]

INFECTION VERSUS DISEASE

As diagnostic assays become more sensitive in detecting viruses and rickettsiae by antibody, antigen, or nucleic acid–based tests, the distinction must be made between the diagnosis of a disease and the detection of an infectious agent with potential to cause disease.[28] Most diagnostic assays have been designed to assist in making a disease diagnosis.[31] As interest in screening healthy populations of animals prior to show, sale, breeding, and so forth increases, tests are becoming available to distinguish infection in the absence of disease. Nucleic acid–based assays using PCR (see Applied Molecular Diagnostics) are capable of detecting latently infected cats with FeLV and FHV.[17, 30] The use of such assays requires better understanding of what a positive test result means and greater client education than was necessary with previous tests. An example of the use of nucleic acid–based assays can be seen with tests for FIV.[6] The screening ELISA to detect FIV antibodies determines whether or not the cat has been exposed to the virus, and because the infection is regarded as permanent, the cat is presumed to be infected. No further interpretation is possible.[18] The quantitative competitive reverse transcriptase PCR assay allows for an assessment of the FIV-RNA levels in plasma. This assay distinguishes between cats with rapidly progressive FIV disease and cats that will be long-term survivors.[6]

DIAGNOSTIC TEST INTERPRETATION

Several excellent resources are available for more definitive explanations of test validity and interpretation.[18, 19, 24, 28] In making interpretations, it is important to evaluate the makeup of a diagnostic assay and the limitations of the assay. Two terms used to describe the predictive accuracy of a test are **sensitivity** and **specificity**. Calculation of these values is summarized in Table 1–2. Test sensitivity is defined as the likelihood of a positive test result in an animal known to have a particular disease or infection with a particular agent. The limits of test sensitivity can extend to an animal with a preclinical infection; therefore, the values vary for either disease or infection. One assay may yield false-positive results for disease but true-positive results for infection. Conversely, test specificity is the likelihood of a negative test result in an animal known to be free of disease and/or infection. Knowledge of the specificity of a diagnostic test is very important because more false-positive results will occur with a test of low specificity.

Because of the dichotomy of an assay potentially not being able to distinguish a preclinical carrier-infection status from a true disease status, a test's predictive value becomes very important to the veterinarian.[28] Classically, a **positive predictive value** is the probability of disease in an animal with a positive test result. A **negative predictive value** is the probability that an animal does not have the disease when the test result is negative.

SAMPLE SELECTION AND PRESERVATION

Laboratory diagnosis of viral and rickettsial infections requires proper sample selection, collection, and submission. Detection of definitive disease-causing organisms is best

Table 1–2. Calculation of Sensitivity, Specificity, and Predictive Values

ANIMALS	TEST POSITIVE RESULT	TEST NEGATIVE RESULT	
With disease or infection	TP	FN	TP/TP + FN = sensitivity
Without disease or infection	FP	TN	TN/TN + FP = specificity
	TP/TP + FP	TN/TN + FN	
	Positive predictive	Negative predictive	

TP = true-positive results; FP = false-positive results; TN = true-negative results; FN = false-negative results.

Table 1–3. Collection of Samples for Laboratory Diagnosis of Viral and Rickettsial Diseases

SITE(S) OF CLINICAL SIGNS	ANTEMORTEM[a]	POSTMORTEM[b]
Respiratory and ocular tissues	Nasal swabs, conjunctival scraping, serum, whole blood[c]	Selected tissues[d] and bronchiolar lymph nodes
Gastrointestinal tract	Feces, vomitus, serum, whole blood[c]	Selected sections of small intestine, intestinal contents, mesenteric lymph nodes
Skin and mucous membranes	Swabs, scrapings of lesions, serum, whole blood[c]	Selected tissues[d] and regional lymph nodes
Central nervous system[a, e]	CSF, serum, whole blood, feces	Selected sections from brain
Genitourinary tract	Urogenital swabs, vaginal mucus, urine, serum, whole blood[c]	Selected sections from placenta, fetal lung, liver, kidney, and spleen
Immunosuppression, hematologic abnormalities, blood dyscrasias	Whole blood[c], serum, bone marrow	Selected tissues[d] and lymph nodes

[a]Samples to be kept moist and chilled.
[b]Fresh samples should be fixed (in 10% buffered formalin) for histologic analysis.
[c]Collected in EDTA and kept refrigerated.
[d]Hematogenous organs: lung, liver, kidney, bone marrow, and spleen.
[e]Animals with neurologic signs should be handled with extreme caution and cleared for rabies virus through a public health laboratory before further diagnostic testing (see Chapter 22).
Modified from Fenner F, Bachmann PA, Gibbs EPJ, et al: *Veterinary Virology.* Academic Press, 1987, pp 237–264, with permission.

done when the animal is in the acute phase of the disease. Postmortem samples may be of value in the management of other animals in the susceptible population; however, the degree of diagnostic accuracy is generally reduced owing to degradation of live agents or their antigens. Fresh samples should be promptly refrigerated for short-term (12–24 hours) shipment to a laboratory in close proximity to the clinic. For long-term (2–4 days) shipment, samples should be frozen and shipped to the laboratory on wet ice. Tissues for histopathology should be promptly fixed in buffered formalin. Serology may be of diagnostic value if acute and convalescent sera samples are available for IgG analysis or for IgM if single samples are available. Table 1–3 lists the samples to collect to assist in making a laboratory diagnosis of viral and rickettsial diseases.[5, 31] Of equal importance is specimen preservation and shipment to the testing laboratory. As more in-clinic diagnostic test kits become available, long-term preservation becomes of secondary importance in relation to collecting the appropriate sample. Table 1–4 gives guidelines for specimen collection, processing, and shipment for laboratory diagnosis. Owing to the changing nature of diagnostic assays and the ability to detect some infections earlier, it is suggested that the laboratory be contacted for up-to-date recommendations on sample collection, processing, and shipment.

LABORATORY ANALYSIS

Viral Infections

Table 1–5 presents the five primary methods used in diagnostic virology. Most veterinary hospitals have the capacity for the in-clinic ELISA assays for detection of FeLV and CPV antigens and FIV antibody. Specialized laboratories should be consulted for more in-depth analysis of specimens from a particular case if there is a significant increase in clinically ill

Table 1–4. Specimen Collection, Processing, and Shipment

PROCEDURE (SPECIMEN)	COLLECTION AND PROCESSING	SHIPMENT
Organism isolation, nucleic acid–based testing, ELISA for antigen (tissue, excretions, secretions)	Collect aseptically to prevent bacterial contamination, and store at ≤ 10°C to prevent inactivation; do not freeze or fix.	Use whole blood,[a] tissue biopsy, feces, swabs,[b] commercial transport media, or sterile Hanks' balanced salt solution with 10% bovine albumin or 0.5% lactalbumin hydrolysate with penicillin (100 U/ml) and streptomycin (2 μg/ml) added to inhibit bacterial growth; pack on wet ice to last 48–72 hr.
Serology (serum)	Collect aseptically to prevent contamination and handle gently to prevent hemolysis; remove needle from syringe before dispensing; allow to clot at room temperature; rim clot and centrifuge at 650*g* for 20 min; pipette serum fraction into clean tube; although paired samples (10–14 days apart) are preferred, single samples may be diagnostic (e.g., CDV IgM).	Refrigerate until shipping.
Histology, immunohistochemistry (tissue)	Collect aseptically to prevent contamination, 5 mm thick; fix in 10% buffered formalin (10 × volume).	Ship in leak-proof container with adequate fixative.
Direct FA testing (tissue, tissue impression)	Make tissue impression on clean dry microscope slide, and air dry; fix in alcohol for cytology or in acetone for direct FA[c].	Pack on wet ice and ship as for isolation; smears can be shipped unrefrigerated.
EM		
Tissue	Collect aseptically, 1 × 2 mm thick; fix in 2%–4% glutaraldehyde (10 × volume) for 24 hr at 20°C.	Ship in leak-proof container with adequate fixative.
Feces or body fluids	Collect fresh; do not freeze or fix.	Refrigerate until shipping; pack on wet ice to last 48–72 hr.

[a]Collected in EDTA and kept refrigerated.
[b]Use Culturettes (Becton Dickinson, Cockeysville, MD).
[c]Use Michel's fixative to preserve tissue specimens for antibody testing by indirect FA. For antigen detection, other fixatives may be used.

Table 1–5. Main Methods Used in Diagnostic Virology[a]

DISTINGUISHING CRITERIA FOR THE METHOD	AVAILABILITY OF RESULTS	SPECIAL REQUIREMENTS	SENSITIVITY	SPECIFICITY	ABILITY TO DIFFERENTIATE VACCINE VIRUS FROM VIRULENT VIRUS	CLINICAL UTILITY
EM	Hours	High viral concentration (10^6–10^9 viral particles/g tissue)	Moderate	Moderate	No	Detects viruses that cannot be readily cultured
Immunologic	Hours	Suitable sample and antiserum available	High	High	Usually not[b]	Applicable to in-clinic use
Viral isolation[c]	Days	Susceptible cell culture, specimen free of contaminants, antiserum available	Variable	Variable	Yes	Identify new, emerging infections
Serology	Hours to days	Suitable antigen available; acute and convalescent serum available	Low to moderate	Low	Usually not[d]	IgM assays reveal recent infections; Western blot serology very specific
Nucleic acid	Hours	Conserved specific nucleic acid sequence, PCR equipment and reagents	High	High	Varies with specificity of primer	Detects small quantities of nucleic acid; can be used to detect preclinical infection

[a]Modified from Drs. D. Burger and T. Crawford, Washington State University.
[b]Recent exceptions are assays using monoclonal antibody to strain specific epitopes (rabies and CPV).
[c]ID usually by specific neutralizing or epitope-specific antibody.
[d]Unless vaccine virus has been engineered to provide "markers" (e.g., pseudorabies).

animals, or if there are unusual clinical signs or suspected new variants of pre-existing viruses, such as CPV and CDV.[12, 16, 21, 25, 29, 32] Veterinarians should be on the alert for first-line detection of emerging infections in secondary hosts.[12, 29, 32] The main methods of viral detection are EM; immunologic detection of viral-coded proteins through immunofluorescence; ELISA and immunoperoxidase (immunohistochemistry); virus isolation in cell cultures or embryonating eggs; serologic assays that detect antibodies to specific viral-coded proteins; and nucleic acid–based detection using PCR for amplification of viral nucleic acid.[5, 9, 31]

Rickettsial Infections

Rickettsiae are small obligate intracellular gram-negative bacteria that are often included with viruses because common diagnostic applications are used.[5] Rickettsiae generally require living cells for propagation and are usually cultured in embryonating chicken eggs or in cell culture. Rickettsiae of veterinary importance and common diagnostic assays are listed in Table 1–6. Refer to the respective chapters (Chapters 27 to 30) for further information on these organisms.

APPLIED MOLECULAR DIAGNOSTICS

Molecular diagnostic techniques have brought about tremendous changes in infectious disease testing.[14, 19, 22] These changes are reflected in the sensitivity with which assays are able to detect viruses and rickettsiae in samples from cats and dogs early during the course of the infection-disease process. The techniques that have had a major impact on the molecular detection of infectious agents are the immunoblot or Western blot (WB) assay and nucleic acid–based testing utilizing methods such as hybridization and polymerase chain reaction (PCR).[13, 20]

Table 1–6. Rickettsial Infections of Veterinary Importance

AGENT	HOST(S)	DISEASE	DIAGNOSIS
Neorickettsia helminthoeca and Elokomin fluke fever agents (see Chapter 27)	Dogs, coyotes, foxes, ferrets	Salmon poisoning and salmon fever	1. Observation of fluke eggs (*Nanophyetus salmincola*) in feces 2. Demonstration of the agent in lymph node aspirates
Ehrlichia spp. (see Chapter 28)	Humans, dogs, cats, other domestic animals	Ehrlichiosis	1. Indirect FA test for antibody in serum 2. Giemsa-stained blood smears or marrow
Rickettsia rickettsii (see Chapter 29)	Humans, dogs	RMSF	1. Indirect FA test for antibody in serum 2. Giemsa-stained blood smears
Haemobartonella felis (see Chapter 30)	Cats	Feline infectious anemia	1. Giemsa or FA-stained blood or tissue smears; presence of agent on red blood cells inconsistent

Immunoblotting (Western Blotting)

The WB is a form of serologic assay that offers increased sensitivity and specificity by separating out the seroreactivity to particular antigens of an organism. Proteins extracted from the organism of concern are separated on agar gel using electrophoresis, and these are transferred directly to nitrocellulose paper by WB. Subsequently, the separated antigens can be reacted with test sera. Antibody binding to specific protein bands can be evaluated by staining with peroxidase-labeled conjugates. Specific antibody reactivity to particular organisms can be defined, and nonspecific antibody reactions can be eliminated from consideration; for example, the WB assay to confirm the specificity of serum antibodies in suspect FIV reactor cats following in-clinic ELISA (Fig. 1–2).[26]

PCR

Nucleic acid–based testing with PCR amplification has allowed for a remarkable increase in the sensitivity and specificity of organism detection (Fig. 1–3). PCR is a method of detecting minute quantities of a DNA or RNA sequence, specific to an organism, and amplifying it logarithmically so that it can be detected by visible means in the laboratory. A specific nucleic acid primer reacts with the genomic material of the microorganism in question. It is then amplified to produce a short fragment of DNA specific to the particular organism. To visualize, the amplified products then are subjected to electrophoresis to measure size and migration pattern. Specific complementary nucleic acid probes serve to confirm the identity of the synthesized product. PCR can be used to detect viral latency or carriers (herpesvirus, FIV) viral shedding (coronavirus); to detect fastidious pathogens (*Bartonella, Ehrlichia*) in blood or body fluids; and to study the pathogenesis or to discover the etiologic agents of newly recognized infectious diseases.[10]

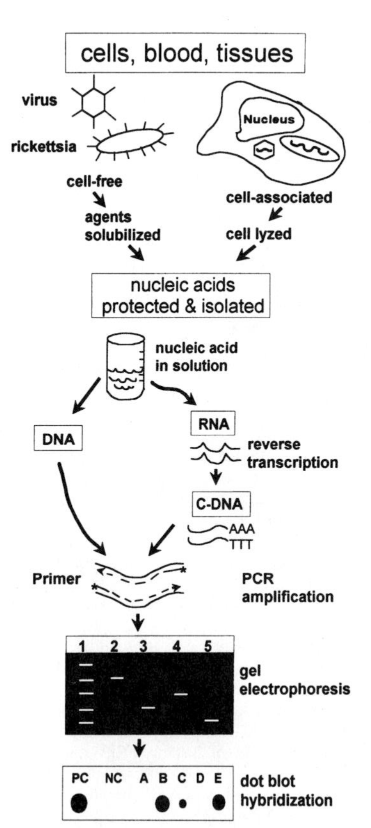

Figure 1–3. Scheme depicting the principles of nucleic acid isolation, amplification by PCR, purification and identification by gel electrophoresis, and/or validation of the PCR products by specific oligonucleotide probes by dot blot hybridization. Dot blot key: PC, positive control; NC, negative control; blots A and D negative; blots B, C, and E positive for viral or rickettsial nucleic acid. Modified from Clontech Laboratories Inc. with assistance from Dr. I. Eriks, Washington State University, 1996, with permission.

Utilization of both the WB assays and nucleic acid–based testing has expanded our capabilities to detect infections during the preclinical stages and to distinguish infections of closely related viruses in expanded host ranges. The employment of WB to study the ecology of the FIV family infecting lions and pumas is an example of the utility of this assay.[3] Studies on the evolution and mutation frequency of viruses affecting cats and dogs have used nucleic acid–based PCR testing. Examples of the use of this technology has been demonstrated by the observation of CPV type 2b in cats and dogs[29] and the divergence of rabies virus in wildlife populations, such as bats.[23, 27] Because of their extreme sensitivity, results of these assays should not be overinterpreted, and precautions and controls must be taken in the laboratory to ensure that specimens have not become contaminated.

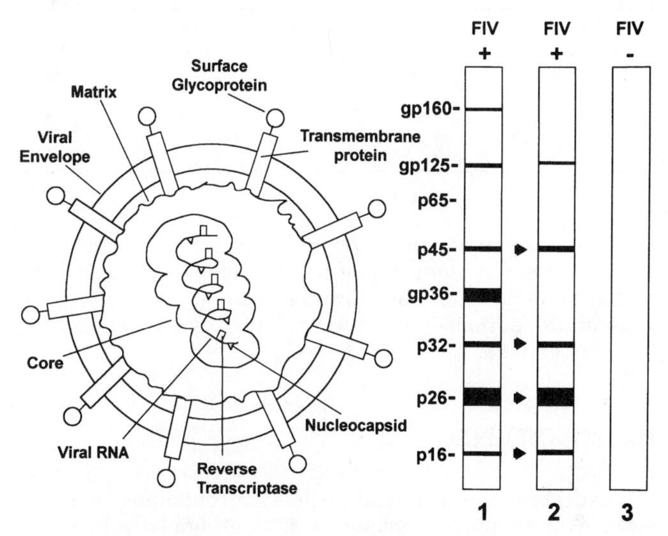

Figure 1–2. Diagram of Western blot (immunoblot) profile using FIV as an example. Cross-section of FIV to the left and three blot profiles to the right. Reactive sera from cat typically contains demonstrable antibodies to envelope glycoproteins (gp125, gp160), to the core proteins (p26, p32, p45), and to reverse transcriptase (p16). The predominant antibodies detected are generally to p16, p26, p32, and p45 *(arrows)*. The numbers indicate the position and size (in kilodaltons) of the FIV protein (p). Blots 1 and 2 represent a FIV-positive cat, and blot 3 represents a negative cat.

References

1. Angulo FJ, Glaser CA, Juranek DD, et al. 1995. Caring for pets of immunocompromised persons. *Can Vet J* 36:217–222.
2. Anvik JD. 1991. Clinical considerations of canine herpesvirus infection. *Vet Med* 86:394–403.
3. Brown EW, Yuhki N, Packer C, et al. 1995. A lion lentivirus related to feline immunodeficiency virus: epidemiologic and phylogenetic aspects. *J Virol* 68:5953–5968.
4. Callanan JJ. 1995. Feline immunodeficiency virus infection: a clinical and pathological perspective, pp 111–130. *In* Willett BJ, Jarrett O (eds): Feline immunology and immunodeficiency. Oxford Science Publishers, Oxford, England.
5. Carter GR, Chengappa MM, Roberts AW. 1995. Some methods used to

study viruses, pp 291–300. *In* Carter GR, Chengappa MM, Roberts AW (eds): Essentials of veterinary microbiology, ed 5. Williams & Wilkins, Baltimore, MD.
6. Diehl LJ, Mathiason-Dubard CK, O'Neil LL, et al. 1996. Plasma viral RNA load predicts disease progression in accelerated feline immunodeficiency virus infection. *J Virol* 70:2503–2507.
7. Evermann JF. 1990. Laboratory diagnosis of viral and rickettsial infections, pp 215–220. *In* Greene CE (ed): Infectious diseases of the dog and cat. WB Saunders, Philadelphia, PA.
8. Evermann JF, Henry CJ, Marks SL. 1995. Feline infectious peritonitis. Clinical update. *J Am Vet Med Assoc* 206:1130–1134.
9. Finlaison DS. 1995. Faecal viruses of dogs: an electron microscope study. *Vet Microbiol* 46:295–305.
10. Gao J-J, Moore PS. 1996. Molecular approaches to the identification of unculturable infectious agents. *Emerg Infect Dis* 2:159–167.
11. Greig B, Asanovich KM, Armstrong PJ, et al. 1996. Geographic, clinical, serologic, and molecular evidence of granulocytic ehrlichiosis, a likely zoonotic disease, in Minnesota and Wisconsin dogs. *J Clin Microbiol* 34:44–48.
12. Harder TC, Kenter M, Vos H, et al. 1996. Canine distemper virus from diseased large felids: biological properties and phylogenetic relationships. *J Gen Virol* 77:397–405.
13. Hardy KJ, Young HA, Lagoo AS. 1994. Molecular diagnostics. *Immunol Allergy Clin North Am* 14:199–223.
14. Herrewegh AP, DeGroot RJ, Cepica A, et al. 1995. Detection of feline coronavirus RNA in feces, tissues, and body fluids of naturally infected cats by reverse transcriptase PCR. *J Clin Microbiol* 33:684–689.
15. Hoskins JD. 1991. Tick-transmitted diseases. *Vet Clin North Am Small Anim Pract* 21:1–199.
16. Houston DM, Ribble CS, Head LL. 1996. Risk factors associated with parvovirus enteritis in dogs: 283 cases (1982–1991). *J Am Vet Med Assoc* 208:542–546.
17. Jackson ML, Haines DM, Taylor SM, et al. 1996. Feline leukemia virus detection by ELISA and PCR in peripheral blood from 68 cats with high, moderate, or low suspicion of having FELV-related disease. *J Vet Diag Invest* 8:25–30.
18. Jacobson RH. 1991. How well do serodiagnostic tests predict the infection or disease status of cats? *J Am Vet Med Assoc* 199:1343–1347.
19. Jacobson RH, Romatowski J. 1996. Assessing the validity of serodiagnostic test results. *Semin Vet Med Surg* 11:135–143.
20. James K. 1990. Immunoserology of infectious diseases. *Clin Microbiol Rev* 3:132–152.
21. Johnson R, Glickman LT, Emerick TJ, et al. 1995. Canine distemper infection in pet dogs. I. Surveillance in Indiana during a suspected outbreak. *J Am Anim Hosp Assoc* 31:223–229.
22. Martinez ML, Weiss RC. 1993. Applications of genetic engineering technology in feline medicine. *Vet Clin North Am Small Anim Pract* 23:213–226.
23. Nadin-Davis SA, Huang W, Alexander S. 1996. The design of strain-specific polymerase chain reactions for discrimination of the raccoon rabies virus strain from indigenous rabies virus of Ontario. *J Virol Methods* 57:1–14.
24. Sackett DL, Haynes RB, Guyatt GH, et al. 1991. Early diagnosis, pp 153–170. *In* Sackett DL et al (eds): Clinical epidemiology. A basic science for clinical medicine, ed 2. Little, Brown, Boston, MA.
25. Scarlett JM. 1995. Companion animal epidemiology. *Prev Vet Med* 25:151–160.
26. Shelton GH, Grant CK, Cotter SM, et al. 1990. Feline immunodeficiency virus and feline leukemia virus infections and their relationships to lymphoid malignancies in cats: a retrospective study (1968–1988). *J Acquire Immune Defic Syndr* 3:623–630.
27. Smith JS. 1996. New aspects of rabies with emphasis on epidemiology, diagnosis and prevention of the disease in the United States. *Clin Microbiol Rev* 9:166–176.
28. Smith RD. 1995. Use of diagnostic tests. Veterinary clinical epidemiology, pp 53–70. *In* Smith RD (ed): A problem oriented approach, ed 2. CRC Press, Boca Raton, FL.
29. Truyen U, Evermann JF, Vieler E, et al. 1996. Evolution of canine parvovirus involved loss and gain of feline host range. *Virology* 215:186–189.
30. Weigler BJ, Babineau CA, Sherry B, et al. 1997. High sensitivity polymerase chain reaction assay for active and latent feline herpesvirus-1 infections in domestic cats. *Vet Rec* 140:335–338.
31. White DO, Fenner FJ. 1994. Laboratory diagnosis of viral diseases, pp 191–218. *In* White DO, Fenner FJ (eds): Medical virology, ed 4. Academic Press, San Diego, CA.
32. Wilbur LA, Evermann JF, Levings RL, et al. 1994. Abortion and death in pregnant bitches associated with a canine vaccine contaminated with bluetongue virus. *J Am Vet Med Assoc* 204:1762–1765.

Chapter **2**

Antiviral Drugs

Craig E. Greene and A. D. J. Watson

The development and clinical use of antiviral drugs have been much slower than those of other antimicrobial agents. It is difficult to achieve selective interference by antiviral chemotherapy because viral replication is more dependent on host cell metabolism than is bacterial replication. Unlike antibacterial therapy, antiviral drug use usually involves prophylactic administration. Viruses are usually inhibited only during their replicative cycle and may be resistant to drugs during latent or nonreplicative phases of infection. Acute viral infections are difficult to treat, partly because diagnosis is often made after the replicative phase of infection is complete. Antiviral agents are often useful, therefore, in treating chronic viral infections and in preventing reactivation of latent infections.

Many antiviral drugs tested are never licensed because they prove too toxic during preliminary screening. All licensed drugs are approved for human use and have limited application for dogs and cats. A number of new drugs specifically intended for treatment of HIV have been omitted in this review. The properties of potentially useful systemic antiviral compounds are summarized in Table 2–1 and later in this chapter. A summary of topical antiviral drugs is presented in Table 93–3. For more information and dosages of systemically administered antiviral drugs, see Drug Formulary, Appendix 8.

IDOXURIDINE

Idoxuridine is a synthetic nucleoside containing deoxyribose. As a thymidine analog, it is incorporated into DNA structure and inhibits the enzymes of DNA synthesis. As with most clinically used antiviral drugs, it does not affect latent virus infections. It is active against herpesviruses, although some strains are resistant. It is applied topically to treat keratitis and dermatitis (see Ocular Infections, Chapter 93). Prolonged topical use may cause irritation or nonhealing corneal ulcers. Because hepatotoxicity is common, it is rarely administered systemically against herpesvirus encephalitis.

Table 2–1. Comparison of Potentially Useful Systemic Antiviral Drugs[a]

DRUG	BRAND NAME (MANUFACTURER)	ANTIVIRAL SPECTRUM	ROUTE OF ADMINISTRATION[b]
Amantadine	Symmetrel (Dupont), Symadine (Reid-Powell)	Influenza virus	PO
Rimantadine	Flumadine (Forest)	Influenza virus	PO
Acyclovir	Zovirax (Burroughs Wellcome)	Herpesviruses[c]	PO, IV
Ganciclovir	Cytovene (Syntex)	Herpesviruses[c]	IV, PO
Ribavirin	Virazole (ICN)	Respiratory syncytial virus	PO, IV
Zidovudine (AZT)	Retrovir (Burroughs Wellcome)	Retroviruses[d]	PO, IV
Foscarnet	Foscavir (Astra)	Herpesviruses, retroviruses	IV
Interferon-α_{2a}	Roferon-A (Roche)	Retroviruses, herpesviruses, other	PO, IV
α_{2b}	Intron A (Schering-Plough)	Retroviruses, herpesviruses, other	PO, IV
Interferon-β_{1b}	Betaseron (Berlex)	Antiviral, immunostimulant	SC
Interferon-γ_{1b}	Actimmune (Genentech)	Biologic response modifier, immunostimulant	SC

[a]For a list of topically applied drugs and their formulations, see Table 93–3. For dosages, formulations, and indications of the drugs listed here, see Drug Formulary, Appendix 8.
[b]IM = intramuscular; IV = intravenous; PO = oral; SC = subcutaneous.
[c]Other antiherpesvirus drugs of this type include famciclovir, Famvir (Smith Kline Beecham); valacyclovir, Valtrex (Burroughs Wellcome).
[d]Other similar antiretroviral nucleoside analog drugs include stavudine, Zerit (Bristol-Meyers Squibb); lamivudine, Epivir (Glaxo); didanosine (dideoxyinosine), Videx (Bristol-Meyers Squibb); zalcitabine (dideoxycytidine), Hivid (Roche). The retroviral protease inhibitors are saquinavir, Invirase (Roche); indinavir, Crixivan (Merck); and ritonavir, Norvir (Abbott).

VIDARABINE

Vidarabine, a purine nucleoside, also inhibits DNA synthesis by being incorporated into nucleic acid and inhibiting DNA-synthetic enzymes. It is effective in vitro against herpesviruses, poxviruses, and oncornaviruses, but clinical use in humans has been restricted to treatment of smallpox and herpesviral keratitis and encephalitis. Vidarabine must be administered IV because of low solubility and must be given in large volumes of fluid over extended periods. Toxic effects include local irritation at infusion sites, nausea, vomiting, and diarrhea. The drug also causes bone marrow suppression, resulting in anemia, leukopenia, and thrombocytopenia. Vidarabine monophosphate, a new form, can be given IM without needing large fluid volumes. However, systemic toxicity restricts its use in veterinary practice to topical ophthalmic treatment (see Chapter 93, Ocular Infections).

AMANTADINE

Amantadine is a highly stable cyclic amine with a narrow spectrum that primarily inhibits penetration and uncoating of RNA viruses. It is rapidly and completely absorbed after oral administration and widely distributed throughout the body. About 90% is excreted unchanged in urine. It has been administered only for prophylaxis of human influenza and is most efficacious when administered during early infection. Commonly encountered side effects include CNS toxicity, nausea, and vomiting in people, although dogs have been given high daily doses for longer than 2 years without ill effects. Rimantadine, a closely related analog, has equal or greater efficacy with reduced CNS side effects but more GI irritation.

ACYCLOVIR AND GANCICLOVIR

Acyclovir, an acyclic purine nucleoside, more potent in vitro against certain herpesviruses than idoxuridine and vidarabine, is becoming the agent of choice for treating herpesvirus infections. Its unique antiviral mechanism involves metabolism by viral-directed enzymes of infected cells to an intermediate that inhibits viral DNA polymerase. It interferes only with actively replicating virus and does not cure latent viral infections. It has been given parenterally, orally, and topically in people to treat genital and mucocutaneous herpesvirus infections and parenterally in people and experimental animals against herpesviral encephalitis. Systemic administration in people is most effective for genital infections. It is incompletely absorbed when administered orally, and more than 45% of the dose appears in the urine unmetabolized. Excretion of the drug is delayed in renal failure.

Acyclovir has a relatively low toxicity because it selectively interferes with viral DNA synthesis. However, when given systemically, it may precipitate in the renal tubules, causing obstructive nephropathy if diuresis is inadequate. This renal failure is reversible with adequate rehydration. IV administration may produce phlebitis and local irritation. Acyclovir has potential benefits for treatment of herpesvirus infections in domesticated animals and has been given to cats.

A number of related derivatives have potent antiviral activity. One, famciclovir, is well absorbed orally and is converted to acyclovir in the body. Its main advantage is high tissue concentrations achievable with oral dosing.

Ganciclovir, another analog, has activity against most of the herpesviruses. Its antiviral effect is greater than acyclovir, but it is also more toxic to bone marrow. Ganciclovir has primarily been used IV to treat immunosuppressed people with cytomegalovirus infection. Resistance of human herpesviruses to acyclovir and ganciclovir occurs.

Bromovinyl arabinosyl uracil (sorivudine) is a halogenated thymidine analog with a mechanism of action similar to acyclovir. It has less toxicity and greater antiviral activity than acyclovir and is currently in clinical trials.

RIBAVIRIN

Ribavirin is a broad-spectrum triazole nucleoside that has marked in vitro antiviral activity against a variety of DNA and RNA viruses. It interferes with protein synthesis, and the strongest antiviral activity in animal studies is against RNA respiratory viruses and herpesviruses. Ribavirin has been effective in HIV infection, and Lassa fever, a human arenovirus infection. This nucleoside is active against a number of canine and feline viruses in vitro (see Drug Formulary, Appendix 8). Ribavirin has also been used in treating people with respiratory syncytial viral infection. By the aerosol route, only low concentrations appear in the systemic circulation. Concentration in respiratory secretions can be much higher when it is given orally. Although not currently marketed for oral use in humans, it has been given orally to cats experimentally infected with calicivirus. Side effects have limited the systemic use of ribavirin in veterinary practice.

TRIFLURIDINE

Trifluridine (trifluorothymidine), a synthetic nucleoside, blocks DNA synthesis through inhibiting enzyme production by becoming incorporated in the structural framework of the viral nucleic acid. When given systemically, it causes many toxic side effects, including leukopenia and GI signs. It has been used most often topically to treat ocular herpesvirus infections.

RETROVIRAL INHIBITORS

In an attempt to control retroviruses affecting people and animals, a number of compounds that interfere with RNA-dependent polymerase (reverse transcriptase, RT) or retroviral proteases have been developed.

Zidovudine (azidothymidine, AZT), an inhibitor of RT, has been extensively used to treat HIV infection in people. It suppresses viral replication and helps slow the onset of progression of AIDS. AZT is 100 times more active against HIV-RT than mammalian cell DNA-RT. It has activity against other mammalian retroviruses as well. AZT has been shown to be somewhat effective in treating cats experimentally infected with FeLV when treatment is initiated less than 3 weeks after infection. When treated less than 1 week after challenge, cats are protected from bone marrow infection and persistent viremia. If the infection is already established, therapy may reduce somewhat the amount of antigen in the blood, although viremia persists. The probability of infection is reduced when treatment is initiated soon after infection and higher dosages of AZT are given. For further information on AZT, see Drug Formulary, Appendix 8. For a listing of other antiretroviral drugs see Table 2–1.

FOSCARNET

This pyrophosphate analog has a wide spectrum of activity against DNA and RNA viruses. It is administered IV and continuously because of its short half-life. Foscarnet accumulates in bone matrix, but the possibility of penetration of the blood-brain barrier is controversial. Most of the drug is excreted in urine. It has been administered to treat HIV infection, but significant nephrotoxicity has limited its use. Certain acyclovir-resistant herpesvirus infections in people have been treated successfully with foscarnet.

IMMUNOGLOBULINS

Immunoglobulins with specific antiviral activity are beneficial in treating viral infections. Improvement has been documented using immunoglobulins for early treatment or prophylaxis of canine and feline parvoviral infections and systemic canine herpesvirus infections. If given as plasma (vs. serum), the IV route can be used; otherwise the IM, SC, and IP routes are possible and are most accessible for puppies and kittens. See also the discussion of passive immunoprophylaxis in Chapter 100.

IMMUNOMODULATORS

These substances modify the responses of immunocompetent cells through cytokines or other mechanisms. They can be used against viruses and other infectious agents. For additional information to that provided next, see the Drug Formulary, Appendix 8, and Immunoprophylaxis and Immunotherapy, Chapter 100. Levamisole, isoprinosine, and transfer factor have been used to treat viral infections, but their effects have never been substantiated by controlled studies; they remain investigational. IFN-α and G-CSF are commercially available and have been given to treat feline retroviral and canine parvoviral infections, respectively. Extracts of *Propionibacterium acnes* (Immunoregulin, Immunovet) and complex carbohydrates (Acemannan, Carrington Labs) are available for veterinary use (see Immunoprophylaxis and Immunotherapy, Chapter 100, and Drug Formulary, Appendix 8).

INTERFERONS

IFNs are polypeptide molecules produced by vertebrate cells in response to viral infections or certain inert substances, such as double-stranded RNA, and other microbial agents. There are at least three types of interferon: IFN-α, formerly leukocyte interferon; IFN-β, formerly fibroblast interferon; and IFN-γ. IFN-α and IFN-β are structurally similar, being produced in response to viral infection or polyribonucleotide administration. IFN-γ is structurally distinct and is produced by T lymphocytes in response to specific antigenic stimulus. Human IFNs have been manufactured by recombinant DNA technology and are available clinically (see Table 2–1). IFN-α and -β have antiviral activity. IFN-α has been licensed for the treatment of people with myelogenous leukemia, papillomatosis, and AIDS-related complications. IFN-β is licensed for adjunctive treatment of various lymphatic and disseminated neoplasms and for treatment of symptomatic AIDS patients. IFN-γ is licensed for the treatment of people with chronic granulomatous diseases and is considered to be an immunostimulant in animals rather than an antiviral drug.

IFN-α and IFN-β bind to specific cell receptors that activate enzymes that inhibit synthesis, assembly, and release of virus. They are not virucidal but merely inhibit viral nucleic acid and protein synthesis. These IFNs are not species specific in their effects, although their biologic activity and toleration are greater in cells of genetically related species. They are active against many DNA and RNA viruses, although in vitro sensitivities vary. Myxoviruses are susceptible, whereas adenoviruses are not. IFNs have been shown to inhibit oncogenic transformation induced by retroviruses.

IFNs are usually given IM and IV to people to achieve therapeutic concentrations because they are not absorbed through GI or other mucosa and are inactivated by gastric acid. They penetrate poorly into the CSF, brain, and eye and are cleared from the circulation rapidly, within 4 hours. In people, high-dose parenteral IFN administration has shown some efficacy against infections such as influenza, rhinoviruses, herpesviruses, and papillomaviruses. IFNs have been given topically, intranasally, and ocularly to control rhinovirus respiratory signs and intralesionally for papillomavirus infections.

Human IFN given parenterally to cats for retroviral infections becomes ineffective after several weeks because of neutralizing antibodies that limit its activity (see Drug Formulary, Appendix 8). When given orally in low doses, human IFN-α has been beneficial in controlled studies in improving the appetite, bone marrow suppression, and clinical well-being of FeLV-infected cats[2] (see Immunotherapy, Chapter 100, and Drug Formulary, Appendix 8).

References

1. Barlough JE, Scott FW. 1990. Effectiveness of three antiviral agents against FIP virus in vitro. *Vet Rec* 126:556–558.

2. Cummins JM, Tompkins MB, Olsen RG, et al. 1988. Oral use of human alpha interferon in cats. *J Biol Response Mod* 7:513–523.
3. Egberink HF, Hartman K, Horzinek MC. 1991. Chemotherapy of feline immunodeficiency virus infection. *J Am Vet Med Assoc* 199:1485–1487.
4. Fogleman RW, Chapdelaine JM, Carpenter RH, et al. 1992. Toxicologic evaluation of injectable acemannan in the mouse, rat and dog. *Vet Hum Toxicol* 34:201–205.
5. Greene CE. 1990. Antiviral chemotherapy, pp 221–225. *In* Greene CE (ed): Infectious diseases of the dog and cat. WB Saunders, Philadelphia, PA.
6. Hart S, Nolte I. 1995. Long term treatment of diseased FIV-seropositive field cats with azidothymidine. *Zentrabl Veterinarmed A* 42:397–409.
7. Hartmann K. 1995. AZT in the treatment of feline immunodeficiency virus infection: part 1. *Feline Pract* 23(5):16–21.
8. Hartmann K. 1995. AZT in the treatment of feline immunodeficiency virus infection: part 2. *Feline Pract* 23(6):13–20.
9. Haschek WM, Weigel RM, Scherba G, et al. 1990. Zidovudine toxicity to cats infected with feline leukemia virus. *Fundam Appl Toxicol* 14:764–775.
10. Hayes KA, Lafrado LJ, Erickson JG, et al. 1993. Prophylactic ZDV therapy prevents early uremia and lymphocyte decline but not primary infection in feline immunodeficiency virus-inoculated cats. *J Acquir Immune Defic Syndr* 6:127–134.
11. Hirschberger J. 1988. Application of acyclovir (virustaticum) to cats. *Tierarztl Prax* 16:427–430.
12. King GK, Yates KM, Greenlee PG, et al. 1995. The effect of acemannan immunostimulant in combination with surgery and radiation therapy on spontaneous canine and feline fibrosarcomas. *J Am Anim Hosp Assoc* 31:439–447.
13. Lafrado JL, Mathes LE, Zack PM, et al. 1990. Biological effects of staphylococcal protein A immunotherapy in cats with induced feline leukemia virus infection. *Am J Vet Res* 51:482–486.
14. Lvov ND, Chekanovskaya LA, Alimbarova LM, et al. 1995. Antiviral activity of vegetan, a new natural immunostimulator, in herpetic meningoencephalitis of mice, genital herpes of guinea pigs and parvoviral enteritis of dogs. *Vopr Virusol* 40:85–89.
15. Macy DW. 1995. Use of antiviral agents in cats. *Feline Pract* 23(5):25–26.
16. Mathes LE, Hayes KA, Swenson CL, et al. 1994. Evaluation of antiviral activity and toxicity of dextran sulfate in feline leukemia virus-infected cats. *Antimicrob Agents Chemother* 35:2147–2150.
17. Remington KM, Chesebro B, Wehrly K, et al. 1991. Mutants of feline immunodeficiency virus resistant to 3′-azido-3′deoxythymidine. *J Virol* 65:308–312.
18. Ritschel WA, Grummich KW, Hussain SA. 1985. Pharmacokinetics of PFA (trisodium phosphonoformate) after IV and PO administration to beagle dogs and rabbits. *Methods Find Exp Clin Pharmacol* 7:41–48.
19. Sheets MA, Unger BA, Giggleman GF, et al. 1991. Studies of the effect of acemannan on retrovirus infections: clinical stabilization of feline leukemia virus-infected cats. *Mol Biother* 3:41–45.
20. Smyth NR, Bennett M, Gaskell RM, et al. 1994. Effect of 3′azido-2′,3′-deoxythymidine (AZT) on experimental feline immunodeficiency virus infection in domestic cats. *Res Vet Sci* 57:220–224.
21. Stiles J. 1995. Treatment of cats with ocular disease attributable to herpesvirus infection: 17 cases (1983–1993). *J Am Vet Med Assoc* 207:599–603.
22. Straw JA, Loo Ti Li, deVera CC, et al. 1992. Pharmacokinetics of potential anti-AIDS agents thiofoscarnet and foscarnet in the cat. *J Acquir Immune Defic Syndr* 5:936–942.
23. Swenson CL, Sams RA, Polas PJ, et al. 1990. Age related differences in pharmacokinetics of phosphonoformate in cats. *Antimicrob Agents Chemother* 34:871–874.
24. Swenson CL, Weisbrode SE, Nagode LA, et al. 1991. Age-related differences in phosphonoformate-induced bone toxicity in cats. *Calcif Tissue Int* 48:353–361.
25. Veda Y, Sakurai T, Kasama K, et al. 1993. Pharmacokinetic properties of recombinant feline interferon and its stimulatory effect on 2′,5′-oligoadenylate synthetase activity in the cat. *J Vet Med Sci* 55:1–6.
26. Weiss RC. 1995. Treatment of feline infectious peritonitis with immunomodulating agents and antiviral drugs–a review. *Feline Pract* 23:103–106.
27. Weiss RC, Cox NR, Boudreaux MK. 1993. Toxicologic effects of ribavirin in cats. *J Vet Pharmacol Ther* 16:301–316.
28. Weiss RC, Cox NR, Martinez ML. 1993. Evaluation of free or liposome-encapsulated ribavirin for antiviral therapy of experimentally induced feline infectious peritonitis. *Res Vet Sci* 55:162–172.
29. Weiss RC, Oostrom-Ram T. 1989. Inhibitory effects of ribavirin alone or combined with human alpha interferon on feline infectious peritonitis virus replication in vitro. *Vet Microbiol* 20:255–265.
30. Weiss RC, Oostrom-Ram T. 1990. Effect of recombinant human interferon-alpha in vitro and in vivo on mitogen-induced lymphocyte blastogenesis in cats. *Vet Immunol Immunopathol* 24:147–157.
31. Whitley RJ, Gnann JW. 1992. Acyclovir: a decade later. *N Engl J Med* 327:782–788.
32. Zeidner NS, Myles MH, Mathiason-DuBard CK, et al. 1990. Alpha interferon (2b) in combination with zidovudine for the treatment of presymptomatic feline leukemia virus-induced immunodeficiency syndrome. *Antimicrob Agents Chemother* 34:1749–1756.
33. Zeidner NS, Rose LM, Mathiason-DuBard CK, et al. 1990. Zidovudine in combination with alpha interferon and interleukin-2 as prophylactic therapy for FeLV-induced immunodeficiency syndrome (FeLV-FAIDS). *J Acquir Immune Defic Syndr* 3:787–796.

Chapter 3

Canine Distemper

Craig E. Greene and Max J. Appel

ETIOLOGY

Canine distemper virus (CDV) is a member of the genus *Morbillivirus* of the Paramyxoviridae and is closely related to other viruses (Table 3–1). CDV is relatively large (150–250 nm) with single-stranded RNA wound in helical symmetry. It is surrounded by a lipoprotein envelope derived from virus glycoproteins incorporated into the cell membrane (Fig. 3–1 and Table 3–2). Viruses such as CDV that code for proteins capable of integrating in the cell membrane make infected cells susceptible to damage by immune-mediated cytolysis. CDV also may induce cellular fusion as a means of direct intercellular spread.

CDV is susceptible to UV light, although protein or antioxidants help to protect it from inactivation. Extremely susceptible to heat and drying, CDV is destroyed by temperatures greater than 50° to 60°C for 30 minutes. In removed tissues it survives for at least an hour at 37°C and for 3 hours at 20°C (room temperature). In warm climates, CDV does not persist in kennels after infected dogs have been removed. Storage and survival times of CDV are longer at colder temperatures. At near-freezing (0°–4°C), it survives in the environment for weeks. Below freezing the virus is stable, surviving at −65°C for at least 7 years. Lyophilization reduces the lability of the virus and is an excellent means of preserving it for commercial vaccine and laboratory use. CDV remains viable between pH 4.5 and 9.0. As an enveloped virus it is susceptible to ether and chloroform, dilute (<0.5%) formalin solution, phenol (0.75%), and quaternary ammonium disinfectant (0.3%). Routine disinfection proce-

Table 3–1. Host Susceptibility to Morbilliviruses[a]

DISEASE (VIRUS ABBREVIATION)	NATURAL HOSTS	EXPERIMENTAL INFECTION
Measles (MV)	Domestic: humans Wild: primates	Macaques, marmosets, mice, hamsters, rats
Rinderpest (RPV)	Domestic: cattle, pigs, goats, sheep Wild: buffalo, eland, giraffe, kudu, warthog, wildebeest, banteng, black buck, gaur, nilgai, sambhar	
Peste des petits ruminants (PPRV)	Domestic: goat, sheep Wild: gazelle, ibex, gemsbok	Goats, cattle, pig, deer
Phocine distemper (PDV)	Seal	Dog, mink, seal
Canine distemper (CDV)	Seal (PDV-2) Canidae (dog, fox, wolf, coyote, etc.) Mustelidae (ferret etc.) Procyonidae (raccoon etc.) Felidae (cat, lion, etc.)	Dog, mouse, rat, hamster, mink, pig, cat, nonhuman primate, ferret
Dolphin distemper (DMV)	Dolphins	Cattle, sheep, goat, dog
Porpoise distemper (PMV)	Porpoises	Cattle, sheep, goat, dog
Equine morbillivirus (EMV)	Domestic: horses, humans Wild: Pteropus bats	Cats

[a]Modified from Osterhaus ADME, de Swart RL, Vos HW, et al: *Vet Microbiol* 44:219–227, 1995, with permission.

dures are usually effective in destroying CDV in a kennel or hospital.

The disease and natural host ranges of CDV include certain species of terrestrial carnivores (see Tables 3–1 and 3–3), and other species can be infected experimentally with varying degrees of susceptibility. CNS signs have been produced in mice and hamsters by intracerebral inoculation. Rabbits and rats are resistant to parenteral inoculation. Inapparent, self-limiting infections, produced in cats, nonhuman primates, and humans by parenteral inoculation of virulent CDV, resemble those in dogs that have been given MLV vaccines. Pigs are subclinically infected, and peccaries that have been naturally infected develop encephalitis.[9] CNS infections in exotic Felidae have been attributed to infection with CDV[9, 63, 81, 92] (see Feline Paramyxovirus Encephalomyelitis, Chapter 18). Encephalitis was documented in a naturally infected monkey.[93] A morbillivirus most closely related to CDV and a strain of CDV has caused severe morbidity in seals (Tables 3–1 and 3–4). It may have spread to them from dogs or other susceptible carnivores. Other closely related but distinct morbilliviruses cause illness in other aquatic mammals.

EPIDEMIOLOGY

CDV, most abundant in respiratory exudates, is commonly spread by aerosol or droplet exposure; however, it can be isolated from most other body tissues and secretions, including urine. Virus can be excreted up to 60 to 90 days after infection, although shorter periods of shedding are more typical. Contact between recently infected (subclinical or diseased) animals maintains the virus in a population, and a constant supply of puppies helps to provide a susceptible population for infection. Although immunity to canine distemper is prolonged, it is not necessarily solid or lifelong. Dogs that do not receive periodic immunizations may lose their protection and become infected after stress, immunosuppression, or contact with diseased individuals. The infection rate is higher than the disease rate, which reflects a certain degree of natural and vaccine-induced immunity in the general dog population. Estimates are that 25% to 75% of susceptible dogs become subclinically infected but clear the virus from the body without showing signs of illness.

The prevalence rate of spontaneous distemper in cosmopolitan dogs is greatest between 3 and 6 months of age, correlating with the loss of maternal antibodies in puppies after weaning. In contrast, in susceptible, isolated populations of dogs, the disease is severe and widespread, affecting all ages.[1, 18, 44, 49, 50, 54, 70] Increased susceptibility among breeds has been suspected but not proved. Brachiocephalic dogs have been reported to have a lower prevalence of disease, mortality, and sequelae compared with dolichocephalic breeds. Breeds most commonly and severely affected include greyhounds, Siberian huskies, Weimaraners, Samoyeds, and Alaskan malamutes.

Viral virulence is another parameter that may affect the severity and extent or type of clinical disease. Certain isolates, such as Snyder Hill, A75/17, and R252 strain, are highly virulent and neurotropic. The first causes polioencephalomyelitis, whereas the latter two cause demyelination. Others vary in ability to cause CNS lesions. Properties of the NP- and M-genes contain the determinants of viral persistence.[81a]

PATHOGENESIS

Systemic Infection

During natural exposure, CDV spreads by aerosol droplets and contacts epithelium of the upper respiratory tract (Fig.

Table 3–2. Structure of Canine Distemper Virus

COMPONENTS	ABBREVIATION	MOLECULAR WEIGHT	FUNCTION
Envelope			
Hemagglutinin	H	76	Structural-viral attachment
Matrix protein	M	34	Structural-penetration
Fusion 1 protein	F_1	40	Structural-penetration
Fusion 2 protein	F_2	20–13	Structural-penetration
Nuclear			
Large protein	L	180–200	Functional-polymerase complex
Polymerase	P	66	Functional-polymerase complex
Nucleocapsid	NP	58	Structural, protects genome

Table 3–3. Order Carnivora Susceptible to Canine Distemper [a]

ORDER	DESCRIPTION
Ailuridae	Lesser and giant pandas
Canidae	Coyote, dingo, raccoon dog, wolf, fox
Hyaenidae	Hyena
Mustelidae	Ferret, marten, mink, other, skunk, wolverine, badger
Procyonidae	Coati, kinkajou, raccoon
Ursidae	Bears
Viverridae	Binturong, fossa, linsang, mongoose, civet
Felidae	Cheetah, lion, jaguar, margay, ocelot

[a]From Appel MJG, Summers BA: *Vet Microbiol* 44:187–191, 1995. Reprinted with permission.

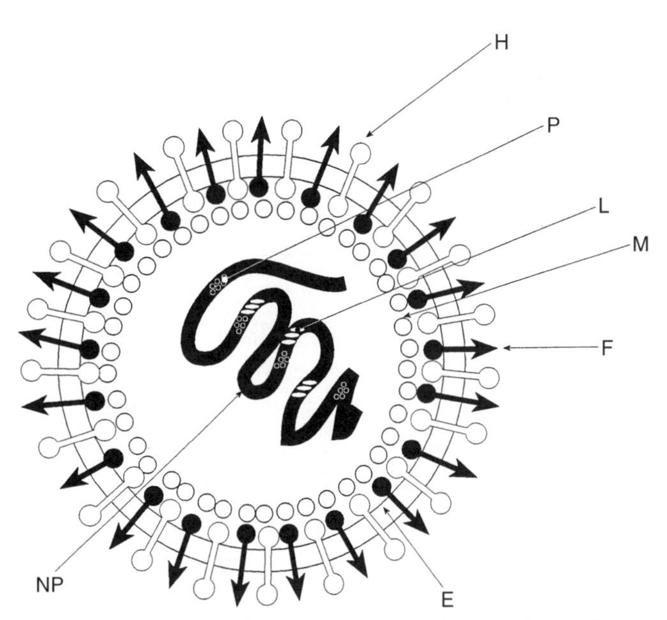

Figure 3–1. Structure of canine distemper virus. (H, hemaglutinin [neuraminidase]; F, fusion protein; M, matrix protein; E, lipoprotein envelope; L, large protein; P, polymerase protein; NP, nucleocapsid.)

3–2). Within 24 hours, it multiplies in tissue macrophages and spreads in these cells via local lymphatics to tonsils and bronchial lymph nodes. By 2 to 4 days postinoculation (PI), virus numbers increase in tonsils and retropharyngeal and bronchial lymph nodes, but low numbers of CDV-infected mononuclear cells are found in other lymphoid organs. By days 4 to 6 PI, virus multiplication occurs within lymphoid follicles in the spleen, in the lamina propria of the stomach and small intestines, in the mesenteric lymph nodes, and in the Kupffer's cells in the liver. Widespread virus proliferation in lymphoid organs corresponds to an initial rise in body temperature and leukopenia. The leukopenia is primarily a lymphopenia caused by viral damage to lymphoid cells, affecting both T and B cells.

Further spread of CDV to epithelial and CNS tissues on days 8 to 9 PI probably occurs hematogenously, as a cell-associated and plasma-phase viremia, and depends on the dog's humoral and cell-mediated immune status. Shedding of virus begins at the time of epithelial colonization and occurs from all body excretions, even in dogs with subclinical infections. By day 14 PI, animals with adequate CDV antibody titers and cell-mediated cytotoxicity clear the virus from most tissues and show no clinical signs of illness. Specific IgG-CDV antibody has been shown to be effective in neutralizing extracellular CDV and inhibiting its intercellular spread.

Dogs with intermediate levels of cell-mediated immunoresponsiveness with delayed antibody titers by days 9 to 14 PI have virus spread to their epithelial tissues. Clinical signs that develop may eventually resolve as antibody titer increases. Virus is cleared from most body tissues as antibody titers increase but may persist for extended periods as complete virus in uveal tissues and neurons and in integument such as footpads. Recovery from CDV infection is associated with long-term immunity and cessation of viral shedding. Protection may be compromised if the dog is exposed to a highly virulent or large quantity of virus or if it becomes immunocompromised or stressed.

Dogs with poor immune status by days 9 to 14 PI undergo virus spread to many tissues, including skin; exocrine and endocrine glands; and epithelium of the GI, respiratory, and genitourinary tracts. Clinical signs of disease in these dogs are usually dramatic and severe, and virus usually persists in their tissues until death. The sequence of pathogenic events depends on the virus strain and may be delayed by 1 to 2 weeks.

Studies on serologic response to CDV in gnotobiotic dogs confirm that serum antibody titers vary inversely with the severity of the disease. Antibody response in dogs has been separated into envelope and core determinants of the virus. Only dogs producing anti-envelope antibodies appear to be able to ward off persistent viral infection of the CNS. The outcome of CNS infection seems to be dependent on the appearance of circulating IgG antibodies to the H glycoprotein.[76] Mortality in gnotobiotic dogs approaches that of naturally infected animals, de-emphasizing the role of secondary bacterial infection in influencing the severity of CNS disease; however, bacteria are probably important in complicating the signs of disease in the respiratory and GI tracts.

CNS Infection

As previously discussed, the spread of virus to the CNS depends upon the degree of systemic immune responses mounted by the host. Virus probably enters the nervous system of many viremic CDV–infected dogs whether or not neurologic signs are observed. Antiviral antibody and resultant immune complex deposition may facilitate the spread of virus to vascular endothelium in the CNS. Virus (free or platelet- or lymphocyte-associated) may enter the vascular endothelial cells in the meninges, the choroid plexus epithe-

Table 3–4. Summary of Aquatic Morbillivirus Infection [a]

VIRUS	DATE	SPECIES	LOCATION
Dolphin morbillivirus (DMV)	1990s	Striped dolphins	Mediterranean
Porpoise morbillivirus (PMV)	Late 1980s	Harbor porpoises	Northwestern Europe
Phocine distemper virus (PDV)	Late 1980s	Harbor seals Gray seals	Northwestern Europe
Canine distemper virus (CDV)	Late 1980s	Baikal seals	Siberia

[a]Data from Osterhaus ADME, De Swart RL, Vos HW, et al: *Vet Microbiol* 44:219–227. Used with permission.

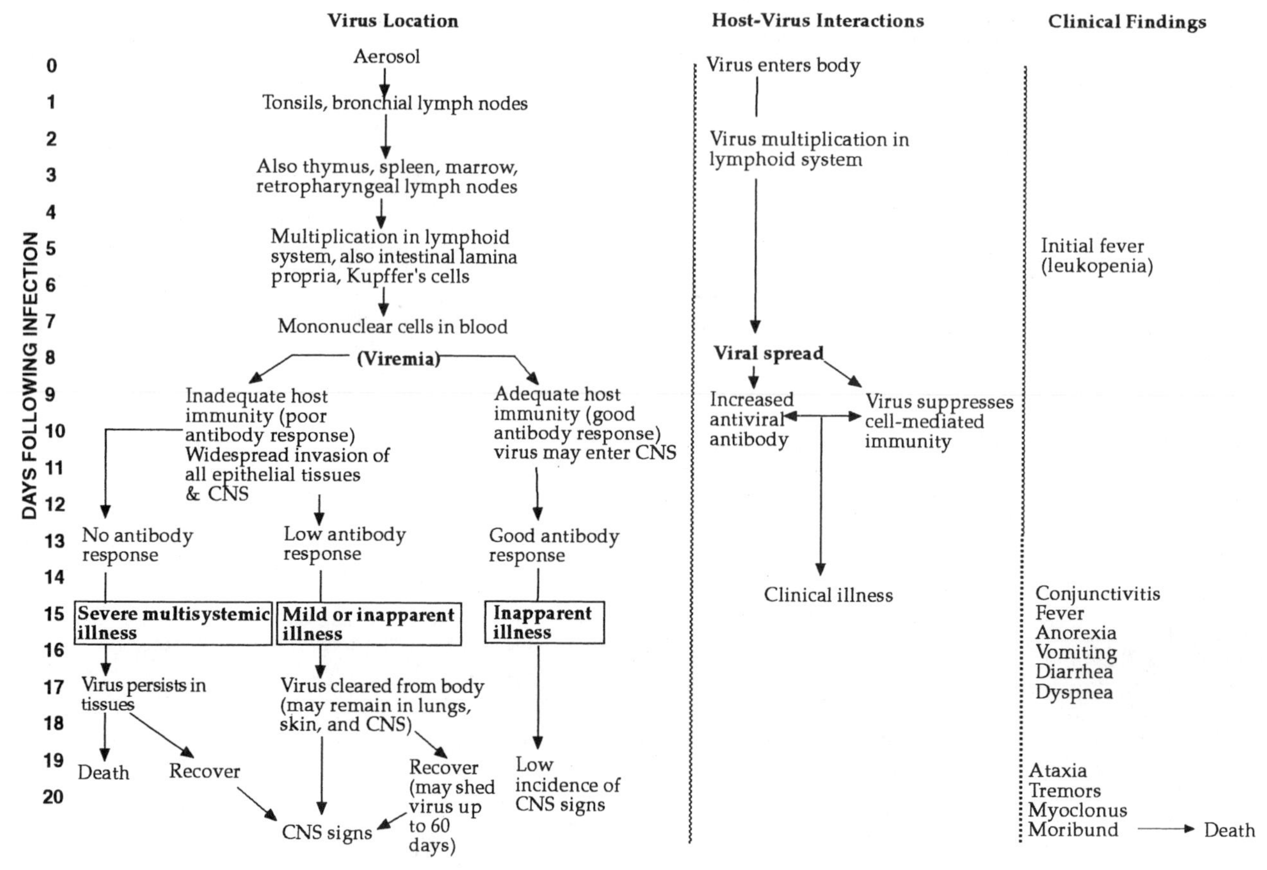

Figure 3–2. Sequential pathogenesis of canine distemper.

lial cells of the fourth ventricle, and the ependymal cells lining the ventricular system. Viral antigen is first detected in CNS capillary and venular endothelium and perivascular astrocytic foot processes. The infection of choroid plexus epithelium has been shown to be productive throughout the course of infection in that virus is continually being produced. From these sites, free or lymphocyte-associated virus may enter the CSF, where it spreads to periventricular and subpial structures. Spread of virus through CSF pathways probably explains the early distribution of lesions in subependymal areas, such as the cerebral cortex (primarily archicortex and paleocortex), optic tracts and nerves, rostral medullary velum, cerebral peduncles, and spinal cord.

The type of lesion produced and the course of infection within the CNS depend upon a number of factors, including the age and immunocompetence of the host at the time of exposure, the neurotropic and immunosuppressive properties of the virus, and the time at which lesions are examined. Either acute or chronic encephalitis can occur independently, or acute-phase lesions may progress to the chronic form in animals that survive.[14]

Acute encephalitis, which occurs early in the course of infection in young or immunosuppressed animals, is characterized by direct viral injury. The virus causes multifocal lesions in the gray and white matter. Gray matter lesions are the result of neuronal infection and necrosis and may lead to predominant polioencephalomalacia. However, neuronal infection can also occur with minimal evidence of cytolysis. White matter lesions, characterized by myelin damage, are associated with replication of CDV in glial cells. Inflammatory changes are minimal, and theories for the lack of inflammation have included immunodeficiency resulting from the physiologic immaturity of the immune system, virus-induced immunosuppression, and the early phase of illness being studied.

Noninflammatory demyelination in acute lesions appears by light and electron microscopy to be associated with viral infection of macrophage and astroglial cells rather than oligodendroglial cells, the myelin-producing cells.[24, 65] Active virus replication occurs in the CNS during this period of unrestricted infection, and lesions contain all CDV-mRNA sequences and viral proteins as detected by in situ hybridization and immunohistochemistry, respectively.[64]

In primary canine brain cell cultures, CDV causes a slow-spreading, noncytolytic infection. CDV viral proteins and nucleocapsids are difficult to detect in oligodendroglia by immunocytochemical or ultrastructural methods. However, using in situ hybridization, the complete viral genome is present.[97] This restricted infection leads to metabolic dysfunction and morphologic degeneration of oligodendroglial cells.[38] Similar alterations of oligodendroglia have been observed in vivo in demyelinating lesions.[16]

In the normal brain expression of the major histocompatibility class II antigen (MHC II) is low. As effector cells, microglia express MHC II when activated, presumably through increases in IFN-γ, a T-cell cytokine. Elevated levels of IFN-γ are seen in the CNS during viral infection and human multiple sclerosis (MS). MHC II is upregulated (expressed) in demyelinating diseases such as experimental allergic encephalomyelitis and MS. In acute CDV encephalitis in dogs, virus was present in a diffuse or multifocal distribution, and MHC II was upregulated throughout the white matter and in CDV infected foci.[4]

Because CDV encephalitis was more chronic, CDV antigen was restricted to a few astrocytes, whereas MHC II expression was prominent in all microglial cells.[4] In later stages, nonviral MHC II expression may be responsible for the continued and more widespread demyelination and perivascular mononuclear cell infiltration.

Chronic CDV encephalitis is also associated with increased concentration of antimyelin antibodies, thought to be a secondary reaction to the inflammatory process. Increased intrathecal virus-neutralizing antibodies are also present.[62] Antibodies to CDV appear to interact with infected macrophages in CNS lesions, causing their activation with release of reactive oxygen radicals. This activity in turn can lead to destruction of oligodendroglial cells and myelin by an "innocent bystander" mechanism.[20, 24]

In surviving animals, CDV is cleared from the inflammatory lesions but can persist in brain tissue in unaffected sites.[64] If the spread through the CNS has been extensive by the time the host responds to the virus, then widespread damage occurs. The unaffected areas of virally infected brain tissue are spared the inflammatory process and immune recognition, presumably because of noncytolytic infections.[88, 94, 96] Reduced expression of CDV proteins on the surface of inflammatory cells has also been implicated as a means of immune avoidance.[2, 3, 64]

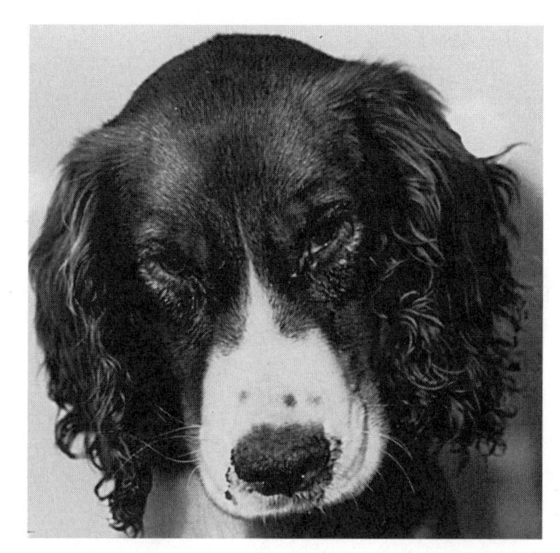

Figure 3–3. Mucopurulent oculonasal discharge in a dog with systemic distemper.

CLINICAL FINDINGS

Systemic Signs

Clinical signs of canine distemper vary depending on virulence of the virus strain, environmental conditions, and host age and immune status. More than 50% to 70% of CDV infections are probably subclinical. Mild forms of clinical illness are also common, and signs include listlessness, decreased appetite, fever, and upper respiratory tract infection. Bilateral serous oculonasal discharge can become mucopurulent with coughing and dyspnea. Many mildly infected dogs develop clinical signs that are indistinguishable from those of other causes of "kennel cough" (see Chapter 6). Keratoconjunctivitis sicca may develop following systemic or subclinical infections in dogs. Persistent anosmia was reported as a sequela in dogs that had recovered from canine distemper.[42]

Severe generalized distemper is the commonly recognized form of the disease. It can occur in dogs of any age with poor immune status, but it most commonly affects unvaccinated, exposed puppies 12 to 16 weeks of age that have lost their maternal immunity or younger puppies that have received inadequate concentrations of maternal antibody. The initial febrile response in natural infections is probably unnoticed. The first sign of infection is a mild, serous-to-mucopurulent conjunctivitis (Fig. 3–3), which is followed within a few days by a dry cough that rapidly becomes moist and productive. Increased lower respiratory sounds from the thorax can be heard upon auscultation. Depression and anorexia are followed by vomiting, which is commonly unrelated to eating. Diarrhea subsequently develops, varying in consistency from fluid to frank blood and mucus. Tenesmus can be present, and intussusceptions may occur. Severe dehydration and emaciation can result from adipsia and fluid loss. Animals can die suddenly from systemic illness, but adequate therapy in many cases can reduce the mortality rate.

Neurologic Signs

These manifestations usually begin 1 to 3 weeks after recovery from systemic illness; however, there is no way to predict which dog will develop neurologic disorders. Neurologic signs can also coincide with multisystemic illness or, less commonly, can occur weeks to months later. Neurologic signs frequently develop in the presence of no or very mild extraneural signs.[86] On an empirical basis, certain features of the systemic disease can be predictive of the incidence of neurologic sequelae. Impetiginous dermatitis in puppies is rarely associated with CNS disease (Fig. 3–4), whereas dogs developing nasal and digital hyperkeratosis usually have various neurologic complications (Fig. 3–5). Mature or partially immune dogs that have been previously vaccinated can develop a sudden onset of neurologic signs without a history of systemic disease.[73] Neurologic signs, whether acute or chronic, are typically progressive. Chronic relapsing neurologic deterioration with an intermittent recovery and a later, superimposed acute episode of neurologic dysfunction can occur.

Neurologic complications of canine distemper are the most significant factors concerning prognosis and recovery from

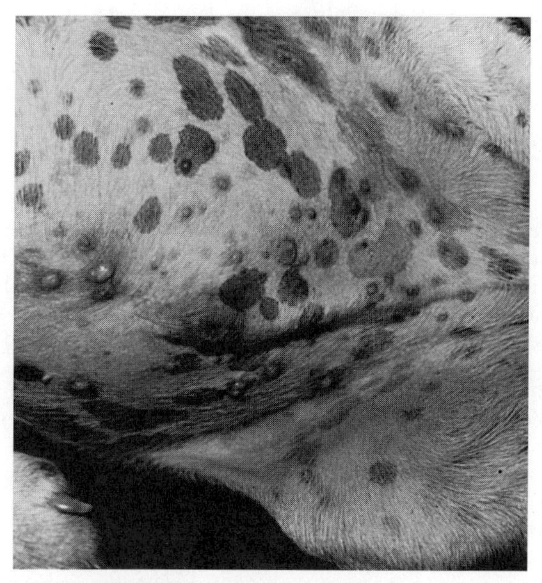

Figure 3–4. Pustular dermatitis in a puppy with canine distemper. Rarely associated with neurologic complications, this is usually a favorable prognostic sign.

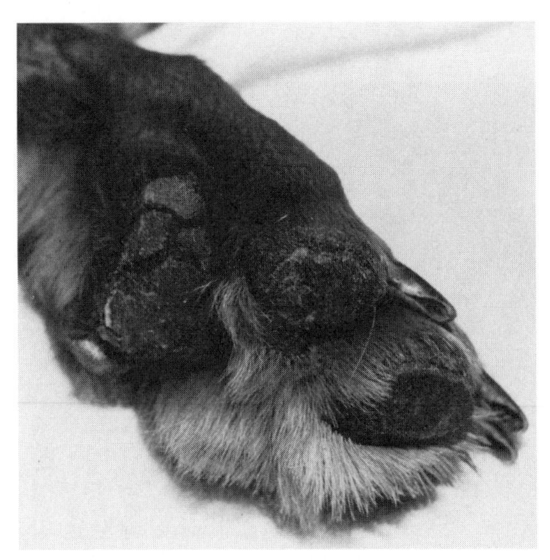

Figure 3–5. Digital hyperkeratosis ("hard pads") in a dog dying of distemper encephalomyelitis.

infection. Neurologic signs vary according to the area of the CNS involved. Hyperesthesia and cervical rigidity can be found as a result of meningeal inflammation, although parenchymal rather than meningeal signs usually predominate. Seizures, cerebellar and vestibular signs, paraparesis or tetraparesis with sensory ataxia, and myoclonus are common. Seizures can be of any type, depending upon the region of the forebrain that is damaged by the virus. The "chewing-gum" type of seizures, classically described for CDV infection, often occurs in dogs developing polioencephalomalacia of the temporal lobes. However, lesions in these lobes from other causes can produce similar seizures.

Myoclonus, the involuntary twitching of muscles in a forceful simultaneous contraction, can be present without other neurologic signs. With more extensive spinal cord damage, there may be upper motor neuron paresis of the affected limb associated with myoclonus. The rhythmic contractions can be present while the dog is awake or, more commonly, while it is sleeping. The neural mechanisms for myoclonus originate with local irritation of the lower motor neurons of the spinal cord or cranial nerve nuclei. Although considered specific for CDV infection, myoclonus can also be seen in other paramyxovirus infections of dogs and cats (see Chapters 7 and 18) and, less commonly, in other inflammatory conditions of the CNS.[84]

Transplacental Infection

Young puppies infected transplacentally may develop neurologic signs during the first 4 to 6 weeks of life. Mild or inapparent infections are seen in the bitch. Depending on the stage of gestation at which infection occurred, abortions, stillbirths, or the births of weak puppies may be noted. Puppies infected in utero that survive such infections may suffer from permanent immunodeficiencies.

Neonatal Infections

Young puppies infected with CDV before the eruption of permanent dentition may have severe damage to the enamel, dentin, or roots of their teeth.[15] An irregular appearance in the enamel or dentin may be noted (Fig. 3–6) in addition to partial eruption, oligodontia, or impaction of teeth. Enamel hypoplasia may be present as an incidental finding in an older dog, with or without neurologic signs, and is relatively pathognomonic for prior infection with CDV.

Neonatal (< 7 days old) gnotobiotic puppies have developed virus-induced cardiomyopathy after experimental infection with CDV. Clinical signs, including dyspnea, depression, anorexia, collapse, and prostration, develop between days 14 to 18 PI. Lesions are characterized by multifocal myocardial degeneration, necrosis, and mineralization, with minimal inflammatory cell infiltration. The clinical significance of this process following natural infection is uncertain at present. Whether there is a relationship with onset of adult cardiomyopathy in dogs remains to be determined.

Bone Lesions

Young growing dogs with experimentally and naturally induced CDV infection develop metaphyseal osteosclerosis of the long bones.[11] Large-breed dogs between 3 and 6 months of age are most commonly affected. Animals with systemic distemper have not shown clinical signs related to the long bone lesions. However, CDV transcripts have been demonstrated in the bone cells of young dogs with hypertrophic osteodystrophy (HOD), a metaphyseal bone disease with differing pathologic features.[59, 61] Juvenile cellulitis and/or HOD has developed in some pups as a result of MLV distemper vaccination[56] (see Chapter 100). Morbilliviral transcripts have also been detected in the bony lesions of people with Paget's disease (see Public Health Considerations).

Rheumatoid Arthritis

Dogs with rheumatoid arthritis had high levels of antibodies to CDV in sera and synovial fluid compared with dogs with inflammatory and degenerative arthritis.[13] CDV antigens were found in immune complexes from synovial fluid of dogs with rheumatoid arthritis but were not found in synovial fluid from dogs with inflammatory or degenerative arthropathies.

Ocular Signs

Dogs with CDV encephalomyelitis often have a mild anterior uveitis that is clinically asymptomatic. More obvious

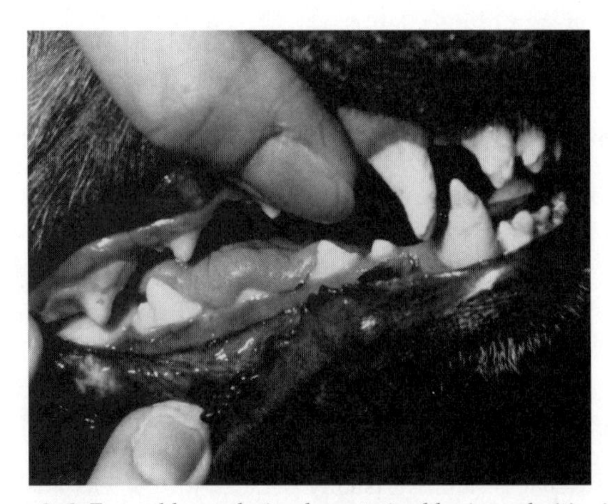

Figure 3–6. Enamel hypoplasia, characterized by irregularities in the dental surface, in an older dog that survived neonatal distemper.

ophthalmologic lesions in canine distemper have been attributed to an effect of the virus on the optic nerve and the retina (see also Canine Distemper, Chapter 93). Optic neuritis can be characterized by a sudden onset of blindness, with dilated unresponsive pupils. Degeneration and necrosis of the retina produce gray-to-pink irregular densities on the tapetal or nontapetal fundus or both. Bullous or complete retinal detachment can occur where exudates dissect between the retina and choroid. Chronic inactive fundic lesions are associated with retinal atrophy and scarring. These are circumscribed, hyperreflective areas termed gold medallion lesions, which are considered characteristic of previous canine distemper infection.

Combined Infections

Immunosuppression caused by or responsible for systemic CDV infection can be associated with combined opportunistic infections. Salmonellosis has been a common complication causing protracted or fatal hemorrhagic diarrhea or sepsis in affected dogs. Combined infections with *Toxoplasma gondii* or *Neospora caninum* have produced lower motor neuron dysfunction from myositis and radiculoneuritis (see Chapter 80).

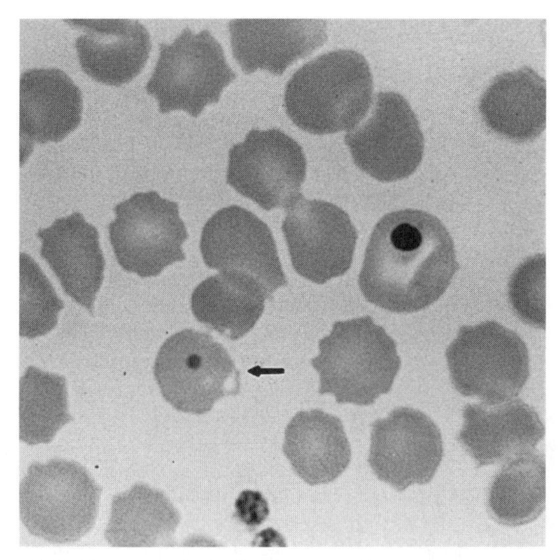

Figure 3–7. Distemper inclusion in an erythrocyte from a peripheral blood film *(arrow)*. Compare its appearance with that of a Howell-Jolly body (Wright's stain × 1000). (Courtesy of Dr. O. W. Schalm, formerly of University of California, Davis, Davis, CA.)

DIAGNOSIS

Practical diagnosis of canine distemper is primarily based on clinical suspicion. A characteristic history of a 3- to 6-month-old unvaccinated puppy with a compatible illness is supportive. Dogs with severe disease in most cases have clinical signs distinctive enough to make a presumptive diagnosis. Missed are the large number of upper respiratory infections in older dogs that are labeled infectious tracheobronchitis. Specific laboratory tests are not always available to confirm the suspicion of CDV infections, and the practicing veterinarian must instead rely on nonspecific findings of routine laboratory procedures.

Clinical Laboratory Findings

Abnormal hematologic findings include an absolute lymphopenia caused by lymphoid depletion that is viral strain dependent. This frequently persists in very young dogs with rapidly progressive systemic or neurologic signs. Thrombocytopenia (as low as 30,000 cells/μl) and regenerative anemia have been found in experimentally infected neonates (< 3 weeks) but have not been consistently recognized in older or spontaneously infected dogs. Distemper inclusions can be detected on examination of stained peripheral blood films; in low numbers in circulating lymphocytes; and with even less frequency in monocytes, neutrophils, and erythrocytes. Wright-Leishman–stained inclusions in lymphocytes are large (up to 3 μm), singular, oval, gray structures, whereas erythrocytic inclusions, most numerous in polychromatophilic cells, are round and eccentrically placed and appear light blue (Fig. 3–7). Erythrocytic inclusions are intermediate in size between metarubricyte nuclei and Howell-Jolly bodies. Buffy coat and bone marrow examination and use of phloxinophilic stains can improve the chances of detecting inclusions. EM has confirmed that these inclusions consist of paramyxovirus-like nucleocapsids.

The magnitude and type of serum biochemistry changes in acute systemic infections are nonspecific. Total protein analysis includes decreased albumin and increased α- and γ-globulin concentration in non-neonates. Marked hypoglobulinemia has been found in puppies infected prenatally or neonatally with CDV from persistent immunosuppression caused by the virus.

Radiology

Thoracic radiography demonstrates an interstitial lung pattern in early cases of distemper. An alveolar pattern is seen with secondary bacterial infection and more severe bronchopneumonia (Fig. 3–8).

CSF

Abnormalities are detectable in dogs with neurologic signs of distemper; however, false-negative results can be anticipated. The CSF may flow more rapidly than normal during collection because of increased intracranial pressure caused by inflammation. Increases in protein (> 25 mg/dl) and cell

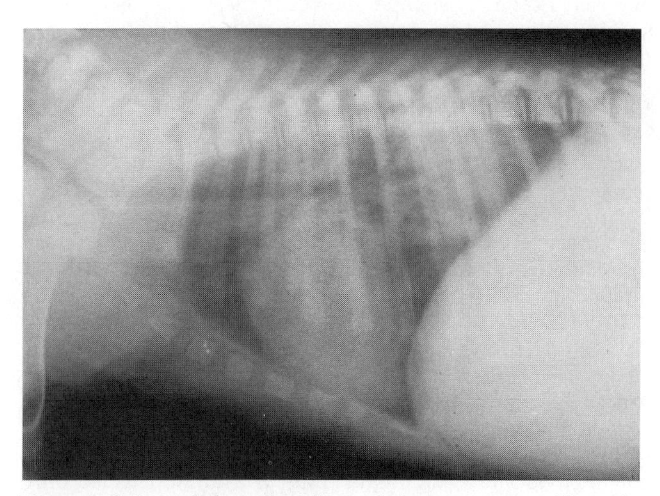

Figure 3–8. Lateral thoracic radiograph from a puppy with canine distemper bronchopneumonia.

count (> 10 cells/μl with a predominance of lymphocytes) have been characteristic of inflammatory forms of CDV encephalomyelitis. Dogs with acute noninflammatory demyelinating encephalomyelitis may have normal CSF analysis. When increased protein is present in CSF, it has been identified primarily as IgG with specific anti-CDV activity. Differences in the humoral immune response in CSF and sera to the H and F envelope proteins (see Table 3–2) have been noted between some dogs with chronic progressive encephalitis and those with other forms of distemper encephalitis.[76]

Increased anti-CDV antibody in CSF offers definitive evidence for distemper encephalitis because antibody is locally produced, and these increases have not been present in vaccinated dogs or in those with systemic distemper without CNS disease. CSF antibody may be artifactually increased owing to traumatic collection procedures causing contamination by whole blood. To help distinguish the effect of nonspecific leakage of distemper-specific IgG into the CSF from serum, an antibody ratio can be determined. Distemper-specific IgG in CSF is divided by that of IgG in serum. This finding is compared with a corresponding CSF–serum antibody ratio for another infectious agent for which serum antibody titers are expected such as CAV. If the ratio for CDV is higher than that for CAV, then de novo production of CSF antibody caused by CNS infection with distemper is expected. Ideally the titer determination for both diseases should use the same methodology (e.g., neutralization, ELISA, indirect FA). Alternatives are to compare the CDV-specific CSF–serum ratio with the ratio of IgG or albumin in CSF and serum,[85] but this approach is less accurate because of the differences in methodology used in these determinations. The CSF IgG antibody concentration is more likely to be increased in dogs with inflammatory demyelinating encephalitis than in younger or immunosuppressed dogs with acute polioencephalitis and noninflammatory virus-induced cellular injury.[80, 86] Although the test for CSF antibodies is sensitive and specific for CDV, it can be performed only by properly equipped diagnostic or research laboratory personnel (see Appendix 5). In acute CNS infections, some mononuclear cells may contain large (15–10 μ) oval homogenous eosinophilic intracytoplasmic inclusions.[5] Increased interferon in CSF has also been used as a marker for CDV encephalitis.

Immunocytology

Immunofluorescent techniques can facilitate a specific diagnosis of canine distemper; however, these tests also require special equipment and are usually handled by regional diagnostic laboratories. In clinically affected dogs, immunofluorescence is usually performed on cytologic smears prepared from conjunctival, tonsillar, and respiratory epithelium. The technique also can be performed on cells in CSF, blood (buffy coat), urine sediment, and bone marrow. Smears should be made on precleaned slides, air-dried thoroughly, and preferably fixed in acetone for 5 minutes before transport to the laboratory. At the laboratory, they are stained directly or indirectly with fluorescein-conjugated CDV antibody and examined by fluorescent microscopy.

Antigen, first detected in buffy coat smears from 2 to 5 days PI, decreases as antibody titer increases by 8 to 9 days PI. Because clinical signs are becoming apparent shortly after this time (day 14), positive results would not be recognized except in dogs that do not mount a sufficient immune response and succumb to infection. Positive fluorescence in conjunctival and genital epithelium is usually detected only within the first 3 weeks PI, when systemic illness is apparent. Virus also disappears in these tissues after the first 1 to 2 weeks of clinical illness (21–28 days PI) as antibody titers rise in association with clinical recovery. Beginning with the recovery stage, antibody may bind and mask antigen in infected cells. Consequently, false-negative results will be obtained. Virus can sometimes be detected for longer periods of time in epithelial cells and macrophages from the lower respiratory tract, and transtracheal washings can be obtained for diagnosis. Virus also persists for periods of at least 60 days in the skin, uveal tissue, footpad, and CNS. Direct fluorescent antibody examination of cells in conjunctival scrapings, CSF, or blood films is helpful in acute phases of illness. In chronic cases it is usually unrewarding because antibody coating of viral antigen interferes with diagnostic immunofluorescence. False-negative results are frequent with these methods. Footpad biopsy has been recommended as a diagnostic technique. Viral antigen is difficult to find in specimens from dogs with neurologic distemper that lack or have recovered from systemic signs.

Fluorescent antibody techniques can also be performed on frozen sections of biopsy or necropsy specimens. Tissues collected from dogs that died from distemper should include spleen, tonsils, lymph nodes, stomach, lung, duodenum, bladder, and brain. Animals dying of generalized infection frequently have abundant quantities of virus in these tissues. Fluorescent antibody techniques can also be adapted to paraffin-embedded sections if special cold (4°C) ethanol (95%) fixation is used.

ELISA has been used to detect viral antigen in serum and CSF of naturally and experimentally infected dogs.[36, 48] A test based on this methodology would be extremely valuable to the practitioner. Other immunochemical techniques have been developed for histologic detection of distemper antigen in formalin-fixed and paraffin-embedded tissues and cell culture.[12, 35] Immunohistochemical demonstration of CDV antigen is superior to reliance on inclusion bodies in brain tissue to confirm distemper encephalitis.[69] Results are more likely to be positive in acute than in chronic infections. Similarly, PCR and nucleic acid hybridization studies, using single-stranded RNA probes, have been performed to detect virulent virus in tissue culture and histologic sections.[95]

Immunologic Testing

A microneutralization method has further simplified neutralizing antibody testing in diagnostic laboratories. The more sensitive ELISA has been used to detect serum IgG and IgM antibodies to CDV. Increased titers of serum IgM–neutralizing antibody can be measured in dogs that survive the acute phase of infection. Although detection of IgM is specific for recent infection or vaccination with CDV, this test is cumbersome and must be performed in specialized laboratories. An IgM-ELISA method has been developed that could simplify the procedure of diagnosis by serum Ig.[17] High serum IgM titers have been more accurate in detecting acute clinical distemper cases (81%) compared with chronic progressive inflammatory encephalitis (60%). Unlike increases in serum IgM titers, high IgG titers are ambiguous and can indicate either past or present infection with or vaccination for CDV. Analysis of CSF-specific IgG levels and determining a CSF-serum ratio is a potentially more reliable use of antibody measurements in detecting chronic CDV infections of the nervous system (see CSF).

Cell-mediated immunosuppression has been documented following CDV infection. Lymphocyte transformation testing of experimentally infected neonates has shown profound depression of lymphocyte response to phytomitogens at a time corresponding to acute viremia and lymphopenia. This depressed response persisted for more than 10 weeks in convalescing puppies and never returned to baseline values in those that died acutely. Prenatal and neonatal distemper infections are causes of immunodeficiency in surviving puppies and may make concurrent infections with other viruses such as parvovirus more severe.

Viral Isolation

Isolation of virulent CDV has been difficult in routine cell cultures. The most successful viral replication occurs during direct cultivation of target tissues from the infected host. Buffy coat specimens taken during the early course of illness provide the best opportunity. Alveolar macrophage cultures detect the virus in 24 to 48 hours. Giant cell (syncytia) formation, a characteristic cytopathic effect of CDV in many tissue cultures, is detected within 2 to 5 days, at which time the virus can be isolated by overlays made on other cells. Macrophage cultures have lately been replaced by dog lymphocyte cultures for isolation of CDV. Buffy coat cells or tissues from infected animals can be cultivated with mitogen-stimulated canine blood lymphocytes, and cultures are examined 72 to 144 hours later by immunofluorescence.[6] A marmoset lymphoid cell line (B95a) has also been used.[52]

Growth in pulmonary macrophages or lymphocytes was once considered an essential feature of virulent CDV isolates; however, some virulent CDV isolates have occasionally been isolated in Vero cells or primary dog kidney and bladder epithelial cell cultures without the need for adaptation or loss of virulence of the virus. However, the success rate is low. In general, titers of vaccine viruses are high in macrophage, lymphocyte, kidney cell, and epithelial cell lines, whereas virulent field strains grow preferentially in macrophages[32] and lymphocytes.[6] Cultures can be examined for virus with fluorescent antibody when cytopathic effects are not observed.

PATHOLOGIC FINDINGS

Young dogs, prenatally or neonatally infected with CDV, usually have thymic atrophy. Pneumonia and catarrhal enteritis are present in postnatally infected puppies with systemic disease. Upper respiratory tract lesions include conjunctivitis, rhinitis, and inflammation of the tracheobronchial tree. Hyperkeratosis of the nose and footpads is common in dogs suffering from neurologic disease. Gross lesions in the CNS are minimal except for occasional meningeal congestion, ventricular dilation, and increased CSF pressure resulting from brain edema.

Lymphoid depletion is a typical histologic finding in a dog with systemic illness. Diffuse interstitial pneumonia is characterized by thickened alveolar septa and proliferation of alveolar epithelium. Alveoli contain desquamated epithelial cells and macrophages; transitional epithelium of the urinary system is swollen. Puppies developing distemper may have defects in enamel of the teeth, and necrosis and cystic degeneration of ameloblastic epithelium are usually present. Ophthalmic lesions are described in Chapter 93. Mild interstitial epididymitis and orchitis are commonly seen in dogs with canine distemper, and this observation may help explain the transient decrease in spermatogenesis, prostate fluid, and testosterone that occurs in recovering animals.

With acute fatal encephalitis of neonates, neuronal and myelin degeneration or primary demyelination can occur without significant perivascular inflammation. In surviving animals, patchy areas of necrosis are replaced by hypertrophic astrocytes that form a network for macrophages' ingesting myelin. The most severe white matter changes in the CNS can be found in the predilection sites of lateral cerebellar peduncles, the dorsolateral medulla adjacent to the fourth ventricle, and the deep cerebellar white matter. Lesions are also present in the midbrain, basal ganglia, and temporal lobes of the cerebral cortex. Superficial areas such as the optic tracts, crus cerebri, cranial nerve pathways, and infundibulum also can be affected. Noninflammatory polioencephalomyelitis, in some dogs, can predominantly affect the cerebrum and thalamus.[83] Acute noninflammatory lesions include demyelination with spongy vacuolation of white matter and reactive gliosis. Intracytoplasmic or intranuclear inclusions can be found predominantly in astrocytes and neurons.

Older or more immunocompetent dogs tend to develop leukoencephalomyelitis with a predominance of lesions in the caudal brain stem and spinal cord. These lesions are usually associated with signs of ataxia and vestibular involvement. Lesions are characterized by widespread perivascular lymphoplasmacytic infiltration with areas of demyelination and neuronal degeneration. They can be more widespread and severe than in the acute encephalitis. In more chronic cases, the lesion may develop into sclerosing panencephalitis characterized by infiltration and replacement of nervous tissue by a dense astrocytic network.

In contrast, lesions of vaccine-induced distemper are typically those of a necrotizing polioencephalitis of the caudal brain stem with preference for the ventral pontine nuclei[87, 91] (see Postvaccinal Complications later and Chapter 100). Inclusions can be found in the nucleus or cytoplasm of astrocytes and neurons.

On histologic examination, CDV inclusions are most commonly cytoplasmic and acidophilic staining. They are 1 to 5 μm in diameter and can be found in epithelial cells of the mucous membranes, reticulum cells, leukocytes, glia, and neurons. Inclusions can be found up to 5 to 6 weeks PI in the lymphoid system and urinary tract. Intranuclear inclusions are most common in lining or glandular epithelium and ganglion cells.

The morphologic significance of distemper inclusions is not completely understood. Histochemically, they are composed of aggregates of viral nucleocapsids and cellular debris as a result of viral infection. Caution must be used when absolutely confirming a diagnosis of canine distemper based on the presence of inclusions alone. Cytoplasmic inclusions typical for CDV infection have been identified in the urinary bladder of normal dogs. Unfortunately, inclusion bodies not only are nonspecific but may appear too late in the disease to be routinely useful. In contrast, inclusion bodies alone to detect CDV infection can lead to a false-negative diagnosis in dogs compared with more sensitive immunocytochemical methods for CDV detection in tissues.

Formation of giant cells primarily in CNS white matter and anterior uvea of the eye and secondarily in lymph nodes, lung, and leptomeninges is peculiar to paramyxoviruses such as CDV. This finding can be used to substantiate CDV infection.

THERAPY

Despite vast advances in research on canine distemper, only minor changes have been made in therapeutic recommendations. Aims in treatment, although supportive and nonspecific, are frequently beneficial in that mortality is reduced. The only reason for refusing to initiate treatment at an owner's insistence is the presence of neurologic signs that are incompatible with life. Even in the absence of neurologic signs, owners should always be warned that such sequelae may develop at a later time. The spontaneous improvement seen in many dogs with symptomatic management of non-neurologic systemic distemper has fostered inappropriate credits to the success of certain treatment regimens. However, unlike the systemic signs, neurologic signs in themselves are not usually reversible unless they are caused by vaccine strains and frequently are progressive.

Dogs with upper respiratory infections should be kept in environments that are clean, warm, and free of drafts. Oculonasal discharges should be cleaned from the face. Pneumonia is frequently complicated by secondary bacterial infection, usually with *Bordetella bronchiseptica*, which requires broad-spectrum antibiotic therapy and expectorants or nebulization and coupage. Good initial antibiotic choices for bronchopneumonia include ampicillin, tetracycline, and chloramphenicol (Table 3–5). However, because of dental staining, tetracycline must be avoided in puppies, and chloramphenicol is less desirable for public health risks. Newer parenteral florfenicol should be considered (see Drug Formulary, Appendix 8). Parenteral therapy is essential when GI signs are present. Antimicrobial therapy should be altered when dictated by sensitivity testing based on transtracheal washing or by lack of response to the initial antibiotics.

Food and water and oral medications or fluids should be discontinued if vomiting and diarrhea are present. Parenteral antiemetics may be required. Supplementation with polyionic isotonic fluids such as lactated Ringer's solution should be given IV or SC, depending on the hydration status of the patient. B vitamins should be administered as nonspecific therapy to replace those lost from anorexia and diuresis and to stimulate the appetite. Historically, benefits have been described with administration of IV ascorbic acid; however, this is controversial and without proven efficacy. Controlled studies have documented morbidity and mortality in children with measles who receive two 200,000-IU (60-mg) doses of vitamin A within 5 days of the onset of systemic illness.[46] Although unproven in distemper, a similar regimen could be tried in acute systemic infection of puppies.

Therapy for neurologic disturbances in canine distemper is less rewarding. Progressive multifocal encephalitis usually leads to tetraplegia, semicoma, and incapacitation so great that euthanasia should be recommended. Despite ineffective therapy, dogs should not be euthanized unless the neurologic disturbances are progressive or incompatible with life. There may be variable or temporary success in halting neurologic signs in some dogs with single anti-CNS edema doses of dexamethasone.

Seizures, myoclonus, or optic neuritis are three neurologic manifestations in dogs that can be tolerated by many owners. Myoclonus is usually untreatable and irreversible; many forms of therapy have been attempted without success. Recommendations have been made to administer anticonvulsants after the onset of systemic disease but before the development of seizures. No evidence shows that anticonvulsants prevent entry of the virus into the CNS; however, they may suppress irritable foci from causing seizures, which, in turn, may prevent seizure circuits from becoming established. Seizures are best treated with parenteral diazepam (5–10 mg/dose rectally or slowly IV) for status epilepticus and phenobarbital for maintenance prevention. Primidone or potassium bromide are alternative choices, and combinations or higher doses may be needed in refractory cases. Glucocorticoid therapy at anti-inflammatory dosages may have variable success in controlling the blindness and pupillary dilation caused by optic neuritis or some of the signs associated with the more chronic inflammatory form of encephalitis.

PREVENTION

Chapter 100 and Appendix 1 should be consulted for overall recommendations on vaccination for canine distemper. The following discussion describes features that are unique to protection against this disease. Immunity to CDV infection is considered long term, and lasting immunity and immunologic homogeneity of the virus have made disease prevention possible through vaccination. Maternal antibodies, received both in utero and in colostrum from the dam, block adequate immunization in puppies for a period of time after birth and weaning, respectively. Maternal antibody to CDV decreases with a half-life of 8.4 days. Three percent of antibody transfer for CDV occurs in utero and 97% in the colostrum, resulting in an initial titer in nursing newborn puppies that is usually equal to 77% of that in the bitch. In the absence of ingestion of colostrum, the puppy is probably protected for at least 1 to 4 weeks. In nursing puppies, nomograms based on the bitch's titer can be used to determine when immunization should be done, although this is not routinely practical. Maternal antibodies are usually absent by 12 to 14 weeks of age. Vaccines for CDV are generally given every 3 to 4 weeks between 6 and 16 weeks of age in puppies that have received colostrum.

***Table 3–5. Drug Therapy for Canine Distemper*[a]**

DRUG	DOSE[b]	ROUTE	INTERVAL (HOURS)	DURATION (DAYS)
Antimicrobial				
Ampicillin/amoxicillin	20 mg/kg	PO, IV, SC	8	7
Tetracycline[c]	22 mg/kg	PO, IV	8	7
Chloramphenicol	15–25 mg/kg	PO, SC	8	7
Florfenicol	25–50 mg/kg	SC, IM	8	3–5
Cephapirin	10–30 mg/kg	IM, IV, SC	6–8	3–5
Anticonvulsive				
Diazepam	5–10 mg total	IV, rectally	1–2	prn
Phenobarbital	2 mg/kg	PO, IV, IM	12	prn
Anti-inflammatory				
Dexamethasone				
CNS edema	1–2 mg/kg	IV	24	1
Optic neuritis[d]	0.1 mg/kg	PO, IV, SC	24	3–5

[a]See Drug Formulary, Appendix 8, for more detailed information on the antimicrobial drugs.
[b]Dose per administration at specified interval.
[c]Avoid in dogs younger than 6 months because of dental staining.
[d]Equivalent glucocorticoid dosage of prednisolone (milligrams per kilogram) is five times this dose.
PO = oral; IV = intravenous; SC = subcutaneous; IM = intramuscular; prn = as needed.

After recovery from natural infection or booster vaccination, immunity can persist for years. This protection may be adequate unless the dog is exposed to a highly virulent or large quantities of virus or becomes stressed or immunocompromised. After a single distemper vaccination, naive puppies do not generally develop immunity that lasts at least 1 year. For this reason, despite the lack of maternal antibody interference, at least two distemper vaccines should be given at 2- to 4-week intervals in first presentation of colostrum-deprived neonates and in dogs older than 16 weeks. Similarly, and because older vaccinated dogs can still develop distemper, periodic boosters are recommended for this disease, despite the relatively long-lived immunity afforded by vaccination.

Humoral immune mechanisms do not totally explain resistance to CDV. Vaccination with attenuated virus appears to protect previously unvaccinated dogs when it is given at least 2 days prior to exposure to virulent distemper virus as compared with at least 5 days with SC vaccination.[28] Because of allergic reactions that may develop, CAV-1 and leptospiral antigens should be avoided with IV vaccination. The IV route should be reserved to protect exposed, unvaccinated dogs. This rapid protection against distemper may be related to immune interference, interferon, or CMI mechanisms. Despite a decrease in antibody titer, immunity to distemper after booster or anamnestic vaccination is known to last as long as 7 years, as demonstrated in isolated, challenged dogs. The duration of protection is much greater than that predicted from antibody titer alone and demonstrates that challenge with virulent organisms is more meaningful than neutralizing antibody titer for predicting the duration of immunity.

Inactivated canine distemper whole-virus vaccines do not produce sufficient immunity to prevent illness after challenge exposure, but vaccinates show an anamnestic immunity response and less severe disease compared unvaccinated controls. Unfortunately, inactivated CDV vaccine must be used in vaccine virus–susceptible wild or exotic species. Whereas inactivated whole-virus vaccines have been unsuccessful, purified (F) surface glycoproteins of CDV (see Table 3–2) have been used to protect dogs against subsequent experimental challenge with virulent virus.[66] Similarly, an inactivated subunit vaccine, containing membrane F antigen and H glycoprotein modified into immune-stimulating complexes, has been effective in protecting dogs from challenge by virulent virus.[31] A vaccine, produced by expressing measles virus H protein in Vaccinia virus, has been effective in producing neutralizing antibody and protecting dogs against challenge with virulent CDV.[82] Experimental vaccines of recombinant pox or canarypox viruses expressing genes for H proteins of measles or CDV have been tested in mice and dogs.[28, 90] A commercial recombinant canarypox-based CDV vaccine is available for dogs (see Chapter 100).[69a]

Despite the success with vaccination in protecting dogs against CDV, vaccine-induced immunity is never as long lasting as the immune response that occurs after natural or experimental infection with virulent virus. Use of MLV vaccines for distemper has led to questions concerning both vaccine stability and safety.

Vaccine Stability

Viability of canine distemper vaccines is an important consideration with respect to vaccination failures. Lyophilized tissue culture vaccines are stable for 16 months under refrigeration (0°–4°C), 7 weeks at 20°C, and 7 days when exposed to sunlight at 47°C. When reconstituted, tissue culture virus remains stable for 3 days at 4°C and 24 hours at 20°C. Vaccine should be used immediately once it is reconstituted for injection, or it should be refrigerated if the delay until usage will be longer than 1 hour.

Postvaccinal Complications

Efficacy and safety of MLV distemper vaccination in dogs with compromised immune systems are important considerations. Dogs on folic acid–deficient diets and methotrexate therapy had no response to MLV distemper vaccine. Although the vaccine virus could be isolated from the lymphoid system, no postvaccinal signs or epithelial tissue infection was detected. In contrast, dogs receiving one dose of antithymocyte serum in conjunction with methotrexate for 5 days developed systemic and neurologic signs of vaccine-induced distemper.[42] Unlike virulent virus, MLV by itself does not appear to suppress measurable CMI. However, when CDV has been combined with CAV-1 or CAV-2, significant suppression in lymphocyte transformation testing response occurred.[71]

Modified live vaccine viruses have not reverted to virulence under natural conditions and do not spread to other dogs. However, reversion to virulence has been experimentally demonstrated in attenuated vaccine virus passed serially in dogs and ferrets or in pulmonary macrophages in tissue culture. There are two major types of MLV distemper vaccines. The Onderstepoort strain was adapted to chicken embryos and chicken cells. This vaccine strain may produce lower measured levels of humoral immunity[67] but no postvaccinal disease. The canine cell–adapted Rockborn strain occasionally in dogs and more commonly in exotic carnivores produces a postvaccinal encephalitis. Vaccine-induced distemper infections have been reported in numerous exotic carnivores, including the lesser panda, black-footed ferrets, and gray foxes. Postvaccinal distemper can be prevented in ferrets by using inactivated virus vaccines or live chicken cell–propagated or recombinant vector vaccines rather than canine cell–propagated vaccines.

Encephalitis has been reported in dogs after vaccination with MLV distemper vaccines[29, 55, 65a] (see also Postvaccinal Encephalomyelitis, Chapter 100). Vaccination of dams in whelp or during the first few days post partum has resulted in systemic infection and/or encephalitis in their pups.[21, 57] CDV vaccine–induced encephalomyelitis has been documented in 3-week-old puppies simultaneously infected with virulent canine parvovirus; however, similar findings could not be reported in 11- to 15-week-old puppies.[42] CDV vaccine–induced disease is usually that of encephalitis, although immunosuppression or neonatal or prenatal infections can result in systemic manifestations. The neurologic signs typically begin 7 to 14 days[29, 30, 91] after receiving a MLV canine distemper vaccine. The clinical signs are variable but often consist of an acute onset of "chewing gum" or generalized motor seizures or paraparesis or tetraparesis and vestibular or sensory ataxia. The seizure form is often progressive and difficult to control with anticonvulsants. The ataxic form can be progressive but may improve in some dogs. Unlike naturally acquired infections from virulent virus, the neurologic signs of vaccine-induced illness may stabilize, improve, or disappear with time and/or anti-inflammatory or supportive therapy. Lesions in the CNS may be multifocal and typically involve the gray matter or white matter but are usually most severe in the pontomedullary gray matter (see Pathologic Findings). CSF findings are indistinguishable from those of virulent CDV infections. The vaccine virus may be distinguished by the ease with which it can be isolated in tissue culture (see Viral Isolation). There are no dramatic genomic differences between virulent and vaccine strains, although some variation in sequences of the NP gene (see Table 3–2) have been detected.[55, 95]

Vaccine Interference

Adverse environmental influences can affect the response to distemper vaccination in dogs. High humidity (85–90%) and high temperature that cause dogs to have rectal temperatures averaging 39.8°C (103.6°F) reduce the immune response after distemper vaccination.[42]

Dogs subjected to anesthesia (barbiturate induction with halothane maintenance) followed by surgery were studied for their response to distemper vaccination.[42] There was no demonstrable impairment in the humoral antibody response to vaccination, although challenge studies were not performed. Some depression of the peripheral blood lymphocyte response to phytohemagglutinin did occur.

Glucocorticoid therapy, given at immunosuppressive doses for 3 weeks, did not suppress the normal humoral response to distemper vaccine, although treated dogs developed depressed responses to phytohemagglutinin stimulation of lymphocytes.[42] These dogs also survived subsequent challenge with virulent CDV.

Concurrent parvoviral infection has been suspected in reducing the antibody response of dogs vaccinated against canine distemper. Simultaneous vaccination against parvoviral infection was suspected of inhibiting the response of dogs to vaccination against CDV infection, although adequate control data were lacking, and this has not been substantiated in older dogs.[42] For a further discussion of canine parvovirus-induced immunologic interference with CDV vaccination, the reader should consult Chapters 8 and 100.

Measles Vaccination

Canine distemper and human measles viruses are antigenically related, and experimental infection of dogs with measles virus protected dogs from subsequent infection with CDV. Distemper virus antibody titers are minimally elevated after measles vaccination despite adequate protection. CMI and other factors are thought to be the primary elements involved in the protective response. Measles vaccine virus produces a self-limiting, noncontagious infection in the lymphoid system of dogs similar to that of MLV-CDV vaccines. There is probably little danger of reversion to virulence and probably no danger to humans when proper vaccination procedures are followed. Only measles vaccines licensed for use in dogs (not human products) should be administered by veterinarians. Higher antigen mass in canine products is required due to the heterologous nature of this product.

Measles vaccination offers the theoretic advantage of protection in young puppies with high concentrations of maternal antibodies to distemper. It should only be used as a replacement for the first vaccination in 6- to 12-week-old puppies. Dogs younger than 6 weeks with very high maternal antibody concentrations do not respond well to either distemper or measles vaccination. If female puppies are vaccinated with measles vaccine after 12 weeks of age, passive transfer of measles antibody will occur to their offspring, especially if they are bred on the first heat cycle.

Immunity to distemper acquired from measles vaccination is not only transient but weaker than that derived from successful vaccination with MLV distemper vaccine. SC inoculation of measles vaccine is not as effective as the initially recommended IM route. However, puppies older than 6 weeks immunized with measles virus vaccine are protected within 72 hours from challenge with CDV despite the lack of increase in distemper virus antibody titer.[27] During an initial vaccination series, measles vaccination alone or in combination with distemper vaccination should be followed by at least two distemper vaccinations to produce adequate long-term immunity of at least 12 months' duration.

Environmental Control

CDV is extremely susceptible to common disinfectants. Infected animals are the primary source of the virus, and they should be segregated from other healthy dogs. Dogs usually shed the virus in secretions for 1 to 2 weeks after the acute systemic illness. Those recovering from systemic illness or with later developing neurologic signs (without systemic disease) may still be shedding some virus.

PUBLIC HEALTH CONSIDERATIONS

Multiple sclerosis (MS) is a neurologic affliction of humans that resembles both subacute sclerosing panencephalitis (SSPE, an encephalitis of humans thought to be caused by a chronic infection with defective or latent measles virus) and chronic progressive distemper encephalitis in dogs. Both of the latter diseases are pathologically similar, with demyelination, glial proliferation, and other findings characteristic of a chronic, persistent nonsuppurative encephalitis. The cause of MS is still uncertain, but there is no substantial evidence for measles or distemper virus involvement. Human herpesviruses have also been implicated.[77] Furthermore there has been no reduction in the incidence of MS since before 1960 despite the widespread reduction of measles and distemper through effective vaccines.

A suggestion has been made that Paget's disease, an inflammatory bone disorder in people, might be related to CDV acquired from exposure to dogs. It is a chronic disease that leads to progressive destruction, remodeling, and deformity of bone. Evidence has accumulated that the disease may be caused by chronic paramyxovirus infection of osteoclasts. Using in situ hybridization, CDV genetic sequences have been found in the bone of 63.5% of untreated Paget's disease patients.[26, 39–41] Ownership of dogs was found to have a high correlation with Paget's disease patients, although the indirect relationship between these factors should not be overstated, because a similar correlation was found with ownership of cats and birds. Other studies have implicated other paramyxoviruses such as measles virus variants as being responsible.[74, 75] Until such viruses are isolated and completely sequenced, the role, if any, of CDV in such infections is questionable.

References

1. Adelus-Neveu F, Saint Gerand AL, Fayet G. 1991. Canine distemper. Conclusions from an outbreak in France. *Prakti Tierarzt* 72:866–871.
2. Alldinger S, Baumgärtner W, Örvell C. 1993. Restricted expression of viral surface proteins in canine distemper encephalitis. *Acta Neuropathol* 85:635–645.
3. Alldinger S, Baumgärtner W, Van Moll P, et al. 1993. In vivo and in vitro expression of canine distemper viral proteins in dogs and nondomestic carnivores. *Arch Virol* 132:421–428.
4. Alldinger S, Wunschmann A, Baumgärtner W, et al. 1996. Up-regulation of major histocompatibility complex class II antigen expression in the central nervous system of dogs with spontaneous canine distemper virus encephalitis. *Acta Neuropathol* 92:273–280.

5. Alleman AR, Christopher MM, Steiner DA, et al. 1992. Identification of intracytoplasmic inclusion bodies in mononuclear cells from the cerebrospinal fluid of a dog with canine distemper. *Vet Pathol* 29:84–85.
6. Appel MJG, Pearce-Kelling S, Summers BA. 1992. Dog lymphocyte cultures facilitate the isolation and growth of virulent canine distemper virus. *J Vet Diagn Invest* 4:258–263.
7. Appel MJG, Reggiardo C, Summers BA, et al. 1991. Canine distemper virus infection and encephalitis in javelinas (collared peccaries). *Arch Virol* 119:147–152.
8. Appel MJG, Summers BA. 1995. Pathogenicity of morbilliviruses for terrestrial carnivores. *Vet Microbiol* 44:187–191.
9. Appel MJG, Yates RA, Foley GL, et al. 1994. Canine distemper epizootic in lions, tigers and leopards in North America. *J Vet Diagn Invest* 6:277–278.
10. Barrett T, Visser IKG, Amaev L, et al. 1993. Dolphin and porpoise morbilliviruses are genetically distinct from phocine distemper virus. *Virology* 193:1010–1012.
11. Baumgärtner W, Boyce RA, Alldinger S, et al. 1995. Metaphyseal bone lesions in young dogs with systemic canine distemper infection. *Vet Microbiol* 44:201–209.
12. Baumgärtner W, Orvell C, Reinacher M. 1989. Naturally occurring canine distemper virus encephalitis: distribution and expression of viral polypeptides in nervous tissues. *Acta Neuropathol* 78:504–512.
13. Bell SC, Carter SD, Bennett D. 1991. Canine distemper viral antigens and antibodies in dogs with rheumatoid arthritis. *Res Vet Sci* 50:64–68.
14. Bernard A, Fevre-Mortange M, Bencsik A, et al. 1993. Brain structures selectively targeted by canine distemper virus in a mouse model infection. *J Neuropathol Exp Neurol* 52:471–480.
15. Bittegko SB, Arnbjerg J, Nkya R, et al. 1995. Multiple dental abnormalities following canine distemper infection. *J Am Anim Hosp Assoc* 31:42–45.
16. Blakemore WF, Summers BA, Appel MG. 1989. Evidence of oligodendrocyte infection and degeneration in canine distemper encephalomyelitis. *Acta Neuropathol* 77:550–553.
17. Blixenkrone-Moller M, Pedersen JR, Appel MJ, et al. 1991. Detection of IgM antibodies against canine distemper virus in dog and mink sera employing ELISA. *J Vet Diagn Invest* 3:3–9.
18. Blixenkrone-Moller M, Svansson V, Appel M, et al. 1992. Antigenic relationships between field isolates of morbilliviruses from different carnivores. *Arch Virol* 123:279–294.
19. Blixenkrone-Moller M, Svansson V, Have P, et al. 1993. Studies on manifestations of canine distemper virus infection in an urban population. *Vet Microbiol* 37:163–173.
20. Botteron C, Zurbriggen A, Griot C, et al. 1992. Canine distemper virus immune complexes induce bystander degeneration of oligodendrocytes. *Acta Neuropathol* 83:402–407.
21. Brix A. 1995. Personal communication. University of Georgia, Department of Pathology, Athens, GA.
22. Brooks R. 1991. Adverse reactions to canine and feline vaccines. *Aust Vet J* 68:342–344.
23. Brugger M, Jungi TW, Zurbriggen A, et al. 1992. Canine distemper virus increases procoagulant activity of macrophages. *Virology* 190:616–623.
24. Burge T, Griot C, Vandevelde M, et al. 1989. Antiviral antibodies stimulate production of reactive oxygen species in cultured brain cells infected with canine distemper virus. *J Virol* 63:2790–2797.
25. Carter SD, May C, Bell SC, et al. 1993. Canine distemper virus and rheumatoid arthritis in dogs. *Vet Immuno Pathol* 35(Suppl):219.
26. Cartwright EJ, Gordon MT, Freemont AJ, et al. 1993. Paramyxoviruses and Paget's disease. *J Med Virol* 40:133–141.
27. Chalmers WSK, Baxendale W. 1994. A comparison of canine distemper vaccine and measles vaccine for the prevention of canine distemper in young puppies. *Vet Rec* 135:349–353.
28. Chappuis G. 1995. Control of canine distemper. *Vet Microbiol* 44:351–358.
29. Coates JR, Carmichael KP, Roberts AW, et al. 1998. Vaccine-associated canine distemper viral encephalomyelitis in 14 dogs. *J Vet Intern Med.* Submitted.
30. Cornwell HJC, Thompson H, McCandlish IAP, et al. 1988. Encephalitis in dogs associated with a batch of canine distemper (Rockborn) vaccine. *Vet Rec* 112:54–59.
31. De Vries P, Uytdehaag FGC, Osterhaus ADME. 1988. Canine distemper virus (CDV) immune-stimulating complexes (iscoms) but not measles virus iscoms protect dogs against CDV infection. *J Gen Virol* 69:2071–2084.
32. Evans MB, Bunn TO, Hill HT, et al. 1991. Comparison of in vitro replication and cytopathology caused by strains of canine distemper virus of vaccine and field origin. *J Vet Diagn Invest* 3:127–132.
33. Gaedke K, Telfke JP, Hardt M, et al. 1995. Detection of distemper virus N protein RNA in the brain of dogs with spontaneous distemper encephalitis using a digoxigenin-labeled, double-stranded DNA probe for in situ hybridization. *Berl Munch Tierarztl Wochenschr* 108:51–54.
34. Gassner G, Baumgartner W, Nolte I. 1996. Atypical form of nervous distemper in two golden retriever bitches. *Tierarztl Umschaw* 51:458.
35. Gathumbi PK. 1993. The retrospective use of a peroxidase technique for confirmation of suspected canine distemper in Kenya. *Vet Res Commun* 17:197–201.
36. Gemma T, Iwatsuki K, Shin Y-S, et al. 1996. Serological analysis of canine distemper virus using an immunocapture ELISA. *J Vet Med Sci* 58:791–794.
37. Gemma T, Watari T, Akiyama K, et al. 1996. Epidemiological observations on recent outbreaks of canine distemper in Tokyo. *J Vet Med Sci* 58:547–550.
38. Glaus T, Griot C, Richard A, et al. 1990. Ultrastructural and biochemical findings in brain cell cultures infected with canine distemper virus. *Acta Neuropathol* 80:59–67.
39. Gordon MT, Anderson DC, Sharpe PT. 1991. Canine distemper virus localized in bone cells of patients with Paget's disease. *Bone* 12:195–201.
40. Gordon MT, Bell SC, Mee AP, et al. 1993. Prevalence of canine distemper antibodies in the pagetic population. *J Med Virol* 40:313–317.
41. Gordon MT, Mee AP, Anderson DC, et al. 1992. Canine distemper virus transcripts sequences from pagetic bone. *Bone Min* 19:159–174.
42. Greene CE, Appel MJ. 1990. Canine distemper, pp 226–241. *In* Greene CE (ed), Infectious diseases of the dog and cat. WB Saunders, Philadelphia, PA.
43. Hamburger D, Griot C, Zurbriggen A, et al. 1991. Loss of virulence of canine distemper virus is associated with a structural change recognized by monoclonal antibody. *Experientia* 47:842–845.
44. Harder TC, Kuczka A, Dubberke M, et al. 1991. An outbreak of canine distemper in dog's home with a vaccinated population of dogs. *Kleintierpraxis* 36:305–314.
45. Holdaway IM, Ibbertson HK, Wattie D, et al. 1990. Previous pet ownership and Paget's disease. *Bone Min* 8:53–58.
46. Hussey GD, Klein M. 1990. A randomized controlled trial of vitamin A in children with severe measles. *N Engl J Med* 323:160–164.
47. Iwatsuki K, Okita M, Ochikubo F, et al. 1995. Immunohistochemical analysis of the lymphoid organs of dogs naturally infected with canine distemper virus. *J Comp Pathol* 113:185-190.
48. Jaggy A. 1996. Enzyme-linked immunosorbent assay for the detection of canine distemper virus. Doctoral dissertation, University of Georgia, Athens, GA.
49. Jarvinen AK, Halonen P, Raha M, et al. 1990. An outbreak of canine distemper in Finland. *Suomen-Elainlaakarilehti* 96:335–341.
50. Johnson R, Glickman LT, Emerick TJ, et al. 1995. Canine distemper infection in pet dogs: I. Surveillance in Indiana during a suspected outbreak. *J Am Anim Hosp Assoc* 31:223–229.
51. Kahn SA, Brennan P, Newman J, et al. 1996. Paget's disease of bone and unvaccinated dogs. *Bone* 19:47–50.
52. Kai C, Ochikubo F, Okita M, et al. 1993. Use of B95a cells for isolation of canine distemper virus from clinical cases. *J Vet Med Sci* 55:1067–1070.
53. Kolbl S, Tschabrun S, Schuller W. 1995. Examination of the humoral immune response in puppies after first immunization with different combination vaccines: 1. Distemper virus component. *Kleintierpraxis* 40:851.
54. Leighton T, Ferguson M, Gunn A, et al. 1988. Canine distemper in sled dogs. *Can Vet J* 29:299.
55. Maes R, Vandevelde M, Zurbriggen A, et al. 1996. Postvaccinal encephalitis in dogs vaccinated with canine distemper vaccine. *Proc Am Assoc Vet Lab Diagn*, Little Rock, AR.
56. Malik R, Dowden M, Davis PE, et al. 1995. Concurrent juvenile cellulitis and metaphyseal osteopathy. An atypical canine distemper virus syndrome. *Aust Vet Pract* 25:62–67.
57. McCandlish IAP, Cornwell HJC, Thompson H, et al. 1992. Distemper encephalitis in pups after vaccination of the dam. *Vet Rec* 130:27–30.
58. McKenna MJ, Kristiansen AG, Haines J. 1996. Polymerase chain reaction amplification of a measles virus sequence from human temporal bone sections with active osteosclerosis. *Am J Otol* 17:827–830.
59. Mee AP, Gordon MT, May C, et al. 1993. Canine distemper virus transcripts detected in the bone cells of dogs with metaphyseal osteopathy. *Bone* 14:59–67.
60. Mee AP, Sharpe PT. 1993. Dogs, distemper and Paget's disease. *Bioessays* 15:783–789.
61. Mee AP, Webber DM, May C, et al. 1992. Detection of canine distemper in bone cells in the metaphyses of distemper-infected dogs. *J Bone Miner Res* 7:829–834.
62. Mitchell WJ, Summers BA, Appel MJG. 1991. Viral expression in experimental canine distemper demyelinating encephalitis. *J Comp Pathol* 104:77–88.
63. Morell V. 1994. Serengeti's big cats going to the dogs. *Science* 264:1664.
64. Muller CF, Fatzer RS, Beck K, et al. 1995. Studies on canine distemper virus persistence in the central nervous system. *Acta Neuropathol* 89:438–445.
65. Multinelli F, Vandevelde M, Griot C, et al. 1989. Astrocytic infection in canine distemper virus-induced demyelination. *Acta Neuropathol* 77:333–335.

65a. Nesseler A, Baumgärtner W, Gaedke K, et al. 1997. Abundant expression of viral nucleoprotein mRNA and restricted translation of the corresponding viral protein in inclusion body polioencephalitis of canine distemper. *J Comp Pathol* 116:291–301.

66. Norrby E, Utter G, Orvell C, et al. 1986. Protection against canine distemper virus in dogs after immunization with isolated fusion protein. *J Virol* 58:536–541.
67. Olson P, Klingeborn B, Bonnett B, et al. 1997. Distemper titer study in Sweden 1995-1996. *J Vet Intern Med* 11:148.
68. Osterhaus ADME, De Swart RL, Vos HW, et al. 1995. Morbillivirus infections of aquatic mammals: newly identified members of the genus. *Vet Microbiol* 44: 219–227.

69. Palmer DG, Huxtable CRR, Thomas JB. 1990. Immunohistochemical demonstration of canine distemper virus antigen as an aid to the diagnosis of canine distemper encephalomyelitis. *Res Vet Sci* 49:177–181.
69a. Pardo MC, Bauman JE, Mackowiak M. 1997. Protection of dogs against canine distemper by vaccination with a canarypox virus recombinant expressing canine distemper virus fusion and hemagglutinin glycoproteins. *Am J Vet Res* 58:833–836.
70. Patronek GJ, Glickman LT, Johnson R, et al. 1995. Canine distemper infection in pet dogs: II. A case-control study of risk factors during a suspected outbreak in Indiana. *J Am Anim Hosp Assoc* 31:230–235.
71. Phillips TR, Jensen JL, Rubino MJ, et al. 1989. Effects of vaccines on the canine immune system. *Can J Vet Res* 53:154–160.
72. Ralston SH, Digiovine FS, Gallacher SJ, et al. 1991. Failure to detect paramyxovirus sequences in Paget's disease of bone using the polymerase chain reaction. *J Bone Miner Res* 6:1243–1248.
73. Raw ME, Pearson GR, Brown PJ, et al. 1992. Canine distemper infection associated with acute nervous signs in dogs. *Vet Rec* 130:291–293.
74. Reddy SV, Singer FR, Mallette L, et al. 1996. Detection of measles virus nucleocapsid transcripts in circulating blood cells from patients with Paget disease. *J Bone Miner Res* 11:1602–1607.
75. Reddy SV, Singer FR, Roodman GD. 1995. Bone marrow mononuclear cells from patients with Paget's disease contain measles virus nucleocapsid messenger ribonucleic acid that has mutations in a specific region of the sequence. *J Clin Endocrinol Metab* 80:2108–2111.
76. Rima BK, Duffy N, Mitchell WJ, et al. 1991. Correlation between humoral immune responses and presence of virus in the CNS in dogs experimentally infected with canine distemper virus. *Arch Virol* 121:1–8.
77. Sanders VJ, Felisan S, Waddell A, et al. 1996. Detection of Herpesviridae in postmortem multiple sclerosis brain tissue and controls by polymerase chain reaction. *J Neuroviral* 2:249–258.
78. Shell LG. 1990. Canine distemper. *Compend Cont Ed Pract Vet* 12:173–179.
79. Shin Y-S, Mori T, Okita M, et al. 1995. Detection of canine distemper virus nucleocapsid protein gene in canine peripheral blood mononuclear cells by RT-PCR. *J Vet Med Sci* 57:439–445.
80. Sorjonen DC, Cox NR, Swango CJ. 1989. Electrophoretic determination of albumin and gamma globulin concentration in the cerebrospinal fluid of dogs with encephalomyelitis attributable to canine distemper virus infection: 13 cases (1980-1987). *J Am Vet Med Assoc* 195:977–980.
81. Spencer LM. 1995. CDV infection in large exotic cats not expected to affect domestic cats. *J Am Vet Med Assoc* 206:579–580.
81a. Stettler M, Beck K, Wagner A, et al. 1997. Determinants of persistence in canine distemper viruses. *Vet Microbiol* 57:83–93.
82. Taylor J, Pincus S, Tartaglia J, et al. 1991. Vaccinia virus recombinants expressing either the measles virus fusion or hemagglutinin glycoprotein protect dogs against canine distemper virus challenge. *J Virol* 65:4263–4274.
83. Thomas WB, Sorjonen DC, Steiss JE. 1993. A retrospective evaluation of 38 cases of canine distemper encephalomyelitis. *J An Anim Hosp Assoc* 29:129–133.
84. Tipold A. 1995. Diagnosis of inflammatory and infectious diseases of the central nervous system in dogs: a retrospective study. *J Vet Intern Med* 9:304–314.
85. Tipold A, Pfister H, Vandevelde M. 1993. Determination of the IgG index for the detection of intrathecal immunoglobulin synthesis in dogs using an ELISA. *Res Vet Sci* 54:40–44.
86. Tipold A, Vandevelde M, Jaggy A. 1992. Neurological manifestations of canine distemper virus infection. *J Small Anim Pract* 33:466–470.
87. Vandevelde M. 1994. Personal communication. University of Bern, Bern, Switzerland.
88. Vandevelde M, Zurbriggen A. 1995. The neurobiology of canine distemper virus infection. *Vet Microbiol* 44:271–280.
89. Vilafranca M, Tello M, Pumarola M, et al. 1996. Neural cells from dogs with spontaneous distemper encephalitis express class II major histocompatibility complex molecules. *J Comp Pathol* 114:43–50.
90. Wild TF, Bernard A, Spehner D, et al. 1993. Vaccination of mice against canine distemper virus-induced encephalitis with vaccinia virus recombinants encoding measles or canine distemper virus antigens. *Vaccine* 11:438–444.
91. Williams K, Cooper B, DeLahunta A, et al. 1992. Postvaccinal canine distemper encephalomyelitis confirmed by virus isolation. *Vet Pathol* 29:440.
92. Wood SL, Thomson GW, Haines DM. 1995. Canine distemper virus-like infection in a captive African lioness. *Can Vet J* 36:34–35.
93. Yoshikawa Y, Ochikubo F, Matsubara Y, et al. 1989. Natural infection with canine distemper virus in a Japanese monkey (Macaca fuscata). *Vet Microbiol* 20:193–205.
94. Zurbriggen A, Graber HU, Vandevelde M. 1995. Selective spread and reduced virus release leads to canine distemper virus persistence in the nervous system. *Vet Microbiol* 44:281–288.
95. Zurbriggen A, Muller C, Vandevelde M. 1993. In situ hybridization of virulent canine distemper virus in brain tissue using digoxigenin-labeled probes. *Am J Vet Res* 54:1457–1461.
96. Zurbriggen A, Vandevelde M. 1994. The pathogenesis of nervous distemper. *Prog Vet Neurol* 5:109–115.
97. Zurbriggen A, Yamawaki M, Vandevelde M. 1993. Restricted canine distemper virus infection oligodenocytes. *Lab Invest* 68:277–284.

Chapter 4

Infectious Canine Hepatitis and Canine Acidophil Cell Hepatitis

Craig E. Greene

Infectious Canine Hepatitis

ETIOLOGY

Infectious canine hepatitis (ICH), caused by canine adenovirus (CAV-1), has worldwide serologic homogeneity as well as immunologic similarities to human adenoviruses. It is antigenically and genetically distinct from CAV-2, which produces respiratory disease in the dog (see Etiology and Pathogenesis, Chapter 6). Genetic variants of CAV-2 have been isolated from the intestine of a puppy with hemorrhagic diarrhea and from kenneled dogs with diarrhea. Human adenoviruses have been used as vectors for recombinant vaccine testing in dogs.[6]

As with other adenoviruses, CAV-1 is resistant to environmental inactivation, surviving disinfection with various chemicals, such as chloroform, ether, acid, and formalin, and is stable when exposed to certain frequencies of UV radiation. CAV-1 survives for days at room temperature on soiled fomites and remains viable for months at temperatures below

4°C. CAV-1 is inactivated after 5 minutes at 50° to 60°C, which makes steam cleaning a plausible means of disinfection. Chemical disinfection has also been successful when iodine, phenol, and sodium hydroxide are utilized.

CAV-1 causes clinical disease in dogs, coyotes, foxes, and other Canidae and in Ursidae (bears). The high incidence of naturally occurring neutralizing antibodies in the unvaccinated feral and wildlife dog population suggests that subclinical infection is widespread.[2, 3] CAV-1 has been isolated from all body tissues and secretions of dogs during the acute stages of the disease. By 10 to 14 days PI, it can be found only in the kidneys and is excreted in the urine for at least 6 to 9 months. Aerosol transmission of the virus via the urine is unlikely insofar as susceptible dogs housed 6 inches apart from virus shedders do not become infected. Viral spread can occur by contact with fomites, including feeding utensils and hands. Ectoparasites can harbor CAV-1 and may be involved in the natural transmission of the disease.

PATHOGENESIS

After natural oronasal exposure, the virus initially localizes in the tonsils (Fig. 4–1), where it spreads to regional lymph nodes and lymphatics before reaching the blood through the thoracic duct. Viremia, which lasts 4 to 8 days PI, results in rapid dissemination of the virus to other tissues and body secretions, including saliva, urine, and feces. Hepatic parenchymal cells and vascular endothelial cells of many tissues are prime targets of viral localization and injury.

Initial cellular injury of the liver, kidney, and eye is associated with cytotoxic effects of virus. A sufficient antibody response by day 7 PI clears the virus from the blood and liver and restricts the extent of hepatic damage. Widespread centrilobular to panlobular hepatic necrosis is often fatal in experimentally infected dogs with a persistently low (<4) antibody titer. Acute hepatic necrosis can be self-limiting and restricted centrilobularly, so that hepatic regeneration occurs in dogs that survive this phase of the disease. Dogs demonstrating a partial neutralizing antibody titer (>16, <500) by day 4 or 5 PI develop chronic active hepatitis and hepatic fibrosis. Persistent hepatic inflammation continues, probably as a result of chronic latent hepatic infection with virus. Dogs with sufficient antibody titers (≥500) on the day of infection usually show little clinical evidence of disease. Dogs immune to parenteral challenge with CAV-1 are still susceptible to respiratory disease via aerosolized viral particles.

Both virulent and modified live strains of CAV-1 produce renal lesions. Virus detected by positive immunofluorescence and ultrastructural evaluation initially localizes in the glomerular endothelium in the viremic phase of disease and produces initial glomerular injury. An increase in neutralizing antibody at approximately 7 days PI is associated with the glomerular deposition of circulating immune complexes (CICs) and transient proteinuria. CAV-1 is not detected in the glomerulus after 14 days PI; however, it persists in renal tubular epithelium. Tubular localization of the virus is primarily associated with viruria, and only a transient proteinuria is noted. A mild focal interstitial nephritis is found in recovered dogs; however, unlike the liver disease, no evidence suggests that chronic progressive renal disease results from ICH.

Clinical complications of ocular localization of virulent CAV-1 occur in approximately 20% of naturally infected dogs and in less than 1% of dogs after SC-MLV CAV-1 vaccination. The development of ocular lesions begins during viremia, which develops 4 to 6 days PI; the virus enters the aqueous humor from the blood and replicates in corneal endothelial cells.

Severe anterior uveitis and corneal edema develop 7 days

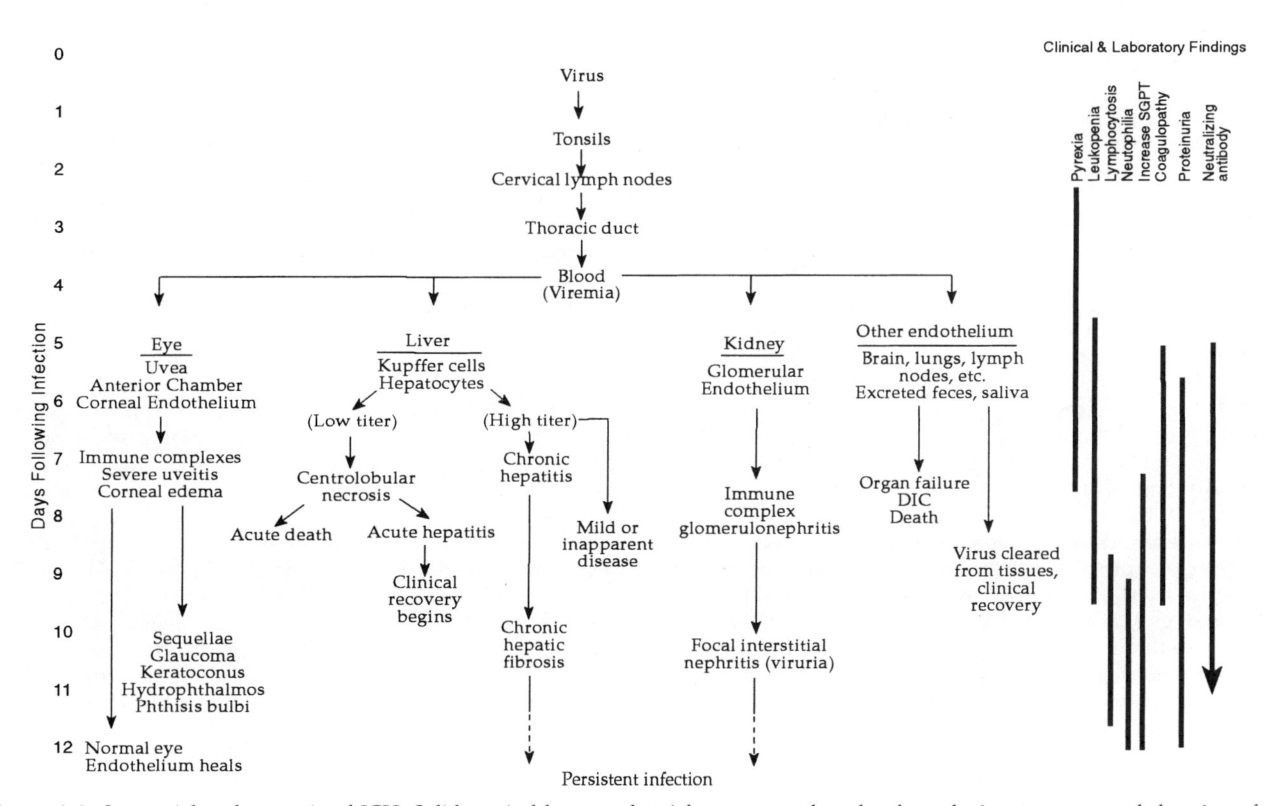

Figure 4–1. Sequential pathogenesis of ICH. Solid vertical bars on the right correspond to the chronologic occurrence and duration of the respective clinical or laboratory findings associated with ICH.

PI, a period corresponding to an increase in neutralizing antibody titer. CIC deposition with CF results in chemotaxis of inflammatory cells into the anterior chamber and extensive corneal endothelial damage. Disruption of the intact corneal endothelium causes accumulation of edematous fluid within the corneal stroma.

Uveitis and edema are usually self-limiting unless additional complications or massive endothelial destruction occurs. Clearing of corneal edema coincides with endothelial regeneration and restoration of the hydrostatic gradient between the corneal stroma and aqueous humor. Normal recovery of the eye is usually apparent by 21 days PI. If the inflammatory changes are severe enough to block the filtration angle, increased intraocular pressure may result in glaucoma and hydrophthalmos.

Complications are often associated with the pathogenesis of ICH. Dogs are more prone to develop pyelonephritis as a result of renal damage after ICH infection. DIC, a frequent complication of ICH, begins in the early viremic phase of the disease and may be triggered by endothelial cell damage with widespread activation of the clotting mechanism or by the inability of the diseased liver to remove activated clotting factors. Decreased hepatic synthesis of clotting factors in the face of excessive consumption compounds the bleeding defect.

Although the cause of death in ICH is uncertain, the liver is a primary site of viral injury. Hepatic insufficiency and hepatoencephalopathy may result in a semicomatose state and death. Some dogs die so suddenly that liver damage with resulting hepatic failure does not have time to occur. Death in these dogs may result from damage to the brain, lungs, and other vital parenchymal organs or from the development of DIC.

CLINICAL FINDINGS

ICH is most frequently seen in dogs younger than 1 year, although unvaccinated dogs of all ages can be affected. Severely affected dogs become moribund and die within a few hours after the onset of clinical signs. Owners frequently believe that their dog was poisoned. Clinical signs in dogs that survive the acute viremic period include vomiting, abdominal pain, and diarrhea with or without evidence of hemorrhage.

Abnormal physical findings in the early phase of infection include increased rectal temperature (39.4–41.1°C [103–106°F]) and accelerated pulse and respiratory rates. Fever may be transient or biphasic early in the course of the disease. Tonsillar enlargement, usually associated with pharyngitis and laryngitis, is common. Coughing and auscultated harsh lower respiratory sounds are manifestations of pneumonia. Cervical lymphadenomegaly is frequently found with SC edema of the head, neck, and dependent portions of the trunk. Abdominal tenderness and hepatomegaly are usually apparent in the acutely ill dog. A hemorrhagic diathesis that is manifested by widespread petechial and ecchymotic hemorrhages, epistaxis, and bleeding from venipuncture sites may occur. Icterus is uncommon in acute ICH, but it is found in some dogs that survive the acute fulminant phase of the disease. Abdominal distention is caused by accumulation of serosanguineous fluid or hemorrhage. CNS signs, including depression, disorientation, seizures, or terminal coma, may develop at any time after infection.

Clinical signs of uncomplicated ICH frequently last 5 to 7 days before improvement. Persistent signs may be found in dogs with a concurrent viral infection such as canine distemper or in dogs that develop chronic active hepatitis.

Corneal edema and anterior uveitis usually occur when clinical recovery begins and may be the only clinical abnormalities seen in dogs with inapparent infection (also see ICH in Chapter 93). Dogs with corneal edema show blepharospasm, photophobia, and serous ocular discharge. Clouding of the cornea usually begins at the limbus and spreads centrally (see Fig. 93–9). Ocular pain, present during the early stages of infection, usually subsides when the cornea becomes completely clouded. However, pain may return with the development of glaucoma or corneal ulceration and perforation. In uncomplicated cases, clearing of the cornea begins at the limbus and spreads centrally.

DIAGNOSIS

Early hematologic findings in ICH include leukopenia with lymphopenia and neutropenia. Neutrophilia and lymphocytosis occur later in dogs with uncomplicated clinical recovery. Increased numbers of dark staining (activated) lymphocytes and nucleated erythrocytes may be found. Serum protein alterations, detectable only on serum electrophoresis, are a transient increase in α_2-globulin by 7 days PI and by a delayed increase in γ-globulin, which peaks 21 days PI.

The degree of increased activities of ALT (formerly SGPT), AST (formerly SGOT), and serum ALP depends on the time of sampling and the magnitude of hepatic necrosis. These enzyme increases continue until day 14 PI, after which they decline, although persistent or recurrent elevations may be found in dogs that develop chronic active hepatitis. Moderate to marked bilirubinuria is frequently found owing to the low renal threshold for conjugated bilirubin in the dog; hyperbilirubinemia is uncommon. BSP retention at 30 minutes may be increased during the acute course of ICH or later in dogs that develop chronic hepatic fibrosis. Hypoglycemia may be found in dogs in the terminal phases of the disease.

Coagulation abnormalities characteristic of DIC are most pronounced during the viremic stages of the disease. Thrombocytopenia with or without altered platelet function is usually apparent. One-stage PT, APTT, and TT are variably prolonged. Early prolongation of the APTT probably results from factor VIII consumption. Factor VIII activity is decreased, and FDPs are increased. Platelet dysfunction and later prolongation of the APTT probably result from increased FDPs. Prolongation of the PT is usually less noticeable.

Proteinuria (primarily albuminuria) is a reflection of the renal damage caused by the virus and can usually be detected on random urinalysis because the concentration is greater than 50 mg/dl. The increase in glomerular permeability can result from localization of the virus in initial stages of infection. Alternatively, as the disease progresses, glomeruli become damaged by CICs or as an effect of DIC. Abdominal paracentesis yields a fluid that varies in color from clear yellow to bright red, depending on the amount of blood present. It is usually an exudate with a protein content ranging from 5.29 to 9.3 g/dl (specific gravity from 1.020 to 1.030).

Bone marrow cytology reflects the dramatic change in leukocytes in the peripheral circulation. Megakaryocytes are absent or decreased during the viremic stage of the disease, and those that are present may have altered morphology.

CSF is normal in dogs with neurologic signs caused by hepatoencephalopathy; it is usually abnormal in dogs that develop a nonsuppurative encephalitis from localization of the virus within the brain. There is an increase in protein concentration (> 30 mg/dl) with mononuclear pleocytosis (> 10 cells/mm^3). The aqueous humor also has increased concentrations of protein and cells associated with anterior uveitis.

Results of laboratory procedures previously discussed are all suggestive of ICH and are the primary means of making a diagnosis in clinical practice. Antemortem confirmation, although not essential for appropriate therapy, can be obtained by serologic testing, virus isolation, and immunofluorescent evaluation. Serologic tests include IHA, CF, immunodiffusion, and ELISA. These tests usually show higher titers after infection with virulent virus in contrast with MLV vaccines.

CAV-1 can be isolated because it readily replicates in cell cultures of several species, including dogs. Typical adenovirus-induced cytopathology includes clustering of host cells and detachment from the monolayers with the formation of intranuclear inclusions. When viremia begins, on day 5 PI, CAV-1 can be cultured from any body tissue or secretion. The virus is isolated in the anterior chamber during the mild phase of uveitis before antibody infiltration and immune complex formation. It is often difficult to culture virus from the liver of dogs because hepatic arginase inhibits viral nucleic acid replication. The virus has not been isolated from the liver later than 10 days PI, even in dogs with chronic active hepatitis, perhaps because viral latency develops. The kidney is the most persistent site of virus localization, and CAV-1 can be isolated from the urine for at least 6 to 9 months after the initial infection.

Immunofluorescent techniques are used experimentally to confirm the presence of virus within various tissues. This method has helped to locate the sites of viral replication, the spread of the virus within the cells, and the presence of viral antigen in inclusion bodies. Immunoperoxidase procedures, applied to formalin-fixed, paraffin-embedded tissues, have detected virus in liver tissues stored for up to 6 years.

PATHOLOGIC FINDINGS

Findings on necropsy or biopsy examination of tissues from dogs can usually confirm a diagnosis of ICH. Dogs that die during the acute phase of the disease are often in good flesh, with edema and hemorrhage of superficial lymph nodes and cervical SC tissue. Icterus is not usually apparent. The abdominal cavity may contain fluid that varies from clear to bright red in color. Petechial and ecchymotic hemorrhages are present on all serosal surfaces. The liver is enlarged, dark, and mottled in appearance, and a prominent fibrinous exudate is usually present on the liver surface and in the interlobar fissures (Fig. 4–2). The gallbladder is thickened and edematous and has a bluish-white opaque appearance. Fibrin may be deposited on other abdominal serosal surfaces, giving them a ground glass–like appearance. Intraluminal GI hemorrhage is a frequent finding. The spleen is enlarged and bulges on the cut surface.

Variable gross lesions in other organs include multifocal hemorrhagic renal cortical infarcts. The lungs have multiple, patchy, gray-to-red areas of consolidation. Hemorrhagic and edematous bronchial lymph nodes are found. Scattered hemorrhagic areas, present on coronal section of the brain, are primarily located in the midbrain and caudal brain stem. Ocular lesions, when present, are characterized by corneal opacification and aqueous humor clouding.

Dogs surviving the acute phase of the disease may have lesions that can be found on subsequent necropsy examination. The liver of those with chronic hepatic fibrosis may be small, firm, and nodular. The kidneys of many dogs that recover are studded with multiple white foci (0.5 cm diameter) extending from the renal pelvis to the outer cortex. Ocular sequelae from the acute disease can include either glaucoma or phthisis bulbi.

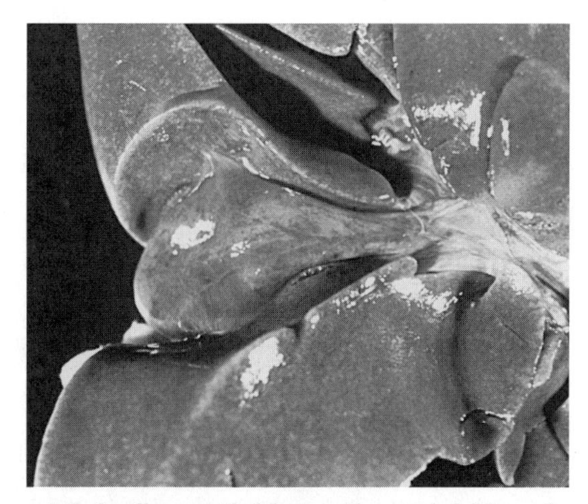

Figure 4–2. Swollen, mottled liver with rounded lobar edges and gallbladder edema characteristic of ICH.

Histologic changes in the liver of dogs that die of acute hepatitis include widespread centrilobular to panlobular necroses. In dogs with mild hepatocellular necrosis, the margin between necrotic and viable hepatocytes is sharply defined within the liver lobule (Fig. 4–3). The preservation of the underlying support stroma allows for eventual hepatic regeneration. Only in severe cases does coagulation necrosis of entire hepatic lobules prevent regeneration of the liver. Neutrophilic and mononuclear cell infiltrates are associated with the removal of underlying necrotic tissue. Bile pigment rarely accumulates in most cases because of the transient nature of hepatocellular necrosis and the frequent lack of peripheral lobular involvement of portal radicles. Intranuclear inclusions are initially found in Kupffer's cells and later in viable hepatic parenchymal cells. Subacute to chronic hepatic disease is marked by sporadic foci of necrosis with neutrophilic, mononuclear, and plasma cell infiltration and is found in dogs with partial immunity that survive initial stages of infection.

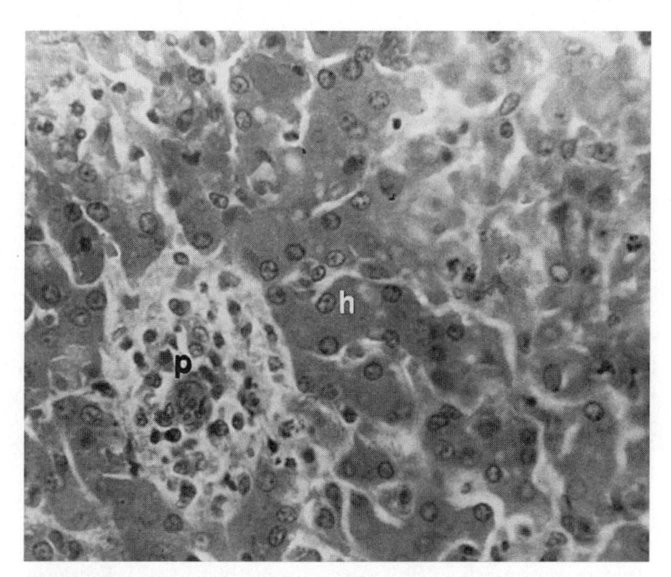

Figure 4–3. Histologic appearance of massive centrolobular necrosis in a fatal case of ICH, showing a few remaining viable hepatocytes (h) around a portal vein (p) in the peripheral lobular area (hematoxylin and eosin, × 250).

Widespread histologic alterations occur in other organs as a result of endothelial injury caused by the virus. The gallbladder has marked subserosal edema, but the epithelium remains intact. Viral inclusions are first found in the renal glomeruli but later are found in renal tubular vascular endothelium. Focal interstitial accumulations of neutrophils and mononuclear cells are found in the renal cortex and medulla. These mild changes often progress to focal interstitial fibrosis. Lymphoid organs, including the lymph nodes, tonsils, and spleen, are congested with neutrophilic and mononuclear cell infiltrates. Lymphoid follicles are dispersed with central areas of necrotic foci. Intranuclear inclusions are present in vascular endothelial cells and histiocytes. The lungs have thickened alveoli with septal cell and peribronchial lymphoid accumulations. Alveoli in consolidated areas are filled with an exudate consisting of erythrocytes, fibrin, and fluid. Mucosal and submucosal edema with focal subserosal hemorrhage are found in the intestinal tract. Widespread vascular degeneration and tissue hemorrhage and necrosis are associated with the presence of intravascular fibrin thrombi.

Swollen, desquamated endothelial cells in meningeal vessels contain intranuclear inclusions. Mononuclear cuffing is present around small vessels throughout the parenchyma of the CNS. Mild endothelial proliferation and mononuclear perivascular infiltration persist for at least 3 weeks after clinical recovery.

Ocular changes are characterized by granulomatous iridocyclitis with corneal endothelial disruption and corneal edema. Iridial and ciliary vessels are congested with inflammatory cells that are also present in the iris and filtration angle.

The **inclusion bodies** seen in ICH have been classified as Cowdry type A and are present in both ectodermal and mesodermal tissues. That they are abundant in the liver makes this the most logical tissue for impression smears obtained by biopsy or at necropsy. Initial hypertrophy of the cell nucleus is followed by peripheral margination of the chromatin network and nucleolus, which forms a central, dark-staining nuclear remnant surrounded by a halo of chromatin. The initial inclusions are acidophilic but become basophilic as the chromatin marginates. Care must be taken to distinguish inclusions from faintly staining hepatocyte nucleoli.

THERAPY

Clinical management of dogs developing ICH is primarily symptomatic and supportive. Fulminant hepatic failure from hepatocellular necrosis is a common cause of death in dogs that do not survive the acute stages of the disease. In the absence of complicating factors, clinical recovery and hepatocellular regeneration can occur with centrilobular necrosis. Therapy is supportive until there is adequate time for hepatocellular repair. Because the dogs are frequently semicomatose, it is impossible to predict whether the neurologic signs are related to hepatoencephalopathy or viral encephalitis. However, this issue can partially be resolved by evaluating blood glucose or ammonia concentrations when therapy is instituted.

Immediate placement of an indwelling IV catheter is a necessity in severely affected dogs, but, because of incoagulability, care must be taken to avoid excessive hemorrhage. Fluid therapy with a polyionic isotonic fluid such as Ringer's solution will correct losses from vomiting and diarrhea and assist in lowering the body temperature. Animals that are too depressed to drink or that continue to vomit must be given daily maintenance fluid requirements (45 ml/kg) by parenteral route.

Treatment of DIC depends on the stage of the clotting deficit. Removal of the inciting stimulus is the initial aim of therapy, but this is not possible in viral diseases. Because of insufficient hepatic synthesis, replacement of clotting factors and platelets by fresh plasma or whole blood may be necessary in conjunction with anticoagulant therapy when marked incoagulability is present.

Because the possibility exists that hypoglycemia is responsible for the comatose state, an IV bolus of 50% glucose (0.5 ml/kg) should be given over a 5-minute period. Hypoglycemia is likely to recur if continuous infusion of hypertonic glucose is not maintained. Hypertonic glucose infusion should be continued at a rate not greater than 0.5 to 0.9 g/kg/hour for efficient utilization. Therapy to decrease the blood ammonia concentration is directed at reducing protein catabolism by colonic bacteria and ammonia resorption in the renal tubules. Ammonia production from protein degradation in the bowel can be reduced by decreasing the quantity of protein intake and by stopping GI hemorrhage. The colon can be evacuated by cleansing and acidifying enemas that relieve bowel stasis and retard ammonia absorption. Nonabsorbable oral antibiotics such as neomycin have been advocated to reduce ammonia-producing bacteria in the intestine, but their effectiveness is questionable. Acidification of the colonic contents can also be achieved by feeding oral lactulose to nonvomiting animals. Renal resorption of ammonia can be reduced by administration of parenteral or oral potassium and correction of the metabolic alkalosis. Urinary acidification with a nontoxic acidifier such as ascorbic acid may greatly reduce ammonia reabsorption by the kidney.

Polyinosinic-polycytidylic acid, an interferon inducer, has been used experimentally to reduce the mortality of dogs experimentally infected with ICH virus, but its clinical application is impractical (see Interferon Inducers, Chapter 100).

PREVENTION

Maternal Immunity

The duration of passively acquired immunity in the pup is dependent on the antibody concentration of the bitch. The half-life of ICH antibodies is 8.6 days compared with 8.4 days for antibodies to distemper virus, and these values correlate well with the half-life for canine globulin (see Maternal Immunity, Chapter 100 and Tables 100–2, 100–3, and 100–4). Immunization for ICH is usually successful when maternal antibody titers decrease below 100, which may occur beginning at 5 to 7 weeks of age. The level of ICH maternal antibodies in the newborn pup declines to negligible concentrations by 14 to 16 weeks.

Vaccinations

Inactivated CAV-1 vaccines do not produce any lesions in vaccinated dogs, but they must be given frequently to equal the protection afforded by MLV vaccines. Adjuvants must be added to inactivated products, making them potentially more allergenic than MLV vaccines. Annual revaccination against ICH with an inactivated CAV-1 vaccine provides continuous protection against infection. These products are not available in the United States.

An inactivated CAV-2 vaccine was tested for use in dogs against challenge infection with CAV-2 infection. Dogs received two doses of vaccine at a 14-day interval and were

Table 4–1. Comparison of Pathogenicity of Modified Live Canine Adenovirus Vaccines

ROUTE ADMINISTERED	CLINICAL SIGNS OBSERVED	
	CAV-1[a]	CAV-2[b]
Intravenous	Fever Uveitis (20%) Urinary shedding	Fever Mild respiratory disease Tonsillitis
Intranasal	None	Mild respiratory disease
Intraocular (anterior chamber)	Uveitis (100%)	Uveitis (100%)
Intramuscular or subcutaneous	Uveitis rare (0.4%), urinary shedding (some strains)	None

[a]Canine adenovirus 1.
[b]Canine adenovirus 2.

challenged 14 days after the second dose. All dogs became seropositive after vaccination but had mild clinical signs of infection compared with challenged unvaccinated dogs. The clinical usefulness of this vaccine remains to be determined, and long-term protection studies are needed.

In contrast to inactivated vaccines, modified live CAV-1 vaccines can produce lifelong immunity with a single dose. A potential disadvantage of MLV vaccines, however, has been that vaccine virus localizes in the kidney and causes mild subclinical interstitial nephritis and persistent shedding of vaccine virus. Increased passage of the virus in cell culture can reduce the incidence of urinary shedding. Ocular localization with associated anterior uveitis occurs in approximately 0.4% of dogs after IV and SC injection. IV CAV-1 vaccination produces a transient systemic illness characterized by pyrexia and tonsillar enlargement and a 20% incidence of anterior uveitis. A summary of the pathogenicity of modified live CAV-1 vaccine and a comparison with that for CAV-2 vaccine are listed in Table 4–1.

Some CAV-1 and CAV-2 strains are known to be oncogenic in hamsters, but those in commercial vaccines do not appear to produce this side effect. Oncogenic reactions in dogs have not been reported in more than 20 years of field use of these products.

CAV-2 vaccines have been developed as an alternative in the prevention of ICH. Modified live CAV-2 vaccine rarely, if ever, produces ocular or renal disease when given IM or SC, although the vaccine virus may localize in and be shed from the upper respiratory tract. The vaccine produces ocular lesions only when experimentally injected into the anterior chamber. Given IV and intranasally (IN), modified live CAV-2 vaccine may produce a mild respiratory disease with associated coughing and tonsillar enlargement, although such an infection has been shown to be subclinical and self-limiting. More severe respiratory signs might develop with CAV-2 vaccine with secondary bacterial infections. Care should be taken to avoid aerosolizing vaccine when it is given by the IM or SC routes. Dogs are adequately protected by the heterotypic antibody titer against CAV-1 infection if CAV-2 vaccine is used; however, the homotypic antibody response is usually greater. CAV-2 vaccine was experimentally given to 3- to 4-week-old pups in an attempt to break through the heterotypic maternal antibodies to ICH virus. Although parenteral vaccination at this age was ineffective, IN vaccination produced a delayed antibody response to CAV-2 and a weak response to CAV-1, 4 to 8 weeks later. Modified live CAV-2 probably localized in the respiratory tract until maternal antibody declined and then spread systemically, stimulating an immune response.

The recommended schedule with any vaccine for ICH involves at least two vaccinations 3 to 4 weeks apart at 8 to 10 and 12 to 14 weeks of age. This is most commonly accomplished through the combination of this antigen with the CDV vaccination protocol (see Immunoprophylaxis, Chapter 100, and Appendix 1). Earlier and more frequent vaccination may be advised in areas of high prevalence. Sporadic ICH infection will be noted in puppies when their vaccinations are delayed. Annual vaccination is often recommended but is probably not essential because of the long-standing immunity produced by MLV vaccines.

Canine Acidophil Cell Hepatitis

A hepatitis distinct from ICH and characterized by acute, persistent, or chronic forms was described in Great Britain. Evidence implying that this syndrome has an infectious nature came from the high prevalence of hepatocellular carcinoma in dogs. The agent, suspected to be a virus, has not been identified, although the disease can be reproduced by inoculating bacteriologically sterile liver homogenates not containing CAV-1 and CAV-2 from spontaneously affected animals into experimental dogs. Presumably, acute infections with this agent lead to acute to chronic hepatitis; cirrhosis with multilobular hyperplasia; and, in some cases, hepatocellular carcinoma.

Clinical findings in the early phase of the illness can be vague and include variable fever, inappetence, vomiting, and abdominal pain, but fever is usually lacking. Terminal clinical signs include abdominal distention with ascites, episodes of seizures, mental status abnormalities, and semicoma.

The only consistent laboratory abnormalities include episodic increased ALT and ALP activities. Diagnosis involves gross and microscopic examination of liver tissue. Gross biopsy or necropsy findings include hepatomegaly with rounded lobe edges and enlarged tonsils, regional lymph nodes, and Peyer's patches. Chronically affected dogs may have reduced hepatic size with exaggerated delineation of the portal radicles or nodular proliferation. Increased fibrous tissue is apparent histologically both centrally and peripherally. Acidophil cells are scattered throughout hepatic lesions and are characterized by angular cytoplasm with acidophil cytoplasm and hyperchromatic nucleus.

Therapy for this condition is uncertain, and it appears to progress with time. Prevention would not seem plausible until the nature of the suspected infectious agent is determined. Although reported only in Great Britain, the disease may be more widespread. It should be suspected when a high frequency of chronic active hepatitis or hepatic fibrous, hepatocellular carcinoma is reported.

References

1. Greene CE. 1990. Infectious canine hepatitis and canine acidophil cell hepatitis, pp 242–251. *In* Greene CE (ed), Infectious diseases of the dog and cat. WB Saunders, Philadelphia, PA.
2. Holzman S, Conroy MJ, Davidson WR. 1992. Diseases, parasites and survival of coyotes in south-central Georgia. *J Wildl Dis* 28:572–580.
3. Johnson MR, Boyd DR, Pletscher DH. 1994. Serologic investigations of canine parvovirus and canine distemper in relation to wolf (*Canis lupus*) pup mortalities. *J Wildl Dis* 30:270–273.
4. Kobayashi Y, Ochiai K, Itakura C. 1993. Dual infection with canine distemper virus and infectious canine hepatitis virus (canine adenovirus type 1) in a dog. *J Vet Med Sci* 55:699–701.
5. Kritsepi M, Rallis T, Psychas D, et al. 1996. Hepatitis in a European brown bear with canine infectious hepatitis-like lesions. *Vet Rec* 139:600–601.
6. Kuo-Hom LH, Lubeck MD, Davis AR, et al. 1992. Immunogenicity of recombinant adenovirus-respiratory syncytial virus vaccines with adenovirus types 4,5, and 7 vectors in dogs and a chimpanzee. *J Infect Dis* 166:769–775.
7. Liu YC, Abouhaidar MG, Sira S, et al. 1988. Characterization of the genome of a vaccine strain of canine adenovirus type 1. *Virus Genes* 2:69–81.
8. Schwendenwein I, Lechner C, Kolbl S, et al. 1989. Hepatitis contagiosa canis (HCC)–2 cases in Austria. *Tierarztl Prax* 17:211–215.
9. Whetstone CA, Draayer H, Collins JE. 1988. Characterization of canine adenovirus type 1 isolated from American black bears. *Am J Vet Res* 49:778–780.

Chapter 5

Canine Herpesvirus Infection

Leland E. Carmichael and Craig E. Greene

ETIOLOGY

Canine herpesvirus (CHV) has biologic and pathogenic properties similar to α-herpesviruses affecting other species. Although an antigenic relationship to human herpes simplex virus has not been confirmed, CHV shares approximately 51% genetic homology with feline herpesvirus type 1 (FHV-1).[11] Antigenic relationship between the canine and feline viruses has also been confirmed in immunoblots with polyvalent or monoclonal antibodies (MAB).[5,13] Less defined immunologic relationships exist between CHV and herpesviruses isolated from harbor seals *(Phoca vitulina)*.[4] Analysis of CHV isolates by restriction endonuclease cleavage of viral DNA revealed differences in the viruses isolated from unrelated individuals, but cleavage patterns of isolates derived from members of the same litter were indistinguishable.[14]

CHV is inactivated by exposure to most disinfectants and to lipid solvents (e.g., ether, chloroform) and to heat (56°C for 5–10 minutes, 37°C for 22 hours). Like other herpesviruses, CHV is readily inactivated at 20°C but is stable at −70°C. It is stable at pH between 6.5 and 7.6 but is rapidly destroyed below pH 5.0.

CHV has a restricted host range and appears to infect only domestic and wild Canidae or canine cell cultures. The virus causes a rapidly spreading, highly destructive cytopathic effect in cell cultures with formation of intranuclear inclusions (see Viral Isolation). Although CHV has not been reported in cats, it is unclear whether an FHV-1 isolate from a pup with a distemper-like syndrome and pancreatic atrophy causes canine infections. Young pups given large ($>10^6$) doses of this FHV-1 virus by multiple routes failed to develop clinical illness or histopathologic changes.[5]

The replication of CHV is similar to that of other α-herpesviruses. Synthesis of viral DNA and nucleocapsids occurs within the host cell nucleus, with the viral envelope being acquired at the nuclear membrane. Virus is transported through the endoplasmic reticulum and Golgi apparatus to the cell surface, where it is released, but most virus remains intracellular. As with other herpesviruses, lifelong latent infections are typical.

PATHOGENESIS

Newborn puppies can acquire CHV infection in utero, from passage through the birth canal, from contact with infected littermates, from oronasal secretions of the dam, or rarely fomites. Neonatal puppies experimentally infected when they are younger than 1 week are particularly susceptible to fatal generalized infections; dogs older than 2 weeks at the time of infection are relatively resistant and generally develop mild or inapparent clinical illness. Virus replication in older dogs is restricted to the nasopharynx, genital tract, tonsils, retropharyngeal lymph nodes, bronchial lymph nodes, and occasionally lungs. Virus may be harbored in the tonsils and parotid salivary gland.[2]

In Utero Infection

Although neonatal infection usually is acquired at or soon after birth, transplacental transmission may also occur during gestation. The effects of transplacental infection with CHV depend on the stage of gestation at which infection occurs. Infertility and abortion of stillborn or weak pups with no clinical signs in the dam have been reported. Although some puppies may survive such in utero infections and appear normal on cesarean section, others harbor the virus inapparently in their tissues. Most pups, however, develop systemic herpesvirus infection within 9 days of birth.

Systemic Neonatal Infection

After oronasal exposure, CHV is first detected in the nasal epithelium and pharyngeal tonsils (Fig. 5–1). Primary replica-

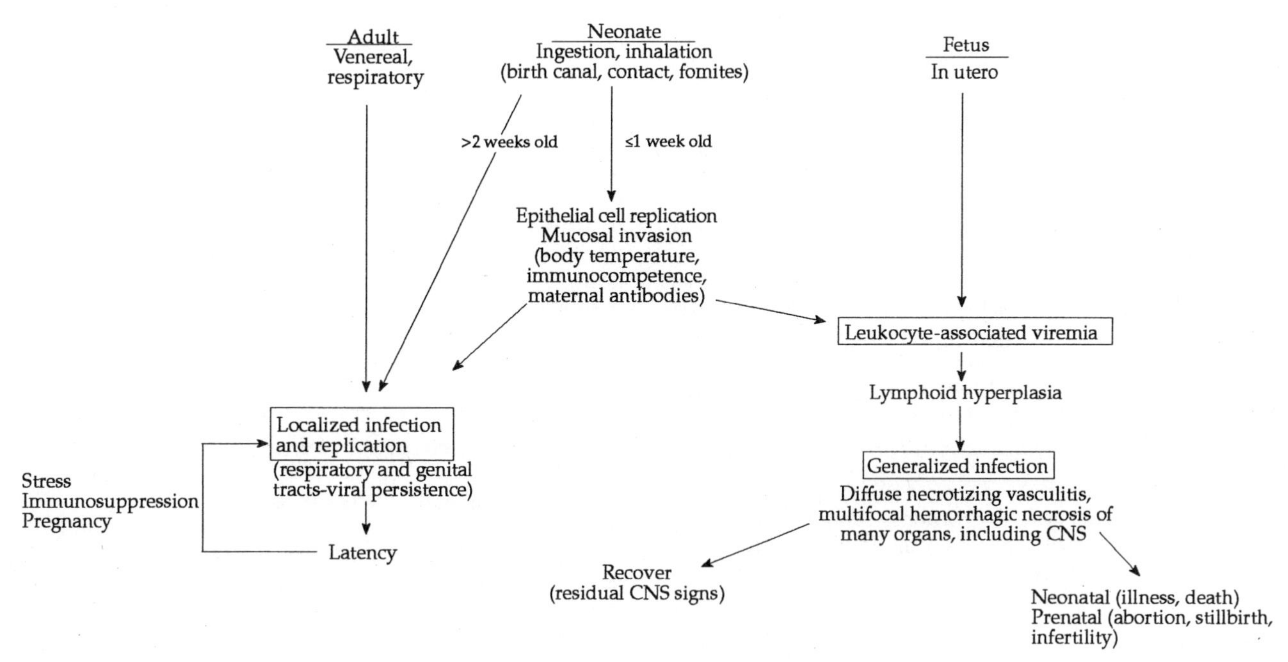

Figure 5–1. Pathogenesis of CHV infection.

tion occurs in epithelial cells and mucosa within 24 hours PI. The virus then enters the blood stream by way of macrophages. Intracellular viremia results in viral spread throughout the body within 3 to 4 days PI. Localization in the mononuclear phagocytic cells of the lymph nodes and spleen results in cell-to-cell spread and lymphoid hyperplasia and necrosis. Progressive multifocal hemorrhagic necrosis occurs in several organs; highest concentrations of virus are found in the adrenals, kidneys, lungs, spleen, and liver. Multifocal hemorrhage associated with necrotic lesions may be related to the marked thrombocytopenia that occurs during infection. Thrombocytopenia may result from DIC associated with widespread vascular endothelial damage and tissue necrosis.

Ganglioneuritis of the trigeminal nerve is a frequent lesion in puppies infected by oronasal exposure. CHV may travel up the nerve axons to the CNS as occurs with human herpes simplex virus. Meningoencephalitis commonly occurs in oronasally infected neonatal puppies, but CNS signs are not always apparent. Under normal circumstances, puppies usually die from systemic illness before neurologic signs are manifest.

Several factors, including temperature regulation and immune status, are involved in the abrupt development of resistance to infection that occurs between 1 and 2 weeks of age. Optimal growth of CHV in cell cultures has been shown to occur between 35° and 36°C. The normal rectal temperature of adult dogs, 38.4° to 39.5°C (101–103°F), is above the critical range. Temperature regulation of the newborn pup is not developed until 2 to 3 weeks of age, and rectal temperature is usually 1° to 1.5°C (2–3°F) lower than that of the adult dog. Besides having a reduced capacity for temperature regulation, neonatal pups are incapable of adequate fever production. Cell-mediated immune functions are also suppressed at temperatures lower than 39°C, rendering hypothermic pups more susceptible not only to CHV but also to vaccinal distemper and CAV. Puppies 4 to 8 weeks of age are normally clinically asymptomatic after infection, but they will develop systemic CHV infection if their body temperatures are artificially reduced. Conversely, elevation of the environmental temperature, and consequently the body temperature of CHV-infected puppies younger than 1 week, results in reduction of the severity of infection. It does not eliminate it.

Immunity acquired from the dam also appears to be important in the survival of infected puppies. Pups nursing seronegative bitches develop a fatal multisystemic illness when they are infected with CHV. In contrast, puppies suckling seropositive bitches become infected but remain asymptomatic, and the virus is recovered primarily from their oropharyngeal region. Maternal antibody or immune lymphocytes acquired through the milk may explain why naturally infected bitches having diseased puppies, with rare exceptions, subsequently give birth to normal litters. Serum antibody titers in previously infected pregnant bitches may also suppress viremia and spread of infection to the fetus.

Adult Genital Infection

Herpesviruses have been isolated occasionally from papulovesicular lesions of the canine genital tract, and such lesions have been described as possible recurrent episodes in previously infected bitches. With CHV, localized genital or respiratory infections and viral shedding can occur in the presence of circulating antibodies. Infection of the genital tract generally appears to be asymptomatic or limited to vaginal hyperemia with hyperplastic lymphoid follicles. Genital localization of the virus in adult dogs may be a means of venereal transmission of the virus, but it is most important as a source of infection for pups at birth. Spread of CHV from seropositive males to susceptible females at the time of breeding does not appear to be a significant mode of transmission, although such a mechanism is believed to occur. PCR has shown persistence of the virus in the lumbosacral ganglion with presumed recrudescence and mucosal replication with subsequent shedding.[2]

Adult Respiratory Infection

Field evidence suggests that CHV might be a cause of respiratory disease, but studies have failed to incriminate

CHV as a primary cause of respiratory illness. Although of uncertain significance, CHV has been recovered from the lungs of dogs with distemper and from dogs with acute conjunctivitis. Neonates that recover from CHV infections or older dogs that have subclinical infections have periodic episodes of viral recrudescence in their oronasal secretions. Viral latency has been demonstrated in intranasally infected dogs for as long as 6 months PI, with recrudescence occurring within 1 week after treatment with glucocorticoids or antilymphocyte serum. Recrudescence of latent virus also has been demonstrated in seropositive adults after being exposed to seronegative juveniles, suggesting a stress mechanism for transmission of CHV in a manner similar to that occurring with FHV infection. Reactivation of latent infections with asymptomatic shedding of virus from nasal, oral, ocular, and vaginal secretions occurred in most bitches given repeated high immunosuppressive doses of glucocorticoids.[9] Recrudescence is a plausible explanation for subclinical persistence and the rare recurrences of abortions, fetal infections, or neonatal illnesses; it also serves as a mode of viral transmission to susceptible dams, especially when they are introduced into a kennel for breeding.

CLINICAL FINDINGS

No premonitory signs of illness or history of neonatal mortality is seen in bitches that lose litters of puppies to CHV. Transplacental infections may occur at mid to late gestation and can result in abortion of mummified or dead fetuses, premature or stillborn pups, or weak or runted newborn puppies. Death of neonatal puppies younger than 1 week appears to be less common and probably indicates in utero infection. Among puppies born alive within a litter, some may not be affected and the gestational age when illness occurred may vary among those that are affected.

CHV infection in postnatally infected puppies is associated with an acutely fatal illness, primarily occurring between 1 and 3 weeks of age. If affected when older than 3 weeks, pups have disseminated herpesvirus infection that is believed to be exacerbated by concurrent infection or immunosuppression. Infected puppies appear dull and depressed; lose interest in nursing; have a decrease in body weight; and pass soft, yellow-green feces. They cry persistently and show discomfort during abdominal palpation. Despite the continued muscular activity associated with crying, restlessness, and shivering, there is no elevation in body temperature. Rhinitis is frequently manifest by serous to mucopurulent or, rarely, hemorrhagic nasal discharges. Petechial hemorrhages are widespread on the mucous membranes. An erythematous rash consisting of papules or vesicles and SC edema of the ventral abdominal and inguinal region are occasionally noted. Vesicles are occasionally present in the vulva and vagina of the female puppies, prepuce of the males, and in the buccal cavity. Puppies lose consciousness and may have opisthotonos and seizures just before death. Rectal temperatures become subnormal before death, which usually occurs within 24 to 48 hours after the onset of clinical illness.

Some puppies develop mild clinical disease with subsequent recovery. Animals that survive the systemic infection are likely to have persistent neurologic signs. Ataxia, blindness, and cerebellar vestibular deficits are most common.

Dogs older than 3 to 5 weeks develop a mild or inapparent upper respiratory infection as a result of CHV. Signs of systemic infection are rare in older pups; however, vomiting, anorexia, depression, serous ocular discharge, hepatomegaly, and sudden death have been reported in naturally infected 8- to 10-week-old coyote pups. For a discussion of ocular lesions, see Chapter 93.

Primary genital infections in older female dogs are characterized by lymphofollicular lesions, variable degrees of vaginal hyperemia, and occasionally petechial or ecchymotic submucosal hemorrhages. No discomfort or vaginal discharge is noted in affected pregnant dogs, even those who had abortions or stillbirths. Vesicular lesions have been noted during the onset of proestrus and regress during anestrus. Male dogs, with similar lesions over the base of the penis and preputial reflection, may have a preputial discharge.

DIAGNOSIS

Clinical Laboratory Findings

The determination of CHV infection in neonatal pups usually depends on information obtained from the clinical history, physical examination, and characteristic pathologic changes seen in affected puppies. Hematologic and biochemical abnormalities are nonspecific, but marked thrombocytopenia may be observed. A marked increase in the ALT activity can be found in infected neonates.

Viral Isolation

CHV can be isolated from several parenchymal organs of puppies' dying of acute systemic infection, but most commonly from the adrenals, kidneys, lungs, spleen, lymph nodes, and liver. In recovered or older animals, growth of CHV is usually restricted to the oral mucosa, upper respiratory tract, and external genitalia. Viral isolation has not been demonstrated longer than 2 to 3 weeks PI. As noted, viral recrudescence may be provoked by immunosuppressive doses of glucocorticoids, and it also has been brought on by stress, such as the introduction of unfamiliar dogs into a kennel.

CHV grows only in cultured cells of canine origin, primarily in dog kidney cells at an optimal temperature range of 35° to 37°C. Infected cells become rounded and detach from the glass surfaces, leaving clear plaques surrounded by necrotic cells. Plaque formation is best observed when monolayers are overlaid with semisolid media such as agar or methylcellulose. Plaque morphology has been used as a marker for virus pathogenicity. CHV produces Cowdry type A intranuclear inclusions, which can be difficult to demonstrate and are best revealed in tissues that have been fixed in Bouin's fluid. Multinucleation of infected cells is unusual with CHV, but it has been observed with one isolate from the canine genital tract. FA techniques, EM, and PCR can be used to detect CHV in tissues and cell cultures (Fig. 5–2). Although not routinely performed, screening of animals for infection is best done by viral detection during recrudescence with respiratory or genital signs. PCR has shown that latent herpesvirus infections are prevalent in asymptomatic dogs.[2]

Serologic Testing

Serologic testing for CHV antibodies is based on VN tests, which rely on reduction in cytopathogenicity or plaque formation. ELISA and an HI assay also have been developed.[8, 12, 14] Neutralizing antibodies increase after infection and may remain high for only 2 months; low titers may be detected for at least 2 years. Seropositivity merely indicates exposure,

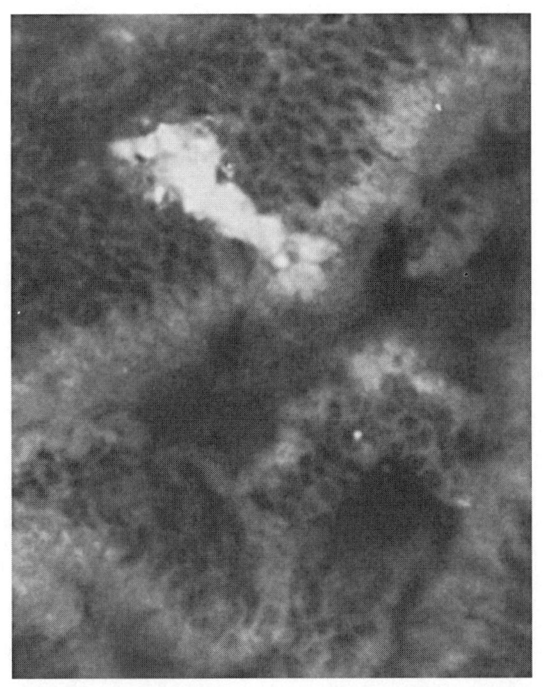

Figure 5–2. Focus of herpesvirus-infected cells in tonsilar crypt epithelium from a 12-week-old pup inoculated with CHV. (FA method, × 125). (From Appel MJG, et al: *Am J Vet Res* 30:2067–2073, 1969. Reprinted with permission.)

not necessarily active infection, although viral persistence and latent infection might be presumed.

PATHOLOGIC FINDINGS

Gross lesions of fatal CHV infection in neonates include diffuse multifocal hemorrhage and gray discoloration in a variety of parenchymal organs, especially the kidney (Fig. 5–3), liver, and lungs. On cut surface, the kidney lesions consist of wedge-shaped hemorrhages radiating outward from the renal pelvis. These wedge-shaped renal lesions are caused by CHV-induced fibrinoid necrosis of interlobular arteries.[16] Serous to hemorrhagic fluid is usually present in the pleural and peritoneal cavities. The lungs are usually firm and edematous with pronounced hyperemia and focal areas of hemorrhage; there also is marked enlargement of the bronchial lymph nodes. Splenomegaly and generalized lymphadenomegaly are consistent findings. Petechial hemorrhages are often distributed throughout the serosal surfaces of the intestinal tract. Icterus has been rarely reported.

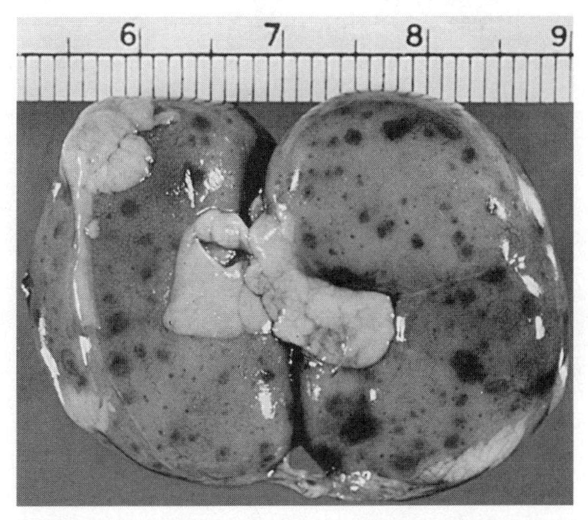

Figure 5–3. Kidney from a puppy inoculated with CHV. Hemorrhagic areas consist of necrotic foci packed with erythrocytes. (From Kakuk TJ, Conner GH: *Lab Anim Sci* 20:69–79, 1970. Reprinted with permission.)

Histologic findings in disseminated infections of neonates are characterized by foci of perivascular necrosis with mild cellular infiltration in the lung, liver, kidney, spleen, small intestine, and brain. Less severe lesions occur in the stomach, pancreas, adrenals, omentum, retina, and myocardium. The lymph nodes and spleen show reactive hyperplasia of mononuclear phagocyte elements. Multifocal necrotizing lesions have been described in the placenta from pregnant bitches and in the pups that acquired infection in utero. Cutaneous or mucosal lesions, which may be seen as the primary lesions in older infected animals, consist of various-sized vesicles produced by profound degeneration of the epithelial cells, resulting in marked acantholysis. Depending on the stage of cellular infection and method of fixation, basophilic or acidophilic inclusions may be noted, but they are less common than those in other herpesvirus infections. Inclusions are more readily seen in the nasal epithelium or kidney than in areas of widespread necrosis, such as occur in the lung or liver.

Lesions in the CNS of recovered puppies are nonsuppurative ganglioneuritis and meningoencephalitis. The parenchymal lesions are multifocal and granulomatous, characterized by increased pericapillary cellular proliferation, and they occur primarily in the brain stem and cerebellum. Cerebellar and retinal dysplasias are frequent findings.

THERAPY

Once a diagnosis has been made, treatment of puppies suffering signs of systemic CHV infection is unrewarding because of the rapidly fatal progression of the disease. In some cases, mortality may be reduced during an epizootic episode by injecting each pup intraperitoneally with 1 to 2 ml of immune sera. Immune sera can be obtained by pooling sera from bitches that had recently lost litters to CHV infection. Only one injection is required because of the short susceptibility period. This empirical treatment seems to be beneficial in reducing losses within an exposed litter, but success depends on the presence of adequate levels of serum antibodies and the administration before the full development of systemic disease.

Elevating the environmental temperature of already affected puppies is ineffective. Newborn puppies maintained under experimental conditions at 36.6° to 37.7°C (98–100°F), and 45% to 55% humidity, have been able to maintain their rectal temperatures at 38.4° to 39.5°C (101–103°F). Under such experimental conditions, in which body temperatures were elevated artificially before exposure to virus, puppies had reduced mortality, less severe clinical signs, and minimal pathologic changes. At elevated temperatures, viral growth in tissues was restricted compared with growth in conventionally reared pups. Pretreatment by raising ambient temperature is obviously not possible in natural CHV infections; however, it could be tried for remaining unaffected puppies in a litter.

Treatment of systemic CHV infection with antiviral drugs such as 5-iodo-2-deoxyuridine has been unsuccessful, and there are only limited studies of newer antiviral agents found to be effective in treating localized and CNS infections of herpes simplex virus in people and in laboratory animals. In one such instance, two 15-day-old pups died of confirmed CHV. Five littermates were given a course of vidarabine as soon as the cause of the deaths was identified, and they all survived. The surviving pups had high (>1:64) neutralizing antibody titers 2 months later, indicating that they had been infected.[3] Antiviral treatment may spare the pups, but residual damage to the CNS and myocardium may occur. This possibility must be discussed with owners before considering antiviral treatment of an infected litter.

PREVENTION

The low frequency of clinical outbreaks and poor immunogenicity of CHV reduce the incentive to produce a commercial vaccine for this disease. Reports from Europe and the United States have demonstrated a prevalence of anti-CHV antibodies in 6% of the random dog population, whereas it may be as high as 100% in some kennels.

Immunization with a commercially inactivated vaccine in Europe has been shown to provoke fourfold increases in VN titers in most vaccinated dogs, but it did not appear to provide long-term protection.[3] Live virus vaccines would probably be required for serviceable immunity in puppies, but such vaccines have the potential disadvantage of establishing latent infection. Experimentally, neutralizing antibodies to CHV have been produced in mice by immunization with anti-idiotypic antibodies.[13] There is no current vaccine that can be claimed to be truly effective.

If a problem exists in a kennel, prevention of disease in exposed puppies may be achieved with the administration of immune serum or globulin during the first few days of life. Other methods have been of little value, although administration of an interferon inducer (avian poxvirus) to bitches before breeding and whelping and to newborn puppies in problem kennels was claimed to induce nonspecific protection against fatal CHV infection.[3] On a practical basis, eradication of CHV from a kennel is not possible. Screening for infected animals also is impractical (see Diagnosis), and owners should be advised that subsequent litters from an affected bitch have a very low risk of developing clinical illness. Accordingly, cesarean delivery or AI is not justified to reduce further spread of infection. AI might be used when a known or suspected infected male is bred to a primiparous bitch, but the benefit of such a practice has not been studied.

As a preventive practice, care should be taken to ensure that the environmental temperature of newborn puppies is kept warm. This can be achieved with heated whelping boxes, heat lamps, or other warming devices that do not cause excessive dehydration.

Inapparent infections are common in recovered CHV-infected dogs with occasional mild rhinitis, vaginitis, or balanoposthitis as the only clinical sign. Such dogs may act as reservoirs of infection for neonates and should be separated from new litters. Clinically affected puppies shed large quantities of virus in their secretions for 2 to 3 weeks after recovery. Virus persists for only short periods of time in respiratory or vaginal secretions, so that spread is most common by way of immediate direct contact with infected animals or through fomites.

References

1. Anvik JO. 1991. Clinical considerations of canine herpesvirus infection. *Vet Med* 86:394–403.
2. Burr PD, Campbell MEM, Nicolson L, et al. 1996. Detection of canine herpesvirus 1 in a wide range of tissues using the polymerase chain reaction. *Vet Microbiol* 53:227–237.
3. Carmichael LE, Greene CE. 1990. Canine herpesvirus infection, pp 252–258. *In* Greene CE (ed), Infectious diseases of the dog and cat. WB Saunders Co, Philadelphia, PA.
4. Harder, TC, Lebich M, Liess, B. 1994. Simplified identification and differentiation of feline, canine and phocine herpesviruses using monoclonal antibodies (German, English abstract). *Tierarzl Prax* 22:408–412.
5. Kramer JW, Evermann JF, Leathers CW, et al. 1991. Experimental infection of two dogs with a canine isolate of feline herpesvirus type 1. *Vet Pathol* 28:338–340.
6. Limbach KJ, Limbach MP, Conte D, et al. 1994. Nucleotide sequence of the genes encoding the canine herpesvirus gB, gC and gD homologues. *J Gen Virol* 75:2029–2039.
7. Limcumpao JA, Horimoto T, Xuan X, et al. 1990. Immunological relationship between feline herpesvirus type 1 (FHV-1) and canine herpesvirus (CHV) as revealed by polyvalent and monoclonal antibodies. *Arch Virol* 111:165–176.
8. Nemoto K, Horimoto, T, Xuan X, et al. 1990. Demonstration of canine herpesvirus-specific hemagglutination. *Jap J Vet Sci* 52:395–398.
9. Okuda Y, Hashimoto A, Yamaguchi T, et al. 1993. Repeated canine herpesvirus (CHV) reactivation in dogs by an immunosuppressive drug. *Cornell Vet* 83:291–302.
10. Okuda Y, Ishida K, Hashimoto A, et al. 1993. Virus reactivation in bitches with a medical history of herpesvirus infection. *Am J Vet Res* 54:551–554.
11. Rota PA, Maes RK. 1990. Homology between feline herpesvirus-1 and canine herpesvirus. *Arch Virol* 115:139–145.
12. Takumi A, Kusanagi K, Tuchiya K, et al. 1989. Serodiagnosis of canine herpesvirus infection—development of an enzyme-linked immunosorbent assay and its comparison with two improved methods of serum neutralization test. *Jap J Vet Sci* 52:241–250.
13. Xuan X, Horimoto T, Limcumpao JA, et al. 1991. Neutralizing determinants of canine herpesvirus as defined by monoclonal antibody. *Arch Virol* 116:185–196.
14. Xuan X, Horimoto T, Limcumpao JA, et al. 1992. Glycoprotein-specific immune response in canine herpesvirus infection. *Arch Virol* 122:359–366.
15. Xuan X, Horimoto T, Ono M, et al. 1990. Restriction endonuclease analysis of canine herpesvirus isolated in Japan. *Jap J Vet Sci* 52:1181–1188.
16. Yamamura T, Minato Y, Kojima A, et al. 1992. Electron microscopy of renal arterial lesions in a pup infected with canine herpesvirus. *Jap J Vet Sci* 54:779–780.

Chapter 6

Canine Infectious Tracheobronchitis

Richard B. Ford and Shelly L. Vaden

ETIOLOGY

Infectious tracheobronchitis, or ITB (synonyms: "kennel cough," "canine cough," "canine croup"), describes an acute, contagious respiratory infection of dogs characterized by sudden-onset, paroxysmal cough with variable expectoration and naso-ocular discharge. Clinical signs are attributed to infection by one or a combination of bacterial and/or viral agents that colonize the epithelium of the upper respiratory tract, trachea, bronchi, bronchioles, and pulmonary interstitium. Vaccines are available for most of the organisms known to be associated with canine ITB, and immunoprophylaxis of puppies and adult dogs is recommended for those considered to be at risk of exposure. Although uncommon, *Bordetella bronchiseptica* pneumonia is reported in humans as a zoonosis (see Public Health Considerations).

Respiratory signs of ITB in dogs known to have single-agent infections are generally mild and frequently self-limiting. However, in the clinical setting, the high prevalence of multiple-agent infections complicates the clinical presentation. CPiV and *B. bronchiseptica* are the most common organisms isolated from dogs with signs of ITB; several other viruses and bacteria are known to influence the clinical course and outcome of infection.

Viruses

CPiV is among the most common viruses isolated from the respiratory tract of dogs with ITB. It appears to have worldwide distribution. CPiV is a single-stranded RNA virus belonging to the family Paramyxoviridae and is closely related to simian virus 5.[4]

CAV-2 (infectious laryngotracheitis virus) and, to a lesser extent, CAV-1 (infectious canine hepatitis virus) are reported to cause signs of acute upper respiratory disease in dogs. These viruses are antigenically related DNA viruses of the family Adenoviridae (see Chapter 4).[3]

Depending on virus strain, CDV can cause acute to subacute systemic infections associated with a high mortality rate among infected dogs throughout the world. CDV is also known to cause respiratory disease in dogs independent of other systemic signs. Although CDV does act synergistically with CPiV and *B. bronchiseptica,* it is not regarded as a primary pathogen in the etiology of ITB (also see Chapter 3).

Other viruses, such as CHV (see Chapter 5) and reovirus-1, -2, and -3, have occasionally been isolated from coughing dogs. However, none of these viruses is regarded as being responsible for ITB.[5]

Bacteria and Mycoplasmas

B. bronchiseptica is a gram-negative bacterium and a principal etiologic agent of ITB in dogs.[6, 11, 12, 22, 34] Hundreds of isolates of *B. bronchiseptica* have been recovered from animals. Several other domestic and wild animal species may become infected with *B. bronchiseptica,* and it may play an important role in kittens with acute viral upper respiratory disease (see Chapter 16).[16] Of the hundreds of isolates, considerable variation exists among individual clones with respect to host distribution and virulence potential.[22]

Other bacteria recovered from the respiratory tract of dogs with ITB include *Streptococcus* sp., *Pasteurella* sp., *Pseudomonas,* and various coliforms.[28] Although these bacteria are regarded as opportunistic invaders, infections can cause serious, life-threatening pneumonia in the patient with ITB.

The mycoplasmas are fastidious, prokaryotic microbes that are distinguished from bacteria by the fact that they are enclosed in a cytoplasmic membrane but lack a distinct cell wall.[6, 17, 25] Yet unclassified groups of mycoplasmas, acholeplasmas, and ureaplasmas are commonly recovered in specimens collected from the nasopharyngolaryngeal mucosa of healthy dogs and cats. The presence of *Mycoplasma* in specimens collected from the lower respiratory tract of dogs (especially *M. cynos*) and cats (*M. felis*) is usually associated with pneumonia (see Chapters 32 and 88).[6, 25, 26]

EPIDEMIOLOGY

Canine ITB is considered to be among the most prevalent infectious respiratory diseases of dogs. Outbreaks of canine ITB are relatively common and can reach epizootic proportions when dogs are housed in high-density population environments such as pet shops, boarding facilities, and commercial kennels.[5, 6] The host range of *B. bronchiseptica* includes wildlife, rodents, and cats; however, most outbreaks are the result of direct dog-to-dog or airborne contact with infectious respiratory secretions. *B. bronchiseptica* has been shown to survive and replicate in natural waters for at least 3 weeks at 37° C.[23]

The common viral agents of ITB are transmitted for up to 2 weeks post-infection. For *Mycoplasma* sp. and *B. bronchiseptica,* however, shedding may occur for 3 months or longer.[5, 6] Although infections are transmitted rapidly and efficiently in high-density populations with high morbidity, death associated with complicating respiratory infection is uncommon, particularly in adult dogs.

PATHOGENESIS

Viruses

Because CPiV does not replicate in macrophages, infections with CPiV are typically restricted to the upper respiratory tract in dogs. Damage to the tracheal epithelium allows for secondary infection by other pathogens (Fig. 6–1). Animals 2

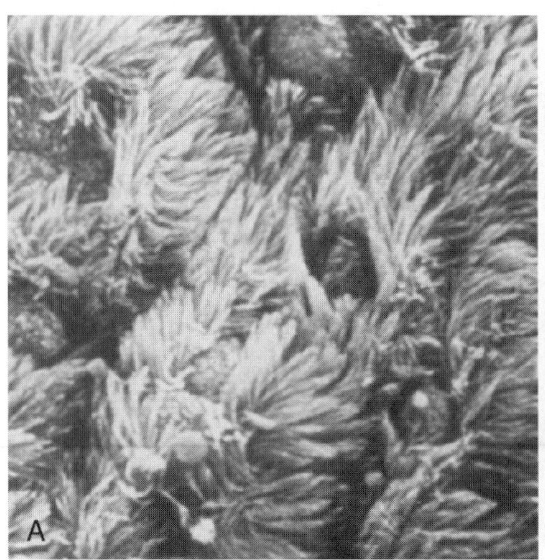

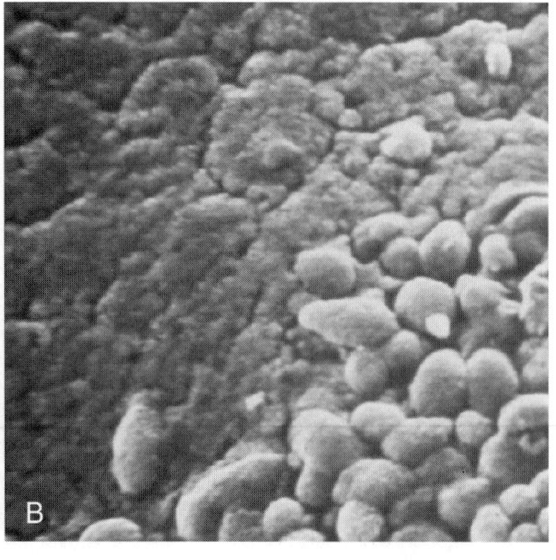

Figure 6–1. *A,* Scanning EM of normal canine tracheal epithelium. *B,* Scanning EM shows mucous hypersecretion and the tracheal epithelium completely denuded of cilia just 72 hours after experimental infection with CPiV.

weeks of age and older are susceptible.[5] Transmission occurs predominantly by aerosolized microdroplets. After a 3- to 10-day incubation period, viral shedding can occur for 6 to 8 days post-infection.[4] In single-agent infections, signs are limited to a dry, hacking cough and serous nasal discharge. After recovery, a CPiV carrier state does not appear to exist. Cats are capable of becoming subclinically infected and shedding the virus.

Infection with CAV-2 occurs after oronasal contact. The virus replicates in the epithelium of the nasal mucosa, pharynx, tonsillar crypts, trachea, and bronchi and in nonciliated bronchiolar epithelium. Replication peaks by day 3 to 6 after inoculation.[3] In immunocompetent animals, infection is typically short lived; virus usually cannot be isolated beyond day 9 of infection. Infection of type 2 alveolar cells has been associated with interstitial pneumonia.[3] Single-agent infections may be associated with tonsillitis and/or lung consolidation.[5] In other dogs, overt clinical signs may not be apparent.

Bacteria and Mycoplasmas

B. bronchiseptica has been associated with respiratory infections in dogs and, of late, in cats (see Chapter 16). The complex pathogenesis of *B. bronchiseptica* infection has been reviewed.[5, 6, 22] Transmission most likely occurs after direct contact or contact with aerosolized microdroplets from infected dogs. During an incubation period of about 6 days, *B. bronchiseptica* preferentially attaches to, and replicates on, the cilia of respiratory epithelium. Because of its ability to colonize the respiratory tract, and to produce a variety of potent toxins that impair phagocytic function and induce ciliostasis, *B. bronchiseptica* is uniquely capable of facilitating colonization of the respiratory tract by opportunistic organisms. Despite the fact that infection elicits production of local antibody, the organisms are not completely cleared from the respiratory tract for an average of 3 months. Although by itself *B. bronchiseptica* can cause rhinitis, mucous nasal discharge, and cough, most naturally occurring illness is associated with other viruses or bacteria. The organism has been isolated primarily from the upper respiratory tract of clinical healthy dogs. In combined infections with CPiV, tracheal mucosal injury is associated with clinically apparent pneumonia.

Several species of *Mycoplasma* and *Ureaplasma* have been associated with pneumonia in dogs.[6, 17, 25] Although endogenous to the nasopharynx of dogs and cats, mycoplasmas are not typically found in the lower respiratory tract. Unlike *B. bronchiseptica,* mycoplasmas colonize both ciliated and nonciliated epithelia. Both natural and experimental infections are characterized by purulent bronchitis and bronchiolitis. Epithelial and lymphoid hyperplasia and interstitial pneumonia may develop. Systemic infection is rare. Once colonized on lower respiratory epithelium, chronic shedding of several months duration is likely.[6]

CLINICAL FINDINGS

B. bronchiseptica and CPV are among the most common agents isolated from affected dogs. Because most natural infections of ITB are caused by multiple agents, it is difficult to associate a distinct set of clinical signs with a particular bacterium or virus.[6, 28]

The classic clinical presentation occurs most commonly during summer and fall. It is seen in animals that have received prior vaccination against CDV and CAV-2.[3, 5, 28] The time between exposure and onset of signs of canine ITB ranges from 3 to 10 days, regardless of the agents involved in the primary infection.[3–5, 22] Paroxysmal coughing episodes, typically associated with retching, in an otherwise healthy, active dog characterize the clinical presentation. A history of exposure to other dogs, particularly in kennel or shelter settings, is common although not a prerequisite. Swollen vocal folds, associated with laryngitis, may result in a loud, high-pitched cough described as a "honking" sound. This is likely to be accompanied by retching behavior. Expectoration of mucus, described as retching or hacking, after cough is commonly misinterpreted by owners as vomiting. The mucus may be foamy or may be unobserved if the animal swallows it. Physical examination is usually unremarkable, although cough may be easily elicited on manipulation of the trachea, particularly at the thoracic inlet. Although secondary bacterial pneumonia can develop in affected dogs, most infections are self-limiting and resolve without treatment.

A second more severe syndrome is described in dogs with no prior natural or vaccine exposure to the various agents that cause ITB or complicating bacterial infection.[5] Affected dogs are more likely to have a history of recent stays in a pet shop, boarding facility, or kennel. The cough may be nonproductive with or without rhinitis and a mucoid to mucopurulent nasal and ocular discharge. Complications associated with bronchopneumonia may become life threatening. On physical examination affected dogs are usually febrile and may be lethargic, anorexic, or dyspneic. Affected dogs are difficult to distinguish from those with CDV infections or other pneumonias. Outbreaks, which occur at any time of the year, may affect more than 50% of dogs in a densely populated environment.

DIAGNOSIS

A clinical diagnosis is based on a history of recent exposure to other dogs, signs, and response to empiric therapy. An uncertain vaccination history can be helpful in determining susceptibility. Routine hematology and biochemistry profiles are not diagnostic but do serve to establish and monitor the health status of affected dogs. A stress leukogram characterized by mature neutrophilia, lymphopenia, and eosinopenia may be evident. An inflammatory leukogram with significant leukocytosis or left shift may be present in dogs with complicating pneumonia. Fluid obtained from transtracheal aspirates may provide evidence of a neutrophilic exudate. Bacterial culture of aspirated fluid may be particularly helpful in confirming bacterial pneumonia and prescribing appropriate therapy.[15]

Because of indigenous microflora, bacterial isolates obtained from swabs of the nasal and oral cavities, oropharynx, and nasopharynx do not necessarily represent primary or secondary pathogens. However, bacteria cultured from transtracheal aspiration fluid, endotracheal or bronchoalveolar lavage, or sterile swabs of tracheal epithelium are more likely to represent disease-causing organisms.

Thoracic radiographs are typically unremarkable in animals with uncomplicated ITB. Dogs with complications associated with ITB may have radiographic signs of pulmonary hyperinflation and segmental atelectasis. Dogs with combined *B. bronchiseptica* and CPiV infections may develop lobar consolidation evident on thoracic radiographs.

Although uncommonly performed on clinical patients, viral isolation of CPiV or CAV-2 can be accomplished on swabs taken from the nasal, pharyngeal, or tracheal epithelium. The ability to inhibit virus growth, cytopathic effect, or hemadsorption with a standardized antiserum confirms the diagnosis.[5]

Acute and convalescent serum neutralizing or HI antibody titers can be used to establish exposure to any of the viral agents involved in canine ITB. The ability to demonstrate a rising titer, however, has little clinical application because of the relatively short duration of viral infection.

THERAPY

Antimicrobials

In uncomplicated cases of ITB, the value of antimicrobial therapy appears limited. However, in at least one study,[29] administration of an oral or a parenteral antibacterial agent reduced the duration of coughing in affected dogs. Drugs found to be particularly effective were trimethoprim-sulfonamide and amoxicillin. Because dogs with clinical signs of ITB may be at increased risk for bacterial bronchopneumonia, administration of empiric antimicrobial therapy is justified even when infections are not complicated by overt bacterial pneumonia.[32]

Systemic antimicrobial therapy is indicated if deeper respiratory or systemic bacterial infection develops, particularly bacterial bronchopneumonia or interstitial pneumonia. Although the antimicrobial prescribed should ideally be based on results of bacterial culture and susceptibility results, in the clinical setting empiric antimicrobial therapy may be most appropriate.[12, 32] Table 6–1 lists those antimicrobials appropriate in the empiric treatment of canine ITB.

Antivirals

Although the availability and potential for clinical application of antiviral compounds in veterinary medicine have increased in the past 3 years, specific antiviral drugs for use against CPiV, CAV-2, or CDV are not available.

Intranasal Vaccine

Unpublished, anecdotal reports from veterinarians have suggested that some animals with ITB may derive therapeutic benefit from the administration of a single dose of IN vaccine. Animals most likely to benefit are those that experience persistent cough beyond the expected recovery time for acute ITB or those that are continuously exposed to other dogs in animal shelters or kennels. Dogs manifesting signs of acute ITB do not appear to benefit therapeutically from vaccination.

Glucocorticoids

Anti-inflammatory doses (see Table 6–1) of orally administered glucocorticoids are effective in ameliorating the cough

Table 6–1. Treatment Options for Canine Infectious Tracheobronchitis

DRUG	DOSE[a] (mg/kg)	ROUTE	INTERVAL (HOURS)	DURATION (DAYS)
Antimicrobials				
Amoxicillin-clavulanate	12.5–25	PO	12	10–14 (minimum)
Trimethoprim-sulfonamide	15	PO	12	10–14 (minimum)
Doxycycline	2.5–5.0	PO	12	10 (minimum)
Antitussives				
Hydrocodone	0.22	PO	6–12	prn
Butorphanol	0.55	PO, SC	6–12	prn
Glucocorticoids				
Prednisolone	0.25–0.5	PO	12	3–5 days
Bronchodilators				
Aminophylline	10	PO	8–12	prn
Terbutaline	2.5	PO, SC	8–12	prn

[a]Dose per administration at specified interval.
PO = oral; prn, as needed.

associated with uncomplicated cases of ITB. Orally administered prednisolone can be used as needed to suppress coughing for periods of up to 5 to 7 days. However, glucocorticoids do not significantly shorten the clinical course.[29] In contrast to previous claims,[30] there are no controlled studies substantiating the value of intratracheal administration of glucocorticoids over oral administration.

Antitussives

Antitussives, alone and in combination with bronchodilators, have been recommended in the treatment of canine ITB. Objectively, these drugs are intended to interrupt the cough cycle; however, certain limitations to antitussive therapy should be noted. Over-the-counter cough suppressant drugs appear to offer little or no relief from the cough associated with ITB. Narcotic cough suppressants, such as hydrocodone, are generally effective in suppressing cough frequency and intensity. However, excessive or prolonged use of these drugs can lead to compromised ventilation and reduced expectoration with subsequent retention of respiratory secretions and diminished clearance of bacteria.[5, 28, 29] In cases of ITB that are complicated by bacterial pneumonia, administration of narcotic antitussives is not recommended.

Bronchodilators

The methylxanthine bronchodilators theophylline and aminophylline (theophylline-ethylenediamine) prevent bronchospasm and, therefore, may be effective cough suppressants in selected conditions, such as occurs in human asthma. However, dogs with signs of ITB are not expected to derive significant benefit from bronchodilator therapy alone.

Aerosol Therapy

In contrast to humidification therapy, aerosol therapy, or nebulization, refers to the production of a liquid particulate suspension within a carrier gas, usually oxygen. Patients with ITB that derive the most benefit from aerosol therapy are those with excessive accumulations of bronchial and tracheal secretions and those with secondary bronchial or pulmonary infections, particularly with *B. bronchiseptica*. Small, disposable, hand-held jet nebulizers are inexpensive and available through hospital supply retailers. From 6 to 10 ml of sterile saline is nebulized over 15 to 20 minutes one to four times daily. Oxygen is delivered at flow rates of 3 to 5 L/min to nebulize the solution. Aerosol therapy must be administered in the hospital. Most patients tolerate aerosol therapy well and generally do not require physical restraint after the first treatment.

There is no value in nebulizing mucolytic agents, which can be irritating and induce bronchospasm. Furthermore, liquefying tenacious respiratory secretions may not be an effective means of facilitating airway clearance. Nebulization of glucocorticoid solutions, such as methylprednisolone sodium succinate, has not been critically studied in veterinary medicine. However, in acute paroxysms of cough that may lead to or predispose the animal to airway obstruction, such therapy may provide short-term benefits.

Dogs that are unresponsive to oral or parenteral administration of antibiotics may respond to nebulized antibiotics. Aerosolized kanamycin, gentamicin, and polymyxin B each have been shown to be effective in reducing the population of *B. bronchiseptica* in the trachea and bronchi of infected dogs for up to 3 days after discontinuation of treatment.[6] Although clinical signs are not eliminated, the severity of signs may be significantly reduced.

Expectorants

Saline expectorants, guaifenesin, and volatile oils that are inhaled as a vapor are intended to stimulate secretion of less viscous bronchial mucus, thereby enhancing clearance of viscous respiratory secretions from the trachea and bronchi. However, the value of expectorant therapy in dogs with ITB has not been established and is not recommended at this time.

Supportive Care

Supportive treatment of the individual dog with ITB is directed at maintaining adequate caloric and fluid intake during the acute infection; preventing secondary or opportunistic bacterial infections, especially pneumonia; suppressing the cough; and reducing exposure to other dogs. When practical, this is best accomplished in the owner's home rather than in a kennel or veterinary hospital. This approach will also reduce the potential spread of infection, because affected animals should be isolated from other dogs.

PREVENTION

Maternal Immunity

Maternal immunity to the viruses known to cause canine ITB provides variable degrees of protection. Maternally derived CPiV antibody does not appear to interfere with parenteral vaccination of puppies that are 6 weeks of age and older.[4] In contrast, maternal antibody interference to parenteral CAV-2 vaccination can persist for as long as 12 to 16 weeks, but it does not protect against infection.[3]

Natural Immunity

The duration of immunity after recovery from CPiV and CAV-2 infection has not been studied, although one unpublished study documented CPiV neutralizing antibody 2 years after infection in dogs that were not re-exposed to virus.[5] Dogs that have recovered from *B. bronchiseptica* infection are highly resistant to reinfection for at least 6 months.[6] It should be expected, however, that the level of protection derived from infection will vary depending on the individual animal, the viruses and bacteria involved, and the opportunity for re-exposure.

Vaccination

Both viral and bacterial vaccines are available against most of the agents having a known pathogenic role in canine ITB (Table 6–2). CDV, CAV-2, and CPiV vaccines are commonly incorporated into routine vaccine protocols recommended for all dogs. *B. bronchiseptica* bacterins are in widespread use throughout the United State; no commercial vaccine is currently in use for protecting dogs against *Mycoplasma* sp.

In the case of *B. bronchiseptica* and CPiV, both parenteral and IN vaccines are available. IN-administered canine ITB vaccines are generally considered to offer superior protection

Table 6–2. Vaccination Options for Canine Infectious Tracheobronchitis[a]

ANTIGEN OPTIONS	TYPE/ROUTE (VOLUME)	PRODUCT NAME (COMPANY)	ADMINISTRATION SCHEDULE
Parenteral Vaccines with Parainfluenza			
Distemper, parainfluenza, adenovirus-2	MLV/SC, IM (1 ml)	Vanguard (Pfizer), Duramune (Ft Dodge), Galaxy (Schering-Plough), RM Canine (Merial), Adenomune (BioCor), D-Vac (Bio-Ceutic), Solo-Jec-7 (Anchor), Performer (AgriLabs)	*Initial*: 6–8 wks of age and older, 2 doses 3–4 wks apart *Revaccination*: If initial dose <16 wks, booster at 16 wks; thereafter annual.
Parenteral Vaccines with *B. bronchiseptica*			
Distemper, parainfluenza, adenovirus-2, *B. bronchiseptica*	All viral antigens MLV; *B. bronchiseptica* is killed SC, IM (1 ml)	Vanguard 5/B (Pfizer)	*Initial*: <16 wks of age, give 3 doses 2–4 wks apart; >16 wks of age, give 2 doses of *B. bronchiseptica* component 2–4 wks apart. *Revaccination*: annual.
Parenteral *B. bronchiseptica* only			
B. bronchiseptica only	AE/SC, IM (ml) WCB/SC, IM (1 ml) AVL/SC, IM (1 ml)	Performer (AgriLabs), Bronchicine (BioCor) Coughguard B (Pfizer)	*Initial*: Two doses 2–4 wks apart. *Revaccination*: If initial dose is given <16 wks of age, booster at 16 wks. Annual booster.
Intranasal Combined Vaccines			
B. bronchiseptica with parainfluenza	*B. bronchiseptica* is AVL; parainfluenza is MLV/IN 1 ml or 0.5 ml (Progard)	Intra-Trac II (Schering-Plough) Naramune-2 (Bio-Ceutic) Bronchi-Shield III[b] (Ft Dodge) Progard-KC (Intervet)	*Initial*: One dose (may be split 0.5 ml/nostril) in dogs at least 2 wks old. *Revaccination*: Annual or prior to potential exposure.
B. bronchiseptica only	AVL/IN (1 ml)	NasaGuard B (Pfizer)	*Initial*: One dose (may be split 0.5 ml/nostril) in dogs at least 2 wks old. *Revaccination*: Annual or prior to potential exposure.

[a]For additional information on vaccines and manufacturers, see Appendix 3.
[b]Also contains MLV adenovirus-2.
MLV = modified live virus; AE = antigenic extract; WCB = whole cell bacterin; AVL = avirulent live; SC = subcutaneous; IM = intramuscular; IN = intranasal.

against both disease and infection compared with parenteral vaccines. IN vaccines induce both local and systemic immunity, are not affected by maternal antibody, and protect against challenge more rapidly than parenterally administered vaccines.[6, 15, 27] Depending on the vaccine, puppies inoculated IN can be immunized as early as 2 weeks of age. Annual revaccination is recommended for those dogs considered to be at risk. Before known or potential exposure to other dogs (e.g., boarding), a single booster vaccination, administered IN, is recommended at least 5 days before exposure[6] in dogs that have not been vaccinated within the preceding 6 months. Vaccination is ineffective in the presence of virulent agents.

The occurrence of adverse reactions after administration of parenteral vaccine for canine ITB is rare and typically is limited to local irritation at the injection site. In contrast, although IN vaccines are capable of inducing both local *and* systemic immunity, they can be associated with development of a cough and/or nasal discharge 2 to 5 days after inoculation. Rarely, postvaccinal signs will be sufficiently severe or persistent that administration of an antimicrobial will be indicated.

Management of Outbreaks

Environments in which transient dogs are housed in adjoining kennels are conducive to efficient and rapid transmission of the agents capable of causing canine ITB. Although important in preventing infections, vaccination may not guarantee protection against development of signs, particularly in high-density populations. Because airborne transmission is common, dogs suspected of having contagious respiratory disease should be isolated when signs first develop in an effort to limit exposure to susceptible dogs. Thorough, routine cleaning of housing facilities, preferably using fresh sodium hypochlorite, chlorhexidine, or benzalkonium solution is necessary to control the spread of ITB. Adequate ventilation from 12 to 20 air exchanges per hour[5, 15] is recommended in kennel or shelter facilities. Although it can be tried, there is no evidence that IN vaccination, administered when clinical signs are first detected, will alter the course of an outbreak.

Once an outbreak has developed, isolating the entire facility for up to 2 weeks may be the only reasonable and the most efficacious method of containing infections. In addition to extensive cleaning, individual dogs are treated as necessary to manage clinical signs.

Animal facilities that maintain large numbers of dogs, especially transient populations, are at considerable risk for canine ITB outbreaks. A reduction in the incidence of ITB has been observed in dogs whose vaccinations for all infections were current. However, attempts to prevent outbreaks through routine, widespread IN vaccines may be ineffective if vaccination and exposure are likely to occur within the same day. Furthermore, postvaccinal coughing/nasal discharge may preclude adoption of otherwise healthy dogs from impoundment facilities. In addition to vaccination, adequate housing, proper cleaning, and adequate ventilation are critical factors in preventing outbreaks of ITB whenever dogs are housed within crowded environments. For further information, see Chapter 98.

PUBLIC HEALTH CONSIDERATIONS

The zoonotic potential of canine *B. bronchiseptica* infection has been reviewed.[10, 35, 36] Human bordetellosis is one of the most common respiratory infections of children and immunocompromised adults. Infections of wounds or other organs can also occur. At greatest risk are individuals whose immunosuppression is related to alcoholic malnutrition, hematologic malignancy, long-term glucocorticoid therapy, concurrent HIV infection, splenectomy, and pregnancy. As expected, individuals subjected to tracheostomy or endotracheal tube intubation are also at risk for infection. Human patients with pre-existing respiratory disease, such as chronic bronchitis and pneumonia, are particularly susceptible. Although human bordetellosis is associated with a variety of domestic and wildlife animal species, transmission of disease from pets to humans is largely circumstantial. In one instance, infection associated with exposure to rabbits was found to persist in a person with bronchopneumonia for at least 2.5 years.[14]

It has been estimated that up to 40% of immunocompromised adults living in the United States today have pets.[2] It is logical, therefore, to assume that these individuals, as pet owners, may be at increased risk of acquiring opportunistic zoonotic infections.[1, 9, 18, 20, 21] The risk of a child or immunocompromised adult becoming infected with pet-associated *B. bronchiseptica* infection must be considered small, particularly when exposure to large numbers of dogs in kennels and animal shelters can be avoided. For further discussion concerning immunocompromised people and pets, see Chapter 99.

References

1. Amador C, Chiner E, Calpe JL, et al. 1991. Pneumonia due to *Bordetella bronchiseptica* in a patient with AIDS. *Rev Infect Dis* 13:771–772.
2. Angulo FJ, Glaser CA, Juranek DD, et al. 1994. Caring for pets of immunocompromised owners. *J Am Vet Med Assoc* 205:1711–1718.
3. Appel M. 1987. Canine adenovirus type 2 (infectious laryngotracheitis virus), pp 45–51. *In* Appel M (ed), Virus infections of carnivores. Elsevier, Amsterdam.
4. Appel M, Binn LN. 1987. Canine parainfluenzavirus, pp 125–132. *In* Appel M (ed), Virus infections of carnivores. Elsevier, Amsterdam.
5. Appel M, Binn LN. 1987. Canine infectious tracheobronchitis: kennel cough, pp 201–211. *In* Appel M (ed), Virus infections of carnivores. Elsevier, Amsterdam.
6. Bemis DA. 1992. *Bordetella* and *Mycoplasma* respiratory infection in dogs and cats. *Vet Clin North Am Small Anim Pract* 22:1173–1186.
7. Burns EH, Norman JM, Hatcher MD, et al. 1993. Fimbriae and determination of host species specificity of *Bordetella bronchiseptica*. *J Clin Microbiol* 31:1838–1844.
8. Dambro NN, Grad R, Witten ML, et al. 1992. Bronchoalveolar lavage fluid cytology reflects airway inflammation in beagle puppies with acute bronchiolitis. *Pediatr Pulmonol* 12:213–220.
9. Decker OR, Lavelle JP, Kumar PN, et al. 1991. Pneumonia due to *Bordetella bronchiseptica* in a patient with AIDS. *Rev Infect Dis* 13:1250–1251.
10. Ford RB. 1995. *Bordetella bronchiseptica* has zoonotic potential. *Top Vet Med* 6:18–22.
11. Ford RB. 1995. Infectious tracheobronchitis, pp 905–908. *In* Bonagura JD (ed), Kirk's current veterinary therapy XII. WB Saunders, Philadelphia, PA.
12. Ford RB. 1996. Pocket guide to antimicrobial therapy, pp 1–8. Veterinary Learning Systems, Trenton, NJ.
13. Ford RB, Vaden SL. 1990. Canine infectious tracheobronchitis, pp 259–265. *In* Greene CE (ed), Infectious diseases of the dog and cat. WB Saunders Co, Philadelphia, PA.
14. Gueirard P, Weber C, LeCoustumier A, et al. 1995. Human *Bordetella bronchiseptica* infection related to contact with infected animals: persistence of bacteria in host. *J Clin Microbiol* 33:2002–2006.
15. Hawkins EC. 1995. Diseases of the lower respiratory tract, pp 767–811. *In* Ettinger SJ, Feldman EC (eds), Textbook of veterinary internal medicine. WB Saunders, Philadelphia, PA.
16. Henik RA, Yeager AE. 1994. Bronchopulmonary diseases, pp 979–1052. *In* RG Sherding (ed), The cat: diseases and clinical management, ed 2. Churchill Livingstone, New York.
17. Kirchner BK, Port CD, Magoc TJ, et al. 1990. Spontaneous bronchopneumonia in laboratory dogs infected with untyped *Mycoplasma* sp. *Lab Anim Sci* 40:625–628.
18. Lecoustumier A, Gueirard P, Guiso N. 1995. Epidemiology of human *Bordetella bronchiseptica* infections. *Medlec Malad Infect* 25:1243–1247.
19. Lemen RJ, Quan SF, Witten ML, et al. 1990. Canine parainfluenza type 2 bronchiolitis increases histamine responsiveness in beagle puppies. *Am Rev Respir Dis* 141:199–207.
20. Meis JFGM, Van Griethuijsen AJA, Muytjens HL. 1990. *Bordetella bronchiseptica* in an immunosuppressed patient. *Eur J Clin Microbiol Infect Dis* 9:366–367.
21. Mesnard R, Guiso N, Michelet C, et al. 1993. Isolation of *Bordetella bronchiseptica* from a patient with AIDS. *Eur J Clin Microbiol Infect Dis* 12:304–306.
22. Musser JM, Bemis DA, Ishikawa H, et al. 1987. Clonal diversity and host distribution in *Bordetella bronchiseptica*. *J Bacteriol* 169:2793–2803.
23. Porter JF, Parton R, Wardlaw AC. 1991. Growth and survival of *Bordetella bronchiseptica* in natural waters and in buffered saline without added nutrients. *Appl Environ Microbiol* 57:1202–1206.
24. Quan SF, Witten ML, Dambro NN, et al. 1991. Canine parainfluenza type 2 and *Bordetella bronchiseptica* infection produces increased bronchoalveolar lavage thromboxane concentrations in beagle puppies. *Prostaglandins Leukot Essent Fatty Acids* 94:171–175.
25. Randolph JF, Moise NS, Scarlett JM, et al. 1993. Prevalence of mycoplasmal and ureaplasmal recovery from tracheobronchial lavages and prevalence of mycoplasmal recovery from pharyngeal swab specimens in dogs with or without pulmonary disease. *Am J Vet Res* 54:387–391.
26. Rosendal S. 1995. *Mycoplasma* infections of dogs and cats, pp 301–302. *In* Bonagura JD (ed), Kirk's current veterinary therapy XII small animal practice. WB Saunders, Philadelphia, PA.
27. Thrusfield MV, Aitken CGG, Muirhead RH. 1989. A field investigation of kennel cough: efficacy of vaccination. *J Small Anim Pract* 30:550–560.
28. Thrusfield MV, Aitken CGG, Muirhead RH. 1991. A field investigation of kennel cough: incubation period and clinical signs. *J Small Anim Pract* 32:215–220.
29. Thrusfield MV, Aitken CGG, Muirhead RH. 1991. A field investigation of kennel cough: efficacy of different treatments. *J Small Anim Pract* 32:455–459.
30. Turner T. 1987. Intratracheal treatment for kennel cough. *Vet Rec* 121:182–183.
31. Ueland K. 1990. Serological, bacteriological and clinical observations on an outbreak of canine infectious tracheobronchitis in Norway. *Vet Rec* 126:481–483.
32. Vaden SL, Papich MG. 1995. Empiric antibiotic therapy, pp 276–280. *In* Bonagura JD (ed), Kirk's current veterinary therapy XII small animal practice. WB Saunders, Philadelphia, PA.
33. Van Oosterhout ICAM, Meij BP, Venker-van Haagen AJ, et al. 1989. Rhinoscopy in small animal clinics: an analysis of the results of 233 rhinoscopies and 97 bacterial cultures from nasal swabs. *Tijdschr Diergeneeskd* 114S1:94–95.
34. Wagener JS, Sobonya R, Minnich L, et al. 1984. Role of canine parainfluenza virus and *Bordetella bronchiseptica* in kennel cough. *Am J Vet Res* 45:1862–1866.
35. Woodard DR, Cone LA, Fostvedt K. 1995. *Bordetella bronchiseptica* infection in patients with AIDS. *Clin Infect Dis* 20:193–194.
36. Woolfrey BF, Moody JA. 1991. Human infections associated with *Bordetella bronchiseptica*. *Clin Microbiol Rev* 4:243–255.
37. Yamamoto S, Shida T, Honda M, et al. 1994. Serum c-reactive protein and immune responses in dogs inoculated with *Bordetella bronchiseptica* (phase 1 cells). *Vet Res Commun* 18:347–357.

Chapter 7

Nonrespiratory Parainfluenza Virus Infection of Dogs

Craig E. Greene

ETIOLOGY

Canine parainfluenza virus (CPiV) is a member of the family Paramyxoviridae, which contains CDV, simian virus 5 (SV-5), and human measles and mumps viruses. Human, simian, and canine type 2 parainfluenza viruses have all been termed SV-5–like viruses because of their close antigenic relationship. Monoclonal antibody studies have shown minor antigenic differences between SV-5 isolates.[11] Whether different SV-5 isolates are transmitted among people, nonhuman primates, and dogs remains to be established. The virus associated with respiratory disease in dogs has been designated CPiV.[5] It causes acute, self-limiting cough in the syndrome of canine infectious tracheobronchitis (ITB, see Chapter 6) and is recognized worldwide as an important cause of respiratory disease in dogs.[1, 10] Serologic studies indicate that the overall prevalence of CPiV in the canine population is high but variable. Experimental inoculation of CPiV in newborn pups can spread to internal tissues. There is evidence that related but distinct paramyxoviruses may cause systemic or nonrespiratory infections in older dogs.[6] A parainfluenza virus also was consistently isolated from the prostatic fluid of a dog.[12]

CLINICAL FINDINGS

A parainfluenza virus variant was isolated from the CSF of a 7-month-old dog with ataxia and paraparesis of 3 to 4 days' duration.[7] The dog had been vaccinated against canine distemper at 7.5 weeks of age. Gnotobiotic puppies inoculated intracerebrally with this virus isolate developed two forms of clinical illness.[3, 4] Some developed acute encephalitis characterized by seizures, myoclonus (involuntary rhythmic muscle contractions), and progressive neurologic signs within a few days PI. Five of six inoculated dogs observed for 6 months PI developed internal hydrocephalus, although clinical signs were not noted at this time. The hydrocephalus was thought to result from ependymitis with decreased absorption of CSF with or without aqueductal obstruction. Seven-week-old seronegative ferrets intracerebrally inoculated have also been found to develop a self-limiting nonsuppurative ependymitis and choroiditis.[2]

A 6-week-old puppy was found in extremis as a result of acute hemorrhagic enteritis.[4] Although a paramyxovirus variant was isolated, it is too early to say it was responsible for the clinical illness.

At present it is uncertain whether the CNS or GI forms of disease caused by paramyxoviral variants occur with any frequency under natural circumstances. Neurologic illness has been more commonly recognized as a complication of other paramyxovirus infections, such as with canine distemper in dogs (see Chapter 3) and in people with measles and mumps viruses (see Chapter 25). In laboratory rodents, other paramyxoviruses have been shown to produce encephalitis and hydrocephalus that are very similar to those that result when the paramyxoviral variant was injected into dogs. Naturally occurring encephalitis, periventriculitis, and hydrocephalus of a suspected bacterial origin have been described in young dogs (see Periventricular Encephalitis, Chapter 84).

DIAGNOSIS

Paramyxovirus-induced encephalitis or hydrocephalus may be confirmed serologically by the HI assay; however, because of the high prevalence of antibody in canine populations and the routine use of a vaccine for CPiV, confirmation requires demonstration of a rising serum antibody titer. CSF antibody titer to this variant virus was shown to remain persistently high in dogs after experimental infection.[7] Viral isolation can be performed on CSF or brain tissue of infected dogs. In addition, direct FA methods can be used to detect viruses in nervous tissue. For cases of enteritis, virus isolation and EM of feces would be most valuable. Serologic techniques such as VN or HI must be utilized to distinguish these variant paramyxoviral strains from CPiV.

PATHOLOGIC FINDINGS

Gross pathologic findings have been identified only in experimentally infected dogs that became hydrocephalic. Moderately enlarged lateral and third ventricles are present. Microscopically, acute meningoencephalitis was characterized by multifocal neuronal necrosis, lymphoplasmacytic cellular infiltrates, and reactive gliosis. Focal ependymitis was also apparent. Flattening and discontinuities of the ependymal cells lining the ventricles were seen in dogs developing hydrocephalus. Ultrastructurally, the virus could not be found in the brains of dogs developing hydrocephalus and encephalitis that were examined 1 to 6 months after experimental infection.

In the puppy with enteritis, the intestinal and gastric contents were blood tinged. Atrophy of small intestinal villi, mucosal congestion, and lymphoid necrosis were noted.

THERAPY AND PREVENTION

The prevalence of paramyxoviral variant diseases is unknown at present. There is no known treatment. It is possible that the CPiV vaccine, developed for ITB (see Chapter 6), may help to prevent these other paramyxoviral diseases.

References

1. Ajiki M, Takamura K, Hiramatsu K, et al. 1982. Isolation and characterization of parainfluenza 5 virus from a dog. *Jpn J Vet Sci* 44:607–618.
2. Baumgärtner W, Krakowka S, Gorham JR. 1989. Canine parainfluenza virus-induced encephalitis in ferrets. *J Comp Pathol* 100:67–76.
3. Baumgärtner WK, Krakowka S, Koestner A, et al. 1982. Acute encephalitis and hydrocephalus in dogs caused by canine parainfluenza virus. *Vet Pathol* 19:79–92.
4. Baumgärtner WK, Krakowka S, Koestner A, et al. 1982. Ultrastructural evaluation of acute encephalitis and hydrocephalus in dogs caused by canine parainfluenza virus. *Vet Pathol* 19:305–314.
5. Binn LN, Eddy GA, Lazar EC, et al. 1967. Viruses recovered from laboratory dogs with respiratory disease. *Proc Soc Exp Biol Med* 126:140–145.
6. Evermann J. 1985. Paramyxovirus infections of dogs. *Vet Rec* 117:450–451.
7. Evermann JF, Lincoln JD, McKiernan AJ. 1980. Isolation of a paramyxovirus from the cerebrospinal fluid of a dog with posterior paresis. *J Am Vet Med Assoc* 177:1132–1134.
8. Greene CE. 1990. Nonrespiratory parainfluenza virus infections of dogs, pp 266–267. *In* Greene CE (ed), Infectious diseases of the dog and cat, ed. 1. WB Saunders, Philadelphia, PA.
9. Macartney L, Cornwell HJ, McCandlish IA, et al. 1985. Isolation of a novel paramyxovirus from a dog with enteric disease. *Vet Rec* 117:205–207.
10. Moloney MB, Pye D, Smith HV, et al. 1985. Isolation of parainfluenza virus from dogs. *Aust Vet J* 62:285–286.
11. Randall RE, Young DF, Goswami KK, et al. 1987. Isolation and characterization of monoclonal antibodies to simian virus 5 and their use in revealing antigenic differences between human, canine and simian isolates. *J Gen Virol* 68:2769–2780.
12. Vieler E, Herbst W, Baumgärtner W, et al. 1994. Isolation of a parainfluenza virus type 2 from the prostatic fluid of a dog. *Vet Rec* 135:384–385.

Chapter 8

Canine Viral Enteritis

Johnny D. Hoskins

Since the late 1970s, viral enteritis has become recognized as one of the most common causes of infectious diarrhea in dogs younger than 6 months. CPV-1 and 2, CCV, and rotaviruses (CRVs) have been incriminated as primary pathogens. Astrovirus, herpesvirus, enteroviruses, calicivirus, parainfluenza viruses, and virus-like particles have been isolated from or identified in feces from dogs with diarrhea, but their pathogenicity is uncertain.[10, 17, 25]

CANINE PARVOVIRAL ENTERITIS

Etiology

CPVs are small, nonenveloped, DNA-containing viruses that require rapidly dividing cells for replication (Fig. 8–1). Like all parvoviruses, CPV-2 and 1 are extremely stable and are resistant to adverse environmental influences. CPV-2 is known to persist on inanimate objects, such as clothing, food pans, and cage floors, for 5 months or longer.

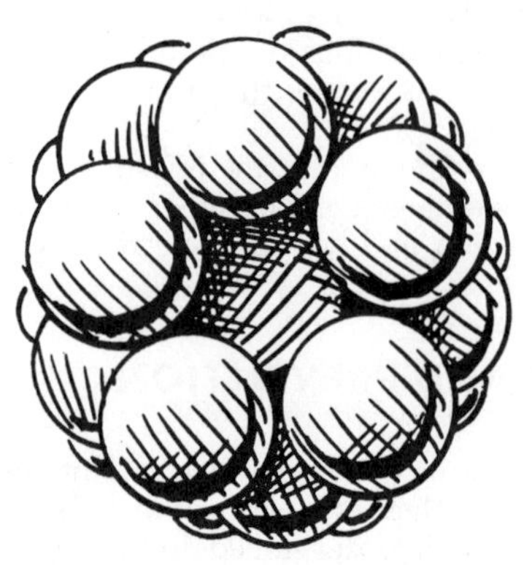

Figure 8–1. Structure of parvovirus.

Most common detergents and disinfectants fail to inactivate CPVs. A noteworthy exception is sodium hypochlorite (1 part common household bleach to 30 parts water), which is an effective and inexpensive disinfectant. It is important that exposure to this disinfectant be prolonged and thorough.

Canine parvoviral enteritis is probably one of the most common infectious disorders of dogs. This highly contagious, often fatal disease is caused by CPV-2. During the past 18 years, CPV-2 has undergone genetic alterations in the dog with development of new strains of the virus.[37, 37a, 38] In 1980, the original strain of CPV-2 evolved into type 2a (CPV-2a), and in 1984 another variant designated type 2b (CPV-2b) appeared. These CPV-2 alterations were associated with a genetic adaptation enabling the parvovirus to replicate and spread more effectively in susceptible dogs. In the United States, CPV-2b has largely replaced those previously isolated strains, whereas in the Far East[6, 29] and Europe[7, 14] both CPV-2a and 2b predominate.

Epidemiology

Natural CPV-2 infections have been reported in domestic dogs, bush dogs, coyotes, crab-eating foxes, and maned wolves, and it is probable that most, if not all, Canidae are susceptible. Experimental infections can be produced in ferrets, mink, and cats; however, the infection is generally self-limiting. The original CPV-2 isolates only produced systemic and intestinal infections in dogs,[52] whereas the newer type 2a and 2b strains may infect felines under experimental[29, 31, 55] and natural[30, 51] circumstances (see Chapter 10). In domestic dogs, CPV-2 infection does not necessarily result in apparent disease; many dogs that become naturally infected never develop overt clinical signs. When it occurs, clinical illness is most severe in young, rapidly growing pups that harbor intestinal parasites, protozoa, and certain enteric bacteria such as *Clostridium perfringens*, *Campylobacter* spp., and

Salmonella spp. In susceptible animals, the incidence of severe disease and death can be very high.

CPV-2 is highly contagious, and most infections occur as a result of exposure to contaminated feces. In addition, humans, instruments (equipment in veterinary facilities or grooming operations), insects, and rodents can serve as vectors. Dogs may carry the virus on their hair coat for extended periods. The incubation period of CPV-2 in the field is 7 to 14 days; experimentally, the incubation period has been found to be 4 to 5 days. With CPV-2a and 2b strains, the incubation period in the field can be as brief as 4 to 6 days.

Acute CPV-2 enteritis can be seen in dogs of any breed, age, or sex. Nevertheless, pups between 6 weeks and 6 months of age, and Rottweilers, Doberman pinschers, Labrador retrievers, American Staffordshire terriers, German shepherds, and Alaskan sled dogs seem to have an increased risk.[13, 22]

Pathogenesis

CPV-2 spreads rapidly from dog to dog via oronasal exposure to contaminated feces (Fig. 8–2). Virus replication begins in lymphoid tissue of the oropharynx, mesenteric lymph nodes, and thymus and is disseminated to the intestinal crypts of the small intestine by means of viremia. Marked plasma viremia is observed 1 to 5 days after infection. Subsequent to the viremia, CPV-2 localizes predominantly in the GI epithelium lining the tongue, oral and esophageal mucosae, and small intestine and lymphoid tissue, such as thymus, lymph nodes, and bone marrow. It may also be isolated from the lungs, spleen, liver, kidney, and myocardium.[61]

Normally, intestinal crypt epithelial cells mature in the small intestine and then migrate from the germinal epithelium of the intestinal crypts to the tips of the villi. Upon reaching the villous tips, the intestinal epithelial cells acquire their absorptive capability and aid in assimilating nutrients. Parvovirus infects the germinal epithelium of the intestinal crypts, causing destruction and collapse of the epithelium. As a result, normal cell turnover (usually between 1 and 3 days in the small intestine) is impaired, and the villi become shortened. CPV-2 also destroys mitotically active precursors of circulating leukocytes and lymphoid cells. In severe infections, the results are often neutropenia and lymphopenia. Secondary bacterial infections from gram-negative and anaerobic microflora cause additional complications related to intestinal damage, bacteremia and endotoxemia, and DIC.[35a, 53, 54] Active excretion of CPV-2 begins on the third or fourth day after exposure, generally before overt clinical signs appear. CPV-2 is shed extensively in the feces for a maximum of 7 to 10 days. Development of local intestinal antibody is most likely important in the termination of fecal excretion of parvovirus. Serum antibody titers can be detected as early as 3 to 4 days after infection and may remain fairly constant for at least 1 year.

Clinical Findings

CPV-2 infection has been associated with two main tissues: GI tract and myocardium. There is a marked variation in the clinical response of dogs to intestinal infection with CPV-2, ranging from inapparent infection to acute fatal disease. Inapparent, or subclinical, infection occurs in most dogs. Severity of the CPV-2 enteritis depends on the animal's age, stress level, breed, and immune status. The most severe infections are usually in pups younger than 12 weeks because these pups lack protective immunity and have an increased number of growing, dividing cells.

Parvoviral Enteritis. CPV-2 enteritis may progress rapidly, especially with the newer strains of CPV-2. Vomiting is often

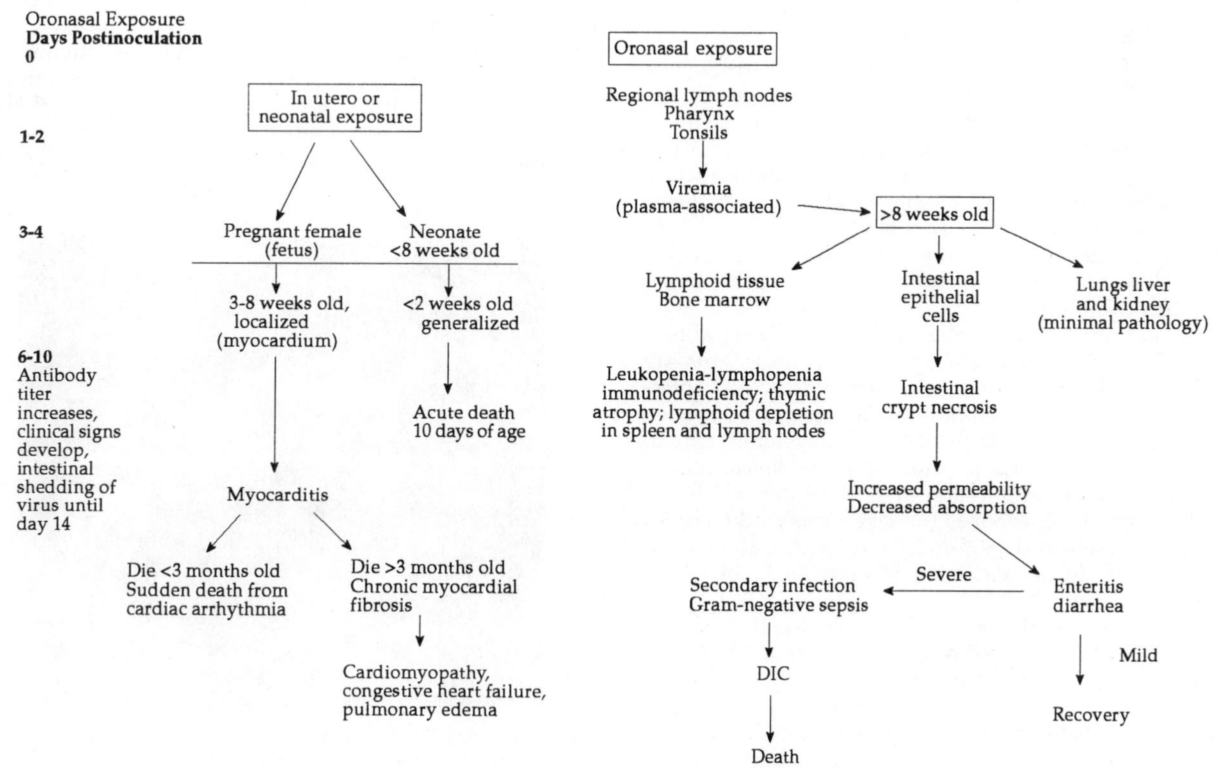

Figure 8–2. Sequential pathogenesis of CPV-2 infection.

severe and is followed by diarrhea, anorexia, and rapid onset of dehydration. The feces appear yellow-gray and are streaked or darkened by blood. Elevated rectal temperature (40–41°C [104–105.8°F]) and leukopenia may be present, especially in severe cases. Death can occur as early as 2 days after the onset of illness and is often associated with gram-negative sepsis and/or DIC. Younger age, absence of vomiting, and monocytopenia have been associated with a poorer chance of survival.[18]

Primary neurologic disease is not caused by CPV-2 but may occur as a result of hemorrhage into CNS from DIC or from hypoglycemia during the disease process, sepsis, or acid-base-electrolyte disturbances. Concurrent infection with viruses such as CDV is also possible. Cerebellar hypoplasia, common in kittens prenatally or neonatally infected with FPV, has not been reported in pups with CPV-2 infection.

CPV-2 Myocarditis. CPV-2 myocarditis can develop from infection in utero or in pups younger than 8 weeks. Usually all pups in a litter are affected. Pups with CPV-2 myocarditis are often found dead, or they succumb after a short episode of dyspnea, crying, and retching. Signs of cardiac dysfunction may be preceded by the enteric form of disease or may occur suddenly without apparent previous illness. The spectrum of myocardial disease in individuals is wide and may include any of the following: acute diarrhea and death without cardiac signs; diarrhea and apparent recovery followed by death, which occurs weeks or months later as a result of congestive heart failure; or sudden onset of congestive heart failure, which occurs in apparently normal pups at 6 weeks to 6 months of age. Myocarditis is still occasionally found in pups born to isolated, unvaccinated bitches[59] in contrast to its frequent occurrence during the widespread epizootic outbreaks of the late 1970s in CPV-naive dogs. Myocarditis, with or without enteritis, has been associated with natural CPV-2a and CPV-2b infections in 6- to 14-week old dogs from Korea.[62]

Diagnosis

The sudden onset of foul-smelling, bloody diarrhea in a young (< 2 years) dog is often considered indicative of CPV-2 infection. However, all dogs with bloody diarrhea (with or without vomiting) are not infected necessarily with CPV-2. Other enteropathogenic bacterial infections should also be considered (see Chapter 39). All clinical signs characteristic of CPV-2 infection are seldom present at any one time. Leukopenia, although not found in all dogs, usually is proportional to the severity of illness and the stage of disease at the time the blood is taken.

Fecal ELISA antigen tests are available for in-hospital testing for CPV-2 infection (see Appendix 6). These tests are relatively sensitive and specific for detecting CPV-2 infection.[21, 44] However, the period of fecal virus shedding is brief; CPV-2 is seldom detectable by 10 to 12 days after natural infection. This corresponds to 5 to 7 days of clinical illness. Positive results confirm infection or may be induced by all attenuated live CPV-2 vaccines (vaccine virus could yield a false-positive result in dogs 5 to 12 days after vaccination); negative results do not eliminate the possibility of CPV-2 infection.

CPV-2 typically produces lesions in the jejunum, ileum, mesenteric lymph nodes, and other lymphoid tissues. CPV-2 can be isolated from these tissues or feces using tissue culture systems, if performed early. Later in the course of disease, virions become coated by antibodies and cleared. Immunochemical methods can also be utilized to detect virus in tissue culture, EM of feces, or tissues (see Pathologic Findings). PCR has been used as a specific and sensitive means of detecting CPV in feces of infected dogs.[29, 31, 56] This method can also help to differentiate between virulent and vaccine CPV strains.[47]

As a general rule, parvoviruses cause hemagglutination of red blood cells. Inhibition of hemagglutination by CPV-2 antisera can be used to demonstrate serum antibody. The presence of high HI titer in a single serum sample collected after the dog has been clinically ill for 3 or more days is diagnostic for CPV-2 infection. Rising titers (seroconversion) can also be demonstrated when acute and 10- to 14-day convalescent serum samples are compared utilizing either canine or feline parvovirus in HI and VN tests. ELISA tests are also available that permit distinction between IgG and IgM.[44] A quantitative, commercially available antibody assay is also available (Immunocomb, Biogal Labs, Megiddo, Israel, see Appendix 6).[60]

Pathologic Findings

Early lesions are most pronounced in the distal duodenum; later the jejunum is more severely affected. The intestinal wall is generally thickened and segmentally discolored, with denudation of intestinal mucosa and the presence of dark, sometimes bloody, watery material within the stomach and intestinal lumen (Fig. 8–3). In mild cases, the lesions are not easy to distinguish from those of nonspecific enteritis. Enlargement and edema of thoracic or abdominal lymph nodes have been observed.

The intestinal lesions are characterized by necrosis of the crypt epithelium in the small intestine. Intranuclear viral inclusion bodies may be seen in these epithelial cells and throughout the squamous epithelia of the upper GI tract.[28] The pathologic changes may range from mild inflammation to diffuse hemorrhagic enteritis. The villi are shortened or obliterated owing to lack of epithelial replacement by maturing crypt cells, resulting in collapse of the lamina propria (Fig. 8–4). Necrosis and depletion of the lymphoid tissue (e.g., Peyer's patches, mesenteric lymph nodes, thymus, and spleen) are present. Pulmonary edema or alveolitis may be observed in dogs dying of complicating septicemia.[54] Histologic examination is usually definitive; however, specific identification of parvovirus in tissue specimens can be done

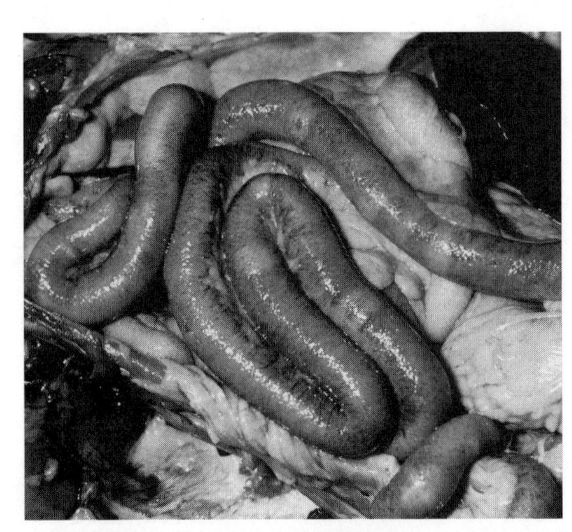

Figure 8–3. Small intestine at necropsy from a dog that died suddenly of parvoviral enteritis. Note the discoloration of the intestinal wall and fibrin on the serosal surfaces.

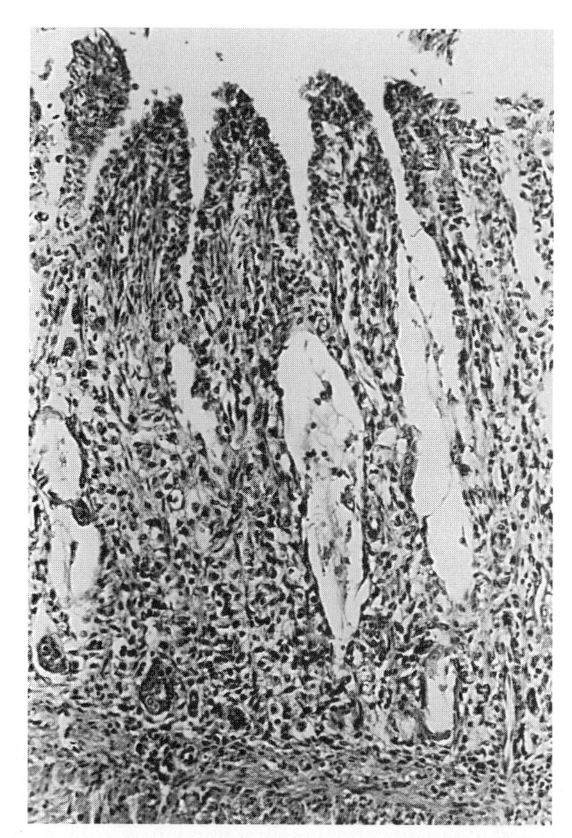

Figure 8–4. Photomicrograph of the small intestine of a dog that died of parvoviral enteritis. Villi are collapsed, and crypt lumina are dilated and filled with necrotic debris (hematoxylin and eosin; × 100). (Courtesy of Dr. Ed Mahaffey, University of Georgia, Athens, GA.)

by immunofluorescence or other immunochemical methods.[57] Using indirect FA, antigen in dogs with lethal CPV enteritis can be found in the dorsal side of the tongue (96.3%), pharynx (81%), esophagus (50%), ventral tongue (20.4%), planum nasale (5.6%), small intestinal mucosa (85.2%), bone marrow (81.6%), spleen (79.6%), thymus (66.7%), mesenteric nodes (50.4%), palatine tonsils (58.5%), and myocardium (1.9%).[61] In situ hybridization is a valuable specific tool for virus identification in formalin-fixed or wax-embedded tissue specimen.[58]

Parvoviral myocarditis, when present, is recognized grossly as pale streaks in the myocardium (Fig. 8–5). The myocardial lesions consist of a nonsuppurative myocarditis with multifocal infiltration of lymphocytes and plasma cells within the myocardium. Basophilic intranuclear inclusion bodies have been observed in cardiac muscle fibers, and parvo-like virus particles have been demonstrated by EM and by in situ hybridization[59] in the inclusion bodies.

Therapy

The primary goals of symptomatic treatment for CPV-2 enteritis are restoration of fluid and electrolyte balance and resting of the GI tract. Antimicrobial agents and possibly motility modifiers and antiemetic agents are given in Table 8–1. Fluid therapy is probably the single most important aspect of clinical management and should be continued for as long as vomiting and/or diarrhea persists. Antimicrobial agents are recommended in most dogs with CPV-2 infections. Antiemetic drugs do little for the primary treatment of CPV-2 enteritis and are indicated only when vomiting is persistent. Metoclopramide hydrochloride has proved helpful in most dogs with persistent vomiting. Drug therapy to alter gut motility is seldom recommended in the treatment of CPV-2 enteritis. If needed, narcotic antispasmodics (e.g., diphenoxylate hydrochloride and loperamide hydrochloride) are preferred when motility modifiers are needed.

In dogs with CPV-2 enteritis, food should be withheld until 24 to 48 hours after cessation of vomiting and reduction of diarrhea. Small amounts of water should be offered over the next 24 hours. If vomiting of water does not occur, small portions of a highly digestible, low-fiber, moderately low-fat diet (e.g., cooked rice or cereal supplemented in a 4:1 ratio with low-fat cottage cheese, boiled lean ground beef, chicken, or commercial baby food) can be given three to six times daily. Commercial low-residue diets specifically formulated for GI disease may also be prescribed. If commercial diets are given, the animal should initially be given one third the amount needed to meet normal maintenance energy needs. Over the next several days, the amount of food should be gradually increased to meet the animal's regular needs.

Table 8–1. Summary of Therapeutic Products Available for Management of Canine Viral Enteritis

DRUG	DOSAGE[a] (mg/kg)	ROUTE	INTERVAL (HR)	DURATION (DAYS)
Antiemetic Agents				
Chlorpromazine	0.5	IM	8	prn
	1.0	Rectally	8	prn
	0.05	IV	8	prn
Metoclopramide	0.2–0.4	SC	8	prn
	1–2	IV[b]	24	prn
Prochlorperazine	0.1	IM	6–8	prn
Antimicrobial Agents				
Ampicillin	10–20	IV, IM, SC	6–8	3–5
Cefazolin	22	IV, IM	8	3–5
Ceftiofur	2.2–4.4	SC	12	3–5
Gentamicin	2	IM, SC	8	3–5
Gastric Protectants				
Cimetidine	5–10	IM, IV	6–8	prn
Ranitidine	2–4	SC, IV	6–8	prn

[a]Dose per administration at specified interval.
[b]Slow infusion can be used for severe vomiting.

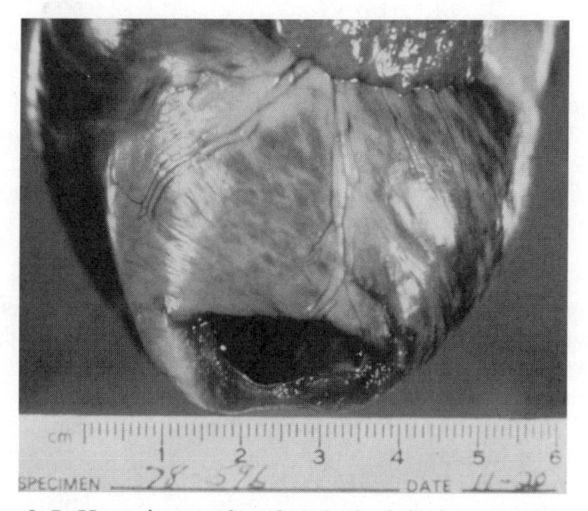

Figure 8–5. Heart from a dog that died of the myocardial form of CPV-2 infection. Pale streaking of the myocardium is apparent. A similar lesion will be noted with CPV-1 infection in puppies younger than 3 weeks. (Courtesy of Pfizer Animal Health, Lincoln, NE.)

After GI signs abate, a broad-spectrum dewormer and treatment for *Giardia* infection should be given. During the initial stage of CPV-2 enteritis, recommended adjunctive therapy has included transfusion of specific hyperimmune plasma, administration of recombinant human G-CSF, or administration of antiendotoxin sera (see Passive Immunization, Chapter 100, and Drug Formulary, Appendix 8). These adjuncts reportedly decrease mortality and the length of hospitalization[8] but are expensive. Recombinant human G-CSF has been advocated for the treatment of severe neutropenias induced by CPV-2 infection.[11] However, supplementing recombinant human G-CSF to neutropenic pups with CPV-2 infection did not change any aspect of their clinical outcome.[43]

Pups that survive the first 3 to 4 days of CPV-2 enteritis usually make a rapid recovery, generally within 1 week in uncomplicated cases. Severely ill pups that develop secondary sepsis or other complications may require prolonged hospitalization.

Prevention

Immunity after Infection. A puppy that recovers from CPV-2 enteritis is immune to reinfection for at least 20 months and possibly for life. Upon re-exposure to the various strains of CPV-2, protected pups will not have an increased serologic titer, show overt signs of illness, or shed virus in the feces. In general, there is a good correlation between serum antibody titer, determined by either HI or VN testing, and resistance to infection. Serum antibody titers remain high for a prolonged period after CPV-2 enteritis, even if re-exposure does not occur. If serum antibody titers become low, a localized infection is possible, but viremia and generalized illness are unlikely to develop. Although it may help in protection against entry of CPV-2, intestinal secretory antibody (IgA) probably does not play a role in the longevity of protective immunity because intestinally derived antibody titers do not persist for longer than 15 days after infection.

Immunization. Inactivated CPV-2 vaccines of sufficient antigenic mass protect dogs against wild-type CPV-2 exposure. If protective immunity is defined as complete resistance to subclinical infection, then that produced by most inactivated CPV-2 vaccines is short lived. Dogs vaccinated with inactivated CPV-2 vaccine can become subclinically infected as early as 2 weeks after vaccination. If a dog is given sequential doses of inactivated CPV-2 vaccine, however, a rapid secondary immune response is mounted and the dog is protected for as long as 15 months.

Commercially prepared attenuated live and inactivated CPV-2 vaccines are available. These vaccines produce varying levels of protective immunity and are safe either alone or in combination with other vaccine components. Transient lymphopenia occurs 4 to 6 days after the administration of some attenuated live CPV-2 vaccines. Most attenuated live CPV vaccine strains replicate in the intestinal tract and are briefly shed in the feces. Although concern has been expressed about the possibility of MLV CPV-2 vaccine undergoing reversion of virulence and causing apparent disease, experimental studies have shown that MLV CPV-2 vaccines are safe.[24] The events following administration of attenuated live CPV-2 vaccines parallel those following wild-type CPV-2 infection. On day 2 after SC administration of vaccine, viremia and systemic distribution occur with shedding from GI tract on days 3 to 10. One difference between vaccine-induced and wild-type infections is that lower quantities of virus are shed after vaccination. Humoral immune responses to attenuated live vaccines that have been studied are similar to those observed with wild-type infection. Serum antibody is usually detectable 3 days after vaccination, with levels rising rapidly to those observed after natural infection. Even if re-exposure does not occur, protective antibody titers may persist for at least 2 years, and dogs exposed during this time should not become infected.

LOW-TITER ATTENUATED LIVE CPV-2 IMMUNIZATION. Contrary to publicized information, vaccination failure is not related to strain differences between field and vaccine strains. The primary causes of failure of vaccines are interfering levels of maternal antibody to CPV-2[35, 41] and lack of sufficient seroconversion to the CPV-2 vaccine administered. The age at which pups can be successfully immunized is proportional to the antibody titer of the bitch, effectiveness of colostral transfer of maternal antibody within the first 24 hours of life, and immunogenicity and antigen titer of the CPV-2 vaccine. Pups from a bitch with low protective titer of antibody to CPV-2 can be successfully immunized by 6 weeks of age, but in pups from a bitch with a very high titer to CPV-2, maternal antibody may persist until 18 weeks of age or longer.[41] With low-titer vaccines approximately 25% of pups will be successfully immunized by 6 weeks of age, 40% by 9 weeks, 60% by 13 weeks, 80% by 16 weeks, and more than 95% by 18 weeks of age.

Without knowledge of the antibody status of each puppy, it is difficult to recommend a practical vaccination schedule that will protect all of them. In addition, there is a problem of pups becoming susceptible to wild-type CPV-2 infection 2 to 3 weeks before they can be immunized. There are no vaccines that completely eliminate this window of susceptibility before pups become immunized.[41] HI titers of 1:10 and higher may interfere with immunization, a situation that is more likely to occur when low-titer attenuated live CPV-2 vaccines are administered.

To maximize the probability of producing protective immunity in individual pups, it has been recommended that pups of unknown immune status be vaccinated with low-titer attenuated live CPV-2 vaccines at 8, 12, 16, and 20 to 22 weeks of age and then revaccinated annually.[20] Some pups with interfering titers of maternal antibody may not be immunized by low-titer vaccines given through 20 to 22 weeks of age necessitating additional vaccinations.

HIGH-TITER ATTENUATED LIVE CPV-2 IMMUNIZATION. In an effort to solve the problems of maternal antibody interference and lack of sufficient seroconversion to some attenuated live and inactivated CPV vaccines, another approach to CPV-2 vaccination programs is a vaccine that contains highly immunogenic, attenuated live CPV-2 strain produced at a high titer.[3, 20, 26, 32, 39, 46] Vaccine studies have demonstrated that a CPV-2 vaccine from a highly immunogenic strain produced at a high titer will actively immunize pups with low to moderate levels of maternal immunity to CPV. With such vaccines, pups are more likely to develop protective antibody titers. Pups of unknown immune status can be vaccinated with a high-titer attenuated live CPV-2 vaccine at 6, 9, and 12 weeks of age and then revaccinated annually. A check for serum antibody level or an additional vaccination could be done at 15 to 16 weeks of age, especially in those breeds at increased risk for CPV-2 enteritis. See discussion of parvoviral infection in Chapter 100 for additional information.

Public Health Considerations

Studies have failed to find any evidence of human infection by CPV-2, even among kennel workers in heavily contaminated premises, although people apparently can act as a passive transport vehicle for the virus between dogs. Although CPV-2 is not itself a human pathogen, extra care should always be practiced in handling fecal materials from diarrheic animals.

CANINE PARVOVIRUS-1 INFECTION

Etiology

In 1967, CPV-1 (also referred to as minute virus of canines or MVC) was first isolated from the feces of military dogs. Physical and chemical properties of CPV-1 are typical of parvoviruses. CPV-1 is distinctly differentiated from CPV-2 by its host cell range, spectra of hemagglutination, genomic properties, and antigenicity.[4]

CPV-1 can be propagated on the Walter Reed canine (WRC) cell line. By HI tests, CPV-1 is serologically distinct from parvoviruses of a number of other species. It appears that CPV-1 and CPV-2 are different viruses; no homology in DNA restriction sites between the two viruses has been demonstrated utilizing several restriction enzymes.

Epidemiology

The domestic dog is the only proven host, although it is likely that other Canidae are susceptible. Before 1985, CPV-1 was considered a nonpathogenic parvovirus of dogs. Since that time clinical infections of CPV-1 in neonatal pups have been encountered by practicing veterinarians and diagnostic laboratory personnel. Serologic evidence indicates that its distribution is widespread in the dog population but is restricted to causing clinical disease in pups younger than 3 weeks.[5] It seems reasonable to assume that spread is similar to that of CPV-2.

Pathogenesis

The virulence of CPV-1 for dogs is uncertain; however, CPV-1 has been identified by immunoelectron microscopy in the feces of pups and dogs with mild diarrhea. Four to 6 days after oral exposure, CPV-1 can be recovered from the small intestine, spleen, mesenteric lymph nodes, and thymus. Histologic changes in lymphoid tissue are similar to those observed in pups infected with CPV-2 but less severe. In addition, CPV-1 is capable of crossing the placenta and producing early fetal death and birth defects.[4] Experimental oronasal infection of neonatal SPF pups, with laboratory isolates from pups dying of enteric illness, produced only mild respiratory disease.[5] Naturally induced disease in young pups has been characterized by enteritis, pneumonia, and myocarditis.[23]

Clinical Findings

CPV-1 has been observed infrequently in field dogs with mild diarrhea as well as in the feces of clinically healthy animals. Primarily, CPV-1 infection is a clinical disease in pups between 5 and 21 days old.[18] Many of these pups have mild or vague symptoms and eventually die, being classified as "fading pups." Affected pups usually have diarrhea, vomiting, and dyspnea and are constantly crying. Sudden death with few premonitory signs has also been observed. Because of transplacental infections, failure to conceive or fetal death or abortion can be caused by this virus.

Diagnosis

CPV-1 infection should be considered in young (< 8-week-old) pups with mild diarrhea that clinically or histologically resemble CPV-2 disease but serologically test CPV-2 negative, or in unexplained fetal abnormalities, in abortions, or in fading pups. CPV-1 has been observed in fecal and rectal swab samples from field dogs by EM. Immunoelectron microscopy is necessary to distinguish CPV-1 from CPV-2. Inhibition of hemagglutinating activity in stool suspensions by specific antiserum also is diagnostic for CPV-1. To determine exposure, sera can be tested for specific antibody with VN or HI tests. Because only the WRC cell line supports growth of CPV-1, the availability of virus isolation and serum VN tests is limited.

Pathologic Findings

Pathologic changes in nursing pups have included thymic edema and atrophy, enlarged lymph nodes, pasty soft stool in the intestinal tract, and pale gray streaks and irregular areas deep within the myocardium as found with CPV-2 (see Fig. 8–5). Histopathologic lesions are predominantly restricted to large intranuclear epithelial inclusions at the tips of the villi in the duodenum and jejunum. These inclusions are eosinophilic and often fill the nuclei. Other intestinal changes noted include crypt epithelial hyperplasia and single-cell necrosis of crypt epithelial cells. Lesions seen in other tissue include moderate to marked depletion and/or necrosis of lymphoid cells of Peyer's patches and thymus, severe pneumonitis with exudate in airways, and mineralized focal to diffuse areas of myocardial necrosis with cellular infiltration.

Therapy and Prevention

Once a diagnosis has been made, treatment of pups suffering CPV-1 infection is unrewarding because of the rapid progression of the disease. However, mortality may be reduced by ensuring that the environmental temperature of newborn pups is kept warm and adequate nutrition and hydration are provided. No vaccine is available at present.

Public Health Considerations

There is no known public health concern; however, extra care should always be practiced in handling sick pups and fecal material from diarrheic animals because other enteropathogens may be present.

CANINE CORONAVIRAL ENTERITIS

Etiology

CCV is a member of the virus family Coronaviridae (Fig. 8–6). Different coronaviruses of this family infect a number of species, including humans, cattle, swine, dogs, cats, horses, poultry, rats, and mice (see Table 11–1). To date, several strains of CCV have been isolated from outbreaks of diarrheal disease in dogs. The virus genome is composed of a

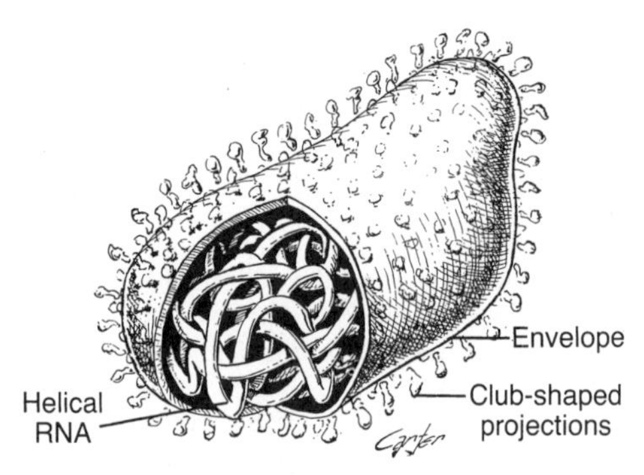

Figure 8–6. Structure of coronavirus.

single-stranded RNA chain; replication occurs in the cell cytoplasm of the host. Coronaviruses are fairly resistant and can remain infectious for longer periods outdoors at frozen temperatures. The virus looses infectivity in feces after approximately 40 hours at room temperature (20°C) and 60 hours when refrigerated (4°C).[48] Coronaviruses can be inactivated by most commercial detergents and disinfectants.

Epidemiology

In 1971, a CCV was isolated from feces of military dogs that were suffering from suspected infectious enteritis. Since then, several outbreaks of contagious enteritis have occurred and a similar coronavirus has been isolated. The true importance of CCV as a cause of infectious enteritis in dogs is unknown. Serologic information suggests that CCV has been present indefinitely in the dog population and is an infrequent cause of infectious enteritis. CCV is highly contagious and spreads rapidly through groups of susceptible dogs. Neonatal pups are more severely affected than those of weaning age and adult dogs. CCV is shed in the feces of infected dogs for 2 weeks or longer, and fecal contamination of the environment is the primary source for its transmission via ingestion.[49]

Pathogenesis

The incubation period is short: 1 to 4 days in the field and only 24 to 48 hours experimentally. CCV generally can be isolated from the feces of infected dogs between 3 and approximately 14 days after infection.

After ingestion, CCV goes to the mature epithelial cells of the villi of the small intestine.[49, 50] After uptake of CCV by the epithelial cell, the virus rapidly reproduces within the cell and accumulates within cytoplasmic vacuoles. Virions from these vacuoles may be released directly into the external environment via the apical plasmalemma, or may be released after lysis of the apical cytoplasm of infected cells. After production of mature virus, infected cells develop severe cytoplasmic changes, and the microvilli of the brush border become short, distorted, and lost. The overall result is that infected cells become lost from the villi at an accelerated rate and are replaced by increased replication rate of immature cells in the crypts of the mucosa. Crypt epithelium is not destroyed; on the contrary, there is hyperplasia. Affected villi become covered by low columnar to cuboidal epithelium, show variable levels of villous atrophy and fusion, and become infiltrated by mononuclear cells in the lamina propria. Unlike CPV infection, villus necrosis and hemorrhage are rare.

Dogs can have CCV and CPV infections simultaneously, and some studies suggest that CCV infection makes CPV infection more severe. Other enteropathogens such as *Clostridium perfringens*, *Campylobacter* spp., *Helicobacter* spp., and *Salmonella* spp. may increase the severity of CCV illness (see Chapter 39).

Clinical Findings

It is difficult to differentiate CCV from other infectious causes of enteritis. It is believed that CCV infection is usually less dramatic than CPV-2 infection. The clinical signs can vary greatly, and dogs of any breed, age, and sex are affected. This finding contrasts with CPV infections in which affected dogs are usually younger than 2 years. Infected dogs usually have a sudden onset of diarrhea preceded sometimes by vomiting. Feces are characteristically orange in color, very malodorous, and infrequently contain blood. Loss of appetite and lethargy are also common signs. Unlike CPV-2 infection, fever is not constant, and leukopenia is not a recognized feature.

In severe cases, diarrhea can become watery, and dehydration and electrolyte imbalances can follow. Concurrent ocular and nasal discharges have been noted, but their relationship to the primary infection is unknown. Most of the dogs affected recover spontaneously after 8 to 10 days. When secondary complicating factors are present (parasites, bacteria, or other viruses), the disease can be significantly prolonged.

Diagnosis

It is difficult to make a definitive diagnosis of CCV-induced disease. The detection of CCV in fresh feces can be done by EM. About 1×10^6 virions are needed in unconcentrated fecal samples for identification of CCV by EM; thus, false-negative findings are possible. Viral isolation is difficult because CCV does not grow well on tissue or cell culture systems. A reverse transcriptase PCR has been developed to detect CCV in fecal specimens.[16] Serum VN and ELISA tests for CCV antibody have been developed.[44] Positive CCV serum titers of affected dogs can only confirm exposure to CCV, and serum IgG titers have no relationship to protection as do intestinal secretory IgA titers.

Pathologic Findings

Mild infections are grossly unremarkable. In severe cases, the intestinal loops are dilated and filled with thin, watery, green-yellow fecal material. Mesenteric lymph nodes are commonly enlarged and edematous.

The intestinal lesions of CCV are characterized by atrophy and fusion of intestinal villi and a deepening of the crypts. There is also an increase in cellularity of the lamina propria, flattening of surface epithelial cells, and discharge of goblet cells. With well-preserved tissues, FA staining can enable specific detection of virus in the intestinal lesions.

Therapy

Deaths associated with diarrheal disease are uncommon and occur in pups as a result of electrolyte and water loss with subsequent dehydration, acidosis, and shock. Management must emphasize supportive treatment to maintain fluid and electrolyte balance as described for CPV-2 infection. Although rarely indicated, broad-spectrum antimicrobial agents can be given to treat secondary bacterial infections. Good nursing care, including keeping the dogs quiet and warm, is certainly essential.

Prevention

Inactivated and MLV vaccines are available for protection against CCV infection.[12, 36] Two doses 3 to 4 weeks apart and annual revaccination are recommended for immunization of dogs regardless of age. They provide incomplete protection in that they reduce but do not eliminate replication of CCV in the intestinal tract after challenge. It is difficult to assess the role of the CCV vaccines in protection against disease because CCV infections are usually inapparent or cause only mild signs of disease. For additional information on vaccination, see Coronaviral Infection, in Chapter 100.

Public Health Considerations

CCV is not believed to infect people. Coronaviruses are not strictly host specific, so the possibility of human infection cannot be excluded. However, extra care should always be practiced in handling sick pups and fecal material from diarrheic animals.

CANINE ROTAVIRAL INFECTION

Etiology

Rotaviruses are recognized as important enteric pathogens in many animal species and in people. They are sometimes referred to as duovirus, reovirus-like, and rota-like virus agents. Currently, rotaviruses are classified as distinct members of the family Reoviridae. Canine rotavirus (CRV) is a double-stranded RNA, nonenveloped virus that is about 60 to 75 nm in diameter (Fig. 8–7). It is resistant to most environmental conditions outside the host.

Rotaviruses have been isolated in tissue cultures or observed by EM of specimens from many species, including mice, monkeys, calves, pigs, foals, lambs, humans, rabbits, deer, cats, and dogs.

Epidemiology

Rotaviruses are transmitted by fecal-oral contamination. The viruses are well adapted for survival outside the host and for passage through the upper GI tract. Serum antibodies to rotavirus have been identified in dogs and cats of all ages.

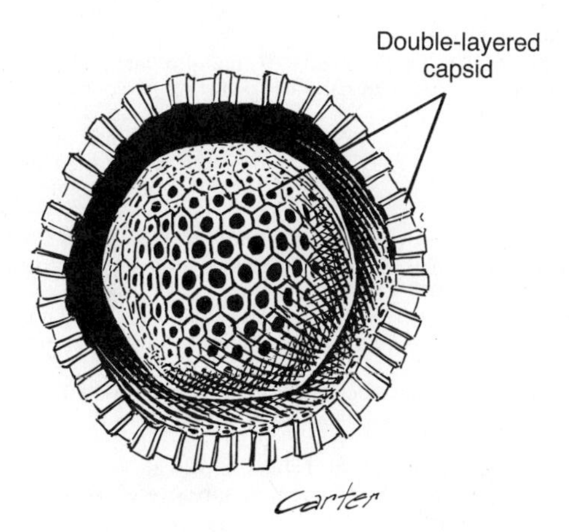

Figure 8–7. Structure of rotavirus.

Pathogenesis

Rotaviruses infect the most mature epithelial cells on the luminal tips of the small intestinal villi that leads to mild to moderate villous atrophy. Infected cells swell, degenerate, and desquamate into the intestinal lumen, where they release large numbers of virions that become sources of infection for lower intestinal segments and for other animals. Necrosis of rotavirus-infected cells is most pronounced 18 to 48 hours after oral infection. Necrotic cells are rapidly replaced by immature crypt epithelium. Clinical signs result primarily from the villous atrophy, leading to mild to moderate maldigestion and malabsorption and osmotic diarrhea.

Clinical Findings

Most clinical rotaviral infections have been demonstrated in the feces of pups younger than 12 weeks with mild diarrhea. Some cases of severe fatal enteritis associated with CRV have been reported to occur in pups as young as 2 weeks. The clinical signs are usually not as severe as those for the other canine enteric viruses (CPV-2 and CCV). A watery to mucoid diarrhea is usual, and this lasts for 8 to 10 days. The pups usually remain afebrile. CRV may contribute to enteric disease in mixed viral infections.

Diagnosis

Most pathogenic rotaviruses share common group-specific internal capsid antigens that can be detected by a number of methods, including commercial fecal ELISA (Rotazyme, Abbott Labs, N. Chicago, IL; Enzygnost, Behring Inst., Marburg, Germany) and latex agglutination (Rotalex, Orion Diag, Helsinki, Finland; Slidex Rota-kit, Biomerieux, Marcy-l'Etoile, France) tests used to diagnose human rotavirus infection (see also Appendix 6).[44] Rotaviruses can also be identified in fecal specimens by EM, although care must be taken to differentiate rotaviruses from the apparently nonpathogenic reoviruses occasionally present in dog feces. EM improves specificity of the test. Testing for seroconversion is possible but not widely available.

Pathologic Findings

Pathologic changes are limited to the small intestine, consisting of mild to moderate villous blunting. Virus can be detected in frozen sections by fluorescent antibody techniques.

Therapy and Prevention

Most dogs recover naturally from their infection. Treatment, if needed, consists solely of symptomatic therapy as described for CPV-2 enteritis. There are no vaccines available for CRV, and current estimates of the frequency and severity of the disease do not appear to justify vaccine development.

Public Health Considerations

Rotaviruses are generally host specific; however, the various strains cannot be easily distinguished, and the possibility of human infection cannot be eliminated. Rotaviral infections in people usually occur in young infants and children (younger than 4 years). Poor sanitation and hygiene, as exist in developing countries, increase the prevalence of infection. Routine precautions should be taken by persons handling feces from diarrheic dogs.

OTHER VIRAL ENTERITIDES

A number of other viruses have been identified in feces of dogs both with and without diarrhea. For the most part, the pathogenicity and importance of these viruses as causes of infectious enteritis remain unknown. On the basis of work in other species, some may be true enteric pathogens, whereas others are most likely incidental findings.

Astrovirus-like particles have been reported in the stools of clinically healthy and diarrheic dogs. Astroviruses are known to cause enteritis in other species, such as swine, but whether this is either true or common in the dog is unknown. The viruses have also been identified in diarrheic cats (see Chapter 12).

A herpesvirus antigenically related to FHV has been isolated from a dog with diarrhea, but Koch's postulates have not been fulfilled.[25] Likewise, the importance of serologic reactivity of some dogs to human echoviruses and coxsackieviruses is unclear (see also Enteroviral Infections, Chapter 24).

An apparently specific canine calicivirus has been isolated on several occasions from the feces of dogs with enteritis, sometimes alone and sometimes in conjunction with other known enteric pathogens.[30a, 45a] Likewise, an antigenically distinct parainfluenza virus, isolated from a dog with bloody diarrhea, was believed to be causal (see Chapter 7).

The study of viral enteritis in dogs is in its infancy; there are undoubtedly other viruses that affect the GI tract of dogs, but they remain to be discovered and characterized.

References

1. Baatz G. 1992. Ten years of clinical experiences with canine parvovirus infection (CPV-2 infection). *Tierarztl Prax* 20:69–78.
2. Buonavoglia C, Tollis M, Buonavoglia D, et al. 1992. Response of pups with maternal derived antibody to modified-live canine parvovirus vaccine. *Comp Immunol Microbiol Infect Dis* 15:281–283.
3. Burtonboy S, Charlier P, Hertoghs J, et al. 1991. Performance of high titre attenuated canine parvovirus vaccine in pups with maternally derived antibody. *Vet Rec* 128:377–381.
4. Carmichael LE, Schlafer DH, Hashimoto A. 1991. Pathogenicity of minute virus of canines (MVC) for the canine fetus. *Cornell Vet* 81:151–171.
5. Carmichael LE, Schlafer DH, Hashimoto A. 1994. Minute virus of canines (MVC, canine parvovirus—type 1): pathogenicity for pups and seroprevalence estimate. *J Vet Diagn Invest* 6:165–174.
6. Chang WL, Chang ACH, Pan MJ. 1996. Antigenic types of canine parvoviruses prevailing in Taiwan. *Vet Rec* 138:447.
7. de Ybañez RR, Vela C, Cortés E, et al. 1995. Identification of types of canine parvovirus circulating in Spain. *Vet Rec* 136:174–175.
8. Dimmitt R. 1991. Clinical experience with cross-protective antiendotoxin antiserum in dogs with parvoviral enteritis. *Canine Pract* 16:23–26.
9. England GCW, Allen WE. 1991. The lack of effect of parvovirus vaccination on the seminal characteristics of dogs. *Vet Rec* 128:611–612.
10. Finlaison DS. 1995. Faecal viruses of dogs—an electron microscope study. *Vet Microbiol* 46:295–305.
11. Fox LM, Bruederle JB. 1996. (Nearly) foolproof parvovirus treatments. *Vet Forum* Apr:36–38.
12. Fulker R, Wasmoen T, Atchison R, et al. 1995. Efficacy of an inactivated vaccine against clinical disease caused by canine coronavirus, pp 229–234. *In* Talbot PJ, Levy GA (eds), Corona- and related viruses. Plenum Press, New York, NY.
13. Glickman LT, Domanski LM, Patronek GJ, et al. 1985. Breed-related risk factors for canine parvovirus enteritis. *J Am Vet Med Assoc* 187:589–594.
14. Greenwood NM, Chalmers WSK, Baxendale W, et al. 1995. Comparison of isolates of canine parvovirus by restriction enzyme analysis, and vaccine efficacy against field strains. *Vet Rec* 136:63–67.
15. Greenwood NM, Chalmers WSK, Baxendale W, et al. 1996. Comparison of isolates of canine parvovirus by monoclonal antibody and restriction enzyme analysis. *Vet Rec* 138:495–496.
16. Ham C, Maes R, Vilnis A, et al. 1996. An RT-PCR assay to detect canine coronavirus and porcine transmissible gastroenteritis infections, p 60. *In* Proceedings of the American Association of Veterinarian Laboratory Diagnoses. Little Rock, AR.
17. Hamilton RC, Drane DP, Smith HV. 1995. Shedding of "virus-like" particles in canine feces. *Vet Microbiol* 46:307–313.
18. Harrington DP, McCaw DL, Jones BD. 1996. A retrospective study of canine parvovirus gastroenteritis: 89 cases. *J Am Coll Vet Intern Med* 10:157.
19. Harrison LR, Styer EL, Pursell AR, et al. 1992. Fatal disease in nursing puppies associated with minute virus of canines. *J Vet Diagn Invest* 4:19–22.
19a. Hoskins JD. 1997. Update on canine parvoviral enteritis. *Vet Med* 92:694–709.
20. Hoskins JD, Gourley KR, Taylor HW, et al. 1995. Challenge trial of Progard-7 vaccine using three field strains of CPV-2. *Intervet's Companion Animal Technical Report* 4:1–4.
21. Hoskins JD, Mirza T, Taylor HW. 1996. Evaluation of a fecal antigen ELISA test for the diagnosis of canine parvovirus. *J Am Coll Vet Intern Med* 10:159.
22. Houston DM, Ribble CS, Head LL. 1996. Risk factors associated with parvovirus enteritis in dogs: 283 cases (1982–1991). *J Am Vet Med Assoc* 208:542–546.
23. Jarplid B, Johansson H, Carmichael LE. 1996. A fatal case of pup infection with minute virus of canines (MVL). *J Vet Diagn Invest* 8:484–487.
24. Kahn DE, Emery JB, Smith MJ, et al. 1983. Safety and efficacy of modified-live canine parvovirus vaccine. *VM/SAC* 78:1739–1746.
25. Kramer JW, Evermann JF, Leathers CW, et al. 1991. Experimental infection of two dogs with a canine isolate of feline herpesvirus type 1. *Vet Pathol* 28:338–340.
26. Larson LJ, Schultz RD. 1996. High-titer canine parvovirus vaccine: serologic response and challenge-of-immunity study. *Vet Med* 90:210–218.
27. Martyn JC, Davidson BE, Studdert MJ. 1990. Nucleotide sequence of feline panleukopenia virus: comparison with canine parvovirus identifies host-specific differences. *J Gen Virol* 71:2747–2753.
28. Matsui T, Matsumoto J, Kanno T, et al. 1993. Intranuclear inclusions in the stratified squamous epithelium in the tongue in dogs and cats with parvovirus infection. *Vet Pathol* 30:303–305.
28a. McCaw DL, Tate D, Dubovi EJ, et al. 1997. Early protection of puppies against canine parvovirus: a comparison of two vaccines. *J Am Anim Hosp Assoc* 33:244–250.
29. Mochizuki M, Harasawa R, Nakatani H. 1993. Antigenic and genomic variabilities among recently prevalent parvoviruses of canine and feline origin in Japan. *Vet Microbiol* 38:1–10.
30. Mochizuki M, Horiuchi M, Hiragi H, et al. 1996. Isolation of canine parvovirus from a cat manifesting clinical signs of feline panleukopenia. *J Clin Microbiol* 34:2101–2105.
30a. Mochizuki M, Kawanishi A, Sakamoto H, et al. 1993. A calicivirus isolated from a dog with fatal diarrhoea. *Vet Rec* 132:221–222.
31. Mochizuki M, San Gabriel MC, Nakatani H, et al. 1993. Comparison of polymerase chain reaction with virus isolation and haemagglutination assays for the detection of canine parvoviruses in faecal specimens. *Res Vet Sci* 55:60–63.
32. Mockett APA, Stahl M. 1995. Comparing how puppies with passive immunity respond to three canine parvovirus vaccines. *Vet Med* 90:430–438.
33. Naveh A, Waner T, Wodowski I, et al. 1995. A rapid self-contained immunoblot ELISA test kit for the evaluation of antibody to canine parvovirus in dogs. *Proc Int Congr Vet Virol* 3:218–221.
34. O'Brien SE. 1994. Serologic response of pups to the low-passage, modified-like canine parvovirus-2 component in a combination vaccine. *J Am Vet Med Assoc* 204:1207–1209.
35. O'Brien SE, Roth JA, Hill BL. 1986. Response of pups to modified-live canine parvovirus component in a combination vaccine. *J Am Vet Med Assoc* 188:699–701.
35a. Otto CM, Drobatz KJ, Soter G. 1997. Endotoxemia and tumor necrosis factor activity in dogs with naturally occurring parvoviral enteritis. *J Vet Intern Med* 11:65–70.
36. Pardo C, Mackowiak M. 1995. Efficacy of a new canine origin, modified live virus vaccine against canine coronavirus. Rhone Merieux, Inc, Athens, GA.
37. Parrish CR. 1990. Emergence, natural history, and variation of canine, mink, and feline parvovirus. *Adv Vir Res* 38:403–450.
37a. Parrish CR. 1997. How canine parvovirus suddenly shifted host range. *ASM News* 63:307–311.
38. Parrish CR, Aquadro CF, Strassheim ML, et al. 1991. Rapid antigenic-type replacement and DNA sequence evolution of canine parvovirus. *J Virol* 65:6544–6552.
39. Phillips TR. 1989. Interactions of canine parvovirus with the immune system of the dog. Doctoral dissertation, University of Wisconsin-Madison, Madison, WI.
40. Phillips TR, Schultz RD. 1988. Failure of vaccine or virulent strains of canine parvovirus to induce immunosuppressive effects on the immune system of the dog. *Viral Immunol* 1:35–143.
41. Pollock RVH, Carmichael LE. 1982. Maternally derived immunity to canine

parvovirus infection: transfer, decline and interference with vaccination. *J Am Vet Med Assoc* 180:37–42.
42. Pollock RVH, Carmichael LE. 1990. Canine viral enteritis, pp 268–287. *In* Greene CE (ed), Infectious diseases of the dog and cat. WB Saunders, Philadelphia, PA.
43. Rewerts JM, Harrington DP, McCaw D, et al. 1996. Effect of rhG-CSF administration on the clinical outcome of neutropenic parvovirus-infected puppies. *J Vet Intern Med* 10:178.
44. Rimmelzwann GF, Groen J, Egberink H, et al. 1991. The use of enzyme-linked immunosorbent assay system for serology and antigen detection in parvovirus, coronavirus, and rotavirus infections in dogs in the Netherlands. *Vet Microbiol* 26:25–40.
45. Rimmelzwann GF, Juntti N, Klingeborn B, et al. 1990. Evaluation of enzyme-linked immunosorbent assays based on monoclonal antibodies for the serology and antigen detection in canine parvovirus infections. *Vet Q* 12:14–20.
45a. SanGabriel MC, Tohya Y, Mochizuki M. 1996. Isolation of a calicivirus antigenically related to feline calicivirus from feces of a dog with diarrhea. *J Vet Med Sci* 58:1041–1043.
46. Schultz RD, Larson LJ, McCoy KP, et al. 1995. An evaluation of canine vaccines for their ability to provide protective immunity against challenge with canine parvovirus, pp 19–24. *In* Proc North Am Vet Conf, Veterinary Learning Systems, Trenton, NJ.
47. Senda M, Parrish CR, Harasawa R, et al. 1995. Detection by PCR of wild-type canine parvovirus which contaminates dog vaccines. *J Clin Microbiol* 33:110–113.
47a. Smith-Carr S, Macintire DK, Swango LJ. 1997. Canine parvovirus: part 1. Pathogenesis and vaccination. *Compend Cont Educ Pract Vet* 19:125–133.
48. Tennant BJ, Gaskell RM, Gaskell CJ. 1994. Studies on the survival of canine coronavirus under different environmental conditions. *Vet Microbiol* 42:255–259.
49. Tennant BJ, Gaskell RM, Jones RC, et al. 1993. Studies on the epizootiology of canine coronavirus. *Vet Rec* 132:7–11.
50. Tennant BJ, Gaskell RM, Kelly DF, et al. 1991. Canine coronavirus infection in the dog following oronasal inoculation. *Res Vet Sci* 51:11–18.
51. Truyen U, Evermann JF, Vieler E, et al. 1996. Evolution of canine parvovirus involved loss and gain of feline host range. *Virology* 215:186–189.
52. Truyen U, Parrish CR. 1992. Canine and feline host ranges of canine parvovirus and feline panleukopenia virus: distinct host cell tropisms of each virus in vitro and in vivo. *J Virol* 66:5399–5408.
53. Turk J, Fales W, Miller M, et al. 1992. Enteric *Clostridium perfringens* infections associated with parvoviral enteritis in dogs: 74 cases (1987–1990). *J Am Vet Med Assoc* 200:991–994.
54. Turk J, Miller M, Brown T, et al. 1990. Coliform septicemia and pulmonary disease associated with canine parvoviral enteritis: 88 cases (1987-1988). *J Am Vet Med Assoc* 196:771–773.
55. Uchida E, Ichijo S, Goto H, et al. 1988. Clinical, hematological and pathological findings in specific pathogen-free cats and conventional cats experimentally infected with canine parvovirus. *Jpn J Vet Sci* 50:597–604.
56. Uwatoko K, Sunairi M, Nakajima M, et al. 1995. Rapid method utilizing the polymerase chain reaction for detection of canine parvovirus in feces of diarrheic dogs. *Vet Microbiol* 43:315–323.
57. Vlemmas I, Wohlsein P, Trautwein G, et al. 1990. Experimental parvovirus infection of puppies. Immunohistochemical findings. *Berl Munch Tierarztl Wochenschr* 103:422–425.
58. Waldvogel AS, Hassam S, Stoerckle N, et al. 1992. Specific diagnosis of parvovirus enteritis in dogs and cats by in situ hybridization. *J Comp Pathol* 107:141–146.
59. Waldvogel AS, Hassam S, Weilenmann R, et al, 1991. Retrospective study of myocardial canine parvovirus infection by in situ hybridization. *Zentralbl Veterinarmed B* 38:353–357.
60. Waner T, Naveh A, Wodovsky I, et al. 1996. Assessment of maternal antibody decay and response to canine parvovirus vaccination using a clinic-based enzyme-linked immunosorbent assay. *J Vet Diagn Invest* 8:427–432.
61. Weissenbock H, Burtscher H. 1991. Fluorescence serologic and histologic studies of antigen distribution in parvovirus infections in dogs and cats. *Zentralbl Veterinarmed B* 38:481–491.
62. Whan-Gook N, Jung-Hyang S, Doster AR, et al. 1997. Detection of canine parvovirus in naturally infected dogs with enteritis and myocarditis by in situ hybridization. *J Vet Diagn Invest* 9:255–260.

Chapter 

Canine Viral Papillomatosis

Clay A. Calvert

ETIOLOGY

Multiple canine papillomas are benign mucocutaneous tumors caused by infectious papillomavirus of the Papovaviridae family. Members of this family are small, ether-resistant, double-stranded DNA viruses that are similar in structure to, but larger than, parvoviruses. Papillomaviruses are naturally oncogenic, producing benign warts, and are usually species and site specific. Serologic cross-reactivity has not been detected among papillomaviruses of different species. Papillomaviruses of humans, cattle, and dogs, although antigenically distinct, share at least one group-specific determinant. Inoculation of COPV into kittens, mice, rats, guinea pigs, rabbits, and nonhuman primates has failed to produce papillomas. Tumors can be transmitted experimentally within their species of origin by scarification with whole cells or cell-free filtrates. A separate papillomavirus has been identified in cutaneous papillomas of cats (see Chapter 21) and dogs.[8a, 8b]

EPIDEMIOLOGY

Papillomas (also referred to as warts or verruca vulgaris) may be either naturally occurring, noninfectious or virus induced, solitary tumors or transmissible, virus-induced, multiple tumors. Infectious papillomas occur in young dogs in oral, ocular, and cutaneous forms. Oral papillomas occur on the oral, labial, and pharyngeal mucosae as well as the tongue and rarely in the esophagus (Fig. 9–1).

Ocular papillomas occur on the conjunctivae, cornea, and eyelid margins (Fig. 9–2). Ocular papillomas are less common than oral papillomas and are caused by a virus that is similar to the oral papillomavirus.

Virus-induced cutaneous papillomas are relatively uncommon and are usually solitary lesions caused by a subtype of the canine papillomavirus. COPV inoculated into the skin of the face may produce papilloma, but attempts to produce a tumor by inoculating the skin of the abdomen or back with COPV have usually failed.

Dogs older than 2 years seldom develop oral papillomas and older dogs are resistant to COPV infection. Ocular papillomas occur most often in dogs 6 months to 4 years of age but have been reported in dogs as old as 9 years. The age range of dogs with cutaneous papillomas is unclear but apparently is broader. In Australia, cutaneous papillomas of the

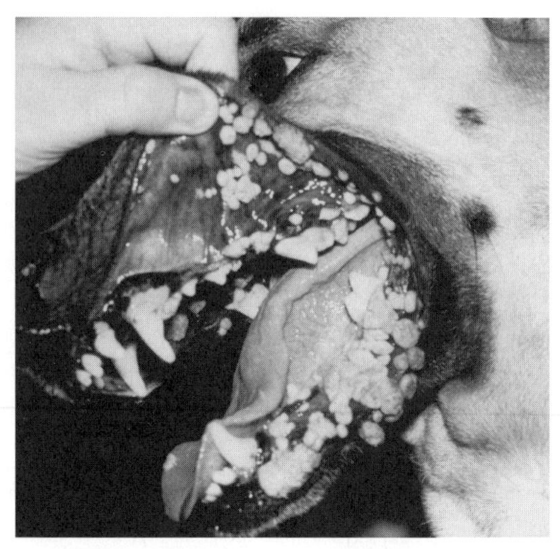

Figure 9–1. Typical canine oral papillomatosis.

distal limbs in racing greyhounds occur in dogs 12 to 18 months of age.

Most infectious papillomas undergo spontaneous regression. Malignant transformation to squamous cell carcinoma has been reported in some species, especially cattle. However, progression to carcinoma has been reported only in a dog with oral papillomatosis and a dog with a corneal papilloma.[13]

PATHOGENESIS

COPV infects the basal cells of the stratum germinativum. The first tissue response to COPV infection is an increase in mitotic activity resulting in acanthosis and hyperkeratosis. As the disease progresses, some infected cells are diverted to a role of virus production. These cells develop inclusion material but do not undergo cytoplasmic differentiation. Cytoplasmic degeneration and cell death ensue with viral persistence in strands of keratin. The majority of basal layer cells, however, differentiate into keratogenetic normal cells. Spontaneous tumor regression is usual.

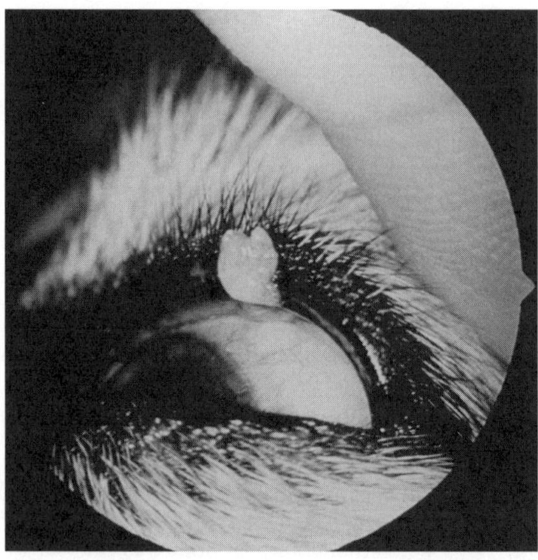

Figure 9–2. Eyelid papilloma in a dog.

The incubation period of COPV is usually 4 to 8 weeks postinoculation. Concentration of COPV in the inoculum may variably influence subsequent tumor growth and regression. Dogs given small doses of virus develop more papillomas, and regression is delayed relative to dogs given larger doses of virus.

Tumor growth usually lasts 1 to 5 months before spontaneous regression begins and subsequent immunity develops. When COPV was inoculated into the eyelid, only 50% of the dogs developed papillomas, the incubation period was longer, and the tumors persisted longer than in the oral cavity.

The mechanisms resulting in spontaneous regression or spread of papillomas are unknown. Virus-neutralizing antibody inactivates COPV in sensitized animals but does not inhibit established virus or papillomas. Serum from dogs whose papillomas have undergone spontaneous regression not only fails to produce tumor regression but enhances tumor growth. This effect may be the result of the induction of blocking antigen-antibody factors that impede cytotoxic lymphocyte action on target cells. Severe oral papillomatosis occurs in beagle dogs with IgA deficiency.[11] Cellular immune mechanisms may be more important in inhibiting the development of early papillomas in dogs. Regression is enhanced by the injection of immune lymphocytes from dogs in which COPV has regressed. In contrast, papillomatosis caused by COPV spread from the oral cavity throughout the haired skin of a Shar pei dog given glucocorticoids.[11] Multiple cutaneous papillomas, caused by a novel papillomavirus, developed in a boxer dog receiving long-term glucocorticoid therapy.[8a] In people, increased prevalence of papillomatosis is associated with defects in the cell-mediated or humoral immune system.

When inoculated into puppies, COPV has produced hyperplastic and neoplastic lesions at sites other than the oropharyngeal mucosa. Lesions have included epidermal hyperplasia, epidermal cysts, squamous papilloma, basal cell epithelioma, and squamous cell carcinoma. However, only a very small number of inoculations were associated with these extraoral lesions.

CLINICAL FINDINGS

Although oral papillomatosis is the clinically relevant disease, there are other forms. Oral papillomatosis is a contagious, self-limiting disease affecting the oral mucosa, labial margins, tongue, palate, pharynx, and epiglottis. Oral papillomas initially are pale, smooth, elevated lesions but soon become cauliflower-like with fine, white, stringy projections. Early tumors appear to "seed" the rest of the susceptible oral tissues. Recognition of the lesions usually occurs while the numbers of tumors are still increasing. Halitosis, ptyalism, hemorrhage, and discomfort are variably observed by the owners of affected dogs. As many as 50 to 100 tumors are often present at the time of diagnosis.

Spontaneous regression is usual, but the time to regression varies from weeks to months. Regression usually begins after 4 to 8 weeks of tumor growth. Occasionally, incomplete regression occurs, and a few papillomas persist indefinitely. Oral papillomatosis may occasionally persist for 6 to 24 months or longer. Dogs affected by persistent papillomas often have many large tumors and may become malnourished. Secondary bacterial infection of large, persistent, and ulcerated tumors is common and is characterized by a purulent discharge.

Ocular papillomas tend to persist longer than oral papillomas. There has been no clinical association of ocular papillomas with oral or cutaneous papillomas under natural conditions.

DIAGNOSIS

The diagnosis of papillomatosis is based on the epidemiology and gross appearance of the tumors. Ocular papillomas are usually examined histologically because they are not as morphologically distinct as oral papillomas. Papillomas microscopically show marked epidermal hyperplasia on fibrovascular stalks. Small intramuscular structures resembling inclusions may be noted. Cutaneous papillomas, usually morphologically distinct, are often excised for aesthetic reasons and examined microscopically. Cutaneous papillomas can occur at many sites, most often on the lower extremities, often in the interdigital areas and footpads and occasionally subungually. The viral cause can be confirmed by immunohistochemistry staining viral antigen, EM findings showing virus, or identification of COPV or its DNA in tissue biopsy specimens.[4, 11]

THERAPY

Treatment is often not recommended if only a few papillomas are present. However, the patient should be re-examined to determine whether tumor numbers are increasing. In such cases, clients often request treatment, although it is usually unnecessary and of unproven efficacy. Spontaneous regression is usual, but treatment may be indicated when tumors persist, when large, multiple tumors produce pharyngeal obstruction, and when aesthetic reasons warrant.

Surgical excision, cryosurgery, and electrosurgery are acceptable modes of treatment of oral tumors. Surgical removal, freezing, or simply crushing 5 to 15 of the tumors may induce spontaneous regression, presumably resulting from antigenic stimulation. Because spontaneous regression is usual, it is difficult to prove a causal relationship between such interventions and regression. Although autogenous vaccines are commonly recommended, their efficacy in dogs is questionable and they are usually not effective against persistent papillomatosis. Cutaneous papillomas that arise as a result of glucocorticoid-induced immunosuppression may regress once this therapy is discontinued.

Surgical excision or cryosurgery is effective for papillomas of the conjunctiva or eyelid. Cryosurgery is not recommended for corneal papillomas. Care should be taken to prevent spread of the virus to adjacent ocular tissues, and cryosurgery offers an advantage in this regard.

Systemic and lesional (bleomycin) chemotherapy using single-agent vincristine, cyclophosphamide, or doxorubicin has been ineffective in the majority of dogs treated. Interferon-α has been administered parenterally to affected humans at a dose of 1×10^6 units daily until regression occurs. Low-dose oral, rather than high-dose parenteral, therapy is more commonly used in pets. Acemannan has been administered intralesionally to cause regression of fibrosarcomas and might offer another alternative to interferon. Dogs recovering from oral papillomatosis are immune, as are most dogs older than 2 years. See Interferons, Chapters 2 and 100, Acemannan, Chapter 100, and the Drug Formulary, Appendix 8, for additional information on administration and precautions of these drugs.

References

1. Belkin PV. 1979. Ocular lesions in canine oral papillomatosis. *Vet Med Small Anim Clin* 74:1520–1524.
2. Bonney CH, Koch SA, Conter AW, et al. 1980. Case report: a conjunctivocorneal papilloma with evidence of a viral etiology. *J Small Anim Pract* 21:183–188.
3. Bonney CH, Koch SA, Dice PF, et al. 1980. Papillomatosis of conjunctiva and adnexa in dogs. *J Am Vet Med Assoc* 176:48–52.
4. Bredal WP, Thoresen SI, Rimstad E, et al. 1996. Diagnosis and clinical course of canine oral papillomavirus infection. *J Small Anim Pract* 37:138–142.
5. Bregman CL, Hirth RS, Sundberg JP, et al. 1987. Cutaneous neoplasms in dogs associated with canine oral papillomavirus. *Vet Pathol* 24:477–487.
6. Calvert CA. 1990. Canine viral papillomatosis, pp 288–290. *In* Greene CE (ed), Infectious diseases of the dog and cat. WB Saunders, Philadelphia, PA.
7. Davis PE, Huxtable CRR, Sabcine M. 1976. Dermal papillomas in the racing greyhound. *Aust J Dermatol* 17:13–16.

7a. Delius H, van Ranst MA, Jenson AB, et al. 1994. Canine oral papillomavirus genomic sequence: a unique 1.5-kb intervening sequence between the E2 and L2 open reading frame. *Virology* 204:447–452.

8. Hare CL, Howard EB. 1977. Canine conjunctiva-corneal papillomatosis. *J Am Anim Hosp Assoc* 13:688–690.

8a. Le Net J-L, Orth G, Sundberg JP, et al. 1997. Multiple pigmented cutaneous papules associated with a novel canine papillomavirus in an immunosuppressed dog. *Vet Pathol* 34:8–14.

8b. Shimada A, Shinya K, Awakura T, et al. 1993. Cutaneous papillomatosis associated with papillomavirus infection in a dog. *J Comp Pathol* 108:103–107.

9. Sundberg JP, O'Banion K, Schmidt-Didier E, et al. 1986. Cloning and characterization of canine oral papillomavirus. *Am J Vet Res* 47:1142–1144.
10. Sundberg JP, Reszka AA, Williams ES, et al. 1991. An oral papillomavirus that infected one coyote and three dogs. *Vet Pathol* 28:87–88.
11. Sundberg JP, Smith EK, Herron AJ, et al. 1994. Involvement of canine oral papillomavirus in generalized oral and cutaneous verrucosis in a Chinese shar pei dog. *Vet Pathol* 31:183–187.
12. Tokita H, Konishi S. 1975. Studies on canine oral papillomatosis: II. Oncogenicity of canine oral papilloma virus to various tissues of dog with special reference to eye tumor. *Jpn J Vet Sci* 37:109–120.
13. Watrach AM, Small E, Case MT. 1970. Canine papilloma: progression of oral papilloma to carcinoma. *J Natl Cancer Inst* 45:915–920.

Chapter **10**

Feline Panleukopenia

Craig E. Greene

ETIOLOGY

Feline panleukopenia is caused by a small, serologically homogeneous parvovirus, with single-stranded DNA. Structurally and antigenically, it is closely related to CPV and MEV.[9] In addition, CPV strains 2a and 2b have been isolated from healthy cats[10] and those with signs of feline panleukopenia (see Chapter 8).[11, 16] In contrast, FPV has not been shown to infect dogs after experimental inoculation.[18] FPV is very stable; it is able to survive for 1 year at room temperature in organic material on solid fomites. It resists heating to 56°C for 30 minutes and remains viable for longer periods at lower temperatures. The virus survives disinfection with 70% alcohol, various dilutions of organic iodines, phenolics, and quaternary ammonium compounds. FPV is inactivated by bleach (6% sodium hypochlorite), 4% formaldehyde, and 1% glutaraldehyde in 10 minutes at room temperature.

EPIDEMIOLOGY

FPV can cause disease in all members of the family Felidae. Some Viverridae, Procyonidae, and Mustelidae, including the binturong, raccoon, coatimundi, ring-tailed cat, and mink, are also susceptible (see Table 100–15). The virus is ubiquitous because of its contagious nature and capacity for persistence in the environment. Virtually all susceptible cats are exposed and infected within the first year of life. Unvaccinated kittens that acquire maternal immunity through colostrum are usually protected for up to 3 months of age. Most infections are subclinical, inasmuch as 75% of unvaccinated, clinically healthy cats have demonstrable antibody titers by 1 year of age. Seasonal variations in the incidence of panleukopenia and disease outbreaks presumably parallel increases in the numbers of susceptible newborn kittens. Although panleukopenia is regarded as a condition of unvaccinated random-source cats, infection has been reported in kittens born into pedigree breeding cats from well-vaccinated queens.[1, 1a]

FPV is most commonly transmitted by direct contact of susceptible animals with infected cats or their secretions. It is shed from all body secretions during active stages of disease but is most consistently recovered from the intestine and feces. Cats shed virus in their urine and feces for a maximum of 6 weeks after recovery. FPV is maintained in the population by its environmental persistence rather than by prolonged viral shedding. In utero transmission occurs. Virus has been isolated for a maximum of 1 year from the kidneys of neonatally infected kittens, but shedding does not occur. Owners who lose a kitten to feline panleukopenia should *not* introduce a new kitten into the household without having it vaccinated.

Fomites play a relatively important role in disease transmission because of prolonged survival of the virus on contaminated surfaces. Vehicles for exposure include contaminated clothing, shoes, hands, food dishes, bedding, and infected cages. Transmission also probably occurs via flies and other insect vectors during warm periods.

PATHOGENESIS

FPV, as a parvovirus, requires rapidly multiplying cells for successful infection, and the distribution of lesions within a prospective feline host occurs in tissues with the greatest rate of mitotic activity (Fig. 10–1). Lymphoid tissue, bone marrow, and intestinal mucosal crypts (intestinal glands) are most commonly invaded in adult animals. Late prenatal and early neonatal infections in cats result in some lymphoid and bone marrow lesions, but the CNS, including the cerebrum, the cerebellum, the retina, and optic nerves, can be affected.

Systemic Infections

Experimental infections have been produced in SPF and germ-free kittens. Clinical severity of infection is milder in these animals compared with that in field cases and in experimentally infected conventional cats, suggesting that copathogenic factors may play a role in the natural disease. The virus undergoes replication in lymphoid tissues of the oropharynx 18 to 24 hours after IN or oral infection. A plasma-phase viremia, occurring between 2 and 7 days, disseminates the virus to all body tissues, although pathologic lesions primarily occur in tissues with the highest mitotic activity. Lymphoid tissue undergoes initial necrosis followed by lymphoid proliferation. Thymic involution and degeneration are found in germ-free and SPF cats infected up to 9 weeks of age. Decreased T-cell responsiveness has been reported in FPV-infected cats, but there is no interference in humoral immune responses. Cats surviving infection have a decrease in viremia corresponding to a rapidly rising VN serum antibody titer by 7 days PI.

During intestinal infection, the virus selectively damages replicating cells deep in the crypts of the intestinal mucosa. Differentiated absorptive cells on the surface of the villi are nondividing and are not affected. Shortening of the intestinal villi results from damage to the crypt cells, which normally migrate up the villi, replacing absorptive cells. Damage to the intestinal villi results in diarrhea caused by malabsorption and increased permeability (see Fig. 89–6C).

SPF cats have more severe intestinal lesions compared with germ-free kittens. The proliferation rate of crypt epithelium is faster in SPF kittens as a result of indigenous microflora or their metabolic by-products, which stimulate the turnover rate of intestinal epithelial cells. The extent of damage throughout the intestinal tract parallels the presence of the virus, and lesions are milder in the colon, where epithelial mitotic rates are slower than in the small intestine. The jejunum and ileum are more affected than the duodenal segment, which may reflect lower numbers of indigenous microorganisms in the proximal small bowel.

SPF and conventional cats with panleukopenia are also susceptible to secondary bacterial infections with enteric microflora. Gram-negative endotoxemia, with or without bacteremia, is a common complication of systemic FPV infection.

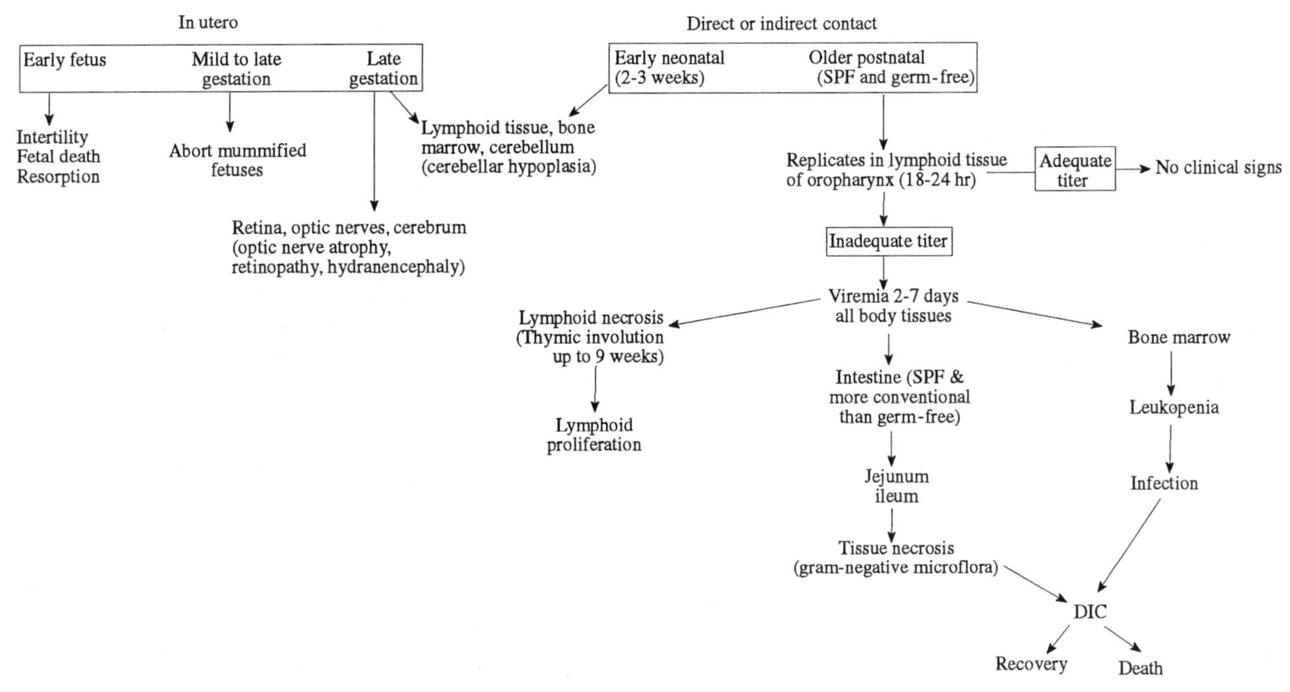

Figure 10–1. Pathogenesis of feline panleukopenia.

DIC, a frequent complication of endotoxemia, can also develop with feline panleukopenia.

In Utero Infection

Early in utero infection can produce a spectrum of reproductive disorders in the pregnant queen, including early fetal death and resorption with infertility, abortions, or the birth of mummified fetuses. Closer to the end of gestation, infections will result in birth of live kittens with varying degrees of damage to the late developing neural tissues. FPV produces variable effects on animals from the same litter. Some kittens are apparently unaffected owing to either innate resistance or the acquisition of maternal antibody, but may harbor virus subclinically for up or 8 to 9 weeks in some cases.

CNS Infection

The CNS, optic nerve, and retina are susceptible to injury by FPV during prenatal or early neonatal development, and, of CNS lesions, cerebellar damage has been most commonly reported. This predilection for cerebellar disease may be explained by the fact that in cats the cerebellum develops during late gestation and early neonatal periods. FPV interferes with cerebellar cortical development, resulting in reduced and distorted cell layers. It can be affected from infections occurring as late as 9 days of age. Other CNS lesions can be produced by earlier prenatal infections. Lesions of the spinal cord and cerebrum, including hydrocephalus, hydranencephaly, and optic nerve and retinal abnormalities, can occur (see Clinical Findings). Purkinje's cell degeneration in the cerebellum was described in one adult feral cat with systemic FPV infection.[4]

CLINICAL FINDINGS

The frequency with which cats show evidence of clinical disease with FPV is much less than the number of cats infected with the virus. This fact is supported by the high prevalence of FPV antibodies in the cat population. Subclinical cases, more common in older susceptible cats, remain unrecognized. Severe clinical illness is the rule in young unvaccinated kittens; the highest morbidity and mortality occurs between 3 and 5 months. Sudden neonatal or adolescent death (fading kittens) has been observed in kittens of 4 weeks to 12 months of age from households of vaccinated pedigree cats.[1a]

The disease has an acute self-limiting presentation, and chronic leukopenia or diarrhea is probably caused by other diseases. In the most peracute form, cats may die within 12 hours, as if poisoned, with little or no premonitory signs. They may be found in terminal stages of septic shock, being hypothermic and comatose.

The acute form is most common, with fever (40–41.6°C [104–107°F]), depression, and anorexia occurring within 3 to 4 days before presentation. Vomiting, which develops during the illness in most cats, is frequently bile-tinged and occurs unrelated to eating. Extreme dehydration, sometimes manifest by the cat crouching with its head over the water dish, may occur as a nonspecific feature of this disease. Diarrhea occurs with less frequency. When it is present, it usually occurs somewhat later in the course of illness.

On abdominal palpation, the intestinal loops have a thickened, ropelike consistency, and discomfort is commonly noted. Mesenteric lymphadenomegaly is usually present, whereas peripheral lymph nodes are not enlarged. Oral ulceration, bloody diarrhea, or icterus may be noted in complicated infections. Petechial and ecchymotic hemorrhages may be found in cats with complicating DIC, although cats do not frequently show overt signs of hemorrhage, even with marked thrombocytopenia.

Severe dehydration associated with anorexia, vomiting, and diarrhea can lead to progressive weakness, depression, and semicoma. Cats become hypothermic during the terminal stages of the illness. They can die suddenly from complications associated with secondary bacterial infection, dehydration, and DIC. Animals that survive infection for longer than 5 days without developing fatal complications usually recover, although frequently it takes several weeks.

Queens infected during pregnancy may show infertility or abortion of dead or mummified fetuses, but there are never any clinical signs in the aborting female. Some kittens in a litter may be born with ataxia, incoordination, tremors, and normal mental status typical of cerebellar disease (Fig. 10–2). They walk with a broad-based stance with hypermetric movements, and they frequently show intention tremors of the head. Tremors and incoordination are absent when kittens are at rest. Not all kittens in a litter are affected or have the same degree of neurologic deficits. Signs of forebrain damage include seizures, behavioral changes, and relatively normal gait despite postural reaction deficits. Affected kittens with minimal cerebellar dysfunction can compensate to a degree with time, and may make suitable pets with subtle residual deficits.

Retinal lesions may be visible on fundic examination of kittens affected with neurologic signs or as an incidental finding in clinically normal cats. These areas of retinal degeneration appear as discrete, gray foci with darkened margins, and retinal folding or streaking may be seen (Fig. 10–3).

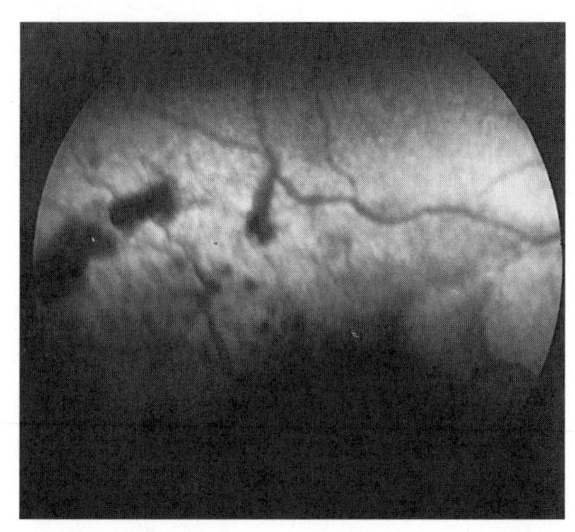

Figure 10–3. Dark foci in the retina from a kitten with hydranencephaly and optic nerve hypoplasia as a result of in utero FPV infection.

DIAGNOSIS

Clinical Laboratory Findings

A presumptive diagnosis of systemic feline panleukopenia is usually made on the basis of clinical signs and the presence of leukopenia. Leukocyte counts during the height of severe infection (days 4–6 of infection) are usually between 50 and 3000 cells/μl. Less affected animals have counts between 3000 to 7000 cells/μl. Leukopenia, from which the disease derives its name, is not pathognomonic for FPV infection alone and may not occur in all cases. The severity of leukopenia usually parallels that of clinical illness, and leukopenia also develops in infected germ-free and SPF cats. Subsequent examination of the leukocyte count in 24 to 48 hours in recovering FPV-infected cats will show a rebound in leukocyte numbers.

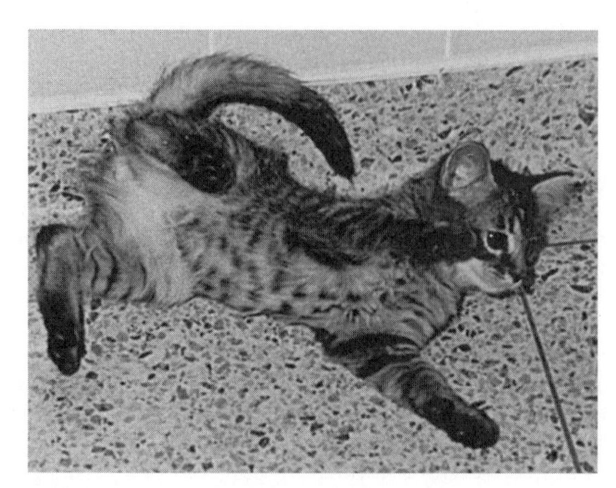

Figure 10–2. Kitten with congenital feline panleukopenia and cerebellar hypoplasia showing marked ataxia.

Repeated examinations should be made because diseases such as feline leukemia cause a more protracted illness and persistent leukopenia. Lymphopenia is less common with FPV infection than is neutropenia, and concurrent lymphopenia and neutropenia are more suggestive of FeLV infection. Feline salmonellosis with overwhelming septicemia may mimic feline panleukopenia with the presence of leukopenia and acute GI illness. Fecal culture may be helpful under these circumstances (see Chapter 39).

A transient decrease in absolute reticulocyte count and a mild (5–10%) decrease in hematocrit have been found during the viremic period in experimentally infected kittens. Because of the sudden onset of the disease and relatively long life span of erythrocytes, marked anemia is also less common in panleukopenia unless intestinal blood loss is severe. A persistent, nonregenerative anemia and leukopenia are more suggestive of FeLV infection (see Diagnosis, Chapter 13).

Thrombocytopenia is a variable feature of feline panleukopenia and may be found with other coagulation abnormalities in cats that develop DIC. Thrombocytopenia, resulting from direct bone marrow injury, can also occur in association with leukopenia early in the course of infection.

Biochemical findings in FPV infections are usually nonspecific. Increases in ALT and AST activities or bilirubin can reflect hepatic involvement, but elevations are mild to moderate and icterus is rare. Azotemia is frequently present from prerenal or nonrenal causes such as dehydration, although the virus can produce minimal renal pathology.

Serologic Testing

These procedures are available for the properly equipped diagnostic and research laboratory, although they are rarely indicated for clinical practice. Serum VN is the most common method. Twofold serial dilutions of antisera are performed against precalculated amounts of FPV. Virus and sera are incubated before inoculation of the cell culture. Cultures can be examined for specific cytopathic changes and inclusion bodies produced by the virus. The first sample is taken as soon as possible during the illness, and the second is taken 2 weeks later. A fourfold rise in titer is indicative of acute infection. CF titers also can be performed. HI and hemagglutination tests can be performed for some strains of FPV. FPV, like CPV, will variably agglutinate porcine erythrocytes at 0°C but at pH 6.4 rather than 7.2. The variation is usually related to individual variation among pig erythrocytes in the test. Direct FA testing can be used to detect virus in cell cultures and from tissues (usually intestine) of infected cats within 2 days after infection. ELISA testing, similar to that for CPV, can detect virus in feces or intestinal contents and is a more sensitive and practical indicator of infection.[1, 1a] Test kits are available for this purpose (see Appendix 6). Monoclonal antibodies can be used to distinguish viral strains, and PCR has also been used.[1a, 6, 12]

Viral Isolation

Feline cells are required to support viral replication in cell cultures, and frequent mitosis is needed to ensure a continuing infection, although FPV has been shown to replicate in cells in which DNA synthesis has been blocked. Cytopathic effects, required to substantiate the presence of the virus, are more easily demonstrated in young, rapidly multiplying cells. Plaque detection methods are possible when certain cell types and cell synchronization are used. Virus can be isolated from the urine and feces of kittens surviving experimental in utero inoculation at 3 and 6 weeks after birth, respectively. Direct culture from trypsinized lung and kidney tissues allows improved isolation of virus for up to 70 days. Virus has been isolated by direct culture for up to 1 year from the lungs and kidneys of prenatally infected kittens, despite a high level of circulating antibody. Virus can be found in the CNS for at least 22 days after neonatal infection and thereafter persists in Purkinje's cells.

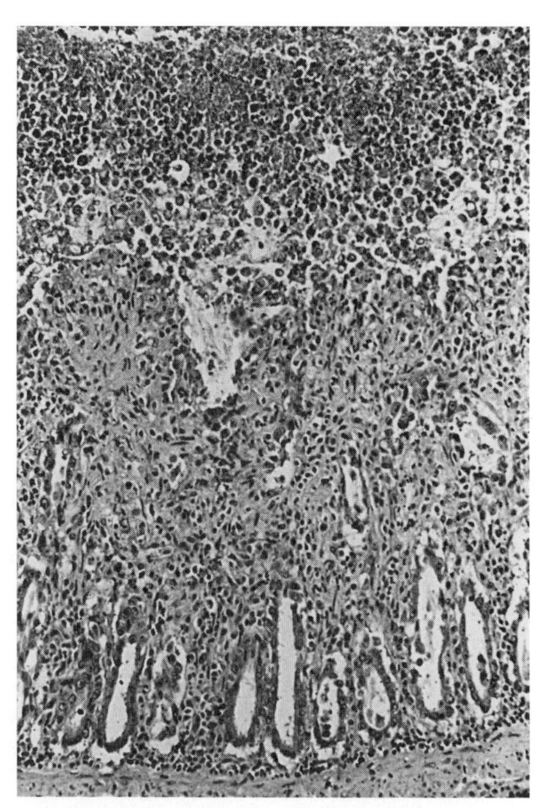

Figure 10–5. Microscopic appearance of the jejunum from a cat with FPV infection. Dilated crypt lumina and collapsed villi are visible in the lower part of the figure; there is sloughing of epithelial cells. Necrotic debris and overlying inflammatory exudate are present in the intestinal lumen in the upper part of the figure (hematoxylin and eosin, × 100).

PATHOLOGIC FINDINGS

Gross pathologic changes in naturally infected cats are usually minimal. The intestinal tract is obviously dilated; the bowel loops are firm and may be hyperemic with petechial and ecchymotic hemorrhages on the serosal surfaces. The feces frequently have a fetid odor when blood is present. Prenatally infected cats may have a small cerebellum, hydrocephalus, or hydranencephaly (Fig. 10–4). Thymic atrophy, present in all neonates, is the only gross finding in germfree kittens.

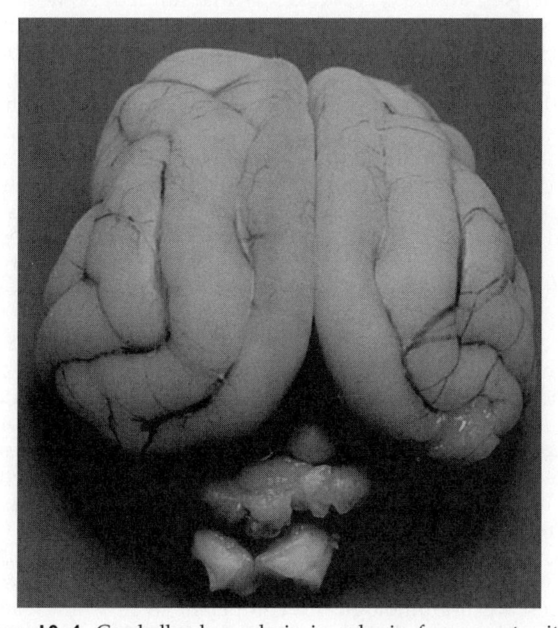

Figure 10–4. Cerebellar hypoplasia in a brain from a cat with in utero FPV invection.

Histologic abnormalities in the intestine include dilated crypts, with sloughing of epithelial cells and necrotic debris into the lumen (Fig. 10–5). Crypt-lining cells may slough completely in some cases so that only the basement membrane remains. Shortening of villi occurs secondary to the necrosis of crypt cells. The most severe histologic lesions are found in the jejunum and ileum; the duodenum and colon are less severely affected. Focal damage is most prominent around lymphoid follicles in the submucosa of the small intestine. Lymphocytic infiltrations are conspicuously absent from all tissues, and lymphocyte depletion is present in the follicles of lymph nodes, Peyer's patches, and spleen. Lymphoid atrophy is present, with concomitant mononuclear phagocyte hyperplasia.

Histologic abnormalities in the cerebrum of prenatally or neonatally infected kittens can include dilation of the ventricles and disruption of the ependymal cells with malacia of subcortical white matter. Cerebellar degeneration is marked by disorientation and reduced population of the granular and Purkinje's cell layers. Myelin degeneration can be found predominantly in the lateral funiculi of the spinal cord.

Eosinophilic intranuclear inclusions can be found in FPV infection, although they are transient and are frequently absent with routine formalin fixation. Bouin's or Zenker's fixatives must be used. EM findings indicate that the inclusions correspond with sites of virus replication. As with CPV infection, EM can detect viral particles in intestine and fecal specimens.

THERAPY

Mortality caused by FPV infection can be avoided with appropriate symptomatic therapy and nursing care. Cats that can be kept alive for several days with supportive measures usually develop adequate immune defense mechanisms to overcome the infection. Parenteral fluid therapy is employed to replace lost electrolytes, counteract dehydration, and replace daily maintenance needs. Oral intake of food and water should be withheld during this time to lessen vomiting and slow the bowel mitotic activity necessary for viral replication. Fluid volumes that must be replaced as a result of vomiting and diarrhea can be calculated by evaluating the cat's state of hydration. Additional maintenance needs from insensible losses are administered at a rate of 44 ml/kg/day. Balanced isotonic fluid replacement with lactated Ringer's solution is desirable, and potassium supplementation may be beneficial. Fluids can be administered SC unless there is severe dehydration associated with reduced peripheral vascular circulation for which IV therapy is required.

Antiemetics (Table 10–1) may be required to control persistent vomiting. The use of anticholinergic medications is controversial and is contraindicated because they produce sustained ileus of the bowel. Metoclopramide given parenterally works best. GI protectants such as Kaopectate and bismuth subsalicylate have been recommended to coat the bowel but cannot be given to vomiting animals. Bismuth compounds have the added theoretic advantage of reducing increased intestinal secretion and resulting diarrhea. Glucocorticoid therapy should not be selected routinely at anti-inflammatory or higher dosages because of its immunosuppressive effects.

Plasma or blood transfusion therapy may be required in cats that develop severe anemia, hypotension, or hypoproteinemia (plasma protein < 5.0 g/dl). A platelet count and activated coagulation time should be evaluated before administration of blood products in cases of ongoing DIC. Low-dose SC heparin therapy (50–100 U/kg given every 8 hours) can be administered simultaneously with transfusion if thrombocytopenia and severe incoagulability are present. Antiserum or high-titer parvoviral antiserum from vaccinated or recovered cats is beneficial if given after exposure and before clinical signs are noted. After signs are observed, it is too late.

Table 10–1. Drug Dosages for Treating Feline Panleukopenia

DRUG	DOSAGE[a] (mg/kg)	ROUTE	INTERVAL (HOURS)	DURATION (DAYS)
Antiemetics				
Metoclopramide[b]	0.2–0.4	PO, SC	6–8	prn
	1–2[c]	IV	24	prn
Thiethylperazine	0.5–5			
Trimethobenzamide				prn
Antimicrobials				
Amp(amox)icillin	15–20	IV, SC	6–8	prn
Cephapirin	10–30	IV, SC, IM	6–8	prn
Gentamicin	2	IV, SC, IM	8	prn[d]

[a]Dose per administration at specified interval.
[b]Should not be given in conjunction with other motility modifiers.
[c]Total dose IV not to exceed 1 to 2 mg/kg/day; this dose may be divided as multiple-bolus infusions throughout the day.
[d]Renal function (blood urea nitrogen, urine casts) should be closely evaluated, and the drug should not be continued for longer than 7 to 10 days at this dosage.
PO = oral; SC = subcutaneous; IV = intravenous; prn = as needed.

Broad-spectrum antibiotics, such as ampicillin or cephalosporin, are administered to control secondary bacterial infection resulting from virus injury to the intestinal mucosa (see Table 10–1). Parenteral therapy is preferred because of continued vomiting. A combination of a penicillin or cephalosporin derivative with parenteral aminoglycosides or quinolones may be required for cats that are septic or moribund. Caution must be taken with aminoglycosides, because of their nephrotoxic potential, and quinolones, because of cartilaginous toxicity in growing animals. One rationale for antibiotic therapy in this disease is to reduce the mitotic activity of the bowel epithelium by decreasing intestinal microflora, because germ-free animals have been shown to have a mild form of disease.

Combination B vitamin therapy should be given parenterally to all cats with feline panleukopenia because of decreased food intake from anorexia, high requirements for B vitamins, and loss in diuresis to prevent development of thiamine deficiency. Low-dose oral or parenteral diazepam (2.5 mg total) can be used intermittently, a few minutes before feeding, to stimulate the appetite of anorectic cats that are not vomiting.

Response to therapy can be followed by monitoring the total and differential leukocyte counts because there is a resurgence of leukopoiesis within 24 to 48 hours. Bizarre forms of leukocytes can be detected in the blood and bone marrow.

After the nursing period, the cat can be started on oral alimentation by frequent feedings of small quantities of bland baby food, broth, or blended food. Eventually, the cat may be fed larger quantities of solid foods. Semimoist foods have lower residue and help to firm the feces of cats with persistent diarrhea. Rarely, cats that refuse to eat after several days should be force-fed by mouth or by pharyngostomy or gastrostomy tube or given diazepam, as indicated previously.

PREVENTION

Colostral antibodies to feline panleukopenia have a half-life of 9.5 days (see Tables 100–2 and 100–4). Both MLV and inactivated TC-origin vaccines are ineffective when maternal-derived antibody VN titers, as measured by some laboratories, are greater than 1:10. Successful vaccination without maternal antibody interference can be achieved by 12 to 14 weeks of age in most cases (range, 6.8–18.8 weeks), depending on the antibody titer in the queen. Kittens with VN titers from 1:10 to 1:30 cannot be successfully vaccinated but are susceptible to infection with FPV. Similar to pups infected with CPV, kittens can still be infected with FPV before the time they are immunized, although this problem has not been as widely recognized. Recovery from natural infection with virulent virus probably results in lifelong immunity.

Therapeutic passive immunity has been utilized to prevent panleukopenia. Homologous antisera from cats with a high titer to infection will provide immunity according to the titer of the product and the amount administered. The recommended dosage is 2 ml per kitten given SC or intraperitoneally. Because administered immunoglobulins persist for up to 2 to 4 weeks, the neonatal vaccination series must be delayed. Passive administration of antisera is recommended for use *only in exposed susceptible* (unvaccinated) cats that require immediate protection or in colostrum-deprived kittens, with subsequent vaccinations at 2 to 3 or 4 to 5 weeks of age with inactivated or MLV vaccines, respectively. Newborn kittens are immunologically competent to FPV and can respond with neutralizing antibodies at 7 to 12 days of age.

Active immunization against FPV has been the most important factor in reducing the incidence of the disease. Both inactivated and MLV products have been effective in preventing this disease. TC–origin inactivated products can break through maternal immunity as early as MLV vaccines. Unlike MLV products, they have the advantage of being safe in pregnant queens and in kittens younger than 4 weeks. Inactivated vaccines may be given to febrile kittens when an effective immune response is doubtful. There is no danger of postvaccinal virus spread or clinical illness as a result of reversion to virulence, although there has been suspicion that inactivated products can contain live virus. The major disadvantage of these products is that, in the absence of maternal antibody, two injections are required to achieve a titer that can be obtained from one injection of MLV product. Protection with inactivated vaccines does not consistently occur until 3 to 7 days after the second vaccination. Antibody titers to inactivated vaccine have been adequate for protection by 2 weeks after the first vaccination but have been greatly boosted by the second injection. CMI responses to FPV were stimulated as early as 3 days after the second of two doses of adjuvant inactivated FPV vaccine. The inactivating agents used in some of these vaccines are also irritating to cats. With cloning of FPV into bacterial plasmids, it may be possible to develop a more purified subunit vaccine against this infection. A raccoon poxvirus-vector, recombinant FPV vaccine has protected cats against challenge infection.[7]

MLV vaccines produce more rapid and effective immunity than do inactivated virus vaccines. In the absence of maternal antibodies, one injection of any of the currently available MLV products for panleukopenia will produce a protective titer greater than 1:8 to 1:10 in a previously unvaccinated cat; however, a second vaccination is recommended. Oral vaccination with MLV vaccine is ineffective, whereas IN or aerosol exposure to vaccine produces an active immune response. MLV vaccines are recommended in contaminated areas such as shelters and infected catteries or in outbreaks to provide faster protection. MLV vaccines should be avoided in immunosuppressed cats because of the risk of vaccine-induced disease (see Chapter 100).

Colostrum-deprived kittens can be vaccinated regardless of age, but MLV products should be avoided in kittens younger than 4 weeks because of the danger of producing cerebellar degeneration. Colostrum-deprived kittens younger than 4 weeks at first presentation should receive at least two inactivated FPV vaccines 2 to 3 weeks apart. If 4 weeks or older, they can receive one MLV-FPV vaccine with an optional one given 2 to 3 weeks later.

Initial vaccinations for nursing kittens are generally begun at 8 to 9 weeks of age and are followed by at least one more MLV product or two more inactivated vaccines, depending on which type of antigen is used. Subsequent vaccines should be given 2 to 4 weeks thereafter; the last vaccine is given at 12 to 14 weeks of age. In situations of apparent vaccine breaks or kitten mortality, subsequent vaccinations in the initial series might be considered.[1a] Panleukopenia vaccines are usually given SC. Combined vaccines that contain FPV and rabies or feline respiratory viruses have been marketed.

Annual vaccination against panleukopenia is recommended and performed by most veterinarians, although it is probably not essential. Actually, one MLV product or two inactivated vaccines may produce lifelong immunity. Two inactivated vaccines given at 8 and 12 weeks to SPF kittens isolated in a barrier-maintained research facility produced high persistent VN antibody titers for at least 6 years.[13, 14] It is probable that revaccination produces an anamnestic response and presumably is not harmful. After the kitten series, and a first booster 1 year later, triennial vaccination in conjunction with the rabies vaccine offers adequate protection.[13] Proper disinfection procedures are essential to prevent or control an outbreak owing to the high resistance of FPV. Household bleach diluted 1:32 (1 oz/gallon) should be used on all cages, feeding dishes, floors, and holding areas along with general cleansing. In cat holding facilities, all new cats should be vaccinated on arrival with MLV products and kept in disinfected cages separate from the resident cats for several days.

References

1. Addie DD, Jarett O, Simpson J, Thompson H. 1996. Feline parvovirus in pedigree kittens. *Vet Rec* 138:119.

1a. Addie DD, Toth S, Thompson H, et al. 1998. Detection of feline parvovirus in pedigree kitten mortality. *Vet Rec,* in press.

2. Buonavoglia C, Cavalli A, Gravino E, et al. 1993. Use of a feline panleukopenia modified live virus vaccine in cats in the primary stage of feline immunodeficiency virus infection. *Zentralbl Veterinarmed (B)* 40:343–346.

3. Carlson ME. 1994. Hydranencephaly and cerebrocortical hypoplasia in a four-month-old kitten. *Feline Pract* 22:10–12.

4. Foley JB. 1993. Concomitant onset of central nervous system and gastrointestinal disease associated with panleukopenia in an adult feral cat. *Feline Pract* 21:12–16.

5. Greene CE, Scott FW. 1990. Feline panleukopenia, pp 291–299. *In* Greene CE (ed), Infectious diseases of the dog and cat. WB Saunders, Phildelphia, PA.

6. Horiuchi M, Yuri K, Soma T, et al. 1996. Differentiation of vaccine virus from field isolates of feline panleukopenia virus by polymerase chain reaction and restriction fragment length polymorphism analysis. *Vet Microbiol* 53:283–293.

7. Hu L, Esposito JJ, Scott FW. 1996. Raccoon poxvirus feline panleukopenia virus VP2 recombinant protects cats against FPV challenge. *Virology* 218:248–252.

8. Martyn JC, Davidson BE, Studdert MJ. 1990. Nucleotide sequence of feline panleukopenia virus: comparison with canine parvovirus identifies host-specific differences. *J Gen Virol* 71:2747–2753.

9. Mochizuki M, Akaboshi T. 1988. Structural polypeptides of feline parvovirus subspecies viruses. *Jpn J Vet Sci* 50:1207–1214.

10. Mochizuki M, Harasawa R, Nakatani H. 1993. Antigenic and genomic variabilities among recently-prevalent parvoviruses of canine and feline origin in Japan. *Vet Microbiol* 38:1–10.

11. Mochizuki M, Horiuchi M, Hiragi H, et al. 1996. Isolation of canine parvovirus from a cat manifesting clinical signs of feline panleukopenia. *J Clin Microbiol* 34:2101–2105.

12. Schunck B, Kraft W, Truyen U. 1995. A simple touch-down polymerase chain reaction for the detection of canine parvovirus and feline panleukopenia virus in feces. *J Virol Methods* 55:427–433.

13. Scott FW. 1995. Feline infectious diseases. *In* Proceedings of the Feline Infectious Disease Symposium, Washington, DC, October 14–17.

14. Scott FW, Geissinger C. 1997. Duration of immunity in cats vaccinated with an inactivated feline panleukopenia, herpesvirus, and calicivirus vaccine. *Feline Pract* 25:12–19.

15. Shell LG. 1996. Viral induced cerebellar hypoplasia. *Feline Pract* 24:28.

16. Truyen U, Evermann JF, Vieler E, et al. 1996. Evolution of canine parvovirus involved loss and gain of feline host range. *Virology* 215:186–189.

17. Truyen U, Gruenberg A, Chang B, et al. 1995. Evolution of the feline-subgroup parvoviruses and the control of canine host range in vivo. *J Virol* 69:4702–4710.

18. Truyen U, Parrish CR. 1992. Canine and feline host ranges of canine parvovirus and feline panleukopenia virus: distinct cell tropisms of each virus in vitro and in vivo. *J Virol* 66:5399–5408.

Chapter 11

Feline Coronavirus Infection

Diane D. Addie and Oswald Jarrett

The clinical condition of feline infectious peritonitis (FIP) was first described in the 1960s.[43] Subsequent studies of the lesions of FIP by EM incriminated a coronavirus labeled FIPV. FIP has become an important disease for veterinarians who treat cats living in populous conditions. A possible explanation for an apparent increase in the prevalence of FIP is that management of the domestic cat has changed.[71, 73] With the introduction of cat litter, more cats are kept permanently indoors, exposing them to large doses of feline coronavirus (FCoV) in the feces, which would previously have been buried outdoors. More and more cats are spending part of their lives in crowded environments such as at cat breeders or shelters, which increases their stress and chance of exposure to pathogens while in such an environment.

ETIOLOGY

FCoVs belong to the same taxonomic cluster of coronaviruses as transmissible gastroenteritis virus (TGEV), porcine respiratory coronavirus, CCV,[36, 53, 58, 59] human bronchitis coronavirus serotype 229E (HCV 229E),[8] and coronavirus-like particles.[14a] A comparison of these viruses and their pathogenicity for cats is summarized in Table 11–1.

Serotypes I and II

The isolation of FCoV in cell culture is very difficult, and only about 20 isolates have been made.[32] Laboratory strains of FCoV can be classified into serotypes I and II according to their growth characteristics in cell culture, cytopathogenicity, and comparative degree of neutralization by antisera to CCV.[45, 73, 102] FCoVs of serotype II are genetically more closely related to CCV than are FCoVs of serotype I,[32, 59, 102] and serotype II FCoVs seem to have arisen by recombination between serotype I FCoV and CCV.[32, 59, 102] Serotype I seems to be the more prevalent serotype in field infections.[32, 38] Each serotype is capable of causing a spectrum of clinical signs in cats ranging from asymptomatic infections to diarrhea to FIP.

Biotypes FECV and FIPV

Laboratory strains of FCoV vary in their ability to cause disease when administered to cats.[8] Some isolates are unable to cause FIP when inoculated intraperitoneally into cats and were named feline enteric coronavirus (FECV). It was believed, therefore, that in nature two biotypes exist of FCoV: FIPV and FECV, with differing potential for causing disease.

In the laboratory, FECV strains can infect and replicate only in enterocytes of living cats, whereas those called FIPV can also grow in macrophages in cell culture.[73, 91] Thus, different cell tropism of each virus was advanced as a possible explanation of different manifestations of disease. Thus, FECV replicated in enterocytes, causing diarrhea or asymptomatic infection, whereas FIPV replicated in macrophages, leading to systemic infection and FIP. Previously it was believed that FECV could not cross the gut mucosa and become systemic.[56] However, FCoV has been detected in the blood of

Table 11–1. Features of Coronaviruses That Infect Cats

VIRUS	HOST	VIRUS INFECTS CATS	CATS DEVELOP FIP	SEROCONVERTS CATS	INFECT HOSTS WITH FCoV	COMMENTS AND REFERENCES
FCoV[a]	Cat	+	±[b]	+	+	Designation for pathogenic coronaviruses that cause either diarrhea or FIP in cats. Previously termed FECV and FIPV. Can infect newborn pigs, producing lesions similar to mild TGEV.[68]
CVLP	Cat	+	–[c]	–	+	Observed in feces of cats.[14a, 45a] Not cross-reactive with FCoV. Not believed to cause disease in cats[45a, 68] but has been associated with diarrhea.[14a] May be excreted for 12 months PI.[45a]
CCV	Dog	+	–[d]	+	–	Causes diarrhea in dogs. Infected cats seroconvert but clinically normal after oronasal exposure.[8] Cats develop effusive FIP after IM or IP inoculation.[53] Shed from oropharynx of experimentally infected cats for 1 week but not feces.[8] CCV vaccines given IM can cause ADE in cats[44, 53] and one caused FIP-like signs in dogs.
TGEV	Pig	+	–	+	+[e]	Causes vomiting and diarrhea in piglets younger than 1 month. Replicates in villus tip epithelium of SI. Mutation in 1980 caused new variant: porcine respiratory coronavirus.[45] Can subclinically infect cats but no ADE with subsequent FCoV infection.[9] Serologic cross-reactive.
HCV-229E	Human	+	–	+	–[8]	Causes common cold in people. Causes asymptomatic feline infection with minimal viral replication and no ADE.[8]

[a]Includes so-called FIPV and FECV strains.[8]
[b]Diarrhea or FIP.
[c]Asymptomatic or diarrhea, may excrete in feces for up to 12 months.
[d]Oronasally infected, shed from oropharynx but not feces for 1 week although asymptomatic; can cause FIP if given parenterally.
[e]Develop diarrhea, lesions indistinguishable from mild TGEV infection; in the 1980s, a new TGEV variant called porcine respiratory coronavirus developed.
FCoV = feline coronavirus; CVLP = coronavirus-like particles; CCV = canine coronavirus; TGEV = transmissible astroenteritis virus; HCV-229E = human coronavirus-229E; ADE = antibody-dependent enhancement; + = occurs; ± = variable occurrence; – = does not occur.

healthy seropositive cats[31, 78] and cats that survived infection with the virulent laboratory strain FIPV-1146,[56] indicating that virus disseminates from the intestine in cats that do not develop FIP.

Comparison of the genomes of FIPV and FECV strains revealed deletion of the 7b open reading frame (ORF) in the FECV strain, which was postulated to account for lack of virulence in the FECV: all 4 FCoV strains with deletions are avirulent.[32] However, subsequent analysis of another FECV strain showed an intact 7b gene, indicating that deletions in ORF7b are not a universal distinguishing property of FECVs.[32] ORF7b deletions readily arise in in vitro passage,[32] but an intact 7b gene was found in all of 16 naturally occurring FCoV isolates. Although unknown, it has been postulated that the glycoprotein coded for by the 7b gene modulates the inflammatory or immune response.[32] An undefined soluble mediator in the ascites of cats with FIP causes T-cell apoptosis in local lymph tissue.[29]

Fed to immunosuppressed cats and given sufficient time, up to 10% of FIV-positive cats with the FECV-RM strain infection developed FIP.[75] Similarly, in natural infections, in households in which the endemic FCoV was thought to be FECV, some cats and kittens developed FIP.[5] Decreased suppression of the virus by the immune system may allow for increased virus replication. This, in turn, predisposes the cat to FIP development through increased virus load or because increased virus replication makes it more likely that a virulent mutation will occur.[73, 75] No specific mutation to account for increased virulence has yet been identified,[75, 102] but that is not unexpected given the large genome of FCoV.

It may simply be that kittens that develop FIP do so because they are subjected to a large virus dose at a time of life when their still undeveloped immune systems are also coping with other infections and the stress of vaccination, rehoming, and neutering.[5, 21b, 32] Furthermore, pedigree kittens and certain of the large cats (cheetahs[10]) may also be genetically predisposed to developing FIP.[21]

Clearly, in natural infections, wherever FCoV infection exists, so does the potential for the development of FIP.[5] In this chapter, the term FCoV is used when discussing the virus, unless it is meaningful to differentiate FECV and FIPV, and FIP is used to denote the disease state.

PATHOGENESIS

Cats become infected with FCoV by ingestion and possibly by inhalation of virus. The receptor for FCoV is an enzyme, aminopeptidase-N, found in the intestinal brush border.[9] The main site of viral replication is probably in the intestinal epithelium. Virus is shed in feces.[7, 31, 90] Virus may replicate in the tonsils[68, 90] and oropharynx[70] and is also shed in the saliva[51] in early infection. Figure 11–1 shows FCoV infection of an intestinal villus from a cat with chronic anorexia and vomiting, stained with anti-FCoV antibody by immunohistochemistry. As in TGEV infection in pigs,[15] humoral immunity associated with secretory IgA may be important in preventing initial infection of epithelial cells.[2]

FIP is an immune complex disease involving virus or viral antigen, antiviral antibodies, and complement. Cats that have no anti-FCoV antibodies do not develop FIP, and if FCoV-seropositive cats are decomplemented using cobra venom factor, FIP does not ensue. Complement fixation leads to the release of vasoactive amines, which cause endothelial cell retraction and thus increased vascular permeability. Retraction of capillary endothelial cells allows exudation of plasma proteins, hence the characteristic protein-rich exudate that develops in effusive FIP.[8] Neutrophils pass through the gaps between the endothelial cells and release lysosomal enzymes, causing necrosis of the vessel wall. The neutrophil is the characteristic cell type encountered in FIP granulomas.

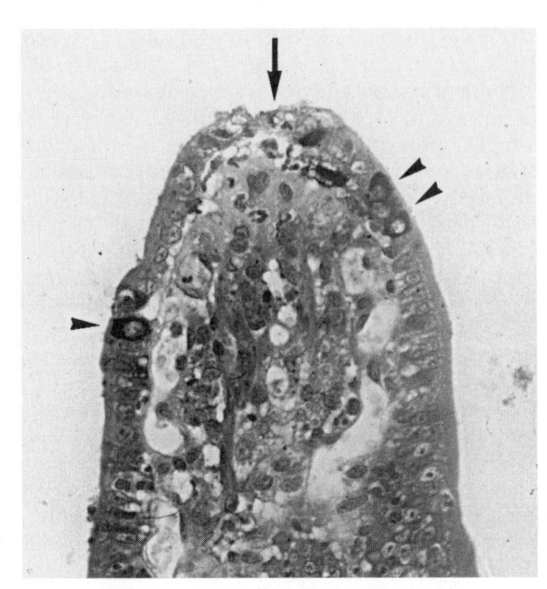

Figure 11–1. Small intestinal villus immunohistochemically stained to show FCoV infected epithelial cells *(arrowheads)* and ulceration of the tip *(arrow)*.

There are two possible explanations for the events following viral dissemination from the intestine. First, FCoV-infected macrophages leave the blood stream and enable virus to enter the tissues.[73] The virus attracts antibodies, complement is fixed, and more macrophages and neutrophils are attracted to the lesion.[73] Noneffusive FIP may be a result of a partially successful CMI response to contain the infection.[73]

The alternative explanation is that FIP occurs as a result of circulating immune complexes (CICs) coming out of circulation onto blood vessel walls, fixing complement,[60] and leading to the development of pyogranulomata. The pathologic consequences of the formation of immune complexes in vivo depend on their size, antibody, and antigen content. Immune complex deposition is most likely the site of high blood pressure and turbulence, and such conditions occur at blood vessel bifurcations. FIP lesions are most common in the peritoneum, kidney, and uvea, all of which are sites of high blood pressure and turbulence. Effusive FIP is usually the more acute form of the disease (although it can occur terminally in cases of noneffusive FIP). In cats that develop effusive FIP, there may be a large quantity of virus present, leading to the formation of great numbers of CICs and the destruction of many blood vessels. Noneffusive FIP may result from the production of fewer CICs or of CICs that neither attach to blood vessel walls nor fix complement efficiently.

The clinical and pathologic signs that occur in FIP are a direct consequence of the vasculitis and the organ damage that results from damage to the blood vessels that supply them. In effusive FIP many blood vessels are affected, hence the exudation of fluid and plasma proteins into the body cavities. In noneffusive FIP the clinical presentation depends on which organ is damaged distal to the blood vessel damage.

Antibody-Dependent Enhancement of FIP

In many infectious diseases, pre-existing antibody protects against subsequent challenge. However, in experimental infections of FCoV, an enhanced form of disease may occur in seropositive cats.[63, 73, 83, 98] The proposed mechanism of antibody-dependent enhancement (ADE) is that antibody facilitates the uptake of FCoV into macrophages.[12, 13, 37, 62, 64, 65] In ADE, a higher proportion of seropositive cats die compared with the seronegative controls, and the seropositive cats develop disease in fewer than 12 days compared with 28 days or more for controls.[83] By contrast, field studies have shown that seropositive pet cats that were naturally reinfected by FCoV showed no evidence of ADE. Indeed, the opposite occurred, because many of the cats that had become seropositive after natural infection appeared to be immune.[5] The mortality rate of in-contact cats at the time of initial FCoV infection was 14% compared with about 8% at the time of reinfection.[5] In practical terms, a seronegative cat introduced into a household in which FCoV was endemic would have a 1 in 6 chance of developing FIP, whereas a seropositive cat would have a 1 in 12 chance. Cats are at greatest risk of developing FIP in the first 6 to 18 months postinfection, and the risk falls to about 4% at 36 months postinfection.[5] Olsen[63] provided an excellent review of ADE of FIP.

Viral Shedding

FCoV is shed mainly in the feces. In early infection it may be found in saliva and possibly the respiratory secretions and urine.[31, 90] Historically, experimental infections of cats using laboratory isolates of FCoV indicated that the virus was shed for fewer than 2 weeks postinfection.[69, 90] Cats that proceeded to develop FIP had a second short burst of virus shedding just before they became symptomatic, and shedding was not detected when they were symptomatic.[90] However, the development of the more sensitive reverse transcriptase polymerase chain reaction (RT-PCR) technique has enabled virus to be detected in naturally infected cats. In this way it has been shown that naturally infected healthy carrier cats may shed FCoV for up to at least 10 months[31] and that 42% to 75% of cats with naturally occurring FIP disease shed virus.[7] Stress of pregnancy and lactation did not cause infected queens to shed virus.[21a] Because RT-PCR cannot measure the viability of the detected organism, the infectivity of the shed virus cannot be absolutely ascertained. However, a correlation between strong RT-PCR results and infectivity has been made.[21a]

It is likely that, when naive cats in a multicat household first encounter FCoV, all become infected (because they seroconvert) and probably most shed virus for a period of weeks or months. Most cats shed virus intermittently, but some become chronic FCoV shedders, reinfecting other cats whose immunity has waned.[21a]

The limitations of serologic testing are discussed later under Diagnosis. It is clear that seronegative cats (as determined by a *reliable* diagnostic test) do not shed FCoV,[2, 21a] whereas approximately one in three FCoV-seropositive cats does shed virus.[2] It is possible that cats with higher antibody titers are more likely to shed virus,[70] although cats with relatively low indirect fluorescent antibody (FA) titers of 40 to 80 have been shown to shed FCoV.[2, 6, 31] Evidence of virus shedding is never a good reason to euthanize a cat because most FCoV shedders stop within a year and less than 10% develop FIP.[6] In addition, if the cat has survived one exposure to FCoV, it may be better to use it for breeding rather than introduce new susceptible animals that may not be resistant, because there may be a genetic element to susceptibility to FCoV infection.[21]

Transmission

Transmission may be direct through virus-containing feces or saliva, by mutual grooming, and through close contact. Sneezed droplet transmission is also a possibility. FCoV is a relatively fragile virus but in dry conditions has been shown to survive for up to 7 weeks outside the cat.[82] Indirect fomite transmission is therefore possible. Probably the major sources of FCoV for the uninfected cat are litter trays and food bowls shared with infected cats.[74] Transmission by lice or fleas is considered unlikely.[8]

Transplacental transmission has been shown to occur because FIP lesions were found in a 4-day-old kitten and in stillborn and weak newborn kittens born to a queen that had FIP during the later stages of pregnancy.[70] However, this means of transmission is probably uncommon because most kittens that are removed from contact with adult virus-shedding cats at 5 to 6 weeks of age do not undergo seroconversion.[2]

Whether or not FCoV transmission significantly occurs at cat shows is unknown. Whereas in one survey showing cats appeared to be of minor significance affecting the incidence of FIP,[47a] in another survey more than 80% of cats at shows in the United Kingdom were found to be seropositive.[87]

CLINICAL FINDINGS

Initial FCoV Infection

There may be a brief episode of upper respiratory tract signs or diarrhea when FCoV first infects cats, although these signs are usually not severe enough to warrant veterinary attention. Kittens infected with FCoV generally have a history of diarrhea, sometimes stunted growth, and occasionally upper respiratory tract signs.[2] Many FCoV-infected cats are asymptomatic.

Coronaviral Enteritis

FCoV can cause a transient and clinically mild diarrhea[73] and/or vomiting in cats. However, occasionally the virus can be responsible for a severe acute or chronic vomiting or diarrhea, with weight loss, which may be unresponsive to treatment and continue for months. See the discussion of colonic or intestinal FIP later.

FIP

Two basic forms, effusive or noneffusive (dry), have been characterized. Approximately half the cats with FIP are younger than 2 years,[30, 34] but cats of any age can be affected. On evaluating the history, cats with FIP typically come from a multicat environment within the previous year, usually from cat breeders or rescue facilities. Occasionally, they have been to a boarding cattery, cat show, or veterinary clinic. Cats that have spent several years in a single-cat environment are extremely unlikely to suffer from FIP. Nevertheless, FIP, especially the noneffusive form, can incubate for months or even years.[95] Cats with FIP may also have a history of stress in the previous few months.[51, 79] Those with effusive FIP are usually presented to their veterinarians within 4 to 6 weeks of arriving in a new home, of elective surgery, or of similar stress, whereas cats with noneffusive FIP develop disease after a greater interval. Clinical signs may reflect the specific organ systems involved.

Effusive FIP. Cats with effusive FIP have ascites (although very few owners notice the abdominal distension[79]) and/or thoracic effusion. The cat may be bright or dull, anorexic or eating normally. Abdominal swelling with a fluid wave, mild pyrexia (39–39.5°C), weight loss, dyspnea, tachypnea, scrotal enlargement, muffled heart sounds, and mucosal pallor or icterus may be noted. In one survey, FIP accounted for 14% of cats with pericardial effusion, second only to congestive heart failure (28%).[81] Abdominal masses may be palpated, reflecting omental and visceral adhesion, and the mesenteric lymph node may be enlarged.

Noneffusive FIP. Signs are often vague and include pyrexia, weight loss, dullness, and depressed appetite. Cats may be icteric. Abdominal palpation may reveal enlarged mesenteric lymph nodes and irregular kidneys or nodular irregularities in other viscera. If the lungs are involved, the cat may be dyspneic, and thoracic radiographs may reveal patchy densities in the lungs.[96]

Cats with noneffusive FIP frequently have ocular lesions. The most common ocular sign in FIP is iritis, manifest by color change of the iris. Usually part or all of the iris becomes brown, although occasionally blue eyes appear green. Iritis may also manifest as aqueous flare, with cloudiness of the anterior chamber, which sometimes can be detected only in a darkened room using focal illumination. Large numbers of inflammatory cells in the anterior chamber settle out on the back of the cornea and cause keratic precipitates, which may be hidden by the nictitating membrane (Fig. 11–2). In some cats there is hemorrhage into the anterior chamber. If there is no sign of iritis, the retina should be checked because FIP can cause cuffing of the retinal vasculature, which appears as fuzzy grayish lines on either side of the blood vessel (Fig. 11–3). Occasionally, pyogranulomata are seen on the retina or the vitreous appears cloudy. Retinal hemorrhage or detachment may also occur.[93] Similar ocular signs can also be caused by infections with *Toxoplasma*, FIV, FeLV, or systemic fungi and are reviewed in Chapter 93 and elsewhere.[49, 93]

Of cats with FIP, 12.5% have neurologic signs.[79] These are variable and reflect the area of CNS involvement. The most common clinical sign is ataxia followed by nystagmus and then seizures.[48] When FIP causes meningitis, the signs reflect damage to the underlying nervous tissue: incoordination, intention tremors, hyperesthesia, behavioral changes,[96] seizures, cranial nerve defects, and unexplained fever. When the FIP lesion is a pyogranuloma on a peripheral nerve or the spinal column, lameness, progressive ataxia, or paresis (tetra-, hemi-, or para-) may be observed. Cranial nerves may be involved, causing visual deficits, loss of menace reflex,[48] and so on, depending on which cranial nerve is damaged.

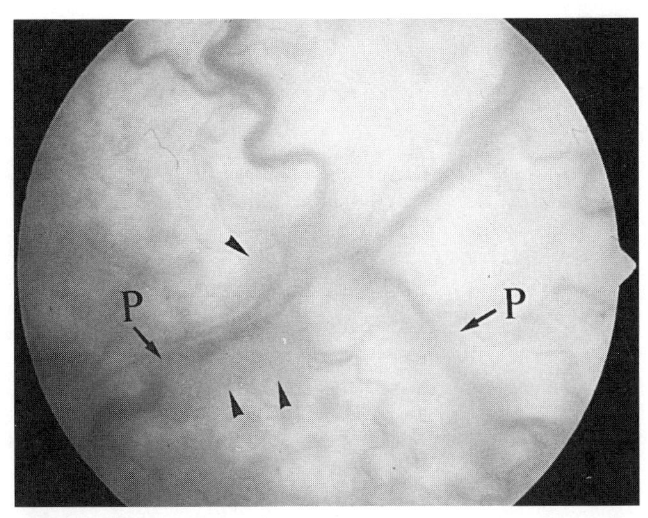

Figure 11–3. The retina of a cat with noneffusive FIP. The photograph is in focus, but appears cloudy because of the high-protein exudate into the vitreous. Cuffing of the retinal blood vessels appears as grayish lines on either side *(arrowheads)*. Retinal blood vessels can be seen disappearing into pyogranulomata (P). (Courtesy of John Mould.)

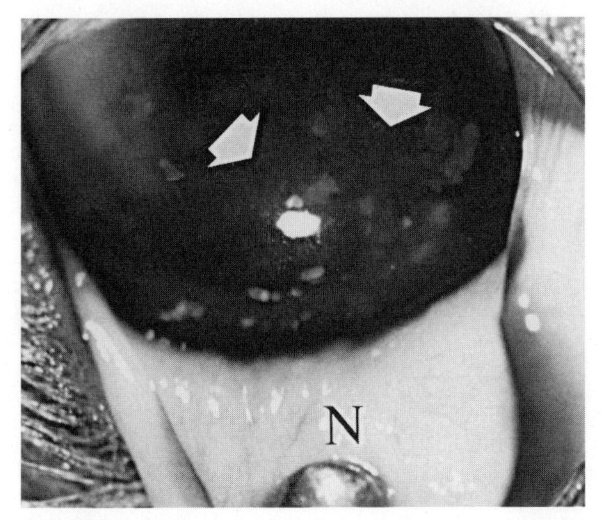

Figure 11–2. Keratic precipitates on the cornea *(arrows)* in noneffusive FIP. The nictitating membrane (N) has been deflected down to enable visualization of the precipitates.

In a study of 24 cats with FIP with neurologic involvement, 75% were found to have hydrocephalus on gross or histologic postmortem examination.[48] Because other diseases such as cryptococcosis, toxoplasmosis, and lymphoma have not been reported to cause hydrocephalus, finding it on a computed tomography scan is highly suggestive of a diagnosis of neurologic FIP.[48]

Colonic or Intestinal FIP. Occasionally, the main or only organ affected by FIP granulomas is the intestine. Lesions are most commonly found in the colon or ileocecocolic junction but may also be in the small intestine.[30, 97] Cats may have a variety of clinical signs as a result of this lesion: usually constipation, chronic diarrhea, or vomiting.[30, 97] Palpation of the abdomen often reveals a thickened intestine. A hematologic finding may be increased numbers of Heinz bodies.

Reproductive Disorders. In the 1970s, FCoV was implicated in various reproductive disorders and in fading kitten syndrome.[8] FCoV is no longer believed to be involved in fading of kittens from birth to 4 weeks of age,[3, 36] but it can cause death, by FIP, in kittens from 7 or 8 weeks of age and older.

DIAGNOSIS

Coronaviral Enteritis

There are no specific tests for this condition, and FCoV can only be assumed to be the cause of diarrhea in FCoV-seropositive or RT-PCR fecal–positive cats in which other infectious or dietary causes have been eliminated. Even biopsy is of limited use, because the histopathologic features of villus tip ulceration, stunting, and fusion are nonspecific.

FCoV infection may only be confirmed if immunohistochemical or immunofluorescent staining of gut biopsies is available.

FIP

At present, there is no single diagnostic test for FIP. Because there are so many organ systems involved, it is probably unlikely that any single specific diagnostic test will be found in the foreseeable future. In no other disease are good clinical skills as important as in the diagnosis of FIP. It is often helpful to consider effusive and noneffusive FIP in different ways, although there is overlap between them, and each may progress to the other. Various schemes and algorithms have been devised that give high predictive positive values of a diagnosis of FIP.[51, 79, 85] An algorithm for the diagnosis of FIP is presented in Table 11–2 and is followed in the rest of this section.

Clinical Laboratory Findings

The typical changes in both effusive and noneffusive FIP are neutrophilia with a left shift. There may also be a nonregenerative anemia associated with chronic inflammation. Many cats that are constipated from granulomatous colitis have an increase in Heinz bodies in the blood.

An important criterion is the albumin-globulin (A:G) ratio, which is especially useful when measured in the effusion. Serum A:G ratio decreases in FIP because, as the albumin level remains normal or falls slightly, globulin levels increase, possibly through stimulation of B cells by interleukin-6, which is produced as part of the disease process.[25] Thus, the total serum protein level is often high. FIP should be suspected when serum protein electrophoresis reveals a polyclonal hypergammaglobulinemia (differential diagnoses include lymphosarcoma, multiple myeloma or other plasma cell neoplasm, chronic infection, or FIV).[48, 55]

Measurement of α1-acid glycoprotein (AGP) may be helpful in the diagnosis of FIP.[16] It is an acute-phase protein that is raised in several infectious diseases of cats and is, therefore, not specific for FIP. However, AGP levels in the plasma or effusions are usually greater than 1500 μg/ml in FIP, a level that helps to distinguish FIP from other clinically similar conditions.

Other biochemical alterations will reflect damage to the organs containing FIP lesions and are not specifically useful for diagnosing FIP, but may help in deciding whether or not treatment is worthwhile. Hyperbilirubinemia may be observed and frequently is a reflection of hepatic necrosis. Despite this fact, the ALP and ALT activities are often not increased as dramatically as they are with cholestatic disorders, such as cholangiohepatitis and hepatic lipidosis. Analysis of CSF from cats with neurologic signs may reveal elevated protein (56–348 mg/dl, normal is less than 25 mg/dl)[48] and pleocytosis (100–10,000 nucleated cells/ml), the latter being neutrophils, lymphocytes, and macrophages.[48] Similar findings may be apparent in aqueous humor of cats with uveitis. CSF may be difficult or impossible to withdraw as a result of inflammatory cell accumulation.[48]

Effusion

The next most useful step in diagnosis is to sample the fluid, which in FIP may be clear, straw colored, and viscous and may froth on shaking because of the high protein content. The effusion may clot when stored refrigerated. If the sample is bloody, pus filled, chylous, or foul smelling, then FIP is unlikely,[79] although rarely it can be pink and chylous in appearance. The effusion in FIP is classified as a modified transudate in that the protein content is usually very high (> 3.5 g/dl), reflecting the composition of the serum, whereas the cellular content approaches that of a transudate (< 5000 nucleated cells/ml).[57] The protein content of the effusion is high because of the raised levels of gamma globulins; thus, a low A:G ratio on an effusion is highly predictive of FIP. An A:G ratio of more than 0.8 almost certainly excludes FIP,[57] and with values between 0.45 and 0.8, FIP remains a possibility.[51, 86] An A:G ratio of less than 0.45[88] in an effusion with greater than 3.5 g/dl of total protein and low cellularity, consisting of predominantly nontoxic neutrophils with or without macrophages and lymphocytes, is diagnostic of effusive FIP.[79] The main diseases with similar fluids are lymphocytic cholangitis and occasional tumors. Cytology of the effusion as well as radiographic and ultrasonographic findings may help to differentiate neoplasia, which, along with cardiomyopathy and liver disease, is the condition most often mistaken for effusive FIP.[34, 85]

Serologic Testing

Although frequently criticized, serologic testing has an important role in the diagnosis and management of FIP when it is done by certain methodologies and results are properly interpreted. Despite all the controversy, serologic testing for FIP can be useful if the laboratory is reliable and consistent, and the test results have been correlated with clinical findings. A single serum sample, divided and sent to five different laboratories in the United States, yielded five different results.[76] Methodologies and antibody titer results may vary between laboratories, but each should have established two levels. One is its least significant level of reactivity (or *low* positive titer) and another is its *high* antibody titer value. Antibody titers expressed in this chapter are those established by the authors' laboratory in Glasgow, Scotland. In searching for a reliable laboratory, repeat samples from the same animal should be sent without warning to the same laboratory and to a FCoV-referenced laboratory for comparison. Serum or plasma samples store well at $-20°C$ without loss of antibody titer. For a listing of some established laboratories for this test, see Appendix 5.

It has been said that more cats have died of FCoV antibody tests than of FIP.[72] At times, clinicians have mistakenly taken a positive titer to equate with a diagnosis of FIP. In addition, FCoV tests are often submitted for inappropriate reasons. There are five major indications to test for FCoV antibodies: (1) for the diagnosis of coronaviral enteritis or FIP; (2) for a healthy cat that has had contact with a suspected or known excretor of FCoV; (3) for a cat breeder; (4) to screen a cattery for the presence of FCoV; and (5) to screen a cat for introduction into a FCoV-free cattery. The specifics for each situation are summarized later.

Diagnosis of Coronaviral Enteritis or FIP. In diarrheic cats seronegativity rules out FCoV as a cause, but in seropositive cats FCoV may or may not be a cause of the diarrhea. In cats with suspected FIP, serologic tests are of limited use for two reasons. First, many healthy cats and cats with conditions other than FIP are seropositive. Second, some cats with effusive FIP appear to have low titers or to be seronegative because of large amounts of virus in the cat's body binding to antibody and rendering it unavailable to bind antigen in the serologic test. Although exceptions have been reported,[48, 89] cats with noneffusive FIP usually have a high FCoV antibody titer and are rarely seronegative; thus, coronavirus serology

Table 11–2. Algorithm for the Diagnosis of FIP

PARAMETER	LIKELIHOOD[a]	PROCEED TO:
A. Presenting Signs		
1. Nonspecific illness, anorexia, chronic recurrent, antibiotic-unresponsive pyrexia, with or without weight loss	3	B
2. Abdominal distention or dyspnea	3	B
B. Environment		
1. Single-cat household	1	C, H
2. Multicat household, cat breeder, humane shelter, in previous 6–12 mos	3	C
3. Stressed in previous 1–12 months (e.g., rehomed, neutered, gave birth, visited veterinarian)	3	C
C. Clinical Signs		
1. Ascites $\pm$ thoracic or pericardial effusion	3	D3, D4, D5
2. No effusion present		
a. Systemic: depression, icterus, renal failure, diarrhea, or constipation; neurologic or ocular signs present	3	D1, D2
b. Neurologic: ataxia, nystagmus, seizures, tremor, paresis or paralysis, circling, menace deficit, behavioral changes, head tilt	3	D1, D2
c. Ocular: iritis, uveitis, keratic precipitates, aqueous flare, retinal vascular cuffing, nystagmus, blindness	4	D1, D2
d. No ocular findings	1	E1, H2
e. CT scan: hydrocephalus	5	G
D. Laboratory Findings		
1. Hematology		
a. Left shift, nonregenerative anemia	4	D2, E1
2. Blood biochemistry		
a. A:G ratio < 0.45 High globulin ($\geq$ 35 g/l or $\geq$ 3.5 g/dl) High α1-acid glycoprotein ($>$ 1500 μg/ml)	5	E1, F3b
b. A:G 0.45-0.8 moderate globulin (25-35 g/l or 2.5-3.5 g/dl)	3	E1, F3b
c. A:G ratio > 0.8 globulin ($<$ 25 g/l or $\leq$ 2.5 g/dl)	0, 1	H
3. Effusion		
a. Clear, straw colored, clots on standing, froths if shaken	4	D4, D5
b. Pus, chyle (milky), or blood	1	H
4. Cytology of effusion		
a. Low cellularity ($<$ 5000 nucleated cells/μl) cells mostly lymphocytes, macrophages, nondegenerate neutrophils (no toxic change)	5	E
5. Biochemistry of effusion		
a. High globulins $>$ 32% A:G $<$ 0.45 α1-acid glycoprotein $>$ 1500 μg/ml	5	E
b. A:G ratio 0.45-0.8	3	E
c. Albumin $>$ 48%, low globulins $<$ 32% A:G $>$ 0.8	1	H
E. Serologic Testing		
1. Antibody titer		
a. High antibody titer	5	G
b. Medium to low antibody titer	2, 0	F
c. Absent antibody titer	2, 0	F2, F3, H
F. Organism-Specific Identification		
1. Histopathology compatible on tissue biopsy	4, 5	F2, F3
2. Immunohistochemistry: fluid or tissues		
a. Immunofluorescence or immunoperoxidase positive	5	G
b. Immunofluorescence or immunoperoxidase negative	1	H
3. Virus detection		
a. Nucleic acid hybridization positive	5	G
b. Effusion RT-PCR positive	5	G
c. Immune complex detection	4, 5	G
G. Final Diagnosis FIP	Done	
H. Consider Similar-Appearing Diseases		
1. Cardiomyopathy: thoracic radiographs, echocardiography; lymphoma (FeLV test, radiography, ultrasound, laparotomy, biopsy); liver disease (hepatic function testing, laparotomy, and biopsy); lymphocytic cholangitis	1	H2
2. Diagnosis uncertain; evaluate for diseases not listed above	Done	

[a]0 = Noneffusive FIP very unlikely; 1 = FIP unlikely; 2 = effusive FIP suspected; 3 = FIP possible; 4 = FIP likely; 5 = FIP very likely.

can usually be utilized to rule out a diagnosis of FIP in suspected noneffusive cases. The presence of a high FCoV antibody titer in a sick cat from a low-risk one- or two-cat household is also unusual and is a stronger indicator of a diagnosis of FIP than the same antibody titer in a cat from a multicat household in which FCoV is likely to be endemic.

Serologic testing should only be performed in the diagnosis of FIP in conjunction with a compatible history, clinical signs, and examination of the effusions or blood for high globulins and low A:G ratio (see Table 11–2). Serologic tests on ascites or thoracic effusions will give the same results as blood samples provided they have high protein concentrations that approximate blood. Seronegative cats with suspected effusive FIP can be examined further for the presence of virus by RT-PCR[17] or immune complex testing[78] when available.

Occasionally, healthy cats are considered to have noneffusive FIP simply because they are seropositive and have no ascites. This assumption is incorrect because cats with noneffusive FIP are clinically ill.

Contact With Suspected or Known Virus Excretor. Testing is usually done for one of two reasons. First, the owner wants to know the prognosis for an exposed cat. Second, the owner wishes to obtain another cat and needs to know whether the exposed cat is shedding FCoV. In either case, it is very likely that the cat will be seropositive because 95% to 100% of cats exposed to FCoV become infected and seroconvert approximately 2 to 3 weeks after FCoV exposure. The owner should be advised of this possibility and reassured that it does not necessarily indicate a poor prognosis. Most cats infected with FCoV will not develop FIP, and many in single- or two-cat households will eventually clear their infection and become seronegative in a few months to years. Adult cats can be retested using the same laboratory every 6 to 12 months until the antibody titer falls three- to fourfold. Kittens and adults that have been exposed only once often have a quicker reduction in antibodies and may be tested every 1 to 2 months. Some cats remain seropositive for years but are not necessarily virus shedders. A rise in antibody titer or maintenance at a high level does not necessarily indicate a poor prognosis for the cat. Thus, of 50 cats tested by the authors, antibody titers remained at 640 or over on at least three occasions, yet only 4 cats died of FIP. However, in a situation of endemic infection, a constant low titer of 20 or less is highly indicative that a cat will not develop FIP.

The aim of serotesting and segregating cats is to stop exposure of cats that have eliminated infection to chronic virus-shedding cats. To test for excretors, the lowest dilution of sample that a laboratory considers positive if reactive in its diagnostic test (least significant level of reactivity [LSLR]) should be ascertained. Laboratories have different techniques, and the LSLR level can vary from 1:10 to 1:100. In a laboratory that uses a LSLR serum dilution of less than 1:100 as negative, some cats that are excreting FCoV will be missed, because FCoV excretors with indirect FA titers of 40 have been identified.[2, 6, 31] Cats with sera that are nonreactive at lower dilutions by the indirect FA test (i.e., dilution $< 1:10$) have been shown not to excrete FCoV. Approximately one third of seropositive cats excrete virus,[2, 6] so if the cat is seropositive it would be unwise to obtain another cat unless it too had antibodies. After 3 to 6 months, the antibody titer can be retested to determine whether the cat has become negative. In a stable, isolated population of fewer than 10 cats that are mixing together, in which half remain seronegative, it is reasonable to infer that the other cats are probably not excreting virus. When RT-PCR becomes widely available, it may become preferable for direct testing for virus infection or excretion rather than inferring infectivity from antibody tests.

Cat Breeder Requests Testing. Cat breeders often request that their cats be screened for FCoV antibodies before mating. Such testing is worthwhile only if a reliable test is used and the laboratory's negative result is low (i.e., less than a titer of 10 or 20). If the cat is seronegative, it can be safely mated with another seronegative cat. If the cat is seropositive, then it can be mated with a seropositive cat, and the resulting kittens should be prevented from becoming infected by isolation and early weaning.[1, 2, 33] Alternatively, a breeder may prefer to isolate the seropositive cat, wait 6 to 12 months, and retest in the hope that it will have become seronegative.

Screening a Cattery for the Presence of FCoV. FCoV infection is highly contagious. If there are many cats housed in a group, then a random sampling of 3 to 4 cats will indicate whether FCoV is endemic. If cats are housed individually, it may be necessary to test them all. Cats in households with fewer than 10 cats that are closed to new cats and in those in which the cats are isolated from each other in groups of 3 or less often eventually lose their FCoV infection.[28] Retesting is worthwhile *only* if the cats are kept in these small groups and are not commingled. Testing every 6 to 12 months will establish when this is occurring because antibody titers fall, and an increasing proportion of cats become seronegative if chronic shedders have been removed.

Screening a Cat for Introduction Into a FCoV-Free Cattery. Once they have been established, seronegative catteries can be maintained free of FCoV by testing and isolating new cats before they are introduced. A seropositive cat should never be introduced; for safety, it should be assumed that they are shedding FCoV.

RT-PCR Testing

PCR is a highly sensitive technique for amplifying and detecting small amounts of DNA (see PCR, Chapter 1 and Fig. 1–3). Because FCoV is an RNA virus, a DNA copy must first be made utilizing the enzyme RT.

Virus detection would be clinically useful to veterinarians in two areas: (1) in confirming the presence of FCoV in cats that appear to have FIP but that are seronegative and (2) in detecting virus shedding for epidemiologic purposes. Virus detection in body tissues or fluids is not a useful prognostic indicator in the healthy cat because FCoV has been detected in the blood of healthy FCoV-seropositive cats.[31] Neither is absence of FCoV in the blood stream indicative that the cat is not going to develop FIP.[20] Furthermore, false-negative results are found. Detection or absence of FCoV in the feces or saliva is not helpful as a prognostic test. Cats that are chronic FCoV shedders are not at special risk of developing FIP.[21a]

Immune Complex Testing

Because FIP is an immune complex disease, detection of immune complexes may be a more accurate method of in vivo diagnosis.[4, 78] With a competitive ELISA, a positive result in an unhealthy cat was 97% predictive of FIP; however, immune complexes were also detected in 8% of healthy cats.[78] Negative test results did not exclude FIP: the test missed 25% of noneffusive FIPs and 42% of effusive cases.[78] The ELISA requires specialized laboratory equipment and is available only from the University of Leipzig.

Antigen Detection in Tissues

Virus detection by direct FA and immunohistochemistry can be applied to effusion cytologic or biopsy specimens but requires a specialized laboratory. Immunofluorescence can confirm the presence of FCoV in macrophages in the effusions of cats with wet FIP.[67] Both tests are commercially available (see Appendix 6) and are confirmatory tests in cases in which the histopathology is not typical of FIP.[94, 103] FCoV antigen has been detected in swabs made from the nictitating membranes of cats with FIP[41]; however, these results have not been confirmed by other laboratories.[94]

PATHOLOGIC FINDINGS

The essential lesion of FIP is the pyogranuloma. In effusive FIP, all the surfaces of the abdominal and/or thoracic contents can be covered in small (1–2 mm) white plaques (Fig. 11–4). Few other diseases have similar lesions, although occasionally miliary tumors or systemic mycoses can appear similarly. In noneffusive FIP, gross pathologic lesions can be much more variable; however, the kidney is frequently affected and should be examined carefully for pyogranulomata in the cortex (Fig. 11–5). In colonic FIP the colon may be thickened and appear grossly like alimentary lymphosarcoma.[30] In some cats, abnormalities are minimal, and a diagnosis can be made only by histopathologic examination. To diagnose FIP definitively, vasculitis must be demonstrated. The lesion consists of an arteriole or venule surrounded by a central area of necrosis that, in turn, is surrounded by a perivascular infiltration of mononuclear cells, proliferating macrophages and lymphocytes, plasma cells, and neutrophils.

For coronaviral diarrhea, FCoV infects the mature columnar epithelium of the tips of the villi of the alimentary tract, resulting in sloughing of the villous tips. FCoV can be demonstrated in the epithelial cells by immunohistochemical staining (see Fig. 11–1) or immunofluorescence.[70] There may be mild to moderate villous atrophy, and villi may be fused.[70]

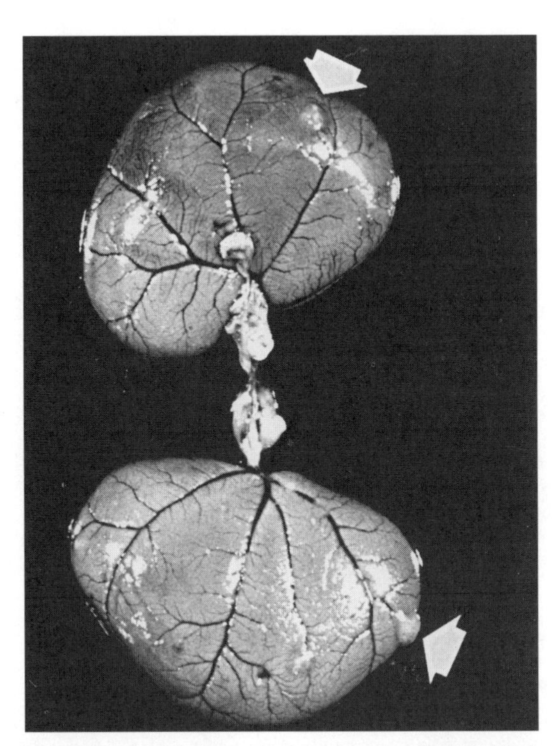

Figure 11–5. Bisected kidney of a cat with noneffusive FIP showing pyogranulomata *(arrows).*

THERAPY

Healthy FCoV-Seropositive Cat

There is no indication that any treatment of the healthy seropositive cat would prevent development of FIP. Treatment with glucocorticoids would conceivably prevent clinical signs from occurring, but immunosuppression might have the opposite effect and precipitate clinical FIP. However, because stress is a common factor in the development of FIP in infected cats,[79] avoidance of unnecessary stress, such as rehoming, elective surgery, or placing in a boarding cattery, may be beneficial.

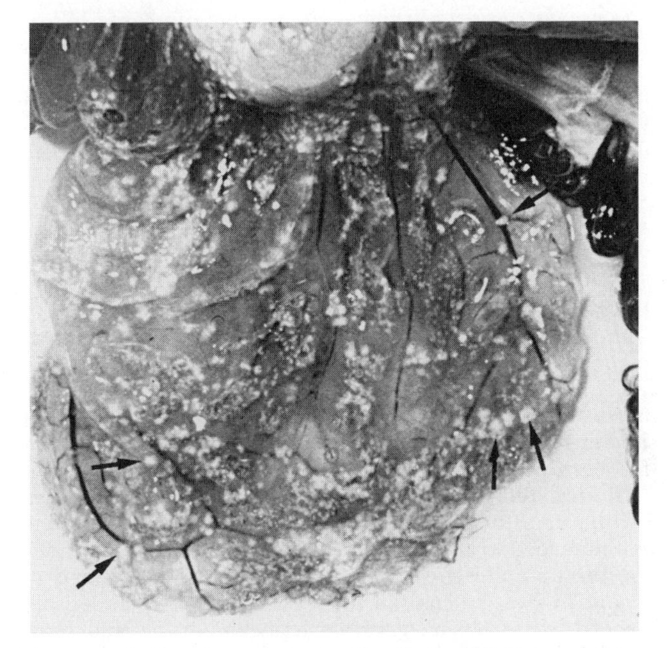

Figure 11–4. Omentum of a cat with effusive FIP. Note gelatinous appearance and small, white perivascular pyogranulomata *(arrows)* typical of effusive FIP on gross postmortem examination.

Coronaviral Enteritis

Most cases of coronaviral diarrhea are self-limiting. Cats with chronic diarrhea in which other possible causes have been eliminated, that are seropositive for FCoV, or in which FCoV has been detected in the feces can only be treated supportively using fluid-electrolyte replacement and restricted caloric oral diet with living natural yogurt as appropriate.[73] No specific antiviral treatment has yet been demonstrated to cure this condition.

Clinical FIP

Treatment for FIP is almost invariably doomed to failure because eventually cats with clinical FIP die. However, some cats with milder clinical signs may survive for several months and enjoy some quality of life with treatment. An exhaustive discussion of treatments outweighs the scope of this review, and readers are referred to an excellent review of the subject by Weiss.[105] A summary of his treatment protocol is presented in Table 11–3. Because FIP is an immune-mediated disease, treatment is aimed at controlling the immune response to FCoV, and the most successful treatments consist of relatively high doses of immunosuppressive and anti-inflammatory drugs.[105] Rest, avoidance of stressful situations, and a high protein diet may also help cats with mild clinical signs.[73]

PREVENTION

More than any other factor, management of kittens determines whether or not they become infected with FCoV.[1, 2, 21b, 33] Kittens of FCoV-shedding queens should be protected from infection by maternally derived antibody until they are at least 5 to 6 weeks old. A protocol for the prevention of

Table 11–3. Treatment for Feline Infectious Peritonitis[a]

DRUG	DOSE	ROUTE
Anti-inflammatory Drugs		
Prednisolone	2–4 mg/kg/day	PO
Cyclophosphamide (Cytoxan)	2.2 mg/kg/day on 4 consecutive days each week **or** 200–300 mg/m^2 every 2–3 weeks[b]	PO
or		
Melphalan (Alkeran)	2 mg/m^2 (1/4 2-mg tab) every 48 hr	PO
or		
Chlorambucil (Leukeran)	20 mg/m^2 every 2–3 weeks*	PO
Human interferon-α (Roferon)	*Effusive FIP*: 2×10^6 IU/kg/day	IM
	Noneffusive FIP: 30 IU/day for 7 days at alternate weeks	PO
Supportive Drugs		
Aspirin	10 mg/kg every 48–72 hrs	PO
Ampicillin	50 mg three times daily	PO
Anabolic steroids	Routine dose	
Ascorbic acid	125 mg twice daily	PO
Vitamin A (not beta-carotene form)	200 IU/kg/day	PO
Vitamin B_1 (thiamine)	100 μg/day	PO

[a]Use of all or a combination of these drugs together is recommended.
[b]Because persistent drug-induced anorexia may be associated with frequent administration of cytotoxic agents (i.e., daily or on 4 consecutive days of each week), some clinicians recommend that cytotoxic drug therapy be given by pulse administration of a large dose of the drug once every 2–3 weeks.
From Weiss R: *In* August JR (ed): Consultations in feline internal medicine. WB Saunders, 1994, pp 3–12. Reprinted with permission.

FCoV infection in kittens is presented in Table 11–4. When reliable serologic tests are available, kittens should be tested when older than 10 weeks to ensure that isolation and early weaning have been effective. Infected kittens younger than 10 weeks may not yet have seroconverted.[2] A protocol for minimizing the spread of FCoV in catteries is presented in Table 11–5.

There have been many attempts to develop effective vaccines, but unfortunately most have failed because of ADE.[44, 83, 98] However, a vaccine was produced (Primucell, Pfizer Animal Health) incorporating a temperature-sensitive mutant of the FCoV strain DF2-FIPV, which could replicate in the cool lining of the upper respiratory tract but not at the higher internal body temperature.[11, 22–24] This vaccine, administered intranasally, produces local immunity at the site where FCoV first enters the body—the oropharynx—and also induces a long-lasting CMI. The vaccine has been available in the United States since 1991 and has been introduced in some European countries.[18] Two concerns of such a vaccine are safety and efficacy.

Table 11–4. Protocol for Prevention of FCoV Infection in Kittens

STEP	DESCRIPTION
Prepare kitten room.	1. Remove all cats and kittens 1 week before putting in queen. 2. Disinfect room using 1:32 dilution of sodium hypochlorite (bleach). 3. Dedicate separate litter trays and food and water bowls to this room, and disinfect with sodium hypochlorite. 4. Introduce single queen 1–2 weeks before parturition.
Practice barrier nursing.	1. Work in the kitten room before tending other cats. 2. Clean hands with disinfectant before going into kitten room. 3. Have shoes and coveralls dedicated to the kitten room.
Wean and isolate kittens early.	1. Test queen for FCoV antibodies either before or after kittening. 2. If queen is seropositive, she should be removed from the kitten room when they are 5–6 weeks old. 3. If the queen is seronegative, she can remain with the kittens until they are older.
Test kittens.	1. Test kittens for FCoV antibodies after 10 weeks of age.

Table 11–5. Protocol for Minimizing FCoV Introduction or Spread in a Cattery[a]

PROTOCOL	DESCRIPTION
Reducing fecal contamination of the environment	Have adequate numbers of litter trays (1 tray per 1–2 cats). Litter trays should be declumped at least daily. Remove all litter and disinfect litter trays at least once a week. Place litter trays away from the food area. Vacuum around litter trays regularly. Clip fur of hindquarters of longhaired cats.
Cat numbers	Ordinary households should have no more than 8–10 cats. Cats should be kept in stable groups of up to 3 or 4. In rescue facilities cats should be kept singly and not commingled. In a FCoV eradication program, cats should be kept in small groups according to their antibody or virus shedding status: seronegative or nonshedding cats together, and seropositive or virus shedding cats together.
Antibody or antigen testing	Incumbent cats should be tested before introducing new cats or breeding. Only seronegative or virus-negative cats should be introduced into FCoV-free catteries. It is safer to introduce seropositive cats than seronegative cats into infected households, but there is still a risk of FIP in both the newcomer and the incumbent cats.
Isolation and early weaning	Both cat breeders and rescuers of pregnant cats should follow the protocol outline in Table 11–4.
Vaccination with Primucell	If new cats must be introduced into a household with endemic infection, they should be vaccinated with *Primucell* before introduction.

[a]Based on recommendations from working groups of the International Feline Enteric Coronavirus and Feline Infectious Peritonitis Workshop.[74]

Safety concerns are whether the vaccine can cause FIP or produce ADE. Although some experimental vaccine trials have recorded ADE on challenge,[54, 84] the overwhelming evidence from field studies is that Primucell is safe.[20, 21b, 77] In two double-blind trials, 609 and 500 cats were vaccinated with either Primucell or a placebo, and in both trials there were fewer FIP deaths in the Primucell-vaccinated group than among those cats receiving the placebo.[20, 77] Clearly, Primucell afforded protection from FIP and did not cause ADE. Furthermore, immediate side effects from vaccination such as sneezing, vomiting, or diarrhea were not statistically different in the vaccinated group and in the placebo group.[20] Primucell vaccination will cause seroconversion. Although this may be at a lower level than natural infection, it can still cause low positive antibody titers. Cats shed vaccine virus oronasally for up to 4 days.[11] Vaccination may stop cats from shedding virulent FCoV after subsequent exposure, although this effect needs further investigation.[46]

The recommendation for vaccination is to give two doses 3 weeks apart from 16 weeks onward. Although Primucell is recommended to be given to cats at least 16 weeks old, it has also been administered to 9-week-old kittens and found to be safe. In these kittens, the vaccine did not prevent infection; however, there was a significant reduction in the amount of FCoV isolated from the gut and mesenteric lymph nodes.[46, 80] Primucell seems to be safe to administer to pregnant cats and does not affect reproductive capability in breeding colonies or kitten mortality.[24, 80] Primucell is also safe to administer along with other vaccines or to FeLV-infected cats or pregnant queens.[24] Annual boosters are recommended. Because mucosal immunity is involved, the duration of protection after natural exposure or vaccination is short lived in most cats after virus is cleared, and reinfection is possible. Vaccine must be given periodically to maintain this immunity.

The efficacy has been questioned because the vaccine strain is a serotype II coronavirus, and the serotype I coronavirus is more prevalent in field isolates. A double-blind trial of 609 16- to 53-week-old vaccinated pet cats was conducted in Switzerland.[20, 52] At the start of the trial 358 cats were seropositive. Up to 150 days after vaccination, there was no significant difference in the number of cats that developed FIP. However, after 150 days there was only one FIP death in the vaccinated group of cats (0.4%) compared with seven FIP deaths in the placebo group (2.7%).[20] RT-PCR of blood from all of the vaccinated cats that developed FIP showed that virus was present in the cat before the vaccine was administered. Thus, many of the cats in which Primucell appeared ineffective had been vaccinated when they were already incubating FIP.[52] Because the vaccine works partly by stimulating local immunity, it is less effective if virus has already crossed the mucosae. Obviously, it follows that Primucell will be more efficacious in cats that have not been exposed to FCoV (or that are seronegative) than in seropositive cats. Clearly, an attempt must be made to prevent kittens from becoming infected with FCoV, by early weaning and isolation, before they are vaccinated.

The efficacy of Primucell, based on preventable fraction (see Vaccine Efficacy, Chapter 100) has been reported to be 50% to 75%.[73] In a survey of 138 cats belonging to 15 cat breeders, in which virtually all of the cats were seropositive, no difference in FIP deaths was found between the vaccinated group and the placebo group.[20] The manufacturers do not specify that FCoV antibody testing should precede vaccination. However, because Primucell will not work in a cat that is incubating the disease, FCoV antibody testing is beneficial. Because Primucell causes seroconversion and low antibody titers, testing before vaccination would be advisable.

References

1. Addie DD, Jarrett O. 1990. Control of feline coronavirus infection in kittens. *Vet Rec* 126:164.
2. Addie DD, Jarrett O. 1992. A study of naturally occurring feline coronavirus infection in kittens. *Vet Rec* 130:133–137.
3. Addie DD, Toth S. 1993. Feline coronavirus is not a major cause of neonatal kitten mortality. *Feline Pract* 21:13–18.
4. Addie DD, Jarrett O. 1993. Isolation of immune complexes in feline infectious peritonitis, p 60. *In* IXth International Congress of Virology Abstracts.
5. Addie DD, Toth S, Murray GD, et al. 1995. Risk of feline infectious peritonitis in cats naturally infected with feline coronavirus. *Am J Vet Res* 56:429–434.
6. Addie DD, Jarrett O. 1995. Control of feline coronavirus infections in breeding catteries by serotesting, isolation and early weaning. *Feline Pract* 23:92–95.
7. Addie DD, Toth S, Herrewegh A, et al. 1996. Feline coronavirus in the intestinal contents of cats with feline infectious peritonitis. *Vet Rec* 139:522–523.
8. Barlough JE, Stoddart CA. 1990. Feline coronaviral infections, pp 300–312. *In* Greene CE (ed), Infectious diseases of the dog and cat. WB Saunders, Philadelphia, PA.
9. Benbacer L, Kut E, Besnardeau L, et al. 1997. Interspecies aminopeptidase-N chimeras reveal species-specific receptor recognition by canine coronavirus, feline infectious peritonitis virus, and transmissible gastroenteritis virus. *J Virol* 1:734–737.
10. Brown EW, Olmsted RA, Martenson JS, et al. 1993. Exposure to FIV and FIPV in wild and captive cheetahs. *Zoo Biol* 12 1:135–142.
11. Christianson KK, Ingersoll JD, Landon RM, et al. 1989. Characterization of a temperature sensitive feline peritonitis coronavirus. *Arch Virol* 109:185–196.
12. Corapi WV, Olsen CW, Scott FW. 1992. Monoclonal antibody analysis of neutralization and antibody-dependent enhancement of feline infectious peritonitis virus. *J Virol* 11:6695–6705.
13. Corapi WV, Darteil RJ, Audonnet J-C, et al. 1995. Localization of antigenic sites of the S glycoprotein of feline infectious peritonitis virus involved in neutralization and antibody-dependent enhancement. *J Virol* 5:2858–2862.
14. Davies C, Forrester SD. 1996. Pleural effusion in cats: 82 cases (1987 to 1995). *J Small Anim Pract* 37:217–224.

14a. Dea S, Roy RS, Elazhary MASY. 1982. Coronavirus-like particles in the feces of a cat with diarrhea. *Can Vet J* 23:153–155.

15. De Diego M, Laviada MD, Enjuanes L, et al. 1992. Epitope specificity of protective lactogenic immunity against swine transmissible gastroenteritis virus. *J Virol* 11:6502–6508.
16. Duthie S, Eckersall PD, Addie DD, et al. 1997. The value of α1-acid glycoprotein in the diagnosis of feline infectious peritonitis. *Vet Rec* 141:299–303.
17. Egberink HF, Herrewegh APM, Schuurman NMP, et al. 1995. FIP: easy to diagnose? *Vet Q* 17:3/4–4/4
18. Eloit M. 1994 La peritonite infectieuse feline. *Rec Med Vet* 170:701–709.
19. Escobar JC, Kochik SA, Skaletsky E, et al. 1992. Immunization of cats against feline infectious peritonitis with anti-idiotype antibodies. *Viral Immunol* 1:71–79.
20. Fehr D, Holznagel E, Bolla S, et al. 1995. Evaluation of the safety and efficacy of a modified live FIPV vaccine under field conditions. *Feline Pract* 23:83–88.
21. Foley JE, Pedersen NC. 1996. The inheritance of susceptibility to feline infectious peritonitis in purebred catteries. *Feline Pract* 1:14–22.

21a. Foley JE, Poland A, Carlson J, et al. 1997. Patterns of feline coronavirus infection and fecal shedding from cats in multiple-cat environments. *J Am Vet Med Assoc* 210:1307–1312.

21b. Foley JE, Poland A, Carlson J, et al. 1997. Risk factors for feline infectious peritonitis among cats in multiple-cat environments with endemic feline enteric coronavirus. *J Am Vet Med Assoc* 210:1313–1318.

22. Gerber JD, Ingersoll JD, Gast AM, et al. 1990. Protection against feline infectious peritonitis by intranasal inoculation of a temperature-sensitive FIPV vaccine. *Vaccine* 8:536–542.
23. Gerber JD, Pfeiffer NE, Ingersoll JD, et al. 1990. Characterization of an attenuated temperature sensitive feline infectious peritonitis vaccine virus. *Adv Exp Med Biol* 276:481–489.
24. Gerber JD. 1995. Overview of the development of a modified live temperature-sensitive FIP virus vaccine. *Feline Pract* 23:62–66.
25. Goitsuka R, Ohashi T, Ono K, et al. 1990. IL-6 activity in feline infectious peritonitis. *J Immunol* 144:2599–2603.
26. Goitsuka R, Tsuji M, Ohashi T, et al. 1991. Characterization of a feline infectious peritonitis virus isolate. *J Vet Med Sci* 2:337–339.
27. Goitsuka R, Furusawa S, Mizoguchi M, et al. 1991. Detection of interleukin 1 in ascites from cats with feline infectious peritonitis. *J Vet Med Sci* 3:487–489.
28. Gonon V, Eloit M, Monteil M. 1995. Evolution de la prevalence de l'infection a coronavirus felin dans deux effectifs adoptant des conduites d'elevage differentes. *Recueil Med Vet* 1:33–38.
29. Haagmans BL, Egberink HF, Horzinek MC. 1996. Apoptosis and T-cell depletion during feline infectious peritonitis. *J Virol* 12:8977–8983.
30. Harvey CJ, Lopez JW, Hendrick MJ. 1996. An uncommon intestinal manifestation of feline infectious peritonitis: 26 cases (1986–1993). *J Am Vet Med Assoc* 209:1117–1120.
31. Herrewegh AAPM, de Groot RJ, Cepica A, et al. 1995. Detection of feline coronavirus RNA in feces, tissue, and body fluids of naturally infected cats by reverse transcriptase PCR. *J Clin Microbiol* 33:684–689.
32. Herrewegh AAPM, Vennema H, Horzinek MC, et al. 1995. The molecular genetics of feline coronaviruses: comparative sequence analysis of the ORF7a/7b transcription unit of different biotypes. *Virology* 212:622–631.
33. Hickman MA, Morris JG, Rogers QR, Pedersen NC. 1995. Elimination of feline coronavirus infection from a large experimental specific pathogen-free cat breeding colony by serologic testing and isolation. *Feline Pract* 3:96–102.
34. Hirschberger J, Hartmann K, Wilhelm N, et al. 1995. Klinik und diagnostik der felinen infektiosen peritonitis. *Tierarztl Prax* 23:92–99.
35. Hohdatsu T, Sasamoto T, Okada S, et al. 1991. Antigenic analysis of feline coronaviruses with monoclonal antibodies (MAbs): preparation of MAbs which discriminate between FIPV strain 79-1146 and FECV strain 79-1683. *Vet Microbiol* 28:13–24.
36. Hohdatsu T, Okada S, Koyama H. 1991. Characterization of monoclonal antibodies against feline infectious peritonitis virus type II and antigenic relationship between feline, porcine and canine coronaviruses. *Arch Virol* 117:85–95.
37. Hohdatsu T, Nakamura M, Ishizuka Y, et al. 1991. A study on the mechanism of antibody-dependent enhancement of feline infectious peritonitis virus infection in feline macrophages by monoclonal antibodies. *Arch Virol* 120:207–217.
38. Hohdatsu T, Okada S, Ishizuka Y, et al. 1992. The prevalence of types I and II feline coronavirus infections in cats. *J Vet Med Sci* 3:557–562.

39. Hohdatsu T, Tokunaga J, Koyama H. 1994. The role of IgG subclass of mouse monoclonal antibodies in antibody-dependent enhancement of feline infectious peritonitis virus infection of feline macrophages. *Arch Virol* 139:273–285.
40. Hohdatsu T, Tatekawa T, Koyama H. 1995. Enhancement of feline infectious peritonitis virus type I infection in cell cultures using low-speed centrifugation. *J Virol Methods* 51:357–362.
41. Hok K. 1991. A comparison between immunofluorescence staining on smears from membrana nictitans (M3 test), immunohistopathology and routine pathology in cats with suspected feline infectious peritonitis (FIP). *Acta Vet Scand* 32:171–176.
42. Hok K. 1993. Morbidity, mortality and coronavirus antigen in previously coronavirus free kittens placed in two catteries with feline infectious peritonitis. *Acta Vet Scand* 34:203–210.
43. Holzworth J. 1963. Some important disorders of cats. *Cornell Vet* 53:157–160.
44. Horsburgh BC, Brown TDK. 1995. Cloning, sequencing and expression of the S protein gene from two geographically distinct strains of canine coronavirus. *Virus Res* 39:63–74.
45. Horzinek MC, Herrewegh A, de Groot RJ. 1995. Perspectives on feline coronavirus evolution. *Feline Pract* 23:34–39.
45a. Hoshino Y, Scott FW. 1980. Coronavirus-like particles in the feces of normal cats. *Arch Virol* 63:147-152.
46. Hoskins JD, Henk WG, Storz J, et al. 1995. The potential use of a modified live FIPV vaccine to prevent experimental FECV infection. *Feline Pract* 23:89–90.
47. Kai K, Yukimune M, Murata T, et al. 1992. Humoral immune response of cats to feline infectious peritonitis virus infection. *J Vet Med Sci* 3:501–507.
47a. Kass PH, Dent TH. 1995. The epidemiology of feline infectious peritonitis in catteries. *Feline Pract* 23:27–32.
47b. Kipar A, Kremendahl J, Addie DD, et al. 1998. Fatal enteritis associated with coronavirus infection in cats. *Comp Pathol*, Accepted for publication.
48. Kline KL, Joseph RJ, Averill DR. 1994. Feline infectious peritonitis with neurologic involvement: clinical and pathological findings in 24 cats. *J Am Anim Hosp Assoc* 30:111–118.
49. Lappin MR, Marks A, Greene CE, et al. 1992. Serologic prevalence of selected infectious diseases in cats with uveitis. *J Am Vet Med Assoc* 7:1005–1009.
50. Lewis EL, Harbour DA, Beringer JE, et al. 1992. Differential in-vitro inhibition of feline enteric coronavirus and feline infectious peritonitis virus by actinomycin D. *J Gen Virol* 12:3285–3288.
51. Lutz H, Fehr D, Rohrer C, et al. 1995. Current knowledge on FIP from a European perspective; current concepts of the disease, current and future research, pp 22–27. *In* Proceedings of the AAFP Symposium on Feline Infectious Diseases, Washington, DC.
52. Lutz H, Fehr D. 1995. FIP vaccine view: evaluation of a modified-live FIP virus vaccine under field conditions in Switzerland, pp 47–50. *In* Proceedings of the AAFP Symposium on Feline Infectious Diseases.
53. McArdle F, Bennett M, Gaskell RM, et al. 1990. Canine coronavirus infection in cats; a possible role in feline infectious peritonitis. *Adv Exp Med Biol* 276:475–479.
54. McArdle F, Tennant B, Bennett M, et al. 1995. Independent evaluation of a modified live FIPV vaccine under experimental conditions (University of Liverpool experience). *Feline Pract* 23:67–71.
55. Mandel NS, Esplin DG. 1994. A retroperitoneal extramedullary plasmacytoma in a cat with a monoclonal gammopathy. *J Am Anim Hosp Assoc* 30:603–608.
56. Martinez ML, Weiss RC. 1993. Detection of feline infectious peritonitis virus infection in cell cultures and peripheral blood mononuclear leukocytes of experimentally infected cats using a biotinylated cDNA probe. *Vet Microbiol* 3:259–271.
57. Meyer DJ, Coles EH, Rich LJ. 1992. Evaluation of effusions, pp 125–130. *In* Veterinary laboratory medicine. WB Saunders, Philadelphia, PA.
57a. McReynolds C, Macy D. 1997. Feline infectious peritonitis. Part 1. Etiology and diagnosis. *Compend Cont Educ Pract Vet* 19:1007–1016.
58. Motokawa K, Hohdatsu T, Aizawa C, et al. 1995. Molecular cloning and sequence determination of the peplomer protein gene of feline infectious peritonitis virus type I. *Arch Virol* 140:469–480.
59. Motokawa K, Hohdatsu T, Hashimoto H, et al. 1996. Comparison of the amino acid sequence and phylogenetic analysis of the peplomer, integral membrane and nucleocapsid proteins of feline, canine and porcine coronaviruses. *Microbiol Immunol* 6:425–433.
60. Nafe LA. 1984. Feline infectious peritonitis. Topics in feline neurology. *Vet Clin North Am: Small Anim Pract* 14:1295–1297.
61. Norsworthy GD. 1993. Feline infectious peritonitis, pp 352–359. *In* Norsworthy D (ed), Feline practice. JB Lippincott, Philadelphia, PA.
62. Olsen CW, Corapi WV, Ngichabe CK, et al. 1992. Monoclonal antibodies to the spike protein of feline infectious peritonitis virus mediate antibody-dependent enhancement of infection of feline macrophages. *J Virol* 66:956–965.
63. Olsen CW. 1993. A review of feline infectious peritonitis virus: molecular biology, immunopathogenesis, clinical aspects, and vaccination. *Vet Microbiol* 36:1–37.
64. Olsen C, Scott F. 1993. Evaluation of antibody-dependent enhancement of feline infectious peritonitis virus infectivity using in situ hybridization. *Microb Pathog* 14:275–285.
65. Olsen CW, Corapi WV, Jacobson RH, et al. 1993. Identification of antigenic sites mediating antibody-dependent enhancement of feline infectious peritonitis virus infectivity. *J Gen Virol* 74:745–749.
66. Panzero RA. 1992. An outbreak of feline infectious peritonitis in a colony of Cornish Rex cats. *Feline Pract* 4:7–8.
67. Parodi MC, Paltrinieri GC, Lavazza A, et al. 1993. Using direct immunofluorescence to detect coronaviruses in peritoneal and pleural effusions. *J Small Anim Pract* 34:609–613.
68. Pedersen NC, Black JW, Boyle JF, et al. 1984. Pathogenic differences between various feline coronavirus isolates. *Adv Exp Med Biol* 173:365–380.
69. Pedersen NC, Evermann JF, McKiernan AJ, et al. 1984. Pathogenicity studies of feline coronavirus isolates 79-1146 and 79-1683. *Am J Vet Res* 45:2580–2585.
70. Pedersen NC. 1984. Feline coronavirus infections, pp 514–526. *In* Greene CE (ed), Clinical microbiology and infectious diseases of the dog and cat. WB Saunders, Philadelphia, PA.
71. Pedersen NC. 1991. Common infectious diseases of multiple-cat environments, pp 163–288. *In* Pedersen NC (ed), Feline husbandry: diseases and management in the multiple-cat environment. CV Mosby, St. Louis, MO.
72. Pedersen NC. 1991. Interpretation of feline infectious peritonitis virus serology, paper synopsis 17. *Presented at the British Small Animal Veterinary Association*, Birmingham, UK.
73. Pedersen NC. 1995. An overview of feline enteric coronavirus and infectious peritonitis virus infections. *Feline Pract* 23:7–20.
74. Pedersen NC, Addie D, Wolf A. 1995. Recommendations from working groups of the International Feline Enteric Coronavirus and Feline Infectious Peritonitis Workshop. *Feline Pract* 23:108–111.
75. Poland AM, Vennema H, Foley JE, Pedersen NC. 1996. Two related strains of feline infectious peritonitis virus isolated from immunocompromised cats infected with a feline enteric coronavirus. *J Clin Microbiol* 12:3180–3184.
76. Postorino Reeves N. 1994. Personal communication. Davis, CA.
77. Postorino Reeves N. 1995. Vaccination against naturally occurring FIP in a single large cat shelter. *Feline Pract* 23:81–82.
78. Reinacher M. 1994. Pathogenesis and diagnosis of naturally occurring feline infectious peritonitis virus infections, pp 9–11. *In* Proceedings of New Perspectives on the Prevention of Feline Infectious Peritonitis Workshop. SmithKline Beecham, Berlin.
79. Rohrer C, Suter PF, Lutz H. 1993. The diagnosis of feline infectious peritonitis (FIP): a retrospective and prospective study. *Kleinterpraxis* 38:379–389.
80. Rosen D. 1995. Overview of a modified live FIP virus vaccine, pp 73–77. *In* Proceedings of the AAFP Symposium on Feline Infectious Diseases, Washington, DC.
81. Rush JE, Keene BW, Fox PR. 1990. Pericardial disease in the cat: a retrospective evaluation of 66 cases. *J Am Anim Hosp Assoc* 26:39–46.
82. Scott FW. 1988. Update on FIP. *Proc Kal Kan Symp* 12:43–47.
83. Scott FW, Olsen CW, Corapi WV. 1995. Antibody-dependent enhancement of feline infectious peritonitis virus infection. *Feline Pract* 23:77–80.
84. Scott FW, Olsen CW, Corapi WV. 1995. Independent evaluation of a modified live FIPV vaccine under experimental conditions (Cornell experience). *Feline Pract* 23:74–76.
85. Shelly SM, Scarlett-Kranz J, Blue JT. 1988. Protein electrophoresis on effusions from cats as a diagnostic test for feline infectious peritonitis. *J Am Anim Hosp Assoc* 24:495–500.
86. Sparkes AH, Gruffydd-Jones TJ, Harbour DA. 1991. Feline infectious peritonitis: a review of clinicopathological changes in 65 cases, and a critical assessment of their diagnostic value. *Vet Rec* 129:202–212.
87. Sparkes AH, Gruffydd-Jones TJ, Howard PE, Harbour DA. 1992. Coronavirus serology in healthy pedigree cats. *Vet Rec* 131:35-36.
88. Sparkes AH, Gruffydd-Jones TJ, Harbour DA. 1994. An appraisal of the value of laboratory tests in the diagnosis of feline infectious peritonitis. *J Am Anim Hosp Assoc* 30:345–350.
89. Speciale J. 1994. Feline infectious peritonitis. *J Am Anim Hosp Assoc* 30:417.
90. Stoddart ME, Gaskell RM, Harbour DA, et al. 1988. Virus shedding and immune responses in cats inoculated with cell culture-adapted feline infectious peritonitis virus. *Vet Microbiol* 16:145–158.
91. Stoddart CA, Scott FW. 1989. Intrinsic resistance of feline peritoneal macrophages to coronavirus infection correlates with in vivo virulence. *J Virol* 1:436-440.
92. Suiter BT, Pfeiffer NE, Jones EV, et al. 1995. Serological recognition of feline infectious peritonitis virus spike gene regions expressed as synthetic peptides and *E. coli* fusion protein. *Arch Virol* 140:687–702.
93. Szymanski C. 1987. The eye, pp 676–723. *In* Holzworth J (ed), Diseases of the cat. WB Saunders, Philadelphia, PA.
94. Tammer R, Evenson O, Lutz H, et al. 1995. Immunohistological demonstration of feline infectious peritonitis virus antigen in paraffin-embedded tissues using feline ascites or murine monoclonal antibodies. *Vet Immunol Immunopathol* 49:177–182.
95. Toomey JM, Carlisle-Nowak MM, Barr SC, et al. 1995. Concurrent toxoplasmosis and feline infectious peritonitis in a cat. *J Am Vet Med Assoc* 31:425–428.
96. Trulove SG, McCahon HA, Nichols R, et al. 1992. Pyogranulomatous pneumonia associated with generalized noneffusive feline infectious peritonitis. *Feline Pract* 3:25–29.

97. Van Kruiningen HJ, Ryan MJ, Shindel NM. 1983. The classification of feline colitis. *J Comp Pathol* 93:275–294.
98. Vennema H, de Groot RJ, Harbour DA, et al. 1990. Early death after feline infectious peritonitis virus challenge due to recombinant vaccinia virus immunization. *J Virol* 3:1407–1409.
99. Vennema H, de Groot RJ, Harbour DA, et al. 1990. Immunogenicity of recombinant feline infectious peritonitis virus spike protein in mice and kittens. *Adv Exp Med Biol* 276:217–222.
100. Vennema H, de Groot RJ, Harbour DA, et al. 1991. Primary structure of the membrane and nucleocapsid protein genes of feline infectious peritonitis virus and immunogenicity of recombinant vaccinia viruses in kittens. *Virology* 181:327–335.
101. Vennema H, Heijnen L, Rottier PJM, et al. 1992. A novel glycoprotein of feline infectious peritonitis coronavirus contains a KDEL-like endoplasmic reticulum retention signal. *J Virol* 8:4951–4956.
102. Vennema H, Poland A, Hawkins KF, et al. 1995. A comparison of the genomes of FECVs and FIPVs and what they tell us about the relationships between feline coronaviruses and their evolution. *Feline Pract* 23:40–44.
103. Watt NJ, MacIntyre NJ, McOrist S. 1993. An extended outbreak of infectious peritonitis in a closed colony of European wildcats (*Felis silvestris*). *J Comp Pathol* 108:73–79.
104. Weiss RC. 1991. The diagnosis and clinical management of feline infectious peritonitis. *Vet Med* 3:308–319.
105. Weiss R. 1994. Feline infectious peritonitis virus: advances in therapy and control, pp 3–12. *In* August JR (ed), Consultations in feline internal medicine. WB Saunders, Philadelphia, PA.
106. Wessling JG, Vennema H, Godeke G-J, et al. 1994. Nucleotide sequence and expression of the spike (S) gene of canine coronavirus and comparison with the S proteins of feline and porcine coronaviruses. *J Gen Virol* 75:1789–1794.
107. Wolf AM. 1997. Feline infectious peritonitis. Part I. *Feline Pract* 25:26–29.

Chapter **12**

Feline Enteric Viral Infections

David A. Harbour

FELINE ASTROVIRAL INFECTIONS

Etiology and Epidemiology

Astroviruses were first described in feces from cases of human infantile gastroenteritis. They have since been identified in several other species, including cats. When negatively stained and examined by transmission electron microscopy, astroviruses appear as unenveloped, spherical particles approximately 28 to 30 nm in diameter, with a characteristic five- or six-point, star-shaped surface pattern, depending on the orientation (Fig. 12–1).

A limited serologic and virologic survey of diarrheic cats from the United Kingdom suggests that the infection is not very common; less than 10% of animals tested have antibody to the Bristol isolate. However, more than one serotype may exist, as in humans, in whom 7 serotypes are known.[6]

Clinical Findings

Only two cases of a natural astrovirus infection in cats have been reported in detail. In both cases, the illness was characterized by persistent green, watery diarrhea; dehydration; and anorexia. No hematologic abnormalities were noted, and the only biochemical abnormalities were mild acidosis and hypokalemia in one of the cats. Other variable signs were gas-distended loops of the small intestine, pyrexia, depression, poor body condition, and vomiting. Vomiting and diarrhea have been reported in another infected cat, although no further clinical details were given.

In an outbreak of diarrhea in a breeding colony, astrovirus was seen by EM in the feces of 25% of affected kittens. Initial signs in these kittens were inappetence, depression, and prolapse of the third eyelid. Other litters in the colony previously had developed a similar syndrome, with diarrhea that persisted 4 to 14 days. A number of adult cats were also affected. Sera from several of these animals had antibody to astrovirus.

Experimental oral administration of an astroviral isolate to specific-pathogen–free kittens resulted in mild diarrhea 11 to 12 days later. This coincided with a period of pyrexia and

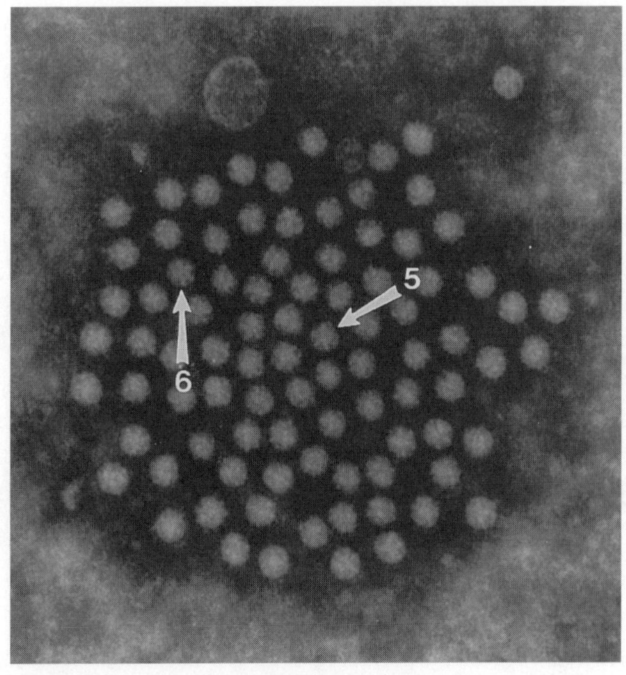

Figure 12–1. Negatively stained astrovirus particles. *Arrows* indicate particles with five- and six-pointed star-shaped surface patterns. (Courtesy of Charles Ashley, Bristol Public Health Laboratory, Bristol, U.K.)

virus shedding with subsequent seroconversion. The kittens remained otherwise well.

Diagnosis

Astrovirus infection is most conveniently diagnosed by EM of negatively stained preparations of diarrheic stools. It is possible to grow some isolates in cell culture, although no cytopathic effect is produced, and virus-infected cells must be located by specific immunofluorescence. Other isolates cannot be grown in cell culture at the present time, so this is not a viable method of diagnosis. Information on the sequence of the viral RNA is becoming available and should lead to improved methods of diagnosis based on molecular techniques, such as polymerase chain reaction (PCR).[1]

Therapy, Prevention, and Public Health Considerations

Treatment of affected animals probably is not necessary, other than to replace lost fluids and electrolytes if the diarrhea is severe or prolonged. No vaccine is available.

Human serum can contain antibody to feline astrovirus, but it is not known whether this finding reflects zoonotic infection or a serologic relationship between human and feline astroviruses.

FELINE ROTAVIRAL INFECTIONS

Etiology and Epidemiology

Rotaviruses are classified as a genus within the family Reoviridae and are of worldwide distribution. They can be distinguished from reoviruses and orbiviruses, when viewed by negative-stain EM by the characteristic morphology of the 70-nm-diameter intact virion. This looks like a wheel with the core in the center forming a hub, the inner layer of capsomeres radiating outward like spokes, and the outer layer giving a sharply defined rim.

Rotaviruses have been isolated from many species of animals and are the major enteric viral pathogens in humans and the main species in domestic livestock, causing significant economic losses. By contrast, although infection of cats is common, with up to 100% of populations being seropositive, clinical disease is rare.

Clinical Findings and Diagnosis

Feline rotavirus was first described in 1979 in kittens of 6 weeks and 8 months old that passed semiformed to liquid stools. The virus isolated from the 6-week-old kitten induced anorexia and diarrhea when given to a 3-day-old colostrum-deprived kitten. Subsequently, feline rotavirus has been recognized more frequently in the stools of normal cats, and a transmission study using a strain isolated from a diarrheic cat failed to produce disease in adult cats or kittens as young as 10 days.

Rotavirus may be readily demonstrated in feces by negative-stain EM or by polyacrylamide gel electrophoresis and silver staining of RNA extracted directly from feces. The latter method is more suitable for screening large numbers of specimens. A PCR method has been described that is considerably more sensitive than either of the other two methods.[7] Other methods, such as ELISA or latex agglutination, have been used, but they have been developed for group A viruses, whereas many feline isolates belong to other groups. Some, but not all, isolates can be grown in cell culture, but this is time consuming.

Pathologic Findings

Histologic findings include swollen intestinal villi with mild infiltration by macrophages and neutrophils. Viral antigen can be detected by FA, and virions by EM, in epithelial cells.

Therapy, Prevention, and Public Health Considerations

Treatment is symptomatic for diarrhea. Signs are mild and transient, and mucosal integrity is not impaired. Fluid therapy can be given IV or SC, depending on the severity of dehydration. There is currently no vaccine available for cats.

Rotaviruses of different hosts can infect other species when inoculated experimentally, but these cross-infections generally are asymptomatic. However, there is evidence from molecular studies[1a, 5] that feline rotaviruses have become established in the human population in Japan.

OTHER VIRAL ENTERITIDES

Torovirus-Like Agent

During the course of a microbiological survey of cats with the syndrome of protruding nictitating membranes and diarrhea, a novel virus was detected that hemagglutinated rat erythrocytes.[3] HI and immune EM suggested that the virus was torovirus-like, but PCR and thin-section EM failed to confirm this finding. The virus could not be grown in cultured cells. Experimental inoculation of SPF kittens induced mild, intermittent diarrhea and pyrexia with hematologic changes (principally neutrophilia, but one kitten also developed lymphocytosis). The agent appears to be ubiquitous, because the majority of cats have antibody against it, but its significance as an enteric pathogen is unclear. In another study, torovirus particles were not detected in the feces of cats with protruding nictitating membranes.[6a]

Feline Reovirus

Mammalian reoviruses all belong to three serotypes, and all three have been isolated from cats. Feline reoviruses have generally been considered to be minor respiratory or ocular pathogens, although they can readily be isolated from both respiratory and enteric tracts. Experimental inoculation of kittens with serotype 2 isolates, however, has resulted in the development of mild diarrhea.[2, 4] Feline reoviruses are widespread in nature as judged by serosurveys.

Other Viruses

A number of other viruses have been detected in the stools of normal and diarrheic cats, but their role as pathogens is unclear. These include parvovirus-like particles (serologically unrelated to feline panleukopenia virus), picornavirus-like particles, coronavirus-like particles (morphologically distinct from FIPV and FECV), calicivirus, "togavirus-like particles," and "thorn apple–like particles."

References

1. Jonassen TO, Monceyron C, Lee TW, et al. 1995. Detection of all serotypes of human astrovirus by the polymerase chain reaction. *J Virol Methods* 52:327–334.

1a. Mochizuki M, Nakagomi T, Nakagomi O. 1997. Isolation from diarrheal and asymptomatic kittens of three rotavirus strains that belong to the AU-1 genogroup of human rotaviruses. *J Clin Microbiol* 35:1272–1275.

2. Mochizuki M, Uchizono S. 1993. Experimental infections of feline reovirus serotype 2 isolates. *J Vet Med Sci* 55:469–470.

3. Muir P, Harbour DA, Gruffydd-Jones TJ, et al. 1990. A clinical and microbiological study of cats with protruding nictitating membranes and diarrhoea: isolation of a novel virus. *Vet Rec* 127:324–330.

4. Muir P, Harbour DA, Gruffydd-Jones TJ. 1992. Reovirus type 2 in domestic cats: isolation and experimental transmission. *Vet Microbiol* 30:309–316.

5. Nakagomi O, Nakagomi T. 1991. Genetic diversity and similarity among mammalian rotaviruses in relation to interspecies transmission of rotavirus. *Arch Virol* 120:43–55.

6. Noel JS, Lee TW, Kurtz JB, et al. 1995. Typing of human astroviruses from clinical isolates by enzyme immunoassay and nucleotide sequencing. *J Clin Microbiol* 33:797–801.

6a. Smith CH, Meers J, Wilks CR, et al. 1997. A survey for torovirus in New Zealand cats with protruding nictitating membranes. *N Z Vet J* 45:41–44.

7. Xu L, Harbour D, McCrae MA. 1990. The application of polymerase chain reaction to the detection of rotaviruses in feces. *J Virol Methods* 27:29–38.

Chapter 13

Feline Viral Neoplasia

Susan M. Cotter

FELINE LEUKEMIA VIRUS INFECTION

Etiology

Feline leukemia virus (FeLV) was first described in 1964 by William Jarrett when virus particles were seen budding from the membrane of malignant lymphoblasts from a cat with naturally occurring lymphoma. The virus was subsequently isolated and shown to produce a similar malignancy when injected into healthy cats. A member of the oncornavirus subfamily of retroviruses, FeLV contains a protein core with single-stranded RNA protected by an envelope. On the basis of similarities in nucleotide sequences, it has been determined that the FeLV evolved from a virus in an ancestor of the rat. FeLV is an exogenous agent that replicates within many tissues, including bone marrow, salivary gland, and respiratory epithelium. The virus is noncytopathic and escapes from the cell by budding from the cell membrane (Figs. 13–1 and 13–2).

Genetic Map and Viral Subgroups. The genetic map of FeLV, similar to that of the murine leukemia viruses, is summarized in Table 13–1. Three viral subgroups have been identified on the basis of interference testing, VN, and ability to replicate in nonfeline tissues (Table 13–2). All viremic cats carry subgroup A either alone or in combination with subgroup B or subgroup C or both. Although subgroup A may cause malignancy by itself, combination with subgroup B may have a synergistic effect on oncogenicity. Groups B and C have evolved by recombination between FeLV-A and endogenous proviral sequences contained in normal feline DNA. Subgroup C has been associated with nonregenerative anemia.

Viral Proteins. Feline viral core proteins, especially p27, are produced within infected cells and are detected by indirect FA testing. They may also circulate free in the plasma or are excreted in tears or saliva, where they can be detected by ELISA techniques. Although proteins are immunogenic, antibodies that are produced are not effective in VN. Core protein is not regularly expressed in the intact virion because it is masked by the presence of the envelope.

Reverse transcriptase (RT) (RNA-dependent DNA polymerase) is an enzyme characteristic of retroviruses, which allows these viruses to enter a cell and make a DNA copy referred to as provirus, which integrates in a stable fashion into a host genome (Fig. 13–3).

The major envelope glycoprotein (gp70) varies with the subgroup (A, B, or C). FeLV-A binds via its presumptive receptor gp70, type A to T lymphocytes.[8] Antibody to gp70 is subgroup specific and results in neutralization of the virus and immunity to reinfection. Thus, gp70 is important in natural resistance and as a target for vaccine production. Only subgroup A is transmitted from cat to cat. If antibody to subgroup A is produced, the cat is protected from all subgroups.

Feline oncornavirus cell membrane antigen (FOCMA) is present on the membrane of malignant cells but absent on all other cells of the body, even those infected with FeLV. Cats with high antibody titers to FOCMA are resistant to the development of leukemia and lymphoma regardless of whether they have positive or negative test results for FeLV. In the presence of complement, FOCMA antibody lyses tumor cells and plays a role in immune surveillance against tumor development.

When virus buds from the cell membrane, some host histocompatibility antigens become incorporated into the viral envelope (see Fig. 13–1). These antigens appear to play some role in the natural immune response when this virus enters a new host. These cellular antigens may serve as targets for neutralization of FeLV.

Epidemiology

FeLV spreads in a contagious manner, with no sex or breed predisposition. Approximately one third of all cancer deaths

Table 13–1. Summary of Genetic Map and Function of FeLV Proteins*

GENE	VIRAL PROTEINS		
	Location	Type	Function
gag	Core	p15 p12 p27 p10	Basis for indirect FA and ELISA tests, immune complex disease, and cytotoxic effects
pol	Core	RT	Copies viral protein into complementary DNA strand
env	Envelope	gp70	Type-specific antigens A,B,C; responsible for neutralizing or protective antibody against viral infection
		p15e	Viral immunosuppression

*As listed in chart, genes are located from 5′ to 3′ end with long terminal repeat sequences at each end. RT = reverse transcriptase.

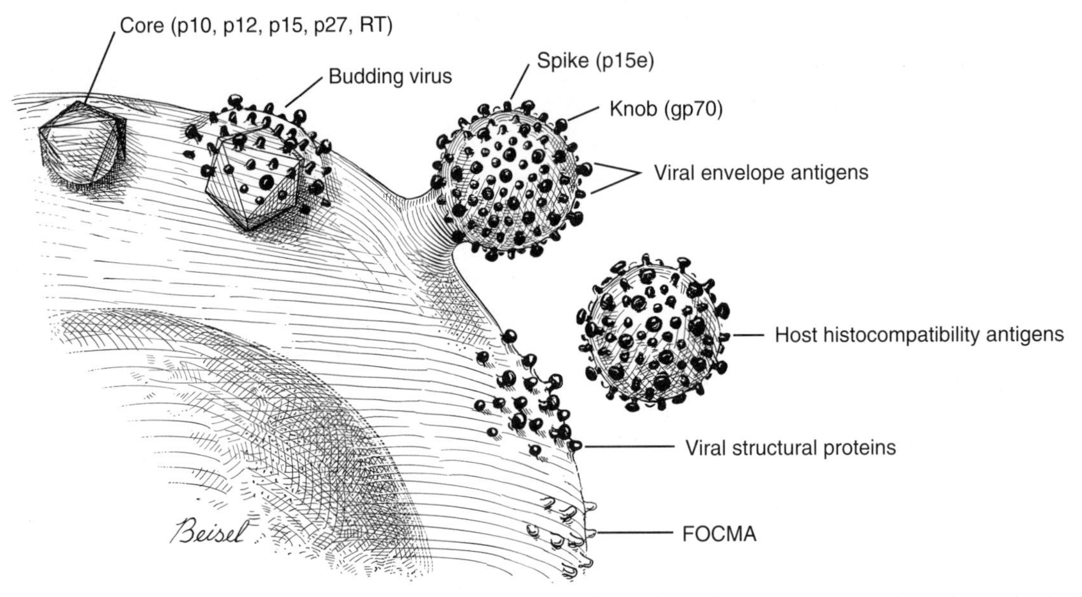

Figure 13–1. Production and release of virus from a feline malignant cell. Viral envelope antigens can be spike or knob shaped. Host histocompatibility antigens may appear on the virus; viral structural proteins may appear on the host cell. Virus replication can also occur in nonmalignant cells, but feline oncornavirus cell membrane antigen (FOCMA) is not on the surface of those cells.

Table 13–2. Subgroups of FeLV

VIRUS SUBGROUPS	FREQUENCY OF ISOLATION IN FeLV-POSITIVE CATS	ASSOCIATED DISEASE	COMPARISON BY SPECIES OF IN VITRO REPLICATION
A	100% viremic cats	Hematopoietic neoplasia, experimentally may cause hemolysis	Cat
B	Occurs with subgroup A in approximately 50% of cats with neoplastic disease	Not pathogenic alone, finding with A may increase virulence	Cat, dog, cow, human
C	Rarely isolated; possibly replication-defective	Nonregenerative anemia	Cat, dog, guinea pig, cow, human

Data from Jarrett O: *In* Hardy WD et al: Feline leukemia virus. Elsevier, 1980, pp 473–479. Used with permission.

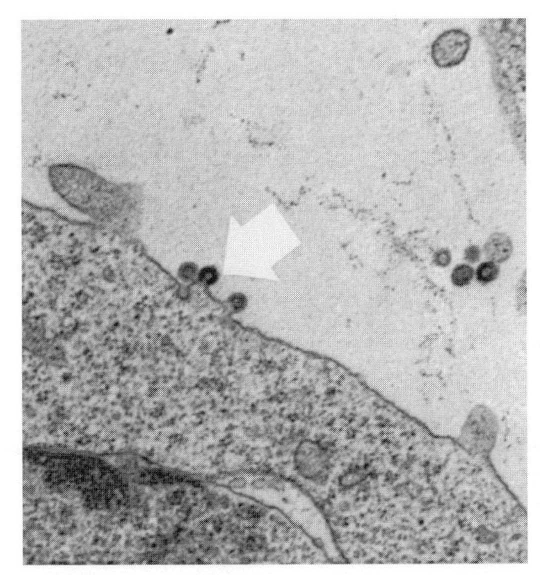

Figure 13–2. Ultrastructural view of FeLV budding from cell surface *(arrow)*. (Courtesy of SmithKline Beecham Animal Health, Exton, PA.)

in cats are caused by FeLV, but an ever greater number of infected cats die of anemia and infectious diseases caused by suppressive effects of the virus on bone marrow and the immune system.

Transmission of FeLV occurs primarily via the saliva, where the concentration of virus is higher than in plasma. Viremic cats shed virus constantly; the concentration in saliva and blood of healthy viremic cats is just as high as in those with signs of illness. Although the virus may enter many tissues, body fluids, and secretions, it is less likely to spread via urine, feces, and fleas. Iatrogenic transmission could occur via contaminated needles, instruments, fomites, or blood transfusion.

The viral envelope is lipid soluble and susceptible to disinfectants, soaps, heating, and drying. Virus is readily inactivated in the environment; if it is kept moist and at room temperature, it may survive for as long as 24 to 48 hours. Close contact, therefore, is required for spread of infection.

FeLV is maintained in nature because viremic cats may live and shed virus for several years. Because of latency, viremia is sometimes detected in middle-aged cats that have lived alone indoors since adopted as kittens. Because of lability, a prolonged waiting period is not needed before introducing a new cat in a household after removal of a viremic cat. FeLV is not a hazard in a veterinary hospital or boarding kennel as long as cats are housed separately and routine cage disinfection and hand washing are performed between cats.

Neonatal kittens may be infected transplacentally, but more are infected when the queen licks them and nurses them. Studies in a household with many viremic cats showed that 7 of 10 kittens placed there at 3 months of age became viremic within 5 months, whereas only 3 of 17 adults in the same house became viremic over a 7-year period.[4] Experimental infection of kittens older than 4 months is difficult to accomplish. Kittens are more susceptible to infection than are adults, possibly because macrophage function matures with age.[18]

Pathogenesis

Sequential pathogenesis of FeLV infection has been determined by experimental studies and is summarized in Figure 13–4.[48] The initial infection may be characterized by malaise and lymphadenopathy from lymphocytic hyperplasia. If the immune response does not intervene, the FeLV spreads to the bone marrow and infects hematopoietic precursor cells.

Latent Infections. Cats that are transiently viremic may develop persistent infection of the bone marrow and clear the viremia because neutralizing antibody prevents viral expression. Virus has been isolated from the marrow of approximately 50% of a group of experimentally infected cats up to 3 months after recovery from viremia. In one study, 5 of 19 previously challenge-exposed cats that tested FeLV negative by ELISA had FeLV-specific antigens detected in tissues, marrow, spleen, lymph node, and small intestine more than 1 year later.[13] Once the marrow has been infected, virus could remain integrated in a small number of cells for a long time, kept in check by a partial immune response. As antibody concentration increases, virus production decreases. When the number of virus-producing cells is small, antibody production decreases, permitting proliferation of virus. Latent infection can be present even though the blood and marrow are negative for virus by FA, ELISA, or viral culture (Table 13–3; see Fig. 13–4). Some infected cats, known as immune carriers, are repeatedly ELISA positive and FA negative. Cats that test as immune carriers early in the postexposure period, before either established bone marrow infection, may clear the viremia to become latent or recovered cats. Immune carriers are more likely to eliminate the infection than are persistently viremic cats that test positive on both ELISA and FA. The presence of latent virus can be demonstrated in research laboratories when the virus is allowed to grow in vitro, thereby bypassing the effects of the immune system. Viral latency helps explain relapsing viremias, protracted incubation periods, and persistent high titers of antiviral and anti-

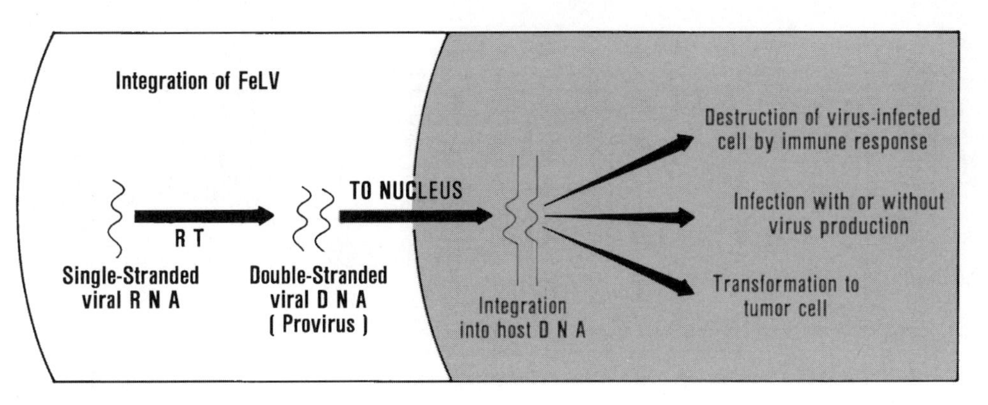

Figure 13–3. Formation of FeLV and integration into cells. (RT, reverse transcriptase.)

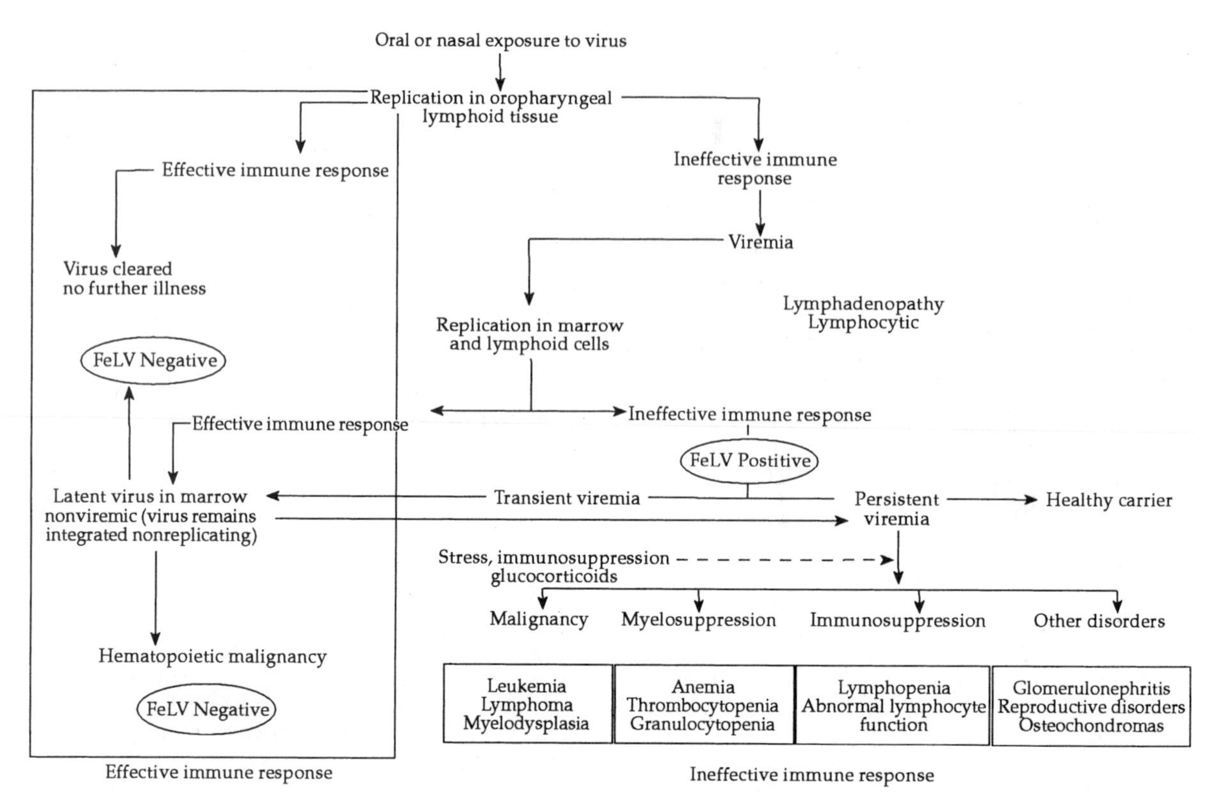

Figure 13–4. Pathogenesis of FeLV infection.

FOCMA antibodies. Latent infections may also explain how myelodysplasia or hematopoietic malignancy could be FeLV related in FeLV-negative cats. Latently infected queens stressed by pregnancy have reverted to overt viremia and have transmitted FeLV to their kittens. Exogenous glucocorticoids produce similar effects. Most latent infections are not clinically significant because viral reactivation is unusual. Latent infections tend to disappear over time. Latency is probably a stage in the elimination process of the virus. Less than 1% of experimentally transiently infected cats had long-term detectable latent infections. So long as the infection remains latent, these cats are not contagious.

Environmental Factors. The prevalence of hematopoietic malignancy, myelosuppression, and infectious diseases is higher in FeLV-infected, multicat households than in the general population. The death rate of healthy persistently viremic cats in multicat households is approximately 50% in 2 years and 80% in 3 years. Survival rates for persistently viremic cats kept indoors in single-cat households is likely to be better than that. As noted previously, immune carrier and latently infected cats have better chances of survival and potential recovery.

Many cats with FeLV in cluster households have antibody titers to FOCMA. Those with the highest titers are most likely to remain healthy. Correlation between FOCMA antibody and VN antibody titers is not absolute; however, many cats immune to FeLV have high FOCMA antibody titers as well. Neither FOCMA nor VN antibodies remain protective indefinitely, so these tests have minimal long-term prognostic significance (Table 13–4). In cluster households, some cats that were initially viremic with a high FOCMA antibody titer have been observed to develop leukemia or lymphoma months to years later after the titer declined.

Prevalence of Viremia. In 1975, approximately 1% to 2% of clinically healthy Boston cats were positive for FeLV based on FA testing; with ELISA testing and inclusion of ill cats, the prevalence would be expected to be higher. Over the past 20 years, a decrease in prevalence of infection has been observed, although comparable populations and methods have not been used.[45, 55] The Tufts Veterinary Diagnostic Lab-

Table 13–3. Classification of FeLV Infection Based on Viral and Immune Testing

FeLV STATUS	FeLV ANTIGENS TEST RESULTS: Blood ELISA	Indirect FA	Marrow Indirect FA	VIRUS-POSITIVE BONE MARROW CULTIVATION	ELEVATED SERUM NEUTRALIZING ANTIBODY	ELEVATED SERUM FOCMA ANTIBODY
Never exposed	−	−	−	−	−	−
Recovered	−	−	−	−	±	±
Latent	−	−	−	+	+	±
Immune carrier	+	−	−	+	+	±
Persistently viremic	+	+	+	+	−	±

+ = results postive; − = results negative; ± = results variable.

Table 13–4. Comparison of Diagnostic Tests Related to FeLV

TEST	SUBSTANCE DETECTED	SIGNIFICANCE	PROGNOSTIC VALUE OF TEST
FeLV test (indirect FA, ELISA)	Antigen p27	Detects viremia	Valuable: positive test indicates increased risk of leukemia, lymphoma, marrow suppression, immunosuppresson
FOCMA antibody test	Antibody against malignant cell	Protects against leukemia, lymphoma	Poor: titer can change with time. FeLV-positive cats with positive titers can die of nonmalignant disease
Neutralizing antibody test	Antibody against virus envelope	Protects against viremia	Poor: titer can change with time

oratory annually evaluates 1500 to 2400 ELISA tests submitted by practitioners on both healthy and ill cats. A gradual but significant decline has occurred in the number of positive test results from 8% in 1989 to 4% in 1995.[6] A major reason is widespread routine testing of kittens, which has also been successful in eradicating FeLV from catteries and shelters. The availability of effective vaccines has been an additional factor.[48a]

In the past 10 years, a similar but even more dramatic reduction in prevalence of viremia has been noted in cats with lymphoma.[39, 42] In 1975 a survey of 74 Boston area cats with lymphoblastic leukemia or lymphoma showed that 70% were viremic, but only 3 cats had the alimentary form.[4] Between 1988 and 1994, 72% of all feline lymphomas treated at the Animal Medical Center were of the alimentary form, and only 8% of affected cats were FeLV positive. The change may be related to a decreased overall prevalence of FeLV rather than a true increase in FeLV-negative tumors. In addition, most viremic cats become infected at a young age and die within 3 years; few survive to develop malignancy, and when they do, they are often viremic. The majority of cats older than 8 years that develop leukemia or lymphoma are not viremic. Furthermore, more than 90% of feline leukemias and lymphomas are of T-cell origin, but those involving the GI tract are usually of B-cell origin and unlikely to be associated with virus.

The prevalence of lymphomas caused by FeLV may be higher than indicated by conventional ELISA or FA testing. Cats from FeLV-cluster households had a 40-fold higher rate of development of FeLV-negative lymphomas than did those from the general population. FeLV-negative lymphomas have also occurred in laboratory cats known to have been infected previously with virus.[47] The FeLV-negative tumor cells are uniformly positive for FOCMA, giving further evidence for a causal role for FeLV. Newer techniques, such as polymerase chain reaction (PCR), detected proviral DNA in formalin-fixed, paraffin-embedded tumor tissue in 7 of 11 FeLV-negative cats with lymphoma.[21] However, another group found evidence of provirus in only 1 of 22 FeLV-negative lymphomas.[51]

Cell Transformation. The mechanism by which FeLV causes malignancy may be by insertion into the genome near a cellular oncogene, most commonly *myc,* resulting in activation and overexpression of that gene. This effect leads to uncontrolled proliferation of that cell (clone). In the absence of an appropriate immune response, a monoclonal malignancy results. The virus may also incorporate the oncogene to form a recombinant virus containing oncogene sequences that are then rearranged and activated. In a study of 119 lymphomas, transduction or insertion of the *myc* locus occurred in 38 (32%).[57]

Clinical Findings

Lymphoma. The incidence of feline leukemia and lymphoma as estimated in the 1960s was 200 cases/100,000 cats/year. Feline lymphomas are most commonly high grade with an immunoblastic or a lymphoblastic morphology, but they may be mixed lymphoblastic and lymphocytic or occasionally low- grade lymphocytic (Fig. 13–5).[58]

Mediastinal lymphoma, previously the most prevalent site in cats, is now seen less frequently. The tumor arises in the area of the thymus and eventually causes a malignant pleural effusion (Figs. 13–6 and 13–7). The fluid-nucleated cell count is usually greater than 8000/μl; the majority are large immature lymphocytes. The most common presenting sign is dyspnea, but sometimes regurgitation from pressure on the esophagus or Horner's syndrome from pressure on sympathetic nerves at the thoracic inlet is present.

Alimentary lymphoma occurs primarily in older cats and is usually FeLV negative. Clinical signs of alimentary lymphoma include vomiting or diarrhea, but many cats present with anorexia and weight loss only.[37] Tumors of the stomach and intestines may be focal or diffuse, and mesenteric lymph nodes are usually involved.

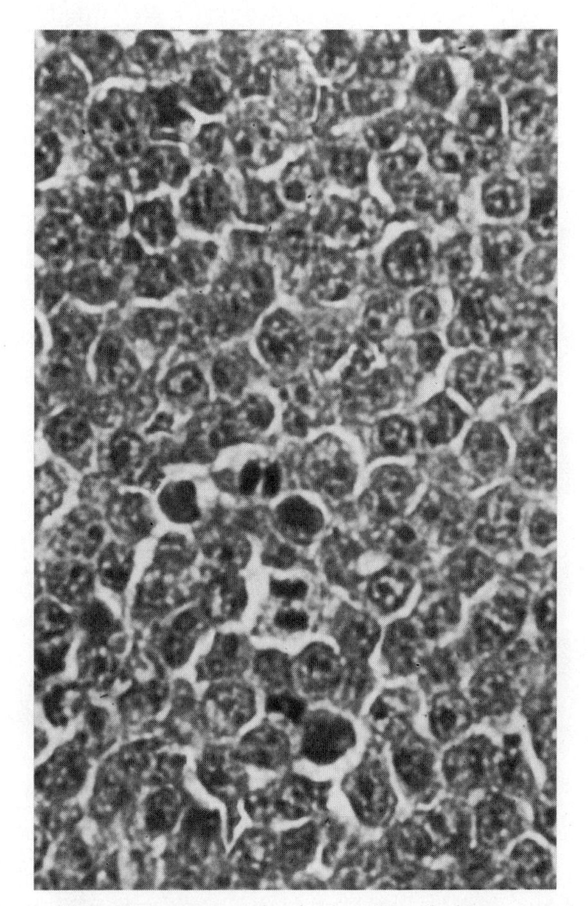

Figure 13–5. Photomicrograph of a lymph node biopsy specimen from a cat with lymphoblastic lymphoma. The architecture of the node has been replaced by a diffuse population of large lymphocytes, many of which contain nucleoli (hematoxylin and eosin, × 400).

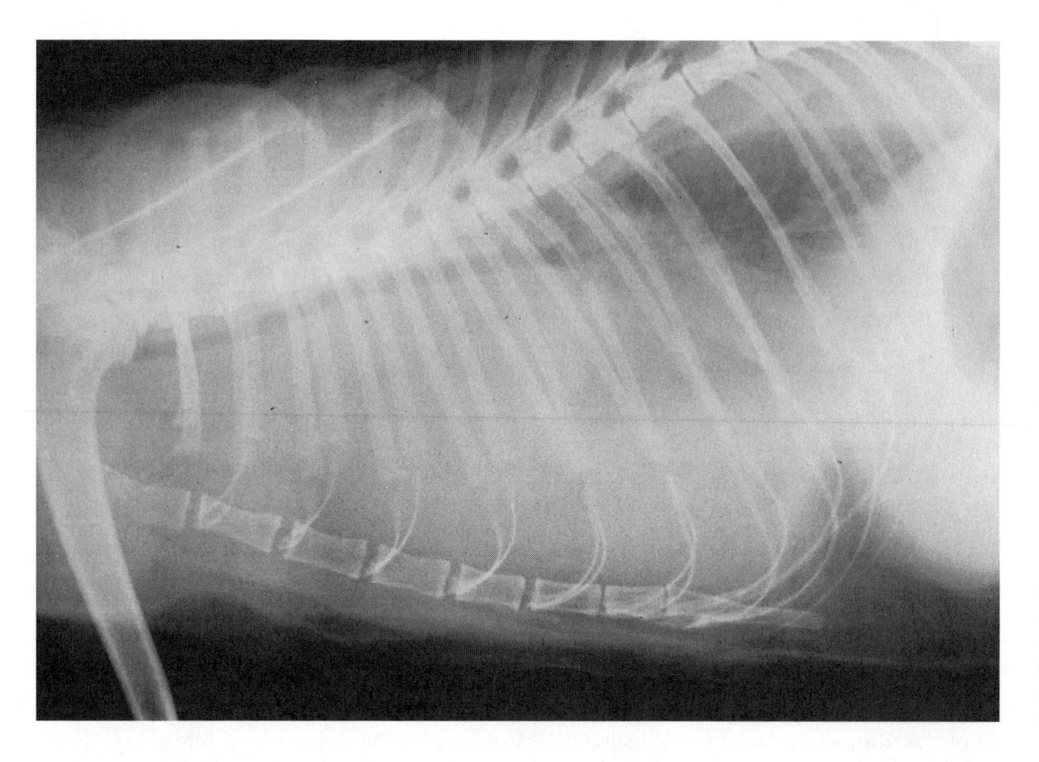

Figure 13–6. Lateral thoracic radiograph of a cat with severe pleural effusion and a mediastinal mass. The trachea is displaced dorsally, and the cardiac shadow is not visualized.

Lymphoma is classified as multicentric if there is major involvement of several sites. Any organ may be involved, such as the retrobulbar area, nasal cavity, gingiva, skin, liver, urinary bladder, brain, and lungs. Renal lymphoma is usually bilateral and does not cause signs of illness until the kidneys are extensively infiltrated so that renal failure occurs. Kidneys are enlarged and usually irregular. Epidural lymphoma may cause sudden or gradual onset of posterior paralysis (Fig. 13–8). The bone marrow is involved in about 70% of these cats even though a CBC may be normal. If the marrow is normal, the diagnosis may be confirmed only by myelography and laminectomy.[29, 53]

Leukemia. All hematopoietic cell lines are susceptible to transformation by FeLV. Thus, lymphoid and myeloid (including granulocytic, erythroid, and megakaryocytic) types occur. In acute leukemia of any type, the marrow is filled with blast cells, and normal hematopoiesis is suppressed. Clinical signs with acute leukemia are related to the loss of normal hematopoietic cells: anemia (lethargy), granulocytopenia (sepsis), and thrombocytopenia (bleeding). Splenomegaly is frequently present, sometimes with malignant infiltration and sometimes with extramedullary hematopoiesis. Diagnosis of acute leukemia is made by CBC and bone marrow examinations. In cats with large numbers of circulating blast cells, the CBC may in itself be diagnostic. Although classifications have been proposed for the acute leukemias, the predominant cell type may be difficult to identify even with histochemical stains. Especially for the nonlymphoid leukemias, transformation occurs at or very close to the stem cell level so that more than one cell line may be affected. The nonlymphoid leukemias are sometimes referred to as myeloproliferative disorders.

Chronic leukemias are rare in the cat and are not known to be associated with FeLV. The chronic leukemias include well-differentiated chronic lymphocytic leukemia (CLL), chronic myelogenous leukemia (CML), polycythemia vera,

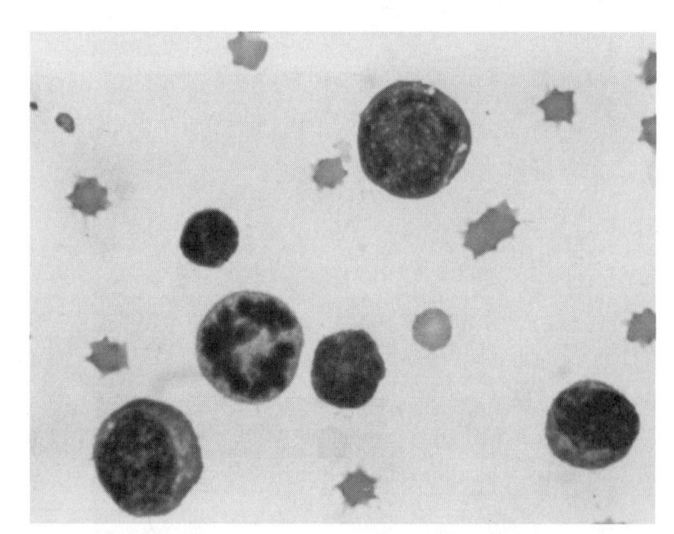

Figure 13–7. Examination of fluid aspirated from the cat in Figure 13–6 showed a pleomorphic lymphoid population composed of blasts, a mitotic figure, and a small lymphocyte. A diagnosis of lymphoma was made (Wright's stain, × 1000). (Courtesy of Gregory O. Freden.)

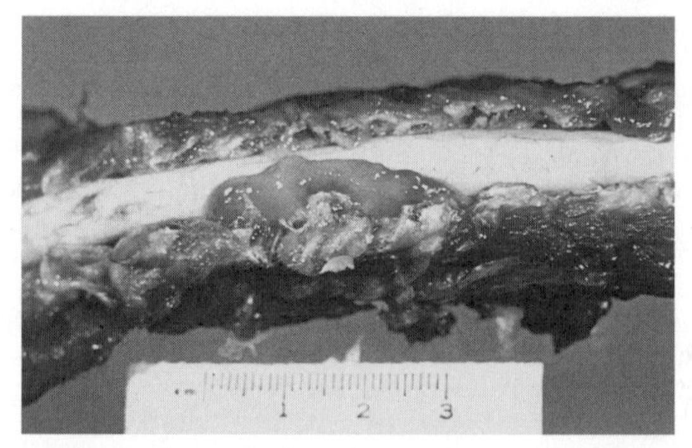

Figure 13–8. Postmortem dissection of the spinal canal reveals a cream-colored gelatinous mass in the epidural space. Histologic findings were diagnostic of lymphoma.

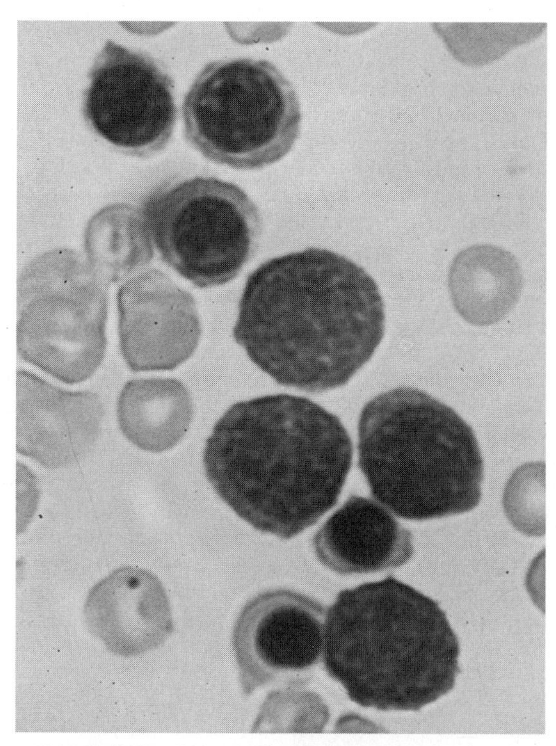

Figure 13–9. Peripheral blood film of a cat with erythroleukemia. At presentation, the cat had severe anemia without reticulocytosis. More than 95% of the circulating nucleated cells were erythroid precursors of varying degrees of maturity. Severe granulocytopenia was noted (Wright's stain, × 1000).

and thrombocythemia. Eosinophilic leukemia may be a subtype of CML and has been described in association with FeLV. The differentiation between severe reactive eosinophilia and malignancy is unclear, because both have been associated with large numbers of morphologically normal eosinophils in the marrow, peripheral blood, and other organs.

ACUTE LYMPHOBLASTIC LEUKEMIA (ALL). Cats with ALL have primary involvement of the bone marrow, often with some circulating lymphoblasts, although the WBC count is usually normal or low. Severe lymphocytosis with large numbers of blast cells is seen occasionally. Anemia is generally severe at the time of diagnosis. Some have gross lesions of lymphoma in other organs, but most have only microscopic infiltration.

ACUTE MYELOGENOUS LEUKEMIA (AML). Cats with AML also have infiltration of the marrow with blast cells, sometimes recognizable as myeloblasts, rubriblasts, or megakaryoblasts. Blast cell counts in blood smears vary from 0 to more than 100,000 cells/μl. The early myeloid cells may show some maturation toward granulocytic or monocytic lineage or sometimes both (myelomonocytic leukemia), because both cell lines share a common blast cell and respond to the same growth factor (granulocyte-macrophage colony-stimulating factor [GM-CSF]). Cats with erythroleukemia are anemic, often with large numbers of circulating nucleated erythrocytes (Fig. 13–9). Evidence of regeneration (reticulocytosis, polychromasia) is absent. The marrow may show megaloblastic changes, characterized by large erythroid cells with asynchrony of nuclear and cytoplasmic maturation and abnormal megakaryocytes or giant granulocytes.

MYELODYSPLASIA (MYELODYSPLASTIC SYNDROME [MDS]). Sometimes called preleukemia, MDS is characterized by nonregenerative anemia, sometimes with granulocytopenia or thrombocytopenia. Examination of the marrow reveals abnormalities of maturation of one or more cell lines, sometimes with nuclear or cytoplasmic atypia or megaloblastosis. A disproportionate number of blast cells may be present but too few to make a diagnosis of leukemia. MDS may evolve into leukemia, but many cats die of persistent anemia or infection. Few will improve with supportive care.

MYELOFIBROSIS. Some cats with peripheral cytopenias also have diffuse fibrosis of the marrow. This diagnosis can be made only by marrow biopsy, not aspiration. Myelofibrosis has been classified as a myeloproliferative disease but more likely represents "end-stage" marrow failure. Most frequently seen in chronically anemic cats, it is usually associated with severe extramedullary hematopoiesis (myeloid metaplasia) of the liver and spleen.

Bone Marrow Suppression Syndromes

Anemia. Anemia secondary to bone marrow suppression is frequently caused by FeLV, especially subgroup C (see Table 13–2). The virus may block differentiation of erythroid progenitors, the burst-forming units, by interfering with signal transduction pathways essential for erythropoiesis.[52] Abnormalities in growth regulation and supportive function of marrow stromal cells or inhibition of the normal effect of helper T cells on erythroid differentiation may also be involved. The virus probably affects precursors near the stem cell level, because leukopenia, thrombocytopenia, or both may accompany the anemia. In some cats, cyclic hematopoiesis, with periodic fluctuation in reticulocytes, leukocytes, and platelets, may be noted. Anemic cats infected with FeLV have increased levels of serum erythropoietin but decreased erythropoiesis on ferrokinetic studies and bone marrow culture. In vitro exposure of normal feline marrow to some strains of FeLV caused suppression of erythrogenesis. Just as FeLV is thought to cause virus-negative lymphoma, approximately 30% of cats with nonregenerative anemia are FeLV negative without another evident cause. Genetic analysis of many of these cats shows the presence of the virus without viremia being manifest.[22, 23] Marrow suppression may be worsened by coinfection with FIV.

Determining the cause of anemia in cats is a common and perplexing problem. When a viremic anemic cat is seen, a reticulocyte count will categorize regenerative and nonregenerative anemias. Either category may have circulating nucleated erythrocytes so that these are not an accurate indication of marrow response. Although regenerative anemia secondary to hemolysis may occur in viremic cats, other causes of hemolysis such as haemobartonellosis, autoimmune hemolytic anemia (AIHA), and toxins must be ruled out even in these cases. An immune-mediated component to FeLV-induced anemias may occur because Coombs' test results are sometimes positive. The relationship between FeLV, *Haemobartonella felis*, and AIHA may be confusing. Haemobartonellosis may occur secondary to FeLV-induced immunosuppression (also see Chapter 30).

Some viremic cats develop a mild anemia (PCV 20–30%), referred to as anemia of chronic disease, after infection or stress. The PCV will often rise spontaneously if the underlying problem is treated successfully, even if the cat remains FeLV positive. If the anemia is more severe (PCV < 20%), a bone marrow aspirate may be indicated to rule out leukemia and to determine whether erythroid precursors are present in adequate numbers with normal maturation. Severe isolated anemia (PCV < 15%) without regeneration (pure RBC aplasia) suggests infection with FeLV subgroup C.[52] Severe pancytopenia or aplastic anemia involves all cell lines, and bone marrow cytology is usually hypocellular. These cats often test FeLV positive, and this may reflect a more advanced stage of FeLV-associated hematologic disease.

FeLV-induced anemia is typically normochromic-normocytic or macrocytic without evidence of reticulocyte response. Whenever macrocytic anemia (MCV $>$ 60 fl) occurs in the cat in the absence of reticulocytosis, FeLV infection should be suspected. These cats are not folate or vitamin B_{12} depleted, and the macrocytosis may represent skipped mitoses during erythropoiesis. The bone marrow is usually normocellular but may be hypocellular with an increased myeloid to erythroid ratio. Anemia in the viremic cat appears to be a distinct syndrome and not a preleukemic manifestation in most cases. In general, regenerative anemia has a better prognosis than does nonregenerative anemia.

Platelet Abnormalities. Thrombocytopenia may occur secondary to decreased platelet production from marrow suppression or leukemic infiltration. The life span of platelets is shortened in some viremic cats. Although the platelet count is low, the mean platelet volume is often increased. Some platelets may approach the size of RBC, falsely raising the RBC count and lowering the platelet count as reported by automated cell counters. In some cats, platelet counts may be increased rather than decreased.

Leukocyte Abnormalities. Viremic cats may have reductions in granulocyte or lymphocyte counts. Cats that have recently become infected with FeLV often have lower WBC counts than those that have been chronically viremic. This occurrence may correlate with a higher rate of illness in recently infected cats than in chronically infected ones. Cats with granulocytopenia are usually seen because of recurrent or persistent bacterial infections, such as gingivitis. The usual signs of inflammation such as hyperemia and purulent exudate may not be evident in oral ulcers, because granulocytes are necessary for the inflammatory response.

A condition known as "panleukopenia-like" syndrome consists of leukopenia with enteritis and destruction of intestinal crypt epithelium. In this syndrome, anemia and thrombocytopenia may be present in contrast to typical cases of panleukopenia in which acute transient leukopenia is usually the only hematologic abnormality. Panleukopenia viral antigen has been demonstrated by FA in intestinal sections of cats that died with this syndrome after being experimentally infected with FeLV.[34] FPV was also demonstrated there by EM despite negative ELISA test results for FPV on the serum. It appears that this syndrome is caused by coinfection with FeLV and FPV.

Immunosuppression. Viremic cats are predisposed to infection primarily because of immunosuppression, sometimes associated with unintegrated cellular viral DNA from replication-defective viral variants. This situation is similar to that in human patients infected with HIV. Cats with recurring or persistent infections should be tested for concurrent FIV infection.

It appears that T-cell function is most disrupted, as evidenced by decreased rejection of skin grafts, suppressed interleukin-2 (IL-2) expression and lymphocyte transformation response, and increased suppressor cell activity. Both primary and secondary humoral antibody responses to specific antigens are delayed and reduced in viremic cats. At the same time, nonspecific increases of IgG and IgM have been noted. T lymphocytes of viremic cats produce significantly lower levels of B-cell stimulatory factors than do those of normal cats.[7] This defect becomes progressively more severe over time. In contrast, B-cell function in viremic cats is normal when cells are stimulated in vitro by uninfected T cells.

Neutrophils of viremic cats have decreased chemotactic and phagocytic function compared with those of normal cats. This abnormality persists for an unknown period of time even if viremia is transient.

Viremic cats are at increased risk for bacterial (stomatitis, pyoderma), rickettsial (haemobartonellosis), viral (FIP, upper respiratory infection), protozoal (toxoplasmosis), and fungal (aspergillosis and cryptococcosis) infections.[30] Some will respond to aggressive treatment despite the presence of FeLV.

Immune Complex Diseases. Circulating immune complexes have been observed after experimental treatment of persistent viremia with monoclonal antibodies to gp70 and in studies of inoculation of complement-depleting factors. Immune complexes predispose cats to such diseases as glomerulonephritis and polyarthritis. Measurement of FeLV antigens has shown that cats with glomerulonephritis have more circulating viral proteins that do other viremic cats. Some cats with glomerulonephritis have circulating antibody to FeLV but are not currently viremic.

Reproductive Disorders. Infertility, resorption or abortion of fetuses, and endometritis have been seen in viremic queens. The apparent infertility might actually be early absorption of fetuses. Abortions usually occur late in gestation, with expulsion of normal-appearing fetuses. Bacterial endometritis has sometimes accompanied these abortions, particularly in cats with leukopenia. Kittens born to an infected queen may become exposed to virus transplacentally, but heavy exposure also occurs at birth and throughout the nursing period. Some kittens become immune, but most become viremic and die at an early age of "fading kitten syndrome," characterized by failure to nurse, dehydration, hypothermia, and thymic atrophy within the first 2 weeks of life.

Lymphadenomegaly. Some viremic cats, especially those younger than 1 year, have peripheral lymphadenopathy, usually most severe in submandibular nodes. This syndrome may be asymptomatic or associated with fever and anorexia. In a few cats, a biopsy is diagnostic of lymphoma, but the majority of cases are classified as lymphocytic hyperplasia. Cultures of hyperplastic nodes are negative for bacteria. Whether this lesion is a response to FeLV or to some as yet undetermined antigenic stimulus is unknown. Transient lymphadenopathy has been reported in kittens experimentally infected with FeLV as well. A few naturally infected cats with lymph node hyperplasia subsequently developed lymphoma, but in most cats the nodes eventually decrease in size. In some young cats, a distinctive form of lymphadenopathy occurs with severe hyperplasia of lymphocytes, plasma cells, and immunoblasts to the point of destroying the architecture of the node. Because the prognosis is good, therapy is not indicated unless the nodes are so large that they interfere with breathing or swallowing. In this situation, anti-inflammatory dosages of glucocorticoids might be helpful in reducing the size of the nodes. In mild cases, glucocorticoids should not be used because they may interfere with an ongoing immune response.

Osteochondromas. Multiple osteochondromas (cartilaginous exostoses) have been described with increased prevalence in viremic cats. Although histologically benign, they may cause significant morbidity if they occur in an area such as a vertebra and put pressure on the spinal cord or nerve roots. The pathogenesis of these is unknown.

Olfactory Neuroblastoma. In three cats with spontaneous feline olfactory neuroblastomas, budding type C retroviral particles were found in the tumors and lymph node metastases.[50] Two of the cats had positive test results for FeLV antigenemia, and the virus in the tumors was identified as FeLV by PCR. The exact role of FeLV in the genesis of these tumors is uncertain.

Diagnosis

Principles for performing and understanding FA and ELISA techniques are discussed in Chapter 1. Both tests detect the FeLV core antigen, p27, and are specific for FeLV (see Tables 13–3 and 13–4). A positive result means that the cat is viremic, not necessarily that the virus is responsible for any observed clinical signs. Some non-neoplastic disorders such as anemia result directly from suppression of the marrow, but the immunosuppressive nature of the virus secondarily predisposes cats to other infectious diseases. A positive test result for FeLV is a presumptive immune function test, although the degree of immunosuppression cannot be determined until a clinical test to enumerate $CD4^+$ cells becomes available to clinicians.[17]

The ELISA test is somewhat more sensitive than the indirect FA test, but some false-positive ELISA results have occurred from technical errors.[9, 35] If performed properly, there is good correlation between the two tests.[33] In experimental FeLV infection, cats become positive by ELISA before they are positive by FA. Cats with transient infections become negative by FA before they are negative by ELISA. Either test is useful clinically, but cats that have positive results only on ELISA are more likely to convert to negative than are cats with positive results on both tests. For prognostication, one or more positive ELISA test results should be followed by FA confirmation to determine whether a cat is persistently viremic. The small number of discordant cats with test results that are persistently ELISA positive and FA negative may have focal infections that are kept localized by the immune system (see Table 13–3, Immune Carrier).[25] It is unusual to find cats that test negative for antigen by ELISA but positive by FA,[9] although some reports suggest differently.[27] One potential error is the use of anticoagulants rather than fresh blood for making smears.[24, 59] Tests available to evaluate tears or saliva are subject to more technical errors and must be used cautiously.[1a, 11] Appendices 5 and 6 list laboratories that perform these tests and commercially available test kits, respectively.

PCR has been used for detection of FeLV long terminal repeat (LTR) sequences in peripheral blood specimens from cats with hematologic abnormalities.[23] Results were comparable to those of ELISA, offering no significant advantage with peripheral blood specimens. In contrast, FeLV LTR sequences can be detected in formalin-fixed, paraffin-embedded neoplastic tissues from cats that have negative test results for virus by immunohistochemical methods.[21]

Therapy

Lymphoma. Untreated lymphoma is usually fatal within 1 to 2 months. Many cats can be helped with chemotherapy, and a few will have remissions that may last several years. Before treatment is considered, a diagnosis of lymphoma must be confirmed by cytology or histology and the condition of the cat evaluated to determine prognosis. The FeLV status does not appear to influence response to treatment.[4, 39, 42] If the cat is in good condition and has a normal bone marrow, the prognosis for complete remission (CR) of lymphoma is relatively good (Table 13–5). Staging of lymphoma in cats has been more difficult than in dogs because cats are more likely to have visceral involvement. For example, cats with alimentary lymphoma generally have a poorer prognosis than cats with lymphoma at other sites because anorexia and debilitation are often present. However, a subgroup with a resectable intestinal mass or well-differentiated histologic features had long survival times after treatment with chemotherapy. Nasal lymphoma seems to remain localized longer than lymphomas in other sites, and radiation alone has significantly prolonged survival. A staging system recommended by Mooney and coworkers is of value in that cats with less advanced disease have a better rate of remission and longer survival.[41]

Combinations of chemotherapeutic drugs offer the best chance for CR. Single-agent glucocorticoids are minimally effective and should be considered for palliation only after clients have been informed about combination chemotherapy and have rejected this option. Drugs most frequently administered in combination include cyclophosphamide (Cytoxan, CTX, Bristol-Myers, Princeton, NJ), vincristine (Oncovin, Eli Lilly, Indianapolis, IN), and prednisone. This combination is abbreviated as COP. These drugs have sometimes been combined with doxorubicin (Adriamycin, Adria Laboratories, Dublin, OH) and called COPA. Less commonly, L-asparaginase (Elspar, Lederle, Wayne, NJ), cytosine arabinoside (ara-C; Cytosar-U, Upjohn, Kalamazoo, MI), and methotrexate (Lederle Laboratories, Wayne, NJ) are included in feline protocols. Detailed descriptions of dosages, efficacy mechanism of action, toxicities, and excretion of these drugs in cats are available.[2, 46]

In a 1983 treatment report of 38 cats with COP, approximately 75% achieved CR with a median duration of remission of 150 days and a 20% chance of still being in remission after 1 year.[4] In this group, most were viremic, and the most frequent site of tumor was the mediastinum. Ten years later, the same number of cats from the same geographic area and treated with the same protocol had a CR rate of only 47%, with a median remission duration of 86 days. In the latter group, few were viremic, and the alimentary form was the most frequent.[42]

At this time, COP is still a reasonable protocol for induction of remission. For maintenance of remission, doxorubicin (COPA) has been more successful than continued COP, with

Table 13–5. Prognostic Indicators in Feline Lymphoma

PROGNOSTIC INDICATOR	DESCRIPTION
Good	Small tumor burden Peripheral lymph nodes, nasal cavity, or mediastinum as primary site Normal major organ function Good appetite, minimal weight loss
Adverse	Anemia, neutropenia, or thrombocytopenia Marrow involvement Prolonged paralysis with spinal lymphoma Fever, sepsis, or focal infection (e.g., gingivitis, chronic rhinitis) Skin or alimentary involvement Emaciation or anorexia
Factors with minimal effect	FeLV status Age, gender Histopathology (lymphoblastic vs. immunoblastic) not known to affect cat's prognosis; immunoblastic more favorable in dogs

a median CR of 243 days (Table 13–6).[42] In contrast, doxorubicin was not effective for induction of remission, with 0 of 10 cats achieving CR.[6]

All these drugs are immunosuppressive, and some are myelosuppressive, so owners must watch for signs of illness. Infections must be treated quickly and aggressively, especially if they occur at the time of the granulocyte nadir. The most frequent problem associated with chemotherapy in cats is anorexia secondary to the malignancy, the treatment, or both. Cyproheptadine (Periactin, Merck Sharp and Dohme, West Point, PA) at a dose of 2 to 4 mg/day divided BID or megestrol acetate (Ovaban, Schering Plough, Kenilworth, NJ) at a dose of 2.5 mg daily for 3 to 4 days may help stimulate the appetite.

In the absence of complications, dosages of drugs must not be decreased nor intervals between treatments lengthened, because either would increase the risk of relapse. The point at which therapy may safely be discontinued is controversial, but there is a trend toward shorter treatment times for cats in continuous CR. Previously, most protocols continued for a year or more; now many stop after 6 months of continuous CR. Some cats can be expected to relapse when treatment ends, so owner awareness and periodic checkups are important.

Acute Leukemia. Cats with acute leukemia are difficult to treat because the marrow becomes filled with neoplastic blast cells, which must be cleared before the normal hematopoietic precursors can repopulate. This process may take 3 to 4 weeks, and therefore granulocytopenia and anemia may not be immediately reversible. Prophylactic antibiotics are not given routinely in the treatment of feline leukemia or lymphoma. Bactericidal antibiotics should be given if fever or other signs of infection occur, especially at the time of the nadir of the leukocyte count. The remission rate for cats with ALL treated initially with vincristine and prednisone is approximately 25%, whereas with AML (treated with doxorubicin or ara-C), it is close to zero. The reason for the very poor response of AML may be that a very early stem cell is involved, and nearly total ablation of the marrow is necessary to clear the malignant clone.

Myelosuppressive Diseases. Blood transfusion is the most important part of treatment of nonregenerative anemia. Most cats that respond will do so after the first transfusion. Of 29 anemic viremic cats (PCV < 20%) treated for more than 2 weeks, the PCV returned to normal in 8, and 1 converted to FeLV-negative status.

Prednisone may increase the life span of erythrocytes if any component of the anemia is immune mediated. It is not likely, however, that immune-mediated hemolysis is a major component of FeLV anemia; therefore, glucocorticoids are only occasionally effective clinically. Anemic cats with treatable infections have the best prognosis because any infection or chronic disease may inhibit hematopoiesis and shorten RBC life span. Because deficiencies of iron, folate, or vitamin B_{12} are rare, replacement therapy is not likely to be helpful.

Even though erythropoietin concentrations are often elevated in cats with FeLV-related anemia or MDS, treatment with human recombinant erythropoietin (Epogen Amgen, Thousand Oaks, CA) at a dose of 100 units/kg, SC, three times weekly is sometimes helpful in raising the PCV. The dose is adjusted to maintain the PCV at about 30%. A response may not be seen for 3 to 4 weeks, and if it does occur, iron supplementation may be required. Iron should not given to cats that have required transfusions because whole blood contains 0.5 mg/ml of iron, and hemosiderosis may occur in the liver.

In some neutropenic, FeLV-positive cats, maturation arrest in the bone marrow may occur at the myelocyte and metamyelocyte stages. Neutrophil counts are corrected in many of these cats by anti-inflammatory to immunosuppressive doses of glucocorticoids, and an immune-mediated mechanism is suspected. In animals with myeloid hypoplasia and absent myeloid precursors, direct effects of FeLV is suspected. Treatment with human recombinant G-CSF has caused transient responses, but antibodies develop within 2 to 3 weeks. Neutrophil counts decrease quickly (see Appendix 8).[52]

Management of the Healthy FeLV-Positive Cat. Studies in cluster households have shown that neither virus-neutralizing nor FOCMA antibody titers are lifelong, so that a previously immune cat may become viremic or develop malignancy if immunity declines. When a viremic cat is identified in a multicat household, the owner must be informed of the potential danger to other cats in the house. A healthy viremic cat need not be removed from the household for the protection of the other cats unless all are tested to be sure that additional carriers are not present. In catteries, a test-and-removal program in which viremic cats are removed has been successful in preventing other cats from becoming infected. The test is repeated every 3 months until all cats have negative test results.

In a household with a few cats, an owner may elect to keep all the cats. The risk of infection in adult FeLV-negative cats is approximately 10% to 15% if they have lived with a viremic cat for more than several months.[5] The viremic cats must be kept indoors not only to protect other cats but also to protect the vulnerable viremic cats from respiratory infections, bite wounds, or other dangers of the outdoors. If the household is closed to new cats, the FeLV-negative cats tend to outlive the infected cats, so that after months to years all remaining cats will be immune. This may be a reasonable alternative to euthanasia for viremic cats, because some can live a normal life span in a protected environment.

The status of healthy viremic cats should be monitored periodically. MLV vaccines against panleukopenia and upper respiratory viruses have been used, although inactivated

Table 13–6. COPA Therapy Protocol for Treatment of Feline Lymphoma

	WEEK NO.															
THERAPY	1	2	3	4	5	6	7	8	9	10	11	12	13	16	19	22
Cyclophosphamide	1			1												
Vincristine	1	1	1	1												
Prednisone	1	....	....	....	....	....	....	....	....	....	....	....	....	....	....	....
Doxorubicin							1			1			1	1	1	1

Outline of the COPA protocol: cyclophosphamide (300 mg/m², PO), round off dose to nearest 25 mg on the low side of dose; vincristine 0.75 mg/m², IV; prednisone 2 mg/kg, PO, daily. Beginning on week 7 doxorubicin (25 mg/m², IV) is substituted for cyclophosphamide and vincristine. Treatment is continued every 3 weeks until relapse or until week 22 of continuous remission. Treatment is then stopped and prednisone tapered over 3 weeks.

ones are available and will not produce postvaccinal disease. Rabies vaccines contain inactivated virus because of increased risk of vaccine-induced encephalitis. There is no benefit to vaccinating viremic cats against FeLV.

Any illness that develops must be diagnosed and treated as would the same infection in a FeLV-negative cat. Elective surgery such as neutering has occasionally preceded episodes of illness; however, the risk-benefit ratio must be considered, and most healthy viremic cats can be neutered without complication. Spread of virus in the hospital is easily prevented by proper hygienic measures (see Chapter 94). Viremic cats can be housed in the same ward as other hospitalized patients. Under no circumstances should they be placed in a "contagious ward" with cats suffering from infections such as viral respiratory disease.

FeLV by itself does not cause fever, so a search for a concurrent infection must be made in febrile cats. Fevers of unknown origin that are unresponsive to antibiotics may have a viral, protozoal, or fungal origin. Neutropenia secondary to FeLV suppression of the marrow may be another reason for difficulties in treating bacterial infections. Glucocorticoids should be avoided unless clearly indicated for a specific problem. They interfere with granulocyte chemotaxis, phagocytosis, and the killing of bacteria, thus compounding the risk of infection. In addition, they may increase the risk of infection with FeLV in FeLV-negative cats living with viremic cats.

Antivirals and Immunotherapy. Currently, no treatment has been proved effective in clearing FeLV infection. Because the virus integrates into the genome, it is not easily eliminated from the body. Because of similarities of FeLV and FIV infections in the cat to HIV infection in people, research has been active in this area. (See Antiviral Therapy, Chapter 2 and Immunotherapy, Chapter 100).

Antibody therapy has been used in an attempt to rid cats of virus. Antibodies were derived from immune cats or were obtained as murine monoclonal antibodies to epitopes of gp70. Antibodies have been successful in experimentally infected cats only when given within 3 weeks of infection. Naturally infected cats showed no response even though the monoclonal antibodies persisted longer in viremic cats than in normal controls. Viremic cats also developed residual circulating immune complexes that could cause adverse reactions.

Attempts to stimulate the immune response against the virus have been made with human IFN-α (Roferon-A, Hoffman LaRoche, Nutly, NJ), diethylcarbamazine (Carbam, Sanofi Animal Health, Overland Park, KS), staphylococcal protein A (SPA, Pharmacia Biotech, Piscataway, NJ), *Propionibacterium acnes* (Immunoregulin, ImmunoVet, Tampa, FL), and acemannan (Carrisyn, Carrington Laboratories, Irving, TX). (See also Antivirals, Chapter 2; Immunotherapy, Chapter 100; and Drug Formulary, Appendix 8). Controlled studies are lacking for all of these agents in large numbers of naturally infected cats.

Prophylactic treatment of experimentally infected cats with oral human IFN-α did not reverse viremia, but was beneficial in preventing disease development and prolonging survival compared with a similar group of control cats. Anecdotal reports of improved appetite and decreased signs of illness are difficult to interpret.[60] A trial of oral IFN-α in human patients with HIV infection did not show a beneficial effect. Studies of human IFN-α given parenterally to cats may be limited by development of neutralizing antibodies.[62] A feline recombinant IFN-α is available in Japan, and preliminary trials of SC injection reversed viremia in small numbers of naturally infected cats.[60] For further information on use of IFN-α in cats see Chapter 100 and Appendix 8.

The efficacies of Immunoregulin and acemannan are currently unknown. Some have described subjective beneficial effects, and others have not observed responses. Because of the difficulties in interpreting responses, double-blind, placebo-controlled studies will probably be the only way to resolve the question.

Some transient responses to extracorporeal SPA therapy have been seen. Because the proposed mechanism of response was that some of SPA eluted from the column and entered the patient, additional cats were treated with direct injection of SPA. A few cats did clear their viremia after this treatment, but the total number of cats treated was small.

Antiretroviral drugs that have been used in cats include zidovudine (AZT, Retrovir, Burroughs Wellcome, Research Triangle Park, NC) and 9-(2-phosphonoyl-methoxyethyl)adenine (PMEA).

RT inhibitors such as AZT will suppress viral replication but not eliminate virus. In experimental infections, AZT (60 mg/kg/day) is effective in preventing viremia, but is given only within 96 hours of the time of exposure to virus.[38] In a similar group of experimentally infected kittens treated with AZT (30 mg/kg/day), antigenemia was inhibited, higher titers of neutralizing antibody were produced, and median survival was greater than 102 weeks compared with controls with a median survival of 35 weeks. Even at the lower dosage, two of six cats in the AZT group experienced myelosuppression with PCV less than 20% and neutrophil nadir of less than 1000 cells/μl.[44] A group of naturally infected cats with stomatitis were treated in a double-blind, placebo-controlled clinical trial with AZT. The oral lesions and the overall health status of the treated cats improved, and a reduction in viral replication was documented.

PMEA was investigated in treatment of stomatitis in cats naturally infected with FeLV, and the efficacy was compared with that of AZT.[10] The PMEA-treated group had a better clinical response but experienced more adverse effects than did the group treated with AZT. Both drugs appeared to reduce, but not eliminate, antigenemia. The dose of AZT used in this study (5 mg/kg BID) was lower than previously recommended, and no significant adverse effects were noted in treated cats.

It may be that combinations of drugs will be required. For example, a combination of SC human IFN-α, AZT, and allogeneic IL-2–activated lymphocytes was successful in reversing experimentally induced viremia 12 weeks after infection. For an agent to be effective in treatment of a retroviral infection, it must inhibit viral replication and allow for recovery of the immune system. Lifelong treatment may be required; thus, the agent should be effective when given orally and should be relatively nontoxic and inexpensive. So far, no such agent has been found.

Prevention

Because most naturally exposed cats produce antibodies to virus and to FOCMA and become immune, it should be possible to produce an effective vaccine. Accomplishment of that task proved to be more difficult than anticipated. Original prototypes of inactivated virus vaccines were not only ineffective but further immunosuppressed the cat. Live virus vaccines produced immunity, but some vaccinated kittens developed clinical disease from "attenuated" virus. There was also concern that the vaccine virus could integrate into the genome and later cause FeLV-negative lymphomas. Early vaccines carried a higher risk of anaphylaxis than did other vaccines that cats routinely received. The emphasis of most manufacturers has been to produce immunity against the gp70 rather than to FOCMA, because viremic cats with FOCMA antibody titers shed infectious virus and are still susceptible to non-neoplastic FeLV-related disorders. Antibody to subgroup A virus is most important because it is the only subgroup that is transmitted naturally, and the other subgroups arise by recombinant events only after a cat is infected. The role of cell-mediated immunity is not as well understood. It is more difficult to measure but important in overall resistance to infection.[12]

Over the past 10 years, several effective vaccines have been developed. Those currently licensed use whole killed virus with or without adjuvant, disrupted virus with adjuvant, or genetically engineered gp70 with adjuvant (see Table 100–11). Vaccination does not interfere with testing for FeLV. Recommendations generally are for two doses SC for initial protection followed by annual boosters. It is not necessary to administer vaccine from the same manufacturer for boosters. Challenge studies to measure efficacy of vaccines have been difficult because of the natural resistance of cats to experimental infection. Some have immunosuppressed both vaccinated and control cats before IN challenge with virulent virus, and others have performed parenteral challenge with large doses of virus without immunosuppression. The relationship of these challenges to natural exposure has been questioned, but no standard challenge protocol has been accepted by all.[3, 16, 19, 31, 32] Some studies have used natural challenge when vaccinated and control cats live together.[28] Efficacy data have generally been reported as preventable fraction (PF), as suggested by Scarlett and Pollock.[49] For further discussion of PF, see Chapter 100.

An epidemiologic association has been made between rabies and FeLV vaccination and later development of soft tissue sarcomas at the injection site.[14, 15, 26, 36] See Postvaccinal Sarcomas, Chapter 100. Fibrosarcomas are the most frequent type, but undifferentiated sarcomas, rhabdomyosarcomas, chondrosarcomas, osteosarcomas, and malignant fibrous histiocytomas are also found. The incidence is somewhat controversial, but estimates range from one tumor per 1000 vaccines to one per 10,000.[36] These may occur as soon as 4 months or as long as 2 years after vaccination, with a median of approximately 1 year.[26] Although no specific vaccine or adjuvant has been incriminated, local irritation from adjuvants might stimulate fibroblasts to the point that malignant transformation occurs. Currently, adjuvants are important because some have questioned the efficacy of nonadjuvanted vaccines.[31] Aluminum has been identified in histologic sections of tumor, but adjuvants that do not contain aluminum have also been implicated in sarcomas.[14]

Until the safety of vaccines improves, care should be taken to weigh the risk of FeLV versus the risk from the vaccine. Cats living in closed households away from other cats and most cats living in open rural environments have minimal risk and should not be vaccinated. Cats in multicat households or shelters with new cats being introduced should be vaccinated. Testing is recommended before vaccination so that only FeLV-negative cats undergo vaccination. It has been suggested that FeLV vaccines be given SC over the lateral aspect of the left (left for leukemia; right for rabies) thigh so that any tumor that might develop could be treated by amputation if local excision is incomplete.[36]

Public Health Considerations

Because FeLV is known to be spread in a contagious manner, concern arose about the possible danger of FeLV to people. A number of facts tend to suggest that human infection might occur. The virus will grow in human marrow cells in culture.[43] Lymphoma has been experimentally induced by injection of large doses of virus into neonatal pups and marmosets. One epidemiologic study linked prior contact with sick cats to subsequent development of childhood leukemia. Cell-bound antibody believed to be directed toward FeLV-RT has been found on malignant cells of people with CML in blast cell crisis. Veterinarians were shown to have a higher death rate from leukemia than a control population of physicians and dentists.[4]

Serologic studies searching for FeLV or antibody to any of its components in people have been confusing and inconclusive. Some investigators have found antibodies to FeLV in human leukemia patients and owners of viremic cats, whereas others utilizing more specific radioimmune assays have obtained negative results. No person has ever been found to be viremic with FeLV. One explanation for the discrepancy between culture of the virus in human cells and the absence of proof of human infection may be related to the lytic action of human complement on the virus and to the fact that subgroup A virus will not grow in human cells. No case of human leukemia has ever been traced to FeLV. Although it is almost impossible to prove a negative hypothesis, it appears that FeLV is *not* a human health hazard.

FELINE SARCOMA VIRUS INFECTION

Etiology

FeSV is the cause of multicentric fibrosarcoma in young cats. Several strains of FeSV have been identified from naturally occurring tumors, and all are defective. They are unable to replicate without the presence of FeLV as a helper virus, which supplies proteins (as those coded by the *env* gene) to FeSV. Through a process of genetic recombination, FeSV acquires one of several oncogenes such as *fes*, *fms*, or *fgr*. As a result, FeSV is an acutely transforming virus, causing a polyclonal malignancy with multifocal tumors arising simultaneously after a short incubation period. The host range for FeSV is dependent on the helper FeLV. By manipulation of the helper virus in the laboratory, FeSV can enter cells of species not naturally infected. Experimental inoculation of FeSV has produced tumors in cats, rabbits, dogs, sheep, rats, and nonhuman primates. Many of these tumors regress spontaneously, even after reaching a large size.

Pathogenesis

Fibrosarcoma cells express FOCMA just as lymphoma cells do. Experimental infection with FeSV causes tumors that progress in some cats and regress in others. The latter group produces high FOCMA antibody titers. In addition to fibrosarcomas, FeSV has experimentally caused melanomas, showing that FeSV can transform cells of ectodermal as well as of mesodermal origin.[4] ID or intraocular inoculation of the virus into kittens produces melanomas in the skin or anterior chamber of the eye. FeSV has not yet been associated with naturally occurring melanomas of cats.

Clinical Findings

Fibrosarcomas caused by various strains of FeSV tend to be rapidly growing, often with multiple cutaneous or SC nodules that are locally invasive and metastasize to the lung and other sites. Solitary fibrosarcomas in old cats are not caused by FeSV. These tumors are often slower growing, locally invasive, slower metastasizing, and sometimes curable by excision. It is not likely that FeSV plays any role in vaccine-induced sarcomas, which behave more like the solitary fibrosarcomas except that they can occur at any age.

Therapy

Treatment of fibrosarcoma is early, wide, and deep surgical excision. If no metastases are present and if microscopic tumors remain after surgery, radiation has been successful in delaying recurrence. Experimentally, FeSV-induced fibrosarcomas in kittens sometimes regress after treatment with anti-FOCMA serum, but this is unlikely to translate into clinical efficacy.

RD114 INFECTION

RD114 is an endogenous xenotropic retrovirus that is present but not replicating in every feline cell. Although there is no evidence of pathogenicity or of any immune response to the virus in cats, the virus may play some role in normal fetal differentiation. The RD114 virus is most closely related to an endogenous baboon retrovirus and only distantly related to FeLV.[4]

References

1. August JR. 1991. Husbandry practices for cats infected with feline leukemia virus or feline immunodeficiency virus. *J Am Vet Med Assoc* 199:1474–1477.

1a. Babyak SD, Groves MG, Dimski DS, et al. 1996. Evaluation of a saliva test for feline leukemia virus antigen. *J Am Anim Hosp Assoc* 32:397–400.

2. Calia CM, Hohenhaus AE, Fox PR, et al. 1996. Acute tumor lysis syndrome in a cat with lymphoma. *J Vet Intern Med* 10:409–411.

3. Clark N, Kushner NN, Barrett CB, et al. 1991. Efficacy and safety field trials of a recombinant DNA vaccine against feline leukemia virus infection. *J Am Vet Med Assoc* 199:1433–1445.

4. Cotter SM. 1990. Feline viral neoplasia, pp 316–334. *In* Greene CE (ed), Infectious diseases of the dog and cat. WB Saunders, Philadelphia, PA.

5. Cotter SM. 1991. Management of healthy feline leukemia-virus-positive cats. *J Am Vet Med Assoc* 199:1470–1473.

6. Cotter SM. 1996. Unpublished data. Tufts University, North Grafton, MA.

7. Diehl LJ, Hoover EA. 1992. Early and progressive helper T-cell dysfunction in feline leukemia virus-induced immunodeficiency. *J Acquir Immune Defic Syndr* 5:1188–1194.

8. Ghosh AK, Bachmann MH, Hoover EA. 1992. Identification of a putative receptor for subgroup A feline leukemia virus on feline T cells. *J Virol* 66:3707–3714.

9. Hardy WD Jr, Zuckerman EE. 1991. Ten-year study comparing enzyme-linked immunosorbent assay with the immunofluorescent antibody test for detection of feline leukemia virus infection in cats. *J Am Vet Med Assoc* 199:1365–1373.

10. Hartzmann K, Donath A, Beer B, et al. 1992. Use of two virustatica (AZT, PMEA) in the treatment of FIV and FeLV seropositive cats with clinical symptoms. *Vet Immunol Immunopathol* 35:167–175.

11. Hawkins EC. 1991. Saliva and tear tests for feline leukemia virus. *J Am Vet Med Assoc* 199:1382–1385.

12. Hawks DM, Legendre AM, Rohrbach BW. 1991. Comparison of four test kits for feline leukemia virus antigen. *J Am Vet Med Assoc* 199:1373–1376.

13. Hayes KA, Rojko JL, Mathes LE. 1992. Incidence of localized feline leukemia virus infection in cats. *Am J Vet Res* 53:604–607.

14. Hendrick MJ, Goldschmidt MH, Shofer FS, et al. 1992. Postvaccinal sarcomas in the cat: epidemiology and electron probe microanalytical identification of aluminum. *Cancer Res* 52:5391–5394.

15. Hendrick MJ, Shofer FS, Goldschmidt MH, et al. 1994. Comparison of fibrosarcomas that developed at vaccination sites and at nonvaccination sites in cats: 239 cases (1991-1992). *J Am Vet Med Assoc* 205:1425–1429.

16. Hines DL, Cutting JA, Dietrich DL, et al. 1991. Evaluation of efficacy and safety of an inactivated virus vaccine against feline leukemia virus infection. *J Am Vet Med Assoc* 199:1428–1430.

17. Hofmann-Lehmann R, Holznagel E, Ossent P. 1997. Parameters of disease progression in long-term experimental feline retrovirus (feline immunodeficiency virus and feline leukemia virus) infections. Hematology, clinical chemistry, and lymphocyte subsets. *Clin Diagn Lab Immunol* 4:33–42.

18. Hoover EA, Mullins JI. 1991. Feline leukemia virus infection and diseases. *J Am Vet Med Assoc* 199:1287–1297.

19. Hoover EA, Perigo NA, Quackenbush SL, et al. 1991. Protection against feline leukemia virus infection by use of an inactivated virus vaccine. *J Am Vet Med Assoc* 199:1392–1401.

20. Ishida T, Uchino T. 1995. Use of feline recombinant interferon in feline viral diseases, pp 430–431. *In* Proceedings of the World Veterinary Congress.

21. Jackson ML, Haines DM, Meric SM, et al. 1993. Feline leukemia virus detection by immunohistochemistry and polymerase chain reaction in formalin-fixed, paraffin-embedded tumor tissue from cats with lymphosarcoma. *Can J Vet Res* 57:269–276.

22. Jackson ML, Haines DM, Misra V. 1996. Sequence analysis of the putative viral enhancer in tissues from 33 cats with various feline leukemia virus-related diseases. *Vet Microbiol* 53:213–225.

23. Jackson ML, Haines DM, Taylor SM, et al. 1996. Feline leukemia virus detection by ELISA and PCR in peripheral blood from 68 cats with high, moderate, or low suspicion of having FeLV-related disease. *J Vet Diagn Invest* 8:25–30.

24. Jarrett O. 1995. Detection of FeLV antigen. *Vet Rec* 137:127.

25. Jarrett O, Pacitti AM, Hosie MJ, Reid G. 1991. Comparison of diagnostic methods for feline leukemia virus and feline immunodeficiency virus. *J Am Vet Med Assoc* 199:1362–1364.

26. Kass PH, Barnes WG, Spangler WL, et al. 1993. Epidemiologic evidence for a causal relation between vaccination and fibrosarcoma tumorigenesis in cats. *J Am Vet Med Assoc* 203:396–405.

27. Kerr MG, Smith KJD. 1995. Detection of FeLV antigen by indirect immunofluorescence in ELISA/CITE negative cats. *Vet Rec* 136:516–518.

28. Lafrado LJ. 1994. Evaluation of a feline leukemia virus vaccine in a controlled natural transmission study. *J Am Vet Med Assoc* 204:914–917.

29. Lane SB, Kornegay JN, Duncan JR, et al. 1994. Feline spinal lymphosarcoma: a retrospective evaluation of 23 cats. *J Vet Intern Med* 8:99–104.

30. Lappin MR. 1995. Opportunistic infections associated with retroviral infections in cats. *Semin Vet Med Surg* 10:244–250.

31. Legendre AM, Hawks DM, Sebring R, et al. 1991. Comparison of the efficacy of three commercial feline leukemia virus vaccines in a natural challenge exposure. *J Am Vet Med Assoc* 199:1456–1462.

32. Legendre AM, Mitchner KL, Potgieter LND. 1990. Efficacy of a feline leukemia virus vaccine in a natural exposure challenge. *J Vet Intern Med* 4:92–98.

33. Lopez NA, Jacobson RH, Scarlett JM, et al. 1989. Sensitivity and specificity of blood test kits for feline leukemia virus antigen. *J Am Vet Med Assoc* 195:747–751.

34. Lutz H, Castelli I, Ehrensperger F, et al. 1995. Panleukopenia-like syndrome of FeLV caused by coinfection with FeLV and feline panleukopenia virus. *Vet Immunol Immunopathol* 46:21–33.

35. Macy DW. 1991. Testing cats for feline leukemia virus. *Vet Med* March:278–288.

36. Macy DW. 1995. The potential role and mechanisms of FeLV vaccine-induced neoplasms. *Semin Vet Med Surg* 10:234–237.

37. Mahony OM, Moore AS, Cotter SM, et al. 1995. Alimentary lymphoma in cats: 28 cases (1988-1993). *J Am Vet Med Assoc* 207:1593–1598.

38. Mathes LE, Polas PJ, Hayes KA, et al. 1992. Pre- and postexposure chemoprophylaxis: evidence that 3'-azido-3'dideoxythymidine inhibits feline leukemia virus disease by drug-induced vaccine response. *Antimicrob Agents Chemother* 36:2715–2721.

39. Mauldin GE, Mooney SC, Meleo RE, et al. 1995. Chemotherapy in 132 cats with lymphoma: 1988–1994, pp 35–36. In *Proceedings of the Veterinary Cancer Society.*

40. McCaw D. 1995. Caring for the retrovirus infected cat. *Semin Vet Med Surg* 10:216–219.

41. Mooney SC, Hayes AA, MacEwen EG, et al. 1989. Treatment and prognostic factors in lymphoma in cats. *J Am Vet Med Assoc* 194:696–699.

42. Moore AS, Cotter SM, Frimberger AE, et al. 1996. A comparison of doxorubicin vs COP for maintenance of remission in cats treated for lymphoma. *J Vet Intern Med.* 10:372–375.

43. Morgan RA, Dornsife RE, Anderson WF, et al. 1993. In vitro infection of human bone marrow by feline leukemia viruses. *Virology* 193:439–442.

44. Nelson P, Sellon R, Novotney C, et al. 1995. Therapeutic effects of diethylcarbamazine and 3'-azido-3'-deoxythymidine on feline leukemia virus lymphoma formation. *Vet Immunol Immunopathol* 46:181–194.

45. O'Connor TP Jr, Tonelli QJ, Scarlett JM. 1991. Report of the National FeLV/FIV Awareness Project. *J Am Vet Med Assoc* 199:1348–1352.

46. Ogilvie GK, Moore AS. 1995. Managing the veterinary cancer patient, pp 228–259. Veterinary Learning Systems, Trenton NJ.

47. Rohn JL, Linenberger ML, Hoover EA. 1994. Evaluation of feline leukemia virus variant genomes with insertions, deletions, and defective envelope genes in infected cats with tumors. *J Virol* 68:2458–2467.

48. Rojko JL, Kociba GJ. 1991. Pathogenesis of infection by the feline leukemia virus. *J Am Vet Med Assoc* 199:1305–1310.

48a. Romatowski J, Lubkin SR. 1997. Use of an epidemiologic model to evaluate feline leukemia virus control measures. *Feline Pract* 25:6–11.

49. Scarlett JM, Pollock R. 1991. Year two of follow-up evaluation of a random-

ized, blind field trial of a commercial feline leukemia virus vaccine. *J Am Vet Med Assoc* 199:1431–1432.
50. Schrenzel MD, Higgins RJ, Hinrichs SH, et al. 1990. Type C retroviral expression in spontaneous feline olfactory neuroblastomas. *Acta Neuropathol* 80:547–553.
51. Sheets RL, Pandey R, Jen WC, et al. 1993. Recombinant feline leukemia genes detected in naturally occurring feline lymphosarcomas. *J Virol* 167:3118–3125.
52. Shelton GH, Linenberger ML. 1995. Hematologic abnormalities associated with retrovirus abnormalities in the cat. *Semin Vet Med Surg* 10:220–233.
53. Spodnick GJ, Berg J, Moore FM, et al. 1992. Spinal lymphoma in cats: 21 cases (1976–1989). *J Am Vet Med Assoc* 200:373–376.
54. Steele KE, Saunders GK, Coleman GD. 1997. T-cell-rich B-cell lymphoma in a cat. *Vet Pathol* 34:47–49.
55. Swango LJ. 1991. Evaluation of feline leukemia virus diagnostic tests available for in-office use by veterinarians. *J Am Vet Med Assoc* 199:1386–1388.
56. Tizard I. 1991. Use of immunomodulators as an aid to clinical management of feline leukemia virus-infected cats. *J Am Vet Med Assoc* 199:1482–1484.
57. Tsatsanis C, Fulton R, Hishigaki K, et al. 1994. Genetic determinants of feline leukemia virus-induced lymphoid tumors: patterns of proviral insertion and gene rearrangement. *J Virol* 68:8296–8303.
58. Valli VE, Jacobs RM, Norris A. 1995. Pathology of feline lymphoma, p 57. *Proceedings of the Veterinary Cancer Society.*
59. Weijer K, van Herwijnen R. 1995. Detection of FeLV antigen. *Vet Rec* 137:127.
60. Weiss RC, Cummins JM, Richards. 1991. Low dose orally administered alpha interferon for feline leukemia virus infection. *J Am Vet Med Assoc* 199:1477–1481.
61. Willemse MJ, Schooneveld SH, Chalmers WS, et al. 1996. Vaccination against feline leukemia using a new feline herpesvirus type-1 vector. *Vaccine* 14:1511–1516.
62. Zeidner NS, Mathiason-DuBard CK, Hoover EA. 1995. Reversal of feline leukemia virus infection by adoptive transfer of activated T lymphocytes, interferon alpha and zidovudine. *Semin Vet Med Surg* 10:256–266.

Chapter 14

Feline Immunodeficiency Virus Infection

Rance K. Sellon

ETIOLOGY

Since its discovery in 1987, much has been learned about feline immunodeficiency virus (FIV), owing to its emergence as an important feline pathogen and model for study of HIV infection. As a lentivirus, FIV shares many virologic properties of other lentiviruses such as HIV. Readers interested in a review of FIV's basic genetic organization, life cycle, and comparisons to other lentiviruses are referred to other sources.[16, 48, 190]

There are clinically important aspects of several FIV genes, especially the FIV envelope *(env)* gene and its proteins.[146] Field isolates of FIV can be divided into several subtypes on the basis of differences in sequences of a hypervariable region of the *env* gene.[144, 210] Three subtypes have been described in naturally infected cats in North America and Europe.[187] In general, cats with subtype A were found in California and Europe, and those with subtype B were found in the central and eastern United States. Subtype C was typically a Canadian isolate. A fourth subtype (subtype D) was subsequently described in Japanese FIV isolates.[94] Naturally infected cats can harbor multiple subtypes,[3a] and, experimentally, superinfection with different subtypes after sequential inoculation has been observed as well, indicating a lack of cross-protection among some subtypes.[97, 137] Additional properties of the viral envelope arise from the incorporation of host cell membrane molecules into the envelope as virions bud from the infected cell, and the virus can induce syncytia formation.[160]

The knowledge of envelope properties is clinically important in cell tropism[78, 95, 144, 182] and pathogenicity.[95, 144, 210] Envelope proteins are targets of immune responses,[37, 62, 82, 181] and differences in, or conservation of, envelope sequences may reflect selection pressures exerted by the immune response of the infected cat.[67, 145, 146a, 170] All of these factors influence the clinical disease observed after infection with a given isolate.[187] Differences in envelope antigenic determinants also represent potential obstacles in the development of FIV vaccines protective against different isolates of FIV[77a, 180, 183] (see Prevention later).

EPIDEMIOLOGY

Prevalence

FIV is common worldwide, and its prevalence varies with geographic location. Across the United States, the seroprevalence of FIV in cats at high risk of exposure and in clinically ill cats ranges from about 4% to 24%, with no apparent regional differences.[32, 132] Seroprevalence outside the United States varies, but approaches 25% to 30% in countries with large populations of free-roaming cats such as Italy and Japan.[5, 150, 190] In the United States and Europe, the prevalence of FIV in healthy cats is lower than in sick cats, with rates commonly at 2% to 3%.[16, 190] Seroprevalence is two to three times higher in males than females. Adult cats (mean age, 6 years) are found infected more often than adolescent cats and kittens. Evidence from retrospective serosurveys suggests that FIV has been present in the domestic feline population since at least 1968.[176]

FIV infection is not limited to the domestic cat population. FIV infection has been reported in Florida panthers and other exotic feline species in U.S. zoos as well as in free-roaming species in Africa and Asia.[11, 23, 138, 155] The degree of genetic divergence observed between isolates from domestic cats and exotic cats suggests that isolates in these two groups of cats are distantly related.[138] Experimental inoculation of lion and puma viral isolates produced persistent infection without disease in domestic cats.[209a]

Transmission

In the natural setting, FIV is transmitted primarily by parenteral inoculation of virus present in saliva or blood, presumably by bite and fight wounds. Supporting evidence for the importance of this route of transmission is the observation that FIV can be found in salivary gland[122] and salivary gland epithelium[147] during acute infection and can be found in saliva, blood lymphocytes, and plasma or serum.[122] Additional support comes from the observation that FIV can be transmitted by experimentally induced bite wounds and that outdoor, intact male cats are at the highest risk of acquiring infection.[32, 190]

Experimentally, FIV is easily transmitted by all parenteral routes (IV, SC, IM, IP) using cell-free or cell-associated virus. In experimental settings, high rates of transmission (>50%), both in utero and postparturition via milk, have been documented in queens with acute and chronic FIV infections.[28, 139, 140, 174, 216] Transmission has also been reported after oral,[127, 174] intrarectal, and intravaginal inoculation with large amounts of cell-associated virus or cell-free viral culture fluid[19, 26a, 127] as well as by laparoscopic insemination of queens with semen from chronically infected males.[92] Inoculation of proviral DNA has also produced infection.[170a] Experimental transmission studies suggest that differences in viral isolates may be an important factor in transmission efficiency. For instance, although high rates of vertical transmission during acute maternal infection have been observed with Colorado and North Carolina isolates of FIV,[139, 140, 174] high rates of transmission from chronically infected queens have been reported only with Colorado isolates.[140, 208]

Despite the experimental evidence of transmission by the routes described, there is no firm evidence that these routes have an important role in maintenance of natural infections. Available epidemiologic and serologic surveys cannot, however, exclude the possibility of occasional transmission by these routes. High kitten mortality in FIV-positive neonates, as observed in some experimental studies,[139, 140] could lead to underestimates of in utero, congenital, and neonatal transmission in natural settings with similar consequences of neonatal infection.

Horizontal transmission of FIV in multiple-cat households is an infrequent event. However, FIV DNA has been found in cats that are seronegative for FIV.[16, 34] The DNA-positive cats had been housed in experimental colonies for long periods of time (months to years) with FIV-seropositive cats. Despite being DNA positive, the cats were asymptomatic and did not develop typical immunologic abnormalities observed in seropositive cats.[34] The clinical consequences, if any, of this latent type of infection are unknown at present.

PATHOGENESIS

Virtually all knowledge of FIV pathogenesis is derived from experimentally induced infections of specific pathogen-free (SPF) cats. After experimental inoculation, a burst of viral replication occurs primarily in cells of lymphoid tissues and salivary glands,[3, 13, 147, 206] with a peak of viremia several weeks PI. The thymus is a site of early viral replication resulting in depletion of the T-cell pool.[221d] Clinical signs of acute infection may be seen during this viremic period, which can last several weeks.[41] Using polymerase chain reaction (PCR) or viral culture, virus is easily detected in plasma or peripheral blood lymphocytes by 2 weeks PI or earlier.[122] Later, FIV spreads to mononuclear cells (lymphocytes, monocytes, and macrophages) in nonlymphoid organs such as the lung, intestinal tract, and kidney.[13] Virus infects follicular dendritic cells in lymph nodes and may serve as a means of infecting naive T cells migrating through the lymph node.[3, 206] During the early acute phase of infection, high levels of FIV are found in circulating $CD4^+$ cells (helper T lymphocytes), and, as the infection progresses, more virus is found in B cells than $CD4^+$ cells.[38, 51] Circulating virus decreases to low levels after the host mounts an immune response to FIV; cats are generally asymptomatic during this period. This is not a period of true viral latency, because FIV production continues in infected cells in tissues, and virus can still be recovered from blood lymphocytes, serum or plasma, CSF, semen, and lymphoid tissues.[3, 16, 44, 49, 93, 186] Plasma levels of virus and viral RNA can increase again during the terminal phase of infection (Fig. 14–1).[41]

FIV infects a wide range of cell types in vitro and in vivo (Table 14–1), but does not use the feline CD4 molecule as a cellular receptor.[85, 130] Antibody blockade of CD9 inhibits FIV infection. Although this molecule was initially considered a possible FIV receptor, later work demonstrates that CD9 blockade inhibits release of virus from infected cells.[36a, 221b] Other receptor molecules or modes of cell entry may be important in establishing productive infections in target cells. Potential candidates include a chemokine receptor,[221a, 221c] immunoglobulin-mediated entry into cells bearing the immunoglobulin Fc receptor (macrophages, B cells), or an intercellular infection through fusion of infected and uninfected cells.

The hallmark of FIV pathogenesis is the progressive disruption of normal immune function, the mechanisms of which are under intense investigation. Early immunologic abnormalities that occur after experimental[2, 6, 203] and natural[77, 131] infection are decreases in both the number and relative proportions of $CD4^+$ cells (see Fig. 14–1). These lymphocyte abnormalities are also found in naturally infected cats.[77, 131] When clinically ill and healthy FIV-infected cats have been compared, $CD4^+/CD8^+$ ratios did not alter with time.[214] Causes of $CD4^+$ cell loss could include decreased production secondary to bone marrow or thymic infection, lysis of infected cells induced by FIV itself (cytopathic effects), destruction of virally infected cells by the immune system, and induction of death by apoptosis.[17, 91, 134, 135, 141a] Apoptosis is a form of cell death that follows receipt of a viral receptor or cytokine-mediated signal at the cell membrane, initiating a series of intracellular events that lead to cell death. In vitro, apoptosis can be induced in FIV-infected lymphocytes.[91, 127a, 134, 135] Ultimately, loss of $CD4^+$ cells impairs immune responses because $CD4^+$ cells have critical roles in promoting and maintaining both humoral and cell-mediated immunity (CMI).

As is seen with HIV infection in people, loss of $CD4^+$ cells leads to inversion of the $CD4^+/CD8^+$ ratio (see Fig. 14–1). The inversion may occur weeks to months after infection depending on the viral isolate studied.[2, 203] Contributing to the inverted ratio in some cases is an increase in the propor-

Table 14–1. In Vivo and in Vitro Cell Tropism of FIV

IN VIVO	IN VITRO
Lymphocytes ($CD4^+$, $CD8^+$, B cells)[25, 37, 51]	Brain endotheial cells[192]
Macrophages[15]	Brain microglial cells[43, 44]
Follicular dendritic cells[3, 206]	Astrocytes[43, 44]
Megakaryocytes[15]	Macrophages[120]
Salivary gland epithelium[147]	

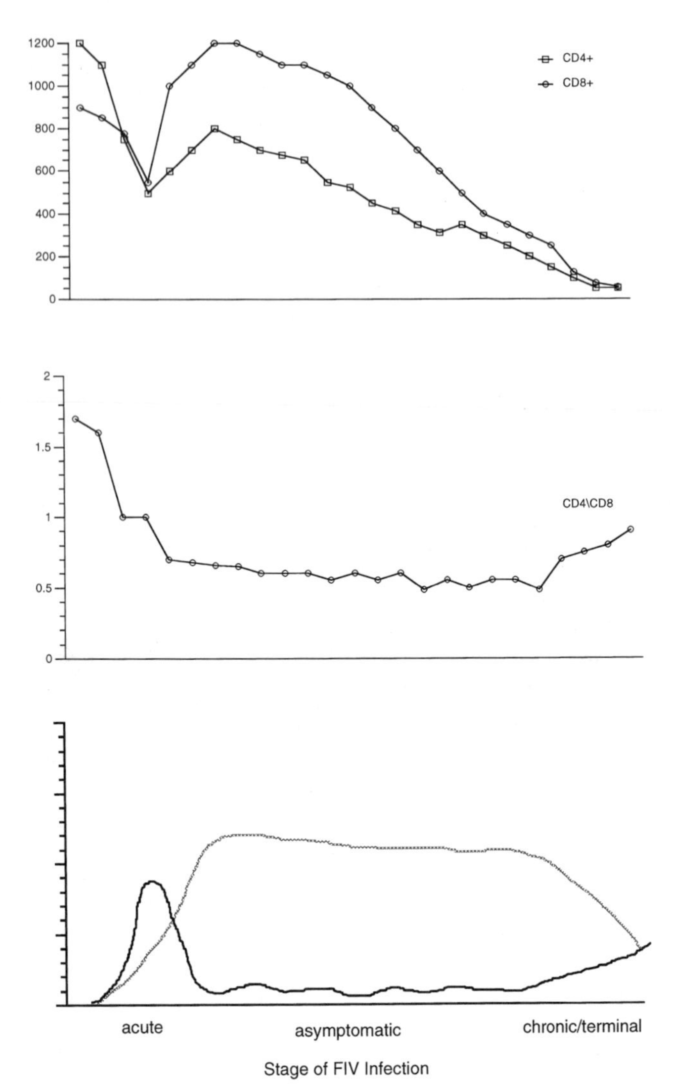

Figure 14–1. Changes in lymphocyte subsets with stage of infection in cats infected with FIV. There is a drop in CD4+ (helper T cells) and CD8+ (cytotoxic T cells) cells early in the course of infection, followed by partial recovery of CD8+ cells and persistent CD4+ lymphopenia (top panel), leading to a decrease in the CD4+/CD8+ ratio (middle panel). Relationship between FIV viremia (dark line) and humoral immune response (light line) with stage of infection in cats infected with FIV (bottom panel).

tion of CD8+ cells (cytotoxic or T lymphocytes).[2, 77, 219] Differences in CD8+ cells are not as consistently observed as CD4+ cell changes, most likely because of differences in behavior among isolates. Although inversion of the CD4+/CD8+ ratio is a consistent feature of both natural and experimental infections, its use as a prognostic tool for cats, as has been demonstrated with HIV-infected people, has not been realized.[21, 213] FIV-infected cats may show severe inversion for prolonged periods of time without developing clinical signs, and available work demonstrates no correlation of the ratio with clinical stage of infection.[77] Despite being a target of viral infection, there have been no reported changes in numbers or proportions of B cells after FIV infection.

Other immunologic abnormalities occur with FIV infection. Over time, lymphocytes from infected cats lose the ability to proliferate in response to stimulation with B- and T-cell mitogens and have impaired priming of T cells by T-dependent immunogens in vitro.[6, 20, 21, 70, 109, 193, 194, 204] The function of lymphocytes may also be impaired by reduced or altered expression of cell surface molecules, such as CD4 and major histocompatibility complex II antigens, and interleukin (IL)-2 receptors,[136, 169, 220] which have critical roles in antigen presentation and amplification of immune responses.

FIV infection is associated with disrupted production of cytokines. Reported abnormalities include both increased[96, 102] and decreased[116] circulating concentrations of tumor necrosis factor-α and increased IL-6.[103, 133] Decreased secretion of IL-1 from lipopolysaccharide-stimulated macrophages has been described.[108] Alterations in function of nonspecific defenses such as neutrophils have also been described in FIV-positive cats.[69] Natural killer cell activity has been reported as diminished[226] or increased[230] in FIV-positive cats, depending on whether the cats were acutely or asymptomatically infected, respectively.

Another manifestation of the immunologic dysregulation observed in many FIV-infected cats is hypergammaglobulinemia primarily resulting from increases in IgG.[2, 61] Hypergammaglobulinemia reflects polyclonal B-cell stimulation because the IgG produced is not FIV specific. It is a direct consequence of FIV infection because healthy FIV-positive SPF cats are also hypergammaglobulinemic.[61] The high concentrations of IL-6 observed by some may be responsible for the immunoglobulin production. In addition to increased IgG production, increased circulating immune complexes (CIC) have been detected in FIV-infected cats.[120a] FIV has also been incriminated as causing a delay in the class shift of antibody isotypes from IgM to IgG on the basis of work in cats infected with both FIV and *Toxoplasma gondii*.[101]

Abnormal neurologic function has been described in FIV-infected cats with mild to moderate histologic evidence of inflammation. Experimental studies in vivo suggest that brain lesions may occur in the absence of massive infection; neurotoxins such as glutamate have been implicated as one cause of neuronal loss.[21a, 160a, 184a] In vitro studies suggest that infection of cells in the CNS, in particular the astrocyte, may impair normal metabolism.[33, 229] Documented abnormalities of astrocyte function include altered intercellular communication, abnormal glutathione reductase activity that could render cells more susceptible to oxidative injury, and alterations in mitochondrial membrane potential that disrupt energy-producing capacities of the cell.

The pathogenesis of some clinical features of FIV remains unexplained but, like neurologic disease, may result from abnormal function of, or inflammation in, affected organs. Wasting disease has been observed in the absence of obvious causes such as diarrhea or neoplasia. Abnormal renal function and nephritis have also been reported in FIV-infected cats.

Secondary infections with resident microflora occur on skin and mucosal surfaces of chronically infected cats. The contribution of other pathogens to the pathogenesis of FIV infection is not entirely clear. SPF cats infected with FIV can develop clinical disease years after infection.[52] However, pet and random-source cats with exposure to numerous feline pathogens can also survive for similar time intervals.[52, 58, 179]

After infection with FIV, there is a vigorous, but ultimately ineffective, humoral immune response mounted against the virus (see Fig. 14–1). Antibodies are made against many FIV proteins,[47, 55, 82, 171] especially those of the viral envelope and capsid. Neutralizing antibodies can be detected with in vitro assays,[4, 142, 207] but whether such antibodies have roles in vivo is unknown.[123] Generally, antiviral antibodies first become detectable in experimental infections 2 to 4 weeks PI, although exposure to lesser amounts of virus may delay the appearance of detectable responses.[16] Delays in detection of

FIV antibody have been described in feline leukemia virus (FeLV)–infected cats experimentally coinfected with FIV.[47]

Stimulation of CMI occurs after experimental FIV infection.[59, 90, 188] Cytotoxic activity against FIV-infected target cells can be detected in the lymphocytes of FIV-positive cats as early as 7 to 9 weeks PI,[188] and cytotoxic cells directed against FIV peptides can be induced in vitro.[60, 107, 189] Stimulation of CMI may be an important aspect in the elimination of virally infected cells or suppression of virus production in that enhanced replication of FIV in $CD8^+$-depleted cell cultures has been described.[90] The persistence of cytotoxic activity and its role in controlling viremia in acute and chronic infections remain to be demonstrated. In vitro studies suggest that nonspecific defenses like complement may also limit viremia and viral spread.[56] Experimentally, the severity of clinical disease is enhanced by inoculation at a young age,[40, 64, 200] inoculation with large amounts of virus,[128] or pre-existing FeLV infection.[149, 205] In congenitally infected kittens, regression of infection has been demonstrated by development of viral latency and disappearance of serum antibody titer to FIV.[140a] Virus was still detected in lymphoid tissues by cell culture or PCR.

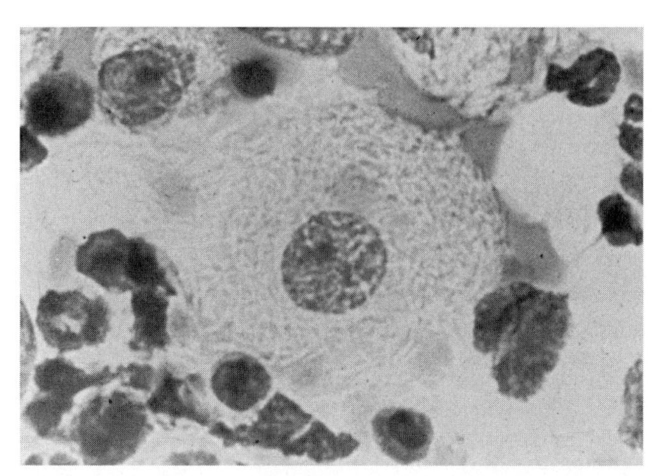

Figure 14–2. Photomicrograph of a mycobacterial laden macrophage from an FIV-positive cat with systemic mycobacterial infection. (Courtesy of Dr. Julie Levy, North Carolina State University, Raleigh, NC.)

CLINICAL FINDINGS

FIV infection progresses through several stages, much like HIV-1 infection in people. Recognized clinical stages in cats include the acute phase, a clinically asymptomatic phase of variable duration, and a terminal phase of infection.[49] Some investigators note two other phases in keeping with the terminology for HIV infection: progressive generalized lymphadenopathy, which follows the asymptomatic phase, followed by AIDS-related complex (ARC).[88, 89, 148] Still others describe a sixth category including miscellaneous diseases such as neoplastic, ocular, and immune-mediated diseases that are observed in some infected cats.[148] Although division of FIV infection into these clinical stages may prove useful from the standpoint of gauging prognosis, there is often no sharp distinction between them, and not all stages will be apparent in some infected cats.

Clinical signs of FIV infection are nonspecific (Table 14–2). During acute experimental infection, cats can exhibit fever and malaise, which may be transient and mild enough so as to go unnoticed, or signs of acute enteritis, stomatitis, dermatitis, conjunctivitis, and respiratory tract disease. Generalized lymph node enlargement is common. It is likely that clinical signs go unobserved in many naturally infected cats. This phase may last several days to a few weeks, after which cats will enter a period in which they appear clinically healthy. The duration of this asymptomatic phase may vary but can last for years. I have heard anecdotal reports of cats that have been seropositive for more than 6 years without developing clinical disease. There is no readily available predictor of the transition from the asymptomatic phase to the ARC (or AIDS) phase, although one study suggested that higher levels of viremia during the acute stage of infection are associated with more rapid progression to the terminal phases of the disease.[42] During the later stages of infection, clinical signs are a reflection of opportunistic infections, neoplasia, or other syndromes such as wasting.

Infections with a number of opportunistic pathogens of bacterial (Fig. 14–2), protozoal, and fungal origin have been reported in FIV-positive cats (Table 14–3). Few studies, however, have compared the prevalence of most of these infections in FIV-positive and FIV-negative cats. There was no correlation between FIV infection and infection with *Cryptococcus* or *Cryptosporidium*.[129, 215] Another study reported a higher prevalence of fungal infections in FIV-positive cats compared with negative cats, but FIV-positive cats had no symptoms of the fungal infections at the time of examination.[118] The role between FIV infection and opportunistic pathogens is complex; however, treatment of secondary infections should not be abandoned simply because of the FIV-positive status.

Stomatitis is a common condition of FIV-positive cats and can occur during any stage of infection. Experimental and naturally occurring coinfection of FIV-positive cats with calicivirus resulted in more severe disease.[167, 195] Similar findings have been described for concurrent FIV and herpesvirus infections.[166]

FIV-positive cats may be presented for ocular disease.[50, 100, 141] Abnormalities may be found in both anterior and posterior segments. Anterior uveitis may result from secondary infections such as toxoplasmosis or may be directly related to FIV infection.[50, 141] Glaucoma, with and without uveitis, has also

Table 14–2. Clinical Signs in Cats With Naturally Acquired Infection[24, 50, 71, 157, 168, 178, 190, 191]

Fever	Weight loss, emaciation
Dermatitis, otitis	Enteritis, diarrhea
Lymph node enlargement	Abscesses
Stomatitis, gingivitis	Chronic renal insufficiency
Neurologic signs	Respiratory tract infection
Uveitis, pars planitis, conjunctivitis	

Table 14–3. Opportunistic Infections and Neoplasms Associated with Naturally Acquired FIV Infection

INFECTIONS	NEOPLASMS
Calicivirus[217]	Lymphoma, leukemia[87]
FeLV[132, 176]	Myeloproliferative disease[176, 190]
Papillomavirus[46]	Squamous cell carcinoma[87]
Poxvirus[22]	Mammary gland adenocarcinoma[178]
Feline syncytium-forming virus[228]	Mast cell tumor[9]
Toxoplasma gondii[76, 141]	Bronchoalveolar carcinoma[170]
Mycobacteria	
Cryptococcus[27, 54]	
Cryptosporidium[129]	
Dermatophytes[190]	
Haemobartonella felis[179]	

been reported.[50, 141] Posterior segment changes that may be seen include pars planitis (an infiltration of leukocytes, mainly plasma cells, into the vitreous behind the lens), focal retinal degeneration, and inner retinal hemorrhages.[50]

Respiratory disease may be observed in FIV-positive cats and can result from bacterial, fungal, and protozoal infections. Experimentally, FIV infection worsens the respiratory disease observed in a model of acute toxoplasmosis.[35]

In the terminal phase of infection, a wasting syndrome is common. Experimentally infected SPF cats have developed a terminal wasting syndrome within 6 to 8 weeks after infection.[40, 42] In contrast, early, rapid wasting has been observed after experimental infection with some Colorado isolates.[40]

Neoplasia is a common reason that FIV-positive cats are brought to a veterinary clinic. Lymphomas, leukemias, and a variety of other tumor types (see Table 14–3) have been reported in association with FIV infection.[9, 26, 30, 58, 87, 154] Most lymphomas in FIV-positive cats are B-cell tumors.[29, 154, 196] FIV is not easily detected in cells from most of these lymphomas, suggesting an indirect role of FIV in lymphoma formation.[48b] Cats dually infected with FeLV and FIV have a higher risk of developing lymphoma than cats infected with FIV alone.[176]

Neurologic signs have been described in both natural and experimental FIV infection.[1, 43, 44, 52, 151, 153] The most common neurologic sign observed is behavior change. Other deficits that have been described include seizures, paresis, multifocal motor abnormalities, and disrupted sleep patterns.[68, 161] Forebrain signs are often a result of direct neuronal injury from the virus. Less commonly, coinfection with opportunistic pathogens such as feline infectious peritonitis virus (FIPV), *Toxoplasma*, or *Cryptococcus* can cause a variety of neurologic deficits. Neurologic disease has been observed during both acute and terminal stages of FIV infection.[52] Neurologic signs may improve if they occur during the acute stage of infection, although residual deficits are possible.

DIAGNOSIS

Clinical Laboratory Findings

A number of clinicopathologic abnormalities have been described in FIV-infected cats, but none are specific or pathognomonic. During the acute phase of infection, cats may exhibit neutropenia and lymphopenia, which resolve as the cat progresses to the asymptomatic phase of infection.[111, 119] During the asymptomatic phase of infection, results of CBC and biochemical analyses are often normal,[111, 113, 119, 179] but intermittent leukopenia may be encountered.[179] Clinically ill, FIV-positive cats may have a variety of cytopenias. Anemia, neutropenia, and lymphopenia are seen in one third to one half of ill cats,[177, 178, 191] although these abnormalities may be as much a reflection of concurrent disease as direct effects of FIV infection itself.[198] Anemia, leukopenia, and less commonly thrombocytopenia[71] have been observed acutely in FIV-infected cats in the absence of other identifiable causes. It is suspected that FIV infection of cells in the bone marrow may decrease the number of progenitor cells and the normal cellular maturation and production kinetics of the various cell lines.[112]

Abnormalities of the biochemical profile of FIV-positive cats typically are few. Some cats will have an increase in total plasma and serum protein that is caused by increased immunoglobulin concentrations. Monoclonal gammopathy has been described in an FIV-positive cat with lymphoma.[172] Azotemia has been reported in infected cats in the absence of other underlying causes of renal disease,[157, 197] but FIV as a definitive cause of renal disease awaits clarification. Other biochemical abnormalities, when found, will usually reflect concurrent disease. When compared with control cats, after 9 months of infection experimentally infected cats had increased serum globulin, glucose, triglyceride, urea, and creatine concentrations and reduced serum cholesterol.[77a] The mechanism of such changes may include altered energy metabolism, subclinical hypercortisolemia, and release of cytokines in infected cats. Prolongations of the activated partial thromboplastin time (APTT) have been reported in FIV-positive cats in the absence of other obvious causes of coagulopathy, although the prolongations were mild and not clinically apparent.[71]

Little has been described of the CSF changes in FIV-positive cats with neurologic disease. Cellular pleocytosis and increases in concentrations of IgG in the CSF have been reported,[44] and it is not unreasonable to expect that there will be increases in cell number and total protein in CSF.

Serologic Testing

A definitive diagnosis of FIV infection is made by detection of FIV-specific antibodies in blood or saliva,[159] most commonly by ELISA-type assays, which are widely available and easy to use (see Appendix 6). ELISA, FA, and Western or immunoblot assays are performed by diagnostic laboratories. Because of the natural history of lentiviral infections, detection of antibody is synonymous with infection. Although anecdotal reports exist, there is as yet no published evidence that a cat may be antibody positive and not be infected, with the exception of kittens with maternally acquired antibody. Cats in the acute phase of infection could be antibody negative, and retesting of suspect cats in 6 to 8 weeks is warranted to establish a diagnosis. The relatively low prevalence of infection will result in occasional false-positive results because tests are not 100% specific. Technical error and use of whole blood rather than serum have been incriminated as causes of weak false-positive test results performed with inhouse assays as have nonspecific reactions to other infectious agents (FeLV, FIPV, *Toxoplasma*) cell culture components in feline vaccines.[8, 10, 16, 57] Cats that have positive results by ELISA should be retested, ideally by Western blot (see Chapter 1), to confirm the diagnosis. Alternatively, other tests (PCR, peptide ELISA viral culture) performed at research laboratories may confirm a positive test result.[94a]

Most cats develop a detectable antibody response within 8 weeks of initial infection; however, in some experimental studies, seroconversion was delayed for 6 months or longer.[148] It may not occur in rapidly progressive infections.[140a]

FIV-specific antibodies are readily detected in blood and saliva of most cats throughout the asymptomatic phase of infection. Asymptomatic kittens with regressive infections became seronegative, and evidence of persistent FIV infection could be only demonstrated by culture of PCR.[140a] In congenitally infected kittens with regressive infections, serologic titer results became negative, and persistent infection was demonstrated only by culture of PCR.[140a] Because of debilitation of the immune system, some cats entering the terminal phase of infection may lose detectable antibody or have reductions in titers to select antibodies identified by Western blot.[41]

Obtaining a definitive diagnosis in some antibody-negative cats in the terminal stage of disease may be a problem. Diagnosis in seronegative cats may be established in research settings by viral culture and detection of FIV provirus by PCR,[202] and practitioners with access to such laboratories may find assistance. Western blots may show FIV-specific antibodies not detected by some ELISAs. Flow cytometric analysis of peripheral blood lymphocytes may demonstrate inverted $CD4^+/CD8^+$ ratios in seronegative cats and is available at many veterinary teaching hospitals. Inverted $CD4^+/CD8^+$ ratios are only consistent with, but not diagnostic of, FIV infection.

Interpretation of antibody test results in young kittens of uncertain background is not straightforward, and sequential testing may be needed. Positive kittens may have maternal antibody, expected in the majority of cases, or may be truly infected. Retesting these kittens after 6 months of age is advised. If the second test is negative, the earlier positive result was likely due to maternal antibody. If still positive, the kitten is likely infected, and, ideally, a confirmatory test such as Western blot should be performed. A kitten of unknown background that is initially antibody negative is likely to be truly negative, but there is a small chance that the kitten has not had time to develop a detectable antibody response. These kittens should be retested after 8 to 12 weeks. If still negative, the kitten is unlikely to be infected. If positive, the kitten is probably infected and should have a confirmatory test performed.

PATHOLOGIC FINDINGS

Numerous pathologic changes may occur after FIV infection. The lymph nodes of FIV-infected cats may be hyperplastic during the acute phase of infection and, in the terminal phase of infection, may have disruption of normal architecture with loss of follicles and cellular depletion. Dysplastic changes have been reported in the bone marrow of infected cats, and inflammation in the GI tract has also been seen. Infected cats develop lymphoid interstitial pneumonitis, characteristic of lentiviral infections in other host species.[27a]

Experimentally infected cats that develop neurologic disease may have lymphocytic infiltration of perivascular areas (Fig. 14–3).[1] Giant cell formation has also been reported.[68] Renal disease includes glomerulosclerosis and tubulointerstitial infiltrates.[157] Some of the common pathologic abnormalities observed in FIV-infected cats are listed in Table 14–4.

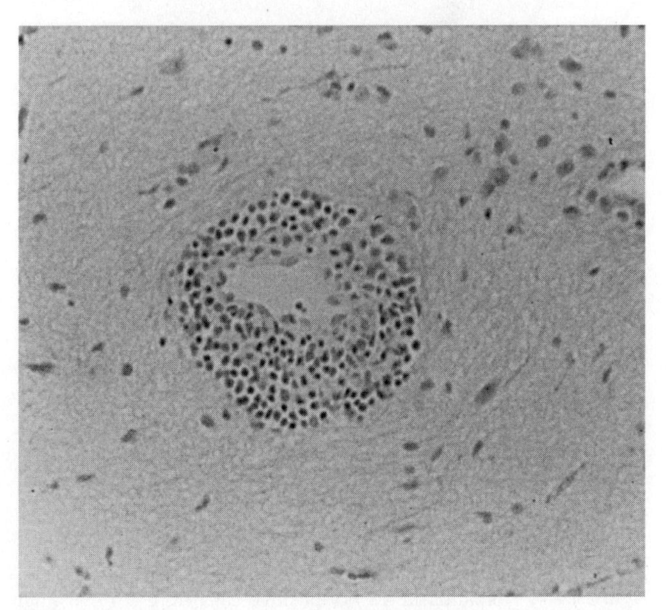

Figure 14–3. Photomicrograph of brain section from a cat experimentally infected with FIV showing prominent perivascular lymphocytic infiltration. (Courtesy of Dr. Bob English, North Carolina State University, Raleigh, NC.)

Table 14–4. Pathologic Abnormalities Described in FIV-Positive Cats[13, 15, 24, 31, 38, 40, 44, 53, 86, 121, 157, 158, 168]

AREA	ABNORMALITY
Lymph node	Follicular involution
	Follicular hyperplasia
	Follicular plasmacytosis
Thymus	Cortical involution, atrophy
Intestinal tract	Villous blunting
	Pyrogranulomatous colitis
	Lymphoplasmacytic stomatitis
Liver	Periportal hepatitis
Bone marrow	Myeloid hyperplasia
Kidney	Interstitial nephritis
	Glomerulosclerosis
Central nervous system	Perivascular cuffing
	Gliosis
	Myelitis
Lung	Interstitial pneumonia

THERAPY

At this time, there is no treatment with proven long-term efficacy specifically directed at the viral infection. Experimentally, treatment with nucleoside analogues such as azidothymidine (AZT) and phosphonylmethoxyethyladenine (PMEA) have been investigated in vitro and in vivo.[45, 72–74, 152, 185, 209] Treatment with either of these drugs before inoculation with FIV does not prevent infection or accumulation of provirus in target tissues, but delays the onset of detectable viremia and some of the immunologic changes.[45, 74, 75, 124, 152] Regression of stomatitis and increased $CD4^+/CD8^+$ ratios have been observed in naturally infected cats treated with AZT or PMEA.[45, 74] PMEA at high doses can cause anemia,[45] which is also a reported side effect of AZT in high doses.[185] As is the case with HIV, there is evidence from in vitro studies that FIV can become resistant to AZT.[65, 163, 164] Other compounds have been investigated, but their clinical efficacy has not been established.[186, 218] For the owner interested in pursuing treatment of a positive cat, AZT can be instituted (Table 14–5). Treatment with AZT is associated with improvement in a cat's clinical condition, immune status and quality of life, and prolonged life expectancy.[73, 73a] Although treatment suppresses viral replication, infection persists. The development of Heinz body anemia, although uncommon, is possible, and treated cats should have a CBC regularly evaluated. (For further information see Drug Formulary, Appendix 8). Treatment with recombinant human insulin-like growth factor with or without AZT increased lymphoid proliferation and T-cell dependent antibody responsiveness but had no effect on infections.[67a]

Immunomodulators such as acemannan have been used in FIV-positive cats,[225] but the reported beneficial effects observed with such agents are not clear. Available studies included cats concurrently treated with antibiotics and other symptomatic or supportive therapies and did not evaluate control (placebo) groups. Because many of the immunomodulators have immunostimulating effects, their use must be considered with extreme caution. In vitro, stimulation of infected immunocyte cultures is consistently associated with enhanced production of FIV.[201]

In the absence of specific antiviral agents, treatment is aimed at managing the complications of FIV infection. Cats not responding to empirical therapy should be carefully screened for the presence of occult infection or neoplasia. In these cases, in addition to a thorough physical examination and minimum data base (CBC and biochemical profiles, urinalysis), thoracic radiographs and abdominal radiographs or

Table 14–5. Therapy of FIV Infection and Its Complications

DRUG	DOSE[a]	ROUTE	INTERVAL (HOURS)	DURATION (WEEK)
Antiviral				
AZT[b]	15 mg/kg	PO, SC[c]	12	
Cytopenias				
Erythropoietin	100 IU/kg	SC	48	2[d]
Granulocyte colony-stimulating factor	5 μg/kg	SC	12	1–2
Stomatitis				
Metronidazole	5 mg/kg	PO	8	2–4
Clindamycin	12.5 mg/kg	PO	8	2–4
Prednisone	5 mg/cat	PO	12	2–4
Bovine lactoferrin	40 mg/kg	Topically to oral cavity	24	prn

[a]Dose per administration at specified intervals. See Drug Formulary, Appendix 8, for additional information.
[b]Monitor CBC regularly for Heinz body anemia.
[c]For PO, administer in gelatin capsules with specific calculated dose; for SC dilute lyophilate in 5 ml sodium chloride.
[d]Until desired PCV is reached.

ultrasonograms may be required to identify disease. Consideration should be given to cytology and culture of pertinent samples (urine, blood, effusions, tracheal wash) as additional diagnostic tests and as guides to pharmacologic choices. Cats with cytopenias may require bone marrow aspiration or biopsy to identify underlying causes. In those cats in which underlying causes of cytopenias are not found, consideration may be given to treating with specific hematopoietic growth factors such as erythropoietin (100 IU/kg, SC every other day until desired packed cell volume is reached, then as needed to maintain the hematocrit) and granulocyte colony-stimulating factor (5 μg/kg, SC, BID). Stomatitis may be treated initially with antibiotics (metronidazole or clindamycin) or prednisone (see Table 14–5). Topical bovine lactoferrin has also been beneficial for FIV-related stomatitis. (See also Chapter 100 and Appendix 8.)[173] Drug treatment should be accompanied by good dental hygiene. In cats that do not respond to drug therapy and teeth cleaning, full-mouth tooth extractions may be of benefit (Fig. 14–4).

When underlying infections are identified, treatment with appropriate antibiotics or antifungals is encouraged because there is no evidence to suggest that the FIV-positive cat is incapable of responding to treatment. Fungal infections in FIV-positive cats should be treated the same as in FIV-negative cats. Itraconazole is useful for cryptococcal infections and is effective for treatment of dermatophytosis. Cats with dermatophyte infections should not be treated with griseofulvin because this drug has been associated with the development of severe neutropenia in cats with naturally acquired FIV infection (see Drug Formulary, Appendix 8).

An important issue for which there are no currently established guidelines is whether FIV-positive cats should be routinely vaccinated for other infectious diseases. Experimental evidence shows that FIV-infected cats are able to mount immune responses to administered antigens[36, 103] except during the terminal phase of infection. FIV-positive cats vaccinated against FeLV early in the asymptomatic phase of infection were less susceptible to challenge infection than unvaccinated FIV-positive cats.[104] FIV-infected cats have developed illness with modified live virus feline panleukopenia vaccine (see Postvaccinal Complications, Systemic Illness, Chapter 100) so that inactivated boosters should be considered. Other studies suggest that immune stimulation helps stabilize $CD4^+$ cell numbers.[165] In contrast, stimulation of FIV-infected lymphocytes is also known to promote virus production in vitro. In vivo, vaccination of chronically infected FIV-positive cats with a synthetic peptide was associated with a decrease in the $CD4^+/CD8^+$ ratio.[106] Thus, the potential tradeoff to protection from infection with vaccination is progression of FIV infection secondary to increased virus production. It is my opinion that only those cats at high risk of exposure to infectious agents should receive vaccinations, and then only inactivated products should be

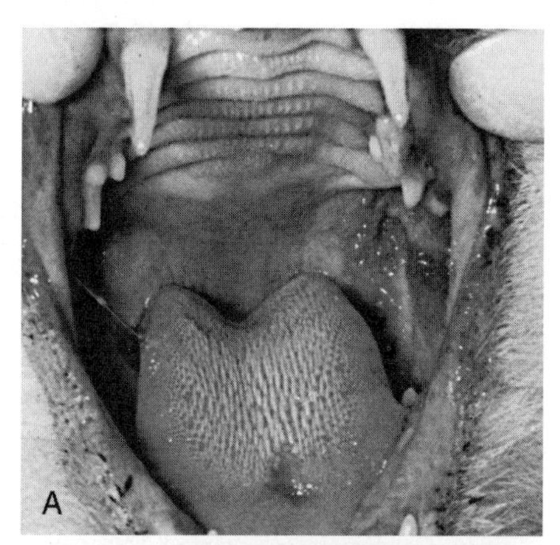

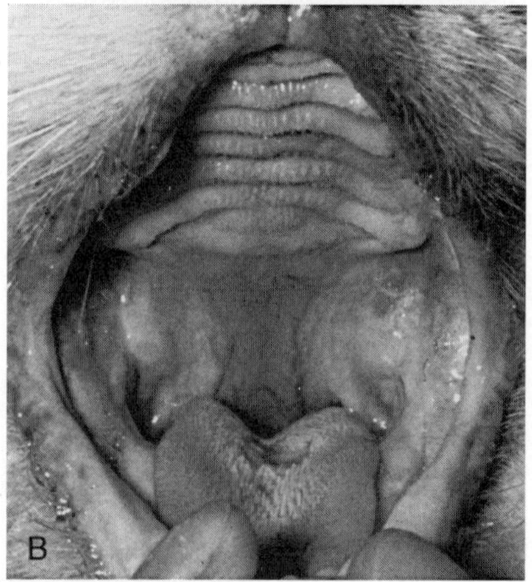

Figure 14–4. Stomatitis in an FIV-positive cat before *(A)* and after *(B)* extraction of all teeth. Note resolution of inflammation and regression of proliferative tissue in the fauces after tooth extraction. (Courtesy of Dr. Julie Levy, North Carolina State University, Raleigh, NC.)

used. The duration of immunity after vaccination of FIV-positive cats with inactivated products is unknown.

PREVENTION

There is currently no effective means of preventing infection other than preventing exposure. For this reason, FIV-positive cats should be segregated from FIV-negative cats. Work toward an FIV vaccine is underway at many laboratories. Developers of effective FIV vaccines face the hurdles of understanding which type of immunity (humoral or cell mediated) is most important in protection and identifying common antigens among the different isolates so that protection against heterologous isolates is achieved. Several different approaches have been taken in attempts to create FIV vaccines.[48a, 66, 198a, 211] There have been encouraging results with inactivated whole-cell or cell-free vaccines that provided some protection against both homologous and heterologous isolates,[81, 84, 223, 224] but duration of immunity is suspect.[123a] Homologous protection has been more effective. However, vaccines utilizing synthetic FIV peptides have not proven as effective.[62, 80, 114, 115, 212] Some concern exists that vaccination against FIV may, in some instances, enhance infection[83, 114, 143, 184] because antibody-bound virus is taken up by FIV target cells, such as macrophages and B cells, that bear Fc receptors. Protection against homologous isolates has been achieved by passive immunization. Kittens may be protected from infection if the queen has a high concentration of FIV-specific antibody, suggesting that stimulation of humoral immunity has a role in protection.[79, 162] Although humoral immunity may be important in early clearance of viremia, CMI is involved in subsequent elimination of virus from infected cells.[81, 194a] Some homologous protection is afforded by transfusion of immune cells to naive cats.[162a] Detection of cytotoxic T lymphocyte activity after vaccination implicates a role for cell-mediated immunity in protection.[62a, 194a] There will undoubtedly be many reports on FIV vaccines appearing in the near future, and, when evaluating the results obtained, it will be critical to note differences in adjuvants, challenge doses, and source of viral challenge (field isolates vs. cell culture isolates).

PUBLIC HEALTH CONSIDERATIONS

FIV is a feline pathogen, and there is no known evidence that it can infect people. Infection of human origin cell cultures has been accomplished in vitro, but only with FIV isolates that had genetically manipulated *env* gene sequences.

References

1. Abramo F, Bo S, Canese MG, et al. 1995. Regional distribution of lesions in the central nervous system of cats infected with feline immunodeficiency virus. *AIDS Res Hum Retroviruses* 11:1247–1253.
2. Ackley CD, Yamamoto JK, Levy N, et al. 1990. Immunologic abnormalities in pathogen-free cats experimentally infected with feline immunodeficiency virus. *J Virol* 64:5652–5655.
3. Bach J-M, Hurtrel M, Chakrabarti L, et al. 1994. Early stages of feline immunodeficiency virus infection in lymph nodes and spleen. *AIDS Res Hum Retroviruses* 10:1731–1738.

3a. Bachmann MH, Mathiason-Dubard C, Learn GH, et al. 1997. Genetic diversity of feline immunodeficiency virus: dual infection, recombination, and distinct evolutionary rates among envelope sequence clades. *J Virol* 71:4241–4253.

4. Baldinotti F, Matteucci D, Mazzetti P, et al. 1994. Serum neutralization of feline immunodeficiency virus is markedly dependent on passage history of the virus and host system. *J Virol* 68:4572–4579.
5. Bandecchi P, Matteucci D, Baldinotti F, et al. 1992. Prevalence of feline immunodeficiency virus and other retroviral infections in sick cats in Italy. *Vet Immunol Immunopathol* 31:337–345.
6. Barlough JE, Ackely CD, George JW, et al. 1991. Acquired immune dysfunction in cats with experimentally induced feline immunodeficiency virus infection: comparison of short-term and long-term infections. *J Acquir Immune Defic Syndr* 4:219–227.
7. Barlough JE, North TW, Oxford CL. 1993. Feline immunodeficiency virus infection of cats as a model to test the effect of certain selection pressures on the infectivity and virulence of resultant lentivirus variants. *Antiviral Res* 22:259–272.
8. Barr MC. 1996. FIV, FeLV and FIPV: Interpretation and misinterpretation of serological test results. *Semin Vet Med Surg* 11:144–153.
9. Barr MC, Butt MT, Anderson KL, et al. 1993. Spinal lymphosarcoma and disseminated mastocytoma associated with feline immunodeficiency virus infection in a cat. *J Am Vet Med Assoc* 202:1978–1980.
10. Barr MC, Pough MB, Jacobson RH, et al. 1991. Comparison and interpretation of diagnostic tests for feline immunodeficiency virus infection. *J Am Vet Med Assoc* 199:1377–1381.
11. Barr MC, Zou L, Holzschu DL, et al. 1995. Isolation of a highly cytopathic lentivirus from a nondomestic cat. *J Virol* 69:7371–7374.
12. Barsanti JA, Brown J, Marks A, et al. 1996. Relationship of lower urinary-tract signs to seropositivity for feline immunodeficiency virus in cats. *J Vet Intern Med* 10:34–38.
13. Beebe AM, Dua N, Faith TG, et al. 1994. Primary stage of feline immunodeficiency virus infection: viral dissemination and cellular targets. *J Virol* 68:3080–3091.
14. Beebe AM, Faith TG, Sparger EE, et al. 1994. Evaluation of in vivo and in vitro interactions of feline immunodeficiency virus and feline leukemia virus. *AIDS* 8:873–878.
15. Beebe AM, Gluckstern TG, George J, et al. 1992. Detection of feline immunodeficiency virus infection in bone marrow of cats. *Vet Immunol Immunopathol* 35:37–49.
16. Bendinelli M, Pistello M, Lombardi S, et al. 1995. Feline immunodeficiency virus: an interesting model for AIDS studies and an important cat pathogen. *Clin Microbiol Rev* 9:87–112.
17. Bishop SA, Gruffydd-Jones TJ, Harbour DA. 1993. Programmed cell death (apoptosis) as a mechanism of cell death in peripheral blood mononuclear cells from cats infected with feline immunodeficiency virus. *Clin Exp Immunol* 93:65–71.
18. Bishop SA, Stokes CR, Gruffydd-Jones TJ, et al. 1996. Vaccination with fixed feline immunodeficiency virus (FIV) infected cells: protection, breakthrough and specificity of response. *Vaccine* 14:1243–1250.
19. Bishop SA, Stokes CR, Gruffydd-Jones TJ, et al. 1996. Vaginal and rectal infection of cats with feline immunodeficiency virus. *Vet Microbiol* 51:217–227.
20. Bishop SA, Williams NA, Gruffydd-Jones TJ, et al. 1992. An early defect in primary and secondary T cell reponses in asymptomatic cats during feline immunodeficiency (FIV) virus infection. *Clin Exp Immunol* 90:491–496.
21. Bishop SA, Williams NA, Gruffydd-Jones TJ, et al. 1992. Impaired T-cell priming and proliferation in cats infected with feline immunodeficiency virus. *AIDS* 6:287–293.

21a. Boche D, Hurtrel M, Gray F, et al. 1996. Virus load and neuropathology in the FIV model. *J Neurovirol* 2:377–387.

22. Brown A, Bennett M, Gaskell CJ. 1989. Fatal poxvirus infection in association with FIV infection. *Vet Rec* 124:19–20.
23. Brown EW, Yuhki N, Packer C, et al. 1994. A lion lentivirus related to feline immunodeficiency virus: epidemiologic and phylogenetic aspects. *J Virol* 68:5953–5968.
24. Brown PJ, Hopper CD, Harbour DA. 1991. Pathologic features of lymphoid tissues in cats with natural feline immunodeficiency virus infection. *J Comp Pathol* 104:345–355.
25. Brown WC, Bissey L, Logan KS, et al. 1991. Feline immunodeficiency virus infects both $CD4^+$ and $CD8^+$ T lymphocytes. *J Virol* 65:3359–3364.
26. Buracco P, Guglielmino R, Abate O, et al. 1992. Large granular lymphoma in an FIV-positive and FeLV-negative cat. *J Small Anim Pract* 33:279–284.

26a. Burkhard MJ, Obert LA, O'Neil LL, et al. 1997. Mucosal transmission of cell-associated and cell-free feline immunodeficiency virus. *AIDS Res Hum Retroviruses* 13:347–355.

27. Cabanes FJ, Abarca ML, Bonavia R, et al. 1995. Cryptococcosis in a cat seropositive for feline immunodeficiency virus. *Mycoses* 38:131–133.

27a. Cadore JL, Steinerlaurent S, Greenland T, et al. 1997. Interstitial lung-disease in feline immunodeficiency virus (FIV) infected cats. *Res Vet Sci* 62:287–288.

28. Callanan JJ, Hosie MJ, Jarrett O. 1991. Transmission of feline immunodeficiency virus from mother to kitten. *Vet Rec* 128:332–333.
29. Callanan JJ, Jones BA, Irvine J, et al. 1996. Histologic classification and immunophenotype of lymphosarcomas in cats with naturally and experimentally acquired feline immunodeficiency virus infections. *Vet Pathol* 33:264–272.
30. Callanan JJ, McCandish IAP, O'Neil B, et al. 1992. Lymphosarcoma in

experimentally induced feline immunodeficiency virus infection. *Vet Rec* 130:293–295.
31. Callanan JJ, Thompson H, Toth SR, et al. 1992. Clinical and pathological findings in feline immunodeficiency virus experimental infection. *Vet Immunol Immunopathol* 35:3–13.
32. Cohen ND, Carter CN, Thomas MA, et al. 1990. Epizootiologic association between feline immunodeficiency virus infection and feline leukemia virus seropositivity. *J Am Vet Med Assoc* 197:220–225.
33. Danave IR, Tiffany-Castiglioni E, Zenger E, et al. 1994. Feline immunodeficiency virus decreases cell-cell communication and mitochondrial membrane potential. *J Virol* 68:6745–6750.
34. Dandekar S, Beebe AM, Barlough J, et al. 1992. Detection of feline immunodeficiency virus (FIV) nucleic acids in FIV-seronegative cats. *J Virol* 66:4040–4049.
35. Davidson MG, Rottman JB, English RV, et al. 1993. Feline immunodeficiency virus predisposes cats to acute generalized toxoplasmosis. *Am J Pathol* 143:1486–1497.
36. Dawson S, Smyth NR, Bennett M, et al. 1991. Effect of primary-stage feline immunodeficiency virus infection on subsequent feline calicivirus vaccination and challenge in cats. *AIDS* 5:747–750.
36a. de Parseval A, Lerner DL, Borrow P, et al. 1997. Blocking of feline immunodeficiency virus infection by a monoclonal antibody to CD9 is via inhibition of virus release rather than interference with receptor binding. *J Virol* 71:5742–5749.
37. De Ronde A, Stone JG, Boers P, et al. 1993. Antibody response in cats to the envelope proteins of feline immunodeficiency virus: identification of an immunodominant neutralization domain. *Virology* 198:257–264.
38. Dean GA, Reubel GH, Moore PF, et al. 1996. Proviral burden and infection kinetics of feline immunodeficiency virus in lymphocyte subsets of blood and lymph node. *J Virol* 70:5165–5169.
39. Del Fierro GM, Meers J, Thomas J, et al. 1995. Quantification of lymphadenopathy in experimentally induced feline immunodeficiency virus infection in domestic cats. *Vet Immunol Immunopathol* 46:3–14.
40. Diehl LJ, Mathiason-Dubard CK, O'Neil LL, et al. 1995. Induction of accelerated feline immunodeficiency virus disease by acute-phase virus passage. *J Virol* 69:6149–6157.
41. Diehl LJ, Mathiason-Dubard CK, O'Neil LL, et al. 1995. Longitudinal assessment of feline immunodeficiency virus kinetics in plasma by use of a quantitative competitive reverse transcriptase PCR. *J Virol* 69:2328–2332.
42. Diehl LJ, Mathiason-Dubard CK, O'Neil LL, et al. 1996. Plasma viral RNA load predicts disease progression in accelerated feline immunodeficiency virus infection. *J Virol* 70:2503–2507.
43. Dow SW, Drietz MJ, Hoover EA. 1992. Feline immunodeficiency virus neurotropism: evidence that astrocytes and microglia are the primary target cells. *Vet Immunol Immunopathol* 35:23–35.
44. Dow SW, Poss ML, Hoover EA. 1990. Feline immunodeficiency virus: a neurotropic lentivrus. *J Acquir Immune Defic Syndr* 3:658–668.
45. Egberink H, Borst M, Niphuis H, et al. 1990. Suppression of feline immunodeficiency virus infection in vivo by 9-(2-phosphonomethoxyethyl) adenine. *Proc Natl Acad Sci U S A* 87:3087–3091.
46. Egberink HF, Berrocal A, Bax HAD, et al. 1992. Papillomavirus associated skin lesions in a cat seropositive for feline immunodeficiency virus. *Vet Microbiol* 31:117–125.
47. Egberink HF, Keldermans EJ, Koolen MJM, et al. 1992. Humoral immune response to feline immunodeficiency virus in cats with experimentally induced and naturally acquired infections. *Am J Vet Res* 53:1133–1138.
48. Elder JH, Phillips TR. 1995. Feline immunodeficiency virus as a model for development of molecular approaches to intervention strategies against lentivirus infections. *Adv Virus Res* 45:225–247.
48a. Elyars JS, Tellier MC, Soos JM, et al. 1997. Perspectives on FIV vaccine development. *Vaccine* 15:1437–1444.
48b. Endo Y, Cho KW, Nishigaki K, et al. 1997. Molecular characteristics of malignant lymphomas in cats naturally infected with feline imunodeficiency virus. *Vet Immunol Immunopathol* 57:153–167.
49. English RV. 1995. Feline immunodeficiency virus, pp 280–286. *In* Bonagura JD (ed), Kirk's current veterinary therapy. WB Saunders, Philadelphia, PA.
50. English RV, Davidson MG, Nasisse MP, et al. 1990. Intraocular disease associated with feline immunodeficiency virus infection in cats. *J Am Vet Med Assoc* 196:1116–1119.
51. English RV, Johnson CM, Gebhard DH, et al. 1993. In vivo lymphocyte tropism of feline immunodeficiency virus. *J Virol* 67:5175–5186.
52. English RV, Nelson P, Johnson CM, et al. 1994. Development of clinical disease in cats experimentally infected with feline immunodeficiency virus. *J Infect Dis* 170:543–552.
53. Femenia F, Crespeau F, Fontaine JJ, et al. 1994. Early haematological and pathological abnormalities of pathogen-free cats experimentally infected with feline immunodeficiency virus (FIV). *Vet Res* 25:544–554.
54. Ferrer L, Ramos JA, Bonavia J, et al. 1992. Cryptococcosis in two cats seropositive for feline immunodeficiency virus. *Vet Rec* 131:393–394.
55. Fevereiro M, Roneker C, De Noronha F. 1991. Antibody response to reverse transcriptase in cats infected with feline immunodeficiency virus. *Viral Immunol* 4:225–235.
56. Fevereiro M, Roneker C, De Noronha F. 1993. Enhanced neutralization of feline immunodeficiency virus by complement virus lysis. *Vet Immunol Immunopathol* 36:191–206.
57. Flagstad A, Jensen AL, Jarrett O. 1997. Evidence of infection with feline immunodeficiency virus among Danish cats between 1970 and 1974. *Vet Rec* 140:99–100.
58. Fleming EJ, McCaw DL, Smith JA, et al. 1991. Clinical, hematologic, and survival data from cats infected with feline immunodeificiency virus: 42 cases (1983–1988). *J Am Vet Med Assoc* 199:913–916.
59. Flynn JN, Beatty JA, Cannon CA, et al. 1995. Involvement of gag- and env-specific cytotoxic T lymphocytes in protective immunity to feline immunodeficiency virus. *AIDS Res Hum Retroviruses* 11:1107–1113.
60. Flynn JN, Cannon CA, Beatty JA, et al. 1994. Induction of feline immunodeficiency virus-specific cytotoxic T cells in vivo with carrier-free synthetic peptide. *J Virol* 68:5835–5844.
61. Flynn JN, Cannon CA, Lawrence CE, et al. 1994. Polyclonal B-cell activation in cats infected with feline immunodeficiency virus. *Immunology* 81:626–630.
62. Flynn JN, Cannon CA, Reid G, et al. 1995. Induction of feline immunodeficiency virus-specific cell-mediated and humoral immune responses following immunization with a multiple antigenic peptide from the envelope V3 domain. *Immunology* 85:171–175.
62a. Flynn JN, Keating P, Hosie MJ, et al. 1996. Env-specific CTL predominate in cats protected from feline immunodeficiency virus infection by vaccination. *J Immunol* 157:3658–3665.
63. Franchini M, Dittmer A, Kottwitz B, et al. 1990. Clinical symptoms and humoral antibody response in cats experimentally infected with FIV and FeLV, pp 201–207. *In* Schellekens H, Horzinek MC (eds), Animal models in AIDS. Elsevier Science, New York.
64. George JW, Pedersen NC, Higgins J. 1993. The effect of age on the course of experimental feline immunodeficiency virus infection in cats. *AIDS Res Hum Retroviruses* 9:897–905.
65. Gobert JM, Remington KM, Zhu YQ, et al. 1994. Multiple-drug-resistant mutants of feline immunodeficiency virus selected with 2',3'-dideoxyinosine alone and in combination with 3'-azido-3'-deoxythymidine. *Antimicrob Agents Chemother* 38:861–864.
66. Gonin P, Fournier A, Oualikene W, et al. 1995. Immunization trial of cats with a replication-defective adenovirus type 5 expressing the ENV gene of feline immunodeficiency virus. *Vet Microbiol* 45:393–401.
67. Greene WK, Meers J, del Fierro G, et al. 1993. Extensive sequence variation of feline immmunodeficiency virus *env* genes in isolates from naturally infected cats. *Arch Virol* 133:51–62.
67a. Gregory CR, Griffey SM, Patz JD, et al. 1997. Effects of insulin-like growth factor-1 and AZT in cats experimentally infected with FIV. *Feline Pract* 25:23–31.
68. Gunn-Moore DA, Pearson GR, Harbour DA. 1996. Encephalitis associated with giant cells in a cat with naturally occurring feline immunodeficiency virus infection demonstrated by in situ hybridization. *Vet Pathol* 33:699–703.
69. Hanlon MA, Marr JM, Hayes KA, et al. 1993. Loss of neutrophil and natural killer cell function following feline immunodeficiency virus infection. *Viral Immunol* 6:119–124.
70. Hara Y, Ishida T, Ejima H, et al. 1990. Decrease in mitogen-induced lymphocyte proliferative responses in cats infected with feline immunodeficiency virus. *Jpn J Vet Sci* 52:573–579.
71. Hart SW, Nolte I. 1994. Hemostatic disorders in feline immunodeficiency virus-positive cats. *J Vet Intern Med* 8:355–362.
72. Hart SW, Nolte I. 1995. Long-term treatment of diseased, FIV-seropositive field cats with azidothymidine (AZT). *Zentralb Veterinarmed* 42:397–409.
73. Hartmann K. 1996. AZT in the treatment of feline immunodeficiency virus infection: part 1. *Feline Pract* 23(5):16–21.
73a. Hartmann K. 1996. AZT in the treatment of feline immunodeficiency virus infection: part 2. *Feline Pract* 23(6):13–20.
74. Hartmann K, Donath A, Beer B, et al. 1992. Use of two virustatica (AZT, PMEA) in the treatment of FIV and FeLV seropositive cats with clinical symptoms. *Vet Immunol Immunopathol* 35:167–175.
75. Hayes KA, Wilkinson JG, Frick R, et al. 1995. Early suppression of viremia by ZDV does not alter the spread of feline immunodeficiency virus infection in cats. *J Acquir Immune Defic Syndr* 9:114–122.
76. Heidel JR, Dubey JP, Blythe LL, et al. 1990. Myelitis in a cat infected with *Toxoplasma gondii* and feline immunodeficiency virus. *J Am Vet Med Assoc* 196:316–318.
77. Hoffman-Fezer G, Thum J, Ackley C, et al. 1992. Decline in $CD4^+$ cell numbers in cats with naturally acquired feline immunodeficiency virus infection. *J Virol* 66:1484–1488.
77a. Hoffman-Lehmann R, Holznagel E, Ossent P, et al. 1997. Parameters of disease progression in long-term experimental feline retrovirus (feline immunodeficiency virus and feline leukemia virus) infections-hematology, clinical chemistry, and lymphocyte subsets. *Clin Diagn Lab Immunol* 4:33–42.
77b. Hohdatsu T, Fujimori S, Maeki M, et al. 1997. Virus neutralizing antibody titer to feline immunodeficiency virus isolates of subtypes A, B and D in experimentally or naturally infected cats. *J Vet Med Sci* 59:377–381.
78. Hohdatsu T, Hirabayashi H, Motokawa K, et al. 1996. Comparative study of the cell tropism of feline immunodeficiency virus isolates of subtypes

A, B, and D classified on the basis of the env gene V3-V5 sequence. *J Gen Virol* 77:93–100.
79. Hohdatsu T, Pu R, Torres BA, et al. 1993. Passive antibody protection of cats against feline immunodeficiency virus infection. *J Virol* 67:2344–2348.
80. Hosie MJ, Dunsford TH, de Ronde A, et al. 1996. Suppression of virus burden by immunization with feline immunodeficiency virus env protein. *Vaccine* 14:405–411.
81. Hosie MJ, Flynn JN. 1996. Feline immunodeficiency virus vacination: characterization of the immune correlates of protection. *J Virol* 70:7561–7568.
82. Hosie MJ, Jarrett O. 1990. Serological responses of cats to feline immunodeficiency virus. *AIDS* 4:215–220.
83. Hosie MJ, Osborne R, Reid G, et al. 1992. Enhancement after feline immunodeficiency virus vaccination. *Vet Immunol Immunopathol* 35:191–197.
84. Hosie MJ, Osborne R, Yamamoto JK, et al. 1995. Protection against homologous but not heterologous challenge induced by inactivated feline immunodeficiency virus vaccines. *J Virol* 69:1253–1255.
85. Hosie MJ, Willett BJ, Dunsford TH, et al. 1993. A monoclonal antibody which blocks infection with feline immunodeficiency virus identifies a possible non-CD4 receptor. *J Virol* 67:1667–1671.
86. Hurtrel M, Ganiere J-P, Guelfi JF, et al. 1992. Comparison of early and late feline immunodeficiency virus encephalopathies. *AIDS* 6:399–406.
87. Hutson CA, Rideout BA, Pedersen NC. 1991. Neoplasia associated with feline immunodeficiency virus infection in cats of Southern California. *J Am Vet Med Assoc* 199:1357–1362.
88. Ishida T, Taniguchi A, Matsumura S, et al. 1992. Long-term clinical observations on feline immunodeficiency virus infected asymptomatic carriers. *Vet Immunol Immunopathol* 35:15–22.
89. Ishida T, Tomoda I. 1990. Clinical staging of feline immunodeficiency virus infection. *Jpn J Vet Sci* 52:645–648.
90. Jeng CR, English RV, Childers T, et al. 1996. Evidence for CD8+ antiviral activity in cats infected with feline immunodeficiency virus. *J Virol* 70:2474–2480.
91. Johnson CM, Benson NA, Papadi GP. 1996. Apoptosis and CD4+ lymphocyte depletion following feline immunodeficiency virus infection of a T-lymphocyte cell line. *Vet Pathol* 33:195–203.
92. Jordan HL, Howard J, Sellon RK, et al. 1996. Transmission of feline immunodeficiency virus in domestic cats via artificial insemination. *J Virol* 70:8224–8228.
93. Jordan HL, Howard J, Tompkins WA, et al. 1995. Detection of feline immmunodeficiency virus in semen from seropositive domestic cats (*Felis catus*). *J Virol* 69:7328–7333.
94. Kakinuma S, Motokawa K, Hohdatsu T, et al. 1995. Nucleotide sequence of feline immunodeficiency virus: classification of Japanese isolates into two subtypes which are distinct from non-Japanese subtypes. *J Virol* 69:3639–3646.
94a. Kania SA, Kennedy MA, Potgieter LND. 1997. Serologic reactivity using conserved envelope epitopes in feline lentivirus-infected felids. *J Vet Diagn Invest* 9:125–129.
95. Kohmoto M, Miyazawa T, Tomonaga K, et al. 1994. Comparison of biological properties of feline immunodeficiency virus isolates using recombinant chimeric viruses. *J Gen Virol* 75:1935–1942.
96. Kraus LA, Bradley WG, Engelman RW, et al. 1996. Relationship between tumor necrosis factor alpha and feline immunodeficiency virus expressions. *J Virol* 70:566–569.
97. Kyaw-Tanner MT, Greene WK, Park H-S, et al. 1994. The induction of in vivo superinfection and recombination using feline immunodeficiency virus as the model. *Arch Virol* 138:261–271.
98. Lappin MR, Gasper PW, Rose BJ, et al. 1992. Effect of primary phase feline immunodeficiency virus infection on cats with chronic toxoplasmosis. *Vet Immunol Immunopathol* 35:121–132.
99. Lappin MR, George JW, Pedersen NC, et al. 1996. Primary and secondary *Toxoplasma gondii* infection in normal and feline immunodeficiency virus-infected cats. *J Parasitol* 82:733–742.
100. Lappin MR, Marks A, Greene CE, et al. 1992. Serologic prevalence of selected infectious diseases in cats with uveitis. *J Am Vet Med Assoc* 201:1005–1009.
101. Lappin MR, Marks A, Greene CE, et al. 1993. Effect of feline immunodeficiency virus infection on *Toxoplasma gondii*-specific humoral and cell-mediated immune responses of cats with serologic evidence of toxoplasmosis. *J Vet Intern Med* 7:95–100.
102. Lawrence CE, Callanan JJ, Jarrett O. 1992. Decreased mitogen responsiveness and elevated tumor necrosis factor production in cats shortly after feline immunodeficiency virus infection. *Vet Immunol Immunopathol* 35:51–59.
103. Lawrence CE, Callanan JJ, Willett BJ, et al. 1995. Cytokine production by cats infected with feline immunodeficiency virus: a longitudinal study. *Immunology* 85:568–574.
104. Lehman R, Franchini M, Aubert A, et al. 1991. Vaccination of cats experimentally infected with feline immunodeficiency virus using a recombinant feline leukemia virus vaccine. *J Am Vet Med Assoc* 199:1446–1452.
105. Lehman R, Joller H, Haagmans BL, et al. 1992. Tumor necrosis factor α levels in cats experimentally infected with feline immunodeficiency virus: effects of immunization and feline leukemia virus infection. *Vet Immunol Immunopathol* 35:61–69.
106. Lehman R, von Beust B, Niederer E, et al. 1992. Immunization-induced decrease of the CD4+:CD8+ ratio in cats experimentally infected with feline immunodeficiency virus. *Vet Immunol Immunopathol* 35:199–214.
107. Li J, Brown WC, Song W, et al. 1995. Retroviral vector-transduced cells expressing the core polyprotein induce feline immunodeficiency virus specific cytotoxic T-lymphocytes from infected cats. *Virus Res* 38:93–109.
108. Lin D-S, Bowman DD. 1992. Macrophage functions in cats experimentally infected with feline immunodeficiency virus and *Toxoplasma gondii*. *Vet Immunol Immunopathol* 33:69–78.
109. Lin D-S, Bowman DD, Jacobson RH. 1990. Suppression of lymphocyte blastogenesis to mitogens in cats experimentally infected with feline immunodeficiency virus. *Vet Immunol Immunopathol* 26:183–189.
110. Lin D-S, Bowman DD, Jacobson RH. 1992. Immunological changes in cats with concurrent *Toxoplasma gondii* and feline immunodeficiency virus infection. *J Clin Microbiol* 30:17–24.
111. Linenberger ML, Abkowitz JL. 1995. Haematological disorders associated with feline retrovirus infections. *Baillieres Clin Haematol* 8:73–112.
112. Linenberger ML, Beebe AM, Pedersen NC, et al. 1995. Marrow accessory cell infection and alterations in hematopoiesis accompany severe neutropenia during experimental acute infection with feline immunodeficiency virus. *Blood* 85:941–951.
113. Linenberger ML, Shelton GH, Persik MT, et al. 1991. Hematopoiesis in asymptomatic cats infected with feline immunodeficiency virus. *Blood* 78:1963–1968.
114. Lombardi S, Garzelli C, Pistello M, et al. 1994. A neutralizing antibody-inducing peptide of the V3 domain of feline immunodeficiency virus envelope glycoprotein does not induce protective immunity. *J Virol* 68:8374–8379.
115. Lutz H, Hofmann-Lehmann R, Leutenegger C, et al. 1996. Vaccination of cats with recombiant envelope glyproprotein of feline immunodeficiency virus. Decreased viral load after vaccine challenge. *AIDS Res Hum Retroviruses* 12:431–434.
116. Ma J, Kennedy-Stoskopf S, Sellon R, et al. 1995. Tumor necrosis factor-α responses are depressed and interleukin-6 responses unaltered in feline immunodeficiency virus infected cats. *Vet Immunol Immunopathol* 46:35–50.
117. Maki N, Miyazawa T, Fukasawa M, et al. 1992. Molecular characterization and heterogeneity of feline immunodeficiency virus isolates. *Arch Virol* 123:29–45.
118. Mancianti F, Giannelli C, Bendinelli M, et al. 1992. Mycological findings in feline immunodeficiency virus-infected cats. *J Med Vet Mycol* 30:257–259.
119. Mandell CP, Sparger EE, Pedersen NC, et al. 1992. Long-term hematological changes in cats experimentally infected with feline immunodeficiency virus (FIV). *Comp Hematol Int* 2:8–17.
120. Martin J-P, Bingen A, Braunwald J, et al. 1995. Evidence of feline immunodeficiency virus replication in cultured Kupffer cells. *AIDS* 9:447–453.
120a. Matsumoto H, Takemura N, Toshimori S, et al. 1997. Serum concentration of circulating immune complexes in cats infected with feline immunodeficiency virus detected by immune adherence hemagglutination method. *J Vet Med Sci* 59:395–396.
121. Matsumura S, Ishida T, Washizu I, et al. 1993. Pathologic features of acquired immunodeficiency-like syndrome in cats experimentally infected with feline immunodeficiency virus. *J Vet Med Sci* 55:387–394.
122. Matteuci D, Baldinotti F, Mazzetti P, et al. 1993. Detection of feline immunodeficiency virus in saliva and plasma by cultivation and polymerase chain reaction. *J Clin Microbiol* 31:494–501.
123. Matteuci D, Pistello M, Mazzetti P, et al. 1996. Vaccination protects against in vivo-grown feline immunodeficiency virus even in the absence of detectable neutralizing antibodies. *J Virol* 70:617–622.
123a. Matteuci D, Pistello M, Mazzetti P, et al. 1997. Studies of AIDS vaccination using an ex vivo feline-immunodeficiency-virus model: protection conferred by a fixed-cell vaccine against cell-free and cell-associated challenge differs in duration and is not easily boosted. *J Virol* 71:8368–8376.
124. Meers J, del Fiero GM, Cope RB, et al. 1993. Feline immunodeficiency virus infection: plasma, but not peripheral blood mononuclear cell virus titer, is influenced by zidovudine and cyclosporine. *Arch Virol* 132:67–81.
125. Meers JM, Robinson WF, del Fierro GM, et al. 1992. Feline immunodeficiency virus: quantification in peripheral blood mononuclear cells and isolation from plasma of infected cats. *Arch Virol* 127:233–243.
126. Miyazawa T, Fukasawa M, Hasegawa A, et al. 1991. Molecular cloning of a novel isolate of feline immunodeficiency virus biologically and genetically different from the original US isolate. *J Virol* 65:1572–1577.
127. Moench TR, Whaley KJ, Mandrell TD, et al. 1993. The cat/feline immunodeficiency virus model for transmucosal transmission of AIDS: nonoxynol-9 contraceptive jelly blocks transmission by an infected cell inoculum. *AIDS* 7:797–802.
127a. Momoi Y, Mizuno T, Nishimura Y, et al. 1996. Detection of apoptosis induced in peripheral blood lymphocytes from cats infected with feline immunodeficiency virus. *Arch Virol* 141:1651–1659.
128. Moraillon A, Barre-Sinoussi F, Parodi A, et al. 1992. In vitro properties and experimental pathogenic effect of three strains of feline immunodeficiency virus isolated from cats with terminal disease. *Vet Microbiol* 31:41–54.
129. Mtambo MMA, Nash AS, Blewett DA, et al. 1991 Cryptosporidium infec-

tion in cats: prevalence of infection in domestic and feral cats in the Glasgow area. *Vet Rec* 129:502–504.
130. Norimine J, Miyazawa T, Kawaguchi Y, et al. 1993. Feline CD4 molecules expressed on feline non-lymphoid cell lines are not enough for productive infection of highly lymphotropic feline immunodeficiency virus isolates. *Arch Virol* 130:171–178.
131. Novotney C, English RV, Housman J, et al. 1990. Lymphocyte population changes in cats naturally infected with feline immunodeficiency virus. *AIDS* 4:1213–1218.
132. O'Connor TP, Tonelli QJ, Scarlett JM. 1991. Report of the national FeLV/ FIV awareness project. *J Am Vet Med Assoc* 199:1348–1353.
133. Ohashi T, Goitsuka R, Watari T, et al. 1992. Elevation of feline interleukin 6-like activity in feline immunodeficiency virus infection. *Clin Immunol Immunopathol* 65:207–211.
134. Ohno K, Nakano T, Matsumoto Y, et al. 1993. Apoptosis induced by tumor necrosis factor in cells chronically infected with feline immunodeficiency virus. *J Virol* 67:2429–2433.
135. Ohno K, Okamoto Y, Miyazawa T, et al. 1994. Induction of apoptosis in a T lymphoblastoid cell line infected with feline immunodeficiency virus. *Arch Virol* 135:153–158.
136. Ohno K, Watari T, Goitsuka R, et al. 1992. Altered surface antigen expression on peripheral blood mononuclear cells in cats infected with feline immunodeficiency virus. *J Vet Med Sci* 54:517–522.
137. Okada S, Pu R, Young E, et al. 1994. Superinfection of cats with feline immunodeficiency virus subtypes A and B. *AIDS Res Hum Retroviruses* 10:1739–1746.
138. Olmsted RA, Langley R, Roelke ME, et al. 1992. Worldwide prevalence of lentivirus infection in wild feline species: epidemiologic and hylogenetic aspects. *J Virol* 66:6008–6018.
139. O'Neil LL, Burkhard MJ, Diehl LJ, et al. 1995. Vertical transmission of feline immunodeficiency virus. *AIDS Res Hum Retroviruses* 1:171–182.
140. O'Neil LL, Burkhard MJ, Hoover EA. 1996. Frequent perinatal transmission of feline immunodeficiency virus by chronically infected cats. *J Virol* 70:2894–2901.
140a. O'Neil LL, Burkhard MJ, Obert LA, et al. 1997. Regression of feline immunodeficiency virus infection. *AIDS Res Hum Retrovir* 13:713–718.
141. O'Neil SA, Lappin MR, Reif JS, et al. 1991. Clinical and epidemiologic aspects of feline immunodeficiency virus and *Toxoplasma gondii* coinfections in cats. *J Am Anim Hosp Assoc* 27:211–220.
141a. Orandle MS, Papadi GP, Bubenik LJ, et al. 1997. Selective thymocyte depletion and immunoglobulin coating in the thymus of cats infected with feline immunodeficiency virus. *AIDS Res Hum Retroviruses* 13:611–620.
142. Osborne R, Rigby M, Siebelink K, et al. 1994. Virus neutralization reveals antigenic variation among feline immunodeficiency virus isolates. *J Gen Virol* 75:3641–3645.
143. Osterhaus ADME, Tijhaar E, Huisman RC, et al. 1996. Accelerated viremia in cats vaccinated with recombinant vaccinia virus expressing envelope glycoprotein of feline immunodeficiency virus. *AIDS Res Hum Retroviruses* 12:437–442.
144. Pancino G, Castelot S, Sonigo P. 1995. Differences in feline immunodeficiency virus host cell range correlate with envelope fusogenic properties. *Virology* 206:796–806.
145. Pancino G, Chappey C, Saurin W, et al. 1993. B epitopes and selection pressures in feline immunodeficiency virus envelope glycoproteins. *J Virol* 67:664–672.
146. Pancino G, Fossati I, Chappey C, et al. 1993. Structure and variations of feline immunodeficiency virus envelope glycoproteins. *Virology* 192:659–662.
146a. Pancino G, Sonigo P. 1997. Retention of viral infectivity after extensive mutation of the highly conserved immunodominant domain of the feline immunodeficiency virus envelope. *J Virol* 71:4339–4346.
147. Park HS, Kyaw-Tanner M, Thomas J, et al. 1995. Feline immunodeficiency virus replicates in salivary gland ductular epithelium during the initial phase of infection. *Vet Microbiol* 46:257–267.
148. Pedersen NC, Barlough JE. 1991. Clinical overview of feline immunodeficiency virus. *J Am Vet Med Assoc* 199:1298–1305.
149. Pedersen NC, Torten M, Rideout B, et al. 1990. Feline leukemia virus infection as a potentiating cofactor for the primary and secondary stages of experimentally induced feline immunodeficiency virus infection. *J Virol* 64:598–606.
150. Peri EV, Ponti W, Dall'ara P, et al. 1994. Seroepidemiologic and clinical survey of feline immunodeficiency virus infection in northern Italy. *Vet Immunol Immunopathol* 40:285–297.
151. Phillips TR, Prospero-Garcia O, Puaoi DL, et al. 1994. Neurological abnormalities associated with feline immunodeficiency virus infection. *J Gen Virol* 75:979–987.
152. Philpott MS, Ebner JP, Hoover EA. 1992. Evaluation of 9-(2-phosphonomethoxyethyl)adenine therapy for feline immunodeficiency virus using a quantitative polymerase chain reaction. *Vet Immunol Immunopathol* 35:155–166.
153. Podell M, Oglesbee M, Mathes L, et al. 1993. AIDS-associated encephalopathy with experimental feline immunodeficiency virus infection. *J Acquir Immune Defic Syndr* 6:678–771.
154. Poli A, Abramo F, Baldinotti F, et al. 1994. Malignant lymphoma associated with experimentally induced feline immunodeficiency virus infection. *J Comp Pathol* 110:319–328.
155. Poli A, Abramo F, Caricchio P, et al. 1995. Lentivirus infection in an African lion: a clinical, pathologic and virologic study. *J Wildl Dis* 31:70–74.
156. Poli A, Abramo F, Matteucci D, et al. 1995. Renal involvement in feline immunodeficiency virus: p24 antigen detection, virus isolation and PCR analysis. *Vet Immunol Immunopathol* 46:13–20.
157. Poli A, Abramo F, Taccini E, et al. 1993. Renal involvement in feline immunodeficiency virus infection: a clinicopathologic study. *Nephron* 64:282–288.
158. Poli A, Falcone ML, Bigalli L, et al. 1995. Circulating immune complexes and analysis of of renal immune deposits in feline immunodeficiency virus-infected cats. *Clin Exp Immunol* 101:254–258.
159. Poli A, Gianelli C, Pistello M, et al. 1992. Detection of salivary antibodies in cats infected with feline immunodeficiency virus. *J Clin Microbiol* 30:2038–2041.
159a. Pontzer CH, Yamamoto JK, Bazer FW, et al. 1997. Potent anti-feline immunodeficiency virus and anti-human immunodeficiency virus effect of IFN-tau. *J Immunol* 158:4351–4357.
160. Poss ML, Dow SW, Hoover EA. 1992. Cell-specific envelope glycosylation distinguishes FIV glycoproteins produced in cytopathically and noncytopathically infected cells. *Virology* 188:25–32.
160a. Power C, Moench T, Peeling J, et al. 1997. Feline immunodeficiency virus causes increased glutamate levels and neuronal loss in brain. *Neuroscience* 77:1175–1185.
161. Prospero-Garcia O, Herold N, Phillips TR, et al. 1994. Sleep patterns are disturbed in cats infected wtih feline immunodeficiency virus. *Proc Natl Acad Sci U S A* 91:12947–12951.
162. Pu R, Okada S, Little ER, et al. 1995. Protection of neonatal kittens against feline immunodeficiency virus infection with passive maternal antiviral antibodies. *AIDS* 9:235–242.
162a. Pu R, Tellier MC, Yamamoto JK. 1997. Mechanisms of FIV vaccine protection. *Leukemia* 11(Supplement 3):98–101.
163. Remington KM, Chesebro B, Wehrly K, et al. 1991. Mutants of feline immunodeficiency virus resistant to 3'-azido-3'-deoxythymidine. *J Virol* 65:308–312.
164. Remington KM, Zhu Y-Q, Phillips TR, et al. 1994. Rapid phenotypic reversion of zidovudine-resistant feline immunodeficiency virus without loss of drug-resistant reverse transcriptase. *J Virol* 68:632–637.
165. Reubel GH, Dean GA, George JW, et al. 1994. Effects of incidental infections and immune activation on disease progression in experimentally feline immunodeficiency virus-infected cats. *J Acquir Immune Defic Syndr* 7:1003–1015.
166. Reubel GH, George JW, Barlough JE, et al. 1992. Interaction of acute feline herpesvirus-1 and chronic feline immunodeficiency virus infections in experimentally infected specific pathogen free cats. *Vet Immunol Immunopathol* 35:95–119.
167. Reubel GH, George JW, Higgins J, et al. 1994. Effect of chronic feline immunodeficiency virus infection on experimental feline calicivirus-induced disease. *Vet Microbiol* 39:335–351.
168. Rideout BA, Lowenstine LJ, Hutson CA, et al. 1992. Characterization of morphologic changes and lymphocyte subset distribution in lymph nodes from cats with naturally acquired feline immunodeficiency virus infection. *Vet Pathol* 29:391–399.
169. Rideout BA, Moore PF, Pedersen NC. 1992. Persistent upregulation of MHC class II antigen expression on T-lymphocytes from cats experimentally infected with feline immunodeficiency virus. *Vet Immunol Immunopathol* 35:71–81.
170. Rigby MA, Holmes EC, Pistello M, et al. 1993. Evolution of structural proteins of feline immunodeficiency virus: molecular epidemiology and evidence of selection for change. *J Gen Virol* 74:425–436.
170a. Rigby MA, Hosie MJ, Willett BJ, et al. 1997. Comparative efficiency of feline immunodeficiency virus-infection by DNA inoculation. *AIDS Res Hum Retrovir* 13:405–412.
171. Rimmelzwaan GF, Siebelink KH, Broos H, et al. 1994. gag- and env-specific serum antibodies in cats after natural and experimental infection with feline immunodeficiency virus. *Vet Microbiol* 39:153–165.
172. Rosenberg MP, Hohenhaus AE, Matus RE. 1991. Monoclonal gammopathy and lymphoma in a cat infected with feline immunodeficiency virus. *J Am Anim Hosp Assoc* 27:335–337.
173. Sato R, Inanami O, Tanaka Y, et al. 1996. Oral administration of bovine lactoferrin for treatment of intractable stomatitis in feline immunodeficiency virus (FIV)-positive and FIV-negative cats. *Am J Vet Res* 57:1443–1446.
174. Sellon RK, Jordan HL, Kennedy-Stoskopf S, et al. 1994. Feline immunodeficiency virus can be experimentally transmitted via milk during acute maternal infection. *J Virol* 68:3380–3385.
175. Sellon RK, Levy JK, Jordan HL, et al. 1996. Changes in lymphocyte subsets with age in perinatal cats, late gestation through 8 weeks. *Vet Immunol Immunopathol* 53:105–113.
176. Shelton GH, Grant CK, Cotter SM, et al. 1990. Feline immunodeficiency virus and feline leukemia virus infection and their relationships to lymphoid malignancies in cats: a retrospective study (1968–1988). *J Acquir Immune Defic Syndr* 3:623–630.

177. Shelton GH, Linenberger ML, Abkowitz JL. 1991. Hematologic abnormalities in cats seropositive for feline immunodeficiency virus. *J Am Vet Med Assoc* 199:1353–1357.
178. Shelton GH, Linenberger ML, Grant CK, et al. 1990. Hematologic manifestations of feline immunodeficiency virus. *Blood* 76:1104–1109.
179. Shelton GH, Linenberger ML, Persik MT, et al. 1995. Prospective ematologic and clinicopathologic study of asymptomatic cats with naturally acquired feline immunodeficiency virus infection. *J Vet Intern Med* 9:133–140.
180. Siebelink KHJ, Bosch ML, Rimmelzwaan GF, et al. 1995. Two different mutations in the envelope protein of feline immunodeficiency virus allow the virus to escape from neutralization by feline serum ntibodies. *Vet Immunol Immunopathol* 46:61–70.
181. Siebelink KHJ, Huisman W, Karlas JA, et al. 1995. Neutralization of feline immunodeficiency virus by polyclonal feline antibody: simultaneous involvement of hypervariable regions 4 and 5 of the surface glycoprotein. *J Virol* 69:5124–5127.
182. Siebelink KHJ, Karlas JA, Rimmelzwaan GF, et al. 1995. A determinant of feline immunodeficiency virus involved in CrFK cell tropism. *Vet Immunol Immunopathol* 46:61–70.
183. Siebelink KHJ, Rimmelzwaan GF, Bosch ML, et al. 1993. A single amino acid substitution in hypervariable region 5 of the envelope protein of feline immunodeficiency virus allows escape from virus neutralization. *J Virol* 67:2202–2208.
184. Siebelink KHJ, Tijhaar E, Huisman RC, et al. 1995. Enhancement of feline immunodeficiency virus infection after immunization with envelope glycoprotein subunit vaccines. *J Virol* 69:3704–3711.
184a. Silvotti L, Corradi A, Brandi G, et al. 1997. FIV-induced encephalopathy: early brain lesions in the absence of viral replication in monocyte/macrophages. *Vet Immunol Immunopathol* 55:263–271.
185. Smyth NR, Bennett M, Gaskell RM, et al. 1994. Effect of 3'azido-2'-3'deoxythymidine (AZT) on experimental feline immunodeficiency virus infection in domestic cats. *Res Vet Sci* 57:220–224.
186. Smyth NR, McCracken C, Gaskell RM, et al. 1994. Susceptibility in cell culture of feline immunodeficiency virus to eighteen antiviral agents. *J Antimicrob Chemother* 34:589–594.
187. Sodora DL, Shpaer EG, Kitchell BE, et al. 1994. Identification of three feline immunodeficiency virus (FIV) *env* gene subtypes and comparison of the FIV and human immunodeficiency virus type 1 evolutionary patterns. *J Virol* 68:2230–2238.
188. Song W, Collisson EW, Billingsley PM, et al. 1992. Induction of feline immunodeficiency virus-specific cytolytic T-cell responses from experimentally infected cats. *J Virol* 66:5409–5417.
189. Song W, Collisson EW, Li J, et al. 1995. Feline immunodeficiency virus (FIV)-specific cytotoxic T lymphocytes from chronically infected cats are induced in vitro by retroviral vector-transduced feline T cells expressing the FIV capsid protein. *Virology* 209:390–399.
190. Sparger EE. 1990. Feline immunodeficiency virus infection, pp 334–345. *In* Greene CE (ed), Infectious diseases of the dog and cat. WB Saunders, Philadelphia, PA.
191. Sparkes AH, Hopper CD, Millard WG, et al. 1993. Feline immunodeficiency infection: clinicopathologic findings in 90 naturally occurring cases. *J Vet Intern Med* 7:85–90.
192. Steffan A-M, Lafon M-E, Gendrault J-L, et al. 1994. Feline immunodeficiency virus can productively infect cultured endothelial cells from cat brain microvessels. *J Gen Virol* 75:3647–3653.
193. Taniguchi A, Ishida T, Konno A, et al. 1990. Altered mitogen response of peripheral blood lymphocytes in different stages of feline immunodeficiency virus infection. *Jpn J Vet Sci* 52:513–518.
194. Taniguchi A, Ishida T, Washizu T, et al. 1991. Humoral immune response to T cell dependent and independent antigens in cats infected with feline immunodeficiency virus. *J Vet Med Sci* 53:333–335.
194a. Tellier MC, Soos J, Pu R, et al. 1997. Development of FIV-specific cytolytic T-lymphocyte response in cats upon immunisation with FIV vaccines. *Vet Microbiol* 57:1–12.
195. Tenorio AP, Franti CE, Madewell BR, et al. 1991. Chronic oral infections of cats and their relationship to persistent oral carriage of feline calici-, immunodeficiency, or leukemia viruses. *Vet Immunol Immunopathol* 29:1–14.
196. Terry A, Callanan JJ, Fulton R, et al. 1995. Molecular anaysis of tumours from feline immunodeficiency virus (FIV)-infected cats: an indirect role for FIV? *Int J Cancer* 61:227–232.
197. Thomas JB, Robinson WF, Chadwick BJ, et al. 1993. Association of renal disease indicators with feline immunodeficiency infection. *J Am Anim Hosp Assoc* 29:320–326.
198. Thomas JB, Robinson WF, Chadwick BJ, et al. 1993. Leukogram and biochemical abnormalities in naturally occurring feline immunodeficiency virus infection. *J Am Anim Hosp Assoc* 29:272–278.
198a. Tijhaar EJ, Siebelink KH, Karlas JA, et al. 1997. Induction of feline immunodeficiency virus specific antibodies with an attenuated *Salmonella* strain expressing the gag protein. *Vaccine* 15:587–596.
199. Tokunaga K, Nishino Y, Oikawa H, et al. 1992. Altered cell tropism and cytopathicity of feline immunodeficiency viruses in two different feline CD4-positive, CD8-negative cell lines. *J Virol* 66:3893–3898.
200. Tokunaga K, Shoda K, Nishino Y, et al. 1995. Maintenance of high virus load even after seroconversion in newborn cats acutely infected wtih feline immunodeficiency virus. *Vaccine* 13:1393–1398.
201. Tomonaga K, Inoshima Y, Ikeda Y, et al. 1995. Temporal patterns of feline immunodeficiency virus transcripts in peripheral blood cells during the latent stage of infection. *J Gen Virol* 76:2193–2204.
202. Tomonaga K, Mikami T. 1996. Detection of feline immunodeficiency virus transcripts by quantitative reverse transcription polymerase chain reaction. *Vet Microbiol* 48:337–344.
203. Tompkins MB, Nelson PD, English RV, et al. 1991. Early events in the immunopathogenesis of feline retrovirus infections. *J Am Vet Med Assoc* 199:1311–1315.
204. Torten M, Franchini M, Barlough JE, et al. 1991. Progressive immune dysfunction in cats experimentally infected with feline immunodeficiency virus. *J Virol* 65:2225–2230.
205. Torten M, Rideout BA, Luciw PA, et al. 1990. Co-infection of cats with feline immunodeficiency virus (FIV) and feline leukemia virus (FeLV) enhances the severity of FIV infection and affects the distribution of FIV DNA in various tissues, pp 209–210. *In* Schellekens H, Horzinek MC (eds), Animal models in AIDS. Elsevier Science, New York.
206. Toyosaki T, Miyazawa T, Furuya T, et al. 1993. Localization of the viral antigen of feline immunodeficiency virus in the lymph nodes of cats at the early stage of infection. *Arch Virol* 131:335–347.
207. Tozzini F, Matteucci D, Bandecchi P, et al. 1993. Neutralizing antibodies in cats infected with feline immunodeficiency virus. *J Clin Microbiol* 31:1626–1629.
208. Ueland K, Nesse LL. 1992. No evidence of vertical transmission of naturally acquired feline immunodeficiency virus infection. *Vet Immunol Immunopathol* 33:301–308.
209. Vahlenkamp TW, de Ronde A, Balzarini J, et al. 1995. (R)-9-(2-phosphonylmethoxypropyl)-2,6-diaminopurine is a potent inhibitor of feline immunodeficiency virus infection. *Antimicrob Agents Chemother* 39:746–749.
209a. Vahlenkamp TW, Verschoor EJ, Schuurman NN, et al. 1997. A single amino acid substitution in the transmembrane envelope glycoprotein of feline immunodeficiency virus alters cellular tropism. *J Virol* 71:7132–7135.
209b. Vandewoude S, O'Brien SJ, Hoover EA. 1997. Infectivity of lion and puma lentiviruses for domestic cats. *J Gen Virol* 78:795–800.
210. Verschoor EJ, Boven LA, Blaak H, et al. 1995. A single mutation within the V3 envelope neutralization domain of feline immunodeficiency virus determines its tropism for CRFK cells. *J Virol* 69:4752–4757.
211. Verschoor EJ, van Vliet ALW, Egberink HF, et al. 1995. Vaccination against feline immunodeficiency virus using fixed infected cells. *Vet Immunol Immunopathol* 46:139–150.
212. Verschoor EJ, Willemse MJ, Stam JG, et al. 1996. Evaluation of subunit vaccines against feline immunodeficiency virus infection. *Vaccine* 14:285–289.
213. Walker C, Canfield PJ, Love DN. 1994. Analysis of leucocytes and lymphocyte subsets for different clinical stages of naturally acquired feline immunodeficiency virus infection. *Vet Immunol Immunopathol* 44:1–12.
214. Walker C, Canfield PJ, Love DN, et al. 1996. A longitudinal study of lymphocyte subsets in a cohort of cats naturally-infected with feline immunodeficiency virus. *Aust Vet J* 73:218–224.
215. Walker C, Malik R, Canfield PJ. 1995. Analysis of leucocytes and lymphocyte subsets in cats with naturally-occurring cryptococcosis but differing feline immunodeficiency virus status. *Aust Vet J* 72:93–97.
216. Wasmoen T, Armiger-Luhman S, Egan C, et al. 1992. Transmission of feline immunodeficiency virus from infected queens to kittens. *Vet Immunol Immunopathol* 35:83–93.
217. Waters L, Hopper CD, Gruffyd-Jones TJ, et al. 1993. Chronic gingivitis in a colony of cats infected with feline immunodeficiency virus and feline calicivirus. *Vet Rec* 132:340–342.
218. Wiggs RB, Lobprise HB, Matthews JL, et al. 1993. Effects of preactivated MC540 in the treatment of lymphocytic plasmacytic stomatitis in feline leukemia virus and feline immunodeficiency virus positive cats. *J Vet Dent* 10:9–33.
219. Willett BJ, Hosie MJ, Callanan JJ, et al. 1993. Infection with feline immunodeficiency virus is followed by the rapid expansion of a CD8$^+$ lymphocyte subset. *Immunology* 78:1–6.
220. Willett BJ, Hosie MJ, Dunsford TH, et al. 1991. Productive infection of T-helper lymphocytes with feline immunodeficiency virus is accompanied by reduced expression of CD4. *AIDS* 5:1469–1475.
221. Willett BJ, Hosie MJ, Jarrett O, et al. 1994. Identification of a putative cellular receptor for feline immunodeficiency virus as the feline homologue of CD9. *Immunology* 81:228–233.
221a. Willett BJ, Hosie MJ, Neil JC, et al. 1997. Common mechanism of infection by lentiviruses. *Nature* 385:587.
221b. Willett BJ, Hosie MJ, Shaw A, Neil J. 1997. Inhibition of feline immunodeficiency virus infection by CD9 antibody operates after virus entry and is independent of virus tropism. *J Gen Virol* 78:611–618.
221c. Willett BJ, Picard L, Hosie MJ, et al. 1997. Shared usage of the chemokine receptor CXCR4 by the feline and human immunodeficiency viruses. *J Virol* 71:6407–6415.
221d. Woo JC, Dean GA, Pedersen NC, et al. 1997. Immunopathologic changes

in the thymus during the acute stage of experimentally induced feline immunodeficiency virus infection in juvenile cats. *J Virol* 71:8632–8641.
222. Yamada H, Miyazawa T, Tomonaga K, et al. 1995. Phylogenetic analysis of the long terminal repeat of feline immunodeficiency viruses from Japan, Argentina and Australia. *Arch Virol* 140:41–52.
223. Yamamoto JK, Hohdatsu T, Holmsted RA, et al. 1993. Experimental vaccine protection against homologous and heterologous strains of feline immunodeficiency virus. *J Virol* 67:601–605.
224. Yamamoto JK, Okuda T, Ackley CD, et al. 1991. Experimental vaccine protection against feline immunodeficiency virus. *AIDS Res Hum Retroviruses* 7:911–922.
225. Yates KM, Rosenberg LJ, Harris CK, et al. 1992. Pilot study of the effect of acemannan in cats infected wtih feline immunodeficiency virus. *Vet Immunol Immunopathol* 35:177–189.
226. Zaccaro L, Falcone ML, Silva S, et al. 1995. Defective natural killer cell cytotoxic activity in feline immunodeficiency virus-infected cats. *AIDS Res Hum Retroviruses* 11:747–752.
227. Zenger E. 1990. Clinical findings in cats with feline immunodeficiency virus. *Feline Pract* 18:25–28.
228. Zenger E, Brown WC, Song W, et al. 1993. Evaluation of cofactor effect of feline syncytium forming virus in feline immunodeficiency virus infection. *Am J Vet Res* 56:713–718.
229. Zenger E, Collisson EW, Barhoumi R, et al. 1995. Laser cytometric analysis of FIV-induced injury in astroglia. *Glia* 13:92–100.
230. Zhao Y, Gebhard D, English R, et al. 1995. Enhanced expression of novel CD57⁺CD8⁺ LAK cells from cats infected with feline immunodeficiency virus. *J Leukoc Biol* 58:423–431.
231. Zhu YQ, Remington KM, North TW. 1996. Mutants of feline immunodeficiency virus resistant to 2′,3′-dideoxy-2′,3′-didehydrothymidine. *Antimicrob Agents Chemother* 40:1983–1987.

Chapter 15

Feline Adenovirus Infection

Frances A. Kennedy

Clinically apparent disease caused by systemic adenoviral infection has been most common in immunologically compromised animals,[1, 2] and there is only one reported case of confirmed disseminated adenovirus infection in a cat.[4] One PCR-confirmed case of adenovirus infection has been documented in the feline species.[6] Serologic studies of cats in Hungary, Scotland, and Denmark showed positive rates of 15%, 20%, and 10%, respectively.[5] Inclusion body hepatitis reported in a black panther was suggestive of adenovirus infections[3]; however, there was no virologic or EM confirmation of the causative agent. In the one confirmed report, a comatose 8-year-old spayed, domestic shorthaired female cat had petechiae on the oral mucous membranes. Abnormal hematologic findings included leukopenia (2100 cells/μl) and thrombocytopenia (73,000/μl). There was no response to treatment with IV lactated Ringer's solution, dexamethasone, and vitamin K. The cat died 4 hours after presentation.

At necropsy, the abdominal cavity and pericardial sac were filled with serous fluid. Serosal and mucosal surfaces of the small and large intestines were diffusely dark red, with scattered serosal petechiae, and the intestinal contents were fluid and dark red. The liver and kidneys were swollen, and the liver had an accentuated lobular pattern.

An undiluted sample of serous abdominal fluid gave a positive test result for the group-specific antigen (p27) of the feline leukemia virus (FeLV) and a negative result for the antibody to feline immunodeficiency virus. A specimen of ileum gave a positive result for feline coronavirus by FA testing. An ELISA test for feline panleukopenia virus was negative on specimens of liver, kidney, ileum, mesenteric lymph node, and spleen. An adenovirus particle was identified by EM examination of the intestinal contents.

Histologically, endothelial cells were detached from intramyocardial coronary arteries, and the sloughed cells were large and spindle shaped with occasional multinucleated cells. Nuclei of these cells were large and pleomorphic with intranuclear inclusion bodies. Multiple round eosinophilic inclusions were present in some nuclei, with amphophilic granular inclusions filling other nuclei. Some nuclei were almost filled with well-delineated basophilic inclusions, with margination of the small amount of surrounding chromatic. Occasional basophilic nuclei had indistinct borders, resulting in the appearance of "smudge cells." Cytoplasm of these cells was eosinophilic. Minimal perivascular infiltrates of lymphocytes were present in the myocardium.

In the stomach there was diffuse, submucosal edema. Diffuse superficial necrotizing and hemorrhagic enteritis with submucosal edema was present in the small intestine. Necro-

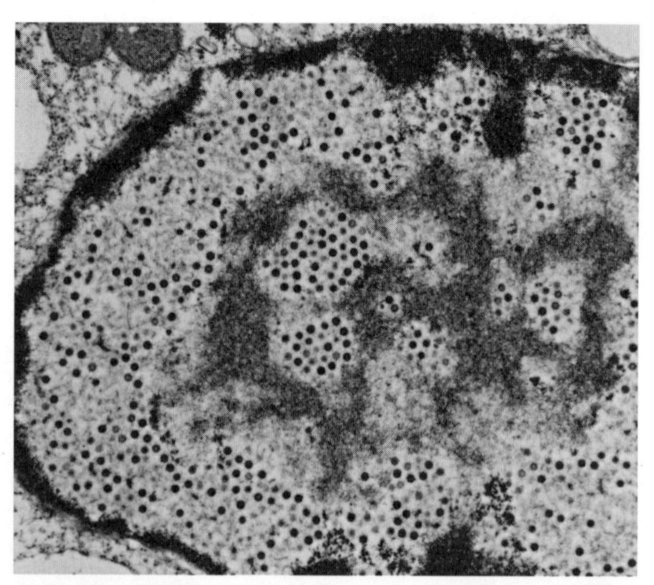

Figure 15–1. Electron micrograph of an endothelial cell with intranuclear viral particles. Moderate autolytic change is responsible for disruption of the adenoviral arrays (× 17,900). (From Kennedy FA, Mullaney TP. 1993. *J Vet Diagn Invest* 5:273–276. Reprinted with permission.)

sis was more severe in the ileum, with full-thickness mucosal necrosis over Peyer's patches. There was moderate lymphoid depletion and peripheral hemorrhage in submucosal lymphoid tissue. Sections of colon were comparably affected, with submucosal edema and particularly severe mucosal necrosis overlying areas of prominent submucosal lymphoid tissue. Submucosal and mesenteric blood vessels at all levels of the GI tract had endothelial lesions as described in the heart. Similar vascular lesions were seen in small hepatic arteries, pulmonary arteries, trachea, thymic remnant, urinary bladder, thyroid gland, adrenal gland, bone marrow, spleen, lymph node, and kidney. There was depletion of lymphoid follicles in spleen and lymph nodes.

EM examination of detached endothelial cells showed intranuclear aggregates of viral particles measuring approximately 65 nm in diameter (Fig. 15–1). Some of these particles were roughly icosahedral with dense central cores. In some areas, viral particles formed loose crystalline arrays.

Overt disease with adenoviruses usually requires an immunodeficient state, whether congenital or acquired.[1, 2] Adenoviruses have relatively narrow ranges of host specificity. Horses, dogs, a goat, and other cats kept on the property with the affected cat appeared clinically normal. The source of infection in this cat was undetermined. It is possible that FeLV infection produced an immunodeficient state in the affected cat, and leukopenia may have been a consequence of FeLV infection and/or terminal endotoxemia. Thrombocytopenia, also seen clinically, was most likely associated with consumption secondary to vascular lesions, because the bone marrow had adequate numbers of megakaryocytes.

The positive FA test for feline coronavirus probably indicated a subclinical infection. There were no gross or histologic lesions typical of feline infectious peritonitis.

References

1. Barker IK, Van Dreumel AA, Palmer N. 1993. The alimentary system, pp 181–184. *In* Jubb KVF, Kennedy PC, Palmer N (eds), Pathology of domestic animals, ed 4, vol 2. Academic Press, San Diego, CA.
2. Dungworth DL. 1993. The respiratory system, pp 626–628. *In* Jubb KVF, Kennedy PC, Palmer N (eds), Pathology of domestic animals, ed 4, vol 2. Academic Press, San Diego, CA.
3. Gupta PP. 1978. Inclusion body hepatitis in a black panther *(Panthera pardus pardus). Zentralbl Veterinarmed B* 25:858–860.
4. Kennedy FA, Mullaney TP. 1993. Disseminated adenovirus infection in a cat. *J Vet Diagn Invest* 5:273–276.
5. Lakatos B, Farkas J, Adam E, et al. 1996. Data to the adenovirus infection of European cats. *Magyar Allatorvosok Lapja* 51:543–545.
6. Lakatos B, Farkas J, Egberink HF, et al. 1997. PCR detection of adenovirus from a cat. *Magyar Allatorvosok Lapja* 52:517–519.

Chapter 16

Feline Respiratory Disease

Rosalind Gaskell and Susan Dawson

ETIOLOGY

Respiratory disease in cats remains a problem despite relatively widespread use of vaccines, although overall the severity of the disease has been reduced. The disease is most commonly seen in cats that are grouped together, as in multicat households, boarding catteries, and breeding establishments. The majority of cases of infectious respiratory disease are due to one of two viruses: feline rhinotracheitis virus (FRV or feline herpesvirus-1, FHV-1) and feline calicivirus (FCV). In the past, both these viruses have been isolated in approximately equal frequency from cases of the disease. Later surveys, however, have found that FCV appears to be relatively more common,[14] possibly because of the antigenic diversity of FCV isolates compared with the single serotype for FRV. Current FCV vaccines may not protect equally well against all strains.

Other agents involved in the syndrome include *Bordetella bronchiseptica*, a feline strain of *Chlamydia psittaci*, feline reovirus, cowpox virus, and other bacteria and mycoplasmas. *B. bronchiseptica* was originally thought to be only a secondary pathogen in cats, and *C. psittaci* is predominantly a conjunctival pathogen.

Feline Rhinotracheitis Virus

FRV is a typical α-herpesvirus, containing double-stranded DNA, with a glycoprotein-lipid envelope. Like most herpesviruses, it is relatively fragile in the external environment and is highly susceptible to the effects of common disinfectants. It can probably survive only for up to 18 hours in a damp environment, less in dry conditions. It is also relatively unstable as an aerosol.

All isolates so far examined are very similar antigenically and belong to one serotype. Although some minor differences have been detected, they are also relatively homogeneous on restriction enzyme analysis of their DNA.[13, 15] Most isolates are of similar pathogenicity, although strains of reduced virulence have been produced for vaccines.

FRV appears to be antigenically unrelated to several herpesviruses tested from other species, and infection appears to be confined to members of the cat family. One group of workers isolated herpesviruses indistinguishable from FRV from dogs with diarrhea, but the significance of this is unclear (see Chapter 8).

Feline Calicivirus

FCV is a small, unenveloped single-stranded RNA virus, a member of the calicivirus family. The name calicivirus is derived from the characteristic cuplike depressions on the surface of the virus particle. FCV is slightly more resistant than FRV, surviving for up to a week in the external environment or possibly longer if conditions are damp. The virus is not as susceptible to the effects of disinfectants as FRV, but both viruses are inactivated by bleach diluted 1 part in 32 in water with added detergent.

A large number of different strains of FCV vary slightly in antigenicity and pathogenicity, although they all show sufficient cross-reactivity to be classified as one serotype. Most isolates are closely related enough to induce some degree of cross-protection, but cats can still be sequentially infected with different strains and show varying degrees of clinical illness.[19, 23]

Some FCV isolates appear to be more immunogenic than others and more broadly cross-reactive. Such strains are obviously ideal candidates for vaccines. F9 was the first vaccine strain shown in the early 1970s to neutralize 50% of isolates tested, and further studies with current field isolates have confirmed that it still cross-reacts with a majority of strains.[7, 23] Other strains of FCV that appear to be useful candidates for vaccine viruses have also been reported.[7, 19a, 23] However, strains of FCV exist that have minimal in vitro cross-reactivity with commonly used vaccine strains, and these could account for some apparent vaccine failures.[6] Vaccine viruses may also alter on passage through the cat, leading to more vaccine-resistant strains.[23]

As far as is known, FCV infects only members of the Felidae,[17a] although caliciviruses antigenically similar to FCV have been recovered from dogs. (See Other Viral Enteritides, Chapter 8.)

Bordetella bronchiseptica

B. bronchiseptica is an aerobic, gram-negative coccobacillus that is a well-known respiratory pathogen in dogs, swine, and rodents. In the past, *B. bronchiseptica* was thought to play only a secondary role in feline respiratory disease, but its status in the syndrome is currently being re-evaluated. The majority of *B. bronchiseptica* isolations were originally associated with cases of bronchopneumonia in laboratory-kept cats, often housed under overcrowded conditions, whose virologic status was unclear. *B. bronchiseptica* has been isolated in association with respiratory disease from pedigree breeding cats and from household pets from various sources.[33, 35]

Whether *B. bronchiseptica* plays predominantly a primary or secondary role is not fully established. However, respiratory disease has been reproduced in *Bordetella*-free, specific pathogen-free (SPF) cats after aerosol or nasal challenge.[2, 17] Clinical respiratory disease has also been reported from laboratory cats suffering from respiratory disease in which the respiratory viruses were known to be absent.[10]

Chlamydia psittaci (var. felis)

Chlamydiae are obligate intracellular bacteria that, unlike viruses, contain both DNA and RNA, have a rigid cell wall, and are susceptible to certain antibiotics. Chlamydiae are relatively unstable outside the host, surviving in conjunctival discharges at room temperature for only several days. They have a lipid-containing cell wall and are inactivated by a number of lipid solvents and detergents. A 1 part in 1000 dilution of a quaternary ammonium compound is recommended for hospital use.

Strains of *C. psittaci* cause respiratory disease, conjunctivitis, abortion, and arthritis in many species. The feline strain of *C. psittaci* is generally thought to infect only cats, causing predominantly conjunctivitis. There are a few isolated reports of its possible involvement in conjunctivitis in humans.

Other Organisms

Reoviruses have been occasionally isolated from cats, and conjunctival and respiratory signs have been induced after experimental inoculation. However, there is no evidence that reoviruses are important as respiratory pathogens in cats in the field.

Cowpox virus infection in cats primarily causes skin lesions, but occasional respiratory or ocular signs may be seen (see Chapter 19). The reservoir hosts of cowpox virus in Europe are small wild mammals, and cats occasionally become infected by contact through hunting. Other orthopoxviruses that may infect cats exist in other parts of the world.

The role of mycoplasmas in feline respiratory disease is not clear. Undoubtedly, they can be important as secondary pathogens, but their role as primary agents is more equivocal (see Chapter 32). Infection is common in both colony cats and household pets, and mycoplasmas have been isolated from both diseased and healthy animals. *M. gateae* is probably a normal commensal, but a higher isolation rate has been found for *M. felis* in some studies on cats with conjunctivitis and respiratory disease compared with clinically healthy animals. Conjunctivitis and other signs have also been induced experimentally, although the implications are not clear because SPF cats were not used and other pathogens may have been involved.

Other bacteria such as *Staphylococcus*, *Streptococcus*, *Pasteurella multocida*, and *Escherichia coli* are thought to play a role as secondary invaders in feline respiratory disease.

EPIDEMIOLOGY

FRV and FCV Infection

FRV and FCV are fairly widespread in the general cat population, but there is a much higher prevalence in colony animals than in household pets. These viruses persist in such populations in three main ways. First, virus passes directly from acutely infected to susceptible animals. This depends on sufficient numbers of susceptible animals in the population and opportunities for contact between them. The second means is environmental persistence. Although this is for only relatively short periods of time, it is long enough for indirect transmission to occur, particularly within the close confines of a cattery. Secretions may contaminate cages, feeding and cleaning utensils, and personnel. Third, virus persists in the cat population because recovered cats may act as carriers. There are no known reservoirs or alternative hosts for these viruses, and in utero transmission does not generally seem to occur.

Despite vaccination, carriers are common in the population and are probably the main reason why these viruses are so successful. An understanding of the FRV and FCV carrier states is important to help determine strategies for control.

Carrier State for FRV

The carrier state is the normal sequel to infection and is characterized by periods of latency with intermittent episodes of detectable virus shedding, particularly after a stress (Fig. 16–1). In the latent phase, virus is undetectable in secretions by normal sampling techniques, but during shedding

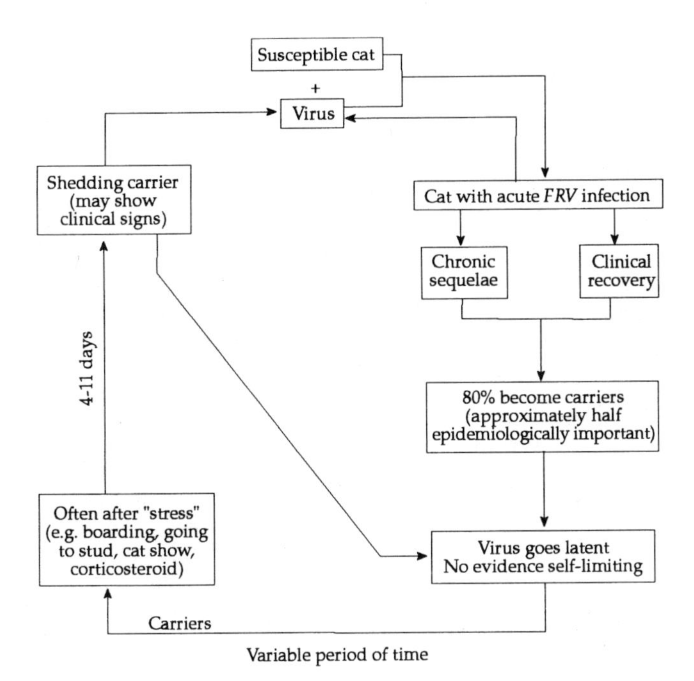

Figure 16–1. FRV (also FHV-1, feline herpesvirus-1) carrier state: epidemiology. From Gaskell RM, Dawson S: *In*: Chandler EA, Gaskell CJ, Gaskell RM (eds): *Feline Medicine and Therapeutics*, ed 2. Blackwell Science, 1994, p 460; Gaskell RM, Bennett M: *Feline and Canine Infectious Diseases*. Blackwell Science, 1996, p 12. Reprinted with permission.

episodes, virus is present in oronasal and conjunctival secretions and cats are infectious to other cats.

Although more than 80% of FRV-recovered cats are carriers, approximately half of these will likely shed virus under natural conditions. Shedding may occur spontaneously but is most likely after stress, for example, after a change of housing such as going into a boarding cattery, to a cat show, or to stud. Glucocorticoid treatment can also induce shedding, but it is inadvisable to use this drug to detect carriers because occasionally severe disease may result.

Shedding does not occur immediately after the stress; there is a lag period of approximately 1 week, followed by a shedding episode of from 1 to 2 weeks. Thus, carrier cats are most likely to be infectious for about 3 weeks after a stress factor. In some cases, carriers show mild clinical signs while they are shedding, which can be a useful indicator that they are likely to be infectious.

The stress of parturition and lactation may also precipitate virus shedding in queens, but the clinical outcome in the kittens depends on their levels of maternally derived antibodies (MDAs) at the time. On some occasions, kittens with MDAs may become subclinically infected and become latent carriers without ever having shown clinical signs. Such a mechanism is obviously ideal for the virus, because it can spread to the next generation without harming its host.

As with some other herpesvirus infections, FRV remains latent in carriers in trigeminal ganglia, although evidence has shown that other tissues may also be involved.[28] The latent carrier state is almost certainly lifelong, but there is a refractory phase of several months after a period of shedding when animals are less likely to experience another episode.

Carrier State for FCV

Unlike FRV, FCV carriers shed virus more or less continuously and are, therefore, always infectious to other cats (Fig. 16–2). The virus persists in tonsillar[9] and other oropharyngeal tissues. In some cats the carrier state appears to be lifelong, but most animals at some point spontaneously recover and appear to eliminate virus. In some experimental studies, most cats were shedding FCV 30 days after infection, and by 75 days approximately 50% of cats were still shedding. This proportion continues to decline, although some animals become long-term carriers. In other studies, carrier animals have been difficult to reproduce, suggesting there may be virus strain differences or other factors involved. There is some evidence that pre-existing feline immunodeficiency virus (FIV) infection may potentiate FCV shedding from carriers either in terms of duration[8] or titer[26] of virus.

FCV carriers have been arbitrarily divided into high-, medium-, and low-level, each shedding a fairly constant amount of virus that fluctuates around a mean for that individual cat. High-level shedders are very infectious and easily detected by oropharyngeal swabbing; low-level shedders are less infectious, and a series of swabs may be necessary to identify them.

FCV carriers are very common despite vaccination. Surveys have shown that approximately 20% of veterinary hospital cases and general practice cases seen for reasons other than oral-respiratory disease[14] and 25% of apparently healthy cats at cat shows[3] were shedding FCV. Experimentally, vaccination protects against disease but not infection or carrier state.[8, 23] The isolation rates in the general cat population are similar to those found in prevaccination surveys, in which

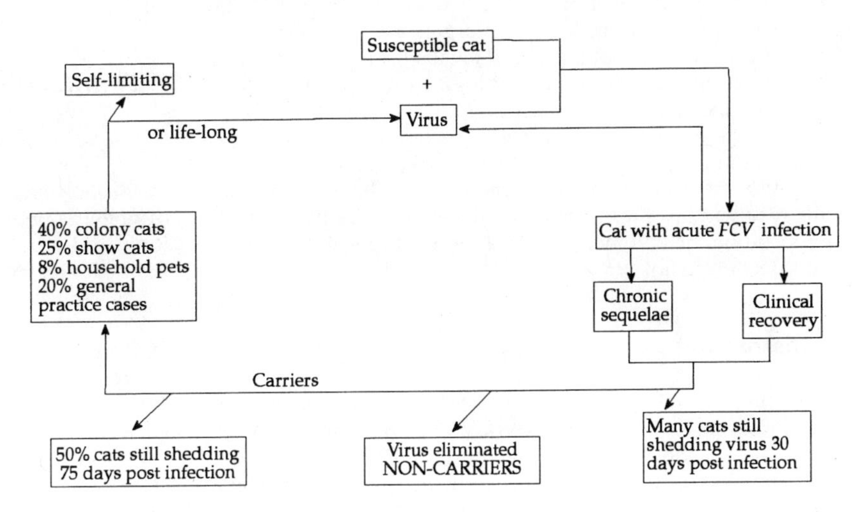

Figure 16–2. FCV carrier state: epidemiology. From Gaskell RM, Dawson S: *In*: Chandler EA, Gaskell CJ, Gaskell RM (eds): *Feline Medicine and Therapeutics*, ed 2. Blackwell Science, 1994, p 462; Gaskell RM, Bennett M: *Feline and Canine Infectious Diseases*. Blackwell Science, 1996, p 13. Reprinted with permission.

approximately 40% of colony cats, 25% of show cats, and 8% of household pets had positive results.

FCV carriers can generally be identified by isolation of virus from a single oropharyngeal swab, although several samples over a 4- to 6-week period are preferable. Because cats can eliminate virus at any time, it is worth retesting if required. Although a positive isolation result usually indicates that the cat is a carrier, some may be undergoing transient reinfection or infection with a nonpathogenic strain or an IN vaccine virus. Thus, results should be interpreted in conjunction with the clinical and vaccination history.

B. bronchiseptica Infection

Studies in the United Kingdom have shown that *B. bronchiseptica* is widespread in the cat population. In a survey of cats with and without respiratory disease, 11% of 740 cats were found to be shedding *B. bronchiseptica* from the oropharynx.[1a] In addition, a high prevalence of antibodies to *B. bronchiseptica* was found, with 72% of 126 sera sampled testing positive.[21] As with the other respiratory agents, it appears that *B. bronchiseptica* infections are probably more common among cats that are kept in colonies or in multicat households.

Epidemiologic evidence suggests that there may be a carrier state with *Bordetella* infection in the cat. Experimental work has shown that *B. bronchiseptica* can be shed from the oropharynx of infected cats for at least 19 weeks after infection.[2] In the same study, two seropositive queens started to shed *B. bronchiseptica* after parturition despite being negative beforehand.

The criteria for cat-to-cat transmission have not yet been established. Some animals may shed higher levels of the bacterium and be of greater epidemiologic significance. Because *B. bronchiseptica* can infect other species such as the dog, it is possible that interspecies transmission may also play a role in this disease.[1b]

C. psittaci Infection

Surveys in the United States have implicated *Chlamydia* with 5% to 10% of all feline respiratory disease. In the United Kingdom, chlamydiae were isolated from 30% of conjunctival swabs from household cats with conjunctivitis.[38] The prevalence was highest in cats between 5 weeks and 9 months old, suggesting that younger kittens are protected by MDA.

C. psittaci is shed predominantly from conjunctival secretions. Shedding has been demonstrated for up to 18 months after experimental infection. The organism has also been demonstrated in vaginal and rectal swabs for several months after infection, but the epidemiologic significance of this finding is unclear.

Chlamydial infection appears to become endemic in infected colonies, and persistent or recurrent signs are common. Whether the organism remains as a latent infection with reactivation after periods of stress, such as parturition and lactation, or whether there is a slowly replicating persistent infection is not yet clear.[36]

Transmission

Transmission occurs mainly by direct cat-to-cat contact via infectious discharges. FRV and FCV are shed primarily in ocular, nasal, and oral secretions, and *Bordetella* can be isolated from both oral and nasal secretions. *Chlamydia* is shed primarily in conjunctival secretions but is also found in nasal and sometimes vaginal secretions and feces.

Indirect transmission may occur in the short term, particularly in catteries. Contaminated secretions may be present on cages, feeding and cleaning utensils, and personnel. Because all the agents are relatively short lived outside the cat, however, the environment is usually not a long-term source of infection.

Aerosol transmission is not thought to be of major importance for the spread of respiratory agents in the cat. Cats do not appear to produce an infectious aerosol for the respiratory viruses during normal respiration, although sneezed macrodroplets may travel over a distance of one to two meters.

Transmission is affected by the length and intimacy of contact between the cats, and for all these agents it is likely that transmission is more successful in overcrowded conditions. Poor ventilation and hygiene will also lead to a buildup of pathogens in the environment. Transmission is thought to be more easily achieved from acutely infected cats rather than carrier cats because the discharges are more copious, but carriers are undoubtedly important, particularly with the close contact seen in multicat environments.

PATHOGENESIS

FRV Infection

The natural routes of infection for FRV are nasal, oral, and conjunctival, and virus replication takes place predominantly in the mucosae of the nasal septum, turbinates, nasopharynx, and tonsils. Virus shedding can be detected in oropharyngeal and nasal swabs as early as 24 hours after infection and generally persists for 1 to 3 weeks.

Viremia is rare because virus replication is normally restricted to areas of lower body temperature like the respiratory tract. However, viremia has occasionally been reported, and generalized disease may be seen particularly in debilitated animals or in neonatal kittens.

Infection leads to areas of multifocal epithelial necrosis with neutrophilic infiltration and exudation with fibrin. In early cases, intranuclear inclusion bodies may be seen. Viral damage can also lead to osteolytic changes in the turbinate bones. Lesions normally take between 2 and 3 weeks to resolve, although the bone damage to the turbinates may be permanent. Primary lung involvement may occur but is rare. Secondary bacterial infection can enhance the pathogenic effect of FRV; thus, bacterial sinusitis or pneumonia is possible.

FCV Infection

Similar to FRV, the natural routes of infection for FCV are nasal, oral, and conjunctival. Virus replication mainly occurs in the oral and respiratory tissues, although there are some differences between strains. Some have a predilection for the lung, and others have been found in the macrophages within the synovial membrane of joints.[4] Virus may also be found in visceral tissues and feces and occasionally in the urine.

Oral ulcers are the most prominent pathologic feature of FCV infection. They begin as vesicles (Fig. 16–3), which subsequently rupture, with necrosis of the overlying epithelium and infiltration of neutrophils at the periphery and the base. Healing takes place over 2 to 3 weeks.

Pulmonary lesions appear to result from an initial focal alveolitis, which leads to areas of acute exudative pneumonia

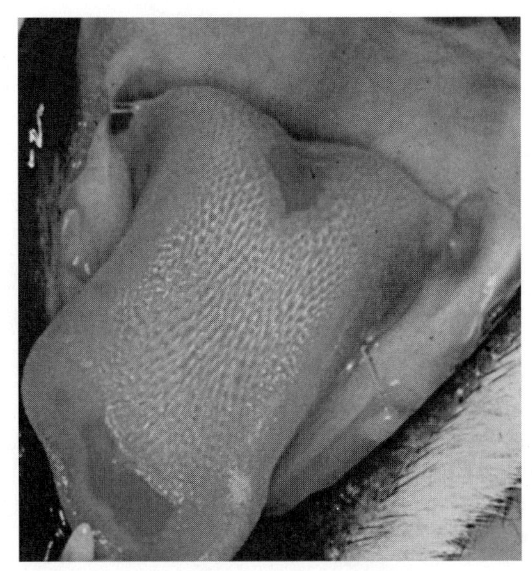

Figure 16–3. Tongue of a cat showing vesicles typical of early FCV infection. From Gaskell RM: *In*: Chandler EA, Gaskell CJ, Hilbery ADR (eds): *Feline Medicine and Therapeutics.* Blackwell Science, 1985, p 260. Reprinted with permission.

and then to the development of a proliferative, interstitial pneumonia. Although primary interstitial pneumonia can occur in FCV infection, particularly with more virulent strains, it has probably been overemphasized in the past as a result of experimental studies using aerosol challenge rather than the more natural oronasal routes.

Lesions seen in FCV-infected joints consist of an acute synovitis with thickening of the synovial membrane and an increased amount of synovial fluid within the joint.[4]

Bordetellosis

In other species such as dogs, *B. bronchiseptica* attaches to the cilia of the respiratory epithelium, thus overcoming the mucociliary clearance and allowing the bacteria to colonize the respiratory tract. The outcome of this in dogs is tracheobronchitis; coughing is the predominant clinical sign. In cats it is presumed that the pathogenesis is similar, although it appears that other parts of the upper respiratory tract may be more commonly involved because coughing is not necessarily the main clinical feature.

Although it appears that *B. bronchiseptica* may be a primary pathogen in cats, undoubtedly other factors such as combined infections with the respiratory viruses and stress factors such as weaning, overcrowding, and poor hygiene and ventilation all play roles. Such factors may account for the severe cases of bronchopneumonia that have been reported in the field.

Chlamydiosis

Conjunctival epithelium is the main target tissue for *C. psittaci*. The organism replicates within an inclusion in the cytoplasm of an infected cell. Within 48 hours, the parasitized cell usually disintegrates, releasing further infectious organisms.

Originally, *C. psittaci* infection in cats was called feline pneumonitis. Despite the name, however, the organism does not normally cause clinical signs of pneumonia: only mild pulmonary lesions may be detected occasionally at necropsy.

C. psittaci appears to generalize, because it has been found in gastric mucosa and in rectal and vaginal swabs. However, no clinical signs seem to be associated with this finding, although rectal and vaginal shedding may well be of epidemiologic significance. Experimentally, genital lesions have been induced but only after artificial routes of inoculation. Although abortion has been noted in some cats infected with *C. psittaci*, in general it appears that the organism is not involved in feline reproductive disease.

CLINICAL FINDINGS

Whatever the respiratory pathogen, the observed clinical signs (Table 16–1) will depend on a number of factors such as the infecting dose and strain of the agent, the general health and husbandry conditions of the cat, the nature of its microbial flora, and any pre-existing immunity. Concurrent infection with immunosuppressive viruses such as FIV and feline leukemia virus may lead to more severe disease.[25, 26]

FRV Infection

In susceptible animals, FRV infection generally causes a severe upper respiratory disease. The incubation period is usually 2 to 6 days but may be longer with lower levels of challenge virus.

Early signs include depression, marked sneezing, inappetence, and pyrexia, followed rapidly by serous ocular and nasal discharges (Fig. 16–4). These initial clinical signs may be accompanied by excessive salivation with drooling. Conjunctivitis, sometimes with severe hyperemia and chemosis, typically develops, and there are copious oculonasal discharges. These gradually become mucopurulent, and crusting of the external nares and eyelids can occur. In severe cases dyspnea and coughing may also develop.

Oral ulceration can occur with FRV infection but is rare. Ulcerative and interstitial keratitis may sometimes be seen, especially in young and immunocompromised animals. Generalized infections and primary viral pneumonia are uncommon, as are other manifestations such as skin ulcers and nervous signs. Abortion has also been reported but is probably due to the debilitating effects of the respiratory disease rather than a direct effect of the virus.

Table 16–1. Essential Features of Clinical Respiratory Disease Related to Pathogen Involved

FEATURE	FRV	FCV[a]	FCh	Bb
Lethargy	+ + +	+	+	+
Sneezing	+ + +	+	+	+ +
Conjunctivitis	+ +	+ +	+ + +[b]	−
Hypersalivation	+ +	−[c]	−	−
Ocular discharge	+ + +	+ +	+ + +	(+)
Nasal discharge	+ + +	+ +	+	+ +
Oral ulceration	+	+ + +	−	−
Keratitis	+	−	−	−
Coughing	(+)	−	−	+ +
Pneumonia	(+)	+	+ / −	+
Lameness	−	+ +	−	−

[a]Strain variation.
[b]Often persistent.
[c]Slight wetness may be seen around the mouth if ulcers present.
FCh = *Chlamydia psittaci* infection; Bb = *Bordetella bronchiseptica* infection; (+) = uncommon but may occur; + / − = lesions may be present but are not usually seen clinically.
Based on a table previously published in Gaskell RM, Bennett M. Feline and canine infectious diseases. Blackwell Science, 1996, p 8.

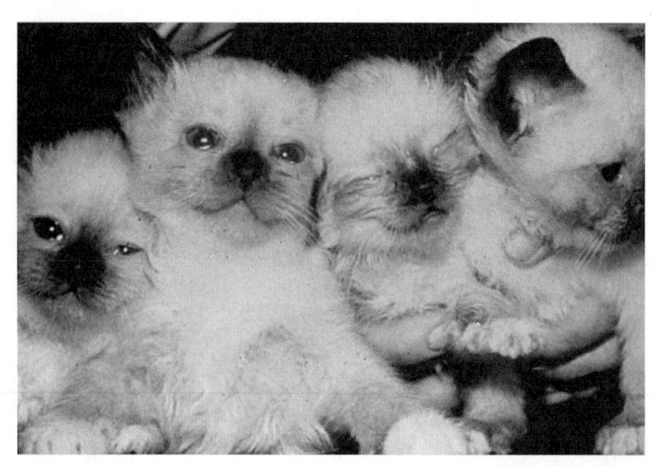

Figure 16–4. A litter of kittens with early FRV infection. From Gaskell RM, Dawson S: *In*: Chandler EA, Gaskell CJ, Gaskell RM (eds): *Feline Medicine and Therapeutics*, ed 2. Blackwell Science, 1994, p 466. Reprinted with permission.

In very young kittens or immunosuppressed cats, the mortality rate may be high, but on the whole mortality with FRV is low. Clinical signs generally resolve within 10 to 20 days. However, in some cats the acute damage may have been severe enough to lead to permanent damage to the mucosae and turbinates, leaving them prone to chronic bacterial rhinitis, sinusitis, and conjunctivitis.

FCV Infection

Strains of FCV can differ in tropism and virulence; therefore, a range of clinical signs may be seen. However, most strains induce a fairly characteristic, mild syndrome characterized by pyrexia, oral ulceration, and mild respiratory and conjunctival signs. Some strains of FCV, however, are nonpathogenic; others are more virulent and may induce more severe disease.

Early signs of infection are depression and pyrexia, although cats typically stay brighter than with FRV. Oral ulceration is very common with FCV infection and may be the only clinical sign present (see Fig. 16–5). Ulceration is usually on the tongue but can occur elsewhere in the mouth, on the lips, and on the nose. Skin ulceration on other parts of the body occurs rarely.

Sneezing, conjunctivitis, and ocular and nasal discharge are generally much less prominent than with FRV. Cats with oral ulcers may show hypersalivation with moisture on the fur around the mouth, but there is no drooling of saliva. Some of the more virulent strains can cause pneumonia with associated dyspnea.

Some FCV strains produce lameness and pyrexia.[4, 31a] The lameness, which is commonly of a shifting nature, may or may not be associated with oral and respiratory signs. Affected cats are often dull and anorexic, and in most cases there is full recovery within 24 to 48 hours. Any possible long-term effects to the joints are as yet unknown. This lameness has also been observed after vaccination (see Postvaccinal Complications, Chapter 100).

Another possible pathogenic role for FCV is in chronic stomatitis-gingivitis. More than 80% of cats with chronic oral disease have been found to shed FCV compared with approximately 20% of controls. FCV infection has been associated with acute faucitis,[27] and it is possible that this may predispose the animal to the development of chronic lesions in this site. However, other agents, in particular FIV, are also involved in the condition. The pathogenesis is not yet fully understood (see Stomatitis, Chapter 89).

Bordetellosis

In experimental studies in cats in which *B. bronchiseptica* is known to be the sole pathogen, the main clinical signs are pyrexia, sneezing, nasal discharge, submandibular lymphadenomegaly, and rales on auscultation.[2, 17] Spontaneous or induced coughing may also occur but is a less consistent sign than in dogs. Signs generally resolve after about 10 days.

In the field, *B. bronchiseptica* infection has been associated with cases of bronchopneumonia, especially in younger cats.[33, 35] Signs included dyspnea and cyanosis, and in such cases mortality is fairly high. In many cases, coughing has been a feature.[33]

Chlamydiosis

After an incubation period of 3 to 5 days or longer, cats develop serous ocular discharge with blepharospasm, chemosis, and hyperemia of the palpebral conjunctivae. The disease may start in only one eye, but eventually both eyes become involved. As the disease progresses, discharges become mucopurulent. Most cases resolve within 3 to 4 weeks, but if left untreated milder clinical signs may persist for some months and recurrent episodes are common.

Mild respiratory disease with sneezing and nasal discharge can accompany the conjunctivitis in the early stages of the disease. Follicular conjunctivitis and corneal involvement have also been described, but it is probable that other agents, such as the respiratory viruses, were involved in such cases.

DIAGNOSIS

Diagnosis may be attempted on the basis of clinical signs alone. For example, predominantly oral ulceration might in-

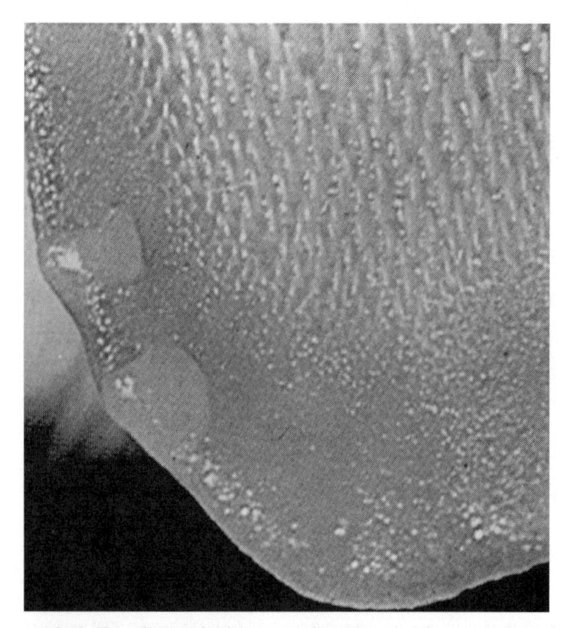

Figure 16–5. Two lingual ulcers on the tongue of a cat infected with FCV. From Gaskell RM, Dawson S: *In*: Chandler EA, Gaskell CJ, Gaskell RM (eds): *Feline Medicine and Therapeutics*, ed 2. Blackwell Science, 1994, p 466. Reprinted with permission.

dicate FCV, whereas marked sneezing with more severe respiratory and conjunctival signs might suggest FRV. With chlamydial infection, the main clinical sign is a marked persistent conjunctivitis.

Confirmatory diagnosis of FRV and FCV can be made by virus isolation in feline cell cultures. Oropharyngeal swabs should be taken from the cat, ideally in the first week of illness, placed in viral transport medium, and sent within 24 hours to the laboratory. FA techniques on conjunctival smears have also been described. Serology is generally not helpful in the diagnosis of FRV and FCV infection because of widespread antibody from vaccination. PCR has also been used on clinical specimens to identify infected cats and, for FCV, to type viral isolates.[12a, 24a, 29a, 29b, 32a]

For diagnosis of *B. bronchiseptica* infection, oropharyngeal or nasal swabs should be taken and placed into charcoal Amies transport medium (Beckton Dickenson, Cockeysville, MD) before plating at the laboratory on appropriate selective medium that prevents overgrowth by other respiratory flora. Transtracheal wash specimens can also be used for the isolation of *B. bronchiseptica* from clinical cases. Serology is not widely available, and many healthy cats are in any case seropositive.

For *Chlamydia* detection, a vigorous conjunctival swab should be placed into *Chlamydia* transport medium and sent within 24 hours to an appropriate laboratory. Some laboratories carry out isolation of *Chlamydia* in cell cultures, whereas others use one of the commercially available ELISA kits (see Appendix 6). ELISA techniques are not as sensitive as cultures in the later stages of disease, but they have the advantage that both viable and nonviable organisms can be detected. In unvaccinated cats serology may be helpful in *Chlamydia* diagnosis: clinically affected animals tend to have high titers. PCR has been used to detect *Chlamydia* in conjunctival swabs from diseased cats[29c] and to type isolates.

When an organism is isolated from an animal with respiratory disease, it is reasonable to assume that the agent has been involved in the disease process. However, especially for FCV and *Bordetella*, relatively large numbers of clinically healthy cats will also be shedding the organisms. Isolation may therefore be a coincidental finding.

THERAPY

No antiviral drugs are in widespread use for the treatment of FRV and FCV. Drugs such as acyclovir, given in human herpesvirus infections, do not seem to have good activity against FRV. However, in cases of ulcerative keratitis associated with FRV infection, other antivirals such as 5-iododeoxyuridine (IUdR) in the form of eyedrops may be used (see Herpesvirus, Chapter 93 and Table 93–3).

In viral respiratory disease, broad-spectrum antibiotic therapy should be given to help control secondary bacterial infection. Because it may be painful for cats to swallow solid tablets, antibiotics can be given as pediatric syrups or long-acting injections. Cats should be re-examined after 4 to 5 days and, if necessary, bacterial culture and susceptibility tests performed.

Good nursing care is essential and is generally best given at home if the owner is conscientious. The cat should be encouraged to eat by offering strongly flavored aromatic foods. If eating is painful, baby foods or specialized proprietary or blended food may be helpful. Diazepam administered just before feeding can stimulate appetite. Severe cases may require fluid therapy, and when anorexia is prolonged a nasogastric or gastrotomy tube may be indicated.[30]

Nasal decongestants (e.g., phenylephrine) in the acute phase and mucolytic drugs (e.g., bromhexine hydrochloride) in the more chronic phase have been suggested to help clear airways, but conventional steam inhalation (e.g., placing the cat in steamy room) or nebulizing saline is probably more useful.

Although several antibiotics have some activity against *Chlamydia psittaci*, tetracyclines are most effective. Because the organism can disseminate, both topical and systemic treatment should be given. Tetracycline ophthalmic ointment is preferable to chlortetracycline. Systemically, doxycycline has a longer half-life than oxytetracycline and only needs to be given orally once a day (5–10 mg/kg). All cats in the household should be treated simultaneously for at least 4 weeks or 2 weeks after the clinical signs have resolved. Systemic tetracyclines are theoretically contraindicated in pregnant cats or young kittens in which dental development is occurring. Erythromycin and tylosin may be effective, but no controlled trials have been carried out in cats.

Tetracyclines are the antibiotic of choice for the treatment of bordetellosis.[29] However, limited experimental evidence suggests that treatment with doxycycline may not eliminate the organism from the cat during the later stages of infection.[2]

PREVENTION

Immunity

For both FRV and FCV, immunity has generally been measured by serum VN antibody levels, although for FRV cell-mediated immunity (CMI) may be a better reflection of immune status. VN antibody was originally thought to be the hallmark of immunity for FCV; however, some cats with no detectable VN antibody have shown immunity to rechallenge with a heterologous strain,[19, 23] and several types of CMI responses have been demonstrated.[32] For both viruses, local immune responses are also likely to be important.[19] The ultimate test of immunity is, of course, response to challenge.

In FRV infection, just after initial infection, cats are generally resistant to challenge, although VN antibody titers are generally low and in some cases undetectable. After 6 months or more, protection may only be partial, and indeed carrier cats may reinfect themselves. After either reactivation or field challenge, VN antibody titers rise to more moderate levels and thereafter remain reasonably stable, independent of virus shedding episodes.

In FCV infection, VN antibody titers are higher than those in FRV, and immunity after natural infection is generally longer lived. However, there is some variation depending on the virus strain involved and whether or not homologous or heterologous protection is being considered. Reinfection with a second strain will generally boost responses to both strains.

MDAs (i.e., essentially colostral) in kittens may persist for 2 to 10 weeks for FRV, with mean levels falling below detectable levels (<1:2) by 9 weeks of age. For FCV, in most kittens MDAs persist for 10 to 14 weeks. However, for both viruses, low levels of MDAs do not necessarily protect against subclinical infection. In contrast, some animals with no detectable FRV antibody appeared to be protected against disease but not infection.

Studies on immunity in *B. bronchiseptica* infection have concentrated on the measurement of IgG levels in serum as measured in an ELISA.[2, 17, 21] After primary infection, antibody levels rise by 4 weeks to reasonably high titers, although no studies on duration of immunity have been done. MDAs for *Bordetella* have been detected in experimental cats, although these appear to be fairly short lived, lasting for only 2 weeks[2] or up to 6 weeks.[17]

Immunity to *C. psittaci* has been measured using immunofluorescence and complement fixation (CF) tests, but the latter are less reliable. CMI responses have also been recorded. After experimental infection with *C. psittaci*, cats are protected against rechallenge 3 months later and there is still partial protection after 18 months.[36] MDAs last in most cases at least until 9 weeks of age and in some cases until 12 weeks of age.[36]

Vaccination

Vaccination has been available for a number of years against the two respiratory viruses and has been relatively successful in controlling disease. However, disease can still be a problem, especially when cats are kept grouped together and when kittens lose their MDAs before vaccination. Both viruses are very widespread in the cat population and carriers are common, ensuring plenty of exposure. Prevention and control, therefore, often require a combined approach of both vaccination and management.

Three types of FRV and FCV vaccines are available: modified live virus (MLV) vaccines administered parenterally or intranasally (IN) and inactivated adjuvanted virus vaccines given parenterally. In addition, genetically engineered vaccines for both FRV and FCV are being developed.[8a, 22, 34]

For routine FRV and FCV vaccination programs, all types of vaccine appear to be suitable. In previously unexposed cats, all vaccines induce reasonable protection against disease but, in general, do not protect against infection or the development of the carrier state.

Several parenteral MLV vaccines are available, the FCV component being based originally on strain F9, but other vaccine strains are now also used.[1, 23] Most vaccines protect against the majority of FCV isolates but not as well against all. Use of a booster vaccine containing a different strain may broaden protection.

Parenteral MLV vaccines should be administered carefully because clinical signs can be induced if the vaccine virus reaches the oral-respiratory mucosa (e.g., if the cat licks the injection site or if an aerosol is made with the syringe). Vaccine virus should not generalize, but spread of MLV-FCV component after parenteral inoculation has been shown to occur, leading to the possibility of cat-to-cat spread.[23] In completely virus-free colonies, therefore, it may be safest to use an inactivated vaccine.

Intranasal MLV vaccine induces better protection but often induces slight side effects, such as sneezing and ocular and nasal discharges. IN vaccines, however, are useful for rapid (2–4 day) onset of protection.

Inactivated adjuvant vaccines can be reasonably effective, although this will depend on the antigen content of the vaccine and the adjuvant (see Chapter 100). However, adjuvants can sometimes cause local reactions. Inactivated vaccines are helpful in virus-free colonies because there is no risk of spread or reversion to virulence. Some inactivated vaccines are licensed for use in pregnant queens, and vaccination during pregnancy can help protect kittens by prolonging MDAs.[16]

Most vaccine manufacturers recommend annual revaccination or semiannual in some circumstances. Possible reasons for vaccine reactions or vaccine failure are reviewed elsewhere.[5, 12] (See Chapter 100.)

For *B. bronchiseptica*, IN MLV vaccines are marketed for dogs and are likely to prove useful in cats. An inactivated fimbrial subunit-based vaccine has also been shown to work experimentally in cats and is licensed for use in some countries.[17]

Vaccination against feline *C. psittaci* has been available in some countries for a long time. Early vaccines were produced in eggs, but cell culture vaccines have now been developed. Such vaccines appear to give reasonable protection against disease, but not infection, for up to a year.[37]

Disease Control

Household Cats. Pets should be vaccinated routinely and given a booster vaccine before entering a high-risk situation, such as a boarding cattery, unless they have been vaccinated within the past 6 months. From the point of view of infectious disease, ideally a friend or neighbor should feed the cat while the owner is on vacation. Individual cats should be protected from stress and social contact as much as possible to avoid exposure.

Boarding Catteries. All cats entering the cattery should have an up-to-date vaccination record, certainly for FRV and FCV. In exceptional circumstances, when there is no alternative and rapid protection is required, IN vaccine may be given. However, clients should be aware that such vaccines themselves may induce mild clinical signs.

However, cattery owners should not rely on vaccination alone for disease control, because pathogens will inevitably be present either from the occasional cat incubating disease or from carriers. Thus, measures should be taken to prevent spread of infection and reduce the concentration of infectious agents in the environment (Table 16–2). Such measures may appear complicated, but in practice they are not difficult to implement and, in our experience, can actually increase the efficiency within a cattery.

Shelter Facilities. In general, the same measures apply as with boarding catteries, but it is often impossible to separate animals to the same extent. However, animals that arrive at a shelter at the same time should stay together and be quarantined, isolated from the general population. Those with clinical signs should be kept apart. Unless animals can

Table 16–2. Recommendations to Prevent the Spread of the Respiratory Viruses in a Boarding Cattery

Admit only fully vaccinated cats.
House cats individually with solid partitions between pens, unless cats are from same household. Ensure frontages are at least 1 m apart.
Put known carriers or cats with history of respiratory disease in a separate section or at least at one end of the cattery, and feed last.
Ensure that surfaces of pen are easily washable and that food and litter bowls can be easily removed without entering the pen (i.e., do not handle cats more than necessary).
Feed cats in same order each day and attend to each pen completely before moving on to the next.
Either disinfect hands between each pen or have individual rubber gloves for each pen, for use only with that pen. Disinfect gloves thoroughly before use with a new boarder.
Wear rubber boots and step into a disinfectant bath if it is necessary to enter a pen.
Either use disposable food trays or have two sets of food bowls used on alternate days. Soak used set in a 1:32 bleach solution with detergent for several hours and then leave rinsed and dried until reuse 24 hours later.
Prepare food in a central area.
Use similar system to food bowls for litter trays.
When a cat goes home, thoroughly disinfect cage, allow to dry, and preferably leave empty for 2 days before reusing.
Reduce concentration of virus in the environment by providing adequate ventilation, low relative humidity, optimal environmental temperatures.

Based on a table previously published in Gaskell RM, Dawson S: *In:* Chandler EA, Gaskell CJ, Gaskell RM (eds): Feline medicine and therapeutics, ed 2. Blackwell Science, 1994, p 468; Gaskell RM, Bennett M: Feline and canine infectious diseases. Blackwell Science, 1996, p 20. Used with permission.

Table 16–3. Feline Respiratory Disease Control Program in a Breeding Cattery With Endemic Disease

Provide regular vaccination programs.
Give booster vaccinations to queens either before mating, or during pregnancy (inactivated vaccine only).
Keep cats as stress free as possible and use good management practices to reduce spread of viruses within the colony.
Avoid breeding queens with a history of oral or respiratory disease in their kittens.
Move queens into isolation at least 3 weeks before term, so that the kittens are not exposed to carriers in the colony and any shedding episode from the queen as a result of the move will end before parturition.
Wean kittens into isolation away from the mother as soon as feasible (ideally at 4–5 weeks before MDAs wane if it is likely she is a carrier).
Vaccinate all kittens as soon as MDAs are at a noninterfering level (normally 9+ weeks) and keep them in strict isolation until a week after the second dose (normally at 12 weeks).
Earlier FRV and FCV vaccination schedules with IN or parenteral vaccines may be used, although these are not always licensed for early use and should be used with care. Parenteral vaccines can be given 3–4 weeks of age, at 3- to 4-week intervals until 12 weeks of age. Intranasal vaccination should be carried out 7–10 days or so before disease has been occurring and then again at 12 weeks. There is some evidence that multiple doses are not necessary, although they were originally advocated.

MDAs = maternally-derived antibodies.

be isolated on arrival for 3 to 4 weeks, parenteral vaccines may not have time to become effective. In these circumstances, it may be advisable to use the IN vaccines.

Breeding Catteries. In disease-free colonies, cats should be vaccinated routinely if there is any contact, direct or indirect, with other cats. Inactivated vaccines are preferable. Care should be taken to avoid bringing virus into the colony: any cat with a history of, or contact with, oral or respiratory disease may be a carrier. Vaccinated cats can be carriers, and kittens can be infected subclinically owing to MDAs. Thus, stud cats and new breeding stock should be from a respiratory disease-free colony. There is a possible risk of infection from cat shows, but the greatest risk of infection to disease-free households is from stud cats and new breeding stock when exposure is prolonged.

Cats entering the disease-free colony should be quarantined for 3 weeks to avoid animals incubating the disease. Virus isolation should be attempted at least twice a week during this time. This practice increases the probability of detecting FRV excretion and low-level shedding FCV carriers. Even so, there is still the risk of importing a latent FRV carrier or a low-level FCV carrier that may be a source of infection. Unvaccinated cats can be screened serologically for FRV and FCV. Conjunctival swabs can be taken for *Chlamydia*, but the necessity to screen for other respiratory pathogens, such as *Bordetella*, is not yet clear.

In colonies with endemic disease, it may be feasible to eliminate FRV and FCV and maintain a virus-free colony with a barrier system. However, FRV and FCV are very widespread, and it might be difficult to ensure that, even with vaccination, the colony would remain virus free. *B. bronchiseptica*–free cats are difficult to obtain because the organism is very widespread, even in SPF cats, but it can be achieved with careful monitoring.[2] For most situations, the only reasonable course is to attempt disease control (Table 16–3).

References

1. Baulch-Brown C, Love DN, Meanger J. 1997. Feline calicivirus: a need for vaccine modification. *Aust Vet J* 75:209–213.
1a. Binns S, Dawson S, Coutts AJ, et al. 1996. *Bordetella bronchiseptica* in cats: risk factors for infection, p 198. Presented at the British Small Animal Veterinary Association Congress, Congress Paper Synopses.
1b. Binns SH, Speakman AJ, Dawson S, et al. 1997. The use of pulsed-field gel electrophoresis to examine the epidemiology of *Bordetella bronchiseptica* isolated from cats and other species. *Epidemiol Infect* In press.
2. Coutts AJ, Dawson S, Binns S, et al. 1996. Studies on the natural transmission of *Bordetella bronchiseptica* in cats. *Vet Microbiol* 48:19–27.
3. Coutts AJ, Dawson S, Willoughby K, et al. 1994. Isolation of feline respiratory viruses from clinically healthy cats at UK cat shows. *Vet Rec* 135:555–556.
4. Dawson S, Bennett D, Carter SD, et al. 1994. Acute arthritis of cats associated with feline calicivirus infection. *Res Vet Sci* 56:133–143.
5. Dawson S, Gaskell RM. 1993. Problems with respiratory virus vaccination in cats. *Compend Cont Educ Pract Vet* 15:1347–1354.
6. Dawson S, McArdle F, Bennett D, et al. 1993. Investigation of vaccine reactions and breakdowns after feline calicivirus vaccination. *Vet Rec* 132:346–350.
7. Dawson S, McArdle F, Bennett M, et al. 1993. Typing of feline calicivirus isolates from different clinical groups by virus neutralisation tests. *Vet Rec* 133:13–17.
8. Dawson S, Smyth NR, Bennett M, et al. 1991. Effect of primary-stage feline immunodeficiency virus infection on subsequent feline calicivirus vaccination and challenge in cats. *AIDS* 5:747–750.
8a. DeSilver DA, Guimord PM, Gibson JK, et al. 1997. Expression of the complete capsid and hypervariable region of feline calicivirus in the baculovirus expression system, pp 131–143. *In* Chasey D, Gaskell RM, Clarke IN (eds), European Society of Veterinary Virology, Symposium Reading. ESVV and Central Veterinary Laboratory, Weybridge.
9. Dick CP, Johnson RP. 1989. Sites of persistence of feline calicivirus. *Res Vet Sci* 47:367.
10. Elliot H. 1991. *Bordetella bronchiseptica* in a closed cat colony. *Vet Rec* 132:474–475.
11. Gaskell RM, Bennett M (eds). 1996. Feline and canine infectious diseases, pp 3–28. Blackwell Science, Oxford, England.
12. Gaskell RM, Dawson S. 1994. Viral-induced upper respiratory tract disease, pp 453–472. *In* Chandler EA, Gaskell CJ, Gaskell RM (eds), Feline medicine and therapeutics. Blackwell Science, Oxford, England.
12a. Geissler K, Schneider K, Platzer G, et al. 1997. Genetic and antigenic heterogeneity among feline calicivirus isolates from distinct disease manifestations. *Virus Res* 48:193–206.
13. Grail A, Harbour DA. 1990. Restriction endonuclease analysis of DNA from isolates of feline herpesvirus type 1. *Jpn J Vet Sci* 52:1007–1013.
14. Harbour DA, Howard PE, Gaskell RM. 1991. Isolation of feline calicivirus and feline herpesvirus from domestic cats 1980 to 1989. *Vet Rec* 128:77–80.
15. Horimoto T, Limcumpao JA, Xuan X, et al. 1992. Heterogeneity of feline herpesvirus type 1 strains. *Arch Virol* 126:283–292.
16. Iglauer F, Gartner K, Morstedt R. 1989. Maternal protection against feline respiratory disease by means of booster vaccinations during pregnancy — a retrospective clinical study. *Kleintierpraxis* 34:235.
17. Jacobs AAC, Chalmers WSK, Pasman J, et al. 1993. Feline bordetellosis: challenge and vaccination studies. *Vet Rec* 133:260–263.
17a. Kadoi K, Kiryu M, Iwabuchi M, et al. 1997. A strain of calicivirus isolated from lions with vesicular lesions on tongue and snout. *Microbiologica* 20:141–148.
18. Knowles JO, Dawson S, Gaskell RM, et al. 1990. Neutralisation patterns among recent British and North American feline calicivirus isolates from different clinical origins. *Vet Rec* 127:125–127.
19. Knowles JO, McArdle F, Dawson S, et al. 1991. Studies on the role of feline calicivirus in chronic stomatitis in cats. *Vet Microbiol* 27:205–219.
19a. Lauritzen A, Jarrett O, Sabara M. 1997. Serological analysis of feline calicivirus isolates from the United States and United Kingdom. *Vet Microbiol* 56:55–64.
20. McArdle F, Dawson S, Carter MJ, et al. 1996. Feline calicivirus strain differentiation using monoclonal antibody analysis in an enzyme-linked immuno-flow assay. *Vet Microbiol* 51:197–206.
21. McArdle HC, Dawson S, Coutts AJ, et al. 1994. Seroprevalence and isolation rate of *Bordetella bronchiseptica* in cats in the UK. *Vet Rec* 135:506–507.
22. Nunberg JH, Wright DK, Cole GE, et al. 1989. Identification of the thymidine kinase gene of feline herpesvirus: use of degenerate oligonucleotides in the polymerase chain reaction to isolate herpesvirus gene homologs. *J Gen Virol* 63(8):3240.
23. Pedersen NC, Hawkins KF. 1995. Mechanisms for persistence of acute and chronic feline calicivirus infections in the face of vaccination. *Vet Microbiol* 47:141–156.
24. Povey RC. 1990. Feline respiratory diseases, pp 346–357. *In* Greene CE (ed), Infectious diseases of the dog and cat. WB Saunders, Philadelphia, PA.
24a. Radford AD, Bennett M, Mcardle F, et al. 1997. The use of sequence-analysis of a feline calicivirus (FCV) hypervariable region in the epidemiologic investigation of FCV related disease and vaccine failures. *Vaccine* 15:1451–1458.
25. Reubel GH, George JW, Barlough JE, et al. 1992. Interaction of acute feline herpesvirus-1 and chronic feline immunodeficiency virus infections in experimentally infected specific pathogen free cats. *Vet Immunol Immunopathol* 35(1-2):95–119.
26. Reubel GH, George JW, Higgins J, et al. 1994. Effect of chronic feline

immunodeficiency virus infection on experimental feline calicivirus-induced disease. *Vet Microbiol* 39:335–351.
27. Ruebel GH, Hoffmann DE, Pedersen NC. 1992. Acute and chronic faucitis of domestic cats, a feline calicivirus induced disease. *Vet Clin North Am* 22:1347–1360.
28. Reubel GH, Ramos RA, Hickman MA, et al. 1993. Detection of active and latent feline herpesvirus 1 infections using the polymerase chain reaction. *Arch Virol* 132:409–420.
29. Speakman AJ, Binns SH, Dawson S, et al. 1997. In vitro antimicrobial susceptibility of *Bordetella bronchiseptica* isolates and comparison using the E-test. *Vet Microbiol* 54:63–72.
29a. Stiles J, McDermott M, Bigsby D, et al. 1997. Use of nested polymerase chain-reaction to identify feline herpesvirus in ocular tissue from clinically normal cats and cats with corneal sequestra or conjunctivitis. *Am J Vet Res* 58:338–342.
29b. Stiles J, McDermott M, Willis M, et al. 1997. Comparison of nested polymerase chain reaction, virus isolation, and fluorescent antibody testing for identifying feline herpesvirus in cats with conjunctivitis. *Am J Vet Res* 58:804–807.
29c. Sykes JE, Studdert VP, Anderson G, et al. 1997. Comparison of *Chlamydia psittaci* from cats with upper respiratory tract disease by polymerase chain reaction analysis of the OMPA gene. *Vet Rec* 140:310–313.
30. Tennant B, Willoughby K. 1993. The use of enteral nutrition in small animal medicine. *Compend Cont Educ Pract Vet* 15:1054.
31. Tenorio AP, Franti CE, Madewell BR, et al. 1991. Chronic oral infections of cats and their relationship to persistent oral carriage of feline calici-, immunodeficiency, or leukaemia viruses. *Vet Immunol Immunopathol* 29:1–14.
31a. TerWee J, Lauritzen AY, Sabara M, et al. 1997. Comparison of the primary signs induced by experimental exposure to either a pneumotrophic or a 'limping' strain of feline calicivirus. *Vet Microbiol* 56:33–45.
32. Tham KM, Studdert MJ. 1987. Antibody and cell-mediated immune responses of feline calicivirus following inactivated vaccine and challenge. *Zentralbl Veterinarmed B* 34:640–654.
32a. Weigler BJ, Babineau CA, Sherry B, et al. 1997. High sensitivity polymerase chain reaction assay for active and latent feline herpesvirus-1 infections in domestic cats. *Vet Rec* 140:335–338.
33. Welsh RD. 1996. *Bordetella bronchiseptica* infections in cats. *J Am Anim Hosp Assoc* 32:153–158.
34. Willemse MJ, Chalmer SK, Cronerberg AM, et al. 1994. The gene downstream of the gC homologue in feline herpesvirus type 1 is involved in the expression of virulence. *J Gen Virol* 75:3107–3116.
35. Willoughby K, Dawson S, Jones RC, et al. 1991. Isolation of *Bordetella bronchiseptica* from kittens with pneumonia in a UK breeding cattery. *Vet Rec* 93:486–487.
36. Wills JM, Gaskell RM. 1994. Feline chlamydial infection, pp 544–551. *In* Chandler EA, Gaskell CJ, Gaskell RM (eds), Feline medicine and therapeutics. Blackwell Science, Oxford, England.
37. Wills JM, Gruffydd-Jones TJ, Richmond S, et al. 1987. Effect of vaccination on infection due to feline *Chlamydia psittaci*. *Infect Immun* 55:2653–2657.
38. Wills JM, Howard PE, Gruffydd-Jones TJ, et al. 1988. Prevalence of *Chlamydia psittaci* in different cat populations in Britain. *J Small Anim Pract* 29:327–339.

Chapter **17**

Feline Syncytium-Forming Virus Infection

Craig E. Greene

ETIOLOGY

Feline syncytium-forming virus (FeSFV) has been classified in the family Retroviridae, subfamily Spumavirinae. The prevalence of FeSFV infection is high in both normal and diseased cats. Virus has been isolated from primary cultures of tissue and body secretions in up to 90% of a population.[4] More typically, the prevalence of infection in a cat population varies between 4% and 50%, depending on the age, geographic location, and local environment of cats.[8] Fifty percent or more of kittens born to FeSFV-infected queens are infected at birth,[8] and 15% of cultures of fetal cats are positive for the virus, suggesting that it can be transmitted vertically.[3] In utero infection probably occurs by the transfer of infected maternal leukocytes across the placenta but not through milk in lactating animals.[8]

In contrast to most feline infectious diseases, the infection rate for FeSFV in cat colonies is actually lower than that in the random cat population. Roaming or outdoor cats have the highest prevalence, suggesting contact through bite wounds.

FeSFV is a nuisance to virologists and manufacturers of feline vaccines because it is found in many normal feline tissues and cell cultures that have been subjected to multiple passages. It is not usually present in primary cell cultures.[6] FeSFV is difficult to distinguish from feline leukemia virus (FeLV), which is visualized only as it buds from the cell. FeSFV forms a recognizable nucleocapsid within the cytoplasm before budding.

FeSFV derives its name from the fact that it produces multinucleated syncytia within 1 to 2 weeks of growth in certain rapidly multiplying tissue cultures. Cell lysis is rarely if ever noted, and intranuclear inclusions are never seen. Malignant transformation has been noted in tissue culture only in some instances.

PATHOGENESIS

FeSFV has not been associated with any disease; many cats were infected both naturally and experimentally without clinical illness. The presence of the virus in 100% of cats affected with chronic progressive polyarthritis has been reported.[10] Concurrent FeLV infection was found in 70% of these cats. The prevalence of infection with both viruses was 2 to 10 times greater than that in age-matched cats not having chronic progressive polyarthritis. By altering the host immune system, FeLV may potentiate the ability of FeSFV to produce disease. Other factors must be involved as well because the disease cannot be induced by inoculation of FeSFV alone. Combined infections with FeSFV and feline immunodeficiency virus (FIV) are also frequently found. Coinfection of FeSFV and FIV showed no enhancement of FIV-induced illness in the early stages of the disease.[12] Combined infection is most likely due to a common mode of transmission rather than a mutual pathogenic mechanism.

Arthritis, thought to result from chronic antigenic stimulation and immune complex deposition, is characterized histologically by lymphoplasmacytic infiltrates and is temporarily responsive to immunosuppressive therapy. An inherent genetic tendency may explain why certain male cats are more prone to develop disease despite the high prevalence of these viral infections in the general population.

CLINICAL FINDINGS

Most infected cats are nonsymptomatic. Chronic progressive polyarthritis of cats generally affects males between 1.5 and 5 years of age.[7, 9–11] Two forms of the disease have been described: one with osteoporosis and periarticular periosteal proliferation; the other with periarticular erosions, collapse of the joint space, and joint deformities. Lymphadenomegaly, swollen joints, and stiff gait are seen in both types.

DIAGNOSIS

Joint fluid abnormalities consist of increased numbers of neutrophils and large mononuclear cells. That FeSFV stimulates antibody production in infected hosts has been used as the basis for immunodiffusion and indirect FA testing for antibody.[1, 10] Serology can be performed in addition to blood cultures to screen cats for infection. Infected kittens can be detected at birth by culturing buffy coat cells from their peripheral blood. Animals are infected for life and develop persistent, nonprotective antibody titers to the virus. For this reason, cats showing a serologic response to the virus are presumed to be infected. Several strains may exist, and the actual prevalence of infection may be higher than indicated by seropositivity. Neonatal kittens born to infected queens lose their maternal antibody by 6 to 8 weeks of age, if they are not infected. Serum antibody titers will increase after this time if they become infected.[3]

Virus can be isolated from most tissues but requires one to four passages in vitro. FeSFV actually is only detected in vivo in cells and secretions of the oropharynx. Despite genetic material being supplied by the host, viral replication is suppressed. Latency can be expressed by cocultivating buffy coat WBC with fetal cat cells or by exposing cells to oropharyngeal secretions.

THERAPY AND PREVENTION

There is no known cure for chronic progressive polyarthritis, and the clinical and pathologic changes it causes usually are temporarily responsive for weeks to months to immunosuppressive therapy such as prednisolone (10–15 mg/cat/day) and cyclophosphamide (Cytoxan, Bristol-Myers Squibb, Princeton, NJ) (7.5 mg/cat/day for 4 days each week). Cats identified as having polyarthritis should be eliminated from research projects and should be removed from vaccine production and specific pathogen-free colonies.

References

1. Gaskin JM, Gillespie JH. 1973. Detection of feline syncytia-forming virus carrier state with a microimmunodiffusion test. *Am J Vet Res* 34:245–247.
2. Greene CE. 1990. Syncytium-forming virus infection, pp 358–359. *In* Greene CE (ed), Infectious diseases of the dog and cat. WB Saunders, Philadelphia, PA.
3. Hackett AJ, Manning JS. 1971. Comments on feline syncytia-forming virus. *J Am Vet Med Assoc* 158:948–954.
4. Hackett AJ, Pfiester A, Arnstein P. 1970. Biological properties of a syncytia-forming agent isolated from domestic cats (feline syncytia-forming virus). *Proc Soc Exp Biol Med* 135:899–904.
5. Kruger JM, Osborne CA. 1993. The role of uropathogens in feline lower urinary tract disease. *Vet Clin North Am Small Anim Pract* 23:101–123.
6. Kukedi A, Bartha A, Nagy B. 1988. Latent infection with feline syncytial virus of cell cultures prepared from the kidneys of newborn kittens. *Vet Microbiol* 16:9–14.
7. Moise NS, Crissman JW. 1982. Chronic progressive polyarthritis in a cat. *J Am Anim Hosp Assoc* 18:965–969.
8. Pedersen NC. 1987. Feline syncytium-forming virus, pp 329–335. *In* Appel MJ (ed), Virus infections of carnivores. Elsevier, New York.
9. Pedersen NC, Pool R, O'Brien T, et al. 1975. Chronic progressive polyarthritis of the cat. *Feline Pract* 5:42–51.
10. Pedersen NC, Pool RR, O'Brien T. 1980. Feline chronic progressive polyarthritis. *Am J Vet Res* 41:522–535.
11. Wilkinson GT, Robins GM. 1979. Polyarthritis in a young cat. *J Small Anim Pract* 20:293–297.
12. Zenger E, Brown WC, Song W, et al. 1993. Evaluation of cofactor effect of feline syncytium-forming virus on feline immunodeficiency virus infection. *Am J Vet Res* 54:713–718.

Chapter 18

Feline Paramyxovirus Infections

Craig E. Greene and Hans Lutz

Viruses of the family Paramyxoviridae (genera *Paramyxovirus* and *Morbillivirus*) have been shown to cause infections in the CNS of domestic and large exotic Felidae, although none of the viruses in this group are known to be primarily feline viruses. These infections differ from commonly known or suspected viral CNS infections of cats, such as feline panleukopenia (see Chapter 10), feline infectious peritonitis (see Chapter 11), and feline polioencephalomyelitis and spongiform encephalopathy (see Chapter 84).

AVIAN NEWCASTLE VIRUS INFECTION

Avian Newcastle disease virus (a *Paramyxovirus*) has been experimentally inoculated into the CNS of domestic adult cats and kittens, producing disseminated encephalomyelitis.[9, 12] Neonatal kittens could also be infected by intraocular or IN exposure to large quantities of virus. The incubation period of oculonasally administered virus was relatively long (11–17 days) compared with that following direct CNS inoculation

(3–4 days). Clinical signs of encephalomyelitis were seizures, head tilt, and myoclonus. Progressive lower motor neuron paralysis developed in limbs and cranial nerve musculature. In some affected animals, behavioral alterations were present. A disseminated nonsuppurative meningoencephalitis was found histologically; virus appeared to spread throughout the nervous system along descending and ascending neuronal pathways.

UNTYPED PARAMYXOVIRUS INFECTION

A paramyxovirus-like agent has also been isolated from the CNS of naturally infected cats that had focal demyelinating encephalitis and inclusion body formation.[6] The virus was isolated from affected cats by cocultivating CNS tissue with fetal feline kidney cell lines. The isolated virus, serologically unrelated to known paramyxoviruses, was inoculated into the CNS of neonatal mice that developed a similar encephalitis 5 months later.

Paramyxovirus-like nucleocapsids have also been observed by EM in explant cultures of CNS tissue from clinically healthy cats or those with demyelinating optic nerve lesions that were cocultured with feline kidney or Vero cell lines.[24] The significance of these ultrastructural findings is uncertain.

Nonsuppurative encephalitis has been reported in an adult Siberian tiger *(Panthera tigris)*, in which intranuclear inclusion bodies detected on light microscopy and nucleocapsid material detected on EM were found to be similar to those of viruses of the family Paramyxoviridae.[8] These observations could represent infections with canine distemper virus (CDV) or a variant, but definitive information is unavailable.

CDV INFECTION

CDV, a *Morbillivirus*, has been shown to infect a wide variety of terrestrial carnivores. Domestic cats were experimentally inoculated, but clinical signs were absent (see Epidemiology, Chapter 3). In contrast to domestic cats, large exotic Felidae appear to be more susceptible to infection with CDV. Isolates appear to be immunologically similar to virulent isolates from other carnivores, but this finding does not exclude differences in viral biotypes.[4] Mutant viral strains, originating from wildlife and domestic dogs in close proximity to the large cats, are the most likely explanation for outbreaks of CDV infection in large cats. A chronic, progressive, nonsuppurative meningoencephalitis, clinically and pathologically similar to that caused by CDV in dogs, has been described in a Bengal tiger *(P. tigris)*.[9] Marked increases in serum and CSF antibodies against CDV were found. Myoclonus was similar to that seen in other paramyxovirus-type infections in dogs and cats. CDV was suspected as the cause of respiratory and neurologic disease in two snow leopards *(Uncina uncina)* that had simultaneous feline panleukopenia.[7] CDV was not isolated; however, histologic lesions, intranuclear inclusions, virus ultrastructure, immunofluorescence, and serologic testing were all positive for CDV infection. Feline panleukopenia virus (FPV)–induced immunosuppression was presumed to have allowed development of CDV infection.

Canine distemper outbreaks have occurred in captive leopards *(Panthera pardus)*, tigers, lions *(P. leo)*, and a jaguar *(P. onca)* in North America.[4, 25] Initial illness was manifest systemically by anorexia, GI and/or respiratory signs followed by CNS signs of ataxia, myoclonus, seizures, and coma. The source of infection for one epizootic was CDV-infected raccoons and skunks having a concurrent outbreak. Viruses isolated from the affected cats were identified as CDV by monoclonal antibody testing and genetic analysis. The isolates were linked to strains from the feral nonfelid hosts and not vaccine virus.[11] CNS lesions were focal and mild, consisting of nonsuppurative polioencephalitis, lymphocytic meningitis, and mild microgliosis in white matter. These lesions were less extensive and severe and did not have the demyelination and perivascular cuffing as typically observed in infected dogs. These features are more typical of acute CDV infection in susceptible carnivores[21] (see Chapter 3).

In 1994, an outbreak of CDV infection occurred in lions in the Serengeti in Tanzania.[14, 17, 19] Clinical signs included seizures, myoclonus, and other neurologic symptoms. Pathology revealed encephalitis and pneumonia. Histopathology typical for CDV infection was seen in 18 of 19 lions examined. Inclusion bodies immunologically cross-reacting with CDV proteins were identified in 14 of 19 lion samples that were available for examination. Of 83 serum samples tested for anti-CDV antibodies, 71 were found to be positive for CDV.[17] To determine the genetic relationship of the virus involved in the disease outbreak with other Morbilliviruses, buffy coat cells collected from 2 lions with neurologic signs were subjected to reverse transcriptase–polymerase chain reaction (PCR), and the nucleotide sequence of the conserved P gene was determined. These tests suggested that the lion CDV isolate was closely related to the Onderstepoort strain of CDV. It is believed that the lion distemper outbreak originated from distemper infections in domestic dogs living around the Serengeti parks. However, for transmission between dogs and lions, hyenas were probably responsible. On the basis of neurologic signs, several hyenas were found to be affected and were also proved to be infected by CDV. In addition, hyenas, in contrast to lions, are known to roam into the villages of the local inhabitants, where they may have come into contact with domestic dogs. To determine whether the presence of other lion viruses may have favored the susceptibility to CDV, serum samples were tested for presence of antibodies to feline immunodeficiency virus (FIV), feline herpesvirus (FHV-1, FRV), feline calicivirus (FCV), FPV, and feline coronaviruses. No relationship between the occurrence of CDV and antibodies to these other pathogens was found.

To reduce the probability of future outbreaks of CDV in these lions, a program to vaccinate the domestic dogs living around the parks has been started in 1995 by the "Project Life Lions," an initiative by U.S. scientists. Inactivated distemper virus vaccine has been recommended to protect large exotic Felidae against infection with this virus.[4] However, the efficacy of inactivated vaccines in dogs and other exotic carnivores, not to mention cats, has not been documented. Because chick embryo–adapted (Onderstepoort strain) vaccines are generally safer than tissue culture–adapted (Rockborn strain) ones, they should be considered for evaluation in large Felidae.[3, 4]

EQUINE MORBILLIVIRUS (EMV) INFECTION

In September 1994, an outbreak of acute respiratory disease in horses occurred in Hendra, a suburb of Brisbane, Queensland, Australia.[15] The horses developed pneumonia clinically characterized by anorexia, depression, pyrexia, tachypnea, and ataxia. Terminally, head pressing and a frothy nasal discharge occurred. A stable hand and horse trainer became ill with an influenza-like illness. The stable hand was ill for 6 weeks, and the trainer died of respiratory distress. A novel *Morbillivirus* was isolated from both the horses and the people. Another episode was retrospectively identified in Mckay, a town in North Coastal Queensland in a farmer who developed an acute progressive encephalitis.[18] The farmer had assisted with treatment and subsequent necropsy of the affected horses. Most interestingly, the horses developed myoclonic twitches similar to those observed in dogs with canine distemper.

The predominant pathologic lesions in horses from the Hendra outbreak were in the lungs, which are congested and edematous. Histologically, interstitial pneumonia with pneumocyte and capillary degeneration was apparent. Virus was immunologically detected in the endothelial cells by FA. In the Mckay episode, virus was detected by positive PCR in CSF and in the Hendra episode, in brain tissue and serum.[16a]

The EMV was unusual in its ability to grow in cell cultures originating from a number of animal species, including submammalian vertebrates. A number of laboratory animal species, including dogs and cats, were experimentally inoculated SC with the virus.[23] The dogs and cats were vaccinated for common viral diseases but notably the dogs for CDV. The dogs did not become ill, but the cats developed inappetence and tachypnea by the fifth day PI and died on the sixth and seventh days PI. The cats had gross lesions of pulmonary edema, hilar lymphadenomegaly, pneumonia, and pleural effusion. Histologic lesions of vasculitis matched those in affected horses. The virus was isolated from the lungs, spleen, kidney, and brain. Surviving cats did not develop specific serum viral neutralizing antibody. Cats have also been experimentally infected via intranasal and oral exposure to virus and by direct contact with previously infected cats.[11a] Because EMV is so genetically distinct from other Morbilliviruses, it is suspected to have existed for a long time and to have been acquired from a mammalian reservoir host. Of all the laboratory species inoculated, cats were most susceptible and developed an illness that matched that in horses and in people. A limited serosurvey of cats in the metropolitan Brisbane area did not reveal detectable antibody to the virus.[23] Subsequent studies in cats have shown that they can be infected by nonparenteral routes and that the virus can spread naturally among cats.[22] Of many wildlife species tested, *Pteropus* bats have serum antibodies to the virus and may be the reservoir species.[26] Transmission from bats to another species, such as the horse, may be required for human exposure.

References

1. Appel MJ. 1987. Canine distemper virus, pp 133–159. *In* Appel MJ (ed), Virus infections of carnivores. Elsevier, New York, NY.
2. Appel M, Sheffy BE, Percy DH, et al. 1974. Canine distemper virus in domesticated cats and pigs. *Am J Vet Res* 35:803–806.
3. Appel MJG, Summers BA. 1995. Pathogenicity of morbilliviruses for terrestrial carnivores. *Vet Microbiol* 44:187–191.
4. Appel MJG, Yates RA, Foley AL, et al. 1994. Canine distemper epizootic in lions, tigers, and leopards in North America. *J Vet Diagn Invest* 6:277–288.
5. Blythe LL, Schmitz JA, Roelke M, et al. 1983. Chronic encephalomyelitis caused by canine distemper virus in a Bengal tiger. *J Am Vet Med Assoc* 183:1159–1162.
6. Cook RD, Wilcox GE. 1981. A paramyxovirus-like agent associated with demyelinating lesions in the CNS of cats. *J Neuropathol Exp Neurol* 40:328.
7. Fix AS, Riordan DP, Hill HT. 1989. Feline panleukopenia virus and subsequent canine distemper virus infection in two snow leopards. *J Zoo Wildl Med* 20:273–281.
8. Gould DH, Fenner WR. 1983. Paramyxovirus-like nucleocapsids associated with encephalitis in a captive Siberian tiger. *J Am Vet Med Assoc* 183:1319–1322.
9. Greene CE. 1990. Feline paramyxovirus encephalomyelitis, pp 360–362. *In* Greene CE (ed), Infectious diseases of the dog and cat. WB Saunders, Philadelphia, PA.
10. Harder TC, Kenter M, Appel MJG, et al. 1995. Phylogenetic evidence for canine distemper viruses in Serengeti's lions. *Vaccine* 13:521–523.
11. Harder TC, Kenter M, Vos H, et al. 1996. Canine distemper virus from diseased large felids: biological properties and phylogenic relationships. *J Gen Virol* 77:397–405.

11a. Hooper PT, Westbury HA, Russell GM. 1997. The lesions of experimental equine morbillivirus disease in cats and guinea pigs. *Vet Pathol* 34:323–329.

12. Luttrell CN, Bang FB. 1958. Newcastle disease encephalomyelitis in cats: I. Clinical and pathological features. *AMA Arch Neurol Psychiatr* 79:646–657.
13. Montali RJ, Bartz CR, Teare JA, et al. 1983. Clinical trials with canine distemper vaccines in exotic carnivores. *J Am Vet Med Assoc* 183:1163–1167.
14. Morell V. 1994. Serengeti's big cats going to the dogs. *Science* 264:1664.
15. Murray K, Rogers R, Selleck P, et al. 1995. A novel *Morbillivirus* pneumonia of horses and its transmission to humans. *Emerging Infect Dis* 1:31–34.
16. Murray PK. 1996. The evolving story of the equine morbillivirus. *Aust Vet J* 74:214–244.

16a. O'Sullivan JD, Allworth AM, Paterson DL, et al. 1997. Fatal encephalitis due to novel paramyxovirus transmitted from horses. *Lancet* 349:93–95.

17. Roelke-Parker ME, Munson L, Packer C, et al. 1996. A canine distemper virus epidemic in Serengeti lions (*Panthera leo*). *Nature* 379:441–445.
18. Rogers RJ, Douglas IC, Baldock FC. 1996. Investigation of a second focus of equine morbillivirus infection in coastal Queensland. *Aust Vet J* 74:243–244.
19. Spencer LM. 1995. CDV infection in large exotic cats not expected to affect domestic cats. *J Am Vet Med Assoc* 206:579–580.
20. Truyen U, Stockhofe-Zurwieden N, Kaaden OR, et al. 1990. A case report: encephalomyelitis in lions. Pathological and virological findings. *DTW Dtsch Tierarztl Wochenschr* 97:89–91.
21. Van Moll P, Alldinger S, Baumgärtner W, et al. 1995. Distemper in wild carnivores: an epidemiological, histological and immunochemical study. *Vet Microbiol* 44:193–199.
22. Westbury HA, Hooper PT, Brouwer SL, et al. 1996. Susceptibility of cats to equine *Morbillivirus*. *Aust Vet J* 74:132–134.
23. Westbury HA, Hooper PT, Selleck PW, et al. 1995. Equine *Morbillivirus* pneumonia: susceptibility of laboratory animals to the virus. *Aust Vet J* 72:278–279.
24. Wilcox GE, Flower RLP, Cook RD. 1994. Recovery of viral agents from the central nervous system of cats. *Vet Microbiol* 9:355–366.
25. Wood SL, Thomson GW, Haines DM. 1995. Canine distemper virus-like infection in a captive African lioness. *Can Vet J* 36:34–35.
26. Young PL, Halpin K, Selleck PW, et al. 1996. Serological evidence in *Pteropus* bats for the presence of a paramyxovirus related to equine moribillivirus. *Emerging Infect Dis* 2:239–240.

Chapter 19

Feline Poxvirus Infection

Malcolm Bennett, Rosalind M. Gaskell, and Derrick Baxby

ETIOLOGY AND EPIDEMIOLOGY

The best described and most common poxvirus infection of cats is cowpox, caused by an *Orthopoxvirus*,[2] but infections with *Parapoxvirus*[12] and uncharacterized poxviruses in India and North America[18] have been reported. Poxviruses are relatively resistant and can remain infective in dry conditions for several months to years. However, they are readily inactivated by many disinfectants, especially hypochlorites.

Cowpox virus is found only in Eurasia.[2] In western and northern Europe, the reservoir hosts are voles (*Clethrionomys* spp. and *Microtus* spp.) and wood mice (*Apodemus* spp.),[8, 9, 14] whereas in Turkmenia and Georgia the reservoir hosts are ground squirrels (*Citellus fulvus*) and gerbils (*Rhombomys opimus* and *Meriones libicus*).[2] Although the domestic cat is the most frequently recognized incidental host,[4, 6, 15, 17] cowpox virus can also infect humans,[3, 10] cattle, and a variety of captive exotic mammals.[2] One case has been reported in a domestic dog.[6] Rats (*Rattus norvegicus*) and house mice (*Mus musculus*) also may be rare incidental hosts.

Feline cowpox is seen mostly in rural cats that hunt rodents. Most cases are seen in autumn.[5, 6] There is no sex or age predisposition to infection. Occasional cat-to-cat transmission occurs, as does cat-to-human transmission.[3]

PATHOGENESIS

The usual route of cowpox infection in cats is skin inoculation, probably through a bite or other skin wound, although oronasal infection is also possible. Local viral replication produces a primary skin lesion, and spread to the draining lymph nodes and a leukocyte-associated viremia give rise to widespread secondary skin lesions. During the viremic period, virus can be isolated from the respiratory tract.

CLINICAL FINDINGS

Feline cowpox virus usually causes widespread skin lesions, but most cats have a history of a single primary skin lesion, generally on the head, neck, or forelimb. Primary lesions often are complicated by concurrent bacterial infection and may vary from a small superficial scabbed-over wound to a large abscess or area of cellulitis.

Secondary skin lesions generally develop 1 to 3 weeks later. First apparent as randomly distributed, small epidermal nodules, the lesions increase in size (1 cm diameter) over 3 to 5 days to form well-circumscribed ulcers, which soon become scabbed (Fig. 19–1). These gradually dry and, after 4 to 5 weeks, exfoliate. New hair growth soon occurs, although some lesions may result in small, permanently bald patches.[4, 6, 15, 17]

Many cats show no clinical signs other than skin lesions. Signs of systemic illness are usually mild and occur during the viremic period just before development of secondary skin lesions. Cats may be pyrexic, inappetent, or depressed; a few may have coryza or transient diarrhea. More severe disease is rare in domestic cats and is often associated with severe bacterial infection or immune dysfunction often resulting from feline leukemia virus (FeLV) or feline immunodeficiency virus (FIV) infection or from glucocorticoid treatment.[4] However, in exotic felids (e.g., cheetahs) a rapidly fatal pneumonia frequently develops. Severely ill cats have a poor prognosis, and euthanasia may be advised.

Feline parapoxvirus, probably orf from sheep or goats, infection also causes multiple crusty skin lesions, which heal over a few weeks. Anecdotal accounts of similar conditions exist in North America.

DIAGNOSIS

Dried scab material can be sent to a laboratory by mail in a sealed container without transport medium. Cowpox virus can be readily isolated in a variety of cell cultures, and virions often can be seen in scab homogenates by EM. EM is the best way to recognize parapoxviruses because of their characteristic morphology and because they are difficult to grow in cell culture. Serum antibodies can be detected by various methods: we routinely use an FA assay for cowpox (see Appendix 5).[9]

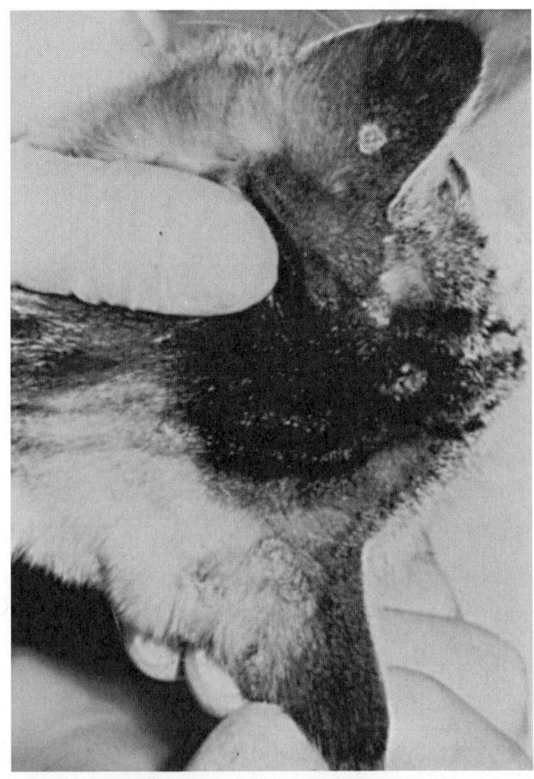

Figure 19–1. Scabbed secondary cowpox lesions on the head of a cat.

PATHOLOGIC FINDINGS

The histologic appearance of feline cowpox includes epithelial hyperplasia and hypertrophy, with multilocular vesicle formation and ulceration. Many infected cells contain intracytoplasmic, eosinophilic inclusion bodies.[4] Immunostaining is a useful aid to histologic diagnosis.

TREATMENT AND PREVENTION

There is no specific treatment for poxvirus infections. Broad-spectrum antibiotics are recommended to control secondary bacterial infections, and general supportive therapy, including fluids, may be necessary. Glucocorticoids are contraindicated because they may exacerbate the condition.

No vaccines are available, but vaccinia virus may be considered for valuable zoo collections at risk for cowpox. Vaccinia virus appears to be of low infectivity and pathogenicity for cats and cheetahs, but its ability to provoke a protective immune response is unknown.

PUBLIC HEALTH CONSIDERATIONS

Cowpox is zoonotic and, in addition to a painful skin lesion, usually causes systemic illness, which may require hospitalization, and rarely causes death.[3, 10] Those with a preexisting skin condition or immune deficiency seem particularly at risk of more severe disease. Human cowpox is rare (one or two cases each year in the United Kingdom), but cats are thought to be the source of more than 50% of these cases.[3] The risk of cat-to-human transmission is small if basic hygienic precautions are taken. With few exceptions, the illness does not warrant euthanasia of the cat.

Even recent smallpox vaccination is unlikely to provide protection for people against the primary cowpox lesions, although it might help prevent more severe disease.[1]

Other poxviruses, including many parapoxviruses, may also be zoonotic, but the risk of cat-to-human transmission of these viruses is unknown.

References

1. Baxby D. 1993. Indications for smallpox vaccination: policies still differ. *Vaccine* 11:395–396.
2. Baxby D, Bennett M. 1994. Cowpox virus, pp 261–267. *In* Webster RG, Granoff A (eds), Encyclopedia of virology. Academic Press, London.
3. Baxby D, Bennett M, Getty B. 1994. Human cowpox: a review based on 54 cases, 1969-93. *Br J Dermatol* 131:598–607.
4. Bennett M, Gaskell RM, Baxby D. 1990. Feline cowpox virus infection, pp 363–364. *In* Greene CE (ed), Infectious diseases of the dog and cat. WB Saunders, Philadelphia, PA.
5. Bennett M, Gaskell CJ, Baxby D, et al. 1990. Feline cowpox virus infection. *J Small Anim Pract* 31:167–173.
6. Bomhard D, von Pfleghaar S, Mahnel H. 1992. Zur epidemiologie, klinik, pathologie und virologie der katzen-pocken-infektion. *Kleintierpraxis* 37:219–230.
7. Boulanger D, Brochier B, Crouch A, et al. 1995. Comparison of the susceptibility of the red fox (*Vulpes vulpes*) to vaccinia-rabies recombinant virus and cowpox virus. *Vaccine* 13:215–219.
8. Boulanger D, Crouch A, Brochier B, et al. 1996. Serological survey of Orthopoxvirus infection of wild animals in areas where a recombinant rabies virus is used to vaccinate foxes. *Vet Rec* 138:247–249.
9. Crouch AC, Baxby D, McCracken CM, et al. 1995. Serological evidence for the reservoir hosts of cowpox virus in British wildlife. *Epidemiol Infect* 115:185–191.
10. Czerny CP, Eis-Hubinger AM, Mayr A, et al. 1991. Animal poxviruses transmitted from cat to man: current event with lethal end. *J Vet Med B* 38:421–431.
11. Czerny CP, Wagner K, Gessler K, et al. 1996. A monoclonal blocking ELISA for detection of orthopoxvirus antibodies in feline sera. *Vet Microbiol* 52:185–200.
12. Hamblet CN. 1993. Parapoxvirus infection in a cat. *Vet Rec* 132:144.
13. Henning K, Czerny C-P, Meyer H, et al. 1995. A seroepidemiological survey for orthopox in the red fox (*Vulpes vulpes*). *Vet Microbiol* 43:251–259.
14. Lvov SD, Gromashevskyi VL, Marennikova SS, et al. 1988. Poxvirus isolation from *Microtus oeconomus* Pal. 1776 in Colsky peninsula. *Vop Virus* 1:92–94.
15. Meenout T, Declercq J, De Keuster T, et al. 1991. Drie gevallenvan Koepokkeninektie bij de Kat in Belgie. *Vlaams Deirgeneeskd Tijdschr* 60:64–67.
16. Naidoo J, Baxby D, Bennett M, et al. 1992. Characterization of orthopoxviruses isolated from feline infections in Britain. *Arch Virol* 125:261–272.
17. Nowotny N, Fischer OW, Schilder F, et al. 1994. Pockenvirusinfektionen bei Hauskatzen: Klinische, Pathohistologische, Virologische und Epizootiologische Untersuchen. *Wien Tierarztl Mschr* 81:362–369.
18. Pedersen NC. 1996. Personal communication. University of California, Davis, CA.

Chapter 20

Hantavirus Infection

Craig E. Greene

ETIOLOGY

Bunyaviridae are enveloped, spherical, RNA viruses containing a nucleocapsid protein that is thought to be the most important immunogen. The family Bunyaviridae has four major genera that can be distinguished genetically, morphologically, and antigenically. Unlike other members of the Bunyaviridae, transmission of hantaviruses does not require arthropod vectors (for comparison, see Chapter 26, Arboviral Infections). The genus Hantavirus comprises at least four known strains: Hantaan, Seoul, Puumala, and Sin Nombre (Table 20–1). The first three viruses cause serious and fatal hemorrhagic diseases in people in the eastern hemisphere, whereas the Sin Nombre strain has been isolated from people in the southwestern United States with pulmonary disease.[1, 3, 5] Another strain producing respiratory distress has been isolated from people in Argentina.[11]

EPIDEMIOLOGY

Aerosol transmission from excreta of infected rodents is the principal means by which these viruses are transmitted; however, bite transmission between rodents has been docu-

Table 20–1. Comparison of Features of Hantavirus Infections

DISEASE	VIRAL STRAIN	GEOGRAPHIC DISTRIBUTION	RESERVOIR HOST	USUAL CONTACT
HFRS	Hantaan	Korea, China, eastern Soviet Republics, Balkans	*Apodemus agrarius* (Striped field mouse)	Agricultural activities
Nephropathia epidemica (milder HFRS)	Puumala	Scandinavia, western Soviet Republics, Europe	*Clethrionomys glariolus* (Bank voles)	Forests and agricultural hedge rows, rural and suburban gardens
Milder HFRS, chronic hypertensive renal failure	Seoul	Worldwide	*Rattus norvegicus* (Norway rat)	Farms and residential areas, laboratory rats outside U.S.
Acute respiratory distress	Sin Nombre	Western and southwestern U.S.	*Peromyscus maniculatus* (Deer mouse)	Human dwellings and outbuilding
Acute respiratory distress	Andes	Southern Argentina	*Oligoryzomys longicaudatus*	Rodent contact, nosocomial(?)

HFRS = hemorrhagic fever with renal syndrome; ? = suspected.

mented. Aerosolized virus is the likely means of spread of infection between rodents and to people.[4] Hantavirus infections of domestic and wild rodents are subclinical. There are species differences among rodents in the length of salivary excretion, with times ranging up to 1 year. Infected rodents are thought to harbor the virus in their lungs and kidneys for life.[3] The disease peaks during seasons and years when population densities of rodent colonies are highest and have a greater chance of contacting human populations. The greatest incidence of infection in people occurs when their work or recreational activities expose them to rodents. Infections occur on farms, in suburbs, or in residential areas, depending on the habitat of the reservoir host. In laboratories in the United States, the disease in rats is of low prevalence because research rats have been derived from cesarean-derived stock maintained under strict barrier conditions.

The role of the cat, if any, in transmission of hantaviruses from rodents to people is uncertain. An epidemiologic study in Asia indicated an increased risk factor of cat ownership for people who developed Puumala virus infection.[12] Serologic studies of outdoor cats in Austria have shown a positive prevalence rate of 5% for Puumala strain with higher titers against Puumala than the Hantaan strain.[9] Serologic studies on cats in Great Britain showed an overall positivity rate of 9.6%.[2] The seropositive rate was much higher (23%) for cats with a variety of chronic illnesses. Cats that are allowed to roam or hunt outdoors have the highest seroprevalence. Among 100 such cats, immunofluorescent detection of Hantavirus antigen in lungs and kidneys showed the virus in specimens of lung from two cats.[10]

CLINICAL FINDINGS

No clinical signs have been attributed to Hantavirus infection in cats. It is likely due to the low carriage and quantities of virus that their infection is asymptomatic.[10]

The signs of Hantaan, Seoul, and Puumala infections in people are fever, headache, abdominal pain, renal dysfunction, and hemorrhagic diathesis. The pulmonary syndrome of Muerto Canyon begins with fever and flulike symptoms, progressing to signs of pulmonary edema and shock. Radiographs reveal acute bilateral pulmonary interstitial infiltrates, which have been attributed to pulmonary vasculitis.

DIAGNOSIS

The diagnosis in people is made by serologic demonstration of antiviral IgM and IgG in serum and CSF. Diagnosis in rodents is made by serologic testing. Culture can be performed since rodents can excrete virus in their saliva, urine, and feces. Whereas some excrete virus in the saliva for short periods, others excrete it in the urine for up to 1 year.

TREATMENT

IV ribavirin has been effective in the treatment of human Hantavirus infections when used early in the illness.[1] Excessive fluid administration must be avoided because it may lead to severe edema and worsening pulmonary edema.

PUBLIC HEALTH CONSIDERATIONS

Most human infections occur by aerosol route, but a few have been documented by contact with urine-contaminated garbage and by rodent bites.[3] Avoidance of contact with rodents and repellents for mosquito and tick vectors are the most effective ways to reduce the prevalence of disease. Rodent-infested structures and soil contaminated with feces must be avoided because harmful aerosols can infect those present. Feral rodents should not be kept in captivity, and care should be taken when entering or cleaning closed buildings infested with rodents. Although cats have been found to be seropositive for the viruses, it is uncertain whether they can excrete hantaviruses or whether cat-to-cat or cat-to-human transmission occurs. Although there has been an epidemiologic link between cat ownership and hantaviral disease in Asia, this link has not been suspected in North America and Europe.[10]

References

1. Anonymous. 1993. Infectious diseases update: outbreak, Hantavirus infection-southwestern United States. *JAMA* 270:25.
2. Bennett M, Lloyd G, Jones N, et al. 1990. Prevalence of antibody to Hantavirus in some cat populations in Britain. *Vet Rec* 127:548–549.
3. Blatt H. 1994. Hantavirus infections—an emerging zoonosis. *J Am Anim Hosp Assoc* 30:418.
4. Dohmae K, Okabe M, Nishimune Y. 1994. Experimental transmission of *Hantavirus* infection in laboratory rats. *J Infect Dis* 170:1589–1592.
5. Eidson M, Ettestad PJ. 1995. Hantavirus. *J Am Vet Med Assoc* 206:851–853.
6. Hughes JM, Peters CJ, Cohen ML, et al. 1993. Hantavirus pulmonary syndrome: an emerging infectious disease. *Science* 262:850–860.
7. Khan AS, Khabbaz RF, Armstrong LR, et al. 1996. Hantavirus pulmonary syndrome: the first 100 US cases. *J Infect Dis* 173:1297–1303.
8. Luo ZZ. 1985. Isolation of epidemic hemorrhagic fever virus from a cat. *Clin J Microbiol Immunol* 1:513–514.
9. Nowotny N. 1994. The domestic cat: a possible transmitter of viruses from rodents to man. *Lancet* 343:921.
10. Nowotny N, Weissenboeck H, Aberle S, et al. 1994. Hantavirus infection in the domestic cat. *JAMA* 272:1100–1101.
11. Wells RM, Young J, Williams RJ, et al. 1997. Hantavirus transmission in the United States. *Emerg Infect Dis* 3:361–365.
12. Xu ZY, Tang YW, Kan LY, et al. 1987. Cats—source of protection or infection? A case control study of hemorrhagic fever with renal syndrome. *Am J Epidemiol* 126:942–948.

Chapter 21

Feline Viral Papillomatosis

Herman F. Egberink and Marian C. Horzinek

ETIOLOGY AND EPIDEMIOLOGY

Papillomaviruses, members of the Papovaviridae family, are small nonenveloped viruses with an icosahedral symmetry and a double-stranded circular DNA genome. They are widespread in nature and infect many species of mammals and birds.[7] They cause benign cutaneous and mucosal proliferations that are usually self-limiting and only rarely progress to malignant tumors.[11] All members of the genus share at least one antigenic determinant[8]; however, papillomaviruses are highly species specific. Transmission has so far been reported within only one animal species or between closely related hosts. In several studies of papillomatous and hyperplastic lesions, papillomaviral antigen was not demonstrated in lesions from cats.[6, 11] There are only a few reports of papillomas in cats that were proved to be related to papillomavirus infection.[1, 2, 4] This occurrence could be due to the inconspicuous nature and uncharacteristic morphology of the lesions, which precludes a clinical diagnosis by analogy.

Serologic studies to determine the incidence of subclinical infections in the feline population have not been reported. A spill-over from another species (e.g., from a prey animal similar to the epidemiology of poxviruses) cannot be excluded but is unlikely. Although the feline isolated papovavirus has not been fully characterized, it was shown to be different from other papillomaviruses. A unique staining pattern using a panel of monoclonal antibodies against papillomavirus capsid protein epitopes could be demonstrated.[3]

PATHOGENESIS

In general, papillomas will develop after introduction of virus through lesions or abrasions of the skin. Experimental infection of healthy cats with material from wartlike lesions of affected cats did not result in papillomas. Papillomaviruses have a specific tropism for squamous epithelial cells. The virus infects the basal cells in the epithelium, and early gene expression can be detected in them. However, the production of viral proteins and the assembly of virions are restricted to the most terminally differentiated keratinocytes at the surface of the papilloma. After infection, hyperplasia of cells of the stratum spinosum occurs, and proliferation of the epithelium becomes clinically evident 4 to 6 weeks PI. There is no reported age resistance in papillomavirus infections; all the feline cases were in older animals (6–13 years old). Papillomas are more prevalent in animals and humans under conditions that impair T-cell functions.[5, 11] Immunodeficiency seems to be a factor of clinical manifestation in cats, because those animals with papillomas were under immunosuppressive therapy[1] or were infected with feline immunodeficiency virus.[2]

CLINICAL FINDINGS

The macroscopic appearance of the lesions is not typical of the papillomas seen in other domestic animals.[1, 2] Although the surface of the lesions is verrucous, they appear as slightly raised plaques rather than warts (Fig. 21–1). The plaques are several millimeters in diameter; sometimes elongated lesions can be noticed. Plaques can be white or pigmented, scaly and greasy to the touch. The wartlike lesions were located on the head, neck, dorsal part of the thorax, and abdomen. Signs of systemic illness have been observed in the cats. These signs are not induced by the papillomavirus infection but are the consequence of concurrent immunodeficiency.

DIAGNOSIS

A full-thickness biopsy of an entire lesion with adjacent normal tissue can be taken and processed for histopathologic, immunohistochemical, or EM examinations.

Histologic examination reveals pigmented, hyperplastic epidermal plaques with defined boundaries. Proliferation of all layers is evident. The epidermal hyperplasia is characterized by acanthosis and hypergranulocytosis with hyperkeratosis. No inflammatory cells are observed in either the plaques or the adjacent stroma. Ballooning degeneration of cells in the stratum spinosum and in the stratum granulosum with nuclear changes can be observed. In the upper part of the former and in the stratum granulosum, solitary cells with large irregularly shaped amphophilic inclusion-like structures occur. These are found in the cytoplasm, but ill-defined, probably intranuclear, inclusions were reported also. By EM, intranuclear papillomavirus-like particles are demonstrated in keratinized cells in the superficial epithelial strata of the plaques. The cytoplasmic inclusions appear as keratohyalin-like granules.

For a definite identification, immunohistology can be per-

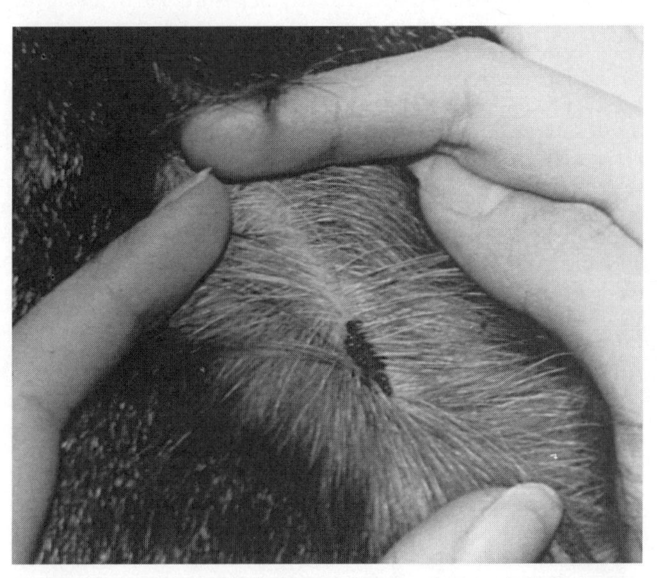

Figure 21–1. Typical skin lesion on the dorsal part of the abdomen. Pigmented, slightly raised plaques with a rough surface are seen.

formed on sections through selected skin lesions using a broad-reactive, genus-specific antiserum (see Appendix 5). Staining of papillomavirus group-specific antigens is found mainly in the stratum granulosum and stratum corneum of the papilloma; some cells in the stratum spinosum also stain positive. Immunoreactivity appears in the nuclei. Sometimes weak staining of the cytoplasm is noticed, possibly after injury of the nuclear membrane.

THERAPY

No specific treatment is known. Often the location and the number of papillomas will not warrant surgical excision. In analogy with papillomas in other species such as dogs, spontaneous regression can be expected (see Chapter 9).

References

1. Carney HC, England JJ, Hodgin EC, et al. 1990. Papillomavirus infection of aged Persian cats. *J Vet Diagn Invest* 2:294–299.
2. Egberink HF, Berrocal A, Bax HAD, et al. 1992. Papillomavirus associated skin lesions in a cat seropositive for feline immunodeficiency virus. *Vet Microbiol* 31:117–125.
3. Lim PS, Jenson AB, Cowsert L, et al. 1990. Distribution and specific identification of papillomavirus major capsid protein epitopes by immunocytochemistry and epitope scanning of synthetic peptides. *J Infect Dis* 162:1263–1269.
4. Lozano-Alarcon F, Lewis TP, Clark EG, et al. 1996. Persistent papillomavirus infection in a cat. *J Am Anim Hosp Assoc* 32:392–395.
5. Matorras R, Ariteca JM, Rementeria A, et al. 1991. Human immunodeficiency virus induced immunosuppression: a risk factor for human papillomavirus infection. *Am J Obstet Gynecol* 164:42–44.
6. Sironi G, Caniatti M, Scanziani E. 1990. Immunohistochemical detection of papillomavirus structural antigens in animal hyperplastic and neoplastic epithelial lesions. *Zentralbl Veterinarmed A* 37:760–770.
7. Sundberg JP. 1987. Papillomavirus infections in animals, pp 41–103. *In* Syrjanen K, Gissmann L, Koss LG (eds), Papillomaviruses and human disease. Springer Verlag, New York, NY.
8. Sundberg JP, Junge RE, Lancaster WD. 1984. Immunoperoxidase localization of papillomaviruses in hyperplastic and neoplastic epithelial lesions. *Am J Vet Res* 45:1441–1446.
9. Sundberg JP, Montali RJ, Bush M, et al. 1994. Feline papillomaviruses: host range, molecular diversity, and epitope conservation. *Vet Pathol* 31:616.
10. Sundberg JP, Montali RJ, Bush M, et al. 1996. Papillomavirus-associated focal oral hyperplasia in wild and captive Asian lions (*Panthera leopersica*). *J Zoo Wildl Med* 27:61–70.
11. Sundberg JP, O'Bannion MK. 1989. Animal papillomaviruses associated with malignant tumors. *Adv Viral Oncol* 8:55–71.

Chapter 22

Rabies

Craig E. Greene and David W. Dreesen

ETIOLOGY

The virus of rabies is the prototype of the genus *Lyssavirus* in the family Rhabdoviridae. They are enveloped, bullet-shaped RNA viruses that usually measure 75 X 180 nm. Rabies viruses have been isolated worldwide and were originally considered to belong to one common antigenic type. However, techniques using monoclonal antibodies (mAB) produced against viral proteins and gene-sequencing techniques have provided evidence for antigenic differences (variants) among various isolates from major wildlife hosts within a given geographic region. Analysis of a nucleotide sequence from the nucleoprotein gene of rabies virus has allowed comparison of isolates from Asia, Africa, Europe, and the Americas.[65] Findings of these studies that support those of mAB typing suggest that rabies may have spread to the Americas, Asia, and Africa from European colonization. Infection in imported domestic dogs may have spread to sylvatic species with establishment of enzootic foci in these areas.

Rabies virus replicates by budding from the host cell membranes, and viral nucleocapsid develops in the cytoplasm. Complete viral particles may be formed at the cell surface, but, more commonly, they bud from intracytoplasmic membranes. Free virus particles infect new or adjacent cells by fusing their envelopes with the host cell membrane, which allows direct entry of viral genetic material.

As an enveloped virus, rabies is destroyed by various concentrations of formalin, phenol, halogens, mercurials, mineral acids, and other disinfectants. It is extremely labile when exposed to UV light and heat.

Rabies virus remains viable in a carcass for fewer than 24 hours at 20°C, although it survives much longer (days) when the body of the victim is refrigerated. Immunofluorescent testing, commonly used for rabies diagnosis, does not depend on the presence of viable viral particles; thus, viral antigen may be detected for 5 to 7 days at 25°C or shorter at 37°C, which are times beyond the presence of viable virus. Virus survival for mouse inoculation can be greatly increased in unrefrigerated tissue by storing it in 50% glycerol in phosphate-buffered saline at room temperature. Preservation can also be enhanced if a 20% suspension of infected tissue or virus culture is made with a solution that is high in protein or amino acids. Storage at ultra-low temperatures (−30° to −80°C) prolongs virus survival for years in untreated fresh-frozen tissue. However, freezing samples in a household-type freezer with subsequent defrosting cycles will damage the tissue and destroy the virus for subsequent detection.

EPIDEMIOLOGY

Susceptibility

All warm-blooded animals are vulnerable to infection with rabies, and susceptibility is affected by factors such as the viral variant, the quantity of virus inoculated, and the bite site. In addition, the degree of species susceptibility varies considerably. Foxes, coyotes, jackals, wolves, and certain rodents are among the most susceptible animal groups. Skunks, raccoons, bats, rabbits, cattle, and some members of the families Felidae and Viverridae have a high susceptibility. Groups with only moderate susceptibility include domestic dogs, sheep, goats, horses, and nonhuman primates. All birds and primitive mammals such as the opossum have low susceptibility. Cats are actually more resistant than dogs to experimental infection with some canine rabies isolates but are much more prone to develop infection with some field isolates from wildlife and with vaccine virus. Younger animals are usually more susceptible to rabies infection than older ones.

Transmission

Rabies infection is nearly always due to the bite of an infected animal that has rabies virus in its saliva. Other modes of transmission to be described are infrequently involved in infections of the dog and cat but may serve to maintain infection in wildlife. Transmission from exhaled or excreted virus has been suggested in large colonies of cave-dwelling bats and in a laboratory outbreak among terrestrial animals.[32] Such air-borne infections are probably important only among highly susceptible animals that live in high-density populations. Rabies can occasionally result from the ingestion of infected tissue or secretions. Transplacental rabies infections in skunks, bats, and a cow also have been reported; however, the ability of such in utero infections to be transmitted in later life is unclear.[32] Environmental transmission by fomites is rarely, if ever, involved. Human rabies has been acquired by corneal transplantation, and the disturbing number of human rabies cases in which no obvious source of exposure can be determined argues against complacency when considering the routes of rabies virus transmission. Latent rabies infections with prolonged salivary shedding of virus do exist rarely among some animal species, so that the absence of neurologic abnormalities cannot be used to rule out absolutely the possibility of rabies infection.

Hosts and Range

More than 27,000 cases of animal rabies are reported yearly in the world; the estimated actual number of cases is many times greater. The World Health Organization reported 31,223 cases of human rabies for 1993 with additional cases from nonreporting countries. Reports suggest that more than 25,000 human rabies deaths may occur in India alone. Antarctica, New Zealand, Taiwan, some of the Caribbean islands, England, Ireland, Spain, Portugal, Norway, Sweden, Iceland, Hawaii, and Japan are currently free of rabies. A rabies-like Lyssavirus has been identified in fruit bats ("flying foxes") in Australia.[30] Fatal infection in one person has been reported.[4]

Throughout the world, in most of the Northern Hemisphere, rabies is predominately a disease of wildlife, whereas in the Southern Hemisphere, the dog is the primary species involved in the transmission of the disease (Fig. 22–1). Despite the fact that all warm-blooded animals are susceptible, rabies virus in a given enzootic area is a distinct variant that usually adapts itself to a single dominant reservoir host. For example, wildlife reservoir species in various geographic

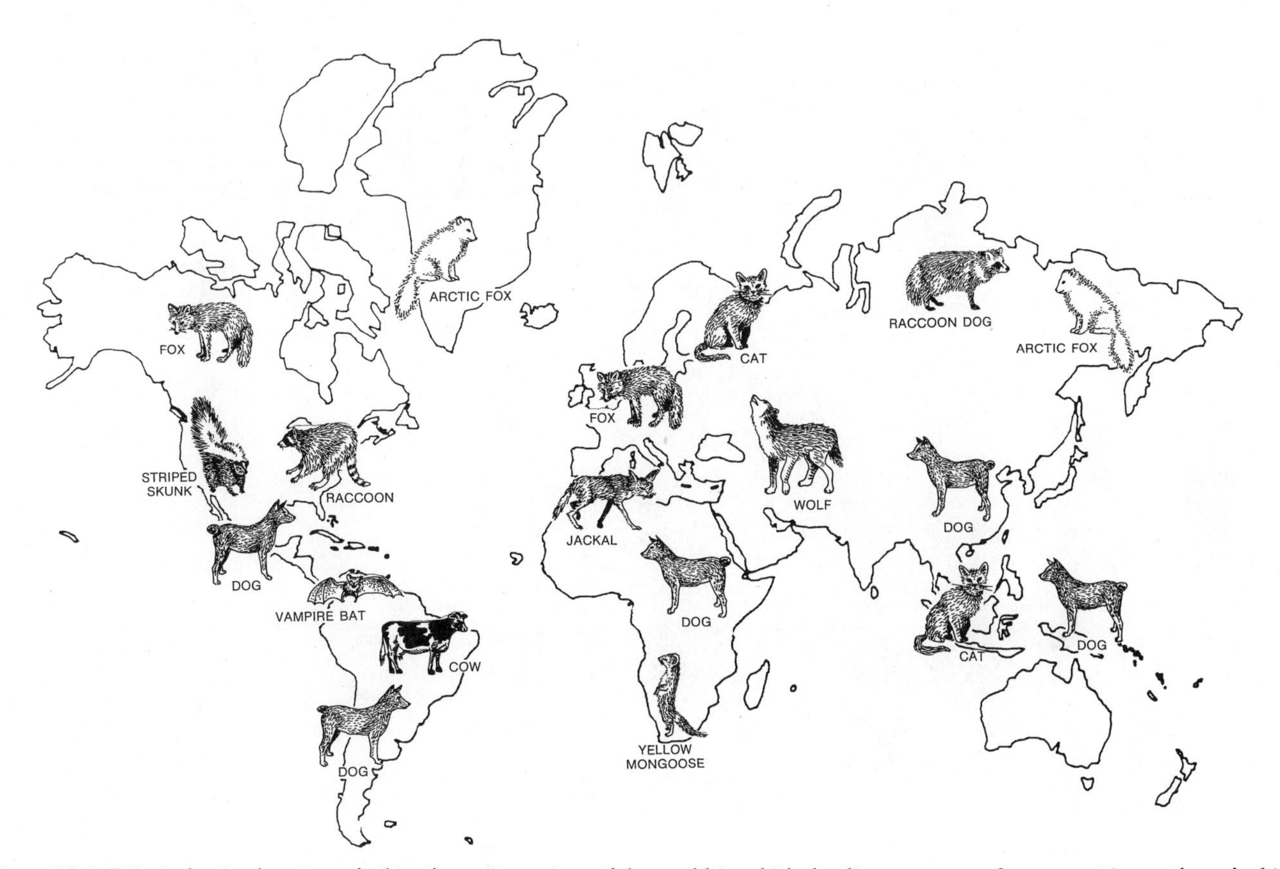

Figure 22–1. Principal animal vectors of rabies for major regions of the world in which the disease appears. Some countries are free of rabies (see Hosts and Range in text).

areas of the United States are raccoons, skunks, foxes, coyotes, and insectivorous bats (Fig. 22–2). In Europe the primary species are foxes and raccoon dogs, whereas in South Africa and certain Caribbean nations mongooses predominate.

Rabies in enzootic areas appears to be cyclic. It spreads into unexposed, susceptible wildlife populations in a region; subsequent decreases and increases in the incidence of disease are caused by population mortality and immunity, which periodically cycles in the wildlife population. These wild animals serve as maintenance hosts for virus transmission to dogs, cats, cattle, and horses. Most human exposures result from contact with these domestic species.

Dogs and Cats. The highest incidence of dog and cat rabies in the United States generally occurs in areas where wildlife rabies is epidemic. Although the incidence of wildlife rabies has been on the increase, cases of canine and farm animal rabies have been decreasing (Fig. 22–3). Vaccination of dogs and animal control programs have been the main factors responsible for this decline. Although the incidence of dog rabies has declined, dogs account for the majority of reported animal bites in the United States. Many of these bites result in people seeking antirabies prophylaxis. Worldwide, dogs account for most of human rabies deaths and postexposure prophylaxis.[16] In less developed nations, where dog rabies has not been controlled, the incidence of canine and human rabies is quite high. Adequate vaccination of at least 70% to 80% of dogs in a given population has been shown to block the occurrence of rabies epidemics.

An increase in feline rabies usually is related to spill-over of infection from wildlife, because there has been no specific virus variant attributed to cats. The relative importance of feline rabies as a source for human exposure in a given geographic area is dependent on whether canine rabies is being controlled by vaccination. In the United States, since 1979, cat rabies cases have shown a slight increase over the previous 7-year period. Beginning in 1981, more cases of rabies in cats than in dogs have been reported annually. This increase probably reflects the low numbers of cats vaccinated for rabies and the epidemics of wildlife rabies in the mid-Atlantic and Northeast regions of the United States. Numerically, cats have been the most important domestic animal affected since 1992.[62] The frequency of human rabies exposures attributed to rabid cats is now increasing at a greater rate than those from dogs. Rabid cats, which usually are reclusive, often become aggressive and may attack humans and other animals when disturbed.[24]

Wildlife Carnivores. The striped skunk *(Mephitis mephitis)*, the most common skunk in the United States, is probably the most important species in perpetuating wildlife rabies in the United States. Studies based on antigenic typing have demonstrated the existence of two distinct variants in skunks: one in the south central states and another in the north central states and California, extending into Canada. Although the spotted skunk *(Spilogale* sp.*)* presented a serious rabies threat in the western United States during the 1800s, the involvement of this small, secretive animal is relatively minor currently.

The threat to people from rabid skunks is based on the animal's increased susceptibility to the virus, the high prevalence of rabies infection in the population, their ability to live in proximity to humans, and the excretion of large quantities of virus in their saliva during the prolonged period (4–18 days) of clinical illness. Rabid skunks often attack anything that moves with extreme fury and frequently roam during daylight hours, which is unusual behavior for this nocturnal animal. Long-term, subclinical rabies in skunks is a major concern with respect to maintenance of the infection in nature. Rabies antibodies have been found in clinically normal skunks. Skunks raised in extended periods of confinement have been found to be clinically infected with rabies. This finding may have resulted from prior infection or from congenital infection combined with a prolonged incubation period.

Foxes are important reservoirs in the ecology of wildlife rabies throughout the Northern Hemisphere, although they account for few human exposures. In North America, fox rabies occurs throughout the range of the red fox *(Vulpes vulpes)*, the gray fox *(Urocyon cinereoargenteus)*, and the Arctic fox *(Alopex lagopus)*, with greatest prevalence in the province

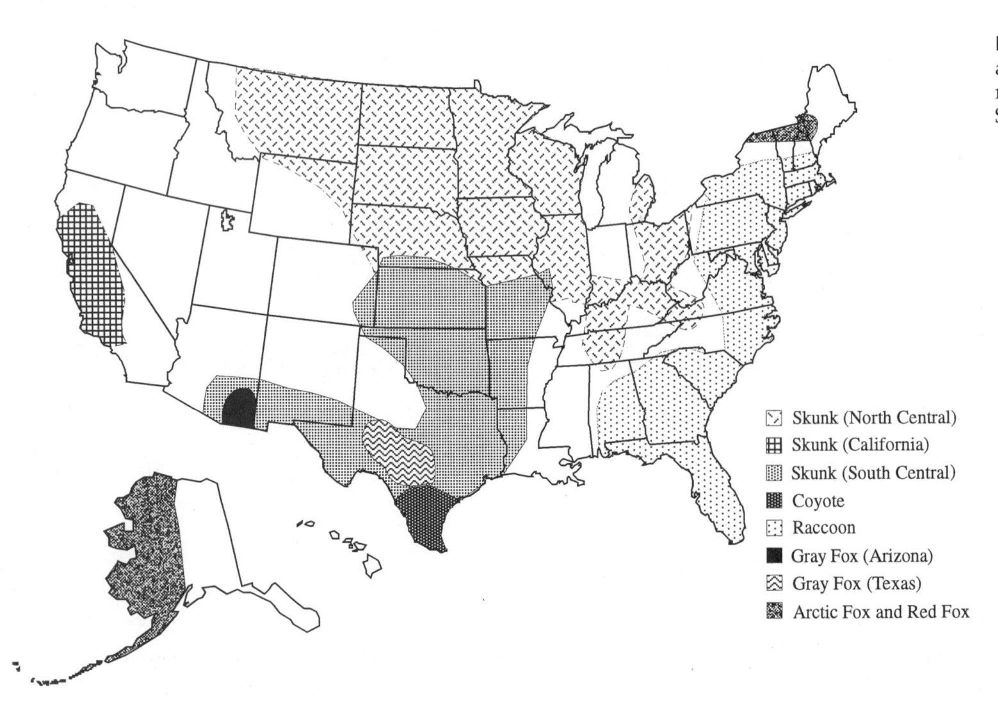

Figure 22–2. Currently recognized areas of endemic rabies in wild terrestrial animals in the United States.

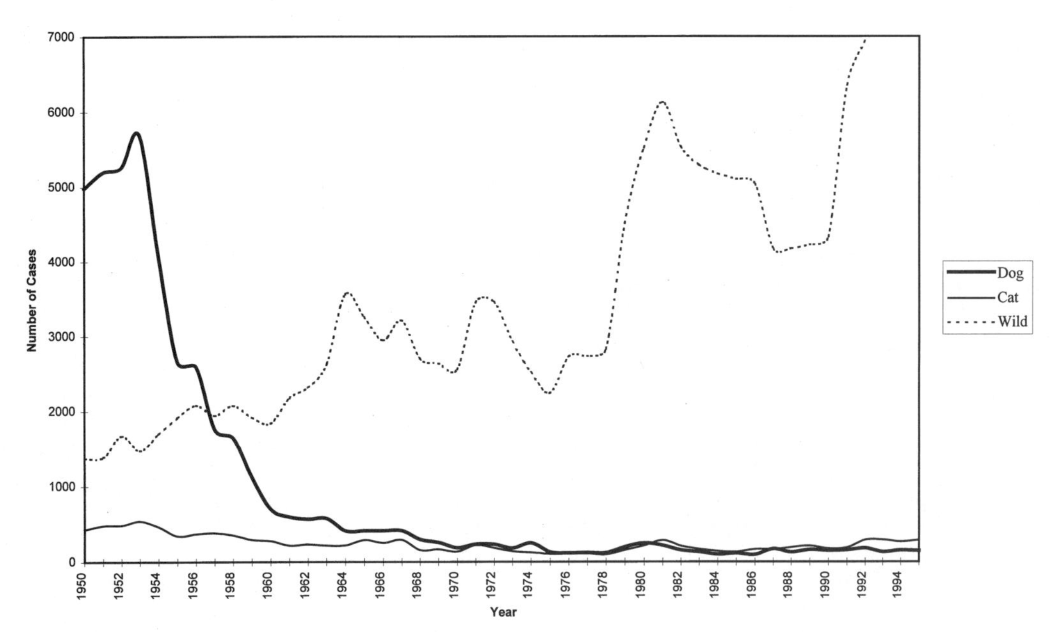

Figure 22–3. Animal rabies cases in the United States from 1950 to 1995. The yearly incidence in dogs has decreased because of vaccination, and cats now have a greater incidence of rabies. Data from records are maintained at the Centers for Disease Control and Prevention and were graphed by Casey S. Greene.

of Ontario in Canada. An outbreak occurring in 1990 in upstate New York is probably an extension of the Canadian fox epidemic. A small focus of rabies in gray foxes has been found in Arizona and Texas. The prevalence of the disease seems to decline when fox populations are reduced to levels in balance with available resources through either natural mortality or fox population–reduction programs. Oral vaccination programs, using modified live virus (MLV) vaccine placed in food bait, have had considerable success in control of red fox rabies in Europe and is now being used to control gray fox rabies in Texas.

Rabid foxes may exhibit either furious or paralytic forms of the disease; however, regardless of form, the disease is invariably fatal. Despite the shorter course of clinical illness, foxes can effectively transmit the virus to other species, but the need for human postexposure prophylaxis from direct exposure to rabid foxes has been extremely low.

Before the mid-1950s, rabies was not a serious problem among raccoons in the United States. However, from 1950 to 1970, the occurrence of rabid raccoons began to rise dramatically in Florida and Georgia and soon spread to Alabama and northward to South Carolina. In the mid-Atlantic Coast states, a major epidemic began in the 1980s owing to the apparent translocation of infected animals from the Southeast. The mid-Atlantic outbreak spread throughout the northeastern states and southward into North Carolina by the mid 1990s. The foci of both epidemics have now merged. The epidemic is spreading westward into Ohio.[5a] Raccoons have adapted well to suburban and semiurban environments; thus, the number of rabies cases in cats and dogs and other domestic animals in the Northeast has dramatically increased. The danger of human exposure to rabid raccoons has also increased, although to date no human deaths associated with rabid raccoons have been confirmed. Exposure of people to rabid domestic animals such as the cat has resulted in the greatest risk.

Bats. Rabies in North American insectivorous bats was first recognized in the early 1950s, but studies suggest that rabid bats were in this region much earlier. The range of bat rabies is widespread throughout North America. The ability of bats to disseminate rabies virus is based on a protracted clinical course rather than a subclinical carrier state. Subclinical infection can progress to more advanced clinical disease during times of stress, changes in metabolic rate (as with the cessation of hibernation), and changes in ambient temperature.

Although there are multiple cocirculating variants of rabies virus in insectivorous bats, most submissions and rabies-positive bats are from only a few of the common species (primarily *Eptesius fuscus*, *Myotis lucifugus*, *Lasiurus borealis*, and *Tadarida brasiliensis*). Phylogenetic studies have shown that bat rabies virus variants found in terrestrial animals are distinct, and variants identified in different bat species are also quite distinct. From 1970 to 1995, 48 persons have died from rabies in the United States. Brain tissues from 39 of them have been examined by mAB and/or gene-sequencing techniques. Variants associated with insectivorous bats were identified in 19 of the 39; 15 of these 19 were associated with the solitary-dwelling, reasonably uncommon silver haired bat *(Lasionycteris noctivagans)*. Only three of the bat-associated cases reported a bite, and in only one of these three reports was the bat identified to species.[64]

There are few authenticated cases of rabies transmission from insectivorous bats *(E. fuscus)* to cats and even fewer cases of transmission to dogs. Rabid bats seldom attack; bat bites usually occur from bats found paralyzed or semiparalyzed or from normal-appearing bats found in buildings.

Vampire bats, which feed exclusively on blood, are a major rabies threat to people and animals in Mexico, Central America, and parts of South America. Approximately 250,000 to 500,000 cases of cattle rabies attributed to vampire bats occur annually in Latin America. Their biting during routine nightly feeding makes them extremely effective in transmitting rabies virus, and the presence of rabies in vampire bats parallels that seen in insectivorous bats and terrestrial animals. Although the vampire bat is not found in North America, except for Mexico, the use of the same cave by rabies-infected vampire bats and North American insectivorous bats on their southward migration may be a major source of infection for bats that spend part of the year in the United States.

Rodents and Lagomorphs. The prevalence of clinical rabies among rats, mice, squirrels, and rabbits and hares is extremely low. Increases, when reported, have been associated with corresponding outbreaks in wild carnivore reservoirs. Rodents and rabbits account for a high percentage of animal bites to people, but no cases of human rabies have ever been associated with these species, probably because they are extremely susceptible to infection and generally will not survive the attack by a rabid carnivore. For such reasons, these species are not routinely examined for rabies in public health laboratories.

PATHOGENESIS

The incubation period is influenced by the age of the bitten individual, the degree of innervation of the bite site, the distance from the point of inoculation to the spinal cord or brain, the variant and amount of virus introduced, postexposure treatment, and other factors. Rabies is unique in that the incubation period, which is relatively prolonged compared with that of other infectious diseases, is primarily a result of the route of virus entry into and spread within the CNS (Fig. 22–4).

Entry of Virus

After IM inoculation, virus may replicate locally in nonnervous tissue and enters neuromuscular junctions and neurotendinal spindles after a variable period of days, weeks, or months.[13a] Virus spreads by intra-axonal flow in peripheral nerves at a rate of up to 100 mm per day. Both motor and sensory fibers may transport virus. The greater the degree of innervation at the site of the bite, the shorter the incubation period. In naturally occurring cases of rabies, ranges of incubation periods before CNS signs have been reported to be 3 to 24 weeks (average, 3–8 weeks) in dogs, 2 to 24 weeks (average, 4–6 weeks) in cats, and 3 weeks to 1 year or more (average, 3–6 weeks) in people.

Although uncommon, infection by other routes is possible. After IN exposure, virus enters the trigeminal nerves and ganglia in its course to the CNS. The cribriform plate and olfactory bulbs have been suggested as a route of spread, but this is not well documented. After being ingested, the virus has been shown to infect cells of the oral mucosa, taste buds, pulmonary system (by aspiration), and intestinal mucosa. From these sites, it migrates up branches of the cranial nerves and spreads to the brain stem.

Spread in CNS

Interneuronal spread of virus corresponds to the progression of clinical signs that are noted. The virus enters the spinal cord or brain stem ipsilateral to the site of initial virus inoculation. Once in the CNS, virus spreads by intra-axonal means to involve the contralateral neurons and ascends rapidly, bilaterally, in the spinal cord or brain stem to the forebrain. Damage to the motor neurons causes progressive lower motor neuron (LMN) disease, which in turn produces the typical flaccid paralysis of rabies infection and an ascending paralysis. Damage to the CNS caused by rabies virus has mainly been attributed to direct viral invasion of the nervous system. Apoptosis, or genetically induced premature cell death, may be important in neuronal necrosis.[39a] Host immune responses to rabies virus may accentuate the inflammation and degeneration of nervous tissue.

Spread From CNS

After replication within the CNS, the virus moves outward to other body tissues via the peripheral, sensory, and motor nerves at a rate of 100 to 400 mm per day. Both visceral and somatic portions of cranial and spinal cord nerves become involved, including the autonomic nervous system. Virus also spreads via cranial nerves to the acinar cells of the salivary glands at this time. The presence of virus in saliva demonstrates that the brain has already been infected. Al-

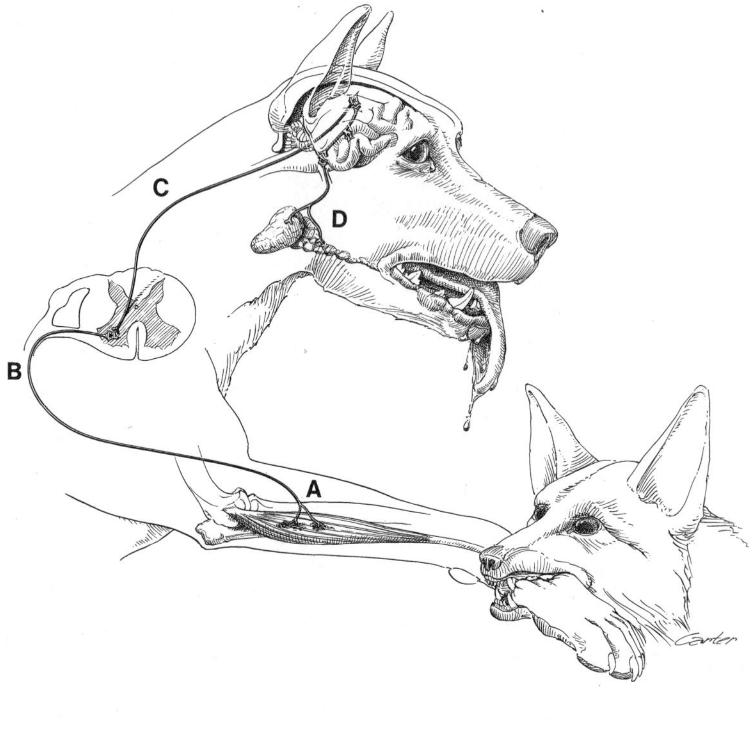

C
D
B
A

Figure 22–4. Pathogenesis of rabies virus infection. Rabies virus replicates in myocytes and spreads to motor nerve endings *(A)*. Retrograde intra-axonal (centripetal) spread to the CNS occurs in peripheral nerves *(B)*. Virus replicates in spinal cord neurons and spreads rapidly (probably by CSF flow) throughout the nervous system, causing progressive lower motor neuron paralysis *(C)*. Virus enters the brain, causing cranial nerve deficits and behavioral changes. Virus spreads centrifugally in peripheral and cranial nerves, from which it enters the saliva *(D)* and other tissues.

though virtually every body tissue may be infected, outward spread in the peripheral nervous system does not occur in all cases. The rate (20–88% positive) of salivary gland infection also varies, depending on the species infected. Death may occur before salivary involvement.

Chronic or Latent Infections

It is now recognized that, in rare instances, the course of rabies can be prolonged and subclinical in nature and that recovery in dogs and in cats is possible.[28] Recovery in people has been exceedingly rare. In many instances, it may be difficult to demonstrate virus and determine whether prolonged incubation, chronic infection with latency, or complete recovery has occurred. Prolonged incubation cannot always be distinguished from latency. During the early incubation period, rabies virus is sequestered at the site of inoculation while replicating in myocytes and nerves. The long period between exposure and clinical signs is due to local replication and recovery or chronic disease after infection and has been associated with high titers of antirabies virus antibody in the CSF and CNS tissue. Adequate serum titers of antirabies virus antibody, acquired by active or passive immunization, have been correlated with protection against infection and restricted viral replication. Effective cell-mediated immunity is essential to the eventual elimination of rabies virus. The chronic or latent rabies states should be regarded as of minor importance in the epidemiology of the disease and not relevant in public health considerations.

Excretion of Virus

Typically, virus excretion occurs for a brief period before the onset of neurologic signs and continues until the animal dies within a few days to weeks. Most public health laws require a 10-day observation period after a bite from a suspected dog or cat because the period of virus shedding before neurologic signs in naturally infected animals is generally between 1 and 5 days. A few studies have shown that rabies-infected dogs shed virus in their saliva up to 13 days before the onset of neurologic signs; thus, some researchers suggest that the 10-day observation period may have to be extended. Dogs that develop neurologic signs and die suddenly actually may have lower concentrations of virus in their brains and salivary glands than those that live longer. At times, experimentally infected dogs have recovered completely from neurologic deficits but have excreted the virus in their saliva as recovered carriers for 2 to 6 months thereafter. However, the amount of virus shed by recovered dogs is exceedingly small. The public health implication of the observation has not been determined and may, in fact, be nonexistent. Excretion of virus in experimentally infected cats has started from 1 to 2 days before to 3 days after the onset of clinical signs.

CLINICAL FINDINGS

Rabies virus infection has classically been divided into two major types: *furious* and *paralytic*. The classification and progression of infection is artificial, because rabies can be quite variable in its presentation and *atypical* signs are commonly seen. Not all animals progress through all the clinical stages, and subclinical, chronic, and recovered infections have been described. The initial history may reveal that the pet has a wound history. Because of the severity of wounds, they may not always be suspected as coming from a bite.

Dogs and Cats

During the prodromal phase in dogs, which usually lasts for 2 to 3 days, apprehension, nervousness, anxiety, solitude, and variable fever may be noted. Friendly animals become shy or irritable and may snap, whereas fractious ones may become more docile and affectionate. Pupillary dilation with or without sluggish palpebral or corneal reflexes may become apparent. Most animals will constantly lick the site of viral inoculation. Some dogs may develop pruritus at the site of exposure and claw and chew at the area until it is ulcerated. The behavior of cats during the prodromal period is similar to that of dogs; however, cats more typically show fever spikes and unusual or erratic behavior for only a day or 2.

The **furious** or psychotic type of the disease in dogs usually lasts for 1 to 7 days and is associated with forebrain involvement. Animals become restless and irritable and have increased responses to auditory and visual stimuli. They frequently become excitable, photophobic, and hyperesthetic and bark or snap at imaginary objects. As they become more restless, they begin to roam, usually becoming more irritable and vicious (Fig. 22–5). Dogs may eat unusual objects, especially wood (pica), which become GI foreign bodies. They may avoid contact with people and prefer to hide in dark or quiet places. When caged or confined, dogs often try to bite or attack their enclosure. They usually develop muscular incoordination, disorientation, or generalized grand mal seizures during this phase. If they do not die during a seizure, they may experience a short paralytic stage and then die.

Cats more consistently develop the furious phase of the disease, showing erratic and unusual behavior. They are described as having anxious, staring, wild, spooky, or blank looks in their eyes.[29] When confined in cages, they may make vicious, striking movements and attempt to bite or scratch at moving objects. In addition, they may have muscular tremors and weakness or incoordination. Some cats may run continuously until they seem to die of exhaustion.

The **paralytic** or dumb type of rabies usually develops within 2 to 4 days (range, 1–10 days) after the first clinical signs are noted. LMN paralysis usually progresses from the

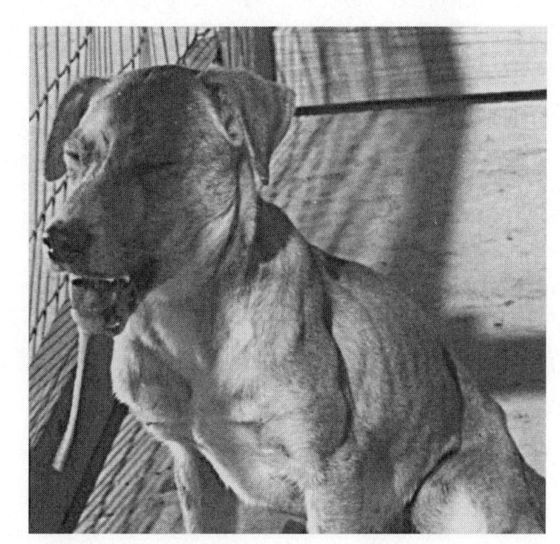

Figure 22–5. Dog with rabies. Note excessive salivary secretions resulting from the inability to swallow.

site of injury until the entire CNS is involved. Cranial nerve paralysis may be the first recognizable clinical syndrome if the bite occurs on the face. When the brain stem becomes affected, a change in the tone of the bark, resulting from laryngeal paralysis, may be observed. Dogs, which more commonly show this type of disease, may begin to salivate or froth excessively as a result of the inability to swallow and the deep labored respiration that occurs (see Fig. 22–5). A "dropped jaw" develops as a result of paralysis of the masticatory muscles. Dogs may make a choking sound, which makes an owner think that something is caught in the animal's throat. Owners or veterinarians may then become exposed to the virus in the saliva while attempting to remove a suspected foreign object. The course of the paralytic phase usually lasts 2 to 4 days. The animal often goes into a coma and dies of respiratory failure.

The paralytic disease in cats often follows the furious form of the disease and begins around the 5th day of clinical illness. Although the total course of illness may last 10 days, rabid cats often die after 3 to 4 days.[62] As in dogs, initial paralysis of the bitten extremity can progress to paraparesis, incoordination, and ascending or generalized paralysis, terminating in coma and death. Mandibular and laryngeal paralysis is less common in cats. Increased frequency of vocalization is a commonly reported sign in cats, and owners often recognize a change in the pitch of the cat's voice.[29] Cats occasionally develop the paralytic form directly after the prodromal phase with little or no signs of excitement.

Atypical, abortive forms of rabies virus infection with recovery may occur but are considered *rare* phenomena. Experimentally infected dogs that developed acute progressive LMN paralysis have shown clinical improvement a few days to months later. Survival with chronic infection has been reported to occur after experimental rabies infection in cats, but clinical recovery from paralysis has not been observed.

People

The clinical syndrome of rabies in people is similar in duration and variability to that in dogs and cats. Fever, headache, anxiety, nervousness, and hyperesthesia at the bite site have been reported. As the syndrome progresses to the excitable phase, clinical signs consist of excitability, restlessness, hyperkinesis, and violent behavior. Humans salivate incessantly and refuse to drink water. They experience painful pharyngeal spasms when attempting to swallow fluids, which gives rise to the term *hydrophobia*. As disorientation and excitability continue, some patients die in convulsive episodes, whereas others develop generalized LMN paralysis and respiratory arrest. Although the rare instance of recovery has been reported after extraordinary efforts, the disease is considered to be invariably fatal after the onset of clinical signs.

DIAGNOSIS

Rabies is often suspected because of the neurologic abnormalities that are present in an affected animal. However, because of the atypical nature of the clinical signs that are now recognized, rabies should be considered in any animal that suddenly develops profound behavioral changes or features of LMN paralysis or both.

No premortem diagnostic tests are sensitive enough to be consistently reliable for rabies diagnosis. Nevertheless, there may be some limited indications for testing serum, CSF, or biopsy specimens before the death of the animal. No hematologic or serum biochemical changes are characteristic or specific for rabies. Biochemical changes in CSF have been minimal in experimentally infected dogs and have been rarely reported in natural infections. Increased CSF protein (110–150 mg/dl) and leukocytes (120–240 cells/μl), with small lymphocytes predominating, have been reported in dogs with postvaccinal rabies encephalomyelitis. Cats with postvaccinal rabies also have had increased CSF protein (55–80 mg/dl) and increased CSF lymphocyte count (5–17 cells/μl).

Direct FA Testing of Dermal Tissues

Because virus enters extraneural tissues via outward spread from the CNS, it arrives at nerve endings in the skin and at the salivary glands simultaneously. Because of the heavy sensory innervation, the skin at the nape of the neck (in humans) and the sensory vibrissae on the maxillary areas (in animals) are most specific for direct FA testing. Direct FA testing of a skin biopsy has a 25% to 50% probability of being positive about the time that clinical rabies develops; accuracy is increased as the course of disease progresses. Rabies vaccines commonly used in dogs and cats do not give false-positive results. The skin biopsy technique should never be done as a substitute for brain examination of an unvaccinated animal with suspect neurologic signs. It has important applications in testing pets that have bitten someone but that have a current vaccination history and normal behavioral and neurologic status. This test appears to be accurate if the virus is present; however, a negative test result does not rule out the possibility that the animal is infected. Its application is restricted at present and has not been approved for routine laboratory diagnosis of rabies.

Serologic Testing

Serologic tests are rarely used for epidemiologic surveys or for diagnosis because of the low percentage of animals surviving the disease that have time to develop PI antibody. Serologic tests are used to determine vaccine efficacy. Some countries require a positive antibody titer for importation.[5] Mouse inoculation has been performed historically for serologic testing but has been replaced by cell culture methods. Indirect FA testing has become a standard, sensitive, and reproducible means of quantifying rabies virus antibody. A modification of the standard FA procedure, the rapid fluorescent-focus inhibition test (RFFIT), can quantify concentrations of specific rabies virus antibody in serum. New tests for rabies virus antibodies, based on ELISA, have been proposed to replace the RFFIT for serodiagnosis.[7, 27, 31, 54]

Testing dogs or cats for serum antibodies to rabies virus to determine recent exposure to rabies can be ambiguous because elevated titers can result from vaccination or from past or recent exposure to virulent virus. Testing for rabies antibody in CSF is a possible means of documenting rabies infection because antibody is locally produced. CSF IgM titers increase 2 to 3 weeks or more after the onset of clinical rabies. Because of this delay, a negative titer result does not eliminate rabies infection as a possibility.

PATHOLOGIC FINDINGS

Submission of Specimens

Selection and submission of proper specimens are critical for accurate rabies diagnosis. Handling live, suspected rabid animals must be done with extreme care. Heavy protective gloves must be worn, and catch poles, cages, and other equipment often facilitate capture and transport of such animals. The animal must be euthanized by a humane method, and the brain must be protected from damage. The use of an ax or power saw should be discouraged when opening the skull, because these may create hazardous aerosols. A procedure to remove the brain of a suspected rabid animal has been published.[68] Small specimens such as mice and kittens may be submitted whole. A technique for retro-orbital removal of brain specimens for collection of material for epidemiologic studies has been described.[56] Complete brain removal is still indicated when human exposure has occurred. When brain tissue has been inadvertently damaged or destroyed, the spinal cord is an alternative but less desirable substitute.

The head (or body) of an animal suspected of having rabies that has died or been euthanized should be cooled immediately and maintained chilled (wet ice) or refrigerated until examined. The head or brain *must not be frozen*, because this delays examination and the thawing process causes brain tissue damage. A complete history should accompany each specimen. Various approved shipping containers are available from public health or animal control facilities and must protect the specimen as well as those handling the container. The container should always indicate that hazardous laboratory specimens are enclosed.

Specimens must be sent to the laboratory as quickly as possible. Postexposure treatment is often delayed while awaiting laboratory results. It is recommended that specimens be delivered personally or by courier whenever possible to minimize delay or potential loss.

Gross and Microscopic Lesions

No gross lesions are detectable in the CNS with rabies infection. Despite the dramatic neurologic signs and high mortality, neuropathologic changes are mild. Pathologic changes depend on the severity and duration of infection at the time of examination. Acute polioencephalitis characterized by minimal neuronophagia, neuronal degeneration, and nonsuppurative inflammation is seen very early in the course of the disease. Necrotizing encephalitis is seen in the next phase of infection and corresponds to a gradually increasing titer in the serum and CSF. Chronic infections are characterized by focal or widespread lymphocytic and plasmacytic perivascular cuffing and focal mononuclear cell infiltrates in the CNS. A ganglioneuritis is usually present. The longer the course of illness, the more pronounced is the nonsuppurative inflammatory response in the brain and spinal cord. In some cats, spongiform lesions appear as vacuolation in the neutrophil of the gray matter, most commonly in the thalamus and inner layers of the cerebral cortex.

Direct FA Testing of Nervous Tissue

This test is both rapid and sensitive and currently is the most widely used and preferred method of diagnosing potential rabies infection. Thin touch impression smears of the medulla, cerebellum, and hippocampus are used for this test. Unless it is completely decomposed, the head should be submitted because specific fluorescence may still be detected. Rabies viral antigen has also been detected by immunoperoxidase techniques on formalin-fixed and paraffin-embedded tissue.[33, 51] It is not necessary that animals show neurologic signs at the time of examination, and all animals excreting virus in the saliva will have detectable virus in the CNS by immunohistochemical examination.

Genetic Detection of Virus

Rabies virus has been detected in nervous tissue by polymerase chain reaction (PCR) with nested primers.[44] This test might be used as a confirmatory test in FA-negative samples or in decomposed brain tissue that is difficult to evaluate with FA methods. Dot hybridization with radiolabeled probes has been performed to detect rabies virus genome in nervous and salivary tissue but requires much greater levels of virus than PCR methods.[70] In situ hybridization can detect rabies virus genomic RNA in paraffin-embedded brain tissues.[40]

Intracellular Inclusions

The classic test for the presence of rabies is to examine the brain for the presence of intracytoplasmic inclusions, known as Negri bodies, in larger neurons. They are most commonly found in the thalamus, hypothalamus, pons, cerebral cortex, and dorsal horns of the spinal cord. Negri bodies are most common in neurons of the hippocampus in carnivores and in Purkinje's cells of herbivores. Negri bodies in tissue sections or impression smears of brain tissue are best demonstrated with Seller's or van Gieson's stains, in which they are magenta. Unfortunately, Negri bodies take time to develop and cannot be found during all stages of infection and in all infected cats. They usually cannot be detected until neurologic signs are apparent, so premature killing of the animal may reduce the chances of finding these inclusions. This test is no longer used in most developed nations for routine diagnosis. Two types of cytoplasmic inclusions that are confused with Negri bodies are found in the brain of healthy cats.[10, 11] They occur in the pyramidal cells of the hippocampus and in neurons of the dorsal part of the lateral geniculate nucleus.

Mouse Inoculation

Intracerebral inoculation of laboratory mice with fresh or fresh-frozen homogenized tissue is a confirmatory test for rabies and is not conducted for routine diagnosis of suspected rabies cases. Specific neutralizing antibody is incubated with extracted tissue before its inoculation to confirm that rabies virus is responsible for the observed neurologic signs. Brains and salivary tissues from proposed infected mice are examined for virus by direct FA. This test does not distinguish between virulent and vaccine viruses because, regardless of attenuation, many of the virus strains produce a similar illness in mice. Replacement of mouse inoculation by viral inoculation into tissue culture (TC) is now feasible because virulent virus can now be grown in various cell lines.[59] When virus isolation or identification attempts fail, PCR can detect and identify rapidly the specific virus strain in salivary tissue, saliva, and CNS of dogs with rabies.[9, 18, 42, 53]

Monoclonal Antibody and Genetic Sequencing

Monoclonal immunoglobulins produced against specific rabies virus nucleocapsid and glycoprotein moieties are able to distinguish the various antigenic variants of rabies virus. Strains of virus to be tested are grown in TC or are found in tissue sections and are stained immunochemically to determine the antigenic composition of the virus. The pattern of staining is compared with that of reference strains of virus. This technique is extremely valuable in distinguishing between vaccine and virulent strains of rabies virus, especially in cases of human exposure to animals with postvaccinal neurologic disease. Direct sequencing of PCR products along with automated gene sequencing can also help to distinguish between virus variants to determine the most probable wildlife reservoir for an isolate from human or animal infection.

THERAPY

Supportive care for rabies-infected animals is not recommended because recovered animals have, on occasion, been shown to excrete the virus in their saliva for extended periods. An asymptomatic dog or cat suspected of contracting rabies should be quarantined as recommended (see Compendium of Animal Rabies Vaccines, Appendix 4) or, as for all other species, humanely euthanized and the brain submitted for examination.

PREVENTION

Vaccine Types

No measure has helped reduce the incidence of human rabies as effectively as the widespread vaccination of the domestic dog population. Early vaccines were developed from virus grown in nervous tissue and later in avian embryos. Low egg passage vaccine virus was produced by approximately 50 serial passages of the virus in chicken embryos (CEOs). The virus lost its viscerotropic properties but retained some of its neurotropic traits. Vaccine-induced rabies was occasionally reported if the product was given to cats. High egg passage CEO vaccine was produced by approximately 180 passages of the virus. It no longer caused neurologic signs in laboratory mice, except when neonates had been injected intracerebrally. The vaccine was safe for dogs and for more susceptible species such as cats and cattle. For this reason, any vaccine for cats must state that it is licensed for such use. Newer MLV vaccines were produced in tissue culture. These products produced fewer allergic reactions compared with CEO vaccines. Despite better immunity produced by MLV compared with inactivated vaccines, postvaccinal rabies is a distinct disadvantage. No MLV rabies vaccines are currently available in the United States, although MLV vaccines are marketed in some other countries.

To develop effective inactivated rabies virus vaccines, the virus had to be produced in high concentrations, which was initially done by growing it in the nervous system of suckling mice. Neonatal mice were chosen because they lacked the antigenic myelin responsible for allergic encephalomyelitis produced by early nervous tissue origin vaccines. An important advance in the development of inactivated rabies vaccines has been the production of less allergenic but more immunogenic products by their production in TC cells so that large quantities of virus can be produced. Newer adjuvants have increased the immune response to the antigen in these products but have also caused some problems with allergenicity and oncogenicity.

Purified subunit rabies vaccines may be the recommended vaccines in the future. With purified glycoprotein vaccines, 5 to 50 times the quantity of purified glycoprotein alone is required to produce an immune response compared with intact virion vaccines. It has been suggested that the glycoprotein is absorbed on lipid complexes, which, if true, would greatly increase the potency of subunit vaccines. Recombinant vaccines, utilizing vaccinia virus, other poxviruses, or adenoviruses as vectors, have been developed that induce the synthesis of rabies virus glycoprotein in infected cells, VN antibodies, and protection in susceptible animals.[22, 73] Such vaccines have been used as experimental vaccines for dogs and cats and are licensed by governmental agencies in various countries to control rabies in wildlife reservoirs. A recombinant parenteral rabies virus vaccine will be commercially available for cats.[12, 66] (See Rabies, Chapter 100.)

Vaccine Recommendations

Many vaccines are currently marketed in the United States for pre-exposure rabies prophylaxis in dogs and cats. All currently licensed products must protect 88% of vaccinates against challenge with virulent virus, whereas at least 80% of those not vaccinated are challenged and develop rabies. In preventing rabies epizootics, the World Health Organization recommends that 70% of dogs in a population should be effectively immunized.[20] Currently available inactivated vaccines have been shown to be safe and effective when administered in neonatal puppies and kittens. However, because of maternal antibody blockade and a relatively poor immune response in the young, the first rabies vaccination is given at a minimum of 3 months of age and then repeated 1 year later (Table 22–1).[1] Subsequent vaccinations are repeated every 1 or 3 years later, depending on the product and local public health regulations. The current Compendium of Animal Rabies Vaccines (Appendix 4) and Appendices 1 and 2 and Chapter 100 should be consulted for canine and feline rabies vaccination protocols. Studies have shown that one injection of inactivated rabies vaccine does not produce a lasting antibody titer in a significant proportion of dogs.[63, 67] However, serum antibody titers can be misleading as a measure of protection, because previously vaccinated dogs usually show an anamnestic response to boosters, even when antibodies are no longer detectable in their sera. Nevertheless, the second vaccination 1 year after the primary inoculation is extremely important. A multiple-dose primary canine rabies vaccination schedule with annual boosters may be considered for dogs in rabies endemic countries where the disease has been a high risk for humans. Booster vaccinations are recommended for dogs and cats whenever vaccination history cannot be established because of the potential for vaccine failures.[21, 29, 42] A small proportion of dogs and cats identified with rabies have had at least one rabies vaccination during their lifetime. No available vaccine is 100% effective; therefore, an immediate booster dose is recommended to the immunized dog or cat after a known rabies exposure.[61] Fortunately, current veterinary vaccines are cross-protective against the *Lyssavirus* identified in Australia.[31a]

Postvaccinal Complications

For additional information on the complications discussed next, the reader should consult Postvaccinal Complications, Chapter 100. Encephalomyelitis in cats and dogs, caused by rabies MLV vaccine, has been commonly observed in the past. As a result, such vaccines are no longer available in many countries. The most frequent non-neurologic complications associated with rabies virus vaccine are local soreness, lameness, and regional lymphadenomegaly in the injected limb. Fever and systemic signs or anaphylaxis are sometimes noted. These signs have been more frequently observed with

Table 22–1. Recommendations for Rabies Vaccination of Animals and People

ANIMAL EXPOSED	RECOMMENDATION
Pre-exposure	
Dogs and cats	Vaccinate at 3 months of age; revaccinate 1 year later and every 1 or 3 years thereafter, depending on product recommendations.
Ferrets	Vaccinate at 3 months of age and revaccinate annually with an approved vaccine.
Wildlife	Discourage ownership; no parenteral vaccine is approved for use.
People	Three doses of an FDA-approved vaccine either 1 ml IM or 0.1 ml ID, based on manufacturer's recommendation, in the upper deltoid on days 0, 7, and 28; booster based on risk group.
Postexposure	
Dogs, cats, and ferrets	Previously unvaccinated: euthanize immediately or quarantine in secure enclosure for 6 months, vaccinate 1 month before release. Vaccine not current: evaluate on case-by-case basis. Vaccination current: revaccinate immediately and keep under owner's control for 45 days.
Wildlife	Regard as rabid and euthanize for examination.
People	Previously unvaccinated: H-RIG, 20 IU/kg, 1/2 or more at site of bite and remainder IM in gluteal muscle on day 0; FDA-approved vaccine at recommended dose IM in the upper deltoid on days 0, 3, 7, 14, and 28. Previously vaccinated: two doses of an approved vaccine at recommended dose IM in upper deltoid on days 0 and 3; no H-RIG

FDA = Food and Drug Administration; H-RIG = human rabies immune globulin.

the newer inactivated TC rabies vaccines because of the need for higher antigenic mass and adjuvants to produce an immune response equal to that of the older attenuated products. Focal cutaneous vasculitis and granulomas have been described in dogs, occurring within 3 to 6 months after inoculation. They consist of well-circumscribed SC inflammatory reactions that involve the overlying dermis. Similar reactions result in palpable nodules in cats that can be detected by clients or veterinarians.[63a]

Sustained inflammatory reactions that develop at vaccine sites are considered to be precursors of sarcoma, which may develop months to years later.[23, 39, 45] Postvaccinal sarcomas can develop in dogs and cats but have been more frequently documented in cats. Sarcomas that develop after vaccination are often aggressive and invasive. For a further discussion, see Vaccination-Site Sarcomas, Chapter 100. Autoimmune polyradiculoneuritis has been observed with inactivated suckling mouse brain–origin rabies vaccines. A small proportion of dogs that were vaccinated with these products developed acute diffuse LMN paralysis with intact pain sensation and hyperesthesia (see Chapter 100).

Control of Epizootics

Where rabies epizootics have occurred, vaccination programs have been shown to reduce greatly the spread of an outbreak. Management of stray and unwanted cats and dogs is essential, and unclaimed animals should be humanely euthanized. Leash laws must be enforced. Reduction in the population of wildlife vectors has been used on a limited scale when epidemics of rabies in dogs and cats have been traced to a particular wildlife reservoir species, but this has been ineffective. Control through trapping and poison baits not only is difficult but may cause public resentment. As previously described, oral vaccination of wild carnivores has worked on a limited basis worldwide and will be expanded in the future.

Postexposure Management

Management of a dog or cat that has been bitten or scratched by a potentially rabid mammal is difficult when the biting animal is not available for testing, because the dog or cat must be considered as having been exposed to a rabid animal (see Table 22–1; and Compendium, Appendix 4). Differences in management depend on whether or not the exposed animal has been previously immunized and local public health laws.[19] The final decision concerning the management of exposed animals generally is made by local or state public health authorities.[43] The current Compendium of Animal Rabies Control (Appendix 4) and local public health officials should be consulted when such circumstances arise.

Disposition of Animals That Bite Humans

Dogs and cats with current rabies vaccinations are of less concern as a transmission risk, although current vaccination status does not remove the need for follow-up (Table 22–2). Any illness or neurologic disease in quarantined animals must be immediately reported to local public health authorities. Management of potentially rabid animals other than dogs or cats depends on the species, the circumstances of the bite, and the epidemiology of rabies in the area.

PUBLIC HEALTH CONSIDERATIONS

Postexposure Prophylaxis

Exposure to rabies is a bite, scratch, or other situation in which saliva or CNS tissue of a potentially rabid animal enters an open wound or a fresh wound or comes in contact with a mucous membrane of the eye, nose, or mouth. Nearly all cases of human rabies (except those attributed to bats) have been acquired by exposure to saliva in bite wounds or, rarely, on abraded or scratched skin. Therapy of bite wounds should be aggressive because immediate, thorough washing of the wound has been shown to be effective in reducing the chance of infection. Ethanol (43% or stronger) can be applied locally to open wounds. Bites should also be irrigated with large quantities of a 20% aqueous soap solution or quaternary ammonium compound (QUAT) under pressure. The optimal concentration of benzalkonium chloride, a QUAT, has been shown to be 1% to 4%; however, most commercial hospital disinfectants have a 0.13% concentration. Deep puncture wounds can be effectively cleaned by irrigation using a 15-ml syringe fitted with a blunted 19-gauge needle that is filled with a sterile saline solution. This provides 20 psi of pressure,

Table 22–2. Postexposure Recommendations for Rabies Exposure of People in the United States[a]

POTENTIAL SOURCE OF INFECTION	SITUATION	ANIMAL DISPOSITION	POSTEXPOSURE PROPHYLAXIS FOR PEOPLE
Rodents[b]	Any episode	Usually not examined.	None, but consult public health officials if circumstances of bite warrant.
Dog, cat, and ferret[c]	Healthy, owned	Confine; observe for at least 10 days, especially if unprovoked attack.	None or consider, if unprovoked; yes, if CNS signs develop in animal.
	Healthy, stray available or escaped	Euthanize immediately; submit head for examination.	Yes; stop if lab results negative, continue if animal unavailable.
	CNS signs or illness	Euthanize immediately; submit head for examination.	Yes; if negative FA result, stop.
Wild carnivore	Any episode	If captured, euthanize immediately; submit head for examination.	Yes, if positive or animal at large; if negative FA result, stop.
Inoculation of attenuated vaccine[d]	Any episode	Not applicable.	No postexposure treatment required.

[a] Other countries have different guidelines.
[b] Squirrels, hamsters, guinea pigs, gerbils, chipmunks, rats, and mice; lagomorphs are also included.
[c] Vaccination status of animal should not be used to make a decision on outcome for prophylaxis.
[d] Accidental inoculation.
FA = fluorescent antibody.

sufficient for cleaning but not so excessive as to cause further tissue damage.

Approximately 20,000 people annually are given antirabies prophylaxis in the United States. Specific antirabies therapy for humans has been most successful in reducing the number of deaths caused by rabies when active immunization is combined with human rabies immune globulin (H-RIG) (see Table 22–1: Postexposure, People). H-RIG is preferable to unpurified γ-globulin because of its greater immunopotency and lesser allergenicity. H-RIG is given simultaneously with the initial dose of vaccine but is not repeated because it interferes with the active immune response to subsequent vaccinations.

Rabies human diploid cell vaccine (HDCV, Pasteur Merieux, Lyon, France) is highly effective and safe for pre- and postexposure immunizations. Rabies vaccine adsorbed (RVA, Michigan Department of Public Health), a fetal rhesus monkey lung cell culture rabies vaccine, which is in very limited supply, and HDCV are the only commercial rabies vaccines currently available in the United States. They are more immunogenic and less allergenic than previously available human rabies vaccines. Postexposure therapy with HDCV or RVA and H-RIG must begin as soon as possible, preferably within 24 hours or less (see Table 22–1: Postexposure, People). Postexposure treatment failures have been noted when the vaccine has been given in the gluteal rather than the deltoid muscle.

The decision to administer postexposure prophylaxis in people must be made immediately and is based on a number of factors concerning the bite incident. The species of animal that inflicts the bite wound is important, because dogs, cats, and especially wild carnivores and bats are more likely to transmit the virus. Many people might have been spared the concern and inconvenience of prophylactic therapy had cats been routinely vaccinated. Bites of rodents such as squirrels, chipmunks, rats, mice, and lagomorphs seldom if ever result in prophylactic vaccination of people (see Table 22–2: Rodents). Despite that fact, postexposure prophylaxis has often been performed unnecessarily.

The epidemiology of the biting incident is also important in determining the need to initiate prophylaxis before laboratory confirmation (see Table 22–2). Bites from rabies-infected animals usually occur without provocation. Animals that show neurologic signs at the time of the bite or soon after should be considered rabid. Bite exposures are much more likely to result in rabies infection than scratches, unless the scratches were contaminated by the animal's saliva. The prevalence of rabies in the geographic area is also important. People accidentally injected with animal rabies vaccines do not require postexposure prophylaxis.

Pre-exposure Prophylaxis

Pre-exposure prophylaxis is warranted in people with a high vocational or recreational risk of contacting rabid animals (see Table 22–1: Pre- and Postexposure, People). Veterinarians, animal health technicians and caretakers, animal control officers, wildlife biologists, laboratory workers, and spelunkers in rabies-endemic and epidemic areas should receive pre-exposure protection. Substitution of 0.1 ml of ID HDCV is also effective for primary immunization. Hypersensitivity reactions have been the main side effects noted in approximately 6% of those receiving booster vaccinations with HDCV after having received the primary series. Local and systemic immune complex–mediated allergic reaction have developed with the use of HDCV, although the reactions are less than those with previously available products. Hives, urticaria, arthralgia, fever, nausea, and vomiting can develop within 1 week of booster vaccinations.

The risk of veterinarians being exposed to rabid animals is more than 300 times greater than that of the general population. In one study, most (230) of the 380 exposures occurred to veterinarians during nonbite contact while they examined rabid animals. Seventy-nine exposures were the result of an animal bite. Seventeen were the result of exposures at necropsy. Many of these potential exposures resulted from contact with infected cattle, although a summary claimed only 13 known confirmed instances of rabies transmission from cattle to people worldwide.

References

1. Aghomo HO, Oduye OO, Rupprecht CE. 1990. The serological response of young dogs to the flury LEP strain of rabies vaccine. *Vet Res Commun* 14:415–425.

2. Aghomo HO, Rupprecht CE. 1990. Antigenic characterization of virus isolates from vaccinated dogs dying of rabies. *Trop Anim Health Prod* 22:275–280.
3. Aghomo HO, Rupprecht CE. 1990. Further studies on rabies virus isolated from healthy dogs in Nigeria. *Vet Microbiol* 22:17–22.
4. Allworth A, Murray K, Morgan J. 1996. A human case of encephalitis due to a Lyssavirus recently identified in bats. *Commun Dis Intel* 25:504.
5. Anonymous. 1996. Vets in support of change call for reform of rabies control policy. *Vet Rec* 139:402–403.
5a. Anonymous. 1997. Update raccoon rabies epizootic—United States, 1996. *Morb Mort Wkly Rep* 45:1117–1120.
6. Aubert MF. 1992. Practical significance of rabies antibodies in cats and dogs. *Rev Sci Tech* 11:735–760.
7. Barton LD, Campbell JB. 1988. Measurement of rabies-specific antibodies in carnivores by an enzyme-linked immunosorbent assay. *J Wildl Dis* 24:246–248.
8. Blancou J, Pastoret PP. 1996. Rabies in cats. *Vlaams Diergeneesk Tijdschr* 65:232–241.
9. Briggs DJ, Hennessy KJ, Kennedy GA, et al. 1993. Rabies in a vaccinated canine exhibiting generalized demodicosis. *J Vet Diagn Invest* 5:248–249.
10. Bunn TO. 1991. Canine and feline vaccines, past and present, pp 416–425. *In* Baer GM (ed), The natural history of rabies. CRC Press, Boca Raton, FL.
11. Bunn TO. 1991. Cat rabies, pp 379–387. *In* Baer GM (ed), The natural history of rabies. CRC Press, Boca Raton, FL.
12. Cadoz M, Strady A, Meignier B, et al. 1992. Immunisation with canarypox virus expressing rabies glycoprotein. *Lancet* 339:1429–1432.
13. Campbell JB. 1994. Oral rabies immunization of wildlife and dogs: challenges to the Americas. *Curr Top Microbiol Immunol* 187:247–266.
13a. Charlton KM, Nadin-Davis S, Casey GA, et al. 1997. The long incubation period in rabies: delayed progression of infection in muscle at the site of exposure. *Acta Neuropathol (Berl)* 94:73–77.
14. Cho HC, Lawson KF. 1989. Protection of dogs against death from experimental rabies by postexposure administration of rabies vaccine and hyperimmune globulin. *Can J Vet Res* 53:434–437.
15. Chomel B, Chappuis G, Bullon F, et al. 1988. Mass vaccination campaign against rabies: are dogs correctly protected? The Peruvian experience. *Rev Infect Dis* 10(Suppl):697–702.
16. Chomel BB. 1993. The modern epidemiological aspects of rabies in the world. *Comp Immun Microbiol Infect Dis* 16:11–20.
17. Claassen IJTM, Osterhaus ADME, Claassen E. 1995. Antigen detection in vivo after immunization with different presentation forms of rabies virus antigen: involvement of marginal metallophilic macrophages in the uptake of immune-stimulating complexes. *Eur J Immunol* 25:1446–1452.
18. Clark KA, Neill SU, Smith JS, et al. 1994. Epizootic canine rabies transmitted by coyotes in south Texas. *J Am Vet Med Assoc* 204:536–540.
19. Clark KA, Wilson PJ. 1996. Postexposure rabies prophylaxis and preexposure rabies vaccination failure in domestic animals. *J Am Vet Med Assoc* 208:1827–1830.
20. Coleman PG, Dye C. 1996. Immunization coverage required to prevent outbreaks of dog rabies. *Vaccine* 14:185–186.
21. Conti LA, Tucker G, Heston S. 1994. Rabies in a dog vaccinated by its owner. *J Am Vet Med Assoc* 205:1250–1251.
22. Desmettre P, Lanquet B, Chappuis G, et al. 1990. Use of vaccinia rabies recombinant for oral vaccination of wildlife. *Vet Microbiol* 23:227–230.
23. Dubielzig RR, Hawkins KL, Miller PE. 1993. Myofibroplastic sarcoma originating at the site of rabies vaccination in a cat. *J Vet Diagn Invest* 5:637–638.
24. Eng TR, Fishbein DB. 1990. Epidemiologic factors, clinical findings, and vaccination status of rabies in cats and dogs in the United States in 1988. *J Am Vet Med Assoc* 197:201–209.
25. Esplin DG, Jaffe MH, McGill LD. 1996. Metastasizing liposarcoma associated with a vaccination site in a cat. *Feline Pract* 24(5):20–23.
26. Esplin DG, McGill L, Meininger AC, et al. 1993. Post vaccination sarcomas in cats. *J Am Vet Med Assoc* 202:1245–1247.
27. Esterhuysen JJ, Prehaud C, Thomson GR. 1995. A liquid-phase blocking ELISA for the detection of antibodies to rabies virus. *J Virol Methods* 51:31–42.
28. Fekadu M. 1991. Latency and aborted rabies, pp 192–198. *In* Baer GM (ed), The natural history of rabies, ed 2. CRC Press, Boca Raton, FL.
29. Fogelman V, Fischman HR, Horman JT, et al. 1993. Epidemiologic and clinical characteristics of rabies in cats. *J Am Vet Med Assoc* 202:1829–1838.
30. Fraser GC, Hooper PT, Lunt RA, et al. 1996. Encephalitis caused by a Lyssavirus in fruit bats in Australia. *Emerging Infect Dis* 2:327–331.
31. Gangadhar NL, Gopal T. 1996. Seromonitoring of antibodies in dogs by indirect ELISA following post-bite rabies vaccination. *Ind J Anim Sci* 66:531–534.
31a. Gleeson LJ. 1997. Australian bat lyssavirus—a newly emerged zoonosis? *Aust Vet J* 75:188.
32. Greene CE, Dreesen DW. 1990. Rabies, pp 365–383. *In* Greene CE (ed), Infectious diseases of the dog and cat. WB Saunders, Philadelphia, PA.
33. Hamir AN, Moser G, Fu ZF, et al. 1995. Immunohistochemical test for rabies: identification of a diagnostically superior monoclonal antibody. *Vet Rec* 136:295–296.
33a. Hanlon CA, Niezgoda M, Shankar V, et al. 1997. A recombinant vaccinia-rabies virus in the immunocompromised host: oral innocuity, progressive parenteral infection, and therapeutics. *Vaccine* 15:140–148.
34. Hemachudha T, Chutivongse S, Wilde H, et al. 1991. Latent rabies. *N Engl J Med* 324:1890–1891.
35. Hendrick MJ, Brooks JJ. 1994. Postvaccinal sarcomas in the cat: histology and immunochemistry. *Vet Pathol* 31:126–129.
36. Hendrick MJ, Dunagan CA. 1991. Focal necrotizing granulomatous panniculitis associated with subcutaneous injection of rabies vaccine in cats and dogs: 10 cases (1988–1989). *J Am Vet Med Assoc* 198:304–305.
37. Hendrick MJ, Goldschmidt MH. 1991. Do injection site reactions induce fibrosarcomas in cats? *J Am Vet Med Assoc* 199:968.
38. Hendrick MJ, Goldschmidt MH, Shofer F, et al. 1992. Postvaccinal sarcomas in the cat: epidemiology and electron probe microanalytical identification of aluminum. *Cancer* Res 52:5391–5394.
39. Hendrick MJ, Shofer FS, Goldschmidt MH, et al. 1994. Comparison of fibrosarcomas that developed at vaccination sites and at nonvaccination sites in cats: 239 cases (1991–1992). *J Am Vet Med Assoc* 205:1425–1429.
39a. Jackson AC, Rossiter JP. 1997. Apoptosis plays an important role in experimental rabies virus infection. *J Virol* 71:5603–5607.
40. Jackson AC, Wunner WH. 1991. Detection of rabies virus genomic RNA and mRNA in mouse and human brains by in situ hybridization. *J Virol* 65:2839–2844.
41. Jacobs FS. 1991. Latent rabies in a cat. *J Am Vet Med Assoc* 199:677.
42. Jay MT, Reilly KF, DeBess EE, et al. 1994. Rabies in a vaccinated wolf-dog hybrid. *J Am Vet Med Assoc* 205:1729–1732.
43. Johnson WB, Walden MB. 1996. Results of a national survey of rabies control procedures. *J Am Vet Med Assoc* 208:1667–1672.
44. Kamolvarin N, Tirawatnpong T, Rattanasiwamoke R, et al. 1993. Diagnosis of rabies by polymerase chain reaction with nested primers. *J Infect Dis* 167:207–210.
45. Kass PH, Barnes WG, Spangler WL, et al. 1993. Epidemiologic evidence for a causal relation between vaccination and fibrosarcoma tumorigenesis in cats. *J Am Vet Med Assoc* 203:396–405.
46. Krebs JW, Holman RC, Hines U, et al. 1992. Rabies surveillance in the United States during 1991. *J Am Vet Med Assoc* 201:1836–1848.
47. Krebs JW, Strine TW, Childs JE. 1993. Rabies surveillance in the United States during 1992. *J Am Vet Med Assoc* 203:1718–1731.
48. Krebs JW, Strine TW, Smith JS, et al. 1994. Rabies surveillance in the United States during 1993. *J Am Vet Med Assoc* 205:1695–1709.
49. Krebs JW, Strine TW, Smith JS, et al. 1995. Rabies surveillance in the United States during 1994. *J Am Vet Med Assoc* 207:1562–1575.
50. Krebs JW, Strine TW, Smith JS, et al. 1996. Rabies surveillance in the United States during 1995. *J Am Vet Med Assoc* 209:2031–2044.
51. Last RD, Jardine JE, Smit MME, et al. 1994. Application of immunoperoxidase techniques to formalin-fixed brain tissue for the diagnosis of rabies in southern Africa. *Onderstepoort J Vet Res* 61:183–187.
52. Lewis VJ, Thacker WL. 1974. Limitations of deteriorated tissue for rabies diagnosis. *Health Lab Sci* 11:8–12.
52a. Lontai I. 1997. The current state of rabies prevention in Europe. *Vaccine* 15(Suppl):S16–S19.
53. McColl KA, Gould AR, Selleck PW, et al. 1993. Polymerase chain reaction and other laboratory techniques in the diagnosis of long incubation rabies in Australia. *Aust Vet J* 70:84–89.
54. Mebatsion T, Sillero-Zubiri C, Gottelli D, et al. 1992. Detection of rabies antibody by ELISA and RFFIT in unvaccinated dogs and in the endangered simian. Jackal (canis simensis) of Ethiopia. *J Vet Med* B39:233–235.
55. Meehan SK. 1995. Rabies epizootic in coyotes combated with an oral vaccination program. *J Am Vet Med Assoc* 206:1097–1099.
56. Montano Hirase JA, Bourhy H, Sureau P. 1991. Retrobulbar route for brain specimen collection for rabies diagnosis. *Vet Rec* 129:291–292.
57. Nicholson KG. 1990. Modern vaccines-rabies. *Lancet* 335:1201–1205.
58. Robinson LE, Fishbein DB. 1991. Rabies. *Semin Vet Med Surg (Small Anim)* 6:203–211.
59. Rudd RT, Trimarchi CV. 1989. Development and evaluation of an in vitro virus isolation procedure as a replacement for the mouse inoculation test in rabies diagnosis. *J Clin Microbiol* 27:2522–2528.
60. Rudmann DG, Vanalstine WG, Doddy F, et al. 1996. Pulmonary and mediastinal metastases of a vaccination site sarcoma in a cat. *Vet Pathol* 33:466–469.
61. Rupprecht CE. 1991. Comments on latent rabies in a cat. *J Am Vet Med Assoc* 199:1686–1687.
62. Rupprecht CE, Childs JE. 1996. Feline rabies. *Feline Pract* 24(5):15–19.
62a. Ruppret CE, Smith JS, Krebs JW, et al. 1997. Molecular epidemiology of rabies in the United States: reemergence of a classical neurotropic agent. *J Neurovirol* 3(Suppl 1):S52–S53.
63. Sage G, Khawplod P, Wilde H, et al. 1993. Immune response to rabies vaccine in Alaskan dogs: failure to achieve a consistently protective vaccine response. *Trans R Soc Trop Med Hyg* 87:593–595.
63a. Schultze AE, Frank LA, Hahn KA. 1997. Repeated physical and cytologic characterizations of subcutaneous postvaccinal reactions in cats. *Am J Vet Res* 58:719–724.
64. Smith JS. 1996. New aspects of rabies with emphasis in epidemiology, diagnosis, and prevention of the disease in the United States. *Clin Microbiol Rev* 9:166–176.
65. Smith JS, Orciari LA, Yager PA, et al. 1992. Epidemiologic and historical

relationships among 87 rabies virus isolates as determined by limited sequence analysis. *J Infect Dis* 166:296–307.
65a. Suliova J, Benisek Z, Svrcek S, et al. 1997. The effectiveness of inactivated, purified and concentrated experimental rabies vaccine for veterinary use: immunogenic activity. *Vet Med (Praha)* 42:51–56.
66. Taylor J, Trimarchi C, Weinberg R, et al. 1991. Efficacy studies on a canarypox-rabies recombinant virus. *Vaccine* 9:190–193.
67. Tepsumethanon W, Polsuwan C, Lumlertdaecha B, et al. 1991. Immmune response to rabies vaccination in Thai dogs: a preliminary report. *Vaccine* 9:627–630.
68. Tierkel ES. 1973. Shipment of specimens and techniques for preparation of animal tissue, pp 29–40, *In* Kaplan MM, Kaprowski H (eds), Laboratory techniques in rabies (monograph series No 23). World Health Organization, Geneva, Switzerland.
69. Uhaa IJ, Mandel EJ, Whiteway R, et al. 1992. Rabies surveillance in the United States during 1990. *J Am Vet Med Assoc* 200:920–929.
70. Vishawapoka U, Hemachudha T, Tepsumethanon W, et al. 1988. Detection of rabies antigen in canine parotid glands by dot-blot technique. *Lancet* 1:881.
71. Weiland F, Cox JH, Meyer S, et al. 1992. Rabies virus neuritic paralysis: immunopathogenesis of nonfatal paralytic rabies. *J Virol* 66:5096–5099.
72. Whitby J. 1996. Rabies diagnosis and the central veterinary laboratory. *Vet Rec* 139:433.
73. Yarosh OK, Wandeler AI, Graham FL, et al. 1996. Human adenovirus type-5 vectors expressing rabies glycoprotein. *Vaccine* 14:1257–1264.
74. Zhu JH, Wang J, Cai B, et al. 1996. Immunogenicity and relative attenuation of different vaccinia-rabies virus recombinants. *Arch Virol* 141:1055–1065.

Chapter 23

Pseudorabies

Marc Vandevelde

ETIOLOGY

Pseudorabies virus (PRV) is an enveloped DNA virus belonging to the α-herpesviruses. As with other herpesviruses, PRV can cause latent infection, with viral DNA being incorporated in the host cell genome. The virus is relatively resistant to environmental factors and can survive outside the host for several months under favorable climatic conditions. Survival of PRV depends on temperature (10 days at 37°C, 40 days at 25°C) and pH (optimum, 7), and it is quickly inactivated by drying and exposure to UV light.[7] The genes of PRV have been cloned and sequenced, and its genetic relationship to other animal herpesviruses has been studied.

EPIDEMIOLOGY

PRV infection (Aujeszky's disease, mad itch, infectious bulbar paralysis) occurs in most countries of the world with the exception of Australia and has been responsible for massive economic losses. Although many mammalian species are susceptible to infection with PRV, it is predominantly a problem in pigs, the main reservoir of the virus. However, cattle, furbearing animals, dogs, and cats are sporadically affected.[7] It does not appear to affect people, because most reports have been circumstantial and not documented. Infection frequently is subclinical in pigs because they have become well adapted to the virus. The disease is spread by commercial movement of infected pigs or contaminated pork products. Venereal transmission occurs because infected boars may shed PRV in semen. Although wild animals, such as raccoons, panthers,[2] and rats, may act as transient reservoirs, they are not important in maintaining the disease in nature. Their role is limited to temporary local spread of virus within enzootic areas. Similarly, PRV infection in dogs and cats only occurs in areas where the disease is enzootic in pigs. In fact, the occurrence of typical pseudorabies signs in pets can be the first indication that the disease is enzootic in the local pig population. Pets almost invariably are infected as a result of consuming contaminated raw pork. Dogs also have developed pseudorabies after having bitten infected pigs. Direct spread from dog to dog has not been shown to occur.[7]

PATHOGENESIS

Naturally acquired infection in dogs and cats occurs after ingestion of the virus, although a similar sequence of events follows parenteral inoculation of virus. PRV enters the nerve endings at the inoculation site and travels in retrograde fashion via the axoplasm of the nerve fibers to the brain. The incubation time in dogs and cats, regardless of inoculation sites, is 3 to 6 days. Experimental studies in orally infected cats have shown that PRV replicates in the tonsils and travels from the oral mucosa via the sensory branches of the 9th and 10th cranial nerves to the nucleus, tractus solitarius, and area postrema in the medulla oblongata.[7] The 5th cranial nerve has been less frequently involved. It has been shown in experimental infections in rats that PRV spreads in a highly specific manner through synaptic connections.[1] Apart from visible damage to the brain tissue associated with inflammatory changes, the virus can cause considerable functional alterations of the nerve cells.[7]

CLINICAL FINDINGS

The majority of dogs and cats that become infected develop severe clinical signs. The onset of clinical illness is hyperacute, and signs progress rapidly until death occurs; the total course rarely lasts longer than 48 hours. With very few exceptions, pseudorabies is always fatal in dogs. Cats may be somewhat more resistant but have rarely recovered from the disease.

The initial sign often noted by the owner is a change in behavior, such as inactivity, lethargy, and indifference, although some animals become aggressive or restless. Dyspnea, diarrhea, and vomiting are occasionally seen. Body temperature may be normal or abnormal, and hypersalivation is common. The most characteristic sign, however, is intense pruritus, which usually occurs in the head region and rarely in other areas, such as the neck and shoulders. The animals violently scratch their faces and ears and rub their heads against the floor or walls. One side of the head and neck may become swollen. Self-mutilation results in erythema, excoriation, and ulceration of the skin and underlying tissues. The scratching becomes increasingly more frantic and may end in a generalized convulsion. An atypical course of the disease has also been observed in cats that died suddenly without developing neurologic signs.[7] Pruritus has been absent in some cases of spontaneous PRV infection in dogs[7] and in experimental oral infection in cats.[7] GI signs have been the predominant feature of some infected dogs.[7] Most of the other neurologic signs that are observed in PRV infection refer to lesions in the lower brain stem and consist of one or several deficits in cranial nerve function. These deficits are usually unilateral and include anisocoria, mydriasis, lack of direct or consensual pupillary light reflexes, trismus, paresis and paralysis of the facial muscles, head tilt, inability to swallow, and vocal changes. Anisocoria and a hoarse voice are considered to be highly consistent signs in the cat.[7] Less commonly observed neurologic signs include behavioral abnormalities such as aggressiveness, generalized hyperesthesia, head pressing, and generalized convulsions. The latter often occur as sequelae to frantic scratching. Paresis and paralysis of the limbs are sometimes noted shortly before death. Less commonly, death has been preceded predominantly by acute GI signs.[8]

DIAGNOSIS

Hematologic or biochemical abnormalities are not found in pseudorabies. CSF may show increased protein concentration and mononuclear pleocytosis. This finding is strongly indicative of viral encephalitis but is not specific for pseudorabies. ECG findings may include cardiac arrhythmias.[7]

Traditionally, the diagnosis of pseudorabies consisted of cutaneous inoculation of infected tissue (usually brain) into a rabbit. Scratching and automutilation of the inoculation site occurred after an incubation time of 5 to 6 days, followed by the rapid death of the animal. Virus can also be propagated in the brains of mice after intracranial inoculation.[7] Pruritus can occur in some mice at the site of inoculation. Newer diagnostic methods, such as direct FA examination for virus, have made animal inoculation studies obsolete. This procedure can detect virus in smears or frozen sections of various tissues. The brain and tonsils are the tissues of choice in such studies. Polymerase chain reaction (PCR) has been used to detect PRV.[6] PCR has been employed successfully to detect the virus in a cat in Japan.[3]

Virus can be isolated in tissue culture from lung and spleen and especially from brain and tonsils of animals with pseudorabies. Although many cell lines have been used, most

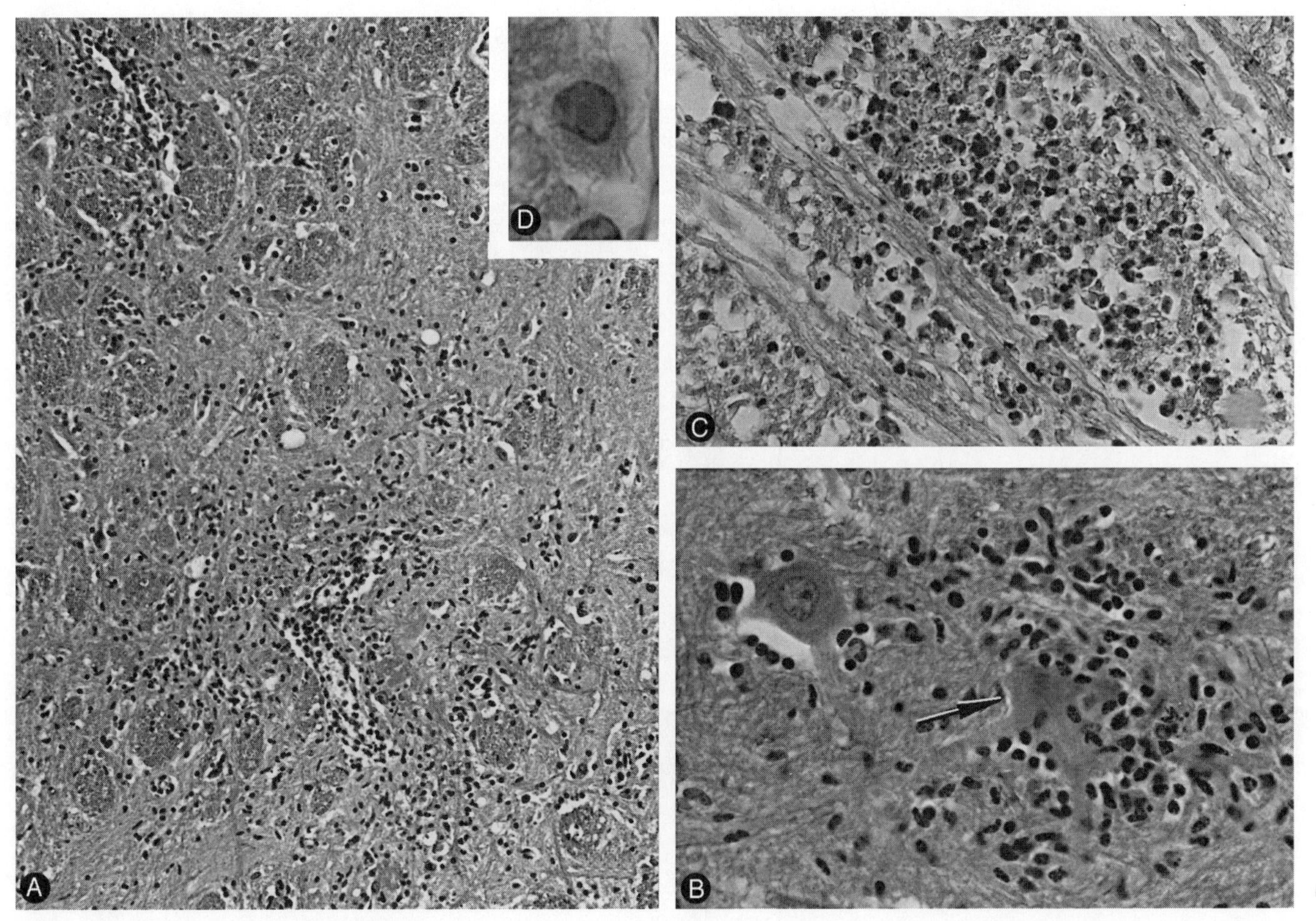

Figure 23–1. Histologic findings of pseudorabies encephalitis. *A*, Disseminated perivascular cuffing and gliosis in the medulla oblongata (H and E, × 100). *B*, Neuronal degeneration *(arrow)* with nodular gliosis (H and E, × 250). *C*, Microabscess (H and E, × 250). *D*, PRV inclusion body in glial cell nucleus (H and E, × 400).

laboratories do use pig kidney epithelial cells. A definite cytopathic effect consisting of syncytial formation is visible after 12 to 24 hours. Virus isolation is not always easy in dogs, even in well-substantiated cases.[7] Pharyngeal washings, tonsillar swabs, and saliva are unsuitable for viral isolation in dogs.[7]

VN, immunodiffusion, and ELISA methods commonly are employed to detect serum antibody to PRV in pigs. Serologic studies have been valuable in determining the incidence of disease in pig populations from an epizootiologic and a disease prevention point of view. PCR has been able to detect latency in the porcine population.[6] Virus neutralizing antibodies have not been found in sera from dogs tested during an outbreak of PRV infection.[7]

PATHOLOGIC FINDINGS

There are no gross lesions diagnostic of pseudorabies, with the exception of the skin lesions that result from intense pruritus. In some cases, abnormal stomach contents have been noted because of pica. Pulmonary edema and congestion have been consistent findings. Focal myocarditis has been found in both dogs and cats. Lesions in the CNS are almost exclusively located in the brain stem and primarily involve cranial nerve nuclei.[7] They may be unilateral and consist of perivascular cuffing with mononuclear cells and pronounced proliferation of astrocytes and microglial cells (Fig. 23–1*A*). The areas of focal gliosis often show degeneration (karyorrhexis) in the center and may progress to the formation of microabscesses (Fig. 23–1*B* and *C*). Severe changes occur in neurons, with chromatolysis and disintegration of the nucleus. A most significant finding is the presence of weak eosinophilic viral inclusion bodies in the nuclei of astrocytes and neurons (Fig. 23–1*D*). Viral antigen can be specifically demonstrated in formalin-fixed, paraffin-embedded tissues with immunocytochemical methods.[7] Inflammatory changes can also be found in the nerves and ganglia associated with the site of viral entry. Severe inflammation of the myenteric plexus in the alimentary canal of dogs naturally infected with PRV has also been reported.[7] Experimentally infected dogs had ganglioneuritis of autonomic nerves of the heart.[7]

THERAPY

Treatment of pseudorabies is generally futile because the disease is almost always fatal. Heavy sedation and anesthesia may lessen or relieve the itching and convulsions; however, nothing can alter the outcome of the disease. Treatment with anti-PRV serum did not improve the condition of a dog with Aujeszky's disease[7] and is considered to be ineffective in the prevention of infection.[7]

PREVENTION

Prevention is the most important means of control of PRV infection in dogs and cats. Contact with pigs and, especially, the use of raw pork from endemic areas as animal food should be avoided. It is possible to vaccinate small animals against PRV, although this is indicated only in endemic areas, where exposure to infected pigs may occur. Natural infection with PRV has not been observed in vaccinated dogs and cats.[7] However, experimental vaccination challenge studies showed that it may be difficult to protect dogs with an inactivated vaccine, although most animals develop serum neutralizing antibodies to PRV.[7] Attenuated PRV vaccines may cause postvaccinal reactions that may be as lethal as the natural infection. PRV deletion mutants have been developed for vaccination of pigs.[4, 5] Such vaccines are safe and very useful to control the disease, because serologic surveys can distinguish between vaccine induced and natural anti-PRV antibodies. To my knowledge, such deletion mutant vaccines have not been systematically tested in dogs and cats.

References

1. Cord JP, Rinaman L, Lynn RB, et al. 1993. Pseudorabies virus infection in the rat central nervous system: ultrastructural characterization of viral replication, transport and pathogenesis. *J Neurosci* 13:2515–2539.
2. Glass CM, McLean RG, Katz JB, et al. 1994. Isolation of pseudorabies (Aujeszky's disease) virus from a Florida panther. *J Wildl Dis* 30:180–184.
3. Hara M, Shimizu T, Nemoto S, et al. 1991. The genome type of Aujeszky's disease virus from a cat in Japan. *J Vet Med Sci* 53:1087–1089.
4. Mettenleitner TC. 1995. New developments in the construction of safer and more versatile pseudorabies virus vaccines. *Dev Biol Stand* 84:83–87.
5. Peeters B, Bouma A, de Bruin, et al. 1994. Non-transmissible pseudorabies gp50 mutants: a new generation of safe live vaccines. *Vaccine* 12:375–380.
6. Schang LM, Osorio FA. 1993. A quantitative technique for the study of the latency of Aujeszky virus. *Rev Sci Tech* 12:505–521.
7. Vandevelde M. 1990. Pseudorabies, pp 384–388. *In* Greene CE (ed), Infectious diseases of the dog and cat. WB Saunders, Philadelphia, PA.
8. Wagnerrietschel H. 1994. Case report—Aujeszky's disease in the dog, an unusual course. *Prakt Tierarzt* 75:767–768.

Chapter 24

Enterovirus Infections

Craig E. Greene

Picornaviridae, the family of the smallest RNA viruses, contains the genus *Enterovirus*. Species in this genus commonly infect humans and have classically been separated into polioviruses, coxsackieviruses, enteric cytopathogenic human orphan (echo) viruses, and as yet unclassified enteroviruses. Newer members of the genus are called enteroviruses and are designated by a sequential numbering system. Enteroviruses are environmentally resistant and infect people primarily via the fecal-oral route. After replication in submucosal lymphatic tissues, the viruses may spread systemically to various other tissues.

Dogs have been tested to determine whether they harbor a variety of human enteroviruses because of the possible zoonotic potential (Table 24–1). Similar information is not available for cats. Dogs have been shown to be exposed to and to chronically shed human enteroviruses; however, serologic evidence of infection does not always correlate with shedding of the viruses. Although dogs appear to become infected with these viruses, clinical signs have not been apparent. The viruses can be found in the stools for a period of months, but whether the extended shedding represents reexposure is uncertain. Enteroviruses recovered from nasopharyngeal or fecal cultures of dogs have been grown and cause cytopathogenic effects, primarily in monkey kidney but not canine cell lines, supporting the fact that they are human viruses. Furthermore, neutralization tests have shown them to be indistinguishable from the human isolates.[7, 8] In some instances, enteroviruses were found in canine feces that were "just passing through," not causing infection. These viruses could have been obtained from sources contaminated by human feces. Alternatively, they could be enteroviruses antigenically related to human enteroviruses or other viruses neutralized by nonspecific substances in the testing sera. Newer techniques to determine viral homogeneity by genetic analysis must be performed on isolates to resolve this issue.

Feeding of echovirus 6 or coxsackievirus B1 to dogs produced minimal signs suggestive of enteric disease. Although the virus could be isolated from the feces, seroconversion could not be demonstrated.[6, 10] Infection seems to be limited to the alimentary tract of dogs and does not spread systemically as such infections do in people. Although dogs shed these viruses in low amounts, viral spread to susceptible dogs has resulted in infection.[10] Whether infected dogs can be a source of human infection is uncertain.

Table 24–1. Human Enteroviruses Recovered From Nonsymptomatic Dogs

VIRUS	SPECIMEN SOURCE	GEOGRAPHIC LOCATION
Poliovirus 1	Feces	West Bengal[2]
	Feces	Costa Rica[4]
Echovirus 6	Feces	California[1]
	Nasopharynx, feces	New Mexico[1, 5, 9]
Echovirus 7	Feces	West Bengal[2]
Coxsackievirus A9, A20	Feces	Costa Rica[4]
Coxsackievirus B_1	Nasopharynx, feces	Texas, New Mexico[1, 5]
Coxsackievirus B_3	Nasopharynx, feces	New Mexico[5]
Coxsackievirus B_5	Nasopharynx, feces	Nex Mexico[5]
Unclassified enteroviruses	Feces	Philippines[11]

References

1. Clapper WE. 1970. Comments on viruses recovered from dogs. *J Am Vet Med Assoc* 156:1678–1680.
2. Graves IL, Oppenheimer JR. 1975. Human viruses in animals in West Bengal: an ecological analysis. *Hum Ecol* 3:105–130.
3. Greene CE. 1990. Enterovirus infections, pp 389–390. *In* Greene CE (ed), Infectious diseases of the dog and cat, ed 1. WB Saunders, Philadelphia, PA.
4. Grew N, Gohd RS, Arguedas J, et al. 1970. Enteroviruses in rural families and their domestic animals. *Am J Epidemiol* 91:518–526, 1970.
5. Lundgren DL, Clapper WE, Sanchez A. 1968. Isolation of human enteroviruses from beagle dogs. *Soc Exp Biol Med* 128:463–466.
6. Lundgren DL, Hobbs CH, Clapper WE. 1971. Experimental infection of beagle dogs with Coxsackievirus type B1. *Am J Vet Res* 32:609–613.
7. Lundgren DL, Meade GH, Clapper WE. 1970. Cross neutralization and gel double diffusion studies of enteroviruses isolated from beagle dogs. *Texas Rep Biol Med* 28:48–58.
8. Lundgren DL, Sanchez A, Magnuson MG, et al. 1970. A survey for human enteroviruses in dogs and man. *Arch Gesamte Virusforsch* 32:229–235.
9. Pindak FF, Clapper WE. 1964. Isolation of enteric cytopathogenic human orphan virus type 6 from dogs. *Am J Vet Res* 25:52–54.
10. Pindak FF, Clapper WE. 1966. Experimental infection of beagle with ECHO virus type 6. *Texas Rep Biol Med* 24:466–472.
11. Steele JH, Arambulo PV, Beran GW. 1973. The epidemiology of zoonosis in the Philippines. *Arch Environ Health* 26:330–338.

Chapter 25

Mumps and Influenza Virus Infections

Craig E. Greene

MUMPS

Mumps virus is a member of the family Paramyxoviridae and genus *Paramyxovirus*. The virus causes illness in humans, its primary natural hosts; however, nonhuman primates and other laboratory animals have been experimentally infected. Clinical signs in affected people include fever, anorexia, and progressive, independent enlargement of the parotid salivary glands. Meningitis, the main complication of infection that sometimes develops, results in headache and nuchal rigidity. Encephalitis, polyarthritis, and pancreatitis may uncommonly develop. Vaccination programs have greatly reduced the prevalence and severity of this infectious disease throughout the world.

Mumps viral antibodies have been identified in the sera of healthy dogs; however, dogs can be infected with canine parainfluenza viruses (similar to but distinct from simian virus 5 of nonhuman primates; see Chapters 6 and 7), which may cross-react with some mumps viral antigens. Interpretation of prior serologic studies may be misleading for this reason. Nevertheless, there are reports of parotid salivary gland enlargement in dogs from households in which children in the family have had concurrent or recent mumpslike infections.[1, 8, 12] Antibody to mumps viral antigen was detected in the serum of some affected dogs.[8, 12] A virus, neutralized by mumps viral antisera, was found in one dog.[8] Early experimental attempts to produce mumps in dogs or cats by inoculation of virus directly in the gland were inconclusive.[8] Although in vivo transmission studies are inconclusive, mumps virus does grow well in primary dog kidney cell culture; this has been a source of producing attenuated vaccine for human use.[7, 13] Veterinarians in practice should be aware of the possible association between mumps in children and pets, although definitive evidence for animal infection is lacking.

INFLUENZA

Influenza viruses are in the family Orthomyxoviridae. Two genera, types A and B, produce an acute self-limiting febrile illness in susceptible people as episodic outbreaks almost every winter. Type C influenza viruses are less closely related and produce similar disease. Fever, myalgia, and signs of upper or lower respiratory tract infections are the most common manifestations. Mortality is the result of pulmonary complications. Pandemic spread of influenza may result periodically when, as a result of genetic alteration of surface glycoproteins, a new virus strain, to which the world population has no immunity, emerges.

Influenza virus spreads from the transfer of virus-containing respiratory secretions from an infected to a susceptible person. Small (<10 μm) aerosols are the important means of spread.

Because of the close association of pets with people, there has been concern that dogs and cats may be important in the spread or maintenance of influenza infection. Many reports exist of serologic evidence of infection of dogs and cats to influenza virus. Experimental IN or IV infection of dogs[6, 10, 11, 14] and cats[10, 11] with influenza virus A strains, of dogs[14] and cats[10] with B strains, and of dogs[9] with type C strains has provided convincing evidence that they do have the infections. Clinical signs in infected animals either were absent or consisted of a mild conjunctivitis, serous nasal discharge, and variable fever. Serologic responses have been inconsistent, although viruses could be recovered from the respiratory secretions. Cats and dogs were also infected in some instances by contact with animals that were infected.

Spontaneous influenza viral infections of dogs and cats have been associated with human populations that are suffering from epidemics of the disease.[2, 11] There is no evidence to suggest that the virus spreads from infected pets back to people. This finding is in contrast to the situation in pigs in which spread from people and birds and back ("mixing vessel hypothesis") probably occurs with genetic recombination and evolution of new viral strains.[16]

References

1. Chandler EA. 1975. Mumps in the dog. *Vet Rec* 96:365–366.
2. Chang CP, New AG, Taylor JF, et al. 1976. Influenza virus isolations from dogs during a human epidemic in Taiwan. *Int J Zoon* 3:61–64.
3. Greene CE. 1990. Mump and influenza virus infections, pp 391–392. *In* Greene CE (ed), Infectious diseases of the dog and cat. WB Saunders, Philadelphia, PA.
4. Manuguerra JC, Hannoun C. 1992. Natural infection of dogs by influenza C virus. *Res Virol* 143:199–204.
5. Manuguerra JC, Hannoun C, Simon F, et al. 1993. Natural infection of dogs by influenza C virus: a serological survey in Spain. *Microbiologica* 16:367–371.
6. Nikitin T, Cohen D, Todd JD, et al. 1972. Epidemiological studies of A/Hong Kong/68 virus infection in dogs. *Bull WHO* 47:471–479.
7. Nöbel B, Glathe H. 1978. Biological particularities of the mumps virus—its behavior in the RCT-marker. *J Hyg Epidemiol Microbiol Immunol* 22:203–207.
8. Noice F, Bolin FM, Eveleth DF. 1959. Incidence of viral parotitis in the domestic dog. *Am J Dis Child* 98:350–352.
9. Ohwada K, Kitame F, Homma M. 1984. Experimental infection of dogs with type C influenza virus. Presented at the Sixth International Congress of Virology, Sendai, Japan, September 1–7.
10. Paniker CK, Nair CM. 1972. Experimental infection of animals with influenza virus types A and B. *Bull WHO* 47:461–463.
11. Romváry J, Rózsa J, Farkas E. 1975. Infection of dogs and cats with the Hong Kong influenza A (H3N2) virus during an epidemic period in Hungary. *Acta Vet Acad Scien Hung* 25:255–259.
12. Smith RE. 1975. Mumps in the dog. *Vet Rec* 96:296.
13. Starke G, Hlinak P. 1974. Requirements for the control of a dog kidney cell–adapted live mumps virus vaccine. *J Biol Stand* 2:143–150.
14. Todd JD, Cohen D. 1968. Studies of influenza in dogs: 1. Susceptibility of dogs to natural and experimental infection with human A2 and B strains of influenza virus. *Am J Epidemiol* 87:426–438.
15. Van Heerden J, Mills MG, van Vuuren MJ, et al. 1995. An investigation into the health status and diseases of wild dogs (Lycano pictus) in the Kruger National Park. *J S Afr Vet Assoc* 66:18–27.
16. Wentworth DE, McGregor MW, Macklin MD, et al. 1997. Transmission of swine influenza virus to humans after exposure to experimentally infected dogs. *J Infect Dis* 175:7–15.

Chapter 26

Arboviral Infections

Arthropod-Borne Encephalomyelitis

Craig E. Greene and Charles A. Baldwin

All arthropod-borne viruses known to infect dogs and cats belong to the families Togaviridae, Flaviviridae, Bunyaviridae, or Orbiviridae (Table 26–1). These RNA viruses are usually maintained in nature by a sylvan cycle involving an arthropod vector and a vertebrate reservoir host (Fig. 26–1). Domesticated animals are usually incidental hosts, but in some cases they serve as reservoirs. As unnatural hosts, domesticated animals may be subclinically affected or show signs of disease (usually nonsuppurative, neurotropic encephalitis). The clinical susceptibility of people, dogs, and cats for each disease also varies. Because serologic cross-reactivity between certain viruses can occur and because dogs and cats can be subclinically infected, the following discussion emphasizes those cases in which virus isolation and consistent pathologic findings have been present or experimental inoculation of dogs or cats has been performed. Results of serologic testing indicate that a large number of these viruses may infect dogs and cats.

TOGAVIRIDAE

Natural and experimental susceptibility of dogs to Venezuelan equine encephalitis (VEE) virus has been well described.[7] In both natural and experimental infections using mosquitoes, viremia and seroconversion occur without clinical illness. For this reason, dogs have been considered good sentinel hosts for human VEE infection. Dogs also have been used to monitor the spread of infection into geographic areas.

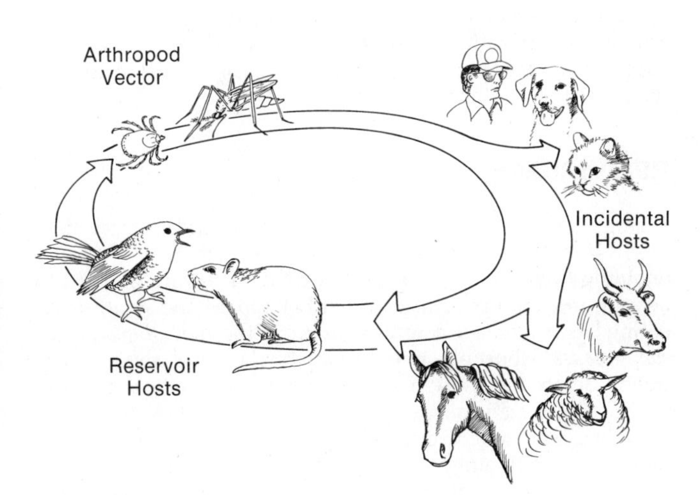

Figure 26–1. Arthropod-borne viral infections have a sylvan cycle involving arthropod vectors that feed on reservoir hosts. Domestic animals and people are usually incidental hosts, but they may serve as reservoirs in some instances (see Table 26–1).

Parenteral inoculation of VEE in dogs has produced fever, leukopenia, and neurologic deficits at the peak of the febrile response. Cerebrovascular hemorrhage and infarction were detected. Naturally occurring VEE was also suspected as causing encephalitis in a puppy.[7] Eastern equine encephalitis (EEE) has been diagnosed in naturally infected dogs from south-central Georgia.[2] All were in pups younger than 6 weeks with signs of diffuse encephalitis manifest by ataxia, tremor, excessive salivation, and seizure.

Petechial hemorrhages have been grossly evident on the surface of the brain at necropsy. Histologic lesions in the brain were inflammation with macrophage infiltration, edema, gliosis, hemorrhage, and multifocal necrosis. Mononuclear and neutrophilic infiltrates have been present in the meninges. Foci of myocardial degeneration and necrosis with mononuclear infiltration have been found in the heart. The viral association has been confirmed by use of an oligonucleotide probe and viral isolation. EEE has also been isolated from the CNS of a litter of dying 6-week-old puppies in which no microscopic lesions could be demonstrated.[3] The infection may have been coincidental. Experimentally, dogs have developed diffuse encephalitis after intracerebral or parenteral inoculation of western equine encephalitis virus.[7]

FLAVIVIRIDAE

Dogs and cats have been more resistant to St. Louis encephalitis, although serosurveys have demonstrated that the animals develop titers during human epidemics. Parenteral inoculation of Japanese encephalitis virus has resulted in subclinical infection, but intracranial inoculation resulted in encephalitis with corresponding neurologic deficits.[7] Louping-ill is described in a separate section of this chapter. Dogs have developed fever, viremia, and serologic response to Powassan virus.[7] Tick-borne encephalitis (TBE) virus inoculated into puppies produced a low-titer viremia but no clinical illness, although naive ticks feeding on the puppies became infected.[7] Natural infections were described occurring in the summer months in four adult dogs from different regions in central Europe.[23, 28] The signs were fever and multifocal neurologic problems consisting of myoclonus, convulsions, hemiparesis to tetraparesis, stupor, and anisocoria. The signs were progressive over 4 to 7 days, and dogs either died or were euthanized. Mononuclear pleocytosis is found in CSF.[23] A nonsuppurative meningoencephalitis with predominant lesions in the brain stem and cerebellum was found. Immunohistochemical staining revealed TBE virus in Purkinje cells, neurons of brainstem nuclei, neuronal cell processes, and macrophage cytoplasm.[27a] Wesselsbron virus was isolated from the CNS of a dog with encephalitis.[7] Inoculation of brain tissue from this case into dogs produced

Table 26-1. Arthropod-Borne Viral Infections Affecting Dogs and Cats

DISEASE	GEOGRAPHIC DISTRIBUTION	ARTHROPOD VECTOR	USUAL HOSTS: RESERVOIR (DOMESTIC)	SUSCEPTIBILITY OF HUMANS, DOGS, AND CATS
Togaviridae				
Eastern equine encephalitis	Eastern U.S., Central America, Caribbean islands, Brazil, Guyana, Argentina	*Culiseta melanura Aedes* spp., *Culex* spp.	Birds (horses, quail, pheasants, cows, sheep)	H, D
Western equine encephalitis	U.S., Canada, Central America, Guyana, Brazil, Argentina	*Culiseta melanura, Culex* spp.	Birds, small mammals, snakes (horses)	H, D
Venezuelan equine encephalitis	Florida, Texas, northern South America, Central America	*Psorophora confinnis, Aedes* spp., *Culex* spp.	Rodents (horses)	H, D, C
Flaviviridae				
St. Louis encephalitis	U.S., Canada, Central America, Caribbean islands, Colombia, Brazil, Argentina	*Culex* spp.	Birds (usually inapparent)	H, D,[a] C[a]
Japanese encephalitis	Siberia, Japan, China, many Far East countries	*Culex* spp.	Birds (pigs, horses)	H, D, C[a]
Louping-Ill	Scotland, Ireland	*Ixodes ricinus*	Sheep?, red grouse (sheep, cattle)	H, D
Powassan	U.S., Canada,	*Ixodes cookei, I. marxi*	Rodents (sheep)	H, D[a]
Tick-borne encephalitis	Europe, Soviet Republics	*Ixodes* spp., *Dermacentor* spp.	Rodents, birds (sheep, goats, cattle)	H, D
Wesselsbron disease	South Africa	*Aedes* spp.	Ungulates, sheep (sheep)	D
Yellow fever	South America, Africa	*Aedes* spp.	Nonhuman primates, humans (none)	H, C[a]
Bunyaviridae				
Tenshaw	Southeastern U.S.	*Anopheles* spp.	Rodents (cattle, dogs)	D, C
Rift Valley fever	East Africa	*Culex theileri, Aedes caballus*	Ungulates (sheep)	H, D,[b] C[c]
La Crosse	Midwestern, eastern, and southern U.S.	*Aedes* spp.	Small mammals (chipmunks)	D[b]
Orbiviridae				
African horse sickness	Africa, Middle East, Mediterranean	*Culicoides* spp., mosquitoes?	Equidae (horse)	D[d]
Bluetongue	Worldwide	*Culicoides* spp.	Ovidae (sheep)	D[e]
Unclassified				
Borna	Europe, Japan	?	Horses, sheep	C[f]

? = uncertain.
[a]Subclinical.
[b]Puppies.
[c]Kittens.
[d]Subclinical, carnivorism.
[e]Parenterally inoculated vaccine contaminant.
[f]In Japan, infections appear to be sublinical.
H = human; D = dog; C = cat.

seroconversion, viremia, and in one dog transient paralysis. Yellow fever virus has produced a transient viremia in cats after inoculation; however, puppies, even when splenectomized, could not be infected.

BUNYAVIRIDAE

Tenshaw virus inoculated into dogs and cats produced nonsymptomatic viremia.[7] Mosquito transmission from infected dogs was also demonstrated. Rift Valley fever virus has produced viremia, severe hepatic necrosis, myocarditis, splenic congestion, meningitis, diffuse petechiae, and death in puppies and kittens younger than 3 weeks.[7] Virus can also be transmitted from puppies to their mother and to other puppies. Older puppies do not succumb to infection but do develop viremias. The virus can cause abortions and stillbirths in pregnant bitches. Inhalation or ingestion of the virus from infected carcasses may occur under natural circumstances. Two litters of puppies younger than 3 weeks developed a sudden onset of seizures and neurologic dysfunction after infection with La Crosse virus.[4] A severe diffuse nonsuppurative meningoencephalitis primarily affecting the cerebral cortex was noted.

REOVIRIDAE

Dogs can be infected subclinically with African horse sickness virus; they develop a serologic response and a viremia enabling them to transmit the infection.[7] They are thought to acquire infection naturally and suffer illness and death from eating dead infected carcasses or from the tick *Rhipicephalus sanguineus*.[9] Abortion in pregnant bitches and their subsequent death have occurred 7 to 9 days after vaccination with a Bluetongue virus–contaminated, modified live virus combination canine vaccine.[1, 6, 30] Lesions in the dam consisted of interstitial pneumonia, myocardial degeneration, hepatic vasculitis, and renal glomerulitis.[6] The natural disease in dogs is probably unlikely due to the low prevalence of seropositivity in dogs in endemic areas.[10]

Borna Disease–Like Meningoencephalitis

Craig E. Greene and Charles A. Baldwin

Borna disease virus naturally infects horses, sheep, ostriches, and several other species, including humans. A spontaneous neurologic disease of cats characterized by behavioral and motor dysfunction (staggering disease) has been described in Europe and attributed to infection with this virus.[11, 15, 16, 19, 21, 29] Clinical signs include paraparesis and ataxia, mental alteration, anorexia, hypersalivation, hypersensitivity to light and sound, visual impairment, and seizure.[13, 15] The signs progress within 1 to 4 weeks despite treatment with anti-inflammatory and antimicrobial therapy.[15] Leukopenia is the only hematologic abnormality, and mononuclear pleocytosis and increased protein typical of viral inflammation are noted with CSF analysis. The inflammatory reaction in the nervous system is characterized by a nonsuppurative meningoencephalitis in the gray matter of the cerebral cortex, hippocampus, basal ganglia, and brain stem.[14] Perivascular mononuclear cell infiltrates consisting of lymphocytes and macrophages accompany neuronal degeneration. Borna disease viral antigen and nucleic acid persist in brain tissue of cats causing chronic inflammatory lesions.[13a]

A large percentage (44%) of affected cats have high serum antibody titers to Borna disease virus compared with unaffected control cats from the same general population.[15, 19] Small numbers of nuclear cells in the perivascular infiltrates have stained positive by immunoperoxidase for Borna virus antigen, and the virus can be isolated.[14, 16] Although some investigators have suggested that lesions of feline Borna disease resemble those of poliomyelitis, there is no evidence that these disorders are related. The histologic and clinical features of Borna disease should be contrasted with feline polioencephalomyelitis, which predominantly affects the spinal cord, causing progressive lower motor neuron dysfunction with milder brain stem involvement (see Neurologic Disease of Suspected Infectious Origin, Chapter 84).[25] Although there are no reports of neurologic dysfunction caused by this virus in Japanese cats, seroprevalence was 8.4%; virus could be detected by PCR in peripheral blood mononuclear cells in 13.3% of tested cats.[18] However, none of the cats tested positive for both the viral RNA and antibodies.

Louping-Ill

Hugh W. Reid

ETIOLOGY

Louping-ill is an acute viral encephalomyelitis transmitted by the sheep tick *Ixodes ricinus*. Although louping-ill occurs most frequently in sheep, it has been reported in people, horses, pigs, cattle, goats, farm-raised deer, and dogs but not in cats.[8, 17]

The causal virus is a member of an antigenically closely related complex of arboviruses (family Flaviviridae) that cause tick-borne encephalitides. These viruses, present throughout the northern temperate latitudes, are primarily associated with disease in people. Infection in domestic animals has been recognized on a regular basis only in the British Isles in areas of rough pastures where sheep ticks are prevalent. However, encephalomyelitis in sheep resulting from infection by either louping-ill virus or closely related viruses has occurred also in Bulgaria, Turkey, Spain, and Norway, suggesting that the disease may be more widespread.[20]

Risk of infection is generally restricted to the periods of tick activity, mainly in the spring and early summer, with a recrudescence in some areas in the fall. However, the precise periods of tick activity vary with latitude and altitude. In dogs, infection has been diagnosed most frequently in working sheepdogs and gun dogs, but any animal visiting enzootic areas during periods of tick activity may become affected.

Infection is assumed to be via the bite of the tick. Alternative routes of transmission should not be overlooked, because disease in people is commonly encountered in abattoir workers. Young goats and pigs can become infected by the ingestion of virus-infected milk and carcasses, respectively.

CLINICAL FINDINGS

The initial systemic phase after infection generally is not associated with clinical signs, but during this period the animal is viremic. The virus invades the CNS. The subsequent course of disease is variable. Many infections are not recognized clinically because virus is eliminated by the immune response that subsequently maintains protection and detectable serum antibody titers, probably for the life of the animals. In animals that do develop clinical disease, initial signs, which are primarily due to cerebellar dysfunction, include mild paresis, ataxia, and tremor that sometimes are associated with difficulty in eating. Within 24 hours, severe incoordination develops. The affected animal is usually in lateral recumbency, paddling its limbs, but this may progress to complete tetraplegia or opisthotonos.

Death may occur at any time, but in dogs that survive, recovery is slow, and locomotor dysfunction may persist for months. On recovery, temperamental and physical changes may be present, the animal being nervous, exercise intolerant, and less tractable.

DIAGNOSIS

Diagnosis relies on the detection of a rising serum antibody response to louping-ill virus during the course of the infection. In fatal cases, histologic examination of the brain accompanied by virus isolation can confirm the disease. Histologic changes include neuronal necrosis and perivascular lymphoid cell accumulations that are particularly prominent

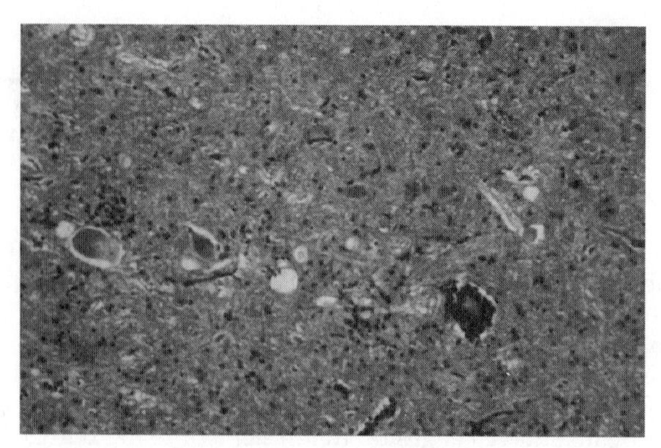

Figure 26–2. Brain stem from an animal clinically affected with louping-ill, showing neurononecrosis, gliosis, and lymphocytic perivascular cuffing (H and E, × 1000). (Courtesy of Dr. D. Buxton, Moredun Research Institute, Edinburgh, Scotland.)

in the spinal cord and cerebellum (Fig. 26–2). Immunohistochemical staining for virus in tissue specimens has been used.[12] Virus may be isolated from a homogenate of brain tissue by intracerebral inoculation of 3-week-old mice or in tissue culture cells.

THERAPY AND PREVENTION

Supportive therapy during the acute phase is beneficial, but no specific therapy is available. An inactivated, tissue culture–propagated vaccine incorporated in an oil adjuvant is available for protection of cattle, sheep, and goats and has been used in dogs. However, dogs appear to require at least two injections to elicit a detectable serum antibody response, and a proportion of them develop painless, fluid-filled swellings at the site of injection that may require surgical drainage.[22]

The ecology of louping-ill virus is largely dependent on a sheep-tick cycle with little involvement of the native fauna. Systematic vaccination of sheep may reduce the prevalence of virus and may, therefore, reduce the risk of infecting other incidental hosts such as dogs.

References

1. Akita GY, Ianconescu M, MacLachlan NJ, et al. 1994. Bluetongue disease in dogs associated with contaminated vaccine. *Vet Rec* 134:283–284.
2. Baldwin CA. 1992. Eastern equine encephalomyelitis virus infection in dogs. Georgia Veterinary Diagnostic Laboratories Newsletter, Tifton, GA.
3. Baldwin CA. 1997. Unpublished observations. Veterinary Diagnostic Laboratory, Tifton, GA.
4. Black SS, Harrison LR, Pursell AR, et al. 1994. Necrotizing panencephalitis in puppies infected with LaCrosse Virus. *J Vet Diagn Invest* 6:250–254.
5. Calisher CH. 1994. Medically important arboviruses of the United States and Canada. *Clin Microbiol Rev* 7:89–116.
6. Evermann JF, McKeirnan AJ, Wilbur LA, et al. 1994. Canine fatalities associated with the use of a modified live vaccine administered during late stages of pregnancy. *J Vet Diagn Invest* 6:353–357.
7. Greene CE. 1990. Arthropod-borne encephalomyelitis, pp 393–394. *In* Greene CE (ed), Infectious diseases of the dog and cat. WB Saunders, Philadelphia, PA.
8. Hobson G. 1973. Louping ill in a working collie. *Vet Rec* 92:436.
9. House JA. 1993. African horse sickness. *Vet Clin North Am* 9:355–365.
10. Howerth EW, Dorminy M, Dreesen DW, et al. 1995. Low prevalence of antibodies to bluetongue and epizootic hemorrhagic disease viruses in dog from southern Georgia. *J Vet Diagn Invest* 7:393–394.
11. Kronevi T, Nordström M, Moreno W, et al. 1974. Feline ataxia due to nonsuppurative meningoencephalomyelitis of unknown etiology. *Nord Vet Med* 26:720–725.
12. Krueger N, Reid HW. 1994. Detection of louping ill virus in formalin-fixed, paraffin wax-embedded tissues of mice, sheep, and a pig by the avidin-biotin-complex immunoperoxidase techniques. *Vet Rec* 135:224–225.
13. Lundgren AL, Czech G, Bode L, et al. 1993. Natural Borna disease in domestic animals other than horses and sheep. *J Vet Med B* 40:298–303.

13a. Lundgren AL, Johannisson A, Zimmermann W, et al. 1997. Neurological disease and encephalitis in cats experimentally infected with Borna-disease virus. *Acta Neuropathol* 93:391–401.

14. Lundgren AL, Lindberg R, Ludwig H, et al. 1995. Immunoreactivity of the central nervous system in cats with a Borna disease-like meningoencephalomyelitis (staggering disease). *Acta Neuropathol* 90:184–193.
15. Lundgren AL, Ludwig H. 1993. Clinically diseased cats with nonsuppurative meningoencephalitis have Borna disease virus-specific antibodies. *Acta Vet Scand* 34:101–103.
16. Lundgren AL, Zimmermann W, Bode L, et al. 1995. Staggering disease in cats. Isolation and characterization of the feline Borna-disease virus. *J Gen Virol* 76:2215-2222.
17. Mackenzie CP. 1982. Recovery of a dog from louping ill. *J Small Animal Pract* 23:233–236.
18. Nakamura Y, Asahi S, Nakaya T, et al. 1996. Demonstration of Borna disease virus RNA in peripheral blood mononuclear cells derived from domestic cats in Japan. *J Clin Microbiol* 34:188–191.
19. Nowotny N, Weissenbock H. 1995. Description of feline nonsuppurative meningoencephalomyelitis ("staggering disease") and studies of its etiology. *J Clin Microbiol* 33:1668–1669.
20. Reid HW. 1990. Louping ill, pp 395–396. *In* Greene CE (ed), Infectious diseases of the dog and cat. WB Saunders, Philadelphia, PA.
21. Ström B, Andrén B, Lundgren AL. 1992. Idiopathic nonsuppurative meningoencephalomyelitis (staggering disease) in the Swedish cat: a study of 33 cases. *Eur J Compan Anim Pract* 3:9–13.
22. Thomson JR, Reid HW, Pow I. 1987. Louping-ill vaccination of dogs. *Vet Rec* 120:94.
23. Tipold A, Fatzer R, Holzmann H. 1993. Central European tick-borne encephalitis in dogs. *Kleintier Praxis* 38:619–628.
24. Truyen U, Stockhofe-Zurwieden N, Kaaden DR, et al. 1990. A case report: encephalitis in lions. Pathological and virological findings. *DTW Dtsch Tierarztl Wochenschr* 97:89–91.
25. Vandevelde M. 1996. Personal communication. University of Bern, Bern, Switzerland.
26. Vandevelde M, Braund KG. 1979. Polioencephalomyelitis in cats. *Vet Pathol* 16:420–427.
27. Van Rensburg IBJ, DeClerk J, Groenewald HB, et al. 1981. An outbreak of African horse sickness in dogs. *J S Afr Vet Assoc* 52:323–325.

27a. Weissenbock H, Holzmann H. 1997. Immunohistochemical diagnosis of tick-borne encephalitis in Austrian dogs. *Wein Tierarztl Mnsch* 84:34–38.

28. Weissenbock H, Holzmann H. 1996. Tick-borne encephalitis in Austrian dogs. *Vet Rec* 139:575–576.
29. Weissenbock H, Nowotny N, Zoher J. 1994. Feline meningoencephalomyelitis (staggering disease) in Austria. *Wien Tierarztl Monatsch* 81:195–201.
30. Wilbur LA, Evermann JF, Levings RL, et al. 1994. Abortion and death in pregnant bitches associated with a canine vaccine contaminated with bluetongue virus. *J Am Vet Med Assoc* 204:1762–1765.

Chapter 27

Salmon Poisoning Disease

John R. Gorham and William J. Foreyt

ETIOLOGY

Salmon poisoning disease (SPD), a highly fatal, helminth-transmitted, rickettsial disease of domestic and wild Canidae, occurs on the western slopes of the Cascade Mountains from northern California to central Washington (Fig. 27–1). Occasionally, cases of SPD occur outside the indigenous range of the disease in areas where infected fish migrate or are transported. Cases in British Columbia may indicate that the indigenous range of the disease is greater than previously reported.[1]

Salmon Disease Agent

The etiologic agent of SPD is *Neorickettsia helminthoeca*, a coccoid or coccobacillary rickettsia, which is approximately 0.3 μm in size. Pleomorphic rods, up to 2 μm in length, sometimes bent in rings or crescents, have been observed. The gram-negative rickettsial organisms appear purple with Giemsa stain, red with Macchiavellos stain, black or dark brown with Levaditi's method, and pale blue with hematoxylin and eosin. The rickettsiae almost fill the cytoplasm of cells of the mononuclear phagocytic system (MPS) that they primarily infect (Fig. 27–2). The rickettsiae have been grown in canine monocytes, in canine leukocytes and sarcoma cells, in mouse lymphoblasts, and in a macrophage cell line.[12] Antigenically and genetically, *N. helminthoeca* is closely related to *Ehrlichia* spp., and based on Western blot analysis and FA labeling results, *N. helminthoeca* is most closely related to *E. risticii*, the agent of Potomac horse fever, and *E. sennetsu*, the agent of human Sennetsu fever in Japan (see Table 28–1).[11] All three agents are likely in the same genus.

In dead fish, rickettsiae in metacercariae (encysted trematode larvae) of *N. salmincola* do not survive 30 days at 4°C. In lymph nodes, organisms resist freezing at −20°C for 31 to 158 days; they remain viable in leukocytes at 4.5°C and 52.5°C for 48 hours and 2 minutes, respectively, but not at 60°C for 5 minutes. At −80°C, the agent can be maintained in cell culture fluid for up to 3 months.[8, 12]

Elokomin Fluke Fever Agent

It is highly likely that the Elokomin fluke fever (EFF) agent is another strain of *N. helminthoeca*. The disease in dogs associated with the EFF agent results in high morbidity but a lower mortality than SPD. It appears that metacercariae can harbor both EFF and SPD agents simultaneously. EFF is rarely recognized as a distinct entity in naturally occurring disease. Histologically, EFF infections in dogs are similar to but less severe than those of SPD. In a survey of 331 practitioners in endemic areas, 35% reported that they had diagnosed SPD in dogs that had been treated previously for SPD.[7] Although it has been generally accepted that dogs that survived SPD infection had a solid immunity, the data now suggest that other strains such as EFF may be pathogenic under field conditions, or there was a failure of the initial SPD infection to evoke a durable immunity.

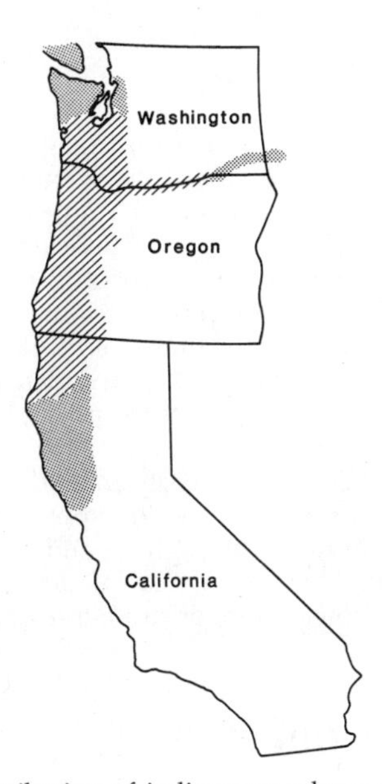

Figure 27–1. Distribution of indigenous salmon poisoning disease. Area indicated by slashed lines represents the distribution of *Oxytrema silicula* and the usual distribution of salmon poisoning disease. Shaded area indicated by dots represents occasional cases of salmon poisoning disease usually resulting from infected migrating fish.

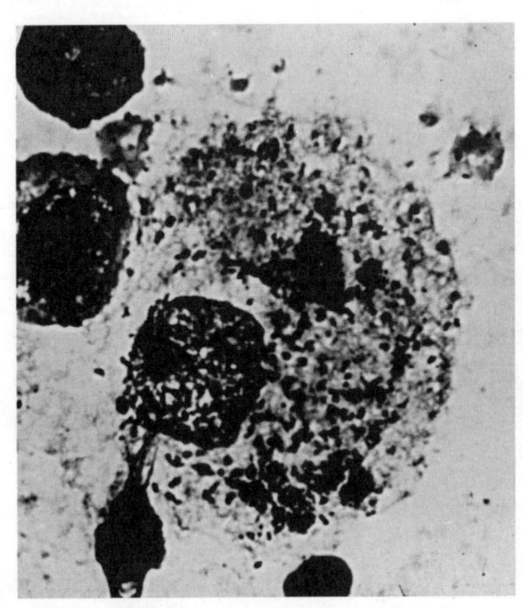

Figure 27–2. *Neorickettsia helminthoeca* in a lymph node smear (Giemsa stain, × 1000).

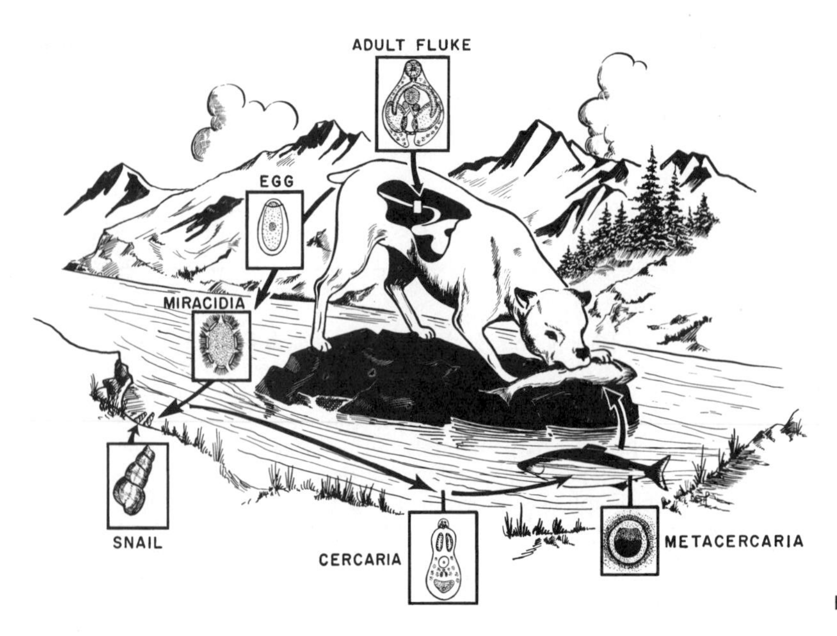

Figure 27–3. Life cycle of *Nanophyetus salmincola.*

EPIDEMIOLOGY

The vector of SPD is a trematode, *Nanophyetus salmincola*, which harbors the rickettsiae throughout its life cycle stages from egg to adult.[9] Three different hosts are required for the completion of the trematode life cycle: snails, fish, and mammals or birds (Fig. 27–3). Lists of intermediate and definitive hosts of the fluke can be found elsewhere.[9] The pleurocerid snail intermediate host, *Oxytrema silicula*, inhabits fresh or brackish stream water in coastal areas of Washington, Oregon, and northern California. Areas of trematode infection, therefore, depend on the distribution of *O. silicula*. Cercariae (free-swimming trematode larvae) leave the snail and penetrate the second intermediate host, which is usually a salmonoid fish, certain species of nonsalmonoid fish, or the Pacific giant salamander *(Dicamptodon ensatus)*. The metacercariae usually localize in the kidneys of fish (Fig. 27–4) but can be found in any tissue. Fish are infected in fresh water and retain the trematode and the rickettsia infection throughout their ocean migration before returning to fresh water up to 3 years later.

Adult trematodes develop in the intestine approximately 6 days after the ingestion of metacercariae-infected fish by dogs and certain other fish-eating mammals, such as bears and raccoons, and birds, which serve as definitive hosts.

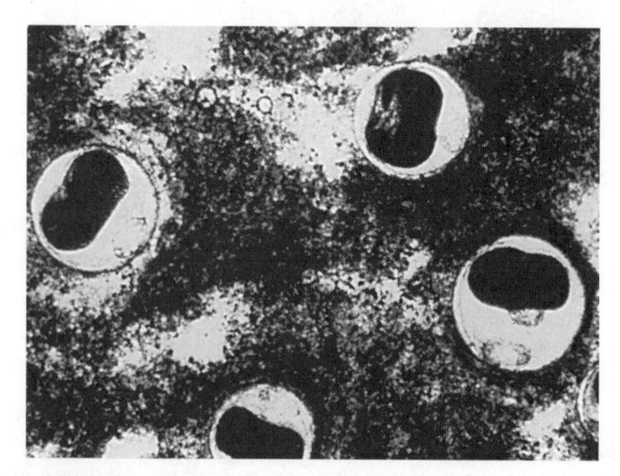

Figure 27–4. Squash preparation of salmon kidney containing numerous metacercariae of *Nanophyetus salmincola* (× 200).

Clinical signs of rickettsial disease occur in Canidae, primarily dogs and coyotes. However, two captive polar bears receiving long-term glucocorticoid therapy for skin conditions succumbed to an SPD-like disease after eating inadequately frozen salmon.[14] Cats are not susceptible to SPD, but trematodes will develop when infected fish are ingested.[9]

SPD also has been transmitted by parenteral injection of infected blood, spleen and lymph suspensions, adult flukes, helminth-infected snail livers, and helminth eggs. Partial transmission success was obtained by allowing ticks (*Haemaphysalis leachi* and *Rhipicephalus sanguineus*) that had fed on infected dogs to subsequently feed on susceptible dogs and by parenteral injection of suspensions of *R. sanguineus* into dogs.[8] Susceptible dogs also have been experimentally infected with aerosolized lymph node suspensions from infected dogs, and on rare occasions direct transmission of infection between dogs has been suspected.[8]

PATHOGENESIS

After ingestion of raw, metacercariae-infected salmonoid fish by a susceptible dog, the fluke matures, and the adult stage attaches to the mucosa of the intestine and by some unknown mechanism inoculates the rickettsiae (Fig. 27–5). Initial replication of rickettsiae probably takes place in the epithelial cells of the villi or in the intestinal lymphoid tissue. Inflammation of the solitary lymphoid follicles and Peyer's patches along the intestinal tract contributes to enteritis. Mild enteritis may be observed in dogs infected only with the flukes, without rickettsiae.

Rickettsiae enter the blood early in the course of the disease and spread to the lymph nodes, spleen, tonsils, thymus, liver, lungs, and brain.[6] Although secondary bacterial infections often occur, the exact cause of death in SPD is unknown. Investigations to demonstrate a toxin have been limited.

CLINICAL FINDINGS

Salmon Poisoning Disease

The signs of infection are consistent in all Canidae with SPD. The usual incubation period after the ingestion of para-

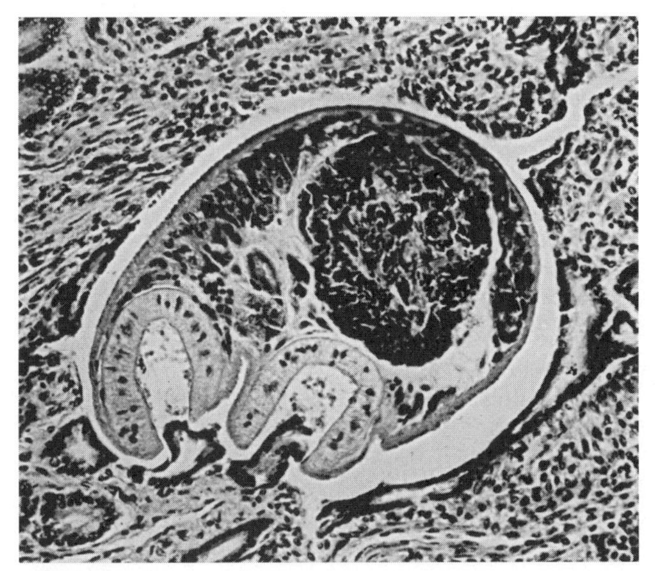

Figure 27–5. *Nanophyetus salmincola* ingesting intestinal mucosa and initiating *Neorickettsia helminthoeca* infection in a dog (H and E, × 300).

sitized fish is 5 to 7 days, although some dogs have incubation periods as long as 19 to 33 days. The first sign usually is a sudden febrile response, which typically reaches a peak of 40° to 42°C (104°–107.6°F) (Fig. 27–6). The temperature gradually decreases to normal or below normal over the next 4 to 8 days. Dogs are frequently hypothermic when death occurs 7 to 10 days after the initial clinical evidence of infection. Some animals show only a slight increase in temperature or a shortened febrile period; however, they may still die if untreated.

Anorexia frequently accompanies or follows the onset of fever and may be marked and complete. Affected animals often continue to have inappetence throughout the course of the disease. Marked weight loss, weakness, and depression usually follow. Within 14 days of eating infected fish, coyotes on a controlled experiment lost approximately 58% of their body weight compared with uninfected coyotes.[8] Diarrhea and vomiting may occur; the diarrhea becomes progressively worse and often consists primarily of blood at the time of death. The animal will occasionally exhibit extreme thirst and will drink copious quantities of water. A serous nasal discharge may be recorded early in the febrile period. Later a mucopurulent conjunctival exudate may be seen. Enlarged cervical and prescapular lymph nodes can be palpated as early as 5 days PI.

SPD-infected dogs may show severe GI signs that are often clinically indistinguishable from canine parvovirus enteritis. Distemper and SPD can also occur concurrently, and appropriate laboratory tests can be conducted to determine which agent is involved in a particular animal.

Elokomin Fluke Fever

The incubation period is generally 5 to 12 days. The febrile period, which differs from that of SPD, is marked by a plateau of elevated temperature lasting 4 to 7 days, followed by a decline, usually to subnormal temperature. Other signs are similar to those of SPD.

DIAGNOSIS

Operculated trematode eggs appear in dog feces 5 to 8 days after the ingestion of infected fish. The light brown egg is approximately 87 to 97 μm × 35 to 55 μm in size, with a small, blunt point on the end opposite the indistinct operculum (Fig. 27–7). Eggs can be detected on direct smears or by a washing-sedimentation technique.[2] In addition, we have routinely recovered *N. salmincola* eggs with the standard sugar flotation technique (specific gravity, 1.27). Eggs recovered by this latter method are somewhat deformed but recognizable. Diagnosis of the rickettsial disease cannot be based entirely on the presence of trematode eggs in feces, because trematode infection does not necessarily indicate rickettsial infection. In addition, animals that have recovered from the rickettsial disease may be reinfected with the trematode. The trematode infection can remain patent for 60 to 250 days.[5]

Fluid aspirated from enlarged lymph nodes can be air dried on a microscope slide, fixed, defatted for 1 minute with a mixture of equal parts of ether and absolute alcohol, and then stained by Giemsa or Macchiavellos stain. In addition, a rapid-staining Giemsa technique can be used that involves staining the fixed smears for 2 minutes with equal parts of stock Giemsa and buffered water at pH 7.2 and then washing

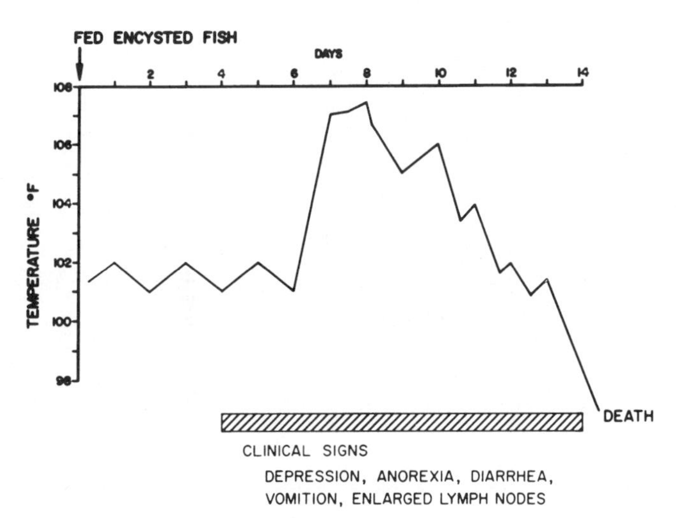

Figure 27–6. Clinical course of salmon poisoning disease in a dog.

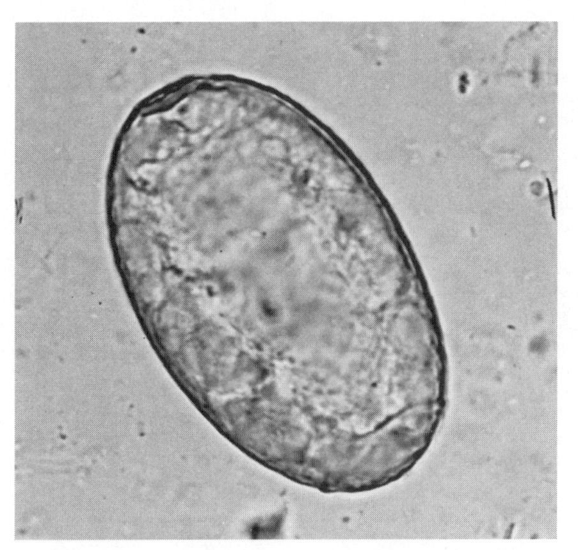

Figure 27–7. Egg of *Nanophyetus salmincola* (× 480).

the slides.[8] Typical intracytoplasmic rickettsial bodies are characteristically seen in MPS cells (see Fig. 27–2). Extracellular organisms are not easily separated from artifacts and should not be considered diagnostic for SPD.

Hematologic and biochemical findings of SPD-infected domestic dogs are often nonspecific, and total leukocyte counts have ranged from those for leukopenia to leukocytosis. Laboratory results[10] of 45 dogs representing 17 breeds and various mixed breeds that were naturally infected with SPD are listed in Table 27–1. Among the dogs tested, the most consistent findings were thrombocytopenia (88%), lymphopenia (77%), eosinophilia (77%), increased alkaline phosphatase (ALP) (64%), and reduced serum albumin (49%).[10] In experimentally infected coyotes, significantly higher numbers of band cells, lower numbers of eosinophils, and lower concentrations of serum creatinine, glucose, calcium, inorganic phosphorus, albumin, and ALP were detected compared with uninfected coyotes.[5]

PATHOLOGIC FINDINGS

The principal gross findings at necropsy are changes in lymphoid tissues. The tonsils, thymus, and visceral and somatic nodes are markedly enlarged. The most pronounced swelling occurs in the ileocecal, colic, mesenteric, portal, and lumbar nodes. The nodes are usually yellowish, with prominent white foci representing the cortical follicles. Occasionally, nodes show diffuse petechiae, and edema is often observed.

The spleen frequently ranges from slightly swollen to nearly twice the normal size. Splenic follicles, which often appear as grayish-white nodules in foxes, are unaffected in dogs. The spleens of animals that die of SPD are typically a dark bluish-red, smooth, soft, and blood filled. Livers of dogs are usually normal, although those of foxes are usually soft and pale yellowish-brown. Hemorrhages may appear in the gallbladder wall. Petechiae may be the only change in the pancreas. The kidneys of dogs are grossly normal, whereas those of foxes may have a slight color change toward a pale yellowish-brown. The mucosa of the urinary bladder may show petechiae.

Along the intestinal tract, petechiae may be apparent in the mucosae of the lower esophagus, large intestine, ileocolic valve, distal colon, rectum, and gastric serosa. There may be bleeding ulcers in the pylorus. Intussusception of the ileum in the colon may also occur. The intestinal contents frequently contain free blood. Some blood may also appear in the colon and rectum. The intestines are typically empty except for some bile-stained mucus. Flukes in the intestinal tissue, primarily found in the duodenum, cause some tissue damage.

Microscopically, a characteristic pattern is observed in lymphocytic tissues. The lymph nodes show a marked and consistent depletion in the number of mature lymphocytes, with hyperplasia of the MPS cells in the cortex and medulla. In most foxes and dogs, there are foci of necrosis in the MPS cells. The CNS is usually involved with nonsuppurative meningitis or meningoencephalitis.

THERAPY

All patients should be hospitalized so that they can receive adequate monitoring and nursing care. Control of the rickettsia can be achieved with oral or parenteral sulfonamide, penicillin, chlortetracycline, chloramphenicol, doxycycline, or oxytetracycline. Aminoglycosides are ineffective. The preferred treatment schedule is parenteral oxytetracycline given for at least 3 days (Table 27–2). Oral doxycycline or tetracycline therapy, used for most rickettsial diseases, may be contraindicated because of the severe vomiting and diarrhea that are usually present.

Relief of dehydration, emesis, and diarrhea is also important. Fluid therapy with appropriate electrolytes should

Table 27–1. Results of Initial Laboratory Tests in Dogs With Salmon Poisoning (N = 45)

	NORMAL RANGE	MAXIMUM	MINIMUM	MEAN	SD	NO. ABOVE NR*	NO. BELOW NR*	NO. OF DOGS
Leukocytes/μl	6000–17,000	66,000	4200	12,800	10,600	6	6	44
Mature neutrophils/μl	3000–11,500	62,604	1792	10,908	10,296	13	1	44
Band neutrophils/μl	0–300	2548	0	168	430	8	0	44
Lymphocytes/μl	1000–4800	3776	92	791	667	0	34	44
Eosinophils/μl	100–1250	891	0	77	202	0	34	44
Monocytes/μl	150–1350	4137	0	824	811	10	0	44
Packed cell volume (%)	37–55	54	25	43	7	1	8	43
Platelet counts $\times 10^3$/dl	200–500	377	16	113	108	0	14	16
Fibrinogen (mg/dl)	200–400	700	100	400	160	14	3	38
Serum sodium (mEq/L)	145–154	159	126	141	8	1	13	16
Serum potassium (mEq/L)	4.1–5.3	5.3	3.4	4.4	.5	0	3	16
Serum chloride (mEq/L)	105–116	134	84	106	12	1	4	14
Total carbon dioxide	16–26	24	15	18	3	0	4	10
Serum calcium (mg/dl)	9.9–11.4	10.8	7.3	9.1	0.9	0	30	37
Serum phosphorus (mg/dl)	3.0–6.2	7.9	3.0	4.8	1.5	7	0	36
Creatinine (mg/dl)	0.8–1.6	1.7	0.5	1.1	.5	2	2	17
Blood urea nitrogen (mg/dl)	8–31	90	9	22	19	6	0	37
Serum glucose (mg/dl)	70–118	133	44	92	17	4	2	37
Alanine aminotransferase (IU/L)	19–102	499	21	92	83	9	0	37
Aspartate aminotransferase (IU/L)	15–66	274	24	90	60	17	0	35
Alkaline phosphatase (IU/L)	15–150	2098	60	254	339	23	0	36
Total protein (g/dl)	5.4–7.4	8.2	3.9	5.9	1.1	4	11	37
Albumin (g/dl)	2.5–3.5	3.3	1.6	2.5	0.4	0	18	37
Total bilirubin (mg/dl)	0–0.4	2.0	0	0.4	0.6	4	0	37
Globulins (mg/dl)	2.9–3.9	5.8	1.9	3.4	0.9	9	10	37
Cholesterol (mg/dl)	135–300	408	99	215	85	8	6	37
Age (years)		12	0.3	5.0	3.7			

*NR = normal range.

From Mack RE, Becovitch MG, Ling GV, et al: *Calif Vet* 44:42–45, 1990. Reprinted with permission.

Table 27–2. Therapy for Salmon Poisoning Disease

DRUG	DOSE[a] (mg/kg)	ROUTE	INTERVAL (HOURS)	DURATION (DAYS)
Oxytetracycline[b]	7	IV[c]	8	3–5
Doxycycline[b]	10	IV,[c] PO	12	7
Tetracycline[b]	22	PO	8	3–5
Praziquantel[d]	10–30	PO, SC	Once	—

[a]Dose per administration at specified interval.
[b]For rickettsial infection.
[c]Parenteral therapy preferred because of GI signs.
[d]For fluke infection.

be administered IV. In cases of hemorrhagic diarrhea, transfusion of whole blood may be necessary. Other antidiarrheal treatments include fasting followed by gradual introduction of a bland, high-calorie diet. In addition, the most supportive treatment consists of keeping the dog dry, clean, and warm.

Praziquantel, when given as one dose at appropriate dosages (see Table 27–2), is highly effective against the fluke in coyotes and dogs.[4] Elimination of the fluke from infected animals will minimize the diarrhea associated from trematode infections alone and will minimize or eliminate fluke eggs from feces.

PREVENTION

Vaccines have not been developed against SPD; therefore, keeping dogs from feeding on infected fish is the best means of preventing infection. Because metacercariae can remain viable for months in rotting fish carcasses, dogs will become infected with the fluke if they eat decomposed fish; however, they may not develop SPD. In many areas, metacercariae apparently contain nonpathogenic rickettsiae. Freezing fish at −20°C for 24 hours or thoroughly cooking infected fish will kill both the metacercariae and rickettsiae.[8] Supplemental prevention methods include isolation of dogs with SPD and sterilization of equipment used around infected dogs.

Infection of fish in hatcheries can be prevented by using water that snails do not inhabit. However, this practice is not possible in most hatcheries except those that use drilled well water rather than stream water. Other control techniques such as snail elimination are impractical.

References

1. Booth AJ, Stogdale L, Grigor JA. 1984. Salmon poisoning disease in dogs on southern Vancouver Island. *Can Vet J* 25:2–6.
2. Bosman DD, Farrell RK, Gorham JR. 1970. Non-endoparasite transmission of salmon poisoning disease of dogs. *J Am Vet Med Assoc* 156:1907–1910.
3. Farrell RK, Ott RL, Gorham JR. 1955. The clinical laboratory diagnosis of salmon poisoning. *J Am Vet Med Assoc* 127:241–244.
4. Foreyt WJ, Gorham JR. 1987. Evaluation of praziquantel against induced *Nanophyetus salmincola* infections in coyotes and dogs. *Am J Vet Res* 48:563–565.
5. Foreyt WJ, Gorham JR, Green JS, et al. 1987. Salmon poisoning disease in juvenile coyotes: clinical evaluation and infectivity of metacercariae and rickettsiae. *J Wildl Dis* 23:412–417.
6. Frank DW, McGuire TC, Gorham JR, et al. 1974. Lymphoreticular lesions of canine rickettsiosis. *J Infect Dis* 129:163–171.
7. Gorham JR. 1996. Unpublished data. Washington State University.
8. Gorham JR, Foreyt WJ. 1990. Salmon poisoning disease, pp 397–403. *In* Greene CE (ed), Infectious diseases of the dog and cat. WB Saunders, Philadelphia, PA.
9. Knapp SE, Millemann RE. 1981. Salmon poisoning disease, pp 376–387. *In* Davis JW (ed), Infectious diseases of wild mammals. Iowa State University Press, Ames, IA.
10. Mack RE, Becovitch MG, Ling GV, et al. 1990. Salmon disease complex in dogs—a review of 45 cases. *Calif Vet* 44:42–45.
11. Rikihisa Y. 1991. Cross-reacting antigens between *Neorickettsia helminthoeca* and *Ehrlichia* spp. shown by immunofluorescence and Western immunoblotting. *J Clin Microbiol* 29:2024.
12. Rikihisa Y, Stills H, Zimmerman G. 1991. Isolation and continuous culture of *Neorickettsia helminthoeca* in a macrophage cell line. *J Clin Microbiol* 29:1928.
13. Schalm OW. 1978. Leukocyte counts and lymph node cytology in salmon poisoning of dogs. *Canine Pract* 5:59–63.
14. Schmidt M. 1982. Personal communication. Portland, OR.

Chapter 28

Ehrlichiosis

Canine Monocytic and Granulocytic Ehrlichiosis

T. Mark Neer

ETIOLOGY AND EPIDEMIOLOGY

Ehrlichiosis is a tick-borne disease caused by obligate intracellular parasites of the genus *Ehrlichia* of the family Rickettsiaceae (Fig. 28–1). Table 28–1 summarizes the ehrlichial species known to cause disease in animals throughout the world. These species can be tentatively divided into three classes based on the host cells they infect: mononuclear, granulocytic, and thrombocytic elements. Species such as *E. chaffeensis*, *E. risticii*, and *E. phagocytophila* may infect more than one cell type. The arthropod vectors and domestic animal hosts are known for many species, but epidemiologic information, including potential wild or domestic animal reservoir hosts, remains to be elucidated. The following discussion focuses on *E. canis* for which there is the most information.

Vertebrate hosts for *E. canis* have been limited to members of the family Canidae. The coyote, fox, and jackal, in addition

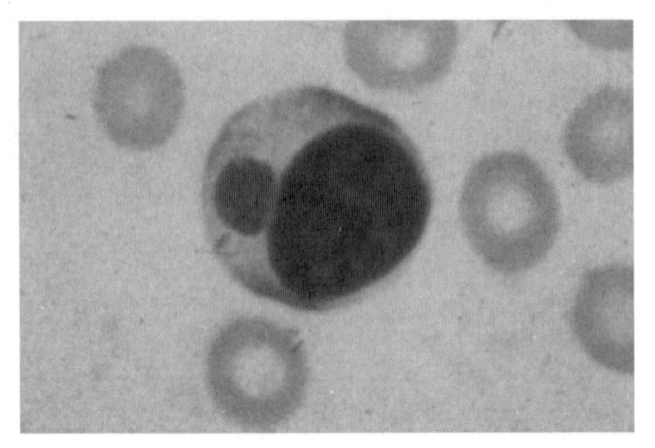

Figure 28–1. A mononuclear leukocyte containing a compact *E. canis* morula in the cytoplasm.

to the domestic dog, are considered reservoir hosts. The arthropod vector of *E. canis* is the brown dog tick, *Rhipicephalus sanguineus*, with strict transstadial transmission. Because transovarial spread does not occur, the vector tick cannot be a true reservoir. Ticks acquire *E. canis* by feeding, as either larvae or nymphs, on rickettsemic dogs and transmit the infection as nymphs or adults. Adult ticks can survive for up to 568 days and transmit infection to susceptible dogs for at least 155 days after infection. This permits the vector and pathogen to overwinter and then infest and infect susceptible dogs the next spring. The minimal time required for tick attachment to transmit infection has not been established, although it is less likely for ticks to become infected by feeding on a dog in the chronic phase of the disease.

PATHOGENESIS

The majority of information concerning pathogenesis is also related to *E. canis*. Infection of the vertebrate host occurs when an infected tick ingests a blood meal and salivary secretions contaminate the feeding site. Blood transfusions from infected donors can also transmit the organism. The subsequent course of ehrlichiosis has been divided into three phases — acute, subclinical, and chronic — based on clinical signs and clinicopathologic abnormalities. However, with

Table 28–1. Ehrlichial Species Infecting People and Domestic or Laboratory Animals

SPECIES (DISEASES)	GEOGRAPHIC DISTRIBUTION	VECTOR	LEUKOCYTES INFECTED	NATURALLY INFECTED HOST	EXPERIMENTALLY INFECTED HOST
Monocytic					
E. canis (canine monocytic ehrlichiosis)	Worldwide, tropical and temperate	*Rhipicephalus sanguineus*	Mononuclear cells, lymphocytes	Canidae	None
E. chaffeensis (human monocytic ehrlichiosis)	U.S. (primarily southern)	*Amblyomma americanum, Dermacentor variabilis*	Mononuclear cells, neutrophils, lymphocytes	Humans, dogs, deer	Dogs, white-tailed deer, white-footed mice
Venezuelan human ehrlichiosis agent	Venezuela	?	Mononuclear cells	Humans, dogs?	Mice
E. sennetsu (Sennetsu fever)	Western Japan, Malaysia	?	Mononuclear cells	Humans	Mice, dogs, nonhuman primates
E. risticii (equine monocytic ehrlichiosis)	U.S., Canada	?	Monocytes	Horses	Dogs, cats, mice, nonhuman primates
E. risticii (subsp. *atypicalis*)	U.S.	?	Monocytes, mast cells, enterocytes	Dogs	?
E. bovis (bovine ehrlichiosis)	Middle East, Africa	*Hyalomma* spp., *Rhipicephalus* spp.	Monocytes, macrophages	Cattle	?
Granulocytic					
E. ewingii (canine granulocytic ehrlichiosis)	U.S.	*A. americanum*?, *Otobius megnini*?	Neutrophils, eosinophils	Dogs	?
E. equi[a] (equine granulocytic ehrlichiosis)	U.S. (West Coast)	*Ixodes pacificus*	Neutrophils, eosinophils	Horses, dogs, humans, llamas	Burros, sheep, dogs, goat, cats, nonhuman primates
Human granulocytic ehrlichiosis agent (*E. microti?*)[a]	U.S. (upper Midwest, Northeast)	*I. scapularis* (northern)	Neutrophils	Humans, horses, dogs, white-footed mice, chipmunks, voles	Mice, deer
E. phagocytophila[a] (tick-borne fever)	Great Britain, Europe,[b] Africa, Asia	*I. ricinus*	Neutrophils, eosinophils, monocytes	Sheep, cattle, bison, dogs, deer, llamas, humans	Guinea pigs, mice
Thrombocytic					
E. platys (infectious canine cyclic thrombocytopenia)	Southern U.S., Southern Europe	*R. sanguineus*?	Platelets	Dogs	Dogs
Other					
Cowdria ruminantium[c] (Heartwater)	Sub-Saharan Africa	*A. hebraeum*	Endothelial cells, macrophages, neutrophils	Cattle	Dogs

? = uncertain.

[a]May all be geographic variants of the same species. Granulocytic ehrlichiosis has been also identified in horses in Florida and deer in the southeastern U.S.

[b]Reports of human granulocytic ehrlichiosis (from serologic and PCR detection) from Sweden, Switzerland, Great Britain, Belgium, Spain, in countries where Lyme borreliosis transmitted by *I. ricinus* is also present.[51]

[c]Genetic relatedness to *E. canis* indicates reconsidered classification in the tribe *Ehrlichiae.*

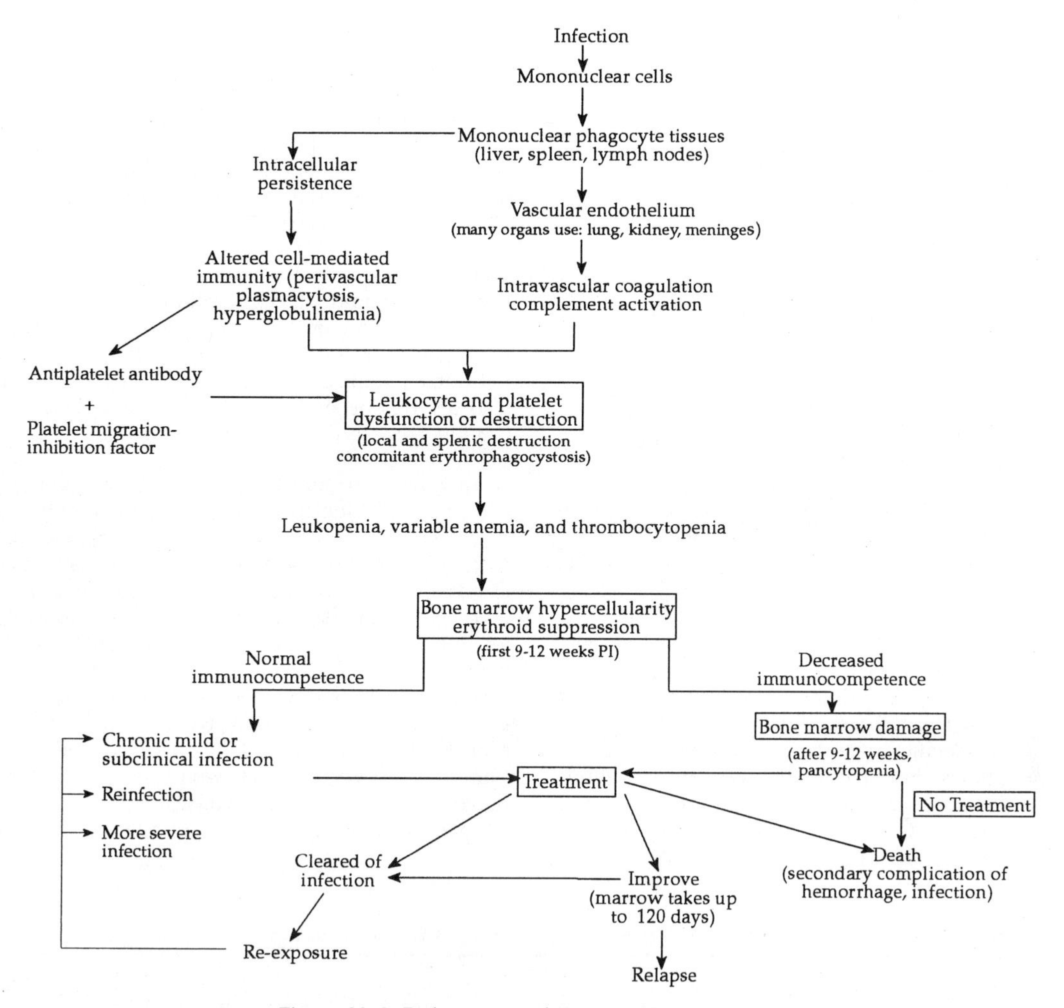

Figure 28–2. Pathogenesis of *E. canis* infection in dogs.

naturally occurring cases, accurate staging of the disease is difficult.

The *acute phase* begins after an incubation period of 8 to 20 days and lasts 2 to 4 weeks, during which the organisms multiply in mononuclear cells by binary fission, spreading throughout the body (Fig. 28–2). Hematologic changes are associated with immune and coagulatory processes triggered by the infection. Nonspecific signs such as fever, oculonasal discharge, anorexia, depression, weight loss, and lymphadenomegaly may be seen. Laboratory abnormalities include thrombocytopenia and variable mild leukopenia and anemia. The acute phase usually resolves spontaneously, and then the *subclinical phase* of 40 to 120 days begins. During this phase, the dog's weight normalizes and the pyrexia resolves; clinically, the dog appears normal.[136, 137] In naturally infected dogs, the subclinical phase has the potential to persist for years. If infected dogs are immunocompetent, they may be able to eliminate *E. canis*. If not, the *chronic phase* of infection develops. This phase can be mild, appearing as vague illness and weight loss with less severe hematologic changes. The severe chronic form is characterized by impaired bone marrow production of blood elements, resulting in pancytopenia. The severity of the disease is greater with certain strains of the organism, concomitant disease, breed (e.g., German shepherd), and younger animals.

Various mechanisms exist for the thrombocytopenia and thrombocytopathy that occur. In the acute phase, immunologic and inflammatory mechanisms are involved with increased platelet consumption, and platelet half-life is decreased, probably as a result of splenic sequestration. Platelet-associated IgG and antibodies that recognize platelet proteins in dogs with *E. canis* infection may play a role in the thrombocytopenia.[61, 71] In addition, a serum cytokine, called platelet migration–inhibition factor (PMIF), has been found to exist in dogs with ehrlichiosis, and its level is related inversely to the platelet count.[1] Higher levels of PMIF are associated with more virulent strains of *E. canis* (Fig. 28–3). PMIF inhibits platelet migration and is produced by lymphocytes when they are exposed to infected monocytes. Platelet function, as measured by aggregation responses, is decreased in conjunction with the low platelet count, contributing to the hemorrhage.[69–71] Gammopathy may result in thrombocytopathia in some infected dogs.[134a]

CLINICAL FINDINGS

Canine ehrlichiosis is a multisystemic disorder that is now known to be caused by a variety of rickettsial species. In the past, all clinical reports of this disease confirmed by cytologic or serologic means have been attributed to *E. canis* infections. Cases diagnosed cytologically as "granulocytic strain" infections in the United States may have been caused by the human granulocytic ehrlichiosis (HGE) agent, by *E. equi*, or by *E. ewingii*. Because of cross-reactivity with *E. canis*, serologically confirmed cases could have been caused by *E.*

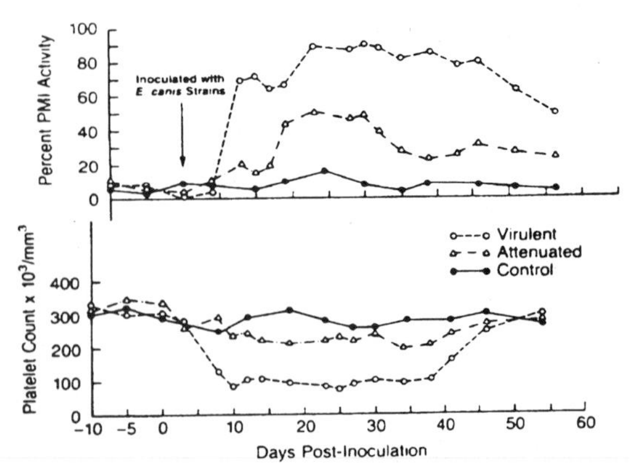

Figure 28–3. Graphs showing the temporal relationship between platelet counts and platelet migration inhibition (PMI) activity after infection with different strains of *E. canis* (From Abeygunawardena I, Kakoma I, Smith RD: *In* Williams JC, Kakoma I (eds): *Ehrlichiosis.* Dordrecht, 1990, pp 78–92. Reprinted with permission from Kluwer Academic Publishers.)

chaffeensis or *E. ewingii*. For this reason, the following discussion first categorizes previously published clinical features based on body systems and primarily focuses on *E. canis* infection. It then describes clinical features that have now been attributed to specific organisms other than *E. canis*. Table 28–2 differentiates clinical and laboratory abnormalities of individual ehrlichial species based on experimental and clinical observations.

Multisystemic Signs. A common presentation is depression, lethargy, mild weight loss, and anorexia with or without hemorrhagic tendencies. If present, the bleeding is usually manifested by dermal petechiae and/or ecchymoses. Although bleeding can occur from any mucosal surface, epistaxis is most frequent. Physical examination of these patients may also reveal lymphadenomegaly and splenomegaly in 20% and 25% of the patients, respectively.[145]

Ocular Signs. Dogs may show changes in eye color or appearance or may develop blindness. Anterior uveitis and retinal disease (such as chorioretinitis, papilledema, retinal hemorrhage, retinal perivascular infiltrates, and bullous retinal detachment) are the more common findings. Uveitis has also been associated with *E. platys* infection in the dog (see Canine Thrombocytic Ehrlichiosis).

Neuromuscular Signs. The neurologic signs of ehrlichiosis are primarily due to meningitis from inflammation and/or bleeding. Neurologic dysfunction occurs with damage to the adjacent central or peripheral nervous tissue. Infections with *E. canis* and granulocytic strains have been most common,[93, 133] and signs are indistinguishable from those of RMSF (see Chapter 29). Seizures, stupor, ataxia with upper or lower motor neuron dysfunction, acute central or peripheral vestibular dysfunction, anisocoria, cerebellar dysfunction, intention tremor, and generalized or localized hyperesthesia have been observed. Morulae have been found in cells from the CSF in some instances.[93, 101] Two dogs that were seropositive for *E. canis* had polymyositis, and the signs consisted of acute-onset progressive tetraparesis, hyporeflexia, and muscle wasting.[29] Skeletal mus-

Table 28–2. Comparison of Naturally Occurring Canine Disease Caused by Various Ehrlichial Species

SPECIES	REPORTED GEOGRAPHIC ISOLATIONS	CLINICAL FEATURES	LABORATORY ABNORMALITIES	REFERENCES
Monocytic				
E. canis	Worldwide	Fever, anorexia, weight loss, hemorrhagic diathesis, CNS signs, lymphadenomegaly	Anemia, leukopenia, marked thrombocytopenia, hyperglobulinemia, pancytopenia, proteinuria	67a, 68, 133
E. risticii (subsp. *atypicalis*)	U.S.	Fever, lethargy, hemorrhagic diathesis, edema, polyarthritis	Anemia, thrombocytopenia	81, 82
Granulocytic				
E. ewingii	Southern and lower mideastern U.S., Missouri	Fever, anorexia, lameness, polyarthritis	Mild thrombocytopenia Mild nonregenerative anemia	129, 130
Human granulocytic ehrlichiosis agent[a]	Upper midwestern U.S. (Minnesota, Wisconsin), northeastern U.S., Switzerland[b]	Fever, lethargy, splenomegaly hepatomegaly, CNS signs, lameness	Thrombocytopenia, mild hypoalbuminemia, increased serum ALP activity, increased serum amylase, proteinuria, occasional neutropenia or regenerative left shift	65, 80
E. phagocytophila[a]	Sweden, Great Britain, Switzerland[b]	Fever, anorexia, depression, lameness, lymphadenomegaly, limb edema	Thrombocytopenia	37, 54, 54a, 74, 80, 94a, 113b
E. equi[a]	California, Oklahoma	Fever, anorexia, limb edema, CNS signs	Leukopenia, thrombocytopenia	89, 90
Thrombocytic				
E. platys	U.S., Greece, France, Italy, Israel[c]	Mild fever, uveitis, petechia and ecchymoses, skin and mucosal hemorrhage	Thrombocytopenia	67, 72

[a]May all be geographic variants of the same species. It has been termed the *E. phagocytophilia* genogroup.
[b]Genetic analysis of Swiss isolates from two dogs showed 100% homology to HGE agent;[113b] similar isolates have been detected in people in Europe.[112a]
[c]Clinical manifestations of infected dogs in Israel were more severe than in other reports.[67]
ALP = alkaline phosphatase.

cles were atrophic and characterized histologically by lymphoplasmacytic and immature lymphoreticular cellular infiltrates within areas of necrosis. Unfortunately, the histopathology of peripheral nerves was not reported.

Polyarthritis. Dogs with ehrlichiosis may develop lameness with a stiff gait secondary to polyarthropathy. Joint disease may occur from hemarthrosis or immune complex deposition with resultant arthritis and neutrophilic effusion into the joint. Most instances of polyarthritis have been associated with infection by granulocytic strains or *E. risticii*.[40, 129, 130] When titers have been determined, approximately 81% of the dogs with the granulocytic strain had titers to *E. canis* (which cross-reacts with antibodies to *E. ewingii*), and 8% had titers to *E. equi*.[129]

Species-Specific Signs. Table 28–2 summarizes the clinical and laboratory findings of the various ehrlichial infections in dogs.

E. risticii infection can be experimentally established in dogs and cats, producing minimal clinical illness.[42, 45, 121] In two of eight cats inoculated with *E. risticii*, mild, self-limiting disease consisting of intermittent diarrhea was seen in one cat, and lymphadenomegaly, acute depression, and anorexia was seen in another.[42] Even though this ehrlichial species appears to cause little if any clinical disease in the dog and cat experimentally, whether this is the same with natural infections has yet to be determined.

In 100 cases of serologically atypical canine ehrlichiosis, with three deaths, the indirect FA test was negative for *E. canis* and *E. sennetsu* but positive for *E. risticii*. Subsequent genetic sequencing techniques characterized an isolated agent to be *E. risticii*.[82] Clinicopathologic findings included vomiting, lethargy, anemia, thrombocytopenia, polyarthropathy, and/or fever. The 100 cases were distributed geographically as follows: California (32), Texas (26), Arizona (16), Illinois (10), Washington State (9), Florida (5), and Michigan (2). A new species name *E. risticii* subsp. *atypicalis* was proposed.[82] If typical signs of ehrlichiosis are present in a dog and it is seronegative for *E. canis*, one should consider evaluation for the presence of antibody titers to *E. risticii*.

E. ewingii causes clinically significant disease in naturally and experimentally infected dogs. The main clinical signs are lameness and joint swelling with stiff gait, all characteristic of polyarthritis.[3, 129] The most common hematologic abnormality is thrombocytopenia.

The **HGE agent**, which is closely related to *E. phagocytophila* and *E. equi*, causes clinical illness in naturally infected dogs, horses, and people.[65–67, 80] In dogs, fever, lethargy, anorexia, splenomegaly, hepatomegaly, lymphadenomegaly, and CNS signs have been most common. The most consistent laboratory findings in HGE agent–infected dogs are thrombocytopenia, lymphopenia, hypoproteinemia, hypoalbuminemia, high serum alkaline phosphatase (ALP) and amylase activities, and proteinuria.

E. equi infections in cats experimentally and dogs both naturally and experimentally have been described. Signs include fever, anorexia, depression, limb edema, and CNS problems.[92] Laboratory findings include leukopenia and thrombocytopenia.

E. phagocytophila has been described to infect dogs and horses in Europe.[80, 94a] Signs include those for *E. equi* and HGE agent such as fever, anorexia, depression, lameness, lymphadenomegaly, and limb edema, and this signalment may reflect the similarity of these ehrlichial species, which may actually be subspecies or strain variants.

E. chaffeensis has been experimentally inoculated into pups, and signs were mild compared with corresponding *E. canis*–inoculated animals.[45] Only fever was apparent. This finding contrasts to the clinical syndrome observed in humans infected with *E. chaffeensis*, which may be related to species differences or attenuation of the agent in cell culture. The clinical significance of natural infections in dogs or cats is unknown. Clinical signs in infected people mimic those of RMSF. Serologic and PCR testing suggested that dogs in animal shelters and kennels in southeastern Virginia are naturally infected.[44]

DIAGNOSIS

The diagnosis of ehrlichiosis is usually made on the basis of a combination of clinical signs, hematologic abnormalities, thrombocytopenias, and serology findings.

Hematology. Hematologic changes are best documented for infections caused by *E. canis* and include anemia (82%), which is usually nonregenerative, thrombocytopenia (82%), and leukopenia (32%, of which 20% had neutropenia).[133, 135] Pancytopenia is usually a result of hypoplasia of all bone marrow precursor cells and occurs in the severe chronic phase (18% of the cases) and more often in German shepherd dogs.[145]

Thrombocytopenia has been a consistently reported finding in all stages of *E. canis* ehrlichiosis; however, because it is often a screening test for ehrlichiosis, this proportion may be overestimated. Ehrlichiosis should never be ruled out simply because the platelet count is normal. Serology should be performed if other clinical signs are compatible.

Granular lymphocytosis has been observed with *E. canis* infection.[139] Affected dogs had absolute lymphocyte counts ranging from 5200 to 17,200 cells/μl and granularity to their cytoplasm typical of well-differentiated lymphocytic leukemia. Some of these dogs had monoclonal gammopathies, which could further mislead one to a diagnosis of lymphocytic leukemia.

Biochemistry. The most frequent serum chemistry abnormalities have included hyperproteinemia (33%), hyperglobulinemia (39%), hypoalbuminemia (43%), and elevated alanine aminotransferase and ALP activities (43% and 31%, respectively). The hyperproteinemia results from elevated globulin levels, but there is no direct correlation between the levels of serum globulins and serum antibodies. The serum electrophoresis generally shows a polyclonal hyperglobulinemia,[68] although monoclonal gammopathies occur. An *E. canis* antibody titer should be performed in all dogs in which a diagnosis of benign monoclonal gammopathy is contemplated or in which definitive evidence of myeloma, leukemia, or macroglobulinemia is lacking. Infected dogs with pancytopenia generally have lower serum γ-globulin concentrations compared with nonpancytopenic dogs.[68] Dogs with *E. canis* often have plasmacytosis in the bone marrow or sometimes other tissues, which can be confused with plasma cell myeloma.

Other clinicopathologic findings include proteinuria, hematuria, prolonged bleeding time (even in some dogs that have normal platelet counts), and pulmonary interstitial radiopacity ranging from a mild linear pattern to marked interstitial infiltration with peribronchial opacities. Experimentally, peak urine protein loss, consisting principally of albumin, is observed 2.5 to 3.5 weeks after inoculation and resolves by 6 weeks after infection.[38, 39] During the peak loss, urine protein/creatinine ratios ranged from 4.5 to 23.2 (normal ratio < 1.0). There was a corresponding drop in serum albumin concentrations (mean 2.1 g/dl). CSF analysis in dogs with signs of CNS disease has revealed increased protein level and predominant lymphocytic pleocytosis similar to that found in viral infection. Comparable CSF findings have been noted in human ehrlichiosis.[114]

A definitive diagnosis of ehrlichial disease can be made by demonstration of morulae in leukocytes from blood smears or tissue aspirates such as spleen, lung, and lymph node. The finding of morulae is difficult and time consuming, but may be optimized by performing buffy coat smears or examining thin blood smears made from a peripheral capillary bed of the ear margin. Morulae may be visualized within neutrophils present in peripheral blood smears and/or within synovial fluid (Fig. 28–4).

Serology. A diagnosis of ehrlichiosis is usually based on positive results of the indirect FA test. This test detects serum antibodies as early as 7 days after initial infection, although some dogs may not become seropositive until 28 days after infection begins. Serum antibody levels in untreated dogs peak at 80 days after infection. During the first 7 days PI the titer consists of IgA and IgM, and by 20 days the majority is IgG. Most laboratories measure this antibody. An IgG titer of 20 or greater is generally considered to be evidence of infection and/or exposure, but this finding may vary with each laboratory's methods. Conversely, because of measurable titer persistence after treatment or potential recovery, a positive titer does not necessarily mean that the animal's disease or clinical symptoms are strictly due to ehrlichiosis, especially in endemic areas where there are animals with titers to *E. canis* and no clinical signs.

In one study, 20.3% of healthy kennel dogs had antibody titers to *E. canis*. I have dealt with at least 12 dogs during the last 10 years in which platelet counts were less than 50,000/μl, each had positive titers to *E. canis* and no increase in platelet numbers with tetracycline therapy, but all had dramatic platelet count increases in response to immunosuppressive doses of glucocorticoids. These dogs most likely had immune-mediated thrombocytopenia coincidentally or as a result of exposure to *E. canis*. They developed antiplatelet antibodies, but at the time were not clinically affected by the *Ehrlichia* infection.

After treatment, in most dogs, the titer progressively declines and generally becomes negative in 6 to 9 months. Some dogs may become asymptomatic after therapy, but yet retain very high titers to *E. canis* for years.[15, 111] Whether the organism or antibody persistence is occurring cannot always be determined.[15] Clinically treated dogs are assumed to have eliminated the organism if hyperglobulinemia and other clinical and laboratory abnormalities resolve progressively after treatment.

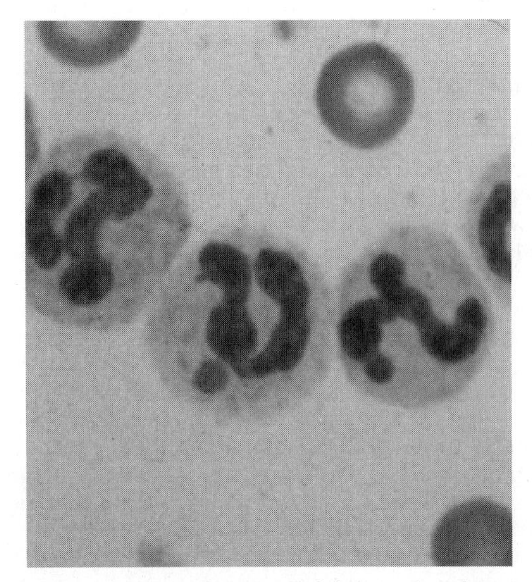

Figure 28–4. A segmented neutrophil from a dog that contains a morula of a granulocytic species of *Ehrlichia.*

Antigenic cross-reactivity exists with *E. canis* organisms in different regions of the world.[73a] Differences can be detected in serologic response by Western immunoblotting. There is also some cross-reactivity between ehrlichial species, which could pose problems in the interpretation of indirect FA serology in certain geographic areas (Table 28–3). Little, if any, cross-reactivity occurs between *E. canis* and *Rickettsia rickettsii*, the etiologic agent of RMSF. Because the clinical presentation of these two diseases is similar, dogs with clinical signs of ehrlichiosis in the absence of a titer to *E. canis* should be tested for RMSF by collecting serum for paired IgG titers, acute and 2-week convalescent serums (see Chapter 29). *Neorickettsia helminthoeca* will cause cross-reactions to *E. canis*, *E. risticii*, and *E. sennetsu* (see Chapter 27).[115] Titers to other *Ehrlichia* should be examined depending on the geographic area and clinical signs. Antibodies to *E. ewingii* cross-react with *E. canis* and *E. chaffeensis*, and the use of one of these antigens will detect infection with either of the three. *E. ewingii* cannot be cultured in vitro beyond isolation in primary cells; therefore, a specific serologic test is not available. Cross-reactive antigens are also present between *E. chaffeensis* and HGE agent using human but not dog sera.[120] *E. equi* will detect infection with HGE agent, or *E. phagocytophila*, and some cross-reactivity exists between *E. risticii* and *E. sennetsu*. In addition to indirect FA, ELISA has been developed to detect antibodies in dogs to *E. canis* and circulating antigen.[59]

Immunoblotting and PCR. On a research basis, Western immunoblotting and PCR have been used to characterize and distinguish between different organisms causing ehrlichiosis and may prove clinically helpful in the future.[24, 44, 73a, 76, 78, 82, 97, 115, 118, 151] The immunoblots for *E. canis* show a number of reacting antigens, the most prominent being those separating in a broad band at 27 kd (22–29 kd).[73a, 97] Western immunoblotting will detect *E. canis* antibodies as early as 2 to 8 days after exposure, and PCR tests have positive results as early as 4 to 10 days after exposure to *E. canis* in experimental studies.[76, 140a] The indirect FA test also becomes positive within a similar time frame. From a practical clinical standpoint, the indirect FA test will continue to be the initial screening test of choice. Western immunoblotting has also been useful in distinguishing between infections with *E. canis* and *E. ewingii*.[118] This characteristic is beneficial because most dogs with *E. ewingii* infection will have positive indirect FA titers to *E. canis*, and there is no indirect FA test available for *E. ewingii*.

PCR has been shown to be a sensitive method for detection of acute *E. canis* infection in dogs.[56, 100] PCR testing has also been used to determine that HGE is caused by *E. phagocytophila*, *E. equi*, or a closely related *Ehrlichia* sp.[11, 36] In addition, if PCR becomes more refined, it may prove useful in distinguishing some treated animals with persistent *E. canis* infection from those with persistent high indirect FA titers after successful treatment.[78, 140a]

PATHOLOGIC FINDINGS

Gross pathologic findings of *E. canis*–infected dogs include petechial and ecchymotic hemorrhages on the serosal and mucosal surfaces of most organs, including the nasal cavity, lung, kidney, urinary bladder, GI tract, and SC tissue. Gener-

***Table 28–3. Serologic Cross-Reactivity of* Ehrlichia *in Indirect FA Testing*[a]**

ANTIGEN	DEGREE OF REACTIVITY	SOURCE OF ANTIBODY — Organism Exposure (Type Infection-Host)
Granulocytic		
HGE agent[b]	High	*E. equi* (N-human[120], X-horse[8a])
E. phagocytophila[b]	None	*E. chaffeensis* (N-human)[49]
	High	*E. equi* (X-horse), HGE (N-human)[49]
E. equi[b]	None	*E. risticii* (X-horse), *E. sennetsu* (X-mouse), *Bartonella henselae* (X-mouse), *E. ewingii* (X-dog), *E. canis* (X-dog), *E. chaffeensis* (N-human), *R. rickettsii* (N-human)[49]
	High	HGE agent (N-human,[8a, 142a] N-deer[18a]), *E. phagocytophia* (N-cow)[49]
Monocytic		
E. chaffeensis	None	*E. equi* (X-horse, X-dog), *E. phagocytophila* (N-cow)[49] *R. rickettsii* (N-human), HGE agent (N-human)[49, 142a]; *E. muris* (X-mouse)[110a]
	Low	*E. ewingii* (X-dog, acute)[118, 110a]; *E. canis* (X-dog, acute)[118]
	Intermediate	*E. canis* (X-dog, chronic)[45, 110a]
	High	*E. ewingii* (X-dog, chronic)[44, 49, 118]; VHE agent (N-human)[110a]
E. canis	None	*E. muris* X-mouse[110a]; *E. ewingii* (X-dog, acute)[110a]; atypical agent (N-dog)[82]; *E platys* (N-dog)[94a]
	Low	*E. muris* (X-mouse)[83]; *E. risticii* (X-horse), *E. sennetsu* (X-Horse)[115]; E. ewingii (X-dog, acute)[118], *E. equi* (N-dog, high > 5120 titers)[92a]
	Intermediate	VHE (N-human)[110a]; *E. chaffeensis* (X-dog, acute[118], N-human)[24, 45, 110a]; *Cowdria ruminantium* (X-dog)[85]; *Neorickettsia helminthoeca* (X-dog)[115]
	High	*E. ewingii* (N-dog)[44]; *E. ewingii* (X-dog, chronic)[118], *E. chaffeenis* (X-dog)[45]
VHE agent	None	*E. sennetsu* (X-rabbit), *E. muris* (X-mouse)[110a]
	Low	*E. ewingii* (X-dog), *E. muris* (X-mouse)[110a]
	High	*E. canis* (X-dog), *E. chaffeensis* (N-human)[110a]
E. muris[c]	High	VHE agent (N-human), *E. chaffeensis* (N-human), *E. canis* (X-dog), *E. ewingii* (X-dog)[110a]
E. risticii	Low	*E. canis* (X-dog)[24, 115]; *E. sennetsu* (X-horse)[115]
	High	Atypical canine ehrlichial agent (N-dog)[82] *Neorickettsia helminthoeca* (X-dog)[115]
E. sennetsu	None	*E. phagocytophila* (N-cow), *E. canis* (X-dog), *E. equi* (X-horse), *E. ewingii* (X-dog), HGE agent (N-human), *E. chaffeensis* (N-human), *Rickettsia rickettsii* (N-human)[49]
	Low	*E. canis* (X-dog)[24, 115]; *E. equi* (N-horse)[49]
	High	*E. risticii* (X-horse)[24, 49, 115]; *Neorickettsia helminthoeca* (X-dog)[115]
Thrombocytic		
E. platys	Unknown	Unknown
Other		
Neorickettsia helminthoeca	None	*E. risticii* (horse)[115]
	Low	*E. canis* (X-dog), *E. sennetsu* (X-horse)[115]
Cowdria ruminantium[d]	High	*E. canis* (X-dog)[52, 85]

The assistance of J. Dawson and Y. Rikihisa was appreciated in reviewing this table.
[a]Immunoblotting may help discriminate cross-reactivity.[24, 49, 73a, 82, 118]
[b]These may represent variants of the same or closely-related species (genogroup).
[c]Isolated from a mouse in Japan and has antigenic and genetic similarity to *E. chaffeensis*.
[d]Genetic relatedness to *E. canis* indicates reconsidered classification in the tribe Ehrlichiae.
N = natural; X = experimental infections; all human sera is from naturally occurring disease; HGE = human granulocytic ehrlichiosis; VHE = Venezuelan human ehrlichia.

alized lymphadenomegaly, splenomegaly, and hepatomegaly are present most often during the acute phase.[64] All lymph nodes may be enlarged and have a brownish discoloration. Emaciation with loss of overall body condition is an additional finding in chronic cases. Bone marrow is hypercellular and red in color in the acute phase but, with chronic disease, becomes hypoplastic and pale owing to fatty discoloration.

One of the more characteristic histopathologic findings is a perivascular plasma cell infiltrate in numerous organs, including the lungs, brain, meninges, kidney, lymph nodes, bone marrow, spleen, and sometimes skin or mucosa. The degree of plasma cell infiltrate appears to increase in chronically affected dogs.[133]

In the CNS, there is a multifocal, nonsuppurative meningoencephalitis involving the brain stem, midbrain, and cerebral cortex. Most lesions are located ventrally in the brain stem and around the periventricular gray and white matter.[133] Only a very mild encephalitis of the cerebellum occurs. There may be a marked lymphoplasmacytic cell infiltrate into the meninges, especially around veins. Microscopic meningeal lesions are present in nearly all dogs at necropsy, yet few dogs demonstrate clinical signs of meningitis.

Pulmonary changes in ehrlichiosis are consistent with interstitial pneumonia. Initially, there is subendothelial accumulation of mononuclear cells, and interstitial and alveolar hemorrhages may be present. *E. canis* organisms may be found in septal mononuclear cells and macrophages of the pulmonary vascular endothelium.

Renal lesions include a vasculitis with plasma cell infiltrate localized in the corticomedullary junction. Glomerulonephritis and interstitial plasmacytosis occur in dogs with ehrlichiosis and may account for the proteinuria of some cases. After experimental infection with *E. canis*, there are minimal histologic changes in the kidneys, but ultrastructural examination shows fusion of podocyte processes that coincide with development of proteinuria.[38]

Ehrlichia organisms are difficult to detect histologically in tissues fixed in either formalin or Bouin's solution. Morulae are infrequently observed in mononuclear phagocytic cells of tissues stained with hematoxylin and eosin.[64] The difficulty with which organisms are found histologically may explain why the disease is not frequently diagnosed at necropsy.

Ultrastructurally, morulae in blood monocytes are intracytoplasmic inclusions made up of numerous organisms (Fig.

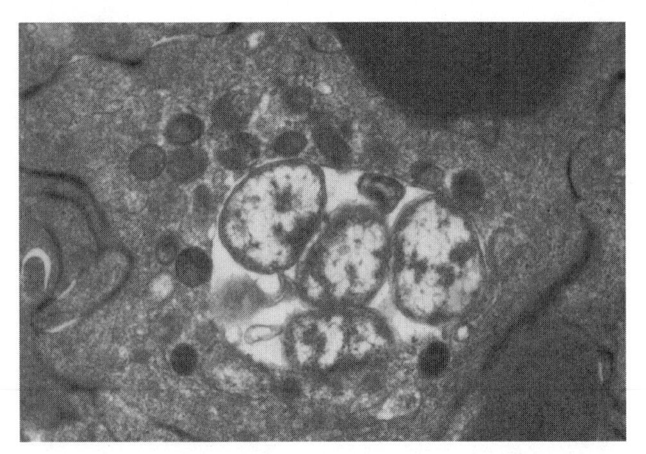

Figure 28–5. Ultrastructure of *E. canis* morula in a monocyte showing that the intracytoplasmic inclusion is made up of numerous organisms.

28–5). The organisms are round, ovoid, or elongated and are surrounded by a double membrane.

THERAPY

The treatment of canine ehrlichiosis consists of antirickettsial agents and supportive care. Successful drugs have included tetracycline, chloramphenicol, imidocarb dipropionate, and amicarbalide (Table 28–4). Generally, the earlier treatment is initiated in the disease process, the more favorable the prognosis and outcome, because dogs in the severe chronic stage are difficult to cure.

Tetracycline and oxytetracycline have been considered the initial drugs of choice in the past and still work well, but doxycycline and minocycline are used more frequently now. Doxycycline and minocycline are semisynthetic, lipid-soluble tetracyclines that are readily absorbed to produce high blood, tissue, and intracellular concentrations. They can be given for shorter duration than tetracycline and still be effective. The suggested duration of therapy with doxycycline is 7 to 10 days, although one study found that doxycycline (10 mg/kg daily) for 7 days was ineffective in eliminating *E. canis* from 3 of 5 dogs.[78] In other studies, doxycycline (5 mg/kg twice daily) used for 10 or 14 days was effective in eliminating *E. canis* from 13 of 13 and 12 of 12 acutely infected dogs.[23, 106] Dramatic clinical improvement generally occurs within 24 to 48 hours after initiation of tetracycline therapy in dogs with acute-phase or mild chronic-phase disease. The platelet count correspondingly begins to increase during this time and is usually in the normal range by 14 days after treatment. Recovery is not equated with permanent immunity, and dogs can become reinfected with *E. canis* after a previous effective treatment. Experimental reinfection with heterologous strains has caused more severe disease manifestations than those with homologous strains.[23]

Chloramphenicol has been recommended for puppies younger than 5 months to avoid yellow discoloration of erupting teeth. It should be used in dogs that have persistent infections despite therapy with tetracyclines.[133] However, because of the public health risks associated with chloramphenicol and because it directly interferes with heme and bone marrow synthesis, its administration in anemic or pancytopenic dogs should be avoided when possible.

The quinolones have some known antirickettsial activity. *E. sennetsu* is susceptible to ciprofloxacin in vitro.[25] Enrofloxacin has been shown to be effective for the treatment of experimental RMSF in dogs[22] (see Chapter 29). In contrast, *E. chaffeensis* was resistant to ciprofloxacin but sensitive to doxycycline and rifampin in vitro.[26] In addition to doxycycline, rifampin and fluoroquinolones have in vitro activity against the HGE agent.[86b] The effectiveness of enrofloxacin for treatment of experimentally induced *E. canis* infection has been evaluated.[106] At a dose of 5 mg/kg twice daily, and 10 mg/kg twice daily PO for 21 days, 6 of 7 and 5 of 5 dogs, respectively, remained blood culture positive and thrombocytopenic after each treatment regimen. All 12 dogs were then treated with doxycycline (5 mg/kg twice daily, PO, for 10 days) and had blood culture–negative results and platelet counts returned to normal. On the basis of these results, enrofloxacin does not seem to be effective against *E. canis*.

Imidocarb has been successful in treating resistant *E. canis* infections and is available for use in North America (see Chapter 71 and Drug Formulary, Appendix 8).[96] When imidocarb was given as a single IM injection, 83.9% of dogs with ehrlichiosis recovered. Transient, dose-dependent side effects of imidocarb dipropionate include excessive salivation, serous nasal discharge, diarrhea, and dyspnea. These signs may be the result of an anticholinesterase effect.

In addition to antimicrobial therapy, supportive therapy with fluids for dehydration or blood transfusions if the dog is severely anemic may be justified. Blood transfusions will not significantly increase platelet number; therefore, platelet-rich plasma may be needed in an emergency situation. No clinical studies have been published regarding the use of colony-stimulating factors for the treatment of the severe chronic ehrlichiosis, but they might be useful. These would include such products as erythropoietin (Epogen, Amgen, Thousand Oaks, CA) and granulocyte colony-stimulating factor (G-CSF, Neupogen, Amgen, Thousand Oaks, CA). See Drug Formulary, Appendix 8.

Table 28–4. Antimicrobial Therapy for Ehrlichiosis

DRUG[a]	SPECIES	DOSE[b] (mg/kg)	ROUTE PREFERRED (ALTERNATIVE)	INTERVAL[c] (HOURS)	DURATION (DAYS)
Tetracycline	D	22	PO	8	14–21
Oxytetracycline	D	25	PO (IV)	8	14–21
Doxycycline	D	5–10	PO (IV)	12–24	10–21
	C	10	PO	12	21
Minocycline	D	10	PO (IV)	12	10
Chloramphenicol	D	15–25	PO (IV, SC)	8	14
Imidocarb dipropionate	B	5	IM	Once	Repeat in 2–3 wks
Amicarbalide	D	5–6	IM	Once	Repeat in 2–3 wks

[a]See Drug Formulary, Appendix 8 for additional information.
[b]Dose per administration at specified interval.
[c]Expressed in hours unless otherwise stated.
D = dog; C = cat; B = both dog and cat.

Short-term (2–7 days) therapy with glucocorticoids may be beneficial early in the treatment period when severe or life-threatening thrombocytopenia is present. An immune-mediated mechanism is partially responsible for the thrombocytopenia and decreased platelet function. The rationale for prednisone therapy has some scientific basis. Some clinicians prefer to use glucocorticoids and tetracycline in combination initially, because of the difficulty in distinguishing between canine ehrlichiosis and immune-mediated thrombocytopenia and because of the lag time before serologic test results are available. When serologic testing will not be performed, it is better to use tetracyclines alone first to allow for a therapeutic diagnosis by clinical improvement in 24 to 48 hours. Glucocorticoids should not be excluded in these situations if the hemorrhage is life threatening because they help reduce the tendency for hemorrhage in various causes of primary thrombocytopenic disorders.

Glucocorticoids may also be helpful in the treatment of other "immune-mediated" conditions associated with ehrlichiosis such as polyarthritis, vasculitis, and meningitis. In one dog with meningitis secondary to granulocytic ehrlichiosis, glucocorticoids were required in addition to doxycycline before clinical resolution of signs was achieved.[93]

PREVENTION

A vaccine is not currently available; therefore, chemotherapy, chemoprophylaxis, and tick control measures are the primary means of prevention. Tetracycline has been shown to be an effective prophylactic drug against initial infection or reinfection when administered PO at 6.6 mg/kg/day. Control in endemic areas can be accomplished by maintaining strict tick control programs for dogs and premises; using the indirect FA test to identify infected dogs; and treating all infected dogs with the therapeutic regimen of tetracycline. When these measures fail, then maintenance of all susceptible and successfully treated dogs on prophylactic levels of tetracycline may be the only recourse. If these guidelines are followed, the cycle of *E. canis* infection in the tick should be broken, because transovarian transmission of *E. canis* does not occur in the domiciled, one-host *Rhipicephalus* tick. For the other ehrlichial species, ticks are outdoors and have multiple, as yet unidentified wildlife reservoir hosts. Tick control measures are the only solution.

PUBLIC HEALTH CONSIDERATIONS

Before 1986, the only *Ehrlichia* sp. recognized as infecting people was *E. sennetsu* (see Table 28–1). This agent, first isolated in Japan, is responsible for a mild mononucleosis-like syndrome. Two new ehrlichial agents have been reported to cause disease in humans in the United States. The first is *E. chaffeensis*, the causative agent for human monocytic ehrlichiosis (HME),[2, 127, 123] which manifests as an acute flulike illness characterized by fever, headache, malaise, and sometimes death in severely affected people.

E. chaffeensis is closely related to *E. canis*, and although dogs can be experimentally infected, they do not develop clinical disease.[45] The role dogs may play as carriers of *E. chaffeensis* in endemic geographic regions requires further study. HME, which is predominant in the south-central and southeastern United States, likely involves a sylvan cycle in nature, with deer and/or rodents as reservoir hosts and *Amblyomma americanum* (or possibly *Dermacentor variabilis*) being the most likely vectors.

A similar clinical syndrome in people, known as HGE, occurs in the western United States and is caused by *E. equi*,[62, 91] in the north-central and northeastern United States tentatively *E. microti*[11, 12, 51, 90, 102, 108, 120, 131] is the causative agent, and in Europe HGE is caused by *E. phagocytophila*.[51, 103, 113] Dogs or cats and other domestic animals can be experimentally and/or naturally infected with *E. equi*,[89, 90] HGE agent,[65–67] and *E. phagocytophila*.[80] It is likely that these granulocytic species are the same or closely related, having a broad range of incidental mammalian hosts. The role, if any, of domestic animals in the human disease is yet to be determined. Wildlife hosts such as rodents are probably the maintenance reservoirs, with immature tick stages as vectors; deer may become infected or involved in vector maintenance. The vectors for the three HGE agents are *Ixodes* spp. ticks, which also transmit *Borrelia* spp. (see Chapter 45) explaining the superimposed worldwide geographic distribution of these diseases. Coinfections with *Borrelia* and *Ehrlichia* spp. may result in more severe disease in infected hosts. In addition to tick exposure, it is possible that some individuals had been infected by handling deer carcasses and by contacting associated engorged ticks or infected blood.[12, 131] The affected individuals had butchered large numbers of deer carcasses and sustained numerous cuts during the process. They also used an electric saw, which did not control aerosolized blood particles.

Canine Thrombocytic Ehrlichiosis

John W. Harvey

ETIOLOGY

Infectious cyclic thrombocytopenia of dogs is caused by a small rickettsial parasite classified as *Ehrlichia platys*.[58, 73] This organism was first reported in the United States and subsequently has been reported in Greece,[87] France,[17] and Italy.[110] *E. platys* has been shown to be related to other ehrlichial species using PCR amplification and sequencing of the 16S rRNA gene,[3, 5, 82] but it infects platelets rather than leukocytes. *E. platys* organisms appear as blue inclusions in platelets when blood films are stained with Giemsa or new methylene blue (Fig. 28–6).

Ultrastructurally, organisms range from 350 to 1250 nm in diameter; are round, oval, or bean shaped; and are surrounded by a double membrane. Infected platelets may contain one to three single membrane–lined vacuoles with one to eight organisms per vacuole (Fig. 28–7). Organisms appear to enter platelets by endocytosis after adherence. The vacuolar membrane probably is derived, therefore, from the external platelet membrane. Repetitive binary fission of organisms within the vacuole results in the formation of a small morula.

Megakaryocytes in bone marrow have not been observed to contain organisms either before or during parasitemia. *E. platys* antigen has been identified in macrophages using

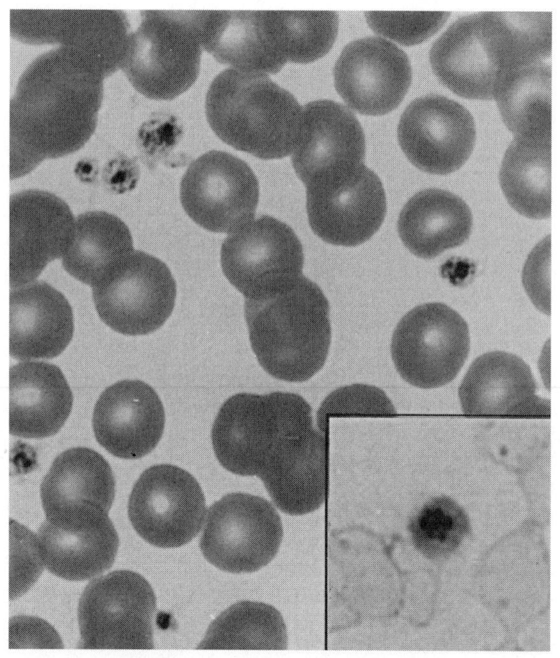

Figure 28–6. *E. platys* organisms in platelets from a dog with infectious cyclic thrombocytopenia (Giemsa stain, original magnification × 1400). *Inset:* Platelet containing morula of *E. platys* (new methylene blue, × 1500).

immunofluorescent staining of frozen tissues 14 days after experimental infection, but this finding may represent the fate of infected platelets rather than a site of replication.

Attempts to culture the organism have been unsuccessful. An attempt to infect a cat by IV inoculation was also unsuccessful. Some human sera have been shown to contain antibodies reactive to *E. platys*; however, these same sera also reacted with *E. canis* antigens in a similar test.[58] Consequently, it is unknown whether humans can become infected with this agent or are infected with a related organism that results in cross-reacting antibodies.

PATHOGENESIS

The incubation period after experimental IV infection in dogs is 8 to 15 days. The natural mode of transmission has not been demonstrated, but it likely involves a tick vector, although attempts to transmit the agent with *Rhipicephalus sanguineus* were not successful.[126] The highest percentage of parasitized platelets occurs during the initial parasitemic episode (Fig. 28–8). Within a few days after the appearance of parasitized platelets, there is a precipitous decrease in platelet count (generally 20,000 cells/μl or less), and organisms are usually no longer seen. After the disappearance of microorganisms, platelet counts increase rapidly, reaching normal values within 3 to 4 days.

Parasitemias and subsequent thrombocytopenias recur at 1- to 2-week intervals (see Fig. 28–8). Although the percentage of infected platelets decreases to as low as 1% or less with subsequent parasitemias, thrombocytopenic episodes are as severe as those after the initial parasitemia. Whereas initial thrombocytopenia may develop primarily as a consequence of injury to platelets by replicating organisms, immune-mediated mechanisms of platelet removal may be more important in subsequent thrombocytopenic episodes.[58] The cyclic nature of the parasitemias and thrombocytopenias diminishes with time, resulting in mild, slowly resolving thrombocytopenias in association with sporadically occurring organisms in blood platelets.

In some instances, transient decreases in total leukocyte counts have occurred concomitantly with parasitemia, but values are usually not below the reference range for dogs. Mild normocytic normochromic anemias may occur during the first month of infection. On the basis of serum iron and bone marrow studies, decreases in packed cell volume may be attributed to the syndrome of anemia of inflammation. Slight to moderate increases in acute-phase proteins and immunoglobulins and slight decreases in albumin may be present in serum samples.

CLINICAL FINDINGS

Minimal clinical signs have been recognized in experimentally infected dogs in the United States. A slight increase in

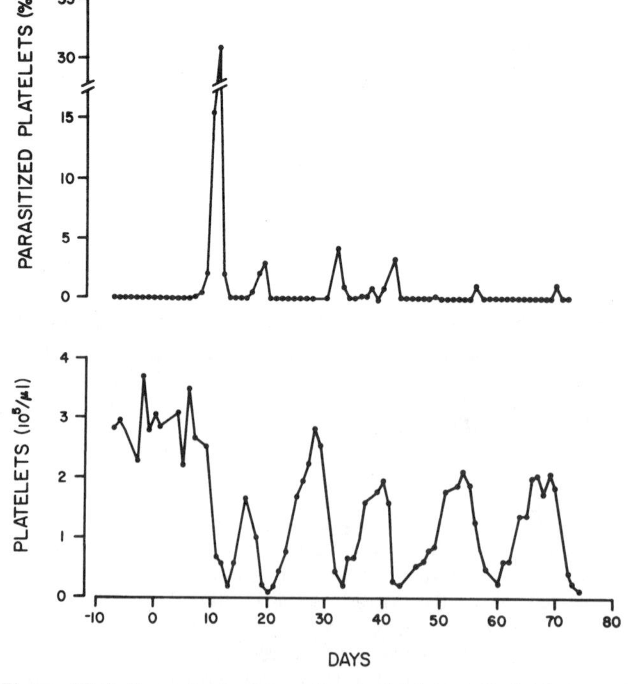

Figure 28–8. Percentage of parasitized platelets and platelet counts from a dog inoculated IV with *E. platys;* 0 on the abscissa represents the day of inoculation. (From Harvey JW et al: *J Infect Dis* 137:182–188, 1978. Reprinted with permission from the University of Chicago.)

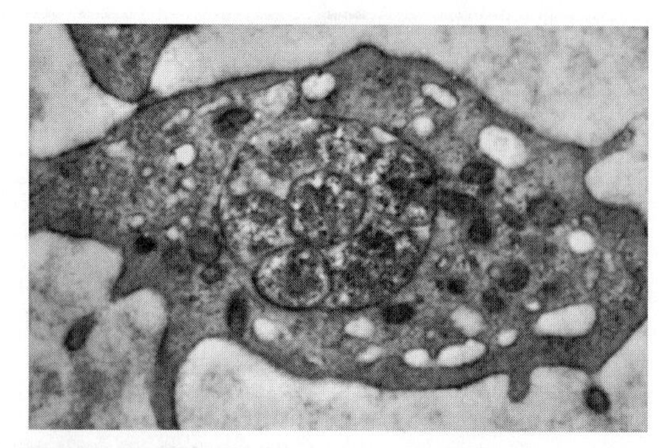

Figure 28–7. Ultrastructure of *E. platys.* Platelet with a membrane-lined vacuole containing seven visible organisms. (From Harvey JW et al: *J Infect Dis* 137:182–188, 1978. Reprinted with permission from the University of Chicago.)

rectal temperature has sometimes been noted during initial parasitemias, and slight hematochezia has been recognized in some thrombocytopenic dogs. Splenectomy before experimental infection results in higher initial platelet counts but does not alter the periodicity of the parasitemias or the severity of the disease. The age of the animal does not appear to have a significant effect on the course of infection; clinical and hematologic findings in a group of three weanling pups were similar to those in mature dogs.[58] More severe clinical signs, including fever and uveitis in one dog and petechial and ecchymotic hemorrhages of gums, sclera, and skin and epistaxis in another dog, have been reported in natural cases.[141]

More pathogenic strains of *E. platys* have been reported outside the United States.[87] Clinical signs including fever, pale mucous membranes, petechial hemorrhages of skin and oral mucosa, decreased appetite, and weight loss have been reported in both experimental and natural studies of dogs infected with a Greek strain of *E. platys*.[87]

The occurrence of *E. platys* with other infectious agents (e.g., *E. canis* and *Babesia canis*) may potentiate the clinical disease produced by either of these agents. As with *E. canis*, certain breeds of dogs or individual animals may be more severely affected than the dogs studied experimentally. Dogs with thrombocytopenia may bleed after trauma or surgery. Even if *E. platys* infection seldom produces clinical illness in the United States, it must be considered in the differential diagnosis of thrombocytopenia in dogs.

DIAGNOSIS

A diagnosis of *E. platys* infection may be made by finding organisms within platelets on stained blood films. In most instances, this method of diagnosis is not reliable because the parasites are either absent or present in very low numbers. An avidin-biotin immunocytochemical staining procedure has been described that can specifically identify *E. platys* morulae in platelets, assisting in the differentiation of organisms from large platelet granules or remnants of megakaryocyte nuclei.[125]

An indirect FA test for detection of serum antibodies to *E. platys* is commercially available (see Appendix 5). Sera of dogs experimentally infected with *E. platys* change from negative to positive coincident with or shortly after the peak of the first parasitemia.[48a, 58] On the basis of serologic studies, it appears that *E. platys* infection is widely distributed in the United States. As many as 33% of thrombocytopenic dogs in Florida and Louisiana have positive titers. More than 50% of dogs seropositive for *E. canis* also have positive titers to *E. platys*. Evidence for positive serologic reactions to both organisms in serum samples from some dogs probably represents combined infections inasmuch as other dogs have positive titers to either agent alone. Conditions necessary to establish a PCR-based diagnostic test have been reported.[5, 82] Western immunoblotting assays should also be helpful in diagnosing *E. platys* infections. PCR has been used to detect *E. platys* in infected dogs.[32, 32a, 94a]

PATHOLOGIC FINDINGS

Generalized lymph node enlargement was the only gross finding at necropsy in an experimental study of dogs euthanized during the early weeks of infection. Histologic lesions were generally mild and included lymphoid hyperplasia and plasmacytosis in lymph nodes and spleen, crescent-shaped perifollicular hemorrhages in the spleen, and multifocal Kupffer cell hyperplasia in the liver. Megakaryocyte numbers in the bone marrow were normal or increased.

THERAPY AND PREVENTION

On the basis of preliminary studies, it appears that tetracyclines at dosages recommended for *E. canis* infections are effective against this agent (see Table 28–4).[58] Inasmuch as ticks and possibly other arthropods are probably responsible for natural transmission of the disease, adequate vector control is recommended to prevent its spread.

Feline Ehrlichiosis

Michael R. Lappin

ETIOLOGY AND EPIDEMIOLOGY

The species of *Ehrlichia* that infect cats after natural exposure have not been determined. *Ehrlichia*-like bodies or morulae have been detected in peripheral blood cells of naturally exposed cats in the United States,[20] Kenya,[28, 30] France,[18, 35] and Thailand.[79] Morulae have been found in mononuclear cells or neutrophils of naturally infected cats (Table 28–5). EM assessment of an isolate from feline mononuclear cells revealed organisms from 0.54 to 1.3 μm, intermediate in size between *E. canis* and *E. sennetsu*.[28]

Cats can be experimentally infected with *E. equi*[89] and *E. risticii*[42] after IV inoculation. Although clinical abnormalities were not reported, two of five cats inoculated with *E. equi* developed morulae in eosinophils and eosinophilia. Morulae of *E. risticii* were detected in mononuclear cells from two of six cats inoculated IV; diarrhea developed in one cat, and depression, anorexia, and lymphadenomegaly developed in the other.

Sera from some cats have been evaluated for the presence of antibodies against *Ehrlichia* spp. using indirect FA tests. Antibodies to *E. risticii* were detected in serum of 26.4% and 16.6% of the cats tested in Maryland[42] and Virginia,[112] respectively. In a neighborhood in Colorado from which a cat with a mononuclear form of *Ehrlichia* was identified, 14 of 17 cats (82.4%) and 9 of 17 cats (52.9%) had serum antibodies against *E. canis* and *E. risticii*, respectively.[20] Cats with antibodies against both species generally had higher titers to *E. canis*. A national seroprevalence study of cats found antibodies against *E. canis* or *E. risticii* in 33.1% of the 583 cats tested.[88] *E. risticii*–seropositive cats were detected in all regions of the continental United States. Cats with antibodies against *E. canis* morulae were detected in all regions, excluding the Midwest. Antibodies against *E. risticii* were detected by indirect FA and Western immunoblot in five cats in a

Table 28–5. Clinical Ehrlichiosis in Cats With Morulae Morphologically Consistent With Ehrlichia spp.

SIGNALMENT (COUNTRY)	CLINICAL FINDINGS	LABORATORY FINDINGS	DIAGNOSIS	TREATMENT/ RESPONSE	REFERENCE
10 yr, FS, DSH (U.S.)	Fever, anorexia, hyperesthesia	Nonregenerative anemia, hyperglobulinemia	Morulae in mononuclear cells *E. canis* and *E. risticii* seropositive	Doxycyline/ excellent	20
10 yr, M, DSH (Kenya)	Fever, anorexia, dyspnea, splenomegaly, pale mucous membranes	Nonregenerative anemia, hyperglobulinemia, interstitial lung disease	Morulae in mononuclear cells, rarely in neutrophils	Tetracycline/ excellent	28
4 yr, M, DSH (Kenya)	Fever, anorexia, splenomegaly, pale mucous membranes	Nonregenerative anemia	Morulae in mononuclear cells, rarely in neutrophils	Imidocarb/ excellent	28
2 yr, F. DSH (Kenya)	Fever, anorexia, dyspnea, splenomegaly, lymphadenomegaly, pale mucous membranes	Nonregenerative anemia, neutropenia, interstitial lung disease	Morulae in mononuclear cells, rarely in neutrophils	Imidocarb/ excellent	28
Adult lioness (Kenya)	Lethargy, emaciation, lymphadenomegaly	Neutrophilic leukocytosis	Morulae in mononuclear cells	Not treated	30
6 y r, MC, DSH (France)	Fever, anorexia, pale mucous membranes, depression	Regenerative anemia, *H. felis*, leukocytosis, lymphocytosis, monocytosis, hyperbilirubinemia	Morulae in mononuclear cells	Tetracycline/ euthanasia	35
11 yr, FS, DSH (France)	Fever, weight loss, anorexia, depression, joint pain	Nonregenerative anemia, leukopenia, hypoalbuminemia, hyperglobulinemia	Morulae in lymphocytes, *E. canis* seropositive	Doxycycline/ glucocorticoids/ euthanasia	18
9 yr, MC, DSH (France)	Anorexia, gingivitis, pale mucous membranes, polyuria, polydipsia, weight loss	Anemia, FeLV positive, FIV positive, hyperglobulinemia	Morulae in lymphocytes, *E. canis* seropositive	Euthanasia	18
14 yr, MC, DSH (France)	Dyspnea, pale mucous membranes, weight loss, lethargy	Pleural effusion, hyperglobulinemia	Morulae in lymphocytes, *E. canis* seropositive	Euthanasia/ lymphosarcoma	18

M = male; DSH = domestic shorthair; F = female; MC = male, castrated; FS = female, spayed; FeLV = feline leukemia virus; FIV = feline immunodeficiency virus.

household in California.[109] Antibodies against an *Ehrlichia* spp. were detected in sera from some cats in Sweden,[5] 12% of cat sera from southern Africa,[99] and in sera from 16 cats with clinical illness in France.[17a]

Experimental transmission of *E. risticii* to cats was successful by IV, but not SC, inoculation.[42] It is unknown how the clinically ill, naturally exposed cats described in the literature were infected. Exposure to arthropods was not documented in two of the four cases reported from France or the case from the United States.[18, 20, 35] *Haemaphysalis leachi* was found on each of four cats with clinical ehrlichiosis in Kenya.[28, 30] A novel species, *E. muris*, has been isolated from a wild mouse in Japan.[83, 140] It is possible that mice may be involved with infection of cats.

PATHOGENESIS

Pathogenesis of disease associated with ehrlichiosis in cats is unknown. On the basis of clinical, laboratory, and radiographic findings, it is likely that pathogenesis of disease is similar to that for *E. canis* infection of dogs.

CLINICAL FINDINGS

Ehrlichia spp. infection of cats has been presumptively diagnosed based on the combination of positive *E. canis* or *R. risticii* serology, clinical or laboratory findings consistent with ehrlichial infection, and response to doxycycline in two cats from Colorado,[20] five cats from California,[109] and seven cats from France.[17a] When these cases are combined with the nine cases with morulae documented in circulating leukocytes (see Table 28–5), there have been 23 reported cases of clinical feline ehrlichiosis. All cats for which age was reported were older than 2 years. Most cats were domestic shorthaired, and both males and females have been affected.

Fever was documented in at least eight cats. Most cats had nonspecific signs of lethargy, inappetence, and weight loss. Hyperesthesia, joint pain, or irritable disposition was also common. Splenomegaly (three cats), lymphadenomegaly (three cats), dyspnea (three cats), and pale mucous membranes (seven cats) were other reported physical examination abnormalities. Concurrent diseases detected in some cats included *Haemobartonella felis*, feline leukemia virus and feline immunodeficiency virus infections, and lymphosarcoma.

DIAGNOSIS

Hematology. Complete or partial blood cell evaluations were available for 18 of 23 cats. Anemia was reported in 7 cats; 5 were nonregenerative. The cat with a known regenerative anemia was infected with *H. felis*.[35] Leukopenia was reported in 7 cats; leukocytosis characterized by neutrophilia, lymphocytosis, or monocytosis was reported in three cats. Thrombocytopenia was reported in six cats.[17a, 109]

Biochemistry. Biochemical abnormalities were infrequently reported in cats with suspected clinical ehrlichiosis. Hyperproteinemia was reported for eight cats; protein electrophoresis documented polyclonal gammopathy in the four cats assayed.[17a, 18] A cat with hyperbilirubinemia also had hemolytic anemia most likely resulting from *H. felis* infection.[35]

Radiographic Findings. Of the three cats with respiratory abnormalities, two had interstitial lung patterns. The third cat had pleural effusion resulting from lymphosarcoma. Thoracic and abdominal radiographs were made in six other cats; findings were considered within normal limits.

Serology. Results of indirect FA for antibodies against *E. canis* or *E. risticii* were reported for some cats with suspected clinical ehrlichiosis. The three cats in Colorado had antibodies against *E. canis* and *E. risticii*[20]; the five cats in California using Western immunoblotting had antibodies against *E. risticii* alone.[109] The ten cats serologically evaluated in France were positive for antibodies against *E. canis*; the cats were not tested for antibodies against *E. risticii*. Positive serologic test results can occur in healthy cats as well as clinically ill cats.[88] A diagnosis of clinical ehrlichiosis, therefore, should not be based on serologic test results alone. A tentative diagnosis of feline clinical ehrlichiosis can be based on the combination of positive serologic test results, clinical signs of disease consistent with *Ehrlichia* infection, exclusion of other causes of the disease syndrome, and response to antirickettsial drugs.

Organism Demonstration. Morulae were reported in leukocytes in 9 of 16 cases. All 9 cats had morulae in mononuclear cells; 3 domestic cats from Kenya had morulae rarely in neutrophils.[28] Infected cells were reported to be more common in blood collected from an ear vein than a large vein.[18] Infection by *Ehrlichia* spp. can be confirmed by cell culture or PCR. The organism was isolated from whole blood on monocyte cultures in the domestic cat cases[28] but not from a lioness[30] from Kenya. Monocyte cultures failed to document an *Ehrlichia* spp. in the cats from California, but morulae were not seen in circulating blood of these cats.[109] PCR of blood using *E. risticii*–specific primers proved negative in the cats tested in California.[8]

PATHOLOGIC FINDINGS

Pyogranulomatous lymphadenitis was detected in a mesenteric lymph node from a cat from Colorado with antibodies against *E. canis* and *E. risticii*.[20] Perivascular plasma cell and lymphocyte infiltrates were detected in the lungs, kidneys, and liver of the untreated lioness in Kenya.[30]

THERAPY

Therapy with tetracycline, doxycycline, or imidocarb dipropionate was attempted in 20 of the 23 cases with suspected clinical feline ehrlichiosis. Administration of doxycycline at 5 mg/kg, twice daily, PO for 21 days resulted in resolution of clinical signs of disease in three cats.[20] One cat was seropositive 180 days after discharge but seronegative 1365 days after discharge. Serologic follow-up was available for six of the seven cats with presumptive ehrlichiosis in France.[17a] Of these cats, four were serologically negative and two had increasing titers. Recurrence of disease and serum antibodies was reported in the five California cats treated with doxycycline.[109] The authors recommended treatment with doxycycline at 10 mg/kg, PO, twice daily for 21 days (see Table 28–4). Imidocarb dipropionate administered at 5 mg/kg, IM, and repeated in 14 days resulted in clinical resolution of disease of two cats in Kenya.[28] Tetracycline (dose not listed) given twice daily PO for 7 days resulted in clinical resolution of disease in one cat.[28] Euthanasia was chosen in two cats with documented morulae because of tetracycline[35] or doxycycline[18] treatment failures. Some cats with suspected ehrlichiosis based on clinical signs and positive serologic test results failed to respond to doxycycline administration.[17a] However, since ehrlichiosis was not definitively diagnosed by organism demonstration techniques, it is unknown whether these cases represent treatment failures.

PREVENTION

Because routes of transmission for naturally infected cats are unknown, definitive statements concerning prevention cannot be made. Exposure of cats to potential arthropod vectors and ingestion of rodents should be avoided. It is apparent that *Ehrlichia* spp. can be transmitted by blood; therefore, cats used as blood donors should be screened for antibodies against *E. canis* and *E. risticii*, and seropositive cats should be excluded as donors.

PUBLIC HEALTH CONSIDERATIONS

There are currently no known public health risks associated with the *Ehrlichia* spp. infecting cats. Since some species of *Ehrlichia* cross-infect, it is possible that cats could be a reservoir for species that infect people.

References

1. Abeygunawardena IS, Kakoma I, Smith RD. 1990. Pathophysiology of canine ehrlichiosis, pp 79–92. *In* Williams JC, Kakoma I (eds), Ehrlichiosis. Kluwer, Dordrecht, Netherlands.
2. Anderson BE, Dawson JE, Jones DC, et al. 1991. *Ehrlichia chaffeensis*, a new species associated with human ehrlichiosis. *J Clin Microbiol* 29:2838–2842.
3. Anderson BE, Greene CE, Jones DC, et al. 1992. *Ehrlichia ewingii* sp. nov. the etiologic agent of canine granulocytic ehrlichiosis. *Int J Syst Bacteriol* 42:299–302.
4. Anderson BE, Sims KG, Olson JG, et al. 1993. *Amblyomma americanum*: a potential vector of human ehrlichiosis. *Am J Trop Med Hyg* 49:239–244.
5. Anderson BE, Summer JW, Dawson JE, et al. 1992. Detection of the etiologic agent of human ehrlichiosis by polymerase chain reaction. *J Clin Microbiol* 30:775–780.
6. Anziani OS, Ewing SA, Barker RW. 1990. Experimental transmission of a granulocytic form of the tribe Ehrlichieae by *Dermacentor variabilis* and *Ambylomma americanum* to dogs. *Am J Vet Res* 51:929–931.
7. Arraga de Alvarado CM. 1992. Canine ehrlichiosis in Maracaibo, Venezuela. Report of 55 cases. *Rev Cientif* 11:30–40.
8. Artursson K, Malmqvist M, Olsson E, et al. 1994. Diagnosis of borreliosis and granulocytic ehrlichiosis of horses, dogs, and cats in Sweden. *Svensk Veterinartidning* 45:331–336.

8a. Asanovich KM, Bakken JS, Madigan JE, et al. 1997. Antigenic diversity of granulocytic *Ehrlichia* isolates from humans in Wisconsin and New York and a horse in California. *J Infect Dis* 176:1029–1034.

9. Atwill ER, Mohammed HO. 1996. Benefit-cost analysis of vaccination of horses as a strategy to control equine monocytic ehrlichiosis. *J Am Vet Med Assoc* 208:1295–1299.
10. Atwill ER, Mohammed HO. 1996. Evaluation of vaccination of horses as a strategy to control equine monocytic ehrlichiosis. *J Am Vet Med Assoc* 208:1290–1294.
11. Bakken JS, Dumler JS, Chen SM, et al. 1994. Human granulocytic ehrlichiosis in the upper mid west United States: a new species emerging. *JAMA* 272:212–218.
12. Bakken JS, Krueth JK, Lund T, et al. 1996. Exposure to deer blood may be a cause of human granulocytic ehrlichiosis. *Clin Infect Dis* 23:198.

12a. Bakken JS, Kreuth JK, Wilson-Nordskog C, et al. 1996. Clinical and laboratory characteristics of human granulocytic ehrlichiosis. *J Am Med Assoc* 275:199–205.

13. Baneth G, Waner T, Koplah A, et al. 1996. Survey of *Ehrlichia canis* antibodies among dogs in Israel. *Vet Rec* 138:257–259.

13a. Bark H, Harrus S, Keysary A, et al. 1997. Splenic function in canine monocytic ehrlichiosis. *J Vet Intern Med* 11:132.

14. Barlough JE, Madigan JE, DeRock E, et al. 1995. Protection against *Ehr-*

lichia equii is conferred by prior infection with the human granulocytotropic *Ehrlichia* (HGE Agent). *J Clin Microbiol* 33:3333–3334.
14a. Barlough JE, Madigan JE, Kramer VL, et al. 1997. *Ehrlichia phagocytophilia* genogroup rickettsiae in ixodid ticks from California collected in 1995 and 1996. *J Clin Microbiol* 35:2018–2021.
14b. Barlough JE, Madigan JE, Turoff DR, et al. 1997. An *Ehrlichia* strain from a llama (*Lama glama*) and llama-associated ticks (*Ixodes pacificus*). *J Clin Microbiol* 35:1005–1007.
15. Bartsch RC, Greene RT. 1996. Post-therapy antibody titers in dogs with ehrlichiosis: follow-up study on 68 patients treated primarily with tetracycline and/or doxycycline. *J Vet Intern Med* 10:271–274.
16. Bauer J. 1995. Infection with *Ehrlichia platys* and *Ehrlichia canis* in a dog. *Kleintierpraxis* 40:947.
17. Beaufils JP. 1985. Un syndromes accompagnant d'inclusions plaquettaires chez le chien, dans la region de Montpellier. Description et comparaison aux affections engendrées par *Ehrlichia canis* et *Ehrlichia platys*, thesis, Toulouse, France.
17a. Beaufils JP. 1997. Ehrlichiosis: clinical aspects in dogs and cats. *Compend Cont Educ Pract Vet* 19:57–61.
17b. Beaufils JP, Martin-Granel J, Jumelle PH. 1997. Ehrlichiose feline: a propos de deux cas. *Bull Acad Vet France* 70:73–80.
18. Beaufils JP, Martin-Granel J, Jumelle P. 1995. *Ehrlichia* infection in cats: a review of three cases. *Prat Med Chir Animal Compagnie* 30:397–402.
18a. Belongia EA, Reed KD, Mitchell PD, et al. 1997. Prevalence of granulocytic *Ehrlichia* infection among white-tailed deer in Wisconsin. *J Clin Microbiol* 35:1465–1468.
19. Botros BAM, Elmolla MS, Salib AW, et al. 1995. Canine ehrlichiosis in Egypt. Sero-epidemiological survey. *Onderstepoort J Vet Res* 62:41–43.
20. Bouloy RP, Lappin MR, Holland CH, et al. 1994. Clinical ehrlichiosis in a cat. *J Am Vet Med Assoc* 204:1475–1478.
21. Braund KG, Blagburn BL, Tovio-Kinnucan M, et al. 1988. *Toxoplasma* polymyositis/polyneuropathy—a new clinical variant in two mature dogs. *J Am Anim Hosp Assoc* 24:93–97.
22. Breitschwerdt EB, Davidson MG, Aucoin DP, et al. 1991. Efficacy of chloramphenicol, enrofloxacin, and tetracycline for treatment of experimental Rocky Mountain spotted fever in dogs. *Antimicrob Agents Chemother* 35:2375–2381.
23. Breitschwerdt EB, Hegarty BC, Hancock SI. 1997. Doxycycline treatment and challenge infection with two *Ehrlichia canis* strains. Abstract 116. *J Vet Intern Med* 11:133.
24. Brouqui P, Dumler JS, Raoult D, et al. 1992. Antigenic characterization of ehrlichiae: protein immunoblotting of *Ehrlichia canis*, *Ehrlichia sennetsu* and *Ehrlichia risticii*. *J Clin Microbiol* 30:1062–1066.
25. Brouqui P, Raoult D. 1990. In vitro susceptibility of *Ehrlichia sennetsu* to antibiotics. *Antimicrob Agents Chemother* 34:1593–1596.
26. Brouqui P, Raoult D. 1992. In vitro antibiotic susceptibility of the newly recognized agent of ehrlichiosis in humans. *Ehrlichia chaffeensis*. *Antimicrob Agents Chemother* 36:2799–2803.
27. Brouqui R, Raoult D. 1994. Human ehrlichiosis. *N Engl J Med* 330:1760–1761.
28. Buoro IBJ, Atwell RB, Kiptoon J, et al. 1989. Feline anemia associated with *Ehrlichia*-like bodies in three domestic short-haired cats. *Vet Rec* 125:434–436.
29. Buoro IBJ, Kanui TI, Atwell RB, et al. 1990. Polymyositis associated with *Ehrlichia canis* infection in two dogs. *J Small Anim Pract* 31:624–627.
30. Buoro IBJ, Nyamwange SB, Kiptoon JC. 1994. Presence of *Ehrlichia*-like bodies in monocytes of an adult lioness. *Feline Pract* 22:36–37.
31. Cadman HF, Kelly PJ, Matthewman LA, et al. 1994. Comparison of the dot-blot enzyme linked immunoassay with immunofluorescence for detecting antibodies to *Ehrlichia canis*. *Vet Rec* 135:362.
32. Chang WL, Pan MJ. 1996. Specific amplification of *Ehrlichia platys* DNA from blood specimens by 2 step PCR. *J Clin Microbiol* 34:3142–3146.
32a. Chang WL, Su WL, Pan MJ. 1997. 2-step PCR in the evaluation of antibiotic-treatment for *Ehrlichia platys* infection. *J Vet Med Sci* 59:849–851.
33. Chang YF, Kim JB, Dubovi E, et al. 1996. Detection of agent of human granulocytic ehrlichiosis in *Ixodes scapularis* by polymerase chain reaction. Presented at the meeting of the American Association of Veterinary Laboratory Diagnosticians, Little Rock, AR, October 1996.
34. Chang YF, Kim JB, Dubovi E, et al. 1996. Detection of DNA of agent of human granulocytic ehrlichiosis in *Ixodes scapularis* by polymerase chain reaction. Presented at the meeting of the American Association of Veterinary Laboratory Diagnosticians, Little Rock, AR, October 1966.
35. Charpentier F, Groulade P. 1986. Probable case of ehrlichiosis in a cat. *Bull Acad Vet France* 59:287–290.
36. Chen SM, Dumler S, Bakken JS, et al. 1994. Identification of a granulocytotropic *Ehrlichia* species as the etiologic agent of human disease. *J Clin Microbiol* 32:589–595.
36a. Chen SM, Yu XJ, Popov VL, et al. 1997. Genetic and antigenic diversity of *Ehrlichia chaffeensis*: comparative analysis of a novel human strain from Oklahoma and previously isolated strains. *J Infect Dis* 175:856–863.
37. Clark AM, Hopkins GE, MacLean IA. 1996. Tick-borne fever in dogs. *Vet Rec* 139:268.
38. Codner EC, Caceci T, Saunders GK, et al. 1992. Investigation of glomerular lesions in dogs with acute experimentally induced *Ehrlichia canis* infection. *Am J Vet Res* 53:2286–2291.
39. Codner EC, Maslin WR. 1992. Investigation of renal protein loss in dogs with acute experimentally induced *Ehrlichia canis* infection. *Am J Vet Res* 53:294–299.
40. Cowell RL, Tyler RD, Clinkenbeard KD, et al. 1988. Ehrlichiosis and polyarthritis in three dogs. *J Am Vet Med Assoc* 192:1093–1095.
40a. Daniels TJ, Falco RC, Schwartz I, et al. 1997. Deer ticks (*Ixodes scapularis*) and the agents of Lyme disease and human granulocytic ehrlichiosis in a New York City park. *Emerg Infect Dis* 3:353–355.
41. Dawson JE. 1996. Personal communication. Centers for Disease Control, Atlanta, GA.
42. Dawson JE, Abeygunawardena I, Holland CJ, et al. 1988. Susceptibility of cats to infection with *Ehrlichia risticii*, causative agent of equine monocytic ehrlichiosis. *Am J Vet Res* 49:2096–2100.
43. Dawson JE, Anderson BE, Fishbein DB, et al. 1991. Isolation and characterization of an *Ehrlichia* sp from a patient diagnosed with human ehrlichiosis. *J Clin Microbiol* 29:2741–2745.
44. Dawson JE, Biggie KL, Warner CK, et al. 1996. Polymerase chain reaction evidence of *Ehrlichia chaffeensis*, an etiologic agent of human ehrlichiosis, in dogs from southeast Virginia. *Am J Vet Res* 57:1175–1179.
45. Dawson JE, Ewing SA. 1992. Susceptibility of dogs to infection with *Ehrlichia chaffeensis*, causative agent of human ehrlichiosis. *Am J Vet Res* 53:1322–1327.
46. Dawson JE, Fishbein DB, Eng TR, et al. 1990. Diagnosis of human ehrlichiosis with the indirect florescent antibody test: kinetics and specificity. *J Infect Dis* 162:91–95.
47. Dawson JE, Stallknecht DE, Howerth EW, et al. 1994. Susceptibility of white-tailed deer (*Odocoileus virginianus*) to infection with *Ehrlichia chaffeensis*, the etiologic agent of human ehrlichiosis. *J Clin Microbiol* 32:2725–2728.
48. Dawson JE, Warner CK, Standaert S, et al. 1996. The interface between research and the diagnosis of an emerging tick-borne disease, human ehrlichiosis due to *Ehrlichia chaffeensis*. *Arch Intern Med* 156:137–142.
48a. Dealvarado CM, Parra OD, Palmar M, et al. 1997. *Ehrlichia platys*—antigen-processing and use of the indirect fluorescent-antibody test (IFA) in canines and humans. *Rev Client-Fac Clien Vet* 7:99–109.
49. Dumler JS, Asanovich KM, Bakken JS, et al. 1995. Serologic cross reaction among *Ehrlichia equi*, *Ehrlichia* phagocytophilia and human granulocytic *Ehrlichia*. *J Clin Microbiol* 33:1098–1103.
50. Dumler JS, Chen SM, Asanovich K, et al. 1995. Isolation and characterization of a new strain of *Ehrlichia chaffeensis* from a patient with nearly fatal monocytic ehrlichiosis. *J Clin Microbiol* 33:1704–1711.
51. Dumler JS, Dotevall L, Gustafson R, et al. 1997. A population-based seroepidemiologic study of human granulocytic ehrlichiosis and Lyme borreliosis on the west coast of Sweden. *J Infect Dis* 175:720–722.
52. Du Plessis JL, Fourie N, Nel PW, et al. 1990. Concurrent babesiosis and ehrlichiosis in the dog: blood smear examination supplemented by the indirect fluorescent antibody test, using *Cowdria ruminantium* as antigen. *Onderstepoort J Vet Res* 57:151–155.
53. Dykstra EA, Slater MR, Teel PD. 1997. Perceptions of veterinary clinics and pest control companies regarding tick-related problems in dogs residing in Texas cities. *J Am Vet Med Assoc* 210:360–365.
54. Egenvall A, Hedhammar A, Bjoersdorff A. 1994. Tickborne infections in dogs in Sweden. *Svensk Veterinaer* 46:321–329.
54a. Egenvall A, Hedhammar A, Bjoersdorff A. 1997. Clinical features and serology of 14 dogs affected by granulocytic ehrlichiosis in Sweden. *Vet Rec* 140:222–226.
55. Elias E. 1991. Diagnosis of ehrlichiosis from the presence of inclusion bodies in morulae of *E. canis*. *J Small Anim Pract* 33:540–543.
56. Engvall EO, Petterson B, Persson M, et al. 1996. A 16S rRNA-based PCR assay for detection and identification of granulocytic *Ehrlichia* species in dogs, horses and cattle. *J Clin Microbiol* 34:2170–2174.
56a. Everett ED, Evans KA, Henry RB, et al. 1994. Human ehrlichiosis in adults after tick exposure. Diagnosis using polymerase chain reaction. *Ann Intern Med* 120:730–735.
56b. Ewing SA, Dawson JE, Mathew JS, et al. 1997. Attempted transmission of human granulocytotropic *Ehrlichia* (HGE) by *Amblyomma americanum* and *Amblyomma maculatum*. *Vet Prasitol* 70:183–190.
56c. Fishbein DB, Dawson JE, Robinson LE. 1994. Human ehrlichiosis in the United States, 1985 to 1990. *Ann Intern Med* 120:736–743.
57. Fishbein DB, Dennis DT. 1995. Tick-borne diseases—a growing risk. *N Engl J Med* 333:452–453.
58. French TW, Harvey JW. 1993. Canine infectious cyclic thrombocytopenia (*Ehrlichia platys* infection in dogs), pp 195–208. *In* Woldehiwet Z, Ristic M (eds), Rickettsial and chlamydial diseases of domestic animals. Pergamon Press, New York, NY.
58a. Fritz CL, Kjemtrup AM, Conrad PA, et al. 1997. Seroepidemiology of emerging tickborne infectious diseases in a Northern California community. *J Infect Dis* 175:1432–1439.
59. Futch RR, Corstvet RE. 1996. Diagnosis *Ehrlichia canis* infection in dogs using enzyme-linked immunosorbent assays for antibody and antigen. Presented at the meeting of the American Association of Veterinary Laboratory Diagnosticians, Little Rock, AR, November 1996.
60. Gaunt SD, Cortsvet RE, Berry CM, et al. 1996. Isolation of *Ehrlichia canis* from dogs following subcutaneous inoculation. *J Clin Microbiol* 34:1429–1432.

61. Gaunt SD, Cortsvet RE, Brennan RE, et al. 1996. Platelet-associated IgG and antibodies to platelet proteins in dogs with *Ehrlichia canis* infection. Abstract 29. *Vet Pathol* 33:557.
62. Gewirtz AS, Cornbleet PJ, Vugia DJ, et al. 1996. Human granulocytic ehrlichiosis: report of a case in northern California. *Clin Infect Dis* 23:653–654.
63. Goodman JL, Nelson C, Vitale B, et al. 1996. Direct cultivation of the causative agent of human granulocytic ehrlichiosis. *N Engl J Med* 334:209–215.
64. Greene CE, Harvey JW. 1984. Canine ehrlichiosis, pp 545–561. *In* Greene CE (ed), Clinical microbiology and infectious diseases of the dog and cat. WB Saunders, Philadelphia, PA.
65. Greig B, Asanovich KM, Armstrong PJ, et al. 1996. Geographic, clinical, serologic, and molecular evidence of granulocytic ehrlichiosis, a likely zoonotic disease in Minnesota and Wisconsin dogs. *J Clin Microbiol* 34:44–48.
66. Greig B, Frigo E, Nelson PM, et al. 1996. Seroprevalence of a newly emerging zoonotic granulocytic ehrlichial disease in Minnesota and Wisconsin dogs (abstract 126). *J Am Coll Vet Intern Med* 10:180.
67. Harrus S, Aroch I, Lavy E, et al. 1997. Clinical manifestations of infectious canine cyclic thrombocytopenia. *Vet Rec* 141:247–250.
67a. Harrus S, Bark H, Waner T. 1997. Canine monocytic ehrlichiosis: an update. *Compend Cont Educ Pract Vet* 19:431–443.
68. Harrus S, Kass PH, Klement E, et al. 1997. Canine monocytic ehrlichiosis: a retrospective study of 100 cases, and an epidemiological investigation of prognostic indicators for the disease. *Vet Rec* 141:360–363.
69. Harrus S, Waner T, Eldor A, et al. 1996. Platelet dysfunction associated with experimental acute canine ehrlichiosis (abstract 174). *J Am Coll Vet Intern Med* 10:192.
70. Harrus S, Waner T, Eldor A, et al. 1996. Platelet dysfunction associated with experimental acute canine ehrlichiosis. *Vet Rec* 139:290–293.
71. Harrus, Waner T, Weiss DJ, et al. 1996. Kinetics of serum antiplatelet antibodies in experimental acute ehrlichiosis. *Vet Immunol Immunopathol* 51:13–20.
72. Harvey JW. 1990. *Ehrlichia platys* infection, pp 415–418. *In* Greene CE (ed), Infectious diseases of the dog and cat. WB Saunders, Philadelphia, PA.
73. Harvey JW, Simpson CF, Gaskin JM. 1978. Cyclic thrombocytopenia induced by a *Rickettsia*-like agent in dogs. *J Infect Dis* 137:182–188.
73a. Hegarty BC, Levy MG, Gager RF, et al. 1997. Immunoblot analysis of the immunoglobulin G response to *Ehrlichia canis* in dogs: an international survey. *J Vet Diagn Invest* 9:32–38.
74. Henschen A. 1994. Ehrlichiosis in the dog. *Svensk Veterinaer* 46:337–341.
75. Hess PR, English RV, Hegarty BC, et al. 1997. Immunologic consequences of experimental *Ehrlichia canis* infection in the dog. Abstract 117. *J Vet Intern Med* 11:33.
75a. Ijdo JW, Zhang Y, Hodzic E, et al. 1997. The early humoral response in human granulocytic ehrlichiosis. *J Infect Dis* 176:687–692.
76. Iqbal Z, Chaichansiriwithaya W, Rikihisa Y. 1994. Comparison of PCR with other tests for early diagnosis of canine ehrlichiosis. *J Clin Microbiol* 32:1658–1662.
77. Iqbal Z, Rikihisa Y. 1994. Application of the polymerase chain reaction for the detection of *Ehrlichia canis* in tissues of dogs. *Vet Microbiol* 42:281–287.
78. Iqbal Z, Rikihisa Y. 1994. Reisolation of *Ehrlichia canis* from blood and tissues of dogs after doxycycline treatment. *J Clin Microbiol* 32:1644–1649.
78a. Jafari S, Gaur SN, Hashemi A. 1997. Prevalence of *Ehrlichia-canis* in dog-population of Shiraz, Fars Province of Iran. *J Appl Anim Res* 11:19–23.
79. Jittapalapong S, Jansawan W. 1993. Preliminary survey on blood parasites of cats in Bangkhen District Area. *Kasetsart J Nat Sci* 27:330–335.
80. Johansson KE, Pettersson M, Uhlen M, et al. 1995. Identification of the causative agent of granulocytic ehrlichiosis in Swedish dogs and horses by direct solid phase sequencing of PCR products. *Res Vet Sci* 58:109–112.
81. Kakoma I, Hansen R, Liu L, et al. 1991. Serologically atypical canine ehrlichiosis associated with *Ehrlichia risticii* infection. *J Am Vet Med Assoc* 199:1120.
82. Kakoma I, Hansen RD, Anderson BE, et al. 1994. Cultural, molecular, and immunological characterization of the etiologic agent for atypical canine ehrlichiosis. *J Clin Microbiol* 32:170–175.
83. Kawahara M, Suto C, Rikihisa Y, et al. 1993. Characterization of ehrlichial organisms isolated from a wild mouse. *J Clin Microbiol* 31:89–96.
84. Kelly PJ, Carter SD, Bobade PA, et al. 1994. Absence of antinuclear antibodies in dogs infected with *Ehrlichia canis*. *Vet Rec* 134:382.
85. Kelly PJ, Matthewman LA, Mahan SM, et al. 1994. Serological evidence for antigenic relationships between *Ehrlichia canis* and *Cowdria ruminantium*. *Res Vet Sci* 56:170–174.
86. Keysary A, Waner T, Rosner M, et al. 1996. The first isolation, in vivo propagation, and genetic characterization of *Ehrlichia canis* in Israel. *Vet Parasitol* 62:331–340.
86a. Klein MB, Miller JS, Nelson CM, et al. 1997. Primary bone marrow progenitors of both granulocytic and monocytic lineages are susceptible to infection with the agent of human granulocytic ehrlichiosis. *J Infect Dis* 176:1405–1409.
86b. Klein MB, Nelson CM, Goodman JL. 1997. Antibiotic susceptibility of the newly cultivated agent of human granulocytic ehrlichiosis: promising activity of quinolones and rifamycins. *Antimicrob Agents Chemother* 41:76–79.
86c. Kolbert CP, Bruinsma ES, Abdulkarim AS, et al. 1997. Characterization of an immunoreactive protein from the agent of human granulocytic ehrlichiosis. *J Clin Microbiol* 35:1172–1178.
87. Kontos VI, Papadopoulos O, French TW. 1991. Natural and experimental canine infections with a Greek strain of *Ehrlichia platys*. *Vet Clin Pathol* 20:101–105.
88. Lappin MR, Holland CH, Thrall MA. 1996. Regional distribution of *Ehrlichia canis* and *E risticii* seropositive cats in the United States. *J Vet Intern Med*. In review.
89. Lewis GE, Huxsoll DL, Ristic M, et al. 1975. Experimentally induced infection of dogs, cats, and nonhuman primates with *Ehrlichia equi*, etiologic agent of equine ehrlichiosis. *J Am Vet Med Assoc* 36:85–88.
89a. Lockhart JM, Davidson WR, Stallknecht DE, et al. 1997. Isolation of *Ehrlichia chaffeensis* from wild white-tailed deer (*Odocoileus virginianus*) confirms their role as natural reservoir hosts. *J Clin Microbiol* 35:1681–1686.
90. Madigan JE, Barlough JE, Dumler JS, et al. 1996. Equine granulocytic ehrlichiosis in Connecticut caused by an agent resembling the human granulocytotropic ehrlichia. *J Clin Microbiol* 34:434–435.
91. Madigan JE, Richter PJ, Kimsey RB, et al. 1995. Transmission and passage in horses of the agent of human granulocytic ehrlichiosis. *J Infect Dis* 172:1141–1144.
92. Madwell BR, Gribble DH. 1982. Infection in two dogs with an agent resembling *E. equi*. *J Am Vet Med Assoc* 180:512–514.
92a. Magnarelli LA, Ijdo JW, Anderson IF, et al. 1997. Antibodies to *Ehrlichia equi* in dogs from the Northeastern United States. *J Am Vet Med Assoc* 211:1134–1137.
93. Maretzki CH, Fisher DJ, Greene CE. 1994. Granulocytic ehrlichiosis and meningitis in a dog. *J Am Vet Med Assoc* 205:1554–1556.
94. Mathew JS, Ewing SA, Barker RW, et al. 1996. Attempted transmission of *Ehrlichia canis* by *Rhipicephalus sanguineus* after passage in cell culture. *Am J Vet Res* 57:1594–1598.
94a. Mathew JS, Ewing SA, Murphy GL, et al. 1997. Characterization of a new isolate of *Ehrlichia platys* (order rickettsiales) using electron microscopy and polymerase chain reaction. *Vet Parasitol* 68:1–10.
95. Matthewman LA, Kelly PJ, Bobade PA, et al. 1993. Infections with *Babesia canis* and *Ehrlichia canis* in dogs in Zimbabwe. *Vet Rec* 133:344–346.
96. Matthewman LA, Kelly PJ, Brouqui P, et al. 1994. Further evidence for the efficacy of imidocarb dipropionate in the treatment of *Ehrlichia canis* infection. *J S Afr Vet Assoc* 65:104–107.
97. Matthewman LA, Kelly PJ, Mahan SM, et al. 1993. Western blot and indirect fluorescent antibody testing for antibodies reactive with *Ehrlichia canis* in sera from apparently healthy dogs in Zimbabwe. *J S Afr Vet Assoc* 64:111–115.
98. Matthewman LA, Kelly PJ, Mahan SM, et al. 1994. Reactivity of sera collected from dogs in Mutare, Zimbabwe to antigens of *Ehrlichia canis* and *Cowdria ruminantium*. *Vet Rec* 134:498–499.
99. Matthewman LA, Kelly PJ, Wray K, et al. 1996. Antibodies in cat sera from southern Africa react with antigens of *Ehrlichia canis*. *Vet Rec* 138:364–365.
100. McBride JW, Corstvet RE, Gaunt SD, et al. 1996. PCR detection of acute *Ehrlichia canis* infection in dogs. *J Vet Diagn Invest* 8:441–442.
101. Meinkoth JH, Hoover JP, Cowell RL, et al. 1989. Ehrlichiosis in a dog with seizures and nonregenerative anemia. *J Am Vet Med Assoc* 195:1754–1755.
102. Mitchell PD, Reed KD, Hofkes JM. 1996. Immunoserologic evidence of coinfection with *Borrelia burgdorferi*, *Babesia microtic*, and human granulocytic *Ehrlichia* species in residents of Wisconsin and Minnesota. *J Clin Microbiol* 34:724–727.
103. Morais JD, Dawson JE, Greene C, et al. 1991. First European case of ehrlichiosis. *Lancet* 338:633–634.
104. Moreland KJ, Wilson EA. 1990. Concurrent *Ehrlichia canis* and *Borrelia burgdorferi* infections in a Texas dog. *J Am Anim Hosp Assoc* 26:635–639.
104a. Mott J, Rikihisa Y, Zhang Y, et al. 1997. Comparison of PCR and culture to the indirect fluorescent-antibody test for diagnosis of Potomac horse fever. *J Clin Microbiol* 35:2215–2219.
105. Munderloh UG, Madigan JE, Dumler JS, et al. 1996. Isolation of the equine granulocytic ehrlichiosis agent, *Ehrlichia equi* in tick cell culture. *J Clin Microbiol* 34:664–670.
106. Neer TM. 1995. Unpublished data. Louisiana State University, Baton Rouge, LA.
106a. Nicholson WL, Comer JA, Sumner JW, et al. 1997. An indirect immunofluorescence assay using a cell culture-derived antigen for detection of antibodies to the agent of human granulocytic ehrlichiosis. *J Clin Microbiol* 35:1510–1516.
107. Nyindo MBA, Kakoma I, Hansen R. 1991. Antigenic analysis of four species of the genus *Ehrlichia* by use of the protein immunoblot. *Am J Vet Res* 52:1225–1230.
107a. Paddock CD, Sumner JW, Shore GM, et al. 1997. Isolation and characterization of *Ehrlichia chaffeensis* strains from patients with fatal ehrlichiosis. *J Clin Microbiol* 35:2496–2502.
108. Pancholi P, Kolbert CP, Mitchell PD, et al. 1995. *Ixodes dammini* as a potential vector of human granulocytic ehrlichiosis. *J Infect Dis* 172:1007–1012.
109. Peavy GM, Holland CJ, Dutta SK, et al. 1997. Suspected ehrlichial infection in 5 cats from a household. *J Am Vet Med Assoc* 210:231–234.
110. Pennisi MG, French TW, Catarsini O. 1989. Infectious cyclic thrombocyto-

penia (*Ehrlichia platys*) of dogs in Italy. *Atti della Società Italiana delle Scienze Veterinarie* XLIII:1341–1344.

110a. Perez M, Rikihisa Y, Wen B. 1996. *Ehrlichia canis*-like agent from a man in Venezuela: antigenic and genetic characterization. *J Clin Microbiol* 34:2133–2139.

111. Perille AL, Matus RE. 1991. Canine ehrlichiosis in six dogs with persistently increased antibody titers. *J Vet Intern Med* 5:195–198.

112. Perry BD, Schmidtmann ET, Rice EM, et al. 1989. Epidemiology of Potomac horse fever: an investigation into the possible role of non-equine mammals. *Vet Rec* 125:83–86.

112a. Petrovec M, Furlan SL, Zupanc TA, et al. 1997. Human disease in Europe caused by a granulocytic *Ehrlichia* species. *J Clin Microbiol* 35:1556–1559.

113. Pierard D, Levtchenko E, Dawson JE, et al. 1996. Ehrlichiosis in Belgium. *Lancet* 346:1233–1234.

113a. Pusteria N, Braun U, Wolfensberger C, et al. 1997. Intrauterine infection with *Ehrlichia phagocytophila* in a cow. *Vet Rec* 141:101–102.

113b. Pusteria N, Huder J, Wolfensberger C, et al. 1997. Granulocytic ehrlichiosis in two dogs in Switzerland. *J Clin Microbiol* 35:2307–2309.

114. Ratnasamy N, Everett ED, Roland WE. 1996. Central nervous system manifestations of human ehrlichiosis. *Clin Infect Dis* 23:314–319.

115. Rikihisa Y. 1991. Cross-reacting antigens between *Neorickettsia helminthoeca* and *Ehrlichia* species, shown by immunofluorescence and Western immunoblotting. *J Clin Microbiol* 29:2024–2029.

116. Rikihisa Y. 1991. The tribe Ehrlichiae and ehrlichial diseases. *Clin Microbiol Rev* 4:286–308.

117. Rikihisa Y, Ewing SA, Fox JC. 1994. Western immunoblot analysis of *Ehrlichia chaffeensis*, *E. canis*, or *E. ewingii* infections in dogs and humans. *J Clin Microbiol* 32:2107–2112.

118. Rikihisa Y, Ewing SA, Fox JC, et al. 1992. Analyses of *Ehrlichia canis* and a canine granulocytic *Ehrlichia* infection. *J Clin Microbiol* 30:143–148.

119. Rikihisa Y, Yamamoto S, Kwak I, et al. 1994. C-reactive protein and α1-acid glycoprotein levels in dogs infected with *Ehrlichia canis*. *J Clin Microbiol* 32:912–917.

120. Rikihisa Y, Zhi N, Wormser GP, et al. 1997. Ultrastructural and antigenic characterization of a granulocytic ehrlichiosis agent directly isolated and stably cultivated from a patient in New York State. *J Infect Dis* 175:210–213.

121. Ristic M, Dawson JE, Holland CJ, et al. 1988. Susceptibility of dogs to infection with *E. risticii*, the causative agent of equine monocytic ehrlichiosis (Potomac horse fever). *Am J Vet Res* 49:1497–1500.

122. Rodgers SJ, Morton RJ, Baldwin CA. 1989. A serological survey of *Ehrlichia canis*, *Ehrlichia equi*, *Rickettsia rickettsii* and *Borrelia burgdorferi* in dogs in Oklahoma. *J Vet Diagn Invest* 1:154–159.

122a. Rosenfeld-Aguero ME, Horowitz HW, Wormser GP, et al. 1996. Human granulocytic ehrlichiosis: a case series from a medical center in New York State. *Ann Intern Med* 125:904–908.

122b. Sainz A, Delgado S, Amusategui I, et al. 1996. Seroprevalence of canine ehrlichiosis in Castilla-Leon (North-West Spain). *Prev Vet Med* 29:1–7.

123. Schaffner N, Standaert SM. 1996. Ehrlichiosis—in pursuit of an emerging infection. *N Engl J Med* 334:262–263.

123a. Schwartz I, Fish D, Daniels TJ. 1997. Prevalence of the rickettsial agent of human granulocytic ehrlichiosis in ticks from a hyperendemic focus of Lyme disease. *N Engl J Med* 337:49–50.

124. Shankarappa B, Dutta SK, Mattingly-Napier BL. 1992. Antigenic and genomic relatedness among *Ehrlichia risticii*, *Ehrlichia sennetsu* and *Ehrlichia canis*. *Int J Syst Bacteriol* 42:127–132.

125. Simpson RM, Gaunt SD. 1991. Immunocytochemical detection of *Ehrlichia platys* antigens in canine blood platelets. *J Vet Diagn Invest* 3:228–231.

126. Simpson RM, Gaunt SD, Hair JA, et al. 1991. Evaluation of *Rhipicephalus sanguineus* as a potential biologic vector of *Ehrlichia platys*. *Am J Vet Res* 52:1537–1541.

127. Standaert SM, Dawson JE, Schaffner W, et al. 1995. Ehrlichiosis in a golf-oriented retirement community. *N Engl J Med* 333:420–425.

128. Stith DM, Telford SR III, Dawson JE. 1996. Diagnosing ehrlichiosis. *Ann Intern Med* 124:854.

129. Stockham SL, Schmidt DA, Curtis KS. 1992. Evaluation of granulocytic ehrlichiosis in dogs of Missouri, including serologic status to *Ehrlichia canis*, *Ehrlichia equi*, and *Borrelia burgdorferi*. *Am J Vet Res* 53:63–68.

130. Stockham SL, Tyler JW, Schmidt DA, et al. 1990. Experimental transmission of granulocytic ehrlichial organisms in dogs. *Vet Clin Pathol* 19:99–104.

130a. Sumner JW, Nicholson WL, Massung RF. 1997. PCR amplification and comparison of nucleotide sequences from the groESL heat shock operon of *Ehrlichia* species. *J Clin Microbiol* 35:2087–2092.

131. Telford SR. 1997. Risk for acquiring human granulocytic ehrlichiosis: exposure to deer blood or deer ticks. *Clin Infect Dis* 24:531.

132. Telford SR, Lepore TJ, Snow P, et al. 1995. Human granulocytic ehrlichiosis in Massachusetts. *Ann Intern Med* 123:277–279.

133. Troy GC, Forrester SD. 1990. Canine Ehrlichiosis, pp 404–418. *In* Greene CE (ed), Infectious Diseases of the Dog and Cat. WB Saunders, Philadelphia, PA.

134. Troy GC, Vulgamott JC, Turnwald GH. 1980. Canine ehrlichiosis: a retrospective study of 30 naturally occurring cases. *J Am Anim Hosp Assoc* 16:181–187.

134a. Varela F, Font X, Valladares JE, et al. 1997. Thrombocytopathia and light-chain proteinuria in a dog naturally infected with *Ehrlichia canis*. *J Vet Intern Med* 11:309–311.

135. Waddle JR, Littman MP. 1988. A retrospective study of 27 cases of naturally occurring canine ehrlichiosis. *J Am Anim Hosp Assoc* 24:615–620.

135a. Walls JJ, Greig B, Neitzel DF, et al. 1997. Natural infection of small mammal species in Minnesota with the agent of human granulocytic ehrlichiosis. *J Clin Microbiol* 35:853–855.

136. Waner T, Harrus S, Bark H, et al. 1996. Subclinical canine ehrlichiosis (*Ehrlichia canis*) in experimentally infected Beagle dogs (abstract 175). *J Am Coll Vet Intern Med* 10:192.

137. Waner T, Harrus S, Bark H, et al. 1997. Characterization of the subclinical phase of canine ehrlichiosis in experimentally infected beagle dogs. *Vet Parsitol* 69:307–317.

138. Waner T, Harrus S, Weiss DJ, et al. 1995. Demonstration of serum antiplatelet antibodies in experimental acute canine ehrlichiosis. *Vet Immunol Immunopathol* 48:177–282.

139. Weiser MG, Thrall MA, Fulton R, et al. 1991. Granular lymphocytosis and hyperproteinemia in dogs with chronic ehrlichiosis. *J Am Anim Hosp Assoc* 27:84–88.

140. Wen B, Rikihisa Y, Mott J, et al. 1995. *Ehrlichia muris* sp. nov., identified on the basis of 16S rRNA base sequences and serological, morphological, and biological characteristics. *Int J Sys Bacteriol* 45:250–254.

140a. Wen B, Rikihisa Y, Mott JM, et al. 1997. Comparison of nested PCR with immunofluorescent-antibody assay for detection of *Ehrlichia canis* infection in dogs treated with doxycycline. *J Clin Microbiol* 35:1852–1855.

141. Wilson JF. 1992. *Ehrlichia platys* in a Michigan dog. *J Am Anim Hosp Assoc* 28:381–383.

142. Winkler GC, Arnold P, DePlazes, et al. 1990. Clinical and serological diagnosis of ehrlichiosis in Switzerland. *European J Companion Anim Pract* 1:49–54.

142a. Wong S, Brady G, Dumler J. 1997. Serological responses to *Ehrlichia equi*, *Ehrlichia chaffeensis*, and *Borrelia burgdorferi* in patients from New York State. *J Clin Microbiol* 35:2198–2205.

143. Wong S, Grady LJ. 1996. *Ehrlichia* infection as a cause of severe respiratory distress. *N Engl J Med* 334:273.

144. Woody BJ. 1985. Clinicopathologic findings in 135 cases of naturally occurring canine ehrlichiosis. Presented at the Workshop on Diseases Caused by *Leucocytic Rickettsiae* of Man and Animals. University of Illinois, Champaign-Urbana, IL.

145. Woody BJ, Hoskins JD. 1991. Ehrlichial diseases of dogs. *Vet Clin North Am Small Anim Pract* 21:75–98.

146. Yamane I, Gardner IA, Ryan CP, et al. 1994. Serosurvey of *Babesia canis*, *Babesia gibsoni* and *Ehrlichia canis* in pound dogs in California, USA. *Prev Vet Med* 18:293–304.

147. Yeh MT, Mather TN, Coughlin RT, et al. 1997. Serologic and molecular-detection of granulocytic ehrlichiosis in Rhode Island. *J Clin Microbiol* 35:944–947.

148. Yu X, Crocquet-Valdes P, Cullman LC, et al. 1996. The recombinant 120-kilodalton protein of *Ehrlichia chaffeensis*, a potential diagnostic tool. *J Clin Microbiol* 34:2853–2855.

149. Yu X, Crocquet-Valdes P, Walker DH. 1997. Cloning and sequencing of the gene for a 120-kDa immunodominant protein of *Ehrlichia chaffeensis*. *Gene* 184:149–154.

150. Yu X, Piesman IF, Olson JG, et al. 1997. Short report: geographic distribution of different genetic types of *Ehrlichia chaffeensis*. *Am J Trop Med Hyg* 56:679–680.

151. Zhi N, Rikihisa Y, Kim HY, et al. 1997. Comparison of major antigenic proteins of six strains of the human granulocytic ehrlichiosis agent by Western immunoblot analysis. *J Clin Microbiol* 35:2606–2611.

Chapter 29

Rocky Mountain Spotted Fever, Q Fever, and Typhus

Craig E. Greene and Edward B. Breitschwerdt

Rocky Mountain Spotted Fever

ETIOLOGY AND EPIDEMIOLOGY

Rocky Mountain spotted fever (RMSF) is a tickborne, rickettsial disease of the Americas that affects dogs and people. Although cats and other domestic animals can be seropositive, knowledge concerning the occurrence of disease in these other animals is minimal. RMSF was recognized primarily in the western United States before 1930. RMSF is known to occur throughout the contiguous United States with the exception of Maine. It has been reported in western Canada, Mexico, Panama, Costa Rica, Honduras, Nicaragua, Colombia, and Brazil. Overall, the reported prevalence of the human disease appears to have increased since its discovery; the highest yearly incidence is now reported from the eastern United States (Fig. 29–1). Presumably, this increase reflects increased recognition and reporting rather than geographic spread of the disease.

Deciduous forests, increased humidity, and warmer temperatures are factors associated with the high prevalence of this tick-transmitted disease in these areas.

Rickettsia rickettsii, the etiologic agent of RMSF, is an obligate intracellular parasite in the family Rickettsiaceae (Fig. 29–2). Members of the spotted fever group (SFG), such as *R. rickettsii*, are most closely related to the typhus group of rickettsiae (Table 29–1) but are distinct from other rickettsial genera. Serologically, genetically, and pathogenically distinct strains of SFG rickettsiae have been described throughout the world.[15, 23] Four main SFG species, *R. rickettsii*, *R. montana*, *R. rhipicephali*, and *R. bellii*, are isolated from ticks on dogs in the United States.[15] *R. rickettsii* is the only SFG species in the Western Hemisphere known to be pathogenic for people and animals. However, serologic evidence supports potential infection with *R. canada* or other as yet uncharacterized rickettsiae in dogs and people.[9] In addition, the role of nonpathogenic SFG rickettsiae in immunocompromised individuals has not been clarified. *Rhipicephalus sanguineus* and *Amblyomma cajennense* are the most commonly implicated ticks in transmission of *R. rickettsii* to people in Mexico and South America, respectively. *R. conorii*, the etiologic agent of boutonneuse or Mediterranean spotted fever, is an analogous organism predominating in the Eastern Hemisphere. It is primarily transmitted by dog ticks of the genus *Rhipicephalus*.[37–39, 58] Queensland tick typhus (*R. australis*), Japanese spotted fever (*R. japonica*), North Asian tick typhus (*R. sibirica*), and rickettsialpox (*R. akari*) are analogous diseases caused by other SFG rickettsiae and transmitted by arthropods in

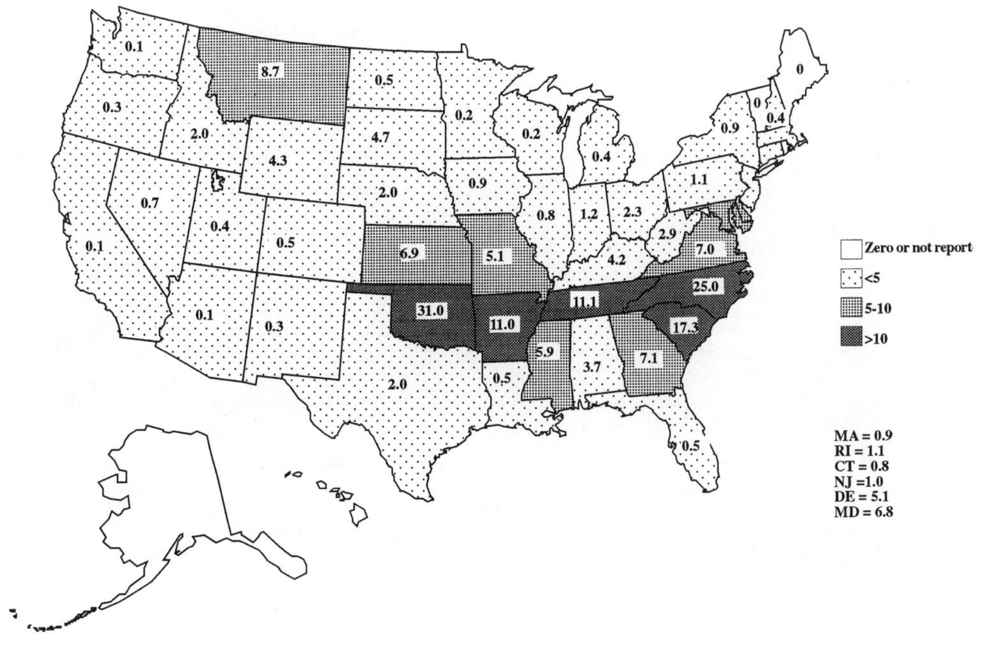

Figure 29–1. Distribution of cases of RMSF in people in the United States from 1981 to 1992 reported as average yearly incidence per million population. (Data compiled from Dalton MJ et al: *Am J Trop Med Hyg* 52:405–413, 1995, with permission.)

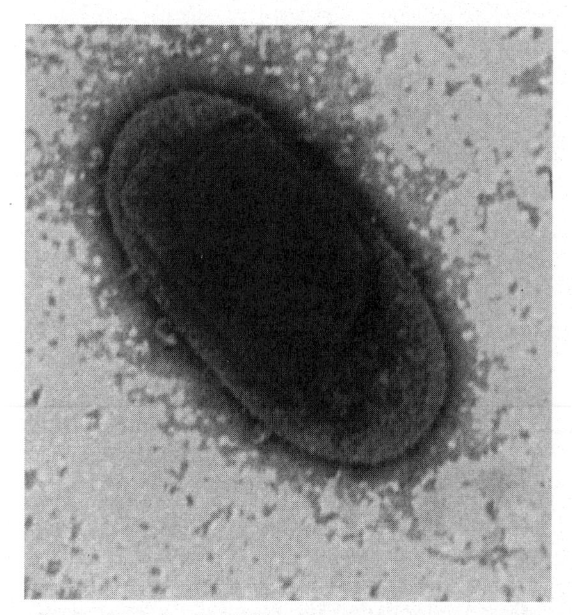

Figure 29–2. *R. rickettsii* in yolk sac culture (× 15,000).

geographically distinct regions. In this chapter, RMSF, as it occurs in the United States, is emphasized as the model disease.

The natural history and distribution of RMSF in the United States appear to center primarily on the distribution of two ticks, *Dermacentor andersoni* and *D. variabilis*, which serve as natural hosts, reservoirs, and vectors for *R. rickettsii*. *D. andersoni* (the wood tick) is a three-host tick that is found from the Cascades to the Rocky Mountains. It is the principal vector of RMSF in the western United States and is also present in Canada in the provinces of southern British Columbia, Alberta, and Saskatchewan. *D. variabilis* (American dog tick) is a three-host tick found from the Great Plains region eastward to the Atlantic Coast of the United States and southern Canada. It has also been reported in California, southwestern Oregon, southern Washington, and Idaho.

Three other ticks have been incriminated in the United States in the transmission of RMSF to animals and people, but their significance is uncertain. The Lone Star tick (*Amblyomma americanum*) occurs in the United States from Texas eastward to the Atlantic Coast. The brown dog tick, *Rhipicephalus sanguineus*, is found throughout the United States, southern Canada, Mexico, and South America. Unlike the other vector ticks, *R. sanguineus* feeds on dogs during all three stages and has rarely been reported to feed on people. *Haemaphysalis leporispalustris*, the rabbit tick, resides throughout the Western Hemisphere. Although some rickettsiae recovered from this tick have been antigenically similar to *R. rickettsii*, they do not produce disease in laboratory animals.

Ticks become infected by two means (Fig. 29–3). First, horizontal transmission can occur during feeding of noninfected ticks on small mammals, including chipmunks, voles, and ground squirrels, that have developed sufficient rickettsemia during acute infection. The primary sylvan cycle, which maintains the transmission cycle in nature, occurs between these small rodents and immature (larval and nymphal) tick stages, and it is possible that medium-sized mammals such as raccoons, opossums, and foxes are additional sources for infecting ticks. Although of minor importance, birds are a means by which infected ticks can be transported into new areas.

Second, ticks can be infected transtadially and also vertically by transovarial passage between generations. *R. rickettsii* initially replicates in the epithelial cells of the tick midgut, enters the hemocoel, and from there spreads to and multiplies in other tick tissues, including the salivary glands and ovaries. Ticks must ingest numerous rickettsiae for successful transovarial transmission, which is the primary means by which *R. rickettsii* is maintained in nature.

Table 29–1. Comparison of Some Pathogenic Rickettsiae Affecting Dogs and Cats[a]

DISEASE (AGENT)	GEOGRAPHIC LOCATION	INSECT VECTOR	INCIDENTAL HOST	RESERVOIR HOST
Spotted Fever Group[b]				
Rocky Mountain spotted fever (*Rickettsia rickettsii*)	Western Hemisphere	*Dermacentor* ticks	People, dogs, cats	Rodent, dogs
Boutonneuse fever (*R. conorii*)	Africa, India, Black Sea countries, Mediterranean region	*Rhipicephalus* ticks	People	Rodent, dogs
Typhus Group[c]				
Epidemic typhus (*R. prowazekii*)	South America, United States?, Africa, Asia	*Pediculus* body louse	Domestic animals	People, flying squirrels
Murine (endemic) typhus (*R. typhi*)	Foci worldwide	Rat flea *Xenopsylla*	People	Rats, cats
R. felis	Texas, California, Oklahoma	Cat flea *Ctenocephalides*	People	Opossum, cats
Scrub Typhus				
(*Orientia tsutsugamushi*)	Southeastern Asia	Mites, *Leptotrombidium*	People, dogs (subclinical)	Rats, birds
Other				
Q fever (*Coxiella burnetii*)[d]	Worldwide	Aerosols, ixodid ticks	People, dogs	Cattle, sheep, goats, cats
Salmon poisoning[e] (*Neorickettsia helminthoeca*)	U.S. Pacific Northwest	Fluke	People (rare)	Dogs, foxes

[a]For Ehrlichiosis and other related rickettsiae, see Table 28–1.
[b]Also includes Queensland tick typhus (*R. australis*; Australia), North Asian (Siberian) tick typhus (*R. sibirica*; Siberia, Mongolia), rickettsialpox (*R. akari*; Soviet Republics, United States, Africa, Korea), Japanese spotted fever (*R. japonica*; Japan), African tick bite fever (*R. africae*; Africa), Indian and Thai tick typhus rickettsiae, and Flinders Island spotted fever (*R. honei*, Tasmania). Astrakhan fever *Rickettsia* is closely related to Israel tick typhus *Rickettsia*, and both are genotypes in the *R. conorii* complex. Unnamed spotted fevers have been identified as *R. slovaca* (Slovakia, Armenia, Russia, France, Switzerland, Portugal) and *R. mongolotimonae* (Inner Mongolia, France).
[c]Also includes *R. canada*.
[d]*Coxiella* is now classified as a member of the *Proteobacteria* but is included in this section for clinical and historical reasons.
[e]See Chapter 27.

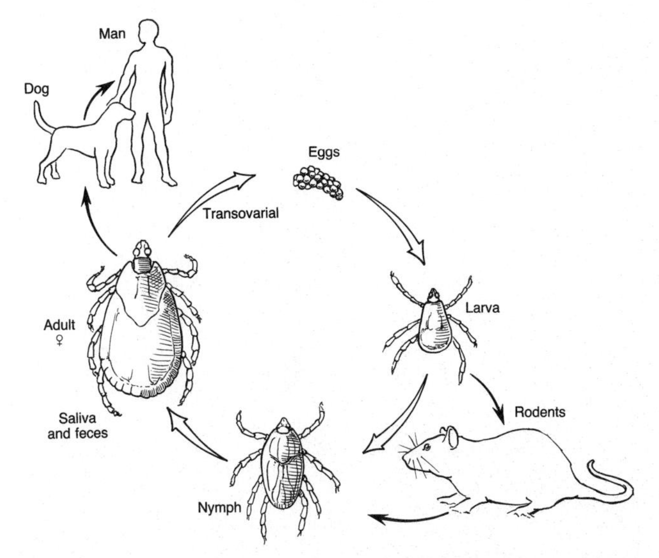

Figure 29–3. Relationship of ticks and their host in transmission of RMSF.

Several restrictions may explain why RMSF is limited to geographic islands in the Americas. The overall low prevalence of infection in ticks, less than 2% even in areas with a high prevalence of RMSF, suggests that most mammalian hosts of adult ticks, such as dogs, rarely develop rickettsemias of sufficient magnitude and duration to infect large numbers of ticks. Furthermore, rickettsial infection of ticks is not an ideal symbiotic relationship, and tick reproduction may be impaired or death may occur. Last, resistance to infection with *R. rickettsii* develops in ticks and possibly mammalian hosts as a result of infection with the other common nonpathogenic SFG rickettsiae.

For reasons that are not completely understood, ticks do not usually infect a new host until they have been attached for a minimum of 5 to 20 hours. A reactivation period within the tick with an apparent increased rickettsial virulence is thought to occur after ticks reattach and take their first blood meal of the season. A period of feeding also may be needed for the continued replication of infective rickettsiae in the salivary glands. Delayed transmission may also relate to the ticks' need to produce a cement collar around their mouth parts before they begin feeding. Although infections that people acquire from tick bites require extended attachment, those acquired from contact of mucous membranes with feces or hemolymph from pre-engorged ticks on animals or contact with laboratory-infected cultures or mammalian blood do not appear to involve extended contact periods.

PATHOGENESIS

R. rickettsii usually enter the body through the bite of infected ticks (Fig. 29–4). Rickettsiae are disseminated via the circulatory system and invade and replicate in endothelial cells of smaller arteries and venules. Phospholipase and proteases have been incriminated as mechanisms for rickettsial damage to cell membranes. Subsequent endothelial cell damage initiates a vasculitis with platelet activation and activation of the coagulation system accompanied by decreased plasma levels of antithrombin III and plasminogen and increased fibrinogen degradation products (FDPs). These hematologic changes are consistent with simultaneous activation of the fibrinolytic and coagulation systems. Coagulation factor consumption is not usually extensive enough to cause hypofibrinogenemia or disseminated intravascular coagulation (DIC).[70] Results of coagulation factor analysis suggest activation of both the extrinsic and intrinsic pathways. Progressive necrotizing vasculitis may be caused sequentially by complement activation, cellular chemotaxis, and subsequent vascular necrosis and extravasation of blood. Organs with endarterial circulation, such as the skin, brain, heart, and kidneys, are frequently affected.

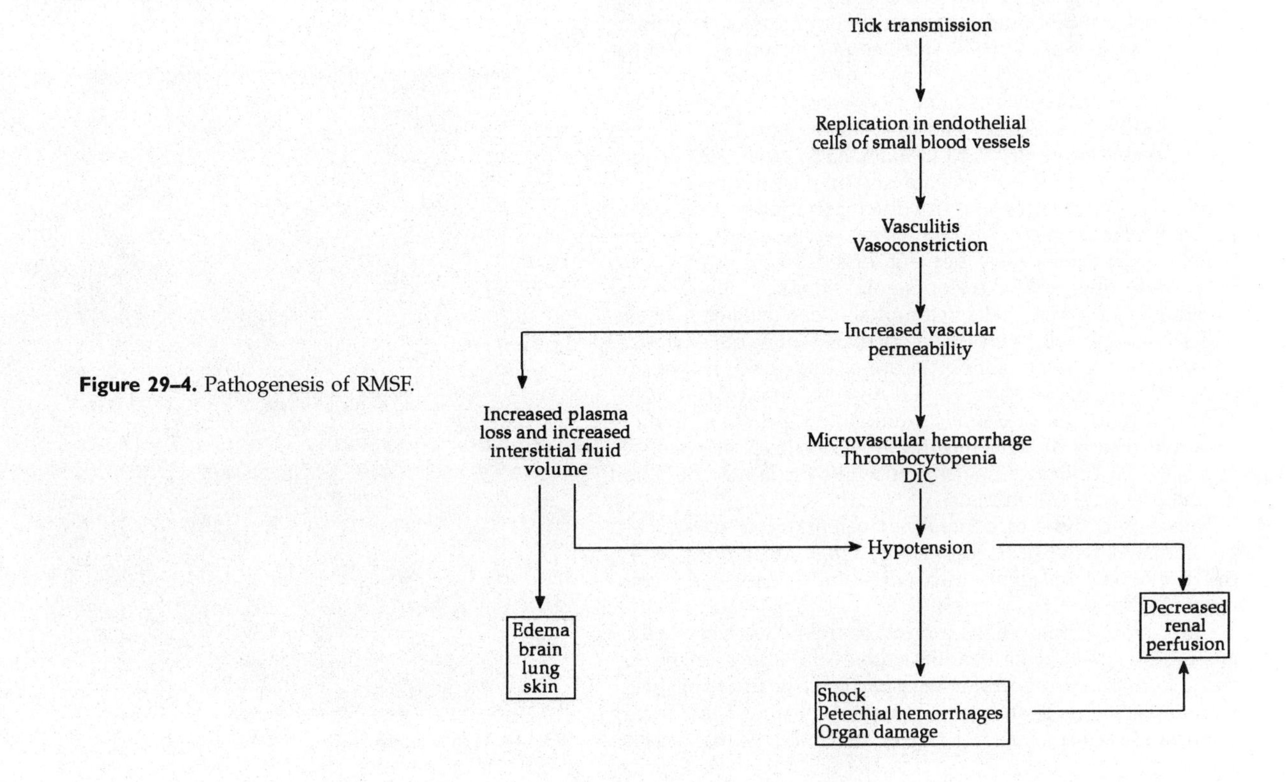

Figure 29–4. Pathogenesis of RMSF.

Significantly increased plasma and extracellular fluid volume have been described in experimental infections of nonhuman primates. Accumulation of extracellular fluid and electrolytes, renal water retention, and edema were correlated with increased concentrations of aldosterone and antidiuretic hormone (ADH) in people. Hyponatremia, which occurs in both dogs and people, may be related to the syndrome of inappropriate ADH release. Fluid overload in the circulation and edema of the medulla oblongata in experimental animals suggest that IV fluid therapy be used sparingly in the management of dogs with RMSF. CNS signs and death may relate to cardiorespiratory depression through edema involving medullary centers. Fulminant infection may result in peripheral vascular collapse and death in the first week of infection, before proliferative and thrombotic lesions occur. Acute renal failure, a fatal complication of RMSF in people, has been infrequently reported in dogs.

CLINICAL FINDINGS

Both clinical and subclinical illnesses have been reported in dogs with naturally occurring and experimentally produced RMSF. Naturally acquired immunity has an important role in protection against clinical illness. Anti-SFG rickettsial antibodies can be found in the healthy canine population in endemic areas. This observation may be a consequence of subclinical infections or the result of exposure to nonpathogenic SFG in ticks. Immunogenic contact with *R. rickettsii* induces a protective response in experimental dogs to reinfection for up to 3 years.[10] These factors may explain the propensity of infection in dogs younger than 2 years. Most dogs are presented for examination of illness during the months of March to October. Purebred dogs appear to be more prone to develop clinical illness compared with mixed breed dogs, and the German shepherd dog has a particularly high prevalence of disease. People with glucose-6-phosphate dehydrogenase deficiency and English springer spaniels with suspected phosphofructokinase deficiency have a more fulminant course of illness and are more likely to develop dermal necrosis.[72] Clinical signs of illness in dogs are similar to those in cases of naturally infected people and are summarized in Table 29–2.

Fever, one of the earliest and most consistent findings, can occur within 2 to 3 days after tick attachment. The range of the incubation period is 2 to 14 days. Early cutaneous lesions in some dogs consist of edema and hyperemia of the lips, penile sheath, scrotum, pinna, other extremities, and rarely the ventral abdomen. Discrete clear vesicles and focal erythematous macules have been observed on the buccal mucosa. Male dogs that develop scrotal edema or epididymal swelling often have a stiff gait and show reluctance to walk.

Petechial and ecchymotic hemorrhages may develop subsequent to the acute illness in some dogs and, if present, occur on ocular, oral, and genital mucous membranes rather than the skin. Funduscopic examination provides a more sensitive means of detecting these hemorrhagic lesions (see Fig. 93–12).[18] Epistaxis, melena, and hematuria may be noted in severely affected animals.

Neurologic signs of generalized cerebral and spinal cord involvement have been found (see Table 29–2). Focal or localizing neurologic signs, such as vestibular disease, are common.

Infected dogs may make a rapid complete recovery if they are mildly affected or if antimicrobial therapy is instituted early. Permanent organ damage, particularly resulting in residual neurologic dysfunction, may occur within 1 to 2 weeks of onset of clinical signs in severely affected dogs that survive the acute stages of illness. Necrosis of the extremities and previously hyperemic or edematous portions of the body may occur at this time (Fig. 29–5). Dogs may die in the acute stages of illness as a result of hemorrhagic diathesis or from

Table 29–2. Frequency of Clinical Findings in People and Dogs With RMSF

CLINICAL FINDINGS	PEOPLE (N = 262)	DOGS (N = 79)
Low fever	99 (>37.8°C)	67 (>39.2°C)
High fever	90 (>38.9°C)	54 (>40°C)
Headache	91	NR
Rash, petechiae	88	19
Myalgia, arthralgia	83	49
Anorexia	NR	51
Known tick exposure	67	52
Nausea, vomiting	60	18
Abdominal/lumbar pain	52	30
Conjunctivitis, scleral congestion	30	34
Lymphadenomegaly	27	43
Stupor, depression, altered mental status	26	83
Vestibular deficits[a]	18	41
Cervical pain, nuchal rigidity	18	8
Coma, unconsciousness	9	4
Seizures	8	10
Diarrhea	19	16
Edema of face, extremities	18	25
Polydipsia, polyuria	NR	5
Splenomegaly	16	3
Hepatomegaly	12	3
Pneumonitis, dyspnea, cough	12	39
Jaundice	9	4
Cardiac arrhythmias	7	8
Death	4	3

Data from Helmick CG et al: *J Infect Dis* 150:480–488, 1984; Greene CE: *J Am Vet Med Assoc* 19:666–671, 1987; and Greene CE, University of Georgia, unpublished observations, 1989.
[a]Deficits include vestibular signs of nystagmus, head tilt, circling, and incoordination.
NR = not reported.

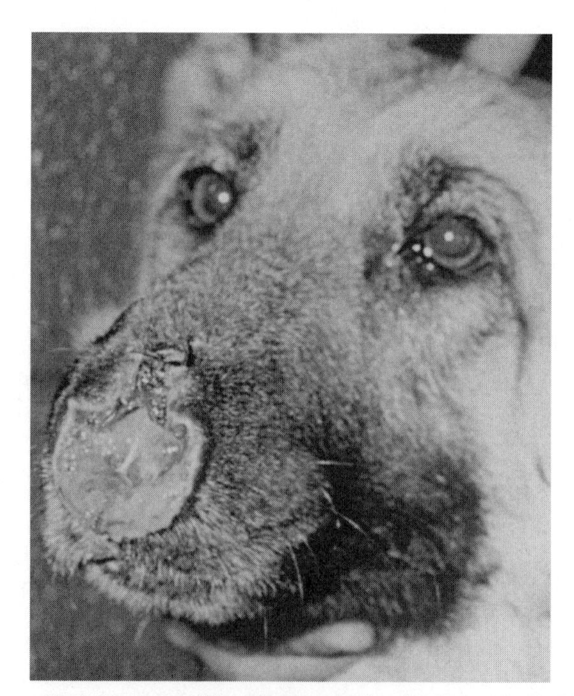

Figure 29–5. Necrosis of the planum nasale of a dog with RMSF.

thrombosis of vital organs. Cardiovascular, neurologic, and renal damage are the most consistent causes of death or permanent organ dysfunction. Death in some severely affected dogs has been caused by disseminated, rapidly progressing meningoencephalitis. Shock, cardiovascular collapse, and oliguria become apparent in the terminal stages of illness.

DIAGNOSIS

Clinical Laboratory Findings

Mild leukopenia, which may develop early in the course of illness, is followed by a moderate leukocytosis generally characterized by stress leukogram or accompanied by a minimal left shift. The longer the duration of clinical signs before diagnosis, the more pronounced is the leukocytosis. A normocytic normochromic anemia and elevated erythrocyte sedimentation rate are nonspecific hematologic changes. Fibrinogen concentration, which increases as a result of an acute-phase reaction in mildly to moderately affected dogs, may be decreased in severely affected dogs as a result of rapid consumption secondary to vasculitis.

Thrombocytopenia is one of the most consistent hematologic abnormalities in infected dogs. Platelet counts generally range from 23,000 to 220,000/μl. Megathrombocytosis is usually detectable in a majority of cases. Platelet enumeration may be preferable to microscopic examination of a few fields on blood smears because the thrombocytopenia in RMSF is often not less than 75,000/μl. A mild prolongation of the ACT may be the only coagulation abnormality.[16, 17] Rarely, DIC characterized by prolongation of the activated coagulation time, prothrombin time, activated partial thromboplastin time, and thrombin time with elevated FDPs occurs in dogs.[18]

Biochemical abnormalities may include mildly increased serum glucose concentration and elevated serum alkaline phosphatase, alanine aminotransferase, and aspartate aminotransferase activities. Hypercholesterolemia has been one of the more consistent findings in affected dogs. Hypoalbuminemia is often observed and probably is caused by leakage associated with generalized vascular endothelial damage. Hyponatremia, hypochloremia, and metabolic acidosis are variable findings. The blood urea nitrogen may increase in terminal stages of the disease corresponding with oliguria and renal failure. Proteinuria and hematuria occur as a result of incoagulability or glomerular and tubular injury. Bilirubinuria and hyperbilirubinemia occur in some dogs. Serum creatine kinase has been mildly to moderately increased in some dogs. CSF analysis is frequently normal; however, mildly increased protein (> 25 but < 100 mg/μl) and polymorphonuclear or mononuclear cells may be found. Analysis of synovial fluid in dogs with accompanying polyarthritis has shown inflammatory changes, with a predominant increase in neutrophils. Results of lupus erythematosus cell, rheumatoid factor, antinuclear antibody, platelet autoantibody, and Coombs' testing and of bacterial blood culture results are usually negative.

ECG abnormalities, if present, consist of sinoatrial node dysfunction, ST-segment and T-wave depressions, and premature ventricular contractions. Thoracic radiography reveals diffuse increased interstitial density, especially in dogs presented for dyspnea and coughing.[19a]

Serologic Testing

A wide variety of mammals have detectable antibodies to SFG rickettsiae. The high prevalence of serologic reactivity in these animals compared with the low prevalence of disease may reflect infection by antigenically related avirulent rickettsiae or subclinical infections. Mammalian hosts differ in regard to the specificity of their immune response to rickettsiae. Well-adapted hosts, such as mice, develop highly specific antibody titers against each species of organism. Human serologic responses generally react strongly with group-reactive antibodies, but do not consistently distinguish between typhus group and SFG rickettsiae. Seroreactivity of dogs appears to be intermediate between that of rodents and people. Cross-reactions in dog sera develop between SFG antigens; however, the titer is generally highest to the specific rickettsial species causing infection. There is generally minimal reaction to typhus group or other *Rickettsia*. Clinically healthy dogs on the Atlantic seaboard have between 5% and 15% seropositivity to SFG rickettsiae. Some ill dogs have shown stronger reactivity to nonpathogenic *R. bellii* and typhus group antigens than *R. rickettsii,* suggesting that another yet unidentified *Rickettsia* may be pathogenic.[9]

Several serologic tests have been developed to detect antibodies to RMSF in humans, including Weil-Felix, complement fixation microscopic immunofluorescence (Micro-IF), microagglutination, indirect hemagglutination, ELISA, and latex agglutination.[35] The Micro-IF, ELISA, and LA tests appear to be the best suited to examine canine sera.

The Micro-IF test, an indirect FA test, and the ELISA have the advantages of requiring small amounts of sera and reagents, having high sensitivity, and classifying antibodies to *R. rickettsii* as IgM or IgG. Measurement of IgG antibodies to *R. rickettsii* using the Micro-IF method is used by most diagnostic laboratories that test canine sera. Acute and convalescent IgG titers have been generally less than 64 in uninfected dogs and in those with ehrlichiosis, although titers will vary among laboratories. Actively infected dogs may or may not have increased titers (≥64) by the time clinical signs are apparent and the first sample is taken. IgG titers in experimentally infected dogs with disease manifestations by 3 to 6 days PI have not increased until 2 to 3 weeks PI. Therefore, seronegative results do not discount the possibility of RMSF, and a convalescent sample should be tested at a later date. An IgG titer increase of fourfold or greater is required to document active infection definitively. High IgG titers that develop in actively infected dogs generally decrease after 3 to 5 months, although some may remain positive (≥128) for at least 10 months.[24, 27] Thus, unless single titers are markedly increased (≥1024), active infection cannot be absolutely ascertained and paired samples must be obtained. Differences can be found among laboratories performing the test and within laboratories testing the same sample at a later date. Therefore, it is recommended that acute and convalescent serum samples be submitted together. Simultaneous assessment of IgM and IgG titers can provide more accurate assessment as to the time course of infection when evaluating a single serum sample.

A modification of the test that allows for measurement of IgM has advantages in permitting more specific diagnosis of recent infection with a single convalescent titer, and IgM titers can be increased before increases in IgG titers. The IgM titers in naturally and experimentally infected dogs only increase (≥8) during the first week after infection and decrease after 4 weeks to 8 or less. The maximum measured titers are generally of two to four dilutions lower in magnitude than the corresponding IgG titers in the same animal.

The LA test appears to be a rapid and specific assay for recent *R. rickettsii* infection in dogs.[27] Because the sensitivity is lower than the Micro-IF test, false-negative results occur, although a single increased titer (≥32) appears diagnostic for RMSF in dogs.

Direct Immunodetection

Direct FA staining of infected tissues is a valuable test for rapid clinical or postmortem diagnosis of RMSF. Direct FA procedures have been used to detect organisms in embryonated eggs or tissue culture, tissues at necropsy, ticks, and skin biopsies from acutely infected people and dogs. Full-thickness skin biopsies should be surgically removed from visible lesions on the skin or mucosae and placed in isotonic saline on melting ice or in formalin at room temperature until they are processed. Rickettsiae can be found in approximately 75% of specimens taken from affected lesions and are rarely found in unaffected skin. Formalin fixation causes some decrease in sensitivity of rickettsial detection. Trypsin digestion and deparaffinization are needed to examine specimens that have been processed for light microscopy. Tissue sections are stained by anti–*R. rickettsii* fluorescent antibody for the presence of coccobacillary organisms in endothelial cells and vascular walls of the dermis.

The advantages of the direct FA procedure on tissue is that it potentially can confirm the diagnosis as early as the third or fourth day of disease on a single sample. Direct FA procedures can be performed by veterinary or human laboratories without regard to host species differences. Few false-positive results are found with the direct FA test, but many (30–40%) false-negative reactions can occur and are usually due to prior therapy with chloramphenicol or tetracycline or failure to obtain a sample through an area of vasculitis. Specimens should be obtained early in the course of infection because organisms are eliminated from the tissue within a few days, especially after antimicrobial therapy. Owing to the usual absence of cutaneous petechiae in dogs, biopsy specimens could be obtained from mucosal hemorrhages or from vesicles that may develop in the buccal mucosa. Adaptation of this method using immunoperoxidase staining increases the test sensitivity and specificity.[43a]

Genetic Detection

PCR has made it possible to detect DNA from low numbers of rickettsiae in whole blood or tissue specimens and for comparison of isolates.[60, 69] Amplification of a unique region of the 16S rRNA gene sequence of *R. rickettsii* facilitates acute-phase diagnosis of RMSF, but with current techniques it has not been highly sensitive.

Rickettsial Isolation

Bioassays involving isolation of *R. rickettsii* in susceptible species of laboratory animals have been a research laboratory means of diagnosing RMSF.[15] Fresh- or deep-frozen (−80°C) tissue such as liver, spleen, or brain or clotted blood from biopsy or necropsy specimens can be inoculated into meadow voles or guinea pigs. Their serum may be tested for the presence of antibody to *R. rickettsii*. Tissues or blood of the affected or laboratory animal may be inoculated into embryonated chicken eggs or tissue culture to isolate and purify the agent. A described shell vial method involves using concentrated inoculum to infect a small number of cells, and permits detection in cell culture in as few as 24 to 48 hours.[51] A staining technique using carbol basic fuchsin is widely used for the identification of SFG and typhus group rickettsiae. Rickettsiae may replicate sufficiently within several days with in vitro isolation procedures, whereas bioassays often require a month to complete. Isolation of *R. rickettsii* requires an appropriate tissue culture system and a biosafety level 3 laboratory, and poses a risk of infecting laboratory workers by inadvertent parenteral or aerosol inoculation.

PATHOLOGIC FINDINGS

When RMSF proves fatal, gross lesions, if present, consist of widespread petechial and ecchymotic hemorrhages in all tissues. Generalized hemorrhagic lymphadenomegaly and splenomegaly are usually found.

Microscopic findings consist of necrotizing vasculitis with perivascular polymorphonuclear and lymphoreticular cell infiltrations. Vascular lesions are most prominent in the skin, epididymis, testicle, GI tract, pancreas, kidneys, urinary bladder, myocardium, meninges, retina, and skeletal muscle. Acute meningoencephalitis with vasculitis and small focal nodular gliosis is found in brain parenchyma of dogs with acute infections (Fig. 29–6). Focal myocardial and hepatic necrosis and acute interstitial pneumonia are common lesions. Rickettsiae can be detected in many tissues by previously described staining and isolation procedures but not by routine histologic methods.

THERAPY

Mortality in dogs with RMSF usually relates to incorrect diagnosis and treatment or to rapidly progressive shock or severe CNS infections. Antibody titers are generally not available when the dog is admitted, and even then, results from the first sample may not be diagnostic, because it may

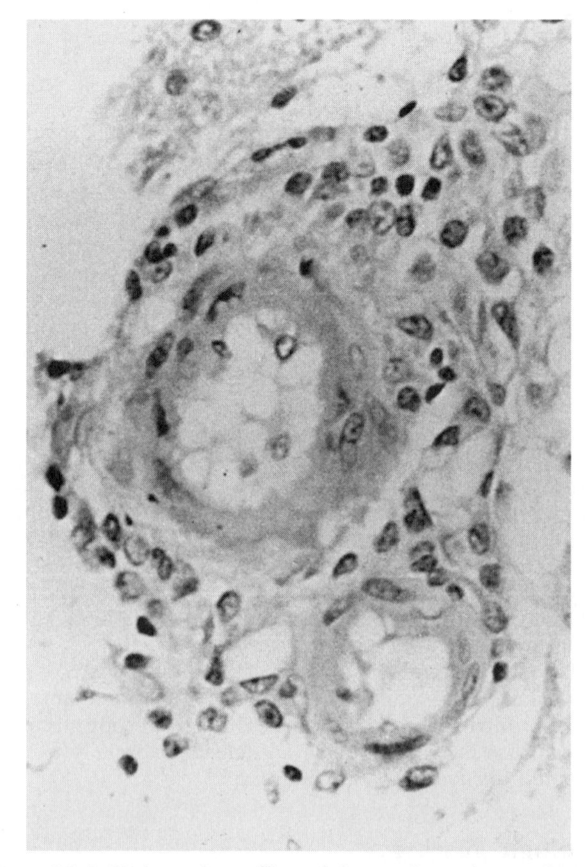

Figure 29–6. Perivascular cuffing of the meninges from a dog that died of rapidly progressive RMSF associated with meningoencephalitis.

Table 29–3. Therapy for Rocky Mountain Spotted Fever

DRUG	DOSE[a] (mg/kg)	ROUTE PREFERRED (ALTERNATE)	INTERVAL (HOURS)	DURATION (WEEKS)
Tetracycline	22–30	PO (IV)	8	1
Chloramphenicol	15–30	PO (IV, SC, IM)	8	1
Doxycycline	10–20	PO (IV)	12	1
Enrofloxacin	3	PO (SC)	12	1

[a]Dose per administration at specified interval.

take 1 to 3 weeks for maximal IgG response. For this reason, a response to therapy is used to increase the index of suspicion. It is judicious to begin treatment immediately after obtaining samples for diagnostic testing. Presumptive diagnosis of RMSF can be made based on the seasonal occurrence and clinical and laboratory abnormalities. The antibiotics used to treat RMSF are considered to be rickettsiostatic (Table 29–3). Although slightly prolonging the duration of rickettsemia, anti-inflammatory and immunosuppressive doses of glucocorticoids do not increase the severity of disease in experimentally infected dogs.[8] Tetracycline or oxytetracycline should be given for at least 7 days. Lipid-soluble tetracyclines, such as minocycline or doxycycline, have been shown to be as effective in treating rickettsial infections in people when they have been used for periods of fewer than 7 days. Chloramphenicol is equally effective and is indicated in pregnancy or in young (< 6 months old) puppies to avoid dental staining. Fluoroquinolones such as enrofloxacin are also effective,[7] but their use must be restricted to older animals. A newer macrolide antimicrobial, josamycin, has been used successfully in treating pregnant women with *R. conorii* infection.[19] Parenteral administration of these drugs may be required in patients that are semicomatose or have nausea or are vomiting. Dogs treated early in the course of illness have rapid clinical improvement, generally within 24 to 48 hours after therapy is instituted. Defervescence within 12 hours is not unusual. Delayed or incomplete recovery is associated with organ failure or with CNS damage. Some dogs treated with chloramphenicol and, less commonly, with tetracycline develop depression, nausea, and vomiting, which can appear to delay their clinical recovery. Antibiotics are only effective in reducing the severity of the illness if they are given before the development of advanced pathologic changes, such as thrombosis and tissue necrosis. Dogs that develop acryl gangrene and recover will have eventual healing of their extremities with permanent scarring or disfigurement.

Supportive care must be used in dogs with shock, coagulation disorders, and clinical or laboratory evidence of organ failure. IV fluid therapy must be used with caution because increased vascular permeability and expanded extracellular fluid volume can give rise to pulmonary and cerebral edema.

PREVENTION

Dogs recovering from infection with *R. rickettsii* have been immune to reinfection when challenged 6 to 36 months later. Experimentally, infection with nonpathogenic rickettsiae such as *R. montana* does not seem to protect dogs from subsequent infection with the more virulent *R. rickettsii*. Naturally infected dogs that recover from RMSF have never been shown to be reinfected.

No vaccines are available for use in dogs or people. Challenge infection in people after vaccination with inactivated products has been associated with a prolonged incubation period, a shorter and milder course of illness, and reduced prevalence of relapses, but reinfection is not prevented. Experimental, inactivated, tissue culture–origin vaccines appear to offer protection against infection in experimental animals. Specific antigenic components of *R. rickettsii* responsible for producing protective antibody response were identified. Inactivated vaccine containing a 190-kDa surface antigen of *R. rickettsii* produced by recombinant DNA technology has been shown to be immunoprotective in rodents.[2, 67]

The best means of prevention of RMSF in dogs is avoidance of tick-infested areas and rapid, safe removal of attached ticks. Pets should be dipped repeatedly if they frequent areas inhabited by ticks. Tick eradication in the environment is impossible because of the maintenance of the life cycle by rodents and other reservoir hosts. Elimination of small ground rodents is difficult if not impossible to achieve. Some reduction in tick numbers has been achieved locally in the eastern and southern United States by application of insecticides in the form of aqueous suspension or dust to surrounding vegetation.

PUBLIC HEALTH CONSIDERATIONS

SFG rickettsial infections are important zoonotic diseases because of their endemic nature, their high prevalence, and their severity when mistreated or misdiagnosed. Of the more than 1000 cases of rickettsial diseases reported each year in the United States, approximately 90% are RMSF. Mortality in people remains between 2% and 10%.[14] The yearly incidence rate probably reflects a summation of factors, including encroachment of people on undeveloped wooded areas, improved recognition and reporting of disease, and a periodic cyclicity of infection. The prevalence of seropositive reactions in dogs within a given area usually parallels human risk of infection.

The seasonal occurrence of RMSF in people parallels that in dogs.[14] The rate of infection is highest in children and young adults and is higher in males. Patients from rural areas have a greater proportion of confirmed diagnoses compared with those from suburban and urban areas. Approximately 60% of infected people have reported a tick bite, and 30% more said that they were in a wooded area just before clinical illness. The lack of known exposure does not eliminate tick involvement in infection, especially because small larval and nymphal stages can feed transiently and remain undetected. Most exposures in the eastern United States occur at the place of residence, but a number have been related to an outdoor recreational activity. Approximately 10% of reported human cases follow only known exposure to dogs or their ticks, but this should not imply an absolute association, because common exposure to the same tick population is a more likely source of infection.

Dogs are a potential source for human infections because they carry infected ticks into nonendemic environs or into closer proximity to people, who become exposed by transfer of unattached ticks from dogs to themselves or by their contact with the engorged tick's hemolymph during tick removal or by contact with tick excreta with the person's abraded skin or conjunctivae.[58] It is not the secretions from infected dogs but the effluents from engorged, infected ticks that pose the greatest danger. Aerosol exposure from an infected dog's secretions is unlikely under natural conditions because the organism does not survive outside host or tick cells. Aerosol exposure has only occurred in the laboratory, where inadvertent inoculation of infected tissues may also occur.

The clinical manifestations in affected people closely parallel those signs seen in dogs (see Table 29–2). Early signs in people are vague and may mimic an upper respiratory tract infection. Although the rash is considered typical of RMSF, it never develops in up to 12% of people, and when it does develop, it is seen in less than 50% of the cases within the first 3 days of illness. Not all people develop all manifestations of RMSF, although fever and headache are most consistent. Neurologic signs usually develop later in the course of illness. Death appears to be more of a problem in people who develop severe hepatomegaly, jaundice, stupor, and azotemia (serum urea >25 mg/dl). Cardiac arrhythmias from myocarditis, meningoencephalitis, and DIC often are detected in terminal patients. Subclinical infections in people have been suspected, but the role of nonpathogenic rickettsiae in causing the observed serologic responses has not been determined.

Ticks should be removed by applying constant traction with curved forceps or less desirably with tweezers or fingers protected with facial tissue placed as close as possible to the point of insertion. Ticks should not be squeezed or crushed with bare fingers because the organism can be transmitted via tick feces or hemolymph. Hands should be washed thoroughly with soap and water after removal of the tick.

The most effective measures to prevent tick-induced infections have been to wear permethrin-treated clothing and to tuck trouser legs into boots when spending time in tick-infested areas.[75] Wearing clothing that is tight around the ankles and wrists when walking through wooded areas is advised. After outdoor activities, the skin along the hairline and clothing around the cuffs and collars should be examined. Bathing in a tub of water with a cup of added bleach is recommended after leaving tick-infested areas. Consult the chapter on Lyme borreliosis (Chapter 45) for additional information on tick control.

Q Fever

ETIOLOGY AND EPIDEMIOLOGY

Q (query) fever is caused by the bacteria *Coxiella burnetii* (see Table 29–1). It is an endemic zoonosis worldwide except in Sweden, Norway, Iceland, and New Zealand, where reports of the disease are rare. Reservoir hosts vary, depending on the geographic location, and include domestic and wild animals and their ectoparasites. Approximately 40 species of ticks and many other arthropods are naturally infected with *C. burnetii*. The tick facilitates a sylvan cycle with reservoir animals. Resultant infection of humans and domestic animals may occur when infected ticks feed on them. However, domestic animals and people are more commonly infected by inhalation or ingestion of environmentally resistant organisms. Cattle, sheep, and goats are the most common domestic animal reservoirs for human infection. Wildlife species may be the reservoir hosts for domestic pets. Typically, animals are subclinically infected and shed environmentally resistant organisms in their urine, feces, milk, and parturient discharges. The placenta in late gestation may contain the greatest concentration of *C. burnetii* organisms (10^9 per gram of tissue). Within the herd, infection is probably maintained by inhalation of infected dusts and aerosols or by fomites.

This organism sporulates and is highly resistant, maintaining viability in spite of elevated temperatures, dessication, osmotic shock, UV light, and chemicals.[57] Hypochlorite (0.5%), phenolics (15%), formalin (5%), and quaternary ammonium compounds (2%) were not completely effective in killing the organism after 24 hours. After 30 minutes, solutions of alcohol (70%) or chloroform (5%) were effective in destroying *C. burnetii*.

Serologic and organism isolation studies indicate that dogs and cats can be infected (Table 29–4). Dogs and cats may acquire infection under natural circumstances by tick bites or by ingestion or inhalation of organisms while feeding on infected body tissues, milk, placentas, or carcasses. Inhalation of infected aerosols is also possible in contaminated environments. *C. burnetii* has been found in the blood of experimentally infected cats for 1 month and in their urine for 2 months. It has been isolated from the uteri of postpartum cats. Bitches can shed coxiellae in their milk for 1 month and in urine for at least 70 days. Infected (especially parturient) dogs and cats can be a source of infection for people. The organism was isolated from dogs and from *Rhipicephalus sanguineus* ticks, which were feeding on them, on farms where human outbreaks of Q fever occurred. People have become infected via contact with pets that have acquired their infection from exposure to herbivores. There have been frequent reports of people becoming infected after exposure of aerosols from contaminated environment or fomites with parturient or aborted tissues from infected cats[42, 45–47, 52] and a dog.[11]

PATHOGENESIS

After inhalation in people, the lungs appear to be the main portal of entry of the organism to the systemic circulation. If the organism is ingested, the liver is prone to develop more severe lesions. The incubation period is shorter and severity of disease greater when people are exposed to increasing numbers of organisms; after exposure to highly virulent strain; or when the organism is inhaled rather than ingested. This bacterium has a predilection for replication in the vascular endothelium and respiratory, renal tubular, and serosal epithelia. Widespread vasculitis results in focal necrotizing hemorrhagic pneumonitis and necrosis and hemorrhage of many other organs, including the liver, CNS, and mononuclear phagocyte system. After recovery, people can be latently infected with *C. burnetii* for extended periods. During chronic

Table 29–4. Prevalence of Serum Antibodies to* Coxiella burnetii *in Dogs and Cats

ANIMAL	GEOGRAPHIC LOCATION	SEROPOSITIVITY (%)	REFERENCE
Pound cats	Southern California	20	52a
Dogs	Northern California	48	41
Stray dogs	Northern California	66	41
Cats	Maritime Canada	20	31
Dogs	Japan	15	34
Cats	Japan	16	34
Dogs	Egypt	15.9	41
Pet dogs	Bologna, Italy	0.87	5
Stray dogs	Sicily, Italy	32	41
Dog	Central Italy	24.5	41
Stray dogs	Czechoslovakia	23.7	40
Farm dogs	Czechoslovakia	13.6	40
Dogs	Switzerland	31.4	41
Dogs	West Germany	13	41

infection, immune complex phenomena can develop. In chronically infected people and in subclinically infected animals, the organism remains latent until parturition, at which time large numbers enter the placenta, parturient fluids, feces, urine, and milk.

CLINICAL FINDINGS

Infections in dogs and cats are usually subclinical. Splenomegaly was the only clinical finding in an infected dog. Fever, anorexia, and lethargy beginning 2 days after inoculation and lasting for 3 days occurs in experimentally infected cats. Abortion has occurred in some of the cats and has also been associated with human outbreaks, but the organism has also been isolated from cats having normal parturition. A dog that transmitted infection to people delivered pups that died within 24 hours of birth. For clinical signs in people, see Public Health Considerations.

DIAGNOSIS

Lymphocytosis and thrombocytopenia are the main nonspecific hematologic changes in infected people. Definitive diagnosis of Q fever is made by serologic testing or by isolation of the organism. Although information concerning human exposure can be obtained by examining a single serum sample, it is recommended that a second sample be submitted 4 weeks later. A fourfold increase in *C. burnetii*–specific IgG titer is diagnostic.

Two separate serologic antigens are used in detecting antibodies. Phase I antigens are isolated from organisms taken directly from animals or their parasites. Phase II antigens are found in organisms that have been passed serially in embryonated eggs. During acute illness, antibody to phase II antigen increases, whereas that to phase I antigen is low. In chronic infections, antibody to phase I antigen equals or is greater than that of the phase II type.[21] Titers from cats involved in outbreaks have shown a similar pattern of reactivity to phase I and phase II antigens. Newer diagnostic tests that can provide a convincing diagnosis on a single sample involve measurement of specific IgM to phase II antigen or of IgA to phase I antigen using immunofluorescent or ELISA methods.[13, 64] Organism isolation is usually performed by inoculation of tissue samples into laboratory rodents whose serum and lymphoid tissues are examined for evidence of infection. PCR can be used for detection of *C. burnetii* in tissue culture or in specimens of tissue derived from patients.[66]

THERAPY

Rickettsiostatic drugs, such as tetracyclines and chloramphenicol, are as effective in the treatment of Q fever as when treating RMSF (see Table 29–3). Use of erythromycin and trimethoprim-sulfonamide has been variably successful in treating infected people. Newer erythromycin derivatives such as clarithromycin may be more effective.[11] Because many affected people recover spontaneously from their acute illness, interpretation of recovery is difficult without an untreated control population. The most successful in vitro combinations have included rifampin combined with doxycycline or trimethoprim. Quinolones are active in vitro against this organism as with related organisms. Chronic infections in people with endocarditis have been treated effectively with a combination of quinolones and doxycycline for 3 years.[44]

PREVENTION

Q fever vaccines are not available for animals or people. Experimentally, dogs have been vaccinated with formalin-inactivated phase I and phase II antigens and have developed humoral and cell-mediated immunity responses to *C. burnetii*.[73] Unfortunately, the vaccines or their adjuvants caused significant reactions at the inoculation sites.

PUBLIC HEALTH CONSIDERATIONS

Human Q fever is usually contracted by inhalation of infected aerosols such as occurs after parturition or by ingestion of raw or poorly cooked foodstuffs from livestock. Inhalation has been the suspected means of infection in outbreaks associated with parturient cats[42, 45–47] and a dog.[11] Because of occupational exposure, abattoir workers, wool sorters, tanners, farm workers (shepherds, dairy workers), and veterinary and laboratory personnel are particularly susceptible to infection from livestock. Investigational inactivated vaccines are available in the United States for such high-risk exposure groups. Children, who are commonly infected from ingestion of raw milk, are usually nonsymptomatic, regardless of the source of infection.

Dogs have been reported to transmit infection to people on a few occasions. These have usually been rural exposures associated with farm dogs that have had exposure to sheep or their offal. Some of the previously reported outbreaks of Q fever in urban settings have related to exposure to environments contaminated by infected cats. In cat-associated Q fever, the incubation period, from time of contact until the first signs of illness, ranges from 4 to 30 days. The radiographic appearance of pneumonia in people infected from cats is more often associated with rounded pulmonary opacities.[47] Common source exposure is likely under such circumstances because the organism can be spread on clothing, dust, and other fomites to other people. Direct person-to-person transmission is uncommon but can occur because the organism is present in the body secretions of infected people.

After a prolonged incubation period (14–39 days), acute systemic manifestations consist of headache, fever (≥40°C [104°F]), chills, and myalgia. Less commonly, nausea, vomiting, diarrhea, arthralgia, or erythematous macules are noted. Although the respiratory tract is the usual source of infection and clinical or radiographic findings of interstitial pneumonitis may develop, respiratory signs occur infrequently. Signs of acute hepatitis may also occur. The acute illness generally lasts 15 days, and mortality rates are low, except in older or immunosuppressed individuals. A diagnosis is often made in infected people by measuring serum antibodies (see Diagnosis).

Only a small number (<1%) of patients with acute Q fever develop chronic illness. Chronic Q fever is a potentially fatal, multisystemic disorder that may develop up to 20 years after an acute episode. Signs of chronic endocarditis or hepatitis, such as fever, lethargy, dyspnea, cardiac murmurs, hepatomegaly, thrombocytopenia, and occasional thromboembolism or jaundice, occur. More than 50% of chronic Q fever patients have sera that cross-react at measurable but lower levels with *Bartonella henselae*, another zoonotic agent of cats (see Chapter 54).[43]

Typhus

Humans are the primary reservoirs of louse-borne or epidemic typhus, a sporadic illness caused by *Rickettsia prowazekii.* It occurs when events favor proliferation and spread of lice, such as unsanitary conditions and natural disasters. Human cases of recrudescent or recently introduced typhus are thought to initiate outbreaks. The organism in the louse infects its alimentary tract and is excreted in the feces. Irritation from biting lice causes the person to scratch their skin, thereby contaminating the abraded site with infected louse feces. Lice are affected by *R. prowazekii* such that they die within 1 to 3 weeks after ingestion of infected blood. Lice do not transmit the infection transovarially to their progeny. Another reservoir for this infection in people in the United States appears to be the southern flying squirrel. The clinical signs of disease in people are generally similar to those of spotted fever. Reactivity to typhus group rickettsiae has been observed in dogs suspected of having rickettsial disease.[9] *R. prowazekii* caused no illness or sustained infection in experimentally inoculated immunocompetent dogs.[9] There is no information as to whether this organism infects cats.

Murine or endemic typhus has a more worldwide distribution and is caused by *Rickettsia typhi*, which is transmitted by fleas. It is most prevalent in temperate and subtropical climates where the reservoir rodent hosts and their fleas are found. The disease is transmitted by scratching of infected flea feces into a pruritic bite wound. Some transovarial transmission occurs so that direct bites from fleas can also produce illness. The clinical signs in people are very similar to those of spotted fever.

In the United States, typhus has been reported most frequently in southern Texas and California.[20, 65] Opossums have been implicated as reservoir hosts in these areas, and the vector is the cat flea (*Ctenocephalides felis*). A newly described rickettsial agent, named *Rickettsia felis* (previously ELB),[32] which is serologically indistinguishable from *R. typhi* and *R. prowazekii*, has been identified by PCR in infected fleas, opossums, and people in the same area of the United States reported to be endemic for *R. typhi*.[55, 56] Of five people examined with typhus from Texas, *R. typhi* was identified using PCR and restriction fragment length polymorphism (RFLP) in four people, and *R. felis* was found in the remaining person.[55] In addition to opossums, cats (but not dogs, or rats) have been seropositive to *R. typhi* antigen in these areas.[56, 65] The newly recognized *R. felis* agent is the predominant rickettsiae (over *R. typhi*) in the cat fleas that are feeding on opossums in these endemic regions.[56, 74] *R. felis* has been shown to be transmitted transovarially and trans-stadially in successive generations of *C. felis*.[3, 33] Cats may be likely hosts to transport infected fleas into human habitats. The reservoir potential of cats for this organism, or pathogenicity for cats, has not been determined. Prior experimental infection of cats has produced subclinical infection with seroconversion. *R. felis* has been detected in cat fleas from California, Florida, Georgia, Louisiana, New York, North Carolina, Oklahoma, Tennessee, and Texas, and is probably even more widespread.[2a]

Scrub typhus is a rickettsial disease caused by *Orientia* (previously *Rickettsia*) *tsutsugamushi* in southeastern Asia, the South Pacific, and Australia. It is transmitted by the chigger mite, and wild rodents and birds are reservoir hosts. Dogs have been experimentally infected with *O. tsutsugamushi* without signs of clinical illness.

References

1. Adams JR, Schmidtman ET, Azad AF. 1990. Infection of colonized cat fleas *Ctenocephalides felis* (Bouché) with a *Rickettsia*-like microorganism. *Am J Trop Med Hyg* 43:400–409.
2. Anderson BE, McDonald GA, Jones DC, et al. 1990. A protective protein antigen of *Rickettsia rickettsii* has been tandemly repeated, near identical sequences. *Infect Immun* 58:2760–2769.

2a. Azad AF, Radulovic S, Higgins JA, et al. 1997. Flea-borne rickettsioses: ecologic considerations. *Emerg Infect Dis* 3:319–327.

3. Azad AF, Sacci JB, Nelson WN, et al. 1992. Genetic characterization and transovarial transmission of a typhus-like *Rickettsia* found in cat fleas. *Proc Natl Acad Sci U S A* 89:43–46.
4. Azad AF, Traub R, Sofi M, et al. 1984. Experimental murine typhus infection in the cat flea, *Ctenocephalides felis* (Siphonoptera: Pulicidae). *J Med Entomol* 21:675–680.
5. Baldelli R, Cimmino C, Pasquinelli M. 1992. Dog transmitted zoonoses: a serological survey in the province of Bologna. *Ann 1st Super Sanita* 28:493–496.
6. Beard CB, Butler JF, Hall DW. 1990. Prevalence and biology of endosymbionts of fleas (Siphonaphera: Pulicidae) from dogs and cats in Alachua County Florida. *J Med Entomol* 27:1050–1061.
7. Breitschwerdt EB, Davidson MG, Aucoin DP, et al. 1991. Efficacy of chloramphenicol, enrofloxacin, and tetracycline for treatment of experimental Rocky Mountain spotted fever in dogs. *Antimicrob Agents Chemother* 35:2375–2381.
8. Breitschwerdt EB, Davidson MG, Hegarty BC, et al. 1997. Prednisolone at anti-inflammatory or immunosuppressive dosages in conjunction with doxycycline does not potentiate the severity of *Rickettsia rickettsii* infection in dogs. *Antimicrob Agents Chemother* 41:141–147.
9. Breitschwerdt EB, Hegarty BC, Davidson MG, et al. 1995. Evaluation of the pathogenic potential of *Rickettsia canada* and *Rickettsia prowazekii* organisms in dogs. *J Am Vet Med Assoc* 207:58–63.
10. Breitschwerdt EB, Levy MG, Davidson MG, et al. 1990. Kinetics of IgM and IgG responses to experimental and naturally acquired *Rickettsia rickettsii* infection in dogs. *Am J Vet Res* 51:1312–1316.
11. Buhariwalla F, Cann B, Marrie TJ. 1996. A dog-related outbreak of Q fever. *Clin Infect Dis* 23:753–755.
12. Cooksey LM, Haile DG, Mount GA. 1990. Computer simulation of Rocky Mountain spotted fever transmission by the American dog tick (Acari: Ixodidae). *J Med Entomol* 27:671–680.
13. Cowley R, Fernandez F, Freemantle W, et al. 1992. Enzyme immunoassay for Q fever: comparison with complement fixation and immunofluorescence tests and dot immunoblotting. *J Clin Microbiol* 30:2451–2455.
14. Dalton MJ, Clarke MJ, Holman RC, et al. 1995. National surveillance for Rocky Mountain spotted fever 1981–1992: epidemiologic summary and evaluation of risk factors for fatal outcome. *Am J Trop Med Hyg* 52:405–413.
15. Dasch GA, Weiss E, Balouss A. 1992. The genera *Rickettsia, Rochalimaea, Ehrlichia, Cowdria* and *Neorickettsia*, pp 2407–2470. *In* Schleifer KH (ed), The Prokaryotes—a handbook on the biology of bacteria: ecophysiology, isolation, identification, applications, vol III, ed 2. Springer Verlag, New York, NY.
16. Davidson MG, Breitschwerdt EB, Nasisse MP, et al. 1989. Ocular manifestations of Rocky Mountain spotted fever in dogs. *J Am Vet Med Assoc* 194:777–781.
17. Davidson MG, Breitschwerdt EB, Walker DH, et al. 1989. Identification of rickettsiae in cutaneous biopsy specimens from dogs with experimental Rocky Mountain spotted fever. *J Vet Intern Med* 3:8–11.
18. Davidson MG, Breitschwerdt EB, Walker DH, et al. 1990. Vascular permeability and coagulation during *Rickettsia rickettsii* infection in dogs. *Am J Vet Res* 51:165–170.
19. Drancourt M, Raoult D. 1989. In vitro susceptibilities of *Rickettsia rickettsii* and *Rickettsia conorii* to roxithromycin and pristinamycin. *Antimicrob Agents Chemother* 33:2146–2148.

19a. Drost WT, Berry CR, Breitschwerdt EB, et al. 1997. Thoracic radiographic findings in dogs infected with *Rickettsia rickettsii. Vet Radiol Ultrasound* 38:260–266.

20. Dumler JS, Taylor JP, Walker DH. 1991. Clinical and laboratory features of murine typhus in south Texas 1980 through 1987. *JAMA* 266:1365–1370.
21. Embil J, Williams JC, Marrie TJ. 1990. The immune response in a cat-related outbreak of Q fever as measured by the indirect immunofluorescence test and the enzyme-link immunosorbent assay. *Can J Microbiol* 36:292–296.
22. Eremeeva M, Balayeva N, Roux V, et al. 1995. Genomic and proteinic characterization of strain S, a *Rickettsia* isolated from *Rhipicephalus sanguineus* ticks in Armenia. *J Clin Microbiol* 33:2738–2744.
23. Eremeeva M, Yu X, Raoult D. 1994. Differentiation among spotted fever group rickettsiae species by analysis of restriction fragment length polymorphism of PCR-amplified DNA. *J Clin Microbiol* 32:803–810.

24. Espejo E, Alegre MD, Font B, et al. 1993. Antibodies to *Rickettsia conorii* in dogs—seasonal differences. *Eur J Epidemiol* 9:344–346.
25. Graves SR, Stewart L, Stenos J, et al. 1993. Spotted fever group rickettsial infection in southeastern Australia: isolation of rickettsiae. *Comp Immunol Microbiol Infect Dis* 16:223–233.
26. Greene CE, Breitschwerdt EB. 1990. Rocky mountain spotted fever and Q fever, pp 419–433. *In* Greene CE (ed), Infectious diseases of the dog and cat. WB Saunders, Philadelphia, PA.
27. Greene CE, Marks MA, Lappin MR, et al. 1993. Comparison of latex agglutination indirect immunofluorescent antibody, and enzyme immunoassay methods for serodiagnosis of Rocky Mountain spotted fever in dogs. *Am J Vet Res* 54:20–28.
28. Grindem CB, Corbett WT, Levy MG, et al. 1990. Platelet aggregation in dogs experimentally infected with *Rickettsia rickettsii*. *Vet Clin Pathol* 19:25–28.
29. Gudiol F, Pallares R, Carratala J, et al. 1989. Randomized double-blind evaluation of ciprofloxacin and doxycycline for Mediterranean spotted fever. *Antimicrob Agents Chemother* 33:987–988.
30. Herrero C, Pelaz C, Alvar J, et al. 1992. Evidence of the presence of spotted fever group rickettsiae in dogs and dog ticks of the central provinces in Spain. *Eur J Epidemiol* 8:575–579.
31. Higgins D, Marrie TJ. 1990. Seroepidemiology of Q fever among cats in New Brunswick and Prince Edward Island. *Ann NY Acad Sci* 590:271–274.
32. Higgins JA, Radulovic S, Schriefer ME, et al. 1996. *Rickettsia felis*: a new species of pathogenic *Rickettsia* isolated from cat fleas. *J Clin Microbiol* 34:671–674.
33. Higgins JA, Sacci JB, Schriefer ME, et al. 1994. Molecular identification of *Rickettsia*-like organisms associated with colonized cat fleas (*Ctenocephalides felis*). *Insect Mol Biol* 3:27–33.
34. Htwe KK, Amano K, Sugiyama Y, et al. 1992. Seroepidemiology of *Coxiella burnetii* in domestic and companion animals in Japan. *Vet Rec* 131:490.
35. Jones D, Anderson B, Olson J, et al. 1993. Enzyme-linked immunosorbent assay for detection of human immunoglobulin G to lipopolysaccharide of spotted fever group rickettsiae. *J Clin Microbiol* 31:138–141.
36. Kelly PJ, Beati L, Mason PR, et al. 1997. *Rickettsia africae* sp nov, the etiologic agent of African tick bite fever. *Int J Syst Bacteriol* 46:611–614.
37. Kelly PJ, Mason PR. 1990. Serological typing of spotted fever group *Rickettsia* isolates from Zimbabwe. *J Clin Microbiol* 28:2302–2304.
38. Kelly PJ, Mason PR. 1991. Tick bite fever in Zimbabwe: a survey for antibodies to *Rickettsia conorii* in man and dogs and *Rickettsia*-like organisms in dog ticks. *S Afr Med J* 80:233–236.
39. Kelly PJ, Matthewman LA, Mason PR, et al. 1992. Experimental infection of dogs with a Zimbabwean strain of *Rickettsia conorii*. *J Trop Med Hyg* 95:322–326.
40. Kocianova E, Lisak V, Kopcok M. 1992. *Coxiella burnetii* and *Chlamydia psittaci* infection in dogs. *Vet Med Praha* 37:177–183.
41. Lang GH. 1990. Coxiellosis (Q fever) in animals, pp 33–34. *In* Marrie TJ (ed), Q fever, vol 1: the disease. CRC Press, Boca Raton, FL.
42. Langley JM, Marrie TJ, Covert A, et al. 1988. Poker player's pneumonia. An urban outbreak of Q fever following exposure to a parturient cat. *N Engl J Med* 319:354–356.
43. LaScola B, Raoult D. 1996. Serological cross-reactions between *Bartonella quintana*, *Bartonella henselae*, and *Coxiella burnetii*. *J Clin Microbiol* 24:2270–2274.
43a. LaScola B, Raoult D. 1997. Laboratory diagnosis of rickettsioses: current approaches to diagnosis of old and new rickettsial diseases. *J Clin Microbiol* 35:2715–2727.
44. Levy PY, Drancourt M, Etienne J, et al. 1991. Comparison of different antibiotic regimens for therapy of 32 cases of Q fever endocarditis. *Antimicrob Agents Chemother* 35:533–537.
44a. Mahara F. 1997. Japanese spotted fever: report of 31 cases and review of the literature. *Emerg Infect Dis* 3:105–111.
45. Marrie TJ, Durant H, Williams JC, et al. 1988. Exposure to parturient cats: a risk factor for acquisition of Q fever in Maritime Canada. *J Infect Dis* 158:101–108.
46. Marrie TJ, Langille D, Papukna V, et al. 1989. Truckin' pneumonia—an outbreak of Q fever in a truck repair plant probably due to aerosols from clothing contaminated by contact with newborn kittens. *Epidemiol Infect* 102:119–127.
47. Marrie TJ, MacDonald A, Durant H, et al. 1988. An outbreak of Q fever probably due to contact with a parturient cat. *Chest* 93:98–103.
48. Morita C, Katsuyama J, Yanase T, et al. 1994. Seroepidemiological survey of *Coxiella burnetii* in domestic cats in Japan. *Microbiol Immunol* 38:1001–1003.
49. Morita C, Tsuboi Y, Iida A, et al. 1989. Spotted fever group *Rickettsia* in dogs in Japan. *Jpn J Med Sci Biol* 42:143–147.
50. Okada T, Tange Y, Kobayashi Y. 1990. Causative agent of spotted fever group rickettsiosis in Japan. *Infect Immunol* 58:887–892.
51. Peter O, Raoult D, Gilot B. 1990. Isolation by a sensitive centrifugation cell culture system of 52 strains of spotted fever group rickettsiae from ticks collected in France. *J Clin Microbiol* 28:1597–1599.
52. Pinsky RL, Fishbein DB, Greene CR, et al. 1991. An outbreak of cat-associated Q fever in the United States. *J Infect Dis* 164:202–204.
52a. Randhawa AS, Dieterich WH, Jolley WB, et al. 1974. Coxiellosis in pound cats. *Feline Pract* 4:37–38.
52b. Raoult D, Roux V. 1997. Rickettsioses as paradigms of new or emerging infectious diseases. *Clin Microbiol Rev* 10:694–719.
53. Regnery RL, Spruill CL, Plikaytis BD. 1991. Genotypic identification of rickettsiae and estimation of intraspecies sequence divergence for portions of two rickettsial genes. *J Bacteriol* 173:1576–1589.
54. Ruys TA, Schrijver M, Ligthelm R, et al. 1994. Boutonneuse fever caught in the Netherlands: a traveling dog as a source of *Rickettsia conorii*. *Ned Tijdschr Geneeskd* 183:2592–2594.
55. Schriefer ME, Sacci JB, Dumler JS, et al. 1994. Identification of a novel rickettsial infection in a patient identified with murine typhus. *J Clin Microbiol* 32:949–954.
56. Schriefer ME, Sacci JB Jr, Taylor JP, et al. 1994. Murine typhus: updated roles of multiple urban components and a second typhus-like *Rickettsia*. *J Med Entomol* 31:681–685.
57. Scott GH, Williams JC. 1990. Susceptibility of *Coxiella burnetii* to chemical disinfectants. *Ann NY Acad Sci* 590:291–296.
58. Senneville E, Ajana F, Lecocq P, et al. 1991. *Rickettsia conorii* isolated from ticks introduced to northern France by a dog. *Lancet* 337:676.
59. Sexton DJ, Banks, Graves S, et al. 1991. Prevalence of antibodies to spotted fever group rickettsiae in dogs from southeastern Australia. *Am J Trop Med Hyg* 45:243–248.
60. Sexton DJ, Kanj SS, Wilson K, et al. 1994. The use of a polymerase chain reaction as a diagnostic test for Rocky Mountain spotted fever. *Am J Trop Med Hyg* 50:59–63.
61. Sexton DJ, King G, Dwyer B. 1990. Fatal Queensland tick typhus. *J Infect Dis* 162:779–780.
62. Sexton DJ, Muniz M, Corey GR, et al. 1993. Brazilian spotted fever in Espirito Santo, Brazil: description of a focus of infection in a new endemic region. *Am J Trop Med Hyg* 49:222–226.
63. Soliman AK, Botros BAM, Ksiazek TG, et al. 1989. Seroprevalence of *Rickettsia typhi* and *Rickettsia conorii* infection among rodents and dogs in Egypt. *J Trop Med Hyg* 92:345–349.
64. Soliman AK, Botros BAM, Watts DM. 1993. Evaluation of a competitive enzyme immunoassay for detection of *Coxiella burnetii* antibody animal sera. *J Clin Microbiol* 30:1595–1597.
65. Sorvillo FJ, Gondo B, Emmons R, et al. 1993. A suburban focus of endemic typhus in Los Angeles County: association with seropositive cats and opossums. *Am J Trop Med Hyg* 48:269–273.
66. Stein A, Raoult D. 1992. Detection of *Coxiella burnetii* by DNA amplification using polymerase chain reaction. *J Clin Microbiol* 30:2462–2466.
67. Sumner JW, Sims KG, Jones DC, et al. 1995. Protection of guinea pigs from experimental Rocky Mountain spotted fever by immunization with baculovirus-expressed *Rickettsia rickettsii* rOmpA protein. *Vaccine* 13:29–35.
68. Tylewska-Wierzbanowska SK. 1990. Q-fever–sexually transmitted infection. *J Infect Dis* 161:368–369.
69. Tzianabos T, Anderson BE, McDade JE. 1989. Detection of *Rickettsia rickettsii* DNA in clinical specimens by using polymerase chain reaction technology. *J Clin Microbiol* 27:2866–2868.
70. Walker DH. 1989. Rocky Mountain spotted fever: a disease in need of microbiological concern. *Clin Microbiol Rev* 2:227–240.
71. Warner RD, Jemelka ED, Jessen AE. 1996. An outbreak of tick-bite associated illness among military personnel subsequent to a field training exercise. *J Am Vet Med Assoc* 209:78–81.
72. Weiser IB, Greene CE. 1989. Dermal necrosis associated with Rocky Mountain spotted fever in four dogs. *J Am Vet Med Assoc* 195:1756–1758.
73. Williams JC, Peacock MG, Race RE. 1993. Immunization of dogs with Q fever vaccines: comparison of phase I, II, and phase I CMR *Coxiella burnetii* vaccines. *Rev Elev Med Vet Pays Trop* 46:87–94.
74. Williams SG, Sacci JB Jr, Schriefer ME, et al. 1992. Typhus and typhus-like rickettsiae associated with opossums and their fleas in Los Angeles County, California. *J Clin Microbiol* 30:1758–1762.
75. Yevich SJ, Sanchez JL, DeFraites RF, et al. 1995. Seroepidemiology of infections due to spotted fever group rickettsiae and *Ehrlichia* species in military personnel exposed to areas of the United States where such infections are endemic. *J Infect Dis* 171:1266–1273.

Chapter **30**

Haemobartonellosis

John W. Harvey

ETIOLOGY

Haemobartonella is a genus of gram-negative, non–acid-fast, epicellular parasites of erythrocytes, currently classified in the family Anaplasmataceae, but genetic evidence suggests it is a mycoplasma.[1, 12a] The host range of *H. felis* and *H. canis* appears to be restricted to cats and dogs, respectively, although experimental subclinical infections of cats with *H. canis* have been reported. *Haemobartonella* organisms appear to contain both DNA and RNA and replicate by binary fission. These organisms have not been cultivated outside the hosts and are distinctly different from *Bartonella* organisms, which are bacteria that can be cultured in cell-free media. *Bartonella* (*Rochalimaea*) *henselae* organisms have been described within cat erythrocytes using transmission EM, but they have not been definitively visualized by light microscopy in routinely stained blood films (see Chapter 54). Comparison of 16S ribosomal RNA gene sequences shows a relationship of isolates to either *H. muris* from mice or *Eperythrozoon suis* depending on their geographic origin.[14a]

Haemobartonella felis

In polychrome-stained blood films, *H. felis* organisms appear as small, blue-staining cocci, rings, and rods that are usually attached to erythrocytes (Fig. 30–1). In thick blood films or thick areas of thin films, nearly all organisms appear as cocci. Ring- and rod-shaped organisms are seen more readily in thin blood films or in the feathered edges of thick blood films.

The epicellular nature of *H. felis* on erythrocytes is readily apparent by scanning EM examination (Fig. 30–2). Organisms are approximately 0.5 μm in diameter and appear to be partially buried in indented foci on the surface of the erythrocytes. Discoid, conical, coccoid, rod-shaped, and doughnut-shaped organisms have been observed. Parasitized erythrocytes, for the most part, lose the normal biconcave shape and become spherocytes or stomatospherocytes.

The epicellular nature of *H. felis* parasites is also readily apparent by transmission EM (Fig. 30–3).[3] A single membrane surrounds the organisms. The cytoplasm of organisms is composed of granules of varying size and density. No cytoplasmic organelles have been recognized. Electron-lucent areas (vacuoles) appear to be present in some organisms. Organisms appear to adhere to the erythrocytic membrane by intermittent contact points. Although smudging of the erythrocytic membrane in association with organisms has been reported, complete erosion of the membrane has not been documented.

Haemobartonella canis

H. canis differs from *H. felis* in that it more commonly forms chains that extend across the surface of affected erythrocytes (Fig. 30–4). However, individual organisms may also appear as small dots, rods, and rings.

Results of scanning and transmission EM studies of *H. canis* indicate that it is ultrastructurally similar to *H. felis*. Although single organisms dimple the surface of the host

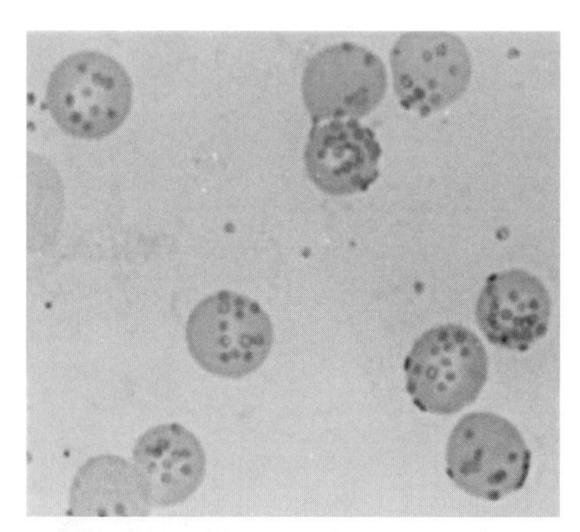

Figure 30–1. *H. felis* organisms parasitizing feline erythrocytes. Some free organisms displaced during blood film preparation are also present. (Wright-Giemsa stain, × 1600.)

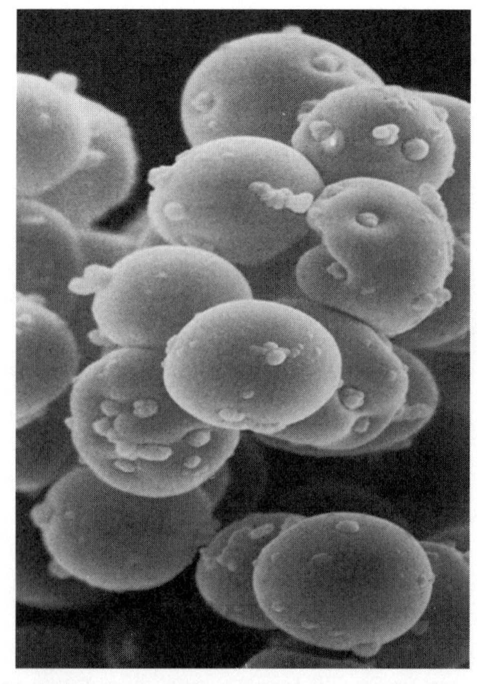

Figure 30–2. Scanning electron photomicrograph of erythrocytes from a cat infected with *H. felis* (× 5000). (Courtesy of Dr. Dallas Hyde, University of California, Davis, CA.)

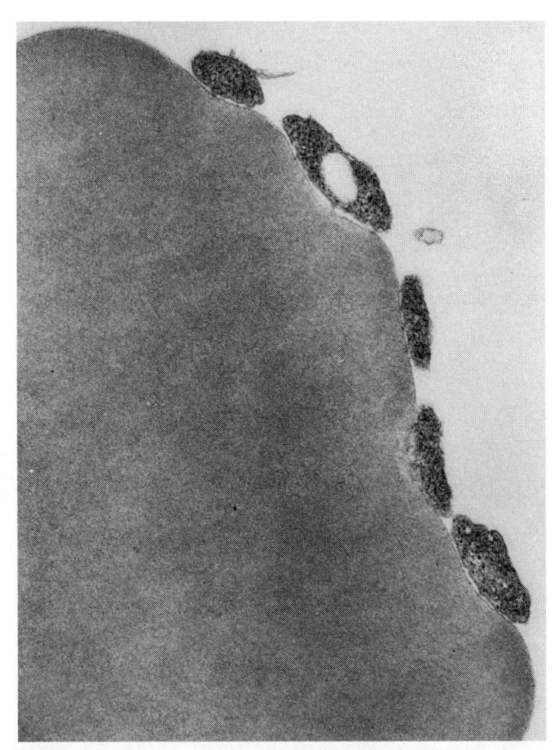

Figure 30–3. Transmission electron photomicrograph of five *H. felis* organisms in intermittent contact with the plasmalemma of a parasitized erythrocyte (× 17,000). (From Simpson CF et al: *J Parasitol* 64:504–511, 1978. Reprinted with permission.)

erythrocytes in a manner similar to that described previously for *H. felis*, chains of organisms frequently occur in grooves or deep infoldings that can markedly distort the erythrocyte shape.

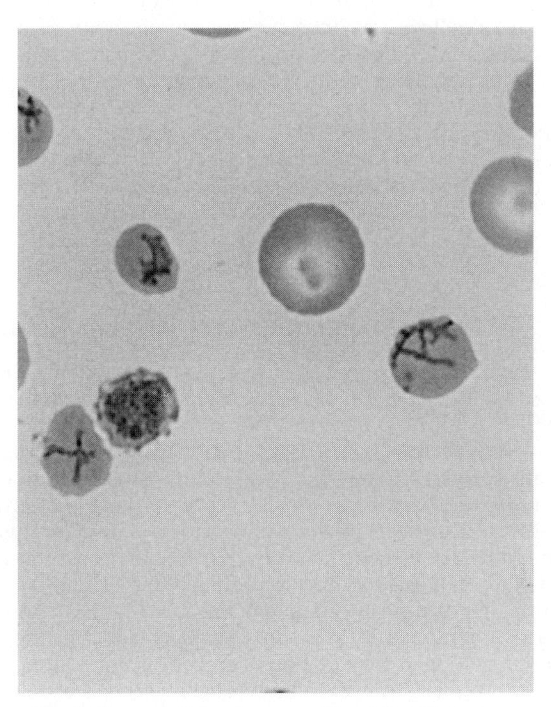

Figure 30–4. Four erythrocytes parasitized by *H. canis* organisms (Wright-Giemsa stain, × 1500).

PATHOGENESIS

Cat

Experimentally, *H. felis* infection has been transmitted by the IP and IV injection and PO administration of infected blood. Saliva and urine are not believed to be infective. Dissemination of infection by blood-sucking arthropods, such as fleas, is considered by many to be the primary mode of transmission, although such transmission has not been established experimentally in cats. *H. felis* can be transmitted from female cats with clinical disease to their newborn offspring in the absence of arthropod vectors. It is not known whether transmission occurs in utero, during parturition, or via nursing. Iatrogenic transmission of *H. felis* can occur by the transfusion of blood from normal-appearing carrier cats.

The severity of disease produced by *H. felis* varies from cats that are mildly anemic and without clinical signs to cats that are markedly depressed and die as a result of severe anemia. To facilitate the understanding of feline haemobartonellosis, the disease has been divided into preparasitemic, acute, recovery, and carrier phases or stages (Fig. 30–5).[2] The preparasitemic phase is generally about 1 to 3 weeks after IV injection.

The acute phase of disease represents the time from the first to last major parasitemia. This phase often lasts a month or more, but occasionally cats die quickly after the occurrence of massive parasitemias and precipitous decreases in packed cell volume (PCV) early in the course of the disease. Parasites generally appear in the blood in a cyclical manner within discrete parasitemic episodes (see Fig. 30–5). The number of parasites generally increases to a peak value over 1 to 5 days followed by a rapid decline. The synchronized disappearance of organisms from the blood can occur in 2 hours or less. Few, if any, parasites are seen in blood films for several days following parasitemic episodes.

In many instances, a rapid decrease followed by a rapid increase in PCV occurs in association with the appearance and disappearance of organisms from the blood. These fluctuations in PCV appear to be associated with splenic sequestration of parasitized erythrocytes and with later release of nonparasitized erythrocytes. In other instances, the PCV remains decreased or continues to decline for 1 or more days after a parasitemic episode, probably as a result of erythrocyte destruction.

Repetitive parasitemic episodes appear to result in progressive erythrocyte damage and shortened erythrocyte life spans. Some damage to erythrocytes may be caused directly by the parasite, but immune-mediated injury appears to be more important. Direct Coombs' tests may have positive results within a week after the first parasitemia. Coombs' test results remain positive during the acute stage of disease whether or not parasites are present. It is postulated that the attachment of organisms to erythrocytes either exposes hidden erythrocyte antigens or results in altered erythrocyte antigens, to which the host responds by producing antierythrocyte antibodies. Inasmuch as antibodies are made against *H. felis* organisms, another possible mechanism of immune-mediated injury should also be considered: if complement fixation occurs, the erythrocytic membrane may be damaged as an "innocent bystander." Minimal intravascular hemolysis occurs in this disorder. The anemia occurs primarily as a result of extravascular erythrophagocytosis by macrophages in the spleen, liver, lungs, and bone marrow.

As a lymphocyte- and macrophage-rich blood filter, the spleen is of primary importance in the clearance of blood-borne particulate antigens and the elaboration of specific immune responses to these antigens. In animals other than

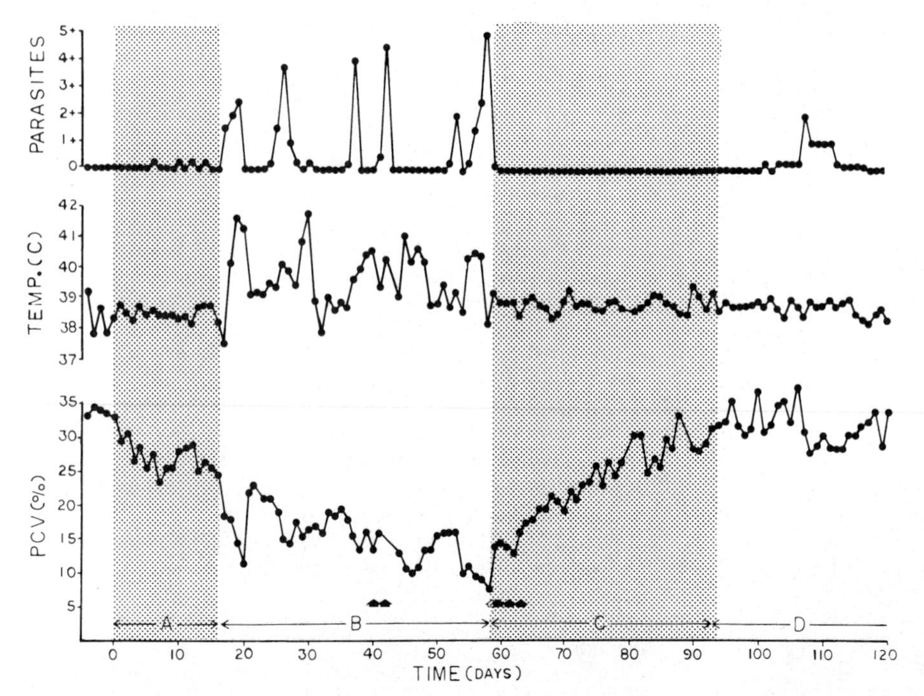

Figure 30–5. Daily measurements of packed cell volume (PCV), rectal temperature, and blood parasite value in a cat following IV inoculation with *H. felis*–infected blood on day 0. *Closed arrows* indicate intravenous administration of thiacetarsamide sodium (1 mg/kg). *Open arrow* at day 60 indicates a 25-ml IV whole blood transfusion. Phases of disease are indicated by letter and shading, with A being the preparasitemic phase, B the acute phase, C the recovery phase, and D the carrier phase. (From Harvey JW, Gaskin JM: *J Am Anim Hosp Assoc* 13:28–38, 1977. Reprinted with permission.)

the cat, splenectomy is generally required before clinical disease is produced by the various species-specific *Haemobartonella* organisms. *Haemobartonella* organisms are removed less readily in splenectomized cats, resulting in parasitemias lasting about twice as long as those in intact cats, but splenectomy performed before infection does not appear to affect the incubation period or severity of disease in cats. Splenectomy after cats have recovered results in the transient reappearance of blood parasites, but in most cases the PCV does not drop to a clinically significant level.

Without therapy, approximately one third of the cats with uncomplicated acute haemobartonellosis die as a result of severe anemia. Cats that mount both a sufficient immune response to the organism and a regenerative bone marrow response in excess of the rate of erythrocyte destruction will recover from the disease. The recovery phase, the time from the last major parasitemia until the PCV has stabilized within or close to the reference range, often takes a month or more. In untreated cats, organisms are commonly observed in low numbers in the blood during the recovery phase but do not usually occur as discrete parasitemic episodes.

Cats that recover from acute infections with *H. felis* remain chronically infected for months to years, if not for life. Although an extracellular parasite should be eliminated by immune mechanisms, intact organisms have been reported within phagocytic vacuoles of spleen and lung macrophages. Possibly some organisms survive within the cells and account for the indefinite, chronically infected state. Chronically infected "carrier" cats appear clinically normal. They may have normal PCV or mild regenerative anemia. Low numbers of organisms are regularly observed in some cats, but in others no organisms may be visible in blood films for weeks. Carrier cats appear to be in a balanced state in which replication of organisms is balanced by phagocytosis and removal.

H. felis may be an opportunistic agent that exists commonly in healthy cats and produces disease when the cat is stressed by other diseases or surgical procedures; however, some cats with haemobartonellosis do not have identifiable predisposing disease or stress conditions. Cat-bite abscesses appear to be the most frequent disorder recognized to precede haemobartonellosis by a few weeks. Although an abscess is undoubtedly stressful, the possibility of transmission of the disease through a bite has not been ruled out. Other factors associated with increased risk of *Haemobartonella* infection include lack of vaccinations, outdoor roaming, and positive feline leukemia virus (FeLV) test result.[21]

Of particular interest is the possible interrelationship between *H. felis* and FeLV-produced disease. About half of the cats with clinical haemobartonellosis are FeLV positive.[10, 21] Inasmuch as FeLV can suppress the normal immune response to unrelated antigens, this virus might increase the susceptibility of cats to haemobartonellosis or convert a latent *H. felis* infection into clinical disease. However, experimental studies have demonstrated that the opposite can also occur (i.e., haemobartonellosis can increase the susceptibility of cats to FeLV infection).[16] Regardless of how the concurrent infections occur, infection with both agents generally results in more severe anemia and clinical signs than occurs with infection of either agent alone.[16, 20] In contrast, concurrent infection with feline immunodeficiency virus (FIV) and *H. felis* does not appear to cause more anemia than does *H. felis* infection alone.[22]

Dog

Transmission of *H. canis* by the brown dog tick (*Rhipicephalus sanguineus*) has been demonstrated experimentally. Transstadial and transovarial transmission in ticks has also been described, indicating that the tick may be an important reservoir as well as a vector of infection. Iatrogenic transmission of *Haemobartonella* organisms by blood transfusion from clinically normal carrier dogs can also occur but is of less concern than it is in cats because the recipient dog generally must be splenectomized before clinically significant disease occurs. Haemobartonellosis has been recognized in a litter of 4-week-old pups, causing the death of two animals. Experimental studies to demonstrate transmission to puppies in utero or through nursing have not been successful, but indirect evidence for in utero transmission has been given. Transmission by PO administration of infected blood has also been reported.

In contrast to haemobartonellosis in cats, the majority of nonsplenectomized dogs infected with *H. canis* do not develop clinical evidence of disease and probably do not become anemic or have sufficient numbers of organisms present in the blood to be recognized on routine blood film examination.

The prepatent period after IV injection of infected blood into splenectomized dogs has been reported to range from 1 or 2 days to 2 weeks or more. Some cases have been characterized by a rapidly developing anemia associated with nearly constant parasitemia. Death generally occurs in these dogs within a month after inoculation. In other dogs, the development of anemia is more gradual as a result of repetitive parasitemic episodes. Parasites are generally observed in large numbers in the blood for a week or more, with a few intervening days when organisms are not observed. One to 2 months are generally required for the PCV and hemoglobin concentration to drop to minimum values and an equal time for them to return to normal. Although immunologic evaluation of infected dogs has been limited, it appears that antibodies are produced against erythrocytes.

Although splenectomy is generally required before clinically significant haemobartonellosis occurs in dogs,[6, 9] cases have been described in nonsplenectomized dogs with concurrent *Ehrlichia*, *Babesia*, bacterial, and viral infections.[18] Haemobartonellosis has also occurred in dogs given immunosuppressive drugs[11] and in dogs with splenic disease. Rare cases have occurred in spleen-intact dogs in which no evidence for immunosuppression was found.

CLINICAL FINDINGS

Cat

Acute haemobartonellosis occurs in cats of all ages. Some studies have reported an increased incidence in adult males and attributed it to their increased roaming and fighting behavior, with greater exposure to cats infected with *H. felis*. Feline haemobartonellosis is usually a disease of individual cats, although multiple infections in multicat households have been reported.[6]

No clinical signs may be recognized in cats with subclinical infections and mild anemia.[6] The most common clinical signs in ill cats are depression, weakness, anorexia, weight loss, paleness of mucous membranes, and, at times, splenomegaly. Icteric mucous membranes are occasionally noted. Clinical signs depend on the stage of disease and the rapidity with which anemia develops. If anemia develops gradually, a cat may exhibit weight loss but remain bright and alert. In contrast, a precipitous drop in PCV early in the disease in association with a severe parasitemia causes little weight loss, but marked mental depression occurs.

The rectal temperature generally is normal except during the acute phase of disease, when it is increased approximately 50% of the time. Subnormal temperatures may be present in moribund cats.

Dog

Unless other diseases are also present, clinical signs are rarely apparent in nonsplenectomized dogs infected with *H. canis*. Splenectomized experimental dogs become listless and have pale mucous membranes as the anemia develops but generally have normal rectal temperatures and appetites.

DIAGNOSIS

Cat

H. felis organisms are present in sufficient numbers to be easily recognized in stained blood films only about 50% of the time during the acute phase of disease. The PCV is usually below 20% and frequently below 10% before clinical signs of disease are apparent to the client. The PCV is not always a good indicator of total erythrocyte mass in cats with haemobartonellosis. Parasitized erythrocytes that are primarily sequestered in the spleen and other organs may return to the general circulation after the removal of organisms.

If the PCV decreases rapidly, mean corpuscular volume (MCV) may be normal with little polychromasia and few reticulocytes present. In most instances, by the time clinical signs of disease are apparent, there is a regenerative anemia with polychromasia and reticulocytosis. Erythrocytes are usually macrocytic, with an MCV greater than 50 fl, and frequently hypochromic, with a mean corpuscular hemoglobin concentration (MCHC) less than 32%. Although anisocytosis, nucleated erythrocytes, and increased number of Howell-Jolly bodies are consistently observed in the circulation during the acute phase of feline haemobartonellosis, these findings are not reliable indicators of regenerative response in the cat. Howell-Jolly bodies are often observed in normal cats, nucleated erythrocytes may appear in a wide variety of feline diseases, and marked anisocytosis without polychromasia has been reported in cats with myeloproliferative disease. Cats with latent infections (carriers) occasionally have low numbers of parasites visible in the blood. The PCV fluctuates over time and may be normal or slightly to moderately decreased (never below 20%). Slight polychromasia and reticulocytosis and increased MCV are present at times.

Because two morphologic forms of reticulocytes have been described in cats, it is important to know the criteria that a reference laboratory uses to count reticulocytes. Aggregate reticulocytes occur in a low proportion (0–0.4%) of the erythrocytes in blood from normal cats. The percentage of this form correlates well with the percentage of polychromatophilic erythrocytes. A greater proportion (up to 10%) of circulating erythrocytes in normal cats contains punctate reticulocytes, which contain punctate inclusions of precipitated ribosomes. Reticulocyte counts are not valid in blood heavily parasitized with *H. felis*, because organisms also stain as blue inclusions with reticulocyte stains.

Total and differential WBC counts are quite variable and of limited diagnostic assistance.[10] Platelet counts are usually normal. Erythrophagocytosis by monocytes or macrophages may be observed if blood films are scanned at low magnification.

Phagocytosis of erythrocytes by mononuclear cells in the circulation appears to occur as a result of antibodies and/or complement on the erythrocyte surface. Autoagglutination is frequently observed in refrigerated blood samples during early stages of acute haemobartonellosis,[4] but the clinical significance of these IgM cold agglutinins is unclear.[8] The direct Coombs' test (37°C) is often positive by the time a patient is presented for diagnostic evaluation. Only reagents made specifically for cats can be used in this test.

Bone marrow myeloid to erythroid (M:E) ratios are normal in the early stages of disease but are generally decreased later in the disease. Erythroid hyperplasia is evident not only by an increase in the total number of erythroid cells but also by an increased proportion of immature stages. Slight to marked erythrophagocytosis by macrophages is often present.

Icteric plasma is not consistently observed in feline haemobartonellosis but may be present within 1 to 2 days after a rapid decrease in PCV. That icterus index values and bilirubin content are not always increased subsequent to rapid decreases in PCV is probably due to the fact that erythrocytes can be sequestered in capillaries and vascular spaces within the spleen without being destroyed. Plasma protein concentrations are usually in the reference range (6–8 g/dl) but may be increased in some cats. Moribund cats may be hypoglycemic.

Presently, the only readily available method for the diagnosis of *H. felis* infection is the demonstration of organisms in the blood. Thin, well-stained blood films, without artifacts caused by improper drying or fixation or by precipitated stain, are required. A number of Romanowsky-type blood stains (e.g., Wright-Giemsa) may be used, although low numbers of organisms are difficult to recognize using the Diff-Quik stain (Baxter Scientific Products, McGraw Park, IL). Blood films must be examined before therapy is begun, because organisms are absent while cats are being treated with tetracyclines. Organisms may detach from erythrocytes during storage; consequently, it is advisable to make blood smears as soon as possible after sample collection. One must be able to differentiate *H. felis* organisms from Howell-Jolly bodies, basophilic stippling, and *Cytauxzoon* parasites, which are small protozoa with both a nucleus and cytoplasm (see Chapter 76). New methylene blue wet preparations and reticulocyte stains should not be used to diagnose *H. felis* infections, because even normal cats have up to 10% punctate reticulocytes, and precipitated ribosomal material in reticulocytes cannot be accurately differentiated from *H. felis* organisms.

Owing to the cyclic nature of the parasitemias, the absence of *H. felis* organisms from blood does not rule out a diagnosis of haemobartonellosis. A regenerative anemia with a positive Coombs' test result, the presence of autoagglutination in refrigerated blood samples, or erythrophagocytosis by blood monocytes is suggestive of haemobartonellosis, but other diseases such as primary autoimmune hemolytic anemia (AIHA) or FeLV-induced hemolytic anemia should also be considered.

The mere presence of *H. felis* organisms in the blood does not necessarily indicate that the clinical illness present was produced by this agent, because parasites may be incidentally observed in carrier cats with other diseases. On the other hand, one should not automatically discount the significance of organisms in cats because the anemia appears nonregenerative. If the PCV drops precipitously after infection, a cat can be depressed and anemic for several days before a substantial regenerative bone marrow response is evident in the peripheral blood. However, a persistent nonregenerative anemia should make one pursue other causes of anemia, such as FeLV infection.

Acridine orange and direct FA staining techniques are reported to be more sensitive than standard Romanowsky-type stains for demonstrating *H. felis*. These procedures are not generally available and have definite limitations. Diagnosis using these staining techniques is limited by the presence of organisms in the blood. Both procedures require a fluorescent microscope (not available to most practicing veterinarians) and a person trained in fluorescent microscopy (staining techniques are more difficult than routine blood stains and nonspecific fluorescence might give false-positive results). A PCR test has been developed to detect the organism in blood as an aid to diagnosis (see Appendix 5).[1, 15]

Dog

Organisms are usually present when clinical evidence of anemia is recognized in dogs. Although the anemia has varied from mild to severe in studies of splenectomized experimental dogs, the PCV has generally been below 20% before clinical signs of haemobartonellosis were observed. Organisms may be found incidentally on hematologic screening when an animal is examined early in the disease because of clinical signs attributable to other concurrent disorders.

In most cases, sufficient time has elapsed between the development of anemia and initial recognition of the disease for there to be peripheral blood evidence of a regenerative bone marrow response. Hematologic findings include reticulocytosis, increased polychromasia and anisocytosis, circulating nucleated erythrocytes, and frequent Howell-Jolly bodies. Macrocytosis takes more time to develop and, therefore, may not be present when dogs are initially presented.

No consistent leukogram abnormalities are recognized in canine haemobartonellosis. Neither icteric plasma nor hemoglobinemia is generally recognized in uncomplicated cases, but substantial bilirubinuria may occur.[6] Spherocytosis and positive direct Coombs' test results occur in some cases. Dogs with latent infections generally have normal hemograms.

The diagnosis of canine haemobartonellosis depends on the recognition of organisms in the blood. One must be able to differentiate between organisms and staining artifacts, basophilic stippling, and Howell-Jolly bodies. The most useful criterion is the tendency of *H. canis* to form chains of organisms across the erythrocyte surface. Blood films should be inspected closely if an anemia develops or becomes worse in a dog after splenectomy.

PATHOLOGIC FINDINGS

Gross necropsy findings in cats include pale-appearing tissues in all cases, emaciation in approximately 75% of the cats, slight to marked splenomegaly in approximately 50%, and slight to moderate icterus in some instances.

Abnormal histologic findings are variable and include erythroid and at times myeloid hyperplasia of bone marrow and passive congestion, extramedullary hematopoiesis, follicular hyperplasia, erythrophagocytosis, and increased hemosiderin in the spleen. In some cases, fatty degeneration and centrilobular necrosis of the liver are recognized.

Necropsy findings in canine haemobartonellosis have not been thoroughly reported. The blood appears thin and tissues are pale. The bone marrow is red and gelatinous. Hyperplasia of the mononuclear phagocyte system may be present.

THERAPY

Cat

Blood transfusions are probably not needed in cats if the PCV is 15% or greater. The necessity of a blood transfusion is related to the rapidity of the onset of the hemolytic crisis. The physical appearance of the patient is an important consideration when one must decide whether a transfusion is needed. If the cat is comatose, parenteral glucose may be indicated.

Cats should be treated orally for 3 weeks with a tetracycline antibiotic (Table 30–1). Some tetracycline products appear to produce fever, anorexia, and liver injury as adverse side effects in some cats.[13] If adverse side effects occur, a lower dosage or a different tetracycline product may be used, or the drug may be discontinued altogether. Doxycycline reportedly has fewer side effects than tetracycline or oxytetracycline.[5] Tetracycline antibiotics do not appear to totally eliminate organisms from infected cats; consequently,

Table 30–1. Drug Dosages for Canine and Feline Haemobartonellosis

DRUG	SPECIES	DOSE[a] (mg/kg)	ROUTE	INTERVAL (HOURS)	DURATION (DAYS)
Tetracyline	B	20	PO (IV)	8	21
Oxytetracycline	B	20	PO (IV)	8	21
Doxycycline	B	5	PO	12	21
Chloramphenicol	D[b]	20	PO (IV)	12	9
Prednisolone	B	1–2	PO	12	prn

[a]Dose per administration at specified interval.
[b]Can cause erythroid hypoplasia in bone marrow, more severe in cats, so reserved for use in dogs.
B = dog and cat; D = dog.

"recovered" animals remain chronically infected. Persistence of infection after treatment has been documented with PCR.[1, 15]

In addition to tetracycline therapy, treatment with an orally administered glucocorticoid such as prednisolone (see Table 30–1) is indicated in severely anemic cats. The immediate benefit of prednisolone is to inhibit erythrophagocytosis. The glucocorticoid dosage should be decreased gradually as desired increases in PCV are measured. Unless parasites are present in the circulation, it is impossible to differentiate haemobartonellosis from AIHA. Consequently, the same therapeutic approach to both diseases is indicated.

Thiacetarsamide sodium IV has been recommended in the past, but recent studies indicate a lack of effectiveness of this drug. Chloramphenicol has also been recommended for the treatment of haemobartonellosis. Unfortunately, this drug produces significant (albeit reversible) erythroid hypoplasia and clinical signs of illness at therapeutic dosages recommended for cats, and its efficacy has been questioned.

The long-term prognosis of cats after recovery from uncomplicated haemobartonellosis appears to be good. Although carrier cats are believed to be prone to relapse into clinical disease after periods of "stress" when body defenses are weakened, experimental studies thus far have not been able to verify this phenomenon.

Dog

Experimental studies evaluating therapy for canine haemobartonellosis have been limited. Blood transfusions should be administered when the anemia is considered to be life threatening. Oxytetracycline, administered orally, is reported to be effective in treating *H. canis* infections (see Table 30–1).

Successful treatment has been reported in three experimentally infected dogs with thiacetarsamide sodium IV and in one experimentally infected dog with chloramphenicol IV (see Table 30–1). Dogs that recover from haemobartonellosis probably have latent infections.

PREVENTION

Elimination of blood-sucking arthropods from dogs and cats is recommended because they may transmit infectious diseases, including haemobartonellosis. Iatrogenic transmission of canine haemobartonellosis is usually of concern only if the recipient has had a splenectomy. Iatrogenic transmission can be prevented in both cats and dogs by splenectomizing blood donor animals and examining blood films for organisms for 10 days thereafter to make sure they do not have latent infections.

References

1. Berent LM, Messick JB, Cooper SK. 1997. Use of a PCR test to detect a fragment of the 16SrRNA of *Haemobartonella felis* in the blood of acutely parasitemic and steroid challenged cats (abstract). *Vet Pathol* 34:515.
2. Bobade PA, Nash AS, Rogerson P. 1988. Feline haemobartonellosis: clinical haematological and pathological studies in natural infections and the relationship with feline leukaemia virus. *Vet Rec* 122:32–36.
3. Bücheler J, Giger U. 1991. Cold agglutinins in feline haemobartonellosis. *J Am Vet Med Assoc* 198:740.
4. Carney HC, England JJ. 1993. Feline hemobartonellosis. *Vet Clin North Am Small Anim Pract* 23:79–90.
5. Grindem CB, Corbett WT, Tomkins MT. 1990. Risk factors for *Haemobartonella felis* infection in cats. *J Am Vet Med Assoc* 196:96–99.
6. Handcock WJ. 1989. Clinical haemobartonellosis associated with use of corticosteroid. *Vet Rec* 125:585.
7. Harvey JW. 1990. Haemobartonellosis, pp 434–442. *In* Greene CE (ed), Infectious diseases of the dog and cat. WB Saunders, Philadelphia, PA.
8. Harvey JW, Gaskin JM. 1977. Experimental feline haemobartonellosis. *J Am Anim Hosp Assoc* 13:28–38.
9. Hoskins JD. 1991. Canine haemobartonellosis, canine hepatozoonosis, and feline cytauxzoonosis. *Vet Clin North Am Small Anim Pract* 21:129–140.
10. Kaufman AC, Greene CE. 1993. Increased alanine transaminase activity associated with tetracycline administration in a cat. *J Am Vet Med Assoc* 202:628–630.
11. Kociba GJ, Weiser MG, Olsen RE. 1983. Enhanced susceptibility to feline leukemia virus in cats with *Haemobartonella felis* infections. *Leuk Rev Int* 1:88–89.
12. Kordick DL, Breitschwerdt EB. 1995. Intraerythrocytic presence of *Bartonella henselae. J Clin Microbiol* 33:1655–1656.
13. Lester SJ, Hume JB, Phipps B. 1995. *Haemobartonella canis* infection following splenectomy and transfusion. *Can Vet J* 36:444–445.
14. Messick JB, Berent LM, Cooper SK. 1998. Development and evaluation of a PCR based assay for detection of *Haemobartonella felis* infection in cats and differentiation using restriction fragment length polymorphism. *J Clin Microbiol,* in press.
15. Mrljiak V, Modrick Z, Bedrica L, et al. 1995. *Haemobartonella felis* as a cause of infectious anemia in a cat in Croatia. *Kleinterpraxis* 40:403.
16. Nash AS, Bobade PA. 1993. Haemobartonellosis, pp 89–110. *In* Woldehiwet Z, Ristic M (eds), Rickettsial and chlamydial diseases of domestic animals. Pergamon Press, New York, NY.
17. Pennisi MG. 1992. Feline haemobartonellosis (feline infectious anemia): a review. *Vlaams Diergeneesk Tijdsch* 61:2–5.
18. Reubel GH, Dean GA, George JW, et al. 1994. Effects of incidental infections and immune activation on disease progression in experimentally feline immunodeficiency virus-infected cats. *J Acquir Immune Defic Syndr* 7:1003–1015.
19. Rikihisa Y, Kawahara M, Wen BH, et al. 1997. Western immunoblot analysis of *Haemobartonella muris* and comparison of ribosomal RNA gene sequence of *H. muris, H. felis,* and *Eperythrozoon suis. J Clin Microbiol* 35:823–829.
20. Simpson CF, Gaskin JM, Harvey JW. 1978. Ultrastructure of erythrocytes parasitized by *Haemobartonella felis. J Parasitol* 64:504–511.
21. VanSteenhouse JL, Taboada J, Millard JR. 1993. Feline hemobartonellosis. *Compend Cont Educ Pract Vet* 15:535–545.
22. Zulty JC, Kociba GJ. 1990. Cold agglutinins in cats with haemobartonellosis. *J Am Vet Med Assoc* 196:907–910.

Chapter **31**

Chlamydial Infections

Craig E. Greene

ETIOLOGY

The genus *Chlamydia* is a member of the class Microtatobiotes, order Chlamydiales, and family Chlamydiaceae. Chlamydiae are obligate intracellular parasites that, like bacteria, have a cell wall, DNA, and RNA but lack the metabolic machinery required for autonomous survival and replication. They multiply within membrane-band cytoplasmic vacuoles of host cells. They have an unusual developmental cycle that involves both extracellular and intracellular forms (Fig. 31–1).

Elementary bodies are small (0.3 μm), resistant particles with rigid cell walls. They undergo a transient extracellular migration to infect new cells, where they subsequently grow into larger (0.5–1.5 μm) initial bodies that lack cell walls and are noninfectious. The initial bodies proliferate by means of budding and fission within a cytoplasmic vesicle, or phagosome, of the host cell. This proliferation is followed by a phase of rapid division, in which the initial bodies divide to become a large, membrane-bound population of elementary bodies (reticulate body). These are released from the cell after lysis, and free elementary bodies are able to infect new host cells.

Chlamydiae persist as commensal flora on the ocular, respiratory, GI, and genitourinary mucosae. They produce inapparent to overt infections in a variety of hosts. Immunity to these organisms involves cellular and hormonal mechanisms. Their tendency to cause chronic, relapsing, or latent infections indicates that only a partial host immune response is evoked. *C. trachomatis, C. pneumoniae, C. pereorum,* and *C. psittaci* are the four recognized species within this genus.[6a] *C. trachomatis* and *C. pneumoniae* are parasites of people that produce ocular, urogenital, and pulmonary infections. *C. trachomatis* forms compact rigid cell wall inclusions, containing glycogen, that stain with iodine, a characteristic distinguishing it from *C. psittaci*. *C. psittaci* has many host-adapted strains that can be differentiated by monoclonal antibody reactivity. Each strain preferentially infects one animal species, sometimes producing respiratory, genital, and systemic illness. PCR followed by restriction enzyme digestion of chlamydial DNA has shown that strains of *Chlamydia* from different hosts may be distinct species. Isolates from cats worldwide are genetically similar with at least two subtypes.[9b, 10] Serologic relationships may be more diverse.[9a] The following discussion concentrates on those infections in dogs and cats.

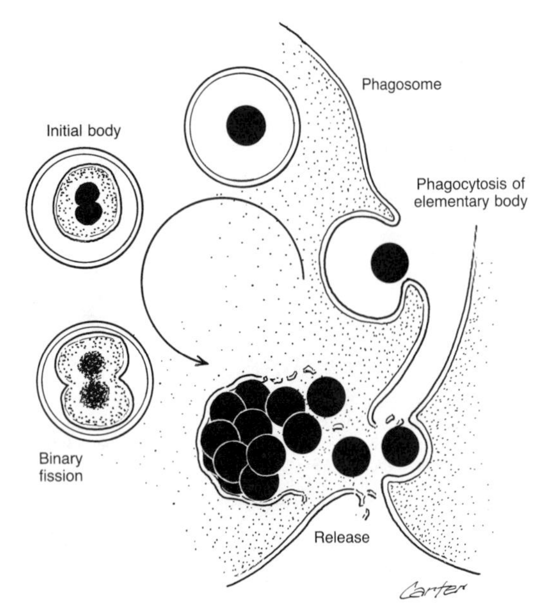

Figure 31–1. Reproduction and development of *Chlamydia*.

CLINICAL FINDINGS

Dogs

Chlamydiosis has not been well documented as a spontaneously occurring entity in dogs. Serologic surveys have detected antibodies to chlamydiae in up to 50% of healthy dogs. Chlamydiae have been suggested as a cause of chronic superficial keratitis in dogs; however, they can be found as ocular flora in clinically healthy animals. Although never established as the cause, chlamydiae were isolated from dogs with encephalitis and systemic illness. A *Chlamydia* isolated from a sheep with polyarthritis produced fever, anorexia, depression, pneumonia, joint pain, and diarrhea in experimentally inoculated dogs. The organism has been reisolated from parenchymal tissues, the intestinal tract, and synovial fluid; lesions were focal hepatitis, lymphoid hyperplasia, fibrinopurulent polyarthritis, and meningitis. Although chlamydiosis was a presumptive diagnosis, a dog developed coughing and a radiographically consolidated lung lobe after being exposed to an aviary of budgerigars suffering from an epidemic of psittacosis. Chlamydiosis was diagnosed in a febrile dog with shifting leg lameness.[1] The organisms were demonstrated in the cytoplasm of macrophages of thoracic fluid, which cultured positive for an avian strain and the dog seroconverted.

Cats

Positive antibody titers to chlamydiae have been detected in as many as 9% of healthy, laboratory-reared cats and 45% of farm cats. Despite this high prevalence of seropositivity, *Chlamydia* were isolated from conjunctival or rectal swabs from only 6% and 4%, respectively, of clinically healthy cats. Isolation rates of up to 30% of household cats with conjunctivitis were reported. Chlamydiae have been well recognized as a cause of ocular, nasal, and lower respiratory tract infections of cats (see Chapters 16 and 93). Acute, chronic, and recurrent conjunctivitis have been the most documented clinical illness.[8] Clinical signs are conjunctival hyperemia, blepharospasm, and mucopurulent to serous ocular discharge. Experimental ocular infection of specific pathogen-free cats with the feline pneumonitis strain of *C. psittaci* produced acute conjunctivitis and persistent genital and GI infections in some cats. They also colonize the GI and genital mucosae.

Chlamydiae were isolated from the superficial mucus-producing cells of the gastric mucosa. There has been no consistent association of GI-infected cats with GI or respiratory signs, which may represent subclinical carrier infection. Experimental inoculation of the gastric chlamydiae into the respiratory tract produced upper respiratory tract infection similar to that caused by the feline pneumonitis agent. Inoculation of the feline conjunctivitis agent directly into feline oviducts produced chronic salpingitis, and the organism was isolated for up to 2 months after inoculation. This infection was similar to that produced by *C. trachomatis* in people, although anatomic differences would limit the spread of genital chlamydiae up the oviducts. Whether chlamydiae are responsible for reproductive disorders in cats is uncertain. Genital infections may be a means by which the organism is spread from queens to their kittens.

Concurrent (feline immunodeficiency virus [FIV]) infection in cats prolonged the duration of conjunctivitis and clinical signs noted after ocular inoculation of *C. psittaci*.[9] Prolonged (270 days) excretion of *Chlamydia* was noted in FIV infected cats compared with control cats (70 days). Peritonitis also was attributed to chlamydial infection in cats.

DIAGNOSIS

Swab specimens of surface tissues or aspirations or washings from deeper tissues are inoculated in McCoy cell tissue culture in the laboratory. Vigorous swabbing of mucosal surfaces is essential to obtain enough epithelial cells that contain the organism. Cotton swabs are best; Dacron swabs or those with wooden sticks should not be used. Swabs should be placed immediately in a chlamydial transport medium such as 2SP (0.2 *M* sucrose and 0.02 *M* phosphate). Routine viral transport media contain antibiotics that will inactivate the organisms. The sample should be refrigerated (4°C) if it is not immediately sent to the laboratory; however, the specimens ideally should be frozen at −70°C. Examination of the amino acid nutritional requirements can help to differentiate the strains of *C. psittaci*. For cytology, swabs or conjunctival spatulas are swiped across the inferior cul-de-sac and cells are smeared on glass slides. The slides are air dried and fixed in acetone. Intracytoplasmic inclusions composed of clusters of coccoid (0.5-μm diameter) bodies are usually 10 μm in diameter in phagocytes or epithelial cells and stain basophilic.

Giemsa is the traditional stain for demonstrating chlamydiae, but artifacts in the cytoplasm may stain similarly. FA techniques using monoclonal antibodies make identification highly specific. ELISA methodology can detect antigen directly in patient specimens. Cross-reaction with all the members of the genus occurs with these tests as currently utilized commercially (Chlamydiazyme, Abbott Labs, Chicago IL; IDEIA Chlamydia Test, Boots-Celltech Diagnostics Inc, East Hanover, NJ). ELISA methods are relatively specific but less sensitive than cell culture in detecting feline infections. See Appendix 6 for further information on test kits. Serologic testing for antibodies to chlamydiae is of limited diagnostic benefit in determining active infection because the IgG antibody titer increase is variable or prolonged and IgM antibody titers are inconsistently elevated. However, highest antibody titers are generally associated with symptomatic cats. Chlamydial infections persist in the presence of high serum antibody levels; therefore, serologic testing only documents exposure and cannot be used to evaluate protection afforded by vaccines.

THERAPY

Treatment of chlamydial infections primarily involves tetracyclines. Oral administration is usually preferred at a dosage of 22 mg/kg three times daily for 3 to 4 weeks or doxycycline at 5 to 10 mg/kg, twice daily for the same time period. Ocular infections respond best to tetracycline eye ointment applied three times daily. In cat colonies with chlamydial infection, treatment may have to be continued for up to 6 weeks. The entire population may have to be treated simultaneously.

PREVENTION

Kittens acquire maternal antibodies to *C. psittaci* that usually protect them from infection until 7 to 9 weeks of age. Both inactivated and modified live vaccines have been available to protect cats from chlamydial respiratory disease (see Prevention, Chapter 16, and Feline Respiratory Disease, Chapter 100). Even modified live vaccines, which provide the best protection, do not entirely prevent colonization of mucosae and shedding of chlamydiae after challenge. They minimize the replication of the organism and hence reduce the clinical signs in subsequently infected cats. A delayed postvaccinal reaction of transient fever, anorexia, lethargy, and occasional limb soreness 7 to 21 days after use of combined vaccines containing modified live *Chlamydia* has been reported (see Postvaccinal Reactions, Chapter 100).[10]

PUBLIC HEALTH CONSIDERATIONS

Chlamydia of feline origin has been suspected as the cause of human conjunctivitis on several occasions. In one instance, chlamydiae isolated from an infected person were inoculated into experimental cats and produced acute conjunctivitis and persistent chlamydial infection, attesting to their potential feline origin. Although these associations are difficult to document, people should take precautions in medicating cats with conjunctivitis, and infected cats may have to be treated simultaneously in households where people develop chlamydial conjunctivitis. *Chlamydia* causing conjunctivitis in a cat was suspected to have been acquired from a pet macaw in the same household.[5] The *C. psittaci* strain causing infection in birds is known to cause human psittacosis. In another household[4] three humans and three dogs developed infection attributed to psittacosis from a cockatiel. Although the bird was euthanized, the affected people and dogs had clinical recovery with treatment. I am aware of a dog living in a house with many psittacine birds that developed fever, lymphadenomegaly, and respiratory signs. These signs resolved with doxycycline therapy.

References

1. Arizmendi F, Grimes JE, Relford RL. 1992. Isolation of *Chlamydia psittaci* from pleural effusion in a dog. *J Vet Diagn Invest* 4:460–463.

1a. Blanchart JM. 1994. Feline chlamydiosis. *Reucueil Med Vet* 170:715–729.

2. Dorin SE, Miller WW, Goodwin J-K. 1993. Diagnosing and treating chlamydial conjunctivitis in cats. *Vet Med* 88:322–330.

3. Greene CE. 1990. Chlamydial infections, pp 443–445. *In* Greene CE (ed), Infectious diseases of the dog and cat. WB Saunders, Philadelphia, PA.

4. Gresham ACJ, Dixon CE, Bevan BJ. 1996. Domiciliary outbreak of psittacosis in dogs: potential for zoonotic infection. *Vet Rec* 138:622–623.

4a. Kik MJ, Vanderhage MH, Greydanusvanderputten SW. 1997. Chlamydiosis in a fishing cat (*Felis veverrina*). *J Zoo Wildl Med* 28:212–214.
4b. Kocianova E, Lisak V, Kopcok M. 1997. Seroprevalence of *Coxiella burnetii* and *Chlamydia psittaci* in dogs. *Vet Med* 37:177–183.
5. Lipman NS, Yan L-L Y, Murphy JC. 1994. Probable transmission of *Chlamydia psittaci* from a macaw to a cat. *J Am Vet Med Assoc* 204:1479–1480.
6. Matsuno H, Fukushi H, Yamaguchi T, et al. 1991. Antigenic analysis of feline and bovine *Chlamydia psittaci* with monoclonal antibodies. *J Vet Med Sci* 53:173–179.
6a. Martin JL, Cross GF. 1997. Comparisons of the *omp* I gene of *Chlamydia psittaci* between isolates in Victorian koalas and other animal species. *Aust Vet J* 75:579–582.
6b. May SW, Kelling CL, Sabara M, et al. 1996. Virulence of feline *Chlamydia psittaci* in mice is not a function of the major outer membrane protein. *Vet Microbiol* 53:355–368.
7. McClenaghan M, Inglis NF, Herring AJ. 1991. Comparison of isolates of *Chlamydia psittaci* of ovine, avian and feline origin by analysis of polypeptide profiles from purified elementary bodies. *Vet Microbiol* 26:269–278.
8. Nasisse MP, Guy JS, Stevens JB, et al. 1993. Clinical and laboratory findings in chronic conjunctivitis in cats: 91 cases (1983–1991). *J Am Vet Med Assoc* 203:834–837.
9. O'Dair HA, Hopper CD, Gruffyd-Jones TJ, et al. 1994. Clinical aspects of *Chlamydia psittaci* infection in cats infected with feline immunodeficiency virus. *Vet Rec* 134:365–368.
9a. Pudjiatmok O, Fukushi H, Ochiai Y, et al. 1996. Seroepidemiology of feline chlamydiosis by microimmunofluorescence assay with multiple strains as antigens. *Microbiol Immunol* 40:755–759.
9b. Pudjiatmok O, Fukushi H, Ochiai Y, et al. 1997. Diversity of feline *Chlamydia psittaci* revealed by random amplification of polymorphic DNA. *Vet Microbiol* 54:73–83.
10. Sikes JE, Studdert VP, Anderson G, et al. 1997. Comparison of *Chlamydia psittaci* from cats with upper respiratory tract disease by polymerase chain reaction of the ompA gene. *Vet Rec* 140:310–313.
11. Starr RM. 1993. Reaction rate in cats vaccinated with a new controlled-titer feline panleukopenia-rhinotracheitis-calicivirus-*Chlamydia psittaci* vaccine. *Cornell Vet* 83:311–323.
12. Ts'ao YC, Magee WE. 1994. Monoclonal antibody to a major outer membrane protein of feline *Chlamydia psittaci* antibody specificity and anti-idiotype antibody production. *Vet Microbiol* 42:1–13.

Chapter 32

Mycoplasmal, Ureaplasmal, and L-Form Infections

Craig E. Greene

Mycoplasmal and Ureaplasmal Infections

ETIOLOGY

Mycoplasmas, the smallest free-living microorganisms, are prokaryotes, within the class Mollicutes. They have replicating cells as small as 300 nm and a DNA molecule expressing as few as 700 genes (Fig. 32–1). Although this molecule is enough for an extracellular existence, it restricts their metabolic capacity. Mycoplasmas, therefore, depend on nourishment from a rich environment, which they find on mucosal membranes of the respiratory and urogenital tracts of their warm-blooded hosts. The lack of a rigid protective cell wall makes the mycoplasmas rather fragile outside the host but resistant to lysozyme and cell wall–inhibiting antibiotics, such as penicillin, cephalosporin, vancomycin, and bacitracin.

Mycoplasmas of the genera *Mycoplasma*, *Ureaplasma*, and *Acholeplasma* are represented in the natural mucosal flora of dogs and cats (Table 32–1). The term *Mycoplasma* in this chapter refers to any of these organisms. Many species may have a role in diseases by virtue of being isolated from disease processes, but few have been conclusively proved to be pathogenic. Table 32–1 also contains a list of diseases of dogs and cats in which mycoplasmas may be causal factors. These diseases most often involve inflammation of mucosal or serosal surfaces of the respiratory tract, urogenital tract, joints, mammary glands, and conjunctiva.

Studies in experimental mycoplasmal infections have shown that these organisms may induce T-cell responses, which cause both beneficial and adverse immunologic consequences. Increased cytokines promote antimicrobial clearance and increased tissue injury. Mycoplasmal products may act as superantigens (SAg), which may stimulate chronic immune-mediated diseases such as rheumatoid arthritis. In addition, some mycoplasmas may become intracellular, resulting in chronic persistent infections.

CLINICAL FINDINGS

Ocular. It has been considered that *M. felis* is a significant pathogen in conjunctivitis of cats. Experimental inoculation of *Mycoplasma* has only produced conjunctivitis when cats are young or when a large inoculum is used. Spontaneously observed conjunctivitis usually occurs when infected cats are housed in groups and develops soon after weaning with loss of maternal immunity. The incidence of *M. felis* in cats with conjunctivitis is 25%, and it is not isolated from clinically healthy cats, although it may be present in levels below the sensitivity of culture.[9] The clinical signs for mycoplasmal conjunctivitis have been described as serous discharge followed by mucoid and sticky exudate. The conjunctiva is initially hyperemic and edematous and later becomes indurated. Untreated cats may show signs as long as 60 days, but the cornea is usually not involved.

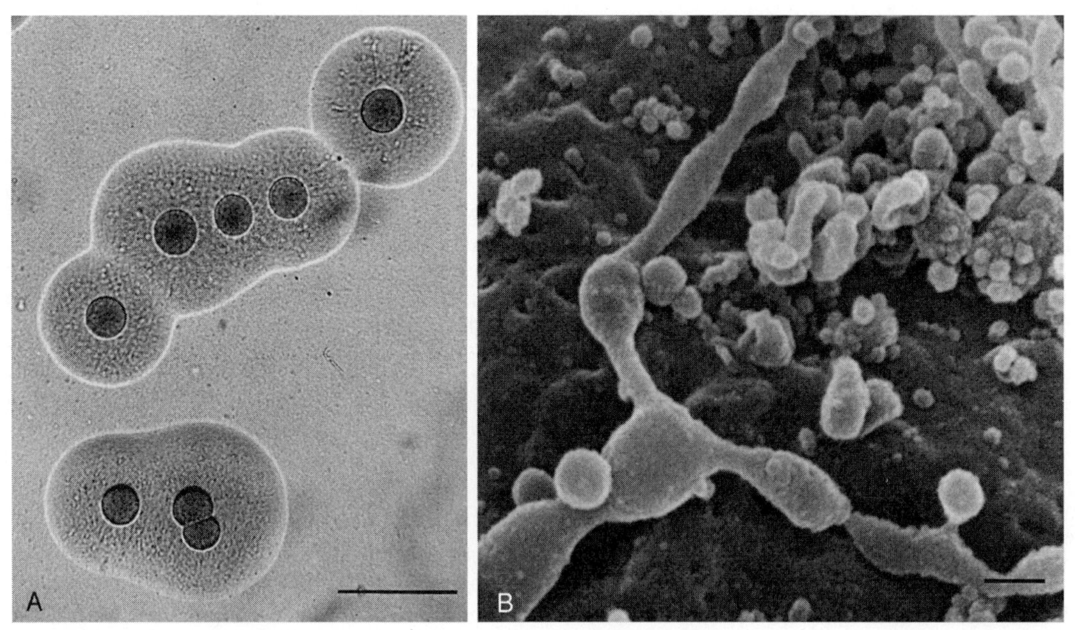

Figure 32–1. *A,* Colonies of mycoplasmas grown for 4 days on solid substrate and viewed in a dissecting microscope (bar = 1 mm). *B,* Scanning electron micrograph of mycoplasmas colonizing the surface of epithelial cells (bar = 200 mm). (Courtesy of V. Bermudez, Ontario Veterinary College, Guelph, ON.)

Respiratory. Most *Mycoplasma* spp. normally appear in the upper respiratory tract. They have also been isolated at necropsy from lungs of dogs and cats with various types of pneumonia but are not generally present in the lungs of healthy animals, especially cats.[18, 19] Isolation of *Mycoplasma* from tracheobronchial lavage specimens of clinically healthy animals was 0% for cats and 25% for dogs, whereas animals with pulmonary disease had a 21% isolation rate.[19, 20] Ureaplasmas are rarely, if ever, isolated from the respiratory tract of healthy or diseased animals.[19, 20] In animals with impaired pulmonary clearance resulting from viral infection, mycoplasmas inhaled from the upper respiratory tract may establish an infection in the lung and/or pleural cavity as a secondary opportunistic pathogen.[7, 16] Chronic pulmonary mycoplasmosis has been observed in dogs with primary ciliary dyskinesia.[1] These bacteria have the tendency to produce prolonged suppurative infection of the conducting airways.[1] Histopathology consists of purulent bronchitis and bronchiolitis with bronchiectasis early, followed by bronchial and bronchiolar epithelial hyperplasia, mononuclear infiltration, lymphoid hyperplasia, interstitial pneumonia, and bronchiolitis obliterans.[12] When a number of mycoplasmal species isolated from lungs of dogs with distemper pneumonia were evaluated for virulence by experimental exposure of healthy puppies, only one strain of *M. cynos* induced pulmonary disease. Although it is not likely to play a primary role, it undoubtedly contributes to the multifactorial cause of canine pneumonia. It is possible that *M. felis* in the cat should be viewed in a similar manner because pneumonia has been found with experimental challenge of kittens. A kitten with

Table 32–1. Species of* Mycoplasma, Acholeplasma *and* Ureaplasma *Isolated From Dogs and Cats

SITUATION	DOGS	CATS
Upper respiratory tract (oropharynx, nasopharynx, larynx) of clinically healthy animals	Three unclassified, *M. canis, M. spumans, M. maculosum, M. opalescens, M. edwardii, M. cynos, M. molare, M. feliminutum, M. gateae, M. arginini, M. bovigenitalium, Acholeplasma laidlawii, Ureaplasma* spp., *Mycoplasma* spp.[20]	*M. felis, M. gateae, M. feliminutum, M. arginini, Acholeplasma* spp., *Ureaplasma* spp., *M. pulmonis, M. arthritidis, M. gallisepticum*[19]
Lower respiratory tract (lung and tracheobronchial secretions) of healthy animals	Rarely isolated[20]	Usually more, *M. felis, M. gateae*[18, 19]
Lower respiratory tract of pneumonic animals	*M. canis, M. spumans, M. cynos, M. edwardii, M. gateae, M. feliminutum, M. bovigenitalium, Mycoplasma* spp., *Ureaplasma* spp.[10, 12, 20]	*M. felis, M. arginini*[16]
Pleuropulmonary abscesses	NR	*Mycoplasma* spp.[15]
Conjunctiva of healthy animals	NR	None[9]
Conjunctivitis	NR	*M. felis*[9, 17]
Peritoneal cavity	NR	NR
Genital tract	*M. canis, M. cynos, M. felis, Ureaplasma* spp., *Mycoplasma* spp.[14]	*M. felis, M. gateae*[5]
Urinary tract	*M. canis, M. spumans, M. cynos*	NR
Epididymoorchitis	*M. canis*	NR
Abscesses	NR	*Mycoplasma*-like organisms: cat bites[a]; *M. canis, M. spumans:* dog bite[23]

[a]These may represent L-form infections.
NR = not reported

congenital mitral valve dysplasia developed pneumonia and pyothorax associated with *M. felis* infection.[15]

Genitourinary. It is not uncommon to isolate mycoplasmas in large numbers from the urine of dogs with urinary tract infection (UTI). Although in most situations they are in mixed culture with bacteria, they are also occasionally isolated alone. The same conditions, such as tumors and urinary calculi, predisposing the animal to bacterial infection may promote *Mycoplasma* infection. The source of the mycoplasmas in the urinary tract is undoubtedly the abundant microflora in the distal urogenital tract. Collection of urine by voiding or catheterization will result in contamination of the urine specimen. Conditions causing obstruction and urine stasis of the urethra will allow ascending contamination of the urinary system so that they may be isolated with cystocentesis. *M. felis* and *M. gateae* have not been able to survive under osmotic conditions present in normal feline urine,[5] indicating that mycoplasmas are unlikely candidates for urinary disorders of cats. *Ureaplasma* spp. are more resistant to osmotic damage by urine and are more likely candidates for UTIs in dogs and cats.[5] No features can be used to distinguish *Mycoplasma* UTI from other bacterial urinary infections.

Mycoplasma of the reproductive tract is currently considered to be opportunistic. *M. canis* has been isolated from dogs with endometritis. The assumed opportunistic role of mycoplasmas in endometritis is probably overlooked in many cases of mixed infection when conventional bacteria are cultured. Alternatively, opportunistic bacterial infections may be responsible for the reproductive disorders in kennels where both mycoplasmas and bacteria are found. Vaginal and preputial swabs and semen samples are often submitted for mycoplasmal culture in dogs with infertility problems. Very often, these give positive results; however, their significance as pathogens are uncertain. It is important to weigh the culture results in relation to other diagnostic findings and judge whether antibiotic treatment for mycoplasmas will solve the infertility problem. Deep vaginal or semen cultures are the most accurate means of determining the presence of the organisms.

A survey of dogs with infertility and fertile dogs showed that infertile dogs had ureaplasmas in vaginal and preputial samples more often than fertile dogs. This difference was statistically significant in male dogs but not in female dogs. Because ureaplasmas are associated with infertility in other animals, research work is urgently needed to evaluate the role of these organisms in dogs and cats. The percentages of dogs culturing positive for *Mycoplasma* from the vagina or semen has not been statistically different between fertile and infertile dogs.[8]

Systemic. It is generally assumed that microorganisms from the natural flora cross the mucosal barrier with regularity, but healthy individuals eliminate these invaders by specific and nonspecific defense reactions. Mycoplasmas originating from the natural flora may, therefore, occasionally be isolated from parenchymatous organs of dogs and cats with debilitating diseases, such as malignancies and immunosuppression.

Dysgammaglobulinemia has been a predisposing cause of mycoplasmal polyarthritis and sepsis in people.[13] A reported *M. gateae* case of polyarthritis in a cat should probably be viewed in this light. Cats injected IV developed polyarthritis, thus confirming the potential virulence of this organism. Predisposing conditions were not identified in a young greyhound with polyarthritis caused by *M. spumans*.

GI. Mycoplasmas are occasionally isolated from rectum and colon biopsy samples of dogs with colitis, but there is no conclusive evidence for their etiologic role in the inflammatory condition.

Abscesses. Organisms with the characteristics of mycoplasmas have been isolated from cats with abscesses, most likely introduced by bite-inflicted wounds. Unfortunately, the isolates have been difficult to adapt to in vitro conditions and, therefore, have been impossible to classify. In one cat with multiple abscess wounds from a dog bite, *M. canis* and *M. spumans* were isolated.[23] In one report, three cats had mycoplasmal abscesses in subcutaneous and muscle tissue and another cat was diagnosed with a cervical and a pulmonary abscess. Mycoplasmal abscesses are characterized by nonodorous, nondegenerate neutrophilic exudates in which bacteria cannot be visualized with Gram-stained smears. In all situations, the abscesses did not respond to surgical debridement or to cell wall–inhibiting antibacterials, but they did respond to treatment with tetracycline or tylosin (see also L-Form Infections).

DIAGNOSIS

Mycoplasmas are often recovered as commensals from mucosal surfaces. To determine whether mycoplasmas are causative agents, they should be isolated from animals with disease in greater frequency than in healthy animals. Antibody responses should also be more prevalent in diseased animals, and clinical improvement should occur with *Mycoplasma*-susceptible antibiotics.

Exudates from draining lesions, inflamed mucosae, or body cavity effusions usually contain intact nondegenerate neutrophils but no bacteria are noted. Organisms can be visualized by examining exudate or colony cultures by negative staining with transmission EM. The clinician should be aware of the fragile nature of mycoplasmas. Special requests should be made of the laboratory if mycoplasmosis is suspected. Cotton swabs placed in Hayflicks broth medium or commercially available swabs with either Amies medium (without charcoal) or modified Stuart bacterial transport medium can be submitted to the diagnostic laboratory for *Mycoplasma* culture. The specimens should be cooled and shipped with an ice pack if transport time is less than 24 hours but must be frozen and shipped with dry ice if longer transport time is expected. Mycoplasmas from dogs and cats grow best on special media prepared according to Hayflicks formula and can be identified quite easily, provided specific reference antisera are available. An immunobinding assay using polyclonal antisera has been utilized to distinguish *M. felis* and *M. gateae* isolated from cats and from other species.[2, 4] The PCR can help to detect *Mycoplasma* in clinical specimens.[11]

THERAPY

Susceptibility testing to antimicrobial agents is not available for mycoplasmas on a routine basis. They are generally susceptible to the macrolides (tylosin, erythromycin, tiamulin), tetracycline, chloramphenicol, spiramycin, lincomycin, clindamycin, nitrofurantoin, and aminoglycoside in vitro. Since no agents are bactericidal, it is necessary to treat for an extended period of time (see the Drug Formulary, Appendix 8, for dosages). The immune system must be competent to eradicate the infection. Because tetracycline and chloramphenicol should not be used in pregnant animals; erythromycin and lincomycin, although less effective, are safer. The fluoroquinolones have been shown to be effective against mycoplasmas in vitro and in vivo.[6, 24] No vaccines are available to prevent mycoplasmal infections in dogs and cats or other species. Attempts to protect animals against challenge with these agents have been discouraging.

PUBLIC HEALTH CONSIDERATIONS

Mycoplasmal infections of dogs and cats have not been considered as major public health risks. A veterinarian developed suppurative tenosynovitis 1 week after being scratched on a finger by a cat being treated for colitis. The infection was resistant to erythromycin, cloxacillin, and penicillin but was cured with doxycycline. This was the first report of mycoplasmal infection as a zoonosis and of *Mycoplasma* producing an abscess in people. Subsequently, *M. felis* has produced septic arthritis of the hip and knee in a person with common variable immunodeficiency syndrome that was receiving glucocorticoid therapy.[3]

L-Form Infections

ETIOLOGY

L forms of bacteria represent cell wall–deficient forms and are morphologically similar to *Mycoplasma*. They are distinguishable from the latter by their variable size (1 to 4-μm diameter), their greater pleomorphism, and their penicillin-binding affinities. Cell wall deficiencies can be induced in vitro or in vivo in many bacteria by exposing them to cell wall–damaging chemicals, antimicrobials, or host immune responses.

Cell wall–deficient bacteria have been isolated from cats with a syndrome of fever and persistently draining, spreading cellulitis and synovitis that often involve the extremities. The usual source of infection has been contamination of penetrating bite wounds or surgical incisions. Cats have also presumably been infected from wound exudates from other cats. Infection begins at the point of inoculation, and lesions spread, drain, dehisce, and do not permanently heal. Bacteremic spread of infection can occur, and polyarthritis or distant abscess formation may develop as a sequela. Progressive polyarthritis, unresponsive to antibiotics and glucocorticoids, occurred in a dog infected with an L form of *Nocardia asteroides*.

CLINICAL FINDINGS

Clinical laboratory abnormalities in cats with polyarthritis may include leukocytosis (> 25,000 cells/μl) with a mature neutrophilia and monocytosis, lymphocytosis, and eosinophilia. Hyperfibrinogenemia and hyperglobulinemia may be found. The exudates contain predominantly macrophages and neutrophils with a few lymphocytes. Erythrophagia may be present; organisms *cannot* be detected by numerous cytologic stains. Radiographic abnormalities include periarticular soft tissue swelling and periosteal proliferation. In severe cases, damage occurs to the articular cartilage and subchondral bone.

DIAGNOSIS

Diagnosis is difficult because these organisms are difficult to demonstrate by light microscopy. The organisms are also difficult to culture on bacterial or mycoplasmal media. Infection has been transmitted experimentally by SC inoculation with cell-free material from tissues or exudates of affected cats. EM evaluation of tissues may show the characteristically pleomorphic, cell wall–deficient organisms in phagocytes.

THERAPY

Cell wall–deficient organisms found in cats have been most responsive to tetracycline at 22 mg/kg given three times daily. Erythromycin and chloramphenicol have been used in canine infections, but these infections do not respond to most antimicrobials. They are characteristically resistant to cell wall–synthesis inhibitors such as the β-lactam antibiotics or many other broad-spectrum antimicrobials often chosen for persistent multifocal infections. Response to therapy should occur within 2 days, and therapy should continue for at least 1 week after discharges have stopped.

PUBLIC HEALTH CONSIDERATIONS

The public health risk of L-form infections in dogs and cats is uncertain, because all of the cell wall–deficient organisms have not been adequately characterized. Instances of L-form infections in people are rare. In one report, a person developed an L-form infection at the site of a permanent indwelling catheter used for hemodialysis. The L-form isolate was characterized as *Streptococcus sanguis* of animal origin. The same strain of this organism was also isolated from the person's pet dog.

References

1. Bemis DA. 1992. Bordetella and *Mycoplasma* respiratory infections in dogs and cats. *Vet Clin North Am Small Anim Pract* 22:1173–1186.
2. Bencina D, Bradburg JM. 1992. Combination of immunofluorescence and immunoperoxidase techniques for serotyping mixtures of *Mycoplasma* species. *J Clin Microbiol* 30:407–410.
3. Bonilla HF, Chenoweth CE, Tally JG, et al. 1997. *Mycoplasma felis* septic arthritis in a patient with hypogammaglobulinemia. *Clin Infect Dis* 24:222–225.
4. Brown MB, Gionet P, Senior DF. 1990. Identification of *Mycoplasma felis* and *Mycoplasma gateae* by an immunobinding assay. *J Clin Microbiol* 28:1870–1873.
5. Brown MB, Stoll M, Maxwell J, et al. 1991. Survival of feline mycoplasmas in urine. *J Clin Microbiol* 29:1078–1080.
6. Cooper AC, Fuller JR, Fuller MK, et al. 1993. In vitro activity of danofloxacin, tylosin, and oxytetracycline against mycoplasmas of veterinary importance. *Res Vet Sci* 54:329–334.
7. Dhein CR, Prieur DJ, Riggs, MW, et al. 1990. Suspected ciliary dysfunction in Chinese shar pei pups with pneumonia. *Am J Vet Res* 51:439–446.
8. Ellington JE. 1993. *Mycoplasma* and infertility. A little fact, a little fiction and a lot of unknown. *AKC Gazette* 110:75–78.
9. Haesebrouck F, DeVriese LA, van Rijssen B, et al. 1991. Incidence and significance of isolation of *Mycoplasma felis* from conjunctival swabs of cats. *Vet Microbiol* 26:95–101.
10. Jameson PH, King LA, Lappin MR, et al. 1995. Comparison of clinical signs, diagnostic findings, organisms isolated, and clinical outcome in dogs with bacterial pneumonia: 93 cases (1986–1991). *J Am Vet Med Assoc* 206:206–209.
11. Jensen JS, Uldum SA, Søndergard-Andersen J, et al. 1991. Polymerase chain reaction for detection of *Mycoplasma genitalium* in clinical samples. *J Clin Microbiol* 29:46–50.
12. Kirchner BK, Port CD, Magoc TJ, et al. 1990. Spontaneous bronchopneumonia in laboratory dogs infected with untyped *Mycoplasma* spp. *Lab Anim Sci* 40:625–628.
13. Lee AH, Ramanujan T, Ware P, et al. 1992. Molecular diagnosis of *Ure-*

aplasma urealyticum septic arthritis in a patient with hypogammaglobulinemia. *Arthritis Rheum* 35:443–448.
14. Lein DH. 1989. *Mycoplasma* infertility in the dog: diagnosis and treatment. *Proc Soc Theriogenol* 9:307–313.
15. Malik R, Love DN, Hunt GB, et al. 1991. Pyothorax associated with a *Mycoplasma* species in a kitten. *J Small Anim Pract* 32:31–34.
15a. Mimouni P. 1997. Mycoplasma in canine reproductive pathology. *Point Veterinaire* 28:41–44.
16. Moise NS, Wiedenkeller D, Yeager AE, et al. 1989. Clinical, radiographic, and bronchial cytologic features of cats with bronchial disease: 65 cases (1980–1986). *J Am Vet Med Assoc* 194:1467–1475.
17. Nasisse MP, Guy JS, Stevens JB, et al. 1993. Clinical and laboratory findings in chronic conjunctivitis in cats: 91 cases (1983–1991). *J Am Vet Med Assoc* 203:834–837.
18. Padrid PA, Feldman BF, Funk K, et al. 1991. Cytologic, microbiologic, and biochemical analysis of bronchoalveolar lavage fluid obtained from 24 healthy cats. *Am J Vet Res* 52:1300–1307.
19. Randolph JF, Moise NS, Scarlett JM, et al. 1993. Prevalence of mycoplasmal and ureaplasmal recovery from tracheobronchial lavages and of mycoplasmal recovery from pharyngeal swab specimens in cats with or without pulmonary disease. *Am J Vet Res* 54:897–900.
20. Randolph JF, Moise NS, Scarlett JM, et al. 1993. Prevalence of mycoplasmal and ureaplasmal recovery from tracheobronchial lavages and prevalence of mycoplasmal recovery from pharyngeal swab specimens in dogs with or without pulmonary disease. *Am J Vet Res* 54:387–391.
21. Rosendal S. 1990. Mycoplasmal infections, pp 446–454. *In* Greene CE (ed), Infectious diseases of the dog and cat. WB Saunders, Philadelphia, PA.
22. Slavik MF, Beasley JN. 1992. Mycoplasmal infection of dogs. *Canine Pract* 17:15–16.
23. Taylor-Robinson D. 1996. Infections due to species of *Mycoplasma* and *Ureaplasma*: an update. *Clin Infect Dis* 23:671–674.
24. Walker RD, Walshaw R, Riggs CM, et al. 1995. Recovery of two *Mycoplasma* species from abscesses in a cat following bite wounds from a dog. *J Vet Diagn Invest* 7:154–156.

Section II

BACTERIAL DISEASES

Chapter 33

Laboratory Diagnosis of Bacterial Infections

Robert L. Jones

The purpose of clinical bacteriology is to provide information rapidly and accurately concerning the presence or absence of a bacterial agent in an infectious disease process. It usually requires at least 24 to 72 hours for bacteria to be isolated, but the clinician can seldom wait that long to institute therapy. Knowledge of the prevalence of specific pathogens responsible for defined clinical syndromes and trends in antimicrobial susceptibility patterns provides the basis for making early rational treatment decisions and selecting the antimicrobial agent most likely to be effective. This knowledge can only be developed and updated by submission of specimens to the laboratory for isolation, identification, and antimicrobial susceptibility testing. The use of the laboratory, therefore, builds a data base that can guide the design of treatment plans for future patients as well as the current animal.

Use of the microbiology laboratory is subject to unique pitfalls posed by the diversity of bacterial agents, each with unique requirements for identification: multiple and often poorly accessible sites for collection of specimens and contamination of specimens with indigenous flora, and the necessity for subjective interpretation of results. Problems in communication may occur between the microbiology laboratory and the clinician regarding the suitability of the specimen for laboratory examination, uncertainty of the significance of bacterial isolates, incorrect interpretation of reports, and length of delay between the submission of the specimen and the production of needed information. Special efforts by the clinician to provide history and signalment information along with the specimen assist the laboratory in recognizing and reporting significant results.

Major technologic advances have changed the way microbiology laboratories function. Bacterial identification is now achieved largely through the use of miniaturized packaged systems, many of which are automated. Antimicrobial susceptibility testing is commonly accomplished with a commercial microdilution system or with some form of instrumentation. Immunodiagnostic methods for both antigen and antibody detection have benefitted greatly from RIA, FA, ELISA, latex agglutination, and immunoblotting, and the development of monoclonal antibody technology. Nucleic acid technology is leading the clinical microbiology laboratory into a new era of molecular diagnostics for both detecting and identifying microorganisms. Cost constraints for all this new technology increasingly limit the scope of services that can reasonably be provided by any one laboratory. It is unreasonable, therefore, to expect equal diagnostic capabilities from all microbiology laboratories. With increasing frequency, specimens must be sent to reference laboratories that perform specialized diagnostic tests.

DIAGNOSTIC METHODS

Microbiologic tests complement clinical judgment, enhance the clinician's ability to select specific antimicrobial drugs, and ultimately improve patient care through detection and identification of the etiologic agents.

Direct Microscopic Examination

Direct microscopic examination of exudates or infected body fluids is the single most important and cost-effective laboratory procedure that can be done for diagnosis and management of bacterial infections. Evaluations can be done in a variety of clinical settings to obtain immediate information on the number, morphology, and Gram-staining properties of microorganisms (Table 33–1) and the host cellular response. Purulent inflammatory responses are most suggestive of bacterial infection. Microscopic examination also gives an indication of the suitability of the specimen for culture, the likelihood of the presence of infection, the likely pathogens, and the predominant organisms in a mixed infection.

Table 33–1. Appearance of Clinical Material in Gram-Stained Preparations

COMPONENT	STAINING REACTION
Gram-positive bacteria	Organisms retain the crystal-violet iodine complex and appear dark blue or purple.
Gram-negative bacteria	Organisms lose the primary complex, take up the secondary dye safranin, and appear red.
Fungi (yeasts)	Appear gram positive.
Inflammatory cells	Appear gram negative; epithelial cells may appear gram positive and/or gram negative depending on the thickness of the smear.
Backgrounds	Usually appear gram negative but may appear gram positive. Fibrin, mucus, and erythrocytes often stain gram negative.

This information may be used as a basis for interpretation of the significance of subsequent culture results.

Bacteria are readily observed in a smear from a specimen when they occur in a concentration of about 10^4 to 10^5/ml. Examination of specimens such as blood or CSF for bacteria is usually unrewarding because, even when present, the bacteria are too few in number to be detected. Some bacteria, such as spirochetes and mycoplasmas, do not stain well with Gram's stain. Dark-field microscopy allows visualization of spirochetes, but mycoplasmas are too small for observation by light microscopy. Background material and artifacts can interfere with interpretation. Mucus or other proteinaceous matter that stains gram negative may make slender, weakly staining bacilli blend into the background, thus making them difficult to visualize. Differential staining techniques that enhance visualization of gram-negative bacteria include methylene blue, Giemsa, and Wright's stains.

Isolation and Identification

Whether isolation and identification are attempted depends on many factors; chief among them are the source of the specimen and whether or not a presumptive diagnosis can be made microscopically. Most commonly encountered pyogenic bacteria readily grow on routinely inoculated blood agar plates. Liquid media provide enrichment for recovery of organisms present in small numbers and facilitate isolation of fastidious organisms. In some cases, selective media must be used to suppress growth of contaminants and normal flora while allowing growth of the pathogen.

Certain infectious diseases may be more efficiently diagnosed by direct detection of antigens, nucleic acids, or toxins. For diagnosis of some clostridial diseases, such as botulism (Chapter 42), tetanus (Chapter 43), and *Clostridium difficile* enterocolitis, it is imperative that the toxin be identified in the specimen rather than relying solely on isolation. Direct or indirect FA stains are extremely helpful for the rapid presumptive diagnosis of infection with some bacteria. Because *Yersinia pestis* (Chapter 47) and *Francisella tularensis* (Chapter 48) are hazardous to laboratory personnel, antigen detection by FA staining of exudate or tissue is the best tool for their rapid and specific identification. DNA probes and nucleic acid amplification techniques are useful for identification of microorganisms for which culture and serologic methods are difficult, extremely expensive, or unavailable.

Specimen Collection

Specimens must be collected from the actual site of infection with a minimum of contamination from adjacent tissues, organs, or secretions (Fig. 33–1). They must then be transported to the laboratory without further contamination or change in the relative numbers of bacteria. Some specimens are likely to become contaminated with indigenous flora during the collection process. Great care must be taken to use aseptic technique when collecting specimens to reduce the amount and likelihood of contamination. Some specimens are simply inaccessible except by aspiration or biopsy of deeper tissues. Skin decontamination should be performed as for surgery for all specimens obtained by biopsy or fine-needle aspiration. Specimens should be collected as early in the course of the disease process as possible. As the disease progresses and necrosis of tissue occurs, some microorganisms may die or be overgrown by other bacteria.

Whenever possible, specimens should be obtained before the administration of antimicrobials. However, their use does not necessarily preclude the recovery of bacteria from selected tissues in which low antimicrobial concentrations are achieved or from those cases with antimicrobial resistant bacteria. If it is not possible to collect the specimen before any antimicrobials are administered, the specimen should be collected just before the next dose is given. If antimicrobials are concentrated at the sampling site, such as urine, it is best to wait 48 hours after the last dose before collecting a specimen.

An adequate (several millimeters or grams) quantity of material should be obtained for appropriate laboratory tests. All too frequently, an inadequate amount of material is obtained with a swab, making it nearly impossible for the laboratory to make appropriate smears and inoculate adequate culture media. A swab should *never* be submitted in lieu of curettings, biopsy material, fluid (especially urine), or surgically removed tissue.

Multiple specimens should be submitted when lesions are present at several sites or when more than one laboratory procedure is requested. Multiple blood samples are necessary for detection of bacteremia. Multiple fecal samples are also indicated for detection of enteric pathogens such as salmonellae.

Collection Devices and Transport. Appropriate collection devices and specimen transport systems are needed to ensure survival of the microorganism without overgrowth and for optimal isolation and identification. A variety of containers are commercially available, ranging from simple swab and plastic tube combinations to complicated specimen collection devices (Fig. 33–2). Swabs must be made of noninhibitory materials and transported in a sterile container. Many bacteria are susceptible to desiccation during transport. Swabs are only acceptable for transport of specimens when provided with a humidified transporting chamber or placed in trans-

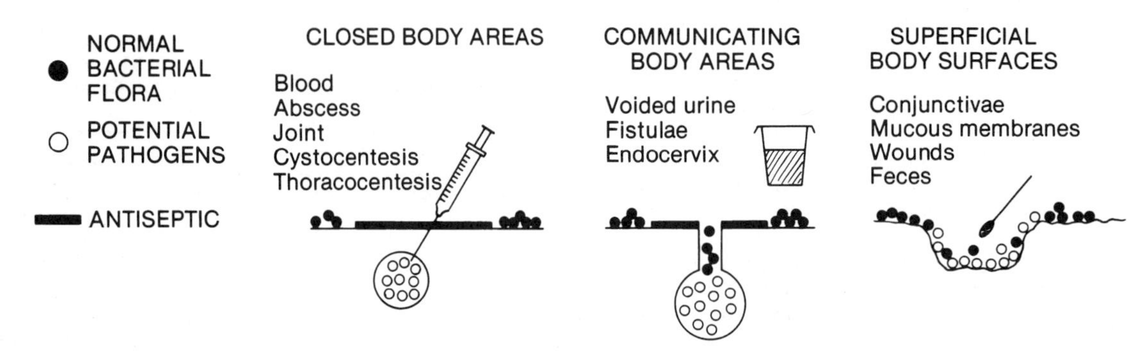

Figure 33–1. Collection of bacterial culture specimens from various sites, illustrating approaches used to avoid excessive contamination of the specimen and probable sources of contamination. (From Jones RL: *In* McCurnin DM (ed): Clinical Textbook for Veterinary Technicians. WB Saunders, 1985, pp 110–147. Reprinted with permission.)

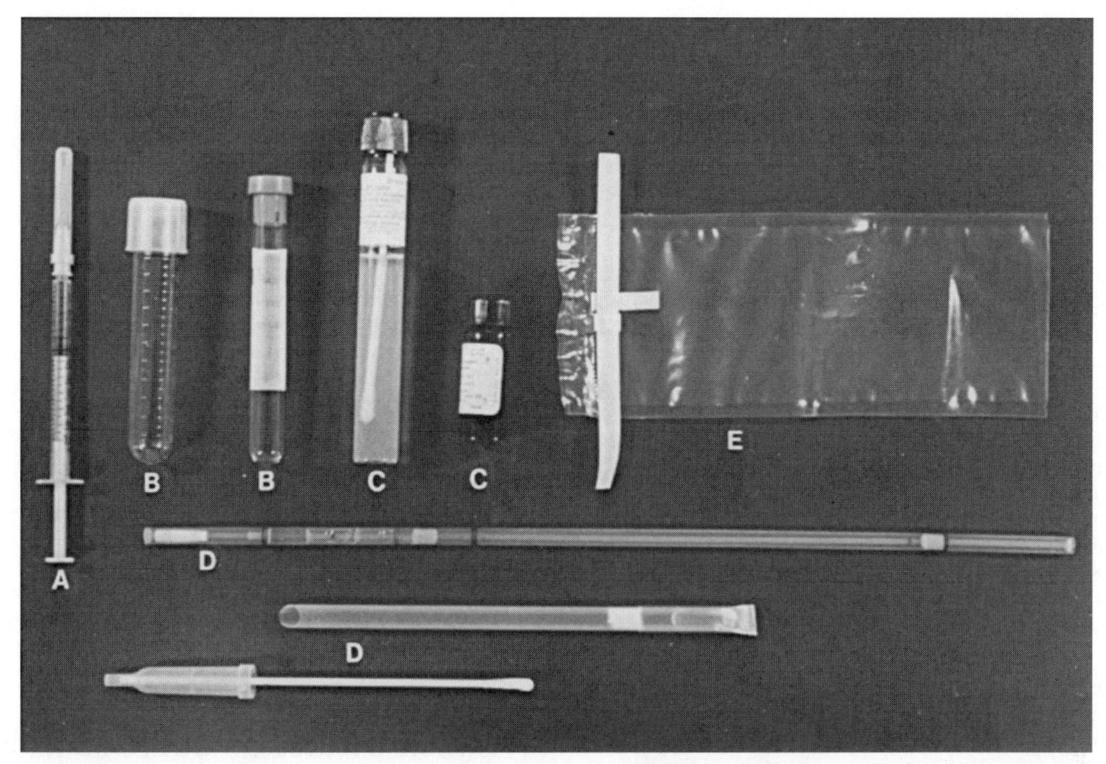

Figure 33–2. Specimen collection devices include swabs, syringes, tubes, and plastic bags. Fluid specimens can be transported in syringes (A) or tubes (B). Swabbed specimens can be transported in transport media (C) or special chambers (D). Tissues and fecal specimens can be placed in plastic bags (E).

port medium. Several swab–transport medium systems are available and are often available from the clinical laboratory. Tissue, exudate, feces, or fluid should be submitted in an appropriate closed (leak-proof), sterile container. Self-sealing plastic food storage bags and blood collection tubes that do not contain anticoagulants or preservatives are examples of recommended specimen containers. Each tissue or specimen must be placed in a separate container. Direct aspiration into a syringe is often a convenient and satisfactory means for collection of tissues and fluids. However, the needle must be removed to avoid injuries, and the syringe should be capped.

A variety of media may be utilized for transporting specimens to the laboratory. Transport media, such as Stuart's, Cary-Blair, Amies, and anaerobic devices (frequently available from the microbiology laboratory), are buffered, nonnutritive formulations that preserve the viability of fastidious organisms in the specimen as well as minimize overgrowth by rapid-growing bacteria that may be present. Use of transport media eliminates the need to refrigerate or chill most specimens for shipment to the laboratory. Ordinary nutrient-type broth such as that in blood culture bottles may be used only when swabs or aspirates are collected from normally sterile body sites (e.g., CSF, synovia) and when great care has been taken to avoid any contamination. Special anaerobic transport devices must be utilized to prevent exposure of obligate anaerobes to lethal concentrations of oxygen (Chapter 41). Because reduced oxygen is not lethal for the aerobes and facultative anaerobes, they can be transported in the same anaerobic transport devices. Tissue in formalin, dry swabs, urine collected several hours earlier and not refrigerated, and selective swabs for isolation of mycobacteria are unsuitable for bacterial culture.

Blood. Successful isolation of microorganisms from blood requires an understanding of the intermittence and low order of magnitude of most bacteremias (see Blood Culture, Chapter 87, for the appropriate technique). Several specimens must be collected for culture over a period of time. If possible, the first blood culture specimen should be drawn at the onset of fever. Another suggestion is to take three or four cultures within 1 1/2 to 3 hours; if more than one culture yields the same organism, it is probably significant.

Urine. The collection, transport, and storage of urine specimens are important adjuncts to the reliability of culture results. Urine is an excellent growth medium for some organisms, allowing small insignificant numbers of bacteria to multiply rapidly to large numbers unless proper precautions are taken. Culture results from a voided specimen taken without cleansing are useful only if there is no growth; growth may be from urethral contamination, infection, or both. Contamination of a midstream-voided sample must be considered when less than 10^5 colony-forming units/ml are isolated, although total counts of viable bacteria may be reduced in some infections. Gram's staining of a drop (allowed to dry without spreading) of well-mixed urine not only will provide a means of determining the adequacy of collection but will also provide the findings for the diagnosis of significant bacteriuria ($> 10^5$ colony-forming units/ml) when at least two bacteria per oil immersion (1000 magnification) field are found.

Urine collection for culture by urethral catheterization is seldom indicated, except in those cases in which catheterization must otherwise be performed for diagnostic or therapeutic reasons. Contamination of the urine by urethral flora is best avoided by cystocentesis, a relatively safe and simple procedure in experienced hands (Chapter 91). This procedure will solve the problem of equivocal counts and the risk of nosocomial urinary tract infections (UTIs) associated with catheterization.

Urine must be collected and stored in a sterile capped syringe or a capped container or tube, not in a "clean" cup or swab. If urine cannot be cultured within 1 to 2 hours after its collection, it must be refrigerated for a maximum of 8 hours. For longer storage or transport and storage, a urine preservation tube (*B-D Urine Tubes*, Becton-Dickinson, Rutherford, NJ) allows for analysis and culture of specimens held for up to 48 hours at room temperature and for quantitative culture for up to 72 hours refrigerated.

Transudates and Exudates. A sterile syringe and needle should be used to collect a generous quantity of liquid material from unopened abscesses and body cavities after antiseptic has been applied to the surface. After aspiration, air remaining in the syringe should be expelled and the end capped or the specimen transferred immediately into an anaerobic transport device. When a wash solution is used to aid in collection of a specimen such as a tracheal aspirate, it is imperative to have a solution that does not contain a bacteriostatic preservative. Best results can be expected when a buffered solution such as lactated Ringer's solution is utilized instead of isotonic saline solutions, which tend to be acidic.

Feces. Proper collection and preservation of feces are frequently neglected but important requirements for the isolation of pathogenic bacteria contributing to intestinal disease. Unless the specimen can be taken immediately to the laboratory and properly handled on delivery, salmonellae may not survive because of the pH changes that occur with a reduction from body temperature. A small quantity of feces (2–3 g) is the preferred specimen; a rectal swab specimen is less satisfactory, yielding fewer positive results. Portions of the feces containing mucus and blood may harbor a larger number of the pathogenic organisms. Fecal specimens should be collected in clean containers that can be sealed for leak-proof transport to the laboratory.

Repeated cultures are often required for screening fecal specimens, because some pathogens may be shed only several days after onset of diarrhea, whereas other organisms may be few or absent later in the disease. Although the number three is not inviolate, repeated cultures are indicated if the clinical picture suggests GI infection by pathogenic bacteria and the first cultures are unrewarding.

Tissue Samples. Surgical biopsy specimens are of considerable importance for culture and may represent the entire pathologic process. They are usually obtained at considerable expense and some risk to the patient. They should be handled carefully, therefore, to avoid contamination or desiccation, which would reduce their diagnostic value. A portion of the tissue rather than a swabbed specimen should be submitted. When the lesion is large or when there are several lesions, multiple specimens from different sites should be collected. Samples from an abscess should include pus and a portion of the wall of the abscess. When collecting necropsy specimens, it is best to anticipate which specimens will be needed for microbiologic analysis before starting the necropsy and then to collect these first, before excessive tissue handling and exposure cause further contamination. Samples from the GI tract should be taken last to avoid contaminating other tissues. When collecting fluid from a body compartment (joints, CSF, pericardial fluid), a syringe and needle should be used rather than a swab. The fluid sample should be aseptically aspirated. Tissue specimens should be placed (unfixed and without preservative) in sealed, leak-proof sterile containers to prevent contamination or desiccation. If there will be a delay in delivering specimens to the laboratory, they should be refrigerated.

Specimen Submission, History, and Signalment

Ideally, the microbiology laboratory should provide the clinician with directions for collecting and transporting specimens and guidance in ordering tests. In turn, the clinician should provide the laboratory with sufficient history and signalment from the case and description of the specimen source for proper processing of the specimen and interpretation of the results. Information about the case will aid in the selection of appropriate media to inoculate and additional tests to be performed, and will increase the probability of significant results being recognized, properly interpreted, and reported to the clinician. Spending extra time and effort to submit adequate information to the laboratory is the best way to ensure better quality results and to avoid the necessity of collecting repeat specimens.

In most cases of infection of unknown cause that do not yield results after initial culturing attempts, consultation between the microbiologist and clinician is recommended. Simply repeating culture after culture is expensive and often unsuccessful.

INTERPRETATION OF CULTURE RESULTS

Specimens that have been properly collected, carefully transported to the laboratory, and processed for bacteriologic culture and antimicrobial susceptibility testing frequently yield important information about the cause of the infection and the antimicrobials expected to be most effective. However, laboratory identification of a bacterium is not necessarily indisputable evidence of disease. The findings must be interpreted by evaluating the clinical signs or lesion, the site of collection of the specimen, the presence of normal flora or other contaminants, the method of handling and transporting the specimen to the laboratory, and the number of different bacteria isolated and the quantitative recovery of the agents.

Normal Flora

All mucous membranes and external body surfaces are potentially colonized with bacteria as part of the normal flora. These bacteria may be pathogenic if they are invading the tissue and causing inflammation, or they may be just colonizing the surfaces. Culture results, therefore, must be correlated with clinical signs. Quantitation of culture results is often an aid to evaluating the significance of the findings. Isolation of a mixture of four or more aerobic microorganisms in light or moderate numbers is typical of normal flora.

Quantitation of Growth

The amount of bacterial growth can aid in interpreting the significance of isolates, although the number of bacteria can be related to the vigor of swabbing to collect the specimen and subsequent handling. The laboratory report should indicate whether growth is light, moderate, or heavy. Finding large numbers of a single microorganism in nearly pure culture is a strong indication of significance. Light growth, including growth from broth enrichment alone, is often typical of normal flora, insignificant contaminants, or suppression of growth by antimicrobials. Such culture results usually have limited significance unless the sample was taken from a normally sterile body site and knowledge exists that the specimen was properly collected.

Absence of Specified Pathogens

Sometimes it is more important to know that the laboratory sought to isolate specific pathogens but was unable to find them rather than to receive a report identifying the microorganisms that were present. For example, a culture report on a fecal sample stating that no *Salmonella* or *Campylobacter* were isolated is much more useful than a report that names several species of normal fecal flora, because this indicates that a specifically directed effort was made to identify these pathogens in the specimen.

No-Growth Cultures

Failure to isolate bacteria may be a false-negative result for a number of reasons, including sampling and transporting mistakes, such as desiccation or inappropriate transport media; previous antimicrobial therapy; and infections caused by fastidious microorganisms for which proper culture procedures were not performed, such as mycoplasmas, obligate anaerobes, spirochetes, and rickettsias. If microscopic examination of the specimen reveals microorganisms but comparable microorganisms are not isolated, transporting and culturing procedures should be evaluated in consultation with the clinical microbiologist. Innovative techniques of molecular detection and immunochemistry are now being developed for direct application to specimens to identify microorganisms that are difficult to cultivate.

MOLECULAR DETECTION AND IDENTIFICATION

Direct nucleic acid hybridization probe and gene amplification protocols have a tremendous potential for detecting microbial pathogens, and there has been significant progress in the development of these assays. Many improvements have occurred in specificity and sensitivity as well as in protocols for processing samples. DNA probe assays are particularly well suited for in situ hybridization in tissue in which the location and distribution of the organisms must be ascertained, for identification of slow-growing bacterial cultures, and for identification of toxicogenic strains of bacteria that cannot be differentiated from nontoxicogenic strains by conventional methods.[3] Nucleic acid amplification assays that can be performed in situ or on specimens employ primers and PCR to provide specificity and sensitivity able to detect as few as one organism or between 1 and 10 copies of the specific gene sequence (see Chapter 1).

Ultimately, the goal of these molecular techniques is the direct determination of identities of microorganisms in clinical specimens for prediction of their antimicrobial susceptibility patterns. As the technology for nucleic acid amplification currently stands, application of the procedure is limited to referral and research laboratories. Partial or full automation and improved technology are reducing costs and increasing access to these assays. Specimen handling and preparation remain the most critical limiting steps. Specimen preparation must release the nucleic acids from the target organism, prevent degradation of the free nucleic acids, remove any substances inhibitory to nucleic acid amplification or hybridization, concentrate the nucleic acids into a small volume, place the nucleic acids in amplification or hybridization buffer, and prevent false-positive results caused by contaminating nucleic acids. Various samples have to be processed differently to extract the nucleic acids from their matrix. Clinicians must consult with the laboratory, therefore, when collecting specimens in order to obtain useful results.

Despite their sensitivity and specificity, molecular detection procedures will never totally replace conventional cultural and serologic procedures because the results of nucleic acid amplification procedures and the results of culture or serology have different purposes. Nucleic acid detection procedures determine whether DNA or RNA from a particular organism is present in the specimen. They cannot determine whether the organism is involved in an infectious process, and they reveal nothing about the viability of the organism because they can detect DNA from dead organisms. Culture, by comparison, clearly demonstrates the viability of the organism, and a rise in titer of antibody to a specific organism strongly suggests active infection.

ANTIMICROBIAL SUSCEPTIBILITY TESTS

Testing bacteria for their susceptibility to antimicrobials is one of the laboratory procedures that has significant impact on the prescribing of antimicrobials. To improve the predictive value of susceptibility tests, the indications for these tests and their limitations must be understood. Susceptible and resistant are relative terms (and somewhat arbitrarily defined) because a microorganism within the animal may be susceptible in one location as a result of attainable antimicrobial concentrations but may be resistant in another. Susceptibility tests measure the lowest concentration of antimicrobial required to macroscopically inhibit growth of the microorganism, called the minimum inhibitory concentration (MIC). The concentration of antimicrobial that inhibits the infectious agent, either by killing it outright or by slowing its growth sufficiently so that normal body defense mechanisms can take over, is assumed to be similar to the in vitro MIC. Comparison of the MIC with the concentration of antimicrobial that can be attained in various body compartments allows one to predict the susceptibility or resistance of the organism to the drug at the infection site.

Indications

Some microorganisms are known to be susceptible to a highly effective antimicrobial and there is no need for testing. Susceptibility testing is indicated for any microorganism contributing to an infectious process if its susceptibility cannot be reliably predicted or resistance is anticipated based on knowledge of the organism's identity. Generally, isolates from normally sterile body sites should be tested, although questions have been raised about the cost effectiveness of routine testing of all urinary tract isolates. Susceptibility testing of multiple bacterial isolates from abscesses and wounds or normal flora is meaningless. Testing the susceptibility of anaerobes remains a technical problem and an unsettled issue; most anaerobes except those that produce β-lactamases are predictably susceptible.

Test Methods

The reference method of antimicrobial susceptibility testing measures the MIC in micrograms per milliliter by incorporat-

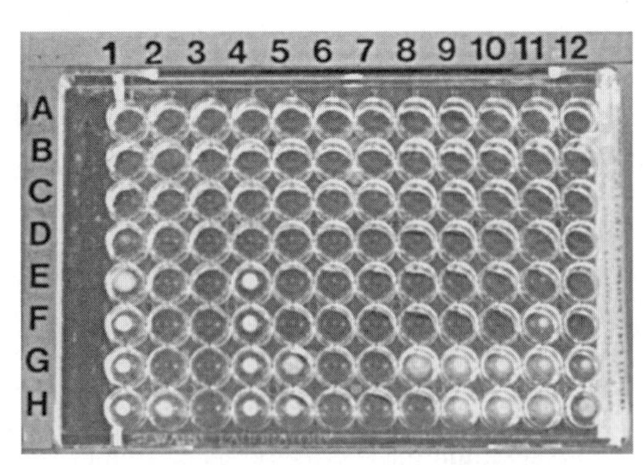

Figure 33–3. Antimicrobial susceptibility testing by the microdilution method. Each column of microwells contains serial twofold dilutions of an antimicrobial. The lowest concentration of drug that inhibits growth of the bacteria is defined as the MIC. For example, the first column contains ampicillin (32 μg/ml in well A1, decreasing to 0.25 μg/ml in well H1). The pellet of bacteria in the lower four wells (E1–H1) indicates that 4 μg/ml (well D1) is the MIC. Susceptibility to 11 other drugs has also been tested in this microwell plate.

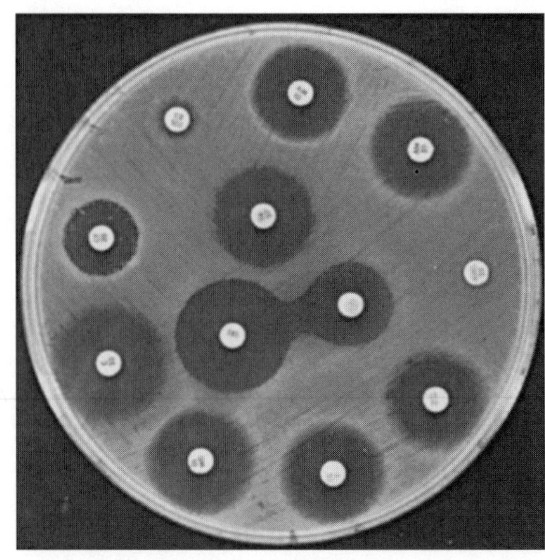

Figure 33–4. Antimicrobial susceptibility testing by the agar diffusion method using disks containing antimicrobials. The diameter of the zone of inhibited microbial growth correlates inversely with the susceptibility of the microorganism.

ing serial twofold dilutions of antimicrobials in a bacteriologic growth medium (Fig. 33–3). These dilutions can be made in microdilution wells, a procedure used by many larger laboratories. The clinical significance is determined by interpreting the results according to the criteria in Table 33–2.

In contrast to the dilution method, the most common antimicrobial susceptibility test performed in small laboratories and veterinary practices is the agar diffusion test. This method uses antimicrobial-impregnated paper disks applied to the surface of agar that have been inoculated with pure cultures of the test organism (Fig. 33–4). The diameter of the zone of inhibition of growth around the disk correlates inversely with the MIC. The disk diffusion technique is not difficult to perform; however, strict guidelines must be followed to use the standard zone size interpretive chart for each drug. Any variation in technique changes the relationship between the zone size and the MIC, leading to possible misinterpretation of the test result.

Interpretations

In general, in vitro susceptibility testing is useful and reliably applied only to common, rapidly growing microorganisms such as staphylococci, enterococci, Enterobacteriaceae, and *Pseudomonas aeruginosa*. Infections caused by fastidious bacteria are usually treated more reliably on the basis of published guidelines. A helpful guide to empiric therapy can be compiled by monitoring susceptibility trends of microorganisms recently isolated from animals within the practice region.

Table 33–2. Interpretation Categories for Antimicrobial Susceptibility Tests

CATEGORY	DEFINITION
Susceptible	Infection caused by a strain may be appropriately treated with the standard dosage of antimicrobial recommended for that type of infection and infecting species unless otherwise contraindicated.
Intermediate	Infection caused by a strain with antimicrobial MICs that approach usually attainable blood and tissue levels. Therapeutic response rates may be lower than for susceptible isolates. Selected drugs should be physiologically concentrated (e.g., quinolones and β-lactams in urine) or given at a high dosage without toxicity (e.g., β-lactams).
Resistant	Infection caused by a strain not inhibited by the usually achievable systemic concentrations of the antimicrobial at usual dosages. Specific microbial resistance mechanisms are likely, and clinical efficacy has not been reliable in treatment studies.

Susceptibility test results are a prediction of the expected response to treatment, not a guarantee. Most susceptibility tests employ class-representative drugs rather than each possible antimicrobial. Furthermore, the interpretative criteria are based on the average blood levels of antimicrobials that are expected to be achieved with a standard dose. Extralabel drug use in patients of other species, ages, and body sizes or modified dosages may significantly alter drug distribution. Levels of drug in tissues usually differ from levels in serum, such as low levels in CSF or high in urine. Although in vitro susceptibility testing predicts effectiveness, the drug may not be able to penetrate to the site of infection. The predictive value of susceptibility tests for a favorable response, therefore, is moderate at best. Their value in predicting failure is much better but is still not totally accurate. An MIC result, for example, that is interpreted as resistant according to blood levels may not have taken into account that the organism was recovered from urine, where the drug is concentrated, or that topical treatment is being applied where drug concentrations are milligrams per milliliter rather than micrograms per milliliter.

SEROLOGIC TESTING

Detection of specific antibodies in the serum of an animal can be an indication of previous exposure, infection, vaccination, or passively acquired antibody. It is not always easy to discern the origin of these antibodies. Serology is most effective, therefore, as a diagnostic tool when the prevalence of antibodies in a population is low or when paired serum samples are collected to evaluate changes in antibody titers. The more common bacterial infections for which serologic tests are useful include brucellosis (Chapter 40), leptospirosis (Chapter 44), and borreliosis (Chapter 45).

For best results from serologic tests, serum should be transferred to a sterile tube as soon as possible after complete clotting and centrifugation to separate it from cellular elements. Excessive hemolysis interferes with some tests. Bacterial growth in serum may alter the immunoglobulin molecules. Once separated, serum samples should be refrigerated until testing is commenced, if within 72 hours. For longer periods of storage, serum may be preserved for extended periods by storage in a freezer (−20°C). Frozen serum samples should be packaged and shipped with adequate insulation and ice to prevent thawing before arrival at the laboratory.

References

1. Isenberg HD (ed). 1992. Clinical microbiology procedures handbook. American Society for Microbiology, Washington, DC.
2. Jones RL. 1990. Laboratory diagnosis of bacterial infections, pp 453–460. *In* Greene CE (ed), Infectious diseases of the dog and cat. WB Saunders, Philadelphia, PA.
3. Lou Q, Chong SKF, Fitzgerald JF, et al. 1997. Rapid and effective method for preparation of fecal specimens for PCR assays. *J Clin Microbiol* 35:281–283.
4. Murray PR (ed). 1995. Manual of clinical microbiology, ed 6. American Society for Microbiology, Washington, DC.
5. National Committee for Clinical Laboratory Standards. 1994. Performance standards for antimicrobial disk and dilution susceptibility tests for bacteria isolated from animals: proposed standard (NCCLS document M31-P). NCCLS, Villanova, PA.

Chapter 34

Antibacterial Chemotherapy

Craig E. Greene and A.D.J. Watson

Antibacterials, among the most widely used drugs in veterinary practice, are often administered without adequate documentation that an infection exists. Although this practice may not immediately harm the patient, routine and irrational use of antimicrobials may cause several undesirable consequences for the future. Unrestricted use encourages the selection of resistant strains of bacteria, which subsequently limits the choice of effective agents. Long-term treatment with antimicrobials may suppress the animal's resident microflora, thereby allowing the overgrowth of more resistant microorganisms.

This chapter presents a review of the general properties of antibacterial drugs by pharmacologic groupings. Information on specific drugs used in the dog and cat can be found in the Drug Formulary at the end of this book. Because of space limitations, a discussion of general principles of antibacterial chemotherapy has been omitted here. Antibacterial drug resistance and prophylaxis are discussed in Chapter 94. The administration of antibacterial drugs in treating infections of various organ systems is covered in Chapters 35 through 55. Dosage charts are listed in each of these chapters, in addition to Appendix 8, which also contains a list of appropriate antibacterial drugs for particular types and locations of infections.

PENICILLINS AND β-LACTAM DERIVATIVES

Penicillins

Natural Penicillins. Penicillin G (benzyl penicillin) is a naturally occurring bactericidal antibiotic produced by certain molds of the genus *Penicillium*. It primarily inhibits synthesis of the gram-positive bacterial cell wall, causing osmotic fragility of susceptible bacteria. Penicillin G has three significant therapeutic limitations: it is degraded by gastric acid, which reduces absorption via the oral route; it is inactivated by β-lactamase, produced by certain staphylococci and many gram-negative organisms; and at usual therapeutic dosages, it is active mainly against gram-positive organisms (Table 34–1). Newer semisynthetic penicillins have been produced that overcome the disadvantages of penicillin G. Penicillins are thought to work synergistically with aminoglycosides (AGs) in vivo.

Despite the production of newer derivatives, penicillin G is still the most active against many gram-positive aerobic bacteria. Most streptococci, with the exception of enterococci (see Chapter 35), are susceptible. Many gram-positive bacilli and anaerobic bacteria with the exception of β-lactamase–producing *Bacteroides fragilis* are susceptible. Staphylococci, because of β-lactamase production, are frequently resistant. Procaine penicillin and benzathine penicillin are poorly soluble compounds that slowly dissolve at the site of injection, liberating penicillin G.

Penicillin V (phenoxymethyl penicillin) is an acid-stable derivative that is better absorbed from the GI tract, although the resulting blood concentration is much lower than that produced by parenteral administration of the same dose of penicillin G. Therapeutic effects equivalent to those obtained with penicillin V may be achieved at less expense by giving oral penicillin G to fasting animals at four times the usual parenteral dosage.

β-Lactamase–Resistant Penicillins. Methicillin, the first semisynthetic penicillin developed, resists β-lactamase, but is inactivated by gastric acid and must be administered parenterally, which limits its clinical usefulness. Isoxazolyl derivatives, which include cloxacillin, dicloxacillin, flucloxacillin, and oxacillin, are β-lactamase resistant and can be administered orally with reasonable absorption from the GI tract. These drugs might be considered to treat patients with infections caused by β-lactamase–producing staphylococci, as in pyoderma or osteomyelitis.

Aminopenicillins. Ampicillin, amoxicillin, and hetacillin are susceptible to β-lactamase, but can be given orally or paren-

Table 34–1. Properties of Penicillins and Associated β-Lactam Derivatives[a]

GENERIC NAME (TRADE NAME)	ROUTE OF ADMINISTRATION	Gastric Acid Stability	Staphylococcal β-Lactamase Resistance	ANTIMICROBIAL SPECTRUM Gram Positive	Gram Negative	Anaerobic	*Pseudomonas*
Natural Penicillins							
Penicillin G (many)	IM, IV	–	–	+	–	+	–
Penicillin V (many)	PO[b]	+	–	+	–	+	–
β-Lactamase–Resistant Penicillins							
Methicillin (Staphcillin, Celbenin)	IM, IV	–	+	+	–	–	–
Nafcillin (Unipen, Nafcil)	IM, IV	±	+	+	–	–	–
Cloxacillin (Tegopen)	PO	+	+	+	–	–	–
Dicloxacillin (Veracillin, Pathocil, Dynapen)	PO	+	+	+	–	–	–
Oxacillin (Prostaphylin, Bactocil)	PO, IM, IV	+	+	+	–	–	–
Aminopenicillins[c]							
Ampicillin (many)	PO, SC, IM, IV	+	–	+	±	±	–
Amoxicillin (Omnipen)	PO[b], IM	+	–	+	±	±	–
Hetacillin (Hetacin)	PO	+	–	+	±	±	–
Extended-Spectrum Carboxypenicillins[d]							
Carbenicillin (Pyopen, Geopen)	IM, SC, IV	–	–	±	+	+	+
Ticarcillin (Ticar)	IM, SC, IV	–	–	±	+	+	+
Ureidopenicillins[d]							
Mezlocillin (Mezlin)	IM, IV	–	–	+	+ +	±	+ +
Piperacillin (Pipracil, Pipral)	IM, IV	–	–	+	+ +	±	+ +
Other β-Lactams							
Aztreonam (Azactam)	IM, IV	–	+ +	–	+ +	–	+ +
Imipenem-cilastatin (Primaxin)	IV	–	+ +	+ +	+ +	+ +	+ +
β-Lactamase Inhibitors							
Clavulanate (CA)[e]	PO, IV	+	+ +	–	–	–	–
CA + amoxicillin (Clavulox, Clavamox, Augmentin)	PO[b]	+	+ +	+ +	+ +	+	–
CA + ticarcillin (Timentin)	IV	–	+ +	±	+	+	+
Sulbactam (SB)[e]	IV	–	+ +	+	±	±	–
SB + ampicillin (Unasyn, Synergistin)	IV	–	+ +	+	+	+	+
Tazobactam (TZ)[e]	IV	–	+ +	+	+	±	±
TZ + piperacillin (Zosyn)	IV	–	+ +	+	+ +	±	+ +

[a]See Appendix 8 for dosages.
[b]For best results, administer on empty stomach.
[c]Also includes bacampicillin (Spectrobid), cyclacillin (Cyclapen), epicillin, pivampicillin, and talampicillin. Bacampicillin has good oral absorption.
[d]Also includes azlocillin (Azlin).
[e]Susceptibility data indicate efficacy of inhibitor alone, although the drug is not available by itself.
PO = oral; IM = intramuscular; IV = intravenous; – = none; + = good; + + = excellent; ± = variable.

terally and have wider spectra of action against gram-negative aerobic bacteria than previously discussed penicillins. *Escherichia*, *Proteus*, and *Salmonella* are more susceptible. Amoxicillin has antibacterial spectrum identical to ampicillin but is better absorbed orally and has more rapid and longer action. Hetacillin is an inactive derivative of ampicillin, is more stable in gastric acid, and is hydrolyzed rapidly to ampicillin in vivo. Bacampicillin, pivampicillin, and talampicillin are similar derivatives.

Carboxypenicillins. Carbenicillin and ticarcillin have increased activity against gram-negative aerobes, including *Acinetobacter*, *Proteus*, *Enterobacter*, some *Klebsiella*, *Pseudomonas* (especially ticarcillin), and some anaerobes. Carboxypenicillins are destroyed by β-lactamase and are less effective against gram-positive organisms. The minimum inhibitory concentrations (MICs) for these organisms are relatively high, and therefore large dosages of the drugs must be administered. Coadministration with an aminoglycoside improves efficacy against *Pseudomonas* and reduces development of drug resistance. They are not well absorbed orally and must be given parenterally. Two esters of carbenicillin (carindacillin, carfecillin) are available for oral administration. Expense limits systemic use of carboxypenicillins.

Ureidopenicillins. Azlocillin, mezlocillin, and piperacillin have acid instability and β-lactamase resistance similar to those of the carboxypenicillins, with greater activity against gram-negative aerobes including *Pseudomonas* and less activity against some anaerobes. The main area of interest is their antipseudomonal activity, and piperacillin is one of few drugs consistently effective against enterococci and *Bacteroides fragilis*. Cost is a limiting factor in ureidopenicillins, but coadministration with a cephalosporin or quinolone might be considered when treating patients with difficult gram-negative aerobic bacterial infections.

Pharmacokinetics

Absorption and duration of activity of penicillins depend on the dosage administered, the vehicle containing the drug, and the solubility of the salt formulation. The potassium and sodium salts are soluble and can be given PO, IM, SC, IV, and topically, whereas insoluble trihydrates are absorbed less rapidly by PO, IM, and SC routes. Soluble penicillin derivatives are absorbed from serous and mucosal surfaces but not through unbroken skin. Food in the stomach can adversely affect bioavailability of orally administered penicillins. All penicillins are eliminated by the kidney through active tubular secretion. As a result, soluble penicillin derivatives must be given at least every 4 hours to maintain therapeutic blood concentrations. Probenecid inhibits this rapid elimination. Activity can also be prolonged by delaying release of penicillins from injection sites by placing them in water-insoluble vehicles or combining them with organic salts. Examples are procaine penicillin and benzathine penicillin.

In general, penicillins are widely distributed into most body fluids and bone. Brain and CSF are exceptions, but concentrations in CSF are higher when meninges are inflamed. Penetration of body fluids and tissues by the highly protein-bound isoxazolyl derivatives is more limited. The dosage of penicillins may not have to be adjusted in patients with renal failure, despite impaired excretion, because of the low inherent toxicity and the increased biliary secretion obtained with the semisynthetic penicillins. Potassium-containing penicillins should not be given IV to oliguric patients because of the risk of hyperkalemia.

Most aqueous solutions of penicillins are unstable, especially at higher temperatures. They should be maintained at a pH of 5.5 to 7.5 and not added to solutions containing bicarbonate or other alkalinizing ingredients. PO suspensions of penicillins must be kept refrigerated after reconstitution. They generally remain stable for only 1 week. IV solutions should be used within 24 hours of preparation.

Penicillins should never be mixed with blood, plasma, or other proteinaceous fluids or with other antibiotics before administration. They might display in vivo antagonism with tetracycline and chloramphenicol; variable interactions with erythromycin, novobiocin, and lincomycin; no antagonism with sulfonamides; and possible synergism with AGs, cephalosporins, and polymyxins. As a matter of course, penicillins should not be mixed in the same syringe with AGs because of potential inactivation of both drug types.

Toxicity

Toxic reactions are relatively rare with penicillin derivatives, which generally have a high margin of safety. Rapid IV infusion or occasional IM injections may cause neurologic signs and convulsions. Hypersensitivity reactions such as hives, fever, joint pain, and acute anaphylaxis have been noted immediately after administration to dogs and cats. Administration of any penicillin derivatives should be avoided in known sensitized animals because of cross-reactivity.

Bleeding, presumably caused by interference with coagulation factors, has been an important side effect in human patients treated with antipseudomonal and extended-spectrum penicillins. This side effect has been attributed to various factors, including delayed fibrin polymerization, suppression of vitamin K–dependent procoagulants, and platelet dysfunction. Acute postoperative (within 5 days) azotemia has been ascribed to administration of nafcillin to dogs during surgery.[121]

Other β-Lactam Drugs

Monobactams. Aztreonam is the only clinically available member of this group. It is resistant to β-lactamase and active against a wide range of aerobic and facultative gram-negative bacteria, including many strains resistant to other drugs, but has no useful activity against gram-positive or anaerobic pathogens. It is given parenterally and enters many body tissues and fluids of dogs, including the CSF. Adverse effects are minimal and include diarrhea and vomiting. Its primary use has been to treat patients with serious gram-negative infections in which resistance or toxicity to AGs is anticipated.

Carbapenems. The first drug in this broad-spectrum series of atypical β-lactams was imipenem; newer members are panipenem, biapenem, and meropenem. Imipenem is active against a very wide range of gram-positive and gram-negative aerobes and anaerobes. It is primarily indicated for treatment of infections caused by cephalosporin-resistant members of the family Enterobacteriaceae and some anaerobes. Emergence of resistant *Pseudomonas* isolates has occurred during therapy. Breakdown of imipenem by dehydropeptidase-1 in the kidney and other tissues produces nephrotoxic metabolites and decreases the urine concentration of active drug. Coadministration of cilastatin, a metabolic inhibitor of dehydropeptidase-1, increases urine drug concentrations and decreases potential nephrotoxicity. Panipenem is combined with betamipron for the same reason. Biapenem and meropenem are more stable and do not require that inhibitors be given concurrently. Parenteral administration is necessary because neither imipenem nor cilastatin is absorbed orally. Dosage of the combination must be reduced in renal failure. Adverse effects have included nausea, vomiting, diarrhea, phlebitis at the infusion site, fever, and seizures.

β-Lactamase Inhibitors

Clavulanate. Some naturally occurring β-lactam products have low antibacterial activity by themselves but cause irreversible binding and inactivation of β-lactamase. Concurrent administration of these agents increases the activity of penicillins and decreases the in vitro MIC required to inactivate many β-lactamase–producing organisms, such as staphylococci, *Escherichia*, *K. pneumoniae*, some *Proteus* species, *B. fragilis*, *Salmonella*, and *Campylobacter* (Table 34–2). Organisms such as *Enterobacter*, *Serratia*, *Citrobacter*, and *Pseudomonas* are still resistant. For additional information on any of the β-lactam drugs, refer to the formulary, Appendix 8.

Clavulanate has weak antibacterial activity against a wide range of organisms but is a potent inhibitor of β-lactamase. It is rapidly absorbed, unaffected by food, and widely distributed in extravascular sites with the exception of the CNS. It is excreted rapidly in unchanged form in urine.

An orally administered product combining amoxicillin with potassium clavulanate is licensed for small animal use. A parenteral formulation of ticarcillin with potassium clavulanate is licensed for human and equine use. This combination is best suited to treat resistant infections caused by members of the family Enterobacteriaceae (except some *Pseudomonas*) and anaerobes. It is given commonly to treat infections of the skin, lower respiratory tract, soft tissue, middle ear, and sinuses. The primary side effect has been diarrhea.

Sulbactam. This drug, an irreversible β-lactamase inhibitor, has weak intrinsic antibacterial activity against most gram-positive and some gram-negative organisms, with best activ-

Table 34–2. Comparison of Antibacterial Activity of Selected β-Lactam–Inhibitor Combinations[a]

		BACTERIAL SUSCEPTIBILITY			
PENICILLIN	INHIBITOR	Gram Positive	Gram Negative	Anaerobes	*Pseudomonas*
Amoxicillin	Clavulanate	+	+	+	−
Ticarcillin	Clavulanate	++	++	+++	+
Ampicillin	Sulbactam	+	+	+	−
Piperacillin	Tazobactam	++	+++	++	++

[a]See Appendix 8 for further drug information and dosages.
+++ = excellent; ++ = very good; + = good; − = poor.

ity against *Neisseria* and *Bacteroides*. It extends the bacterial spectrum of ampicillin to include *Staphylococcus, Bacteroides,* and most *Escherichia*. It has been given with ampicillin to treat resistant bacterial meningitis in people and to treat those with intra-abdominal, pelvic, skin, soft tissue, bone, and joint infections.

Tazobactam. This β-lactamase inhibitor has been provided in combination with piperacillin to enhance the antibacterial spectrum of piperacillin. It is active against many resistant Enterobacteriaceae, *Staphylococcus*, and *Bacteroides*.

CEPHALOSPORINS

The cephalosporins are a group of antibiotics derived chemically from a substance produced by the fungus *Cephalosporium acremonium*. A number of related compounds can also be considered in the cephalosporin group because they have similar antibacterial activity, pharmacology, and indications. This group includes cefoxitin and cefotetan (both cephamycins), loracarbef (a carbacephem), and latamoxef (an oxacephem).

Like penicillins, cephalosporins are bactericidal β-lactam antibiotics that inhibit bacterial cell wall synthesis, resulting in osmotic fragility. These drugs are generally more effective than penicillin in penetrating the outer cell wall of gram-negative bacteria and are less susceptible to inactivation by bacterial β-lactamase.

Cephalosporins have been separated into three generations, or classes, based on the chronology of discovery, chemical structure, and therapeutic activity. The characteristics of the classes are compared in Table 34–3, and important features of common cephalosporins are presented in Table 34–4. For further information on specific drugs and dosage, see the Drug Formulary (Appendix 8).

First Generation

The first-generation cephalosporins are primarily active against gram-positive bacteria, with the exception of some resistant *Staphylococcus*, and some gram-negative aerobes, such as *Escherichia, Klebsiella,* and *Proteus mirabilis*. The activity against susceptible aerobes and facultative anaerobes exceeds that of penicillin G. The cephalosporins are relatively ineffective against anaerobes such as *Bacteroides*. First-generation cephalosporins can be administered orally or parenterally, depending on the drug, and they have variable protein binding with wide distribution into pleural, pericardial, peritoneal, and synovial fluids and most soft tissues. They enter the CSF only in the presence of meningeal inflammation. Most are excreted unchanged in the urine. Many cephalosporins interfere with glucose oxidase methods for determining urine glucose with test strips.

Two members of this group are of historic significance but are no longer used. Cephalothin is found in susceptibility disks, but it is of limited use because of pain and sterile abscesses produced on IM injection. Cephaloridine produces similar complications and is nephrotoxic. It is the only first-generation drug to penetrate CSF well. First-generation agents available for parenteral use include cefazolin, cephapirin, and cephradine. Oral drugs include cefadroxil and cephalexin.

Cefadroxil has been marketed for veterinary practice. It has uses for treating gram-negative urinary and gram-positive skin infections in dogs and skin and soft tissue infections in cats. Both cefadroxil and cephalexin reach effective blood concentrations after oral dosing of dogs and cats.

Second Generation

Second-generation cephalosporins have a broader spectrum of antibacterial activity and greater efficacy against gram-negative aerobic bacteria and anaerobes than the first generation. This activity is largely due to their greater resistance to β-lactamases. They are slightly inferior to the first group but are equal to penicillin in efficacy against gram-positive bacteria. They are more effective than first-generation drugs against *Proteus* other than *P. mirabilis, Escherichia, Klebsiella, Enterobacter,* and anaerobic bacteria. As with first-generation drugs, second- and third-generation cephalosporins are relatively ineffective against *Bacteroides*. Exceptions are cefoxitin, cefotetan, and moxalactam, which are effective against most obligate anaerobes. Cefoxitin is also effective

Table 34–3. Comparison of Antimicrobial Activity of Cephalosporins

	BACTERIAL SUSCEPTIBILITY				
GENERATION	Gram Positive	Gram Negative	Anaerobic	β-Lactamase Resistant	SELECTED SUSCEPTIBLE ORGANISMS
First	+++	+	−	−	*Staphylococcus*
Second	++	++	+	+	*Proteus*
Third	+	+++	++	++	*Pseudomonas*[a]

[a]Variable activity is noted depending on the third-generation drug. See Table 34–4 for antipseudomonal efficacy of selected cephalosporins.
+++ = excellent; ++ = very good, + = good; ± = variable; − = poor.

Table 34–4. Properties of Cephalosporins[a]

GENERIC NAME (TRADE NAME)	ROUTE OF ADMINISTRATION	COMMENTS
First Generation[b]		
Cephalexin (Keflex)	PO	Less active against *Staphylococcus.*
Cefazolin (Ancef, Kefzol)	IV, IM	Achieves greatest blood concentration; longest half-life; most protein-bound; more active against *Escherichia, Klebsiella, Enterobacter* than others in its class.
Cephapirin (Cefadyl)	IV, IM	Resists β-lactamase; high dosages for life-threatening infections when causative organism shows susceptibility to first-generation drugs.
Cefadroxil (Duricef, Cefa-Tabs)	PO	Rapid and complete oral absorption even with food; enters prostate.
Cephradine (Velosef, Anspor)	IV, IM, PO	Spectrum similar to cephalexin; less active against some gram-negative organisms.
Second Generation[c]		
Cefaclor (Ceclor)	PO	Similar spectrum but more active than first generation against *Proteus, Escherichia, Enterobacter,* and *Klebsiella;* adequate soft tissue concentrations; minor amount excreted in urine unchanged.
Cefoxitin (Mefoxin)[d]	IV, IM	Pain on IM injection; active against *Bacteroids fragilis* and *Serratia;* particularly effective against most anaerobes.
Cefuroxime (Zinacef, Kefurox)	IV, IM	Crosses blood-brain barrier, good for lower respiratory tract and CNS infections.
Third Generation[e]		
Cefixime (Suprax)	PO	For urinary and respiratory infections caused by resistant bacteria. Not active against *Pseudomonas.*
Ceftiofur (Naxcel)	IV, IM	Licensed for treatment of bovine respiratory disease. Good for broad-spectrum treatment of systemic infections. Low activity against *Staphylococcus.*
Cefotaxime (Claforan)	IV	Activity against *Leptospira* and gram-negative aerobes except *Pseudomonas;* metabolized in liver to active drug; good CNS penetration.
Ceftriaxone (Recephin)	IV, IM	Longest duration for once-daily dosing; active against resistant gram-negatives except *Pseudomonas;* good against *Borrelia.*
Antipseudomonal Third Generation[f]		
Ceftazidime (Fortaz, Tazidime, Tazicef)	IV	Primarily active against gram-negative aerobes and best of cephalosporins against *Pseudomonas.*
Cefoperazone (Cefobid)	IV	Less active than other third-generation drugs against gram-positive and negative aerobes; second best of its class against *Pseudomonas;* can produce coagulation deficiencies, erratic CNS penetration; predominant (80%) biliary excretion.

[a]See Appendix 8 for appropriate dosages.
[b]Also includes cephaloglycin, cephalothin, cephaloridine.
[c]Also includes cefuroxime axetil (Ceftin), cefmetazole, cefonicid (Monocid), and cefotetan (Cefotan) and three more given orally: cefprozil, cefpodoxime (Vantin), and loracarbef.
[d]Cefoxitin and cefotetan are cephamycins, moxalactam (Latamoxef) is an oxacephem, and loracarbef is a carbacephem, but they are included with cephalosporins because of similar attributes.
[e]Also includes ceftriaxone (Rocephin), ceftrizoxime (Cefizox), flomoxef, ceftibuten (Cedax), cefmenoxime, ceftiofur (Naxcel), and moxalactam (Moxam, Lactoxacef).
[f]Also includes cefsulodin, cefpiramide.

against *Serratia.* They have generally been given parenterally, but orally effective drugs include cefaclor, cefuroxime axetil (a pro-drug), cefprozil, cefpodoxime, and loracarbef.

Third Generation

The third-generation cephalosporins have longer duration of activity than the other two classes. Excretion in either urine or bile is variable, depending on the drug, although most undergo some inactivation and excretion by the liver. Third-generation drugs, except for latamoxef, moxalactam, ceftriaxone, and cefotaxime, do not usually penetrate CSF. Third-generation cephalosporins have marked activity against anaerobes and aerobic gram-negative organisms and less effectiveness against aerobic gram-positive organisms. They are more active than second-generation drugs against *Citrobacter, Acinetobacter, Pseudomonas,* and *Serratia.* Unlike other cephalosporins, cefoperazone and ceftazidime are among the most effective drugs against *P. aeruginosa.* However, most third-generation cephalosporins are not as effective against *Pseudomonas* as the newer extended-spectrum penicillins. Third-generation cephalosporins when given IV have been recommended for use in septicemia, bacteremia, intra-abdominal infection, and endocarditis. Second- and third-generation drugs have had good efficacy against drug-resistant *Salmonella* isolated from people.

Indications

The varied indications for use of cephalosporins include treatment of bacterial infections of respiratory, urinary, and genital tracts; soft tissues; bones and joints; and skin. Cephalosporins are effective when given prophylactically for polymicrobial intra-abdominal infections after bowel surgery. In addition, they have also been recommended for prophylactic purposes in biliary surgery and for treating biliary infections, because many are excreted unchanged in bile. However, they do not enter the biliary tract when complete biliary obstruction and jaundice are present. Failure of cephalosporins to prevent postoperative staphylococcal infections has been associated with strains that hydrolyze cephalosporins.[75] Cefotaxime, moxalactam, and ceftriaxone are very effective for meningitis caused by drug-resistant bacteria.

Most oral cephalosporins administered in small animal practice are first-generation drugs but oral second- and third-generation products are available (see Table 34–4). Cefazolin and cephapirin are the most commonly used parenteral first-generation cephalosporins. The second-generation drugs, such as cefoxitin, have increased efficacy against anaerobic infections. Of the second-generation drugs, cefuroxime has a high degree of penetration into the CNS and CSF for treatment of meningitis.

Toxicity

The toxicity of cephalosporins is minimal compared with that of other antibiotics. In this regard, the cephalosporins are similar to the penicillin derivatives.[109] Allergic skin reactions have been reported with cephalosporins in dogs. A greater incidence of diarrhea is associated with agents undergoing biliary excretion. Cephaloridine is nephrotoxic, but this is not characteristic of the newer drugs. Because most cephalosporins are excreted by the kidney, blood concentrations are increased and half-lives are prolonged in renal failure or when probenecid, loop diuretics, or AGs are used. All parenteral formulations of cephalosporins may cause phlebitis and myositis after IV and IM administration, respectively. GI irritation may cause vomiting and diarrhea with oral administration. Bleeding disorders in people resulting from vitamin K antagonism, platelet dysfunction, and immune-mediated thrombocytopenia have been associated with third-generation cephalosporins, most frequently cefamandole, cefoperazone, and moxalactam. Cephalosporin-induced blood dyscrasias, a result of immune-mediated destruction of blood cells and direct marrow toxicity, have occurred in dogs given high-dose, long-term cephalosporins.[30] Myelosuppression resolves when therapy is withdrawn. For individual drug characteristics, consult the Drug Formulary (Appendix 8).

AMINOGLYCOSIDES

These bactericidal antibiotics interfere with the synthesis of bacterial protein. They are relatively small, primarily basic, water-soluble molecules that are active against certain gram-negative and gram-positive aerobic and facultative anaerobic bacteria, including mycobacteria. They are particularly effective against aerobic gram-negative bacilli such as *Escherichia*, *Klebsiella*, *Proteus*, and *Enterobacter*, and some are effective against *Pseudomonas*. AGs are *not* active against fungi or obligate anaerobic bacteria and should *not* be used to treat abscesses or granulomatous infections. Their uptake by bacteria requires the presence of oxygen. When used alone, they are relatively ineffective against *Streptococcus* but are effective against *Staphylococcus intermedius*. The properties and indications for the various AGs are summarized in Table 34–5.

Dihydrostreptomycin, streptomycin, neomycin, and kanamycin have been extensively used for many years. However, with such frequency, extensive bacterial resistance has developed. The first two are no longer commercially available in many countries. Amikacin and gentamicin are more effective and routinely given. Amikacin is generally more effective than gentamicin against resistant strains. Tobramycin and netilmicin have been developed to increase antibacterial activity and reduce toxicity. Sisomicin, isepamicin, and dactimicin are newer AGs being evaluated for clinical purposes. The latter two have broad-spectrum activity against gram-positive and gram-negative aerobes.

Antimicrobial synergy is often observed when AGs are combined with β-lactam drugs. The β-lactams may also enhance AG activity under conditions of reduced oxygen tension.

The pharmacokinetics of many of the AGs have been studied in dogs and cats. AGs are poorly absorbed from the GI tract and must be administered parenterally to achieve therapeutic blood concentrations; however, some (such as neomycin and paromomycin) are administered orally for the local treatment of bacterial or protozoal enteritis or to suppress the levels of enteric microflora in hepatic coma. They are poorly absorbed through intact skin, but may cross damaged squamous, mucosal, or visceral epithelium resulting in potential toxicity. Topical AG creams and solutions can help to control bacterial growth and facilitate healing of open

Table 34–5. Properties of Aminoglycosides

GENERIC NAME (TRADE NAME)	ROUTE OF ADMINISTRATION	COMMENTS
Streptomycin (many)[a]	IM, SC	Occasional parenterally/IM? for bacteremias, *Brucella canis, Leptospira* carriers; limited availability
Dihydrostreptomycin (many)	IM, SC	As for streptomycin; many resistant strains; limited commercial availability
Neomycin (Biosol, Mycifradin)[a]	PO, topical	PO for local GI effect; topical use in solutions, ointments, etc; spectrum similar to kanamycin; absorbed and toxic if bowel wall damaged
Kanamycin (Kantrim, Kantrex, Klebcil)	PO, IM, SC	PO for local GI effect; useful in UTI and superficial and systemic infections; spectrum similar to gentamicin, but resistant strains much more common; effective against *Staphylococcus*
Gentamicin (Gentocin, Garamycin Apogen, Bristagen, U-Gencin)	IM, SC, IV, aerosol, topical	Bacteremia; in aerosol for respiratory infections caused by *Escherichia, Pasteurella, Pseudomonas, Proteus, Staphylococcus, Enterobacter, Serratia, Klebsiella, Bordetella*
Paromomycin (Humatin)	PO	PO for local GI effect; used for susceptible *Staphylococcus, Escherichia, Salmonella,* and protozoa (*Entamoeba, Balantidium, Cryptosporidium*)
Tobramycin (Nebcin)[a]	IM, SC	Gram-negative spectrum similar to gentamicin, effective against some *Pseudomonas* resistant to gentamicin; less nephrotoxic than gentamicin
Amikacin (Amikin, Amiglyde)	IM, SC	Widest antibacterial spectrum of currently used aminoglycosides; effective against *Pseudomonas* and many gram-negative bacilli resistant to gentamicin and tobramycin (e.g., *Klebsiella*)
Sisomicin (Sisomin)	IM, SC	More active than gentamicin against many bacteria, especially *Pseudomonas* and *Escherichia;* not effective against organisms resistant to gentamicin; toxicity parallels gentamicin
Netilmicin (Netromycin)	IM, SC	*Staphylococcus* highly susceptible; active against some organisms resistant to gentamicin, more active than sisomicin or tobramycin, slightly less active than amikacin against *Pseudomonas,* less toxic than tobramycin
Framycetin (Sulframycin, Neomycin B)	PO, topical	PO for local GI effect, topical in ointment drops, etc; gram-negative spectrum similar to neomycin
Dactinomycin[b]	IM, SC	Intra-abdominal infections; wide activity against gram-positive and gram-negative aerobes; may combine with metronidazole for anaerobic spectrum; most active AG against *Acinetobacter* and *Staphylococcus*
Isepamicin[b]	IV, IM, SC	Exceptional activity against Enterobacteriaceae and *Pseudomonas*

[a]See Drug Formulary (Appendix 8) for appropriate dosages.
[b]Not available commercially.
UTI = urinary tract infection; AG = aminoglycoside; IM = intramuscular; SC = subcutaneous; PO = oral; IV = intravenous.

wounds. They are rapidly absorbed following IM or SC administration.[180] After intraoperative IV administration, they enter surgical wounds for a time that parallels blood concentrations. They are minimally bound to plasma proteins, but, because they are poorly lipid soluble and highly ionized, they penetrate little beyond extracellular fluid compartments, including synovial, peritoneal, and pleural spaces. They also diffuse poorly into CNS, prostate, amniotic fluid, and eyes, even in the presence of inflammation. Obese cats have smaller volumes of distribution of AGs than lean cats, warranting dosage reductions in obese animals.[182] There is little excretion into bile and feces, but unchanged AG is eliminated rapidly in urine. Within 1 hour after administration, urine AG concentrations are 25 to 100 times greater than peak blood concentrations and remain above therapeutic levels for several days. AGs are eliminated slowly from renal tissue; once daily dosing produces less renal accumulation than thrice daily dosing with higher peak tissue concentrations. The pH at which optimum antibacterial activity occurs is 7.5 to 8.0. Streptomycin may produce spuriously high results with measurements of urine glucose by glucose oxidase strips. AGs such as gentamicin have been effective in treating canine bronchopulmonary infections when administered as aerosols: drug concentration in the airway lumen is increased and toxicity is reduced because of poor absorption from this site.

Individual variability in distribution and elimination of AGs accounts for unpredictable variability in blood and tissue concentrations. Consequently in human medicine, the monitoring of blood concentration is common. Liposomal encapsulation of AGs has been used in an attempt to increase therapeutic efficacy and decrease toxicity.[159]

Bacteria are likely to develop resistance to AGs by one of three mechanisms: alteration of the receptor sites on bacterial ribosomes, decreased bacterial cell penetrability, and plasmid-associated production of enzymes that inactivate AGs. Bacterial resistance to AGs is greater with the older drugs and less with newer compounds. Cross-resistance is not uniform among all members of the class. For example, although many *Klebsiella* are resistant to kanamycin and gentamicin, they are susceptible to amikacin, a derivative of kanamycin. In general, there is a high degree of cross-resistance between gentamicin and other AGs, except for amikacin and tobramycin.

Toxicities with AG antibiotics are relatively common and are a result of the individual drug and dosage, duration of therapy, state of patient hydration, presence of upper urinary tract infection (UTI), and pretreatment of renal function. Nephrotoxicity can be attributed to the uptake of AGs by proximal renal tubular cells and drug retention in lysosomes of these cells in the cortex. Above a certain concentration, cell necrosis occurs. Although species differences exist, nephrotoxicity in decreasing order is as follows: neomycin, kanamycin, gentamicin, tobramycin, amikacin, and streptomycin. Nephrotoxicity has been associated with high trough blood concentrations (> 2.0 μg/ml for gentamicin and 5.0 μg/ml for amikacin). Frequent administration of small doses to maintain constant blood AG concentrations is more toxic than less frequent administration of larger dosages. Frequent (three to four times daily) dosing is recommended for treatment of systemic infections in animals, but renal function must be closely monitored with such protocols. AGs may be given at higher doses and less frequent intervals than commonly recommended. Pulse administration of large (10 mg/kg) doses of gentamicin at 5-day intervals has been shown to maintain effective tissue concentrations in dogs. Pulse administration should be less nephrotoxic than frequent dosing because blood concentrations decrease sufficiently during the longer treatment interval; however, documentation of the efficacy of such regimens is uncertain.[46] AGs, in contrast to some other antibiotics, show marked concentration-dependent killing of bacteria. After bacterial killing, a bacteriostatic phase without regrowth, known as postantibiotic effect, is observed.

Renal proximal tubular dysfunction is the most common and serious side effect of AG administration. Higher protein diets have been protective to dogs in the development of gentamicin-induced nephrotoxicity.[47] Inadvertent absorption of gentamicin administered topically when lavaging an abscess produced nephrotoxicity in a cat.[100] Use of AGs should be restricted in puppies and kittens because they are more prone to develop renal failure than older animals.

The best method of detecting early renal tubular dysfunction in practice is to examine the urine for casts and proteinuria. Blood urea and creatinine concentrations are primarily measures of glomerular filtration and are less sensitive indications of AG nephrotoxicity. Although mainly a research tool, the most sensitive way to detect AG toxicity in dogs and cats is to measure urinary concentrating ability and urinary enzyme activities.[48] Acute renal failure typically develops several days after therapy is initiated but may develop several days after the drug is discontinued. Because AGs accumulate in renal tubular cells, the insult persists even after administration ceases. The prognosis for recovery from AG-induced renal failure is very poor in dogs and cats. In human hospitals, AG concentrations are monitored to avoid toxicity; dosages are modified so that blood levels are high enough 1 hour after administration to be bactericidal but are below toxic threshold levels 30 minutes later.

Clinical reports from human hospitals have noted increased nephrotoxicity when AGs are given with cephalosporins. However, studies in rats indicated the combination may actually be protective. Similarly, combinations of piperacillin with gentamicin or cephaloridine have been shown to have reduced nephrotoxicity. Furosemide may enhance nephrotoxicity and ototoxicity of AGs. Toxicity is thought to result from decreased extracellular fluid volume with decreased drug excretion and increased blood AG concentration. Other diuretics may have similar effects and should be avoided in combination with AGs. Cats and dogs should be well hydrated whenever AG therapy is instituted. Other nephrotoxic drugs such as amphotericin B and cisplatin should be avoided because they may potentiate nephrotoxicity.

Gentamicin-impregnated methyl methacrylate beads and methyl methacrylate cement have been applied successfully for prophylaxis in orthopedic surgery.[158] Local release of the gentamicin into the surrounding bone, soft tissue, and synovial fluid allowed for long-term therapy, an effective cure, and no side effects. AGs have also been incorporated into liposomes to reduce systemic toxicity.

Irreversible ototoxicity has been a problem with AG therapy; both vestibular and auditory impairment from damage to the sensory end-organs have been reported. High concentrations of AGs remain in the perilymph fluid of the ear for extended periods compared with blood. AGs are potentially ototoxic when instilled directly into the external ear canal of dogs and cats, especially if the tympanic membrane has been ruptured. However, ototoxicity has not been found at concentrations present in commercial otic preparations.[153] Table 34–6 summarizes relative otic and renal toxicities of AGs for dogs and cats. In cats the ototoxicity of AGs in decreasing order was streptomycin, dihydrostreptomycin, gentamicin, tobramycin, and netilmicin, with vestibular damage more likely than auditory damage.

AGs, associated with underlying risk factors, may produce neuromuscular blockade by competitive antagonism of ace-

Table 34–6. Relative Toxicity of Aminoglycosides[a]

DRUG	KIDNEY	VESTIBULAR	AUDITORY
Streptomycin	−	+	−
Dihydrostreptomycin	?	−	+
Neomycin	+	−	+
Gentamicin	+	+	±
Kanamycin	+	−	+
Tobramycin	+	+	+
Amikacin	±	−	+
Netilmicin	±	±	±

[a]See Appendix 8 for appropriate dosages.
− = lesions have not been detected; + = lesions have been detected; ? = information concerning lesions is lacking; ± = milder lesions than +.
Adapted from data from Conzelman GM: *J Am Vet Med Assoc* 176:1078–1080, 1980; McCormick GC et al: *Toxicol Appl Pharmacol* 77:478–489, 1985; Pickrell JA et al: *Semin Vet Med Surg Small Anim* 8:42–49, 1993.

tylcholine at the myoneural junction. In addition to their own neuromuscular blocking effects, they enhance the actions of other neuromuscular blocking agents and general anesthetics.[44] Irrigation of body cavities or parenteral administration of AGs, therefore, should be avoided during surgery that requires general anesthesia.

Circulatory depression, manifest by decreased systemic blood pressure and heart rate, has been found in cats, dogs, and nonhuman primates given AGs during pentobarbital anesthesia. Cardiac arrest has been reported in humans overdosed with kanamycin. If possible, AG administration should be avoided in animals in shock or with cardiovascular insufficiency. Calcium gluconate, given IV, may reverse AG-induced neuromuscular blockade or myocardial depression and restore blood pressure.

Prolonged high oral dosages of neomycin or paromomycin may produce diarrhea and malabsorption owing to overgrowth of resistant indigenous intestinal flora. Hypersensitivity and allergic reactions have been reported rarely in humans receiving AGs. AGs should not be administered to pregnant animals because they can cross the placenta and may produce fetal intoxication. Penicillins and AGs should never be mixed in the same solution before administration. Depending on the type and concentration of penicillin, mixing can cause inactivation of the AGs. They should not be administered IV with solutions containing calcium, other antimicrobials, heparin, or sodium bicarbonate. For individual drug characteristics and dosages consult the Drug Formulary (Appendix 8).

SPECTINOMYCIN

Aminocyclitol antibiotics, composed of a basic cyclic structure with an amino group, include spectinomycin and its derivatives and the aforementioned AGs. Spectinomycin shares many properties with the AGs, including low plasma protein binding, high water solubility, poor GI absorption, primary renal excretion, bacterial ribosomal protein synthesis inhibition, and optimum antibacterial activity at pH 8.

Spectinomycin has bacteriostatic activity, mainly against gram-negative aerobic pathogens such as *Escherichia, Klebsiella, Salmonella, Enterobacter,* and *Proteus* as well as the mycoplasmas. The antibiotic has low efficacy against gram-positive aerobes, most pseudomonads, and chlamydiae. Obligate anaerobes are resistant. Parenteral administration of spectinomycin may be useful for treatment of bacteremia associated with infectious gastroenteritis caused by susceptible enteropathogenic bacteria and for treatment of intra-abdominal sepsis (see Intra-abdominal Infections, Chapter 89). As with some AGs, development of resistant bacteria is a problem with spectinomycin. Trospectomycin is an analog of spectinomycin with similar activity against enterobacteria but increased activity against gram-positive aerobes.

PEPTIDES

Vancomycin

This is a complex glycopeptide molecule that has bactericidal activity. In susceptible replicating bacteria, it inhibits cell wall formation and RNA production and alters cytoplasmic membranes. Vancomycin is active primarily against gram-positive organisms, mainly *Staphylococcus,* including methicillin-resistant strains, *Streptococcus,* and *Clostridium.* The majority of gram-negative bacteria are resistant.

Vancomycin can be administered orally to treat susceptible enteric pathogens. It is absorbed poorly from the GI tract and must be given IV for systemic infections. The drug distributes well into body cavities and across inflamed meninges. Excretion is largely by glomerular filtration, with small amounts entering the bile.[186]

The most frequent side effects with vancomycin in people have been fever, chills, and phlebitis at injection sites. These can be reduced if the drug is administered slowly in a large volume of fluid. Leukopenia and eosinopenia have been reported.

Possible uses for vancomycin in animals are limited. It might be considered for treating severe, persistent staphylococcal infections and colitis associated with overgrowth of *Clostridium difficile.* See the Drug Formulary (Appendix 8) for further information. In the United States, restrictions have been placed upon the use of glycopeptides in food producing animals.[1a]

Teicoplanin

This complex glycopeptide has similar structure, activity, and other properties to vancomycin. It is primarily active against aerobic and some anaerobic gram-positive organisms. Teicoplanin is more protein bound and lipophilic than vancomycin. Its half-life in plasma is much longer, which may allow once daily administration. Possible indications for veterinary use are as for vancomycin. Further information is given in Appendix 8.

POLYMYXINS

These agents form a group of closely related, cationic, cyclic peptides. Of the types A through E, polymyxin B and polymyxin E (colistin) are therapeutically most important. Polymyxins appear to exert their bactericidal effects as cationic detergents by binding to cell membrane phospholipids and increasing cell permeability of gram-negative bacteria. Most gram-negative organisms, such as *Pasteurella, Escherichia, Shigella, Salmonella, Bordetella,* and some *Klebsiella* and *Pseudomonas,* are susceptible, whereas *Brucella* and *Proteus* are frequently resistant. Resistance is also a factor of increased usage, and although emergent strains develop during usage, they become susceptible again once polymyxin therapy is stopped.

Polymyxins are poorly absorbed when given orally and topically. They do not produce high blood concentrations after parenteral administration, presumably because of their affinity for host cell membranes. They diffuse poorly through biologic membranes and are excreted unchanged in the urine.

These drugs are provided chiefly as topical preparations for treating localized infections in the ear canal, eye, bowel, and urinary tract. Respiratory therapy may be achieved by means of nebulization. Intrathecal administration has been performed with aqueous preparations; however, they are highly irritating. For topical use, polymyxins have been combined with neomycin and bacitracin or tetracycline to widen antibacterial activity.

Polymyxins have been given systemically (IM) to treat infections that are resistant to AGs and as such have shown some synergism with sulfonamide and trimethoprim. Colistin sulfomethate (sodium colistimethate) is the least toxic parenteral preparation. The major side effect of the polymyxins is nephrotoxicity, although pain at the injection site, CNS signs, and neuromuscular blockade have also been noted. Toxicity has limited the usefulness of these drugs for systemic therapy.

CHLORAMPHENICOL

Chloramphenicol is a highly lipid-soluble, broad-spectrum antibiotic that is predominantly bacteriostatic and inhibits microbial protein synthesis. It is effective against a variety of pathogens, including *Mycoplasma, Rickettsia, Ehrlichia, Chlamydia, Staphylococcus, Streptococcus, Pasteurella, Bordetella, Haemophilus*, and Enterobacteriaceae, including many *Escherichia, Proteus*, and *Salmonella*. This antibiotic has good activity against most obligate anaerobic bacterial pathogens.

Administration

Chloramphenicol can be administered orally or parenterally, and absorption depends on formulation. The drug is usually given orally in capsular form but can be bitter tasting, causing salivation and anorexia if capsules are not swallowed intact. Oral film-coated tablets may overcome this problem. Chloramphenicol palmitate is an oral suspension that requires hydrolysis by digestive enzymes before absorption can occur. Blood concentrations are lower initially with this dosage form in cats and poor in those that are not eating. Capsules or tablets, therefore, may be preferable in cats. Chloramphenicol sodium succinate, a water-soluble ester, is recommended for systemic use. Otic, ophthalmic, and topical preparations are also available.

Pharmacokinetics

Less than 50% of the drug is bound to plasma protein. In dogs and cats, most of the drug is metabolized by the liver to inactive metabolites excreted in urine, and a minor amount is excreted in bile, from where it undergoes enterohepatic circulation. Chloramphenicol diffuses rapidly and well into most tissues. Highest concentrations are found in liver, kidney, bile, spleen, lung, pancreas, and urine, and it penetrates all body fluids. It takes several hours for the brain concentration to approximate that of the blood concentration; however, brain tissue concentration remains adequate for up to 12 hours, although blood concentration diminishes before that time. The concentration of active chloramphenicol in urine is usually sufficient to be effective against susceptible bacteria.

Indications

Chloramphenicol is effective against most aerobic and anaerobic bacterial pathogens in dogs and cats. It is a preferred antibiotic for treating *Salmonella* and *Escherichia* infections in the GI tract and has been recommended for prophylaxis before intestinal surgery or dental procedures but is contraindicated with pentobarbital anesthesia. Chloramphenicol is considered helpful in the treatment of UTIs in dogs with subnormal renal function, because the drug is unlikely to accumulate in dogs unless renal failure is advanced.

Chloramphenicol penetrates the cornea well because it is lipid soluble and has low molecular weight. Systemic administration is required for treatment of intraocular and orbital infections and deep corneal lesions.

Toxicity

The most common side effects of chloramphenicol administration in dogs and cats are depression, anorexia, dysphagia, salivation, nausea, vomiting, and sporadic diarrhea. Reversible bone marrow suppression and severe irreversible bone marrow failure have been reported in humans. The persistent pancytopenia is idiosyncratic and not dose related. However, only reversible bone marrow changes have been demonstrated in dogs and cats, with variable suppression of erythropoiesis and granulopoiesis. Chloramphenicol is more toxic to cats than to dogs, perhaps because of their inability to conjugate glucuronic acid, which is an important step in elimination of chloramphenicol in other species. Bone marrow changes in cats can occur after only 1 week of therapy. Toxic changes do not develop if cats are given the drug on an intermittent basis or at low doses. Clinical improvement and resolution of hematologic changes usually occur within several days after cessation of therapy. A normal hemogram does not rule out toxicosis, because bone marrow changes precede those in peripheral blood.

The small public health hazard associated with inadvertent contact with chloramphenicol has limited its use in food-producing species and may increase the veterinarian's liability to owners handling the drug intended for their pets. Thiamphenicol, an analog of chloramphenicol, has been widely provided in Europe as a substitute. It has similar antibacterial properties, is associated with enhanced renal excretion of active drug, and is said not to cause irreversible marrow failure in people. Another related drug, florfenicol, is licensed for cattle. For further information on chloramphenicol and florfenicol, and dosage regimens, consult the Drug Formulary (Appendix 8).

TETRACYCLINES

Tetracycline antibiotics are bacteriostatic and interfere with protein synthesis of bacterial RNA. As a group, they have a broad spectrum of activity that includes certain aerobic and anaerobic gram-positive and gram-negative bacteria, mycobacteria, spirochetes, mycoplasmas, rickettsiae, chlamydiae, and some protozoa (Table 34–7). The newer lipid-soluble tetracyclines, doxycycline and minocycline, have increased activity against anaerobes and several facultative intracellular bacteria like *Brucella canis*. For further information on susceptibility of pathogens to individual tetracyclines consult the Drug Formulary (Appendix 8). Bacterial resistance to tetracyclines is usually mediated by plasmids, although it may occur following genetic mutation. Resistance has been a major problem with conventional tetracyclines but occurs less often with doxycycline and minocycline.

The tetracyclines vary markedly in their lipid solubility, a factor that determines their relative GI absorption, and tissue penetration. Highly lipid-soluble doxycycline and minocy-

Table 34–7. Properties of Tetracyclines[a]

GENERIC NAME (TRADE NAME)	ROUTE OF ADMINISTRATION	COMMENTS AND SPECIFIC INDICATIONS
Short Acting, Water Soluble		
Tetracycline (Panmycin, Achromycin, Tetracyn)	PO, IV, IM	Therapeutic or prophylactic use for *Ehrlichia;* IM injections painful; do not inject intra-articularly
Oxytetracycline (Terramycin)	PO, IV, IM	Reaches high concentration in lung, liver, kidney, and mononuclear phagocyte system; better tolerated orally by cats
Chlortetracycline (Aureomycin)	PO	pH is very important for activity
Intermediate Acting[b]		
Demeclocycline[c] (Declomycin)	PO	Photosensitivity may occur; dosage-dependent diabetes insipidus
Long Acting, Lipid Soluble		
Minocycline (Minocin, Vectrin)	PO, IV	More effective against *Ehrlichia, Babesia, Brucella;* greater activity against *Nocardia, Staphylococcus,* and anaerobes; wide distribution in tissues
Doxycycline (Vibramycin, Doxychel)	PO, IV	Same as for minocycline; tetracycline of choice for extrarenal infections with concurrent renal failure; more active against *Bacteroides;* prophylaxis for bowel surgery; used to treat chronic prostatitis

[a]See Appendix 8 for appropriate dosages.
[b]Also includes methacycline.
[c]Formerly demethylchlortetracycline.

cline show better absorption and wider tissue distribution although they are more protein bound. Absorption, a passive process that occurs primarily in the duodenum, is interfered with by sodium bicarbonate and by divalent and trivalent cations in food, milk, aluminum hydroxide gels, calcium and magnesium salts, and iron preparations. Because absorption of doxycycline and minocycline is somewhat less affected than other tetracyclines by food or cations, these two agents are often given with meals to reduce GI irritation. However, tetracyclines undergo enterohepatic circulation, and intraintestinal multivalent cations can still chelate and reduce the bioavailability of parenterally administered drug.

Tetracyclines inhibit the activity of neutral matrix metalloproteinases, perhaps related to their chelation of multivalent cations. These enzymes are involved in the progression of cartilage degeneration in osteoarthritis. Dogs with experimentally induced anterior cruciate ligament injuries had reduced severity of osteoarthritis when they were treated with doxycycline.[185] This nonspecific protective effect should be considered in dogs that improve with tetracycline-responsive polyarthritis, which is often considered to have an infectious cause.

Tetracyclines enter most tissues, including the eye and CNS of dogs. They even penetrate well into the paranasal sinuses and secretions, so they are good for treating bacterial sinusitis. Tetracyclines are less active in alkaline media, especially in the case of chlortetracycline.

The less lipid-soluble agents tetracycline and oxytetracycline are primarily excreted unchanged in the urine: 60% is recoverable as unchanged drug in urine, whereas 40% is excreted by the liver and found in feces. In contrast, lipid-soluble minocycline is primarily eliminated by hepatic metabolism, and only 10% of the administered dose enters the urine. The excretion of doxycycline is not controlled by hepatic or renal excretion; this drug is unique in that the major means of elimination appears to be diffusion across the intestinal wall. Minocycline and doxycycline may not reach high enough concentrations in the urine to be effective against some pathogens, although doxycycline has been given to eliminate the carrier state of *Leptospira* in renal tissues.

Numerous side effects have been associated with tetracyclines. GI disturbances result from esophageal, gastric, and intestinal irritation and changes in enteric microflora. Because doxycycline and minocycline are well absorbed in the upper GI tract, they are less likely to alter the lower intestinal flora. Orally administered tetracyclines frequently produce fever in cats with or without severe GI upsets from local irritation. As with chloramphenicol, tetracyclines inhibit hepatic microsomal enzymes and may delay elimination of hepatically metabolized drugs. Hepatotoxicity (including increased blood alanine aminotransferase activity) has been found in dogs and cats that are receiving tetracyclines.[74]

Except for doxycycline, tetracyclines should be avoided in patients with renal failure because drug excretion is delayed and azotemia may worsen. The use of tetracyclines in dogs has been associated with direct nephrotoxicity from acute tubular necrosis; and in people the use of outdated tetracyclines or the drug's breakdown products have produced a Fanconi's syndrome–like disorder with reversible renal tubular dysfunction. Findings on urinalysis have included glucosuria, phosphaturia, and aminoaciduria with or without proteinuria. The nephrotoxicity occasionally produced by methoxyflurane anesthesia is accentuated by tetracyclines given before surgery.

Anaphylactic reactions to parenterally administered tetracyclines or their vehicles have occasionally been noted in dogs and cats. Phototoxic reactions, characterized by erythema and edema of the skin, have been associated with certain tetracyclines after exposure to UV light. Demeclocycline has been shown to induce acute reversible nephrogenic diabetes insipidus in humans.

Tetracyclines become fixed in growing osseous structures. Staining of deciduous teeth of neonates and enamel hypoplasia may occur when tetracyclines are given to a bitch or queen during the last 2 or 3 weeks of pregnancy. The deciduous teeth of puppies or kittens may also be affected if they are given these drugs during the first months of life.

Thrombophlebitis frequently occurs after IV injections of tetracyclines and is seen more frequently with the less lipid-soluble agents. IM administration of nonrepositol tetracyclines is discouraged because it causes pain and necrosis.

Tetracyclines may cause false-positive urine test results for glucose if copper sulfate reagents are employed (Clinitest, Ames Laboratories, Elkhart, IN), and false-negative test results may occur with glucose oxidase reagents. Leukocytosis, atypical lymphocytes, toxic granulation, and immune hemolytic anemia have been reported with tetracyclines in humans. Interference of tetracycline with coagulation factors has also been noted.

MACROLIDES AND LINCOSAMIDES

Erythromycin is the parent drug of the macrolides. Oleandomycin and troleandomycin, two older members of the group, are less active and more toxic than erythromycin and are rarely administered. Rosamicin is similar to erythromycin in antibacterial spectrum and usage. Josamycin is better absorbed and less toxic and is less likely to lead to bacterial resistance than erythromycin. Rokitamycin achieves higher blood concentrations after oral administration and causes fewer GI side effects than erythromycin. Dirithromycin is a potent erythromycin derivative that has been shown to produce higher and longer lasting blood concentrations than erythromycin base. This pro-drug is hydrolyzed during intestinal absorption to the active moiety erythromycylamine.

A number of macrolides including erythromycin, azithromycin, clarithromycin, and tylosin are discussed briefly later and more extensively in the Drug Formulary (Appendix 8). Because of its antiprotozoal efficacy, spiramycin is discussed in Chapter 71. The lincosamide antibiotics are structurally unrelated to macrolides but have similar antibacterial and pharmacokinetic attributes. Lincomycin and clindamycin are discussed later, and further information is given in the formulary (Appendix 8).

Erythromycin inhibits protein synthesis in bacterial cells and is bacteriostatic for susceptible organisms at usual dosages. Because its mechanism of action resembles that of chloramphenicol and lincosamides, erythromycin can compete with these drugs for binding sites.

Erythromycin is a weak base, unstable in the presence of gastric acid, which inhibits its bioavailability after oral administration. Different formulations of erythromycin have been made to circumvent destruction of erythromycin by digestive enzymes, incorporating enteric coating, acid-stable salts (stearate), esters (ethylsuccinate), and salts of esters (estolate) (Table 34–8). GI absorption of erythromycin base and stearate is impaired by ingesta and gastric acid. Lactobionate and gluceptate esters of erythromycin can be administered parenterally but are relatively expensive. Topical preparations are also available for general use and as ophthalmic ointments to treat chlamydial and mycoplasmal conjunctivitis.

Erythromycin diffuses readily into most tissues and extracellular fluid compartments, with the exception of CSF, and therapeutic concentrations are reached within 2 to 3 hours. It is concentrated by the liver and excreted in bile in high concentration, undergoing enterohepatic circulation and final excretion in feces. High concentrations are found in most body fluids and secretions, with the exception of urine.

Erythromycin, which has a primarily gram-positive spectrum, is most effective against *Streptococcus, Staphylococcus, Erysipelothrix, Clostridium, Bacteroides, Borrelia,* and *Fusobacterium.* It is also effective against a few gram-negative organisms, such as *Pasteurella* and *Bordetella,* but not against aerobic enteric bacteria unless the environmental pH is alkaline. Erythromycin has exceptional activity against *Campylobacter, Legionella, Mycoplasma, Chlamydia,* rickettsiae, spirochetes, some atypical mycobacteria, *Leptospira,* and amebae. Resistance to some bacteria has developed with increased usage. Erythromycin is rarely selected as a first-choice drug, except for treating *Campylobacter* or *Legionella* infections, but it is selected more often as an alternative.

Erythromycin has relatively low toxicity; the most frequent side effect is GI irritation manifested as nausea, vomiting, and diarrhea. Water or dilute antacid solution, given with the drug, may decrease irritation and facilitate absorption. Erythromycin estolate and occasionally erythromycin ethyl succinate have been associated with increased risk of cholestasis and hepatotoxicity, which may cause increased blood bilirubin concentration and hepatic enzyme activity. All parenteral preparations are irritating at injection sites.

Azithromycin and Clarithromycin

These azalides are derivatives of erythromycin with better enteral absorption and increased resistance to destruction by gastric acid. They reach high concentrations in phagocytic cells throughout the body and are slowly released over several days after a single dose. They are widely distributed to tissues in high concentrations except for the brain and eye.[172] They are less active than erythromycin against gram-positive bacteria but more active against gram-negative aerobes and anaerobes. Azithromycin and clarithromycin have strong activity against *Mycoplasma, Borrelia,* and *Leptospira.* Clarithromycin has been suggested as an alternative treatment against *Toxoplasma* and atypical *Mycobacterium.* For further information on these drugs, see Drug Formulary, Appendix 8.

Tylosin

Like other macrolides, tylosin is generally bacteriostatic against susceptible bacteria. Gram-positive bacteria, *Campylobacter,* and *Mycoplasma* are particularly susceptible to its effects, as are most organisms that are susceptible to erythromycin. Oral absorption of tylosin is variable, depending on the product formulation. The drug is metabolized by the liver and excreted in both urine and bile. Tylosin has been suggested also for the management of clostridial enteritis (see Chapter 39) and chronic colitis in dogs and cats and in the supportive treatment of systemic coronaviral diseases in cats. Proof of efficacy in the latter disorder, however, is lacking. The drug is effective in the treatment of staphylococcal

Table 34–8. Comparison of Erythromycin Formulations for Oral Use[a]

GENERIC NAME (TRADE NAME)	ABSORBED AS FREE BASE	ABSORPTION AFFECTED BY GASTRIC ACID/INGESTA	FORMULATION	ROUTE OF ADMINISTRATION COMMENTS
Erythromycin base (Erythromycin, Ilotycin, Robimycin, E-Mycin, Eryc)	+	+ / ±	PO tablets	Enteric coating reduces irritation.
Erythromycin stearate (Erythrocin, Ethril, Erypar, Wyamycin)	+	± / +	PO tablets	Absorption increased by drinking large amounts of water.
Erythromycin estolate (Ilosone)	−	− / −	PO drops	Tablets, suspension; associated with increased risks of cholestasis and hepatotoxicity.
Erythromycin ethylsuccinate (Pediamycin, Eryped, E.E.S.)	−	± / ±	PO drops	Capsules, tablets, suspension; milk enhances absorption.

[a]See text for properties and indications for each product. See Drug Formulary, Appendix 8 for appropriate dosages.
+ = yes; ± = variable; − = no; PO = oral.

pyoderma in dogs.[142, 143] (For additional information consult the Drug Formulary, Appendix 8.)

Lincomycin and Clindamycin

Lincosamides bind to 50S ribosomal subunits and inhibit protein synthesis in susceptible bacteria. Their mode of action resembles that of chloramphenicol and the macrolides. Depending on the concentrations achieved, lincomycin is bacteriostatic to bactericidal. Clindamycin, a chlorosubstituted lincomycin, has increased bactericidal activity and rate of absorption and has shown less toxicity in animals than lincomycin.

Lincomycin and clindamycin are widely distributed in body tissues and fluids, including bile, peritoneal and pleural fluid, milk, placenta, prostatic fluid, and bone. Neither drug enters the CSF or ocular structures unless inflammation is present. Both drugs accumulate in neutrophils, macrophages, and abscesses. These features make them useful in treating infections caused by anaerobic or persistent intracellular pathogens.

Both agents are primarily indicated to treat infections caused by gram-positive aerobes and by gram-positive and gram-negative anaerobes. Lincomycin has been recommended for use in a variety of respiratory, GI, soft tissue, and bone infections, especially when gram-positive organisms are involved. Clindamycin is known to be effective against a greater variety of organisms, including anaerobic bacteria and protozoa such as *Toxoplasma* (see Therapy, Chapter 41; Therapy, Chapter 80; and the Drug Formulary, Appendix 8).

Toxicity of these drugs has been relatively low in dogs that received supratherapeutic dosages for relatively long periods. GI irritation, vomiting, and diarrhea may occur with oral administration.

Pseudomembranous colitis, a complication in some humans treated with either drug, is manifested by abdominal pain, fever, and mucus or blood in the stools. Overgrowth of resistant, toxin-producing strains of *C. difficile* is believed responsible. Diarrhea in treated dogs and cats does not seem to be caused by *C. difficile* toxin.[51] If this side effect occurs, one should discontinue the drug and substitute vancomycin or metronidazole.

NOVOBIOCIN

This antibiotic has an antibacterial spectrum similar to, but not as consistent as, that of penicillin G. Many gram-positive aerobic bacteria, including *Streptococcus* and *Staphylococcus*, are susceptible to it. Variable effectiveness has been found against *Proteus* and *Pasteurella*. Novobiocin inhibits bacterial DNA and subsequent RNA and protein synthesis, and antibacterial resistance to this drug does not transfer to other antibiotics.

Novobiocin is absorbed well after oral administration and is predominantly excreted in the bile and feces. The antibiotic has been marketed in the United States mainly in fixed combination with tetracycline. In vitro studies have suggested possible inhibition reactions between these compounds. However, a subjective evaluation reported more clinical improvement in upper respiratory tract infections in dogs treated with novobiocin plus tetracycline than in dogs treated with either drug alone.

NITROFURANS

These synthetic antibacterial compounds are chemical derivatives of 5-nitrofuraldehyde. Their exact mechanism of action is uncertain, although they are known to interfere with many cellular enzymes. Nitrofurans are bacteriostatic or bactericidal, depending on the susceptibility of the organisms and the amount of drug at the site of infection. The nitrofurans as a group have a relatively broad spectrum of activity, although they are generally more effective against gram-negative organisms. *Escherichia, Salmonella, Staphylococcus*, and *Streptococcus* are usually susceptible, whereas *Pseudomonas* and some *Proteus* and *Klebsiella* are resistant. *Pseudomonas* can actually grow in many preparations of nitrofurazone, which may lead to nosocomial wound infection. Resistance rarely develops during therapy with nitrofurans. Table 34–9 summarizes the uses of nitrofurans in veterinary practice.

Nitrofurantoin is rapidly absorbed after oral ingestion, but the low concentrations achieved in blood are insufficient to treat systemic infections. Most of the drug is excreted rapidly in the urine, which makes it helpful in UTIs. However, treatment with nitrofurantoin is probably not warranted if other drugs have failed. Nitrofurantoin in urine may cause a spuriously positive test result for glucose when glucose oxidase test strips are used. Alkalinization of the urine, which increases the amount of nitrofurantoin excreted, should be avoided because the drug is more effective at acid pH. A macrocrystalline form of nitrofurantoin was developed to decrease the rate of absorption, thereby minimizing the irritating effect on the GI mucosa and prolonging its effect. Nifuratel is an analog with a similar pattern of absorption; however, it is unaffected by urine pH and has a wider spectrum of activity, including efficacy against *Candida*.

Furazolidone is not absorbed by the GI mucosa after oral administration and has been administered to treat local infections caused by enteric pathogens. Nitrofurazone is a nonabsorbable, topically applied antimicrobial powder, cream, or spray solution. Evidence exists that the spray preparation may be carcinogenic. Nitrofurazone is frequently incorpo-

Table 34–9. Comparison of Properties of Nitrofurans[a]

GENERIC NAME (TRADE NAME)	ROUTE OF ADMINISTRATION (FORMULATION)	USES/COMMENTS
Nitrofurantoin (Furadantin, Macrodantin)	PO (tablet, suspension) IM (solution)	UTI; avoid in renal failure; macrocrystalline is absorbed slower and is less toxic.
Nifuratel (Magmilor)	PO (tablet)	UTI; also effective against *Candida* at any urine pH.
Furazolidone (Furoxone)	PO (tablet, suspension)	For enteric pathogens, not absorbed PO; used for *Salmonella* and coccidia.
Nitrofurazone (Furacin)	Topical (ointment, powder, solution, cream, suppository)	For skin and mucosal infections; *Pseudomonas* can contaminate.
Nifuroxime (Micofur)	Topical (suppository, cream)	Antifungal properties; used together with other nitrofurans.

[a]See Appendix 8 for appropriate dosages of systemically administered drugs.
UTI = urinary tract infection.

Table 34–10. Properties of Sulfonamides Commonly Used in Small Animal Practice[a]

GENERIC NAME (TRADE NAME)	ROUTE OF ADMINISTRATION	INDICATIONS AND COMMENTS
Short Acting[b]		
Sulfadiazine (Suladyne, Debenal)	PO, IM	Systemic and UTIs and nocardiosis; frequently combined as triple sulfa to minimize renal tubular precipitation; sulfadiazine and sulfamethoxazole may be combined with trimethoprim (see below).
Sulfamethazine (Sulmet, Sulfamezathine)	PO, IM	As above.
Sulfamethoxazole (Gantanol, Methoxal)	PO, IM	As above.
Intermediate Acting[c]		
Sulfisoxazole (Gantrisin, Soxisol, Sulfasox)	PO	UTI
Sulfadimethoxine (Sudine, Bactrovet, Albon, Madribon)	PO	UTI
GI Preparations[d]		
Succinylsulfathiazole (Sulfasuxidine)	PO	Local antibacterial effects on GI tract; administer with kaolin-pectin.
Phthalylsulfathiazole (Sulfathalidine)	PO	*Shigella* enteritis, preoperative prophylaxis for GI surgery; mineral oil, laxatives, and purgatives interfere with action.
Special/Combination		
Sulfasalazine (Azulfidine)	PO	Colitis; salicylate component may help in therapy.
Mafenide (Sulfamylon cream)	Topical	Burns; prophylaxis only.
Trimethoprim and sulfamethoxazole (Septra, Bactrim)	PO	Systemic, respiratory, UTI, *Pneumocystis* pneumonia, *Brucella;* must be given to dogs at least twice daily for systemic infections; effective once daily for UTI, coccidiosis.
Trimethoprim and sulfadiazine (Tribrissen, Di-Trim)	PO, IM	As for trimethoprim-sulfamethoxazole.
Ormetoprim and sulfadimethoxine (Primor)	PO	Skin and UTI, wounds, coccidiosis.
Baquiloprim and sulfadimethoxine (Zaquilan)	PO, IM	Skin, respiratory, urogenital, GI, and soft tissue infections.

[a]Most of these drugs are licensed for human use. See the Drug Formulary (Appendix 8) for specific information and dosages.
[b]Rapidly absorbed and rapidly excreted.
[c]Rapidly absorbed and slowly excreted.
[d]Poorly absorbed.
UTI = urinary tract infection.

rated in an oil base rather than a water-soluble cream; however, this practice reduces its antibacterial efficacy and can delay healing by causing maceration of the wound.

Adverse reactions to nitrofurans are not uncommon. Nitrofurantoin frequently causes nausea and emesis in dogs and cats. Acute polyneuropathy/myopathy developed in a dog as a complication of nitrofurantoin. For more information on nitrofurantoin and furazolidones consult the Drug Formulary (Appendix 8).

SULFONAMIDES

Sulfonamides were the first drugs developed early in the antibacterial chemotherapy era and have been superseded by a variety of newer antimicrobial agents. However, there has been a resurgence in sulfonamide therapy since the introduction of several diaminopyrimidine compounds that enhance the antimicrobial efficacy. Sulfonamides are derivatives of sulfanilamide and act by interfering with bacterial synthesis of folic acid from para-aminobenzoic acid (PABA). They are bacteriostatic compounds that are ineffective in the presence of pus, necrotic tissue, or blood containing PABA. Organisms that are highly susceptible to sulfonamides include *Streptococcus, Bacillus, Corynebacterium, Nocardia, Campylobacter, Pasteurella,* and *Chlamydia. Pseudomonas, Serratia,* and *Klebsiella* are generally resistant. Caution must be exercised in interpreting disk susceptibility test results with these drugs because they frequently do not correlate with in vivo susceptibility. An increasing number of organisms are becoming resistant to sulfonamides. Resistance appears to develop more commonly with long-term therapy.

Except for a few compounds, most sulfonamides are readily and rapidly absorbed and reach bacteriostatic concentrations in blood. Blood concentrations attained depend on the route of administration and the dosage. They are variably bound to plasma protein and undergo wide distribution to all tissues and pleural, peritoneal, synovial, and ocular fluids. They cross the placenta and readily enter CSF. Sulfonamides are generally metabolized in the liver and excreted in small amounts in the bile. Most of the metabolized drug is excreted in urine.

The orally absorbed sulfonamides can be divided into three groups on the basis of their duration of action (Table 34–10). The short-acting drugs, rapidly absorbed and excreted, require doses at 8-hour intervals. These are given for systemic infections and UTIs. The intermediate-acting sulfonamides are excreted more slowly, administered every 12 to 24 hours, and mainly used for treating UTIs. Sulfisoxazole is the most often provided member of the group. Long-acting sulfonamides, such as sulfadoxine, are excreted slowly and require administration every few days. These have been given in some countries to treat infections in cattle and swine in combination with trimethoprim.

Some sulfonamides, poorly absorbed from the GI tract, will alter enteric microflora but will not disrupt the balance of microflora and rarely cause superinfection. Phthalylsulfathiazole has been administered to reduce coliform flora, stool bulk, and gas before colonic surgery.

Although marketed for topical application, sulfonamides are relatively ineffective in the presence of exudates. Mafenide, the only exception, is helpful for prophylaxis in burn patients because of its ability to inhibit *Pseudomonas.*

Certain sulfonamides have been administered for specific indications. Sulfapyridine, which is relatively toxic, is given only for treating dermatitis herpetiformis. Sulfasalazine (salicyl azosulfapyridine) is used to treat colitis in dogs.

Toxic reactions to sulfonamides are relatively uncommon in dogs and cats. Acute hemolytic complications and precipitation of sulfonamide metabolites in renal tubules seen in humans have not been seen in dogs. Failure of insoluble acetylated metabolites to cause renal problems in dogs may be explained by the fact that deacetylation of metabolites occurs more rapidly than their formation. Dogs given high dosages of sulfonamides can develop cystic sulfonamide uroliths. Sulfonamide crystalluria and neurologic signs, including convulsions, occurred in a dog ingesting sulfonamide cream.[45] However, cats may develop azotemia and renal failure during sulfonamide or trimethoprim-sulfonamide therapy. Keratitis sicca can develop in dogs on acute or long-term treatment.[32] Dogs should perhaps have Schirmer's tear tests performed before administering these drugs. Sulfonamides should be avoided in dogs with low values. The prognosis for return of lacrimation is poor, but topical cyclosporine appears to be effective in some cases.[32] For additional information, refer to the following discussion of trimethoprim-sulfonamides and to the Drug Formulary (ormetoprim or baquiloprim combined with sulfonamide) in Appendix 8.

TRIMETHOPRIM-SULFONAMIDES

Sulfonamides inhibit bacterial synthesis of dihydrofolic acid. Trimethoprim and related compounds (ormetroprim, baquiloprim) interfere with dihydrofolate reductase, preventing the conversion of dihydrofolic acid (folic acid) to tetrahydrofolic acid (folinic acid), which is essential for synthesis of purines and pyrimidines and thus of DNA. Mammals, unlike microorganisms, acquire most folic acid preformed in the diet, which explains the selective action of sulfonamides against microbes. Trimethoprim has less affinity for dihydrofolate reductase in mammals than in microorganisms, which accounts for the reduced toxicity of the drug for mammalian cells. Each drug alone is generally bacteriostatic; however, when trimethoprim and sulfonamide are coadministered in a 1:5 ratio, a synergistic interaction is expected, with bactericidal activity whenever the optimum in vivo ratio of 1:2 is achieved.

Trimethoprim is rapidly and completely absorbed and widely distributed after oral administration. Therapeutic concentrations are achieved in CSF, brain, eye, prostate, bone, and joints. It is not necessary to reduce the dosage in renal failure unless it is severe. Sulfadiazine has been chosen for administration with trimethoprim in dogs. Sulfamethoxazole is used in human preparations. Trimethoprim is available by itself in some countries, but offers little advantage because it is less active and just as toxic as the combined product.

Trimethoprim-sulfonamide has been recommended for treatment of respiratory infections and UTIs caused by *Escherichia*, *Streptococcus*, *Proteus*, *Salmonella*, and *Pasteurella*. Lesser and more variable activity is noted against *Staphylococcus*, *Klebsiella*, *Corynebacterium*, *Clostridium*, and *Bordetella*. *Moraxella*, *Nocardia*, and *Brucella* are moderately susceptible. Trimethoprim-sulfonamide has been administered simultaneously with AGs to enhance activity against gram-negative organisms. Bacterial resistance has developed with continued usage. Because of good CNS penetrability, it is an excellent choice for gram-negative pathogens producing meningitis.

All the side effects noted previously with sulfonamides can be seen with the drug combination (see trimethoprim-sulfonamide, adverse reactions, in the Drug Formulary, Appendix 8). Trimethoprim-sulfonamide causes greater adverse reactions and has a smaller margin of safety in cats than in dogs. Cats are more likely to develop anorexia, vomiting, azotemia, anemia, and leukopenia.

Other toxicities have been reported in dogs and cats. Ataxia has sometimes been observed when higher therapeutic dosages are given. Reversible cholestatic hepatitis has been observed in dogs with pre-existing hepatic disease.[50] Fatal hepatic necrosis resulting in hepatic failure has been reported as an idiosyncratic reaction in dogs.[162, 168] Dose and duration of therapy were not related. Aplastic anemia was associated with trimethoprim-sulfadiazine and fenbendazole administration in a dog.[179] Anemia resolved after withdrawal of the drugs and may have reflected drug idiosyncrasy or immune hypersensitivity rather than inhibited folate metabolism.

Treatment with the trimethoprim-sulfadiazine combination has been associated with allergic immune complex reactions in dogs specifically as a result of the sulfonamide. Polyarthritis, lymphadenomegaly, fever, polymyositis, glomerulonephritis, urticaria, focal retinitis, anemia, leukopenia, and thrombocytopenia have been noted. Doberman pinschers may be predisposed to these reactions. Immune-mediated, cutaneous drug eruptions have occurred in dogs treated with trimethoprim-sulfamethoxazole (see Drug Formulary, Appendix 8). Similarly, a presumed immune-mediated meningitis has been described in people given trimethoprim-sulfamethoxazole.

QUINOLONES

Pharmacokinetics

The quinolones (fluoroquinolones) are a diverse group of bactericidal naphthyridine derivatives that prevent bacterial DNA synthesis by partly inhibiting bacterial DNA gyrase. Compared with the rarely used first-generation compounds nalidixic acid and cinoxacin, the newer second-generation quinolones (Table 34–11), such as ciprofloxacin, marbofloxacin, and enrofloxacin, have improved antibacterial spectrum, increased bioavailability, favorable pharmacokinetics, and less toxicity and bacterial resistance. Third-generation quinolones, including levofloxacin, clinafloxacin, sparfloxacin, grepafloxacin, trovafloxacin, and DU-6859a, have enhanced pharmacokinetics and increased activity against important pathogens.

Variable GI absorption occurs with quinolones. Food and antacids inhibit their absorption. Absorption is also impaired by concurrent administration of preparations containing multivalent cations (magnesium, bismuth, iron, zinc, aluminum), such as antacids, and by sucralfate-containing preparations. Sparfloxacin is more slowly absorbed and excreted and can be given less frequently. To improve serum concentrations in dogs and cats in these circumstances, giving quinolones at least 2 hours before these preparations or parenteral administration may be preferable. With higher blood concentrations, quinolones penetrate into body fluids, secretions, and other harder-to-enter tissues, including CSF, prostate, and bone. The distribution volumes of third-generation quinolones may exceed those of the second-generation drugs. They are partially metabolized by the liver and excreted in bile or urine as parent drug and/or metabolites, most of which have antibacterial activity. Concentrations achieved in bile and urine are 10 to 20 times higher than those in blood. Urine recovery varies from 30% to 70%, depending on the drug.

Indications

The quinolones are primarily active against gram-negative aerobic and facultative anaerobic bacteria and are more effective in alkaline pH (> 7.4). Although many gram-positive bacterial pathogens are susceptible, MIC ranges usually are higher than those for gram-negative organisms. Second-gen-

Table 34–11. Quinolones Licensed for Human and Veterinary Use[a]

DRUG	GENERIC	TRADE NAME	ORAL BIOAVAILABILITY (%)	FORMULATIONS
First Generation[b]				
	Nalidixic acid	NegGram (Sandofi)	95	Tablets: 250 mg, 1 g Suspension: 250 mg/5 ml
	Cinoxacin	Cinobac (Oclassen)	95	Tablets: 250 mg, 500 mg
Second Generation[c]				
Human	Norfloxacin	Noroxin (Merck)	30–50	Tablets: 400 mg
	Ciprofloxacin	Cipro (Bayer)	75–80	Tablets: 250 mg, 500 mg, 750 mg Injection: 200-mg and 400-mg vials
	Ofloxacin	Floxin (Ortho)	>95	Tablets: 200 mg, 300 mg, 400 mg Injection: 200-mg and 400-mg vials
	Lomafloxacin	Maxaguin (Searle)	>95	Tablets: 400 mg
	Enoxacin	Penetrex (Rhone-Poulenc)	90	Tablets: 200 mg, 400 mg
	Fleroxacin	Megalone, Quinodis (Roche)	>80	Tablets: 200 mg, 400 mg
	Amifloxacin	Investigational (Sterling Winthrop)	>90	Tablets: 200 mg
Veterinary[a]	Enrofloxacin[d]	Baytril (Bayer)	>80	Tablets: 5.7 mg, 22.7 mg, 68 mg Injection: 22.7 mg/ml
	Marbofloxacin	Marbocyl (Vetoquinol)	>90	Tablets: 5 mg, 20 mg, 80 mg
	Orbifloxacin	Orbax (Schering-Plough AH)	97	Tablets: 5.7 mg, 22.7 mg, 68 mg
	Difloxacin	Dicural (Fort Dodge)	>80	Tablets: 11.4 mg, 45.4 mg, 136 mg
Third Generation[e]				
	Levofloxacin	Levaquin (Ortho-McNeil)	~100	Tablets: 250 mg, 500 mg Injection: 250-mg and 500-mg vials
	Sparfloxacin	Zogam (Rhone-Poulenc)	~100	Tablets: 200 mg
	Pefloxacin[f]	Peflacine, Peflox (Rhone-Poulenc)	~100	Tablets and injection; investigational

[a]Only second-generation drugs are licensed for veterinary purposes. The three listed veterinary preparations are licensed for dogs and cats. In some countries, sarafloxacin, benofloxacin, enrofloxacin, and ofloxacin are licensed for poultry; onrofloxacin, danofloxacin, and orbifloxacin are licensed for cattle and swine. See the Drug Formulary (Appendix 8) for more specific information and dosages.
[b]Restricted for use in gram-negative urinary infections; not recommended owing to high toxicity.
[c]Primarily active against gram-negative aerobic bacteria, *Mycoplasma, Chlamydia,* some *Mycobacterium,* Rickettsiae.
[d]Metabolized to ciprofloxacin. Bioavailability is extrapolated from absorption of ciprofloxacin.
[e]Same as second generation with more activity against staphylococci, streptococci, and obligate anaerobes. Also includes grepafloxacin, clinafloxacin, trovafloxacin, and DU-6859a.
[f]Metabolized to norfloxacin.

eration quinolones are not suitable for treating infections caused by obligate anaerobes or *Streptococcus.* Activity against *Staphylococcus* is variable, but some staphylococci resistant to many other drugs may be susceptible to quinolones. Third-generation quinolones are broad-spectrum antimicrobials with excellent in vitro activity against gram-positive and gram-negative bacteria, including obligate anaerobes and intracellular pathogens. They have more consistent activity against *Streptococcus* and *Staphylococcus.*[124] Some rickettsiae are susceptible to quinolones. Some of the drugs have activity against *Chlamydia, Mycoplasma, Bartonella,* and some mycobacteria.[156] Ciprofloxacin, enrofloxacin, and ofloxacin are active against *M. tuberculosis* and some atypical mycobacteria but not against *M. avium* complex. Quinolones have good activity against bacterial enteropathogens, such as *Salmonella, Shigella, Campylobacter, Yersinia enterocolitica,* and *Escherichia.* Third-generation drugs have good activity against anaerobes such as *Bacteroides, Clostridium, Fusobacterium, Porphyromonas, Bilophila,* and *Prevotella.* They kill bacteria at concentrations close to inhibitory concentrations and have marked postantibiotic inhibitory effect in vivo. The postantibiotic effect refers to their ability to inhibit bacterial growth for 4 to 8 hours after drug elimination from the body. High concentrations, which exceed those in blood are achieved in prostate, kidney, liver, and lung, with lower but therapeutic concentrations in respiratory secretions, saliva, and prostatic fluid. Urine concentrations are well above the MICs of most urinary pathogens, and CSF concentrations are adequate if inflammation is present. Fecal levels are adequate to inhibit most GI enteropathogens. Recurrent UTIs caused by organisms that are difficult to eliminate, such as *Pseudomonas, Proteus,* and *Klebsiella,* are the primary indications for quinolones. They are very effective in the treatment of bacterial prostatitis. They have also been used to treat enteric and respiratory infections caused by organisms resistant to other agents. Bone concentrations of quinolones are adequate to treat osteomyelitis provided the organism is susceptible. Oral administration is advantageous for long-term therapy. When mixed flora are present in intra-abdominal infections, quinolones have been effective against aerobic or facultative bacteria when given in combination with a drug effective against anaerobes, such as clindamycin or metronidazole.

A common misconception is that bacteria do not become resistant during treatment with quinolones. Being chromosomal rather than plasmid mediated, resistance most commonly occurs during treatment of infections caused by *Pseudomonas, Klebsiella, Acinetobacter, Serratia, Enterococcus,* and *Staphylococcus.* Bacteria may become cross-resistant to several quinolones at one time but not necessarily to antimicrobials in other classes. The quinolones have been restricted from use in food-producing animals in the United States to help prevent the development of drug-resistant strains of zoonotic pathogens.[1a]

Toxicity

Quinolones are relatively safe at routine oral and parenteral dosages. Prokaryotic DNA gyrase is partially affected by these compounds. Extremely high concentrations of fluoroquinolones, therefore, can cause systemic toxicity. Rapid IV administration of 10 to 30 mg/kg of certain quinolones to anesthetized dogs or cats produces systemic hypotension, presumably related to histamine release. Hypotension and tachycardia have also been seen after oral administration. Abnormal EEG activity has been observed in dogs and cats after IV administration of 25 mg/kg or greater.[26] Seizures have been precipitated by administration of parenteral doses of quinolones with concurrent administration of nonsteroidal anti-inflammatory drugs such as fenbufen and ibuprofen.

Toxic effects were noted in the eyes, kidneys, and joints of juvenile animals given oral dosages. Dogs given high dosages had subcapsular lenticular cataract formation and associated inflammation after treatment for 8 to 12 months.

Quinolones have limited solubility at alkaline pH and may crystallize. Therapeutic dosages may cause increased serum hepatic enzyme activities. At high dosages in dogs, renal toxicity developed from crystalluria and crystal deposition in tubular lumens, especially at alkaline urine pH. Nephrotoxicity has also occurred uncommonly in people and dogs treated with usual therapeutic dosages. Quinolones inhibit mitochondrial dehydrogenase activity and proteoglycan synthesis, resulting in cartilaginous damage.[61] Quinolones also chelate magnesium resulting in altered chondrocyte surface integrin receptors and cartilage matrix integrity.[22a] These findings are accentuated by magnesium deficiency. Cartilaginous defects in growing cartilage of young dogs[21, 22] were accentuated by exercise and prevented by exercise restriction. Nevertheless, quinolones are contraindicated in dogs during the rapid-growth phase, between 2 to 8 months in small and medium breeds, to 1 year in large breeds, and to 18 months in giant breeds. Cats given high doses of ciprofloxacin developed pinnae erythema, vomiting, and clonic muscle spasms. Dogs consistently vomited when given high doses and, therefore, did not show other manifestations of toxicity. Because of effects on DNA synthesis and known fetal toxicity in other species, these drugs should not be given to young (< 6 months of age) or pregnant dogs or cats. High doses have been fetotoxic to animals. Because these drugs are excreted in milk, their use in lactating animals should be avoided. High doses (100 mg/kg) for longer than 3 months have been associated with impaired spermatogenesis and testicular atrophy in dogs. Phototoxicity has developed in some people.

URINARY ANTISEPTICS

Methenamine (hexamethylenetetramine), a highly water-soluble organic compound, decomposes at an acid pH to form formaldehyde. It is dispensed in an enteric-coated tablet to prevent degradation by gastric acid and is given only for long-term treatment and prophylaxis of UTIs. Methenamine is rapidly absorbed after oral administration and excreted primarily in urine. Formulations containing organic acids (mandelic, hippuric, sulfosalicylic salts) have been prepared to facilitate formaldehyde production by lowering urine pH when these substances are simultaneously excreted. Antibacterial activity is largely confined to the bladder, because transit in the upper tract is brief and time is required to generate formaldehyde.

ANTITUBERCULOUS DRUGS

Isoniazid

This hydrazide derivative of isonicotinic acid is one of the most active compounds against *Mycobacterium tuberculosis*. It interferes with synthesis of mycolic acids in mycobacterial cell walls and acts only against replicating bacteria, leaving slow-growing or inactive organisms unaffected. Absorption of isoniazid from the intestine is rapid but inhibited by antacids, and much of the dose is excreted unchanged in the urine within 24 hours. Isoniazid penetrates most tissues well. CSF concentration is 20% of that of blood but increases to 100% in the presence of CNS inflammation. Most strains of *M. tuberculosis* are sensitive to isoniazid, but resistance usually develops during therapy. Drug susceptibility testing, therefore, is recommended.

The principal side effects of isoniazid, hepatotoxicity and hepatic enzyme elevation, are reversed if therapy is discontinued immediately. Peripheral neuropathy and CNS excitability may be caused by monoamine oxidase antagonism. Seizures, tremors, and hyperexcitability were noted in dogs that were overdosed. Immune-mediated thrombocytopenia was also noted in a dog treated with isoniazid. GI irritation, allergic skin reaction, and vasculitis have also been reported in people.

Rifampin

This semisynthetic hydrazone derivative of rifampin B interferes with RNA synthesis. It is well absorbed from the GI tract. Rifampin is lipid soluble and is bound 75% to 90% to serum protein. It penetrates all body tissues and reaches higher than blood concentrations in lung, liver, bile, cholecystic wall, and urine. Therapeutic concentrations of rifampin are attained in pleural exudate, ascites, milk, urinary bladder wall, soft tissue, and CSF. Much of the drug is metabolized by the liver and excreted in the bile. Only 6% to 30% appears in the urine.

Rifampin has antibacterial, antichlamydial, and some antiviral activity. It is primarily given to treat infections caused by *M. tuberculosis*. It is also one of the most active antibiotics against *Staphylococcus* and is effective against some gram-negative pathogens. This antibiotic is frequently helpful in combination with β-lactam drugs in the treatment of resistant staphylococcal endocarditis or osteomyelitis. The drug has been combined with vancomycin and with cephalosporin to achieve increased efficacy against *Staphylococcus*. Rifampin was superior to tetracycline for treatment of experimental *Brucella* infection in laboratory animals. It was not as successful as minocycline for treating naturally occurring canine brucellosis. Rifampin has similar effectiveness in treatment of feline bartonellosis (see Chapter 54). Although ineffective against fungi when administered alone, rifampin has been shown to enhance the effect of amphotericin B and miconazole against *Candida*.

Resistance to rifampin may develop rapidly when it is used alone, but can be hindered by combining it with other drugs. Side effects of rifampin include orange-colored urine, tears, saliva, and sweat. Rash, GI signalment, and increased liver enzymes may be associated with long-term daily administration. Many other side effects have been noted at higher doses, and it should always be reformulated to the calculated dose when given to dogs and cats. Rifampin accelerates the hepatic metabolism of other drugs and reduces the activity of concurrently administered glucocorticoids, digoxin, quinidine, barbiturates, isoniazid, dapsone, and theophylline.

Rifabutin

This drug is structurally similar to rifampin but is more lipid soluble. It has better tissue distribution but lower oral bioavailability. Rifabutin is extensively metabolized to active intermediates. It can be used as a substitute for rifampin and has less effect on hepatic metabolism of other drugs.

Ethambutol

This tuberculostatic drug interferes with RNA synthesis and is active only against dividing organisms. It is well absorbed from the GI tract and is widely distributed in body tissues, including CSF. Most of the drug is excreted unmetabolized in urine, and the dose should be reduced in patients with renal failure. Its primary toxic effect is optic and peripheral neuritis.

Miscellaneous Drugs

Para-aminosalicylic acid is an analog of PABA that is mycobacteriostatic, interfering with folic acid synthesis. It potentiates the effect of isoniazid by delaying its metabolism. Pyrazinamide, a tuberculostatic drug with an unknown mode of action, is relatively hepatotoxic. Cycloserine inhibits bacterial cell wall synthesis and is excreted primarily by the kidneys. Ethionamide inhibits protein synthesis and has widespread tissue distribution. PABA is combined in therapy when resistance is found to other drugs. Viomycin, capreomycin, kanamycin, and amikacin have all been shown to be effective against mycobacteria when combined with other drugs. See Chapter 50 for a discussion of tuberculosis in dogs and cats.

AGENTS AGAINST RAPIDLY GROWING OPPORTUNISTIC MYCOBACTERIA

Certain antituberculous drugs, such as isoniazid, rifampin, and AGs, are effective in treating other mycobacteria. Other antimicrobials, including erythromycin, clarithromycin, doxycycline, minocycline, enrofloxacin, clofazimine, and trimethoprim-sulfonamide, have also been successful in some cases, as have drugs to treat human leprosy (see Therapy sections, Chapter 50).

Dapsone is a sulfone derivative that is bacteriostatic to bactericidal against *M. leprae*. It is completely absorbed from the bowel, metabolized in the liver, and primarily eliminated by renal excretion. Toxic effects in dogs have consisted of hemolytic anemia, leukopenia, thrombocytopenia, and increased liver enzyme activities. Acedapsone is another derivative with a longer duration of action. Clofazimine is a dye with antiprotozoal and antifungal activity. It is active against *M. leprae*, *M. avium*-complex organisms, and opportunistic mycobacteria. This drug should always be given in combination with other drugs. For additional information on dapsone and clofazimine see Chapter 50 and Appendix 8.

TOPICAL ANTIBACTERIALS

Bacitracin

This mixture of cyclic peptides has bactericidal activity against many gram-positive pathogens, including *Staphylococcus*, *Streptococcus*, *Corynebacterium*, *Clostridium*, and *Actinomyces*. It is not absorbed to any extent after topical or oral administration and is nephrotoxic when given parenterally. Accordingly, its use is limited to surface application for treating infections of skin, ear, and eye. It is often given in conjunction with an AG (usually neomycin) and polymyxin. Toxicity of bacitracin is primarily through a hypersensitivity associated with topical application.

Mupirocin

This novel antibiotic, unrelated in structure and action to other known antimicrobials, inhibits bacterial protein synthesis. It is bactericidal against *Staphylococcus*, *Streptococcus*, and some gram-negative aerobic pathogens. The drug is available commercially as a topical ointment. The only side effect observed has been a local dermal hypersensitivity reaction at the site of application in some animals.

Table 34–12. Improved Formula for Buffered EDTA Solution

1. Dissolve 1.2 g of ethylenediaminetetraacetate (EDTA) in 1 L of 0.05 M (6.05 g) tromethamine (hydroxymethyl)aminomethane (TRIS) and 1.9 g/L sodium dodecyl sulfate[a]
2. Adjust pH to 8.0 (usually requires concentrated NaOH)
3. Sterilize in autoclave (121°F for 20 min) or filter with 0.22-μm filter
4. Store in sterile bottles at room temperature. Stable for 1 year.
5. Can add gentamicin (3 mg/ml) or amikacin (9 mg/ml)

[a]Sodium dodecyl sulfate is added to improve efficacy.

Fusidic Acid

The principal interest in fusidic acid lies in its excellent activity against *Staphylococcus*, including β-lactamase–producing and methicillin-resistant strains. It is available in some countries in enteral, parenteral, and topical preparations.

Topical Buffered EDTA Solution

Many gram-negative bacteria are susceptible to chelating agents such as EDTA. The bactericidal effect appears to occur by removal of cations from the bacterial cell wall, which results in leakage of cell solutes. Alkaline pH appears to facilitate bactericidal activity. Research has proved EDTA to be safe when applied topically to animal tissues. Appropriate pH is maintained by combining it with stable amino buffers, such as tromethamine (TRIS) hydrochloride at a pH of 8. Administration of this combination (Wooley's solution) is restricted to topical application or irrigation because of toxicity that results from removal of blood cations such as calcium and production of nephrocalcinosis. The buffered EDTA solution can be made with easily obtainable ingredients (Table 34–12). Incorporation of sodium dodecyl sulfate, an ionic detergent, improves efficacy.

Buffered EDTA solutions have been administered alone and in combination with several antimicrobial agents to treat various resistant bacterial infections in dogs and cats. A prime use has been against *Pseudomonas* organisms, which are resistant to many antibacterial drugs; use with lysozyme, gentamicin, or oxytetracycline has been attempted to increase the potency of these drugs and to decrease the incidence of antimicrobial resistance.[43, 43a, 148] Buffered EDTA solutions may help by increasing gram-negative bacterial cell wall permeability, facilitating drug penetration and antimicrobial activity. Overgrowth of fungi may occur during such treatment unless an antifungal drug is administered simultaneously. Such overgrowth may be more likely when treating infections in body regions that lack a normal competitive microflora, as in the urinary bladder. Repeated catheterization and flushing with these solutions may also favor introduction and persistence of resistant bacterial strains.

ANTIBACTERIAL DRUG SAFETY

A listing of the safety factors of various antimicrobial drugs in various medical conditions is provided in Table 34–13.

Table 34–13. Comparison of Safety of Antimicrobial Drugs in Various Clinical Conditions

	RENAL DYSFUNCTION	HEPATIC DYSFUNCTION	PREGNANCY	NEONATE
Probably safe	Chloramphenicol, doxycycline, griseofulvin, macrolides, penicillins (including clavulanate)	Aminoglycosides, cephalosporins, penicillins	Cephalosporin, erythromycin, lincomycin, penicillins (including clavulanate)	Cephalosporin, macrolides, penicillins (including clavulanate)
Consider dosage adjustment	Fluoroquinolones, lincomycin, trimethoprim-sulfonamide (dog)	Clindamycin, metronidazole	Nitrofurantoin, sulfonamides, trimethoprim-sulfonamide, tylosin	Lincomycin
Use caution, can accumulate	Chloramphenicol (cat), flucytosine, nitrofurantoin, tetracyclines (not doxycycline)	Chloramphenicol, lincomycin, macrolides, metronidazole, sulfonamides, tetracyclines	Aminoglycosides, amphotericin B, chloramphenicol, fluconazole, flucytosine, ketoconazole, metronidazole	Aminoglycosides, polymyxins
Potentially toxic, avoid use	Aminoglycosides[a], amphotericin B, polymyxins, trimethoprim-sulfonamide (cat)	Chlortetracycline, erythromycin isolate, griseofulvin, ketoconazole, trimethoprim-sulfonamide (dog)	Fluoroquinolones, griseofulvin, nalidixic acid, tetracycline	Fluoroquinolones, nitrofurans, chloramphenicol, sulfonamides, tetracycline, trimethoprim-sulfonamide

[a]If any aminoglycosides must be used in renal failure, maintain the dose but lengthen the interval by multiplying the usual interval in hours by patient creatinine divided by the higher reference value for creatinine.

References

1. Acar JF, Goldstein FW. 1997. Trends in bacterial resistance to floroquinolones. *Clin Infect Dis* 24(Suppl):S67–S73.
1a. Anonymous. 1997. Extralabel use of fluoroquinolones prohibited. *J Am Vet Med Assoc* 211:1106.
2. Anwar H, Costerton W. 1992. Effective use of antibiotics in the treatment of biofilm-associated infection. *ASM News* 58:665–668.
3. Aucoin DP. 1990. Fluoroquinolone antibiotics: use in companion animal medicine, pp 13–23. *In* Proceedings of the Symposium on Quinolones, Eastern States Veterinary Conference, Orlando, FL 13–23.
4. Aucoin DP, Hardie L, Bissonette K, et al. 1991. Disposition and efficacy study of enrofloxacin in 18 canine patients with multiresistant bacterial infections (abstract 99). *J Am Coll Vet Intern Med* 5:138.
5. Barbhaiya RH, Wang L, Shuy WC, et al. 1992. Absolute bioavailability of cefprozil after oral administration in Beagles. *Antimicrob Agents Chemother* 36:687–689.
6. Bark H, Perk R. 1995. Fanconi syndrome associated with amoxicillin therapy in a dog. *Canine Pract* 20:19–22.
7. Berger SL, Scagliotti RH, Lund EM. 1995. A quantitative study of the effects of tribrissen on canine tear production. *J Am Anim Hosp Assoc* 31:236–241.
8. Bialer M, Wu WH, Look ZM, et al. 1987. Pharmacokinetics of cefixime after oral and intravenous doses in dogs: bioavailability assessment for a drug showing nonlinear serum protein binding. *Res Commun Chem Pathol Pharmacol* 56:21–32.
9. Boeckh M, Lode H, Deppermann KL, et al. 1990. Pharmacokinetics and serum bactericidal activities of quinolones in combination with clindamycin, metronidazole, and ornidazole. *Antimicrob Agents Chemother* 34:2407–2414.
10. Bone RC. 1991. A critical evaluation of new agents for the treatment of sepsis. *JAMA* 266:1686–1691.
11. Boothe DM. 1989. The practical aspects of treating bacterial infections in cats. *Vet Med* 84:884–904.
12. Boothe DM. 1996. Antimicrobial therapy in the critically ill patient. *Compend Cont Educ Pract Vet* 18(Suppl):66–83.
13. Boothe DM, Brown SA, Fate GD, et al. 1996. Plasma disposition of clindamycin microbiological activity in cats after single oral doses of clindamycin hydrochloride as either capsule or aqueous solution. *J Vet Pharmacol Ther* 19:491–494.
14. Brandt KD. 1995. Modification by oral doxycycline administration of articular cartilage breakdown in osteoarthritis. *J Rheumatol* 22(Suppl 43):149–151.
15. Brogan JC. 1992. Sorting out the cephalosporins. *Postgrad Med* 91:301–315.
16. Brown SA, Arnold TS, Hamlow PJ, et al. 1995. Plasma and urine disposition and dose proportionality of ceftiofur and metabolites in dogs after subcutaneous administration of ceftiofur sodium. *J Vet Pharmacol Ther* 18:363–369.
17. Brown SA, Dieringer TM, Hunter RP, et al. 1989. Oral clindamycin disposition after single and multiple doses in normal cats. *J Vet Pharmacol Ther* 12:209–216.
18. Budsberg SC, Gallo JM, Starliper CE, et al. 1991. Comparison of cortical bone and serum concentrations of clindamycin achievable by direct local infusion and intravenous administration. *J Orthop Res* 9:594–599.
19. Budsberg SC, Kemp DT. 1990. Antimicrobial distribution and therapeutics in bone. *Compend Cont Educ Pract Vet* 12:1758–1763.
20. Budsberg SC, Walker RD, Slusser P, et al. 1989. Norfloxacin therapy in infections of the canine urogenital tract caused by multiresistant bacteria. *J Am Vet Med Assoc* 25:713–716.
21. Burkhardt JE, Hill MA, Carlton WW, et al. 1990. Histologic and histochemical changes in articular cartilages of immature Beagle dogs dosed with difloxacin, a fluoroquinolone. *Vet Pathol* 27:162–170.
22. Burkhardt JE, Hill MA, Turek JJ, et al. 1992. Ultrastructural changes in articular cartilages of immature Beagle dogs dosed with difloxacin, a fluoroquinolone. *Vet Pathol* 29:230–238.
22a. Burkhardt JE, Walterspiel JN, Schaad UB. 1997. Quinolone arthropathy in animals versus children. *Clin Infect Dis* 25:1196–1204.
23. Carlotti DN. 1996. New trends in systemic antibiotic therapy of bacterial skin disease in dogs. *Compend Cont Educ Pract Vet* 18:40–47.
24. Carson JL, Strom BL, Duff A, et al. 1993. Acute liver disease associated with erythromycins, sulfonamides, and tetracyclines. *Ann Intern Med* 119:576–583.
25. Cassell GH. 1995. ASM task force urges broad program on antimicrobial resistance. *ASM News* 61:116–120.
25a. Cester CC, Schneider M, Toutain PL. 1996. Comparative kinetics of 2 orally administered fluoroquinolones in dog—enrofloxacin versus marbofloxacin. *Revue De Medecine Veterinaire* 147:703–716.
26. Christ W. 1990. Central nervous system toxicity of quinolones: human and animal findings. *J Antimicrob Chemother* 26:219–225.
27. Cotard JP, Gruet P, Pechereau D, et al. 1995. Comparative study of marbofloxacin and amoxicillin-clavulanic acid in the treatment of urinary tract infection in dogs. *J Small Anim Pract* 36:349–353.
28. Cribb AE. 1989. Idiosyncratic reactions to sulfonamides in dogs. *J Am Vet Med Assoc* 195:1612–1614.
29. Cribb AE, Spielberg SP. 1990. An in vitro investigation of predisposition to sulphonamide idiosyncratic toxicity in dogs. *Vet Res Commun* 14:241–252.
29a. Dalvie DK, Khosla NB, Navetta KA, et al. 1996. Metabolism and excretion of trovalfloxacin. *Drug Metabol Dispos* 24:1231–1240.
30. Deldar A, Lewis H, Bloom J, et al. 1988. Cephalosporin-induced changes in the ultrastructure of canine bone marrow. *Vet Pathol* 25:211-218.
31. Delmage DA, Payne-Johnson CE. 1991. Erythema multiforme in a Dobermann on trimethoprim-sulphamethoxazole therapy. *J Small Anim Pract* 32:635–639.
32. Diehl KJ, Roberts SM. 1991. Keratoconjunctivitis sicca in dogs associated with sulfonamide therapy: 16 cases (1980–1990). *Prog Comp Ophthalmol* 1:276–282.
33. DiNubile MJ. 1990. Antibiotics: the antipyretics of choice. *Am J Med* 89:787–788.
34. Dodds WJ. 1990. Side effects associated with trimethoprim-sulfa drugs. *Adv Small Anim Med Surg* 3:5–7.
35. Dodds WJ. 1990. Sulfonamides and blood dyscrasias. *J Am Vet Med Assoc* 196:681–682.
36. Dodds WJ. 1993. Hemorrhagic complications attributable to certain drugs (letter, comments). *J Am Vet Med Assoc* 202:702–703.
37. Dorfman M, Barsanti J, Budsberg SC. 1995. Enrofloxacin combinations in

dogs with normal prostate and dogs with chronic bacterial prostatitis. *Am J Vet Res* 56:386–390.
38. Dow SW, Papich MG. 1991. An update on antimicrobials: new uses, modifications and developments. *Vet Med* 86:707–715.
39. Dowling PM. 1996. Rational antimicrobial therapy. *Can Vet J* 37:246–249.
40. Duval JM, Budsberg SC. 1995. Cortical bone concentrations of enrofloxacin in dogs. *Am J Vet Res* 56:188–192.
41. El Bahri L, Blouin A. 1991. Fluoroquinolones: a new family of antimicrobials. *Compend Cont Educ Pract Vet* 13:1429–1434.
42. Eriksson A, Rauraama V, Happonen I, et al. 1990. Feeding reduces the absorption of erythromycin in the dog. *Acta Vet Scand* 31:497–499.
43. Farca AM, Nebbia P, Re G. 1993. Potentiation of the in vitro activity of some antimicrobial agents against selected gram-negative bacteria by EDTA-tromethamine. *Vet Res Commun* 17:77–84.
43a. Farca AM, Piromalli G, Maffei F, et al. 1997. Potentiating effect of EDTA-Tris on the activity of antibiotics against resistant bacteria associated with otitis, dermatitis, and cystitis. *J Small Anim Pract* 38:243–245.
44. Forsyth SF, Ilkiw JE, Hildebrand SV. 1990. Effect of gentamicin administration on the neuromuscular blockade induced by atracurium in cats. *Am J Vet Res* 51:1675–1678.
45. Frank A, Egenvall A. 1994. Sulphanilamide toxicity and crystalluria in a dog after suspected ingestion of a wound treatment ointment. *J Small Anim Pract* 35:531–534.
46. Gilbert DN. 1991. Once-daily aminoglycoside therapy. *Antimicrob Agents Chemother* 35:399–405.
47. Grauer GF, Greco DS, Behrend EN, et al. 1994. Effects of dietary protein conditioning on gentamicin-induced nephrotoxicosis in healthy male dogs. *Am J Vet Res* 55:90–97.
48. Grauer GF, Greco DS, Behrend EN, et al. 1995. Estimation of quantitative enzymuria in dogs with gentamicin-induced nephrotoxicosis using urine enzyme/creatinine ratios from spot urine samples. *J Vet Intern Med* 9:324–327.
49. Gray A. 1990. Trimethoprim-sulphonamide hypersensitivity in dogs (letter, comments). *Vet Res* 127:459–460.
50. Greene CE, Ferguson DC. 1990. Antibacterial chemotherapy, pp 461–493. *In* Greene CE (eds), Infectious diseases of the dog and cat. WB Saunders, Philadelphia, PA.
51. Greene CE, Lappin MR, Marks AM. 1992. Clindamycin in cats. *J Am Anim Hosp Assoc* 28:323–326.
52. Gruet P, Richard P, Thomas E, et al. 1997. Prevention of surgical infections in dogs with a single intravenous injection of marbofloxacin: an experimental model. *Vet Rec* 140:199–202.
53. Gunn-Moore DA, Jenkins JA, Lucke VM. 1996. Feline tuberculosis: a literature review and discussion of 19 cases caused by an unusual mycobacterial variant. *Vet Rec* 138:53–58.
54. Hall IA, Campbell KL, Chambers MD, et al. 1993. Effect of trimethoprim/sulfamethoxazole on thyroid function in dogs with pyoderma. *J Am Vet Med Assoc* 202:1959–1962.
55. Harari J, Besser TE, Gustafson SB, et al. 1993. Bacterial isolates from blood cultures of dogs undergoing surgery (comments). *Vet Surg* 22:327–329.
56. Harari J, Besser TE, Gustafson SB, et al. 1993. Bacterial isolates from blood cultures of dogs undergoing dentistry. *Vet Surg* 22:27–39.
57. Harari J, Lincoln J. 1989. Pharmacologic features of clindamycin in dogs and cats. *J Am Vet Med Assoc* 195:124–125.
58. Hariharan H, McPhee L, Heaney S, et al. 1995. Antimicrobial drug susceptibility of clinical isolates of *Pseudomonas aeruginosa*. *Can Vet J* 36:166–168.
59. Harvey RG. 1987. Possible sulphadiazine-trimethoprim induced polyarthritis (letter). *Vet Rec* 120:537–538.
59a. Harvey RG. 1996. Tylosin in the treatment of canine superficial pyoderma. *Vet Rec* 139:185–187.
60. Harvey RG, Noble WC, Ferguson EA. 1993. A comparison of lincomycin hydrochloride and clindamycin hydrochloride in the treatment of superficial pyoderma in dogs. *Vet Rec* 132:351–353.
61. Hildebrand H, Kempka G, Schluter G, et al. 1993. Chondrotoxicity of quinolones in vivo and in vitro. *Arch Toxicol* 67:411–415.
62. Hirsh DC. 1995. Antimicrobial drugs: a strategy for rational use and the ramifications of misuse. *Small Anim Med Digest* 1:188–194.
63. Hirsh DC, Jang SS. 1994. Antimicrobial susceptibility of selected infectious bacterial agents obtained from dogs. *J Am Anim Hosp Assoc* 30:487–494.
64. Hirsh DC, Jang SS, Biberstein EL. 1990. Lack of supportive susceptibility data for use of ampicillin together with trimethoprim-sulfonamide as broad spectrum antimicrobial treatment of bacterial disease in dogs. *J Am Vet Med Assoc* 197:594–596.
65. Hogan RW. 1989. Therapeutics. *JAMA* 261:1652.
66. Hooper DC, Wolfson JS. 1991. Drug therapy: fluoroquinolone antimicrobial agents. *N Engl J Med* 324:384.
67. Hoskins JD. 1993. Feline neonatal sepsis. *Vet Clin North Am Small Anim Pract* 23:91–100.
68. Houston DM, Cochrane SM, Conlon P. 1989. Phenobarbital toxicity in dogs concurrently treated with chloramphenicol. *Can Vet J* 30:598.
69. Hunter RP, Lynch MJ, Ericson JF, et al. 1995. Pharmacokinetics, oral bioavailability and tissue distribution of azithromycin in cats. *J Vet Pharmacol Ther* 18:38–46.
70. Ihrke PJ. 1996. Experiences with enrofloxacin in small animal dermatology. *Compend Cont Educ Pract Vet* 18:35–39.
70a. Intorre L, Mengozzi G, Maccheroni M, et al. 1995. Enrofloxacin theophylline interaction—influence of enrofloxacin on theophylline steady-state pharmacokinetics in the Beagle dog. *J Vet Pharmacol Ther* 18:352–356.
71. Jackson MW, Panciera DL, Hartmann F. 1994. Administration of vancomycin for treatment of ascending bacterial cholangiohepatitis in a cat. *J Am Vet Med Assoc* 204:602–605.
71a. Jang SS, Breher JE, Dabaco LA, et al. 1997. Organisms isolated from dogs and cats with anaerobic infections and susceptibility to selected antimicrobial agents. *J Am Vet Med Assoc* 210:1610–1614.
72. Jones RL, Godinho KS, Palmer GH. 1994. Clinical observations on the use of oral amoxycillin/clavulanate in the treatment of gingivitis in dogs and cats and anal sacculitis in dogs. *Br Vet J* 150:385–388.
73. Jung AC, Paauw DS. 1994. Management of adverse reactions to trimethoprim-sulfamethoxazole in human immunodeficiency virus-infected patients. *Arch Intern Med* 154:2402–2406.
74. Kaufman AC, Greene CE. 1993. Elevated alanine aminotransferase activity associated with tetracycline administration in a cat. *J Am Vet Med Assoc* 202:628–630.
75. Kernodle DS, Classen DC, Burke JP, et al. 1990. Failure of cephalosporins to prevent *Staphylococcus aureus* surgical wound infections. *JAMA* 263:961–966.
76. Kietzmann M, Mischke R, Albrecht N, et al. 1990. Vertraglichkeit und pharmakokinetik von cephalaxin (Cefaseptin) beim Hund. *Kleintierprax* 35:390–398.
77. Kietzmann M, Strothmann-Luerssen A, Grünau B, et al. 1992. Tolerance and pharmacokinetics of cephalexin in cats after oral administration. *J Small Anim Pract* 33:521–525.
78. Klemens SP, Cynamon MH, Swenson CE, et al. 1990. Liposome-encapsulated-gentamicin therapy of *Mycobacterium avium* complex infection in beige mice. *Antimicrob Agents Chemother* 34:967–970.
79. Klesel N, Adam F, Limbert M, et al. 1992. RU 29 246, the active compound of the cephalosporin prodrug-ester HR 916 III. Pharmacokinetic properties and antibacterial activity in vivo. *J Antibiot (Tokyo)* 45:922–931.
80. Kobayashi H. 1995. Biofilm disease: its clinical manifestation and therapeutic possibilities of macrolides. *Am J Med* 99(Suppl 6A):26–30.
81. Krol van Staaten MJ, Landheer JE, de Maat CE. 1990. Beware of the dog: meningitis in splenectomised woman. *Neth J Med* 36:301–303.
82. Küng K, Hauser B, Wanner M. 1995. Effect of the interval between feeding and ampicillin absorption in dogs. *J Small Anim Pract* 36:65–68.
83. Küng K, Riond JL, Wanner M. 1993. Pharmacokinetics of enrofloxacin and its metabolite ciprofloxacin after intravenous and oral administration of enrofloxacin in dogs. *J Vet Pharmacol Ther* 16:462–468.
84. Küng K, Wanner M. 1994. Bioavailability of different forms of amoxicillin administered orally to dogs. *Vet Rec* 135:552–554.
85. Kunkle GA, Sundlof S, Keisling K. 1995. Adverse side effects of oral antibacterial therapy in dogs and cats: an epidemiologic study of pet owners' observations. *J Am Anim Hosp Assoc* 31:46–55.
86. Lavy E, Goldstein R, Shem-Tov M, et al. 1995. Disposition kinetics of ampicillin administered intravenously and intraosseously to canine puppies. *J Vet Pharmacol Ther* 18:379–381.
87. Lavy E, Ziv G, Aroch I, et al. 1995. Clinical pharmacologic aspects of cefixime in dogs. *Am J Vet Res* 56:633–638.
88. Lavy E, Ziv G, Shem-Tov M, et al. 1995. Minimal inhibitory concentrations for canine isolates and oral absorption of roxithromycin in fed and fasted dogs. *J Vet Pharmacol Ther* 18:382–384.
89. Light RW, O'Hara VS, Moritz TE. 1990. Intrapleural tetracycline for the prevention of recurrent spontaneous pneumothorax. Results of a Department of Veterans Affairs Cooperative study. *JAMA* 264:2224–2230.
90. Liu CX, Wang JR, Lu YL. 1990. Pharmacokinetics of sulbactam and ampicillin in mice and dogs. *Acta Pharm Sinica* 25:406–411.
90a. Lloyd DH, Carlotti DN, Koch HJ, et al. 1997. Treatment of canine pyoderma with co-amoxyclav: a comparison of two dose rates. *Vet Rec* 141:439–441.
91. MacGregor RR, Graziani AL. 1997. Oral administration of antibiotics: a rational alternative to the parenteral route. *Clin Infect Dis* 24:457–467.
92. Malik R, Hunt GB, Goldsmid SE, et al. 1994. Diagnosis and treatment of pyogranulomatous panniculitis due to *Mycobacterium smegmatis* in cats. *J Small Anim Pract* 35:524–530.
93. Mandsager RE, Clarke CR, Shawley RV, et al. 1995. Effects of chloramphenicol on infusion pharmacokinetics of propofol in Greyhounds. *Am J Vet Res* 56:95–99.
94. Mansfield PD. 1990. Ototoxicity in dogs and cats. *Compend Cont Educ Pract Vet* 12:331–337.
95. Marcellin-Little DJ, Papich MG, Richardson DC, et al. 1996. Pharmacokinetic model for cefazolin distribution during total hip arthroplasty in dogs. *Am J Vet Res* 57:720–723.
96. Marco-Algarra J, Honrubia V. 1991. Comparative study of the effect of gentamicin on the vestibulo-ocular and visual vestibulo-ocular reflexes in the cat. *Acta Otolaryngol Stockh* 111:162–168.
97. Matsubayashik, Shintani Y, Yoshioka M. 1992. Metabolic disposition of DQ-2556, a new cephalosporin in rats, rabbits, dogs, and monkeys. *Antimicrob Agents Chemother* 36:966–972.
98. Mattie H, van Dokkum AM, Brus-Weijer L, et al. 1990. Antibacterial activity of four cephalosporins in an experimental infection in relation to in vitro effect and pharmacokinetics. *J Infect Dis* 162:717–722.

99. McEwan NA. 1992. Presumptive trimethoprim-sulphamethoxazole associated thrombocytopenia and anemia in a dog. *J Small Anim Pract* 33:27–29.
100. Mealey KL, Boothe DM. 1994. Nephrotoxicosis associated with topical administration of gentamicin in a cat. *J Am Vet Med Assoc* 12:1919–1921.
101. Medleau L, Shanley KJ, Rakich PM. 1990. Trimethoprim-sulfonamide-associated drug eruptions in dogs. *J Am Anim Hosp Assoc* 26:305–311.
102. Meinen JB, McClure JT, Rosin E. 1995. Pharmacokinetics of enrofloxacin in clinically normal dogs and mice and drug pharmacodynamics in neutropenic mice with *Escherichia coli* and staphylococcal infections. *Am J Vet Res* 56:1219–1224.
103. Merchant SR, Neer TM, Tedford BL, et al. 1993. Ototoxicity assessment of a chlorhexidine otic preparation in dogs. *Prog Vet Neurol* 4:72–75.
104. Messinger LM, Beale KM. 1993. A blinded comparison of the efficacy of daily and twice daily trimethoprim-sulfadiazine and daily sulfadimethoxine-ormetoprim therapy in the treatment of canine pyoderma. *Vet Dermatol* 4:13–18.
105. Metchock B, Lonsway DR, Carter GP. 1991. *Yersinia enterocolitica*: a frequent seasonal stool isolate from children at an urban hospital in the southeast United States. *J Clin Microbiol* 29:2868–2869.
106. Metchock B, McGowan JE. 1991. Evaluation of the vitek GPS-TA card for laboratory detection of high-level gentamicin and streptomycin resistance in *Enterococci*. *J Clin Microbiol* 29:2870–2872.
107. Moon YSK, Chung KC, Gill MA. 1997. Pharmacokinetics of neoplasm in animals, healthy volunteers, and patients. *Clin Infect Dis* 24(Suppl):S249–S255.
108. Muir P, Gruffydd-Jones TJ, Cripps PJ, et al. 1996. Breath hydrogen excretion by healthy cats after oral administration of oxytetracycline and metronidazole. *Vet Rec* 138:635–639.
109. Neu HC. 1990. Third generation cephalosporins: safety profiles after 10 years of clinical use. *J Clin Pharmacol* 30:396–403.
110. Neu HC. 1992. New macrolide antibiotics: azithromycin and clarithromycin. *Ann Intern Med* 116:517–519.
111. Nielsen OS, Møller NF, Maigaard S, et al. 1981. Nitroimidazoles in the canine prostates, vagina and urethra. *Prostate* 2:71–78.
112. Norden CW, Shinners, Niederriter K. 1986. Clindamycin treatment of experimental chronic osteomyelitis due to *Staphylococcus aureus*. *J Infect Dis* 153:956–959.
113. Nossaman BC, Amouzadeh HR, Sangiah S. 1990. Effects of chloramphenicol, cimetidine and phenobarbital on and tolerance to xylazine-ketamine anesthesia in dogs. *Vet Hum Toxicol* 32:216–219.
114. Novotny MJ, Shaw DH. 1991. Effect of enrofloxacin on digoxin clearance and steady-state serum concentrations in dogs. *Can J Vet Res* 55:113–116.
115. Orsini JA, Perkons S. 1994. New beta-lactam antibiotics in critical care medicine. *Compend Cont Educ Pract Vet* 16:183–186.
116. Ostro MJ, Cullis PR. 1989. Use of liposomes as injectable-drug delivery systems. *Am J Hosp Pharm* 46:1576–1587.
117. Page SW. 1991. Chloramphenicol: 1. Hazards of use and the current regulatory environment. *Aust Vet J* 68:1–2.
118. Papp JR, Muckle CA. 1991. Antimicrobial susceptibility testing of veterinary clinical isolates with the sceptor system. *J Clin Microbiol* 29:1249–1251.
119. Paradis M, Lemay S, Scott DW, et al. 1990. Efficacy of enrofloxacin in the treatment of canine bacterial pyodermas. *Vet Dermatol* 1:123–127.
120. Parpia SH, Nix DE, Hejmanowski LG, et al. 1989. Sucralfate reduces the gastrointestinal absorption of norfloxacin. *Antimicrob Agents Chemother* 33:99–102.
121. Pascoe PJ, Ilkiw JE, Kass PH, et al. 1996. Case control study of the association of intraoperative administration of nafcillin and acute postoperative development of azotemia. *J Am Vet Med Assoc* 208:1043–1047.
122. Petersen SW, Rosin E. 1993. In vitro antibacterial activity of cefoxitin and cefotetan and pharmacokinetics in dogs. *Am J Vet Res* 54:1496–1499.
123. Pickrell JA, Oehme FW, Cash WC. 1993. Ototoxicity in dogs and cats. *Semin Vet Med Surg Small Anim* 8:42–49.
124. Piddock LJV. 1993. Newer fluoroquinolones and gram-positive bacteria. *AMS News* 59:603–608.
125. Pohlenz-Zertuche HO, Brown MP, Gronwall R, et al. 1992. Serum and skin concentrations after multiple-dose oral administration of trimethoprim-sulfadiazine in dogs. *Am J Vet Res* 53:1273–1276.
126. Prescott JF, Yielding KM. 1990. In vitro susceptibility of selected veterinary bacterial pathogens to ciprofloxacin, enrofloxacin and norfloxacin. *Can J Vet Res* 54:195–197.
127. Riond JL, Riviere JE. 1990. Allometric analysis of doxycycline pharmacokinetic parameters. *J Vet Pharmacol Ther* 13:404–407.
128. Riond JL, Vaden SL, Riviere JE. 1990. Comparative pharmacokinetics of doxycycline in cats and dogs. *J Vet Pharmacol Ther* 13:415–424.
129. Riviere JE. 1991. Handbook of comparative pharmacokinetics and residues of veterinary antimicrobials. CRC Press, Boca Raton, FL.
130. Rosin E. 1990. Empirical selection of antibiotics in small animal surgery. *Compend Cont Educ Pract Vet* 12:231–232.
131. Rosin E, Ebert S, Uphoff TS, et al. 1989. Penetration of antibiotics into the surgical wound in a canine model. *Antimicrob Agents Chemother* 33:700–704.
132. Rosin E, Uphoff TS, Schultz-Darken NJ. 1993. Cefazolin antibacterial activity and concentrations in serum and the surgical wound in dogs. *Am J Vet Res* 54:1317–1321.
132a. Rothstein E, Scott DW, Riis RC. 1997. Tetracycline and niacinamide for the treatment of sterile pyogranuloma/granuloma syndrome in a dog. *J Am Anim Hosp Assoc* 33:540–543.
133. Rowland PH, Center SA, Dougherty SA. 1992. Presumptive trimethoprim-sulfadiazine–related hepatotoxicosis in a dog. *J Am Vet Med Assoc* 200:348–350.
134. Rubenstein E, Meissel D, Klein E, et al. 1988. Effect of pancreatitis on moxalactam excretion in pancreatic fluids of dogs and man. *World J Surg* 12:411-414.
135. Rutgers HC, Stepien RL, Elwood CM, et al. 1994. Enrofloxacin treatment of gram-negative infections. *Vet Rec* 135:357–359.
136. Salmon SA, Watts JL, Yancey RJ. 1996. In vitro activity of ceftiofur and its primary metabolite desfuroylceftiofur against organisms of veterinary importance. *J Vet Diagn Invest* 8:332–336.
137. Sarkiala E. 1992. Penetration of tinidazole into the gingival crevicular fluid in dogs. *Res Vet Sci* 52:391–393.
138. Sarkiala EM. 1993. Treatment of periodontitis in dogs with tinidazole. *J Small Anim Pract* 34:90–94.
139. Sarkiala E, Harvey C. 1993. Systemic antimicrobials in the treatment of periodontitis in dogs. *Semin Vet Med Surg Small Anim* 8:197–203.
140. Sarkiala E, Järvinen A, Valttila S, et al. 1991. Pharmacokinetics of tinidazole in dogs and cats. *J Vet Pharmacol Ther* 14:257–262.
141. Sarkiala-Kessel EM, Jarvinen A, Nokelainen M, et al. 1996. Concentrations of tinidazole in gingival crevicular fluid and plasma in dogs after multiple dose administration. *J Vet Pharmacol Ther* 19:171–175.
142. Scott DW, Miller WH, Cayatte SM, et al. 1994. Efficacy of tylosin tablets for the treatment of pyoderma due to *Staphylococcus intermedius* infection in dogs. *Can Vet J* 35:617–621.
143. Scott DW, Miller WH, Rothstein SE, et al. 1996. Further studies on efficacy of tylosin tablets for the treatment of pyoderma due to *Staphylococcus intermedius* infection in dogs. *Can Vet J* 37:617–618.
144. Scott DW, Miller WH, Wellington JR. 1993. The combination of ormetoprim and sulfadimethoxine in the treatment of pyoderma due to *Staphylococcus intermedius* infection in dogs. *Canine Pract* 18:29–33.
145. Shepard RM, Falkner FC. 1990. Pharmacokinetics of azithromycin in rats and dogs. *J Antimicrob Chemother* 25(Suppl A):49–60.
146. Shiba KA, Saito A, Shimada J, et al. 1990. Renal handling of fleroxacin in rabbits, dogs, and humans. *Antimicrob Agents Chemother* 34:58–64.
147. Smith IM, Mackie A, Lida J. 1991. Effect of giving enrofloxacin in the diet to pigs experimentally infected with *Actinobacillus pleuropneumoniae*. *Vet Rec* 129:25.
148. Sparks TA, Kemp DT, Wooley RE, et al. 1994. Antimicrobial effect of combinations of EDTA-tris and amikacin or neomycin on the microorganisms associated with otitis externa in dogs. *Vet Res Commun* 18:241–249.
149. Speer BS, Shoemaker NB, Salyers AA. 1992. Bacterial resistance to tetracycline: mechanisms, transfer and clinical significance. *Clin Microbiol Rev* 5:387–399.
149a. Spreng M, Deleforge J, Thomas V, et al. 1995. Antibacterial activity of marbofloxacin—a new fluoroquinolone for veterinary use against canine and feline isolates. *J Vet Pharmacol Ther* 18:284–289.
150. Stampley AR, Brown MP, Gronwall RR, et al. 1991. Serum concentrations of cefepime (BMY-28142), a broad-spectrum cephalosporin, in dogs. *Cornell Vet* 82:69–76.
151. Stegemann M, Heukamp U, Scheer M, et al. 1996. Kinetics of antibacterial activity after administration of enrofloxacin in dogs serum and skin: in vitro susceptibility of field isolates. *Compend Cont Educ Pract Vet* 18:30–34.
152. Sterner KE. 1991. An overview of new guidelines on the use and dispensing of veterinary drugs. *J Am Vet Med Assoc* 198:825.
153. Strain GM, Merchant SR, Neer TM, et al. 1995. Ototoxicity assessment of a gentamicin sulfate otic preparation in dogs. *Am J Vet Res* 56:532–537.
154. Ström B, Linde-Forsberg C. 1993. Effects of ampicillin and trimethoprim-sulfamethoxazole on the vaginal bacterial flora of bitches. *Am J Vet Res* 54:891–896.
155. Strube W, Thein P, Kretzdorn D, et al. 1989. Baypamun: new possibilities for the control of infectious diseases in domestic animals. *Vet Med Rev* 60:3–15.
156. Studdert VP, Hughes KL. 1992. Treatment of opportunistic mycobacterial infections with enrofloxacin in cats. *J Am Vet Med Assoc* 201:1388–1390.
157. Sullivan PS, Arrington K, West R, et al. 1992. Thrombocytopenia associated with administration of trimethoprim/sulfadiazine in a dog. *J Am Vet Med Assoc* 201:1741–1744.
158. Swalec-Tobias KM, Schneider RK, Besser TE. 1996. Use of antimicrobial-impregnated polymethyl methacrylate. *J Am Vet Med Assoc* 208:841–845.
159. Swenson CE, Stewart KA, Hammett JL, et al. 1990. Pharmacokinetics and in vivo activity of liposome-encapsulated gentamicin. *Antimicrob Agents Chemother* 34:235–240.
160. Teng RL, Girard D, Gootz TD, et al. 1996. Pharmacokinetics of trovafloxacin (CP-99,219) a new quinolone in rats, dogs, and monkeys. *Antimicrob Agents Chemother* 40:561–566.
160a. Tenover FC. 1992. Bauer and Kirby meet Watson and Crick. Antimicrobial susceptibility testing in the molecular era. *ASM News* 58:669–672.
161. Ten Voorde G, Broeze J, Hartman EG, et al. 1990. The influence of the injection site on the bioavailability of ampicillin and amoxicillin in beagles. *Vet Q* 12:73–79.

162. Thompson GW. 1990. Possible sulfamethoxazole/trimethoprim–induced hepatic necrosis in a dog. *Can Vet J* 31:530.
162a. Thornton JR, Martin PJ. 1997. Pharmacokinetics of cephalexin in cats after oral administration of the antibiotic in tablet and paste preparations. *Aust Vet J* 75:439–440.
163. Tilley BC, Trentham DE, Leisen JCC, et al. 1995. Minocycline in rheumatoid arthritis. *Ann Intern Med* 122:81–89.
164. Tomasz A. 1994. Multiple-antibiotic-resistant pathogenic bacteria. A report on the Rockefeller University workshop. *N Engl J Med* 330:1247–1251.
165. Trettien AL, Kram MA. 1994. Primor once-a-day canine antibacterial has important advantages. *SmithKline Beecham Animal Health Technical Bulletin* 1–5.
166. Tretien AL, Kram MA. 1994. Primor once a day canine antibacterial has important advantages. *Top Vet Med* 5:4–8.
167. Trudel JL, Wittnich C, Brown RA. 1994. Antibiotics bioavailability in acute experimental pancreatitis. *J Am Coll Surg* 178:475–479.
168. Twedt DC, Diehl KJ, Lappin MR, et al. 1997. Association of hepatic necrosis with trimethoprim sulfonamide administration in 4 dogs. *J Vet Intern Med* 11:20–23.
169. Ubeeva IP, Nikolaev SM, Sambueva ZG. 1989. Effect of antihepatotoxic tea on the course of drug-induced hepatitis. *Antibiot Khimioter* 34:859–862.
170. Vancutsem PM, Babish JG, Schwark WS. 1990. The fluoroquinolone antimicrobials: structure, antimicrobial activity, pharmacokinetics, clinical use in domestic animals and toxicity. *Cornell Vet* 80:173–186.
171. Villar D, Knight MK, Holding J, et al. 1995. Treatment of acute isoniazid overdose in dogs. *Vet Hum Toxicol* 37:473–477.
172. Vilmanyi E, Kung K, Riond J-L, et al. 1996. Clarithromycin pharmacokinetics after oral administration with or without fasting in crossbred Beagles. *J Small Anim Pract* 37:535–539.
173. Walker RD, Stein GE, Budsberg SC, et al. 1989. Serum and tissue fluid norfloxacin concentrations after oral administration of the drug to healthy dogs. *Am J Vet Res* 50:154–157.
174. Walker RD, Stein GE, Hauptman JC. 1990. Serum and tissue cage fluid concentrations of ciprofloxacin after oral administration of the drug to healthy dogs. *Am J Vet Res* 51:896–900.
175. Walker RD, Stein GE, Hauptman JG, et al. 1992. Pharmacokinetic evaluation of enrofloxacin administered orally to healthy dogs. *Am J Vet Res* 53:2315–2319.
176. Watson ADJ. 1991. Chloramphenicol: 2. Clinical pharmacology in dogs and cats. *Aust Vet J* 68:2–5.
177. Watson ADJ. 1992. Bioavailability and bioinequivalence of drug formulations in small animals. *J Vet Pharmacol Ther* 15:151–159.
178. Watts JL, Yancey RJ. 1994. Identification of veterinary pathogens by use of commercial identification systems and new trends in antimicrobial susceptibility testing of veterinary pathogens. *Clin Microbiol Rev* 7:346–356.
179. Weiss DJ, Adams LG. 1987. Aplastic anemia associated with trimethoprim-sulfadiazine and fenbendazole administration in a dog. *J Am Vet Med Assoc* 191:1119–1120.
179a. White SD, Rosychuck RAW, Reinke SI. 1992. Use of tetracycline and niacinamide for treatment of autoimmune skin disease in 31 dogs. *J Am Vet Med Assoc* 200:1497–1500.
180. Wilson RC, Duran SH, Horton CR, et al. 1989. Bioavailability of gentamicin in dogs after intramuscular or subcutaneous injections. *Am J Vet Res* 50:1748–1750.
181. Wolfson JS, Hooper DC. 1989. Fluoroquinolone antimicrobial agents. *Clin Microbiol Rev* 2:378–424.
182. Wright LC, Horton CR Jr, Jernigan AD, et al. 1991. Pharmacokinetics of gentamicin after intravenous and subcutaneous injection in obese cats. *J Vet Pharmacol Ther* 14:96–100.
183. Yabe K, Yoshida K, Yamamoto N, et al. 1997. Diagnosis of quinolone-induced arthropathy in juvenile dogs by use of magnetic-resonance (MR) imaging. *J Vet Med Sci* 59:597–599.
184. Yoshida K, Matsubayashi K, Sekiguchi M, et al. 1997. Toxicological evaluation and disposition of DV–7751A, a new quinolone antimicrobial agent, administered orally to dogs and monkeys. *Chemotherapy* 43:332–339.
185. Yu LP, Smith GN, Brandt KD, et al. 1992. Reduction in the severity of canine osteoarthritis by prophylactic treatment with oral doxycycline. *Arthritis Rheumat* 35:1150–1159.
186. Zaghlol HA, Brown SA. 1988. Single- and multiple-dose pharmacokinetics of intravenously administered vancomycin in dogs. *Am J Vet Res* 9:1637–1640.
187. Zetner K, Thiemann G. 1993. The antimicrobial effectiveness of clindamycin in diseases of the oral cavity. *J Vet Dent* 10:6–9.

Chapter 35

Streptococcal and Other Gram-Positive Bacterial Infections

Craig E. Greene and John F. Prescott

STREPTOCOCCAL INFECTIONS

Streptococci are gram-positive nonmotile, facultatively anaerobic cocci that cause localized to widespread pyogenic infections in animals and people. Although a number are pathogenic, many species are commensal microflora of the oral cavity, nasopharynx, skin, and genital and GI tracts. Species differences among streptococci are responsible for the varying host ranges and virulence. Several classification systems exist for streptococci based on cultural characteristics, antigenic composition, and biochemical features. Because it tends to correlate with pathogenicity, Lancefield classification based on antigenic differences in cell wall carbohydrates is used to distinguish the groups. The action on erythrocytes in culture medium has also been employed to distinguish different groups of streptococci. β Hemolysis is characterized by complete lysis of erythrocytes and clearing around the colonies. α Hemolysis is characterized by a greenish-colored zone and intact erythrocytes in the discolored region. Some are nonhemolytic. β-Hemolytic strains tend to be most pathogenic. Lancefield groups A, B, C, E, G, L, and M are usually β hemolytic. Group D is usually α hemolytic or sometimes nonhemolytic and contains a number of species that have been reclassified as *Enterococcus* (see Enterococcal Infections). Organisms in the α-hemolytic and nonhemolytic categories are found on mucous membranes and skin of clinically healthy animals. If present in an infectious process, they are usually regarded as contaminants or unimportant invaders. When they do cause illness, it may take the form of valvular endocarditis or embolic abscess. The precise species classification of streptococci in a number of the disease processes described next is in doubt, especially in the older literature. Increasingly, Lancefield grouping combined with detailed phenotypic characterization by commercial identification systems will classify streptococci correctly and will define more clearly the streptococci causing significant infections in dogs and cats.

Group A Streptococcal Infections of Dogs and Cats

Humans are the principal natural reservoir hosts of group A streptococci, and most human infections are caused by this group. Dermatitis, pharyngitis, and scarlet and rheumatic fevers are the main syndromes caused by *Streptococcus pyogenes* (Table 35–1). Rarely these organisms produce perianal cellulitis, vaginitis, and localized abscesses. Certain strains produce pyrogenic exotoxins, which may cause toxic shock–like syndrome. Of all the streptococcal groups, group A organisms have the greatest virulence for human adults, whereas organisms of the other groups, such as B, C, D, F, and G, cause the most severe manifestations in neonates.

Streptococcus pyogenes. The sites of greatest carriage of group A streptococci in humans are the caudal aspects of the pharynx and tonsillar region. Group A streptococci can survive extremes in environmental temperature and humidity; however, most infections are associated with direct or close contact among susceptible individuals (Fig. 35–1). As is true with many streptococcal infections, some individuals can harbor the infection for extended periods in the absence of clinical illness. Prevalence rates for group A streptococci are higher in young children, especially those in day-care or classroom situations. The prevalence of positive throat culture findings in such circumstances may approach 50%, even in the absence of an obvious epidemic.[17] Symptomatic rather than carrier children are most likely to bring infection into the home. Under such circumstances, the isolation rate in other humans in the household approaches 25% to 50%. If the child is nonsymptomatic, the rate is only 9%.[17] Dogs and cats have been suggested as possible sources of reinfection of treated household members, but there is no convincing evidence that dogs and cats represent significant reservoirs of infection for humans. Veterinarians may, however, be consulted on this topic.

Whenever streptococcal typing has been performed on the oropharyngeal region of dogs and cats, groups G, C, L, and M have been present (in order of decreasing frequency). However, screening for group A streptococcal colonization of the tonsils of dogs and cats from random households in urban environments has shown the apparent prevalence to range between 1% and 10%. In one study in which recurrent group A streptococcal pharyngitis occurred in people, the prevalence for households was said to be 42% for dogs and 36% for cats. However, because only bacitracin susceptibility was used to distinguish group A from non-group A strains

Table 35–1. Summary of Streptococcal Infections of People, Dogs, and Cats

SPECIES	SEROGROUP	HOST SPECIES	MICROFLORAL DISTRIBUTION	DISEASE SYNDROME(S)[a]
Streptococci				
S. pyogenes	A	H	Tonsils	Tonsillitis, pharyngitis, otitis, impetigo, bacteremia, toxemia, toxic shock, necrotizing fasciitis
		B	None (human reservoir)	Nonsymptomatic
S. pneumoniae	A	H	Tonsils	Pneumonia, otitis, bacteremia, polyarthritis, meningitis
		C	None (human reservoir)	Polyarthritis, bacteremia
S. agalactiae	B	H	Anorectum, vagina	Neonate: sepsis Immunosuppressed: bacteremia, meningitis, endocarditis Postparturient: metritis; septic arthritis; pharyngitis; respiratory, skin, and wound infection
		D	Urogenital	Fatal septicemia in pups, necrotizing pneumonia, bacteremia, endocarditis, pyelonephritis[28]
		C	Urogenital	Peritonitis, septicemia, placentitis
S. equi subsp. *zooepidemicus*, *S. dysgalactiae* subsp. *equisimilis*	C	D	Skin, genitourinary tract	Endocarditis, septicemia,[32] fibrinopurulent bronchopneumonia, acute death, UTIs
		H	None (animal reservoir)	Pharyngitis, glomerulonephritis, pericarditis
S. suis	D or none	C	Oropharynx	Dermatitis, fibrinonecrotic pleuropneumonia[13]
S. dysgalactiae	G	H	Tonsils, vagina	Pharyngitis, tonsillitis, wound infections, neonatal and puerperal sepsis, endocarditis
S. canis	G	C	Nasopharynx, genitalia, skin	Abscesses, neonatal sepsis, umbilical infections
		D	Tonsils, anorectum, genitalia	Otitis media, neonatal sepsis (fading puppy?), umbilical infections, polyarthritis, abscesses, dermatitis, mastitis, genital infections: infertility, anestrus, abortion, failure to conceive, UTI; streptococcal toxic shock syndrome/necrotizing fasciitis
Streptococcus sp.	L	D	Genitalia	Abortion, fading puppy, sterility in bitch, endometritis
Streptococcus sp.	M	D	Tonsils	Nonsymptomatic colonization
Streptococcus sp.	E	D	Skin, upper respiratory tract	Nonsymptomatic colonization found as mixed flora in mucosal inflammation
Enterococci[b]				
E. faecalis, E. avium, E. faecium	D	D, H, C	Intestine, feces, tonsils	Nonsymptomatic colonization, UTI, nosocomial surgical infections
E. hirae	D	D	Intestine, feces	Diarrhea, symptomatic upper intestinal colonization[13]

[a]For additional citations see Table 56–1, Greene.[17]
[b]Also includes *E. cecorum, E. durans,* and *E. zymogenes.*
H = human; B = dog and cat; C = cat; D = dog; UTI = urinary tract infection.

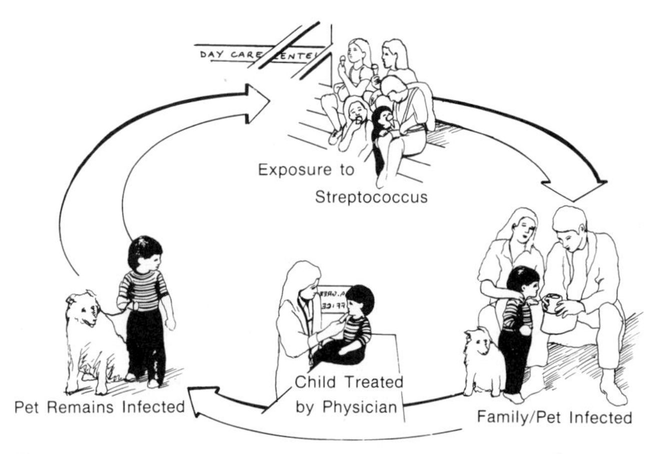

Figure 35–1. Zoonotic aspects of group A streptococcal infection in pets. Children usually acquire infection at school. When the child is treated, reinfection may result if the household pet has acquired infection and is not simultaneously treated. Treatment of additional family contacts is as important in breaking the cycle.

in a number of these studies, the findings of high prevalence must be regarded as unproven at best and fictitious at worst. When Lancefield typing has been done, the prevalence of true group A streptococcal carriage has varied from 0 to 3% of dogs and has not correlated with the presence of infection in the owner.[9, 44] Biochemical testing of isolates from dogs and cats cannot accurately distinguish between those from groups A and G.[33]

Domestic pets that come into close contact with infected individuals can sometimes apparently develop pharyngeal colonization with group A streptococci. Infected pets show no clinical illness or tonsillar enlargement. Because clinical symptomatology is absent in these animals, the main consideration is their potential public health risk. If they were overlooked during treatment, they might serve as possible reservoirs for reinfection of family members. Pets, however, usually lose their infection within 2 to 3 weeks after they are removed from the household. Infected humans are carriers of group A streptococci for much longer periods. It is not acceptable to consider culturing and treating the dog and cat in a household in which reinfection occurs without doing so for the human contacts.

The recovery of group A streptococci is affected by the method utilized in swabbing the throat, because overgrowth by indigenous microflora can result in the death of group A streptococci. Sedation may be needed, because sterile swabs should be rubbed over the surface of the exposed tonsils in their crypts. Swabs that will be unrefrigerated during transport should be kept dry; otherwise overgrowth by contaminating microflora will occur. Latex agglutination and ELISA tests are available for rapid detection of group A streptococci in children. Their value in detection of asymptomatic group A infections in dogs and cats is likely to be low.

The antimicrobial spectrum for group A streptococcal infection in pets is the same as that for human strains. It is judicious to treat pets when they may be a source of recurrent infection of household members. Isolates of group A streptococci from dogs have shown the greatest susceptibility to penicillin, erythromycin, and chloramphenicol. Recommended total daily dosages are listed in Table 35–2. Resistant strains can be treated with cephalosporins.

Streptococcus pneumoniae. *S. pneumoniae* (formerly *Diplococcus pneumoniae*) can produce pneumonia, bacteremia, otitis media, endocarditis, and meningitis in humans, but is of no significance in dogs and cats. A single report of bacteremia and septic arthritis in a cat attributed the infection to transmission of *S. pneumoniae* from a human infant in the same household.[36]

Group B Streptococcal Infections of Dogs and Cats

Group B streptococci *(Streptococcus agalactiae)* have been associated mainly with neonatal septicemia and postpartum metritis in humans and mastitis in cows. Skin, pharyngeal, and wound infections can occur. Immunosuppressed individuals can develop disease in many tissues (see Table 35–1). Group B streptococci are more frequently isolated than group G from people with these syndromes. Factors at the time of delivery, such as low birth weight or difficult delivery, precipitate the development of clinical illness.

Group B streptococcal infections are rare in dogs and cats. They have been reported to cause septicemia in a dog, endometritis, and fading puppy syndrome, symptoms of which include bacteremia, pyelonephritis, and necrotizing pneumonia. Group G streptococci have been far more commonly isolated than group B as causes of neonatal sepsis. Similarly, peritonitis with septicemia and parturient endometritis and placentitis have been described in cats. Whether canine and feline strains are indigenous or of human or other animal origin is uncertain. Therapy is similar to that for group A streptococcal infections (see Table 35–2).

Group C Streptococcal Infections of Dogs and Cats

Disease associated with group C streptococci has been described only in dogs, although both dogs and cats may carry these organisms as commensal flora, in lower frequency than group G. Acute hemorrhagic and purulent pneumonia

Table 35–2. Drug Therapy for Streptococcal Infections in Dogs and Cats[a]

DRUG	SPECIES	DOSE[b]	ROUTE	INTERVAL (HOURS)	DURATION (DAYS)
Penicillin G	B	10,000–20,000 U/kg	IM, SC	12–24	5–7
Penicillin V	B	8–30 mg/kg	PO	8	5–7
Erythromycin	D	3–20 mg/kg	PO	12–24	5–7
Chloramphenicol	D	15–25 mg/kg	PO, IV, SC	8	5–7
	C	10–15 mg/kg	PO, IV, SC	12	5–7
Cephalexin	B	10–40 mg/kg	PO	12	5–7

[a]For specific dosages for perinatal group G infections in cats, see Table 35–4. For additional information on each drug, see Appendix 8.
[b]Dose per administration at specified interval.
B = dog and cat; D = dog; C = cat.

has been described, primarily in racing greyhounds or research dogs.[17] Weakness, coughing, dyspnea, fever, hematemesis, and red urine have been the predominant clinical signs. Many of the dogs developed septicemia, and some died suddenly without signs of clinical illness. Gross lesions at necropsy of fatally affected animals consisted of widespread petechial and ecchymotic hemorrhages and pulmonary congestion with mediastinal and free pleural hemorrhage. Microscopically, streptococci were found in clusters intracellularly throughout the lung parenchyma and in the spleen. The circumstances leading to group C streptococcal septicemia or pneumonia in adult dogs kept in kennels or groups are unclear, and these infections appear to be rare. The isolates have been identified as *S. equi zooepidemicus*, although more details of the bacterial characterization are needed to determine whether this finding is correct (see later discussion of streptococcal toxic shock syndrome [STSS]). Other group C streptococci isolated from less severe infections (urinary tract infections or abscesses) in dogs have been identified as *S. dysgalactiae equisimilis*, although this subspecies also has caused serious losses through septicemia and pneumonia in captive coyotes.[15] Drugs and dosages recommended for treatment are similar to those for group A infections (see Table 35–2).

Group G Streptococcal Infections

Cats. β-Hemolytic streptococci are commensal microflora of the skin, pharynx, and upper respiratory and genital tracts of cats. The majority of β-hemolytic streptococcal infections in cats are caused by Lancefield group G streptococci and are apparently *S. canis*. Whether more virulent disease-producing strains of this organism exist is uncertain, but these organisms can cause severe infections in kittens. For neonatal kittens, the source of streptococci is the vagina of the queen. Streptococci can gain entrance via the umbilical vein and can spread by direct extension into the peritoneal cavity or through the ductus venosus and portal circulation of the liver, resulting in bacteremia. In juvenile kittens (3–7 months old), cervical lymphadenitis may follow a subclinical episode of pharyngitis and tonsillitis. Group G infections of older cats are often opportunistic and follow wounds, trauma, surgical procedures, viral infections, and immunosuppressive conditions. These suppurative infections can result in septicemia and embolic lesions, most often in the lung and heart.

Although infections in juveniles and older cats are generally sporadic, several kittens in a litter can be affected at one time, but most frequently in the first litter of queens younger than 2 years. Young queens that become infected carry higher numbers of organisms in the vagina, and the carrier state persists throughout pregnancy, whereas older, multiparous queens can eliminate the carrier state by midgestation.

The prevalence of infection is low in kittens born to older or multiparous queens. A higher prevalence of infection occurs in grouped cats. Occasional outbreaks of neonatal infections with high mortality can occur in breeding catteries, especially after the introduction of group G streptococci into a naive population. Approximately 50% of female household cats younger than 2 years and 70% to 100% of similarly aged queens in breeding catteries may carry group G streptococci in the vagina. Queens in endemically affected catteries can develop protective levels of antibodies by 8 months of age. Kittens receive levels of antibodies equivalent to those of the dam via the colostrum.

Group G streptococci also can be found in the tonsils and pharynx. The tom can carry the organism in the prepuce. Age, exposure, and immune responses are all important in determining whether this commensal organism causes illness.

The clinical signs vary with the site of infection and host immunocompetence. Sites of streptococcal infections in cats are listed in Table 35–3. Although cats of any age may be affected, most cases involve neonatal kittens (< 2 weeks of age). Most infected kittens gain less weight than littermates, and occasionally an affected kitten has a swollen, infected umbilicus. Death usually occurs by 7 to 11 days of age, but kittens born to queens with minimal prior exposure may die suddenly at younger than 3 days of age with overwhelming sepsis. In kittens with septicemia, the febrile response is transient, occurs within 24 hours before death, and frequently remains undetected. Older kittens are febrile and anorexic with swelling and purulent exudate at the site of infection. Cervical lymphadenitis is a unilateral or bilateral swelling in the ventral cervical lymph nodes (Fig. 35–2). Abscess, pharyngitis, pneumonia, diskospondylitis, osteomyelitis, and arthritis are other localizations of the infectious process in this age group.[19] Animals with respiratory localization will

Table 35–3. Anatomic Distribution of β-Hemolytic Streptococcal Isolates[a] from Lesions in Cats[b]

SOURCE	NUMBER OF ISOLATES	NUMBER OF PURE ISOLATES[c]
Integumentary	57	23
Respiratory	38	11
Genital (female)	28	12
Urinary	17	4
Serous cavities	22	9
Neonatal sepsis	12	6
Other[d]	34	13
Total	208	78

[a]Thirty-four of 38 isolates tested were Lancefield group G positive.
[b]Data compiled from cases during a 17-year period at the Veterinary Medical Teaching Hospital, University of California, Davis.
[c]Number of times isolated in pure culture (only organism isolated).
[d]Other sites include oral cavity, lymph node, CNS, eye, ear, joint, and mammary gland.

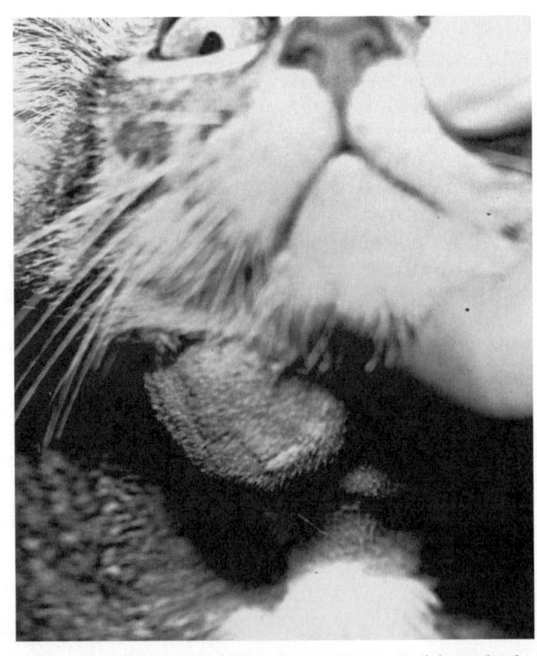

Figure 35–2. Unilateral *Streptococcus canis* cervical lymphadenitis in a 4-month-old kitten. From Timoney JF, et al (eds): Hagan and Bruner's microbiology and infectious diseases of domestic animals, 8th ed. Cornell University Press, 1988. Reprinted with permission.

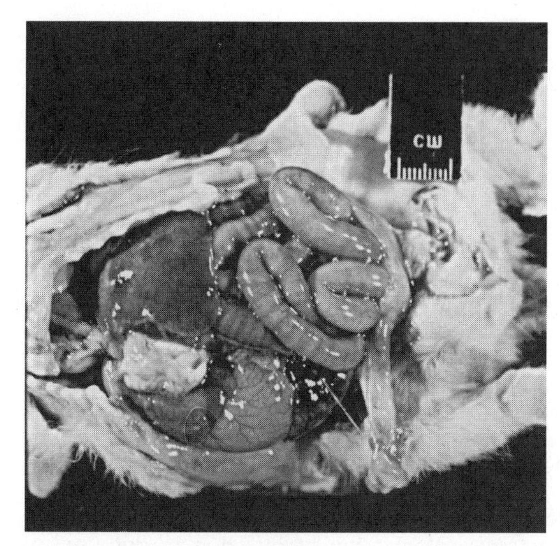

Figure 35–3. Peritonitis and umbilical vein abscess with extension into the liver in a 7-day-old kitten.

have fever, anorexia, coughing, and dyspnea. Those with diskospondylitis have fever, paraspinal hyperesthesia, and progressive paresis. Fever, joint swelling, and lameness are characteristic of arthritis and may involve one or more joints or extremities.

The leukogram shows a typical neutrophilic inflammatory response with a left shift. Neonatal kittens (< 2 weeks of age) usually have a degenerative left shift in the leukogram owing to the limited bone marrow storage pool. With overwhelming sepsis, cocci may be found in the cytoplasm of circulating neutrophils.

Gram staining of exudates from affected tissues reveals single and chains of gram-positive cocci. Confirmation is based on bacteriologic culture of the affected tissues. Aerobic culture of exudates or needle aspirates of enlarged lymph nodes yield β-hemolytic, gram-positive cocci on sheep and bovine blood agar plates. In fatally affected neonates, the organism is found most consistently in the liver, lung, umbilicus, and peritoneal cavity (Fig. 35–3).

Necropsy findings in affected neonatal kittens with septicemia include omphalophlebitis, peritonitis, and, less frequently, embolic hepatitis, pneumonia, diskospondylitis, and myocarditis. Untreated cases of cervical lymphadenitis in juvenile cats can progress to pleuritis, embolic myocarditis, and embolic pneumonia with secondary pulmonary infarction (see also later discussion of STSS). Older cats are less susceptible to systemic spread of streptococci.

Group G streptococci are very sensitive to penicillin and its derivatives. Juvenile and older cats with lymphadenitis should be treated immediately with oral or parenteral therapy (Table 35–4). Draining and flushing the abscesses hasten recovery. These cats should be examined for predisposing conditions such as feline leukemia, feline infectious peritonitis, feline immunodeficiency virus or viral respiratory infections, feline urologic syndrome, and wounds.

For prevention of infection in newborn kittens, dipping the navel and umbilical cord in 2% tincture of iodine and treatment of all kittens at birth with ampicillin, amoxicillin, or procaine and benzathine penicillin combined have been successful. A much higher dosage of combined procaine and benzathine penicillin should be given immediately to the queen of an infected litter or as a single preventive dose at parturition. Although the population of group G streptococci can be temporarily suppressed by antimicrobial therapy, the carrier state cannot be eliminated.

Treatment of infected juvenile or adult cats with lymphadenitis or arthritis can be accomplished with parenteral or oral therapy (see Table 35–4). Doses are higher than normally recommended because the organism can be harbored in the tonsillar crypts and a considerable amount of pus forms in the abscess. Cats with diskospondylitis have required up to 6 months of therapy. Parenteral therapy can be instituted in the veterinarian's office, and medication can be dispensed for subsequent oral administration.

Group G streptococci have received increasing attention as a cause of pharyngitis, tonsillitis, wound infection, cellulitis, neonatal and puerperal septicemia, and endocarditis in people. Group G streptococci in cats appear to be *S. canis* and to be distinct from human group G streptococci.[33] In a review of all reported human group G infections in Great Britain, a majority of the patients had underlying immunosuppressive illness, and in only one was there even suspected infection from a dog.[19]

Dogs. Group G streptococci are the major streptococcal type isolated as commensal flora from the skin and mucosa of dogs.[3, 4] The majority of group G isolates from dogs are *S. canis*. Nevertheless, some group G isolates have the biochemical characteristics of human group G streptococci. More work is needed to define the biotypic variation within *S. canis* and the identity of unusual group G streptococci isolated from dogs. Historically, the veterinary literature contains numerous reports of diseases in dogs caused by these organisms, including abortion, infertility, sterility, and neonatal death. In addition, cellulitis, mastitis, pharyngitis, tonsillitis, and genital infection have been described (see Table 35–1). Some of these historical descriptions of disease, especially pharyngitis, tonsillitis, infertility, and sterility, caused by group G

Table 35–4. Therapy for Group G Streptococcal Infections in Cats[a]

DRUG	AGE	DOSE[a]	ROUTE	INTERVAL (hours)	DURATION (days)
Prevention at Parturition					
Ampicillin (amoxicillin)	N	25 mg/kg	PO, SC	8	5–7
Procaine and benzathine penicillin	N	6250 IU[b]	SC	48–72	3–5[c]
	Q	150,000 IU[b]	SC	48–72	3–5[c]
Infected (Lymphadenitis or Arthritis)					
Procaine and benzathine penicillin	J, A	75,000–150,000 IU[b]	SC	48–72	3–5[c]
Procaine penicillin	J, A	50,000 IU[b]	SC	24	5
Penicillin V	J, A	20 mg/kg	PO	8	5

[a]Dose per administration at specified interval. For additional information on each drug, see Appendix 8.
[b]Total dose needed for each drug in a fixed combination, based on a 2- to 3-kg cat.
[c]Only one or two doses usually given during this treatment regimen.
N = neonates; Q = queens; J = juveniles; A = adults.

streptococci should be treated with suspicion because of the frequency with which these organisms are isolated from clinically healthy animals and the lack of clear description of the microbiology of the infections. It is, however, also likely that streptococcal infections have declined in importance in the last 50 years with the widespread use of penicillin and its derivatives in dogs.

S. canis is generally an opportunist pathogen of dogs and is isolated from an array of nonspecific infections, including genitourinary tract, wound, mammary gland, and skin (especially otitis externa). In addition, it may cause bacteremia or septicemia in neonatal puppies, forming part of the fading puppy syndrome, in which the pup is predisposed owing to lack of warmth, improper navel disinfection, and lack of nursing. It has also been associated with a rapidly progressive systemic infection in older dogs (see later discussion of STSS) *S. canis* is a common commensal of the genital tract. It may be an opportunistic infection in vaginitis, but its historical role in infertility in bitches is not supported by current findings. There are historical but no current accounts of the association of this organism with acute tonsillitis and suppurative cervical lymphadenitis in dogs in kennels and other settings. Treatment is similar to that for group A streptococcal infections (see Table 35–2).

STSS and Necrotizing Fasciitis (NF). During the last decade there has been a resurgence of severe group A streptococcal infections in humans characterized by septic shock associated with multiple-organ failure with or without NF. There is one report of this syndrome in a person caused by group G streptococci.[41] This dramatic and severe infection has been dubbed "flesh-eating" bacterial infection in the popular media. A similar clinical picture caused by various isolates of *S. canis* or other group G streptococci has been identified in dogs[25, 29–31] and cats.[43] In most cases affected animals were previously healthy adult dogs or cats younger than 1 year. The dogs had a history of mild trauma, bite wound, or respiratory or urinary tract disease. Affected kittens had suppurative lymphadenomegaly, typical of group G infection. In addition, they had multifocal purulent ulcerative skin lesions. They were generally depressed but afebrile.[43] All the dogs were febrile (40–41°C [104–105.8°F]) at admission. With NF, the dogs had severe, rapidly developing cellulitis, usually of a limb but in one case of the ventral thorax. The most consistent clinical sign in the history and on physical examination was intense, excruciating pain localized around the affected area but sometimes involving the whole body. Localized heat and swelling were identified at presentation or within 2 days of hospitalization. Once evident, the cellulitis developed rapidly. Chains of streptococci would be readily demonstrated in fluid aspirated from the cellulitis or in underlying tissues by histopathology. Dogs with NF were extremely depressed on presentation and eventually went into shock. They had extensive exudate accumulation along fascial planes. The fascia required surgical debridement. In two dogs, acute onset of posterior paresis with lower motor neuron deficits developed because of the presence of septic emboli in blood vessels of the gray matter of the spinal cord and because of extension of infection into the surrounding connective tissue and peripheral nerves.

Other dogs with severe invasive *S. canis* infection developed STSS without clinically apparent NF. The dogs with STSS had severe depression, fever, and rapidly developing hypotension and shock. In most, the lungs were considered the primary site of infection, and acute infection appeared to be superimposed on chronic pre-existing pulmonary infection. One dog had a urinary infection as the presumed source.[29]

The majority of kittens having NF responded favorably to treatment with amoxicillin-clavulanate supportive care and wound management with topical antibiotic application.[43] The dogs with STSS died or were euthanized within 48 hours of hospitalization but those with NF survived. All dogs had full-thickness skin sloughs and required debridement of necrotic tissue, appropriate antibiotic treatment, and intensive supportive medical care (crystalloids, colloids, plasma, low-dose heparin) aimed at treating shock with disseminated intravascular coagulation. Interestingly, most of the dogs had received enrofloxacin in the early stages of disease, but this approach was without apparent effect despite in vitro susceptibility in some cases. Less commonly, glucocorticoid treatment was used. More appropriate antibiotics for treatment of this condition are penicillin G, aminopenicillins (ampicillin, amoxicillin), erythromycin, and clindamycin. In human STSS or NF, clindamycin is regarded as the drug of choice.

Public Health Considerations. In general, public health risks from *S. canis* colonization of infection in dogs or cats are low. When veterinarians drain and debride NF lesions, they should recognize the severe hazard of inadvertent cuts on their hands. Risk to humans can probably be contained by the wearing of latex gloves and protective clothing when handling dogs with STSS or NF. Group G streptococci are normal inhabitants of the skin, oropharynx, GI tract, and female genital tract of people. Human strains generally belong to the species *S. dysgalactiae* rather than *S. canis*. Nonsymptomatic pharyngeal carriage of group G streptococci is found in up to 23% of people. The organisms commonly colonize human skin, and approximately 5% of nonsymptomatic puerperal women harbor them on the genital mucosa. Group G streptococcal infections in people are not common and involve primarily dermatitis and pharyngitis; however, bacteremia and septicemia, endocarditis, peritonitis, peripheral sepsis, soft tissue infection, and septic arthritis are unusual.

There is little evidence that dogs are a significant source of human infection. In one report,[5] dogs were mentioned as a possible source of group G streptococcal arthritis in people, but the association was speculative. The source of infection was more likely autogenous. In one report of meningitis,[21] the isolate was not completely characterized. In another report, *S. canis* was isolated from the blood of a person with septicemia.[1] The organism was specifically typed on the basis of biochemical and genetic analysis. It was presumably transmitted from the family dog and colonized the varicose ulcers of the legs of the person. The occurrence of such infections probably involves close contact between the animal and open skin wounds. Routine hand washing after animal contact and not allowing dogs to lick people, especially their wounds, are always advisable.

Other Streptococcal Infections of Cat and Dogs

Group L streptococci have been similarly associated with syndromes that parallel some of those reported historically for group G streptococci (abortion, infertility, and septicemia in puppies), although their frequency of isolation from normal and diseased dogs has been low (see Table 35–1). Groups M and E have been found as normal microflora of dogs, although they are isolated with very low frequency from the oral, urogenital, and respiratory mucosae. Group D streptococci are considered normal GI flora of dogs, and many of these species have been classified as enterococci (see following discussion). These enteric cocci are often found in urinary tract or nosocomial tissue infections of dogs. *S. suis* has been isolated rarely from pleuropneumonic conditions in cats but appears to be of little significance.

ENTEROCOCCAL INFECTIONS

Enterococci are gram-positive cocci that grow into short chains and are impossible to distinguish morphologically from streptococci. They were initially classified as group D streptococci but now have their own genus that contains the species such as *Enterococcus faecalis*, *Enterococcus faecium*, and *Enterococcus hirae*. These organisms can survive under more adverse environmental conditions than the less robust streptococci. In addition to being saprophytes, their major habitat in the host is the GI tract, where they are normal microflora (Table 35–5).[11] Enterococci are not as virulent as other streptococci, but their resistance to many antimicrobials allows them to persist in host tissues despite antimicrobial therapy. In people and pets, they have predominantly caused infections in hospitalized patients as nosocomial complications. Systemic infections such as bacteremia and endocarditis and localized infections of the abdominal cavity, genitourinary tract, soft tissue, or respiratory tract have been most frequent. The multiple antibiotic resistance of some isolates, including notably resistance to vancomycin in rare cases, has led to the increasing prominence of these poorly virulent bacteria.

Vancomycin-resistant enterococci (VRE) are becoming a major threat to human health. People often become infected in hospital settings or their home environments. In Europe, community-acquired infections are presumably more common because a vancomycin-related glycopeptide, avoparcin, has been used extensively as a growth promoter for food-producing animals.[25a] VRE have been recovered from dog food sold in the United States.[13b] VRE with the same genotype as in people has been recovered from the feces of pet dogs and cats.[13a, 39a]

Although we have primarily observed resistant nosocomial enterococcal infections in the veterinary hospital, published reports have implicated *E. hirae* as a cause of diarrhea in dogs. *E. hirae* was isolated from the small intestine of an 11-day-old pup.[7, 12] The pup was one of three that died in a litter affected with acute diarrhea. Microscopically, bacterial colonization of the apical surfaces of the enterocytes in the jejunum was diffuse with mild inflammatory infiltrates. A mixed growth of *Escherichia coli* and *E. hirae* was cultured. Although bacterial attachment has been seen in the ileum and colon of healthy pups, it is not usually found in the upper small intestine. Although enterococci have been associated with malabsorption and diarrhea in other animals, their exact role in the diarrhea or death of these three puppies is uncertain. Concurrent infection with an undetected organism may have been possible. Bacterial adhesion has also been reported in two other mature dogs with diarrhea.[22] *E. faecium* was one of many floral organisms isolated from feces of one of these affected dogs. Replication and adherence of bacteria in the upper small intestine must be distinguished from bacterial overgrowth because it can develop as a result of other small intestinal disorders.

Enterococci are generally resistant to a variety of antimicrobials used to treat gram-positive organisms. Nevertheless, penicillin, ampicillin, and rarely vancomycin combined with aminoglycosides are the treatments of choice. Trimethoprim-sulfonamide is not effective, despite in vitro susceptibility, because these organisms can circumvent the block in folate synthesis in vivo.

Table 35–5. Enterococcal and Streptococcal Species Isolated From the Anal and Tonsillar Mucosae of Dogs and Cats

SPECIES		DOGS Anus	DOGS Tonsils	CATS Anus	CATS Tonsils
Enterococci					
E. faecalis		45	48	60	40
E. hirae		37	8	15	4
E. faecium		12	20	15	19
E. avium		12	0	0	0
E. avium-like		13	12	0	0
E. raffinosis		2	0	0	27
E. durans		2	0	0	0
E. cecorum		2	8	14	12
Streptococci (Lancefield Group)					
S. canis	(G)	12	32	30	19
S. bovis	(D)	10	8	32	12
S. suis	(S, R)	0	20	5	12
S. alactolyticus	(D)	2	8	5	0
S. dysgalactiae	(G)	0	8	0	0

Data adapted from Devriese LA, et al: *J Appl Bacteriology* 73:421–425, 1992, with permission.

RHODOCOCCUS EQUI INFECTION OF CATS

R. equi (previously *Corynebacterium equi*) is a soil-borne, pleomorphic, gram-positive bacillus that has been primarily associated with suppurative infections in domestic livestock, especially foals. Reports of infections in cats are rare but increasing and are probably associated with immunosuppressive illness such as that caused by retrovirus infection. Cats with *R. equi* infection should be examined for predisposing immunocompromising viral infections.

R. equi commonly produces purulent pneumonia in foals, suppurative lymphadenitis in pigs, and granulomatous lymphadenitis in cows. *R. equi* has also been isolated from lesions in dogs, but isolation from abscesses in cats have been most commonly reported. It is increasing in prominence in humans because immunocompromised people, particularly those infected with HIV, have been affected. Pulmonary lobar infiltration with cavitation, similar to that observed with tuberculosis, has been the most frequently observed syndrome in AIDS patients.[39, 40] *R. equi*, a saprophyte, can commonly be recovered from herbivore-manured soil and from feces of herbivores. The organism may sometimes enter the body by a penetrating wound contaminated from the environment and subsequently spread via lymphatics to regional lymph nodes and via the blood to the liver, spleen, and visceral lymph nodes. It is commonly inhaled in dust. *R. equi* is a facultative intracellular parasite that invades lymphatic tissues and macrophages, resulting in granulomatous inflammation. Underlying immunosuppression is usually thought to be responsible for this hematogenous dissemination. The organism grows readily in air and has distinctive colonial characteristics, but laboratories not familiar with horse isolates may fail to identify it correctly.

Pyogranulomatous lesions are the characteristic finding, and most cats have had primary involvement of an extremity. Localized swelling with ulcerations or fistulas and purulent drainage have been found. Pyothorax from mediastinal lymphadenitis is manifest by anorexia, weight loss, and dyspnea. Abdominal distention with a palpable fluid wave, hepatomegaly, and mesenteric lymphadenomegaly may be found.

Hematologic abnormalities may consist of leukocytosis with a left shift. Gram staining of the purulent discharge will show large pleomorphic gram-positive bacilli, which may be found inside macrophages. Thoracic or abdominal effusions are typically exudates with high protein (>3.5 g/dl) and nucleated cell counts (>10,000 cells/μl); the majority of cells are lymphocytes or nondegenerate neutrophils. Organisms may not be apparent.

Peripheral abscesses often have many sinus tracts with purulent drainage. Lymph nodes may be enlarged and necrotic with a similar discharge on sectioning. Histologically, the lesions have been pyogranulomatous or granulomatous with necrotic foci. Macrophages contain phagocytized gram-positive bacteria.

Surgical removal of extremity lesions is only temporarily effective, and new lesions commonly develop even after limb amputation. In cats, treatment with lincomycin and gentamicin has been most effective, and results with erythromycin have been variable (Table 35–6). A poor response has been seen in cats treated with penicillin and streptomycin, because the organism is poorly susceptible to these drugs, and in cats with lesions disseminated to many organs. In people with pneumonia, only long-term treatment with erythromycin, combined with either rifampin or vancomycin, has been the effective chemotherapy.[40] The standard, highly effective treatment in foals is prolonged oral administration of erythromycin and rifampin, and this combination can be recommended for cats although with greater toxicity. Infected cats have not been considered a source of infection for people, who usually acquire the infection from environmental exposure. Nevertheless, infected cats with discharges may pose some theoretical risk to immunocompromised owners.

LISTERIOSIS

Listeria monocytogenes is a pathogenic, β-hemolytic, gram-positive, rod-shaped facultative anaerobe that is morphologically indistinguishable from diphtheroids and may be mistaken for a contaminant in tissues. It is capable of growing over a wide temperature range. Although at least 16 serotypes of the organism exist, most infections are caused by only a few serotypes. As a ubiquitous saprophyte, *L. monocytogenes* can be isolated from soil, water, sewage, dust, and decaying vegetation. Commonly, it can be found in farm animal feed and silage. A study of fecal specimens from animals in Japan found a prevalence of 0.9% in dogs but no isolation in cats.[20]

L. monocytogenes differs from nonpathogenic species in that it possesses a hemolytic toxin, a factor that has been implicated in its virulence. This species is also able to persist as a facultative intracellular organism indefinitely in macrophages and to escape humoral immune responses. Underlying host immunosuppression, especially of cell-mediated immunity, appears to be an important factor in the intracellular persistence of the organism and in the development of clinical listeriosis.

Natural infection usually results from ingestion of contaminated foodstuffs; damage to the intestinal mucosal integrity is not necessary. Food-borne epidemics are associated with ingestion of contaminated feed or silage by domestic herbivores or of contaminated meat and dairy products by people. *Listeria* in dogs and cats is uncommon; when it occurs it is usually associated with ingestion of contaminated meat or meat by-products. Reports of septicemic listeriosis in dogs and cats after oral ingestion of contaminated foodstuffs have been rare. Pathogenic strains of *L. monocytogenes* can be recovered from the GI tracts of nonsymptomatic animals. Exposure in itself does not always produce disease. After penetration of the intestinal mucosa, *L. monocytogenes* produces a blood-borne bacteremia, localization in mononuclear phagocyte tissues, and septic embolization of many organs, including the CNS.

Clinical signs are due to the degree of intestinal inflammation and the sites of embolic microabscess formation. Fever, diarrhea, and vomiting have been most frequent. Neurologic signs have been apparent in some cases. Abortion was suspected in one bitch. Localized infections have also been infrequently reported. Peritonitis was reported in one cat as a result of a plant awn migrating through the bowel into the peritoneal cavity. Another cat developed an abscess of the front paw 2 weeks after an insect bite at the same location.

Cytologic evaluation of bone marrow from one dog with septicemia had coccobacilli within macrophages and neutrophils.[35] In the case of CNS infection, the organism may be recognized premortem with gram-stained sediment of CSF. Organisms appear as short intracellular and extracellular gram-positive bacilli to coccobacilli. Diagnosis of infection has usually been made at necropsy, because infected animals often succumb to the septicemia. Microabscess formations and focal necrotic lesions may be grossly or microscopically visible in many organs, especially the liver and spleen. Immunohistochemical staining of formalin-fixed, paraffin-embedded brain sections has been used to confirm infection.[42] In the absence of contaminating organisms, *L. monocytogenes* can grow and be identified within 36 hours on routine media at incubation temperature. Laboratory cultivation of the organism from a nonsterile site is difficult unless special precautions are taken. Selective media and cold cultivation (4°C) have been utilized to isolate the organism, but weeks of cold enrichment are needed owing to the slow growth at this temperature. Because the organism can be commonly isolated from the GI tract of nonsymptomatic animals, rectal cultures may not be meaningful.

Antimicrobial agents effective against *Listeria* are penicillin and ampicillin, erythromycin, chloramphenicol, rifampin, tetracycline, trimethoprim-sulfonamide, and aminoglycosides. The latter two drugs are bactericidal, and they are recommended as the first choices for clinical use. Gentamicin and tobramycin have more activity than the other aminoglycosides. The combination of gentamicin and ampicillin is considered the most desirable therapy, although high doses or alternative, widely distributed drugs such as trimethoprim-sulfonamide and rifampin may be needed to reach the CNS or to treat resistant infection.

Listeria in animals has not always been considered a public health risk because animals and people have exposure to the same source of environmental contamination. Nevertheless, human outbreaks have been associated with contact with food-producing animals or their products. Direct transmission from animals has occurred in veterinarians and farm workers through contact of unprotected skin or mucous membranes with infected animal tissues.[27] Most outbreaks occur in urban areas, where food-borne contamination is suspected. As a reverse zoonosis, listerial gastroenteritis was suspected in a litter of puppies and a newborn infant that received *Listeria*-infected milk discarded from the human mother's mammary gland.[17]

Table 35–6. Drug Therapy for* Rhodococcus equi *Infection in Cats

DRUG	DOSE[a] (mg/kg)	ROUTE	INTERVAL (hours)	DURATION (days)
Gentamicin	2	SC	12	5[b]
Lincomycin	20	PO	12	7–10[b]
Erythromycin	10	PO	8	14

[a]Dose per administration at specified interval.
[b]A second course of therapy may be used with a 1-week interval between courses.

ANTHRAX

Bacillus anthracis is a large (1 μm × 3–6 μm), gram-positive, spore-forming bacillus that causes anthrax, a soil-borne systemic disease of domestic animals. Tropical and subtropical regions of the world have alkaline soils with a high nitrogen content, which allows vegetative growth of spores released into the soil from carcasses of animals that died of anthrax.

Although peracute, fatal infections usually occur in herbivores. Carnivores such as the dog and cat are usually infected by ingesting raw meat of contaminated carcasses or animal by-products. Dogs are relatively resistant to infection.[8]

The infection in dogs and cats is usually manifest initially by local inflammation, necrosis, and edema of tissues of the upper GI tract, which first contact the swallowed organism. Swelling of the head and neck tissues is usually apparent. Subsequent spread to the local and mesenteric lymph nodes, spleen, and liver usually occurs.

Anthrax is a notifiable disease; however, necropsy of affected carcasses is not advisable, because resistant aerobic spores are released into the environment. Examination of stained smears of blood from a peripheral vein or of fine-needle aspirates is the most effective and safest means of making a diagnosis. The organisms can be isolated from these samples on routine media, provided materials are fresh.

The organism is very sensitive to penicillin, the treatment of choice if the infection is detected early (see Appendix 8 for dosages). From a public health standpoint, care must be taken in handling infected tissues or carcasses, because the organism can penetrate cuts in the skin, resulting in localized infection with subsequent dissemination. Infection in humans is almost always from infected animals or their by-products.

ERYSIPELOTHRIX INFECTIONS

Erysipelothrix rhusiopathiae (insidiosa) and *E. tonsillarum* are small gram-positive nonmotile, nonsporulating pleomorphic facultatively anaerobic rods. These organisms, distributed worldwide, are associated with swine production. *E. rhusiopathiae* is the causative agent of swine erysipelas and other diseases in animals such as joint-ill in sheep and cattle and septicemia in turkeys, ducks, and laboratory mice. The anaerobes can be cultured from the tonsils of clinically healthy swine, from the skin of freshwater and saltwater fish, and from the decomposing plant and animal matter in this environment. People occupationally exposed to these sources of bacteria may develop localized cutaneous or systemic infections.

Initially, the genus *Erysipelothrix* was thought to have a single species, *rhusiopathiae*, but biochemical and genetic analyses have identified *E. tonsillarum*, a nonpathogenic commensal of the tonsils of swine.[37] In dogs, endocarditis and septicemia were initially thought to be caused by *E. rhusiopathiae* after natural[18] and experimental[16] inoculation. However, all available isolates from endocarditis reported in dogs have been now reclassified as serovar 7 of *E. tonsillarum* and have been nonpathogenic for swine.[23, 37] Clinical signs of fever, shifting-leg lameness, and recent-onset heart murmur have been characteristic of infected dogs.

The isolated strains have been susceptible to penicillin and ampicillin in vitro but resistant to aminoglycosides and sulfonamides.[37] Most cases of *Erysipelothrix* bacteremia are associated with endocarditis; therefore, high doses of antimicrobials are recommended for at least a 6- to 8-week period. Relapses and reinfection are common in infected animals and people. Most human infections are acquired through occupational exposure among slaughterhouse workers, food handlers, and animal trappers.[27] Infected dogs do not seem to pose a public health hazard.

References

1. Bert F, Lambert-Zechovsky N. 1997. Septicemia caused by *Streptococcus canis* in a human. *J Clin Microbiol* 35:777–779.
2. Bjurstrom L. 1993. Aerobic bacteria occurring in the vagina of bitches with reproductive disorders. *Acta Vet Scand* 34:29–34.
3. Bjurstrom L, Linde-Forsberg C. 1992. Long term study of aerobic bacteria of the genital tract in breeding bitches. *Am J Vet Res* 53:665–669.
4. Bjurstrom L, Linde-Foresberg C. 1992. Long term study of aerobic bacteria of the genital tract in stud dogs. *Am J Vet Res* 53:670–673.
5. Bradlow A, Mitchell RG, Mowat AG. 1982. Group G streptococcal arthritis. *Rheumatol Rehab* 21:206–210.
6. Brückler J, Wibawan IWT, Lammler CH. 1990. Camp-reaction among skin isolates obtained from a dog with an acute squamous eczema. *J Vet Med* 37:769–770.
7. Collins JE, Bergeland ME, Lindeman CJ, et al. 1988. *Enterococcus (streptococcus) durans* adherence in the small intestine of a diarrheic pup. *Vet Pathol* 25:396–398.
8. Creel S, Marusha-Creel N, Matovelo JA, et al. 1995. The effects of anthrax on endangered African wild dogs. *J Zool* 236:199–209.
9. Crowder HR, Dorn CR, Smith RE. 1978. Group A *Streptococcus* in pets and group A streptococcal disease in man. *Int J Zoon* 5:45–54.
10. Devriese LA. 1991. Streptococcal ecovars associated with different animal species: epidemiological significance of serogroups and biotypes. *J Appl Bacteriol* 71:478–483.
11. Devriese LA, Cruz-Colque JI, DeHerdt P, et al. 1992. Identification and composition of the tonsillar and anal enterococcal and streptococcal flora of dogs and cats. *J Appl Bacteriol* 73:421–425.
12. Devriese LA, Haesebrouck F. 1991. *Enterococcus hirae* in different animal species. *Vet Rec* 129:391–392.
13. Devriese LA, Haesebrouck F. 1992. *Streptococcus suis* infections in horses and cats. *Vet Rec* 130:380.

13a. Devriese LA, Ieven M, Goossens H, et al. 1996. Presence of vancomycin-resistant enterococci in farm and pet animals. *Antimicrob Agents Chemother* 40:2285–2287.

13b. Dunne WM, Dunne BS, Smith D. 1996. Watch out where the huskies go. *Am Soc Microbiol News* 62:283.

14. Farca AM, Nebbia P, Re G. 1994. Potential of antibiotic activity by EDTA-tromethamine against three clinically isolated gram-positive resistant bacteria. An in vitro investigation. *Vet Res Commun* 18:1–6.

14a. Fischetti VA. 1997. The streptococcus and the host: present and future challenges. *Am Soc Microbiol News* 63:541–545.

15. Gates NL, Green JS. 1979. Epizootic streptococcal pneumonia in captive coyotes. *J Wildl Dis* 15:497–498.
16. Goudswaard J, Hartman EG, Jannaat JA, et al. 1973. *Erysipelothrix rhusiopathiae* strain 7, a causative agent of endocarditis and arthritis in the dog. *Tijdschr Diergeneeskd* 9:416–423.
17. Greene CE. 1990. Streptococcal and other gram-positive bacterial infections, pp 599–610. *In* Greene CE (ed), Infectious diseases of the dog and cat. WB Saunders, Philadelphia, PA.
18. Hoenig M, Gilletti DM. 1980. Endocarditis caused by *Erysipelothrix rhusiopathiae* in a dog. *J Am Vet Med Assoc* 176:326–327.
19. Iglauer F, Kunstyr I, Moerstedt R, et al. 1991. *Streptococcus canis* arthritis in a cat breeding colony. *J Exp Anim Sci* 34:59–65.
20. Iida T, Kanzaki M, Maruyama T, et al. 1991. Prevalence of *Listeria monocytogenes* in intestinal contents of healthy animals in Japan. *J Vet Med Sci* 53:873–875.
21. Jacobs JA, deKrom MCT, Kellens JTC, et al. 1993. Meningitis and sepsis due to group G streptococcus. *Eur J Clin Microbiol Infect Dis* 12:224–225.
22. Jergens AE, Moore FM, Prueter JC, et al. 1991. Adherent gram-positive cocci on the intestinal villi of two dogs with gastrointestinal disease. *J Am Vet Med Assoc* 198:1950–1952.
23. Kucsera G. 1979. Serological typing of *Erysipelothrix rhusiopathiae* strains and the epizootiological significance of the typing. *Acta Vet Acad Sci Hung* 27:19–28.
24. Makino S, Iinuma-Okada Y, Maruyama T, et al. 1993. Direct detection of *Bacillus anthracis* DNA in animals by polymerase chain reaction. *J Clin Microbiol* 31:547–551.
25. Mathews K. 1995. Personal communication. Ontario Veterinary College, Guelph, Ontario, Canada.

25a. McDonald LC, Kuehnert MJ, Tenover FC, et al. 1997. Vancomycin-resistant enterococci outside the health-care setting: prevalence, sources and public health implications. *Emerg Infect Dis* 3:311–317.

26. McGee ED, Fritz DL, Ezzell JW, et al. 1994. Anthrax in a dog. *Vet Pathol* 31:471–473.
27. McLauchlin J, Low JC. 1994. Primary cutaneous listeriosis in adults: an occupational disease of veterinarians and farmers. *Vet Rec* 135:615–617.

28. Messier S, Daminet S, Lemarchand T. 1995. *Streptococcus agalactiae* endocarditis with embolization in a dog. *Can Vet J* 36:703–704.
29. Miller CW, Prescott JF, Mathews KA. 1996. Further evidence of streptococcal toxic shock syndrome in pets. The author's response. *J Am Vet Med Assoc* 209:1995.
30. Miller CW, Prescott JF, Mathews KA, et al. 1996. Streptococcal toxic shock syndrome in dogs. *J Am Vet Med Assoc* 209:1421–1426.
30a. Prescott JF, DeWinter L. 1997. Canine streptococcal toxic shock syndrome and necrotizing fascitis. *Vet Rec* 140:263.
31. Prescott JF, Mathews K, Gyles CL, et al. 1995. Canine streptococcal toxic shock syndrome in Ontario: an emerging disease? *Can Vet J* 36:486–487.
32. Ramos-Vara JA, Briones V, Segales J, et al. 1994. Concurrent infection with *Streptococcus equisimilis* and Leishmania in a dog. *J Vet Diag Invest* 6:371–375.
33. Reitmeyer JC, Guthrie RK, Steele JH. 1991. Biochemical properties of Group G streptococci isolated from cats and man. *J Med Microbiol* 35:148–151.
34. Sager M, Remmers C. 1990. Some aspects of perinatal mortality in the dog. A clinical, bacteriological and pathological study. *Tierarztl Prax* 18:415–419.
35. Schroeder H, van Rensburg IBJ. 1993. Generalised *Listeria monocytogenes* infection in a dog. *J S Afr Vet Assoc* 64:133–136.
35a. Soedarmanto I, Lammler C. 1996. Comparative studies on streptococci of serological group G isolated from various origins. *Zentrabl Vet Med [B]* 43:513–523.
36. Stallings B, Ling GV, Lagenaur LA, et al. 1987. Septicemia and septic arthritis caused by *Streptococcus pneumoniae* in a cat: possible transmission from a child. *J Am Vet Med Assoc* 191:703–304.
37. Takahashi T, Fujisawa T, Tamura Y, et al. 1992. DNA relatedness among *Erysipelothrix rhusiopathiae* strains representing all twenty-three serovars and *Erysipelothrix tonsillarum*. *Int J Syst Bacteriol* 42:469–473.
38. Takahashi T, Tamura Y, Yoshimura H, et al. 1993. *Erysipelothrix tonsillarum* isolated from dogs with endocarditis in Belgium. *Res Vet Sci* 54:264–265.
39. Takai S, Sasaki Y, Ikeda T, et al. 1994. Virulence of *Rhodococcus equi* isolates from patients with and without AIDS. *J Clin Microbiol* 32:457–460.
39a. VanBelkum A, vanden Braak N, Thomassen R, et al. 1996. Vancomycin-resistant enterococci in cats and dogs. *Lancet* 348:1038–1039.
40. Vestbo J, Lundgren JD, Gaub J, et al. 1991. Severe *Rhodococcus equi* pneumonia: case report and literature review. *Eur J Clin Microbiol* 10:762–768.
41. Wagner JG, Schlievert PM, Assimacopoulos AP, et al. 1996. Acute group G streptococcal myositis associated with streptococcal toxic shock syndrome: a case report review. *Clin Infect Dis* 23:1159–1161.
42. Weinstock D, Horton SB, Rowland PH. 1995. Rapid diagnosis of *Listeria monocytogenes* by immunohistochemistry in formalin-fixed brain tissue. *Vet Pathol* 32:193–195.
43. White S. 1996. Further evidence of streptococcal toxic shock syndrome in pets. *J Am Vet Med Assoc* 209:1994–1995.
44. Wilson KS, Maroney SA, Gander RM. 1995. The family pet as an unlikely source of group A beta-hemolytic streptococcal infection in humans. *Pediatr Infect Dis J* 14:372–375.

Chapter **36**

Staphylococcal Infections

Hollis Utah Cox

ETIOLOGY

Staphylococci are facultatively anaerobic, gram-positive cocci. Their principal habitats are the skin and some mucous membranes of mammals and birds.[22] Staphylococci are classified into 28 species and several subspecies on the basis of genotypic differences and consideration of habitat or pathogenic processes.[18, 22] There is good evidence that the species of *Staphylococcus* have evolved together with their hosts.[22] Although geographic differences between the distribution of *Staphylococcus* species in apparently similar human populations have been demonstrated, studies comparing dog and cat populations have not been reported.[22] All species of staphylococci isolated from normal animals are potentially pathogenic. However, individual species display a wide spectrum of virulence, host preference, and site specificity, and relatively few species are commonly isolated from infections of dogs and cats.[17, 26, 32, 34] Host-adapted species may transiently colonize another host species when contact between hosts is frequent or infections are present. Staphylococci are readily acquired from environments (e.g., fomites, soil, air, and water) associated with animals and from a variety of animal products. Staphylococci are halophilic bacteria that survive well in the environment because they are among the more resistant of the nonsporulating bacteria to drying and disinfection.

Staphylococci are not inherently invasive and colonize the intact epithelium of healthy animals without causing disease. In this sense, normal animals are subclinical carriers of both transient or resident colonizing staphylococci. Rather, as opportunistic pathogens, they invade epithelium damaged by traumatic insult (e.g., incisions, wounds), other infections (e.g., demodicosis, dermatophytosis), or clinical conditions (e.g., seborrhea, thyroid dysfunction). Disease, therefore, results from a disturbance in the natural host-parasite balance. Immunocompromised hosts are more susceptible to clinical illness as a result of infection. German shepherd dogs develop severe recurrent staphylococcal pyoderma.

Knowledge of the pathogenesis of staphylococcal infections is limited. Although many underlying causes are known to predispose animals to canine pyoderma, the specific host defect that allows staphylococci to proliferate and the bacterial factors that contribute to lesion development and tissue damage are not known. Virulence is often equated with the presence of specific cell envelope components and extracellular toxins and enzymes that potentially produce a wide variety of biologic effects on the host after tissue invasion. None of these virulence factors alone has been consistently implicated in clinical infections, although intradermal injections of staphylococcal extracts and protein A produce epidermal lesions and histologic changes similar to those observed in clinical cases of canine superficial pyoderma and pustular dermatitis.[19] Attempts to determine whether subpopulations of virulent and nonvirulent staphylococci reside on dogs are inconclusive. Staphylococci can produce various exotoxins that may have immunologic effects. On the basis of analysis of digests of DNA after restriction endonuclease treatment, *Staphylococcus intermedius* isolates from canine pyoderma differ from *S. intermedius* isolates from normal dogs but do not differ in recognized virulence factors or exoproteins.[1] If dogs are colonized by more than one strain of *S. intermedius*, it appears that the recognized toxins are not important virulence markers and an as yet unrecognized factor may be involved.[1]

Coagulase, an enzyme present in most clinically significant staphylococci, polymerizes fibrinogen and clots plasma. Although it is not toxic itself, its presence in a strain correlates with the presence of the other recognized virulence factors or extracellular products. *S. aureus*, *S. intermedius*, and some *S. hyicus* produce coagulase and are generally more pathogenic than *S. epidermidis*, *S. xylosus*, and *S. felis*, which lack this enzyme. Although coagulase-negative staphylococci are constituents of the normal microflora, they are capable of producing infections in hosts that are immunosuppressed by the host factors or invasive techniques. Protein A, an extracellular or a cell-bound protein produced by some canine and feline strains of *S. intermedius*, may enhance virulence by activating complement and by nonspecifically binding to immunoglobulins. These and other biologic effects may provoke various inflammatory and allergic responses, particularly delayed hypersensitivity, that intensify the pyogenic process and heighten the damage produced by staphylococcal infections. Some of these responses may be related to the high concentrations of circulating immune complexes that are found in dogs with recurrent pyoderma and pyoderma secondary to generalized demodicosis.[8, 21] Complex polysaccharide capsules and slime layers (glycocalyx) produced by many strains of staphylococci may also enhance virulence by promoting bacterial adherence, inhibiting host phagocytosis, and resisting antibacterial drugs.

Transmissible plasmids are common in human strains of *S. aureus*. They may carry genes for virulence factors and for antimicrobial resistance to penicillin, ampicillin, amoxicillin, lincomycin, erythromycin, tetracycline, chloramphenicol, cephalosporin, kanamycin, and gentamicin. Strains of *S. intermedius* infrequently carry similar plasmids, and most antibiotic resistance resides in chromosomal genes.[10, 23, 30] The antimicrobial susceptibility patterns of clinically important isolates of staphylococci from dogs have not changed considerably. However, the potential exists for transfer of virulence and antimicrobial resistance genes from human strains of *S. aureus* to animal strains of *S. intermedius*. Although not common, multiresistant staphylococci are sometimes isolated from dogs with deep pyoderma or a history of antibiotic therapy. Nosocomial transfer is known to modify the staphylococcal flora because nasal carrier rates for coagulase-positive staphylococci increase considerably with prolonged hospitalization of humans and dogs.

Humans are the natural hosts for *S. aureus*, which colonizes the nasal passages of up to 40% of healthy adults and rarely other body sites in the absence of dermatoses. Although variants adapted to other hosts (ruminants, horses, and pigs) occur, *S. aureus* comprises less than 10% of clinical isolates from normal dogs and cats and apparently is not indigenous or site specific in these hosts.

The predominant staphylococcal species of the resident bacterial microflora of dogs is *S. intermedius*. Specific biotypes have been persistently isolated in temporal studies from the hair coat and mucous membranes of individual dogs. However, the subpopulations at these two sites cannot be differentiated on the basis of antibiotic or phage susceptibility profiles, ribotyping, or other techniques.[1, 9, 11–14, 24] Although agreement as to the natural anatomic habitat for *S. intermedius* is still not reached, cultural studies have clarified the situation. After birth, puppies acquire staphylococcal flora gradually from their dam over the first few weeks of life.[2] The oral cavity is the predominant site to be colonized, followed by abdominal skin and nasal and anal mucosae. Large populations in adult dogs reside at moist sites such as the nasal, anal, and oral mucosae and in rather occluded areas of the interdigital spaces and the ear canal.[3, 6, 11] *S. intermedius* is found on the genital mucosae of breeding bitches almost exclusively after parturition.[2, 5] Lesser populations found at the skin surface and the distal hair coat probably indicate contamination or transient colonization rather than true resident status.[4, 28] Because staphylococci can survive in inhospitable areas that are drier, more salty, and less humid, they are able to displace less tolerant species.[6] Other studies have suggested the possibility of a resident population within the pilosebaceous units from which secondary surface colonization can occur. The staphylococci on the distal hair shaft are contaminants whose origin is the resident population on the mucosae.[11] A temporal study compared the carriage of *S. intermedius* on normal dogs with that of atopic dogs in clinical remission and concluded that atopic lesions had become secondarily colonized from mucous membrane sites (nares, oral cavity, and anus).[28] When secondary staphylococcal infections were resolved, significant differences in isolation of *S. intermedius* at any single site of the two groups of dogs was not evident. Dogs with pyoderma had significantly denser populations of *S. intermedius* at mucosal sites than did healthy household pets, a further indication that mucosal sites are the sources for skin contamination. However, results from one study indicated that nasal carriage was dependent on skin colonization.[12]

The predominant resident staphylococcal species of cats are *S. felis* and *S. xylosus*.[17] *S. intermedius* and *S. aureus* are isolated primarily from the hair coat of household cats and rarely from mucous membranes or from cats confined in a cattery. Apparently, they are transient residents acquired from contact with people or other animals. In general, a less heterogeneous population of staphylococci is associated with cattery cats when compared with household cats or dogs.

CLINICAL FINDINGS

Coagulase-positive staphylococci are most frequently isolated from pyogenic infections of dogs and, less commonly, cats. As significant pathogens, they can affect every organ system independently or concurrently, but are most common in abscesses and infections of the skin, eyes, ears, respiratory and genitourinary tracts, skeleton, and joints. In dogs, *S. intermedius* is the most common staphylococcal species isolated from pyoderma, otitis externa, diskospondylitis, bacteremia, conjunctivitis, and urolithiasis. The infection sites are similar for cats; however, *S. felis* is the most frequent (45%) species, whereas *S. aureus* (13%) and *S. intermedius* (10%) are less common.[17]

DIAGNOSIS

Staphylococcal infections can be diagnosed presumptively by direct microscopy. Staining of a clinical specimen with Gram's stain or rapid cytologic stain will reveal neutrophils and cocci arranged singly or in pairs, short chains, or, rarely, irregular clusters. For culture, collection methods other than swabbing should be used whenever possible and should be designed to avoid superficial contamination. Surfaces of intact pustules, furuncles, or abscesses should be gently cleaned with alcohol, and exudate directly aspirated or expressed onto a sterile swab without touching the skin (see Specimen Collection, Chapter 33). Punch biopsies are suitable procedures for both superficial and deep skin infections. Ear specimens are best obtained with a swab protected by a sterile otoscope cone inserted to the level of the horizontal ear canal. Before obtaining blood by venipuncture or urine by cystocentesis for culture, hair should be shaved and skin scrubbed as if for surgery. Respiratory tract specimens should be taken by transtracheal aspiration technique, bronchoscopic wash, or percutaneous transthoracic aspiration to bypass the oral flora. Specimens from deep-seated infections are often taken by direct biopsy or during surgery, such as aspirates or bone fragments curetted in cases of diskospondylitis.

Staphylococci in clinical specimens survive for up to 48 hours when kept cool (4°C [39.2°F]), particularly on commercial swabs containing a holding medium. Clinically significant staphylococci and normal flora contaminants grow best aerobically and may overgrow other pathogens when specimens are cultured on general-purpose nonselective media.

Serologic assays, especially for antibodies reactive with teichoic acid or nucleases, are used as clinical aids in the diagnosis and management of bacteremia, endocarditis, and other deep-seated staphylococcal infections in people. However, their use and interpretation of results are controversial. Dogs with deep recurrent staphylococcal skin infections have high serum antistaphylococcal IgG levels compared with clinically unaffected dogs.[21, 31a] Dogs with superficial pyoderma secondary to atopy had high IgE levels. Despite these findings, it is unlikely that serotesting will be adapted for clinical use in animal infections.[16] High titers are more a reflection of bacterial hypersensitivity that perpetuates the inflammatory response.

THERAPY

Dosages for antimicrobials used to treat staphylococcal infections are listed in the Drug Formulary (Appendix 8) and Table 85–3. Staphylococci are rarely resistant (< 5% of isolates) to first-generation cephalosporins (cephalexin, cefadroxil), β-lactamase–resistant synthetic penicillins (oxacillin, dicloxacillin, and clavulanate–potentiated amoxicillin), gentamicin, tobramycin, enrofloxacin, bacitracin, and polymyxin B.[25] These should be the drugs of first choice when culture and susceptibility results are unavailable and staphylococcal infection is suspected. Resistance to trimethoprim-sulfonamide combinations, chloramphenicol, and tylosin is relatively infrequent (6–19% of isolates).[31] Resistance to lincomycin, clindamycin, and erythromycin is relatively frequent (20–37% of isolates). Clinical isolates of staphylococci from dogs and cats are most frequently resistant (40–83%) to penicillin, ampicillin, amoxicillin, neomycin, and tetracycline.[18a, 18b, 23a] Antimicrobials for which resistance is common should not be given for staphylococcal infections unless an isolate is shown to be susceptible by antimicrobial testing or by lack of β-lactamase production. Deep pyoderma or a history of antimicrobial therapy for staphylococcal infection indicates a need to culture regardless of the antimicrobial agent being considered for therapy.[23] Increased resistance of *S. intermedius* to chloramphenicol, clindamycin, and erythromycin has been associated with previous unspecified antimicrobial therapy of canine pyoderma. However, during a 1-year study in which dogs with recurrent folliculitis were treated with repeated courses of cephalexin, antimicrobial susceptibility patterns of *S. intermedius* from lesions and noninfected body sites were unchanged. Clindamycin has been shown to be efficacious in the treatment of experimentally induced *S. aureus* osteomyelitis in dogs.[7]

References

1. Allaker RP, Garrett N, Kent L, et al. 1993. Characterisation of *Staphylococcus intermedius* isolates from canine pyoderma and from healthy carriers by SDS-PAGE of exoproteins, immunoblotting and restriction endonuclease digest analysis. *J Med Microbiol* 39:429–433.
2. Allaker RP, Jensen L, Lloyd DH, et al. 1992. Colonization of neonatal puppies by staphylococci. *Br Vet J* 148:523–528.
3. Allaker RP, Lloyd DH, Bailey RM. 1992. Population size and frequency of staphylococci at mucocutaneous sites on healthy dogs. *Vet Rec* 130:303–304.
4. Allaker RP, Lloyd DH, Simpson AI. 1992. Occurrence of *Staphylococcus intermedius* on the hair and skin of normal dogs. *Res Vet Sci* 52:174–176.
5. Bjurstrom L, Linde-Forsberg C. 1992. Long-term study of aerobic bacteria of the genital tract of breeding bitches. *Am J Vet Res* 53:665–669.
6. Chesney CJ. 1996. Mapping the canine skin: a study of coat relative humidity in Newfoundland dogs. *Vet Dermatol* 7:35–41.
7. Cox HU, Hoskins JD. 1990. Staphylococcal infection, pp 611–613. *In* Greene CE (ed), Infectious disease of the dog and cat. WB Saunders, Philadelphia, PA.
8. DeBoer DJ. 1994. Immunomodulatory effects of staphylococcal antigen and antigen-antibody complexes on canine mononuclear and polymorphonuclear leukocytes. *Am J Vet Res* 55:1690–1696.
8a. Edwards VM, Deringer JR, Callantine SD, et al. 1997. Characterization of the canine type C enterotoxin produced by *Staphylococcus intermedius* pyoderma isolates. *Infect Immun* 65:2346–2352.
9. Greene RT, Lammler C. 1993. *Staphylococcus intermedius*: current knowledge on a pathogen of veterinary importance. *Zentralbl Veterinarmed B* 40:206–214.
10. Greene RT, Schwarz S. 1992. Small antibiotic resistance plasmids in *Staphylococcus intermedius*. *Int J Med Microbiol Virol Parasitol Infect Dis* 276:380–389.
11. Harvey RG, Lloyd DH. 1994. The distribution of *Staphylococcus intermedius* and coagulase-negative staphylococci on the hair, skin surface, within the hair follicles and on the mucous membranes of dogs. *Vet Dermatol* 5:75–81.
12. Harvey RG, Noble WC, Ferguson EA. 1993. A comparison of lincomycin hydrochloride and clindamycin hydrochloride in the treatment of superficial pyoderma in dogs. *Vet Rec* 132:351–353.
13. Hesselbarth J, Schwarz S. 1995. Comparative ribotyping of *Staphylococcus intermedius* from dogs, pigeons, horses, and mink. *Vet Microbiol* 45:11–17.
14. Hesselbarth J, Witte W, Cuny C, et al. 1994. Characterization of *Staphylococcus intermedius* from healthy dogs and cases of superficial pyoderma by DNA restriction endonuclease patterns. *Vet Microbiol* 41:259–266.
15. Hoekstra KA, Paulton RJ. 1996. Antibiotic sensitivity of *Staphylococcus aureus* and *Staphylococcus intermedius* of canine and feline origin. *Lett Appl Microbiol* 22:192–194.
16. Hoie S, Fossum K. 1989. Antibodies to staphylococcal DNase in sera from different animal species, including humans. *J Clin Microbiol* 27:2444–2447.
17. Igimi S, Atobe H, Tohya Y, et al. 1994. Characterization of the most frequently encountered *Staphylococcus* species in cats. *Vet Microbiol* 39:255–260.
18. Igimi S, Takahashi E, Mitsuoka T. 1990. *Staphylococcus Schleiferi subsp. coagulans subsp. nov.*, isolated from the external auditory meatus of dogs with external ear otitis. *Int J Syst Bacteriol* 40:409–411.
18a. Kruse H, Hofshagen M, Thoresen SI, et al. 1996. The antimicrobial susceptibility of staphylococcal species isolated from canine dermatitis. *Vet Res Commun* 20:205–214.
18b. Lloyd DH, Lamport AI, Feeney C. 1996. Sensitivity to antibiotics amongst cutaneous and mucosal isolates of canine pathogenic staphylococci in the UK 1980–1996. *Vet Dermatol* 7:171–175.
19. Mason IS, Lloyd DH. 1995. The macroscopic and microscopic effects of intradermal injection of crude and purified staphylococcal extracts on canine skin. *Vet Dermatol* 6:197–204.
20. Mason IS, Mason KV, Lloyd DH. 1996. A review of the biology of canine skin with respect to the commensals *Staphylococcus intermedius*, *Demodex canis* and *Malassezia pachydermatis*. *Vet Dermatol* 7:119–132.
21. Morales CA, Schultz, DeBoer DJ. 1994. Antistaphylococcal antibodies in dogs with recurrent staphylococcal pyoderma. *Vet Immunol Immunopathol* 42:137–147.
22. Noble WC. 1993. Staphylococci on the skin, pp 135–152. *In* Noble WC (ed), The skin microflora and microbial skin disease. Cambridge University Press, Cambridge, England.
23. Noble WC, Kent LE. 1993. Antibiotic resistance in *Staphylococcus intermedius* isolated from cases of pyoderma in the dog. *Vet Dermatol* 3:71–74.
23a. Oluoch AO, Weisiger R, Siegel AM, et al. 1996. Trends of bacterial infections in dogs. Characterization of *Staphylococcus intermedius* isolates (1990-1992). *Canine Pract* 21:12–19.
24. Overturf GD, Talan DA, Singer K, et al. 1991. Phage typing of *Staphylococcus intermedius*. *J Clin Microbiol* 29:373–375.
25. Paradis M, Lemay S, Scott DW, et al. 1990. Efficacy of enrofloxacin in the treatment of canine bacterial pyoderma. *Vet Dermatol* 1:123–127.
26. Pedersen K, Wegener HC. 1995. Antimicrobial susceptibility and rRNA gene restriction patterns among *Staphylococcus intermedius* from healthy dogs and from dogs suffering from pyoderma or otitis. *Acta Vet Scand* 36:335–342.
27. Reiman KA, Evans MG, Chalifoux LV, et al. 1989. Clinicopathologic characterization of canine juvenile cellulitis. *Vet Pathol* 26:499–504.
28. Saijonmaa-Koulumies LE, Lloyd DH. 1995. Carriage of bacteria antagonistic towards *Staphylococcus intermedius* on canine skin and mucosal surfaces. *Vet Dermatol* 6:187–194.

29. Saijonmaa-Koulumies LE, Lloyd DH. 1996. Colonization of the canine skin with bacteria. *Vet Dermatol* 7:153–162.
30. Schwartz S, Werckenthin C, Pinter L, et al. 1995. Chloramphenicol resistance in *Staphylococcus intermedius* from a single veterinary centre: evidence for plasmid and chromosomal location of the resistance genes. *Vet Microbiol* 43:151–159.
31. Scott DW, Miller WH, Cayatte SM, et al. 1994. Efficacy of tylosin tablets for the treatment of pyoderma due to *Staphylococcus intermedius* infection in dogs. *Can Vet J* 35:617–621.
31a. Shearer DH, Day MJ. 1997. Aspects of the humoral immune response to *Staphylococcus intermedius* in dogs with superficial pyoderma, deep pyoderma, and anal furunculosis. *Vet Immunol Immunopathol* 58:107–120.
32. Shimizu A, Berkhoff HA, Kloos WE, et al. 1996. Genomic DNA fingerprinting using pulsed-field gel electrophoresis of *Staphylococcus intermedius* isolated from dogs. *Am J Vet Res* 57:1458–1462.
33. Wegener HC, Pedersen K. 1992. Variations in antibiograms and plasmid profiles among multiple isolates of *Staphylococcus intermedius* from pyoderma in dogs. *Acta Vet Scand* 33:391–394.
34. Woldehiwet Z, Jones JJ. 1990. Species distribution of coagulase-positive staphylococci isolated from dogs. *Vet Rec* 126:485.

Chapter 37

Gram-Negative Bacterial Infections

Stephen A. Kruth

ETIOLOGY

Gram-negative bacteria fall into a number of heterogenous phylogenetic groups that are, in some cases, distantly related. In addition to the cytoplasmic membrane and peptidoglycan cell wall, gram-negative bacteria have an outer membrane composed of lipoprotein. The outer surface of this membrane contains a lipopolysaccharide (LPS), which has a lipid portion (lipid A) embedded in the membrane with a polysaccharide portion protruding out from the bacterial surface (O antigen) (Fig. 37–1). These structures are important virulence determinants for gram-negative bacteria.

Many gram-negative bacteria can be pathogenic in dogs and cats. Several of these bacteria are discussed in other chapters (*Pasteurella* [Chapters 52 and 53], *Bordetella* [Chapters 6 and 16], and *Salmonella* [Chapter 39]). This chapter focuses on *Escherichia coli, Proteus, Klebsiella,* and *Pseudomonas. E. coli, Proteus,* and *Klebsiella* are members of the family Enterobacteriaceae, facultative anaerobic gram-negative bacteria that are natural inhabitants of the intestinal tract of mammals. *Pseudomonas* is a ubiquitous gram-negative bacterium that is found in soil, water, decaying vegetation, and animals.

Classification

There are 28 genera of Enterobacteriaceae, with more than 100 well-defined species. Important species include *E. coli, Proteus mirabilis, P. vulgaris,* and *Klebsiella pneumoniae.* The most common pseudomonad in North America is *Pseudomonas aeruginosa.* Two other species are of importance in tropical regions. *Pseudomonas pseudomallei* is a soil organism found in the Far East, central Africa, and Australia. In dogs and cats it can cause syndromes ranging from a benign pulmonary form to a lethal systemic form (see Chapter 46). *P. mallei* is the cause of glanders in horses living in Asia, eastern Europe,

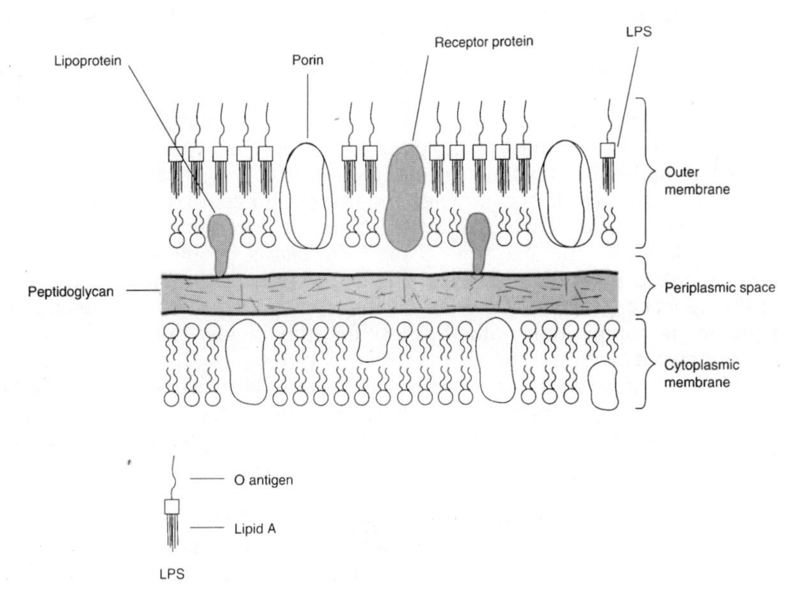

Figure 37–1. Structure of the cell surface of a gram-negative bacterium. (From Salyers AA, Whitt DD: Bacterial pathogenesis: a molecular approach. ASM Press, 1994, p 342. Reprinted with permission.)

and Africa. The cat is especially prone to infection from the horse reservoir (see Chapter 46).

Antigenic Structure

An internationally recognized serologic classification scheme has been developed for the Enterobacteriaceae on the basis of antigenic differences in highly variable bacterial surface molecules. The *serogroup* is determined by the *O antigens*, sugars on the most external part of LPS. The *serotype* is determined by the flagellar *H antigens*. Additionally, *K antigens* can be identified in strains with a capsule. The antigenic formula of the strain indicates the presence of specific antigens (e.g., 055:K5:H21). However, for most strains, only O and H antigens are determined. At least 170 different serogroups have been identified for *E. coli*, and there is some correlation between serogroup and virulence.

EPIDEMIOLOGY

These bacteria are commonly isolated from spontaneously arising infections of several different organ systems of dogs and cats. Isolates can be endogenous or exogenous to the individual. They can be the cause of sepsis, nosocomial infections, and opportunistic infections in immunocompromised animals.[37] These types of infections are increasing in frequency with the use of new antibiotics, invasive procedures, and immunosuppressive therapies.

PATHOGENESIS

Some strains of *E. coli* are true enteropathogens; however, most *E. coli, Klebsiella, Proteus*, and *Pseudomonas* are opportunistic pathogens. The pathogenicity of the Enterobacteriaceae depends on the presence of various *virulence factors* being expressed by the organism. It is the set of virulence genes carried by the organism that make it pathogenic, not its genus or species designation. Examples of virulence factors follow.

The establishment of infection depends on bacteria adhering to an epithelium. *Adhesins* are located on bacterial pili (or fimbriae)—slender, proteinaceous external structures that facilitate attachment to host cells. Colonization factor antigens I and II (CFA-I, CFA-II) are specific pilus adhesins-hemagglutins that promote colonization by some enteropathogens. Another fimbrial antigen is the vir antigen, which is associated with septicemia in some species. Bacterial *capsules* are polysaccharides, which protect the outer membrane from the membrane attack complex of the complement cascade and inhibit the attachment of phagocytic cells. Colonization with *Pseudomonas* occurs when the fibronectin coat covering host cells is disrupted by infection or mechanical trauma. The pili and exozyme S of *Pseudomonas* promote attachment to epithelial cells, and the extracellular slime is antiphagocytic. *Siderophores*, such as aerobactin, aid the bacterium in its competition with the host for iron in low-iron environments.

The production of a variety of toxins is important in the pathogenesis of gram-negative infections. Secreted α-hemolysin damages host cell membranes. *Endotoxins* (LPS) activate the complement cascade and stimulate various cytokine cascades. Excessive activation of these systems leads to the systemic response of endotoxic shock (see Chapter 38). *Pseudomonas* variably produces collagenase, lecithinase, lipase, proteases (elastase, LasA protein, and alkaline protease), hemolysins, fibrinolysin, leukocidin (also called cytotoxin), and enterotoxin. Many stains also secrete *exotoxin A*, a cytotoxin that causes tissue necrosis, allowing the organism to colonize deep tissues in burn and trauma cases. As in the Enterobacteriaceae, *Pseudomonas* LPS can act as a relatively weak endotoxin.

Virulence Factors Associated With *E. coli* Intestinal Infections

The virulence factors of *E. coli* have been especially well characterized. The cytotoxins and enterotoxins have been comprehensively reviewed by Gyles.[11]

Enteropathogenic *E. coli* (EPEC). EPEC adhere to mucosal cells of the small and large bowel, causing loss of microvilli ("effacement" or "attaching and effacing" lesions) and formation of filamentous actin pedestals or cuplike structures under the organisms. An inflammatory response is associated with the changes in microvillous morphology. EPEC also occasionally invade mucosal cells. Clinically, EPEC cause watery diarrhea as a result of invasion of host cells and alteration of signal transduction systems rather than as a result of production of toxin. Normal canine intestinal epithelium can undergo attaching and effacing changes when infected with EPEC 0111 or EPEC 0118 in tissue culture.[13, 31] EPEC infections have been reported in dogs[3, 6, 9, 31] and cats.[24]

Enterotoxigenic *E. coli* (ETEC). ETEC adhere to small intestinal mucosal cells and produce symptoms by elaborating toxins. There are no histologic changes in mucosal tissues to which the bacteria are attached, and there is little inflammation. Heat-labile toxins (LT) and heat-stable (ST) toxins have been well characterized. Heat-labile toxins (LT-I, LT-II) alter adenyl cyclase activity in epithelial cells of the small intestine, resulting in inhibition of absorption of sodium and chloride in villous epithelial cells and in active secretion of chloride by crypt cells, causing extensive loss of water and chlorides. LT toxin was identified in two dogs with enteritis[21] and in 1 of 13 dogs with *E. coli*--associated enteritis[9]; however, other investigators were unable to find LT genes in *E. coli* isolated from a large number of normal and diarrheic dogs.[12]

Heat-stable toxins (STa, STb) are a family of small toxins, some forms of which deregulate guanylyl cyclase, with resultant fluid secretion in similar fashion to that induced by LT. Other forms stimulate cyclic nucleotide–independent secretion. ST secreting *E. coli* have been isolated from dogs and cats with enteritis,[1a, 33] and one case series comparing the rate of isolation from normal and diarrheic dogs supports a causal association.[12]

Enterohemorrhagic *E. coli* (EHEC). These forms bind tightly to epithelial cells and produce the same type of attachment-effacement lesions as seen with EPEC. EHEC are minimally invasive but do incite an inflammatory response and preferentially localize in the large intestine. EHEC produce *verotoxins* (VT or Shiga-like toxins), of which there are two major antigenic forms (VT-I and VT-II). VT inhibit protein synthesis by interfering with 28S ribosomal RNA, leading to damage of vascular endothelium in target organs. In humans, EHEC infections have been associated with diarrhea, hemorrhagic colitis, and hemolytic-uremic syndrome (HUS). *E. coli* secreting VT-II have been isolated from stools of normal dogs,[4] and a case-control study suggested that VT-II–positive isolates may be causally associated with diarrhea in dogs, while VT-I–positive isolates are carried, but do not appear to cause diarrhea.[12] In humans, HUS is associated with 0157:H7 serotype of *E. coli*. Holloway and colleages[17] described a syndrome similar to HUS in three dogs with acute renal failure after an episode of hemorrhagic gastroenteritis. There was evidence of microangiopathic hemolytic anemia in these dogs. Isolation of *E. coli* was attempted in only one dog; however, it was untypable and did not produce VT.[17] VT producing *E. coli* may be responsible for the glomerular lesions characteristic of cutaneous and renal glomerular vasculopathy of greyhounds ("Alabama rot").[14] *E. coli* isolates were evaluated from 113 cats with diarrhea and 66 normal cats for VT toxins and genes. The prevalence of verocytotoxigenic *E. coli* in the total population was 5%; there was no difference between normal cats and cats with diarrhea, suggesting that cats carry VT-producing strains but that these strains are not pathogenic in cats.[28]

Enteroinvasive *E. coli*. These bacteria actively invade colonic cells and spread laterally to adjacent cells and lymphatics, ultimately leading to septicemia and endotoxemia, especially in neonates. Diagnosis is made by isolating *E. coli* from normally sterile sites, such as bone marrow, spleen, or blood.

Cytotoxic Necrotizing Factors (CNFs). CNFs are protein toxins originally called vir toxin. CNF1 and CNF2 have been associated with diarrhea, bacteremia, and urinary tract infections (UTIs) in humans. Hemolytic *E. coli* strains isolated from the stools of healthy cats produced CNF1,[5] and Prada and colleagues[25] described dogs with gastroenteritis from which strains of *E. coli* that elaborated CNF1 were isolated.

Uropathogenic *E. coli* and *P. mirabilis*

Most urinary infections result from complications of urinary stasis and the ascension of coliform bacteria from the periurethral region. Nonpathogenic and opportunistic organisms that lack virulence factors are involved. In contrast, some strains of *E. coli* are uropathogenic in dogs and cats. These organisms have little difficulty in colonizing the urethra ascending the urinary tract. The major determinant of their pathogenicity is the ability to adhere to the uroepithelium with special pili. LPS and pili can also recruit neutrophils and induce release of cytokines into the bladder lumen, leading to a marked inflammatory response and characteristic signs of urgency, discomfort, and hematuria. Exotoxins, especially hemolysins, may also be important in the development of clinical signs. Iron acquisition is also an important virulence factor, as are bacterial capsules and antiphagocytic systems. CNF1 has been found in strains associated with severe UTI in dogs.[23] Senior and coworkers[27] studied the serotype, hemolysin production, and adherence characteristics of 82 strains of *E. coli* isolated from dogs with UTIs. These strains were found to differ from human uropathogenic strains with regard to clonotype, variety, and proportion of various receptors that expressed adhesions attached to uroepithelial cells.[27] *E. coli* from dogs with pyometra and/or UTIs are derived from the endogenous fecal flora.[32] The presence of any adherence factors among these strains was not determined. *P. mirabilis* strains isolated from the urine of dogs have been characterized and found to be similar to human uropathogenic *P. mirabilis* strains.[10]

CLINICAL FINDINGS

All of these organisms can colonize normal tissues and maintain a commensal relationship in dogs and cats (Table 37–1). Most of these bacteria are opportunists, requiring alterations in local or systemic immune functions for disease to develop. However, clinical disease cannot develop unless the colonizing strain carries at least some virulence factors. Examples of clinically significant infections with these organisms are listed in Table 37–1.

Some important clinical associations have been reported for these bacteria. For instance, *E. coli* septicemia and lesions consistent with adult respiratory distress syndrome were diagnosed in a high percentage of canine parvovirus cases examined by necropsy.[30] *E. coli* and *Klebsiella* neonatal septicemia have been identified in puppies, with signs of failure to gain weight, dyspnea, cyanosis, hematuria, and sloughing of extremities, or acute death.[22] *Klebsiella* produces urease, which splits urea to ammonia; this can damage the uroepithelium and alter urine pH, favoring the development of struvite uroliths. *Klebsiella* is also associated with extensive, necrotizing, consolidating pneumonias. Gastroenteritis and fatal sepsis caused by *K. pneumoniae* have been observed in dogs fed a commercially frozen, meat dog food.[25a] *Pseudomonas* is pathogenic only when it colonizes areas devoid of normal

***Table 37–1. Examples of Sites of Isolation of Enterobacteriaceae and* Pseudomonas**

NORMAL TISSUES[a]	*E. COLI* INFECTIONS	*KLEBSIELLA* INFECTIONS	*PROTEUS* INFECTIONS	*PSEUDOMONAS* INFECTIONS
Gut Nasal cavity Mouth, tonsils, oral pharynx Trachea, bronchi (*Klebsiella* only) Distal urethra, prepuce, semen, vagina Conjunctiva	Gut (enteropathogenic strains) Small intestine bacterial overgrowth Cholecystitis, cholangitis, cholelithiasis, hepatic abscess Peritonitis Metritis, pyometra Mastitis, deep pyoderma, anal sacculitis Osteomyelitis Conjunctivitis, keratitis Tonsillitis, pharyngitis Urinary tract infections (lower, prostatitis, and pyelonephritis) Endocarditis Pneumonia, pleuritis Septicemia, including neonatal septicemia	Lower urinary tract infections, prostatitis Pneumonia, pleuritis Cholelithiasis, cholangiohepatitis Enteritis Septicemia, including neonatal septicemia	Deep pyoderma, otitis externa, media, and interna Conjunctivitis, keratitis Lower urinary tract, pyelonephritis, prostatitis Osteomyelitis Pneumonia, pleuritis Cholelithiasis Septicemia	Corneal ulcers Deep pyoderma Otitis externa, media, interna Lower urinary tract infections, prostatitis Osteomyelitis Chronic rhinitis (cats) Pneumonia, pleuritis Septicemia Bacterial endocarditis

[a]From which *E. coli, Klebsiella, Proteus,* and *Pseudomonas* can be cultured.

defenses. Debilitated patients are at risk for infection, as are those with malignancies, immunodeficiencies, urinary or IV catheters, traumatized tissues, or altered normal flora secondary to the administration of antibiotics.[7] *Pseudomonas* is associated with rapidly progressive corneal ulcers caused by proteolytic enzymes secreted by the bacteria.

Cholestasis associated with nonhepatic bacterial infections, including *E. coli* UTI and *E. coli*, *Klebsiella*, and *Proteus* soft tissue infections, is described in humans and dogs. Characteristic findings include hyperbilirubinemia, slight increases in liver enzyme activities, marked bile retention within canaliculi, hepatocytes and/or Kupffer's cells, and minimal hepatocellular inflammation or necrosis. The mechanism is not clearly delineated, and the prognostic significance is controversial.[29]

DIAGNOSIS

Clinical samples such as urine, blood, exudate, spinal fluid, airway samples, and so forth should be submitted in a routine manner. Special transport media are not necessary.

By direct microscopy, the Enterobacteriaceae are gram-negative, medium-sized short rods that can be motile. Stained morphology is highly variable in clinical specimens. Capsules are large and regular in *Klebsiella*. *Pseudomonas* is a motile rod occurring as single bacteria, in pairs, or in short chains. Capsules or slime may be produced.

The Enterobacteriaceae grow well on ordinary nonenriched media. On blood agar these bacteria look similar, typically with circular, smooth colonies with distinct edges. *Klebsiella* colonies are large and mucoid and tend to coalesce with prolonged incubation. *Proteus* are actively motile, resulting in swarming on solid media. Some strains of *E. coli* produce hemolysis on blood agar. Selective media such as MacConkey's or triple sugar iron agar contain specific dyes and carbohydrates, which may be utilized for rapid preliminary identification. The IMViC reactions (indole, methyl red, Voges-Proskauer, citrate) can be used to further differentiate *E. coli*, *Klebsiella*, and *Proteus*.

Pseudomonas is an obligate aerobe that also grows on ordinary nutrient media. Some strains are hemolytic, and some produce a sweet or grapelike odor caused by the production of aminoacetophenone. *P. aeruginosa* forms smooth, round colonies with a fluorescent greenish color, and a variety of pigments can be produced. A single strain can form multiple colony types on the same plate, giving the impression that mixed species are present. *Pseudomonas* can grow at 42°C, a feature that is employed to differentiate it from other bacteria.

The metabolic characteristics of these bacteria are commonly used in their identification. In general, the Enterobacteriaceae ferment glucose with the production of acid or acid and gas, are catalase positive and oxidase negative, and reduce nitrate to nitrite. Many biochemical tests can help to evaluate the carbohydrate fermentation patterns and the activity of amino acid decarboxylases and other enzymes. Several test kits are commercially available.

Several schemes have been developed to differentiate *E. coli* strains, including serotyping, biotyping, phage-susceptibility typing, electrophoretic typing of enzymes, and colicin typing.

The routine culture and identification of *E. coli* from blood or deep tissue samples are all that is required to diagnose septicemia and soft tissue infection. Quantitative culture is necessary to diagnose UTIs. Enteric pathogens can be differentiated from enteric commensals by evaluating cultured isolates for surface antigens O, H, and K and by testing for production of enterotoxins. Several cell culture–based bioassays are available, as are ELISA and other binding techniques.[18] Cytotoxin (verotoxin) assays can be performed on fecal specimens when EPEC and EHEC strains are suspected. When a toxin is demonstrated, specific neutralization by antisera is employed for confirmation. Isolates can also be tested for toxin or other virulence encoding genes by DNA hybridization or polymerase chain reaction.[38] Infected animals develop rising levels of VT-neutralizing antibodies, which can be identified serologically.[18] Histologic examination is necessary to describe attaching and effacing lesions.

Pseudomonas is typically catalase and oxidase positive and splits sugars by oxidation, not fermentation. It is citrate and indole negative and reduces nitrate. Strains can be identified by serotyping, immunotyping with cross-protection studies in mice, pyocin typing, or phage typing.

Further descriptions of the isolation and identification of these bacteria can be found elsewhere in standard veterinary microbiology texts.

PATHOLOGIC FINDINGS

All of these organisms induce a pyogenic rather than a granulomatous response. The histopathologic lesions associated with EPEC and EHEC have been described previously in this chapter. Holloway and colleagues[17] have described the lesions of hemolytic uremia syndrome in dogs. Local lesions caused by *Pseudomonas* typically have inflammation and necrosis as well as invasion of vascular walls and degenerative changes in epithelial and endothelial cells.

THERAPY

These bacteria have some inherent resistance to antibiotics because of the presence of a gram-negative cell wall. An important outer cell wall protein group is the porins (Fig. 37–1), which create small channels across the outer membrane that admit low-molecular-weight nutrients. Large molecules do not diffuse through these channels. Thus, the peptidoglycan is protected against many antibiotics. This protection gives minor resistance advantage to all gram-negative bacteria, which can be increased by porin mutations, which further limit diffusion of antibiotics. Multiple-drug resistance is common and is under the control of resistance (R) plasmids, which are transferred by conjugation. There is great variation in acquired antibiotic susceptibility, and laboratory testing of isolates for specific susceptibility is always indicated.

Empiric recommendations for suspected soft tissue infections with the Enterobacteriaceae vary, and most are not substantiated by susceptibility data. However, the antibiotic susceptibilities of large numbers of isolates obtained from dogs in a teaching hospital are presented in Table 37–2.[15] My experience is in agreement, with the exception of the effectiveness of enrofloxacin and gentamicin against *Pseudomonas* and amoxicillin-clavulanate against *E. coli* and *Klebsiella*. The Enterobacteriaceae have not been susceptible to chloramphenicol, tetracycline, ampicillin, or trimethoprim-sulfonamide. Clinically stable animals with non–life threatening infections, which are suspected to be caused by gram-negative rods, can be treated with amoxicillin-clavulanate or first- or second-generation cephalosporins until susceptibility results are known. Amikacin, a third-generation cephalosporin, or enrofloxacin should be administered to animals with more life-threatening bacteremia.

Renal excretion results in high urine concentration of anti-

Table 37–2. Guidelines for Initial Antibiotic Therapy for Infections with Gram-Negative Bacteria[a]

DRUG	DOSE[c] (mg/kg)	ROUTE[d]	INTERVAL (HOURS)	ORGANISM (% SUSCEPTIBILITY)[b] *E. coli*	*Klebsiella*	*Proteus*	*Pseudomonas*[e]
Amikacin	5–10	IV, IM, SC	8–12	99	95	96	97
Amoxicillin-clavulanate	11–22	PO	8	NR[d]	NR	95	NR
Carbenicillin	20–30	PO	8	—	—	—	High
	30–100	IV, IM	6–8				
Cefotaxime	20–80	IV, IM, SC	8 (dog) 6 (cat)	99	100	98	NR
Ceftazidime	25	IM, SC	8–12	—	—	—	High
Ciprofloxacin	10–15	PO	12	—	—	—	High
Enrofloxacin	2.5–5	IV, PO	12	95	90	91	NR
Gentamicin	2–4	IV, IM, SC	8	92	NR	NR	NR
Imipenem-cilastatin	2–5	IV	8	—	—	—	High
Ticarcillin	40–75	IV, IM	6–8	—	—	—	High
Ticarcillin-clavulanate	30–50	IV	6–8	NR	NR	96	92
Tobramycin	1	IV, IM, SC	8 (dog)	—	—	—	High
	2	SC	8 (cat)				

[a]Specific therapy should be based on sensitivity testing results. For additional information on each drug, see Appendix 8.
[b]Data from Hirsh and Jang.[15]
[c]Dose per administration at specified interval.
[d]Oral routes not recommended for the initial therapy of serious infections.
[e]High = generally > 80% to 90% unless very resistant hospital strain.
IV = intravenous; IM = intramuscular; SC = subcutaneous; PO = oral; NR = not recommended.

biotics, which facilitates the management of cystitis caused by gram-negative rods. Eighty percent of *E. coli* lower UTIs (LUTIs) can be treated effectively with trimethoprim-sulfadiazine, approximately 90% of *Klebsiella* infections can be treated effectively with cephalexin, and 80% percent of *Proteus* infections, ampicillin.[19] See Chapter 91 for a complete discussion of the management of UTI.

Therapy of *Pseudomonas* infections can be difficult because natural and acquired resistance are common. Gentamicin, amikacin, tobramycin, carbenicillin, ticarcillin, ceftazidime, or ciprofloxacin (isolates may be resistant to enrofloxacin) can be used for initial empirical therapy. Life-threatening infections should be treated with ticarcillin or carbenicillin in combination with an aminoglycoside. Imipenem-cilastatin is another antibiotic active against *P. aeruginosa*. *Pseudomonas* is usually resistant to penicillin, ampicillin, tetracycline, first- and second-generation cephalosporins, chloramphenicol, and trimethoprim-sulfadiazine. Eighty percent of LUTIs can be treated effectively with tetracycline.[19] The management of *Pseudomonas* otitis externa has been reviewed elsewhere (see Chapter 85).[26]

PREVENTION

Sunlight and desiccation kill the Enterobacteriaceae readily; freezing does not. *E. coli* can survive in feces, dust, and water for months. The mode of infection and transmission is almost always by ingestion, and fomite transmission is important. Routine hand washing and disinfection of fomites are mandatory parts of prevention. *Pseudomonas* is an important nosocomial pathogen that survives well in hospital environments, including water faucets, utensils, floors, instruments, humidifiers, baths, and respiratory care equipment. It can also survive in disinfectant solutions, antiseptics, and liquid fluorescein drops.

Orally administered autogenous vaccines have been utilized to prevent and treat kennel-acquired enteric *E. coli* infections in dogs and cats, with significant decreases in morbidity and mortality.[2, 34, 35]

PUBLIC HEALTH CONSIDERATIONS

Most *E. coli*, *Klebsiella*, and *Proteus* are opportunistic pathogens; however, some enteropathogenic *E. coli* (EPEC, EHEC) could potentially be carried by dogs or cats and transmitted to humans (or vice versa). R plasmids are transmitted between gram-negative organisms, and multiple drug resistance could be a potential human health problem. Zoonotic transmission from cattle is thought to occur because of epidemiologic associations of hemorrhagic colitis and HUS with ingestion of poorly cooked ground beef or of raw milk contaminated with *E. coli* 0157:H7.[8, 36]

References

1. An H, Fairbrother JM, Dubreuil JD, et al. 1997. Cloning and characterization of the *eae* gene from a dog attaching and effacing *Escherichia coli* strain 4221. *FEMS Microbiol Lett* 148:239–245.

1a. Awad-Masalmeh M, Youssef U, Silber R. 1990. Properties of haemolytic *Escherichia coli* strains from dogs and cats affected by, or dead from diarrhoea or enteritis. Virulence factors and sensitivity to antibiotics. *Wien Tierarztl Monatsschr* 77:254–258.

2. Baljer G, Hinsch F, Mayr B. 1990. Clinical experience with kennel-specific oral *E. coli* vaccines in puppies and dogs. *Tierarztl Prax* 18:65–68.

3. Beaudry M, Zhu C, Fairbrother J, et al. 1996. Genotypic and phenotypic characterization of *Escherichia coli* isolates from dogs manifesting attaching and effacing lesions. *J Clin Microbiol* 34:144–148.

4. Beutin L, Geier D, Zimmermann S, et al. 1995. Virulence markers of shiga-like toxin producing *Escherichia coli* strains originating from healthy domestic animals of different species. *J Clin Microbiol* 33:631–635.

5. Blanco J, Blanco M, Wong I, et al. 1993. Hemolytic *Escherichia coli* strains isolated from stools of healthy cats produce cytotoxic necrotizing factor type 1 (CNF1). *Vet Microbiol* 38:157–165.

6. Broes A, Drolet M, Jacques M, et al. 1988. Natural infection with an attaching and effacing *Escherichia coli* in a diarrheic puppy. *Can J Vet Res* 52:280–282.

7. Court EA, Watson ADJ, Martin P. 1994. *Pseudomonas aeruginosa* bacteremia in a dog. *Aust Vet J* 71:25–27.

8. Dorn CL. 1995. *Escherichia coli* 0157:H7. *J Am Vet Med Assoc* 206:1583–1585.

9. Drulet R, Fairbrother JM, Harel J, et al. 1994. Attaching and effacing and enterotoxigenic *Escherichia coli* associated with enteric colibacillosis in the dog. *Can J Vet Res* 58:87–92.

10. Gaastra W, Vanoosterom RAAA, Pieters EWJ, et al. 1996. Isolation and characterization of dog uropathogenic *Proteus mirabilis* strains. *Vet Microbiol* 48:57–71.

11. Gyles CL. 1992. *Escherichia coli* cytotoxins and enterotoxins. *Can J Microbiol* 38:734–746.

12. Hammermueller J, Kruth S, Prescott J, et al. 1995. Detection of toxin genes in *Escherichia coli* isolated from normal dogs and dogs with diarrhea. *Can J Vet Res* 59:265–270.
13. Hart CA, Embaye H, Getty B, et al. 1990. Ultrastructural lesions to the canine intestinal epithelium caused by enteropathogenic *Escherichia coli*. *J Small Anim Pract* 31:591–594.
14. Hertzke DM, Cowan LA, Schoning P, et al. 1995. Glomerular ultrastructural lesions of idiopathic cutaneous and renal glomerular vasculopathy of greyhounds. *Vet Pathol* 32:451–459.
15. Hirsh D, Jang SS. 1994. Antimicrobial susceptibility of selected infectious bacterial agents obtained from dogs. *J Am Anim Hosp Assoc* 30:487–494.
16. Hoffman WD, Pollack M, Banks SM, et al. 1994. Distinct functional activities in canine septic shock of monoclonal antibodies specific for the O polysaccharide and core regions of *Escherichia coli* lipopolysaccharide. *J Infect Dis* 169:553–561.
17. Holloway S, Senior D, Roth L, et al. 1993. Hemolytic uremic syndrome in dogs. *J Vet Intern Med* 7:220–227.
18. Karmali MA. 1989. Infection by verocytotoxin producing *Escherichia coli*. *Clin Microbiol Rev* 2:15–38.
18a. Kim DH, Back NJ, Park KH, et al. 1997. Subacute toxicity of a *Pseudomonas* vaccine prepared from outer membrane fraction of *Pseudomonas aeruginosa* in beagle dogs. *Arzneimittelforsch* 47:80–83.
19. Lulich JP, Osborne CA. 1995. Bacterial infections of the urinary tract, pp 1775–1788. *In* Ettinger SJ, Feldman EC (eds), Textbook of veterinary internal medicine, disorders of the dog and cat, ed 4. WB Saunders, Philadelphia, PA.
20. Meinen JB, McClure JT, Rosin E. 1995. Pharmacokinetics of enrofloxacin in clinically normal dogs and mice and drug pharmacodynamic in neutropenic mice with *Escherichia coli* and staphylococcal infections. *Am J Vet Res* 56:1219–1224.
21. Olson P, Hedhammar A, Wadstrom T. 1984. Enterotoxigenic *Escherichia coli* infection in two dogs with acute diarrhea. *J Am Vet Med Assoc* 184:982–983.
22. Poffenbarger EM, Olson PN, Ralston SL, et al. 1991. Canine neonatology: part II. Disorders of the neonate. *Compend Cont Educ Pract Vet* 13:25–31.
23. Pohl P, Mainil J, Devriese LA, et al. 1993. *Escherichia coli* from dogs and cats, producing cytotoxic necrotizing factor type 1 (CNF1). *Ann Med Vet* 137:21–25.
24. Pospischil A, Mainil JG, Baljer G, et al. 1987. Attaching and effacing bacteria in the intestines of calves and cats with diarrhea. *Vet Pathol* 24:330–334.
25. Prada J, Baljer G, De Ryche J, et al. 1991. Characteristics of α hemolytic strains of *Escherichia coli* isolated from dogs with gastroenteritis. *Vet Microbiol* 29:59–73.
25a. Roberts D, Howerth E. 1998. University of Georgia, unpublished data.
26. Rosychuk RAW, Luttgen P. 1995. Diseases of the ear, pp 533–550. *In* Ettinger SJ, Feldman EC (eds), Textbook of veterinary internal medicine, diseases of the dog and cat, ed 4. WB Saunders, Philadelphia, PA.
27. Senior D, deMan P, Svanborg C. 1992. Serotype, hemolysin production, and adherence characteristics of strains of *Escherichia coli* causing urinary tract infections in dogs. *Am J Vet Res* 53:494–498.
28. Smith KE. 1996. Personal communication. University of Guelph, Guelph, Ontario, Canada.
29. Taboada J, Meyer DJ. 1989. Cholestasis associated with extrahepatic bacterial infection in five dogs. *J Vet Intern Med* 3:216–221.
30. Turk J, Miller M, Brown T, et al. 1990. Coliform septicemia and pulmonary disease associated with canine parvovirus enteritis: 88 cases (1987–1988). *J Am Vet Med Assoc* 196:771–772.
31. Wada Y, Kondo H, Nakaoka Y, et al. 1996. Gastric attaching and effacing *Escherichia coli* lesions in a puppy with naturally occurring enteric colibacillosis and concurrent canine distemper virus infection. *Vet Pathol* 33:717–720.
32. Wadas B, Kuhn I, Langerstadt A-S, et al. 1996. Biochemical phenotypes of *Escherichia coli* in dogs: comparison of isolates isolated from bitches suffering from pyometra and urinary tract infection with isolates from feces of healthy dogs. *Vet Microbiol* 52:293–300.
33. Wasteson Y, Olsvik O, Skancke E, et al. 1988. Heat-stable enterotoxin producing *Escherichia coli* strains isolated from dogs. *J Clin Microbiol* 26:2564–2566.
34. Weber A, Gobel D. 1996. Treatment of chronic diarrhea in dogs and cats under field conditions using oral *Escherichia coli* vaccines. *Tierarztl Prax* 23:80–82.
35. Weiss HE, Bertl F. 1991. Treatment of enteritis caused by antibiotic resistant *Escherichia coli* in dogs and cats by orally administered autogenous vaccines. *Prakt Tierarztl* 72:12–14.
36. Whipp SC, Rasmussen MA, Cray WC. 1994. Animals as a source of *Escherichia coli* pathogenic for human beings. *J Am Vet Med Assoc* 204:1168–1175.
37. Wise LA, Jones RL, Reif JS. 1990. Nosocomial canine urinary tract infections in a veterinary teaching hospital. *J Am Anim Hosp Assoc* 26:148–152.
38. Woodard MJ, Kearsley R, Wray C, et al. 1990. DNA probes for the detection of toxin genes in *Escherichia coli* isolated from diarrhoeal disease in cattle and pigs. *Vet Microbiol* 22:277–290.

Chapter **38**

Endotoxemia

Stephen A. Kruth

ETIOLOGY

Bacteremia, the presence of live bacteria in the blood, is a relatively common event. It may occur with the diagnostic or therapeutic manipulation of any site heavily colonized by bacteria, as with dentistry, rectal palpation, or intestinal endoscopy or surgery. Animals with known sites of infection such as peritonitis, mastitis, prostatitis, pneumonia, pulmonary abscess, pyothorax, pyometra, pyelonephritis, intra-abdominal abscess, biliary tract infection, and bite wounds are likely to develop systemic spread or effects of infection. Indwelling venous or arterial catheters may also allow bacteria to enter the blood. Normally, circulating bacteria are rapidly cleared by the mononuclear-phagocyte system. Occasionally, however, focal infections will result. Disease is caused by the presence of vegetating bacteria, and a local inflammatory response is invoked. The *systemic inflammatory response syndrome* (SIRS) is a host response to a wide variety of insults, including those of infectious origin.[12, 29] The primary lesion of SIRS is widespread vascular endothelial inflammation, which leads to the initial clinical signs of fever, tachycardia, tachypnea, and neutropenia. Sepsis and endotoxemia are mediated through SIRS. *Sepsis* is diagnosed when SIRS occurs in a patient with an infectious disease, and is associated with the presence of bacteria and their toxins in the blood or tissues.

Endotoxemia exists when lipopolysaccharide (LPS; endotoxin), originating from gram-negative bacteria, is present in the blood. LPS is derived from the outer membrane of gram-negative bacteria, which consists of lipid A and polysaccharides. It is the lipid A portion of LPS that is believed to be the toxic component (see Fig. 37–1). Endotoxemia is usually associated with members of the Enterobacteriaceae family (*Escherichia, Klebsiella, Enterobacter, Proteus*) and *Pseudomonas*.

The term "endotoxemia" implies only that toxin is present; in some cases, bacteria are present in the circulation, whereas in others they remain compartmentalized in the gut or tissues, with only toxin being absorbed. Animals have evolved to recognize and respond to the LPS of gram-negative bacteria. *Endotoxic shock* is the extreme host response to endotoxemia. Approximately 25% of humans with gram-negative aerobic bacteremia develop endotoxic shock, with a 50% to 80% mortality rate. Predisposing conditions for endotoxic shock include diabetes mellitus, hepatic cirrhosis, burns, cancer, surgery, irradiation, cytotoxic drug therapy, administration of glucocorticoids, and blood transfusions.

Although endotoxemia is a life-threatening syndrome, the prevalence of endotoxemia in small animals has not been determined. Endotoxemia appears to occur more commonly in dogs than in cats and has been associated with hemorrhagic enteritis[32] (especially canine parvovirus [CPV] enteritis[7, 17, 25a]), GI accidents with compromised vascular perfusion to the gut (especially gastric dilatation–volvulus[5]), pyometra,[8a] and mastitis[6] and other invasive gram-negative infections. It has also occurred as a complication of surgery or heatstroke. Endotoxemia can also be noted when hepatic clearance of LPS is reduced, as in primary hepatic insufficiency and portosystemic shunts.[16a, 26] Additionally, obstructive biliary disease can lead to the development of endotoxemia, because bile salts bind endotoxin in the gut. Endotoxemia is recognized as a cause of neonatal death in puppies and kittens.[27]

PATHOGENESIS

Endotoxin is released into the intestinal lumen when gram-negative bacterial cell walls break down, as occurs with rapid bacterial replication or with bactericidal action of effective antibiotics. Within the intestinal lumen, most endotoxin is bound by bile acids and contained by the mucosal barrier. Small amounts are absorbed into the portal circulation and cleared by hepatic macrophages. Endotoxin absorbed through lymphatics is cleared in regional lymph nodes. Thus, endotoxin levels in systemic circulation are usually extremely low. Clinical signs of endotoxemia occur only when these binding and clearance mechanisms are overwhelmed.

Circulating endotoxin is bound in plasma by specific lipoproteins, which subsequently attach to monocytes and macrophages via CD14 cell receptor.[31] Endotoxin has direct cytotoxic activity, especially against hepatocytes; however, endotoxin per se is not the culprit that leads to the clinical state of endotoxemia. Macrophage-derived cytokines are responsible for many of the pathophysiologic consequences. The macrophage response to endotoxin is release of various biochemical mediators, which are potent stimuli to neutrophils, platelets, and vascular endothelium. *Interleukin-1* (IL-1) and *tumor necrosis factor* (TNF) are multifunctional proinflammatory cytokines that are the primary autocrine and paracrine mediators of the local responses to gram-negative infections. SIRS occurs when IL-1 and TNF are released from macrophages in exaggerated amounts, with resultant systemic activation of several enzyme cascades.[3, 19, 29, 30]

TNF levels increase over baseline within 15 minutes of exposure to LPS, peak at 2 hours,[21] and return to baseline levels in 4 hours. IL-1 is released in similar burst fashion secondarily to TNF. These cytokines are thus released early and transiently in response to endotoxin.[21a] Both cytokines have myriad effects, including increasing cytokine release from T lymphocytes; increasing antibody production in B lymphocytes; activating neutrophils; stimulating hematopoiesis; increasing release of prostaglandins, cytokines, and other mediators from macrophages; increasing lipolysis and decreasing lipoprotein lipase activity in adipocytes; increasing prostaglandin and cytokine activity in fibroblasts; inducing acute-phase reactants (C-reactive protein, serum amyloid A protein, α1-acid glycoprotein, and fibrinogen) in hepatocytes; increasing prostaglandin release and procoagulant activity in vascular endothelium; inducting fever, somnolence, and inappetence; and enhancing production of insulin, glucagon, catecholamines, and glucocorticoids.[3] Other cytokines, such as IL-6 and IL-8 are becoming recognized as additional mediators in endotoxemia.[9, 29] Macrophage-derived glucocorticoid-antagonizing factor inhibits gluconeogenesis, and mediators from macrophages with insulin-like activity contribute to the hypoglycemia associated with endotoxemia.

Several lipid mediators are also important in the genesis of endotoxic shock. Platelet-activating factor (PAF) is released from leukocytes, platelets, and endothelial cells. It causes platelet activation and aggregation; neutrophil activation, aggregation, and chemotaxis; increased activity of plasma proteases; vasodilation and systemic hypotension; vasoconstriction in the heart and lungs; increased vascular permeability; and GI ulceration. Additionally, both the cyclooxygenase (leukotriene) and lipoxygenase (prostaglandin) pathways are activated. Prostaglandins (PGs; thromboxane, prostacyclin, $PGF_{2\alpha}$, and PGE) and leukotrienes have a variety of vascular and other effects that add to the syndrome of endotoxemia.

Other secondary mediators amplify the initial response; these include β-endorphin, histamine, serotonin, vasopressin, angiotensin II, and catecholamines. Activation of Hageman factor (factor XII) induces the coagulation, fibrinolytic, complement, and kallikrein-kinin cascades. Lysosomal enzymes such as elastase and chymotrypsin deplete fibronectin and activate blood clotting, triggering disseminated (excessive) intravascular coagulation (DIC). Direct cellular toxins are also important in the genesis of endotoxemia. Oxygen free radicals oxidize membrane lipids, and nitric oxide induces vasodilation.

Endotoxin results in structural and metabolic changes in vascular endothelial cells, causing increased permeability. The vascular endothelium becomes "sticky," and the neutrophils and platelets are sequestered in target organs (gut and liver in dogs, lung in cats). The endothelium also becomes leaky, and plasma proteins move from the intravascular space to the interstitium. Reviews by Hardie are available with in-depth discussions of the pathophysiology of SIRS and endotoxemia.[13, 14]

CLINICAL FINDINGS

Dogs

The dog has been frequently studied as a model for endotoxemia; however, the actual clinical presentation is modified by intercurrent disorders and duration of exposure to and dose of endotoxin. The clinical presentation is variable, but tachypnea, vomiting, mucoid bloody diarrhea, weakness, fever, and chills are classic features. Early (within minutes) signs of SIRS are related to portal hypertension, hepatosplanchnic pooling of blood, decreased central venous pressure, increased cardiac output, normal or decreased arterial blood pressure, and low systemic vascular resistance. Blood flow to most tissues is diminished. Warm skin, brick-red mucous membranes, tachycardia, and diminished to bounding arterial pulses can be observed. These signs may resolve but are followed by later changes, which include falling cardiac output and arterial blood pressure, pooling of blood in the viscera, and myocardial failure. Clinical signs include cold extremities, pale mucous membranes, weak pulses, and prolonged capillary refill times.[21, 23–25] In survivors, cardiovascular abnormalities peak at 2 to 3 days and do not return to normal for 7 to 10 days. In others, myocardial damage is progressive, and death from heart failure can occur up to 7 days after presentation.

Clinical pathologic findings include rapidly developing hemoconcentration followed by leukocytosis, thrombocytopenia, lactic and hyperchloremic acidosis, hypoxemia, hypo- or hyperglycemia, prolonged coagulation times and elevated fibrin degradation products, and increased serum alkaline phosphatase and alanine aminotransferase activities. Increased vascular permeability leads to plasma protein loss and hypoproteinemia—and potential edema. Signs consistent with acute renal failure may also be present. The pervasive histologic abnormality is marked vascular endothelial damage. Mild pulmonary edema, marked hepatic congestion and necrosis, subendocardial hemorrhage, renal congestion, adrenal hemorrhage, and marked hemorrhage and sloughing of the GI mucosa can be identified.

Cats

Endotoxemia is less well described in cats as a clinical syndrome; the major difference is that respiratory signs predominate in cats. Severe pulmonary hypertension and bronchoconstriction cause respiratory failure (respiratory distress syndrome) manifested by pulmonary edema. Hyperglycemia is more common than in dogs.

DIAGNOSIS

The *Limulus* amebocyte lysate assay is the most commonly described definitive assay for endotoxin[26, 32]; however, assays are not available for routine clinical practice. A clinical diagnosis depends on recognition of risk factors along with the clinical signs outlined previously. The clinician should attempt to identify the sites of infection by radiology, ultrasonography, and centesis as needed. At this time, an IV access should be established and a urinary catheter placed. It is also important to establish baseline hemodynamic and perfusion indices, including rectal and toe web temperature, heart rate, mucous membrane color, pulse character, arterial blood pressure, and arterial blood gases when available. Testing for serum electrolyte, glucose, serum urea nitrogen, creatinine, and liver enzyme activities should be performed along with a CBC and platelet counts and coagulation parameters. Culture specimens of wounds, urine, and blood should be taken so that antibiotic therapy can be instituted as necessary.[8] For a review of specimens collection, see Chapters 33, 87, and 91. When an external wound, an abscess, or a fracture is identified, the area should be shaved and cleaned and lanced, drained, or debrided as necessary.

After initial diagnostic and therapeutic management is instituted and the patient is more stable, one should search for the origin of endotoxemia. Diagnostic modalities may include radiography of the thorax and abdomen. When available, echocardiography and abdominal ultrasonography may be helpful in locating sources of sepsis. Additional procedures that involve anesthesia or sedation include diagnostic peritoneal lavage, tracheal or bronchoalveolar lavage, arthrocentesis, and CSF collection.

THERAPY

Empiric therapy should be initiated as soon as clinical signs of endotoxemia are observed. The management is primarily supportive, with emphasis on the maintenance of tissue perfusion. Management of complications of SIRS is essential even when the site of infection cannot be determined.

A shock dose of an isotonic crystalloid solution should be infused and careful monitoring performed. If the animal does not respond adequately within the first hour, fresh or fresh-frozen plasma should be administered, along with a synthetic colloid. Fluid support should be aggressive and adjusted as dictated by the animal's response. If blood pressure cannot be maintained, dopamine or dobutamine should be infused.[5a, 12, 20, 24] Several aspects of fluid therapy are under investigation, including the use of hypertonic solutions.[28]

Once fluid therapy has been initiated, infected sites should be drained and debrided. Antibiotic therapy should be directed toward the primary site of infection. In endotoxemia from any source, there is increased translocation of bacteria from the GI lumen to the portal circulation; antibiotic therapy should also be directed against these flora. As initial combination antibiotic therapy for endotoxemia, I use one of three options: metronidazole with a first-generation cephalosporin (e.g., cefazolin) and enrofloxacin; clindamycin with enrofloxacin; or imipenem-cilastatin as a single agent (Table 38–1).

GI ulceration is a common sequela to endotoxemia, and management should include cimetidine or ranitidine, sucralfate, and misoprostol as necessary. Nutritional support is important in animals with SIRS; however, optimum nutritional management has not been determined. Enteral alimentation with nasoesophageal, gastrotomy, or jejunostomy tubes is preferable to partial or total parenteral nutrition.

DIC is treated supportively with fluids and plasma to replace antithrombin III. The efficacy of heparin in the treatment of DIC secondary to endotoxemia has not been well established.

Other complications such as noncardiogenic pulmonary edema, acute renal insufficiency, and cardiac failure should be managed as discussed in other sources.

Chronic low-level endotoxemia can complicate portosystemic shunts and other forms of hepatic insufficiency.[26] Inflammatory bowel disease in these cases could increase endotoxin absorption. Lactulose, ursodeoxycholic acid, and neomycin potentially lower portal endotoxin levels.

A number of experimental therapeutic modalities have been investigated, most of which are designed to block pathways in the generation of endotoxic shock. Drugs include glucocorticoids, calcium channel blockers, glucagon, aspirin, indomethacin, flunixin meglumine, naloxone, PAF blockers, tyrosine kinase inhibitors, free radical scavengers and antioxidants, and lazaroids.[5, 14, 15, 28a] Because animals are presented clinically *after* inflammatory mediators have been released, the benefits of these drugs is debatable. Because of the high rate of complications associated with most of these drugs, their use in the management of SIRS is not recommended.

Plasma exchange, extracorporeal activated charcoal hemoperfusion, and hemoperfusion or plasmapheresis over polymyxin B will decrease LPS concentration in peripheral blood. Novel therapies that may eventually be used in the management of endotoxic shock include antiproteases, specific eicosanoid blockers, IL-1 and TNF receptor antagonists, anti-TNF monoclonal antibodies, and soluble TNF receptors.[1, 4, 33]

Antiendotoxin antibodies have been reported as having variable efficacy in the management of human endotoxemia.[2] Plasma endotoxin levels have been shown to increase over several days in dogs with CPV enteritis and remain elevated for as long as 10 to 30 days.[17] An equine-origin polyclonal antiendotoxin serum (SEPTI-serum, Immunovet, Columbia, MO) has been reported to improve the survival rate in dogs

Table 38–1. Drug Dosages for Endotoxemia

DRUG	SPECIES	DOSE[a]	ROUTE	INTERVAL (HOURS)
Volume expanders				
Isotonic crystalloid solutions				
(Plasma-Lyte 148, lactated Ringer's,	D	90 ml/kg	IV	1[b]
normal saline)	C	60 ml/kg	IV	1[b]
Colloids				
(fresh or fresh-frozen plasma, pentastarch, hetastarch 120, dextran 70)	B	20 ml/kg	IV	24
Sympathomimetic drugs				
Dopamine	B	1–10 μg/kg	IV	1 min
Dobutamine	B	5–20 μg/kg	IV	1 min
Antibacterial drugs				
Metronidazole	B	10 mg/kg	IV, PO	8
	B	15 mg/kg	IV, PO	12
Cefazolin	B	5–15 mg/kg	IV, IM	6–8
Enrofloxacin	B	2.5–5 mg/kg	IV	12
Clindamycin	B	5–11 mg/kg	IV, IM, PO	8
Imipenem-cilastatin	B	2–5 mg/kg	IV	8
Antiulcer drugs				
Cimetidine	B	5–10 mg/kg	IV, IM, PO	6–8
Ranitidine	B	2 mg/kg	IV	8–12
Sucralfate	C	250 mg total	PO	8–12
	D (<20 kg)	500 mg total	PO	8–12
	D (>20 kg)	1 g total	PO	8–12
Misoprostol	B	2–5 μg/kg	PO	8–12
Portosystemic shunt therapy				
Lactulose	B	0.5 ml/kg	PO	8
Ursodeoxycholic acid	B	5–7.5 mg/kg	PO	12
Neomycin	B	2.5–20 mg/kg	PO	8–12

[a]Dose per administration at specified interval. For additional information on each antibacterial drug, see Appendix 8.
[b]Reassess perfusion and hemodilution after first hour before continuing.
D = dog; B = dog and cat; C = cat.

with CPV enteritis[7] (see Chapter 8, and the Drug Formulary, Appendix 8).

PREVENTION

Immunization against CPV and proper management of large- and giant-breed dogs to lessen the occurrence of gastric dilatation–volvulus will help prevent endotoxemia of intestinal origin. Appropriate surgical technique and postsurgical management, limited perioperative administration of antibiotics, and careful management of vascular access devices and urinary catheters will minimize iatrogenic and nosocomial infections. Finally, animals at risk for endotoxemia, especially those with established infections, should be managed appropriately for the primary disorder and monitored for signs of SIRS.

References

1. Abraham E, Raffin TA. 1994. Sepsis therapy trials: continued disappointment or reason for hope? *N Engl J Med* 271:1876–1878.
2. Baumgartner JD, Glauser MP. 1993. Immunotherapy of endotoxemia and septicemia. *Immunobiology* 187:464–477.
3. Beutler B, Grau GE. 1993. Tumor necrosis factor in the pathogenesis of infectious diseases. *Crit Care Med* 21:S423–S435.
4. Bodmer M, Fournel MA, Hinshaw LB. 1993. Preclinical review of anti-tumor necrosis factor monoclonal antibodies. *Crit Care Med* 21:S441–S446.
5. Davidson JR, Lantz GC, Salisbury SK, et al. 1992. Effects of flunixin meglumine on dogs with experimental gastric dilatation-volvulus. *Vet Surg* 21:113–120.
5a. DeBacker D, Zhang H, Manikis P, et al. 1996. Regional effects of dolbutamine in endotoxic shock. *J Surg Res* 65:93–100.
6. Dernell WS, Kreeger J. 1992. Peracute, necrotizing mastitis as a cause of fatal septicemia and endotoxemia in a dog. *Canine Pract* 17:25–29.
7. Dimmitt R. 1991. Clinical experience with cross-protective anti-endotoxin antiserum in dogs with parvoviral enteritis. *Canine Pract* 16:23–26.
8. Dow SW, Jones RL. 1989. Bacteremia: pathogenesis and diagnosis. *Compend Cont Educ Pract Vet* 11:432–443.
8a. Fransson B, Lagerstedt AS, Hellmen E, et al. 1997. Bacteriological findings, blood-chemistry profile and plasma endotoxin levels in bitches with pyometra or other uterine diseases. *Zentralbe Vet Med (A)* 44:417–426.
9. Giroir BP. 1993. Mediators of septic shock: new approaches for interrupting the endogenous inflammatory cascade. *Crit Care Med* 21:780–789.
10. Green EM, Adams HR. 1992. New perspectives in circulatory shock: pathophysiologic mediators of mammalian response to endotoxemia and sepsis. *J Am Vet Med Assoc* 200:1834–1841.
11. Hardie EM. 1990. Endotoxemia, pp 494–497. *In* Greene CE (ed), Infectious diseases of the dog and cat. WB Saunders, Philadelphia, PA.
12. Hardie EM. 1995. Life-threatening bacterial infection. *Compend Cont Educ Pract Vet* 17:763–777.
13. Hardie EM, Kruse-Elliot K. 1990. Endotoxic shock: part I. A review of causes. *J Vet Intern Med* 4:258–266.
14. Hardie EM, Kruse-Elliot K. 1990. Endotoxic Shock: part II. A review of treatment. *J Vet Intern Med* 4:306–314.
15. Hardie EM, Rawlings CA, Shotts EB, et al. 1987. *Escherichia coli*-induced lung and liver dysfunction in dogs: effects of flunixin meglumine treatment. *Am J Vet Res* 48:56–62.
16. Hoffman WD, Pollack M, Banks SM, et al. 1994. Distinct functional activities in canine septic shock of monoclonal antibodies specific for the O polysaccharide and core regions of *Escherichia coli* lipopolysaccharide. *J Infect Dis* 169:553–561.
16a. Howe LM, Boothe DM, Boothe HW. 1997. Endotoxemia associated with experimentally induced multiple portosystemic shunts in dogs. *Am J Vet Res* 58:83–88.
17. Isogai E, Isogai H, Onuma M, et al. 1989. *Escherichia coli* associated endotoxemia in dogs with parvovirus infection. *Jpn J Vet Sci* 51:597–606.
18. LeGrand EK. 1990. Endotoxin as an alarm signal of bacterial invasion: current evidence and implications. *J Am Vet Med Assoc* 197:454–456.
19. Livingston DH, Mosenthal AC, Deitch EA. 1995. Sepsis and multiple organ dysfunction syndrome: a clinical-mechanistic overview. *N Horiz* 3:257–266.
20. Mathews KA. 1996. Personal communication. University of Guelph, Guelph, Ontario, Canada.
21. Miyamoto T. 1993. Changes of cytokine activities and other parameters in experimentally induced endotoxin shock in dogs. *Jpn J Vet Res* 41:32.
21a. Miyamoto T, Fujinaga T, Yamashita K, et al. 1996. Changes of serum cytokine activities and other parameters in dogs with experimentally induced endotoxic shock. *Jpn J Vet Res* 44:107–118.
22. Morris DD. 1991. Endotoxemia in horses. A review of cellular and humoral mediations involved in its pathogenesis. *J Vet Intern Med* 5:167–181.

23. Natanson C, Eichenholz PW, Danner RL, et al. 1989. Endotoxin and tumor necrosis factor challenges in dogs simulate the cardiovascular profile of human septic shock. *J Exp Med* 169:823–832.
24. Nostrandt AC. 1990. Bacteremia and septicemia in small animal patients. *Prob Vet Med* 2:348–361.
25. Novotny M, Laughlin MH, Adams HR. 1988. Evidence for lack of importance of oxygen free radicals in *Escherichia coli* endotoxemia in dogs. *Am J Physiol* 254:H954–H962.
25a. Otto CM, Drobatz KJ, Soter C. 1997. Endotoxemia and tumor-necrosis-factor activity in dogs with naturally occurring parvoviral enteritis. *J Vet Intern Med* 11:65–70.
26. Peterson SL, Koblik PD, Whiting PG, et al. 1991. Endotoxin concentrations measured by a chromogenic assay in portal and peripheral venous blood in ten dogs with portosystemic shunts. *J Vet Intern Med* 5:71–74.
27. Poffenbarger EM, Olson PN, Ralston SL, et al. 1991. Canine neonatology: part II. Disorders of the neonate. *Compend Cont Educ Pract Vet* 13:25–37.
28. Schertel ER, Tobias TA. 1992. Hypertonic fluid therapy, pp 471–485. *In* DiBartola SP (ed), Fluid therapy in small animal practice. WB Saunders, Philadelphia, PA.
28a. Sevransky JE, Shaked G, Novogrodsky A, et al. 1997. Tryphostin AG 556 improves survival and reduces multiorgan failure in canine *Escherichia coli* peritonitis. *J Clin Invest* 99:1966–1973.
29. Strieter RM, Kunkel SL, Bone RC. 1993. Role of tumor necrosis factor-α in disease states and inflammation. *Crit Care Med* 21:S447–S463.
30. Tracey KJ, Cerami A. 1993. Tumor necrosis factor: an updated review of its biology. *Crit Care Med* 21:S415–S422.
31. Ulevitch RJ, Mathison JC, Schumann RR, et al. 1990. A new model of macrophage stimulation by bacterial lipopolysaccharide. *J Trauma* 30:S189–S192.
32. Wessels BC, Gaffin SL, Wells MT. 1987. Circulating plasma endotoxin (lipopolysaccharide) concentrations in healthy and hemorrhagic enteric dogs: antiendotoxin immunotherapy in hemorrhagic enteric endotoxemia. *J Am Anim Hosp Assoc* 23:291–295.
33. Wherry JC, Pennington JE, Wenzel RP. 1993. Tumor necrosis factor and the therapeutic potential of anti-tumor necrosis factor antibodies. *Crit Care Med* 21:S436–S440.

Chapter 39

Enteric Bacterial Infections

Campylobacter *Infections*

James G. Fox

ETIOLOGY

Campylobacter is a genus of gram-negative, slender, curved, motile rods (1.5–5 μm × 0.2–0.5 μm) that occur singularly, in pairs, or in chains with three to five spirals (Fig. 39–1). The cells can also be curved, S, or gull shaped. *Campylobacter* spp. have a single polar flagellum and microaerobic growth requirements. *C. jejuni* is the organism routinely associated with diarrheal disease in dogs, cats, and humans as well as other domestic, wild, and laboratory animals. *C. coli*, distinguished from *C. jejuni* on the basis of hippurate hydrolysis, is also isolated from diarrheic animals and people. In addition, a catalase-negative species, *C. upsalensis*, has been isolated from asymptomatic and diarrheic dogs as well as asymptomatic cats.[36, 56a]

EPIDEMIOLOGY

Privately owned adult dogs and cats generally have a lower isolation rate of the *C. jejuni* organism than strays or those maintained in kennels or catteries, laboratories, and animal shelters.[36] It has been isolated from 21% and 29% of diarrheic cats and dogs, respectively, compared with 4% of clinically healthy cats and dogs.[36] In other studies, the isolation rate from feces of mature dogs and cats, with and without diarrhea, has varied from 0% to 50%. Puppies and kittens appear more likely to acquire *C. jejuni* and show clinical disease probably because of a lack of previous exposure and development of protective antibody. Studies of pups show that shedding of *Campylobacter* spp. ranges from less than 5% to a high of 90%.

As with most enteric microbial pathogens, fecal-oral spread, with food-borne and water-borne transmission, appears to be the principal avenue for infection. Sources of the organism include contaminated meat products, particularly poultry and unpasteurized milk. Nosocomial infection of hospitalized animals is possible, as is exposure from other pets in a household (ferrets, hamsters, birds, rabbits) and rural farm animals that may shed the organism.

PATHOGENESIS

Severity of the disease is dependent on the number of organisms ingested by the host as well as previous exposure and development of protective antibody. Other enteric pathogens, such as parvovirus and coronavirus, *Giardia*, or *Salmonella*, may play a synergistic role.[36] Environmental, physiologic, and surgical stress may also exacerbate the severity of the disease. A variety of virulence factors, such as enterotoxins, cytotoxins, or adherence or invasion properties, are expressed by different *C. jejuni–coli* isolates. Blood and leukocytes in the feces, congestion, edema, mucosal ulcers, and occasional sepsis in people suggest that the organism can be invasive. Experimental challenge in laboratory animals also indicates that the organism can be isolated several days after blood challenge. Experimental infections of puppies and kittens with strains isolated from humans with diarrhea are less severe. Animals appear to be more resistant or better adapted

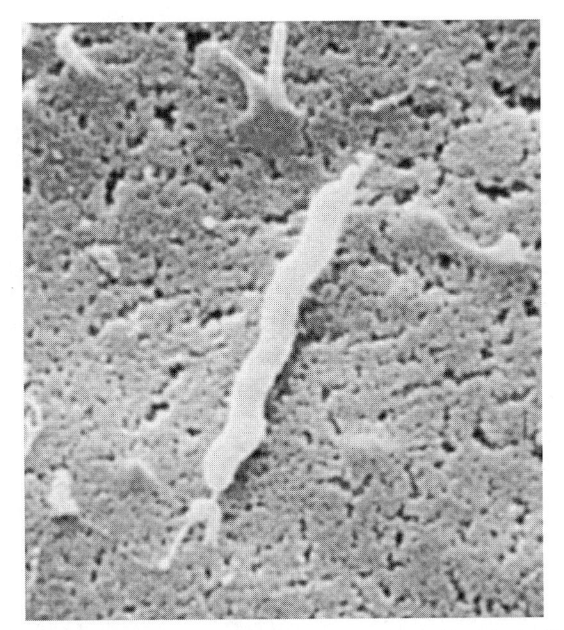

Figure 39–1. Scanning electron microscopy view of *C. jejuni* adhered to chick embryo cell (× 15,900).

to withstand the pathogenic effects of different *C. jejuni* strains and usually develop watery mucoid diarrhea.[36]

CLINICAL FINDINGS

Dog

In many cases, dogs are asymptomatic carriers of *Campylobacter* spp. The clinical syndrome, when present, occurs most frequently in dogs younger than 6 months. Animals may be more susceptible to clinical disease when stressed by hospitalization, concurrent disease, pregnancy, shipment, or surgery. *Campylobacter*-associated diarrhea has a wide clinical spectrum in dogs as well as humans, ranging from mild, loose feces to watery diarrhea to bloody mucoid diarrhea. Acute campylobacteriosis that develops in puppies and some adult dogs is manifest by mucus-laden, watery, or bile-streaked diarrhea (with or without blood and leukocytes) of 5 to 15 days duration, partial anorexia, and occasional vomiting.[36] Elevated temperature and leukocytosis may also be present. In certain cases, diarrhea can be chronic of 2 or more weeks' duration, can be intermittent, or in some cases can be present for several months.[36]

C. jejuni has been isolated from two dogs with bacteremia and cholecystitis.[98] Presenting signs included anorexia, fever, and icterus. On ultrasonography, a fluid-filled, abnormally thickened gallbladder wall was observed in both dogs. In humans with cholecystitis, *C. jejuni* and *C. fetus* are also recovered infrequently from the bile.[144, 146] Insofar as *Helicobacter* spp. are present in liver and bile of various hosts (see Intestinal and Hepatic Helicobacters), detailed biochemical and phenotypic descriptions are necessary to fully characterize and validate whether microaerophilic organisms isolated from the hepatobiliary tract of dogs are *Campylobacter* or *Helicobacter* species.

Cat

In cats, clinical signs of campylobacteriosis are poorly documented in the absence of other pathogens. As with dogs, campylobacteriosis is usually nonsymptomatic. If clinical signs are evident, the animal generally is younger than 6 months. In a prevalence survey of 159 cats from pounds, 17 shed *C. jejuni* in the feces, but of these only 2 had bloody mucus-laden diarrhea. *Giardia* spp. was present in both, combined with *Isospora* spp. in one cat and *Toxocara* spp. in the other. Another cat concurrently infected with *Salmonella* spp. and *C. jejuni* was depressed and anorectic but not diarrheic. Culture results from the two cats' feces after antibiotic therapy and clinical improvement were negative for *C. jejuni*.[36] Chronic diarrhea in another cat that had serum antibodies to *C. jejuni*, plus positive culture results for the organism, abated when treated with chloramphenicol. *C. jejuni* could not be recultured from the stool after therapy.[36]

DIAGNOSIS

Microscopic Examination

Rapid presumptive diagnosis is possible using either dark-field or phase-contrast microscopy. Fresh fecal samples are examined for curved bacteria with the characteristic darting motility of *C. jejuni*. This method is especially sensitive in people (and perhaps dogs and cats) during the acute stage of clinical diarrhea. With Gram's stain, faintly staining, gram-negative, gull wing–shaped slender rods are apparent. Maintaining the safranin counterstaining improves their visualization.[84] Presence of fecal WBCs should be ascertained, because they may be found in enteritis caused by natural or experimental infections with *C. jejuni*.

Cultural Identification

Rectal swab specimens can be obtained or fresh feces can be collected. For diagnosis of *C. jejuni* cholecystitis and bacteremia, appropriate diagnostic testing, including abdominal ultrasonography, gallbladder aspiration with bile culture, and blood culture, should be performed.[98] Transport of fecal specimens usually does not present isolation difficulties because *C. jejuni–coli* remain viable in feces at room temperature for at least 3 days and at refrigeration temperatures for at least 1 week. However, higher rates of isolation can be achieved with shorter time delays.

Swabs obtained from fresh feces are streaked onto *Campylobacter* blood agar plates (Campy BAP), which are then placed in an oxygen-reduced atmosphere. The standard method for culture uses commercially available selective medium that inhibits fecal flora; however, it may not be necessary for isolating thermophilic *Campylobacter* strains from acute cases of enteritis. Similarly, broth enrichment procedures have not been more effective than direct plating methods on Campy BAP for isolation of *C. jejuni* from canine feces.

Plates are incubated at 42°C and examined at 72 to 96 hours. Colonies composed of curved gram-negative rods are round, raised, translucent, and sometimes mucoid. Isolates are identified as *C. jejuni* on the basis of positive oxidase and catalase reactions, susceptibility to nalidixic acid, resistance to cephalothin, and inability to grow at 42°C under aerobic conditions. *C. upsalensis* is catalase negative, and isolation is enhanced by selective filtration of feces to be cultured through a 0.45-μ filter.[51]

Various procedures have been used, especially in outbreaks, to identify different serotypes of *C. jejuni–coli* by using thermostabile and thermolabile surface antigens.[36] Isolates from people and various animal species have shown that extensive serologic heterogeneity exists within *C.*

jejuni–coli. Many of the isolates frequently found in diarrheic and normal dogs and cats have had serotypes frequently encountered in human patients.[36] For example, serotype 4 (commonly associated with outbreaks of *C. jejuni*–associated diarrhea in humans) was also a common serotype isolated from commercially reared beagles.[36, 136] Plasmid characterization, restriction enzyme analysis, and ribotyping can also be used for strain identity, but these techniques require specialized methodologies. The technique of restriction enzyme analysis of whole genomic DNA allowed verification of *C. jejuni* zoonotic transmission to personnel in vivaria caring for wild but caught and captive coyotes.[46]

Serologic Testing

A variety of techniques can detect serum antibodies to various antigens of *Campylobacter*. A specific bactericidal assay has been used to demonstrate a rising antibody titer in both people and animals. Other serologic assays, such as ELISA, have been developed to survey human populations during outbreaks of campylobacteriosis and to ascertain previous exposures to the organism. Unfortunately, no systematic studies have been performed in dogs and cats to ascertain the importance of antibody titers as an indicator of infection in animals with or without diarrhea.

PATHOLOGIC FINDINGS

Grossly visible findings in naturally and experimentally infected canine neonates are abnormally fluid colonic contents and thickening, congestion, and edema of the colonic mucosa.[36] Microscopically, the colon and cecum show decreases in epithelial cell height, brush borders, and numbers of goblet cells. Hyperplasia of epithelial glands results in a thickened mucosa. Subepithelial congestion, hemorrhage, and inflammatory infiltrates have also been seen. Findings in adult animals inoculated with *C. jejuni* were similar to those in some dogs with natural campylobacteriosis: stunting of intestinal villi, infiltration of lamina propria with inflammatory cells, and hyperplastic Peyer's patches.[36] Naturally occurring intestinal lesions in adult dogs have consisted of mucosal hyperplasia in the colon, characterized by immature hyperchromatic, hyperplastic epithelial cells with a high mitotic index, and deep and irregular crypts.[36] With Warthin-Starry stain, *Campylobacter*-like organisms have been demonstrated attached to, but not within, colonic epithelium. However, in experimentally produced *C. jejuni* colitis in macaques, intraepithelial invasion of *C. jejuni* was demonstrated by EM.[116] A relative increase had been noted in the number of lymphocytes infiltrating the lamina propria. Ileal lesions consisted of focal, shallow crypts and blunt, irregular villi, which occasionally fused. There has been mild congestion and dilatation of lacteals. Stunting and fusing of intestinal villi and mononuclear cell infiltrates in lamina propria have also been noted in subacute stages of parvovirus infection and in a dog with protracted *Campylobacter*-associated diarrhea.[36]

THERAPY

Efficacy of antibiotic therapy and treatment of *Campylobacter*-associated diarrhea in the dog and cat is not known, nor is it known whether antibiotics indeed effectively alter the course of enteric disease. However, in some cases of severe diarrhea in dogs and cats, antibiotic therapy may be warranted. Antibiotic treatment of infected animals may be instituted to minimize exposure to humans and other pets in the household. Fortunately, strains of *Campylobacter* isolated from animals and people are susceptible to several antimicrobial agents (Table 39–1). Erythromycin, the drug of choice for *Campylobacter*-induced diarrhea in humans, may also be effective in the treatment of the disease in animals. Treatment of clinically affected cats and dogs has resulted in resolution of the illness and elimination of the organism as determined by *Campylobacter*-negative fecal cultures. It must be cautioned, however, that failure to eliminate *C. jejuni* with oral erythromycin from ferrets housed in a research environment has also been noted.[36] Erythromycin can also cause gastric irritation and vomiting in some animals.

Chloramphenicol has been given with mixed results to treat *Campylobacter*-associated diarrhea in dogs and cats. Treatment in dogs has resulted in abatement of clinical signs. However, the same organism has been reisolated after therapy has been completed. It is possible that these dogs developed an antibiotic-induced carrier state, as recognized in enteric *Salmonella* infections, experienced a protracted period of shedding of the *Campylobacter* spp., or became rein-

Table 39–1. Drug Therapy for Nonenteric Salmonellosis and Other Enteric Bacterial Infections in Dogs and Cats

DRUG	SPECIES	DOSE[a] (mg/kg)	ROUTE	INTERVAL (HOURS)	DURATION (DAYS)	INDICATED INFECTIONS
Erythromycin	D	20	PO	12	5–21	Campylobacterosis, nongastric helicobacteriosis
	C	10	PO	8	5	
Trimethoprim-sulfonamide	B	12–15	PO, IV	12	7–10	Salmonellosis, shigellosis, yersiniosis
Amoxicillin/ampicillin	B	10–20	PO, IV	8	7–10	Salmonellosis, shigellosis
Chloramphenicol	D	15–25	PO, SC, IV	8	5–7	Salmonellosis, shigellosis, campylobacteriosis, nongastric helicobacteriosis
	C	10–15	PO, SC	12	8	
Metronidazole	B	8–10	PO	8	5–10	Bacterial overgrowth, nongastric and gastric helicobacteriosis
Tetracycline	B	10–20	PO	8	42	Shigellosis, yersiniosis, bacterial overgrowth
Gentamicin[b]	D	2	IM, SC	12	5	Yersiniosis, salmonellosis, nongastric helicobacteriosis
Tylosin	B	11	PO	8	42	Bacterial overgrowth
Cephalosporins (1st gen.)	B	20	PO	8	7	Yersiniosis
Cephalosporins (2nd gen.)	B	22	IV	8	21	Campylobacteriosis, nongastric helicobacteriosis
Enrofloxacin[c]	B	5	PO, SC	12	5–7	Campylobacteriosis, salmonellosis

[a]Dose per administration at specified interval. For additional information on each drug, see Appendix 8.
[b]Monitor for renal failure.
[c]Other quinolones such as ciprofloxacin, difloxacin, or marbofloxacin, although dosages vary, are alternatives.
B = both dog and cat; C = cat; D = dog.

fected. A diarrheic cat treated with chloramphenicol showed clinical improvement, and fecal cultures after completion of the treatment were negative for *C. jejuni*. *C. jejuni*–associated bacteremia and cholecystitis have been successfully treated with IV cefoxitin, a second-generation cephalosporin, or oral erythromycin at dosages listed in Table 39–1, for a 21-day period, which resulted in complete resolution of all clinical and laboratory abnormalities.[98]

Several other antibiotics are active against *Campylobacter* strains isolated from dogs and cats. These strains show in vitro susceptibility to furazolidone as well as gentamicin, neomycin, clindamycin, and tetracycline. However, many strains may carry plasmids that confer resistance to a variety of tetracyclines. Antimicrobial agents that are usually ineffective in treatment include penicillin, ampicillin, polymyxin B, trimethoprim, and vancomycin. In vitro resistance is also found to metronidazole and sulfadimethoxine.[36] Many *Campylobacter* strains produce β-lactamase, which accounts for the resistance to penicillin and ampicillin.

PUBLIC HEALTH CONSIDERATIONS

It is now recognized that *C. jejuni–coli* is a leading cause of enteric disease in people and that puppies and kittens can serve as sources of infection for humans. The infectious dose of *C. jejuni* for humans is as low as a few hundred organisms. The disease is often severe in people and, in addition to diarrhea, may be characterized by vomiting, fever, and abdominal discomfort. Usually the incriminated pets have been suffering from diarrhea and have been recently acquired from pet stores or kennels.[36] However, asymptomatic dogs and cats can also be a source of infection to people.[36] A survey conducted in Seattle, Washington, indicated that 6% of sporadic *C. jejuni* infections were linked to exposure to diarrheic kittens.[2] The association of *C. jejuni* with zoonotic transmission to humans, especially children handling young puppies and kittens, strengthens the argument that dogs may be responsible for zoonotic infection of intestinal helicobacters in humans.[130] Another study reported that 30% of the cases in university students were associated with healthy cats.[36] However, the major risk factors for acquiring *C. jejuni* enteritis is the consumption of raw or undercooked meat, particularly chicken.[36] Nevertheless, veterinary practitioners should alert owners of the zoonotic implication of *Campylobacter* infection for other household members and stress the importance of exercising appropriate hygienic measures, especially when pets have diarrhea. An additional zoonotic risk is the Guillain-Barré syndrome, a demyelinating polyradiculoneuritis in people, which may follow infection with *C. jejuni*. The antigens of peripheral nerves may share epitopes with those of these bacteria.[96a]

C. upsalensis has been isolated from a human with bloody diarrhea as well as his pet dog, which also had diarrhea. The plasmid profile of the two strains were identical, suggesting that *C. upsalensis* infection may also be a zoonosis.[51] The isolation of *C. upsalensis* from the blood and fetoplacental tissue of a diarrheic woman 18 weeks' pregnant, who had contact with a cat having a similar strain of *C. upsalensis* isolated from its feces, is suggestive of zoonotic transmission.[55] Others have also reported *C. upsalensis* gastroenteritis in humans who had contact with pets.[103] Human and canine isolates of *C. upsalensis* have distinct ribotypes and plasmid profiles, suggesting that host-specific genotype differences may exist among strains of *C. upsalensis*.[129] However, these analyses or other molecular fingerprinting techniques must be used on suspected pet-associated *C. upsalensis* zoonoses before the definitive transmission can be defined.

Gastric Helicobacters

James G. Fox

ETIOLOGY

Gram-negative, microaerophilic, curved to spiral-shaped bacteria isolated from gastric mucosa of humans and animals have created a great deal of interest because of their causal role in gastric disease.[80] To date, the genus *Helicobacter* includes 14 formally named species as well as other unnamed closely related organisms.[20, 39, 41, 47, 82, 96, 130, 131, 144] Once considered a predominantly sterile organ, protected from microbial colonization by low gastric pH, the euchlorhydric stomach is now known to be colonized with gastric bacteria belonging to the newly named genus *Helicobacter* (Table 39–2). The type species *H. pylori* colonizes the stomach of 20% to 95% of human adult populations worldwide.[52] *H. pylori* causes persistent, active, chronic gastritis and peptic ulcer disease in humans and has been linked to the development of gastric adenocarcinoma and gastric mucosa–associated lymphoma.[100, 101] *H. pylori* has also been isolated from inflamed gastric tissue of cats in a commercial cattery.[57]

Other gastric helicobacters have been linked to gastritis in a variety of mammalian hosts.[37] Additional species of gastric *Helicobacter* have been isolated from stomachs of various mammalian hosts, including dogs, cats, ferrets *(H. mustelae)*, cheetahs *(H. acinonyx)*, and nonhuman primates.

Historically, these *Helicobacter* in dogs and cats have been described histologically as gastric "spirilla."[37] Three morphologically distinct forms have been described in dogs and cats.[83, 152a, 153] More than one of these morphologic types of bacteria can be seen in the stomach of one animal. Lockard type 1 is a bacterium with multiple bipolar, sheathed flagella entwined with periplasmic fibers, which appear to cover the entire surface of the organism. A similar organism was isolated from aborted ovine fetuses and was classified as "*Flexispira rappini*."[74, 96] This bacterium, classified as a *Helicobacter* spp. based on 16sRNA sequencing, has been isolated from the feces of asymptomatic mice and dogs as well as from the stomach of dogs.[83, 119] Lockard type 2 also has periplasmic fibers, but they are most sparsely distributed on the organism and can appear singly or in groups of two, three, or four. This organism has been cultured from the cat stomach and has been named *H. felis*.[102] The third type of organisms, termed gastrospirilla, are the bacteria most commonly found in animal stomachs. These are also very tightly spiraled, but there are no periplasmic fibrils. On the basis of morphology, it appears that the Lockard type 2 organism primarily is restricted to cats and dogs, whereas type 3 has been seen in cats, dogs, nonhuman primates, cheetahs, swine, and humans. The type 3 bacterium has been given various names

Table 39–2. Comparative Features of **Campylobacter** *spp. and* **Helicobacter** *spp. That Infect Dogs or Cats*

ORGANISM (OLDER TERMINOLOGY)	MORPHOLOGY/DISTINCTIONS	HOST	CLINICAL FEATURES
Campylobacters			
C. jejuni/C. coli	Slender-curve motile rods; singular, pairs, chains 3–5 spirals curved S or gull shaped, single polar, nonsheathed flagella/*C. coli* hippurate negative	Dogs, cats Humans	Neonatal diarrhea, adults asymptomatic carriers Diarrhea, systemic manifestations
C. upsalensis	Catalase negative	Dogs Humans	Asymptomatic Diarrhea in immunocompetent
Gastric Helicobacters			
H. pylori	Small 2–4 μ, curved to spiral shaped	Humans, nonhuman primates Cats	Gastritis, peptic ulcer, gastric neoplasia Gastritis in catteries
H. (Flexispira) rappini (Lockard type 1)	Fusiform shape, entwined with multiple periplasmic fibers; multiple bipolar sheathed flagella	Sheep Humans and animals Dogs	Abortion, hepatic necrosis Intestinal disease Asymptomatic, gastric & fecal isolate
H. felis (Lockard type 2)	7–10 μ length, superficial periplasmic fibers, sparse, singly or in groups, multiple bipolar flagella with sheaths	Cats, dogs, humans	Cultured from stomach subclinical (histologic) gastritis
H. bizzozeronii (Lockard type 3, *Gastrospirillium hominis, H. heilmannii*)	7–10 μ length, tightly spiraled, no periplasmic fibers/difficult to culture deep in gastric glands and parietal cell canaliculi	Dogs and cats, humans, swine, nonhuman primates	Common gastric colonizer
Intestinal and Hepatic Helicobacters			
H. cinaedi and *H. fennelliae*	Single bipolar sheathed flagella	Dogs and cats Nonhuman primates Humans	Fecal isolate Experimental infection Often asymptomatic, colitis and proctitis if immunosuppressed
H. canis	Sheathed bipolar flagella, resists bile, resists polymyxin B, cannot reduce nitrate	Dogs Humans	Liver with multifocal hepatitis Diarrhea or asymptomatic

in different hosts, including *Gastrospirillum hominis, H. heilmannii,* and *H. bizzozeronii.*[59, 123] *H. bizzozeronii* from dogs is the only formal name, based on defined biochemical and genetic analysis.[59] *H. bizzozeronii* has also been cultured from the inflamed gastric tissue of humans.[1] By EM, this organism lacks periplasmic fibers in contrast to *H. felis*. This morphologic distinction is confounded with the observation of two gastric *Helicobacter*-like organisms (GHLOs). These GHLOs from dog stomachs lacking periplasmic fibers had genetic analysis compatible with *H. felis.*[28]

EPIDEMIOLOGY

Although infected animals and humans mount a significant systemic IgG response to gastric organisms, the antibodies are not protective and the organisms persist in the mucous layer or closely adhere to the gastric epithelium, protected from the gastric acidic milieu. The mechanisms of transmission are poorly understood. Gastric helicobacters have specific enteric tissue tropism and colonize only gastric and not intestinal epithelium. Fecal-oral transmission has been suggested, but gastric helicobacters have rarely been isolated from feces of animals or humans. *H. mustelae* was isolated from feces of ferrets, particularly when ferrets had drug-induced hypochlorhydria.[44] *H. pylori* has been isolated from feces of children from a third-world country as well as adults from a more developed country that were infected with *H. pylori.*[70, 139] House flies have been shown to harbor the organism[53a]; however, their role, if any, in transmission is uncertain.

Oral-oral transmission is more likely and is supported by clinical observations of humans being infected by exposure to gastric secretions; isolation of *H. pylori* from dental plaque and tissue; and nosocomial infection from improper disinfection of gastric pH probes and endoscopic equipment. Similar transmission routes are also probable for gastric *Helicobacter* in animals. Vomitus containing gastric *Helicobacter* is another likely source for transmission.[31] Cats, naturally infected with *H. pylori*, were screened by culture and polymerase chain reaction (PCR) for the organism in salivary secretions, gastric juices, gastric tissues, and feces.[45] *H. pylori* was cultured in cats from salivary secretions in 50% and from gastric fluid samples in 91%. A PCR product specific for an *H. pylori* surface protein was amplified in feline specimens from dental plaque in 42% and from feces in 80%. Isolation of *H. pylori* from feline mucosal secretions suggests a zoonotic risk from exposure to personnel handling *H. pylori*--infected cats in vivaria.[57] In comparison, the infection was not detected in stray cats,[29a] which may reflect an anthroponosis. Additional studies using molecular, cultural, and histologic techniques are needed to ascertain whether *H. pylori* naturally colonizes dogs and cats.

The prevalence of gastric *Helicobacter* infections in colony-raised animals with high population density routinely approaches 100%, indicating the organisms' unique ability to colonize the stomach of numerous hosts selectively and efficiently. In laboratory reared beagles, *H. felis* and other spiral helicobacters were observed in greater numbers in the gastric glands of the fundic-pyloric junction and the cardia. These organisms were associated with lymphoid hyperplasia and parietal cell degeneration.[62, 83] In pet dogs and cats, a series of gastric biopsy samples were examined for the presence of GHLOs.[63] GHLOs were observed in 82% of dogs and 76% of cats; the bacteria were present in the mucus of foveolar epithelia, gastric pits, and parietal cells. An increase of lymphoid follicles in the stomachs of older pound cats with high numbers of GHLOs in their gastric mucosa has been observed compared with younger cats with lower numbers of GHLO colonization.[99]

PATHOGENESIS

To date, chronic or chronic active gastritis resulting from oral inoculation of *Helicobacter* spp. has been experimentally produced in humans, germ-free pigs, germ-free dogs, cats, mice, and nonhuman primates with *H. pylori*; in the ferret with *H. mustelae*; in kittens with *H. acinonyx* and *H. heilmannii*; and in germ-free dogs, mice, and rats with *H. felis*.[37] The *H. pylori*–associated gastritis in humans consists of polymorphonuclear cells as well as mononuclear cell infiltrates and is classified as active chronic gastritis. Persistent *H. pylori* infection in humans (particularly children) and the domestic cat also is often characterized by lymphoid aggregates and gastric lymphoid follicles.[38, 58] Inflammation and associated lymphoid follicles were primarily located in the antrum, which corresponded to the heaviest concentration of *H. pylori*.[57] Ultrastructurally, the organisms were numerous in the gastric mucus and, less frequently, adhered tightly to gastric epithelia and formed pedestals between bacterial membranes and the epithelial microvilli.[57] In the past, gastric lymphoid elements were considered a normal histologic finding in dogs and cats. However, experimental and clinical evidence suggests that they are the result of host responses to *Helicobacter* antigens. The presence of GHLOs is often associated with a reduction in mucus content of surface epithelia, occasional intraepithelial leukocytes, and some degenerating glands. Eosinophils in gastric mucosa of animals can also be a major component of the inflammation, particularly in the acute phase of the infection.[38, 81, 110]

The degree of GHLO colonization and lymphoid follicles correlated well in cats but not in dogs. If the number of GHLOs in dogs was classified as high, then lymphoid follicles were more likely to be present. In high-grade GHLO infection, glandular degeneration was more pronounced in cats than dogs.[63] In other dogs,[78] the severity of gastritis correlated that of infection but not with the clinical sign of vomiting. In other studies[27] 100% of laboratory and shelter dogs and 67% of pet dogs were colonized with GHLOs morphologically consistent with *H. heilmannii* or *H. felis*. Regardless of the colonization intensity, all dogs had mild to moderate gastritis, and *H. pylori* was not isolated.

Competitive inhibition may occur in gastric helicobacteriosis. *H. pylori*–infected cats did not have large gastric spiral organisms colonizing the gastric mucosa. This phenomenon has also been suggested to account for the rare occurrence of concurrent infection in humans and nonhuman primates with large gastric spiral organisms and *H. pylori*.[23, 24, 61, 80, 132] Experimental inoculation of the feline *H. pylori* strain into naive cats without gastric infection caused by GHLOs confirmed that *H. pylori* produces a persistent gastritis identical to that noted in cats naturally infected with *H. pylori*.[38] *H. pylori* was isolated on serial biopsies and at necropsy 7 months after inoculation from all cats.[38] Additional studies are required to ascertain whether duodenal and gastric ulcers have an infectious component in dogs and cats.[40]

CLINICAL FINDINGS

Although gastric helicobacters produce gastritis in humans and animals, they usually cause asymptomatic infection in their hosts.[27, 57] Clinical signs in pet animals, however, attributable to *Helicobacter*-associated gastritis, do occur. Signs include chronic vomiting, weight loss, and, in some cases, severe emaciation or diarrhea.[28, 63] Vomiting in dogs with chronic superficial gastritis attributed to gastric spiral organisms has been characterized as intermittent, consisting of mucus or gastric secretions, sometimes containing bile. Pica, belching, anorexia, and weight loss also are occasionally noted. Signs attributed to gastric helicobacteriosis have been based on finding these organisms in gastric biopsy samples from animals with GI illness. Because these organisms can be present in clinically healthy animals, the direct cause-and-effect relationship to clinical illness cannot always be ascertained.

DIAGNOSIS

A diagnosis of chronic gastritis in animals, as in humans, cannot be made by gross visual examination of the gastric mucosa by endoscopy. Histologic evaluation of gastric biopsy samples is required utilizing a special silver stain or modified Giemsa stain to reveal the presence of GHLOs (Fig. 39–2). A definitive diagnosis requires culture and isolation of the specific species of *Helicobacter*. Unfortunately, *H. bizzozeronii* is the most common spiral organism in dogs and cats, and it has been extremely difficult to culture on artificial media.[59] *H. felis* is also difficult to isolate. In practice, histologic findings of inflammatory changes accompanied by gastric spiral organisms on the gastric mucosa or in the gastric mucous layer have been used for diagnosis. *H. felis* cannot be distinguished from *H. heilmannii* by histologic examination; EM evaluation is necessary.

Because oral bacteria and bacteria refluxed from the duodenum (e.g., Enterobacteriaceae, diphtheroids, streptococci, and anaerobes) may overgrow the fastidious *Helicobacter* species, selective media are available for isolation. Media consist of *Brucella* agar with 10% horse blood containing vancomycin (10 mg/L), polymyxin B (2500 U/L), and trimethoprim (5 mg/L). Fresh media are recommended for optimal growth. Various *Helicobacter* spp. have different antibiotic susceptibilities, and selection of the type and quantity of antibiotics in culture media may determine success of isolation. Helicobacters, like campylobacters, require special environmental and cultural conditions for their growth. The organisms are thermophilic and grow at 37°C, and some species at 42°C. Growth on chocolate or blood agar takes 3 to 5 days. For *H. bizzozeronii* isolation, incubation requires 5 to 10 days.[59] Helicobacters

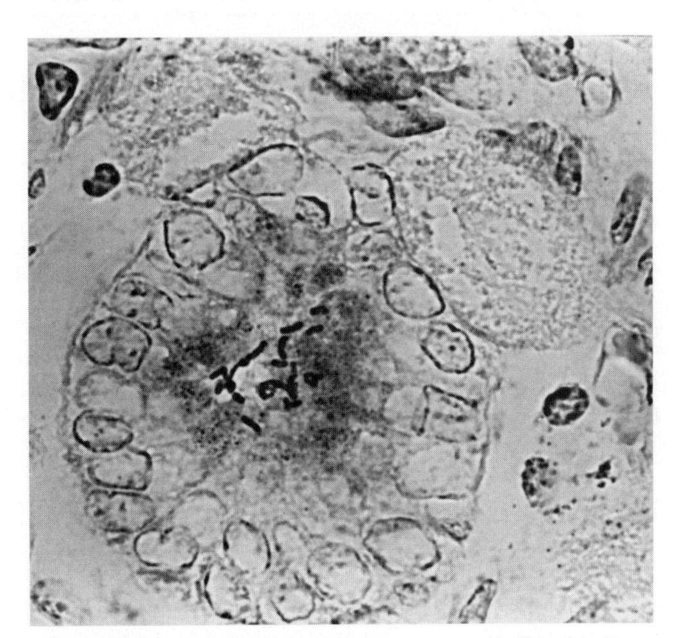

Figure 39–2. *H. pylori* in the crypt of a cat stomach (Warthin-Starry stain, × 1000).

will not grow under aerobic or anaerobic conditions but achieve optimum growth in a high humidity with microaerobic conditions (10% carbon dioxide, 80% nitrogen, 5% hydrogen).

Isolation of helicobacters is enhanced by proper processing of gastric tissue. Mincing the gastric tissue with sterile scalpel blades or using a tissue homogenizer enhances isolation. If immediate processing of the biopsy sample is not possible, the tissue can be placed in sterile 30% glycerol in *Brucella* broth and placed at 4°C for at least 5 hours. Specimens in this media can also be frozen for longer periods for subsequent culture of the biopsy sample or transport of previously characterized organisms.

A provisional diagnosis of gastric helicobacters takes advantage of a biochemical feature of these organisms: the ability to produce large quantities of urease. Gastric biopsy samples can be placed in a urea broth containing a pH indicator (phenol red) and a preservative (sodium azide). A similar test is available commercially, or a microtiter tray with a measured amount of urea test solution delivered to each well can be used very effectively and economically. Other urease tests for humans, but not perfected in other than research animals, are the urea breath test, which measures expired radiolabeled carbon dioxide, a by-product of a carbon-labeled urea test meal that is ingested by the patient.[150] An alternative but less accurate method would be direct measurement of ammonia in gastric juice utilizing a colorimetric assay.

Serologic assays are being employed to diagnose *H. pylori* in humans and *H. mustelae* infection in ferrets.[40, 128] However, they currently do not provide a reliable, noninvasive diagnostic test for gastric *Helicobacter* infection in dogs and cats. Analyses of serum and mucosal secretions by ELISA in *H. pylori*, naturally infected cats revealed an *H. pylori*–specific IgG response and elevated anti-*H. pylori* IgA levels in salivary and local gastric secretions.[45] This assay probably cannot be used clinically in cats because of the high prevalence of the large spiral GHLOs in pet cats and the cross-reactive antigens shared by these bacteria and *H. pylori*.

THERAPY

Various clinical trials using different antimicrobial treatments were initially conducted in people to assess their ability to eradicate *H. pylori*. A triple-therapy regimen consisting of amoxicillin and metronidazole or tetracycline and metronidazole in combination with bismuth subsalicylate given for 2 to 3 weeks has proved to be the most efficient in eradication of *H. pylori*. Indeed, this antimicrobial regimen, plus ranitidine, has proved successful in treating patients with *Helicobacter*-induced gastric ulcers. In studies comparing this treatment with ranitidine alone, ulcers not only healed faster, but the recurrence was significantly less than in those receiving only antibiotics. Therapy regimens using proton pump inhibitors (e.g., omeprazole) in combination with antibiotics (e.g., amoxicillin) also have shown considerable efficacy in eradicating *H. pylori*. Whether antimicrobial therapy should be instituted in domestic dogs and cats with gastritis or ulcer disease has not been consistently evaluated. Suggested combination drug regimens based on those that are effective for *H. pylori*–infected humans[150] with dosages for dogs and cats are listed in Table 39–3. Studies in ferrets indicate that the triple therapy consisting of amoxicillin, metronidazole, and bismuth subsalicylate three times a day for 3 to 4 weeks has successfully eradicated *H. mustelae* from ferrets. Omeprazole, given in ferrets once daily, effectively induces hypochlorhydria and can be given in conjunction with antibiotics to treat *H. mustelae*–associated duodenal or gastric ulcers. Cases of acute bleeding ulcers must be treated as emergencies, and fluid and blood transfusions are essential.

The duration of treatment of dogs and cats with helicobacteriosis has not been well substantiated. Cats naturally infected with *H. pylori* have received a 21-day course of oral amoxicillin, metronidazole, and omeprazole.[106] All six treated cats were culture negative at several sites (saliva, gastric juice, and gastric mucosa) for *H. pylori*. However, as determined by PCR, the majority of cats at 2 and 4 weeks after treatment had gastric biopsy samples positive for *H. pylori*. At 6 weeks after treatment, all six cats had *H. pylori*–negative

Table 39–3. Therapy for Gastric Helicobacteriosis in Dogs and Cats

DRUG	SPECIES	DOSE[a]	ROUTE	INTERVAL (HOURS)	DURATION (DAYS)
A. Triple therapy regimen					
Bismuth[b]	D	0.5–2 ml/kg	PO	4–6	14–28
	C	0.5–1 ml/kg	PO	4–6	14–28
Metronidazole	C	62.5 mg total	PO	24	14–28
	D	15 mg/kg	PO	12–24	14–28
Amoxicillin	B	15–20 mg/kg	PO	8	14–28
B. Antimicrobial substitute for amoxicillin in A					
Tetracycline	B	22 mg/kg	PO	8	14–28
C. Antisecretory substitute for bismuth in A					
Cimetidine[c]	B	5–10 mg/kg	PO	8	28
	B	5–6 mg/kg	IM, IV	8[d]	28
Ranitidine	D	1–2 mg/kg	PO, IV	12	28
	C	2.5 mg/kg	IV	12	28
		3.5 mg/kg	PO	12	28
Omeprazole	B	0.5–1 mg/kg[e]	PO	24	28
	D > 20 kg	20 mg total	PO	24	28
Misoprostol	D	1–5 μg/kg	PO	8	28
D. Antimicrobial substitute for metronidazole[f] in A					
Clarithromycin	B	7.5 mg/kg	PO	12	14–28

[a]Dose per administration at specified interval. For additional information, see Appendix 8. Treatment duration in people has been up to 8 weeks for successful resolution.
[b]Bismuth subsalicylate, original formula (Procter). Dose is 17.5 mg/kg when using other products. Salicylate compounds must be used judiciously in cats, and other substitutes should be considered.
[c]Cimetidine inhibits absorption of ketoconazole; metoclopramide inhibits cimetidine absorption.
[d]Not as a bolus but by slow infusion.
[e]Available as 20-mg capsule; granules must be fractionated and placed in gelatin capsules for lower dosages.
[f]Metronidazole resistance has been noted in *H. pylori* infections in people with increasing frequency.[144a]
B = both dog and cat; C = cat; D = dog.

cultures for samples from several gastric sites taken at necropsy, and only one cat had *H. pylori* cultured from gastric juice. PCR analysis revealed that five of six cats still had *H. pylori* DNA amplification products from plaque, saliva, or gastric biopsy samples. Persistence of *H. pylori* at extragastric sites may allow subsequent recolonization of the stomach after cessation of therapy. Antibiotics may also induce formation of viable but nonculturable coccoid forms of *H. pylori* that can still be detected by PCR.

In people with severe GHLO infection (i.e., *H. heilmannii* or *H. felis*), bismuth subsalicylate, amoxicillin, tetracycline, and metronidazole in various combinations successfully eradicated GHLOs from the gastric mucosa with resolution of gastritis.[61, 140] In two separate reports, prolonged treatment with bismuth subsalicylate (4 weeks) or bismuth subcitrate (8 weeks) successfully eradicated the GHLOs from patients.[61, 88] No systematic antibiotic trials have been conducted in dogs and cats to test for efficacy in eradicating either *H. heilmannii* or *H. felis* from gastric mucosa.

PUBLIC HEALTH CONSIDERATIONS

Because *H. heilmannii* (currently *H. bizzozeronii*) and to a lesser extent *H. felis* colonize a small percentage of humans with gastritis, and no environmental source for these bacteria has been recognized, pets have been implicated in zoonotic transmission. In one report of *H. heilmannii* infection in a child, the household had two cats. A gastric biopsy from one cat indicated it was infected with gastric spiral organisms with similar morphology to that detected in the child's stomach.[79] In another, a girl moving to a rural environment developed an 18-month history of epigastric pain, nausea, vomiting, and anorexia. An antral active chronic gastritis associated with *H. heilmannii* was present.[140] Institution of various anti-*Helicobacter* antimicrobial treatment was only temporarily successful. She had two dogs: one with chronic intermittent vomiting that frequently licked her face and an asymptomatic dog. The symptomatic dog had active chronic gastritis associated with large numbers of *H. heilmannii,* whereas the asymptomatic dog had a mild gastritis associated with fewer *H. heilmannii.* The girl and the dogs were simultaneously placed on a 6-week course of amoxicillin and bismuth. The symptoms in the dog resolved, but the girl required additional therapy with omeprazole. Without DNA analysis of the *H. heilmannii* strains to confirm identity, the zoonotic association is highly suggestive.

In Germany, a survey of 125 individuals infected with GHLOs provided information in a questionnaire regarding animal contact. Of these patients, 70.3% had contact with one or more animals compared with 37% in the clinically healthy control population.[132] More than a threefold preponderance of males over female patients with GHLOs was recorded. Because *H. bizzozeronii* can be cultured on artificial media, a comparison is needed between the various species infecting cats and their genetic markers. A researcher performing physiologic studies with cat stomachs developed an acute gastritis presumably resulting from *H. felis* on the basis of EM.[77] Similar gastric spiral bacteria were demonstrated in gastric mucosa of cats being used by this scientist.

If *H. pylori,* as demonstrated in commercially reared cats,[45, 57] is isolated from pet cats, the zoonotic potential of helicobacteriosis from cats would obviously increase substantially. *H. pylori* infection is an important cause of human gastritis. Most epidemiologic studies do not incriminate pet contact with human infection.

In serologic studies of people with *H. pylori* infection, owning pets was inversely related to *H. pylori* IgG antibody titers; however, pet ownership in these studies was associated with a higher socioeconomic status.[31, 52] Furthermore, pet ownership was not segregated by whether the pets were dogs or cats, by the number and age of pets, or the length of pet ownership. In another study, even though the number of patients with pets was small, exposure to cats or dogs in the preceding year was not statistically associated with *H. pylori* infection.[145] An epidemiologic survey conducted in Germany did not show an increased risk of *H. pylori* because of cat ownership.[3] In a serologic survey measuring antibodies to *H. pylori,* lower socioeconomic status, and not pet ownership or day care, was associated with seropositivity.[128] In a survey of male employees in England, pet ownership as a child was marginally associated with current *H. pylori* infection; however, overcrowding plus person-to-person contact was found to be the major risk factor.[152] Only one study suggested an epidemiologic risk. IgG anti-*H. pylori*–seropositive farm workers were more likely to report contact with cats and to report less contact with dogs.[138]

Intestinal and Hepatic Helicobacters

James G. Fox

ETIOLOGY

In addition to their association with the gastric mucosae, an increasing number of other *Helicobacter* spp. have been isolated from the lower intestinal tract of mammals and birds[41, 47, 121, 130, 131] (see Table 39–2). Some of these (e.g., *H. cinaedi* and *H. fennelliae*) have been linked to proctitis and colitis in immunocompromised humans.[72, 141] In addition, *H. hepaticus* and *H. bilis* have been isolated from livers of mice with hepatitis as well as from intestines of asymptomatic mice.[41, 47] *H. bilis* has been isolated from a gastric sample of a dog.[27]

One of these gram-negative spiral organisms with sheathed bipolar flagella was given the name *Helicobacter canis* group because it evidenced weak DNA homology to *H. cinaedi* and *H. fennelliae,* but was distinguishable from these organisms because it was resistant to polymyxin B and was unable to reduce nitrate. The organism was named *H. canis,* and, like *H. hepaticus, H. bilis,* and *H. pullorum,* its marked resistance to bile probably enables the organism to colonize the liver.[41, 47, 130, 131]

Also of interest is the isolation, on the basis of cellular fatty acid analysis, of *H. cinaedi* from the feces of dogs and a cat.[72] *H. fennelliae* has also been identified in the feces of a dog and macaque monkey. Like *H. cinaedi, H. fennelliae* (previously known as *Campylobacter fennelliae* or *Campylobacter*-like organisms [CLO]-2), was first isolated from HIV-infected homosexuals with colitis and proctitis.[141] However, unlike *H. cinaedi,* this enteric *Helicobacter* does not often cause bacteremia in adult humans.[71, 93]

EPIDEMIOLOGY

In epidemiologic studies regarding incidence of CLOs in 1000 dogs, 4% of the animals had an organism, later to be determined as *H. canis*, isolated from their feces.[12, 130] The organism was also isolated from the feces of a child with gastroenteritis during a similar survey of children to determine prevalence of CLOs.[14]

H. canis has also been identified, on the basis of 16S rRNA data, from the liver of a puppy diagnosed as having an active, multifocal hepatitis.[42] Whether this organism is capable of experimentally inducing hepatitis in dogs or occurs as a natural liver infection in humans requires further study. The pathogenic potential is strengthened by isolation of *H. canis* from a bacteremic human[96] and by studies that demonstrate that *H. hepaticus*, an intestinal *Helicobacter* of mice, can experimentally induce hepatitis in both inbred and germ-free mice.[43, 48, 151]

PATHOGENESIS

The mechanism whereby certain species of helicobacters, whose normal ecologic niche is the lower intestine, colonize the liver is unknown. Like another intestinal enteropathogen, *Salmonella typhi*, the organism may gain access to the liver by initial enterocyte or M-cell uptake in the intestine, with spread to the liver via the portal circulation; finally the bacteria are discharged from the liver into the biliary tract.[65] Alternatively, helicobacters may migrate retrograde from the lumen of the gut into the bile duct. Whether the presence of intestinal parasites facilitates the ability of *H. canis* (and other helicobacters) to colonize the liver and to cause hepatitis is unknown. Organisms compatible with *H. bilis* morphology have been noted previously in bile canaliculi of rats experimentally infected with *Fasciola hepatica*.[35] Also *Flexispira (Helicobacter) rappini* has been associated with abortion in sheep, necrotic hepatitis in the aborted fetuses, and intestinal disease in animals and humans. Experimentally, *F. rappini* causes similar abortions and necrotic hepatitis in guinea pigs.[4, 74, 113] It is conceivable but certainly not proven that puppies can be infected in utero. However, its importance as a pathogen in pet animals has not been determined.

Pigtail macaques (*Macaca nemistrina*) were experimentally challenged orally with *H. cinaedi* and *H. fennelliae*.[33] Although infection occurred in these monkeys and caused abnormal feces and focal large-bowel lesions, only one of five monkeys infected with *H. fennelliae* had acute proctitis, whereas *H. cinaedi* induced only lymphoid hyperplasia.[33]

CLINICAL FINDINGS

It is not known whether intestinal *Helicobacter* can cause primary diarrheal disease in immunocompetent companion pet animals or whether they have to be immunocompromised. *H. hepaticus* is linked to severe inflammatory bowel disease in immunocompromised mice,[151] and select germ-free mice inoculated with the organism develop segmental enteritis.[41, 43, 48] Similarly, if helicobacters are determined to be a common cause of hepatitis in dogs and cats, appropriate liver function tests as well as microaerobic culture of liver biopsies should provide insight.

DIAGNOSIS

Many hospital laboratories have difficulty in isolating these organisms. For example, because of the slow growth of *H. cinaedi*, laboratory diagnosis is unlikely if blood culture procedures that rely on visual detection of the culture media are used.[72, 73] In a retrospective study of humans with *H. cinaedi*–associated illness, most of the patients had the organism isolated from blood using automated blood culture system.[73] Dark-field microscopy or use of acridine orange staining of blood culture media, rather than Gram's stain, increases the likelihood of seeing the organism. Likewise, fecal isolation is difficult; selective antibiotic media are required, and recovery is facilitated by passing fecal homogenates through a 0.45-μ filter.[50, 122] Also some strains of both *H. cinaedi* and *H. fennelliae* are inhibited by concentrations of cephalothin and cefazolin used frequently in selective media for isolation of enteric microaerophilic bacteria.[72] These organisms also require an environment rich in hydrogen for optimum in vitro growth. *H. canis* can be distinguished from *H. fennelliae* by its ability to grow at 42°C, its failure to produce catalase, and its marked tolerance to bile.

PATHOLOGIC FINDINGS

Although the normal ecologic niche of *H. canis* and *H. hepaticus* is the crypts of the intestine, these organisms can also colonize the liver. The best characterized liver lesion caused by a *Helicobacter* is *H. hepaticus*–associated hepatitis in A/JCr mice. In infected mice, the organism causes a multifocal hepatic lesion with cholangitis and vasculitis, which progresses in severity to include bile duct hyperplasia, hepatomegaly, oval cell hyperplasia, hepatocellular proliferation, and, in aged A/JCr mice, hepatoma or hepatocellular carcinoma.[41, 43, 151] The *H. canis*–associated liver lesion noted in a young dog consisted of an acute multifocal necrotizing hepatitis.[42] Interestingly, *Helicobacter*-like organisms were present at the periphery of the hepatic lesion and appeared to be located in bile canaliculi. This pattern of colonization is also noted in *H. hepaticus*– and *H. bilis*–infected livers.[41, 43, 47, 151]

THERAPY

Antimicrobial susceptibility testing of *H. cinaedi* indicates that tetracycline, chloramphenicol, and various aminoglycosides should be effective in treating infections with *H. cinaedi*.[73] See Table 39–1 for appropriate dosage information. Apparent relapses of *H. cinaedi* bacteremia have occurred in people treated with ciprofloxacin despite its previous use to treat *H. cinaedi* infection successfully. The occurrence of in vitro resistance of *H. cinaedi* isolates to ciprofloxacin suggests that fluoroquinolones should be used with caution.[72, 73]

PUBLIC HEALTH CONSIDERATIONS

Because *H. cinaedi* has been isolated from normal intestine flora of hamsters, it was suggested that pet hamsters could serve as a reservoir for transmission to humans.[50] *H. cinaedi* was isolated from the blood and feces of a neonate with septicemia and meningitis.[97] The mother of the neonate, who had worked with hamsters during her first two trimesters of pregnancy, had a diarrheal illness during the third trimester of pregnancy; the newborn was likely infected during the birthing process, although this was not proven. Further studies are needed to confirm zoonotic risk of handling *H. cinaedi*–infected hamsters and possibly other animals as well.[50]

Even though *H. canis*, *H. cinaedi*, *H. fennelliae*, and *H. rappini* have been isolated from both dogs and humans, additional investigations will be required to ascertain whether these helicobacters in dogs constitute a potential reservoir for zoonotic transmission to people. Although *H. canis* and *H. pullorum* have been isolated from diarrheic children and adults with gastroenteritis, evidence that either organism can cause hepatitis in humans is indirect. *H. canis* has been isolated from the blood of humans, which increases the likelihood that liver infection with *H. canis* in humans also occurs.[21a, 96] Also a patient with *H. pullorum*–associated diarrhea had persistent increases in three liver enzymes as well as hepatomegaly on abdominal ultrasonography.[13] With the use of appropriate diagnostic media and microaerobic culture conditions, various other *Helicobacter* species will also be isolated from cases of hepatitis in humans and companion pet animals.

Salmonellosis

Craig E. Greene

ETIOLOGY

Salmonella are primarily motile, non-spore-forming, gram-negative bacilli of the family Enterobacteriaceae. Members of the genus *Salmonella* are ubiquitous pathogens that infect a wide variety of mammals, birds, reptiles, and even insects. Although they occur primarily as intestinal parasites, they can cause systemic disease and can be isolated from other organs and blood. Salmonellae from animals have important public health implications because they are capable of causing mild to severe gastroenteritis in humans.

The taxonomy of salmonellae has undergone many changes, with classification schemes being based on both biochemical and serologic differences. Because the salmonellae are related, they are thought to belong to a single species: *S. enterica*. The practice of substituting serovar names as species is commonly accepted. Serovars of *S. enterica* are identified by agglutination reactions of their somatic (O) and flagellar (H) antigens. The species (serovars) recognized to be of major pathogenic significance in veterinary and human microbiology include *S. choleraesuis*, *S. arizonae* (formerly *Arizona arizonae*), *S. enteritidis*, and *S. typhimurium*. *S. typhī*, which is extremely important as the cause of typhoid fever in people, is not normally pathogenic for animals and is of little, if any, zoonotic importance. *S. enteritidis* has been further divided into more than 1700 bioserotypes, each with a distinguishing name such as *S. enteritidis dublin*. Again, the species name is omitted in favor of using the bioserotype alone, that is, *S. dublin*.

Some species of salmonellae show a preference for certain animal hosts, and each domesticated farm animal species appears to have an adapted *Salmonella* spp. (horse—*S. abortus equi*, cow—*S. dublin*, sheep—*S. abortus ovis*, pig—*S. choleraesuis*, fowl—*S. pullorum* and *S. gallinarum*). Rarely, *S. choleraesuis* and *S. dublin* produce disease in humans or other animals.

The remaining serotypes of *Salmonella* show little or no specific host adaptation and are equally pathogenic for people and other animals. Many have been isolated from vertebrates and invertebrates and the environment. These *Salmonella* serotypes or individual isolates of certain serotypes vary widely in their ability to infect and produce disease within a given animal host, and more virulent serotypes appear to be able to multiply intracellularly. Mucoid and encapsulated strains are more pathogenic than other strains; *S. typhi*, which produces prolonged and systemic infections in its human hosts, is noted for these features. The species most commonly isolated from diseased animals and humans is *S. typhimurium*.

EPIDEMIOLOGY

Source of Infection

Most serotypes of *S. typhimurium* are ubiquitous in nature and are readily transmitted among animals and people and the environment (Fig. 39–3). The most common source of

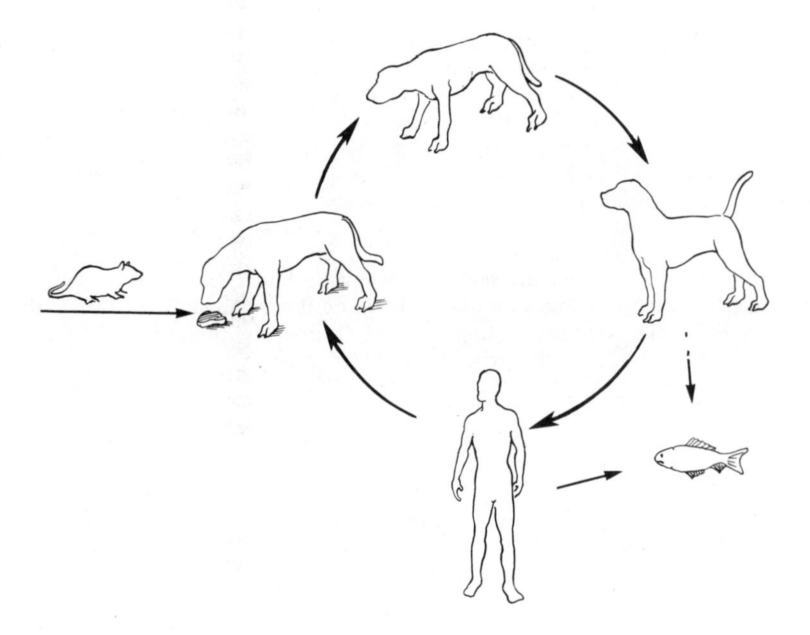

Figure 39–3. Epidemiology of salmonellosis.

infection, which occurs through the GI route, is contact with contaminated food, water, or fomites. Air-borne transmission, which produces respiratory infection, may occur occasionally, because the organism is able to survive on dried air-borne particles in the absence of organic material.

Salmonellae can survive for relatively long periods outside the host. Finding *Salmonella* in the environment usually indicates direct or indirect fecal contamination. A large portion of the aquatic biosphere is now contaminated with *Salmonella* organisms, probably as a result of pollution of streams and lakes with untreated sewage, garbage, and other refuse. Fish and shellfish living in previously infected waters are microbiologic monitors, because they can harbor the organisms in their digestive tracts for extended periods after direct isolation from the water is no longer possible. Dogs and cats may acquire their infections by drinking contaminated water, although this is less of a problem in areas where pets drink from chlorinated municipal water supplies.

Another source of infection for dogs and cats, as well as for their human owners, is contamination of foodstuffs. This was a major problem in the past because pets were fed uncooked or unprocessed foods. Meat and meat by-products, especially those from contaminated horse meat, were the foods most commonly incriminated. Isolation of *Salmonella* from infected animals has been most common from swine, cattle, turkeys, and horses, in that order. *S. typhimurium* was by far the most common isolate. Raw, dehydrated, or improperly cooked cat or dog food products prepared from these sources have a higher prevalence of contamination than pelleted and heat-processed foods, which are less likely to be infected because they are adequately sterilized during preparation. Even commercially processed foods can become contaminated if they are exposed to infected mammals, birds, reptiles, amphibians, or insects or to unsanitary conditions. Salmonellae can multiply quickly in moistened foodstuffs left at room temperature. Supplementation of processed foods with uncooked food scraps or meat by-products is another common source of infection. In the United States, raw meat (4-D meat) used to feed racing greyhounds is highly contaminated with *Salmonella*.[18, 133, 156]

Contaminated fomites such as food dishes, hospital cages, endoscopic equipment, and bathtubs can spread the disease throughout a veterinary hospital. Salmonellae can occasionally be transmitted by means of contaminated pharmacologic or diagnostic preparations of animal origin, such as pancreatic extracts, liver extracts, bile salts, gelatin, vitamins, and hormonal extracts. Free-roaming dogs and cats have ample opportunity for exposure to *Salmonella* because they are carnivorous and occasionally coprophagous. Such animals may be infected with and shed a number of strains simultaneously.[11, 135, 153, 158] Cats may have greater resistance to infection than dogs, as suggested by the less frequent isolation of *Salmonella* from them.

Infected animal handlers may also be a source of *Salmonella* in a hospital, kennel, or cattery. Human infections with nontyphoid salmonellae are usually self-limiting, and shedding of the organism is usually not a persistent problem. Animal infections are more important in maintaining the organism in animal-holding facilities. Human carriers chronically infected with typhoid fever-producing salmonellae pose no health hazard for animals.

Prevalence

Salmonellosis in the dog and the cat is more common than the prevalence of clinical disease would suggest, with numerous serotypes being isolated from each species. The frequency of fecal isolation from clinically healthy or hospitalized dogs is reported to be 1% to 36% and from healthy cats, 1% to 18%. The actual prevalence of infection is probably higher than that estimated on the basis of fecal swab culture results and routine isolation procedures, because culture of intestinal lymph node specimens taken at necropsy yields a much higher prevalence of *Salmonella* organisms. Currently, the prevalence is probably decreasing because an increasing number of pets are now fed commercially processed foods. The problem still exists in exotic carnivores in zoologic gardens where raw meat diets are fed.

Host Resistance

The ability to experimentally infect animals with *Salmonella* and to establish clinical illness depends on many factors. Age is an important variable. Puppies and kittens younger than 1 year are more susceptible to infection and clinical illness than adult animals. Neonates may acquire infections from contaminated secretions of their dams. In utero transmission may result in death and abortion of the fetuses or birth of weak or ill puppies and kittens.

Nutritional considerations are also important in the establishment of salmonellosis. Obesity and overfeeding decrease the resistance of experimentally infected dogs to salmonellosis. Dietary deficiencies of methionine or choline in pregnant animals increase the susceptibility of their offspring to salmonellosis.

Stress caused by hospitalization, anesthesia, surgical and medical therapy, and overcrowding has been correlated with an increased risk of salmonellosis in dogs and cats. Thiamylal anesthesia enhanced the virulence of *Salmonella* endotoxin for experimentally infected animals.

The impairment of host immune defenses that occurs with malnutrition, malignancy, and glucocorticoid therapy may increase the prevalence of clinically severe salmonellosis. Immunosuppression associated with diabetes mellitus and feline leukemia virus infection may have contributed to the development of salmonellosis in two cats.[22] An increased postoperative prevalence of clinical salmonellosis in dogs given high-dosage glucocorticoid therapy for intervertebral disc and intraocular surgery has been noted. Salmonellosis has also been reported as a complication of anticancer chemotherapy in dogs and one cat[64] with multicentric lymphosarcomas and in a dog with cyclic hematopoiesis.[87] The severity of salmonellosis is increased in people with chronic or severe hemolytic anemia when the mononuclear-phagocyte system is overwhelmed by erythrophagocytosis.

The intestinal tract normally is protected against colonization by enteric pathogens, which explains why the clinical prevalence of gastroenteritis is lower than the frequency of *Salmonella* isolation from the pet population. Normal intestinal motility propels ingested *Salmonella* to the cecum and colon. There the resident bacterial population produces volatile fatty acids, including acetic and butyric acids, which limit further replication of the pathogens. Thus, any factor that alters the animal's indigenous microbial population increases its susceptibility to infection by *Salmonella*. Intestinal mucus by itself is not bactericidal; however, it contains humoral and cellular immune factors that are important in protection against salmonellosis.

Antibiotic therapy both reduces resistance to salmonellosis and prolongs the course of the illness in experimental animals. A single dose of penicillin or streptomycin greatly increases the susceptibility of mice to salmonellosis by altering the normal intestinal microflora that protects the bowel against colonization by enteric pathogens. Dogs developing salmonellosis in a hospital outbreak were at high risk if they had received antimicrobials, especially GI flora–altering drugs such as ampicillin.

PATHOGENESIS

Experimentally, a large number of organisms (10^6–10^9) must be ingested to produce GI colonization by *Salmonella* with or without clinical illness. Because a large proportion of ingested organisms are destroyed by the low pH of the stomach, reducing the amount of gastric acidity by administration of buffered compounds or by performing vagotomy or partial gastrectomy induces a greater risk of salmonellosis in experimental animals. The organisms that survive passage through the stomach are able to colonize the middle portions of the ileum on the day of ingestion. Here they attach preferentially to the tips of villi, which they invade and in which they multiply. Strains of *Salmonella* within a given species vary in their virulence, which is partially determined by their ability to invade nonphagocytic host cells.[7] Localization and persistence of the organisms in the intestinal epithelium and lymph nodes account for shedding, which occurs for 3 to 6 weeks in most cases. The shedding is continual for the first week but then becomes intermittent. Phagocytic cells in the intestinal lymph nodes, liver, or spleen may harbor the organism persistently, even in the absence of shedding. Reactivation of shedding or clinical illness may occur after stress, immunosuppression, concurrent systemic viral infections, and crowding.

Mucosal invasion, host inflammatory response, and resultant GI epithelial injury and sloughing are more common with salmonellosis than with bacterial diarrhea resulting from other kinds of infections. *Salmonella* strains differ in their pathogenicity, which correlates with their ability to attach to and invade mucosa, a property associated with their pili and flagella.[90] However, the extent of injury is not sufficient to explain the amount of fluid loss associated with diarrhea. There is adequate evidence that some salmonellae produce heat-labile enterotoxins, which increase adenyl cyclase, thereby stimulating secretion of fluid by the intestinal mucosa, as in other diarrheas associated with noninvasive enterotoxigenic bacteria (see Fig. 89–6*A*).

Endotoxemia or bacteremia may occur during overt enteric infection or in the absence of signs of intestinal illness. Fever, leukopenia, endotoxic shock, and death may result. In surviving animals, focal suppuration with localization of organisms can occur in the biliary tract, kidneys, heart, spleen, meninges, joints, and lungs. A decrease in bacteremia and clearance of organisms from the blood are associated with a rising antibody titer to cell wall (somatic, O) antigen; the flagellar (H) antigen has no role in protection. Prolonged bacteremia or overwhelming sepsis is usually indicative of compromised host defense mechanisms. Prolonged intermittent bacteremia following salmonellosis is not as common a problem in animals as it is with *S. typhi* in humans. The K or capsular antigen (termed Vi for *S. typhi*) of this organism allows it to persist intracellularly for long periods despite adequate host defenses. Virulence plasmids found in some *Salmonella* serotypes enhance their extraintestinal growth and production of bacteremia.[32, 75]

Endotoxemia from overwhelming salmonellosis is associated with a variety of effects on the host and is related to the lipopolysaccharide composition of their cell wall (see Endotoxemia, Chapter 38). Pooling of leukocytes, erythrocytes, and platelets in the peripheral vasculature; hypoglycemia; complement activation; release of vasoactive amines; and development of disseminated intravascular coagulation (DIC) may occur.

CLINICAL FINDINGS

Clinical findings in salmonellosis vary according to the number of infecting organisms, the immune status of the host, and the complicating factors or concomitant diseases. The syndromes can be artificially divided into gastroenteritis, bacteremia and endotoxemia, organ localization, and persistence of an asymptomatic carrier state.

Gastroenteritis

The clinical signs associated with *Salmonella* gastroenteritis are variable. Most acute episodes begin within 3 to 5 days of exposure to the organism or after stress in carriers. Very young or old animals show the most severe clinical signs. Fever of 40° to 41.1°C (104–106°F), malaise, and anorexia are noted initially followed by vomiting, abdominal pain, and diarrhea. Cats frequently hypersalivate as a result of persistent vomiting. The diarrhea varies in consistency from watery to mucoid, and fresh blood is present in severe cases. Weight loss and dehydration become evident within several days after the onset of illness. Severely affected animals have pale mucous membranes, weakness, marked dehydration, cardiovascular collapse, shock, and icterus just before death. CNS signs in some animals include hyperexcitability, incoordination, posterior paresis, blindness, and convulsions. Pneumonia can be associated with acute *Salmonella* gastroenteritis. Coughing, dyspnea, and epistaxis are seen in affected animals.

Bacteremia and Endotoxemia

These are usually transient subclinical features of *Salmonella* gastroenteritis and become clinically significant in either very young or immunosuppressed dogs and cats. Other dogs and cats may have bacteremia and persistent fever in the absence of GI signs. Affected kittens and puppies younger than 7 weeks may not show a febrile response despite bacteremia or endotoxemia. In severe cases, mental depression, pale mucosae, weakness, tachycardia, hypothermia, and cardiovascular collapse may be seen with or without GI signs. Organ dysfunction from thrombosis or hemorrhagic tendencies can occur from DIC.

Organ Localization

Metastatic infection may occur after clinical or subclinical bacteremia. Organisms may localize in particular organ systems for a period of time before producing overt clinical signs. Localization is most likely to occur in tissues previously damaged or devitalized but may spread to involve healthy structures. The clinical signs are referable to the organ system of localization. For example, a cat developed pneumonia caused by *S. choleraesuis* without enteric manifestations or positive fecal culture results.[112] Abscesses, pyothorax, meningitis, osteomyelitis, and cellulitis are other examples of focal disease.

Other Syndromes

Abortions, stillbirths, and birth of weak puppies or kittens may result from in utero infection.[111] Vaginal discharges, placentas, and meconia usually contain *Salmonella*. The bitch or queen generally has prolonged vaginal discharges and delayed postpartum involution. Puppies that survive are weak, unthrifty, and emaciated, and *Salmonella* can be isolated from various organs. Conjunctivitis has been a major manifestation in some infected cats that also have regional lymphadenomegaly and persistent fecal shedding of salmonellae. For a further discussion of ocular lesions, see Chapter 93.

Songbird Fever

Seasonal bird migrations in the northeastern United States have been associated with *S. typhimurium* and an acute febrile illness in cats that usually lasts 2 to 7 days. Affected cats have primarily been outdoors and have preyed on birds or frequented bird feeders. Clinical signs include acute depression, anorexia, fever (40–40.6°C [104–105°F]), diarrhea, which is often hemorrhagic, and variable vomiting. Recovery usually is rapid, but in some cases normal feeding behavior does not return for several weeks. Mortality may be as high as 10%, and other diseases causing immunosuppression may increase this rate. Therapy and prevention of this syndrome are the same as for other *Salmonella* infections.

Subclinical Infections and Clinical Recovery

Only a small proportion (<10%) of infected animals die during the acute stages of salmonellosis. Dogs and cats infected with few organisms and those that have otherwise normal defense mechanisms will have transient or no clinical illness. Some cats may have a persistent chronic febrile illness, characterized by anorexia and lethargy without diarrhea. Animals affected by acute diarrhea usually recover after 3 to 4 weeks. Rarely, diarrhea of a chronic or intermittent nature for up to 8 weeks is reported.[22] Recovered and clinically normal animals usually shed the organisms for up to 6 weeks.

DIAGNOSIS

Salmonellosis should be suspected with any acute or chronic GI illness. It has frequently been overlooked in favor of the more notorious viral enteritis caused by canine parvovirus or coronavirus and feline panleukopenia virus. The clinical and pathologic features of these diseases may be indistinguishable from those of salmonellosis. Refer to Clinical Findings in Chapters 8 and 10, respectively.

Clinical Laboratory Findings

Hematologic abnormalities are variable depending on the stage of illness. Nonregenerative hypochromic anemia, lymphopenia, thrombocytopenia, neutropenia with a left shift, and toxic leukocytes are found in animals with systemic disease and endotoxemia. Bacterial rods may be found in the leukocytes of dogs or cats with overwhelming sepsis. A mature neutrophilic leukocytosis is more characteristic of chronically infected animals or animals with localization of infection in a particular organ system. Prolonged coagulation test times will be apparent in animals with severe DIC.

Biochemical abnormalities are usually present only in animals with severe clinical illness. These abnormalities include hypoproteinemia, especially hypoalbuminemia, hypoglycemia, and moderate prerenal azotemia. Dogs with salmonellosis have had electrolyte abnormalities, hyponatremia, and hyperkalemia typical of primary hypoadrenocorticism.

Bacterial Isolation

Isolation of *Salmonella* organisms is the most definitive means of confirming infection. However, mere isolation from the oral cavity, vomitus, or feces does not indicate that the organisms are causing clinical disease, because the prevalence of subclinical carriers in dog and cat populations is high. Animals recovering from clinical salmonellosis shed organisms for at least 4 to 6 weeks, and shedding can be reactivated by stress or recurrent illness.

Finding organisms in samples of normally sterile secretions or body fluids, such as blood, urine, synovial fluid, transtracheal washings, CSF, and bone marrow, may allow a definitive diagnosis of systemic salmonellosis to be made from chronically febrile animals or during the acute phases of illness. Samples for culture should be taken from the liver, spleen, bone marrow, lung, mesenteric lymph nodes, and intestinal tract at necropsy. The gallbladder and bile do not appear to be consistent sites of localization of infection in animals, although they are in humans infected with *S. typhi*.

Negative culture results do not necessarily eliminate the possibility of infection, because it is difficult to isolate *Salmonella* in the presence of other organisms. Specimens from normally sterile tissues, such as blood, bone marrow, joint fluid, and CSF, can be cultured on ordinary media. Samples taken from the oral cavity or bowel, both of which have a high concentration of commensal organisms, must be cultured on special media. Treated animals should not be considered free of infection during monitoring until at least three successive attempts at culture have been made over 2- to 3-week intervals. To avoid loss of organisms in shipment to a laboratory, fresh fecal specimens should be placed in Amies transport medium with charcoal.

Enrichment broths (e.g., selenite and tetrathionate) are used to increase the yield and to inhibit growth of competing organisms. A number of improved plating media have been developed.[26, 114] After 24 hours, subculturing is performed on an inhibitory medium such as deoxycholate, which favors the growth of *Salmonella*. After isolation, salmonellae are identified by Gram's staining, motility, and biochemical reactions. They ferment certain sugars, including glucose (but not lactose), and react positively with substances such as urea, indole, and methyl red.

Other nonculture methods can help to identify infected hosts. The PCR method has been used to detect salmonellae in canine fecal specimens.[133, 134] In addition, an ELISA with monoclonal antibody has been utilized to detect *Salmonella* antigens in urine of bacteremic people.[16]

Serologic Testing

Demonstration of a rise in serum antibody titer to O and H antigens has been used in human medicine as a less specific means of detecting clinical illness. Not all subclinically infected dogs and cats have positive serologic titers; thus, serologic testing is not an accurate means of detecting carriers. Cats respond consistently with increased titers only when they are clinically ill. For these reasons, culture of body fluids or secretions is a simpler and more definitive means of making a diagnosis.

Cytology

Cytologic examination is helpful in detecting invasive GI pathogens in diarrheal illnesses. The presence of leukocytes in feces can identify diseases that cause disruption of the intestinal mucosa. A wet mount is prepared by mixing small flecks of mucus with a drop of new methylene blue on a microscope slide and covering the mixture with a coverslip. The absence of fecal leukocytes indicates a viral, mild bacterial, or nonspecific diarrhea that does not require extensive therapy. The presence of large numbers of leukocytes is typical of acute salmonellosis and other forms of diarrhea that cause extensive mucosal disruption. These cases usually require intensive parenteral fluid and antibiotic therapy.

PATHOLOGIC FINDINGS

Gross lesions are found at necropsy in only a small percentage of infected animals that develop severe clinical illness. Pale mucous membranes and dehydration accompany a diffuse mucoid to hemorrhagic enteritis. Lesions in the intestinal mucosa vary from catarrhal inflammation to mucosal sloughing with extensive denudation of the gut. GI lesions may be extensive but are usually confined to the distal small bowel, cecum, and colon. Diffusely scattered petechial to ecchymotic hemorrhages present throughout most organ systems are associated with focal thrombosis and necrosis. A serohemorrhagic effusion may be present in the abdominal cavity with fibrin adhered to inflamed viscera. The lungs are frequently edematous or consolidated, and mesenteric and peripheral lymph nodes are enlarged and hemorrhagic.

Histologically, variable lesions are a fibrinous to fibropurulent pneumonia, multifocal necrotizing hepatitis and splenitis, and suppurative meningitis, all of which are associated with necrotic intestinal lymphadenitis and hemorrhagic ulcerative gastroenteritis. Histologic or cytologic examination may reveal that bacteria have disseminated to many organs, including the bone marrow, spleen, and lymph nodes.

THERAPY

Appropriate therapy for canine and feline salmonellosis varies according to the type and severity of clinical illness. Acute *Salmonella* gastroenteritis, without systemic signs, is best treated with parenteral polyionic isotonic fluids to replace losses from vomitus and diarrhea. Fluids can be administered orally when vomiting is not a problem. Hypertonic glucose-containing solutions have been effective in reversing fluid loss in infectious diarrhea (see Chapter 89). Transfusion of plasma may be more beneficial than fluid therapy when mucosal disruption and increased GI permeability lower serum albumin concentration to less than 2.0 g/dl.

Prostaglandin inhibitors such as indomethacin have been effective in reducing fluid losses in animals with experimentally induced *Salmonella* gastroenteritis. Increased net water loss in the lower bowel results from increased intestinal secretion induced by bacterial endotoxin and mediated through prostaglandin synthesis. Prostaglandin inhibitors must be used early in the disease to be effective and must be used cautiously if GI hemorrhage is severe. Flunixin meglumine has been more commonly administered in dogs and cats, but GI bleeding and renal failure have been associated factors.

Paradoxically, osmotically active laxatives such as lactulose have been recommended for treating acute *Salmonella* gastroenteritis. A nonabsorbable sugar, lactulose, produces osmotic diarrhea through the formation of acid metabolites in the distal small bowel and colon. Shortened transit time and an acid environment are deleterious to the survival of *Salmonella* organisms. Such therapy should be used only in unresponsive cases in which fluid deficits have already been corrected.

Routine antibiotics reported to be effective against *Salmonella* include chloramphenicol, trimethoprim-sulfonamide, and amoxicillin. Aminoglycosides such as gentamicin and amikacin may be considered when bacterial resistance is anticipated, but the risk of renal toxicity precludes their routine use. Isolates are generally sensitive to the quinolones and imipenem[117]; however, high cost and the desire to reduce the development of antimicrobial resistance make these second choices unless overwhelming sepsis is apparent. Variable resistance to erythromycin, clindamycin, ampicillin, cephapirin, sulfonamides, or nitrofurans is reported.[18] Resistance is greatest to streptomycin, tetracycline, and sulfonamides alone.[157] Unfortunately, the in vivo response of *Salmonella* to antibiotics does not always correlate with the results of in vitro testing. For example, a cat with salmonellosis that did not respond to amoxicillin or cephapirin was effectively treated with cephalexin.[22]

Antibiotic therapy has not been advocated for treating animals with uncomplicated *Salmonella* gastroenteritis but, rather, has been recommended for animals with concurrent signs of systemic infection or histories of immunosuppression (see Table 39–1). Studies in human patients have indicated that routine antimicrobial use in treating salmonellosis induces drug-resistant strains and prolongs the convalescent excretion period. However, this widely held view has been questioned in studies that demonstrate effective eradication of *Salmonella* from humans and animals by combined antibiotic therapy.

Another inherent problem with routine antibiotic administration for *Salmonella* gastroenteritis is that infecting organisms may acquire transferable (plasmid-mediated) resistance. An increased prevalence of transferable resistance has been demonstrated among *Salmonella* isolates from dogs, cats, and humans. The fluoroquinolones have reduced tendency to produce plasmid-mediated resistance in bacteria compared with other antibacterials and their efficacy against *Salmonella* has been reviewed.[117, 125] Other disadvantages of routine antibiotic therapy for salmonellosis are that it may enhance susceptibility to infection or activate clinical illness in the latent carrier state.

Animals with more severe signs of endotoxemia or bacteremia should be treated differently from those with simple gastroenteritis. Plasma transfusions of at least 250 ml for dogs larger than 15 kg have reduced mortality in those dogs that had been given *Salmonella* endotoxin. Equal volumes of isotonic fluid or smaller volumes of plasma were not helpful. Plasma-treated dogs developed leukopenia, thrombocytopenia, and extensive tissue injury, as did untreated dogs, but had better survival rates. Dogs with experimentally induced endotoxic shock were protected by infusion of monoclonal antibodies directed against the endotoxic lipid A cell wall component of *Salmonella*.[115] A commercially available polyclonal antiserum is available for this purpose (see Therapy, Chapters 8 and 38).

PREVENTION

Prevention of salmonellosis in dogs and cats can be frustrating because of the tendency of some animals to develop a chronic subclinical carrier state or latent infection. Nontyphoid salmonellae that infect pets are also harbored by many other animals and persist in the environment, making eradication difficult.

Hygiene and isolation of individual pets should be enforced during hospitalization because of the highly infectious and contagious nature of salmonellosis, should it occur. Infection from food sources can be minimized by using commercially available heat-processed products. Proper sanitation during handling and storing of processed foods is also important, because they frequently become contaminated by contact with utensils, rodents, or insects. Meat, eggs, and dairy products given as food should be stored or thawed at temperatures lower than 4.4°C (40°F) and should be cooked to internal temperatures of at least 74°C (165°F).

Cages in hospitals, kennels, or catteries should be routinely cleaned and disinfected between uses by different animals (see Chapter 94). Phenolic compounds or household bleach (diluted 1:32 or 4 oz/gal of water) can be applied as surface disinfectants, but their contact with cats should be avoided. Animals brought into group confinement should be segregated if they have or develop diarrhea or vomiting. Food dishes and utensils should be cold disinfected or, preferably, autoclaved between uses. Disposable dishes eliminate this requirement. Endoscopic equipment, shown to be a source of infection in human hospitals, should also be properly disinfected, that is, subjected to ethylene oxide gas or immersed in glutaraldehyde (2%) or formalin (20%) for a minimum of 1 hour. The equipment must be thoroughly aerated or rinsed before use (see Chapter 94).

Human carriers of nontyphoid *Salmonella* may transmit the infection as a reverse zoonosis, and this possibility should not be overlooked if there is a recurrent problem with salmonellosis in an animal-holding facility. Long-term boarders or blood donors should not be housed with the transient hospital population because the former may become exposed and then act as future sources of salmonellae.

PUBLIC HEALTH CONSIDERATIONS

Clinical signs of animal-acquired salmonellosis in people include abdominal tenderness, nausea, vomiting, and diarrhea accompanied by fever, myalgia, headache, and dehydration. As in animals, people may develop localized or septicemic forms of illness depending on their immunocompetence.

Salmonellosis is a disease of major zoonotic importance. All *Salmonella* infections, except those causing human typhoid fever (*S. typhi* and *S. paratyphi*) infect both humans and animals. Considerable emphasis has been placed on food-borne outbreaks of nontyphoid salmonellosis in humans by means of contaminated products of animal origin. Food such as meat, eggs, or milk products that has been improperly stored, prepared, or handled before consumption is most incriminated. Sporadic, pet-associated infections have not received as much attention. Dogs have been recognized as important vectors for non-food-borne infections of people because of the canine habit of coprophagy or ingesting carrion, coupled with long-term shedding of organisms and close proximity to people. Dogs and horses have the greatest zoonotic potential for the occupationally exposed. Contact with feces from infected pets has been an inadvertent but important source of exposure for young children. Cats, proved to be important but less frequently infected reservoirs, shed organisms orally, conjunctivally, and fecally. Thus, they may contaminate their food, fur, or water source, any of which may serve as a source of infection for humans. Persons handling raw-meat diets, or the feces of domestic or wild dogs or cats being fed such diets, are at increased risk of exposure.[19a] Multiresistant *S. typhimurium* strain DT 104, which has been a prevalent strain in people in the United Kingdom and the United States, has also been found in cats, dogs, and other nonfood and food animals.[1a, 147–149]

To reduce the risk of infection from pets, hands should be thoroughly washed with soap and water after handling animals or fomites such as animal bedding, footwear, or clothing contaminated with feces.[105] Detergents and household bleach added to the laundry will eliminate the organisms in these fomites.

Of increasing concern is the frequency with which antibiotic-resistant *Salmonella* strains have been isolated from dogs and cats.[115, 147–149] Most of the resistance is plasmid mediated and is intensified by indiscriminate or frequent administration of antibiotics by veterinarians. Antibiotic resistance has made recently acquired salmonellosis more difficult to treat in people. Quinolone resistance has been feared and reported in *Salmonella* in the United States necessitating the restricted use of these drugs in food animals.[62a] *Salmonella* infections have been more frequent and severe in people infected with HIV.

Shigellosis

Craig E. Greene

ETIOLOGY

Shigella is a genus of nonmotile gram-negative bacteria, morphologically indistinguishable from other enterobacteria, that cause a diarrheal condition known as bacillary dysentery in apes and people.[53] On the basis of biochemical and serologic properties, they are divided into four serogroups: *S. dysenteriae*, *S. flexneri*, *S. boydii*, and *S. sonnei*. Each group is further divided into a number of subserotypes that vary in pathogenicity. Shigellae are not as environmentally resistant as salmonellae; they cannot survive a temperature of 55°C for longer than 1 hour, and they are destroyed by dilute (1%) phenol within 30 minutes. They are susceptible to inactivation by sunlight and acid pH but can remain viable for a few days in nonacidic stools maintained in the dark. Shigellae survive best in dried fecal matter on cloth that is kept in a dark, moist place. Because of this short survival, the carrier host is most important in maintaining these organisms in nature.

EPIDEMIOLOGY

Shigellae are principally primate pathogens, causing severe hemorrhagic enteritis (dysentery). The disease, which spreads primarily via fecal-oral contact, is most commonly a problem in nonhuman primate colonies in which substandard sanitation or hygiene is practiced. Water-borne outbreaks in people, although rare, may occur with sewage contamination of domestic water supplies.

Dogs may become infected after contamination of their food or water supplies with infected human feces. Because of their coprophagous habits, pets may become exposed in areas where there is improper sewage disposal. Once they contract infection, dogs are probably not carriers but only transient excreters of organisms. Cats have not been reported to be naturally infected.

PATHOGENESIS

Shigella may cause damage in the body because of the gram-negative endotoxin that is produced. Shiga toxin is one of the most toxic biologic agents when given systemically. Certain organisms (e.g., *S. dysenteriae* type 1) produce enterotoxins that increase intestinal fluid secretions and can cause ulceration. Shigellae probably produce diarrhea both by means of intestinal epithelial cell invasion with resultant necrosis and hemorrhage and by effects of the Shiga toxin. Shiga toxin is also synthesized by and may be an important virulence factor of other pathogenic bacterial species. Systemic manifestations of the toxin in infected people include DIC with renal failure, thrombocytopenia, and microangiopathic hemolytic anemia.

CLINICAL FINDINGS

In primates, the organism causes a severe hemorrhagic, mucoid, large-bowel diarrhea. Lesions are usually ulcerative, and they spread from the distal to the proximal colon with time. In children and rarely in adults, septicemia may develop with or without diarrhea. Unlike primates, dogs are relatively resistant and cats are highly resistant to infection with *Shigella*. Organisms have been isolated from a small number of clinically normal dogs, but they have not been directly implicated as a cause of diarrhea in this species.

DIAGNOSIS

Demonstration of organisms in cultures is essential to differentiate *Shigella* enterocolitis from diarrhea caused by other bacteria. Owing to the fastidious nature of the organism, samples collected on swabs should be transported to the laboratory immediately and should not be exposed to sunlight. Cytologic examination of the stool will reveal large numbers of inflammatory cellular exudates associated with invasion of the bowel wall by *Shigella*.

THERAPY

Symptomatic treatment with parenteral fluids and antimicrobial therapy are similar to those in salmonellosis and enteropathogenic diarrhea (see Table 39–1). Unlike *Salmonella*, many shigellae are still sensitive to ampicillin, sulfonamide, tetracycline, and streptomycin. Antimotility therapy was detrimental to people with experimentally induced shigellosis.[53]

PREVENTION

Control measures are very similar to those outlined for *Salmonella*. Shigellosis is easier to prevent in dogs and cats than salmonellosis because the reservoir of *Shigella* organisms is restricted to the primate host.

Yersiniosis

Craig E. Greene

ETIOLOGY AND EPIDEMIOLOGY

Three major pathogenic members of the genus *Yersinia* infect dogs and cats. *Y. enterocolitica* and *Y. pseudotuberculosis* are discussed later and *Y. pestis*, the cause of plague, is discussed in Chapter 47. *Y. enterocolitica* is a motile, gram-negative, facultative coccobacillus, measuring 0.5 to 1.0 × 1.0 to 3.0 μm, that causes an enterocolitis in people. An unusual feature of this bacterium is that it replicates in culture at refrigeration temperatures, which allows its selective growth in the laboratory and refrigerated foodstuffs. Heating food at 60°C for a few minutes kills the organism. The bacterium, isolated from the feces of a variety of domestic and wild animal reservoirs and the environment, has a worldwide distribution. The prevalence of isolation of this organism from animals increases in colder months, perhaps because of its affinity for colder temperatures. The organism causes illness by invasion of many body tissues and through the elaboration of a heat-stable enterotoxin. Virulence-related factors of the organism appear primarily at lower temperatures, making human acquisition of infection more likely through contamination of the environment or food rather than directly from the carrier host. People appear to be unnatural hosts for this organism because they develop fever, diarrhea, abdominal pain, septicemia, or skin rashes, all signs that closely mimic those of acute appendicitis. Nonsuppurative arthritis may develop as a sequela after recovery from GI illness. Conditions associated with iron overload appear to predispose the host to systemic spread of the organism.[53]

Y. pseudotuberculosis is a cause of enteritis in many animals especially during the wet, cold winter and spring months.[8] A variety of animals, including birds, rodents, cats, and pigs, have been incriminated as reservoir hosts.[49, 118] People are more severely affected and develop mesenteric lymphadenitis and septicemia.[49]

CLINICAL FINDINGS

Because *Y. enterocolitica* has been isolated from feces of clinically normal dogs and cats, it is thought to be a commensal organism.[30, 53, 118] It has also been isolated from people with clinical illness who presumably contracted the organisms from contact with the excreta of infected household pets.[53, 56] Experimental infections in adult dogs have produced no clinical illness despite periodic fecal shedding for 52 days and recovery of the organism from mesenteric lymph nodes and other tissues.[53, 60] Infected dogs have developed resistance to reinfection.[60] *Y. enterocolitica* has also been cultured from the feces of young dogs with symptomatic GI illness.[53] The syndrome has been characterized by a several-week history of diarrhea associated with increased frequency of stools, tenesmus, blood, and mucus. In contrast to infected humans, dogs were not systemically ill. Dogs and cats may be asymptomatic carriers of *Y. pseudotuberculosis*. A Persian cat, infected with *Y. pseudotuberculosis*, developed anorexia, abdominal discomfort and weight loss, and dehydration.

DIAGNOSIS

Diagnosis of yersiniosis has been based on culture of the organism from the feces or deeper tissues of affected animals. As with other enteropathogenic bacterial infections, mere isolation from the intestinal tract may not be diagnostic of pathogenicity because the organism can be found in clinically healthy animals. Isolation of the organism from deeper tissues such as blood, urine, lymph nodes, wounds, or abscesses is more meaningful. *Yersinia* are not usually cultivated on conventional media because they produce small colonies that are later overgrown by normal floral organisms. A selective medium containing cefsulodin, irgasan, and novobiocin greatly improves the ability to isolate *Yersinia* from enteric specimens.[53] Serotyping of strains of this organism is similar to that of *Salmonella*. In systemically affected individuals, small pale-yellow abscesses are scattered on the surface and throughout the parenchyma of the liver and spleen. Histologic examination in one clinically affected dog with *Y. enterocolitica* infection revealed a chronic enteritis with mononuclear and plasma cell infiltrates in the intestinal mucosa and mesenteric lymph nodes.[53] In a cat with *Y. pseudotuberculosis* infection, there was focal microabscesses with microthrombosis in the liver and spleen.[66]

THERAPY

Therapy of yersiniosis should be attempted in younger dogs or cats, from whose feces the organism has been isolated, that have diarrhea or contact with people with confirmed infections. The organism is usually sensitive to routine dosages of chloramphenicol, tetracycline, gentamicin, cephalosporins, and trimethoprim-sulfonamides (see Table 39–1). Penicillin and its derivatives are not usually effective at routine dosages. As with other enteropathogenic bacteria, feeding of raw dairy or meat products or consumption of wildlife carcasses predisposes the animals to infection and should be avoided.

PUBLIC HEALTH CONSIDERATIONS

Outbreaks of gastroenteritis have been reported in people exposed to infected pet dogs.[56] Young children drinking water from puddles and playing in a sandbox frequented by a stray cat became infected with *Y. pseudotuberculosis*.[49] The organism could be isolated from the water, sand, and soil. Precautions should be taken to avoid such exposures in young children.

Tyzzer's Disease

Boyd R. Jones and Craig E. Greene

ETIOLOGY

Tyzzer's disease is caused by *Clostridium piliforme* (formerly *Bacillus piliformis*), a spore-forming, gram-negative obligate intracellular parasite measuring 0.5 × 10 to 40 μm that moves by means of peritrichous flagella. RNA sequences of this organism are now known to be more closely related to those of the clostridia, and the new name, *C. piliforme*, has been proposed and now adopted by most investigators.[25] Originally described as a disease of mice, it is now known to affect a wide range of animals. Reports of spontaneous disease have been described for dogs and cats.[8a, 68, 91, 106a, 109]

EPIDEMIOLOGY

C. piliforme, which appears to be a commensal organism of the intestinal tracts of laboratory rodents, is found on fecal cultures of normal and diseased animals. Clinical illness in rodents seems to be precipitated by stress, such as crowding, unsanitary conditions, weaning, transportation, irradiation, glucocorticoid therapy, or other forms of immunosuppression.

Dogs and cats may acquire infection by contact with or ingestion of rodent feces containing bacterial spores, although such interspecies transmission has never been reported. Experimental disease has been difficult to produce in healthy dogs and cats. Most feline cases have occurred in laboratory-reared cats, some with known contact with rodents. It is possible that dogs and cats harbor the organism.

A majority of infected animals have had naturally or experimentally induced immunosuppressive diseases such as

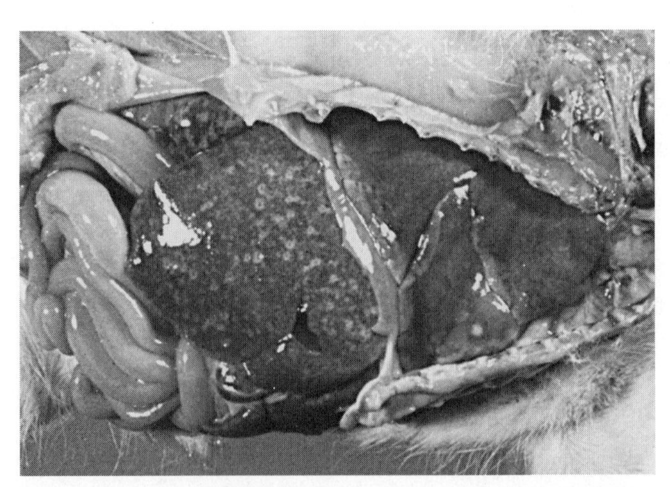

Figure 39–4. Tyzzer's disease in a kitten showing multifocal white spots on the liver from hepatocellular necrosis. Similar-appearing lesions visible through the pericardial sac are caused by focal myocarditis. (From Jones BR et al: *J Small Anim Pract* 26:411–419, 1985. Reprinted with permission.)

feline leukemia, feline panleukopenia, and canine distemper.[67, 68] One group of affected kittens had familial lipoprotein lipase deficiency and were persistently lipidemic.[68]

In experimental studies the severity of the disease was enhanced by overcrowding, administration of glucocorticoids or cyclophosphamide, splenectomy, irradiation, partial hepatectomy, and mononuclear-phagocyte blockade.[94, 155]

PATHOGENESIS

The pathogenesis is uncertain. The mechanisms by which *C. piliforme* attaches to and enters host cells are unknown. Endogenous or exogenous infection is followed by local proliferation of organisms in the intestinal epithelial cells. After stress or immunosuppression of the host, organisms spread by portal circulation to the liver. Colonization in the hepatic parenchyma results in multifocal periportal hepatic necrosis, presumably as the result of an unidentified toxin.

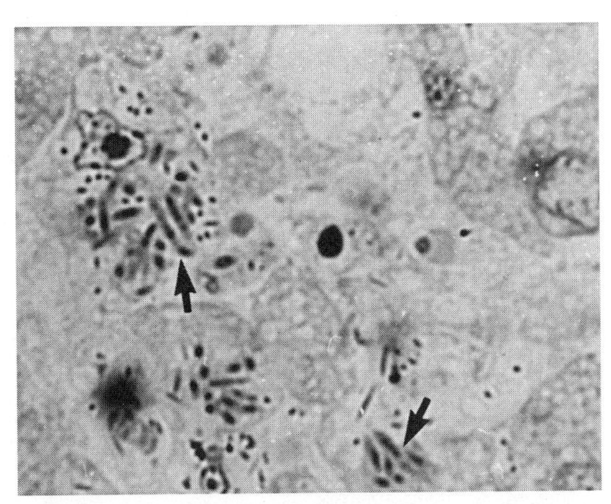

Figure 39–5. Hepatocytes at the margins of a necrotic focus in Tyzzer's disease. Bacteria resembling *C. piliforme (arrows)* are present within viable cells and extracellularly on necrotic tissue (toluidine blue; × 1500). (From Jones BR et al: *J Small Anim Pract* 26:411–419, 1985. Reprinted with permission.)

CLINICAL FINDINGS

Clinical signs have been relatively consistent among dogs and cats in which the disease has been reported. There is a very rapid onset of lethargy, depression, anorexia, and abdominal discomfort. Hepatomegaly and abdominal distention are followed by hypothermia, with the animal becoming moribund, resulting in death within 24 to 48 hours. Diarrhea has been infrequent; scant amounts of pasty feces are more characteristic. Icterus has been apparent in some animals, especially cats.

DIAGNOSIS

Because of the rapidly fatal course of the disease, diagnosis usually has been made by gross examination of specimens collected at necropsy. Just before death, marked elevations of alanine aminotransferase activity have been found. Characteristically, there are multiple, whitish-gray to hemorrhagic foci, 1 to 2 mm in diameter, on the capsule and cut surface of the liver (Fig. 39–4). Similar lesions may be apparent on other viscera. The intestinal mucosa may be thickened and congested in the region of the terminal ileum and proximal colon. Foamy, dark-brown feces are usually present in the lumen, and mesenteric lymph nodes are generally enlarged.

Histologic findings usually include multifocal periportal hepatic necrosis and necrotic ileitis or colitis; other tissues, such as the myocardium, may be affected in some animals.[68, 159, 160] Infiltrates of neutrophils and mononuclear cells are usually present at the margins of necrotic lesions. There are numerous intracellular filamentous organisms, only faintly visible by hematoxylin and eosin stain, in the hepatocytes at the margins of necrotic lesions and in the intestinal epithelial cells. Special stains, such as Giemsa stain or Warthin-Starry or Gomori silver stain, must be used to confirm the morphology of the organisms, which have a characteristic beaded appearance (Fig. 39–5). The organisms also can be demonstrated in methylene blue–stained impression smears made from lesions in fresh tissues. Both filamentous and spore forms of *C. piliforme* have been found.[69] *C. piliforme* cannot be isolated on artificial medium that lacks living cells and has so far been cultured only in eggs or cell cultures.[126]

Serologic methods have become a common tool for diagnosing latent infections in rodent colonies.[17] Monoclonal antibody–based tests have aided investigation of the disease. Flagellar antigens have been purified from *C. piliforme* from different species.[89, 126] There are significant antigenic differences. Nevertheless, such serologic tests could be applied to investigations of the dog and cat.

THERAPY AND PREVENTION

Thus far, treatment has not been successful, because affected animals die before it can have an effect. Antibiotic efficacy is undetermined. Success has been achieved with formalin-inactivated vaccines, which produce immunity to infection in mice. Whenever possible, predisposing factors that have been associated with infection in dogs and cats should be identified and avoided.

Clostridium perfringens Infection

Craig E. Greene

ETIOLOGY AND EPIDEMIOLOGY

The anaerobic gram-positive rod *Clostridium perfringens* is a normal inhabitant of the skin, skeletal muscle, and large bowel of animals and people. Nonenteric infections can involve skeletal muscles or connective infections with gas gangrene. Isolated cases of clostridial metritis or emphysematous cystitis have been reported in dogs. Severe diarrhea from hemorrhagic gastroenteritis has been associated with specific strains of enterotoxigenic *C. perfringens* in a number of domestic species, including dogs and cats.[19, 34, 76, 107, 143] The toxin binds to the intestinal epithelial cells, increases membrane permeability, and decreases synthesis, resulting in fluid and ion secretion with eventual death and sloughing of epithelial cells. Normally existing in the vegetative state within the intestinal tract, these *C. perfringens* strains can undergo sporulation, releasing their enterotoxin. Similar sporulation occurs in the environment. Exogenous enterointoxication results when foodstuffs containing toxin produced by contaminated bacteria are ingested. Endogenous sporulation of *C. perfringens* follows antimicrobial therapy, alkaline conditions, viral enteritis, and dietary alterations and immunosuppression. *C. perfringens* can also be associated with enterotoxemia and rapid death in dogs with intestinal strangulation or bowel stasis. Less documented infections have been reported in dogs and cats ingesting spoiled meat or carrion. Sporadic infections generally occur; however, nosocomial outbreaks can result from cross-contamination in hospitalized or grouped animals. After initial diarrheal illness, the organism can be shed for weeks to months. As a resistant spore-forming bacteria, *C. perfringens* is very stable in the environment, being resistant to disinfection for months or longer.

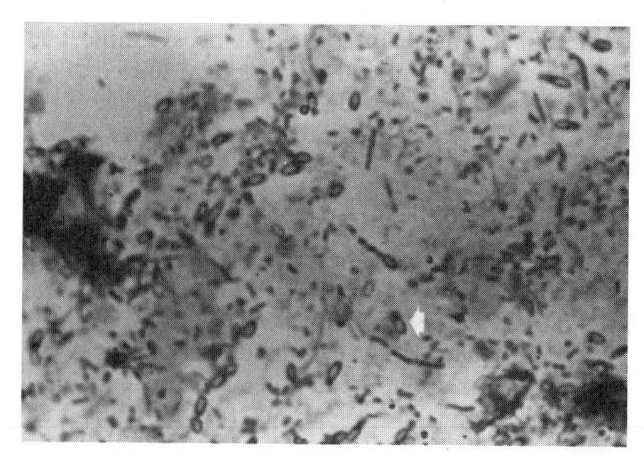

Figure 39–6. Diff-Quick stained fecal smear on oil imersion showing numerous *Clostridium perfringens* spores *(arrow)* found in a dog positive for enterotoxin. (From Twedt DC: *In Current Veterinary Therapy XI*. WB Saunders, 1992. Reprinted with permission.)

CLINICAL SIGNS

Diarrhea is a hallmark of clostridial infection. It typically develops in a few days after naive animals are exposed by ingestion or are introduced into an endemic environment such as a kennel or cattery. Diarrhea can vary from watery to mucohemorrhagic. Tenesmus may be present. Anal tissues may become severely inflamed, and some sloughing of intestinal mucosa may be noted in the stool. Diarrhea often lasts for a few days but can persist and become chronic for weeks to months. Signs may be intermittent and cyclic in chronically affected animals. Some animals may show additional findings of depression, vomiting, and anorexia.

DIAGNOSIS

C. perfringens is a normal bowel commensal; as such, the mere culture of an isolate from the stool is not definitive proof of its pathogenic nature (see also Epidemiology, Chapter 41).[134a] In dogs, numbers of this organism are known to increase with advancing age.[6] The organism may be found in clinically healthy animals from the stomach to the anus; the largest and most consistent isolations are made in the more distal intestinal regions. Clinical laboratory data, including hematologic and biochemical parameters, are usually unaffected in diarrheic or asymptomatic carrier animals.

With typical clinical signs, the organism should be demonstrated in stool with its associated enterotoxin for a definitive diagnosis. Large numbers of gram-positive clostridial spores (> 5 per oil immersion field) may be found on Gram's stain of fecal material or offending food that is suspected of causing an outbreak. Thin smears of feces on a slide are air dried or heat fixed and stained with Wright's-type stains or malachite green spore stains. The spores are larger than most bacteria and have a "safety-pin" appearance (Fig. 39–6). In comparing affected and unaffected animals in an outbreak, the feces will have higher fecal spore counts and rates of enterotoxin detection than in animals without diarrhea. Fecal spore counts can also be made by heat-inactivating vegetative bacteria in the specimen before culture. Clostridial spore colony counts per gram of greater than 10^6 are found in affected animals, whereas less than 10^3 are found in clinically healthy animals. Microbiologic and biochemical testing (e.g., lecithinase production) can be used on isolates for species identification. Fecal spore detection is not as specific as enterotoxin analysis, and some asymptomatic animals can have large numbers of spores (from nonenterotoxigenic strains) in the feces in the absence of clinical signs. Reverse passive latex agglutination (RPLA Kit, Oxoid, Columbia, MO) or ELISA (Pet RPLA, Unipath, Japan) assays are commercially available for specific identification of toxin. PCR has also been utilized for detection of specific enterotoxigenic strains in animal feces and meat.[86]

Carrier animals may also be identified by testing of their feces for enterotoxin. Approximately 1 g of stool is needed for the tests, which are not host specific, so that specimens can be submitted to human and veterinary diagnostic laboratories equipped for this analysis. Specimens of feces can be refrigerated or frozen for analysis. False-negative test results may be related to watery diarrhea causing dilution of fecal specimens; taking specimens later in the course when lower numbers of organisms may be shed; and interfering substances in the specimen.[143]

Endoscopic examination of clinically affected animals will reveal hemorrhagic or hyperemic and, less commonly, ulcerated colonic mucosa. Biopsy findings are a catarrhal or suppurative colitis, but they can be normal in the asymptomatic carrier. At laparotomy or necropsy, the stomach and intestines contain watery blood-stained fluid. The mucosal surface may be a dark-red color, and serosal roughening and hyperemia are found. Erosions and ulcerations are rare. Mesenteric lymph nodes may be enlarged and edematous. Histologically, in intestinal biopsy specimens, villi are blunted with shortened irregular profiles. Neutrophils may be apparent in capillaries of the lamina propria. Scattered foci of hemorrhage and neutrophil accumulation may be seen at the tips of villi, with small foci of epithelial necrosis overlying these sites. Large numbers of neutrophils and necrotic debris may cover the luminal surface. Gram-positive bacilli can be found adhering to the necrotic epithelial surfaces of the intestinal tract.

TREATMENT

Reducing oral intake to bland diets and parenteral fluid therapy are imperative for severely affected animals with acute diarrhea. Antimicrobial susceptibility testing of isolated strains is often misleading. Treatment is often given for 5 to 7 days, and most animals improve within 3 to 5 days. Clinical improvement may be variable or often lacking with metronidazole, despite in vitro susceptibility results, although it is often selected first (Table 39–4). More consistent clinical bene-

Table 39–4. Antimicrobial Therapy for **Clostridium perfringens***–Associated Diarrhea*[a]

DRUG	SPECIES	DOSE[b]	ROUTE	INTERVAL (HOURS)[c]	DURATION (DAYS)
Metronidazole	D	10 mg/kg	PO	8–12	5–7
	C	62.5 mg total	PO	12	5–7
Tylosin	B	10–20 mg/kg	PO	12–24	5–7
Ampicillin	B	22 mg/kg	PO	8–12	5–7
Amoxicillin-clavulanate	B	22 mg/kg	PO	12	5–7
Clindamycin	B	10 mg/kg	PO	12	5–7
Tetracycline	D	22 mg/kg	PO	8	5–7

[a]For additional information on selected drugs, see Drug Formulary, Appendix 8.
[b]Dose per administration at specified interval.
[c]For chronic recurring signs, animals may be given the indicated dose every 12 to 24 hours.
B = both dog and cat, C = cat, D = dog.

fits may be noted with ampicillin, amoxicillin-clavulanate, tylosin, clindamycin, or tetracycline.

Animals with chronic, recurring illness will have relapses shortly after antimicrobial therapy is discontinued or at variable time intervals thereafter. Less frequent administration at a maintenance dose may be enough to suppress bacterial proliferation and sporulation. Dietary recommendations are also beneficial (see following discussion) and may obviate the need for long-term prophylaxis.

PREVENTION

High fiber–containing diets or bulk additives (psyllium) greatly reduce the proliferation of clostridial organisms in the stool. These diets are recommended to help prevent the disease in hospitalized or congregated animals in a contaminated environment and in animals with chronic recurrences. Short-chain fatty acids produced by fiber fermentation may protect the colonic epithelium and produce an acid environment or alter microbial flora, thus inhibiting bacterial sporulation. Experimentally, administration of nondigestible sugars, such as lactulose and lactulosucrose, may temporarily increase the fluidity of the stool but also greatly decrease the numbers of enteric *C. perfringens*.[137]

As in any diarrheal outbreak, reducing the spread of infection involves judicious care by animal handlers. Hand washing, improved cage cleaning, and isolating symptomatic animals to reduce the spread of infection are needed. Animals should be handled in isolation wards where gowns, gloves, and boots must be worn.

References

1. Andersen LP, Norgaard A, Holck S, et al. 1996. Isolation of a *Helicobacter heilmannii*–like organism from the human stomach. *Eur J Clin Microbiol Infect Dis* 15:95–96.
1a. Anonymous. 1997. Federal agencies collaborate to control dangerous new *Salmonella* strain. *J Am Vet Med Assoc* 210:1712–1716.
2. Anonymous. 1984. Surveillance of the flow of *Salmonella* and *Campylobacter* in a community. Seattle—King County Department of Public Health, CDC Control Section, Seattle, WA.
3. Ansorg R, Vonheinegg EH, Vonrecklinghausen G. 1995. Cat owner's risk of acquiring a *Helicobacter pylori* infection. *Zentralbl Bakteriol* 283:122–126.
4. Archer JR, Romero S, Ritchie AE. 1988. Characterization of an unclassified microaerophilic bacterium associated with gastroenteritis. *J Clin Microbiol* 26:101–105.
5. Bartlett ML, Walker HW, Ziprin R. 1972. Use of dogs as an assay for *Clostridium perfringens* enterotoxin. *Appl Microbiol* 23:196–197.
6. Benno Y, Nakao H, Uchida K, et al. 1992. Impact of the advances in age on the gastrointestinal microflora of Beagle dogs. *J Vet Med Sci* 54:703–706.
7. Betts J, Findlay BB. 1992. Identification of *Salmonella typhimurium* invasiveness loci. *Can J Microbiol* 38(8):852–857.
8. Black SS, Austin FW, McKinley E. 1996. Isolation of *Yersinia* pseudotuberculosis and *Listeria monocytogenes* serotype 4 from a gray fox (*Urocyon cinereoargenteus*) with canine distemper. *J Wildl Dis* 32:362–366.
8a. Boschert KR, Allison N, Allen TLC, et al. 1988. Tyzzer's disease in an adult dog. *J Am Vet Med Assoc* 192:791–792.
9. Brett MM, Rodhouse JC, Donovan TJ, et al. 1992. Detection of *Clostridium perfringens* and its enterotoxin in cases of sporadic diarrhoea. *J Clin Pathol* 45:609–611.
10. Bryner JH, Ritchie AE, Pollet L, et al. 1987. Experimental infection and abortion of pregnant guinea pigs with a unique spirillum-like bacterium isolated from aborted ovine fetuses. *Am J Vet Res* 48:91–97.
11. Buogo C, Burnens AP, Perrin J, et al. 1995. Presence of *Campylobacter* spp, *Clostridium difficile*, *Clostridium perfringens* and *Salmonella* in some litters and in a kennel population of adult dogs. *Schweizer Arch Tierheilkunde* 137:165–171.
12. Burnens AP, Angeloz-Wick B, Nicolet J. 1992. Comparison of *Campylobacter* carriage rates in diarrheic and healthy pet animals. *Zentralbl Veterinarmed* 39:175–180.
13. Burnens AP, Stanley J, Morgenstern R, et al. 1994. Gastroenteritis associated with *Helicobacter pullorum* (letter). *Lancet* 344:1569–1570.
14. Burnens AP, Stanley J, Schaad UB, et al. 1993. Novel *Campylobacter*-like organism resembling *Helicobacter fennelliae* isolated from a boy with gastroenteritis and from dogs. *J Clin Microbiol* 31:1916–1917.
15. Burrows GI, Morton RJ, Fales WH. 1993. Microdilution antimicrobial susceptibilities of selected gram-negative veterinary bacterial isolates. *J Vet Diagn Invest* 5:541–547.
16. Chaicumpa W, Ruangkunaporn Y, Burr D, et al. 1992. Diagnosis of typhoid fever by detection of *Salmonella typhi* antigen in urine. *J Clin Microbiol* 30:2513–2515.
17. Chanter N. 1995. Infection of horses by Tyzzer's bacillus. *Equine Vet J* 27:1–3.
18. Chengappa MM, Staats J, Oberst RD, et al. 1993. Prevalence of *Salmonella* in raw meat used in diets of racing greyhounds. *J Vet Diagn Invest* 5:372–377.
19. Citino SB. 1995. Chronic, intermittent *Clostridium perfringens* enterotoxicosis in a group of cheetahs (*Acinonyx jubatus jubatus*). *J Zoo Wildl Med* 26:279–285.
19a. Clyde VL, Ramsay EC, Bemis DA. 1997. Fecal shedding of *Salmonella* in exotic felids. *J Zoo Wildl Med* 28:148–152.
20. Dewhirst FE, Seymour C, Fraser GJ, et al. 1994. Phylogeny of *Helicobacter* isolates from bird and swine feces and description of *Helicobacter pametensis* sp. nov. *Int J Syst Bacteriol* 44:553–560.
21. Dillon AR, Boosinger TR, Blevins WT. 1987. *Campylobacter* enteritis in dogs and cats. *Compend Cont Educ Pract Vet* 9:1176–1183.
21a. Domellöf L. 1996. Personal communication. Örebro Medical Center Hospital, Örebro, Sweden.
22. Dow SW, Jones RL, Henik RA, et al. 1989. Clinical features of salmonellosis in cats: six cases (1981–1986). *J Am Vet Med Assoc* 194:1464–1466.
23. Dubois A, Fiala N, Heman-Ackah LM. 1994. Natural gastric infection with *Helicobacter pylori* in monkeys: a model for spiral bacteria infection in humans. *Gastroenterology* 106:1405–1417.
24. Dubois A, Tarnawski A, Newell DG, et al. 1991. Gastric injury and invasion of parietal cells by spiral bacteria in rhesus monkeys: are gastritis and hyperchlorhydria infectious diseases? *Gastroenterology* 100:884–891.
25. Duncan AJ, Carman RJ, Olsen GJ, et al. 1993. Assignment of the agent of Tyzzer's disease to *Clostridium piliforme* comb-nov on the basis of 16S ribosomal-RNA sequence analysis. *Int J Syst Bacteriol* 43:314–318.
26. Dusch H, Altwegg M. 1995. Evaluation of five new plating media for isolation of *Salmonella* species. *J Clin Microbiol* 33:802–804.
27. Eaton KA, Dewhirst FE, Paster BJ, et al. 1996. Prevalence and varieties of *Helicobacter* species in dogs from random sources and pet dogs: animal and public health significance. *J Clin Microbiol* 34:3165–3170.
28. Eaton KA, Radin MJ, Kramer L, et al. 1993. Epizoonotic gastritis associated with gastric spiral bacilli in cheetahs (*Acinonyx jubatus*). *Vet Pathol* 30:55–63.
29. El-Sanousi SM, El Shazly MO, Al-Dughyem A, et al. 1992. An outbreak of enterotoxemia in cats. *Zentralbl Veterinarmed B* 39:403–409.
29a. El-Zaatari FA, Woo JS, Badr A, et al. 1997. Failure to isolate *Helicobacter*

pylori from stray cats indicates that *H. pylori* in cats may be an anthroponosis—an animal infection with a human pathogen. *J Med Microbiol* 46:372–376.
30. Fenwick SG, Madie P, Wilks CR, et al. 1994. Duration of carriage and transmission of *Yersinia enterocolitica* biotype-4, serotype 0/3 in dogs. *Epidemiol Infect* 113:471–477.
31. Fiedorek SC, Malaty HM, Evans DL, et al. 1991. Factors influencing the epidemiology of *Helicobacter pylori* infection in children. *Pediatrics* 88:578–582.
32. Fierer J, Krause M, Tauxe R, et al. 1992. *Salmonella typhimurium* bacteremia: association with the virulence plasmid. *J Infect Dis* 166:639–642.
33. Flores BM, Fennell CL, Kuller L, et al. 1990. Experimental infection of pig-tailed macaques (*Macaca nemestrina*) with *Campylobacter cinaedi* and *Campylobacter fennelliae*. *Infect Immun* 58:3947–3953.
34. Foley J, Hirsh DC, Pedersen NC. 1996. An outbreak of *Clostridium perfringens* enteritis in a cattery of Bengal cats and experimental transmission to specific pathogen free cats. *Feline Pract* 24:31–35.
35. Foster JR. 1984. Bacterial infection of the common bile duct in chronic fascioliasis in the rat. *J Comp Pathol* 94:175–181.
36. Fox JG. 1990. Campylobacteriosis, pp 538–542. *In* Greene CE (ed), Infectious disease of the dog and cat. WB Saunders, Philadelphia, PA.
37. Fox JG. 1996. In vivo studies of emergent issues in gastric *Helicobacter* pathogenesis and epidemiology, pp 11–33. *In* Hunt R, Tytgat G (eds), *Helicobacter pylori*: basic mechanisms to clinical cure. Kluwer Academic Publishers, Lancaster, United Kingdom.
38. Fox JG, Batchelder M, Marini RP, et al. 1995. *Helicobacter pylori* induced gastritis in the domestic cat. *Infect Immun* 63(7):2674–2681.
39. Fox JG, Chilvers T, Goodwin CS. 1989. *Campylobacter mustelae*, a new species resulting from the elevation of *Campylobacter pylori subsp. mustelae* to species status. *Int J Syst Bacteriol* 39:301–303.
40. Fox JG, Correa P, Taylor NS, et al. 1990. *Helicobacter mustelae* associated gastritis in ferrets: an animal model of *Helicobacter pylori* gastritis in humans. *Gastroenterology* 99:352–361.
41. Fox JG, Dewhirst FE, Tully JG, et al. 1994. *Helicobacter hepaticus* sp. nov, a microaerophilic bacterium isolated from livers and intestinal mucosal scrapings from mice. *J Clin Microbiol* 32:1238–1245.
42. Fox JG, Drolet R, Higgins R, et al. 1996. *Helicobacter canis* isolated from a dog liver with multifocal necrotizing hepatitis. *J Clin Microbiol* 34:2479–2482.
43. Fox JG, Li X, Yan L, et al. 1996. Chronic proliferative hepatitis in A/JCr mice associated with persistent *H. hepaticus* infection: a model of *Helicobacter* induced carcinogenesis. *Infect Immun* 64:1548–1558.
44. Fox JG, Paster BJ, Dewhirst FE, et al. 1992. *Helicobacter mustelae* isolation from feces of ferrets: evidence to support fecal-oral transmission of a gastric *Helicobacter*. *Infect Immun* 60:606–611.
45. Fox JG, Perkins S, Yan L, et al. 1996. Local immune response in *Helicobacter pylori* infected cats and identification of *H. pylori* in saliva, gastric fluid and feces. *Immunology* 88:400–406.
46. Fox JG, Taylor NS, Penner JL, et al. 1989. Investigation of zoonotic acquired *Campylobacter jejuni* enteritis with serotyping and restriction endonuclease DNA analysis. *J Clin Microbiol* 27:2423–2425.
47. Fox JG, Yan L, Dewhirst FE, et al. 1995. *Helicobacter bilis* sp. nov., a novel *Helicobacter* isolated from bile, livers, and intestines of aged, inbred mouse strains. *J Clin Microbiol* 33:445–454.
48. Fox JG, Yan L, Shames B, et al. 1996. Persistent hepatitis and enterocolitis in germfree mice infected with *Helicobacter hepaticus*. *Infect Immun* 64:3673–3681.
49. Fukushima H, Gomyoda M, Ishikura S, et al. 1989. Cat-contaminated environmental substances lead to *Yersinia pseudotuberculosis* infection in children. *J Clin Microbiol* 27:2706–2709.
50. Gebhart CJ, Fennell CL, Murtaugh MP, et al. 1989. *Campylobacter cinaedi* is normal intestinal flora in hamsters. *J Clin Microbiol* 27:1692–1694.
50a. Goodwin CS. 1997. Antimicrobial treatment of *Helicobacter pylori* infection. *Clin Infect Dis* 25:1023–1026.
51. Goossens H, Ulaes L, Butzler JP, et al. 1991. *Campylobacter upsalensis* enteritis associated with canine infections. *Lancet* 337:8755.
52. Graham DY, Malaty HM, Evans DG, et al. 1991. Epidemiology of *Helicobacter pylori* in an asymptomatic population in the United States. *Gastroenterology* 100:1495–1501.
53. Greene CE. 1990. Enteric and other bacterial infections, pp 538–557. *In* Greene CE (ed), Infectious disease of the dog and cat. WB Saunders, Philadelphia, PA.
53a. Grubel P, Hoffman JS, Chong FK, et al. 1997. Vector potential of houseflies *(Musca domestica)* for *Helicobacter pylori*. *J Clin Microbiol* 35:1300–1303.
54. Gruenewald R, Henderson RW, Yappow S. 1991. Use of Rambach propylene glycol containing agar for identification of *Salmonella* spp. *J Clin Microbiol* 29:2354–2356.
55. Gurgan T, Diker KS. 1994. Abortion associated with *Campylobacter upsalensis*. *J Clin Microbiol* 32:3093–3094.
56. Gutman LT, Ottesen EA, Quan TJ, et al. 1973. An inter-familial outbreak of *Yersinia enterocolitica* enteritis. *N Engl J Med* 288:1372–1377.
56a. Hald B, Madsen M. 1997. Healthy puppies and kittens as carriers of *Campylobacter* spp. with special reference to *Campylobacter upsaliensis*. *J Clin Microbiol* 35:3351–3352.
57. Handt LK, Fox JG, Dewhirst FE, et al. 1994. *Helicobacter pylori* isolated from the domestic cat: public health implications. *Infect Immun* 62:2367–2374.
58. Handt LK, Fox JG, Stalis IH, et al. 1995. Characterization of feline *Helicobacter pylori* strains and associated gastritis in a colony of domestic cats. *J Clin Microbiol* 33:2280–2289.
59. Hanninen ML, Happonen I, Saari S. 1996. Culture and characteristics of *Helicobacter bizzozeronii*, a new canine gastric *Helicobacter* sp. *Int J Syst Bacteriol* 46:160–166.
60. Hayashidani H, Kaneko K, Sakurai K, et al. 1995. Experimental infection with *Yersinia enterocolitica* serovar 0:8 in beagle dogs. *Vet Microbiol* 47:71–77.
61. Heilmann KL, Borchard F. 1991. Gastritis due to spiral shaped bacteria other than *Helicobacter pylori*: clinical, histological, and ultrastructural findings. *Gut* 32:137–140.
62. Henry GA, Long PH, Burns JL, et al. 1987. Gastric spirillosis in beagles. *Am J Vet Res* 48:831–836.
62a. Herikstad H, Hayes P, Mokhtar M, et al. 1997. Emerging quinolone-resistant *Salmonella* in the United States. *Emerg Infect Dis* 3:371–372.
63. Hermanns W, Kregel K, Breuer W, et al. 1995. *Helicobacter*-like organisms: histopathological examination of gastric biopsies from dogs and cats. *J Comp Pathol* 112:307–318.
63a. Hill JE, Khanolkar SS, Stadtlander CT. 1997. Gastric ulcer associated with a *Helicobacter*-like organism in a cougar *(Felis concolor)*. *Vet Pathol* 34:50–51.
64. Hohenhaus AE, Rosenberg MP, Moroff SD. 1990. Concurrent lymphoma and salmonellosis in a cat. *Can Vet J* 31:38–40.
65. Hornick RB. 1995. Enteric fever, pp. 325–332. *In* Blaser MJ, Smith PD, Ravdin JI, et al (eds), Infections of the gastrointestinal tract. Raven Press, New York, NY.
66. Iannibelli F, Caruso A, Castelluccio A, et al. 1991. *Yersinia pseudotuberculosis* in a Persian cat. *Vet Rec* 129:103–104.
67. Iwanaka M, Orita S, Mokuno Y, et al. 1993. Tyzzer's disease complicated with distemper in a puppy. *J Vet Med Sci* 55:337–339.
68. Jones BR, Greene CE. 1990. Tyzzer's disease, pp 552–555. *In* Greene CE (ed), Infectious disease of the dog and cat. WB Saunders, Philadelphia, PA.
69. Jones BR, Johnstone AC, Hancock WS. 1985. Tyzzer's disease in kittens with familial primary hyperlipoproteinaemia. *J Small Anim Pract* 26:411–419.
70. Kelly SM, Pitcher MCL, Farmery SM, et al. 1994. Isolation of *Helicobacter pylori* from feces of patients with dyspepsia in the United Kingdom. *Gastroenterology* 107:1671–1674.
71. Kemper CA, Mickelson P, Morton A, et al. 1993. *Helicobacter (Campylobacter) fennelliae*-like organisms as an important but occult cause of bacteremia in patient with AIDS. *J Infect* 26:97–101.
72. Kiehlbauch JA, Brenner DJ, Cameron DN, et al. 1995. Genotypic and phenotypic characterization of *H. cinaedi* and *H. fennelliae* strains isolated from humans and animals. *J Clin Microbiol* 22:2940–2947.
73. Kiehlbauch JA, Tauxe RV, Baker CN, et al. 1994. *Helicobacter cinaedi*-associated bacteremia and cellulitis in immunocompromised patients. *Ann Intern Med* 121:90–93.
74. Kirkbride CA, Gates CE, Collins JE. 1985. Ovine abortion associated with an anaerobic bacterium. *J Am Vet Med Assoc* 186:789–791.
75. Kowarz L, Coynault C, Robbe-Saule V, et al. 1994. The *Salmonella typhimurium* katF(rpoS) gene: cloning, nucleotide sequence, and regulation of spvR and spvABCD virulence plasmid genes. *J Bacteriol* 176(22):6852–6860.
76. Kruth SA, Prescot JF, Welch MK, et al. 1989. Nosocomial diarrhea associated with enterotoxigenic *Clostridium perfringens* infection in dogs. *J Am Vet Med Assoc* 195:331–334.
77. Lavelle JP, Landas S, Mitros FA, et al. 1994. Acute gastritis associated with spiral organisms from cats. *Dig Dis Sci* 39:744–750.
77a. Lecoindre P, Chevalier M, Peyrol S, et al. 1997. Pathogenic role of gastric *Helicobacter* sp. in domestic carnivores. *Vet Rec* 28:207–215.
78. Lecoindre P, Chevalier M, Peyrol S, et al. 1995. A study of dog stomach *Helicobacter* spp. and their pathogenicity. *Rev Med Vet* 146:671–678.
79. Lee A. 1992. *Helicobacter pylori* and *Helicobacter*-like organisms in animals: overview of mucus-colonizing organisms, pp 259–275. *In* Rathbone BJ, Heatley RU (eds), *Helicobacter pylori* and gastroduodenal disease, ed 2. Blackwell Scientific Public, London.
80. Lee A, Fox JG, Hazell S. 1993. Pathogenicity of *Helicobacter pylori*: a perspective. *Infect Immun* 61:1601–1610.
81. Lee A, Krakowka S, Fox JG, et al. 1992. Role of *Helicobacter felis* in chronic canine gastritis. *Vet Pathol* 29:487–494.
82. Lee A, Philips MW, O'Rourke JL, et al. 1992. *Helicobacter muridarum* sp. nov., a microaerophilic helical bacterium with a novel ultrastructure isolated from the intestinal mucosa of rodents. *Int J Syst Bacteriol* 42:27–36.
83. Lockard VG, Boler RK. 1970. Ultrastructure of a spiraled microorganism in the gastric mucosa of dogs. *Am J Vet Res* 31:1453–1462.
84. McDonough PL, Simpson KW. 1996. Diagnosing emerging bacterial infections: salmonellosis, campylobacteriosis, clostridial toxicosis, and helicobacteriosis. *Semin Vet Med Surg* 11:187–197.
85. McDonough PL, Timoney JF, Jacobson RH, et al. 1989. Clonal groups of *Salmonella typhimurium* in New York State. *J Clin Microbiol* 27:622–627.
86. Miwa N, Nishina T, Kubo S, et al. 1996. Nested polymerase chain reaction

for detection of low levels of enterotoxigenic *Clostridium perfringens* in animal feces and meat. *J Vet Med Sci* 58:197–203.
87. Moazed TC, Deeb BJ, DiGiacomo RF. 1990. Subcutaneous abscess due to *Salmonella adelaide* in a grey collie with cyclic hematopoiesis. *Lab Anim Sci* 40:639–641.
88. Morris A, Ali MR, Thomson L, et al. 1990. Tightly spiral shaped bacteria in the human stomach: another cause of active chronic gastritis. *Gut* 31:139–143.
89. Motzel SL, Riley LK. 1991. *Bacillus piliformis* flagellar antigens for serodiagnosis of Tyzzer's disease. *J Clin Microbiol* 29:2566–2570.
90. Murray MJ. 1986. *Salmonella*: virulence factors and enteric salmonellosis. *J Am Vet Med Assoc* 189:145–147.
91. Myerslough N. 1988. Tyzzer's disease in puppies. *Vet Rec* 122:238.
92. Nakayama H, Nii A, Oguihara S, et al. 1986. Effect of reticuloendothelial system blocking on Tyzzer's disease of mice. *Jpn J Vet Sci* 48:211–217.
93. Ng VL, Hadley WK, Fennell CL, et al. 1987. Successive bacteremias with "*Campylobacter cinaedi*" and "*Campylobacter fennelliae*" in a bisexual male. *J Clin Microbiol* 25:2008–2009.
94. Nii A, Nakayama H, Fujiwara K. 1986. Effect of partial hepatectomy on Tyzzer's disease of mice. *Jpn J Vet Sci* 48:227–235.
95. Nora PF, Mousavipour M, Mittelpunkt A, et al. 1966. Brain as a target organ in *Clostridium perfringens* exotoxin toxicity. *Arch Surg* 92:243–246.
96. On SL, Holmes B. 1995. Classification and identification of Campylobacters and Helicobacters and allied taxanumerical analysis of phenotypic characters. *Syst Appl Microbiol* 18:374–390.
96a. Oomes PG, Jacobs BC, Hazenberg MP, et al. 1995. Anti-GM1 IgG antibodies and *Campylobacter* bacteria in Guillain-Barré syndrome: evidence of molecular mimicry. *Ann Neurol* 38:170–175.
97. Orlicek SL, Welch DF, Kuhls TL. 1993. Septicemia and meningitis caused by *Helicobacter cinaedi* in a neonate. *J Clin Microbiol* 31:569–571.
98. Oswald GP, Twedt DC, Steyn P. 1994. *Campylobacter jejuni* bacteremia and acute cholecystitis in two dogs. *J Am Anim Hosp Assoc* 30:165–169.
99. Otto G, Hazell SH, Fox JG, et al. 1994. Animal and public health implications of gastric colonization of cats by *Helicobacter*-like organisms. *J Clin Microbiol* 32:1043–1049.
99a. Papasouliotis K, Gruffydd-Jones TJ, Werrett G, et al. 1997. Occurrence of gastric *Helicobacter*-like organisms in cats. *Vet Rec* 140:369–370.
100. Parsonnet J, Friedman GD, Vandersteen DP, et al. 1991. *Helicobacter pylori* infection and the risk of gastric carcinoma. *N Engl J Med* 325:1127–1131.
101. Parsonnet J, Hanson S, Rodriguez L. 1994. *Helicobacter pylori* infection and gastric MALT lymphoma. *N Engl J Med* 330:1267–1271.
102. Paster BJ, Lee A, Fox JG, et al. 1991. Phylogeny of *Helicobacter felis* sp. nov., *Helicobacter mustelae*, and related bacteria. *Int J Syst Bacteriol* 41:31–38.
103. Patton CM, Shaffer N, Edmonds P, et al. 1989. Human disease associated with "*Campylobacter upsalensis*" (catalase negative or weakly positive *Campylobacter* species) in the United States. *J Clin Microbiol* 27:66–73.
104. Pelkonen S, Romppanen E, Siitonen A, et al. 1994. Differentiation of *Salmonella* serovar infantis isolates from human and animal sources by fingerprinting IS200 and 165 rrn loci. *J Clin Microbiol* 32:2128–2133.
105. Pelzer KD. 1989. Salmonellosis. *J Am Vet Med Assoc* 195:456–463.
106. Perkins SE, Yan LL, Shen Z, et al. 1996. Use of PCR and culture to detect *Helicobacter pylori* in naturally infected cats following triple antimicrobial therapy. *Antimicrob Agents Chemother* 40:1486–1490.
106a. Poonacha KB. 1997. Naturally occurring Tyzzer's disease in a serval *(Felis capensis)*. *J Vet Diagn Invest* 9:82–84.
107. Prescott JF, Johnson JA, Patterson JM. 1978. Hemorrhagic gastroenteritis in the dog associaed with *Clostridium welchii*. *Vet Rec* 103:116–117.
108. Pritchett SJ. 1991. Enterotoxaemia in dogs. *Vet Rec.* 129:391.
109. Qureshi SR, Carlton WW, Olander HJ. 1988. Tyzzer's disease in an adult dog. *J Am Vet Med Assoc* 168:602–604.
110. Radin JM, Eaton KA, Krakowka S, et al. 1990. *Helicobacter pylori* infection in gnotobiotic Beagle dogs. *Infect Immun* 58:2606–2612.
111. Reilly GA, Bailie NC, Morrow WT, et al. 1994. Feline stillbirths associated with mixed *Salmonella typhimurium* an *Leptospira* infection. *Vet Rec* 135:608.
112. Rodriguez CO, Moon ML, Lieb MS. 1993. *Salmonella choleraesuis* pneumonia in a cat without signs of gastrointestinal tract disease. *J Am Vet Med Assoc* 202:953–955.
113. Romero S, Archer JR, Hamacher ME. 1988. Case report of an unclassified microaerophilic bacterium associated with gastroenteritis. *J Clin Microbiol* 26:142–143.
114. Ruiz J, Nunez M, Diaz J, et al. 1996. Comparison of five plating media for isolation of *Salmonella* species from human stools. *J Clin Microbiol* 34:686–688.
115. Rumiantsev AG, Kasatakin VN, Blokhim BM, et al. 1993. The use of monoclonal antibodies to lipid A for the correction of the hemodynamic disorders in endotoxemia. *Gematol Transfuziol* 38:31–33.
116. Russell RG, O'Donnoghue M, Blake DC, et al. 1993. Early colonic damage and invasion of *Campylobacter jejuni* in experimentally challenged infant *Macaca mulatta* (note). *J Infect Dis* 168:210–215.
117. Rutgers HC, Stepien RL, Elwood CM, et al. 1994. Enrofloxacin treatment of gram-negative infections. *Vet Rec* 135:357–359.
118. Salamah AA. 1994. Occurrence of *Yersinia-enterocolitica* and *Yersinia-pseudotuberculosis* in rodents and cat feces from Riyadh area, Saudia Arabia. *Arab Gulf J Sci Res* 12:547–557.
119. Schauer DB, Ghori N, Falkow S. 1993. Isolation and characterization of "*Flexispira rappini*" from laboratory mice. *J Clin Microbiol* 31:2709–2714.
120. Seddon ML, Barry SJ. 1992. Clostridial myositis in dogs. *Vet Rec* 131:84.
121. Seymour C, Lewis RJ, Kim M, et al. 1994. Isolation of *Helicobacter* strains from wild bird and swine feces. *Appl Environ Microbiol* 60:1025–1028.
122. Shames B, Fox JG, Dewhirst FE, et al. 1995. Identification of widespread *H. hepaticus* infection in feces in commercial mouse colonies by culture and PCR assay. *J Clin Microbiol* 33:2968–2972.
123. Solnick JV, O'Rourke J, Lee A, et al. 1993. An uncultured gastric spiral organism is a newly identified *Helicobacter* in humans. *J Infect Dis* 168:379–385.
124. Song JH, Cho H, Park MY, et al. 1993. Detection of *Salmonella typhi* in the blood of patients with typhoid fever by polymerase chain reaction. *J Clin Microbiol* 31:1439–1443.
125. Sonstein SA, Burnham JC. 1993. Effect of low concentrations of quinolone antibiotics on bacterial virulence mechanisms. *Diagn Microbiol Infect Dis* 16:277–289.
126. Spencer TH, Ganaway JR, Waggie KS. 1990. Cultivation of *Bacillus piliformis* (Tyzzer) in mouse fibroblasts (3T3 cells). *Vet Microbiol* 22:291–297.
127. Spier C. 1990. Treatment of *Yersinia* infection with tetracyclines. *Aust Vet J* 67:471.
128. Staat MA, Kruszon-Moran D, McQuillan GM, et al. 1996. A population-based serologic survey of *Helicobacter pylori* infection in children and adolescents in the United States. *J Infect Dis* 174:1120-1123.
129. Stanley J, Jones C, Burnens A, et al. 1994. Distinct genotypes of human and canine isolates of *Campylobacter upsalensis* determined by 16S rRNA gene typing and plasmid profiling. *J Clin Microbiol* 32:1788–1794.
130. Stanley J, Linton D, Burens AP. 1993. *Helicobacter canis* sp. nov., a new species from dogs: an integrated study of phenotype and genotype. *J Gen Microbiol* 139:2495–2504.
131. Stanley J, Linton D, Burens AP. 1994. *Helicobacter pullorum* sp.nov.—genotype and phenotype of a new species isolated from poultry and from human patients with gastroenteritis. *Microbiology* 140:3441–3449.
132. Stolte M, Wellens E, Bethke B. 1994. *Helicobacter heilmannii* (formerly *Gastrospirillum hominis*) gastritis: an infection transmitted by animals? *Scand J Gastroenterol* 29:1061–1064.
133. Stone GG, Chengappa MM, Oberst RD, et al. 1993. Application of the polymerase chain reaction for the correlation of *Salmonella* serovars recovered from greyhound feces with their diet. *J Vet Diagn Invest* 5:378–385.
134. Stone GG, Oberst RD, Hays MP, et al. 1995. Detection of *Salmonella typhimurium* from rectal swabs of experimentally infected Beagles by short cultivation and PCR hybridization. *J Clin Microbiol* 33:1292–1295.
134a. Struble AL, Tang YJ, Kass PH, et al. 1994. Fecal shedding of *Clostridium difficile* in dogs: a period prevalence survey in a veterinary medical teaching hospital. *J Vet Diagn Invest* 6:342–347.
135. Sugiyama Y, Sugiyama F, Yagami K. 1993. Isolation of *Salmonella* from impounded dogs introduced in a laboratory. *Exp Anim* 42:119–121.
136. Taylor NS, Ellenberger MA, Wu PY, et al. 1989. Diversity of serotypes of *Campylobacter jejuni* and *Campylobacter coli* isolated in laboratory animals. *Lab Anim Sci* 39:219–221.
137. Terada A, Hara H, Kato S, et al. 1993. Effect of lactosucrose on fecal flora and fecal putrefactive products of cats. *J Vet Med Sci* 55:291–295.
138. Thomas DR, Salmon RL, Meadows D, et al. 1995. Incidence of *Helicobacter pylori* in farmworkers and the role of zoonotic spread (abstract). *Gut* 37(Suppl 1):A24.
139. Thomas JE, Gibson GR, Darboe MK, et al. 1992. Isolation of *Helicobacter pylori* from human feces. *Lancet* 340:1194–1195.
140. Thomson MA, Storey P, Greer R, et al. 1994. Canine-human transmission of *Gastrospirillum hominis* (note). *Lancet* 343:1605–1607.
141. Totten PA, Fennel CL, Tenover FC. 1985. *Campylobacter cinaedi* (sp. nov.) and *Campylobacter fennelliae* (sp. nov.): two new *Campylobacter* species associated with enteric disease in homosexual men. *J Infect Dis* 151:131–139.
142. Tschirdewahn B, Notermans S, Wernars K, et al. 1991. The presence of enterotoxigenic *Clostridium perfringens* strains in feces or various animals. *Int J Food Microbiol* 14:175–178.
143. Twedt DC. 1993. *Clostridium perfringens* associated diarrhea in dogs, pp 121–125. *In* Proceedings of the 11th ACVIM Forum, Washington, DC.
144. Vanderhoop AG, Veringa EM. 1993. Cholecystitis caused by *Campylobacter jejuni*. *Clin Infect Dis* 17:133.
144a. Van der Wouden EJ, van Zwet AA, Thijs JC, et al. 1997. Rapid increase in the prevalence of metronidazole-resistant *Helicobacter pylori* in the Netherlands. *Emerg Infect Dis* 3:385–389.
145. Veldhuyzen van Zanten SJO, Pollak PT, Best LM, et al. 1994. Increasing prevalence of *Helicobacter pylori* infection with age: continuous risk of infection in adults rather than cohort effect. *J Infect Dis* 169:434–437.
146. Verbruggen P, Creve U, Hubens A, et al. 1986. *Campylobacter fetus* as a cause of acute cholecystitis. *Br J Surg* 73:46.
147. Wall PG, Davis S, Threlfall EJ, et al. 1995. Chronic carriage of multidrug resistant *Salmonella typhimurium* in a cat. *J Small Anim Pract* 36:279–281.
148. Wall PG, Morgan D, Lamden K, et al. 1994. A case controlled study of infection with an epidemic strain of multiresistant *Salmonella typhimurium* DT104 in England and Wales. *Commun Dis Rep* 11:R130–R135.
149. Wall PG, Threllfall EJ, Ward LR, et al. 1996. Multiresistant *Salmonella typhimurium* DT104 isolated from cats: a public health risk. *Lancet* 348:471.

150. Walsh JH, Peterson WL. 1995. The treatment of *Helicobacter pylori* infection in the management of peptic ulcer disease. *N Engl J Med* 333:984–991.
151. Ward JM, Fox JG, Anver MR, et al. 1994. Chronic active hepatitis and associated liver tumors in mice caused by a persistent bacterial infection with a novel *Helicobacter* species. *J Natl Cancer Inst* 86:1222–1227.
152. Webb PM, Knight T, Greaves S, et al. 1994. Relation between infection with *Helicobacter pylori* and living conditions in childhood: evidence for person to person transmission in early life. *BMJ* 308:750-753.
152a. Weber A, Schmittdiel EF. 1962. Electron microscopic and bacteriologic studies of spirilla isolated from the fundic stomach of cats and dogs. *Am J Vet Res* 23:422–426.
153. Weber A, Wachowitz R, Weigl U, et al. 1995. Occurrence of *Salmonella* in fecal samples of dogs and cats in northern Bavaria from 1975 to 1994. *Berl Munch Tierarztl Wochenschr* 108:401–404.
154. Werdeling F, Amtsberg G, Tewes S. 1991. The occurrence of enterotoxigenic *Clostridium perfringens* strains in the feces of dogs and cats. *Berl Munch Tierarztl Wochenschr* 104:228–233.
155. Wilkie JSN, Barker IK. 1985. Colitis due to *Bacillus piliformis* in two kittens. *Vet Pathol* 22:649–652.
156. Williams LP. 1992. More concern about "4-D meat." *J Am Vet Med Assoc* 200:1057–1058.
157. Wray C, Beedell YE, McLaren IM. 1991. A survey of antimicrobial resistance in salmonellae isolated from animals in England and Wales 1984–1987. *Br Vet J* 147:356–369.
158. Yokoyama E, Katsube Y, Maruyama S, et al. 1991. Occurrence of cross-infection of *Salmonella* sp in detained dogs. *J Vet Med Sci* 53:929–930.
159. Yong CW, Nutting G, Hupka-Butz D. 1992. Tyzzer's disease in a dog. *Can Vet J* 33:827.
160. Young JK, Baher DC, Burney DP. 1995. Naturally occurring Tyzzer's disease in a puppy. *Vet Pathol* 32:63–65.

Chapter **40**

Canine Brucellosis

Leland E. Carmichael and Craig E. Greene

ETIOLOGY AND EPIDEMIOLOGY

Brucella canis is a small (1.0–1.5 μm), gram-negative, aerobic, coccobacillary organism. Its rough colonial morphology and differences in biochemical and antigenic reactions distinguish it from other members of the genus *Brucella*. Unlike the smooth *Brucella* organisms that infect several domestic animal species, *B. canis* has a limited host range; only dogs and wild Canidae have been found to be susceptible. Cats can be infected experimentally but are relatively resistant, having a transient bacteremia. Rabbits and nonhuman primates also have been found to be susceptible to experimental infections. No other animal species has developed significant agglutination titers. Human cases have been reported as a result of laboratory accidents and contact with infected dogs, but people appear to be relatively resistant (see Public Health Considerations).

Dogs also are susceptible to infection with *B. abortus*[7, 22] and *B. suis*.[2] Natural infection is thought to occur after ingestion of contaminated placentas and aborted fetuses from livestock. Dogs usually harbor the organisms in the lymph nodes of the GI tract for extended periods. Dogs are not believed to be important in the spread and maintenance of these infections. Testing and removal of affected dogs from infected farms are the optimal preventive measures for eradication.

B. canis infects a susceptible host by penetrating the mucous membranes, especially those of the oral cavity, vagina, and conjunctiva. The minimum oral infectious dose for dogs is about 10^6 bacteria, and the conjunctival dose is 10^4 to 10^5 organisms. Because they contain the highest concentration of organisms, vaginal discharges and semen are the most likely sources for infection by mucosal contamination.

Natural transmission of canine brucellosis occurs by several routes. Infected female dogs apparently transmit *B. canis* only during estrus, at breeding, or after abortion through oronasal contact with vaginal discharges. Transmission is most common by oronasal contact with aborted materials because they contain up to 10^{10} organisms per milliliter. Shedding of *B. canis* may occur for periods up to 6 weeks after an abortion. Milk of infected bitches contains lower concentrations of organisms and appears to be less important in transmitting infection to surviving pups; most have already been infected in utero.

Seminal fluid and urine have been incriminated as sources of infection from male dogs that harbor the organisms in the prostates and epididymides. The rate of isolation of *B. canis* from the semen of infected dogs is usually high for the first 6 to 8 weeks PI. Intermittent shedding of the organism in low numbers has been noted for up to 60 weeks PI and may continue for at least 2 years. Urinary excretion begins a few weeks after the onset of bacteremia and continues for at least 3 months. Concentrations of 10^3 to 10^6 organisms per milliliter of urine have been found in male dogs, with lesser numbers of bacteria in the urine of females. At one time, urine of infected males was thought to contain too few organisms to be infectious by the oronasal route; however, studies have demonstrated that *B. canis* can be transmitted from infected to uninfected mature male dogs after several weeks or months of close contact.[3] The propensity of males to shed the organism in the urine is probably related to its localization in the prostate and epididymis, which are in close association with the urinary bladder.

Alternative means of transmission occur less frequently under natural circumstances. In utero or congenital transmission becomes important as a means of spread of infection to live-born puppies. Transmission via fomites has been reported after vaginoscopy, blood transfusion, artificial insemination, and use of contaminated syringes. *B. canis* is relatively short lived outside the dog and is readily inactivated by common disinfectants.

The prevalence of infection varies according to the animal's age, housing conditions, breed, and geographic location. Pet dogs in suburban environments have a lower prevalence compared with stray dogs in economically depressed areas, which may reflect increased population density and uncon-

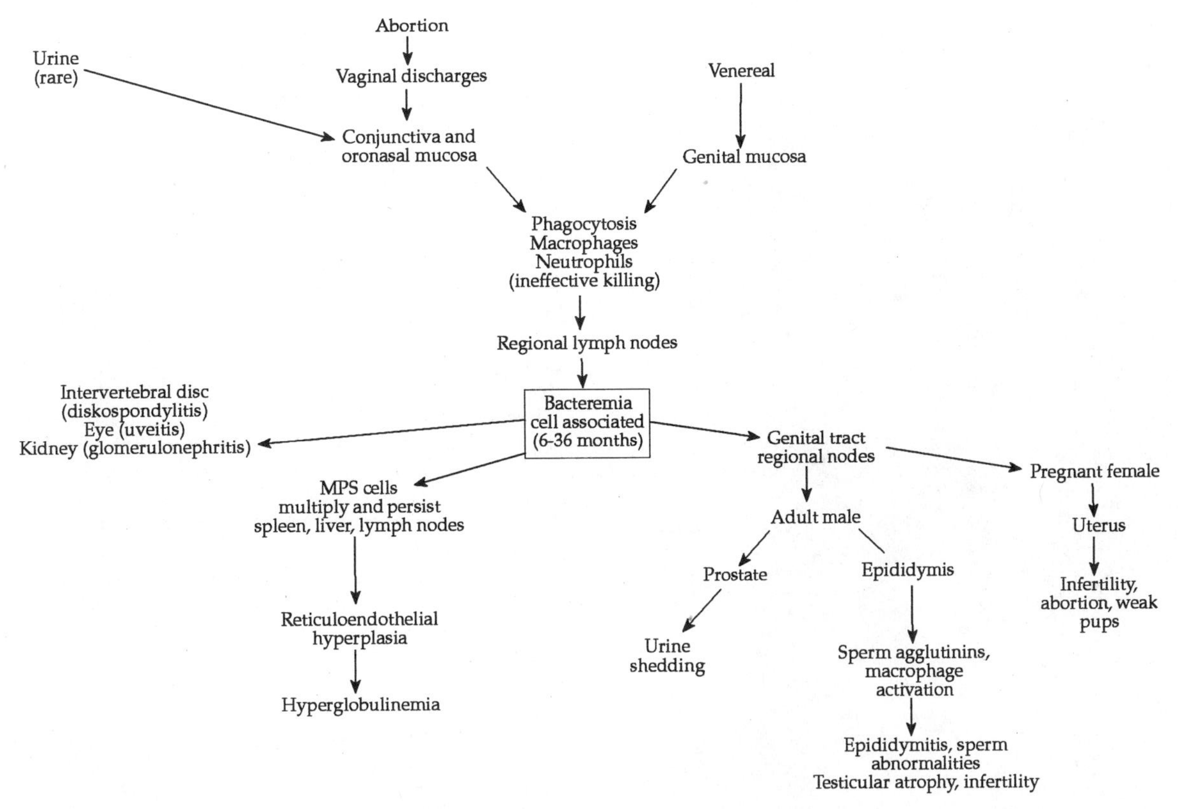

Figure 40–1. Sequential pathogenesis of canine brucellosis. MPS = mononuclear phagocyte system.

trolled breeding of dogs. A relatively low prevalence has been reported in the United States and Japan (range, 1–18%) compared with rates as high as 28% in Mexico and Peru.[3] Cases have also been identified in other countries in Central and South America and in Germany, Spain, Czechoslovakia, and Tunisia.[5] The disease also appears to be prevalent in regions of the People's Republic of China.[9] The southern United States appears to have a relatively higher (approximately 8%) prevalence of infection. Among breeds in this region, beagles and Labrador retrievers have a higher prevalence of infection. Determination of seroprevalence is strongly influenced by the means of testing and interpretation.

PATHOGENESIS

The general sequence of events after infection by *Brucella* is summarized in Figure 40–1. The bacteria are probably phagocytized at contaminated mucosal sites by tissue macrophages and other phagocytic cells and transported to lymphatic and genital tract tissues, where they multiply. They persist intracellularly within mononuclear phagocytes. A leukocyte-associated bacteremia occurs beginning 1 to 4 weeks PI and can last 6 to 64 months. Generalized lymphoreticular hyperplasia (Fig. 40–2) and development of hyperglobulinemia occur during the course of infection. As with other intracellular parasites, cell-mediated immunity is probably the most important defense mechanism against *B. canis*. Persistent nonprotective antibody titers are characteristic of such infections and appear to have little influence on the level of bacteremia or number of organisms in tissues. The greatest numbers of *B. canis* organisms are found in the lymph nodes, spleen, and tissues of gonadal steroid dependency. Although usually confined to mononuclear phagocytes, they may enter other cells such as placental epithelium. In fact, the uterus is not a favored site of growth in the nongravid or diestral female. Inflammation of the epididymides and testes in males causes sperm leakage, which provokes the immune system to produce a complex of antisperm agglutinating antibodies and delayed-type hypersensitivity reactions against sperm

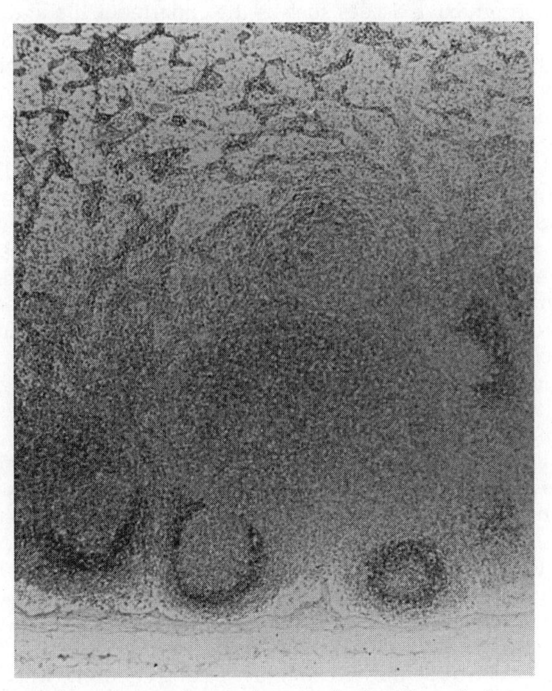

Figure 40–2. Follicular hyperplasia in the lymph node from a dog with chronic *B. canis* infection (H and E; × 40).

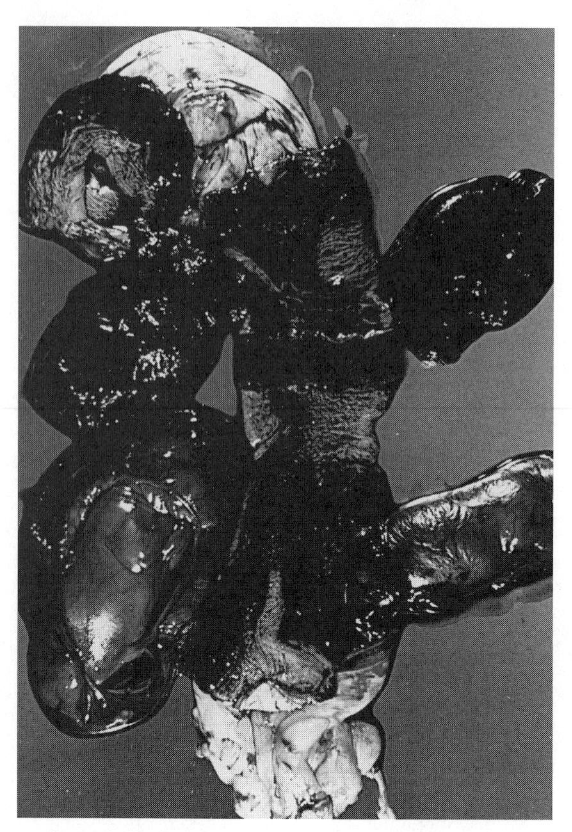

Figure 40–3. Partially autolyzed fetuses with placenta and uterus from a dog infected with *B. canis* that was neutered at 45 days gestation.

that are unrelated to the antibodies against *B. canis*. The immune responses produced against spermatozoa contribute to the epididymitis, infertility, and eventual spermatogenic arrest seen in most infected male dogs.

B. canis, like other blood-borne bacteria, may localize in nonreproductive tissues such as the endarterial circulation of the intervertebral disc, causing diskospondylitis. Other tissues that filter blood-borne organisms or immune complexes may become involved, including the eye (anterior uveitis), kidney (glomerulopathy), and meninges (meningoencephalitis).

Spontaneous recovery from infection may occur within 1 to more than 5 years PI. Therapy accelerates the recovery process. Some dogs may have persistent bacteremia throughout this time, whereas others can harbor bacteria in tissues for several months after the bacteremia ceases. The prostate gland may be a site of this persistence in male dogs. Despite tissue persistence, when *B. canis* is no longer detected in the blood, serum agglutination titers decrease.

Dogs that recover naturally have low or negative agglutination titers and yet are immune to reinfection, suggesting that protective immunity is cell mediated. Recovered dogs challenged PO or IV as long as 4 years after spontaneous recovery from experimental infection were completely immune.[3] However, chronically infected dogs that were successfully treated with antibiotics were found to be fully susceptible to oronasal challenge 12 weeks after treatment had been halted. Natural recovery from *B. canis* infection appears to be a requirement to sustain protective immunity. Immunosuppression with glucocorticoids and antilymphocyte serum appears to increase the susceptibility of dogs to initial infection, but it does not augment the severity of the disease or alter the course of infection in experimentally infected dogs.

CLINICAL FINDINGS

Despite generalized systemic infection with *B. canis*, adult dogs rarely are seriously ill. Fever is uncommon and, with the exception of males who commonly have epididymitis, most infections will not be diagnosed by routine history or physical examination. Dry, lusterless coats, loss of vigor, and decreased exercise tolerance are occasionally reported by owners of working dogs. Nongravid females show no signs of illness other than lymphadenomegaly, which occurs in both sexes.

Overt clinical signs usually involve reproductive disturbances in sexually mature animals. Bitches usually abort dead pups between 45 and 60 days of gestation but show no other clinical signs. Pups are usually partially autolyzed, with subcutaneous edema and congestion and hemorrhage of the abdominal subcutaneous region (Fig. 40–3). Moderate quantities of serosanguineous peritoneal effusions are found. Their appearance suggests fetal death in utero some time before abortion. Decomposed fetuses are not usually found because they are ingested by the bitch. Abortion is characterized by a brown or greenish-gray vaginal discharge that lasts for 1 to 6 weeks. Brucellosis should be suspected under any circumstance when apparently healthy bitches abort 2 weeks before term.

Although abortion of dead puppies is the primary clinical sign reported with brucellosis, conception failures can occur at any time after breeding. In utero death with fetal resorption or abortion and ingestion of fetuses may be suspected if a bitch fails to conceive after an apparently successful mating. Embryonic death may occur as early as 20 days after mating, although most conception failures are actually undetected abortions. Less commonly, bitches may carry infected puppies to term and whelp both live and dead puppies within a single litter. Most pups that are born alive will die within a few hours or days, but those that survive or that are infected

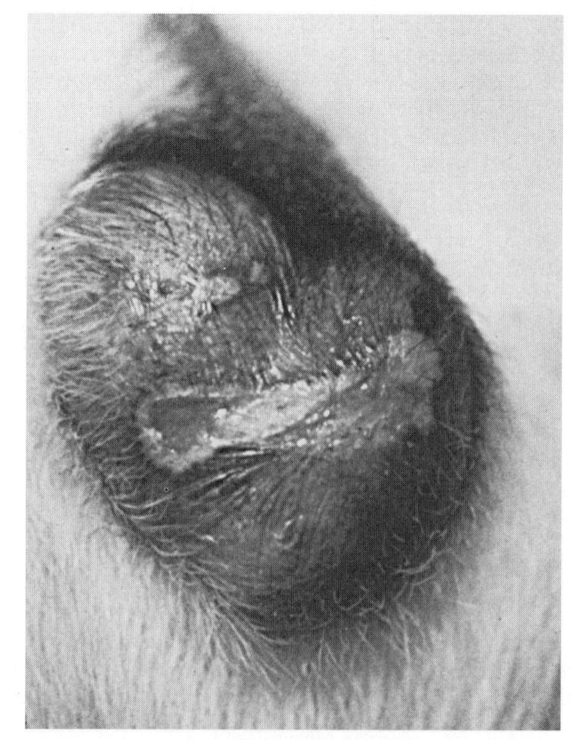

Figure 40–4. Testicular enlargement and scrotal dermatitis in an experimentally infected dog 35 weeks PI.

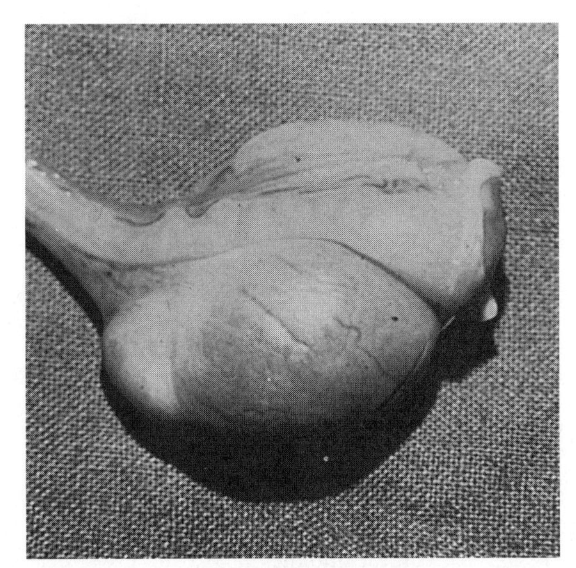

Figure 40–5. Enlargement of the tail of the epididymis on the testicle from an experimentally infected dog 60 weeks PI.

as neonates usually have generalized peripheral lymphadenomegaly as the primary clinical manifestation of disease until they reach sexual maturity. Such puppies usually have persistent hyperglobulinemia, and some may have transient fever, leukocytosis, or seizures as the systemic manifestations of their infections.

As with brucellosis in other species, infections with *B. canis* do not interfere with normal estrous cycles. A high proportion of bitches that abort may have normal litters subsequently. However, even after having normal litters, some infected bitches experience intermittent reproductive failures.

Because of the prominent testicular abnormalities, male dogs are presented for examination more often than are females, even though impairment of male reproductive performance often is less noticed. Nevertheless, infertility occurs. Males appear to be in good health but may have an enlarged scrotum because of accumulation of serosanguineous fluid in the tunica. Scrotal dermatitis is the result of constant licking and secondary infection with nonhemolytic staphylococci (Fig. 40–4). A major cause of testicular swelling is enlargement of the tail of the epididymis (Fig. 40–5); orchitis and primary testicular enlargement are rarely apparent. In fact, chronically infected males usually develop unilateral or bilateral testicular atrophy. A decreased volume of ejaculate without loss of libido is usually present. Acute pain is not usually evident on scrotal or testicular palpation, but discomfort may be seen at the time of ejaculation.

Nonreproductive abnormalities have been noted less frequently. Splenomegaly may accompany the diffuse lymphadenomegaly in some dogs. Dogs with diskospondylitis initially experience spinal pain and later paresis and ataxia if spinal cord compression develops. Osteomyelitis of the appendicular skeleton causes lameness of the affected limb. Meningoencephalitis has been reported after experimental and natural infections; however, neurobrucellosis in dogs, as in humans, is uncommon.[19] One of the authors observed a male dog that had confirmed *B. canis* infection with behavioral changes, anisocoria, ataxia, hyperesthesia, head tilt, and circling. Neurologic signs began within 3 weeks after the dog's first breeding. Chronic multifocal pyogranulomatous dermatitis that resembled lick granuloma lesions also has been reported in an infected dog, but a direct causal relationship was not established. Recurrent anterior uveitis with corneal edema has been detected in infected dogs either alone or in combination with other signs (see Chapter 93). Endophthalmitis has resulted in secondary glaucoma or phthisis bulbi.

DIAGNOSIS

Clinical Laboratory Findings

Hematologic and biochemical values are either unaltered or nonspecific in canine brucellosis. Hyperglobulinemia (β and γ) with concomitant hypoalbuminemia has been the most consistent finding in chronically infected dogs. An increased incidence of positive Coombs' test findings in the absence of anemia has been reported. Examination of aspirates or biopsy samples from enlarged lymph nodes usually reveals lymphoid hyperplasia with large numbers of plasma cells. CSF analysis results are pleocytosis, primarily consisting of neutrophils, and increased protein concentration with meningoencephalitis, but they are unremarkable when diskospondylitis alone is present. Urinalysis is usually normal despite the variable presence of bacteriuria. Radiographic demonstration of intervertebral disc infection should always be followed by serologic testing and, when possible, bacteriologic confirmation of *B. canis* (Fig. 40–6).

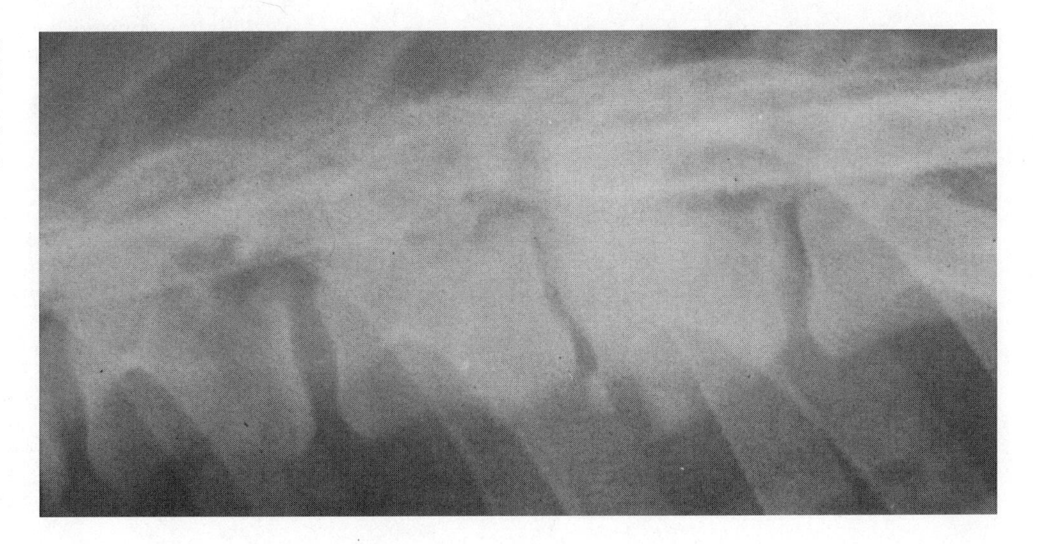

Figure 40–6. Myelogram of a dog with diskospondylitis showing thoracic and abdominal hyperesthesia and pelvic limb paralysis. Note obstruction of the flow of radiographic contrast medium over the affected disc space.

Semen Examination

Semen abnormalities, evident by 5 weeks PI, become pronounced by 8 weeks PI. Abnormalities include immature sperm, deformed acrosomes, swollen midpieces, and retained protoplasmic droplets. By week 15 PI, there are bent tails, detached heads, and head-to-head agglutination. Large aggregates of inflammatory cells, usually consisting of neutrophils, surround adherent macrophages containing phagocytized sperm (Fig. 40–7). More than 90% of the sperm is abnormal by 20 weeks PI. Aspermia without inflammatory cells corresponds with the development of bilateral testicular atrophy. Semen morphology should always be evaluated in dogs with infertility because of the obvious abnormalities that occur with brucellosis.

Serologic Testing

Serologic testing is the most frequently used diagnostic method for detecting canine brucellosis. These tests are subject to considerable interpretive error because lipopolysaccharide (LPS) antigens of several bacterial species cross-react with *B. canis*.[15, 17] The problem of false-positive cross-reactions, therefore, is more common than that of false-negative reactions. All sera should be free of hemolysis because hemoglobin causes false-positive agglutination of the tube test antigen.

Serologic test results often are negative during the first 3 to 4 weeks PI despite the presence of bacteremia by 2 weeks PI. For this reason, newly acquired animals should be tested sequentially at least twice at 30-day intervals before introduction into a breeding kennel. Low or intermediate titers may mean previous disease or very recent infection, and testing should be repeated or attempts made to isolate the organism by hemoculture. Male dogs may harbor the organism in the prostate glands and epididymides for extended periods after bacteremia ceases and agglutination titers have declined.

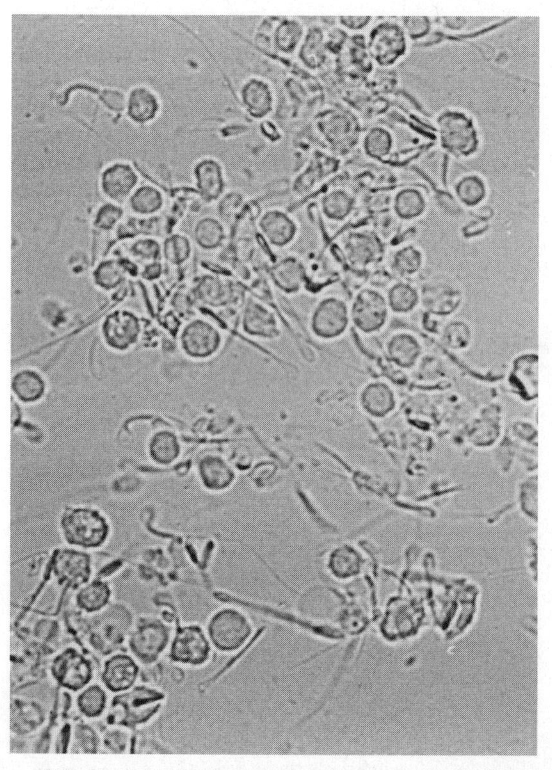

Figure 40–7. Unstained saline smear of semen sample from a dog 35 weeks PI. Large numbers of inflammatory cells are present.

Chronically infected female dogs may have diagnostically equivocal antibody titers and negative blood cultures. In females, recrudescence of bacteremia and increased antibody titers develop during proestrus, estrus, pregnancy, or abortion. These are the most reliable times to screen female dogs for infection.

Antibiotic therapy may suppress bacteremia and the associated serologic response, possibly contributing to false-negative serology and failure to isolate the organism from infected dogs. Antibacterials should not be given until diagnostic tests have been completed. Tetracycline drugs cause abacteremia and a corresponding decrease in antibody titer that may rebound after treatment is discontinued because tetracyclines are not bacteriocidal.

Table 40–1 compares the serologic tests described next. Consult Appendices 5 and 6 for information concerning commercially available testing. Serologic tests should be evaluated in light of clinical findings in the dog being evaluated (Fig. 40–8). A single high agglutination titer to *B. canis* usually indicates active infection, but this should be substantiated by further tests. Dogs that are asymptomatic but have positive results on agglutination procedures should never be condemned as infected until blood culture results or the more specific cytoplasmic antigen (CPAg) agar gel immunodiffusion (AGID) test results confirm the positive findings. All tests, with the exception of the CPAg-AGID method, measure antibodies to LPS antigens and may give nonspecific test results.

Rapid Slide Agglutination Test. The 2-mercaptoethanol (ME) rapid slide agglutination test (ME-RSAT) is preferred as an in-office screening procedure because it is inexpensive, rapid, and sensitive and detects antibodies early (D-Tec CB, Synbiotics, San Diego, CA). A 99% correlation exits between a negative test and lack of infection. The test kit used rose bengal–stained *B. ovis* because its growth is less mucoid than *B. canis*. *B. canis* cross-reacts with all rough *Brucella* and with certain other bacterial species, such as mucoid strains of *Pseudomonas*, *Bordetella bronchiseptica*, and *Actinobacillus equuli*, to which serum antibodies may be present. Most causes of cross-reactions, however, have not been identified. Some breeds (e.g., Irish wolfhounds and Old English sheepdogs) have an exceptionally high false-positive test result rate for unknown reasons.[5] The ME-RSAT substantially reduces false-positive reactions by eliminating less specifically reacting IgM antibodies. ME is labile and must be kept in a dark, tightly stoppered bottle at 4°C; use of inactivated ME gives false-positive results. A modification of the RSAT, utilizing a less mucoid (M–) variant of *B. canis*, further reduces the rate of false-positive results.[15, 17] The ME-RSAT with the *B. canis* M– antigen, therefore, can be employed for confirmation of positive results of screening tests.

Tube Agglutination Test. The tube agglutination test (TAT) has been the most widely used serodiagnostic procedure for confirmation of infection in ME-RSAT–positive dogs. However, availability of antigen formerly provided by the U.S. Department of Agriculture is currently erratic. As with the RSAT, the TAT also is troubled by heterospecific reactions with other infectious agents and by equivocal titers in chronically infected animals; therefore, the ME modification is used. Unfortunately, the ME-TAT also suffers from lack of specificity, and the increase in ME-TAT antibody titers usually lags 1 to 2 weeks behind those of the TAT and 2 to 4 weeks behind those of the ME-RSAT. Nevertheless, results of the

Table 40–1. Comparison of Serologic Procedures for Canine Brucellosis

SEROLOGIC TEST	ANTIGEN USED	EARLIEST TITER[a] (WEEKS PI)	ADVANTAGES	DISADVANTAGES
ME-RSAT	Cell wall	3–4	Quick, high sensitivity, few (1%) false-negative results	False-positive results common; must confirm by other tests
TAT	Cell wall	3–6	Semiquantitative determination	False-positive results similar to RSAT
ME-TAT	Cell wall	5–8	Same at TAT, somewhat increased specificity	Longer to get positive titer compared with TAT
AGID cell wall (somatic) antigen	Cell wall (LPS)	5–10	Very sensitive, positive earlier than with CPAg	Procedure and interpretation complex, nonspecific reactions
CPAg-AGID	CPAg	8–12	Most specific (confirmatory) test, detects chronic cases when other tests are negative; detects infections by other *Brucella* species	Complex procedure, least sensitive for initial screening, variable duration of time with positive; may stay positive for up to 1 year after recovery from infection
Indirect FA	Cell wall (LPS)	Unknown	Available and convenient for diagnostic laboratories	May be less sensitive than ME-TAT as screening test Not extensively evaluated
ELISA	Cell wall (LPS) or CPAg	Unknown	Good results with mutant (M-) *B. canis* for cell wall extracts or *B. abortus* for CPAg	Antigen purity and preparation critical

[a]First significant titer to appear. Data based on adult dog.
ME = mercaptoethanol; RSAT = rapid slide agglutination test; TAT = tube agglutination test; AGID = agar gel immunodiffusion; CPAg = internal cytoplasmic protein antigen; LPS = lipopolysaccharide.

ME-RSAT correlate well with the ME-TAT, both of which should be considered as screening tests.

Lack of standardized reagents or methods makes absolute ME-TAT titer comparisons difficult. Nevertheless, a 50 titer may indicate either very early (< 3 weeks) or recovering infections. Titers of 50 to 100 should be considered suspect for infection; and titers of 200 or greater are highly presumptive of active infection because they often correlate with positive hemocultures. However, sera from noninfected dogs have been found to have titers from 50 to 100 and occasionally higher. As a semiquantitative test, the ME-TAT is best in control programs to quantitate serologic responses of dogs over months to determine whether infection has been eliminated with chemotherapy.

AGID Test. This has been developed as a sensitive procedure

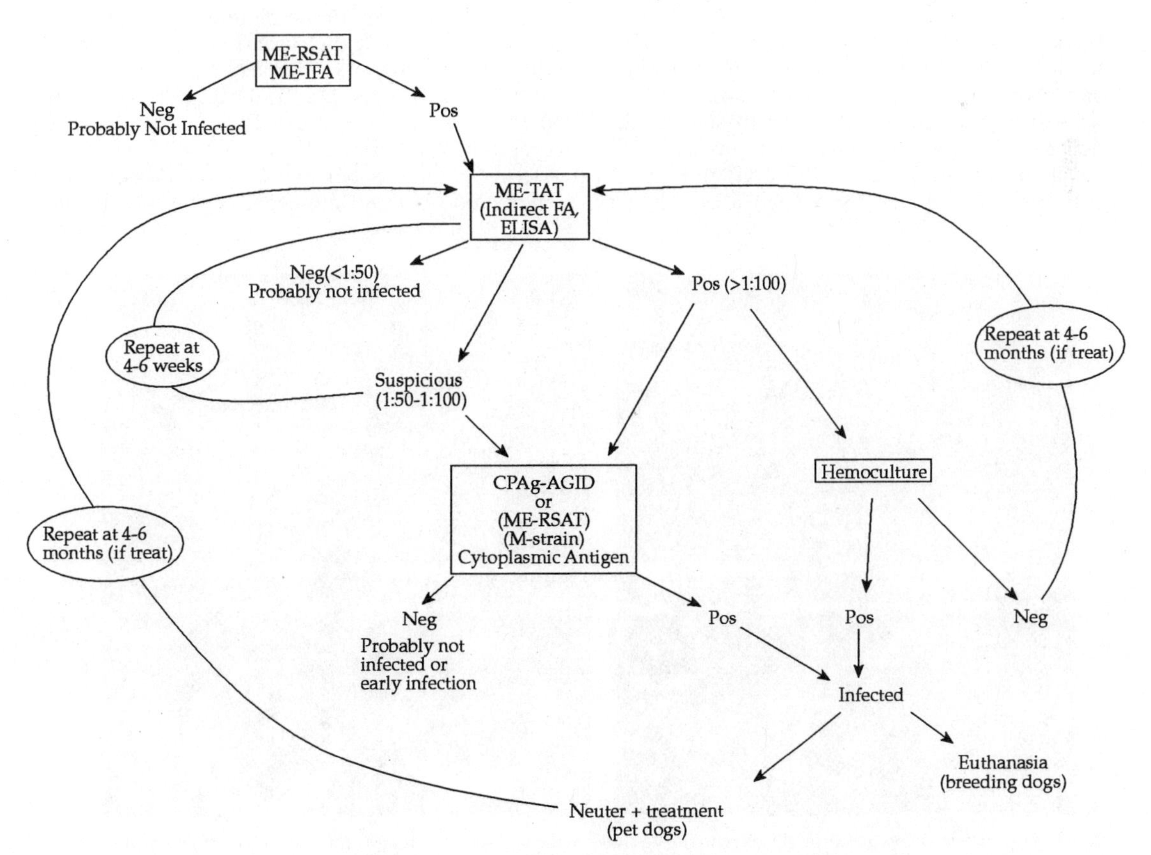

Figure 40–8. Diagnostic algorithm for canine brucellosis. The indirect FA and ELISA test are being used more as screening tests because of unavailability of ME-RSAT and ME-TAT test antigens (see text). Titer is equal to numeral of the dilution ratio following the colon.

for the serodiagnosis of canine brucellosis. AGID tests reveal precipitins in the sera of infected dogs 5 to 10 weeks PI, and antibodies persist for several weeks or months after the bacteremia has ceased. The AGID test, using cell wall (somatic) LPS antigen, suffers from the same problems of cross-reactions as agglutination tests, but positive sera may be distinguished from false-positive sera by a distinct precipitin band for *B. canis* (Fig. 40–9*A*). The somatic LPS antigen is seldom employed in the diagnostic regimen because of the lack of standardization and difficulty of interpreting test results.

The CPAg-AGID test, which is highly specific for *Brucella*, utilizes internal (cytoplasmic protein) antigens liberated by sonication of *B. canis* (Fig. 40–9*B*) or *B. abortus*.[1] This test has been able to specifically detect precipitins in the sera from dogs after other tests have become equivocal or even negative. It should be used as a confirmatory test following other serologic methods. A high proportion of sera sent to a reference laboratory for CPAg-AGID testing that are positive or suspect in the commercial ME-RSAT or the ME-TAT are found to be false-positive reactions.[5]

A disadvantage of tests with CPAg is the longer period between infection and the presence of detectable precipitins[4] (see Table 40–1). Furthermore, one or more precipitin lines may persist up to 12 months after bacteremia has ceased. In contrast to LPS antigens, both rough and smooth *Brucella* share the internal protein antigens. Thus, the possibility of infection with other *Brucella* (e.g., *B. suis* or *B. abortus*) must be considered when CPAg is used. False-positive reactions have not been observed with non-*Brucella* species. False-negative results can occur in some dogs, presumably with early infections, whose sera are RSAT positive and AGID negative. Hemoculture is the only definitive way to resolve these differences.

Indirect FA Testing. As a result of a production shortage in the RSAT test kit and the unavailability of TAT reagents, many diagnostic laboratories have switched to indirect FA or ELISA tests for serologic screening. Although these tests are being performed more widely, they have not been as consistently evaluated as have the ME-RSAT, ME-TAT, and AGID methods. The indirect FA allows for visualization of the organism in the test procedure, eliminating some of the nonspecific reactions that can develop with ELISA procedures. With any test the purity and specificity of the antigen are critical. The sensitivity of the FA method is uncertain but may be lower than that of the ME-TAT and ELISA, meaning some infected dogs may be missed during screening.

ELISA. As with other assays, the antigen source is critical in establishing test specificity. An antigen-specific, sandwich ELISA using highly purified *B. canis* cell wall antigen has been developed as a serologic test for *B. canis* infection.[23] It is very specific but may be less sensitive than the TAT in screening for infected dogs. Cytoplasmic proteins of *B. abortus* have also been utilized.[1, 1a] The sensitivity of the ELISA has been improved by a hot saline extract of the less mucoid (M–) variant strain of *B. canis*.[18] Because of their convenience, ELISA methods are being further evaluated as screening tests and for quantitating serologic responses in naturally and experimentally infected dogs.[1, 14]

Bacterial Isolation

Isolation of *B. canis* is time consuming but not difficult, because the organism grows well aerobically on conventional media used for other *Brucella*. Blood is the most practical tissue or fluid for isolating the organism. Isolation of the organism from blood is the most definitive diagnostic procedure. Hemoculture should not be the sole criterion for infection, because the bacteremia, although generally sustained, may be absent in more chronically infected animals. Blood culture can be helpful if serologic tests are ambiguous. Whole blood must be taken for culture because the organisms are associated with the leukocyte fraction. Bacteremia is detected 2 to 4 weeks after oronasal infection, and if untreated, it persists for long (> 1–2 years) periods of time. Experimentally infected dogs have remained blood culture positive for as long as 5.5 years. Bacterial numbers in the blood exceed 10^3/ml after 4 to 5 weeks PI and remain high for many (generally > 6) months.[3]

Urine culture is positive in some dogs, especially males, when blood cultures are negative; however, unless cystocen-

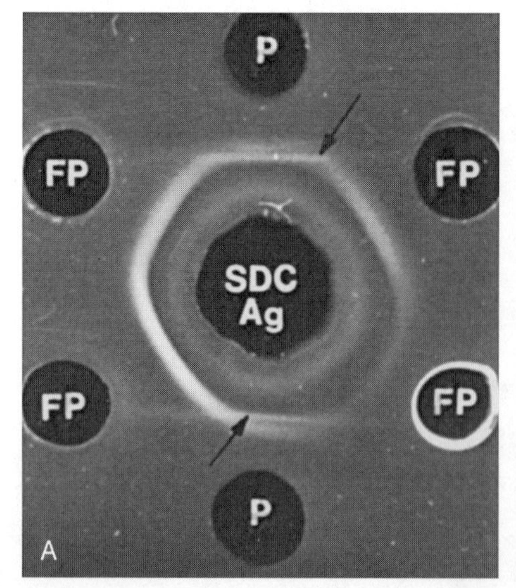

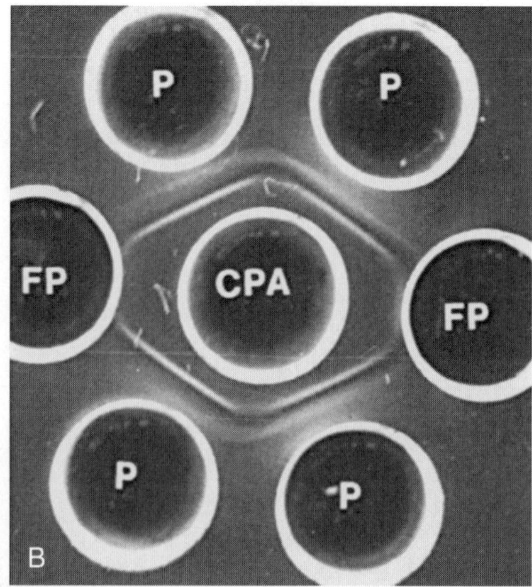

Figure 40–9. *A*, AGID patterns using sodium desoxycholate (SDC)–extracted somatic (LPS) antigens reacted with positive (P) and false-positive (FP) sera. Cross-reactions are evident. Arrows indicate *B. canis*–specific precipitin line. *B*, Cytoplasmic protein antigen (CPA). Precipitin lines occur only with sera from *Brucella*-infected dogs using the CPA.

tesis is performed, urinary isolation of *B. canis* may be difficult because of overgrowth by contaminants. Collection of semen by ejaculation is valuable for culture during the first 3 months of infection, when the concentration of organisms is greatest.

B. canis can be isolated at necropsy from several tissues of hemoculture-positive dogs. The lymph nodes, spleen, liver, bone marrow, and male reproductive organs are the most common sources, even though gross lesions are seldom present. In females, the gravid or estrual uterus, the placenta, and the vaginal or uterine fluids are most consistent tissues for isolation. Polymerase chain reaction (PCR) has also been utilized to detect *Brucella* species in tissues and fluids.[13, 21a]

Laboratory Cultivation

Contamination of specimens for culture of *B. canis* should be avoided because of overgrowth by faster-growing bacteria. Antibiotics such as bacitracin, polymyxin, and cycloheximide are usually added to the media before cultivation. Whole blood or fluid samples usually are cultured for 4 to 5 days at 37°C in Albimi, Trypticase soy, or Tryptose broth (Difco Labs, Detroit, MI), with citrate added as anticoagulant. After 4 to 7 days of growth, cultures are streaked on solid media such as Brucella broth (BBL, Cockeysville, MD), Tryptose agar, horse or cow blood agar, Trypticase soy agar (BBL, Cockeysville, MD), or Thayer-Martin media (Difco Labs, Detroit, MI). Tissue swabs or specimens may be streaked directly onto solid media and incubated aerobically at 37°C. Growth is not usually seen before 48 hours. Initially, colonies appear small and translucent but become mucoid after several days of incubation. Biochemical and immunologic methods and phage typing help identify isolates of *B. canis*.

PATHOLOGIC FINDINGS

Macroscopic changes in adults or surviving pups are usually confined to lymphadenomegaly and splenomegaly. Histologic changes are relatively uniform. Lymph node enlargement is the result of diffuse lymphoreticular hyperplasia. In dogs with chronic bacteremia, lymph node sinusoids and the spleen are filled with plasma cells and macrophages containing phagocytized bacteria. Special stains (e.g., Brown-Brenn stain) must be used to detect intracellular organisms.

Diffuse submucosal lymphocytic infiltration occurs in all genitourinary organs. A necrotizing vasculitis occurs in the target tissues of gonadal steroids, including the prostate, scrotum, sheath, or vulva. Lesions are most prominent in the prostate, epididymis, and uterus, whereas milder changes are observed in the renal pelvis, testes, ductus deferens, urinary bladder, and ureters. Extensive necrosis of the prostatic parenchyma and seminiferous tubules is caused by inflammatory cell infiltration, which eventually results in atrophy or fibrosis (Fig. 40–10). There is a chronic to subacute endometritis in the uterus, with glandular hyperplasia and reticular cell nodules. Focal hepatic necrosis, myocarditis, and meningoencephalitis also have been described. Renal abnormalities occur in some dogs and consist of hyaline thickening of the basement membrane of glomeruli with minimal cellular infiltration or proliferation. A mild interstitial nephritis has been noted. Ocular disease includes granulomatous iridocyclitis and exudative retinitis, consisting of diffuse infiltration of lymphocytes, plasmacytes, and neutrophils. Corneal endothelium has vacuolated cytoplasm with variable plasma cell infiltration; exudates with leukocytes are present in the anterior chamber (see Systemic Bacterial Infections, Chapter 93).

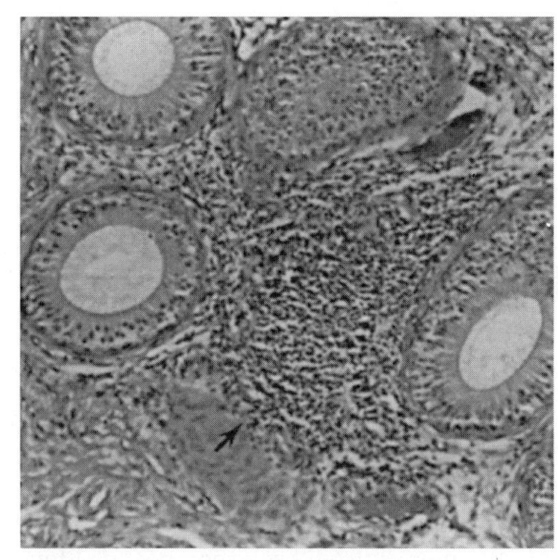

Figure 40–10. Early focal inflammatory cell cluster *(arrow)* in the head of the epididymis from a dog infected with *B. canis* (H and E; × 40).

THERAPY

Because of the intracellular location of *B. canis*, the outcome of antibiotic therapy of canine brucellosis is uncertain. The organism is susceptible to several antibiotics, but the ineffectiveness of in vivo therapy commonly leads to failures or relapses. Unfortunately, the most studied regimen (tetracycline plus dihydrostreptomycin) is unobtainable because of the restricted availability of dihydrostreptomycin. Bacteremia often recurs days to months after treatment is discontinued, making follow-up evaluation essential because animals can still harbor infection in certain tissues.

In breeding kennels, it is strongly recommended that infected animals be isolated and eliminated from breeding programs as soon as a diagnosis is confirmed.[10] Treatment should be considered only under exceptional circumstances, because therapy is expensive and often unsuccessful, especially in chronically infected animals. Aborting females may subsequently produce normal litters, but even in those cases the success of therapy is uncertain. Clinically normal, infected bitches may transmit infection to their surviving offspring. Despite treatment, intact males frequently develop irreversible sterility, making their prognoses as breeding animals poor. Limited studies suggest inability to clear infection in the prostate gland in most instances. Infected female dogs have been reinstated in breeding programs, but only after prolonged isolation and therapy and with great risk of failure. The risk of infecting males when breeding with previously infected females has been minimized by judicious artificial insemination. Breeding of such animals should be done only under exceptional circumstances when it is considered essential (e.g., the loss of a valuable blood line) and after the risk is explained to an owner.

Infected pets should, minimally, be neutered and given a regimen of antibiotic therapy to reduce the chance of infecting family members via genital secretions. The organism can persist in tissues of neutered animals, but shedding is believed less likely. Repeated courses of antibiotic therapy are recommended on the basis of follow-up serologic testing and blood cultures.

Cures of brucellosis must not be assumed, because bacteremia may recur weeks or months after antibiotics are discontinued. Attempted culture of bacteria or serologic testing immediately after treatment is halted is deceiving. Reports of successful cures should be viewed with caution unless subsequent cultures and serology have been performed for at least 6 months.

Antibiotic Therapy

Several drugs have been used to treat canine brucellosis, but the organism is rarely eliminated if the appropriate antibiotic combination and regimen are not used.[20] Single antibiotic therapy is not efficacious to eradicate *Brucella* species. By mean inhibitory concentration, in vitro susceptibility has been demonstrated for tetracycline, chloramphenicol, aminoglycosides, spectinomycin, rifampin, ampicillin, and fluoroquinolones. Synergy has been noted in vitro among tetracycline and fluoroquinolones and aminoglycosides and sulfonamides.[16] Infected dogs respond poorly or not at all to those drugs when they are given alone or for a single course of therapy. Relapse occurs within a short period of time after therapy is discontinued. Partial in vitro susceptibility occurs with erythromycin, penicillin, novobiocin, and lincomycin. Decreased susceptibility to cephalosporins, nalidixic acid, and cycloserine exists. None of the antibiotics in these last two groups should be given to treat canine brucellosis. Quinolones such as ciprofloxacin, norfloxacin, and enrofloxacin have been shown to be effective in vitro against *Brucella* species,[12] but limited in vivo studies have not. Fluoroquinolone monotherapy has been associated with treatment failures and relapses, especially in cases of uveitis or diskospondylitis.

High-dose oral minocycline or doxycycline therapy combined with IM streptomycin (Table 40–2) has given the highest rate of success in experimentally infected dogs. Lower dosages of this combination or other antibiotics alone or in combination were not as effective. Because of the unavailability of streptomycin and its derivatives, gentamicin has been substituted for streptomycin, but efficacy was less than with dihydrostreptomycin.[21] Unfortunately, the cost of minocycline treatment may be high for larger dogs, but prices of minocycline and doxycycline have decreased. Treatment regimens that are less expensive but generally less effective have been described (see Table 40–2). A longer treatment regimen of tetracycline for 28 days combined with streptomycin for 14 days has had success, especially in treating dogs infected for less than 1 to 2 months.[20]

Localized infections in hard-to-reach areas such as in the intervertebral disc or uveal tract should be treated with two or more 4-week courses of antimicrobial therapy after neutering. Recurrence of hyperesthetic episodes is common in dogs with canine brucellosis diskospondylitis. Owners of infected animals should be cautioned about the potential need for repeated treatment. Decompressive surgery should be avoided in paraparetic dogs when possible by first evaluating the clinical response to antimicrobial therapy. Sequential radiography and titers at 3- to 6-month intervals are used to monitor progress.

CONTROL IN INFECTED KENNELS

Control of canine brucellosis in a kennel with cases confirmed by serologic tests and isolation of the organism is a difficult, time-consuming, and agonizing experience for both dog owners and their veterinarians. Difficulties are compounded if antibiotic therapy is instituted when brucellosis is suspected, but not confirmed, because isolation of *B. canis* becomes uncertain and serologic tests results are questionable. A clear and reasoned discussion of control procedure in infected kennels has been published.[10] A kennel should be quarantined as soon as the diagnosis of *B. canis* is ascertained, and infected animals should be promptly eliminated. Appropriate disinfection procedures should be implemented to arrest spread of infection via fomites. All dogs and discharges or secretions in an infected kennel should be handled with gloves until serotesting can be done to determine the extent of the infection. Animals should not be admitted to or released from the kennel until the disease is eradicated. Movement of dogs within a colony also should be restricted to removal of proven and suspect cases to isolation quarters. New additions are at high risk for infection, especially if dogs are not individually penned, which also increases the number of animals requiring repeated testing during the eradication process. Animals must not be released for sale or any other purpose, because they may spread the disease. All dogs in an infected kennel should be serotested for at least 3 months after seronegative status is achieved, especially before each breeding, even by artificial insemination. If animals are retained as pets or working dogs, or if treatment is contemplated, they should be neutered and moved to separate housing. Although it is important to determine the origin of infections, this has proved difficult because of the reluctance of owners to reveal actual or suspected sources.

Carrier dogs are important in maintaining *B. canis* in the dog population because its survival outside the host is short lived, and disinfection with quaternary ammonium com-

Table 40–2. Recommended Tetracycline and Aminoglycoside Combination Therapy for Canine Brucellosis[a]

DRUG	DOSE[b] (mg/kg)	ROUTE	INTERVAL (HOURS)	DURATION (WEEKS)
Tetracyclines				
Minocycline[c,6]	25	PO	24	4
	12.5	PO	12	4
Tetracycline[20]	30	PO	12	4
Aminoglycosides				
Dihydrostreptomycin[d,6]	10	IM, SC	12	2 (treatment weeks 1 & 4)
	20	IM, SC	24	2 (treatment weeks 1 & 4)
Gentamicin	2.5	IM, SC	12	2 (treatment weeks 1 & 4)
	5.0	IM, SC	24	2 (treatment weeks 1 & 4)
Streptomycin[d,20]	20	IM, SC	24	2 (treatment weeks 1 & 4)

[a]Combination therapy is *always* indicated. One tetracycline and one aminoglycoside should be chosen and administered over a 4-week interval as indicated, with the aminoglycoside being given for 2 of the weeks. Dogs should be tested at the end of treatment and again 1 and 3 months later. If treatment unsuccessful, improved therapeutic efficacy has been reported by repeating the regimen. Fluoroquinolones, alone and in combination, have not been as efficacious as this recommended combination.
[b]Dose per administration at specified interval. For additional information, see Appendix 8.
[c]Generic doxycycline may be substituted at the same dose at a lower cost.
[d]Dihydrostreptomycin and streptomycin are not currently available to veterinarians in the United States. Gentamicin may be substituted at the dose indicated, but its efficacy is uncertain.
PO = oral; IM = intramuscular; SC = subcutaneous.

pounds or iodophors has been effective in killing the bacterium.

PREVENTION

Preventive measures are particularly important in large breeding kennels or wherever large numbers of dogs are kept, but there are no legally mandated control measures, and canine brucellosis is not a reportable disease in most states. Prevention is accomplished by quarantine of all new acquisitions until two serotest results at a 1-month interval are negative. Animals from kennels known to have had breeding problems should be rejected unless test results are negative.[10] Animals with any clinical sign of canine brucellosis should be rejected. Animals used for breeding should be tested 3 to 4 weeks before each mating to allow time for test results to be reported. Brood bitches should not be mated to stud dogs unless they have been tested and certified negative. If dogs leave a colony, they should be tested before readmission. There is no vaccine, and results of experimental studies have been unsatisfactory. The desirability of a vaccine is questionable, especially when diagnostic testing is available, because an effective vaccine would be required to provide serviceable immunity but not confound the serodiagnosis.

PUBLIC HEALTH CONSIDERATIONS

More than 35 cases of human infection caused by *B. canis* exist in the literature.[3] Natural and laboratory-acquired infections have been reported in several countries; however, the actual number of cases is unknown because human infections are often misdiagnosed. Contact with aborting bitches was the source of infection for the majority of infected pet owners, whereas male dogs and undetermined sources were present in other cases.

People are relatively resistant to infection with *B. canis*, and the disease is relatively mild compared with infections caused by other *Brucella*. A proportion of cases are asymptomatic, as determined by serotesting, but the overall rate of infection is low. Fever, chills, fatigue, malaise, lymphadenomegaly, and weight loss have been present in symptomatic patients. Rare complications include endocarditis, meningitis, arthritis, hepatitis, and visceral abscesses. Diagnosis of human infections should include bacteriologic examination by blood culture and serologic evaluation. Antibodies to *B. canis* in human sera will react in serologic tests used in dogs and, as in dogs, they do not cross-react with *B. abortus* antigen used in routine testing for human brucellosis. Titers of 200 or more, utilizing the ME-TAT, are seen in most active cases. Human infections can be readily and effectively treated with tetracycline therapy. As with infected dogs, people have suffered relapse with ampicillin.

Clients should always be informed of the potential health hazard in keeping *B. canis*–infected pets. Caution should be taken in the laboratory when handling or pipetting samples submitted for diagnostic testing. Veterinarians should practice good hygiene when examining suspected dogs, especially aborting bitches.

References

1. Baldi PC, Wanke MM, Loza ME, et al. 1994. *Brucella abortus* cytoplasmic proteins used as antigens in an ELISA potentially useful for the diagnosis of canine brucellosis. *Vet Microbiol* 41:127–134.

1a. Baldi PC, Wanke MM, Loza ME, et al. 1997. Diagnosis of canine brucellosis by the detection of serum antibodies against an 18 kDa cytoplasmic protein of *Brucella* spp. *Vet Microbiol* 51:273–281.

2. Barr SC, Eilts BE, Roy AF, et al. 1986. *Brucella suis* biotype 1 infection in a dog. *J Am Vet Med Assoc* 189:686–687.

3. Carmichael LE, Greene CE. 1990. Canine brucellosis, pp 573–584. *In* Greene CE (ed), Infectious diseases of the dog and cat. WB Saunders, Philadelphia, PA.

4. Carmichael LE, Joubert JC, Jones L. 1989. Characterization of *Brucella canis* protein antigens and polypeptide antibody responses of infected dogs. *Vet Microbiol* 19:373–387.

5. Carmichael LE, Shin SJ. 1996. Canine brucellosis: a diagnostician's dilemma. *Semin Vet Med Surg* 11:161–165.

6. Flores-Castro R, Carmichael LE. 1977. Canine brucellosis: current status of methods for diagnosis and treatment. *Gaines Vet Symp* 27:17–24.

7. Forbes LB. 1990. *Brucella abortus* infection in 14 farm dogs. *J Am Vet Med Assoc* 196:911–916.

8. Gómez JM, Villalba EJ, Pasamontes B, et al. 1992. Utilizacion de la technica ELISA para detectar anticuerpos frenti a *Brucella canis* en sueros caninos. *Med Vet* 7:531–534.

9. Jian H. 1992. Identification and characterisation of 200 strains of *Brucella canis* under test from China. *Wei Sheng Wu Hseuh Pao* 32:370–375.

10. Johnson CA, Walker RD. 1992. Clinical signs and diagnosis of *Brucella canis* infection. *Compend Cont Educ (Small Anim)* 14:763–772.

11. Katami M, Sato H, Yoshimura Y, et al. 1991. An epidemiological survey of *Brucella canis* infection of dogs in the Towada area of Aomori prefecture. *J Vet Med Sci* 53:1113–1115.

12. Kerwin SC, Lewis DD, Hribernik TN, et al. 1992. Diskospondylitis associated with *Brucella canis* infection in dogs: 14 cases (1980–1991). *J Am Vet Med Assoc* 201:1253–1257.

12a. Kulakova IK, Zheludkov MM, Dranosvskaia EA. 1997. Comparative study of the antigenic composition of *Brucella canis* strains by immunoblotting. *Mol Gen Mikrobiol Virusol* 3:15–17.

13. Leal-Klevezas DS, Martinez-Vazquez IO, Lopez-Merino A, et al. 1995. Single step PCR for detection of *Brucella* spp. from blood and milk of infected animals. *J Clin Microbiol* 33:3087–3090.

14. Martin BM, Henderson LM, Walden OM, et al. 1996. An ELISA for the detection of canine antibodies specific for *Brucella canis*, p 100. *In* Proceedings of the American Association of Laboratory Diagnosticians, Little Rock, AR.

15. Mateu de Antonio EM, Martin M. 1993. Encuesta seroepidemiologica frente a *Brucella canis* y brucellas de tipo leso en perros. *Med Vet* 10:241–246.

16. Mateu de Antonio EM, Martin M. 1995. In vitro efficacy of several antimicrobial combinations against *Brucella canis* and *Brucella melitensis* strains isolated from dogs. *Vet Microbiol* 45:1–10.

17. Mateu de Antonio EM, Martin M, Casal J. 1994. Comparison of serological tests used in canine brucellosis diagnosis. *J Vet Diagn Invest* 6:257–259.

18. Mateu de Antonio EM, Martin M, Soler M. 1993. Use of indirect enzyme-linked immunosorbent assay with hot saline solution extracts of a variant (M-) strain of *Brucella canis* for diagnosis of brucellosis in dogs. *Am J Vet Res* 54:1043-1046.

19. McLean DR, Russell N, Kahn MY. 1992. Neurobrucellosis: clinical and therapeutic features. *Clin Infect Dis* 15:582–590.

20. Nicoletti P. 1991. Further studies on the use of antibiotics in canine brucellosis. *Comp Cont Educ (Small Anim)* 13:944–946.

21. Nicoletti P, Carmichael LE. 1995. Unpublished data. Florida State University, Gainesville, FL, and Cornell University, Ithaca, NY.

21a. Queipo-Ortuno MI, Morata P, Ocon P, et al. 1997. Rapid diagnosis of human brucellosis by peripheral blood PCR assay. *J Clin Microbiol* 35:2927–2930.

22. Scanlan CM, Pidgeon GL, Richardson BE, et al. 1989. Experimental infection of dogs with *Brucella abortus*: effect of exposure dose on serologic responses and comparison of culture methods. *Cornell Vet* 79:93–107.

23. Sirikawa T, Iwaki S, Mori M, et al. 1989. Purification of a *Brucella canis* cell wall antigen using immunosorbent colums and use of the antigen in enzyme-linked immunosorbent assay for specific diagnosis of canine brucellosis. *J Clin Microbiol* 27:837–842.

24. Van Duijkeren E. 1992. Significance of the vaginal bacterial flora in the bitch—a review. *Vet Rec* 131:367–369.

Chapter 41

Anaerobic Infections

Dwight C. Hirsh and Spencer S. Jang

ETIOLOGY

Obligate anaerobic bacteria (anaerobes) cannot grow in the presence of molecular oxygen because they do not make superoxide dismutase, and most do not produce catalase. These enzymes are necessary for breakdown of reactive oxygen intermediates (e.g., superoxide anion and hydrogen peroxide) that are normally generated when bacteria grow in the presence of oxygen. Obligate anaerobes are either gram-positive or gram-negative rods or cocci (Table 41–1). Only species of the genus *Clostridium* form endospores anaerobically, distinguishing them from the genus *Bacillus*, which forms spores under aerobic conditions. The most commonly encountered anaerobes are listed in Table 41–2.

Anaerobes make up a significant portion of the normal bacterial flora of dogs and cats.[6, 30] The predominant microorganisms living on most mucosal surfaces are anaerobes, and metabolic by-products produced by this group of microorganisms are important in the regulation of the numbers of aerobic species (facultative and obligate) that also compose the normal flora. Thus, anaerobic bacteria play an important role in protection of mucosal surfaces from interactions involving other microorganisms with pathogenic potential. For example, approximately 10^6 salmonellae are needed to produce disease in animals with intact anaerobic flora, whereas fewer than 10 salmonellae are needed to produce disease in animals with depressed numbers of anaerobes. The importance of this observation is seen clinically, wherein dogs are more prone to develop salmonellosis when they are medicated with antibiotics, especially those effective in reducing the anaerobic component of the normal flora (e.g., ampicillin).[48]

Aside from being responsible for a significant portion of innate immunity (the normal flora), anaerobes may be important participants in clinical disease.[18, 21, 23a, 28, 29] Compromise of a mucosal surface by perforation or compromise of a surface or locale contiguous to a mucosal surface may lead to inoculation of members of the normal flora into a normally sterile site. At this point, introduced anaerobes become clinically relevant along with other members of the normal flora. These are important facts to be aware of because antibiotic therapy is almost always started before results of microbiologic analysis of exudative material are received. Therefore, an educated guess has to be made as to the microorganisms present. If anaerobic bacteria are present in an infectious process, there are, on average, two different species, almost always admixed with aerobic bacteria. The most commonly associated aerobic bacteria are enterics (mainly *Escherichia coli*), members of the genus *Pasteurella*, and coagulase-positive staphylococci (Table 41–3). See also Bite Infections, Chapter 53.

Anaerobic bacteria, if they contain the appropriate virulence factors, may also produce disease at a mucosal surface. Aside from periodontal disease (see Chapter 89), anaerobes are associated with disease of the GI tract. The most important anaerobes playing a role in this regard are *Clostridium difficile* and *C. perfringens*.[42, 46] Both of these species may be a part of the normal flora of dogs and cats, although there is evidence that both may be passed to previously uncolonized animals.[27, 35, 37]

EPIDEMIOLOGY

Infectious processes involving a normally sterile site are usually a consequence of "contamination" by a members of the normal flora. The composition of the normal flora of the contiguous surface usually mirrors what is found in the infectious process. In human patients, infectious processes involving structures above the diaphragm are more likely to contain anaerobes originating in the mouth compared with below the diaphragm where different anaerobes most often come from the intestinal tract.[43] In animal patients, there does not appear to be a differing predilection in the species of anaerobes for a particular site or location.[24]

Although disease produced by *C. difficile* is the result of proliferation of this microorganism in the enteric tract of the host after a "trigger event" (e.g., certain antibiotics and chemotherapeutic agents), epidemiologic evidence from human hospitals suggests that the agent can be spread from patient to patient, resulting in outbreaks of *C. difficile*–associated disease (see Chapter 39).[41] Such observations imply contagiousness or at least the potential to be so. However, whether *C. difficile* is truly a "contagious" pathogen is confounded by the fact that it is also observed in the enteric tract of clinically healthy animals.[37, 42]

It is unclear whether toxigenic *C. perfringens* has contagious potential. Proliferation of this agent in the intestinal tract with production of enterotoxin is probably how the disease progresses. What stimulates the proliferation is unknown. The question is whether the source of the agent is endogenous, acquired from another infected animal, or acquired from the environment. The report of outbreaks of *C. perfringens*–associated diarrhea in small animal hospital settings suggests a contagious potential, although it is important to keep in mind that low numbers of *C. perfringens* are present in the enteric tract of clinically healthy dogs.[27, 46] Detectable levels of *C. perfringens* enterotoxin are not often found in the feces of asymptomatic animals.[46]

PATHOGENESIS

Anaerobic bacteria are not able to live in healthy tissue. On mucosal surfaces (e.g., intestinal tract, gingival crevice, and genital tract), they live with other microorganisms that "scavenge" molecular oxygen, resulting in a local environ-

Table 41–1. Characteristics of Obligate Anaerobic Bacteria Isolated From Dogs and Cats

MICROORGANISM	GRAM REACTION	SHAPE
Bacteroides	Negative (pale)	Rod
Prevotella	Negative (pale)	Rod (coccobacillus)
Porphyromonas	Negative (pale)	Rod (coccobacillus)
Fusobacterium	Negative (pale)	Rod (usually thin)
Peptostreptococcus	Positive	Coccus
Clostridium	Positive	Rod (spores)

Table 41–2. Species of Obligate Anaerobic Bacteria Isolated From Dogs and Cats[a]

ORGANISM	NO.	PERCENT OF ISOLATES (n = 316)
Bacteroides spp.	74	23
B. fragilis group[b]	38	12
Other *Bacteroides*	36	11
Peptostreptococcus spp.[c]	57	18
Fusobacterium spp.[d]	43	14
Porphyromonas spp.[e]	34	11
Clostridium spp.[f]	28	9
Prevotella[g]	16	5
Miscellaneous	39	12

[a]Data compiled from cases from Veterinary Medical Teaching Hospital, University of California, Davis, 1991–1995.
[b]*B. fragilis* was most commonly isolated.
[c]*P. anaerobius* was most commonly isolated.
[d]*F. nucleatum* was most commonly isolated.
[e]*P. asaccharolyticus* was most commonly isolated.
[f]*C. perfringens* was most commonly isolated.
[g]*P. heparinolyticus* was most commonly isolated.

ment with very low eH (a measure of oxygen tension). Likewise, in compromised tissue, inflammatory cells as well as coinoculated aerobic microorganisms lower the eH sufficiently for anaerobes to grow.

Components of anaerobic bacteria have been shown to elicit potent inflammatory responses. Gram-negative anaerobes possess lipopolysaccharides with endotoxic activity, the same as their aerobic counterparts. The peptidoglycan of gram-positive anaerobes incites the same inflammatory response as do gram-positive aerobic microorganisms. Some anaerobic bacteria produce capsules (e.g., *Bacteroides fragilis*, pigmented *Prevotella*, and *Porphyromonas*), which incite inflammatory responses that result in abscess formation (i.e., capsule without viable bacteria will induce abscess formation).[47] There is some evidence that coinoculated aerobic microorganisms induce anaerobe capsule formation. Capsules also play the more traditional role by discouraging association with phagocytic cells.[4, 20]

Synergy occurs between aerobic and anaerobic microorganisms.[4] Aside from helping to trigger capsule formation, aerobic organisms not only scavenge oxygen but also possess the capacity to curtail phagocytosis of the anaerobic component of the sample and vice versa.[49] Enzymes such as β-lactamase produced by one member of the "partnership" will protect susceptible microorganisms in the vicinity from being killed by β-lactam antibiotics. These synergistic interactions are important to keep in mind when designing therapeutic regimens, because antibiotic therapy should be directed at both populations for optimal resolution of the infectious process.

Some anaerobic bacteria produce toxins. *Fusobacterium necrophorum* produces a toxin that forms pores in leukocyte membranes.[20] *C. difficile* produces toxins (A and B) that disrupt the cytoskeletal elements of the intestinal epithelial cell, resulting in cell death.[1, 40] *C. perfringens* produces an enterotoxin that interacts with the target cell membrane, resulting in the formation of "pores" made in part by the enterotoxin and by the target cell.[40] Electrolytes are lost through these "pores," resulting in reversal of ion and water flow (diarrhea) and, finally, death of the cell.

Some species of anaerobes produce adhesin molecules (pili or fimbriae).[20] These proteins are usually associated with more virulent anaerobes. However, adhesins probably do not play a role other than association with specific sites or locations on mucosal surfaces. Adhesin molecules probably are not expressed and do not have an important role when exposed to phagocytic cells to which they might adhere—an event that leads to phagocytosis and the demise of the anaerobe. In keeping with this model, it has been shown that blood or abscess isolates of *B. fragilis* are rarely piliated, whereas those found on the mucosal surface are almost always so.[4]

Table 41–3. Most Commonly Isolated Aerobic Microorganisms From Dogs and Cats Associated With Anaerobic Infections[a]

MICROORGANISM	% ISOLATES FROM	
	Dogs (505 Isolates)	Cats (85 Isolates)
Enterics[b]	29	18
Pasteurella spp.[c]	12	28
Coagulase-positive *Staphylococcus*	11	7

[a]Data compiled from cases from Veterinary Medical Teaching Hospital, University of California, Davis, 1991–1995.
[b]Most common isolate was *E. coli*, accounting for 70% of the enteric isolates from dogs and 53% of the enteric isolates from cats.
[c]Most common isolate was *P. canis*, accounting for 48% of the isolates from dogs, and *P. multocida*, accounting for 75% of the isolates from cats.

Table 41–4. Relative Frequency of Obligate Anaerobic Bacteria With Respect to Disease Process or Anatomic Site in Dogs and Cats[a]

DISEASE PROCESS OR SITE	SPECIES (D/C)	RANKING	% CULTURE POSITIVE	% WITH ANAEROBES
Draining tract	D	1	79	39
Pleural fluid	D	2	43	31
	C	1	44	40
Abscess	D	3	81	30
	C	2	82	40
Bone	D	6	22	6
	C	3	46	36
Abdominal fluid	D	4	52	19
	C	4	50	27
Respiratory tract	D	5	50	9
	C	5	70	17

[a]Data compiled from cases from Veterinary Medical Teaching Hospital, University of California, Davis, 1991–1995.
D = dog; C = cat.

CLINICAL FINDINGS

Conditions involving anaerobic bacteria infecting a normally sterile site vary according to location, but all involve the formation of a pyonecrotic process. This process stems primarily from the inflammatory response triggered by anaerobe capsule material, cell wall constituents of both the anaerobic and aerobic microorganisms that may be present, and thwarted attempts of phagocytosis, leading to deposition of lysosomal contents into surrounding tissue. The most commonly encountered sites of anaerobic isolation are listed in Table 41–4. The clinical findings of such infections are listed in Tables 41–5 and 41–6. Another clue is that exudate from infectious processes that contain anaerobes are often malodorous.

Table 41–5. Clinical Findings Suggestive of Anaerobic Infection

Fever, pain, and swelling
Bite or puncture wound
Foul-smelling wounds or discharges
Gas present in tissues or body cavities
Abscess formation
Contiguous to mucosal surface with anaerobic microflora
Necrotic or devitalized tissue
Gangrenous tissue
Dark, discolored exudates
Presence of sulfur granules in exudate
Mixed population of organisms or filamentous forms with microscopy
Failure to culture organisms with routine methods

Table 41–6. Comparative Clinical Features of Anaerobic Infections

SITE	PARTICULAR CLINICAL FEATURES	SOURCES
Head & neck	Cranial or cervical abscesses, exophthalmos, pain on opening mouth, subauricular swelling, anorexia, difficulty swallowing, gingivitis and stomatitis, para-aural abscesses, tonsillar abscesses, brain abscess, panophthalmitis	Traumatic ear canal separations,[32] pharyngeal foreign body penetration (stick injuries),[36] dental infections, chronic sinusitis,[50] tonsillar abscess, chronic otitis media, bite wounds
Intrathoracic		
Pulmonary	Coughing, fever, dyspnea, lobar or multifocal consolidation (abscesses), hypertrophic osteopathy	Pneumonia, endocarditis,[11] aspiration pneumonia[16]
Intrapleural or mediastinal	Fever, dyspnea, muffled heart sounds, leukocytosis, pyothorax	Penetrating chest injuries, inhaled foreign bodies, esophageal foreign body perforation[39]
Intra-abdominal		
Peritoneal	Fever, abdominal distention, anorexia, intra-abdominal abscess, adhesions	Postoperative foreign suture materials (silk, multifilament nylon, braided), ovariohysterectomy, bowel leakage, genital tract infections, actinomycosis
Hepatic	Anorexia, lethargy, vomiting, diarrhea, fever, dehydration, hepatomegaly, mucosal bleeding	Bacteremia, hepatic neoplasia, ascending biliary infection, immunosuppression in diabetes mellitus[9]
Enteric	Chronic diarrhea, blood, mucus	Intestinal stasis, blind loop syndrome, colitis, colonic ulceration
Retroperitoneal	Swelling in lumbar flank, sinus tracts or drainage, pain, fever, anorexia, reluctance to walk	Osteomyelitis of lumbar vertebrae from plant awns, ovarian or uterine ligatures,[26] actinomycosis, ruptured urethra and perirenal abscess
Paraspinal	Pain, reluctance to walk, fever, paresis or paralysis	Usually epidural from local penetration or extension of paraspinal infection, bite wounds, meningitis less likely anaerobic and often from hematogenous sources
Subcutaneous	Fever, swelling, discharge, leukocytosis	Bite wounds, penetrating injuries (see Chapter 53)

DIAGNOSIS

The standard for determining the presence of anaerobic bacteria in an infectious process is the isolation from clinical samples. This is difficult to achieve in clinical practice unless precautions are taken. If attempts are to be made in isolating anaerobic bacteria, care should be taken in how samples are handled before receipt by laboratory personnel (Table 41–7). As mentioned, anaerobes are sensitive to oxygen and, because of their slow growth, are also easily overgrown in samples containing aerobic microorganisms (> 70% will be mixed). Transport media, transport time, and temperature, therefore, become important issues (see also Chapter 33). Refrigeration has been shown to be detrimental to recovery of anaerobic bacteria; thus, samples should not be placed at temperatures lower than 4°C. In comparison, aerobic microorganisms in samples held at 25°C increase in numbers and will, in some cases, overgrow the anaerobic component. However, at 15°C aerobes do not increase to any extent, nor do the anaerobes die. Because of their tendency to dry out and become oxygenated, the use of swabs should be discouraged. The amount of time between sample collection and culture depends on the type of sample, whether transport medium is used, and the volume of the sample. Anaerobic microorganisms in large pieces of tissue or quantities of fluid (>2 ml) are relatively protected from toxic interaction with oxygen, and these microorganisms will survive for up to 24 hours before culture, whereas anaerobes in smaller samples will probably not. Anaerobic transport media greatly increase the survival of anaerobes and discourage the growth of aerobes. Anaerobic media are available for transport of aspirated material, tissue or biopsy material, and material collected on swabs.[31]

Isolation of anaerobes is time consuming and expensive. For example, the isolation and demonstration of an anaerobe in a sample containing only one species of anaerobe will take

Table 41–7. Specimen Collection for Anaerobic Isolation

Percutaneous needle aspiration into deeper tissues
Surgical curettage or scraping of mucosal surface
Tissue biopsy (soft or bony)
Body fluid aspiration (synovia, peritoneal, plural, bile, urine)

Inject fluids via syringe directly into anaerobic transport media.
Infected tissue pieces preferably stored in sterile capped containers in anaerobic bags.
Keep at room temperature, not refrigerated.

Do not submit:
- Specimens of tissue with abundant microflora
- Pus
- Contents in plastic syringes
- Swabs

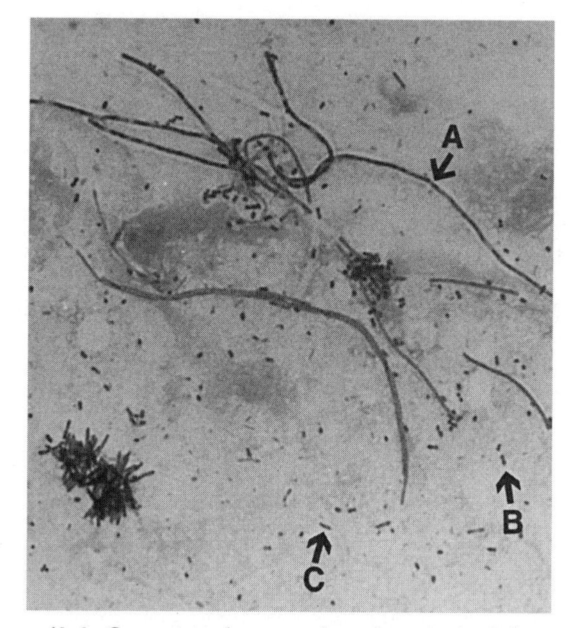

Figure 41–1. Gram-stained smear of exudate obtained from a cat with pyothorax. The filamentous microorganism (A) is probably *Filifactor (Clostridium) villosus*,[5, 29, 44] the cocci are probably *Peptostreptococcus* (B), and the rods are either an enteric microorganism (e.g., *E. coli*), a nonenteric microorganism (e.g., *Pasteurella*), or an anaerobe (*Bacteroides, Prevotella, Porphyromonas, Fusobacterium*) or a combination. Filamentous microorganisms (C) in the chest of a dog would most likely be microaerophilic members of the genus *Actinomyces*.

Table 41–8. Percent Susceptibility of Selected Infectious Bacterial Agents Obtained From Dogs[a]

DRUG	*Bordetella bronchiseptica*	*Escherichia coli*	*Klebsiella pneumoniae*	*Pasteurella* spp.	*Pseudomonas aeruginosa*	Coagulase-positive *Staphylococcus*
Amikacin	90	99	95	100	97	100
Ampicillin	45	57	7	100	1	54
Amoxicillin-clavulanate	95	67	52	100	1	99
Ceftizoxime	5	99	100	100	2	100
Ceftiofur	5	91	80	100	1	96
Cephalothin	35	32	48	100	2	99
Chloramphenicol	90	67	54	100	0	92
Enrofloxacin	–	95	90	100	2	94
Erythromycin	0	0	0	38	0	85
Gentamicin	90	92	71	100	70	99
Tetracycline	95	64	59	100	0	71
Ticarcillin/clavulanate	–	65	42	100	92	–
Trimethoprim/sulfamethoxazole	75	74	72	97	6	94

[a]Data excluding that from *Enterococcus* spp., *Enterobacter* spp., and *Proteus mirabilis.*
Data from Hirsh DC, Jang SS. Antimicrobial susceptibility of selected infectious bacterial agents obtained from dogs. 1994. *J Am Animal Hosp Assoc* 30:487–494.

at least 4 days. The cost is approximately $10 (U.S. currency) in media alone. Because most infectious processes contain on average two different species of anaerobes and at least one aerobe, the amount of effort is significantly increased, as is the cost.

Diagnosis, therefore, can be made by other methods. Depending on the site, condition, characteristics of the exudate (e.g., odor), and contents observed in stained smears, a presumptive diagnosis of anaerobic bacterial involvement can be made (see Tables 41–5 and 41–6 and Fig. 41–1). When viewed microscopically, some gram-negative anaerobic rods are pale staining and have shapes that suggest that an anaerobe is present—often being thin, sometimes misshapen, and occasionally displaying pointed ends.

Disease produced by anaerobes while on a mucosal surface make the diagnosis somewhat more difficult to make. For *C. difficile*, this process entails using cycloserine-cefoxitin-fructose agar for isolation, immunologic tests to determine the presence of microorganism or toxin in feces or in broth culture, or polymerase chain reaction for toxin genes in feces or in isolates.[34] A major clue that *C. perfringens* may be involved with observed clinical disease of the intestinal tract is the presence of increased numbers of spore-forming rods in fecal smears (spore formation and enterotoxin production are coregulated genes) or demonstration of the presence of toxin in fecal extracts.[34, 38, 46] Demonstration of five or more spore-forming rods per oil immersion field in fecal smears stained with a Romanovsky-type stain (Wright's or Giemsa) or with Gram's stain is presumptive evidence of *C. perfringens*–associated diarrhea.[46]

THERAPY

Successful treatment of infectious processes containing an anaerobic microorganism involves both medical and surgical intervention (e.g., correction of fluid and electrolyte imbalances, drainage) combined with appropriate antimicrobial therapy. Antimicrobial therapy in the absence of surgical drainage is usually unsuccessful. Antimicrobial therapy of infectious processes containing an anaerobic component should be aimed at both the anaerobic and the presumed aerobic component. The susceptibility of these microorganisms to aerobic antimicrobial agents is shown in Table 41–8.

It is difficult and expensive to determine susceptibility of anaerobes to antimicrobial agents. For this reason, few laboratories perform such assays, with the possible exception of the disk test used for therapeutic predictions to determine whether an isolate produces a β-lactamase (Nitrocefin Disc, Difco Laboratories, Detroit, MI). In this test, a portion of an isolated colony is smeared onto a disk containing a substrate that will change color if a β-lactamase is present. The most common anaerobe β-lactamases are cephalosporinases, active on first-generation cephalosporins such as cephalexin and cefazolin, as well as penicillin G, ampicillin, and amoxicillin. Clavulanate will irreversibly bind to these enzymes.

Antimicrobial treatment aimed at the anaerobic component is most often empiric and is based on retrospectively acquired data. Certain antibiotics exist to which anaerobic bacteria are inherently resistant (e.g., the aminoglycosides and the quinolones), although there are third-generation quinolones—levofloxacin, grepafloxacin, trovafloxacin, cinafloxa-

Table 41–9. Susceptibility of Selected Isolates of Obligate Anaerobes Obtained From Dogs and Cats to Antimicrobial Agents[a]

		% SUSCEPTIBLE				
MICROORGANISM	NO.	Mz	Cm	A/C	Ap	Cl
Bacteroides	41	100	100	100	68	81
B. fragilis—group	26	100	100	100	65	77
Other *Bacteroides*	15	100	100	100	73	87
Peptostreptococcus	9	100	100	100	100	100
Fusobacterium	25	100	100	100	100	100
Porphyromonas	4	100	100	100	100	100
Clostridium	5	100	100	100	100	80
Prevotella	13	100	100	100	100	100

[a]Data compiled from cases from Veterinary Medical Teaching Hospital, University of California, Davis, 1994–1995. Determined by use of the E-test (Epsilometer, AB Biodisk, Solna, Sweden). Results interpreted using the interpretive categories and correlative minimum inhibitory concentrations as described by the National Committee for Clinical Laboratory Standards.
NO. = number of isolates; Mz = metronidazole; Cm = chloramphenicol; A/C = amoxicillin-clavulanate; Ap = ampicillin; Cl = clindamycin.

Table 41–10. Dosages of Drugs for Anaerobic Infections [a]

DRUG	SPECIES	DOSE[b]	ROUTE	INTERVAL (HOURS)
Penicillin G	B	20,000 U/kg	IM, IV	6–8
Amoxicillin-clavulanate[c]	B	20 mg/kg	PO, IV	8–12
Cephalexin	B	10–20 mg/kg	PO	8
Cefoxitin	B	10–20 mg/kg	IV, IM	8
Clindamycin	B	5–10 mg/kg	PO, IV	12
Chloramphenicol	D	15–25 mg/kg	PO, SC, IV	8
Metronidazole	B	10 mg/kg	PO, IV	8

[a]For specific information on each drug, see Drug Formulary, Appendix 8.
[b]Dose per administration at specified interval.
[c]Recommended to use amoxicillin with clavulanate for anaerobic infections.
B = dog and cat; D = dog.

cin, sparfloxacin, and DU-6859a—with activity toward anaerobic bacteria.[3, 13, 14] The most active antimicrobials for anaerobic bacteria are metronidazole, amoxicillin-clavulanate, chloramphenicol, and clindamycin (Tables 41–9 and 41–10). Ticarcillin-clavulanate, although not tested for veterinary isolates, has been shown to be very active for human anaerobic isolates.[2] Although anaerobes may test susceptible to trimethoprim-sulfonamides in vitro, inhibitors (mainly thymidine) are found in vivo that make this drug combination unpredictable as a treatment modality for anaerobic microorganism infections.[23] The tetracyclines are unpredictable as well.[18] Isolates of *C. difficile* are susceptible to metronidazole and vancomycin in vitro, and disease produced by this microorganism responds to either drug.[51] Isolates of *C. perfringens* are susceptible to and respond to treatment with the macrolides (tylosin, erythromycin), metronidazole, and ampicillin.[46]

PUBLIC HEALTH CONSIDERATIONS

It is estimated that several million humans are bitten by dogs and cats every year.[12] Although most of the wounds resulting from animals bites will contain aerobic microorganisms, approximately one third will contain anaerobes. All are thought to be members of the normal flora of the mouth of dogs and cats. The most common anaerobes belong to the same genera as the anaerobes found in disease processes in dogs and cats.[12] Some members of the oral flora of dogs and cats produce serious disease in immunocompromised individuals and those that are asplenic or that have liver disease (see Chapter 53).

C. difficile is an important cause of disease in human beings. Data indicate that strains of *C. difficile* found in animals are not the ones found in human patients.[17, 35] There are no data concerning the communicability of *C. perfringens* from dogs and cats to humans. However, because it appears that this microorganism can be acquired from contaminated environments, it seems likely, but as yet unproven, that *C. perfringens* of any source can infect dogs, cats, or humans. Whether disease results would depend on a "trigger" event, which remains undetermined.

References

1. Aktories K, Just I. 1995. Monoglucosylation of low-molecular-mass GTP-binding rho proteins by clostridial cytotoxins. *Trends Cell Biol* 5:441–443.
2. Appelbaum PC, Spangler SK, Jacobs MR. 1990. Beta-lactamase production and susceptibilities to amoxicillin, amoxicillin-clavulanate, ticarcillin, ticarcillin-clavulanate, cefoxitin, imipenem, and metronidazole of 320 non-*Bacteroides fragilis Bacteroides* isolates and 129 fusobacteria from 28 U.S. centers. *Antimicrob Agents Chemother* 34:1546–1550.
3. Borobio MV, Conejo MDC, Ramirez E, et al. 1994. Comparative activities of eight quinolones against members of the *Bacteroides fragilis* group. *Antimicrob Agents Chemother* 38:1442–1445.
4. Brook I. 1995. Pathogenesis and management of polymicrobial infections due to aerobic and anaerobic bacteria. *Med Res Rev* 15:73–82.
5. Collins MD, Lawson PA, Willems A, et al. 1994. The phylogeny of the genus *Clostridium*: proposal of five new genera and eleven new species combinations. *Int J Syst Bacteriol* 44:812–826.
6. Delles EK, Willard MD, Simpson RB, et al. 1994. Comparison of species and numbers of bacteria in concurrently cultured samples of proximal small intestinal fluid and endoscopically obtained duodenal mucosa in dogs with intestinal bacterial overgrowth. *Am J Vet Res* 55:957–964.
7. Dow SW. 1990. Anaerobic Infections, pp 530–537. *In* Greene CE (ed), Infectious diseases of the dog and cat. WB Saunders, Philadelphia, PA.
8. Dunn DL, Barke EAA, Ewald DC, et al. 1985. Effects of *Escherichia coli* and *Bacteroides fragilis* on peritoneal host defenses. *Infect Immun* 48:287–291.
9. Farrar ET, Washabau RJ, Saunders HM. 1996. Hepatic abscesses in dogs: 14 cases (1982–1994). *J Am Vet Med Assoc* 208:243–247.
10. Finegold SM, Wexler HM. 1996. Present status of therapy for anaerobic infections. *Clin Infect Dis* 23(Suppl):S9–S14.
11. Forrester SD, Fossum TW, Miller MW. 1992. Pneumothorax in a dog with a pulmonary abscess and suspected infective endocarditis. *J Am Vet Med Assoc* 200:351–354.
12. Goldstein EJC. 1992. Bite wounds and infection. *Clin Infect Dis* 14:633–640.
13. Goldstein EJC. 1993. Patterns of susceptibility to fluoroquinolones among anaerobic bacterial isolates in the United States. *Clin Infect Dis* 16:S377–S381.
14. Goldstein EJC. 1996. Possible role for new fluoroquinolones (levofloxacin, grepafloxacin, trovafloxacin, clinafloxacin, sparfloxacin, and DU-6859a) in the treatment of anaerobic infections: review of current information on efficacy and safety. *Clin Infect Dis* 23(Suppl):S25–S30.
15. Goldstein EJC, Citron DM. 1993. Comparative susceptibilities of 173 aerobic and anaerobic bite wound isolates to sparfloxacin, temafloxacin, clarithromycin, and older agents. *Antimicrob Agents Chemother* 37:1150–1153.
16. Hesselink JW, van den Twell JG. 1990. Hypetrophic osteopathy in a dog with chronic lung abscess. *J Am Vet Med Assoc* 196:760–762.
17. Hirsh DC. 1996. Unpublished observations, University of California—Davis, Davis, CA.
18. Hirsh DC, Indiveri MC, Jang SS, et al. 1985. Changes in prevalence and susceptibility of obligate anaerobes in clinical veterinary practice. *J Am Vet Med Assoc* 186:1086–1089.
19. Hirsh DC, Jang SS. 1994. Antimicrobial susceptibility of selected infectious bacterial agents from dogs. *J Am Anim Hosp Assoc* 30:487–494.
20. Hofstad T. 1989. Virulence determinants in nonsporeforming anaerobic bacteria. *Scand J Infect Dis Suppl* 62:15–24.
21. Hoshuyama S, Kanoe M, Amimoto A. 1996. Isolation of obligate and facultative anaerobic bacteria from feline subcutaneous abscesses. *J Vet Med Sci* 58:273–274.
22. Hsu H, Finberg RW. 1989. Infections associated with animal exposure in two infants. *Rev Infect Dis* 11:108–115.
23. Indiveri MC, Hirsh DC. 1992. Tissues and exudates contain sufficient thymidine for growth of anaerobic bacteria in the presence of inhibitory levels of trimethoprim-sulfamethoxazole. *Vet Microbiol* 32:235–242.
23a. Jang SS, Breher JE, Dabaco LA, et al. 1997. Organisms isolated from dogs and cats with anaerobic infections and susceptibility to selected antimicrobial agents. *J Am Vet Med Assoc* 210:1610–1614.
24. Jang SS, Hirsh DC. 1991. Identity of *Bacteroides* isolates and previously named *Bacteroides* spp in clinical specimens of animal origin. *Am J Vet Res* 52:738–741.
25. Jang SS, Hirsh DC. 1994. Characterization, distribution, and microbiological associations of *Fusobacterium* spp. in clinical specimens of animal origin. *J Clin Microbiol* 32:384–387.
26. Johnston DE, Christie BA. 1990. The retroperitoneum in dogs: retroperitoneal infections. *Compend Cont Educ Pract Vet* 12:1035–1045.
27. Kruth SA, Prescott JF, Welch MK, et al. 1989. Nosocomial diarrhea associated with enterotoxigenic *Clostridium perfringens* infection in dogs. *J Am Vet Med Assoc* 195:331–333.

28. Love DN, Johnson JL, Moore LVH. 1989. *Bacteroides* species from the oral cavity and oral-associated diseases of cats. *Vet Microbiol* 19:275–281.
29. Love DN, Jones RF, Bailey M, et al. 1982. Isolation and characterisation of bacteria from pyothorax (empyaemia) in cats. *Vet Microbiol* 7:455–461.
30. Love DN, Vekselstein R, Collings S. 1990. The obligate and facultatively anaerobic bacterial flora of the normal feline gingival margin. *Vet Microbiol* 22:267–275.
31. Mangels J. 1994. Anaerobic transport systems: are they necessary? *Clin Microbiol Newslett* 16:101–104.
32. McCarthy PE, Hosgood G, Pechman RD. 1995. Traumatic ear canal separations and para-anal abscessations in three dogs. *J Am Anim Hosp Assoc* 31:419–424.
33. Methods for antimicrobial susceptibility testing of anaerobic bacteria, 3rd ed. Approved standard M11-A3, supplement M100-S5. 1994. National Committee for Clinical Laboratory Standards, Villanova, PA.
34. Onderdonk AB, Allen SD. 1995. *Clostridium*, pp 574–586. *In* Murray PR, Baron EJ, Pfaller MA, et al (eds), Manual of clinical microbiology, ed 6. American Society for Microbiology Press, Washington, DC.
35. O'Neill G, Adams JE, Bowman RA, et al. 1993. A molecular characterization of *Clostridium difficile* isolates from humans, animals and their environments. *Epidemiol Infect* 111:257–264.
36. Peeters ME. 1992. The treatment of recurrent abscessation in the neck region of the dog, evaluation of 35 patients. *Tijdschr Diergeneeskd* 117(Suppl 1):305.
37. Riley TV, Adams JE, O'Neill GL, et al. 1991. Gastrointestinal carriage of *Clostridium difficile* in cats and dogs attending veterinary clinics. *Epidemiol Infect* 107:659–665.
38. Rood JI, Cole ST. 1991. Molecular genetics and pathogenesis of *Clostridium perfringens*. *Microb Rev* 55:621–648.
39. Salisbury SK, Forbes S, Blevins WE. 1990. Peritracheal abscess associated with tracheal collapse and bilateral laryngeal paralysis in a dog. *J Am Vet Med Assoc* 196:1273–1275.
40. Sears CL, Kaper JB. 1996. Enteric bacterial toxins: Mechanisms of action and linkage to intestinal secretion. *Microbiol Rev* 60:167–215.
41. Silva J, Tang YJ, Gumerlock PH. 1994. Genotyping of *Clostridium difficile* isolates. *J Infect Dis* 169:661–664.
42. Struble AL, Tang YJ, Kass PH, et al. 1994. Fecal shedding of *Clostridium difficile* in dogs: a period prevalence survey in a veterinary medical teaching hospital. *J Vet Diagn Invest* 6:342–347.
43. Styrt B, Gorbach SL. 1989. Recent developments in the understanding of the pathogenesis and treatment of anaerobic infections (second of two parts). *N Engl J Med* 321:298–302.
44. Summanen P. 1995. Microbiology terminology update: clinically significant anaerobic gram-positive and gram-negative bacteria (excluding spirochetes). *Clin Infect Dis* 21:273–276.
45. Talan DA, Staatz D, Staatz A, et al. 1989. Staphylococcus intermedius in canine gingiva and canine inflicted human wound infections: laboratory characterization of a newly recognized zoonotic pathogen. *J Clin Microbiol* 27:78–81.
46. Twedt DC. 1992. *Clostridium perfringens*–associated enterotoxicosis in dogs, pp 602–604. *In* Kirk RW, Bonagura JD (eds), Current veterinary therapy XI. WB Saunders, Philadelphia, PA.
47. Tzianabos AO, Onderdonk AB, Rosner R, et al. 1993. Structural features of polysaccharides that induce intra-abdominal abscesses. *Science* 262:416–419.
48. Uhaa IJ, Hird DW, Hirsh DC, et al. 1988. Case-control study of risk factors associated with nosocomial *Salmonella krefeld* infection in dogs. *Am J Vet Res* 49:1501–1505.
49. Vel WAC, Namavar F, Verweij-VanVught A, et al. 1985. Killing of *Escherichia coli* by human polymorphonuclear leucocytes in the presence of *Bacteroides fragilis*. *J Clin Pathol* 38:86–91.
50. Visser CJ. 1990. Chronic maxillary sinus abscessation in the canine. *J Vet Dent* 7:10–12.
51. Wenisch C, Parschalk B, Hasenhundl M, et al. 1996. Comparison of vancomycin, teicoplanin, metronidazole, and fusidic acid for the treatment of *Clostridium difficile*–associated diarrhea. *Clin Infect Dis* 22:813–818.

Chapter 42

Botulism

Jeanne A. Barsanti

ETIOLOGY

Clostridium botulinum is a gram-positive, spore-forming, saprophytic, anaerobic rod that is distributed in soil worldwide. Botulism is an intoxication caused by a neurotoxin produced by the organism. To produce disease, either the organism or its spores must contaminate a food source.

Seven types (A, B, C, D, E, F, and G) of *C. botulinum* have been identified on the basis of their antigenically distinct neurotoxins. All have similar structure and the same neurotoxic effect. Types A, B, E, and F are associated with human disease.[2, 7] Most cases of botulism in animals are caused by types C and D, which are related immunologically.[7] All canine cases to date have been caused by type C toxin, with the exception of two cases of type D reported from Senegal.[1]

Although the disease has been experimentally produced in cats,[1] no natural cases have been reported. A cat that ate contaminated yogurt did not become ill even though two humans eating the same yogurt did.[4] Type C botulism has been reported in lions, but jaguars and coatis eating the same food as the lions did not become affected.[1, 3] The present discussion is limited to dogs, but if it occurred in cats, the disease should be similar because botulinal neurotoxins cause similar signs in all species studied to date.

Clostridial spores are resistant to heat, light, drying, and radiation, but specific conditions are necessary for germination. The organism grows best under anaerobic conditions and with warmth (15–45°C), although some strains can grow at temperatures as low as 6°C. Mildly alkaline pH stimulates growth of some types, but pH 5.7 may be optimal for type C–producing strains.

Botulinal toxin is a protein released mainly from vegetative cells by lysis of the cell or by diffusion through the cell wall. The amount of toxin in spores is only about 1% of that found in vegetative cells, but the intrasporal toxin is resistant to heat denaturation. The type C toxin is stable at a pH range from 2.7 to 10.2.[9] Vegetative cells produced by germinating spores begin to produce toxin within several days after germination. All the different serotypes of botulinal toxin are inactive when initially released by bacterial lysis. Bacterial or tissue proteases cleave them to generate the active dichain neurotoxin. All the botulinal neurotoxins are composed of a heavy (H) chain of 100,000 molecular weight and a light (L) chain of 50,000 molecular weight, bridged by a single interchain disulfide bond (Fig. 42–1).[10]

PATHOGENESIS

Botulism is usually due to ingestion of the preformed toxin, although a variant of the disease in people, infant

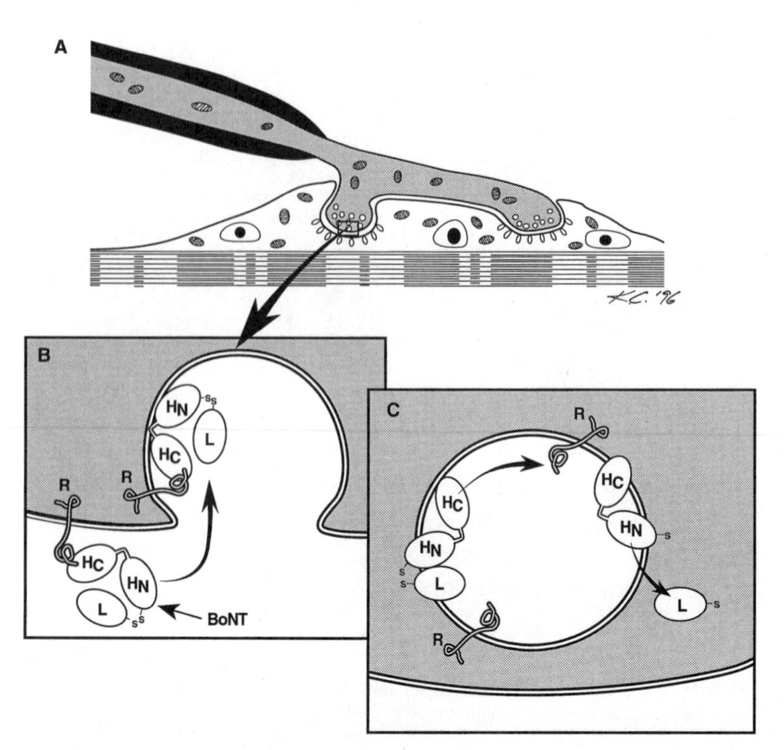

Figure 42–1. Schematic drawing of the binding of botulinal toxin by a membrane receptor (R) at the neuromuscular junction *(A)*. The toxin is composed of a heavy chain with carboxyl (HC) and amino (HN) terminal ends and a light (L) chain containing zinc. The carboxyl end of the heavy chain binds to the receptor at the nerve ending *(B)*. The HN terminal end is thought to be involved in the membrane translocation of the L chain into the nerve cell by inserting itself into the membrane lipid bilayer *(C)*. The L chain, free in the cytosol and by its zinc-endopeptidase activity, selectively cleaves proteins involved in the exocytosis of acetylcholine *(C)*.[10] Whether the intact double-chain toxin or only the L chain enters the cytosol is debated.[5, 7, 10]

botulism, is due to ingestion of spores, usually in honey.[2] Normal adults are resistant to intestinal colonization with *C. botulinum*, largely because of intestinal microflora, because colonization can be induced in adult animals or humans only if they are germ free or are being treated with antibiotics.[1] Persistent intestinal colonization in adults with *C. botulinum* rarely causes clinical illness.[1] Intestinal colonization was established experimentally in 8- to 11-day-old puppies, but no intoxication occurred.[1] Intestinal colonization has been found in a natural case of botulism in a 6-month-old dog.[1] However, the dog recovered without antibiotic therapy, even though intestinal colonization continued for several months.

The source of botulinal toxin is rarely found in reported canine cases. Type C toxin has been isolated from fly larvae (maggots) and from carrion,[7, 12] and most canine cases are thought to be associated with ingestion of carrion.[1] Others are associated with wetlands during warm weather—the areas associated with avian botulism epizootics.[16]

Once ingested, types C and D toxins are absorbed primarily from upper small bowel into lymphatics via endocytosis similar to nutrient proteins. Some toxin is denatured by digestive processes. Toxin can continue to be absorbed from the lower small bowel and colon, but this process proceeds more slowly. Type C toxin is often found in a complex with one other nontoxic protein of similar molecular weight.[10] The function of this nontoxic protein is unknown. Such proteins do seem to protect the neurotoxin from degradation in the intestine or enhance its absorption, because the toxin combined with nontoxic protein complexes is more toxic than neurotoxin alone when administered orally.[10] The mechanism of transport of the toxin to the neuromuscular junction is unknown.[7]

The toxin, a metalloproteinase similar to tetanus toxin, prevents the presynaptic release of acetylcholine at the neuromuscular junction. Both the spontaneous release of acetylcholine and its release caused by a nerve action potential are inhibited.

The carboxyl-terminal end of the H chain seems to be responsible for the binding to the presynaptic membrane (see Fig. 42–1).[10, 14] Binding occurs very quickly and is irreversible, unaffected by temperature and independent of neural activity. The cell membrane receptors for the toxin must have very high affinity for it because only minute quantities ($< 10^{-12}$ mol) of botulinal toxin are sufficient to cause death, making it the most potent toxin known.[7, 10] Variations in receptor affinity for different types of toxin explain the different sensitivities of animal species to the different botulinal toxins.[7, 10, 14] However, the nature of the receptor molecules is still unknown.[7] During this stage the toxin is susceptible to inactivation by antitoxin, and paralysis does not result.

Because acetylcholine is released from the nerve ending, the toxin passes through the cell membrane by receptor-mediated endocytosis.[2] The amino-terminal end governs cell penetration (see Fig. 42–1).[12] This process is temperature and energy dependent.[14] Once inside the cell, the toxin is resistant to inactivation by antitoxin.

Whether the intact double-chain toxin or just the L chain must reach the cytosol to inhibit acetylcholine release is debated.[7, 10, 14] However, the L chain is most responsible for blockade of acetylcholine release.[7, 10, 14] The blockage of acetylcholine release may be due to zinc-dependent cleavage of protein components of the neuroexocytosis apparatus.[14] Several different membrane proteins are involved in the vesicles important in acetylcholine release. Different types of botulinal toxin cleave different bonds within this membrane protein system. Type C toxin targets the protein syntaxin.[14]

Botulinal neurotoxins do not cause death of the affected neuron. They only cause paralysis and degeneration of the intoxicated synapse. Under light microscopy, no lesions are apparent at the neuromuscular junction. However, changes in terminal axons, synaptic clefts, and adjacent muscle fibers have been noted by EM of neuromuscular junctions from human cases.

The blockage of acetylcholine release results in generalized lower motor neuron (LMN) and parasympathetic dysfunction. Blockage of neurotransmission can cause the death of the affected animal from inability to breathe. If the animal survives, recovery occurs by development of new terminal

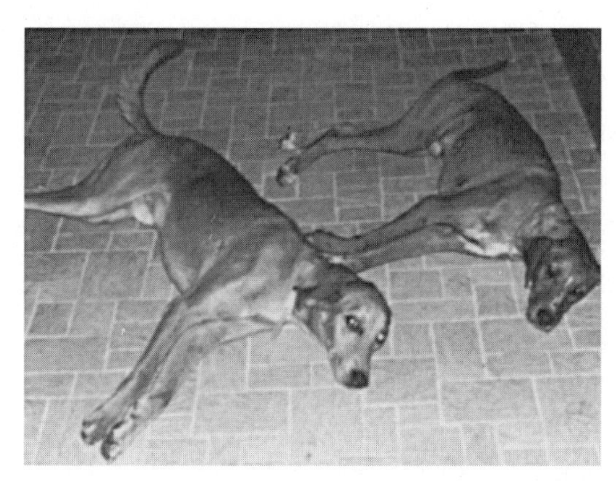

Figure 42–2. Dogs with quadriplegia resulting from botulism.

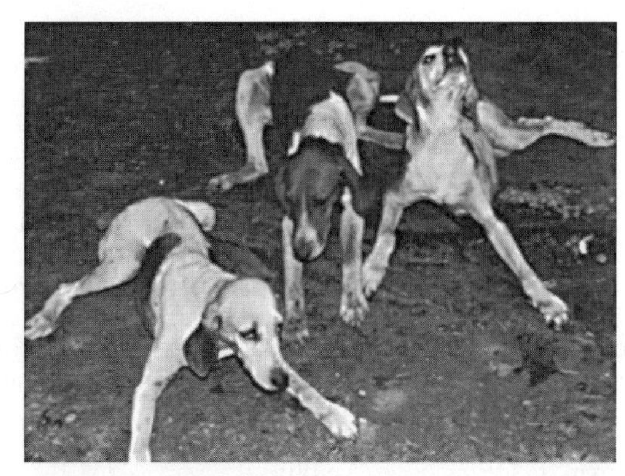

Figure 42–4. Dogs recovering from botulism, having regained the ability to resume sternal recumbency and move the head and neck.

axons with functional neuromuscular junctions.[1] Thus, the effect of botulinal neurotoxin always has the potential of a complete reversal.

CLINICAL FINDINGS

The reported clinical signs in canine botulism type C have been the same whether experimentally or naturally induced.[1, 16, 19] The severity of the signs varies with the amount of toxin ingested and individual susceptibility. The first sign is a progressive, symmetric, ascending weakness from the rear to the forelimbs that can result in quadriplegia (Fig. 42–2). Tail wag is maintained. A complete neurologic examination will show hyporeflexia and hypotonia, indicating generalized LMN dysfunction. Cranial nerves are often affected: mydriasis with sluggish pupillary responses, decreased jaw tone, decreased gag reflex with excess salivation, diminished palpebral reflexes, and weak vocalization have been found in affected dogs. Pain perception and alert mental attitude are maintained (Fig. 42–3). In severely affected dogs, there may be decreased abdominal muscle tone and primarily diaphragmatic respiration.

The heart rate is variable (increased or decreased), and constipation and urinary retention may develop. Megaesophagus has been noted in six affected dogs. Muscle atrophy is variable. There is no hyperesthesia. Conjunctivitis and ulcerative keratitis may develop because of the weak palpebral reflex. Bilateral keratoconjunctivitis sicca has been noted. Death may result from respiratory paralysis or from secondary respiratory or urinary infections. On necropsy there are no gross or light microscopic abnormalities in the nervous system.

The progression of signs is explained by differences in affected muscles, the diaphragm being much more resistant than skeletal muscle to paralysis with progressive neuromuscular blockade.

The incubation period after ingestion of contaminated food in dogs has been from hours to 6 days. The earlier the signs appear, the more serious is the disease. The duration of illness in dogs that recovered has ranged from 14 to 24 days. Cranial nerve, neck, and forelimb functions tend to return first in affected dogs. If recovery occurs, it is complete (Fig. 42–4).

In cases of type D botulism, the dogs died suddenly with signs of generalized hemorrhage and without observed neurologic deficits.[1] The signs were probably due to a different toxin, C2 toxin, which increases vascular permeability and induces hemorrhage and edema.[15]

DIAGNOSIS

All results of routine laboratory work (CBC, blood chemistry profile, urinalysis) are normal unless a secondary infection develops.[1, 16] CSF is normal in affected dogs and humans.

Electromyography (EMG) shows that LMN dysfunction in clinically affected dogs is due to a problem at the neuromuscular junction and perhaps to peripheral nerve conduction.[1, 20] When a motor nerve is stimulated, motor unit potentials are subnormal in amplitude but not polyphasic (Fig. 42–5). Decrements in motor unit potentials are variable after repeti-

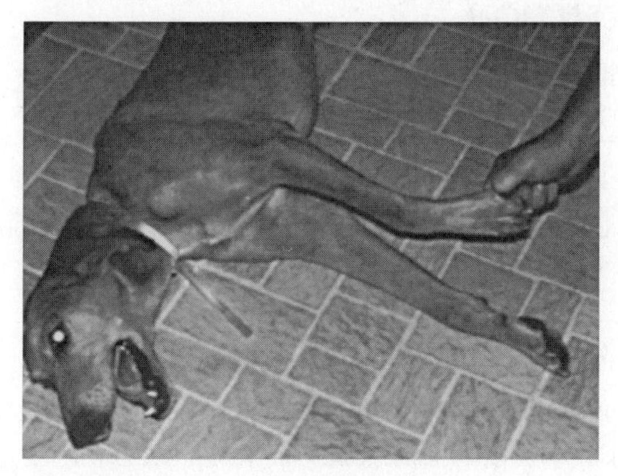

Figure 42–3. Dog with botulism showing normal pain perception but lack of a withdrawal reflex.

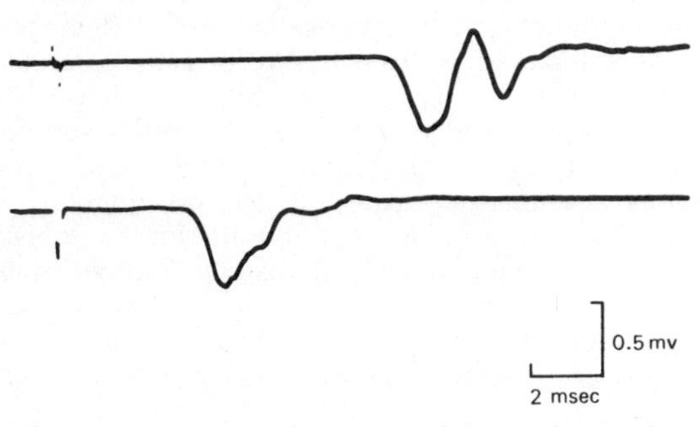

Figure 42–5. Electromyographic tracing after stimulation of the right tibial nerve of a dog with botulism. The upper tracing is the response to stimulation at the level of the femoral trochanter, and the lower tracing is the response to stimulation at the popliteal fossa. The amplitudes of the evoked potentials are markedly subnormal.

tive stimulation. Fibrillation potentials have been noted in one study but not in another,[1] which may be related to the difference in the time of performance of EMGs (mean of 16 and 12 days, respectively). Nerve conduction velocity was mildly decreased in one report, even with correction for hypothermia. As the dogs recovered, increased electrode insertional activity and positive sharp waves were found. The main EMG findings in affected humans are decreased compound muscle action potentials with normal nerve conduction.[16] In some patients there is a decremental pattern to low-frequency repetitive nerve stimulation. As in dogs, EMG findings in affected people vary and sometimes lead to incorrect initial diagnoses.[4]

Confirmatory diagnosis of botulism is based on the finding of the toxin in serum, feces, vomitus, or samples of the food that was ingested. Serum should be collected as early in the disease course as possible and when clinical signs are maximal. About 10 ml of serum or 50 g of feces, vomitus, or food is needed to conduct the test.

The preferred method of identifying the toxin is the neutralization test in mice. In this test, serum or an extract of feces, vomitus, or food is injected alone and in combination with type-specific antitoxin into the peritoneal cavity of mice. The mice are then observed for signs of botulism. Survival of one group protected with one type of antitoxin and death of the other groups with signs consistent with botulism confirm the presence of botulinal toxin.

Newer in vitro tests have been developed to identify botulinal toxin. These tests include radioimmune assay (RIA), passive hemagglutination, ELISA, and polymerase chain reaction (PCR). To date, these tests have not replaced the mouse test.[8, 11, 13, 18]

The diagnostic importance of isolation of the organism *C. botulinum* from feces is controversial. The organism can be isolated from feces of only 60% of humans with botulism.[1] Although isolation of the organism in association with clinical signs provides some evidence for the diagnosis, it is not as conclusive as toxin identification. The type C organism is one of the most difficult types to culture because it is a strict anaerobe. Often the presence of toxin in an extract of cultured feces is used as evidence of the organism's presence.[1, 4]

THERAPY

Supportive Care

Supportive treatment is most important because spontaneous recovery will occur if the amount of toxin ingested is not too large and if respiratory and urinary tract infections can be avoided. Affected animals should be assisted to eat, drink, and move about. Water beds or cage padding will reduce the incidence of decubital sores. Ability to urinate should be monitored and the bladder expressed as needed. Enemas and stool softeners should be given for constipation. Parenteral fluids should be used as necessary to avoid dehydration, especially if swallowing is impaired. Antibiotics should be provided if infection develops, but aminoglycosides should be avoided because they also have the potential to block neuromuscular transmission. To avoid altering the intestinal microflora, which might allow *C. botulinum* to grow, antibiotics should be given only when necessary.[1] Nonmedicated or antibiotic ophthalmic ointments should be provided to prevent exposure keratitis in dogs with poor palpebral function.

Antitoxin

Antitoxin is not effective after the toxin has penetrated the nerve endings, which occurs rapidly after the toxin enters the blood stream. Antitoxin may prevent further toxin binding if intestinal absorption and circulation are still occurring. Because most cases in dogs to date have been type C, type C antitoxin should be given. The recommended dose for treating dogs (10,000 to 15,0000 U, IV or IM, two doses 4 hours apart) is that for treating adult people. The antitoxin will remain in circulation for 40 days after administration, so there is no need for further administration. Five milliliters of polyvalent antitoxin (types A, B, C, D, E, F, Statens Serum Institute, Copenhagen, Denmark) administered IV or IM has been administered in dogs treated to date. Anaphylaxis is a potential risk. ID skin testing can be performed with 0.1 ml of antitoxin 20 minutes before IV injection. Any immediate reaction at the test site is a warning that an allergic response may occur.

Antibiotics

Penicillin or metronidazole has been administered in dogs and people in an attempt to reduce any potential intestinal population of *C. botulinum*.[1] The efficacy of these drugs is doubted because disease is usually due to ingestion of preformed toxin and because neither drug is certain to eradicate *C. botulinum* from the intestine.[1] The possibility that these drugs could make the disease worse by releasing more toxin through bacterial lysis or by promoting intestinal infection has also been raised.[1] Even in infant botulism, which may involve intestinal colonization with *C. botulinum*, penicillin has no effect on recovery.[7]

Neuromuscular Potentiators

Three drugs, guanidine hydrochloride, 4-aminopyridine, and 3,4 diaminopyridine, have been used without demonstrable efficacy in clinical cases in humans or animals.[1, 4, 5] Side effects of guanidine hydrochloride in people include GI upset and muscle twitching. Administration of guanidine hydrochloride to an affected lion resulted in seizures and pyrexia with death 2 days after drug administration.[1] 4-Aminopyridine caused severe, repetitive convulsions in two of four treated people without improvement in respiratory function and is not recommended. Diaminopyridine was ineffective in a human case, but no side effects were noted. Diaminopyridine was given to two lions, with improvement in signs for only 30 minutes. Current research is focused on finding specific inhibitors of the toxin's action on the proteins involved in acetylcholine release.[14]

PREVENTION

Botulinal toxin is destroyed by heating food to 80°C for 30 minutes or to 100°C for 10 minutes. Preventing access to carrion and thorough cooking of any food fed to dogs will prevent the disease. Foxhounds appear predisposed to the disease because they may be fed raw meat. Vaccination with a toxoid has been successful in cattle[3] and in exposed laboratory workers.[11, 13]

References

1. Barsanti JA. 1990. Botulism, pp 515–520. *In* Greene CE (ed), Infectious diseases of the dog and cat. WB Saunders, Philadelphia, PA.
2. Bleck TP. 1995. *Clostridium botulinum*, pp 2178–2181. *In* Mandell GL, Bennett JE, Dolin R (eds), Principles and practice of infectious diseases. Churchill Livingstone, New York, NY.

3. Critchley EM. 1991. A comparison of human and animal botulism: a review. *J R Soc Med* 84:295–298.
4. Critchley EM, Hayes PJ, Isaacs RE. 1989. Outbreak of botulism in north-west England and Wales, June, 1989. *Lancet* 2:849–853.
5. Davis LE, Johnson JK, Bickell JM, et al. 1992. Human type A botulism and treatment with 3,4-diaminopyridine. *Electromyogr Clin Neurophysiol* 32:379–383.
6. Doellgast GJ, Brown JE, Koufman JA, et al. 1997. Sensitive assay for measurement of antibodies to *Clostridium botulinum* neurotoxins A, B and E: use of hapten-labeled-antibody elution to isolate specific complexes. *J Clin Microbiol* 35:578–583.
7. Ferrari ND, Weisse ME. 1995. Botulism. *Adv Pediatr Infect Dis* 10:81–91.
8. Franciosa G, Fenicia L, Caldiani C, et al. 1996. PCR for detection of *Clostridium botulinum* type C in avian and environmental samples. *J Clin Microbiol* 34:882–885.
9. Halouzka J, Hubalek Z. 1992. Effect of pH on the stability of type-C toxin of *Clostridium botulinum*. *Folia Microbiol* 37:157–158.
10. Hambleton P. 1992. *Clostridium botulinum* toxins: a general review of involvement in disease, structure, mode of action and preparation for clinical use. *J Neurol* 239:16–20.
11. Hatheway CL. 1995. Botulism: the present status of the disease, pp 55–75. *In* Montecucco C (ed), Clostridial neurotoxins. Springer, New York, NY.
12. Hubalek Z, Halouzka J. 1991. Persistence of *Clostridium botulinum* type C toxin in blow fly (*Calliphoridae*) larvae as a possible cause of avian botulism in spring. *J Wildl Dis* 27:81–85.
13. Middlebrook JL, Brown JE. 1995. Immunodiagnosis and immunotherapy of tetanus and botulism neurotoxins, pp 89–122. *In* Montecucco C (ed), Clostridial neurotoxins. Springer, New York, NY.
14. Montecucco C, Schiavo G. 1994. Mechanism of action of tetanus and botulinum neurotoxins. *Mol Microbiol* 13:1–8.
15. Popoff MR. 1995. Ecology of neurotoxigenic strains of clostridia, pp 2–29. *In* Montecucco C (ed), Clostridial neurotoxins. Springer, New York, NY.
16. Read D, Kelly T. 1990. Botulism in dogs associated with a Waikato wetland area. *Surveillance-Wellington* 17:9.
17. Sanders DB. 1993. Clinical neurophysiology of disorders of the neuromuscular junction. *J Clin Neurophysiol* 10:167–180.
18. Thomas RJ. 1991. Detection of *Clostridium botulinum* types C and D toxin by ELISA. *Aust Vet J* 68:111–113.
19. Tjalsma EJ. 1990. Three cases of *Clostridium botulinum* type C intoxication in the dog. *Tijdschr Diergeneeskd* 115:518–521.
20. Zouari N, Choyakh F, Triki C, et al. 1997. Contribution of electromyography to the diagnosis of botulism. *Neurophysiol Clin* 27:220–226.

Chapter 43

Tetanus

Craig E. Greene

ETIOLOGY

Tetanus is caused by the action of a potent neurotoxin formed in the body during the vegetative growth of *Clostridium tetani*. *C. tetani* is a motile, gram-positive, nonencapsulated, anaerobic, spore-forming bacillus. Although strain differences of *C. tetani* exist throughout the world, the toxin produced by all strains is antigenically homogeneous. Resistant spores of the organism can be found in the environment, especially in the soil, where increased moisture, cultivation, and fertilization favor their survival. Organisms are routinely isolated from the feces of many domestic animals, including the dog and cat.[5] Isolation from human feces occurs with greater frequency in those occupationally exposed to farm animals. Spores can survive adverse weather conditions in the absence of direct sunlight for months or years and can be found readily in dust and debris in indoor environments. Spores are resistant to boiling water, phenol, cresol, and mercury bichloride, and they resist an autoclave temperature of 120°C for 15 to 20 minutes. The vegetative phase of *C. tetani*, however, is no more resistant to chemical and physical inactivation than other microorganisms.

EPIDEMIOLOGY

Tetanus develops when spores are introduced into wounds or penetrating injuries. The spores vegetate in response to anaerobic conditions at the site of injury. The presence of a foreign body, tissue necrosis, other microorganisms, or abscess formation contributes to germination. Two toxins have been identified from *C. tetani*. Tetanolepsin causes hemolysis of erythrocytes during rapid in vitro growth of the bacteria; however, it is not considered clinically significant. In contrast, tetanospasmin (molecular weight = 176,000) enters the body from the wound site and produces marked effects on neurologic function. It is not absorbed from the GI tract because it is usually destroyed by digestive juices. Its high molecular weight precludes its entry into the placenta.

The prevalence of the disease in dogs and cats is relatively low compared with that in other domestic animals, which may be related to the natural resistance of dogs and cats to this toxin (Table 43–1). The resistance is related to the inability of the toxin to penetrate and bind to nervous tissue, because direct CNS injections of toxin produce equivalent signs in different species.

PATHOGENESIS

Many experimental studies have been performed with dogs, cats, and other laboratory animals to elucidate the

Table 43–1. Relative Susceptibility[a] of Animals to Tetanus Toxin

ANIMAL	SUSCEPTIBILITY
Horse	1 (most susceptible)
Guinea pig	2
Human	3
Mouse	12
Rabbit	24
Dog	600
Cat	7200
Chicken	360,000 (least susceptible)

[a]The horse is assigned an arbitrary value of 1. Comparison relates to the amount of toxin required to produce clinical illness.

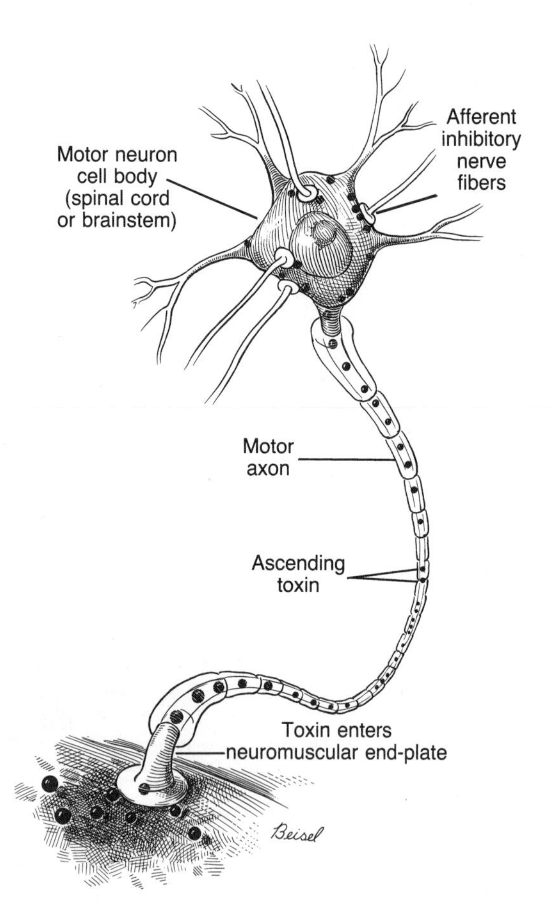

Figure 43–1. Retrograde intra-axonal transport of tetanus toxin into the CNS.

mechanism by which tetanospasmin enters and affects the CNS. The site and route of administration of toxin are important in determining the type of disease that develops. Localized tetanus can be produced by IM or SC injection of toxin at a specific site. Tetanospasmin is a dimer composed of a heavy chain (100 kD) that binds to neuronal cells and transport proteins and a light chain (50 kD) that blocks the release of neurotransmitters.[14] Toxin enters the axons of the nearest motor nerves at the neuromuscular end-plate and migrates by retrograde transport within motor axons, at a rate of 75 to 250 mm per day, to the neuronal cell body within the spinal cord (Fig. 43–1). Within the spinal cord, toxin ascends in a bilateral fashion until it reaches the brain (Fig. 43–2).

Systemic IV administration of large amounts of toxin usually results in intracranial signs, such as convulsions, facial muscle spasms, or respiratory arrest, before development of generalized limb rigidity. Small amounts of blood-borne toxin are thought to enter the CNS through the intact blood-brain barrier. Alternatively, hematogenously disseminated toxin may localize preferentially in the neuromuscular endings of many motor nerves throughout the body, from which it may ascend by retrograde axonal transport simultaneously into many areas of the nervous system. The initial involvement of facial musculature after hematogenous spread of toxin is explained by the fact that cranial nerve motor axons (e.g., facial nerve) are shorter than those of the limbs.

The clinical signs of tetanus intoxication can be explained by the known pathophysiologic effects of tetanus toxin on the nervous system. It inhibits release of glycine and gamma-aminobutyric acid (GABA)—neurotransmitters of inhibitory interneurons of the brain and spinal cord. Presynaptic blockade of synapses of Renshaw cells and 1a fibers of α-motor neurons occurs. Most experimental evidence has confirmed the effect of toxin at the spinal cord; however, brain, neuromuscular junctions, and autonomic nervous system can also be affected. Tetanus toxin has an affinity for gangliosides within the gray matter of the CNS, which may explain the cerebral signs that appear in some cases without obvious spinal cord involvement. Effects of tetanus toxin have also been ascribed to its affinity for binding at the neuromuscular junction, which may induce direct neuromuscular facilitation before the migration of toxin to the CNS. Tetanus toxin may affect sympathetic preganglionic neurons similar to lower motor neurons within the spinal cord and cause signs of autonomic dysfunction. Bradycardia associated with tetanus probably results from vagal-parasympathetic hyperactivity. Tetanus toxin also blocks neurotransmitters in the parasympathetic cardiac inhibitory center of the nucleus ambiguous, resulting in increased vagal tone and pronounced bradyarrhythmias. Increased catecholamine release associated with adrenergic stimulation can also cause episodes of hypertension or tachycardia in tetanus.

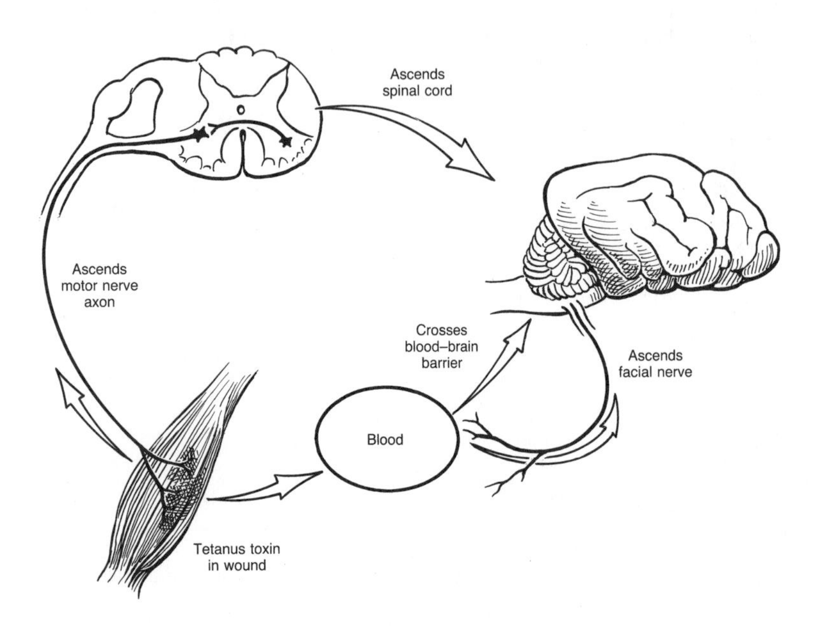

Figure 43–2. Potential routes of spread of tetanus toxin into the CNS.

The binding of tetanus toxin to presynaptic sites of inhibitory neurons is irreversible; recovery depends on sprouting of new axon terminals.[14]

CLINICAL FINDINGS

Clinical signs of tetanus usually occur within 5 to 10 days of wounding, although ranges of 3 to 18 days have been reported.[9] Because of the increased resistance of cats and dogs to intoxication, onset may be delayed for up to 3 weeks. This may account for the absence of a detectable wound at the time of examination. However, because of greater innate resistance of cats, the wound required to produce intoxication is so extensive that it is usually obvious. Wounds nearer the head (brain) are associated with more rapid onset and generalized signs of CNS intoxication than injuries to distant extremities. Tetanus has also been observed as a complication of ovariohysterectomy, pregnancy, or parturition associated with fetal death.[2, 8, 9]

Localized tetanus is more common than generalized tetanus in dogs and cats than it is in humans and other domestic animals because of the relative resistance of carnivores to intoxication. Increased stiffness of a muscle or entire limb is first noted in close proximity to the wound site (Fig. 43–3). In the thoracic limb, the elbow is usually extended and the carpus may be held flexed or extended. The stiffness usually spreads, gradually involving the opposite extremity. This process usually progresses over a variable length of time and eventually involves the entire CNS.[10] Localized tetanus in the pelvic limbs has been commonly associated with the female reproductive tract of dogs and cats. In cases in which a single extremity remains affected, the diagnosis may be confused.

Animals affected with *generalized* tetanus walk with a stiff gait and generally with an outstretched or dorsally curved tail. They have difficulty in standing or lying down in comfortable positions because of the extreme muscle rigidity (Figs. 43–4 and 43–5). Rectal temperature is usually increased due to excessive muscular activity. Postural reaction testing, such as proprioceptive positioning, usually reveals normal initiation but stiff performance of the motor response. Myotactic reflexes are generally accentuated and flexor reflexes depressed, but both may be difficult to elicit because of muscle stiffness.

Intracranial signs develop in the late stages of localized tetanus. They begin earlier in generalized tetanus and usually progress in reverse or descending fashion to produce generalized muscular stiffness. Cranial nerve motor nuclei are affected, causing hypertonicity of respective musculature. Protrusion of the third eyelid and enophthalmos result from retraction of the globe from hypertonus of extraocular muscles (Fig. 43–6). The ears are held erect, the lips are drawn back (risus sardonicus), and the forehead is wrinkled as a result of facial muscle spasm. Trismus (lockjaw) is caused by contraction of masticatory muscles. Increased salivation, heart rate, and respiratory rate; laryngeal spasm; and dysphagia can result from involvement of parasympathetic and somatic cranial nerve nuclei.

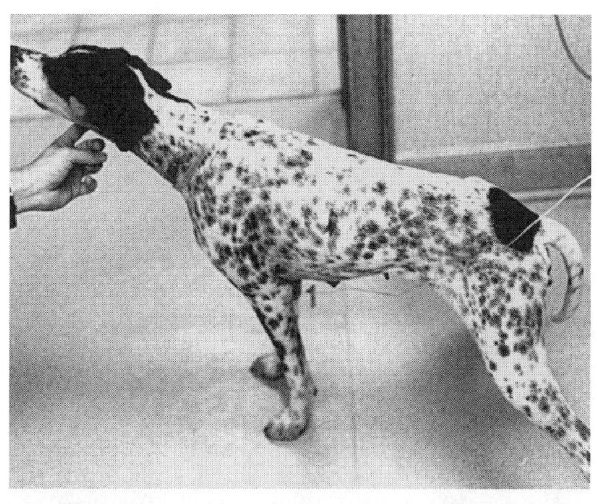

Figure 43–4. Characteristic "sawhorse" stance of a dog with generalized tetanus. (Courtesy of Dr. Wayne Rush, Atlanta, GA.)

Reflex muscle spasms occur in animals with generalized tetanus or intracranial involvement. Animals become apprehensive and react strongly to tactile or auditory stimulation. Mild stimulation may precipitate periodic generalized tonic contraction of all muscles with opisthotonus or precipitate grand mal convulsions. If the tonic contractions are first to occur, the interval between spasms decreases until the animal reaches a convulsive state. Dogs and cats usually remain conscious until they develop convulsions. Reflex muscle spasms are painful, and animals may vocalize during such episodes. Animals with tetanus usually have a desire to eat, but because of jaw stiffness, they may have trouble prehending or swallowing solid food. Regurgitation will develop in animals with complicating hiatal hernia.[3, 18] Dysuria and urine retention, constipation, and gaseous distention are common results of persistent anal and urinary sphincter contractions. The progression of clinical signs culminates in death, which is usually caused by respiratory compromise. This is

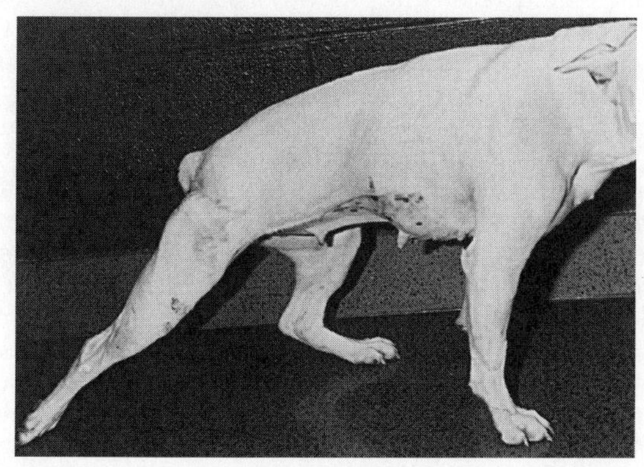

Figure 43–3. Localized tetanus in the rear right limb of a dog with postpartum metritis. Stiffness progressed to involve all four limbs as well as the facial muscles.

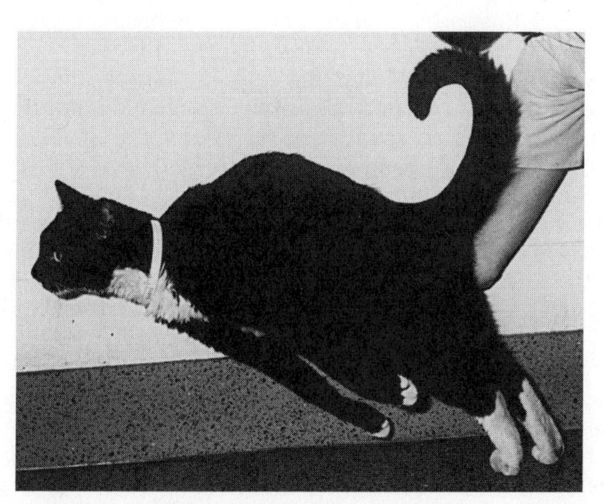

Figure 43–5. Characteristic posture of a cat with generalized tetanus, showing stiff limbs and outstretched tail.

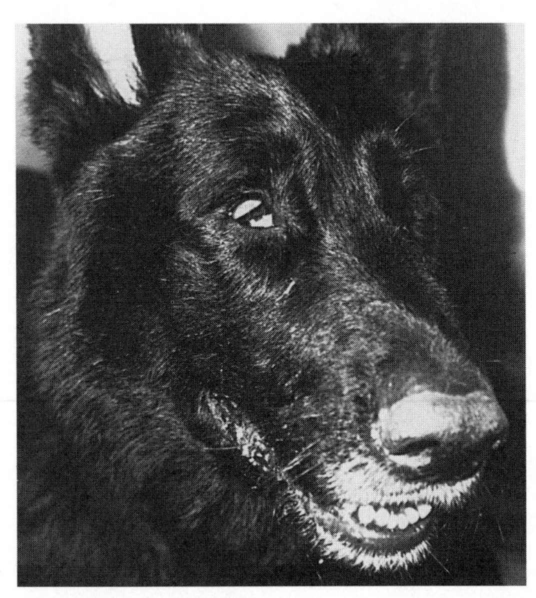

Figure 43–6. German shepherd dog with generalized tetanus, showing protrusion of the third eyelid and contracture of the facial muscles. From Greene CE, Oliver JE. 1983. Neurologic examination, pp 419–460. *In* Ettinger SJ (ed): Textbook of veterinary internal medicine, ed 2. WB Saunders, Philadelphia, PA. Reprinted with permission.

the result of rigidity of the respiratory musculature, reflex spasms of the larynx, increased airway secretions, and central respiratory arrest from medullary intoxication or anoxia.

DIAGNOSIS

History of a recent wound and clinical signs are the primary means of diagnosing tetanus. Hematologic abnormalities, including leukocytosis with neutrophilia and left shift, are the results of wounds that may be present. Serum biochemistry and CSF values are unaffected, except that elevations of muscle enzyme (creatine kinase, aspartate aminotransferase) activities may be present.

Both tachyarrhythmias and bradyarrhythmias can be noted in tetanus. Rapid heart rates are usually associated with sinus tachycardia. Bradycardia (< 70 beats/minute) has been characterized by atrioventricular heart block, sinus arrest, and ventricular escape complexes.

In dogs that develop hiatal hernia and megaesophagus, thoracic radiographic changes occur in the caudal region and include increased density and esophageal dilation.

The muscle spasms that develop in tetanus are usually reduced but not always abolished by general anesthesia. Even when clinically evident relaxation occurs, characteristic electromyographic changes can usually be detected. Insertion of the needle or tapping of the muscles or tendons is followed by persistent electrical motor unit discharges rather than the expected period of electrical silence. Muscle biopsy results are usually normal in acute cases of tetanus, and any observed abnormalities may be attributed to muscle trauma as a result of constant hypertonicity or prolonged recumbency.

Measurement of serum antibody titers to tetanus toxin has been used to substantiate the diagnosis of tetanus. Values must be compared with those for control animals. Such measurements might be helpful in a clinical setting to confirm the cause of undiagnosed muscle stiffness.

Isolation of *C. tetani* from wounds can be a difficult procedure and is unrewarding in a majority of cases. The organisms are usually present in very low concentrations, and although Gram-stained smears may demonstrate gram-positive rods and dark-staining spherical endospores, the morphology is not unlike that of many other anaerobic bacteria. If culture is attempted, it should be done under strict anaerobic conditions at 37°C for 12 days. Biochemical reactions or bioassays can be evaluated in an attempt to classify the organism. Mouse inoculation with isolates is not readily available.

THERAPY

Therapy for tetanus in severely affected animals is costly and time consuming, and owners must be advised of the possibility of complications and lengthy hospitalization. Fortunately, the disease is often localized or mild in dogs and cats because of their innate resistance. However, untreated cases can prove fatal. Because of their natural resistance, dogs and cats are not vaccinated with toxoid as a means of prophylaxis or treatment. Recommended dosages for drugs used in the treatment discussed next are summarized in Table 43–2.

Antitoxin

This consists of antitetanus equine serum (ATS) or human tetanus immune globulin (TIG). In the United States, TIG is approved for IM use, whereas ATS is licensed for IM or IV use. The TIG contains thimerosal and immunoglobulin aggregates and may more likely produce reactions when given by other than the IM route.[1]

The immediate concern in treating tetanus is administration of antitoxin to neutralize any toxin that is unbound to the CNS or is yet to be formed. The timing and route of antitoxin administration are important in determining the effectiveness of detoxification. Use of antitoxin should be a routine measure; however, the elimination of bound toxin by the affected animal is gradual, and the administration of antitoxin does little to hasten the process. Thus, recovery in most cases is slow and progressive. The dosage for prophylaxis is much less than that for treatment.

IV administration of antitoxin is superior to IM or SC administration in producing a rapid and marked increase of circulating antitoxin. It takes 48 to 72 hours for antitoxin to reach therapeutic concentrations when given SC. The dose of equine antitoxin is given slowly over 5 to 10 minutes. Larger animals should receive a proportionally lower dose on the basis of body weight. Total doses greater than 20,000 U do not appear to be more effective, because they increase the antigenic mass, and they are more costly.

Unfortunately, IV antitoxin is associated with a high prevalence of anaphylaxis; therefore, appropriate precautions are warranted during administration. An initial test dose (0.1–0.2 ml) of antitoxin should be given SC or ID 15 to 30 minutes before the administration of the IV dose. A wheal at the site of injection may indicate that an anaphylactic reaction will develop. Epinephrine, glucocorticoid, and antihistamine should be readily available in case of an adverse reaction, or the latter two may be given before an IV injection of antitoxin if a reaction is anticipated. IV 0.1 ml/kg epinephrine (diluted 1:10,000) is the drug of choice in the event that an anaphylactic reaction develops. It is not advisable to repeat the dose at any time during the course of therapy. A therapeutic blood level of antitoxin persists in dogs for 14 days after injection,

Table 43–2. Recommended Drug Dosages for Tetanus

DRUG	SPECIES	DOSE[a]	ROUTE	INTERVAL (HOURS)	DURATION (DAYS)
Antimicrobials					
Penicillin G	B	20,000–100,000 U/kg	IV, IM, SC	6–12	10
Metronidazole	D	10 mg/kg	PO	8	10
	C	250 mg total	PO	12–24	10
Tetracycline	B	22 mg/kg	PO, IV	8	10
Clindamycin	B	3–10 mg/kg	PO, IV, IM	8–12	10
Immunotherapy					
Equine antitoxin[b]	B	100–1000 U/kg	IV, IM, SC[d]		Once
		1000 U/site	Intralesional		Once
		1–10 U/kg	Intrathecal		Once
Sedatives					
Acetylpromazine	B	0.02–0.06 mg/kg[c]	IV	2	prn
	B	0.1–0.25 mg/kg[c]	IM	4	prn
	B	1.0 mg/kg	PO	6–8	prn
Chlorpromazine	B	0.5–2.0 mg/kg	IM, IV, PO	8–12	prn
Diazepam	C	2.5–5.0 mg total	PO	2–4	prn
	D	5.0–10.0 mg total	IV, PO, IM	2–4	prn
	B	0.2–1.0 mg/kg	IV	prn	prn
Methocarbamol	B	15–50 mg/kg	PO	6–12	prn
Pentobarbital	B	3–15 mg/kg	IV, IM	2–3	prn
Phenobarbital	B	1–4 mg/kg	PO, IM	6–12	prn
Autonomic Agents					
Atropine	B	0.05 mg/kg	SC	prn	prn[d]
Glycopyrrolate	B	0.005 mg/kg	SC, IV	prn	prn[d]
		1 mg total	PO	8	prn

[a]Dose per administration at specified interval. Lowest range value applies to animals with greatest body weight. For additional information, see Appendix 8.
[b]IV route is most practical and efficacious. An ID or SC test dose (0.1–0.2 ml) before IV infusion is recommended to detect hypersensitivity.
[c]Maximum dose IV of 3 mg in any dog.
[d]Use as necessary to control bradyarrhythmias.
B = dog and cat; D = dog; C = cat.

and repeated administration increases the chance of an anaphylactic reaction.

Local IM injection of a small dose of antitoxin (1000 units) around and proximal to the wound site has been shown to be beneficial in experimental studies of localized tetanus.

Intrathecal injection of antitoxin in laboratory animals has been shown to be beneficial in treating tetanus under experimental conditions. Use in affected humans has not been proven to be effective.[1, 19] Intrathecal injection of as little as 1% of the recommended IV dose reduced the mortality and morbidity in dogs with mild or moderate tetanus compared with similarly affected animals given IV or lumbar intrathecal injections. Antitoxin injected into the CNS and CSF has an advantage over a similar systemic dose because it need not penetrate the blood-brain barrier and may partially neutralize bound toxin. Being a foreign protein, antitoxin has potential toxicity in the subarachnoid space. For these reasons, intracisternal therapy should be reserved for severely affected animals.

Antimicrobial Therapy

Local and parenteral antibiotic therapy should be instituted in an attempt to kill any vegetative *C. tetani* organisms present in the wound (see Table 43–1). Although antibiotics by themselves may not neutralize circulating toxin, they reduce the amount of antitoxin required to treat experimental tetanus once clinical signs are apparent. Penicillin G, the drug of choice, can be given IV in the form of an aqueous potassium or sodium salt or IM as the procaine salt. A portion of the dosage, in the form of procaine penicillin, can be injected IM in close proximity to an identified wound site. Because the effectiveness of penicillin on the vegetative organisms may vary, tetracycline has been recommended as an alternative. Penicillin derivatives, such as ampicillin, are not as effective against the organism, and their use may cause little or no response. Metronidazole has been shown to be superior to penicillin G and tetracycline in clinical or experimental tetanus, although it has a higher risk for toxicity. Metronidazole may be more active and preferred for treatment of tetanus because it is bactericidal against most anaerobes and achieves effective therapeutic concentrations even in anaerobic tissues. Penicillin is also a known antagonist of GABA as is tetanus toxin.

Sedatives

Various drugs alone or in combination have been given to control the reflex spasms and convulsions associated with tetanus. An ideal agent is one that controls excitability and spasticity without interfering with voluntary motor function or consciousness. Unfortunately, no such drug is available; however, a combination of phenothiazine and barbiturate comes closest to the ideal.

Phenothiazines appear to be highly effective in controlling the hyperexcitable state when provided either alone or in combination with barbiturates. Chlorpromazine is the drug of choice, although acetylpromazine and methotrimeprazine can be given as substitutes. Phenothiazines are ineffective against similar-appearing signs caused by strychnine or other causes of convulsions. Tetanus is one exception when phenothiazines are used in seizure-prone animals. They are thought to work centrally on the brain stem to depress descending excitatory input on the lower motor neurons within the spinal cord.

Barbiturates can be administered successfully to control

grand mal convulsions, generalized body stiffness, and opisthotonus, all of which may occur. Pentobarbital may have to be given every 2 to 3 hours, but the actual dose should be adjusted to coincide with the severity of the clinical signs of the patient, because an overdose may unnecessarily suppress respiration and consciousness. Oral or injectable phenobarbital can be given for a longer duration of action. Combination of phenothiazine and pentobarbital can allow a reduction of the amount of barbiturate needed to control tetany. A complication of the combination of these two drugs is bradycardia. When the heart rate falls below 60 beats/minute, glycopyrrolate can be administered as needed to reverse the bradycardia.

Benzodiazepine derivatives such as diazepam are alternatives to barbiturates in the control of seizures and nervous hyperexcitability. These drugs work by blocking polysynaptic reflexes within the medulla and spinal cord. Methocarbamol is frequently recommended but is less commonly provided as a central-acting muscle relaxant. It has a relatively short duration of action, as does diazepam. Baclofen, a depressant and antispasmolytic that acts as a GABA agonist in the CNS, has been beneficial when given intrathecally to treat severe tetanus in people.[13, 19] Dantrolene, a direct-acting muscle relaxant, has been used to control spasticity in human tetanus.[12, 15] It must be avoided when underlying hepatic disease is present. Respiratory depression has been a complicating factor in some cases.

Narcotics should never be included in tetanus therapy because they depress the respiratory centers and may stimulate other areas of the CNS. Parasympatholytic drugs such as atropine should also be avoided in routine cases; however, bronchospasm, bronchial hypersecretion, and cardiovascular instability have been controlled by continuous atropine infusions in people with severe tetanus.[4]

Severely affected animals with respiratory compromise from uncontrollable tetanic spasms may be sedated or anesthetized, intubated, and placed on positive-pressure ventilation. These measures often become cost prohibitive for veterinary patients.

Surgery

Surgery may be required if tissue necrosis or abscess formation is extensive. Antitoxin should be administered before surgery because of the release of toxin in the circulation during tissue manipulation. General anesthesia is usually required to debride wounds and remove necrotic tissue. Devitalized tissue and visible foreign material should be removed and the wound irrigated. Hydrogen peroxide may be beneficial in flushing the wound because it increases oxygen tension, which inhibits obligate anaerobes. The prognosis for recovery is always greater if the wound site is located and can be debrided.

Autonomic Agents

These are sometimes required to control the cardiac rhythm disturbances that develop. Sympatholytic agents are generally not provided in the management of tachyarrhythmias, because other sedatives usually control this complication. Bradyarrhythmias (< 60 beats/minute) that persist can be controlled by administration of a parasympatholytic agent such as atropine or glycopyrrolate as needed on a short-term basis. These arrhythmias often resolve after a few days in animals that begin to show signs of improvement in their muscle stiffness. Continuous atropine infusion has been used in the management of severe tetanus in people.[4] In addition to assisting with cardiovascular arrhythmias, bronchospasm, bronchial hypersecretion, and hypersalivation are reduced. Clonidine, a central-acting sympathoplegic, reduces autonomic dysfunction in tetanus and might offer benefit in severely affected animals.[17]

Glucocorticoid therapy has never been proven to be beneficial in tetanus and generally should be avoided. In a controlled study of human patients with severe tetanus, betamethasone reduced the need for tracheostomy and ventilation from laryngeal spasm. Hyperbaric oxygenation has been provided in humans and in dogs with tetanus in an attempt to inactivate *C. tetani*; however, there is little proof of benefit to justify the time and cost of such a procedure. Neuromuscular blocking agents have been used in human tetanus in an attempt to control convulsions or to paralyze the patients, who are then placed on artificial respirators. This therapy, however, is impractical in veterinary medicine because of the intensive monitoring required.

Nursing Care

Supportive measures are imperative in the successful management of an animal with tetanus. Constant nursing may be required for severely affected animals. The animal should be placed in a dark, quiet environment with a minimum amount of stimulation. All therapeutic measures should be coordinated for the same time each day so that a minimal amount of handling and stimulation occurs. Soft, comfortable bedding should be provided because tetanus causes incapacitation and animals frequently develop decubital ulcers. Animals should be encouraged to eat and drink on their own. They frequently have difficulty in prehending and swallowing solid foods, but they can usually eat blended foods or fluids by sucking through clenched teeth. A stomach tube may be passed if the animal is reluctant to eat, but this is frequently stressful for conscious animals, and esophageal spasm or hiatal hernia may restrict passage of the tube or cause subsequent regurgitation. Only frequent, small amounts of food should be given in this manner because of the high risk of gastroesophageal reflux or vomiting and resultant aspiration pneumonia. A gastrostomy tube may be required for feeding in severely affected animals. The hematocrit, plasma protein, and body weight should be evaluated daily to determine whether adequate fluid balance is being maintained. Balanced polyionic isotonic fluids should be given parenterally to meet any deficits. Parenteral alimentation requires continual IV administration of special fluids and is expensive.

Complications in dogs and cats with tetanus are numerous. Decubital ulcers may develop over bony prominences of recumbent dogs. These can be prevented by adequate cage padding and rotation of the animal every few hours. Fractures of the long bones, spine, or skull may result from trauma incurred during sudden muscular spasms or convulsions. Other problems include sepsis from IV catheterization and aspiration pneumonia from difficult swallowing. Esophageal hiatal hernia and megaesophagus may result in gastroesophageal reflex and regurgitation. Tracheostomy may be required if obstructive respiration develops from laryngeal spasm. Urinary and fecal retention occurs as a result of hypertonic anal and urethral sphincters. Repeated urinary catheterization may be needed if dysuria or reflex dyssynergia occurs. Simethicone, gastric intubation, and enemas may help relieve gas or obstipation. Hyperthermia from generalized muscle contractions may be controlled by parenteral fluids, fans, and application of alcohol to the footpads and pinnae.

Most dogs and cats have a self-limiting course of tetanus intoxication when rapid and appropriate therapy is instituted. Improvement after institution of treatment is usually noticeable within 1 week, and gradual but complete recovery is noted by 3 to 4 weeks.

PREVENTION

Active immunoprophylaxis with tetanus toxoid is not recommended for dogs and cats; it is used for more susceptible species such as humans and horses. Routine tetanus boosters or postexposure prophylaxis is not required. Appropriate care of infected wounds and rational antibiotic therapy should minimize the occurrence of tetanus. Epizootics have occurred in veterinary hospitals when sterilization of surgical instruments has not been adequate.

References

1. Abrutyn E, Berlin JA. 1991. Intrathecal therapy in tetanus. *JAMA* 266:2262–2267.
2. Bagley RS, Dougherty SA, Randolph JF. 1994. Tetanus subsequent to ovariohysterectomy in a dog. *Prog Vet Neurol* 5:63–65.
3. Dieringer TM, Wolf AM. 1991. Esophageal hiatal hernia and megaesophagus complicating tetanus in two dogs. *J Am Vet Med Assoc* 199:87–89.
4. Dolar D. 1992. The use of continuous atropine infusion in the management of severe tetanus. *Intensive Care Med* 18:26–31.
5. Ebisawa I, Takayanagi M, Kigawa M. 1988. Some factors affecting isolation of *Clostridium tetani* from human and animal stools. *Jpn J Exp Med* 58(6):233–241.
6. Edwards GT. 1989. Tetanus in the dog. *Vet Rec* 125:117.
7. Goodwin RLG. 1985. Tetanus in a cat. *Vet Rec* 116:574.
8. Greene CE. 1990. Tetanus, pp 521–529. *In* Greene CE (ed), Infectious diseases of the dog and cat. WB Saunders, Philadelphia, PA.
9. Lee EA, Jones BR. 1996. Localized tetanus in two cats after ovariohysterectomy. *N Z Vet J* 44:105–108.
10. Malik R, Church DB, Maddison JE, et al. 1989. Three cases of localized tetanus. *J Small Anim Pract* 30:469–473.
11. Mason JH. 1994. Tetanus in the dog and cat. *J S Afr Vet Med Assoc* 35:109–113.
12. Quinio B, Arnaud S, Viviand X, et al. 1992. Dantrolene intraveineux dans le traitement du tetanos. *Presse Med* 21(4):176.
13. Saissy JM, Demaziere J, Vitris M, et al. 1992. Treatment of severe tetanus by intrathecal injections of baclofen without artificial ventilation. *Intensive Care Med* 18:241–244.
14. Sanford JP. 1995. Tetanus—forgotten but not gone. *N Engl J Med* 332:812–813.
15. Sternlo JE, Andersen LW. 1990. Early treatment of mild tetanus with dantrolene. *Intensive Care Med* 16:345–346.
16. Stolleywirth U, Kriegerhuber S. 1993. Tetanus in the dog—a rare case in small animal practice. *Praktische Tierarztl* 74:455–456.
17. Sutton DN, Tremlett MR, Woodcock TE, Nielsen MS. 1990. Management of autonomic dysfunction in severe tetanus: the use of magnesium sulphate and clonidine. *Intensive Care Med* 16:75–80.
18. Van Ham L, Van Bree H. 1992. Conservative treatment of tetanus associated with hiatus hernia and gastroesophageal reflux. *J Small Anim Pract* 33:289.
19. Vitris M, Saissy JM, Demaziere J, et al. 1991. Traitement du tetanos severe par injections intrathecales iteratives de baclofene. *Dekar Med* 36(1):28–29.

Chapter 44

Leptospirosis

Craig E. Greene, Meri A. Miller, and Cathy A. Brown

ETIOLOGY

Leptospirosis, a zoonotic disease of worldwide significance in many animals, is caused by infection with antigenically distinct serovars of the parasitic species *Leptospira interrogans sensu lato,* of which at least eight are of most importance for dogs and cats. The genus has been classified into new species on the basis of genetic relatedness (Table 44–1). Serovars are maintained in nature by numerous subclinically infected wild and domestic animal reservoir hosts that serve as a potential source of infection and illness for humans and other incidental animal hosts. When infected, incidental hosts develop more severe clinical illness and shed organisms for shorter periods. Epidemiologic studies have shown that host preferences can change with time and geographic region of the world.

Leptospires are thin, flexible, filamentous (0.1–0.2 μm wide × 6–12 μm long) bacteria made up of fine spirals with hook-shaped ends (Fig. 44–1). They are composed of a protoplasmic cylinder that is wound around a straight central axial filament. The outer envelope is composed of lipopolysaccharide and antigenic mucopeptide. Leptospires are motile, making writhing and flexing movements while rotating along their long axis.

The most commonly incriminated serovars in canine leptospirosis have been canicola, icterohaemorrhagiae, grippotyphosa, pomona, and bratislava.[10, 20, 36, 44, 44a, 46] The current bivalent canine *Leptospira* vaccines, which are serovar specific, protect against clinical disease associated with serovars canicola and icterohaemorrhagiae. In the United States, the incidence of disease attributed to these serovars has decreased, whereas serologic evidence of more common infection with serovars grippotyphosa, pomona, and bratislava has increased.[11, 20, 34, 41, 44, 46] The prominence of these latter serovars stems from the use of vaccination and the greater exposure of unnatural hosts such as dogs to wildlife reservoir hosts in rural or suburban environments. The duration of shedding and potential spread of these serovars to other dogs or people is uncertain. In serologic surveys, the prevalence of seroreactivity is greater than that of clinical disease, suggesting that subclinical infections occur. In other areas, the prevalence of seroreactivity is low.[35] Despite the presence of leptospiral antibody titers in the feline population, clinical reports of leptospirosis in cats are infrequent. Although cats

***Table 44–1. Range for Common Serovars of* Leptospira interrogans sensu lato *Infecting Animals*[a]**

SPECIES SELECTED SEROVARS[b]	KNOWN PRIMARY RESERVOIR HOSTS	INCIDENTAL HOSTS: Dog	Cat	Human	Other Domesticated Animals	Representative Wild Animals
L. interrogans sensu stricto						
bratislava	Rat, pig, horse?	+	–	+	Cow, horse	Mouse, raccoon, opossum, hedgehog, vole, fox, skunk, bandicoot, weasel, nutria
autumnalis	Mouse	+	–	+	Cow	Rat, raccoon, opossum, bandicoot
icterohaemorrhagiae	Rat	+	+	+	Cow, horse, pig, cavy[c]	Mouse, raccoon, opossum, hedgehog, fox, woodchuck, nutria, ape, skunk, civet, muskrat, mongoose
pomona	Cow, pig, skunk, opossum	+	+	+	Horse, sheep, goat, rabbit, cavy	Mouse, raccoon, hedgehog, wolf, fox, woodchuck, vole, sea lion, deer, civet
canicola	Dog	+	+	+	Cow, horse, pig	Rat, raccoon, hedgehog, armadillo, mongoose, bandicoot, nutria, vole, jackal, skunk
bataviae	Dog, rat, mouse	+	+	+	Cow	Hedgehog, vole, armadillo, bandicoot, shrew, leopard cat
hardjo	Cow	+	–	+	Pig, horse, sheep	Wild bovidae
L. kirschneri						
grippotyphosa	Vole, raccoon, skunk, opossum	+	+	+	Cow, pig, sheep, goat, rabbit, gerbil, cavy	Mouse, rat, fox, bandicoot, squirrel, bobcat, shrew, hedgehog, muskrat, weasel, mole, leopard cat

[a]Classification based on Ramadass et al.[42]
[b]Less common serovars for dogs include hebdomadis, javanica, panama, pyrogenes, and tarassovi; and for cats, javanica and ballum.
[c]Guinea pig.

seroconvert after exposure to leptospires, they appear to be less susceptible than dogs to both spontaneous and experimental infections.[1, 13, 58]

EPIDEMIOLOGY

Leptospires are transmitted between animals by direct or indirect contact. Direct transmission occurs through contact with infected urine, venereal and placental transfer, bite wounds, or ingestion of infected tissues. Direct spread of infection is enhanced by crowding of animals as may occur in a kennel situation. Recovered dogs excrete organisms in urine intermittently for months after infection. Once outside the host, leptospires do not replicate. Indirect transmission occurs through exposure of susceptible animals to contaminated water sources, soil, food, or bedding. Although there is evidence that spirochetes survive in insects and other invertebrate hosts, the significance of this finding with regard to disease transmission is unknown. The indirect transmission of leptospires may increase when those environmental factors favoring the survival of leptospires are optimal.

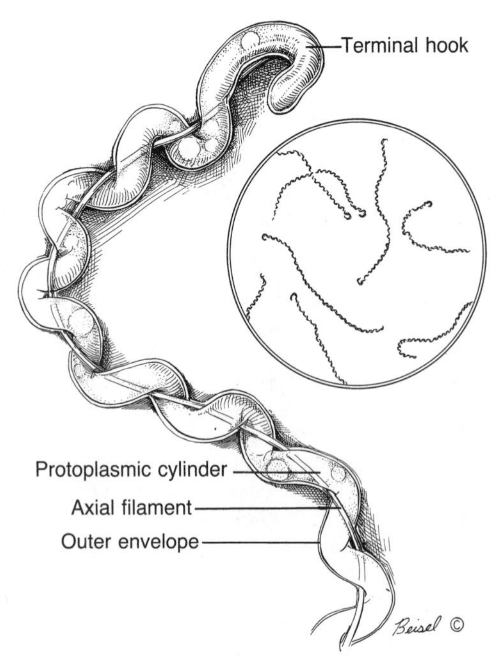

Figure 44–1. Ultrastructure of pathogenic leptospires.

Stagnant or slow-moving warm water, although not essential, provides a suitable habitat for spirochetes. Consequently, disease outbreaks often increase during periods of flooding. In arid areas or during drought conditions, infections of accidental hosts are more common around water sources. Optimum survival in soil is favored by a neutral or slightly alkaline pH. Spirochetes survive only transiently in undiluted acidic urine (pH 5.0–5.5), whereas the opposite conditions provide more suitable habitats. Ambient temperatures between 0° and 25°C favor the survival and replication of leptospires, whereas freezing markedly decreases survival. The temperature and pH requirements for maximal leptospiral survival may explain the apparent increased incidence of canine leptospirosis in the late summer and early fall[11, 34] and in the southern semitropical belt of the United States and similar climatic regions worldwide.

Although the prevalence of clinical leptospirosis in cats is low, they are probably exposed to leptospires excreted by wildlife. Outdoor cats have the highest seroprevalence. Serovars canicola, grippotyphosa, and pomona have been isolated from cats. Cats may also be exposed to urine of cohabitating dogs, and transmission from rodents carrying serovars ballum or icterohaemorrhagiae is suspected.

PATHOGENESIS

Leptospires penetrate mucous membranes or abraded skin and multiply rapidly upon entering the blood vascular space (Fig. 44–2). They then spread and further replicate in many tissues, including the kidney, liver, spleen, CNS, eyes, and

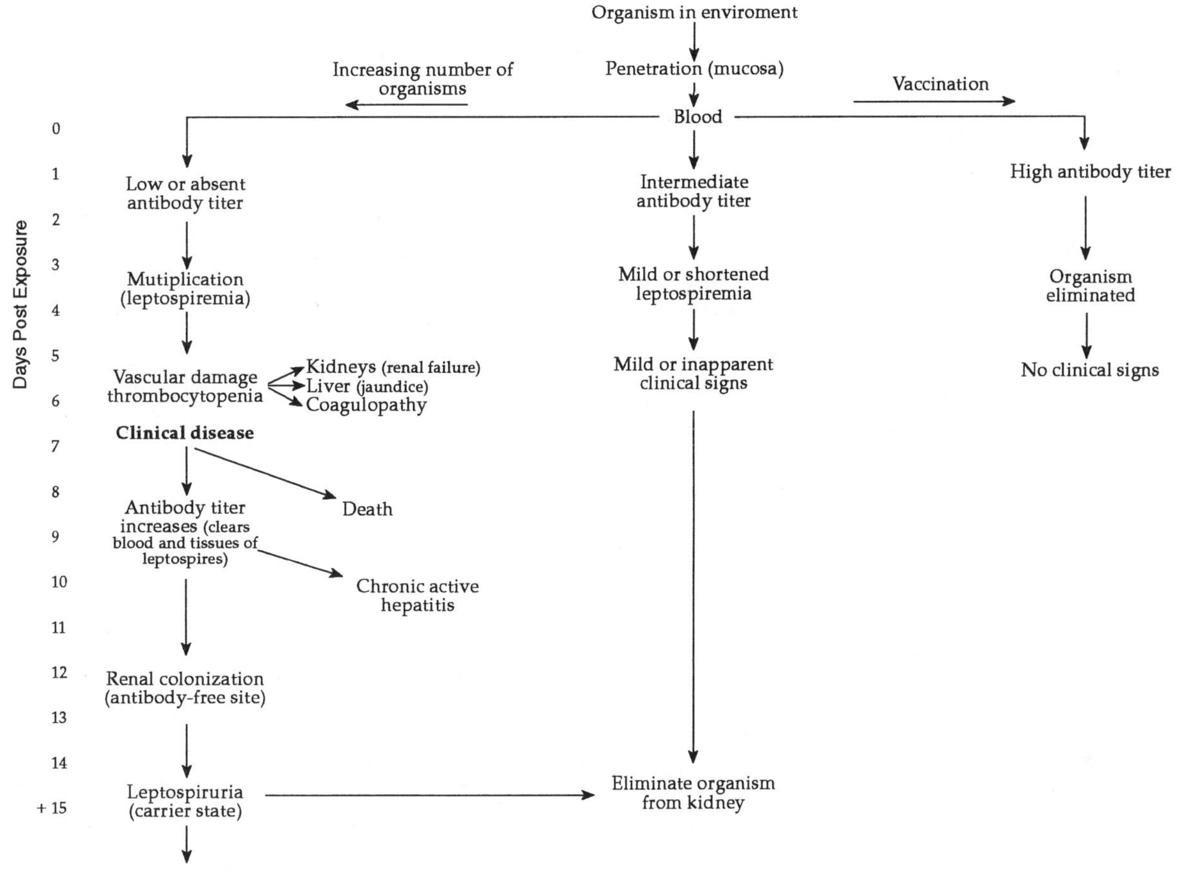

Figure 44–2. Pathogenesis of leptospirosis.

genital tract. Increases in serum antibodies thereafter clear the spirochetes from most organs, but organisms may persist in the kidney and be shed in urine for weeks to months. The extent of damage to internal organs is variable depending on the virulence of the organism and host susceptibility.[33] Certain serovars have the propensity to produce acute hemorrhagic, hepatic, or most commonly renal involvement. More than one form may occur in a given animal, and the clinical manifestations can vary among outbreaks and geographic areas with a given serovar.[11, 20, 44] Tissue edema and disseminated intravascular coagulation (DIC) may occur in rapid and severe infections that result in acute endothelial injury and hemorrhagic manifestations. *Leptospira* lipopolysaccharide stimulates neutrophil adherence and platelet activation,[22c] which may be involved in inflammatory and coagulatory abnormalities that occur.

Generally, infection of dogs with serovars canicola and grippotyphosa has been associated with predominantly renal dysfunction and with minimal liver involvement, whereas serovars icterohaemorrhagiae and pomona produce more hepatic disease. Younger dogs (< 6 months) seem to develop more signs of hepatic dysfunction in any disease outbreak.

Renal colonization occurs in most infected animals because the organism replicates and persists in renal tubular epithelial cells, even in the presence of serum neutralizing antibodies (Fig. 44–3). Acute impairment of renal function may result from decreased glomerular filtration caused by kidney swelling that impairs renal blood perfusion (Fig. 44–4).

Eventual recovery is dependent on increased specific antibody in the circulation within 7 to 8 days after infection. Those animals with adequate functional kidney tissue will recover. Pathologic changes will persist in the severely affected kidney tissue despite clinical improvement (Fig. 44–5). In surviving reservoir hosts, renal colonization will be long term, with shedding in urine for months to years. Although dogs are known to be persistent renal carriers of serovar

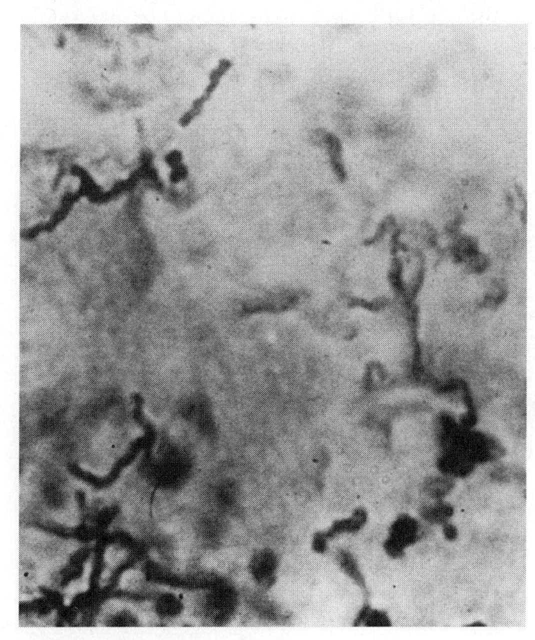

Figure 44–3. Leptospires in renal tubular epithelium from an infected dog (silver stain, × 1800).

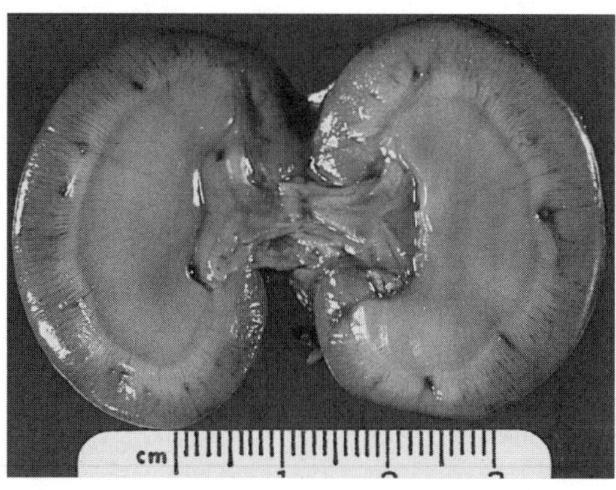

Figure 44–4. Swollen kidney from a dog that died of acute leptospirosis.

canicola, the duration of shedding of other serovars has not been determined.

The liver is the second major parenchymatous organ damaged during leptospiremia. Profound hepatic dysfunction may occur without major histologic changes because of subcellular damage produced by leptospiral toxins. The degree of icterus in both canine and human leptospirosis usually corresponds to the severity of hepatic necrosis. In contrast, icterus, hemoglobinemia, and hemoglobinuria that develop in cattle with leptospirosis result from a serovar-specific hemolytic toxin produced by serovar pomona. Decreased osmotic fragility has been detected in canine leptospirosis,[45] making hemolysis less likely.

Chronic active hepatitis has been a sequela to serovar grippotyphosa infection in dogs. Presumably, initial hepatocellular injury and persistence of the organism in the liver result in altered hepatic circulation, fibrosis, and immunologic disturbances that perpetuate the chronic inflammatory response. Extensive hepatic fibrosis and failure may result from this process.

Other body systems are damaged during the acute phase of infection. A benign meningitis is produced when leptospires invade the nervous system. Uveitis occasionally is present in naturally and experimentally occurring leptospirosis. Abortion or infertility resulting from transplacental transmission of leptospires associated with serovar bataviae infection has occurred in a dog.[18]

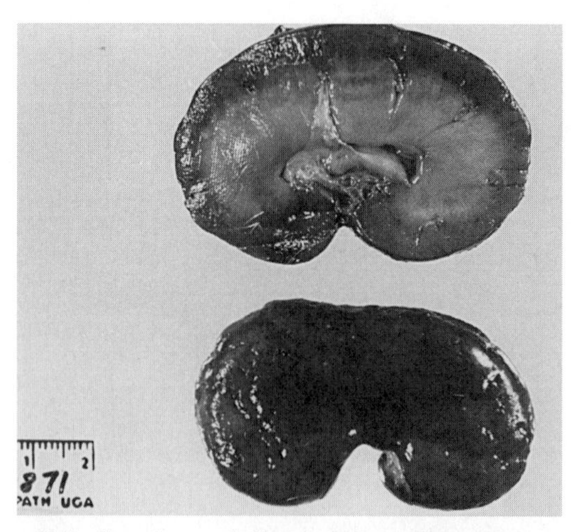

Figure 44–5. Shrunken and fibrotic kidneys from an 8-month-old puppy that had acute icterus and renal failure; the illness had been diagnosed as leptospirosis by serologic testing 5 months previously. The dog was clinically normal until the time of death.

CLINICAL FINDINGS

Dog

Clinical signs in canine leptospirosis depend on age and immunity of the host, environmental factors affecting the organisms, and virulence of the infecting serovar (Table 44–2). Young animals are more severely affected than are adults. Large breed (> 15 kg), outdoor, adult dogs are the most commonly affected.[34] Peracute leptospiral infections can be manifested by massive leptospiremia and death with few premonitory signs. In acute infections, pyrexia (39.5–40°C [103–104°F]), shivering, and generalized muscle tenderness are the first clinical signs. Subsequently, vomiting, rapid dehydration, and peripheral vascular collapse occur. Tachypnea, rapid and irregular pulse, and poor capillary perfusion have been noted. Coagulation defects and vascular injury are apparent with hematemesis, hematochezia, melena, epistaxis, and widespread petechiae. Terminally ill dogs become depressed and hypothermic, and renal and hepatic failure does not have time to develop.

Subacute infections are characterized by fever, anorexia, vomiting, dehydration, and increased thirst. Reluctance to move and paraspinal hyperesthesia in dogs may result from muscular, meningeal, or renal inflammation. Mucous membranes appear injected, and petechial and ecchymotic hemorrhages are widespread. Conjunctivitis, rhinitis, and tonsillitis are usually accompanied by coughing and dyspnea. Progressive deterioration in renal function is manifest by oliguria or anuria. Renal function in some dogs surviving subacute infections may return to normal within 2 to 3 weeks, or chronic compensated polyuric renal failure may develop.

Icterus is more common in dogs affected with the acute form of the disease. Intrahepatic cholestasis from hepatic inflammation may be so complete that fecal color changes

Table 44–2. Historic and Physical Exam Findings of Leptospirosis in Dogs

	SEROREACTIVITY (%)		
CLINICAL SIGN	Predominantly Serovar Grippotyphosa[34] (n = 44[a])	Predominantly Serovars Pomona and Grippotyphosa[20] (n = 17)	Predominantly Serovar Pomona[44] (n = 17)
Lethargy and depression	86	88	88
Anorexia	82	65	88
Vomiting	68	70	88
Fever	52	6	59
Weight loss	41	18	29
PU/PD	39	18	35
Abdominal or lumbar pain	39	35	29
Stiffness, arthralgia, myalgia	27	24	41
Renomegaly	27	0	18
Diarrhea	23	6	24
Icterus	9	24	0
Oculonasal discharge	7	NR	18
Petechiae	5	0	0
Posterior paresis, weakness	NR	NR	24
Labored respiration, cough	NR	NR	18

[a]Includes cases reported by Brown et al.[11]
NR = No data reported.
PU/PD = polyuria/polydypsia.

from brown to gray. Dogs with chronic active hepatitis or chronic hepatic fibrosis as a sequela to leptospirosis may eventually demonstrate overt signs of liver failure, including chronic inappetence, weight loss, ascites, icterus, or hepatoencephalopathy.

Intestinal intussusceptions occur with some frequency in dogs with acute infections presumably associated with GI inflammation. Careful abdominal palpation should be performed in dogs that develop persistent vomiting and diarrhea. Feces becomes scanty in such cases, and hematochezia or melena will be apparent.

Pulmonary manifestations include labored respiration and coughing.[44] Interstitial pneumonia has been documented as the cause in people,[22a] but this problem has not been well studied in dogs.

A majority of leptospiral infections in dogs are chronic or subclinical.[47] Serologic and microbiologic evaluation for leptospirosis should be performed on dogs with fever of unknown origin, unexplained renal or hepatic disease, or anterior uveitis and on healthy dogs in kennels, multidog households, neighborhoods, or other environs where infection in other members has been documented.

Cat

Clinical signs are usually mild or inapparent in feline leptospirosis despite the presence of leptospiremia and leptospiruria and histologic evidence of renal and hepatic inflammation.

DIAGNOSIS

Clinical Laboratory Findings

Hematologic findings in typical cases of canine leptospirosis include leukocytosis and thrombocytopenia. Leukocyte counts fluctuate depending on the stage and severity of infection. Leukopenia, common in the leptospiremic phase, develops into leukocytosis with a left shift. In later stages, WBC counts usually range from 16,500 to 45,000 cells/μl. A majority of dogs with leptospirosis have renal failure on initial examination.

Serum urea and creatinine increases are found in dogs with varying severity of renal failure (Table 44–3). Electrolyte alterations usually parallel the degree of renal and GI dysfunction. Hyponatremia, hypochloremia, hypokalemia, and hyperphosphatemia are present in most cases, whereas hyperkalemia and hyperglycemia develop in those with terminal renal failure. Mild hypocalcemia is related to hypoalbuminemia and decreased concentration of the protein-bound calcium fraction. Blood pH and serum bicarbonate concentration are reduced in severely affected animals, reflecting metabolic acidosis. Hypoglycemia is occasionally present with severe hepatic failure. Hepatic dysfunction may be apparent in some dogs but it usually is less dramatic than renal failure or is associated with concurrent renal failure. Liver damage is demonstrated by increased serum alanine aminotransferase (ALT), aspartate aminotransferase, lactate dehydrogenase, and alkaline phosphatase (ALP) activities and bilirubin concentration. The increase in serum ALP activity is often proportionally greater than that of ALT activity. Marked bilirubinuria usually precedes hyperbilirubinemia. Serum bilirubin peaks by days 6 to 8 after onset of disease. Increased sulfobromophthalein retention (>5%) can be found in acute leptospirosis before the onset of icterus and in dogs that later develop chronic active hepatitis. Increased serum amylase and lipase activities may result from their release from inflamed hepatic and small intestinal tissues and from decreased renal excretion. Dogs with intussusception have the highest serum amylase concentrations. Serum creatine kinase activity is increased when skeletal muscle inflammation occurs. Urinalysis can be characterized by glucosuria, tubular proteinuria, and bilirubinuria and by increased numbers of granular casts, leukocytes, and erythrocytes in the sediment. Leptospires will not be observed without special staining or microscopy.

Table 44–3. Serum Chemical Abnormalities in Dogs With Serologically Confirmed Leptospirosis

SERUM BIOCHEMICAL ALTERATION	PERCENTAGE WITH ABNORMALITIES		
	Miller[34] (n = 36)	Harkin & Gartrell[20] (n = 17)	Rentko et al[44] (n = 17)
Azotemia	94	82	100
Increased creatinine	94	82	100
Hypoalbuminemia	11	NR	18
Hypocalcemia	19	NR	29
Hypercalcemia	14	NR	0
Hyperphosphatemia	83	47	59
High ALP	33	65	59
High ALT	22	35	35
Hyperbilirubinemia	17	47	24
Hyponatremia	14	NR	18
Hypernatremia	3	NR	0
Hypokalemia	14	NR	18
Hyperkalemia	14	NR	18
Hypochloridemia	14	NR	29
Hyperchloridemia	3	NR	6

NR = no data reported; ALP = alkaline phosphatase; ALT = alanine aminotransferase.

Thrombocytopenia and increased fibrinogen degradation products have been found in dogs experimentally infected with serovar icterohaemorrhagiae. In a majority of dogs, other clotting parameters are normal, suggesting compensated hemostatic mechanisms. Severely affected dogs frequently have vascular endothelial damage with hypofibrinogenemia and thrombocytopenia resulting from DIC. With meningitis, increased protein concentration with a predominance of neutrophils can be detected by CSF analysis.

Serologic Testing

Because the microscopic agglutination (MA) test, the standard serologic means to diagnose leptospirosis, requires dark-field microscopy, samples must be sent to commercial laboratories. Organisms grown in liquid media are exposed to serial dilutions of the patient's sera. The end-point is the highest serum dilution that causes 50% of the organisms to agglutinate. It is somewhat serovar specific, so that numerous antigens must be used to identify the serovar causing disease. Sera are usually screened at an initial dilution of 1:100. Further twofold dilutions are done against positive-reacting antigens to determine which antibody is present in highest concentration. The report to the veterinarian will list the various serovars tested and the respective titers. Dogs with positive titers generally have sera that cross-react to a variety of serovars; that with the highest titer is interpreted as the infecting one, and lower titers represent antibody cross-reactivity between serovars. For example, in dogs naturally and experimentally infected with serovar grippotyphosa, the highest titer is against this serovar with lower titers to serovars pomona and bratislava.[11]

Demonstration of a fourfold rise in MA titer is classically required for serologic confirmation of an acute, potentially self-limiting disease such as leptospirosis. Many naturally infected dogs will have titers of 800 or greater, which on a single specimen is presumptive of leptospirosis with compatible clinical illness and knowledge of no recent vaccinations. Because titers can be negative in the first week to ten days of acute illness, a second and sometimes a third serum sample should be obtained within 2- to 4-week intervals. Other affected dogs will have high (≥1600–12,800) titers when they are hospitalized, with no further increases noted. The magnitude of rise in titer does not always parallel the severity of clinical illness. In kenneled foxhounds screened serologically for serovar grippotyphosa, highest titers (≥6400) were found in those dogs that were azotemic, suggesting persistence and replication of the organism.[11] Previous infection or vaccination is usually associated with a titer of less than 300, although high titers are occasionally observed. If higher vaccination titers (≥800) to serovars canicola and icterohaemorrhagiae develop, they generally do not persist for longer than 3 months. Dogs infected with serovar canicola, to which they are well adapted, may be actively infected and excreting organisms with titers less than 100. Antimicrobial therapy very early in the course of disease may decrease the magnitude of the titer rise. Antibody titers will often reduce fourfold over weeks to months after successful antimicrobial therapy of established infections.[20] Antibodies to leptospiral antigens used in the MA test may indicate some exposure to infection with nonleptospiral spirochetes. Dogs exposed to ticks harboring *Borrelia burgdorferi* that developed high titers to that organism did not show significant increases in titers on the MA test.[50] In contrast, leptospiral infections can affect serotest results for borreliosis (see Diagnosis, Chapter 45).

ELISA has been used in dogs to detect IgG or IgM antibodies to leptospires.[18, 59] In comparison, the MA titer appears to parallel the IgM titer more than the IgG titer, although both types of antibodies can cause agglutination. The IgM ELISA becomes increased within 1 week after initial infection, and the maximum titer develops within 14 days, with a subsequent decrease thereafter. The IgM ELISA appears to be more sensitive in detecting antibody and more serovar specific than the MA test for determining very early infection in dogs. Dogs that have died within the first week of illness have had high IgM titers, whereas the MA titer had not had time to increase.

In dogs, increased IgG ELISA titers develop 2 to 3 weeks after infection, with a maximum titer in approximately 1 month. IgG ELISA titers better parallel protection against infection than do MA titers. By using combined IgG and IgM measurements, the ELISA is better suited to distinguish between natural infection and vaccine-induced immunity than is the MA test. ELISA testing in dogs that have received more than one vaccination demonstrates a high IgG titer accompanied by a low or negative IgM titer, even within the first few weeks after vaccination. The ELISA is not widely available for clinical application. IgM ELISA tests have been adapted as a rapid assay system for utilization in human infections.[19]

Isolation

Proper timing and technique are essential for the recovery of leptospires because of their fastidious growth requirements and susceptibility to adverse environmental conditions. Samples should be taken before initiation of antibiotic therapy. Dogs are leptospiremic during the first week of infection, but the numbers of circulating organisms subsequently decrease as serum antibody titers increase. Occurrence of leptospires in CSF parallels that in blood. Urine is the ideal fluid to be cultured thereafter; however, multiple sampling is required because of intermittent shedding of organisms. If animals are adequately hydrated, administration of a low dose of a diuretic such as furosemide (0.5 mg/kg) just before urine collection may facilitate recovery of organisms.

Premortem isolation is preferred because postmortem tissue contaminants will overgrow fastidious leptospires unless selective media are employed. A small volume of tissue (preferably liver or kidney) or body fluid for culture should be collected aseptically in a clean, sterile glass container. Catheterized or voided urine is frequently contaminated by normal flora that interfere with the growth of leptospires; therefore, cystocentesis is preferred. Inhibiting substances such as antibody in host tissues and fluids require dilution of the sample by at least 1:10 (vol/vol) with buffered saline, 1% bovine serum albumin, or culture medium. As an alternative, 0.25 to 0.5 ml of blood, urine, or CSF taken at the appropriate stage of infection can be directly inoculated into 7 to 10 ml of transport media. Blood should be anticoagulated with preservative-free heparin or sodium polyethylene sulfonate (as in blood culture bottles) for transport to the laboratory if it cannot be diluted immediately. Citrate anticoagulants should be avoided because they inhibit leptospires. Urine should be alkalinized to pH 8 or greater during transport because leptospires cannot survive acidic conditions for more than a few hours. Tissue or fluid samples, if shipped, should be kept in transport medium or on ice but not frozen. For research purposes, organisms can be frozen in semisolid or transport media and stored at temperatures of −60°C to −70°C for up to 6 years before culture.

Media for isolation of leptospires are liquid, semisolid, or solid in nature. Ellinghausen, McCullough, Johnson, Harris (EMJH) is a liquid or semisolid medium containing polysorbate 80 and fetal calf serum or bovine serum albumin. Modification of standard medium by adding antibiotics or 5-fluorouracil has produced improved results in isolation of certain leptospiral serovars. Leptospires commonly lose their virulence on culture in artificial media, but this loss can be reversed by passage in susceptible animals. Culture of spirochetes from tissues or body fluids is not by itself diagnostic of clinical illness because leptospires can be recovered from both fluids and tissues of healthy dogs.[4]

Organism Identification

Dark-field examination is necessary for rapid identification of viable leptospires, because they cannot be stained by simple methods with aniline dyes. Wet-mount preparations are also necessary to help characterize their writhing and flexing movements. A variety of bacteria that can be confused with leptospires produce more random movement in wet-mount preparations. Cellular fibrils or extrusions and fibrin strands can be mistaken for organisms. Dark-field microscopy can also fail to detect active infections because approximately 10^5 organisms/ml are required.[9] Centrifugation can be used to concentrate specimens. Because of the inaccuracies of dark-field examination, it should always be followed by cultural or serologic procedures.

Leptospires can be seen by light microscopy in tissue sections or on air-dried smears with Giemsa stain or silver impregnation (see Fig. 44–3).

FA techniques have been adapted to identify leptospiral serovars in tissues imprints of liver and kidney and in body fluids such as blood or urine. FA testing can be used as a screening method to identify animals shedding organisms in urine when culture is impossible or too time consuming. Generally, available conjugates do not discriminate among serovars. Leptospires have been detected in biologic fluids by the very sensitive method of DNA hybridization.

Agglutination-adsorption techniques have been employed in specialized laboratories to serotype isolates. Restriction endonuclease analysis has been shown to be a sensitive and accurate taxonomic means when compared with serotyping. Polymerase chain reaction (PCR) and genetic probes have been used to detect leptospires in blood, CSF, aqueous humor, and urine.[7, 31] Because of higher concentration of leptospires in urine, testing that fluid is most sensitive. Quality control is essential to ensure the accuracy of genetic detection methods.

PATHOLOGIC FINDINGS

External gross lesions vary greatly depending on the severity of the disease, and they may include injected and icteric mucous membranes with diffuse petechiae. Focal ulcerations may be seen on the tongue and in the buccal cavity and are likely secondary to uremia. Tonsillar or lymphoid tissue enlargement may be present. Kidneys are enlarged in animals that die of acute infection. They are pale and yellow-gray in color and bulge on the cut surface (see Fig. 44–4). The renal capsule may be adherent to the surface of the kidneys, and subcapsular hemorrhages are common. In less acute cases, focal, white spotting may be seen in the renal cortex on cut sections and is most prominent along the corticomedullary junction. Leptospires can be cultured from macerated kidney tissue. More commonly, with serovar icterohaemorrhagiae infection, the respiratory tract may be edematous with pulmonary congestion, and spotty, diffuse, pneumonic infiltrates may be present. Petechial and ecchymotic hemorrhages are commonly found on the pleural surface (Fig. 44–6). With hepatic involvement, the liver is enlarged and friable, with pronounced interlobar markings and yellow-brown discoloration. Petechiae and ecchymoses are found throughout the leptomeninges. Ulcerative and hemorrhagic gastritis is often present in uremic animals.

Necrosis and hemorrhage are occasionally present in the bowel with intestinal intussusceptions. Free blood or acholic feces may be found in the colon and rectum of some animals. The spleen may be pale and shrunken.

Histologically, there is a diffuse interstitial inflammatory infiltrate, which is most severe at the corticomedullary junctions. The infiltrate is composed primarily of plasma cells, with lesser numbers of lymphocytes and macrophages. Scattered neutrophils and necrotic epithelial cells are often present within tubular lumina. Kidneys of chronically affected animals have mild to diffuse lymphocytic infiltration, with randomly scattered macrophages. Special stains are needed to visualize leptospires in tissues. With silver staining, globular debris and intact spirochetes can be found in renal tubules. Immunohistochemical stains also facilitate their visualization. Unfortunately, despite the high specificity of this method, organisms are present in such low numbers to make this technique insensitive. Histologic changes in the lung consist of fibrinoid necrosis of blood vessels and perivascular, intra-alveolar, and subpleural hemorrhages. Mononuclear cell infiltrates surround thrombosed pulmonary vessels. Focal necrosis of hepatic parenchyma may be present. Hepatocytes are rounded, with pyknotic nuclei, and contain an eosinophilic granular cytoplasm. Intrahepatic bile stasis and severe hepatocellular injury are usually evident in icteric animals. The clinical severity of hepatic disease parallels the severity of histologic changes in the liver. Subclinical cases usually have mild fatty changes in hepatocytes, whereas moderately ill dogs have fragmented hepatic cords, with lymphocytic infiltrates in areas of necroses, and severely affected dogs have widespread necroses of hepatic parenchyma and disintegration of nuclei. Chronically infected dogs develop chronic active hepatitis and hepatic fibrosis. Organisms may be demonstrated in intercellular locations within hepatic cords.

Neurologic damage includes perivascular hemorrhage (uncommon in the cat), mononuclear cell infiltrate, and, occasionally, vascular thrombosis. When a silver stain is applied, leptospires can be found in pericapillary areas. Although gross lesions are absent in the heart, focal lymphocytic myocarditis is evident on histologic examination.

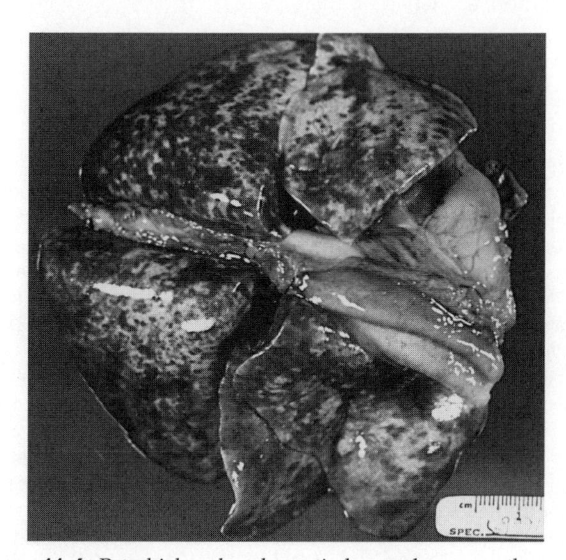

Figure 44–6. Petechial and ecchymotic hemorrhages on the serosal surfaces of the lungs from the dog in Figure 44–4.

THERAPY

Supportive therapy for animals with leptospirosis depends on the severity of infection and the presence of renal or hepatic dysfunction and other complicating factors. Dehydration and shock occur in severely affected animals. Fluid loss results from vomiting and diarrhea, and balanced polyionic IV fluids should be used to correct the deficits. Oral alimentation must be discontinued in vomiting animals. Petechial and ecchymotic hemorrhages indicate thrombocytopenia from vasculitis or DIC in severely affected animals. Plasma or fresh whole blood transfusions should be given, with caution and only with concurrent low-dose heparin, for ongoing DIC or severe hypoalbuminemia.

Oliguria (< 2 ml/kg/hr) and anuria are treated initially with rehydration. Osmotic diuretics, such as 10% glucose (5 ml/kg) or mannitol, should be given IV when impaired renal function persists after rehydration. If treatment with these diuretics fails, dopamine (5 μg/kg/min) may be administered by IV infusion. Tubular diuretics such as furosemide should be administered in conjunction with dopamine to increase urine flow; however, the effect on improving glomerular filtration is debated. It is essential that fluid therapy be adjusted to the individual patient's urine output. Peritoneal dialysis can be considered if oliguria persists, because acute renal dysfunction is potentially reversible. Predicting which dogs will respond to fluid diuresis is not always possible on the basis of laboratory values.

Antibiotics usually reduce fever and bacteremia within a few hours after administration. They immediately inhibit

Table 44–4. Recommended Therapy for Leptospirosis

DRUG	SPECIES	DOSE[a]	ROUTE	INTERVAL (HOURS)	DURATION (WEEKS)
Penicillin G	B	25,000–40,000 U/kg	IM, SC, IV	12	2
Ampicillin	B	22 mg/kg	PO, SC, IV	6–8	2
Amoxicillin	D	22 mg/kg	PO	8–12	2
Doxycycline[b]	D	5 mg/kg	PO, IV	12	2
Tetracycline[c]	B	22 mg/kg	PO	8	2
Erythromycin[d]	D	15–20 mg/kg	PO, IV	8–12	2

[a]Dose per administration at specified interval.
[b]Can be used as primary therapy or to clear renal carriers because excretion not affected by azotemia.
[c]Used to clear the renal carrier once azotemia has resolved. Repositol oxytetracycline (LA-200) has been used to treat large numbers of affected foxhounds at a dose of 20 mg/kg IM once weekly for 4 weeks.
[d]Efficacy of macrolides has not been well studied, although they have an appropriate spectrum. Other alternatives are azithromycin or clarithromycin. See Drug Formulary (Appendix 8) for additional information on these and the tabulated drugs.
B = dog and cat; D = dog.

multiplication of the organism and rapidly reduce fatal complications of infection such as hepatic and renal failure. Penicillin and its derivatives are the antibiotics of choice for terminating leptospiremia (Table 44–4), but they do not eliminate the carrier state. Initially, penicillin or ampicillin can be given parenterally to the vomiting, uremic, or hepatically compromised animal. Once oral alimentation is begun, oral therapy with amoxicillin is recommended because of its superior absorption. Other drugs such as the tetracyclines, aminoglycosides, erythromycins, or fluoroquinolones should be provided after therapy with the penicillins to eliminate the carrier state. Doxycycline can be used for initial therapy or for elimination of the carrier state. It can be given IV or PO depending on the animal's alimentation. The dose does not need to be adjusted in animals with renal failure because it is predominantly excreted in the feces. Aminoglycosides should never be given to clear the carrier state unless results of renal function tests have returned for reference range. In experimental studies in animals, ampicillin and cephalosporins were not effective in eliminating the organisms from tissues and body fluids, whereas tetracyclines and macrolides such as erythromycin and its derivatives were effective.[3] Ineffective drugs include cephalosporins, chloramphenicols, and sulfonamides. Ciprofloxacin is effective in vitro and in vivo against virulent strains of leptospires, but its clinical application has been limited.[49] Orbifloxacin at recommended dosages was not effective compared to oral amoxicillin in treating one dog.[17a]

PREVENTION

Prevention of leptospirosis involves elimination of the carrier state. Unfortunately, wild animal reservoirs and subclinically affected domestic animals continue to harbor and shed organisms. Control of rodents in kennels, maintenance of environmental conditions to discourage bacterial survival, and isolation of infected animals, therefore, are important to prevent spread of the disease. Doxycycline has been given at a low dose (200 mg once weekly) to humans in endemic areas for prophylaxis when vaccination with appropriate serovars is unavailable. Such therapy may result in development of bacterial resistance and is not recommended.

Bivalent bacterins that contain two main serovars, canicola and icterohaemorrhagiae, are available for dogs. Current vaccines are not cross-protective against other significant disease-causing serovars such as grippotyphosa, pomona, hardjo, and bratislava. As a result, serologic evidence for infection with these serovars has been relatively increased.[10, 41, 46] Currently marketed vaccines are chemically inactivated whole cultures, which makes them relatively allergenic in comparison with the tissue culture lines of virus vaccines (see Postvaccinal Complications, Chapter 100). Immunization has been effective in reducing the prevalence and severity of canine leptospirosis, but it does not prevent the carrier state, which is associated with potential zoonotic risk. Adequate initial immunization, employing many of the available products, takes three to four injections 2 to 3 weeks apart to produce immunity to challenge infection that will last 6 to 8 months. Newer vaccines, produced by growing leptospires in synthetic protein-free media, protected against postinfection shedding when dogs were challenged 2 to 4 weeks after two doses of vaccine.

Experimental vaccines have been produced from the outer envelope fraction of leptospires, which is the site of leptospiricidal activity of antibody and complement.[28] Antigenic material has been reduced by culture in a protein-free media, adjuvants have been removed, and up to five *Leptospira* serovars have been included in such vaccines. Maximal antibody titers have been produced in dogs within 2 weeks after a single vaccination, and dogs have been protected against infection and urinary shedding after challenge.

IgG titers, which are primarily responsible for protection, are produced for at least 1 year after the third vaccination in dogs. Because highest titers are produced by multiple injections, yearly (and sometimes biannual) vaccinations should be given to dogs in endemic areas, and all dogs should receive *at least three injections* in their primary vaccination series. For further guidelines concerning leptospirosis vaccination, see Chapter 100.

PUBLIC HEALTH CONSIDERATIONS

The majority of infections in people are among those who engage in water sports activities or who experience occupational exposure to wildlife or domestic animal hosts.[2, 8, 23, 48] In some outbreaks, simultaneous exposure of people and dogs can occur.[56] Contaminated urine is highly infectious for people and for susceptible animal species; therefore, contact with it on mucous membranes or skin abrasions should be avoided. Latex gloves should be worn when handling urine or urine-contaminated items. Face masks and goggles should be worn when hosing contaminated kennel areas. Canine infection and leptospiruria have been found in healthy vaccinated dogs with resultant development of the disease in people. All known or suspected shedders should be treated with aminoglycosides or tetracyclines. Areas contaminated by infected urine should be washed with detergent and then treated with iodophor disinfectants (see Chapter 94) to which the organism is very susceptible.

References

1. Agunloye CA, Nash AS. 1996. Investigation of possible leptospiral infection in cats in Scotland. *J Small Anim Pract* 37:126–129.
2. Alani FSS, Mahoney MP, Ormerod LP, et al. 1993. Leptospirosis presenting as atypical pneumonia, respiratory failure and pyogenic meningitis. *J Infect* 27:281–283.
3. Alt DP, Bolin CA. 1996. Preliminary evaluation of antimicrobial agents for treatment of *Leptospira interrogans* serovar pomona infection in hamsters and swine. *Am J Vet Res* 57:59–62.
4. Anderson JF, Miller DA, Post JE, et al. 1993. Isolation of *Leptospira interrogans* serovar grippotyphosa from the skin of a dog. *J Am Vet Med Assoc* 203:1550–1551.
5. Andre-Fontaine G, Ganiere JP. 1990. New topics on leptospirosis. *Comp Immunol Microbiol Infect Dis* 13:163–168.

5a. Andre-Fontaine G, Monfort P, Buggin-Daubie M, et al. 1995. Fatal disease mimicking leptospirosis in a dog caused by *Aeromonas hydrophila*. *Comp Immunol Microbiol Infect Dis* 18:69–72.

6. Arimitsu Y, Haritani K, Ishiguro N, et al. 1989. Detection of antibodies to leptospirosis in experimentally infected dogs using the microcapsule agglutination test. *Br Vet J* 145:356–361.
7. Bal AE, Gravekamp C, Hartskeerl RA, et al. 1994. Detection of leptospires in urine by PCR for early diagnosis of leptospirosis. *J Clin Microbiol* 32:1894–1898.
8. Belton DJ. 1993. An unusual human case of leptospirosis. *N Z Vet J* 41(1):45.
9. Bolin CA. 1996. Diagnosis of leptospirosis: a reemerging disease of companion animals. *Semin Vet Med Surg* 11:166–171.
10. Brown CA. 1997. Unpublished data, University of Georgia, Athens, GA.
11. Brown CA, Roberts AW, Miller MA, et al. 1996. *Leptospira interrogans* serovar grippotyphosa infection in dogs. *J Am Vet Med Assoc* 209:1265–1267.
12. Champagne MJ, Higgins R, Fairbrother JM, et al. 1991. Detection and characterization of leptospiral antigens using a biotin/avidin double-antibody sandwich enzyme-linked immunosorbent assay and immunoblot. *Can J Vet Res* 55:239–245.
13. Dickeson D, Love DN. 1993. A serological survey of dogs, cats and horses in south-eastern Australia for leptospiral antibodies. *Aust Vet J* 70:389–390.
14. Ellis WA, Montgomery JM, McParland PJ. 1989. An experimental study with a *Leptospira interrogans* serovar bratislava vaccine. *Vet Rec* 125:319–321.
15. Gerritsen MJ, Olyhoek T, Smits MA, et al. 1991. Sample preparation method for polymerase chain reaction-based semiquantitative detection of *Leptospira interrogans* serovar hardjo subtype hardjobovis in bovine urine. *J Clin Microbiol* 29:2805–2808.
16. Gitton X, Andre-Fontaine G, Andre F, et al. 1992. Immunoblotting study of the antigenic relationships among eight serogroups of *Leptospira*. *Vet Microbiol* 32:293–303.
17. Gitton X, Buggin Daubie M, Andre F, et al. 1994. Recognition of *Leptospira interrogans* antigens by vaccinated or infected dogs. *Vet Microbiol* 41:87–97.

17a. Greene CE. 1997. University of Georgia. Unpublished observations.

18. Greene CE, Shotts EB. 1990. Leptospirosis, pp 498–507. *In* Greene CE (ed), Infectious diseases of the dog and cat. WB Saunders, Philadelphia, PA.
19. Gussenhoven GC, Vanderhoorn MA, Goris MG, et al. 1997. Lepto dipstick, a dipstick assay for detection of *Leptospira*-specific immunoglobulin M antibodies in human sera. *J Clin Microbiol* 35:92–97.
20. Harkin KR, Gartrell CL. 1996. Canine leptospirosis in New Jersey and Michigan: 17 cases (1990–1995). *J Am Anim Hosp Assoc* 32:495–501.
21. Heath SE, Johnson R. 1994. Leptospirosis. *J Am Vet Med Assoc* 205:1518–1523.
22. Hilbink F, Penrose M, McSporran K. 1992. Antibodies in dogs against *Leptospira interrogans* serovars copenhageni ballum and canicola. *N Z Vet J* 40:123–125.

22a. Hill MK, Sanders CV. 1997. Leptospiral pneumonia. *Semin Respir Infect* 12:44–49.

22b. Hrinivich K, Prescott JF. 1997. Leptospirosis in 2 unrelated dogs. *Can Vet J* 38:509–510.

22c. Isogai E, Hirose K, Kimura K, et al. 1997. Role of platelet-activating factor (PAF) on cellular responses after stimulation with leptospire lipopolysaccharide. *Microbiol Immunol* 41:271–275.

23. Jackson LA, Kaufmann AF, Adams WG, et al. 1993. Outbreak of *Leptospira interrogans* serovar grippotyphosa associated with swimming. *Pediatr Infect Dis J* 12:48–54.
24. Kashiwase H, Ono E, Yanagawa R, et al. 1994. A neutral sugar is responsible for serovar specificity of the antigenic determinant of *Leptospira interrogans* serovar canicola. *Jpn J Vet Res* 42:103–108.
25. Kogika MM, Hagiwara MK, Baccaro MR. 1992. Metastatic calcification in a dog with leptospirosis. *Canine Pract* 17:35–38.
26. Kreisberg RA. 1993. Clinical problem-solving. *N Engl J Med* 329:413–416.
27. Lindenmayer J, Weber M, Bryant J, et al. 1990. Comparison of indirect immunofluorescent-antibody assay, enzyme-linked immunosorbent assay, and Western immunoblot for the diagnosis of Lyme disease in Dogs. *J Clin Microbiol* 28:92–96.
28. Masuzawa T, Suzuki R, Yanagihara Y. 1991. Comparison of protective effects with tetra-valent glycolipid antigens and whole cell-inactivated vaccine in experimental infection of *Leptospira*. *Microbiol Immunol* 35:199–208.
29. McCormick BM, Millar BD, Monckton RP, et al. 1989. Detection of leptospires in pig kidney using DNA hybridization. *Res Vet Sci* 47:134–135.
30. Merien F, Amouriaux P, Perolat P, et al. 1992. Polymerase chain reaction for detection of *Leptospira* spp. in clinical samples. *J Clin Microbiol* 30:2219–2224.
31. Merien F, Baranton G, Perolat P. 1995. Comparison of polymerase chain reaction with microagglutination test and culture for diagnosis of leptospirosis. *J Infect Dis* 172:281–285.
32. Merien F, Perolat P, Mancel E, et al. 1993. Detection of *Leptospira* DNA by polymerase chain reaction in aqueous humor of a patient with unilateral uveitis. *J Infect Dis* 168:1335–1336.
33. Midwinter A, Vinh T, Faine S, et al. 1994. Characterization of an antigenic oligosaccharide from *Leptospira interrogans* serovar pomona and its role in immunity. *Infect Immun* 62:5477–5482.
34. Miller MA. 1996. Unpublished data, compiled for clinical leptospirosis 1987–1996, University of Georgia, Athens, GA.
35. Myburgh JG, Posnett SJ, Lawrence JV. 1993. Serological survey for canine leptospirosis in the Pretoria area. *J S Afr Vet Assoc* 64:37–38.
36. Nielsen JN, Cochran GK, Cassells JA, et al. 1991. *Leptospira interrogans* serovar bratislava infection in two dogs. *J Am Vet Med Assoc* 199:351–352.
37. Pacciarini ML, Savio ML, Tagliabue S, et al. 1992. Repetitive sequences cloned from *Leptospira interrogans* serovar hardjo genotype hardjoprajitno and their application to serovar identification. *J Clin Microbiol* 30:1243–1249.
38. Poncelet L, Fontaine M, Balligand M. 1991. Polymyositis associated with *Leptospira australis* infection in a dog. *Vet Rec* 129:40.
39. Pope V, Johnson RC. 1991. Effect of heat or formalin treatment of leptospires on antibody response detected by immunoblotting. *J Clin Microbiol* 29:1548–1550.
40. Prescott JF. 1991. Treatment of leptospirosis. *Cornell Vet* 81:7–12.
41. Prescott JF, Ferrier RL, Nicholson VM, et al. 1991. Is canine leptospirosis underdiagnosed in southern Ontario? A case report and serological survey. *Can Vet J* 32:481–486.
42. Ramadass P, Jarvis BDW, Corner RJ, et al. 1992. Genetic characterization of pathogenic *Leptospira* species by DNA hybridization. *Int J Syst Bacteriol* 42:215–219.
43. Raoult D, Bres P, Baranton G. 1989. Serologic diagnosis of leptospirosis: comparison of line blot and immunofluorescence techniques with the genus-specific microscopic agglutination test. *J Infect Dis* 160:734–735.

43a. Reilly GA, Bailic NL, Morrow WT, et al. 1994. Feline stillbirths associated with mixed *Salmonella typhimurium* and leptospira infection. *Vet Rec* 135:608.

44. Rentko VT, Clark N, Ross LA, et al. 1992. Canine leptospirosis: a retrospective study of 17 Cases. *J Vet Intern Med* 6:235–244.

44a. Rubel D, Seijo A, Cernigoi B, et al. 1997. *Leptospira interrogans* in a canine population of Greater Buenos Aires: variables associated with seropositivity. *Rev Panam Salud Publica* 2:102–105.

45. Santoro ML, Kogika MM, Hagiwara MK, et al. 1994. Decreased erythrocyte osmotic fragility during canine leptospirosis. *Rev Inst Med Trop São Paulo* 36:1–5.
46. Scanziani E, Calcaterra S, Tagliabue S, et al. 1994. Serological findings in cases of acute leptospirosis in the dog. *J Small Anim Pract* 35:257–260.
47. Scanziani E, Crippa L, Giusti AM, et al. 1995. *Leptospira interrogans* serovar sejroe infection in a group of laboratory dogs. *Lab Anim* 29:300–306.
48. Schmidt DR, Winn RE, Keefe TJ. 1989. Leptospirosis: epidemiological features of a sporadic case. *Arch Intern Med* 149:1878–1880.
49. Shalit I, Barnea A, Shahar A. 1989. Efficacy of ciprofloxacin against *Leptospira interrogans* serogroup icterohaemorrhagiae. *Antimicrob Agents Chemother* 33:788–789.
50. Shin SJ, Chang YF, Jacobson RH, et al. 1993. Cross-reactivity between *Borrelia burgdorferi* and other spirochetes affects specificity of serotests for detection of antibodies to the Lyme disease agent in dogs. *Vet Microbiol* 36:161–164.
51. Songer JG, Thiermann AB. 1988. Leptospirosis. *J Am Vet Med Assoc* 193:1250–1254.
52. Stamm LV, Gherardini FC, Parrish EA, et al. 1991. Heat shock response of spirochetes. *Infect Immun* 59:1572–1575.
53. Stoianova NA, Semenovich VN, Sergeiko LM, et al. 1993. Dogs as the possible source of leptospirosis in people. *Zh Mikrobiol Epidemiol Immunobiol* Nov-Dec (6):46–48.
54. Van den Broek AH, Thrusfield MV, Dobbie GR, et al. 1991. A serological and bacteriological survey of leptospiral infection in dogs in Edinburgh and Glasgow. *J Small Anim Pract* 32:118–124.
55. Van Eys GJ, Gravekamp C, Gerritsen MJ, et al. 1989. Detection of leptospires in urine by polymerase chain reaction. *J Clin Microbiol* 27:2258–2262.
56. Venkataraman KS, Nedunchelliyan S. 1991. Leptospiral jaundice in dog: a case report. *Indian Vet J* 68:1171–1172.
57. Venkataraman KS, Nedunchelliyan S. 1992. Epidemiology of an outbreak of leptospirosis in man and dog. *Comp Immunol Microbiol Infect Dis* 15:243–247.
58. Watson AD. 1994. Leptospirosis in cats and dogs. *Aust Vet J* 71:59–60.
59. Weekes CC, Everard COR, Levett PN. 1997. Seroepidemiology of canine leptospirosis on the island of Barbados. *Vet Microbiol* 51:215–222.
60. Wohl JS. 1996. Canine leptospirosis. *Compend Cont Educ Pract Vet* 11:1215–1241.

Chapter 45

Lyme Borreliosis

Craig E. Greene, Max J. G. Appel, and Reinhard K. Straubinger

Lyme borreliosis is the most commonly diagnosed vector-borne disease in people. It has been reported from North America, Europe, and Asia. Unconfirmed accounts of the disease have been from Australia, South America, and Africa. This disease is one of a larger group of vector-borne borrelioses that affect mammalian and avian hosts (Table 45–1). Experimentally and spontaneously induced Lyme borreliosis has been described in dogs, cats, and other animals. Because of the difficulty in confirming a diagnosis and the diversity of borrelial species being isolated from ticks, controversy still exists regarding the exact prevalence and geographic distribution of infection.

ETIOLOGY

Like most spirochetes, *Borrelia* are small (0.2 × 30 μm), and dark-field or phase microscopy is needed for proper visualization of live organisms (Fig. 45–1). Isolates of *Borrelia burgdorferi sensu lato,* the causative agent of Lyme borreliosis, have been divided into at least four genomic species groups (see Table 45–1).[20, 36] Analysis of outer surface lipoproteins (Osp) such as OspA and OspB and of genetic and amino acid sequences have been used to subgroup the *Borrelia* spp. Group 1 (*B. burgdorferi sensu stricto*) is the primary isolate seen in the United States. In people, it is associated with annular skin lesions, polyarthritis, and meningitis. In Europe, groups 1, 2, and 3 have been isolated, with groups 2 (*B. garinii*) and 3 (*B. afzelii*) predominating. Meningopolyneuritis (Bannwarth's syndrome) is the primary clinical sign in people with group 2, whereas in Europe group 3 seropositivity has been associated with chronic arthritis and dermatitis (erythema chronicum migrans [ECM]).[31] A new species, *B. japonica* (group 4), has been isolated from ticks found on dogs and people in Japan,[7] and another, *B. andersonii,* has been found in ticks from rabbits in the northeastern United States. Other yet unidentified pathogenic and nonpathogenic strains of *Borrelia* exist.[91] A variant *Borrelia* species has been associated with ECM skin lesions in people in Missouri.[86] The differences in strains or species may account for the regional differences in clinical findings that have been reported.

On the basis of in vitro borreliacidal assay, North American and European isolates of *B. burgdorferi* are divided into at least five seroprotective groups.[75] Although North American isolates have been thought to be more homogeneous than European strains, United States isolates have substantial genetic heterogeneity with regional differences.[88] Many sylvan foci of enzootic infection exist worldwide in wildlife and their associated tick vectors. Clinical disease in people or domestic animals results when stages of ticks feeding on wildlife reservoirs have an affinity for alternate hosts. Breitschwerdt and coworkers[16] described a previously unrecognized borrelial species from dogs in Florida that had visible spirochetemia.

Table 45–1. Borrelial Species of Medical and Veterinary Importance

SPECIES	DISEASE	GEOGRAPHIC LOCATION	VECTOR	WILD ANIMAL RESERVOIR	DOMESTIC HOSTS
B. recurrentis	Epidemic louse borne relapsing fever	Central and East Africa, South America	*Pediculus humanus* (body louse)	None	Human
B. anserina	Avian spirochetosis	Worldwide	*Argas persicus*	Birds	Poultry
B. hermsii, B. turicatae, B. parkeri	Endemic tick-borne relapsing fevers, visible spirochetemia	North America			
B. persica		Asia	*Ornithodoros* spp.	Rodents, small mammals	Human
B. hispanica		Spain			
B. duttonii		East Africa			
B. coriaceae	Enzootic abortion	Western United States	*O. coriaceus*	Deer	Cow
B. burgdorferi sensu lato	Lyme borreliosis, annular skin				
B. burgdorferi sensu stricto (group 1)	lesions (ECM), polyarthritis, meningitis	North America, Europe	*Ixodes ricinus, I. scapularis, I. pacificus*	Larvae & nymphs: rodents, small mammals	Human, dog, cat
B. garinii (group 2)	Meningopolyneuritis, arthritis	Europe, Asia	*I. ricinus, I. persulcatus*	Adults: deer, larger	Humans, dog?,
B. afzelii (group 3)	Chronic dermatitis	Europe, Asia	*I. ricinus, I. persulcatus*	mammals	cat?
B. japonica (group 4)	Arthritis	Japan	*I. persulcatus*		
Borrelia sp.	Visible spirochetemia, lymphadenomegaly, lameness, anterior uveitis, fever	Florida	Unknown	Unknown	Dog

ECM = erythema chronicum migrans.

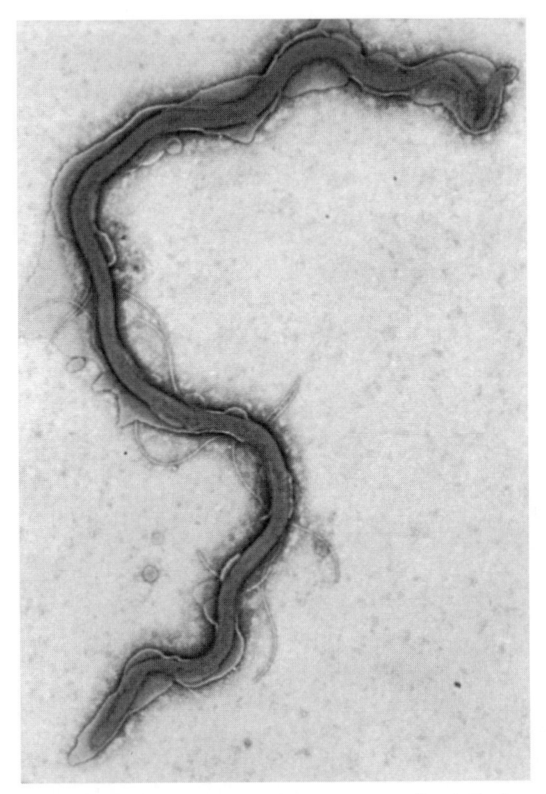

Figure 45–1. Transmission electron micrograph of *B. burgdorferi* showing periplasmic flagella that have been released from the confines of the outer membrane secondary to specimen preparation (phosphotungstic acid, × 7100).

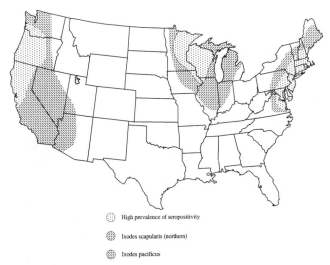

Figure 45–2. In the United States, Lyme borreliosis has been reported to occur in people in a majority of states on the basis of seropositivity. Less is known of the seroprevalence and frequency of canine infections with *B. burgdorferi*. The lighter shaded areas are regions where the highest prevalence of seropositivity have been reported. The dark, superimposed shaded areas show the known geographic distribution of the respective tick vectors.

EPIDEMIOLOGY

Unlike *Leptospira*, the species of *Borrelia* do not survive free living in the environment. They are host associated, being transmitted between vertebrate reservoir hosts and hematophagous arthropod vectors. Those *Borrelia* causing relapsing fevers have limited host ranges and vectors, whereas *B. burgdorferi sensu lato* is more dispersed geographically (see Table 45–1). Within Canada, Lyme borreliosis is endemic in southeastern Ontario. Within the United States, it has been reported in people in 48 states; however, approximately 85% of cases have been from eastern coastal states from Massachusetts to Virginia, 10% were from the upper Midwest (Wisconsin and Minnesota), and 4% were from northern California (Fig. 45–2). Although 1% of the reports have occurred in other states, the organism has never been cultured from people or dogs outside the just-mentioned endemic areas.

The principal vectors of *B. burgdorferi sensu lato* are various species of hard ticks of the *Ixodes ricinus* complex, whose distribution is associated with the prevalence of disease (Table 45–2). *I. ricinus* and *I. persulcatus* are the primary vectors in Europe and Eurasia, respectively. In the United States closely related black-legged ticks, *I. scapularis* (Northeast, Midwest, and Southeast) and *I. pacificus* (West) appear to be involved. There are differences in the northern and southern populations of *I. scapularis* that influence the prevalence of disease in these respective areas. *I. scapularis* in the Northeast has been previously designated *I. dammini*. Debate continues over whether it is distinct from *I. scapularis*.

***Table 45–2. Selected Vectors of* Borrelia burgdorferi**[a]

		FEEDING PREFERENCE		
SPECIES	GEOGRAPHIC LOCATION	Larvae, Nymphs	Adults	Infection Prevalence
Northern *Ixodes scapularis* (previously *I. dammini*)	United States (New England, northern Midwest)	White-footed mouse (*Peromyscus leucopus*), small mammals, birds	Deer, larger mammals	< 1% larvae 10–25% nymphs 10–50% adults
Southern *I. scapularis*	United States (southeastern)	Lizards	Lizards (occas. mammals)	< 1% larvae <1 % nymphs < 1% adults
I. pacificus	United States (western)	Lizards	Lizards (occas. mammals)	1–5%
I. ricinus	Europe (western and central)	Small mammals, birds, mouse (*Apodemus flavicollis, A. sylvaticus, Clethrionomys glareolus*)	Deer, larger mammals	10–25%
I. persulcatus	Eurasia, Soviet Republics	Small mammals, birds	Deer, larger mammals	10–25%

[a]*B. burgdorferi* or related organisms have been recovered from numerous other ticks and arthropods in nature, but the significance is uncertain. Many sylvan cycles exist in nature in which tick vectors do not feed on large mammals. Only the established vectors for human or domestic animals are listed here.
occas. = occasionally.

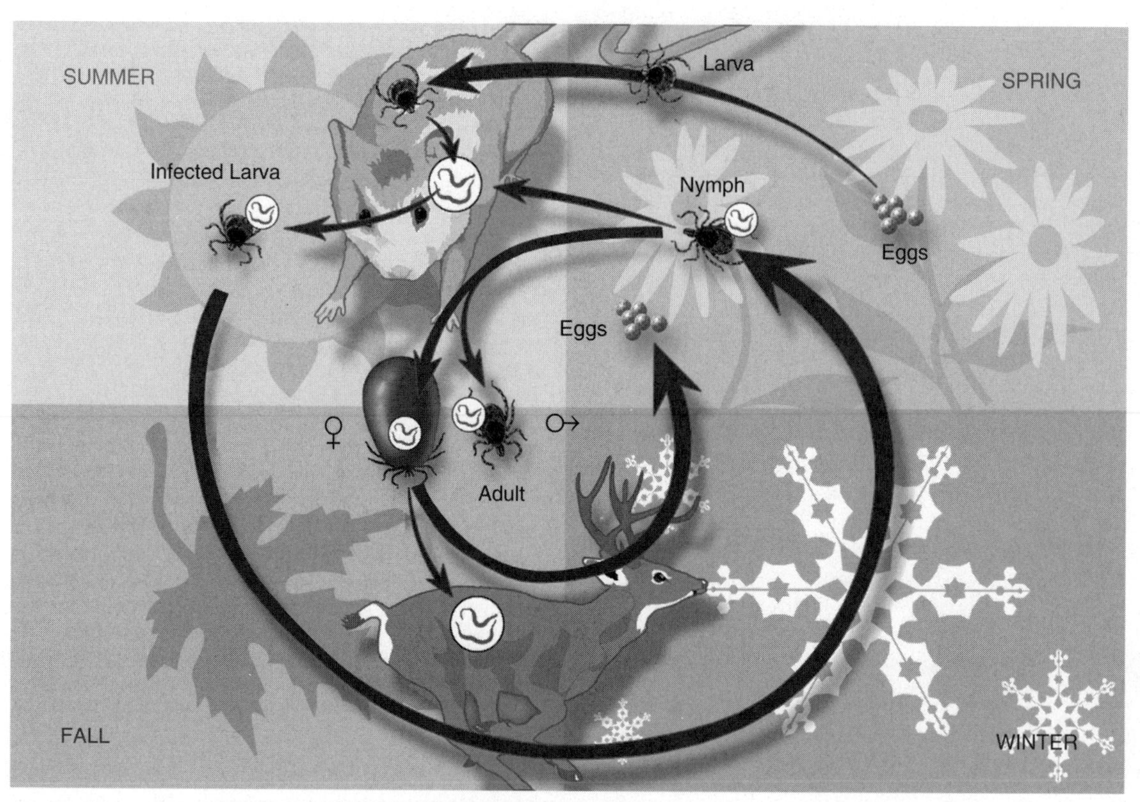

Figure 45–3. The life cycle of northern *I. scapularis (dammini)* lasts 2 years. Eggs are oviposited in the spring, and the larvae emerge approximately 1 month later. They feed once in the summer, usually on small rodents or mammals, and then overwinter. The following spring, the larvae molt into nymphs, which then feed in late spring or early summer. The nymphs feed on mice or larger mammals such as dogs, deer, or human beings and are considered the most likely source of infection for dogs and humans. Nymphs then molt into adults in the fall. The adults usually feed on larger mammals (often the white-tailed deer), where they mate. The females lay their eggs and die in the spring to repeat the 2-year cycle.

In addition to *B. burgdorferi, Ixodes* species ticks are intermediate hosts for granulocytic *Ehrlichia* of the *phagocytophila* group (see Chapter 28 and Table 28–1). People and animals in areas where these ticks reside may become infected with either organism, or in some cases, coinfections have been described.[96a]

These small (< 3.0 mm) ixodid ticks generally feed on more than one host during their life cycle. Larvae and nymphs generally feed on small mammals (*I. scapularis* northern) and reptiles (*I. scapularis* southern), whereas adults feed on deer or larger mammals. Because reptiles are not competent reservoir hosts, the infection rate of southern *I. scapularis* ticks (< 1%) is much lower than that of northern *I. scapularis* ticks (10–50%). Furthermore, because the southern *I. scapularis* ticks do not always feed on mammals, the prevalence of Lyme borreliosis is low in the southern regions.[127a] Infected *Ixodes* ticks may be dispersed to new areas by feeding on migratory birds.

The *Ixodes* species ticks that transmit Lyme borreliosis have a 2-year life cycle and maintain infection in nature by overwintering as infected nymphs (Fig. 45–3). Direct transmission of *Borrelia* between reservoir hosts is unlikely, and transovarial transmission in ticks is relatively nonexistent.[102] When infected nymphs that have overwintered feed in the spring, they transmit organisms to competent reservoir hosts. The larvae from the present year's generation feed later in summer and fall and become infected by feeding on the infected reservoir host. After moulting, they become the nymphs that overwinter for the next tick season (see Fig. 45–3). Nymphs are thought to be primarily responsible for the transmission of infection to domestic animals and people. Adult female ticks feed on deer to maintain the tick population, but deer are not effective reservoir hosts for infection. Despite the zoonotic risk from nymphal ticks, adult ticks appear to have the highest rate of infectivity among stages, presumably because of their longevity and greater chance for exposure.

A number of hematophagous arthropods, including other tick species, fleas, flies, and mosquitoes, have been found to be infected in nature. Whether these infections indicate vector competency is uncertain, but their role is insignificant relative to ticks. Contamination from feeding on infected vertebrates is suspected; however, these other arthropods have not been documented to transfer infection to new hosts.[104a] *Amblyomma americanum* (the Lone Star tick) has been found to harbor spirochetes of unknown virulence similar to *B. burgdorferi* and may be associated with seropositivity in people and animals in areas where *Ixodes* spp. ticks are not found.

Contrary to media reports, Lyme disease is not spreading in epidemic proportions; it is likely being overdiagnosed by those using serologic testing. Nevertheless, it is a significant disease problem in the geographic regions in which it occurs. Although the disease in Connecticut was first recognized in 1975, evidence suggests that *B. burgdorferi* has infected indigenous wildlife and their respective tick vectors for many years. Studies have demonstrated that ear skin samples from museum specimens of the white-footed mouse collected near Dennis, Massachusetts, during 1894 contained DNA positive for *B. burgdorferi.*[85] Similarly, embalmed ticks collected from Long Island, New York, from the 1940s[104] and those from Europe back to the 1880s[90] have also been found to contain borrelial genetic material. The disease has been recognized in Europe since the beginning of the 20th century.

Despite the long-standing presence of the borrelial sylvan cycle, certain environmental conditions have probably caused Lyme disease to become more prevalent in people in the 20th century. Before 1900, the habitat of the eastern United States was heavily deforested by early settlers. Deer and their associated ticks such as *I. scapularis* were reduced. During this time, a sylvan cycle maintaining *B. burgdorferi* most likely existed between *I. muris,* a one-host tick, and rodent species, which were most prevalent in forest-free areas. After the turn of the century, farms were abandoned and reforestation occurred along with a continual increase in the deer population. With an increase in deer, there was a corresponding increase in black-legged ticks of the *I. ricinus* complex. The greater numbers of infected ticks of these species increased the likelihood that people and domestic animals would come in contact with infected ticks. Although Lyme borreliosis is generally associated with forests, it may be acquired in parks in major metropolitan centers. In these areas, rats appear to be the effective reservoir host for feeding ticks.[89]

There is no evidence that infected pet dogs or cats pose a direct risk to humans except by introducing unfed tick stages into a household. The ticks do not survive long indoors, and if fed, tick stages do not reattach without moulting. However, partially fed ticks can refeed and can pose a greater risk of infection because of the shorter required period of attachment. *Ixodes* ticks are extremely small and are detected in only a low percentage of cases of Lyme disease (Fig. 45–4). Unfortunately, pets could be blamed when ticks are not recognized as the source of infection for people. Experimentally, dogs that became infected with *B. burgdorferi* after exposure to infected adult ticks were able to transmit infection to feeding immature ticks.[87] Dogs, therefore, might serve to increase human risk of exposure by being competent reservoirs of infection for ticks, although dogs are not the preferred hosts for these ticks.

Direct horizontal spread from dogs and cats to people is unlikely, and pets merely serve as sentinels for human infection. Most contact studies in which horizontal transmission was achieved in dogs have been performed by exposure coincident to the time of parenteral inoculation.[23] Pregnant bitches were inoculated parenterally every 2 weeks during pregnancy induced by artificial insemination (AI) of semen from infected male dogs.[56] Infection in the offspring was determined by detection of DNA sequences by polymerase chain reaction (PCR). A majority of the females had at least one infected neonate when the pups were tested up to 6 weeks of age. The presence of IgM antibodies in a pup that did not nurse suggested that the infection occurred in utero.

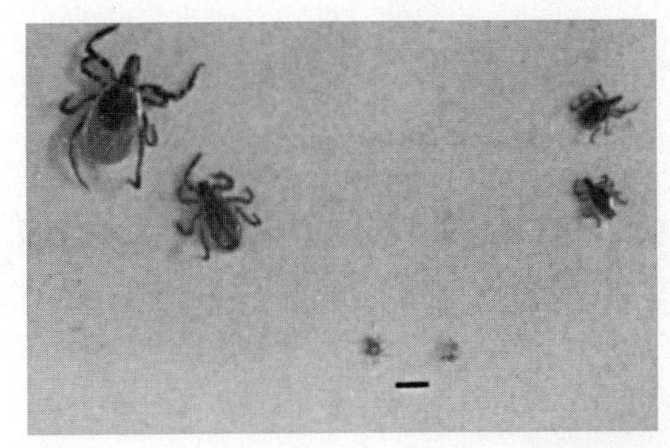

Figure 45–4. Northern *I. scapularis (dammini)* is smaller than other ticks commonly found on dogs. From largest to smallest, two adults (male, female), two nymphs, two larvae (bar = 1 mm). (Courtesy of Mike DeRosa, West Somerville, MA.)

However, infection by parenteral inoculation may have superseded the uterine-placental barrier.

In a more natural infection model with ticks, control dogs in direct contact with infected dogs for up to 1 year did not undergo seroconversion, and organisms could not be isolated from the urine or urinary bladder of infected dogs.[5] Canine urine is an unlikely source of spread. These investigations also could not document any evidence of in utero spread despite seroconversion of the dam. *B. burgdorferi* can survive freezing and storage, making semen intended for AI a potential source of infection.[66] Blood transfusions offer another potential source of infection for dogs and cats.

PATHOGENESIS

Spirochete transmission requires 48 hours of tick attachment, during which time organisms multiply and cross gut epithelium into the hemolymph, disseminate to the salivary glands, and infect the host through tick saliva.[29] It is likely that *Borrelia* proliferate locally in skin at the site of tick inoculation for the duration of infection. From there they replicate and migrate through tissues, beginning in close proximity to the tick bite. Later, they can spread through and infect many tissues, including the joints. Not all animals infected after tick bites develop clinical illness. In fact, evidence suggests that clinical disease in dogs is of very low magnitude (5–10%) relative to the frequency of exposure based on seropositivity (75% in endemic areas) and the rate of infection demonstrated in ticks.[72] Part of this false seropositivity may represent exposure to infectious but nonpathogenic isolates of *Borrelia.*[1] In addition, the development of immune complications such as arthritis is probably related to host immunodeficiency. Humans with certain haplotypes of the major histocompatibility complex are prone to more severe clinical manifestations of the disease.[117]

Once in the body, *B. burgdorferi* may act as a persistent pathogen. Experimental evidence suggests the spirochetes exist extracellularly and, in an undetermined way, can evade immune clearance. Organisms may persist and proliferate in intercellular spaces in the skin at the site of the tick bite. In the intercellular spaces, they act as extracellular pathogens, being more susceptible to the influences of borreliacidal antibodies. They can invade and penetrate many host connective tissues. After a few weeks of infection, *B. burgdorferi* is difficult to detect or isolate from body fluids or internal organs of incidental hosts such as dogs, and numbers in other tissues are exceedingly small.[5, 27, 45] Clinical illness results from the host's own inflammatory response. *B. burgdorferi* seems able to survive for extended periods in the skin, connective tissues, joints, and nervous system. Despite treatment for months or years, *B. burgdorferi* can still persist and be detected by PCR or sometimes culture of blood, spinal fluid, and urine.

PCR studies of synovial fluid are often positive in human patients, whereas results of culture studies are usually negative. In contrast, genetic sequences for plasmid-encoded genes, OspA, OspB, or OspC, are readily detected.[103] The inflammatory response to a small number of spirochetes may be explained by autonomous replications of plasmid DNA. Some of the immunopathologic events may also be related to immune responses generated against specific borrelial antigens. Flagellin, one of the most immunogenic proteins, can elicit an antibody that binds to host neuroaxonal proteins.[114] This sequence may, in turn, stimulate the inflammatory response observed in nervous tissue. Up-regulation of interleukin-8, which recruits neutrophils to inflammatory sites, has been found in the synovial membranes of experimentally infected dogs.[120a] This may be an important mechanism in producing suppurative polyarthritis.

The Jarisch-Herxheimer reaction (JHR) is a severe systemic reaction that is observed after antimicrobial therapy of spirochetal or other bacterial infections. It is associated with the systemic release of cytokines, tumor necrosis factor-α (TNF-α), interleukin-6, and interleukin-8. The JHR has many similarities to severe sepsis. Clinical signs include fever, rapid pulse and respiration, rising blood pressure, and leukopenia. Pretreatment with anti–TNF-α immunoglobulin suppresses the JHR from developing in people.[35]

CLINICAL SIGNS

The clinical features of borreliosis in people include dermatitis, arthritis, meningoencephalitis, and myocarditis. These are discussed further under Public Health Considerations. Diseases documented experimentally and naturally occurring disease in dogs and cats are discussed next.

Cats

Despite evidence for seropositivity in cats, the natural disease has not been described as a distinct clinical entity. Cats examined in endemic areas of the northeastern United States had infestations of *Ixodes*, but a low percentage of attached nymphs were infected.[79] Approximately 13% of cats were seropositive by indirect FA or ELISA; however, there was no difference in positive results from cats with or without lameness. Similarly, cats that were screened as clinical patients in the United Kingdom had a low rate (4.2%) of seroreactivity.[93] The seropositive cats in the latter study were asymptomatic with respect to lameness.

Cats may be more resistant than dogs to development of clinical signs of Lyme borreliosis. As in dogs, inoculation of cultivated *Borrelia* is associated with reduced virulence or immune recognition. Cats inoculated by various routes (parenteral, oral, and conjunctival) with cultivated spirochetes all developed IgG seropositivity; however, organisms were found only in the blood of the IV and ocularly infected cats.[18] The spirochetemia was transient, clearing by day 24, and only one cat had organisms in its tissues at necropsy. In contrast, when cats were inoculated with organisms directly from arthropods, they developed multiple limb lameness and had joint, pulmonary, lymphoid, and CNS inflammation at necropsy.[41, 42] Arthritis or meningitis would seem to be the predominant manifestation to warrant investigation of Lyme borreliosis in cats.

Dogs

Similar to the situation in cats, initial attempts to recreate experimental Lyme borreliosis in dogs using laboratory-derived strains were unsuccessful[17, 51]; however, fever and polyarthritis have been experimentally produced after inoculation or natural exposure to tick-derived *B. burgdorferi*.[5, 23, 45, 126] The use of spirochetes directly inoculated during feeding of field-collected ticks has been most successful.[5] Clinical illness in experimentally infected dogs occurs 2 to 5 months after tick exposure, and the severity and propensity to develop signs of illness seem to vary inversely with the animal's age and immune status.

Systemic Signs. Acute signs consisting of fever (39.5–40.5°C [103.1–104.9°F]), shifting leg lameness, articular swelling, lymphadenomegaly, anorexia, and general malaise, all responsive to antimicrobials, most commonly occur in naturally exposed seropositive dogs.[68, 72, 74, 92] The accuracy of diagnosis in many spontaneously diseased dogs is difficult to determine because limb and joint signs (swelling, lameness, and pain) with fever and inappetence have been observed with equal frequency in seropositive and seronegative dogs.[26, 80, 81]

Arthritis. Polyarthritis is the best experimentally documented syndrome caused by acute *B. burgdorferi* infection in dogs (Fig. 45–5). Despite the transient nature of the arthritis, pathologic changes in the joints are progressive. Chronic nonerosive polyarthritis is the main finding in more prolonged infections, and it may persist despite antimicrobial therapy. Lesions have been most consistent in skin, lymphatic tissues, and joints even though the organism can be isolated from other tissues and body fluids.

Renal Disease. Protein-losing glomerulopathy was described in a few naturally infected dogs.[44, 94] An acute progressive renal failure associated with azotemia, uremia, proteinuria, peripheral edema, and body cavity effusions has been characterized in 49 dogs from *Borrelia*-endemic areas.[27a] A preponderance of Labrador and golden retrievers was affected. The duration of clinical illness was 24 hours to 8 weeks, with a sudden onset of anorexia, vomiting, lethargy, and weight loss. Some dogs had recent or concurrent lameness. All dogs

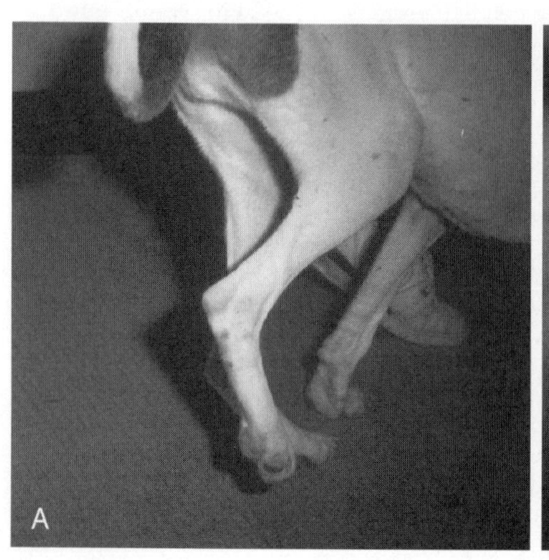

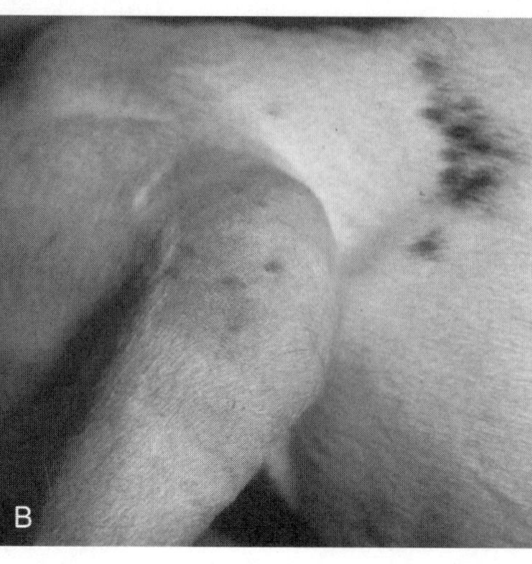

Figure 45–5. Experimentally induced borrelial arthritis in the dog. Shifting leg lameness develops 60 to 90 days after inoculation *(A)*. Joint swelling *(B)* and fever spikes are also transient.

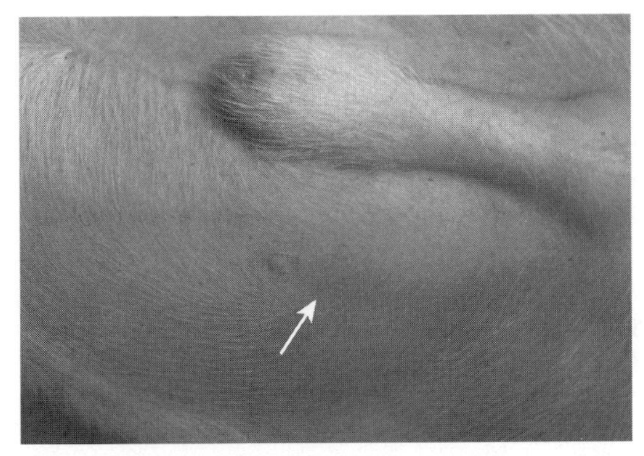

Figure 45–6. Small reddened lesion *(arrow)* in the skin at the site of inoculation of an experimentally inoculated dog.

died or were euthanized as a result of renal failure. Dogs had positive test results for antibody to *B. burgdorferi*. Although natural exposure to *B. burgdorferi* is likely involved, but not yet proven, in rapidly progressing glomerular disease, the role of vaccination, if any, in the development of the lesion is undetermined.

Other Manifestations. A small reddened lesion that develops in the skin at the site of tick attachment disappears within the first week (Fig. 45–6). However, the organism can be isolated from the skin for extended periods. This is not the dramatic lesion of erythema migrans seen in people. The spread of the organism in skin, connective, and muscle tissues may be responsible for some of the observed lameness.

Other nonarthritic syndromes reported in a few spontaneously diseased dogs have been rheumatoid arthritis,[107] neurologic dysfunction,[8, 34, 84, 86a, 100a] and cardiac arrhythmia from myocarditis.[70] These other signs are similar to those that have been reported in people (see Public Health Considerations). Unfortunately, the diagnosis in these naturally diseased dogs has often been circumstantial based on serologic data or microscopic evidence without organism isolation. In humans, conjunctivitis, choroiditis, hepatitis, and myositis or fasciitis have been reported as rare syndromes and have not been documented to occur in dogs. The strain used or the relatively short observation period in experimental studies may be responsible for the failure of the nonarthritic syndromes to be reproduced in experimentally inoculated animals.

Florida Borreliosis. Breitschwerdt and colleagues[16] reported borreliosis in two dogs from Florida caused by a novel borrelial spirochete. Clinical signs included elevated rectal temperature, shifting leg lameness, hepatosplenomegaly, visible spirochetemia, and anterior uveitis similar to the signs of endemic tick-borne relapsing fever. Many of the relapsing fever spirochetes may infect dogs and cats as incidental hosts as they are known to infect people (see Table 45–1).

DIAGNOSIS

Reports of Lyme disease in people often exceed the geographic boundaries of known endemic foci.[21] Although travel accounts for a minor number of disparities, the overestimation results from cross-reactivity to other infectious agents and from the inaccuracies of serologic procedures. Better studies to define the distribution of the disease in nature must be based on examination of ticks and wildlife, because isolation of the organism from ticks or reservoir hosts is more successful than from human and domestic animals.

Clinical Laboratory Findings. There are no specific hematologic or biochemical changes pathognomonic of borreliosis, although CSF, joint fluid, and urine may show inflammatory changes. The synovial fluid changes in dogs have been best substantiated with increased cell counts of 5000 to 100,000 cells/μl with neutrophils predominating (>95%). Protein concentration and turbidity are increased. CSF from human patients with neuroborreliosis demonstrates lymphocytic pleocytosis and mild protein increase. Consistent CSF values have not been found in dogs with suspected neurologic dysfunction.

Serologic Testing. Currently, Lyme borreliosis is probably overdiagnosed in human and veterinary medicine because it has become a "trendy" illness.[118] The presence of an elevated antibody titer to *B. burgdorferi* signifies exposure to the spirochete but does not prove that current clinical illness is caused by the organism. In endemic areas, asymptomatic animals are often seropositive. In addition to seropositive results with a validated assay, the animal should have a history of tick exposure with compatible clinical signs and a rapid response to antimicrobial therapy. Unfortunately, the finding of Lyme disease has become more of a laboratory than a clinical diagnosis. The dependency on serologic testing results from the fact that culture and microscopic detection of the organism from specimens of tissues or body fluids are uncommon. Rather than being a "test for Lyme disease," serology should be viewed more appropriately as "seroreactivity to *B. burgdorferi*."[114]

Various problems have been noted with serologic testing. First, there is no standardization among antigen preparations, techniques, and interpretations by different laboratories. Matched sera sent to 10 commercial laboratories for antiborrelia serology found only 53% agreement of all sera tested.[49] Furthermore, nonspecificity of whole cell borrelial assays is apparent in that other inflammatory conditions in people, such as autoimmune diseases, rheumatoid arthritis, syphilis, and periodontal disease, are known to produce seropositivity, and similar reactivities probably occur in the dog and cat.

Serologic *screening procedures* available for animals are the ELISA and indirect FA techniques. The ELISA and indirect FA utilize whole cells with many cross-reactive proteins present in other bacteria, especially other *Borrelia* and *Leptospira*.[19, 38, 73, 92, 113] The ELISA and indirect FA results have shown that *Leptospira*-positive sera can have low levels of reactivity to *B. burgdorferi*. True seroreactivity likely gives the highest titers, although crossreactions should always be considered with any positive result. False-negative antibody tests results are rare.

Antibodies to the relapsing fever-like organism described from dogs in Florida[16] cross-reacted with *B. burgdorferi*. They caused lower titers than those found when the antigen from the new organism was used in the testing. Some of the reports of human and animal Lyme disease in the western United States, where relapsing fever occurs, may be related to the nonspecificity of whole cell ELISA or indirect FA. An immunoreactive protein, GlpQ, may be able to help distinguish these infections when utilized in immunoassays.[111] Some of the seropositivity noted by testing for antibodies to *B. burgdorferi* probably is due to other pathogenic or nonpathogenic *Borrelia* that exist in nature. Furthermore, in Great Britain, dogs with periodontal disease and presumed oral spirochetosis showed a higher level of seropositivity than clinically healthy dogs from the same hospital population.[109]

The time course of serologic testing is also important in determining whether active or past infection is responsible for seropositivity. Early serodiagnostic results are usually negative because the immune response to *B. burgdorferi* develops gradually. Experimentally, infected dogs had IgG ELISA–positive titers by 4 to 6 weeks after exposure.[5] Titers were at their highest levels by 3 months after exposure and lasted for at least 1 year. Titer increases almost always precede clinical lameness and fever in experimentally infected dogs.[5, 45] High or persistent IgG titers could indicate past exposure or infection and, as such, are difficult to interpret on single specimens. Absolute values of titers can vary widely; therefore, paired titers should always be done on samples submitted simultaneously to the same laboratory. Simultaneous measurements of IgG and IgM in a single specimen would theoretically provide more meaningful information than either titer alone. After experimental inoculation, IgM titers have been the first to increase and remain elevated for 2 months—after which they decline. However, in naturally infected dogs and people, IgM persists for many months so that a positive titer does not help to confirm recent exposure or infection.[58, 59]

In general, data from many laboratories suggest that titers greater than 64 to 128 indicate the least significant level of reactivity. Titers can be much higher in recently exposed, actively infected animals. High serum antibody levels seem to decline or disappear with antibiotic treatment, but increases that occur after 6 months following termination of therapy are associated with proliferation of surviving spirochetes.[121] Vaccinated dogs show seroreactivity for months to years after vaccination, making a diagnosis difficult with whole cell antigen preparations. Although neutralizing antibody titers after vaccination may decrease with time, ELISA and indirect FA titers remain elevated for more extended periods, interfering with serologic testing.

Ongoing infections are characterized by high whole *Borrelia* cell antibody titers. The use of separated or purified protein antigens in ELISA or *confirmation with immunoblotting (Western blotting)* should be the next step to improve specificity of *B. burgdorferi* antibody assays without loss of sensitivity.[5, 12, 77, 82, 113] The pattern of antibody reactivity after natural tick infection also differs from that produced after vaccination. Immunoblotting helps determine the clinical significance of whole cell titers when reactivity to other bacteria such as *Leptospira* occurs.[113] After natural exposure to *B. burgdorferi*, antibodies develop to proteins in the range of 41, 39, and 22 kD, which represent flagellin, p39, and OspC, respectively. A recombinant-produced OspC antigen in ELISA testing of human sera for IgM showed a higher degree of sensitivity in detecting recent infection compared with ELISA of whole cells or immunoblotting.[40, 101]

Reactivity to OspA and OspB (31 and 34 kD, respectively) occurs in vaccinated or parenterally inoculated dogs but is lacking or occurs very late in naturally infected dogs.[5, 52, 54, 71] ELISAs using OspA- and OspB-deficient mutant strains are also able to discriminate natural from vaccine exposure,[129] especially when recombinant vaccine containing OspA was utilized. For example, some dogs develop signs of polyarthritis after vaccination that do not respond to antibiotic therapy. Their immunoblots show a pattern typical of vaccination and not infection.[59] OspC appears to be expressed by the organism in the host at warmer temperatures, and it is lost with in vitro cultivation or arthropod residence of *B. burgdorferi.* It is a prominent protein in the body's immunoreactivity to infection. Newer ELISA tests that incorporate OspC may help improve the accuracy of serodiagnosis.

A number of novel protein antigens may also eventually serve as markers of natural infection because they are not expressed by in vitro derived organisms.[24, 125] With canine sera, good correlation has been observed between purified recombinant proteins in conventional serologic testing and immunoblotting.[82] An immunoblot test kit is available for canine sera (Lyme Immunostrip, Immunetics, Cambridge, MA; see Appendix 6). ELISA test kits containing specific proteins may be available in the future to allow for discriminating antibody titers.

Other tests have been proposed to assist in the diagnosis of borreliosis. Comparing CSF antibody titers with those of serum has been done in human patients in an attempt to diagnose neuroborreliosis. Intrathecal production of specific antibodies to *B. burgdorferi* can be demonstrated if the ratio of CSF or serum *B. burgdorferi* antibody is greater than the CSF or serum albumin, total IgG, or specific IgG to another infectious agent (see Diagnosis of Distemper in Chapter 3 and Toxoplasmosis in Chapter 80). When the same assay method is employed for specific IgG, the specific method has the most reliability.[57, 117]

Increased intrathecal antibody concentration was demonstrated in dogs with neurologic dysfunction.[34, 84] The results of such reports are difficult to assess because the dogs were from endemic areas and no supporting histopathology and no culture findings were supplied.

Isolation. Culture of spirochetes from specimens of a diseased patient is the most definitive means of diagnosis but in most cases is difficult due to the low numbers of organisms present and the insensitivity of isolation methods. Special media are required. Skin appears to be the most consistent tissue for premortem or postmortem culture from dogs when specimens are taken at or near the site of tick attachment. At necropsy muscle and tissues with high fibrocytic and extracellular matrix content, such as fascia, pericardium, peritoneum, meninges, joint capsule, and adrenal glands, give the most consistent positive results.[5]

Heralded as the supreme test for organism detection, PCR has its own limitations. Although most investigators claim high specificity and sensitivity, PCR results can vary according to primer selection. Primers that target conserved DNA sequences can be utilized to detect a variety of strains. Primers targeting DNA in plasmids are much more sensitive because of the multiple copies of cytoplasmic plasmids.[103, 120] Contamination is a possibility, and PCR cannot distinguish live from dead organisms. Research shows that small DNA fragments of *Borrelia* and live organisms may persist in the synovial membranes after treatment.[98, 121] These *Borrelia* fragments may induce false-positive PCR results. PCR has been used to detect *Borrelia* in the CSF of people with acute or chronic neuroborreliosis; however, the sensitivity is limited by false-negative results.[97] PCR has been a valuable experimental tool, but it is not practical for clinical application. Tissue specimens can be examined microscopically for pathogenic spirochetes utilizing specific labeled antibodies. Xenodiagnosis, in which uninfected ticks become infected after feeding on suspect infected hosts, has proved very reliable in the research laboratory setting but can be time consuming otherwise.

PATHOLOGIC FINDINGS

In experimentally infected dogs, lesions have occurred in the lymph nodes, joints, and skin.[5] In addition, blood vessels (vasculitis), peripheral nerves (perineuritis), and meninges (meningitis) have associated inflammation.[121] The joints are grossly swollen in severely affected animals (see Fig. 45–5*B*). Inflammation within the synovial membrane is mild, and the effusion consists of fibrin and neutrophils in acute cases. In more chronic infections, dogs that have undergone seroconversion develop nonsuppurative inflammation within the synovial membrane and joint capsule. Peripheral lymphadenomegaly is present, especially in nodes draining the affected limbs.

Histologically, follicular enlargement and increased size of parafollicular areas are evident. Skin biopsy samples have superficial perivascular lymphoplasmacytic infiltrates with mast cell accumulations. Renal lesions have not been found in experimentally infected dogs but were evident in naturally diseased dogs.[28] Glomerulitis, diffuse tubular necrosis with regeneration, and interstitial inflammation were found. *Borrelia* can be demonstrated in tissues using silver impregnation methods or cytologic specimens with Giemsa stain. Silver stain of the kidneys of these dogs revealed rare spirochetes unrelated to lesion development.

Similar renal lesions have been noted in cats.[27a] Other lesions noted in experimentally infected cats included hepatic degeneration, splenic hyperplasia, regional lymph node plasmacytosis, nonsuppurative meningoencephalitis, and pneumonitis.[41, 42]

THERAPY

Because of the difficulty in obtaining an accurate diagnosis, antibiotics are often given empirically in an attempt to make a therapeutic diagnosis. Many reports exist of successful recovery after institution of antimicrobial therapy in dogs diagnosed with Lyme arthritis. Improvement may often occur within 24 to 48 hours after antimicrobial therapy is instituted. The greatest success is achieved with treatment in the initial phases of clinical illness. Clinical improvement after any therapeutic intervention should be viewed with caution because the acute limb and joint dysfunction is intermittent and often resolves after several days to weeks whether or not antimicrobials are given.[80]

Early treatment is associated with a reduction in antibody titers and organisms in tissues and prevention or cure of joint lesions.[121] Most treatment is instituted for a minimum of 30 days. However, on the basis of research studies, clearance of the organism after 30 days of treatment in dogs and rodents is questionable, and relapse and recrudescence of infection can occur after the antimicrobial is discontinued.[83, 121] In addition to inability to clear the organism, inflammatory changes that occur in various tissues such as the joints may become self-perpetuating. Intra-articular persistence of *B. burgdorferi* nucleic acids occurs despite the inability to culture them, which probably is related to the lower sensitivity of culture methods.[14, 121] The persistence may stimulate chronic immune and inflammatory processes. Those with more chronic borreliosis are less likely to show improvement or have relapses, even if treatment is continued for weeks to months. A difficulty in using a therapeutic response to improve diagnostic accuracy is that fever, joint distention, and lameness may appear and then disappear spontaneously. Doxycycline by itself has been shown to be chondroprotective in noninfectious arthritis produced in dogs.[128]

Antimicrobial therapy, nevertheless, is still the mainstay for treatment of borreliosis (Table 45–3). In vitro antimicrobial susceptibility testing shown to be most to least effective are ceftriaxone, erythromycin, amoxicillin, cefuroxime, doxycycline, tetracycline, and penicillin G.[60] Tetracycline, ampicillin, and erythromycin have been classically used to treat human and animal patients. Doxycycline is the first choice because it is a lipid-soluble tetracycline of relatively low cost. The theoretical advantages of lipid solubility are lower dosage, greater tissue distribution, and improved intracellular penetration compared with conventional tetracycline. Newer erythromycin derivatives, such as azithromycin, or third-generation cephalosporins, such as ceftriaxone, have been administered for more refractory human cases.[28] They are most effective for treatment of chronic established infections. High-dose intravenous penicillin G has been advocated in an attempt to treat unresponsive animals. *Borrelia* are resistant to aminoglycosides and quinolones.

Nonsteroidal compounds offer relief for many of the painful arthritic complications, but judicious use is warranted because of their tendency to produce GI irritation. Glucocorticoids have also been hesitantly provided at very low anti-inflammatory dosages in the management of persistent pain and swelling from chronic arthritis that cannot be completely controlled with one or more courses of antibiotics. Immunosuppressive doses of glucocorticoids should definitely be avoided because of immunosuppression and infection exacerbation.

PREVENTION

Vaccines are being marketed for dogs to prevent borreliosis, and the release of recombinant vaccines for people is imminent.[64] In Europe and other geographic areas, the multiplicity of infecting strains may make protection by vaccination more difficult. The human vaccines to be marketed in the United States are based on recombinant DNA production of Osp products because of the concern about whole cell vaccine safety. Adjuvanted recombinant vaccine with expressed OspA and OspB proteins has protected dogs against tick-induced infection.[27] Unadjuvanted OspA, a lipoprotein, appears to offer equal protection to adjuvanted vaccine in people[64]; this obviates the need for adjuvants in this vaccine. Recombinant protein OspA vaccine and whole cell bacterins are commercially available for dogs (see Appendix 3). The vaccines are recommended for use beginning at 9 and

Table 45–3. Suggested Antibiotic Regimens for Lyme Borreliosis[a]

DRUG	DOSE[b]	ROUTE	INTERVAL (HOURS)	DURATION (DAYS)	PREFERRED USES
Doxycycline	10 mg/kg	PO	12	30	Early, arthritis or neurologic manifestations, not for pups or kittens
Amoxicillin	20 mg/kg	PO	8	30	Early, arthritis, neurologic manifestations, young patients
Azithromycin	5 mg/kg	IV	12	10–20	Early disease
Penicillin G	22,000 U/kg	IV	8	14–30	Persistent arthritis, neurologic or cardiac manifestations
Ceftriaxone	20 mg/kg	IV, SC	12	14–30	Late neurologic or cardiac manifestations, persistent arthritis
Cefotaxime	20 mg/kg	IV	8	14–30	Neurologic manifestations
Chloramphenicol	15–25 mg/kg	PO, SC	8	14–30	Neurologic manifestations

[a]Information on many drugs for particular uses is based on extrapolation from the human literature.
[b]Dose per administration at specified interval. For additional information, see Appendix 8.

12 weeks of age, respectively. Primary vaccination schedules consist of two inoculations 3 weeks apart.

Dogs that are vaccinated with adjuvanted whole cell vaccines or recombinant Osp vaccines before infection develop enhanced resistance to infection as demonstrated by an increased level of antibodies to OspA and OspB and a protective response to infection.[5, 51, 76, 122] This type of protection appears to develop late or not at all in the naturally infected animals. Although OspA is an abundant protein on culture-derived *B. burgdorferi,* vertebrate hosts infected by tick bites or small numbers of organisms rarely seroconvert to OspA.[11, 29] Although OspA is expressed by *Borrelia* in unfed ticks, it is lost during transmission from the vector to the vertebrate host and is not present on spirochetes in engorged ticks. OspC appears to develop on the surface of the spirochete and appears in organisms that infect the feeding host.[29, 110, 119] It appears that antibody to OspA from the host causes an arrest of growth and salivary gland invasion in the ticks that feed on previously vaccinated animals.[28a, 29] In this manner, vaccine-induced immune protection may begin in the tick before spirochetes enter the host. If experimentally infected animals are given passively administered OspA antibodies after tick engorgement, the animals become infected. In parenteral challenge studies, protection is afforded by prior immunization with OspA but not by OspC antigen vaccine.[105] Experimentally, oral administration of a recombinant, vectored OspA vaccine to rodents is protective against systemic infection.[75a]

The disadvantage of vaccination is that these antibodies cause false-positive results on serologic testing for months to years later. Whole cell vaccines might lead to immunologic reactions to cross-reactive host antigens. An additional theoretical disadvantage of the vaccine is the possibility that hypersensitivity reaction may occur if it is given to a dog harboring the organism.[59] There is evidence that vaccination of an already infected animal will not clear the infection or prevent clinical illness.[12] Local and systemic allergic reactions have been noted with whole cell vaccines, but their prevalence rate is relatively low.[71] Vaccines might also be subject to breaks in protection in the future or in various geographic areas because *Borrelia* are known to change their genotypic and phenotypic make-up so they can survive in the presence of organism-specific antibodies. Protection afforded by canine vaccines is not absolute.

Vaccination should not be universally recommended or provided as a replacement for adequate tick control measures. Dogs should be selected for vaccination based on the geographic area in which they reside or travel and by their habits. That is, outdoor, hunting, or field trial dogs that frequent known tick-infested areas should receive the most priority.

Vector control is a supportive measure that can help to reduce the prevalence of infection in people and pets. Environmental insecticides and personal protection methods have received the most attention. Application of insecticides to relatively large environmental areas makes this control both expensive and difficult. *Ixodes* species have a 2-year life cycle, and they become redistributed by various hosts after feeding, making it difficult to treat all stages with one application. Residual environmentally destructive insecticides, such as the chlorinated hydrocarbons, have been the most successful in controlling the ticks, but their disadvantages are obvious.

Another method is to target infested rodents by placing cotton impregnated with permethrin insecticides near entrances to their burrows. To be effective, such insecticides have to target all reservoir hosts in a limited area. Treatment of all deer in a region with insecticides would inhibit the survival and reproduction of adult *I. scapularis;* however, the logistics of such an approach are overwhelming. Even if effective, vaccination of reservoir species would be impossible. Reduction of deer population might help to decrease the number of Ixodid ticks, but other mammalian hosts could still propagate the vectors.

PUBLIC HEALTH CONSIDERATIONS

The case definition of human Lyme disease is an erythematous rash or one objective sign of musculoskeletal, neurologic, or cardiovascular disease and laboratory confirmation of infection.[3] In 1993, 8185 cases were reported nationwide by 44 state health departments; the northeastern United States accounted for 85% of the total cases. Since surveillance was established in 1982, almost 50,000 cases have been reported from 47 states. The sylvan cycle in nature has been found in only 19 states. Errors in reporting are probably due to underreporting, misclassification, and overdiagnosis.

Clinical signs of Lyme disease in people usually begin within several days to 1 month after a tick bite. An expanding nonpruritic ringlike erythematous lesion of at least 5 cm, termed *erythema migrans,* may develop in the vicinity of the bite. Fever, myalgia, arthralgia, and headache (flulike symptoms) may accompany this lesion. A majority of affected people develop recurrent joint swelling and musculoskeletal soreness. Signs of organ system inflammation (arthritis, carditis, meningitis, and uveitis) occur later. Meningeal signs often appear later and include pain, sensory loss, behavioral changes, and recurrent headaches. Myocarditis is characterized by development of symptoms characteristic of atrioventricular conduction disturbances.

Personal protection measures for tick control among humans are not difficult to institute. Avoiding tick habitats; wearing hats, long pants, and long-sleeved shirts; taping socks over cuffs; tucking pants into socks; wearing light clothing; and treating clothing and exposed skin with insect repellents have been most effective. Wearing of light-colored clothing will help one to see the ticks for early removal. Additional measures include walking in areas free of tall grass and dense brush. Prompt tick removal helps prevent transmission of infection. There is a delay in onset of tick feeding and appearance of infectious spirochetes in tick saliva. Studies in animals show little risk of infection within the first 24 hours of attachment, 50% after 48 hours, and 100% infection after 72 hours or if the infected tick feeds until engorgement. The incidence of disease is also greater in people where ticks are attached for 72 hours or more.[116] Agents containing diethyltoluamide (DEET) repel ticks and can be applied to clothing or exposed skin. Those containing permethrin kill ticks on contact but can only be applied to clothing.

Additional information on Lyme disease in humans is available from state and local health departments, from the Centers for Disease Control (CDC) voice information system—(404) 332-4555; from the CDC's Bacterial Zoonoses Branch—(970) 221-6453; and from the office of communications at the National Institutes of Health—(301) 496-5717.

Although Lyme disease is classified as a zoonosis, dogs, cats, and people are incidental hosts for a sylvan cycle that exists in nature. Lyme borreliosis is associated with outdoor activities that result in exposure to tick vectors. Dogs and cats do not appear to be a source for infection in people because they do not excrete the organisms in their body fluids (including urine) to any appreciable extent.[5] Uninfected control dogs kept in direct contact with infected dogs for up to 1 year did not become infected or undergo seroconversion.[5]

Dogs and cats appear to be sentinel hosts but not reservoir hosts for human infection. In the same environment, dogs and cats have a greater risk of exposure than their human counterparts because of their greater likelihood of contacting the tick vector. Pets may bring infected ticks into the household, but ticks do not generally refeed after detachment. As with other tick-borne illnesses, improper handling of ticks, resulting in release of midgut contents onto abraded skin or mucous membranes, might allow percutaneous penetration of infectious material. Even in areas where borreliosis is endemic, the risk of infection after a recognized ixodid tick bite is so low that prophylactic antimicrobial therapy is not routinely indicated.[112]

Immunity to infection may be strain specific and vaccines may not protect against various isolates. Reinfection with borreliosis in a person has been caused by variant strains of *B. burgdorferi*.[98a]

References

1. Anderson JF, Barthold SW, Magnarelli LA. 1990. Infectious but nonpathogenic isolate of *Borrelia burgdorferi*. *J Clin Microbiol* 28:2693–2699.
2. Anonymous. 1989. The ominous spread of *Borrelia burgdorferi* infection. *J Am Vet Med Assoc* 194:1387–1391.
3. Anonymous. 1994. Lyme borreliosis. *Morbid Mortal Wkly Rep* 43:564–565, 571–572.
4. Appel MJG. 1990. Lyme disease in dogs and cats. *Compend Cont Educ Pract Vet* 12:617–626.
5. Appel MJG, Allan S, Jacobson RH, et al. 1993. Experimental Lyme diseases in dogs produces arthritis and persistent infection. *J Infect Dis* 167:651–654.
6. Artsob H, Baarker IK, Fister R, et al. 1993. Serological studies on the infection of dogs in Ontario with *Borrelia burgdorferi*, the etiological agent of Lyme disease. *Can Vet J* 34:543–548.
7. Azuma Y, Isogai E, Isogai H, et al. 1994. Canine Lyme disease: clinical and serological evaluations in 21 dogs in Japan. *Vet Rec* 134:369–372.
8. Azuma Y, Kawamura K, Isogai H, et al. 1993. Neurologic abnormalities in two dogs with suspected Lyme disease. *Microbiol Immunol* 37:325–329.

8a. Banerjee S, Stephen C, Fernando K, et al. 1996. Evaluation of dogs as sero-indicators of the geographic distribution of Lyme borreliosis in British Columbia. *Can Vet J* 37:168–169.

9. Baranton G, Postic D, Saint GI, et al. 1992. Delineation of *Borrelia burgdorferi sensu stricto. Borrelia garinii* sp nov., and group VS461 associated with Lyme borreliosis. *Int J Syst Bacteriol* 42:378–383.
10. Barbour AG, Fish D. 1993. The biological and social phenomenon of Lyme disease. *Science* 260:1610–1616.

10a. Barthold SW, Feng S, Bockenstedt LK. 1997. Protective and arthritis-resolving activity in sera of mice infected with *Borrelia burgdorferi*. *Clin Infect Dis* 25(Suppl 1):S9–S17.

11. Barthold SW, Fikrig E, Bockenstedt LK, et al. 1995. Circumvention of outer surface protein A immunity by host-adapted *Borrelia burgdorferi*. *Infect Immun* 63:2255–2261.
12. Barthold SW, Levy SA, Fikrig E, et al. 1995. Serologic responses of dogs naturally exposed to or vaccinated against *Borrelia burgdorferi* infection. *J Am Vet Med Assoc* 207:1435–1440.
13. Bosler EM, Cohen DP, Schulze TL, et al. 1988. Host responses to *Borrelia burgdorferi* in dogs and horses. *NY Acad Sci* 539:221–234.
14. Bradley JF, Johnson RC, Goodman JL. 1994. The persistence of spirochetal nucleic acids in active Lyme arthritis. *Am Intern Med* 120:487–489.
15. Breitschwerdt EB, Geoly FJ, Meuten DJ, et al. 1996. Myocarditis in mice and guinea pigs experimentally infected with a canine-origin *Borrelia* isolate from Florida. *Am J Vet Res* 57:505–511.
16. Breitschwerdt EB, Nicholson WL, Kiehl AB, et al. 1994. Natural infections with *Borrelia* spirochetes in two dogs from Florida. *J Clin Microbiol* 32:352–357.
17. Burgess EC. 1986. Experimental inoculation of dogs with *Borrelia burgdorferi*. *Zentralbl Bakteriol Hyg (A)* 263:427–434.
18. Burgess EC. 1992. Experimentally induced infection of cats with *Borrelia burgdorferi*. *Am J Vet Res* 53:1507–1511.
19. Burgess EC, Schneider E, Bosler E. 1989. Testing for *Borrelia burgdorferi*. *J Am Vet Med Assoc* 195:844–846.
20. Burkot TR, Piesman J, Wirtz RA. 1994. Quantitation of the *Borrelia burgdorferi* outer surface protein A in *Ixodes scapularis*: fluctuations during the tick life cycle, doubling times, and loss while feeding. *J Infect Dis* 170:883–889.
21. Burkot TR, Schriefer ME, Larsen SA. 1997. Cross-reactivity to *Borrelia burgdorferi* proteins in serum samples from residents of a tropical country nonendemic for Lyme disease. *J Infect Dis* 175:466–469.
22. Canica MM, Nato F, du Merle L, et al. 1993. Monoclonal antibodies for identification of *Borrelia afzelii* sp nov. associated with late cutaneous manifestations of Lyme borreliosis. *Scand J Infect Dis* 25:441–448.
23. Cerri D, Farina R, Andreani R, et al. 1994. Experimental infection of dogs with *Borrelia burgdorferi*. *Res Vet Sci* 57:256–258.
24. Champion CI, Blanco DR, Skare JT, et al. 1994. A 9.0-kilobase-pair circular plasmid of *Borrelia burgdorferi* encodes an exported protein: evidence for expression only during infection. *Infect Immun* 62:2653–2661.
25. Chu HJ, Chaavez LG, Blumer BM, et al. 1992. Immunogenicity and efficacy study of a commercial *Borrelia burgdorferi* bacterin. *J Am Vet Med Assoc* 201:403–411.
26. Cohen ND, Carter CN, Thomas MA, et al. 1990. Clinical and epizootiologic characteristics of dogs seropositive for *Borrelia burgdorferi* in Texas: 100 cases (1988). *J Am Vet Med Assoc* 197:893–898.
27. Coughlin RT, Fish D, Mather TN, et al. 1995. Protection of dogs from Lyme disease with a vaccine containing outer surface protein (Osp) A, OspB and the saponin adjuvant QS21. *J Infect Dis* 171:1049–1052.

27a. Dambach DM, Smith CA, Lewis RM, et al. 1997. Morphologic, immunohistochemical, and ultrastructural characterization of a distinctive renal lesion in dogs putatively associated with *Borrelia burgdorferi* infection: 49 cases (1987–1992). *Vet Pathol* 34:85–170.

28. Dattwyler RJ, Luft BJ, Kunkel MJ, et al. 1997. Ceftriaxone compared with doxycycline for the treatment of acute disseminated Lyme disease. *N Engl J Med* 337:289–363.

28a. De Silva AM, Fish D, Burkot TR, et al. 1997. OspA antibodies inhibit the acquisition of *Borrelia burgdorferi* by *Ixodes* ticks. *Infect Immun* 65:3146–3150.

29. DeSilva AM, Telford SR, Brunet LR, et al. 1996. *Borrelia burgdorferi* OspA is an arthropod-specific transmission-blocking Lyme disease vaccine. *J Exp Med* 183:271–275.
30. Dorward DW, Schwan TG, Garon CF. 1991. Immune capture and detection of *Borrelia burgdorferi* antigens in urine, blood, or tissues from infected ticks, mice, dogs and humans. *J Clin Microbiol* 29:1162–1170.
31. Dressler F, Ackermann R, Steere AC. 1994. Antibody responses to the three genomic groups of *Borrelia burgdorferi* in European Lyme borreliosis. *J Infect Dis* 169:313–318.
32. Eng TR, Wilson ML, Speilman A, et al. 1988. Greater risk of *Borrelia burgdorferi* infection in dogs than in people. *J Infect Dis* 158:1410–1411.
33. Falco RC, Smith HA, Fish D, et al. 1993. The distribution of canine exposure to *Borrelia burgdorferi* in a Lyme disease endemic area. *Am J Public Health* 83:1305–1310.
34. Feder BM, Joseph RJ, Moroff SD, et al. 1991. *Borrelia burgdorferi* antibodies in canine cerebrospinal fluid, p 137. *In* Proceeding of the Annual ACVIM Forum, New York, NY.
35. Fekade D, Knox K, Hussein K, et al. 1996. Prevention of Jarisch-Herxheimer reactions by treatment with antibodies against tumor necrosis factor α. *N Engl J Med* 335:311–315.
36. Filipuzzi-Jenny E, Blot M, Schmid-Berger N, et al. 1993. Genetic diversity among *Borrelia burgdorferi* isolates: more than three genospecies? *Res Microbiol* 144:295–304.
37. Font A, Closa JM, Mascort J. 1992. Lyme disease in dogs in Spain. *Vet Rec* 130:227–228.
38. Frank JC. 1989. Taking a hard look at *Borrelia burgdorferi*. *J Am Vet Med Assoc* 194:1521.
39. Georglis K, Peacocke M, Klempner MS. 1992. Fibroblasts protect the Lyme disease spirochete *Borrelia burgdorferi* from ceftriaxone in vitro. *J Infect Dis* 166:440–444.
40. Gerber MA, Shapiro ED, Bell GL, et al. 1995. Recombinant outer surface protein C ELISA for the diagnosis of early Lyme disease. *J Infect Dis* 171:724–727.
41. Gibson MD, Omran MT, Young CR. 1995. Experimental feline Lyme borrelosis as a model for testing *Borrelia burgdorferi* vaccines. *Adv Exp Med Biol* 383:73–82.
42. Gibson MD, Young CR, Tawfik OM, et al. 1993. *Borrelia burgdorferi* infection of cats. *J Am Vet Med Assoc* 202:1786.
43. Granter SR, Barnhill RL, Hewins ME, et al. 1994. Identification of *Borrelia burgdorferi* in diffuse fasciitis with peripheral eosinophilia: borrelial fasciitis. *JAMA* 272:1283–1285.
44. Grauer GF, Burgess EC, Cooley AJ, et al. 1988. Renal lesions associated with *Borrelia burgdorferi* infection in a dog. *J Am Vet Med Assoc* 193:237–239.
45. Greene CE. 1995. Unpublished data. University of Georgia, Athens, GA.
46. Greene RT. 1989. Lameness and symptomatic *Borrelia burgdorferi* seropositivity in dogs. *J Infect Dis* 160:346–347.
47. Greene RT. 1990. An update on the serodiagnosis of canine Lyme borreliosis. *J Vet Intern Med* 4:167–171.
48. Greene RT. 1990. Lyme borreliosis, pp 508–515. *In* Greene CE (ed), Infectious diseases of the dog and cat. WB Saunders, Philadelphia, PA.
49. Greene RT, Hirsch D, Rottman PL, et al. 1991. Interlaboratory comparison of titers of antibody to *Borrelia burgdorferi* and evaluation of a commercial assay using canine sera. *J Clin Microbiol* 29:16–20.
50. Greene RT, Levine JF, Breitchwerdt EB, et al. 1988. Antibodies to *Borrelia burgdorferi* in dogs in North Carolina. *Am J Vet Res* 49:473–476.
51. Greene RT, Levine JF, Breitschwerdt EB, et al. 1988. Clinical and serologic

evaluations of induced *Borrelia burgdorferi* infection in dogs. *Am J Vet Res* 49:752–757.
52. Greene RT, Walker RL, Burgess EC, et al. 1988. Heterogeneity in immunoblot patterns obtained by using four strains of *Borrelia burgdorferi* and sera from naturally exposed dogs. *J Clin Microbiol* 26:2287–2291.
53. Greene RT, Walker RL, Greene CE. 1991. Pseudospirochetes in animal blood being cultured for *Borrelia burgdorferi*. *J Vet Diagn Invest* 3:350–352.
54. Greene RT, Walker RL, Nicholson WL, et al. 1988. Immunoblot analysis of the immunoglobulin G response to the Lyme disease agent (*Borrelia burgdorferi*) in experimentally and naturally exposed dogs. *J Clin Microbiol* 26:648–653.
55. Greene RT, Walker RL, Nicholson WL, et al. 1991. Comparison of an enzyme-linked immunosorbent assay to an indirect immunofluorescence assay for the detection of antibodies to *Borrelia burgdorferi* in the dog. *Vet Microbiol* 26:179–190.
56. Gustafson JM, Burgess EC, Wachal MD, et al. 1993. Intrauterine transmission of *Borrelia burgdorferi* in dogs. *Am J Vet Res* 54:882–890.
57. Hansen K, Lebech AM. 1991. Lyme neuroborreliosis a new sensitive diagnostic assay for intrathecal synthesis of *Borrelia burgdorferi* specific immunoglobulin G, A, and M. *Am Neurol* 30:197–205.
58. Hilton E, Tramontano A, DeVoti J, et al. 1997. Temporal study of immunoglobulin M seroreactivity to *Borrelia burgdorferi* in patients treated for Lyme borreliosis. *J Clin Microbiol* 35:774–776.
59. Jacobson RH, Chang Y-F, Shin SJ. 1996. Lyme disease: laboratory diagnosis of infected and vaccinated symptomatic dogs. *Semin Vet Med Surg* 11:172–182.
60. Johnson RC, Kodner CB, Jurkovich PJ, et al. 1990. Comparative in vitro and in vivo susceptibilities of the Lyme disease spirochete *Borrelia burgdorferi* to cefuroxime and other antimicrobial agents. *Antimicrob Agents Chemother* 34:2133–2136.
61. Karch H, Huppertz HI, Bohme M, et al. 1994. Demonstration of *Borrelia burgdorferi* DNA in urine samples from healthy humans whose sera contain *B. burgdorferi*–specific antibodies. *J Clin Microbiol* 32:2312–2314.
62. Kaufman AC, Greene CE, McGraw RA. 1993. Optimization of polymerase chain reaction for the detection of *Borrelia burgdorferi* in biologic specimens. *J Vet Diagn Invest* 5:548–554.
63. Kazmierczak JJ, Sorhage FE. 1993. Current understanding of *Borrelia burgdorferi* infection with emphasis on its prevention in dogs. *J Am Vet Med Assoc* 203:1524–1528.
64. Keller D, Koster FT, Marks DH, et al. 1994. Safety and immunogenicity of a recombinant outer surface protein A Lyme vaccine. *J Am Med Assoc* 271:1764–1768.
65. Kuiper H, van Dam AP, Spanjaard L, et al. 1994. Isolation of *Borrelia burgdorferi* from biopsy specimens taken from healthy-looking skin of patients with Lyme Borreliosis. *J Clin Microbiol* 32:715–720.
66. Kumi-Diaka J, Harris O. 1995. Viability of *Borrelia burgdorferi* in stored semen. *Br Vet J* 151:221–224.
67. Levine JF. 1995. Ixodes-borne *Borrelia* spp. infections. *J Am Vet Med Assoc* 207:768–775.
68. Levy SA, Dombach DM, Barthold SW, et al. 1993. Canine Lyme Borreliosis. *Compend Cont Educ Pract Vet Small Anim* 15:833–846.
69. Levy SA, Dreesen DW. 1992. Lyme borreliosis in dogs. *Canine Pract* 17:5–13.
70. Levy SA, Duray PH. 1988. Complete heart block in a dog seropositive for *Borrelia burgdorferi*. *J Vet Intern Med* 2:138–144.
71. Levy SA, Lissman BA, Ficke CM. 1993. Performance of a *Borrelia burgdorferi* bacterin in borreliosis-endemic areas. *J Am Vet Med Assoc* 202:1834–1838.
72. Levy SA, Magnarelli LA. 1992. Relationship between development of antibodies to *Borrelia burgdorferi* in dogs and the subsequent development of limb/joint borreliosis. *J Am Vet Med Assoc* 200:344–347.
73. Lindenmayer J, Weber M, Bryant J, et al. 1990. Comparison of indirect immunofluorescent-antibody assay, enzyme-linked immunosorbent assay, and Western immunoblot for the diagnosis of Lyme disease in dogs. *J Clin Microbiol* 28:92–96.
74. Lissman BA, Bosler EM, Camay H, et al. 1984. Spirochete associated arthritis (Lyme disease) in a dog. *J Am Vet Med Assoc* 185:219–220.
75. Lorvich SD, Callister SM, Lim LCL, et al. 1994. Seroprotective groups of Lyme borreliosis spirochetes from North America and Europe. *Infect Dis* 170:115–121.
75a. Luke CJ, Huebner RC, Kasmiersky V, et al. 1997. Oral delivery of purified lipoprotein OspA protects mice from systemic infection with *Borrelia burgdorferi*. *Vaccine* 15:739–746.
76. Ma J, Bulger PA, Dante S, et al. 1995. Characterization of canine humoral immune responses to outer surface protein subunit vaccines and to natural infection by Lyme disease spirochete. *J Infect Dis* 171:909–915.
77. Magnarelli LA, Anderson JF, Johnson RC, et al. 1994. Comparison of different strains of *B. burgdorferi sensu lato* used as antigens enzyme-linked immunosorbent assays. *J Clin Microbiol* 32:1154–1158.
78. Magnarelli LA, Anderson JF, Kaufmann AF, et al. 1985. Borreliosis in dogs from southern Connecticut. *J Am Vet Med Assoc* 186:955–959.
79. Magnarelli LA, Anderson JF, Levine HR, et al. 1990. Tick parasitism and antibodies to *Borrelia burgdorferi* in cats. *J Am Vet Med Assoc* 197:63–66.
80. Magnarelli LA, Anderson JF, Schreier AB. 1990. Persistence of antibodies to *Borrelia burgdorferi* in dogs of New York and Connecticut. *J Am Vet Med Assoc* 196:1064–1068.
81. Magnarelli LA, Anderson JF, Schreier AB, et al. 1987. Clinical and serologic studies of canine borreliosis. *J Am Vet Med Assoc* 191:1089–1093.
82. Magnarelli LA, Flavell RA, Padula SJ, et al. 1997. Serologic diagnosis of canine and equine borreliosis. Use of recombinant antigens in enzyme-linked immunosorbent assays. *J Clin Microbiol* 35:169–173.
83. Malawista SE, Barthold SW, Persing DH. 1994. Fate of *Borrelia burgdorferi* DNA in tissues of infected mice after antibiotic treatment. *J Infect Dis* 170:1312–1316.
84. Mandel NS, Senker EG, Bosler EM, et al. 1993. Intrathecal production of *Borrelia burgdorferi* specific antibodies in a dog with central nervous system Lyme borreliosis. *Compend Cont Educ Pract Vet* 15:581–585.
85. Marshall WF, Telford SR, Rys PN, et al. 1994. Detection of *Borrelia burgdorferi* DNA in museum specimens of Peromyscus leucopus. *J Infect Dis* 170:1027–1032.
86. Masters EJ, Donnell HD. 1995. Lyme and/or Lyme-like disease in Missouri MO. *Medicine* 92:346–353.
86a. Master EJ, Ellis B. 1995. Unilateral facial paralysis associated with borreliacidal activity against *Borrelia burgdorferi sensu stricto* C-1-11. *J Spirochetal Tick-Borne Dis* 2:42–45.
87. Mather TN, Fish D, Coughlin RT. 1994. Competence of dogs as reservoirs for Lyme disease spirochetes (*Borrelia burgdorferi*). *J Am Vet Med Assoc* 205:186–188.
88. Mathiesen DA, Oliver JH, Kolbert CP, et al. 1997. Genetic heterogenity of *Borrelia burgdorferi* in the United States. *J Infect Dis* 175:98–107.
89. Matuschka F-R, Endepols S, Richter D, et al. 1996. Risk of urban Lyme disease enhanced by the presence of rats. *J Infect Dis* 174:1108–1111.
90. Matuschka F-R, Ohlenbusch A, Eiffert H, et al. 1996. Characteristics of Lyme disease spirochetes in archived European ticks. *J Infect Dis* 174:424–426.
91. Maupin GO, Gage KL, Piesman J, et al. 1994. Discovery of an enzootic cycle of *Borrelia burgdorferi* in *Neotoma Mexicana* and *Ixodes* spinipalpis from northern Colorado, an area where Lyme disease is nonendemic. *J Infect Dis* 170:636–643.
92. May C, Bennett D, Carter SD. 1990. Lyme disease in the dog. *Vet Rec* 126:293.
93. May C, Carter SD, Barnes A, et al. 1994. *Borrelia burgdorferi* infection in cats in the UK. *J Small Anim Pract* 35:517–520.
94. Minkus G, Breuer W, Wanke R, et al. 1994. Familial nephropathy in Bernese mountain dogs. *Vet Pathol* 31:421–428.
95. Moreland KJ, Wilson EA, Simpson RB. 1990. Concurrent *Ehrlichia canis* and *Borrelia burgdorferi* infections in a Texas dog. *J Am Anim Hosp Assoc* 26:635–639.
96. Munger RJ. 1990. Uveitis as a manifestation of Lyme borreliosis. *J Am Vet Med Assoc* 197:811.
96a. Nadelman RB, Horowitz HW, Hsieh T-C, et al. 1997. Simultaneous human granulocytic ehrlichiosis and Lyme borreliosis. *N Engl J Med* 337:27–30.
97. Nocton JJ, Bloom BJ, Rutledge BJ, et al. 1996. Detection of *Borrelia burgdorferi* DNA by polymerase chain reaction in cerebrospinal fluid in Lyme neuroborreliosis. *J Infect Dis* 623–627.
98. Nocton JJ, Dressler F, Rutledge BJ, et al. 1994. Detection of *Borrelia burgdorferi* DNA by polymerase chain reaction in synovial fluid from patients with Lyme arthritis. *N Engl J Med* 330:229–234.
98a. Nowakowski J, Schwartz I, Nadelman RB, et al. 1997. Culture-confirmed infection and reinfection with *Borrelia burgdorferi*. *Ann Intern Med* 127:130–132.
99. Ohlers C. 1991. Tracing the roots of *Borrelia burgdorferi*. *J Am Vet Med Assoc* 199:1249–1250.
100. Oliver JH, Owsley MR, Hutcheson HJ, et al. 1993. Conspecificity of the ticks *Ixodes scapularis* and *I. dammini* (Acari: Ixodidae). *J Med Entomol* 30:54–63.
100a. Overduin LM, van den Bogaard AE. 1997. [Lyme borreliosis in dogs.] Lyme borreliose bij de hond. *Tijdschr Diergeneeskd* 122:7–9.
101. Padula SJ, Dias F, Sampieri A, et al. 1994. Use of recombinant OspC from *Borrelia burgdorferi* for serodiagnosis of early Lyme disease. *J Clin Microbiol* 32:1733–1738.
102. Patrican LA. 1997. Absence of Lyme disease spirochetes in larval progeny of naturally infected *Ixodes scapularis* (Acari Ixodidae) fed on dogs. *J Med Entomol* 34:52–55.
103. Persing DH, Rutledge BJ, Rys PN, et al. 1994. Target imbalance: disparity of *Borrelia burgdorferi* genetic material in synovial fluid from Lyme arthritis patients. *J Infect Dis* 169:668–672.
104. Persing DH, Telford SR, Rys PN, et al. 1990. Detection of *Borrelia burgdorferi* DNA in museum specimens of *Ixodes dammini* ticks. *Science* 249:1420–1423.
104a. Piesman J, Happ CM. 1997. Ability of the Lyme disease spirochete *Borrelia burgdorferi* to infect rodents and three species of human-biting ticks (blacklegged tick, American dog tick, lone star tick) (Acari:Ixodidae). *J Med Entomol* 34:451–456.
105. Probert WS, Crawford M, Cadiz RB, et al. 1997. Immunization with outer surface protein (Osp) A but not OspC, provides cross-protection of mice challenged with North American isolates of *Borrelia burgdorferi*. *J Infect Dis* 175:400–405.

106. Rand PW, Smith RP, Lacombe EH. 1991. Canine seroprevalence and the distribution of *Ixodes dammini* in an area of emerging Lyme disease. *Am J Public Health* 81:1331–1334.
107. Roush JK, Manley PA, Dueland RT. 1989. Rheumatoid arthritis subsequent to *Borrelia burgdorferi* infection in two dogs. *J Am Vet Med Assoc* 195:951–953.
108. Salinas-Metendez JA, Tamez-Gonzalez R, Welsh-Lozano O, et al. 1995. Detection of *Borrelia burgdorferi* DNA in human skin biopsies and dog synovial fluid by the polymerase chain reaction. *Rev Latinoam Microbiol* 37:7–10.
109. Schillhorn Van Veen TW, Murphy AJ, Colmery B. 1993. False positive *Borrelia burgdorferi* antibody titers associated with periodontal disease in dogs. *Vet Rec* 132:512.
110. Schwan TG, Piesman J, Golde WT, et al. 1995. Induction of an outer surface protein on *Borrelia burgdorferi* during tick feeding. *Proc Natl Acad Sci* 92:2909–2913.
111. Schwan TG, Schrumph ME, Hinnebusch BJ, et al. 1996. GlpQ: an antigen for serological discrimination between relapsing fever and Lyme borreliosis. *J Clin Microbiol* 34:2483–2492.
112. Shapiro ED, Gerber MA, Holabird NB, et al. 1992. A controlled trial of antimicrobial prophylaxis for Lyme disease after deer tick bites. *N Engl J Med* 27:1769–1773.
113. Shin SJ, Chang YF, Jacobson RH, et al. 1993. Cross-reactivity between *B. burgdorferi* and other spirochetes affects specificity of serotests for detection of antibodies to the Lyme disease agent in dogs. *Vet Microbiol* 36:161–174.
114. Sigal LH. 1994. The polymerase chain reaction assay for *Borrelia burgdorferi* in the diagnosis of Lyme disease. *Ann Intern Med* 120:520–521.
115. Smith RP, Rand PW, Lacombe EH, et al. 1996. Role of bird migration in the long-distance dispersal of *Ixodes dammini*. *J Infect Dis* 174:221–224.
116. Sood SK, Salzman MB, Johnson BJB, et al. 1997. Duration of tick attachment as a predictor of the risk of Lyme disease in an area in which Lyme disease is endemic. *J Infect Dis* 175:996–999.
117. Steere AC, Berandi VP, Weeks KE, et al. 1990. Evaluation of intrathecal antibody response to *Borrelia burgdorferi* as a diagnostic test for Lyme neuroborreliosis. *J Infect Dis* 161:1203–1209.
118. Steere AC, Taylor E, McHugh GL, et al. 1993. The overdiagnosis of Lyme disease. *JAMA* 269:1812–1816.
119. Stevenson B, Schwan TG, Rosa PA. 1995. Temperature-related differential expression of antigens in the Lyme disease spirochete, *Borrelia burgdorferi*. *Infect Immun* 63:4535–4539.
120. Straubinger RK. 1997. Unpublished observations. Cornell University, Ithaca, NY.
120a. Straubinger RK, Straubinger AF, Härter L, et al. 1997. *Borrelia burgdorferi* migrates into joint capsules and causes an up-regulation of interleukin-8 in synovial membranes of dogs experimentally infected with ticks. *Infect Immun* 65:1273–1285.
121. Straubinger RK, Sumers BA, Yung-Fu C, et al. 1997. Persistence of *Borrelia burgdorferi* in experimentally infected dogs after antibotic treatment. *J Clin Microbiol* 35:111–116.
122. Straubinger RK, Yung-Fu C, Jacobson RH, et al. 1995. Sera from OspA-vaccinated dogs, but not those from tick-infected dogs, inhibit in vitro growth of *Borrelia burgdorferi*. *J Clin Microbiol* 33:2745–2751.
123. Sugiyama Y, Sugiyama F, Yagami K. 1993. Comparative study on cross reaction of leptospiral antibodies in several serological tests to detect antibodies to *Borrelia burgdorferi* in dogs. *J Vet Med Sci* 55:149–151.
124. Torrence ME, Jenkins SR, Levine JF, et al. 1990. Serosurvey of shelter dogs in Virginia for antibodies to *Borrelia burgdorferi*. *Prev Vet Med* 10:41–46.
125. Wallich R, Brenner C, Kramer MD, et al. 1995. Molecular cloning and immunological characterization of a novel linear-plasmid-encoded gene, pG of *Borrelia burgdorferi* expressed only in vivo. *Infect Immun* 63:3327–3335.
126. Wasomen TL, Sebring RW, Blumer BM, et al. 1992. Examination of Koch's postulates for *Borrelia burgdorferi* as the causative agent of limb/joint dysfunction in dogs with borreliosis. *J Am Vet Med Assoc* 201:412–418.
127. Wesson DM, McLain DK, Oliver JH, et al. 1993. Investigation of the validity of species status of *Ixodes dammini* (Acari: Ixodidae) using rDNA. *Proc Natl Acad Sci U S A* 90:10221–10225.
127a. Wright JC, Chambers M, Mullen GR, et al. 1997. Seroprevalence of *Borrelia burgdorferi* in dogs in Alabama, USA. *Prev Vet Med* 31:127–131.
128. Yu LP, Smith GN, Brandt KD, et al. 1992. Reduction of the severity of canine osteoarthritis by prophylactic treatment with oral doxycycline. *Arthritis Rheum* 35:1150–1159.
129. Zhang Y-Q, Mathiesen D, Kolbert CP, et al. 1997. *Borrelia burgdorferi* enzyme-linked immunosorbent assay for discrimination of OspA vaccination from spirochete infection. *J Clin Microbiol* 35:233–238.

Chapter **46**

Miscellaneous Bacterial Infections

Melioidosis

Craig E. Greene

Burkholderia (Pseudomonas) pseudomallei is an aerobic, gram-negative, bipolar-staining, motile bacillus with a single polar flagellum. Prominent in Southeast Asia, northern Australia, and the South Pacific, it causes a chronic nodular or purulent inflammatory disease, melioidosis, in people, dogs, cats, and other animals. A ubiquitous soil saprophyte in endemic regions,[2] it may be inhaled on dust or introduced into wounds or tissues by bites of arthropod vectors or by direct contact with contaminated soil.[5] Infection results in small, caseous nodules that rupture and spread bacilli to the environment and other animals. Infection may disseminate further as a bacteremia in immunosuppressed animals, resulting in embolic abscess formation in many organs.

Military dogs stationed in Vietnam that became infected developed fever, myalgia, dermal abscesses, and epididymitis. Dogs and cats have also been reported to be infected after insect bites or ingestion of contaminated carcasses.[5]

Isolation of the causative agent from blood or lesions is definitive. It grows on routine media used to isolate gram-negative bacteria. Selective media such as Ashdown's agar are needed for isolation from sites such as the respiratory tract where contaminating microflora are present. Serologic testing for antibodies with a hemagglutination assay is supportive but not as definitive for making a diagnosis as culture of the organism from internal tissues. Polymerase chain reaction can detect the organism in the buffy coat and pus of internal organs.[4, 9] Immunohistochemical methods can detect the organism in tissues.[10]

Surgical drainage of large abscesses with systemic antibacterial therapy may be curative, but relapses may also occur.

The organism is susceptible to tetracycline, chloramphenicol, or trimethoprim-sulfonamide, amoxicillin-clavulanate, and novobiocin-tetracycline combinations. The most successful, but expensive, treatment has been 2 weeks of high dosages of parenteral ceftazidime.[3] Imipenem-cilastatin shows preliminary effectiveness.[3] Combinations of penicillins and aminoglycosides are ineffective. Therapy may have to be continued for months. For appropriate dosages see Appendix 8.

Public health risk of infected animals is uncertain because no zoonotic transmission has been documented. People in endemic areas become infected from the environment, as do animals.

Glanders

Craig E. Greene

Pseudomonas mallei is a coccoid to filamentous, non-spore-forming, unencapsulated, nonmotile, gram-negative organism that is a soil saprophyte of worldwide distribution. It primarily affects solipeds that ingest contaminated food or water, or the organism spreads between infected horses via aerosols. Cloven-hoofed animals are relatively resistant. Other animals, such as dogs and cats, and humans have intermediate susceptibility. They are infected by inadvertent contact with diseased horses, by consumption of contaminated horse meat, or occasionally by wound contamination.

After intestinal or local wound infection, the organism produces bacteremia and spreads to the lymph nodes, nasal passages, and lungs, where it produces nodular lesions resembling those of tuberculosis.

The organism grows on laboratory media, a process that can be facilitated by the addition of antimicrobials and growth factors. Serologic testing is used to confirm a diagnosis in solipeds, but accuracy in detecting canine and feline infection is uncertain.

B. mallei is sensitive to sulfonamides and tetracyclines. Dosages are listed in Appendix 8.

Chryseomonas *Infection*

Russell T. Greene

Chryseomonas luteola (formerly Ve-1) has been recognized as a cause of infection in people with bacteremia and of peritonitis from peritoneal dialysis.[3–5] In humans, *C. luteola* is usually associated with infections involving foreign materials, such as central venous catheters or joint prostheses. The 16S rRNA sequence of *C. luteola* supports the close relationship of this genus to *Pseudomonas*[1] and *Flavimonas*.

I have documented infection in a cat. Approximately 1 year after being diagnosed with diabetes mellitus, a 4.8-kg, 8- to 10-year-old domestic shorthaired cat was presented with a 4 × 8 cm swelling with purulent drainage from the right hip. The animal was receiving insulin SC once daily. Pus from the mass was surgically drained, and amoxicillin, 20 mg/kg, was prescribed for 2 weeks. Four days later, the mass was still present, so it was surgically removed and a drain was placed. The mass was submitted for histopathology. Six months later, a smaller mass developed at the lesion site. Cytologic examination of the exudate revealed large gram-negative rods. Biopsy findings were marked suppuration with primarily polymorphonuclear cell infiltration. Within the inflammation, there were very large rod-shaped organisms.

Specimens for bacterial culture yielded a convex, circular, yellow-pigmented colony within 24 hours on sheep blood agar. There was lysis of the red blood cells under the colony. Gram's stain revealed it to be a very large, gram-negative rod. The isolate was identified as *C. luteola*. Kirby-Bauer testing revealed sensitivity to tetracycline, aminoglycosides, trimethoprim-sulfonamide, and enrofloxacin. The isolate was resistant to ampicillin, cephalothin, and oxacillin. The cat was treated with enrofloxacin 22.7 mg (total dose) PO, twice daily for 3 weeks and the lesion resolved.

References

1. Anzai Y, Kudo Y, Oyaizu H. 1997. The phylogeny of the genera *Chryseomonas, Flavimonas,* and *Pseudomonas* supports the synonymy of these three genera. *Int J Syst Bacteriol* 47:249–251.
2. Brook MD, Currie B, Desmarchelier PM. 1997. Isolation and identification of *Burkholderia pseudomallei* from soil using selective culture techniques and the polymerase chain reaction. *J Appl Microbiol* 82:589–596.
3. Chaowagul W. 1996. Melioidosis: a treatment challenge. *Scand J Infect Dis* Suppl 101:14–16.
4. Dharakul T, Songsivilai S, Viriyachitra S, et al. 1996. Detection of *Burkholderia pseudomallei* DNA in patients with septicemic melioidosis. *J Clin Microbiol* 34:609–614.
5. Greene CE. 1990. Enteric and other bacterial infections, pp 553–554. *In* Greene CE (ed), Infectious diseases of the dog and cat. WB Saunders, Philadelphia, PA.
6. Hawkins E, Moriarty RA, Lewis DE, et al. 1991. Serious infections involving the CDC group Ve bacteria *Chryseomonas luteola* and *Flavimonas oryzihabitans*. *Rev Infect Dis* 13:257–260.
7. Kostman JR, Solomon F, Fekete T. 1991. Infections with *Chryseomonas leuteola* (CDC group Ve-1) and *Flavimonas oryzihabitans* (CDC group Ve-2) in neurosurgical patients. *Rev Infect Dis* 13:233–236.
8. Rahav G, Simhon A, Mattan Y, et al. 1995. Infections with *Chryseomonas luteola* (CDC group Ve-1) and *Flavimonas oryzihabitans* (CDC group Ve-2). *Medicine* 74:83–88.
9. Rattanathongkom A, Sermswan W, Wongratanacheewin S. 1997. Detection of *Burkholderia pseudomallei* in blood samples using polymerase chain reaction. *Mol Cell Probes* 11:25–31.
10. Wong KT, Vadivelu J, Puthucheary SD, et al. 1996. An immunohistochemical method for the diagnosis of melioidosis. *Pathology* 28:188–191.

Chapter **47**

Plague

Dennis W. Macy

ETIOLOGY

Plague is caused by *Yersinia pestis*, a nonmotile, non-spore-forming, facultative anaerobic, gram-negative, bipolar-staining coccobacillus of the family Enterobacteriaceae. The organism is nonsaprophytic and is sensitive to desiccation and temperatures above 40°C, which make fomite transmission unlikely. This coccobacillus can survive for several weeks to months in organic material, such as infected carcasses. Cold temperatures or freezing may prolong the viability of this organism for years. Three geographic variants of *Y. pestis* (*orientalis*, *antiqua*, and *mediaevalis*) can be distinguished biochemically but are of identical virulence.

EPIDEMIOLOGY

Humans and domestic animals are alternate hosts for *Y. pestis*, which is maintained in nature by chronic bacteremia in wild rodents and is transmitted among these reservoir hosts by fleas. More than 230 species of rodents and 1500 species of fleas infected with the plague organism have been found. Despite this wide host range, only 30 to 40 rodent species serve as permanent natural reservoirs for plague; other rodent species are considered only temporary or amplifying hosts for the organism. Natural reservoir hosts are relatively resistant to plague infections, but susceptibility varies tremendously within a species and is based on geographic location, flea species, and environmental factors. The dog and cat fleas (*Ctenocephalides* spp.) are considered poor vectors for plague. In the United States, prairie dogs (*Cynomys* species), rock squirrels (*Spermophilus variegatus*), and ground squirrels such as *Spermophilus richardsoni* are commonly infected wild hosts. Mortality approaches 100% in these species.

Plague exists in various areas on every continent except Australia (Fig. 47–1). These foci of plague are most frequently associated with semiarid, cooler climates usually adjacent to deserts. In the United States, plague foci are located throughout an area bounded on the east by the Rocky Mountains and on the west by the Pacific Ocean as well as in Hawaii (Fig. 47–2). During epizootic outbreaks, the geographic area has spread into the high plains of Colorado, western Kansas, Oklahoma, and Texas. These temporary geographic expansions are due to spread of the disease into highly susceptible ground squirrel populations but are usually not maintained for more than several years because of high mortality in these species. High mountain parks in Colorado and grasslands in California are also susceptible to rapid expansion of plague because of the presence of amplifying rodent species.

Transmission of *Y. pestis* between most hosts occurs by flea bite, less commonly by contact of the organism with mucous

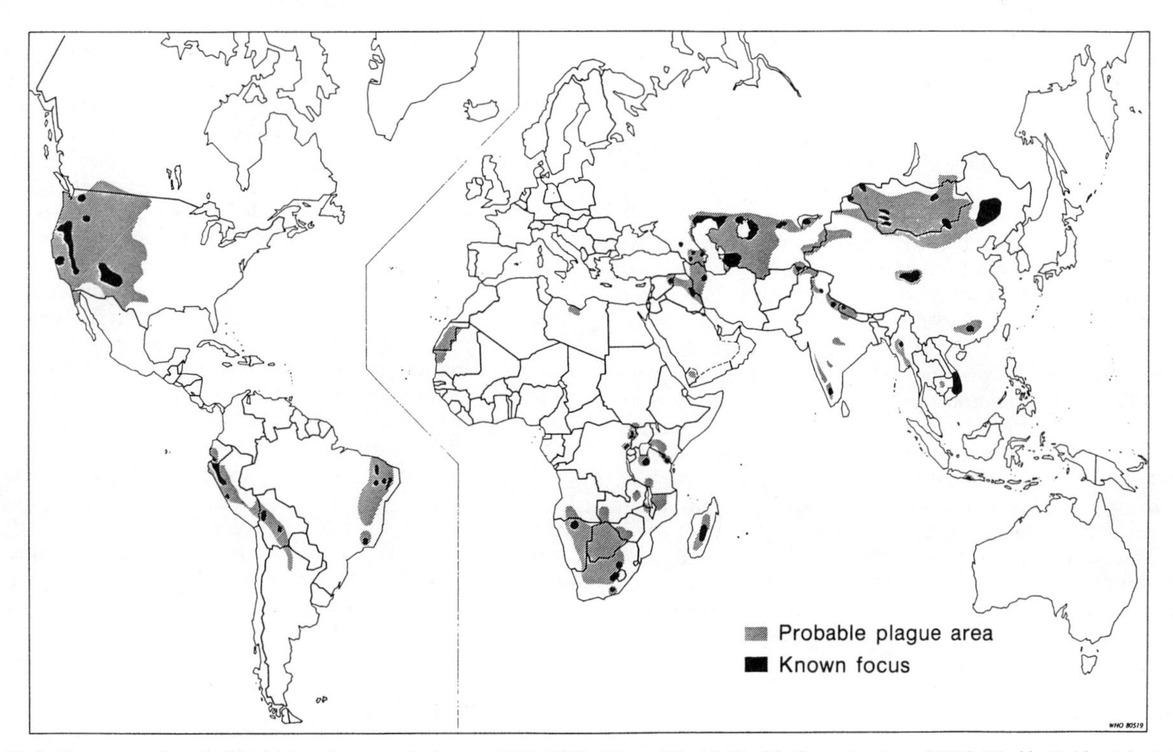

Figure 47–1. Known and probable foci and areas of plague, 1959–1979. (From World Health Organization: *WHO Weekly Epidemiological Record* 32:241–244, 1980. Reprinted with permission.)

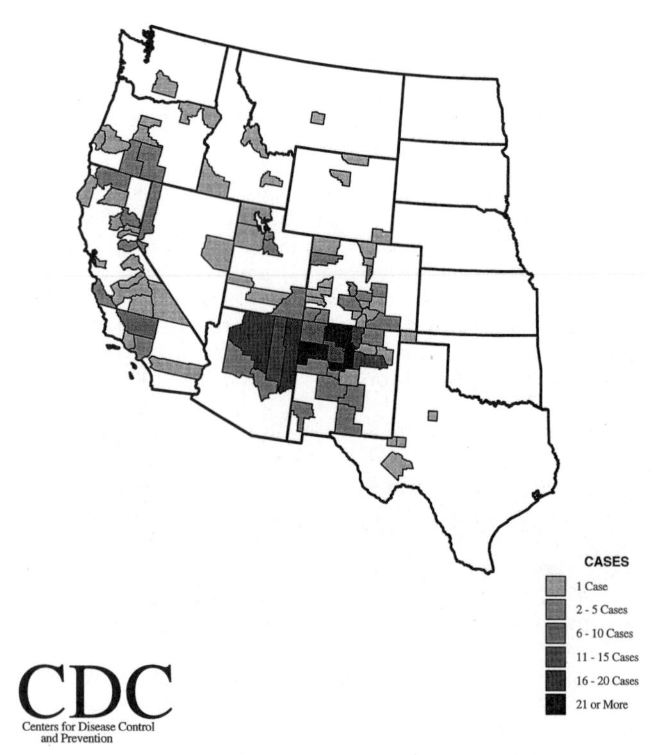

Figure 47–2. Distribution of human plague in the United States from 1970 to 1996. Based on data from the Centers for Disease Control, Atlanta, GA.

membranes or broken skin, or by inhalation of droplets from animals with pneumonic plague (Fig. 47–3). After consumption of a blood meal from an infected host, *Y. pestis* multiplies in the stomach of the flea. While consuming blood from a second host, the flea regurgitates its *Y. pestis*–containing stomach contents, thus transmitting the organism into the new host. The flea may remain infected for more than a year, allowing transmission of the disease long after the death of the host.

Rodent-burrowing systems maintain plague ecosystems by providing a moist environment for flea reproduction and by housing very large numbers of animals such as prairie dogs. Burrows allow the exchange of infected fleas and allow interspecies spread when abandoned burrows are used by another species, such as rabbits, seeking refuge from a predator.

Domestic and wild cats show susceptibility to *Y. pestis* similar to that of people and can be a source of infection for people. Cases in cats have been more common in the summer months; fewer cases are reported in the spring and winter. However, the time of year should not be used to exclude plague from the differential diagnosis. Raptors and other birds; wild carnivores, including black bears, coyotes, badgers, skunks, and raccoons; and domestic dogs are remarkably resistant to *Y. pestis* infection but may transport infected fleas or rodent carcasses. Rabbits, although not considered reservoir hosts, may become infected during enzootic outbreaks and serve sources of infection in hunters.

PATHOGENESIS

Cats and dogs acquire plague by ingestion of infected rodents or lagomorphs or possibly by bites from their prey's plague-infected fleas. Histories in 60 feline plague cases included rodent-hunting activities in 75% of these cats.[7] Ten days after ingestion of *Y. pestis*–infected rodents, plague organisms can be isolated from the oropharynx and blood stream in approximately 50% and 20% of dogs, respectively. Dogs develop only mild clinical symptomatology, including fever and lymphadenomegaly, and undergo seroconversion. Both wild and domestic cats are more susceptible to plague than are dogs or other carnivores. Sixteen healthy cats that were experimentally infected with *Y. pestis* exhibited one of three responses. Thirty-eight percent died within 4 to 9 days after ingestion of the plague-infected mouse. The clinical course included fever (40.7–41.2°C [105–106°F]), depression, and submandibular lymphadenomegaly. Forty-four percent developed transient infections characterized by fever, depression, and lymphadenomegaly. In contrast to cats that maintained elevated body temperature and eventually died of plague, the cats that survived demonstrated a sharp drop in body temperature by day 4 and had clinically recovered by day 14. Nineteen percent of the cats exposed to a plague-infected mouse showed no signs of clinical illness and had no hematologic changes.[8] Most cats fed infected mice had *Y. pestis* cultured from their oropharynx and could have transmitted plague. In the natural environment, the mortality in cats approaches 50%.[11]

Depending on whether the organism enters from a flea bite or through mucous membranes or broken skin, two distinct pathogeneses are possible. First, after a flea bite, the organism is phagocytized by polymorphonuclear cells, in which *Y. pestis* cells are destroyed, and by mononuclear cells, in which *Y. pestis* not only survives but multiplies and is eventually released into the blood stream, delaying bacteremia for 2 to 6 days. Before bacteremia develops, infected mononuclear cells are carried to regional lymph nodes. As *Y. pestis* grows, the lymph nodes become inflamed and swell, forming the bubo. Bubo most frequently develop in the submandibular and sublingual lymph nodes in the cat. Bubo eventually undergo necrosis and abscess formation, with eventual dissemination of the organism via either the lymphatic channels or the blood stream to other organs, including the lungs. Replication in the mononuclear cells results in the production of a capsular envelope, which renders the organism resistant to further phagocytosis. Second, if the organism is ingested or inhaled from contaminated tissues or fluids, which is common in cats and other carnivores, it has already acquired this phagocytosis-resistant capsule from the previous host's mononuclear cells, and it spreads more quickly, resulting in a shorter incubation period of 1 to 3 days.

Lesions at the site of inoculation are usually minimal. The most common visible lesions are in the lymph nodes that drain the site of inoculation. Marked lymphadenomegaly (bubo formation) develops, and nodes may abscess and drain a thick creamy pus through fistulous tracts. Both deep and superficial lymph nodes in other parts of the body may become similarly infected after hematogenous or lymphogenous spread of the organism. In the bacteremic state, other tissues, such as eye, liver, kidney, spleen, brain, and lung, may become infected. *Y. pestis* contains endotoxins that may result in edema, septic shock, and disseminated intravascular coagulation (DIC). The clinical course may last between 6 and 20 days. Cats with previous titers to plague by either vaccination or natural infection generally have a more protracted illness but are not protected from bacteremia or death.

CLINICAL FINDINGS

In both people and cats, three clinical forms of the disease have been recognized: bubonic, septicemic, and pneumonic

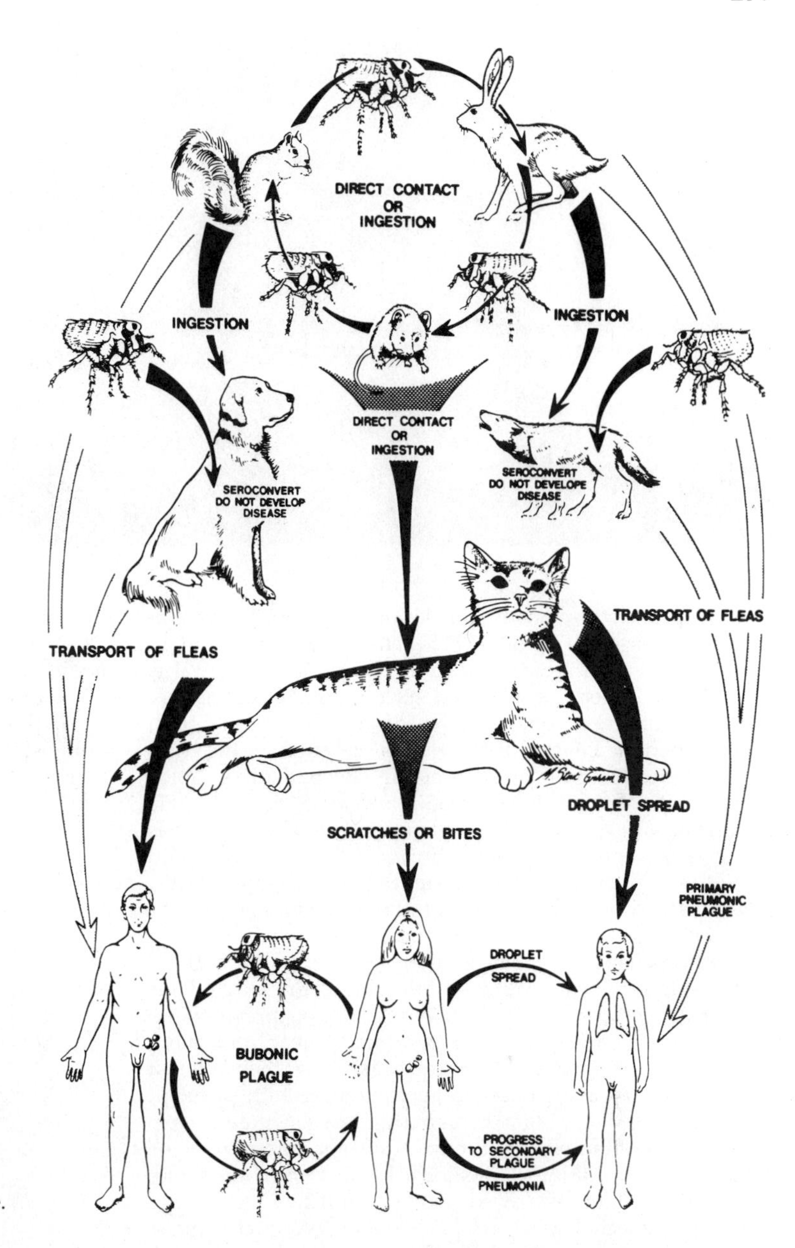

Figure 47–3. Epidemiologic features of plague.

plague. The most common and probably the least fatal form is bubonic plague. In cats, bubonic plague is associated with high (40.6–41.2°C [105–106°F]) temperature, dehydration, and lymphadenomegaly. It is usually acquired by ingesting infected rodents, and the submandibular, retropharyngeal, and cervical lymph nodes in the area of inoculation become enlarged and abscess and may drain. Cats whose abscesses spontaneously drain are more likely to survive. If allowed to progress, the bubonic form may spread hematogenously or through the lymphatics to become the septic form.

Septicemic plague may develop with or without bubo formation. Hematogenous spread may result in involvement of virtually every organ in the body, although the most frequently involved organs are the spleen in people and lungs in cats. Fever, shock, DIC, and marked leukocytosis are characteristic of the septic form of the disease in the cat. The septic form is usually fatal within 1 to 2 days after the presence of bacteremia.

Pneumonic plague in cats develops as a result of hematogenous or lymphogenous spread of the organism and may be seen as a sequel to bubonic or septic forms of the disease rather than primary pneumonic plague, which is contracted through droplet transmission. Although cats normally do not contract primary pneumonic plague, they have been responsible for primary pneumonic plague in people who have contact with them. Pneumonic plague, whether primary or secondary, carries the most severe prognosis. In addition, persistent fevers of greater than 40°C in cats is associated with poor prognoses. In people, untreated pneumonic plague is considered 100% fatal. In summary, plague should be considered when examining any febrile cat in endemic areas. Other atypical clinical signs have included ocular discharge, vomiting, diarrhea, dehydration, weight loss, poor hair coat, swollen tongue, tonsillar enlargement, necrotic stomatitis, facial ulceration, cellulitis, and abdominal distention.[2, 7]

DIAGNOSIS

Although a clinician may have a high degree of suspicion for plague on the basis of clinical and epidemiologic information, the diagnosis must be confirmed. Pneumonic plague

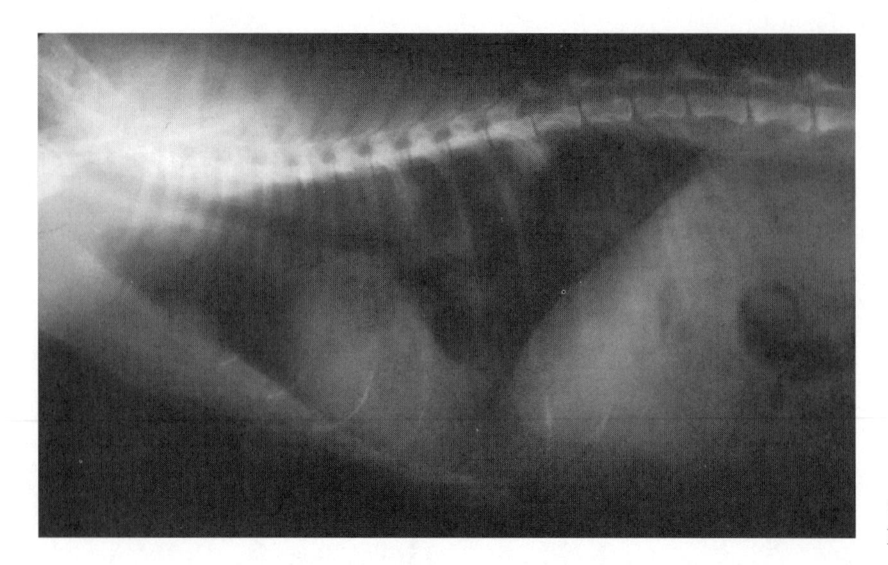

Figure 47–4. Thoracic radiograph of a cat with pneumonic plague.

may be suspected by pneumonic lesions visualized with thoracic radiographs (Fig. 47–4). *Y. pestis* is usually found in large numbers in infected tissues. In the clinical setting it is important to collect samples and start antimicrobial therapy before the disease is confirmed. Needle aspirates from lymph nodes, blood, or infected tissue may be selected on the basis of the clinical form of the disease in the patient. A quick Gram's stain of these tissues usually reveals a monomorphic population of gram-negative organisms (Fig. 47–5), which is in contrast to common cat bite abscesses that usually contain a mixture of organisms found in the oral cavity of cats. Aseptically collected samples of fluids, tissues, or blood should be submitted. Cultures of tonsils from experimentally infected cats have given consistently positive results, and the tonsils may serve as a source of infection of the saliva. Four or more slides for bacterial stains should be prepared by making impression smears or cytologic smears, allowing them to air dry, and then lightly heat fixing them over a flame. Care should be taken to avoid contact with purulent material while obtaining and preparing these samples.

For immunofluorescent testing, fluid specimens may be applied to clean, thin, glass slides. FA tests provide rapid, presumptive diagnosis with good reliability. One or two drops of suspected fluid are placed into two circles made with a wax pencil on the slide. The drops are spread with a loop. With tissue specimens, impression smears are made within each circle. Slides are allow to air dry and should be frozen if they cannot be examined immediately.

Two serum samples, 10 to 14 days apart, should be collected for antibody titers against *Y. pestis*. Because dogs and cats in endemic areas frequently have high titers to *Y. pestis* that persist for a year or longer after exposure, a fourfold rise in titer is needed to distinguish active disease from previous exposure.

Alternatively, specimens for culture may be collected (before antimicrobial therapy) in a sterile syringe by aspiration, placed in blood tubes, or inoculated into transport media (Stuarts [Difco, Detroit, MI] and Cary-Blair [BBL, Cockeysville, MD] are suitable), refrigerated but not frozen, and sent to a reference laboratory for confirmation. Veterinarians should not attempt to culture specimens, because class II precautions are advised in isolating and identifying cultures from plague suspects. Samples should be double-wrapped in plastic and padded to prevent breakage and leakage to conform with federal requirements for transporting hazardous agents. It is recommended that the state veterinarian be contacted before shipping samples to the Division of Vectorborne Infectious Disease, Centers for Disease Control, P.O. Box 2087, Fort Collins, Colorado 80522, (970) 221-6400. A few regional or state laboratories also conduct specialized serologic or cultural testing for plague (see Appendix 5).

At the laboratory, Gram's stains are performed to determine staining characteristics, and Giemsa or Wayson stain is performed to determine the bipolarity "safety pin" appearance suggestive of *Y. pestis*. *Y. pestis* can be cultured on

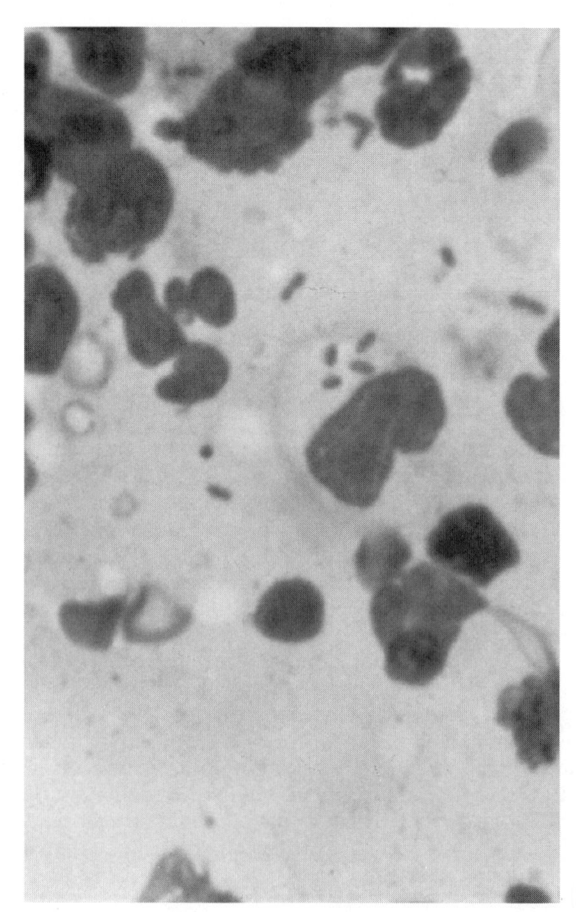

Figure 47–5. Fine-needle aspirate of bubo of a cat with plague. Note the monomorphic population of bipolar staining coccobacillus organisms.

enriched blood agar but grows slowly, requiring 48 hours of incubation to produce colonies 1 to 2 mm in size at an optimum temperature of 28°C. If growth is observed, suspect isolates can be shipped to a reference laboratory. Polymerase chain reaction (PCR) has been developed to identify the presence of the organism in tissues, blood, and fleas.[9]

PATHOLOGIC FINDINGS

Cats, of which 50% die acutely, may have focal necrotic lesions of the spleen and liver, with evidence of secondary pneumonic spread of the disease. Those surviving for longer periods of time develop cervical or submandibular abscesses or bubos. Consistent involvement of the medial retropharyngeal lymph nodes has been apparent in experimentally infected cats. In fatal cases, tonsils and submandibular and cranial thoracic lymph nodes were also affected. The normal nodal architecture was totally replaced by necrosis and hemorrhage. Lymph nodes from cats that were euthanized after clinical recovery showed only lymphoid hyperplasia. Bacterial infiltration of the lung parenchyma, resulting in pneumonia, is characterized by focal areas of hemorrhage with clusters of bacteria. Because experimentally infected dogs develop only transient fever and lymphadenomegaly, no pathologic features have been described.

THERAPY

The decision to treat an animal for plague is seldom based on a definitive diagnosis. When plague is suspected on the basis of clinical or epidemiologic information, specific antimicrobial therapy should be instituted rather than waiting for laboratory confirmation. All plague suspects should be handled by persons wearing gloves, gowns, and high-density surgical masks. Animals with respiratory signs should have thoracic radiographs taken to determine whether they have pneumonic plague. Animals should be examined for fleas. If any are found, patients in surrounding cages and examination rooms should be treated with carbamates or pyrethrins. Bubos should be lanced and flushed with chlorhexidine diacetate (Nolvasan, Fort Dodge, Fort Dodge, IA). Organic material, including tissues or pus-containing gauze pads, should be double bagged and incinerated. Routine disinfectants are effective in killing the plague organism and should be applied as a precautionary measure on cages and examination tables used in the care of infected animals.

Y. pestis is susceptible to a wide variety of antimicrobial agents (Table 47–1). Unfortunately, multiple drug-resistant strains are being isolated with increasing frequency.[5] Although *Y. pestis* appears sensitive in vitro to penicillin, it is resistant to penicillin in vivo. Aminoglycosides such as streptomycin and gentamicin are considered the most effective antibiotics against *Y. pestis*. Treatment efficacy with penicillins or aminoglycosides has been increased in experimentally infected mice by using successive therapy with rifampin.[12] Chloramphenicol is used in the treatment of patients with CNS spread of plague organism. Administration of tetracyclines has been associated with relapse, presumably owing to the development of bacterial resistance or poor absorption from the GI tract. Tetracyclines (doxycycline is preferred) are given primarily for the bubonic form of the disease and for prophylaxis. The fluoroquinolones have been shown to be effective in the treatment of plague in mice and cats.[1] Infected cats should be treated for a minimum of 21 days. Treatment should continue far beyond the resolution of bubos and pneumonic changes.

Prophylactic therapy with tetracycline is indicated in asymptomatic animals exposed to plague and should be continued for a 7-day period. People exposed to plague in the process of caring for plague-infected animals are usually treated in a similar manner under the direction of a physician. The prognosis depends on the clinical form of the disease and the species infected.

Table 47–1. Antimicrobial Therapy for Plague

DRUG	DOSE[a] (mg/kg)	ROUTE	INTERVAL (HOURS)	DURATION (DAYS)
Streptomycin[b]	5	IM	12	21
Kanamycin[b]	5–7.5	IM	12	21
Gentamicin[b]	2–4	IM	12–24	21
Trimethoprim-sulfonamide	15	PO, IV, IM	12	21
Tetracycline	20	PO	8	21
Chloramphenicol	15	PO, SC	12	21

[a]Dose per administration at specified interval. See also Appendix 8.
[b]Renal function must be closely monitored because of potential nephrotoxicity.

PREVENTION

People and domestic animals have intruded into the natural ecosystem in which plague circulates. Elimination of plague in wild rodent populations is generally impossible. Veterinarians should be especially alert in evaluating sick cats in such outbreaks and take appropriate precautions to protect themselves, their employees, and their clients. Examination of fleas taken from patients may quickly determine whether they are of rodent source. Flea control in both dogs and cats should be stressed in enzootic areas, because pets have ample opportunity to share them with their owners. Dogs and cats should not be allowed to come in contact with burrows or have access to carcasses of dead rodents or lagomorphs. Residents in endemic areas should be encouraged to reduce food and habitat, such as rubbish or garbage piles, for peridomestic host species, which may become infected during enzootic outbreaks. Local state and health officials may institute rodent control measures but not before flea control has been instituted in an area.

Both killed and modified live vaccines for *Y. pestis* have been produced for humans, but only the killed formalin-fixed virulent whole-organism preparation is available in the United States. The vaccine requires multiple inoculations to maintain protective titers, and its use is associated with a high degree of local and systemic reactions. Immunization of cats with this vaccine has not protected them against bacteremia or death but has prolonged the clinical course of the disease. Vaccination is recommended for all laboratory and field personnel who are working with *Y. pestis* and for persons engaged in field operations in areas of enzootic plague. Experimental subunit vaccines are being evaluated.[14]

PUBLIC HEALTH CONSIDERATIONS

The incidence of human plague in the United States is increasing. The 105 cases that occurred in eight western states during the 1970s represented the largest number in the continental United States in any decade since 1900 to 1909. Ninety percent of human cases of plague have been reported in California, Arizona, and New Mexico. Since 1949, New Mexico annually has reported more than 50% of plague cases. In one survey, 82% of human plague cases were transmitted by flea bites, 15% by direct contact with infected wild animals, and 3% by contact with infected domestic cats.

From 1977 to 1991, the Centers for Disease Control confirmed 16 human plague cases acquired through inhalation of *Y. pestis*--infected droplets expelled from cats with secondary plague pneumonia. Approximately one half of the cases were fatal and one fourth occurred in veterinarians or their technicians. In people, the overall death rate in treated patients in the United States is 15% to 22%. The major reasons for death in this treatable disease are patient delay in seeking medical attention and lack of recognition of the disease as plague. These factors has been especially true when patients acquire the infection in enzootic areas and travel to areas of the United States where plague has never been seen. The death rates in such instances has been 80%.

All free-roaming cats in an endemic area must be considered at risk of exposure to plague. Veterinarians and their assistants are at increased risk of exposure to plague as a result of their occupations. People may become infected through inhalation of respiratory droplets from animals infected with secondary pneumonic plague, handling infected tissues and body fluids via broken skin or mucous membrane contact, or bites of plague-infected fleas. Patients suspected of having plague should be hospitalized and isolated immediately. Attempts should be made to limit the number of individuals caring for infected animals. These individuals should be informed of the mode of transmission of infection and advised to wear protective clothing and gloves in treating and caring for infected pets. Routine disinfectants should be applied to cages and examination tables, and flea control should be instituted in the area in and around infected animals. After making a diagnosis of plague in cats, veterinarians should advise owners to contact their physicians immediately. Local and state health authorities should be notified early in the management of plague-infected animals.

References

1. Bonacorsi SP, Scavizzi MR, Guiyoule A, et al. 1994. Assessment of a fluoroquinolone, three β-lactams, two aminoglycosides, and a cycline in treatment of murine *Yersinia pestis* infection. *Antimicrob Agents Chemother* 38:481–486.
2. Carlson ME. 1996. *Yersinia pesti* infection in cats. *Feline Pract* 24:22–24.
3. Chomel BB, Jay MT, Smith CR, et al. 1994. Serological surveillance of plague in dogs and cats: California 1979–1991. *Comp Immunol Microbiol Infect Dis* 17:111–123.
4. Craven RB, Maupin GO, Beard ML, et al. 1991. Reported cases of human plague infection in the United States 1970–1991. *J Med Entomol* 30:758–761.
5. Dennis DT, Hughes JM. 1997. Multidrug resistance in plague. *N Engl J Med* 337:702–704.
6. Doll JM, Zeitz PS, Ettestad P, et al. 1994. Cat-transmitted fatal pneumonia plague in a person who traveled from Colorado to Arizona. *Ann J Trop Med Hyg* 5:109–114.
7. Eidson M, Thelsted JP, Rollag OJ. 1991. Clinical, clinicopathologic and pathologic features of plague in cats: 119 cases (1977–1985). *JAVMA* 199:1191–1196.
8. Gasper PW, Barnes AM, Ovan TJ. 1993. Plague (*Yersinia pestis*) in cats: description of experimentally-induced disease. *J Med Entomol* 30:20–26.
9. Hinne Busch J, Schwan TG. 1993. New method for plague surveillance using polymerase chain reaction to detect *Yersinia pestis* in fleas. *J Clin Microbiol* 31:1511–1514.
10. Kilonzo BS, Gisakany DN, Sabun GA. 1993. Involvement of dogs in plague epidemiology in Tanzania: serological observations in domestic animals in Lushoto district. *Scand J Infect Dis* 25:503–506.
11. Macy DW, Gasper PW. 1990. Plague, pp 621–627. *In* Greene CE (ed), Infectious diseases of the dog and cat. WB Saunders, Philadelphia, PA.
12. Makarovskaia LN, Tinker LA, Markovskaia EI, et al. 1996. Enhancement of treatment efficacy in experimental plague by the sequential administration of antibiotics. *Antibiot Khimoter* 41:25–27.
13. Quan TJ. 1992. *Yersinia pestis*, pp 2888–2898. *In* Balows A, Truper HG, Dworkin M, Harder W, Schleifer KH (eds), The prokaryotes, ed 2, vol III. Springer-Verlag, New York, NY.
14. Sharp GJ, Eyles JE, Williamson ED, et al. 1997. Cellular and humoral responses to microencapsulated *Yersinia pestis* subunit vaccines following oral delivery. *Biochem Soc Trans* 25:338S.

Chapter **48**

Tularemia

Arnold F. Kaufmann

ETIOLOGY

Tularemia is an acute bacterial infection of many avian and mammalian species, including the dog and cat and occasionally people, and it occurs throughout the Northern Hemisphere, predominantly between 20° and 70° latitude.[8] The etiologic agent, *Francisella tularensis*, is a small, pleomorphic, gram-negative, non-spore-forming bacillus. The tularemia bacillus has two main biovars: type A *(tularensis)* and type B *(palearctica)*. Type A strains ferment glycerol and are highly virulent for laboratory rabbits *(Oryctolagus cuniculus)*, and type B strains do not ferment glycerol and are avirulent for rabbits. Type A strains are associated with a tick-rabbit cycle of infection and occur only in North America. Type B strains have a more complex epidemiology—involving rodents, ticks, mosquitoes, mud, and water—and occur throughout the Northern Hemisphere. Both type A and B strains have been isolated from cats in the United States.[1] Human illness is generally more severe with type A strain infections.[15]

EPIDEMIOLOGY

Because the epidemiology of tularemia is complex,[8] only those aspects important in its transmission to the dog and cat are discussed here. Various tick species serve as both reservoirs and vectors of tularemia. Infection can pass transovarially in ticks, and infection persists for life. Amplification of the infection rate in a tick population occurs when uninfected ticks feed on bacteremic animals. Although ticks are capable of transmitting tularemia at all three stages of their development, the adult and, less commonly, nymphal stages are most important in transmission to dogs, cats, and people. In the United States, four tick species constitute the primary vectors for dogs and cats: the wood tick *(Dermacentor andersoni)* found in the Rocky Mountain region; the American dog tick *(D. variabilis)* found in the eastern two thirds of the country as well as in the Pacific coastal states; the Pacific Coast tick *(D. occidentalis)* found in California and Oregon; and the Lone Star tick *(Ambylomma americanum)* found in the southern central and southeastern states. Cats and dogs may also be infected when they hunt or eat infected rabbits or rodents.

PATHOGENESIS

The clinical presentation of human tularemia varies by route of infection and initial sites of localization. Typically, a localized infection occurs at the primary inoculation site and is associated with prominent regional lymphadenomegaly. Subsequent bacteremia and multiorgan involvement are common. Bacteremic disease without antecedent localized infection is referred to as typhoidal tularemia. Cell-mediated immunity plays an important role in recovery.

A similar disease pattern appears to occur in dogs and cats. The severity of illness in experimentally infected dogs varies with age; puppies are more susceptible than young adults. Ingestion of infected tissues or intradermal (ID) challenge produced milder disease than intranasal (IN) challenge.[7, 9] When dogs were fed on infected tissues, an acute 5-day illness began after a 48-hour incubation period.[9] Fever (40.2°C [104.4°F]) and a mucopurulent discharge from the nose and eyes were present. Transient ulceroglandular tularemia follows ID challenge with concomitant development of fever, pustules at the inoculation site, and regional lymphadenomegaly.

More serious illness characterized by septicemia and high mortality follows SC or IM inoculation. Draining abscesses develop at the inoculation sites and are associated with regional lymphadenomegaly and high temperature and with systemic dissemination of the disease after 1 week. At this time, the dogs appear obviously ill, have a mucopurulent ocular and nasal discharge, and develop a vesiculopapular skin rash.

Cats have become ill after eating experimentally infected guinea pigs.[16] Although some cats appear unaffected, younger cats primarily succumb to systemic infection characterized by generalized lymphadenomegaly and miliary abscess formation involving the liver and spleen.

After SC inoculation, similar findings have been apparent, and young kittens appear most susceptible.[16] Some SC- and IN-inoculated cats have had areas of bronchopneumonia from which *F. tularensis* was isolated as well as splenomegaly and multifocal hepatic necrosis.

CLINICAL FINDINGS

Despite the ability to produce experimental infections and high seroprevalence, indicating exposure in endemic areas, naturally acquired cases in dogs have been rare.[3, 5, 7, 8, 12] Dogs are considered relatively resistant to tularemia. Typically, a dog develops a brief episode of anorexia, listlessness, and low-grade fever. Sudden death of uncertain cause has occurred in a dog a few days after sniffing a dead infected rabbit. Another dog developed multifocal draining abscesses in the subcutaneous tissue and superficial lymph nodes in addition to fever, anorexia, myalgia, and shivering. Uveitis and conjunctivitis developed in the left eye, with subsequent transient conjunctivitis and corneal clouding in the right eye.

On the basis of the number of reports, cats are more susceptible to tularemia than dogs. The spectrum of illness associated with spontaneous feline tularemia has not been well described. In a series of three typhoidal cases, pertinent clinical signs included marked depression; pharyngeal, cervical, mesenteric, regional, and/or generalized lymphadenomegaly; palpable splenomegaly and hepatomegaly; acute shallow oral and/or lingual ulcers; icterus; and panleukopenia with severe toxic changes of neutrophils.[1] The oral and lingual ulcers were compatible with infection resulting from ingestion of infected rodents or rabbits.

Other cases in cats have been briefly described in epidemiologic reports of human cases.[4, 7a, 8, 11, 13a, 16] Implicated cats had frequently eaten or mouthed wild rabbits before the onset of clinical signs. Variable signs of fever, anorexia, listlessness, lymphadenomegaly, draining abscesses, and, occasionally, icterus and death were reported. Some cats had no signs of illness.

DIAGNOSIS

Testing for serologic evidence of agglutinating antibody is the most commonly used diagnostic procedure. Both dogs and cats develop antibodies, but titers tend to be lower than those observed in people. Titers from 140 to 160 are typical of recent infections in dogs.[9, 15] ELISA techniques have been developed to detect antibodies to specific *F. tularensis* antigens in infected people,[2] but their usefulness for testing canine and feline sera is uncertain. FA methods can be utilized to detect the coccobacillary organisms in exudates and tissues, even with paraffin-embedded tissues.

The isolation of *F. tularensis* from exudates or tissue specimens is the definitive method of diagnosis. This test may be performed by culture on special media, such as supplemented chocolate agar, or by initial inoculation of a susceptible laboratory animal with subsequent culture of the liver and spleen. The infectious dose for humans is less than 100 organisms, inhaled as an aerosol, accidentally inoculated, or splashed in the conjunctival sac. Cultures of *F. tularensis* and necropsies of animals with suspected tularemia should be performed, therefore, only in laboratories with adequate biosafety equipment.

PATHOLOGIC FINDINGS

Gross necropsy findings in affected dogs and cats are similar. Most of this information has been obtained in experimentally infected animals. Lymph nodes in a given anatomic region or more generalized are often markedly enlarged, with multiple foci of necrosis. Draining sinus tracts may arise from the nodes. Hepatomegaly and/or splenomegaly may be present. Multiple small, grayish foci representing necrosis are commonly found in the spleen, liver, lung, and, occasionally, heart. Segmental to diffuse hemorrhage of the small and large intestines has been reported in cats.[1] These same cats had prominent ulceration in Peyer's patches and colonic lymphoid follicles. The causative bacteria are not easily demonstrated in the lesions except by specific FA or other immunohistochemical stains.

THERAPY

No substantial reports have been made on antimicrobial therapy of canine or feline tularemia. In people, the aminoglycosides (streptomycin and gentamicin) are currently considered the drugs of first choice, but streptomycin is available only on a limited case-by-case basis.[6, 13] Tetracycline and chloramphenicol are alternative drugs, but relapses occur frequently with them. Historically, both streptomycin and tetracycline have been given successfully in controlled trials of antibiotic prophylaxis in human tularemia.[14] Fluoroquinolones, ciprofloxacin, and norfloxacin may be effective.[14a, 17] Consult the Drug Formulary, Appendix 8, for dosages and further information on each drug.

PUBLIC HEALTH CONSIDERATIONS

In the United States, the incidence of human tularemia is low: fewer than 225 cases annually in the past 10 years. Most cases have resulted from tick-borne infection and to a lesser extent contact with tissues of wild animals such as rabbits. Of 1041 human cases reported in the southwestern central United States from 1981 to 1987, 17 (1.6%) cases were associated with cat bites and scratches.[18] At least 53 additional cat-associated cases and eight dog-associated cases have been reported in North America, but some of these have not been well substantiated.[4, 8, 11, 19, 20]

Cat-associated cases usually involved people being bitten or scratched, with the initial lesion typically developing at the trauma site. Although the cats often have no obvious illness, a common feature has been a history of hunting or eating wild animals, particularly rabbits.

None of the eight dog-associated cases involved bites or scratches. In one case, a young girl developed typhoidal tularemia 3 days after the onset of a vague illness in her pet puppy, which presumably had contact with rabbits.[8] The dog frequently licked the young girl, and its saliva was considered her probable source of infection. In another instance, a family of seven persons staying at a cottage with their dogs during a 1-week period developed pulmonary tularemia.[19] After the dogs finished hunting for rabbits, they would shake the water from their hair when they entered the cottage. The resultant aerosol was considered the most likely source of infection. The dogs never appeared ill but subsequently were found to have antibodies to *F. tularensis*.

In people, tularemia occurs in two main syndromes: ulceroglandular and typhoidal.[13] Both syndromes have an incubation period of 2 to 10 days followed by acute onset of high temperature, chills, and other nonspecific constitutional symptoms. Ulceroglandular tularemia is characterized by a skin ulcer developing at the portal of infection with associated regional lymphadenomegaly. In typhoidal tularemia, few localizing signs occur, pneumonia is more common, and the case-fatality ratio can exceed 30% if the illness is untreated.

Although no cases have been associated with removing ticks from pets, the finding of infected ticks on dogs does indicate a potential hazard.[15]

References

1. Baldwin CJ, Panciera RJ, Morton RJ, et al. 1991. Acute tularemia in three domestic cats. *J Am Vet Med Assoc* 199:1602–1605.
2. Bevanger L, Maeland JA, Naess AI. 1989. Competitive enzyme immunoassay for antibodies to a 43,000-molecular weight *Francisella tularensis* outer membrane protein for the diagnosis of tularemia. *J Clin Microbiol* 27:922–926.
3. Calhoun EL, Mohr CO, Alford HI Jr. 1956. Dogs and other mammals as hosts of tularemia and of vector ticks in Arkansas. *Am J Hyg* 63:127–135.
4. Capellan J, Fong IW. 1993. Tularemia from a cat bite: case report and review of feline-associated tularemia. *Clin Infect Dis* 16:472–475.
5. Coffee WM, Miller J. 1943. Acute canine tularemia: a case report. *J Am Vet Med Assoc* 102:210–212.
6. Enderlin G, Morales L, Jacobs RF, et al. 1994. Streptomycin and alternative agents for the treatment of tularemia: review of the literature. *Clin Infect Dis* 19:42–47.
7. Ey LF, Daniels RE. 1941. Tularemia in dogs. *JAMA* 117:2071–2072.
7a. Gliatto JM, Rae JF, McDonough PL. 1994. Feline tularemia on Nantucket Island, Massachusetts. *J Vet Diagn Invest* 6:102–105.
7b. Gustafson BW, DeBowes LJ. 1996. Tularemia in a dog. *J Am Anim Hosp Assoc* 32:339–341.
8. Jellison WL. 1974. *Tularemia in North America*. University of Montana Printing Department, Missoula, MT.
9. Johnson HN. 1944. Natural occurrence of tularemia in dogs used as a source of canine distemper virus. *J Clin Lab Med* 29:906–916.
10. Kaufman AF. 1990. Tularemia, pp 628–631. *In* Greene CE (ed), Infectious diseases of the dog and cat. WB Saunders, Philadelphia, PA.11. Liles WC, Burger RJ. 1993. Tularemia from domestic cats. *West J Med* 158:619–622.
11. Liles WC, Burger RJ. 1993. Tularemia from domestic cats. *West J Med* 158:619–622.
12. Martone WJ, Marshall LW, Kaufmann AF, et al. 1979. Tularemia pneumonia in Washington, D.C.: a report of three cases with possible common-source exposures. *JAMA* 242:2315–2317.
13. Penn RL. 1995. *Francisella tularensis* (tularemia), pp 2060—2068. *In* Mandell GL, Bennett JE, Dolin R (eds), Mandell, Douglas, and Bennett's principles and practices of infectious diseases, ed 4. Churchill Livingstone, New York, NY.
13a. Rhyan JC, Gahagan T, Fales WH. 1990. Tularemia in a cat. *J Vet Diagn Invest* 2:239–241.
14. Sawyer WD, Dangerfield HG, Hogge AL, et al. 1966. Antibiotic prophylaxis and therapy of airborne tularemia. *Bacteriol Rev* 30:542–548.
14a. Sheel O, Reiersen R, Hoel T. 1992. Treatment of tularemia with ciprofloxacin. *Eur J Clin Microbiol Infect Dis* 11:447–448.
15. Schmid GP, Kornblatt AN, Connors CA, et al. 1983. Clinically mild tularemia associated with tick-borne *Francisella tularensis*. *J Infect Dis* 148:63–67.
16. Simpson WM. 1929. *Tularemia*. Paul B. Hoeber, New York, NY.
17. Syrjala H, Schildt R, Raisainen S. 1991. In vitro susceptibility of *Francisella tularensis* to fluoroquinolones and treatment of tularemia with norfloxacin and ciprofloxacin. *Eur J Clin Microbiol Infect Dis* 10:68–70.
18. Taylor JP, Istre GR, McChesney TC, et al. 1991. Epidemiologic characteristics of human tularemia in the southwest-central states, 1981–1987. *Am J Epidemiol* 133:1032–1038.
19. Teutsch SM, Martone WJ, Brink EW, et al. 1979. Pneumonic tularemia on Martha's Vineyard. *N Engl J Med* 301:826–828.
20. Von Schroeder HP, McDougall EP. 1993. Ulceroglandular and pulmonary tularemia: a case resulting from a cat bite to the hand. *J Hand Surg* 18:132–134.

Chapter 49

Actinomycosis and Nocardiosis

David F. Edwards

Actinomycosis

ETIOLOGY AND EPIDEMIOLOGY

Actinomycosis is a chronic, pyogranulomatous disease characterized by pleural and peritoneal exudates; dense fibrous masses; frank abscesses; and fistulous tracts with draining sinuses. The disease is caused by members of the family Actinomycetaceae. *Actinomyces viscosus* and *A. hordeovulneris* are the most commonly isolated species in dogs, but most isolates have not been identified to species.[17, 26, 33] *A. viscosus* and *A. meyeri* have been recovered from infected cats.[9, 54, 55] Anaerobic actinomycetes are part of the normal bacterial flora of the oropharynx. *A. viscosus, A. odontolyticus, A. israelii, A. bovis,* and *A. naeslundii* have been cultured from dental plaque in the dog, and *A. viscosus, A. hordeovulneris,* and *A. denticolens* have been cultured from normal feline gingiva.[56] These endogenous oral saprophytes are normally not pathogenic, but if *Actinomyces* spp. are inoculated into tissues with associated bacteria, an insidious pyogranulomatous disease can develop.

Actinomycosis occurs most commonly in young adult to middle-aged large-breed male dogs that are used or kept in an outdoor environment.[36, 43] The highest prevalence of disease is seen in hunting dogs, and in this group the gender bias is not apparent. Actinomycosis in outdoor dogs is related, in large part, to their frequent exposure to grasses.[13, 32, 40, 66] Inhaled or ingested florets or awns contaminated in the oropharynx migrate to various sites and act as the nidus of infection. Although infrequently reported in cats, actinomycosis is often attributed to bite wounds.[54] Because of the difficulty in culturing *Actinomyces* species and their susceptibility to many antibiotics, the true prevalence of actinomycosis in dogs and cats is greater than suggested by the current literature.

PATHOGENESIS

Actinomyces spp. are opportunistic pathogens dependent on mechanical disruption of normal mucosal barriers. Because of the organism's normal habitat, infections are, by necessity, somehow linked to the oropharyngeal area. The disease characteristically spreads by direct extension unimpeded by normal tissue planes; however, rare instances of hematogenous dissemination occur. The most common clinical forms of actinomycosis in cats and dogs involve the cervicofacial region, thorax, abdomen, retroperitoneal space, limbs, and subcutaneous tissue.[9, 26, 32, 36, 40, 43, 54, 55, 66] Infection of the cervicofacial region can develop secondary to bite wounds, perforation of the oropharynx by a foreign body, or chronic gingivitis-periodontitis. A primary pneumonitis can develop after aspiration of organisms. Pleuritis can develop by direct extension of disease or migration of a contaminated grass awn to the pleural surface. Alternative routes of thoracic infection include involvement of the mediastinum from esophageal perforation and direct extension of cervicofacial or abdominal disease. Intra-abdominal actinomycosis develops from swallowed organisms or plant material penetrating the GI mucosa. In people, GI disease, abdominal trauma, or surgery often precedes infection. Penetration of the GI tract by gunshot or other foreign bodies, including plant material, is an additional risk factor for animals. Like thoracic infections, abdominal involvement can occur by direct extension. Infection of the retroperitoneal space in dogs is often associated with grass foreign bodies. Theoretically, contaminated grass florets or awns migrate to this location through the lung, up the diaphragm to its dorsal attachment, or through the intestines, by the attachment of the root of the mesentery. Actinomycosis of the limbs occurs secondary to bite wounds, foreign bodies, and lacerations contaminated by licking. Infection of the subcutaneous tissue in dogs usually represents extension of cervicofacial, thoracic, or retroperitoneal disease, whereas in cats it is caused by bite wounds.

Actinomycosis is characteristically a polymicrobial infection, and the pathogenicity of *Actinomyces* spp. is dramatically increased in mixed infections. The associated bacteria are commensal organisms from the oral cavity or intestinal tract. Inoculation of pure cultures of *Actinomyces* spp. or the associated bacteria alone often do not produce infection. *Actinomyces* fimbriae bind to specific cell surface receptors on other bacteria. This coaggregation markedly inhibits neutrophil phagocytosis of and bactericidal activity on the bacterial complex.[67] If not bound to other bacteria, *Actinomyces* will bind specific receptors on neutrophils, initiating phagocytosis and degranulation. Additionally, *Actinomyces* species induce neutrophil chemotaxis, activate macrophages, and stimulate B-lymphocyte hyperplasia. These bacterial-cellular interactions produce the characteristic lesion in actinomycosis of a dense mat of *Actinomyces* spp. and associated organisms surrounded by neutrophils, macrophages, and plasma cells. Proteolytic enzymes from the macrophages and degranulated neutrophils destroy connective tissue, facilitating extension of the disease through normal tissue planes.

CLINICAL FINDINGS

Dog

Cervicofacial actinomycosis presents as an acute to chronic subcutaneous soft tissue swelling in the head or neck region.[26, 29, 66, 78] The lesion can be fluctuant or firm, sometimes indurated, and can be ulcerated or have draining sinuses. The mandible, submandibular region, and ventral or lateral cervical area are most frequently affected, but infections involving the face, retrobulbar space, and temporal area have been reported. Radiographically, adjacent bone can have peri-

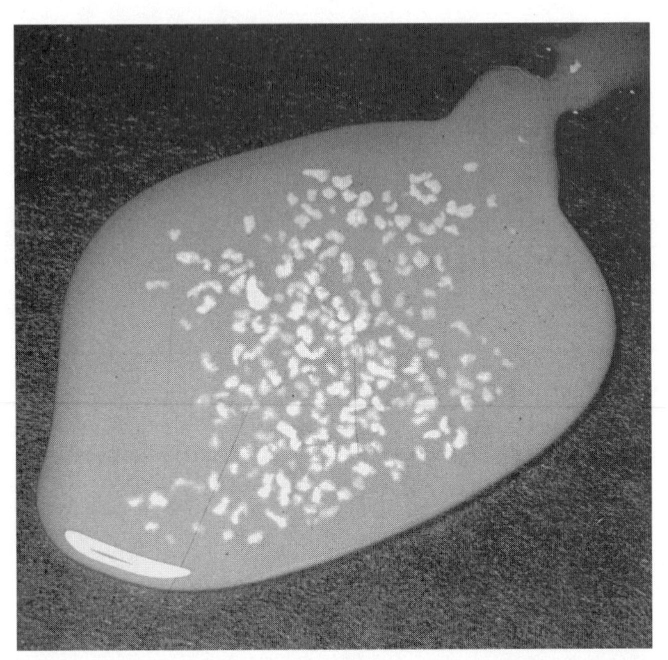

Figure 49–1. Thoracic exudate in Petri dish containing numerous macroscopic sulfur granules.

osteal new bone formation or, with chronic infection, can be characterized by osteomyelitis. Material aspirated from fluctuant masses or discharged from sinuses appears serosanguineous to purulent and may contain macroscopic, yellow-tan granules (i.e., "sulfur granules"), which are small, soft macroscopic colonies of *Actinomyces* that are often present in exudates or infected tissue. The term "sulfur" was derived from the frequently seen yellow pigmentation of the granule; however, granule color can vary from white to tan to gray (Fig. 49–1). Aspiration of firm lesions can yield only a few drops of blood.

Actinomycosis involving the thoracic or abdominal cavity is characteristically chronic and progressive; weight loss, often severe, and fever are the most common clinical signs. **Thoracic actinomycosis** can be limited to the lung parenchyma or can involve multiple structures within the thorax, including the mediastinum, pleura, heart, and chest wall.[12, 21, 26, 30, 32, 36, 53, 70, 78] Other clinical features include cough, tachypnea, dyspnea, decreased lung sounds (empyema or mass lesion), and subcutaneous soft tissue masses on the lateral thorax. Thoracic wall masses often develop a draining sinus. Radiographically, lung disease appears as alveolar and interstitial infiltrates with consolidation. Variable findings include pleural thickening, pleural effusion (often loculated to one side), pericardial effusion, widening of the mediastinum, mass lesions, and periosteal new bone formation or osteomyelitis involving adjacent ribs, vertebral bodies, or sternebrae. Clinical features of **abdominal actinomycosis** include palpable masses and abdominal distention (effusion).[22, 30, 33, 36] Subcutaneous masses, which may have draining sinuses, are rarely present unless the abdominal disease develops from extension of thoracic or retroperitoneal infections. Radiographic manifestations include variable amounts of peritoneal effusion and mass lesions that incorporate or displace adjacent structures. Pleural, pericardial, and peritoneal effusions resemble the exudate from cervicofacial abscesses.

Retroperitoneal actinomycosis is characterized by back pain and rear leg paresis or paralysis.[26, 32, 40, 45] A subcutaneous mass with a draining sinus involving the caudal thorax or flank area is often present. Radiographic findings include periosteal new bone formation involving the ventral aspects of two or three adjacent vertebral bodies (T-13 through L-3 most commonly); involvement of disc spaces is uncommon (Fig. 49–2). With chronicity the vertebral bodies can develop osteomyelitis and compression fractures. This finding should be contrasted with diskospondylitis caused by embolic spread of blood-borne bacteria or fungi to the disc space (see Chapters 40, 65, and 86).

Cutaneous-subcutaneous actinomycosis is characterized by a soft to firm mass, which may have a draining sinus.[26, 32, 43, 66, 78] These infections are typically located in the head and neck area, lateral thoracic wall, and flank region, and usually represent extension of cervicofacial, thoracic, or retroperitoneal actinomycosis. Rare cases of actinomycosis involving the extremities have been reported.[36, 61] Lameness, mass lesions with draining sinuses, and periosteal new bone formation are characteristic.

Cat

Pyothorax and subcutaneous "fight wound" abscesses are the most common disorders in cats from which *Actinomyces* species are isolated.[54, 55] These conditions have a malodorous, yellow to sanguineous exudate without a granulomatous mass, and the *Actinomyces* species is always mixed with two

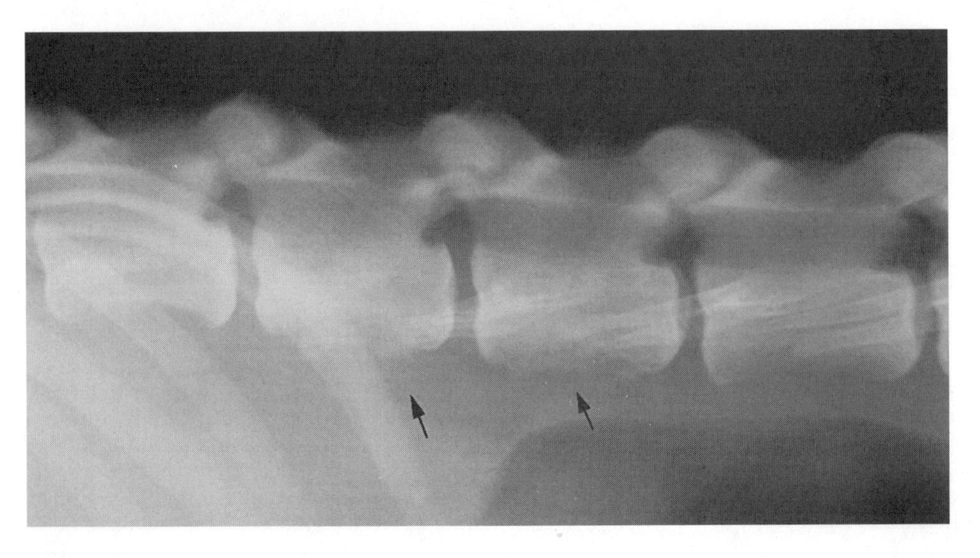

Figure 49–2. Spinal radiograph of an 8-year-old pointer with retroperitoneal actinomycosis. Periosteal new bone growth *(arrows)* is present on the ventral aspect of the vertebral bodies of L-2 and L-3.

to five other pathogens. Actinomycosis, as described in the dog, has been reported infrequently in cats. The cases have involved the cervicofacial region,[23, 49, 88] thoracic cavity,[37] and subcutaneous tissue with extension to the spinal canal.[9, 77]

DIAGNOSIS

Clinical Laboratory Findings

Hematologic test results in animals with actinomycosis vary in the location and duration of disease. Animals with focal lesions (e.g., cervicofacial and limb infections) may have few abnormal results; whereas animals with more extensive, chronic disease have mild to moderate, nonregenerative anemia, leukocytosis with a left shift and monocytosis, hypoalbuminemia, and hyperglobulinemia (sometimes marked). Dogs with body cavity effusions may be hypoglycemic. Aspirates of abscesses or effusions, tracheal lavages, and sinus discharges are suppurative to pyogranulomatous, whereas aspirates of firm masses may reveal only blood. In some specimens, especially effusions, sulfur granules can be visible macroscopically (see Fig. 49–1). Microscopically, mixed bacterial populations containing rods and cocci are common. The actinomycetes appear individually or in dense aggregates (sulfur granules) as gram-positive, non–acid-fast filamentous organisms, which show occasional branching (Fig. 49–3).

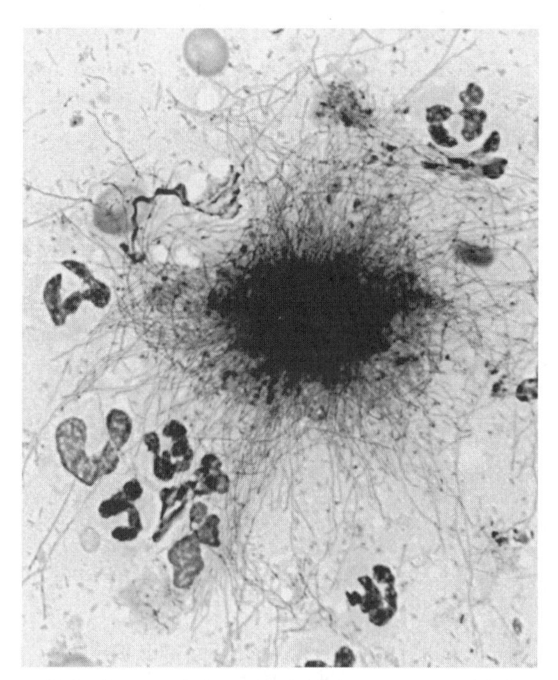

Figure 49–3. Smear of thoracic fluid. Dense mat of infrequently branched, filamentous rods (i.e., sulfur granule). Note the presence of other bacterial species (× 198).

Bacterial Isolation and Identification

The disease is confirmed by culture of the organism, but frequently culture results are negative or contain only associated bacteria. *Actinomyces* species are facultative *(A. denticolens, A. hordeovulneris, A. naeslundii, A. odontolyticus, A. viscosus)* or obligate *(A. bovis, A. israelii, A. meyeri)* anaerobes. Specimens should be collected and processed anaerobically and cultured on blood agar or enriched thioglycolate media in the presence of carbon dioxide (CO_2). Species that are facultatively anaerobic are variably aerotolerant and can grow aerobically. *A. viscosus* actually grows best in aerobic conditions. All species cultured aerobically require CO_2, except *A. naeslundii* and *A. odontolyticus*.[38]

Growth of *Actinomyces* species can be observed within 48 hours but usually requires 5 to 7 days. It may be necessary to hold plates 2 to 4 weeks. Colonies on blood agar are flat to convex, circular with entire or irregular margins, and translucent to opaque and white; surfaces are smooth and moist or rough ("bread crumb" or "molar tooth"). Some strains of *A. israelii* produce aerial filaments resulting in a powdery or "cotton ball" appearance. Microscopically *Actinomyces* spp. are gram-positive, non-acid-fast short rods and filaments. The filaments are less than 1 μm wide, vary considerably in length, may branch, and can stain irregularly, producing a beaded appearance.[12, 22, 30, 36, 43] Species identification is based on physiologic and biochemical characteristics.[38] Cell wall–deficient variants of *A. hordeovulneris* have been produced in culture, suggesting that L forms of *Actinomyces* may be associated with clinical disease; however, because of special culture requirements, these variants would be isolated infrequently.[16]

Actinomycosis is characteristically a mixed bacterial infection.[13, 32, 36, 43, 54, 55, 81] Three to five associated bacteria are typically recovered from properly handled specimens. The most commonly isolated organisms are resident flora of the oral cavity or intestinal tract and include *Bacteroides* spp., *Corynebacterium* spp., *Escherichia coli*, *Eubacterium* spp., *Fusobacterium* spp., *Pasteurella multocida*, *Peptostreptococcus* spp., *Staphylococcus aureus*, and *Streptococcus* spp. Most of the associated bacteria are facultative or obligate anaerobes and, therefore, necessitate appropriate specimen handling for isolation. Unfortunately, the growth of a mixed microflora can impair the isolation of *Actinomyces*.[38]

Because *Actinomyces* spp. are sensitive to many antibiotics, the treatment of animals before obtaining specimens for culture can prevent recovery of the organisms. This fact, compounded by improperly handled specimens and polymicrobial growth, accounts for the frequent failure of bacterial isolation of *Actinomyces* from infected animals. The diagnosis, therefore, is often based on the cytologic or histologic identification of the organism in specimens from animals with appropriate clinical signs. Because *Actinomyces* is a commensal oral bacteria, it is commonly swallowed, inhaled, and transferred by licking; therefore, culture of the organism from the airways, GI tract, or skin does not necessarily constitute infection.

PATHOLOGIC FINDINGS

Actinomycosis is characterized by a poorly defined, often indurated mass that incorporates adjacent structures.[21, 22, 30, 37, 53, 78, 81] The mass may contain one or more pockets of a reddish-brown exudate. Fistulas and sulfur granules are variable findings. Thoracic and abdominal infections produce a diffuse, red, velvety to granular thickening of the parietal pleura and peritoneum and omentum. The visceral pleura and peritoneum may be less affected. A variable amount of a reddish-brown exudate, which may contain sulfur granules, is present. Lung involvement is usually localized and may appear as a consolidation or a mass; infrequently, multiple pulmonary nodules are present. Masses can involve multiple internal structures (e.g., heart, mediastinum, lung, diaphragm, and chest wall) and produce an external subcutaneous swelling, which may have a draining sinus. With abdominal disease only one organ can be affected (e.g., liver), but typically a mass or masses involve multiple adjacent structures.[22, 30, 33] Subcutaneous masses may be ulcerated and, in dogs, are usually an extension of cervicofacial, thoracic, or retroperitoneal disease.[26, 32, 40]

The histologic reaction to *Actinomyces* spp. infection is characterized by a core of neutrophils encapsulated by fibrosing granulation tissue. The granulation tissue contains macrophages, plasma cells, and lymphocytes in a dense, fibrous tissue matrix. The centrally located actinomycotic (sulfur) granule or grain can be very difficult to find, necessitating multiple tissue sections for diagnosis. When associated with appropriate clinical signs, identification of true actinomycotic granules is diagnostic of actinomycosis. In tissue sections stained with hematoxylin and eosin (H and E), the granules appear as round, oval, or scalloped amphophilic solid masses with an outer basophilic band (Fig. 49–4*A*). The granules vary in size (30–3000 μm diameter) and often are rimmed by partially confluent radiate, eosinophilic serrate, or club-shaped structures (i.e., Splendore-Hoeppli phenomenon). Neutrophils frequently contact or appear enmeshed in this material. Individual actinomycete filaments are not delineated by H and E stain or Gridley's fungal or periodic acid–Schiff reactions, whereas tissue Gram's stains (e.g., Brown-Brenn procedure) reveal clumps of tangled, intermittently branched, thin (< 1 μm diameter) filaments that are gram-positive and slightly beaded (Fig. 49–4*B*). Gram-positive or gram-negative nonfilamentous bacteria can be mixed with the *Actinomyces* spp. *Actinomyces* species are non-acid-fast when stained by the Fite-Faraco modification of the Ziehl-Neelsen technique, which uses a weaker decolorizing agent of 1% sulfuric or 1% hydrochloric acid. Although *Nocardia* spp. can be a rare exception, other fungi and bacteria that produce tissue granules can be reliably distinguished from *Actinomyces* by tinctorial and morphologic properties.[20] Features of nocardiosis that distinguish it from actinomycosis are listed in Table 49–1.

THERAPY

Successful treatment of actinomycosis involves prolonged administration of antibiotics; the role of surgery varies with the form of the disease. Large doses of penicillin given for prolonged periods (weeks to months) is the treatment of choice (Table 49–2).[47] No strains of *Actinomyces* spp. have shown in vitro resistance to easily attainable serum concentrations of penicillin, and acquired resistance in vivo has not been confirmed. Poor drug penetration of the dense granulomatous tissue reaction necessitates the prolonged, high-dose therapy. A minimal dose of penicillin G (benzyl penicillin) or

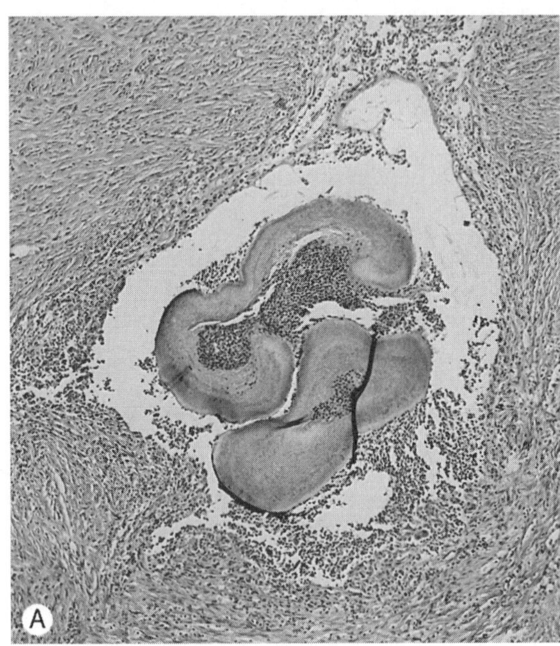

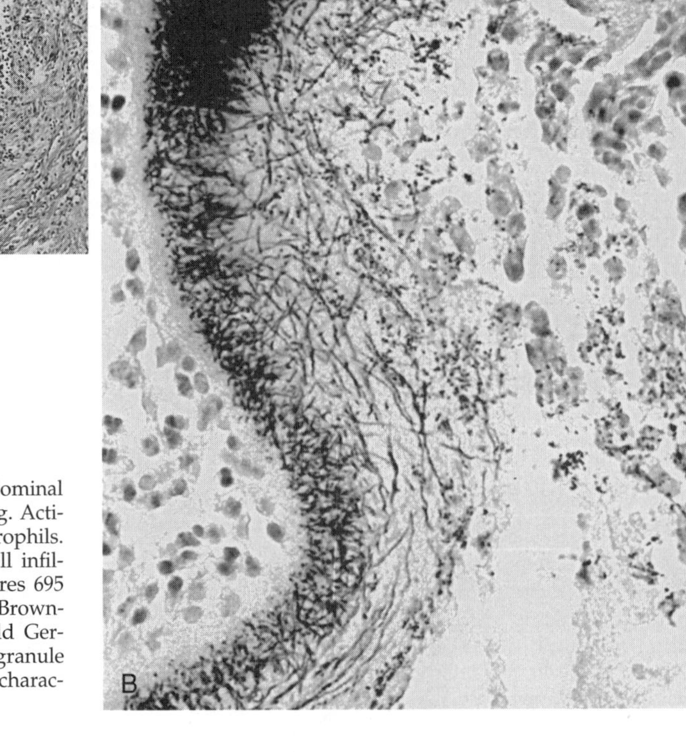

Figure 49–4. *A*, H and E–stained section of an abdominal mass from a 5-year-old neutered female boxer dog. Actinomycotic tissue granule is surrounded by neutrophils. Encapsulating fibrous tissue has mononuclear cell infiltrate. (The long dimension of the granule measures 695 μm; × 13.2.) *B*, Tissue Gram's stained–section (Brown-Brenn) of an intrathoracic mass from a 4-year-old German shorthaired pointer. Actinomycotic tissue granule showing infrequently branched, filamentous rods characteristic of *Actinomyces* (× 132).

Table 49–1. Actinomycosis Versus Nocardiosis

ACTINOMYCES	NOCARDIA
Culture	
1. Facultative or obligate anaerobe	1. Aerobe
2. Fastidious growth requirements; often not cultured	2. Usually cultured
3. Two to 5 associated microbes usually recovered	3. Sole isolate unless from contaminated sample (e.g., tracheal wash, ulcerated skin)
Staining Characteristics	
1. Irregular staining can produce slight beading	1. Irregular staining can produce marked beading
2. Gram-positive and non-acid-fast using Fite-Faraco modification of Ziehl-Neelsen technique	2. Gram-positive and partially acid-fast using Fite-Faraco modification of Ziehl-Neelsen technique
Cytopathology	
1. Suppurative to pyogranulomatous inflammation with a mixed bacterial population; macroscopic and microscopic dense mats of long filamentous bacteria are often present (see Fig. 49–3)	1. Suppurative to pyogranulomatous inflammation; long filamentous bacteria typically are present singly or in loose aggregates (see Fig. 49–6); infrequently macroscopic and microscopic dense mats of long filamentous bacteria are present
Histopathology	
1. Pyogranulomatous inflammation with marked encapsulating fibrosis (see Fig. 49–4*A* and *B*)	1. Pyogranulomatous inflammation; significant fibrosis present only in chronic skin infections (see Fig. 49–7)
2. Variable presence of tissue granules (30–3000 μm diameter)	2. Granules present only in skin infections (15–200 μm diameter)
Clinical Disease	
1. Adult outdoor dogs (especially hunting breeds); fight wounds and pyothorax in cats	1. Dogs < 2 years old; fight wounds in cats
2. Spreads to adjacent structures directly	2. Hematogenous spread; can see lesions at noncontiguous sites
3. Sensitive to high doses of penicillin	3. Variable sensitivity to sulfonamides
4. Low mortality	4. Moderate to high mortality

penicillin V (phenoxymethyl penicillin) of 40 mg/kg every 8 hours is recommended.[30] Units of penicillin equivalency per mg depend upon the formulation (see Appendix 8). The therapeutic advantage of initial parenteral administration is questionable; therefore, if the animal is stable clinically, oral therapy can be started from the outset.[30, 65] Because food reduces the absorption of most penicillins, medication should be given 1 hour before or 2 hours after feeding. Therapy must be extended significantly (weeks to months) beyond resolution of measurable disease to prevent relapse; in some cases treatment can exceed 1 year.[30, 36] Drugs other than penicillin effective against *Actinomyces* include erythromycin, clindamycin, ampicillin, tetracycline, minocycline, doxycycline, chloramphenicol, imipenem, and first-generation cephalosporins.[47, 87] Anecdotal success with ciprofloxacin is reported in a human patient with recalcitrant actinomycosis of 20 years' duration.[57] Oxacillin, dicloxacillin, cephalexin, metronidazole, and aminoglycosides have poor in vitro activity against *Actinomyces* spp. Poor response to appropriate doses of penicillin may be attributable to poor surgical drainage and not eliminating associated bacteria.[47] Infections by these organisms usually resolve with penicillin, but on occasion they may necessitate broader spectrum antibiotics during the initial treatment period followed by long-term administration of penicillin. Cats with pyothorax or subcutaneous abscess that have not developed a granulomatous tissue reaction often can be cured with drainage and a shorter duration of antibiotics.

Surgery has a controversial role in the treatment of actinomycosis. Draining of abscesses and effusions (thoracic, abdominal, and pericardial) should always be used as an adjunct to antibiotic treatments.[36, 37, 70] Continuous suction and intermittent drainage techniques have been utilized for thoracic effusions in dogs.[81] Drain tubes are removed when the purulent exudate changes to a serosanguineous transudate, usually within 4 to 10 days. Daily lavage with fluids containing crystalline penicillin G may be of benefit. The use of sodium penicillin versus potassium penicillin in the lavage fluid will avoid the potential of cardiotoxicity from hyperkalemia (crystalline potassium penicillin G contains 1.7 mEq potassium/10^6 U). Complications of drainage include pneumothorax and subcutaneous abscess formation at the drain tube insertion site. Animals not responding to drainage and appropriate antibiotic therapy warrant exploratory surgery.[70, 81] In animals with pulmonary abscesses, diseased lung lobes may often require removal. The characteristic invasive fibrotic lesions obliterate tissue planes, preventing conservative dissection, and the tissue is well vascularized; therefore, moderate to severe bleeding is common. With diffuse disease involving body cavities, tissue resection should be restricted in order not to compromise the survival of the animal. In dogs with solitary masses involving the thoracic and abdominal walls, radical surgical excision produces a high cure rate, although repeat surgeries may be needed.[32] The masses often can be reduced and better defined by an initial period of antibiotic therapy. Frequently, grass florets or awns are found in these lesions and during surgical exploration of retroperitoneal disease.[32, 40] Surgery should never be performed in lieu of, and should always be followed by, appropriate antibiotic therapy.

Appropriate treatment of dogs with actinomycosis, which can involve extremely prolonged use of antibiotics and surgery, will result in a cure rate of greater than 90%.[30, 32, 36] Because of the infrequent documentation of actinomycosis in cats, a meaningful cure rate is not available, but it should approximate that observed in dogs.

PUBLIC HEALTH CONSIDERATIONS

There are no reports of actinomycosis being transmitted from clinically infected animals to human beings or to other animals; however, persons bitten by dogs, cats, or other humans can develop actinomycosis.[68] Nevertheless, animal care workers handling infected tissues or discharges should wear protective gloves to avoid inadvertent contact by inoculation or through damaged skin.

Table 49–2. Drugs Used to Treat Actinomycosis in Dogs and Cats

DRUG	SPECIES	DOSE[a]	ROUTE	INTERVAL (HOURS)
Penicillin G	B	100,000 U/kg	IV, IM, SC	6–8
Penicillin G[b]	B	40 mg/kg[c]	PO	8
Penicillin V	B	40 mg/kg[c]	PO	8
Clindamycin	B	5 mg/kg	SC	12
Erythromycin	B	10 mg/kg	PO	8
Chloramphenicol	D	50 mg/kg	PO, IV, IM, SC	8
	C	50 mg/kg	PO, IV, IM, SC	12
Rifampin	D	10 mg/kg	PO	12
Minocycline	B	5–25 mg/kg	IV, PO	12
Ampicillin (amoxicillin)[b]	B	20–40 mg/kg	IM, SC, PO	6

[a]Dose per administration at specified interval. For duration, see text.
[b]Give at least 1 hour before or 2 hours after feeding to facilitate GI absorption.
[c]Minimum recommended dose—see text; 1 mg is equivalent to 1600 units (see Appendix 8).
B = dog and cat; D = dog; C = cat.

Nocardiosis

ETIOLOGY AND EPIDEMIOLOGY

Nocardiosis is a suppurative to granulomatous, localized or disseminated bacterial infection caused by members of the family Nocardiaceae, which is uncommon in dogs and rare in cats.[7, 8] *Nocardia asteroides* is the most commonly isolated species in dogs and cats, but infections by *N. brasiliensis* (dog and cat) and *N. otitidiscaviarum* (dog) have been reported.[8] *N. asteroides* and *N. brasiliensis*, as historically defined, consist of several subtypes and/or species, whereas *N. otitidiscaviarum* is taxonomically homogeneous.[76] These aerobic actinomycetes are ubiquitous soil saprophytes that degrade organic matter and are found in soil, water and on plants.[7, 62] Infections are considered opportunistic, occurring by either inhalation of organisms or inoculation through puncture wounds.

In a survey of 53 dogs with nocardiosis, males were infected three times more frequently than females; 65.4% of the dogs were younger than 1 year, 82.7% were younger than 2 years, and only 7.8% were older than 6 years; 26.9% had an underlying condition, most often canine distemper.[8] Apparently in dogs, like humans, predisposing factors (i.e., diseases) increase susceptibility to nocardiosis. Approximately 40% of humans with nocardiosis have primary disorders that involve immunosuppressive drug therapy, obstructive pulmonary disease, metabolic disorders (hyperadrenocorticism, diabetes mellitus), neoplasia (lymphosarcoma, leukemia), immunologic disease (systemic lupus erythematosus, dysgammaglobulinemia), or infectious diseases (AIDS).[7, 62] In 11 case reports of feline nocardiosis, 7 involved males and 3 involved females.[2–4, 6, 19, 27, 46, 58, 80, 86] Ages ranged from 2.5 to 11 years. Five of the cats had draining wounds or abscesses that were associated with scratches or bite wounds.

PATHOGENESIS

Similar to the systemic mycoses, pulmonary nocardiosis probably results from inhalation of soil organisms. Nocardial lesions develop in alveolar spaces and frequently erode into blood vessels, resulting in systemic spread of the disease. Secondary lesions from systemic spread can occur in any tissue. Involvement of contiguous structures within the thorax is also common (pleura, mediastinum, pericardium). Localized cutaneous, subcutaneous, and regional lymph node infections result from inoculation through a puncture wound (e.g., bite, scratch, and foreign body). Other solitary extrapulmonary sites of infection probably represent localization from a transient bacteremia. The primary source may be an inapparent pulmonary infection.[7, 62]

Pathogenicity of *Nocardia* spp. is influenced by the strain and growth phase of the organism and host susceptibility. Normal host response to infection is characterized by an initial neutrophil mobilization that may inhibit growth but not kill the organism. Subsequent cell-mediated immunity consisting of activated macrophages and T lymphocytes is normally bactericidal. Diminished host resistance is a primary factor in nocardiosis, but not all diseased animals have identifiable predisposing conditions. Virulent strains of *Nocardia* are facultative intracellular pathogens that inhibit phagosome-lysosome fusion, neutralize phagosomal acidification, resist oxidative burst, and alter lysosomal enzymes within neutrophils and macrophages. These effects are in part related to the content and structure of mycolic acids within the bacterial cell wall, which vary between strains and during the growth phase. Some strains exhibit organ-specific trophism (e.g., brain) and the filamentous, logarithmically growing organisms are 10 times more virulent than the coccoid stationary-phase cells.[7, 62]

CLINICAL FINDINGS

Dog

Pulmonary nocardiosis can have a peracute onset characterized by inspiratory dyspnea, hemoptysis, hypothermia, collapse, and death[50]; however, a subacute to chronic clinical presentation is more characteristic.[1, 19, 25, 44, 59] The signs are often "distemper like" and include mucopurulent oculonasal discharge, anorexia, weight loss (often emaciation), cough, dyspnea, diarrhea, and hyperthermia. Lung sounds may be increased (bronchopneumonia) or decreased (mass lesion or empyema). Coinfection by the canine distemper virus has been commonly reported. The radiographic lesions are varied and include multiple, diffuse pulmonary nodules, intra- or extrapulmonary solitary masses, focal or diffuse bronchointerstitial to alveolar infiltrates, lobar consolidations, pleural effusions, and often dramatic hilar lymphadenopathy (Fig. 49–5).

Systemic or **disseminated nocardiosis**, defined by lesions at two or more noncontagious sites within the body, is typically associated with pulmonary disease but occurs rarely without obvious pulmonary disease.[1, 5, 41, 42, 44, 59, 69, 73, 79] The most frequently involved extrathoracic organs are skin and subcutaneous tissue, kidney, liver, spleen, lymph nodes, CNS, bone, and joints. The cutaneous-subcutaneous lesions are characterized by firm to fluctuant swellings that may ulcerate or develop fistulous tracts through which a reddish-brown exudate is discharged. Involvement of liver, spleen, and lymph nodes is detected because of organomegaly. CNS lesions may cause seizures. Bone or joint infection results in swelling and lameness; radiographic findings include soft tissue swelling, bone lysis, and periosteal new bone growth.

Solitary extrapulmonary nocardiosis occurs infrequently and usually occurs as a cutaneous-subcutaneous abscess[5] or an actinomycotic mycetoma.[14, 72] A case of humeral osteomyelitis has been reported.[28] Mycetoma is a localized, subcutaneous granulomatous tumor that contains organized aggregates (grains or granules) of free-living or exogenous, geophilic actinomycetes (actinomycotic mycetoma) or fungi (eumycotic mycetoma). Mycetomas usually occur on extremities, may involve underlying bone, and typically form abscesses that result in fistulas to the skin. Because *Actinomyces* is endogenous, tumorous infections of subcutaneous tissues are not classified as mycetomas. Ten dogs with thoracolumbar vertebral osteomyelitis attributed to nocardiosis have been described; however, many of these cases probably represent infection by *Actinomyces* species (see Actinomycosis, Clinical Findings).[11, 64, 74, 75] A *Nocardia*-like organism has been associated with ulcerative urocystitis in a dog.[39]

Cat

The clinical forms of feline nocardiosis (pulmonary, systemic, and solitary extrapulmonary) mirror those described in the dog. In 11 case reports, four cats had cutaneous-subcutaneous lesions (abscesses and actinomycotic mycetoma), four

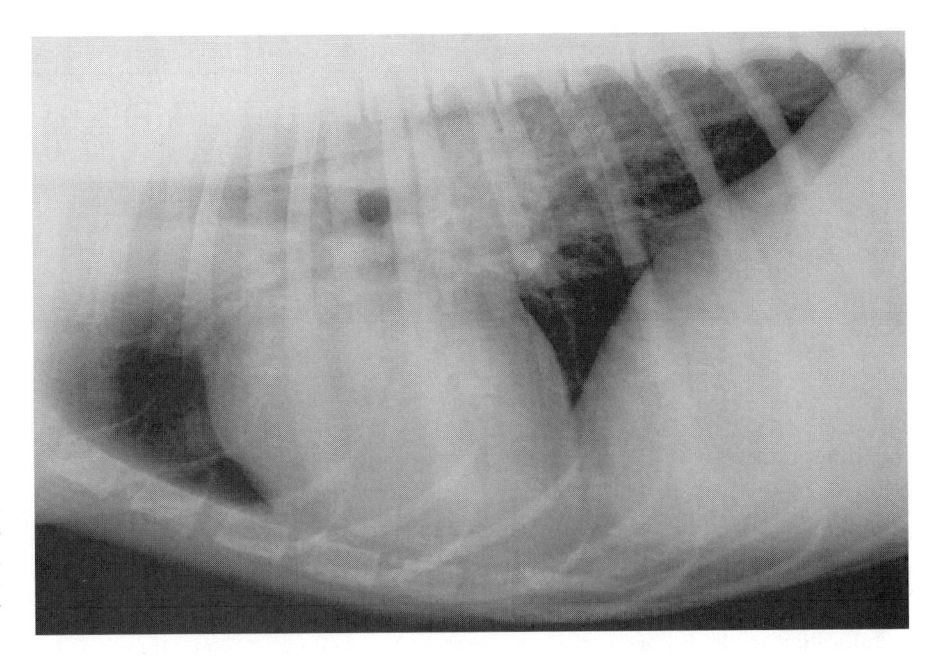

Figure 49–5. Right lateral thoracic radiograph of an 8-month-old male Labrador retriever. Radiographic abnormalities include a bronchointerstitial pattern and marked hilar lymphadenopathy. (Courtesy of Dr. Royce Roberts, University of Georgia Veterinary Teaching Hospital, Athens, GA.)

had pulmonary disease (nodules or empyema), one had peritonitis, and two had systemic nocardiosis.[2–4, 6, 19, 27, 46, 58, 80, 86]

DIAGNOSIS

Clinical Laboratory Findings

Animals with nocardiosis have nonregenerative anemia, neutrophilic leukocytosis with a left shift, monocytosis, and hyperproteinemia. Pleural effusions, bronchial lavages, and aspirates of abscesses are suppurative to pyogranulomatous. Gram-positive, partially or weakly acid-fast, beaded, branching filamentous organisms are often observed individually or in loose aggregates (Fig. 49–6). Macroaggregates (i.e., sulfur granules) have been noted infrequently in effusions. Unlike actinomycosis, mixed bacterial populations from deep tissue sites are rare and probably represent contamination of the sample (e.g., bronchial lavage and ulcerated skin abscess).[1, 5, 44, 59]

Bacterial Isolation and Identification

The presence in clinical specimens of a gram-positive, partially acid-fast, beaded, branched filamentous organism 0.5 to 1 μm in diameter warrants specific therapy for nocardiosis, but the diagnosis is confirmed by culture of the organism. *Nocardia* spp. grow aerobically at a wide temperature range on simple media (e.g., Sabouraud's glucose agar and blood agar). Growth is enhanced by 10% CO_2, modified Thayer-Martin medium, and buffered charcoal-yeast extract agar, but is retarded by inhibitory medium used for fungal isolation. Organisms are usually recovered in pure cultures, and colonies are often visible after 2 days. However, 2 to 4 weeks of incubation may be necessary, especially if samples are from animals receiving antibiotics or contain multiple bacterial species (e.g., bronchial lavage). Colonies can be smooth and moist or rugose with a powdery surface from aerial filaments. Because most *Nocardia* spp. produce carotenoid-like pigments, colony color varies (cream, yellow, orange, pink, or red).[7, 48, 62] Microscopically, *Nocardia* spp. grown on solid media appear as branched filaments that fragment into pleomorphic, rod-shaped, or coccoid elements. *Nocardia* spp. are gram positive and variably acid-fast. In clinical specimens or primary isolates, *Nocardia* spp. are usually partially acid-fast, but a Fite-Faraco modification of the Ziehl-Neelsen tech-

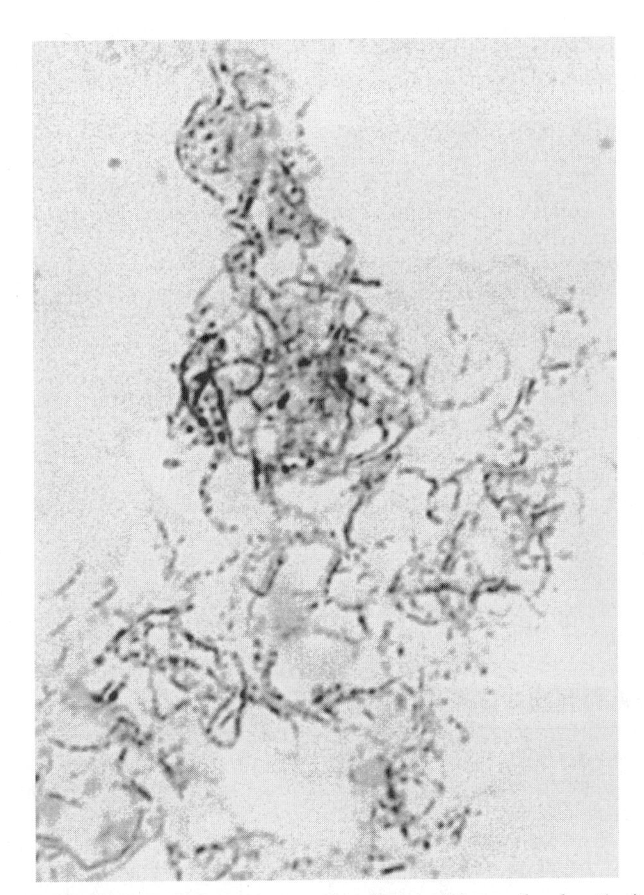

Figure 49–6. Impression smear of a chronic (15 months duration), ulcerated cutaneous lesion on the lateral thorax of a 3-year-old female domestic shorthaired cat. Loose aggregate of infrequently branched, filamentous rods with beading from irregular staining is typical of *Nocardia* (× 330).

Table 49–3. Evolving Nomenclature for Pathogenic Nocardia Species and Characteristic Hydrolysis Reactions[a]

HYDROLYSIS OF	*N. asteroides* COMPLEX			*N. brasiliensis*			
	N. asteroides sensu stricto (Types I, II, IV, VI)	*N. nova*	*N. farcinica*	*N. brasiliensis sensu stricto*	*N. pseudobrasiliensis*	*N. otitidiscaviarum* (Formerly *N. caviae*)	*N. transvalensis*
Adenine	–	–	–	–	+	–	V
Casein	–	–	–	+	+	–	V
Hypoxanthine	–	–	–	V	V	+	V
Tyrosine	–	–	–	+	+	+	V
Xanthine	–	–	–	–	–	–	V

[a]Data from McNeil MM et al: *Clin Microbiol Rev* 7:357–417, 1994; Wallace RJ et al: *J Clin Microbiol* 33:1528–1533, 1995.
+ = ≥ 90% of strains positive; – = ≥ 90% of strains negative; V = 11–89% of strains positive.

nique, decolorized with 1% sulfuric or 1% hydrochloric acid, must be used. Not all pathogenic strains of *Nocardia* spp. are acid-fast, and this characteristic can disappear after subculture.[7, 48, 62]

Traditionally, *N. asteroides*, *N. brasiliensis*, and *N. otitidiscaviarum* have been identified by their differential hydrolysis of casein, hypoxanthine, tyrosine, and xanthine.[62] With this identification method, however, the *N. asteroides* taxon, now referred to as *N. asteroides* complex, is heterogeneous, and infections by *N. farcinica* and *N. nova* are not differentiated (Table 49–3).[76] The distinction is important clinically because *N. farcinica* has a high degree of resistance to various antibiotics and in animal studies is more lethal than isolates of *N. asteroides sensu stricto*.[83, 85] Drug susceptibility patterns and polymerase chain reaction (PCR)–based technology have defined four groups in the *N. asteroides* complex designated as types I, II, IV, and VI (types III and V are now known as *N. nova* and *N. farcinica*, respectively).[76, 84] *N. pseudobrasiliensis*, a new taxon of *N. brasiliensis*, has been identified by susceptibility to ciprofloxacin and hydrolysis of adenine.[82] In human patients, it is usually associated with invasive disease, whereas *N. brasiliensis sensu stricto* most often produces localized cutaneous infections. On the basis of standard hydrolysis reactions, *N. transvalensis* can mimic *N. brasiliensis* or *N. otitidiscaviarum*, but can be distinguished by other biochemical characteristics.[63] PCR-based technology may soon become the laboratory standard for identification of *Nocardia* spp. and subtypes.[76] L-form or cell wall–deficient variants of *Nocardia* spp. have been associated with clinical disease in humans and a dog.[15] These bacteria require special media for isolation and culture (see Chapter 46).

Pathogenic *Nocardia* spp. are not common laboratory contaminants; therefore, the isolation of a single colony from a closed lesion is significant. Because *Nocardia* are ubiquitous in soil and in certain circumstances may act as respiratory saprophytes, the isolation of small numbers of organisms from ulcerated skin lesions or the respiratory tract must be interpreted in conjunction with clinical signs.[7, 48, 62]

PATHOLOGIC FINDINGS

Nocardiosis is characterized by suppurative necrosis and abscess formation and infrequently produces granulomas. Gross lesions of internal organs typically are numerous small (1 mm) to large (1 cm), discrete to coalescing, raised white or gray-white nodules.[41, 69, 73, 79] The nodules are usually subserosal and when cut appear caseous to purulent. Affected lung tissue may appear congested. Lymph nodes are enlarged, often massively, and are firm to fluctuant with a caseous to purulent core.[25, 44, 69] A reddish-brown exudate may be present in the pleural or peritoneal space or within abscesses.[1, 5, 79] Yellow granules in the exudate infrequently have been noted.[44, 80]

The histologic reaction to *Nocardia* spp. infection is characterized by a central region of necrosis and suppuration surrounded by macrophages, lymphocytes, and plasma cells.[69, 73, 79] Clusters of epithelioid macrophages and multinucleated giant cells may be observed. Except with some skin infections, fibrous tissue is usually poorly structured, producing thin or incomplete encapsulation of the lesion. In chronic cutaneous-subcutaneous infections, pyogranulomatous foci can be interspersed within a dense fibrous tissue matrix.[14, 25]

Nocardial organisms are usually present and often abundant in the necrotic and suppurative tissue reactions. Tissue Gram's stains (e.g., Brown-Brenn procedure) are best for demonstrating the filaments, but they are also stained by methenamine silver preparations, especially with prolonged silver nitrate exposure (i.e., 80–100 minutes). *Nocardia* filaments are not visible in tissue sections stained with H and E or with Gridley's fungal or periodic acid–Schiff reactions. The organisms are characteristically, but not invariably, partially acid-fast when a weak decolorizing solution is used

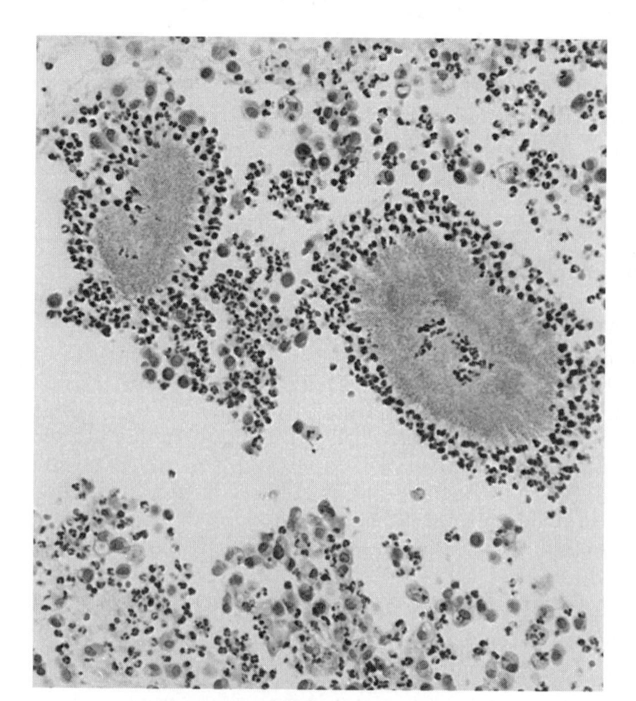

Figure 49–7. H and E–stained section of a chronic ulcerated cutaneous lesion on flank of 3-year-old male domestic longhaired cat. Two *Nocardia* tissue granules are surrounded by pyogranulomatous inflammatory reaction (the long dimension of the largest granule is 110 μm; × 66).

Table 49–4. Drugs Used to Treat Nocardiosis in Dogs and Cats[a]

DRUG	DOSE[b] (mg/kg)	ROUTE	INTERVAL (HOURS)
Triple sulfa no. 4	60[c]	IV	12
Sulfadiazine	80	PO	8
Sulfisoxazole[d]	50	PO	8
Amikacin	8–12	IV, IM, SC	8
Imipenem-cilastatin	2–5	IV	8
Cefotaxime	20–80	IV, IM	6
Minocycline[e]	5–25	IV, PO	12
Erythromycin	10	PO	8
Ampicillin	20–40	IV, IM, SC, PO	6

[a]For duration of therapy, see text; usually there is a minimum of 6 weeks with all drugs.
[b]Dose per administration at specified interval. For duration, see text and Appendix 8.
[c]120 mg/kg IV initially.
[d]Also sulfamethizole.
[e]Doxycycline may be substituted.

(i.e., 1% sulfuric or 1% hydrochloric acid). *Nocardia* spp. appear as beaded, branching filaments, 10 to 30 μm or more in length and 0.5 to 1.0 μm in width. The filaments usually appear individually or in tangled, loose aggregates. In chronic skin infections, tissue granules characterized by colonies arranged in large, rosette-like arrays have been reported (Fig. 49–7). In human nocardiosis tissue granules are uncommon; when present, the granules are small (15–200 μm), are usually not associated with the Splendore-Hoeppli phenomenon, and are most often produced in chronic skin infections by *N. brasiliensis*.

THERAPY

Sulfonamides, including trimethoprim-sulfonamide combinations, are the primary drugs for treating nocardiosis (Table 49–4). Most *Nocardia* spp., with the possible exception of *N. otitidiscaviarum*, are susceptible to sulfonamide therapy, but treatment must be continued for a prolonged period. One to 3 months is recommended in humans with cutaneous infections, up to 6 months for uncomplicated pulmonary infections, and 12 months or longer for systemic infections or infections in immunocompromised patients. Clinical improvement should be observed within 7 to 10 days of starting treatment. Abscesses or empyema usually necessitate surgical drainage to effect a cure.[48, 62]

Antibiotics in addition to or other than sulfonamides may be needed because not all *Nocardia* isolates are sensitive to sulfonamides; in vitro susceptibility may not be associated with clinical response; and resistance can develop during treatment.[48, 62] Adverse drug reactions may prevent prolonged sulfonamide administration; high doses of trimethoprim-sulfadiazine given over long periods to dogs and cats produce myelosuppression (anemia and leukopenia).[24, 52] Drug susceptibility testing of *Nocardia* isolates, which is technically difficult and should be done only at experienced laboratories, has identified relatively characteristic species-associated resistance patterns (Table 49–5). PCR identification and drug susceptibility testing of *Nocardia* spp. can be done at the Department of Microbiology, The University of Texas Health Center at Tyler, 11937 US Highway 271, Tyler, Texas 75708; (903) 877-7680; FAX (903) 871-7652.

Susceptibility studies have led to the use of various antibiotics, other than or in conjunction with sulfonamides, for the treatment of nocardiosis in humans. In vitro, combinations of imipenem with cefotaxime or trimethoprim-sulfamethoxazole and amikacin with trimethoprim-sulfamethoxazole were synergistic, increasing minimum inhibitory concentrations four times or more for the majority of 26 isolates of *N. asteroides* complex. Combinations of amikacin with imipenem or cefotaxime were predominantly additive.[34] Treatment success has been reported with amikacin, ampicillin, broad-spectrum cephalosporin, erythromycin, imipenem, minocycline, and ofloxacin alone or in combination.[48, 62] Nocardiosis in animals that are severely ill, have systemic diseases, or have predisposing conditions may warrant initial combination drug therapy. Ideally, drug selection should be based on susceptibility studies of the isolate, but if that information is not available logical choices can be made from the in vitro data in Table 49–5. Amikacin combined with imipenem has been suggested for initial parenteral treatment of human nocardiosis patients. If, however, *N. otitidiscaviarum* is the cause of infection, an amikacin-minocycline combination is recommended.[48]

In a review of 53 dogs with nocardiosis, 50% of the dogs died and 38.5% were euthanized.[8] Seven of 11 cats with nocardiosis either were euthanized or died.[2–4, 6, 19, 27, 46, 58, 80, 86] The high mortality rate is, in part, attributable to predisposing conditions (distemper in dogs), delayed diagnosis, and inappropriate therapy. With earlier diagnosis and multidrug

Table 49–5. Percentage of Pathogenic Nocardia Species Isolates Susceptible or Moderately Susceptible to Various Drugs in Vitro

DRUG	*N. asteroides sensu stricto*[a]	*N. farcinica*[a]	*N. nova*[b]	*N. brasiliensis sensu stricto*[c]	*N. pseudobrasiliensis*[c]	*N. otitidiscaviarum*[d] (Formerly *N. caviae*)	*N. transvalensis*[e]
Amikacin	100[f]	100	100	100	100	100	82[g]
Amoxicillin-clavulanate	77	71	3	97	19	0	30
Ampicillin	27	0	100[h]	<10	<10	0	10
Cefotaxime	98	18	100	95	78	17	50
Ceftriaxone	98	14	100	92	69		50
Ciprofloxacin	38	68	0	0	95		60
Erythromycin	60	14	100			0	50
Imipenem	77	64	100	<10	<10		90
Minocycline	94	96	97	89	13	100	54
Sulfamethoxazole	100	89	97			0[i]	90
Trimethoprim-sulfamethoxazole	100	93	97	94	82		

[a]Data from McNeil MM et al: *Infect Dis Clin Pract* 4:287–292, 1995.
[b]Data from Wallace RJ Jr et al.[83]
[c]Data from Wallace RJ Jr et al.[82]
[d]Data from Boiron et al: *J Antimicrob Chemother* 22:623–629, 1988; based on only six isolates.
[e]Data from McNeil MM et al.[63]
[f]Wallace RJ Jr et al.[84]; found isolates of *N. asteroides* sensu stricto type IV resistant to all aminoglycosides, including amikacin.
[g]Steingrube VA, et al.[76]; found all isolates of *N. transvalensis* resistant to amikacin.
[h]McNeil MM et al: *Infect Dis Clin Pract* 4:287–292, 1995; found 56% of *N. nova* isolates resistant to ampicillin.
[i]Wallace RJ Jr et al: *Antimicrob Agents Chemother* 23:19–21, 1983; found most isolates of *N. otitidiscaviarum* sensitive to sulfonamides.

therapy, mortality of nocardiosis in animals may approach that reported in people. Only 19.8% of humans with primary infections died, whereas 42.4% of patients with predisposing conditions and more than 50% of patients with either systemic or CNS nocardiosis died.[7]

PUBLIC HEALTH CONSIDERATIONS

There have been no reported cases of human nocardiosis acquired from direct contact with an infected dog or cat; however, there are several documented cases of cutaneous nocardiosis transmitted to humans by a scratch or bite from clinically healthy cats and dogs.[10, 31, 51, 71] *Nocardia* spp., being ubiquitous in the soil, can contaminate the claws and teeth of dogs and cats; however, the risk of contracting nocardiosis by a bite or scratch wound would be no greater in humans than that by a puncture wound while gardening. Special precautions are warranted when a person with suppressed immunity (e.g., immunosuppressive drug therapy and HIV infection) is caring for a dog or cat with nocardiosis.

References

1. Ackerman N, Grain E, Castleman W. 1982. Canine nocardiosis. *J Am Anim Hosp Assoc* 18:147–153.
2. Ajello L, Walker WW, Dungworth DL, et al. 1961. Isolation of *Nocardia brasiliensis* from a cat with a review of its prevalence and geographic distribution. *J Am Vet Med Assoc* 138:370–376.
3. Akün RS. 1952. Nokardiosis bei zwei Katzen in der Turkei. *Dtsch Tierarztl Wochenschr* 59:202–204.
4. Armstrong PJ. 1980. Nocardial pleuritis in a cat. *Can Vet J* 21:189–191.
5. Awad FI, Obeid HM. 1962. Further studies on canine nocardiosis in the Sudan with particular reference to chemotherapy. *Zentralbl Veterinarmed B* 9:257–263.
6. Bakerspigel A. 1973. An unusual strain of *Nocardia* isolated from an infected cat. *Can J Microbiol* 19:1361–1365.
7. Beaman BL, Beaman L. 1994. *Nocardia* species: host-parasite relationships. *Clin Microbiol Rev* 7:213–264.
8. Beaman BL, Sugar AM. 1983. *Nocardia* in naturally acquired and experimental infections in animals. *J Hygiene* 91:393–419.
9. Bestetti G, Bühlman V, Nicolet J, et al. 1977. Paraplegia due to *Actinomyces viscosus* infection in a cat. *Acta Neuropathol (Berl)* 39:231–235.
10. Bottei E, Flaherty JP, Kaplan LJ, et al. 1994. Lymphocutaneous *Nocardia brasiliensis* infection transmitted via a cat scratch: a second case. *Clin Infect Dis* 18:649–650.
11. Bradney IW. 1985. Vertebral osteomyelitis due to *Nocardia* in a dog. *Aust Vet J* 62:315–316.
12. Breitschwerdt EB, Waters JW. 1983. Pulmonary actinomycosis in a dog. *Vet Radiol* 24:186–188.
13. Brennan KE, Ihrke PJ. 1983. Grass awn migration in dogs and cats: a retrospective study of 182 cases. *J Am Vet Med Assoc* 182:1201–1204.
14. Brodey RS, Cole EJ, Sauer RM. 1955. Nocardial mycetoma in a dog. *J Am Vet Med Assoc* 127:433–434.
15. Buchanan AM, Beaman BL, Pedersen NC, et al. 1983. *Nocardia asteroides* recovery from a dog with steroid-and antibiotic-unresponsive idiopathic polyarthritis. *J Clin Microbiol* 18:702–708.
16. Buchanan AM, Scott JL. 1984. *Actinomyces hordeovulneris*, a canine pathogen that produces L-phase variants spontaneously with coincident calcium deposition. *Am J Vet Res* 45:2552–2560.
17. Buchanan AM, Scott JL, Gerencser MA, et al. 1984. *Actinomyces hordeovulneris* sp. nov., an agent of canine actinomycosis. *Int J Syst Bacteriol* 34:439–443.
18. Buoro IBJ, Mande JD, Nyamwange SB. 1993. Isolation of *Nocardia asteroides* from a dog with hemorrhagic cystitis. *J Small Anim Pract* 34:99–102.
19. Campbell B, Scott DW. 1975. Successful management of nocardial empyema in a dog and cat. *J Am Anim Hosp Assoc* 11:769–773.
20. Chandler FW, Kaplan W, Ajello L. 1980. Mycetomas, pp 76–81. *In* Color atlas and text of the histopathology of mycotic diseases. Year Book Medical, Chicago, IL.
21. Chastain CB, Greve JH, Riedesel DH. 1974. Pericardial effusion from granulomatous pleuritis and pericarditis in a dog. *J Am Vet Med Assoc* 164:1201–1202.
22. Chastain CB, Grier RL, Hodge RM, et al. 1976. Actinomycotic peritonitis in a dog. *J Am Vet Med Assoc* 168:499–501.
23. Chastain CB, Grier RL, Mitten RW, et al. 1977. Actinomycotic periodontitis in a cat. *J Am Anim Hosp Assoc* 13:65–67.
24. Craig GR, White G. 1976. Studies in dogs and cats dosed with trimethoprim and sulfadiazine. *Vet Rec* 98:82–86.
25. Cross RF, Nagao WT, Morrison RH. 1953. Canine nocardiosis: a report of two cases. *J Am Vet Met Assoc* 123:535–536.
26. Davenport AA, Carter GR, Schirmer RG. 1974. Canine actinomycosis due to *Actinomyces viscosus*: report of six cases. *Vet Med Small Anim Clin* 69:1442–1447.
27. Davenport DJ, Johnson GC. 1986. Cutaneous nocardiosis in a cat. *J Am Vet Med Assoc* 188:728–729.
28. Ditchfield J. 1961. Nocardiosis in the dog. *Mod Vet Pract* 42:43–45.
29. Donohue DE, Brightman AH. 1995. Cervicofacial *Actinomyces viscosus* infection in a Brazilian Fila: a case report and literature review. *J Am Anim Hosp Assoc* 31:501–505.
30. Edwards DF, Nyland TG, Weigel JP. 1988. Actinomycosis: diagnosis and long term therapy in three dogs. *J Vet Intern Med* 2:184–191.
31. Freland C, Fur JL, Nemirovsky-Trebucq B, et al. 1995. Primary cutaneous nocardiosis caused by *Nocardia otitidiscaviarum*: two cases and a review of the literature. *J Trop Med Hyg* 98:395–403.
32. Frendin J, Greko C, Hellmén E, et al. 1994. Thoracic and abdominal wall swellings in dogs caused by foreign bodies. *J Small Anim Pract* 35:499–508.
33. George LK, Brown JM, Baker HJ, et al. 1972. *Actinomyces viscosus* as an agent of actinomycosis in the dog. *Am J Vet Res* 33:1457–1470.
34. Gombert ME, Aulicino TM. 1983. Synergism of imipenem and amikacin in combinations with other antibiotics against *Nocardia asteroides*. *Antimicrob Agents Chemother* 24:810–811.
35. Hardie EM. 1990. Actinomycosis and nocardiosis, pp 585–590. *In* Greene CE (ed), Infectious diseases of the dog and cat. WB Saunders, Philadelphia, PA.
36. Hardie EM, Barsanti JA. 1982. Treatment of canine actinomycosis. *J Am Vet Med Assoc* 180:537–541.
37. Haywards AHS. 1968. Thoracic effusions in the cat. *J Small Anim Pract* 9:75–82.
38. Hillier SL, Moncla BJ. 1995. *Peptostreptococcus, Propionibacterium, Eubacterium* and other nonsporeforming anaerobic, gram-positive bacteria, pp 587–602. *In* Murray PR, Baron EJ, Pfaller MA, et al (eds), Manual of clinical microbiology, ed 6. ASM Press, Washington, DC.
39. Itkin RJ, Krawiec DR, Cloran JA, et al. 1994. Ulcerative urocystitis in a dog associated with a *Nocardia*-like organism. *J Am Anim Hosp Assoc* 30:296–299.
40. Johnson DE, Summers BA. 1971. Osteomyelitis of the lumbar vertebral in dogs caused by grass-seed foreign bodies. *Aust Vet J* 47:289–294.
41. Kinch DA. 1968. A rapidly fatal infection caused by *Nocardia caviae* in a dog. *J Pathol* 95:540–546.
42. King CB, Sapp CC, Seibold HR. 1955. Systemic nocardiosis with bone lesions in a dog. *Auburn Vet* 11:115–117.
43. Kirpensteijn J, Fingland RB. 1992. Cutaneous actinomycosis and nocardiosis in dogs: 48 cases (1980–1990). *J Am Vet Med Assoc* 201:917–920.
44. Kuttin ES, Feldman M, Perl S, et al. 1980. Canine nocardiosis in Israel. *Refuah Vet* 37:15–23.
45. LaCroix JA. 1973. Vertebral body osteomyelitis: a case report. *J Am Vet Radiol Soc* 14:17–21.
46. Langham RF, Schormer RG, Newman JP. 1959. Nocardiosis in the dog and cat. *Michigan State Univ Vet* 19:102–107, 119.
47. Lerner PI. 1990. *Actinomyces* and *Arachnia* species, pp 1932–1942. *In* Mandell GL, Douglas RG, Bennett JE (eds), Principles and practice of infectious diseases. Churchill and Livingston, New York, NY.
48. Lerner PI. 1996. Nocardiosis. *Clin Infect Dis* 22:891–905.
49. Libke KG, Walton AM. 1974. Actinomycosis-like infection in the mandible of a cat. *Mod Vet Pract* 55:201–202.
50. Lobetti RG, Collett MG, Leisewitz A. 1993. Acute fibrinopurulent pneumonia and haemoptysis associated with *Nocardia asteroides* in three dogs. *Vet Rec* 133:480.
51. Long P, Campana HA. 1966. An unusual mycetoma. *Arch Dermatol* 93:341–345.
52. Lording PM, Bellamy JEC. 1978. Trimethoprim and sulfadiazine: adverse effects of long-term administration in dogs. *J Am Anim Hosp Assoc* 14:410–417.
53. Lorenzana R, Richter K, Ehinger SJ, et al. 1985. Infectious pericardial effusion in a dog. *J Am Anim Hosp Assoc* 21:725–728.
54. Love DN, Jones RF, Bailey M, et al. 1978. Bacteria isolated from subcutaneous abscesses in cats. *Aust Vet Pract* 8:87–90.
55. Love DN, Jones RF, Bailey M, et al. 1982. Isolation and characterization of bacteria from pyothorax (empyaemia) in cats. *Vet Microbiol* 7:455–561.
56. Love DN, Vekselstein R, Collings S, et al. 1990. The obligate and facultatively anaerobic bacterial flora of the normal feline gingival margin. *Vet Microbiol* 22:267–275.
57. Macfarlane DJ, Tucker LG, Kemp RJ. 1993. Treatment of recalcitrant actinomycosis with ciprofloxacin. *J Infect* 29:177–180.
58. Marder MW, Kantrowitz MD, Davis T. 1973. Clinical pathology conference. *Feline Pract* 3:20–22, 29–31.
59. Marino DJ, Jaggy A. 1993. Nocardiosis. A literature review with selected case reports in two dogs. *J Vet Intern Med* 7:4–11.
60. McElhaney LM, Jones MP. 1993. Challenging cases in internal medicine: what's your diagnosis? *Vet Med* 88:1032–1038.
61. McMillan KL, Horne RD, King HA. 1982. Osteomyelitis in a dog caused by an anaerobic actinomycete: a case report. *J Am Anim Hosp Assoc* 18:265–268.

62. McNeil MM, Brown JM. 1994. The medically important aerobic actinomycetes: epidemiology and microbiology. *Clin Microbiol Rev* 7:357–417.
63. McNeil MM, Brown JM, Georghion PR, et al. 1992. Infections due to *Nocardia transvalensis*: clinical spectrum and antimicrobial therapy. *Clin Infect Dis* 15:453–463.
64. Mitten RW. 1974. Vertebral osteomyelitis in the dog due to *Nocardia*-like organisms. *J Small Anim Pract* 15:563–570.
65. Nelson JD, Hermann DW. 1986. Oral penicillin therapy for thoracic actinomycosis. *Pediatr Infect Dis* 5:594–595.
66. Nicholson FR, Horne RD. 1973. Grass awn penetration in the dog. *Auburn Vet* 29:59–65.
67. Ochiai K, Kurita-Ochiai T, Kamino Y, et al. 1993. Effect of coaggregation on the pathogenicity of oral bacteria. *J Med Microbiol* 39:183–190.
68. Reiner SL, Harrelson JM, Miller SE, et al. 1987. Primary actinomycosis of an extremity: a case report and review. *Rev Infect Dis* 9:581-589.
69. Rhoades HE, Reynolds HA, Rahn DP, et al. 1963. Nocardiosis in a dog with multiple lesions of the central nervous system. *J Am Vet Med Assoc* 142:278–281.
70. Robertson SA, Stoddart ME, Evan RJ, et al. 1983. Thoracic empyema in the dog: a report of twenty-two cases. *J Small Anim Pract* 24:103–119.
71. Sachs MK. 1992. Lymphocutaneous *Nocardia brasiliensis* infection acquired from a cat scratch: case report and review. *Clin Infect Dis* 15:710–711.
72. Sapegin G, Cormack GR. 1956. Canine nocardiosis treated with hibitane. *North Am Vet* 37:385–388.
73. Sato Y, Mochizuki A. 1986. A case of canine systemic nocardiosis. *Jpn J Vet Sci* 48:629–732.
74. Scott DW, Barrett RE, Tangorra L. 1976. Drug eruption associated with sulfonamide treatment of vertebral osteomyelitis in a dog. *J Am Vet Med Assoc* 168:1111–1114.
75. Stead AC. 1984. Osteomyelitis in the dog and cat. *J Small Anim Pract* 25:1–13.
76. Steingrube VA, Brown BA, Gibson JL, et al. 1995. DNA amplification and restriction endonuclease analysis for differentiation of 12 species and taxa of *Nocardia*, including recognition of four new taxa within the *Nocardia asteroides* complex. *J Clin Microbiol* 33:3096–3101.
77. Stowater JL. 1978. Actinomycosis in the spinal canal of cat. *Feline Pract* 8:26–27.
78. Swerczek TW, Schiefer B, Nielsen SW. 1968. Canine actinomycosis. *Zentralbl Veterinarmed B* 15:955–970.
79. Swerczek TW, Trautwein G, Nielsen SW. 1968. Canine nocardiosis. *Zentralbl Veterinarmed B* 15:971–978.
80. Tilgner SL, Anstey SI. 1996. Nocardial peritonitis in a cat. *Aust Vet J* 74:430–432.
81. Turner WD, Breznock EM. 1987. Continuous suction drainage for management of canine pyothorax—a retrospective study. *J Am Anim Hosp Assoc* 28:485–494.
82. Wallace RJ Jr, Brown BA, Blacklock Z, et al. 1995. New *Nocardia* taxon among isolates of *Nocardia brasiliensis* associated with invasive disease. *J Clin Microbiol* 33:1528–1533.
83. Wallace RJ Jr, Brown BA, Tsukamura M, et al. 1991. Clinical and laboratory features of *Nocardia nova*. *J Clin Microbiol* 29:2407–2411.
84. Wallace RJ Jr, Steele LC, Sumter G, et al. 1988. Antimicrobiol susceptibility patterns of *Nocardia asteroides*. *Antimicrob Agents Chemother* 32:1776–1779.
85. Wallace RJ Jr, Tsukamura M, Brown B, et al. 1990. Cefotaxime-resistant *Nocardia asteroides* strains are isolates of the controversial species *Nocardia farcinica*. *J Clin Microbiol* 28:2726–2732.
86. Wilkinson GT. 1983. Cutaneous *Nocardia* infection in a cat. *Feline Pract* 13:32–34.
87. Yew WW, Wong PC, Wong CF, et al. 1994. Use of imipenem in the treatment of thoracic actinomycosis. *Clin Infect Dis* 19:984–985.
88. Yovich JC, Read RA. 1995. Nasal *Actinomyces* infection in a cat. *Aust Vet Pract* 25:114–117.

Chapter **50**

Mycobacterial Infections

Tuberculous Mycobacterial Infections

Craig E. Greene and Danielle A. Gunn-Moore

ETIOLOGY

Mycobacterial infections of dogs and cats are caused by bacteria belonging to the family Mycobacteriaceae, order Actinomycetales. *Mycobacterium* is a genus comprising morphologically similar, aerobic, non-spore-forming, and nonmotile bacteria with wide variations in host affinity and pathogenic potential. Historically, they have been subdivided into several groups and individual species, according to characteristic biochemical and cultural reactions (Table 50–1). Genetic sequencing studies have corroborated this taxonomic classification.

Mycobacteria have the distinctive property of retaining hot carbolfuchsin and other stains after subsequent treatment with acid or alcohol. This acid-alcohol fastness is due to the high lipid content of mycolic acid in the cell wall. Cord factor and Wax D, also surface constituents of mycobacterial cells, are partly responsible for the host's granulomatous response to the organism.

Mycobacteria are more resistant to heat, pH changes, and routine disinfection than are other pathogenic non-spore-forming bacteria. Common disinfectants are often added to samples collected for culture of mycobacteria to kill extraneous contaminating organisms. The minimum criteria established for pasteurization and heat disinfection have been developed to kill mycobacteria. Mycobacteria are highly susceptible to dilute (5%) phenol or direct sunlight. Although they are relatively more stable in the presence of organic material, mycobacteria are killed by dilute (5%) household bleach within 15 minutes at room temperature.

Mycobacteria generally produce one of three clinical forms of illness in infected people or animals: internal tubercular granulomas (tuberculosis [TB]); localized cutaneous nodules (leprosy); or spreading, primarily subcutaneous inflammation (opportunistic mycobacterial infections). These are discussed under the respective headings that follow.

M. tuberculosis and *M. bovis*, highly pathogenic tubercle-producing mycobacteria, are facultative or obligate intracellular parasites. They are closely related species that have been difficult to distinguish, except by using a few biochemical

Table 50–1. Characteristics of Selected Species of Mycobacterium of Veterinary Interest

GROUP SPECIES	AFFECTED NATURAL HOSTS (EXPERIMENTAL HOSTS)	MEANS OF EXISTENCE	PECULIAR CULTURAL AND BIOCHEMICAL FEATURES
Tuberculous			
M. tuberculosis	Human, dog, cat, pig (guinea pig, mouse, hamster)	FI	Niacin positive, glycerol enhances
M. tuberculosis–M. bovis variant	Cats, rodents?	OI?	Niacin variable, pyruvate enhances
M. bovis	Human, cat, dog, cow, pig (guinea pig, rabbit, mouse)	FI	Niacin negative, glycerol inhibits
Lepromatous			
M. leprae	Human (armadillo, mouse)	OI	Unable to cultivate
M. lepraemurium	Mouse, cat	OI	Difficult to cultivate, requires complex media
Other			
M. paratuberculosis	Cattle	FI	Requires mycobactin
Opportunistic[a]			
Slow growing			
M. kansasii	Human, dog (hamster, variable in mouse)	S, FI	RC I
M. avium-intracellulare complex[b]	Birds, human, dog, cat (variable in rabbit and mouse)	S, FI	RC III
M. genavense	Birds, human, dog	S, FI	Requires mycobactin
Fast growing			
M. thermoresistible	Cat	S	II
M. xenopi	Cat		III
M. chelonae (M. chelonei)	Dog, cat	S	IV
M. fortuitum	Dog, cat (mouse)	S	IV
M. phlei	Cat	S	IV
M. smegmatis	Cat, dog	S	IV

[a]Older (Runyon's) classification system for atypical mycobacteria based on cultural properties: I: photochromogens—produce yellow pigment on exposure to light, buff color on growth in dark; II: scotochromogens—produce orange pigment, independent of light; III: nonchromogens—filamentous forms, buff or yellow regardless of amount of light; slow growth; IV: nonchromogens—rapid growth, mature colonies in 4–6 days at 37°C, most others require 1–2 weeks.
[b]Included in tuberculous group in this chapter because produces clinically similar disease. Growth enhanced by glycerol and 42°C.
FI = facultative intracellular; OI = obligate intracellular; S = saprophytic; ? = uncertain; RC = Runyon's classification.

tests and nucleic acid probes. To be maintained in nature, they require infection of reservoir mammalian hosts, because environmental survival is limited to a maximum of 1 to 2 weeks on infected fomites. The other members of the *M. tuberculosis* complex are *M. microti*, a rodent pathogen that has been reported to infect cats in earlier literature,[29, 59] and *M. africanum*, a rare cause of human TB in Africa. An unclassified variant with properties intermediate to *M. tuberculosis* and *M. bovis* (*M. tuberculosis–M. bovis* variant) has been identified as a cause of TB in cats in Great Britain.[5, 24, 25]

One of the opportunistic, saprophytic mycobacteria that occurs as a tubercle-producing pathogen is *M. avium*. Considerable overlap occurs between the properties of *M. avium* and a closely related pathogen, *M. intracellulare*. Because of this indistinct separation, *M. avium–M. intracellulare* or *M. avium complex* (MAC) has been used to refer to these organisms. Since they produce tuberculous lesions indistinguishable from *M. tuberculosis* and *M. bovis*, MAC organisms are discussed in this section. Among opportunistic mycobacteria, MAC organisms are most likely to produce bacteremia and multiple-organ disseminated disease.

M. avium and *M. intracellulare* organisms can be distinguished by nucleic acid testing. Serotyping by agglutination reactions has been classically used to differentiate *M. avium* complex isolates. The MAC organisms consist of 28 serovars; 1 through 6 and 8 through 11 are assigned to *M. avium*, and 7, 12 through 17, 19, 20, and 25 are assigned to *M. intracellulare*.[30, 57] Serotypes 1 and 4 have been isolated from cats, and serotypes 1, 2, and 4 have been isolated from dogs.[34]

EPIDEMIOLOGY

M. tuberculosis

Humans are the only reservoir hosts for *M. tuberculosis*. Dogs and cats are susceptible to infections by *M. tuberculosis* and *M. bovis* but are more resistant to infection by MAC organisms. Despite this inherent resistance, the exposure to MAC organisms is much greater because they are ubiquitous in the environment. Canine and feline infections with *M. tuberculosis* are considered an inverse zoonosis; the direction of transmission is from human to animal (Fig. 50–1). Although pets acquire the infection from people, the spread from dogs or cats to people has not been reported. Dogs have had a higher prevalence of infection with *M. tuberculosis* than have cats. Dogs with tuberculous pneumonitis discharge organisms in the sputum as do infected people. Aerosolized droplets are the primary means of transmission of this disease. Air-borne droplet nuclei from respiratory secretions fall to the ground, where they temporarily remain viable but stationary and thus relatively noninfectious for other people and pets. Only small (3–5 μm) diameter particles can successfully bypass upper respiratory clearance mechanisms and deposit in alveoli. Discharges that are not air-borne may potentially be infectious to dogs and cats exposed through close contact. In general, tubercle bacilli are not as infectious as other bacterial pathogens because prolonged, frequent exposure or large inocula are usually required. Because of measures imposed to control infection in people, the overall prevalence of human and animal *M. tuberculosis* infections had been decreasing. Relative increases have occurred in densely populated urban areas and in economically depressed areas. The inter-related factors of homelessness, illicit drug use, and HIV infection have caused unanticipated increases in its prevalence. Multiple-drug–resistant TB has emerged in these so-affected populations because of irregular compliance with drug therapy. Pets in such environments will have an increased risk of becoming infected. The incidence of *M. tuberculosis* infections in the United States is highest in Atlantic Coast metropolitan regions and in the southeastern regions.

M. tuberculosis–M. bovis Variant

Identified in Great Britain, the variant species was predominantly found in rural cats with avid hunting behavior. The source of infection may be a prey species. Some previous reports of this infection from the United Kingdom may have been mistaken for *M. bovis* infections.[5] Currently, the relationship of this variant to *M. microti* is uncertain.

M. bovis

With respect to *M. bovis* infections, the GI tract is the most common portal of entry. Cats and dogs can be potential disseminators of disease when it preferentially localizes in the intestinal and respiratory tracts, respectively. Because of localization of infection, cats usually excrete the organism via feces and dogs via sputum. *M. bovis* does not exist long in the environment, and reservoir hosts are essential for survival of the organism. Outside its hosts, the organism survives for a range of 4 days in summer and less than 28 days in winter.[32] Dogs and cats may be involved in the maintenance of bovine TB on farms, where it is enzootic, and may be rarely responsible for transmission of the bovine bacillus to people (see Fig. 50–1). Subclinically, infected dogs and cats sometimes remain on farms after reactor cattle have been identified and removed from the herd, and farms or families with recurrent TB infections should have their pet animal contacts checked periodically. Rarely, spread of *M. bovis* between humans has been reported.

Cats are more commonly infected with the bovine bacillus than dogs, and on an experimental basis, cats appear to be more susceptible to bovine than to human TB. Part of this affinity is related to the frequent ingestion of contaminated, unpasteurized milk or uncooked meat or offal from infected cattle. Milk is an ideal medium for the organism because it buffers the gastric acid that normally prevents colonization of the lower GI tract with tuberculous bacilli. Dogs and cats may also acquire TB from uncooked, infected meat used as cat and dog foods. Owing to eradication measures, the prevalence of bovine TB is low in the United States. The increasing use of commercial foods and trend to urban living have reduced the prevalence of bovine TB in dogs and cats. In countries such as New Zealand and the Netherlands, where *M. bovis* has become established in the wildlife population, domestic animals such as cattle, cats, and dogs continue to become infected.[14, 15, 50, 60]

M. avium Complex

Infections with avian tubercle bacilli have rarely been reported in dogs and cats owing to innate resistance to the organism. Poultry and swine are primarily susceptible to MAC infection after contact with infected food or water. MAC organisms have been shown to be present in acid (pH 5.0–5.5) conditions and soils high in organic matter.[38] These conditions are met in acidic swamp areas, coastal plains, and brackish coastal waters. Feces of infected birds contain large numbers of bacilli, and infection of dogs and cats occurs from ingestion of infected meat or contact with infected soil or with fomites contaminated by poultry carcasses or feces (see Fig. 50–1). Unlike *M. tuberculosis* and *M. bovis*, MAC organisms remain viable for at least 2 years in the environment, including municipal water supplies, soil, dairy products, and tissues of birds and mammals.

The importance of infection with MAC organisms is that they produce granulomas of deeper tissue and parenchymal organs that are indistinguishable from those caused by mammalian tubercle bacilli. There is no evidence for spread of MAC organisms between or within animals and people. *M. genavense*, a MAC organism, has been the cause of muscle wasting, small-bowel wall thickening, and hepatic granulomatous infiltration in birds and in human AIDS patients.[7] Disseminated infection with *M. genavense* has been found in a dog.[36]

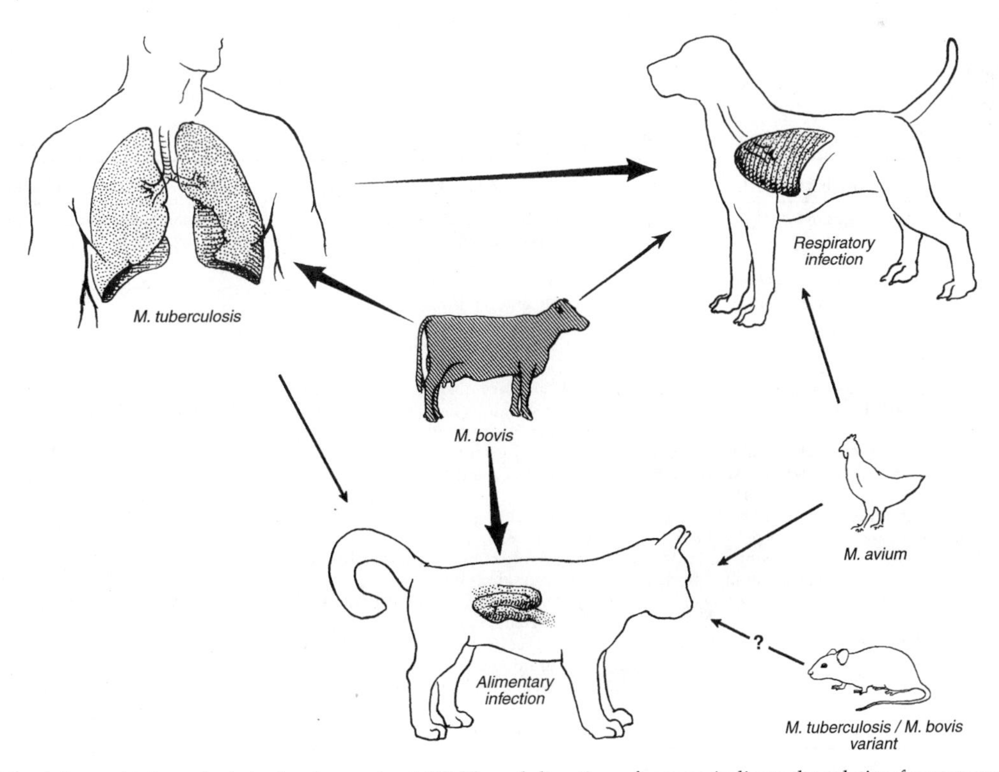

Figure 50–1. Epidemiology of tuberculosis in the dog and cat. Width and direction of arrows indicate the relative frequency and usual sources of infection.

PATHOGENESIS

Tubercle bacilli enter the body through either the respiratory or alimentary tract or skin, depending on the initial route of exposure. Local multiplication of the bacillus at the initial site of deposition—termed a *primary complex*—as well as in the regional draining lymph node may develop. Granuloma formation occurs at both sites. *Incomplete primary complex* refers to infection and localization in the lymph node without lesion formation at the site of deposition. Cats more commonly form incomplete primary complexes whether tonsils, submandibular lymph nodes, or ileocecal lymph nodes are infected; the last are the most common sites of localization and shedding of *M. bovis* organisms. Dogs, which more commonly acquire *M. tuberculosis,* tend to develop respiratory infections with complete primary complex formation and lesions both in the lungs and hilar lymph nodes. *M. tuberculosis* more readily infects the respiratory tract because of its high oxygen requirements. Infections involving MAC organisms in dogs and cats have mainly been disseminated throughout lymphoid and many other tissues, without indications of a primary granuloma at the site of entry.

Not all initial exposure to mycobacteria results in the formation of persistent granulomas, because in most individuals immune responses usually limit further multiplication and spread of the agent. The initial inflammatory response may then subside and resolve, with healing and fibrosis if the remaining tubercle bacilli can be eliminated. The production of persistent focal or disseminated disease is suggestive of defective cell-mediated immunity (CMI). With decreased immunologic resistance, the mycobacteria merely become confined within phagocytic cells, where they continue to multiply intracellularly because of the body's inefficiency in eliminating these intracellular pathogens. Granuloma formation that results is a reflection of the body's attempt to contain remaining organisms. These viable organisms may remain dormant only to break out later and spread as a result of immunosuppression.

In a certain percentage of animals, the mycobacteria may appear to outpace the host defense mechanism, resulting in progressive disease. This increased virulence may result from alterations in the route of exposure, size of inoculum, organism pathogenicity, and CMI defense mechanisms. Having produced primary lesions, the tuberculous mycobacteria may disseminate throughout the body, spreading the infection into adjacent tissue by direct extension or by mechanical means. Aspiration and gravitation of infectious exudates may spread the disease through other areas of lung tissue. Intracellular multiplication of the bacteria is unimpeded as the infection spreads to other tissues by lymphatic or hematogenous means.

A higher prevalence of *M. tuberculosis* infection has been observed in people with AIDS. There has been no association made between feline retroviral infection and mycobacteriosis. Certain breeds, such as the basset hound and possibly the miniature schnauzer and Siamese cat, are over-represented in reports of MAC infection. Siamese cats are similarly predisposed to infections with other persistent intracellular organisms.

It is unclear what factors contribute to mycobacterial resistance by the host.[31] CMI is typically associated with protection against facultative intracellular pathogens such as mycobacteria. Increased resistance seems to be associated with the enhanced capacity of activated macrophages to kill tubercle bacilli or to inhibit their intracellular multiplication.

CLINICAL FINDINGS

Table 50–2 reviews the clinical features of the various mycobacterial diseases. Canine and feline TB is frequently a subclinical disease. Many pets become inadvertently infected with *M. tuberculosis* while living in the same household with tuberculous owners. Farm pets also may serve as subclinical reservoirs of *M. bovis* for susceptible cattle. The ubiquitous distribution of MAC organisms in the environment compared

Table 50–2. Comparison of Mycobacterial Species Infecting Dogs and Cats

ORGANISM	ENVIRONMENTAL FACTORS	CLINICAL FEATURES	DRUG SUSCEPTIBILITY[a]
M. tuberculosis	Urban, close contact affected human	Usually respiratory, pulmonary localization, can disseminate systemically	Isoniazid, rifampin, ethambutol, pyrazinamide
M. tuberculosis/M. bovis variant	Rural, suburban, avid hunter, bite wounds, prey exposure	Nodular cutaneous lesions draining, ulceration, peripheral lymphadenomegaly, local myositis, arthritis, osteomyelitis, can disseminate systemically	Clarithromycin, quinolones, rifampin
M. bovis	Rural cats, ingest raw beef or dairy products	Alimentary disorders, may get respiratory, cutaneous, or lymphatic involvement, disseminate systemically	Rifampin, surgical excision of skin lesions
M. avium complex	Exposure to infected soil, water or dust; acidic soils contaminated with bird feces or carcasses; bassett hounds, miniature schnauzers, and Siamese cats have most prevalence	Dermal granulomas, systemic dissemination	Clarithromycin, clofazimine, doxycycline or minocycline, enrofloxacin, rifabutin, ethambutol
M. lepraemurium	Cooler wet climates, winter months, cats < 3 years old, exposure to infected rodent prey	Multiple cutaneous and subcutaneous dermal nodules on head and extremities, ulcers, fistulas, abscesses regional spread only	Dapsone, clarithromycin, doxycycline or minocycline, clofazamine, rifampin, surgical removal
Opportunistic species	Soil and water exposure, bite, and puncture wounds	Cutaneous and subcutaneous granulomas, especially inguinal region, ulcers, drainage regional spread only	Surgical removal, wide excision, quinolones, aminoglycosides, doxycycline, clofazimine, erythromycin, trimethoprim-sulfonamide, cefoxitin, minocycline

[a]For dosages and detailed information on each, see Tables 50–4 and 50–5 and Drug Formulary, Appendix 8.

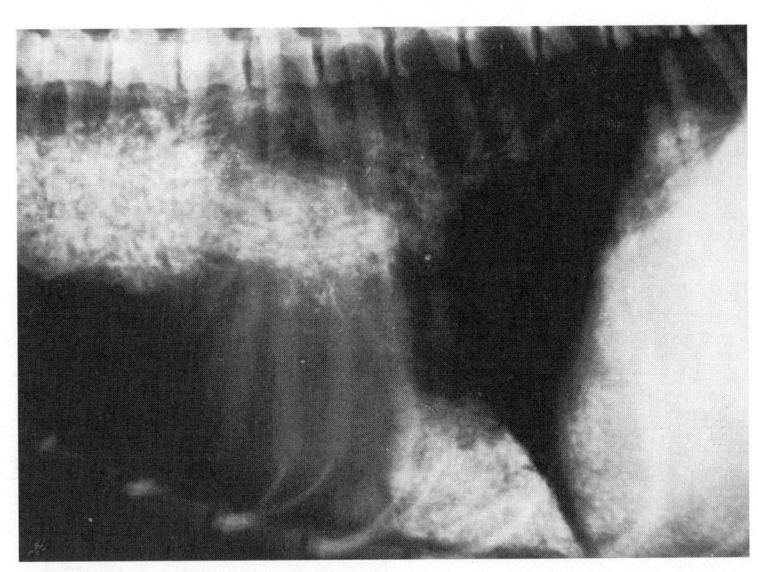

Figure 50–2. Lateral thoracic radiograph of a 3-year-old male Yorkshire terrier with tuberculosis. Note the multiple irregular calcifications of soft tissue in the craniodorsal thorax and cranial abdomen. (From Liu S et al: *J Am Vet Med Assoc* 177:164–167, 1980. Reprinted with permission.)

with the low prevalence of the disease also suggests that subclinical infections are common.

When clinical signs occur in dogs and cats, they reflect the site of granuloma formation. Bronchopneumonia, pulmonary nodule formation, and hilar lymphadenomegaly are most common in dogs, causing fever, weight loss, anorexia, and harsh, nonproductive coughing. Dogs and cats may develop dysphagia, retching, hypersalivation, and tonsillar enlargement, all the result of ulcerated and chronically draining oropharyngeal lesions. Cats, which develop primary intestinal localization more commonly than dogs, exhibit weight loss, anemia, vomiting, and diarrhea as signs of intestinal malabsorption. Mesenteric lymph nodes are palpably enlarged. Abdominal effusion is present in some cases.

A continuum of clinical signs develops with disseminated disease. Direct extension of lung disease has resulted in pleural or pericardial effusion with signs of dyspnea, cyanosis, and right-sided heart failure. Disseminated disease may be the first sign of illness in many dogs and cats, and clinical signs refer to the organ localization in each case. Generalized lymphadenomegaly, anorexia, weight loss, fever, and sudden death may be observed. Masses or enlargement may be detected in many abdominal organs, especially the liver and spleen. Dermal nodules and nonhealing, draining ulcers have been noted commonly in cats and sometimes in dogs. Cats with *M. bovis* infections have developed tuberculous choroiditis and retinal detachments.[17] Granulomatous uveitis and CNS signs have occurred in some cases. Lameness and spontaneous fractures have been observed with bone localization. Additional clinical signs have included hemoptysis, hematuria, and icterus.

DIAGNOSIS

Clinical laboratory findings in TB are frequently nonspecific and include moderate leukocytosis and anemia. The anemia is usually nonregenerative, but in some cats with intestinal infections it has been reported to be macrocytic.[34] Normal to reduced serum albumin levels and hyperglobulinemia are frequently apparent. Organisms may be visualized in leukocytes of blood and bone marrow smears or buffy coat or urine.[11, 58] The lipid-containing cell wall does not stain with Romanovsky's stains, so that bacilli appear as unstained bars within leukocytes. Radiographically visible masses may be apparent in various organ systems. Abnormalities on thoracic radiography can include tracheobronchial lymphadenomegaly and interstitial lung infiltration (Fig. 50–2). Lung consolidation and granuloma formation have been associated with diffuse radiopaque densities in lung lobes. Calcified pulmonary lesions have sometimes been observed in dogs and cats. Metastatic lesions are seen as diffuse miliary densities. Fluid may be present in the pleural or pericardial cavities. Abdominal radiography may reveal enlargement of parenchymal organs such as the liver and spleen or solitary abdominal masses. Fluid may be present in the abdominal cavity, and calcified mesenteric lymph nodes may be noted. Bony lesions consist of small, circumscribed, radiolucent areas. Thoracic involvement may be associated with hypertrophic pulmonary osteoarthropathy. Diskospondylitis or vertebral osteomyelitis may be apparent in the vertebral bodies.

Cytology

The acid-fast stain is the most widely available method for making a rapid presumptive diagnosis of TB. Acid-fast stains will be positive for specimens from many but not all animals with mycobacterial infections. It is more consistent in organisms recovered in culture. Mycobacteria can be stained for acid fastness with carbolfuchsin or fluorescent dyes (i.e., auramine-rhodamine). The fluorochrome stains are more sensitive and technically less difficult to examine than conventional carbolfuchsin stains.

Tuberculin Testing

ID skin testing has been used as an aid in the detection and diagnosis of human TB and to evaluate delayed-type hypersensitivity in animals. The two types of tuberculin utilized for ID testing are summarized in Table 50–3. Depending on whether there is a history of infection or disease, various strengths (1, 5, or 250 TU/0.1 ml) of purified protein derivative (PPD) tuberculin are usually selected in human skin testing. However, the highest concentration is needed to test dogs. ID tuberculin testing in dogs has been reported to be inconsistent and unreliable. However, use of the pinna was shown to be reliable in detecting dogs previously sensitized with bacille Calmette-Guérin (BCG) vaccine, an attenuated mutant strain of *M. bovis* that has been used in people as a vaccine to induce resistance to TB and as a nonspecific immunostimulant. In addition, infected dogs have been shown to respond well to ID skin testing with BCG. A disadvantage of BCG is that it can induce later false-positive reactions in skin testing with PPD. Although not studied in animals, false-positive results have been more common in people utilizing certain brands of PPD.[52] BCG must be handled cautiously to avoid inadvertent inoculation because immunosuppressed people, especially those with AIDS, may develop disseminated disease.[56a]

Tests are performed by injecting BCG or PPD ID on the medial side of the proximal hindlimb or preferably on the inner surface of the pinna. A positive reaction is indicated only if a raised, indurated, and subsequently necrotic swelling appears at the site of injection between 48 and 72 hours later. Necrosis and ulceration may take up to 2 weeks to develop. Mild erythema after ID BCG injection in dogs is considered to be nonspecific. False-positive results caused by cross-reactivity with other bacterial species have been observed.

Another method of tuberculin testing for dogs, recommended by the U.S. Department of Agriculture (USDA), is to take a baseline rectal temperature. If it is in the reference range, inject SC 0.75 ml PPD bovis (as supplied by USDA, see Table 50–3). The rectal temperature is monitored every 2 hours for 12 hours. A 1.1°C (2°F) rise in temperature is a positive test result.

Unlike many species, cats do not react strongly to ID-administered tuberculin. Despite their lack of response to PPD, cats still have adequate immunity to tuberculosis. SC or IV challenge with tuberculin is no more reliable, and cats do not respond well to ID BCG. Cats sensitized to BCG have responded to PPD injected ID in the pinna; unfortunately, the response has usually been inconsistent, infrequent, or transient. The SC method has not been evaluated in cats, and biopsy, culture, and necropsy are more definitive tests.

Table 50–3. Summary of Intradermal Skin Testing for Tuberculosis in Dogs and Cats[a]

SUBSTANCE	PREFERRED SITE	DOSE
PPD	Inner surface pinna	250 TU[b] (0.1 ml)
BCG	Inner surface pinna	0.1–0.2 ml[c]

[a]See text for information on performance and interpretation of the test.

[b]PPD for bovine testing from U.S. Department of Agriculture is 30,000 TU/ml (1 mg/ml). To prepare at least 250 TU/0.1 ml, remove 0.1 ml as supplied; add to 1.1 ml sterile water for injection; mix in sterile glass vial. Diluted solutions of PPD should be made fresh and used soon after preparation. Human (*M. tuberculosis*) or bovine (*M. bovis*) strains can be used for tuberculin source because cross-reactions exist to cell wall components. The human strain might give a stronger reaction to *M. tuberculosis* but bovine is available in higher concentration. Higher concentrations are used to test animals than people when sensitivity rather than specificity is more important when public health risk exists. Note in humans they use 5 TU units in 0.1 ml of solution (50 TU/ml) on volar aspect forearm and read in 48–72 hours. If human tuberculin is supplied in milligrams, the conversion factor is 50,000 U of PPD equals 1 mg of PPD.

[c]BCG vaccine contains 8–26 million colony-forming units/ml of living bacillus. Reconstitute freeze-dried preparation into 1-ml aliquots according to manufacturer's recommendation. BCG may sensitize the animal to false-positive results to further tuberculin testing.

PPD = purified protein derivative of tuberculin; BCG = bacille Calmette-Guérin; TU = tuberculin units.

Serologic Testing

Although unreliable compared with skin testing, serologic testing for antimycobacterial antibodies includes hemagglutination and complement fixation. Serologic testing has been employed to detect infected dogs and cats when skin testing was inconclusive. The serologic response to *M. bovis* BCG vaccination in cats and dogs has been evaluated with immunoblotting against specific protein antigens.[6] Antibody increases were detected 3 to 5 weeks after vaccination and remained increased for 23 weeks and longer than 1 year in dogs and cats, respectively. Serologic testing could potentially detect exposure to mycobacteria similar to ID skin testing.

Bacterial Isolation

For culture, tissue- or mucosa-derived samples are usually treated with 4% sodium hydroxide and another disinfectant such as *N*-acetyl-L-cysteine to eliminate any contaminating microorganisms. Specimens that are usually sterile (internal tissues, CSF, urine, blood) should not be decontaminated because the low numbers of mycobacteria can be lost. When specimens are small and contain acid-fast organisms, the entire sample should be placed in a broth-based culture medium. Broth or liquid media facilitate more rapid growth of mycobacteria. Solid media are still required for optimal isolation of mycobacteria and for detection of more than one species in a specimen. Pathogenic tuberculous mycobacteria are slow growing, often requiring 4 to 6 weeks to establish visible colonies on solid media, and their growth is inhibited unless enrichment media are used. Egg-enrichment media such as Löwenstein-Jensen and agar-based media such as Middlebrook (both from Difco Labs, Detroit, MI) are preferred as solid media for isolating tubercle bacilli. Glycerol, which is added to media such as Löwenstein-Jensen to enhance the growth of *M. tuberculosis*, actually inhibits the growth of *M. bovis*. Stonebrink's or B83 media are used when *M. bovis* is suspected.[13] Growth is more rapid in 5% to 10% carbon dioxide. Pathogenic and saprophytic mycobacteria have been identified and differentiated by colony growth and biochemical characteristics (see Table 50–1).

Commercial methods have been developed that facilitate rapid detection and classification of the mycobacteria. The lysis-centrifugation method (Isolator system, Wampole Labs, Cranbury, NJ) has also been utilized to facilitate culture of intracellular pathogens such as mycobacteria from the blood. Nonradiometric automated methods for broth culture such as the BACTEC system (Becton Dickinson, Towson, MD), ESP-AFB (Difco Labs, Detroit, MI), and MB/Bact (Organon-Teknika, Durham, NC), have reduced initial detection of mycobacterial growth to an average of 10 to 13 days. Final identification can be 4 to 6 weeks longer, but the polymerase chain reaction (PCR) followed by restriction analysis and nucleic acid hybridization has shortened this time to a few days.[9, 49, 57, 61] Commercial kits AccuProbe, Gen-Probe, Inc., San Diego, CA) simplify this identification. PCR has also been used directly on clinical specimens from people, cats, dogs, and other animals to detect mycobacteria.[1a, 8a, 10, 39, 40, 46] A number of commercial direct amplified tests are pending regulatory approval.

Animal inoculation has been performed historically to identify mycobacterial species and those such as *M. leprae* and *M. lepraemurium*, which are difficult to culture. Laboratory animals such as guinea pigs, rabbits, mice, and hamsters have been inoculated intraperitoneally with suspensions of lymph node, spleen, and granulomas from suspected cases.

Mycobacterial components are detectable in body fluids such as CSF using enzyme immunoassay or RIA. The sensitivity of such methods is much greater than acid-fast staining to detect organisms in leukocytes. Detection of mycobacterial antigens in sputum by ELISA is more difficult because they are often lost in the processing of such fluids for analysis.

Tissue Biopsy

Definitive diagnoses can be made by demonstrating acid-fast organisms within a lesion via biopsy and histologic examination of lesions or by direct smears of exudates or fluids. The acid-fast staining method is ideal for aspirates of tissue and granulomas and for identifying organisms in bacterial cultures. Mycobacteria can also be demonstrated by fluorescent dyes on stained preparations. Although often present in low numbers, intracellular tubercle bacilli are recognized by their clubbed shape and beaded appearance.

PATHOLOGIC FINDINGS

In dogs and cats, generalized emaciation is a frequent finding on gross necropsy. Multifocal granulomas are grayish-white to yellow, circumscribed, nodular lesions and appear in many organs. Lung and bronchial lymph nodes are usually the primary lesion sites in dogs, and ileocecal and mesenteric lymph nodes are similarly involved in cats. Generalized spread is more common in dogs than in cats; pleura, pericardium, liver, kidney, heart, intestine, and CNS lesions are the most frequent (Fig. 50–3). The mesenteric lymph nodes, spleen, and skin are more commonly involved in cats. Rarely, bone, joint, and genital lesions may be observed in dogs and cats, and conjunctival lesions have been observed in cats. Unlike larger solitary primary granulomas, metastatic lesions are frequently small (1–3 mm) and multifocal or appear as large clusters of coalescing tubercles in many organs.

Histologically, granulomatous lesions consist of areas of focal necrosis surrounded by infiltrations of plasma cells and macrophages. Evidence of encapsulation is apparent by peripheral layers of densely packed fibroblasts in a thin, fibrous, connective tissue capsule. Calcification of the granuloma is sometimes present; however, liquefaction of the necrotic central portion is rarely if ever observed in carnivores (Fig. 50–4). Epithelioid or histiocytic cells usually border the necrotic zone; giant cell formation, which occurs in other species, is uncommon. Short-chained, beaded, slightly pleomorphic, acid-alcohol–fast bacilli may be detected intracellularly in the periphery of necrotic lesions. Organisms within macrophages and epithelioid cells are usually more numerous in MAC infections than in infections caused by opportunistic mycobacteria or by *M. bovis* and *M. tuberculosis*. Infection with *M. tuberculosis–M. bovis* variant can result in different numbers of intracellular bacilli.

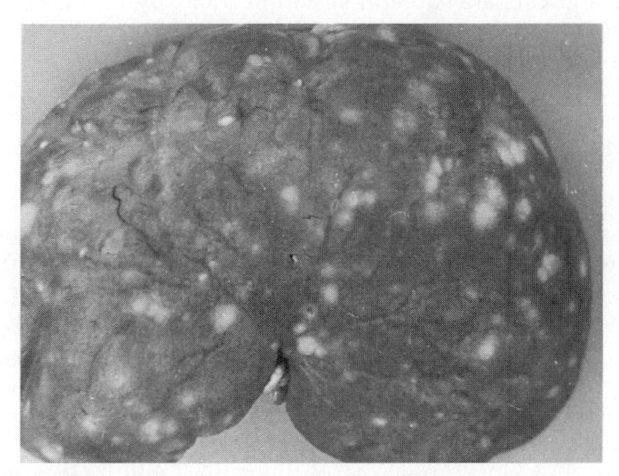

Figure 50–3. Multifocal granulomas in the kidney of a 3 1/2-year-old male boxer with systemic spread of tuberculous infection. (From Liu S et al: *J Am Vet Med Assoc* 177:164–167, 1980. Reprinted with permission.)

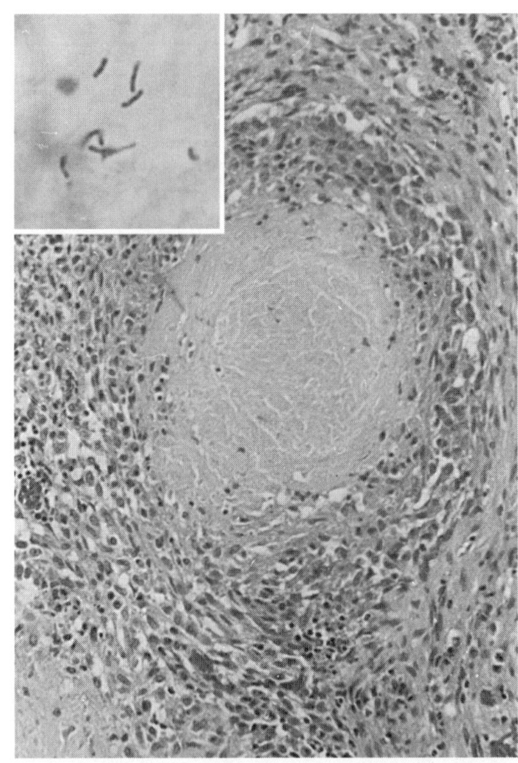

Figure 50–4. Photomicrograph of a liver from a 2-year-old female German shepherd showing a caseous tubercle with central necrosis, proliferation of histiocytes and fibroblasts in the middle zone, and encapsulation in the periphery (H and E, × 100). *Inset:* Beaded bacilli (acid-fast stain, × 1000). (From Liu S et al: *J Am Vet Med Assoc* 177:164–167, 1980. Reprinted with permission.)

THERAPY

Because of the delay in definitive isolation of mycobacteria, treatment should be instituted on the basis of cytologic or histologic diagnosis. Single drug treatment of any mycobacterial infection of animals is *not* advised and, for best efficacy, combination therapy is always needed. Antimicrobial resistant mycobacteria will also develop when single-agent therapy is used.[1]

M. tuberculosis

Treatment of human TB involves several drug regimens, depending on whether the patient has been exposed and whether the subclinical or active disease has been demonstrated. Similar guidelines might apply when considering treatment of pets (Table 50–4). Long-term (6–12 months) sin-

Table 50–4. Dosages of Some Antituberculosis Drugs

DRUG	SPECIES	DOSE (mg/kg)[a]	ROUTE	INTERVAL (HOURS)	TOXICITIES
***M. tuberculosis* Infection**					
Chemoprophylaxis[b]					
Isoniazid	D	10[c]	PO	24	Hepatotoxic
Treatment (minimum of two of the following drugs in combination)[d]					
Isoniazid	D	10–20[e]	PO	24	Hepatotoxic
Rifampin	D	10–20[f]	PO	12–24	Hepatotoxic, discolors tears and urine
Ethambutol	D	15	PO	24	Optic neuritis
Dihydrostreptomycin	D	15	IM	24	Ototoxic
Pyrazinamide[g]	D	15–40	PO	24	Hepatotoxic, GI signs, arthralgia
***M. tuberculosis–bovis* Variant Infection[h]**					
Rifampin	C	10–20	PO	24	Hepatotoxic, pinnal erythema
Enrofloxacin	C	5–10	PO	12–24	Vomiting
Clarithromycin	C	5–10	PO	12	Pinnal erythema?
***M. avium* Complex Infection**					
Enrofloxacin	B	5–10	PO	12–24	Vomiting
Clarithromycin	B	5	PO	12	Pinnal erythema?
Clofazimine	B	4	PO	24	Orange staining
Doxycycline	B	10	PO	12	Vomiting

[a]Dose per administration at specified interval. After daily dosing for weeks to months, switch to twice weekly administration for 6–9 months. See also Appendix 8.
[b]For 6–12 months.
[c]Dosages are extrapolated from human child and adult recommendations. Treatment of *M. tuberculosis* or *M. bovis* infections is not recommended for dogs and cats.
[d]Localized: isoniazid and rifampin daily for 6 months with pyrazinamide added during the first 2 months or isoniazid and rifampin alone for 9 months. Disseminated: isoniazid and rifampin, with ethambutol and/or pyrazinamide initially and treat daily beyond 9 months.
[e]Maximum 300 mg daily.
[f]Maximum 600 mg daily.
[g]Ineffective for *M. bovis* strains.
[h]Treatment for 2 months minimum with all three drugs. Maintenance therapy for 4 months thereafter consists of the same dosages of either enrofloxacin and clarithromycin or rifampin and enrofloxacin (Gunn-Moore DA, personal communication, 1996).
D = dog; C = cat; B = both.

gle-drug (isoniazid) regimens are given prophylactically when exposure with concurrent immunosuppression increases the likelihood of producing active disease. Combination chemotherapy with several agents is used in treating active disease. Treatment of active *M. tuberculosis* infection involves the combination of at least two agents for a minimum of 6 to 9 months. The isoniazid-ethambutol-rifampin combination is the most effective course of therapy, although pyrazinamide is being substituted for ethambutol more frequently. Drugs like these have made human TB a curable disease, and surgical removal of tuberculous granulomas is no longer required. However, increasing resistance to these drugs is cause for concern. Chemotherapy of spontaneous canine TB has been successful in certain cases in which it has been provided. Rapid regression of experimentally produced lesions in dogs has been achieved by combined IV administration of rifampin and isoniazid and IM administration of streptomycin for 23 months. Increases in coagulation times and liver enzyme activities were side effects of this extended therapy.

The decision to treat infected dogs and cats must be taken seriously because of the obvious human health hazard that exists. It is not recommended for confirmed infections. Diagnosis by skin or serologic testing is not as reliable in detecting exposed or latently infected animals, and it may be desirable to place dogs or cats exposed to human or bovine TB on prophylactic chemotherapy.

M. bovis

M. bovis is resistant to pyrazinamide. Cats with *M. bovis* infection have been treated effectively by surgical excision of localized skin lesions and oral rifampin at 4 mg/kg/day for 2 to 5 months.[15] Unfortunately, use of rifampin alone has the potential to induce development of bacterial resistance.

M. tuberculosis–M. bovis Variant

Cats with *M. tuberculosis–M. bovis* variant infections have been treated successfully in some cases with a combination of rifampin, enrofloxacin, and clarithromycin (see Table 50–4).[23]

M. avium Complex

Humans are the only reservoir hosts for *M. tuberculosis*. Dogs and cats are susceptible to infections by *M. tuberculosis* and *M. bovis* but are more resistant to infection by MAC organisms. Despite this inherent resistance, the exposure to MAC organisms is much greater because the MAC organisms may respond to drugs used to treat atypical mycobacterial infections. Unlike opportunistic rapid-growing mycobacteria, MAC strains are resistant in vitro to the quinolones. One dog has been treated with a combination of clofazimine, ciprofloxacin, and rifampin with limited success.[47] Anemia and hepatotoxicity were side effects of rifampin therapy. One cat with a localized MAC granuloma had surgical removal alone, but the mass subsequently returned.[55] A cat with localized MAC infection was successfully treated with surgery followed by a combination of clofazimine and doxycycline.[35] A basset hound with disseminated infection that was on continuous combination therapy of enrofloxacin, clarithromycin, and clofazimine, as outlined in Table 50–4, was in remission for 2 years before experiencing relapse.[4] In human patients with AIDS, the three-drug regimen of rifabutin, ethambutol, and clofazimine is more effective than rifampin, ethambutol, clofazimine, and ciprofloxacin.[54]

PREVENTION

TB is a major human public health problem. Humans are susceptible to *M. bovis*, *M. tuberculosis*, and MAC organisms. This susceptibility is important with respect to control in animals. Identification of cases of *M. tuberculosis* infection in people should be followed by serologic testing or clinical evaluation of pet contacts as possible reservoirs. Outbreaks of *M. bovis* infection in cattle should also be followed by evaluation of dogs and cats on the farm. Feeding of unpasteurized milk or raw offal to pets should be discontinued. Live BCG vaccine has been administered to protect people against infections with *M. tuberculosis*. Live recombinant DNA vaccines have been produced using nonvirulent mycobacteria. The effectiveness of such products is being evaluated on an experimental basis. The attempt to control TB in dogs with modified live vaccines has had moderate success in that some dogs have shown increased resistance to infection, but immunity is partial, and vaccination has not been generally recommended. This approach also can produce false-positive skin test results as it does in other species.

PUBLIC HEALTH CONSIDERATIONS

Although *M. tuberculosis* and *M. bovis* infections are not maintained in canine and feline reservoirs, infected dogs and cats may serve as temporary sources for dissemination of bacteria into the environment. Because respiratory or intestinal secretions may be contaminated, it is recommended that *M. tuberculosis*–infected animals be either treated or euthanized. Where *M. bovis* infections have been frequent in New Zealand, infected cats did not appear to be a major risk to their owners.[14, 15] Nevertheless, owners should be advised that this organism is a known transmitted pathogen. *M. tuberculosis–M. bovis* variant infections in cats are likely acquired from their hunting infected prey species; therefore, restriction of this activity is the only known preventive measure. This species is not known to infect people. Because they are soil saprophytes, MAC organisms are just as likely to be acquired from environmental sources by people as by pets. MAC and *M. tuberculosis–M. bovis* variant infections are the appropriate ones to eliminate in companion animal practice.[25, 34, 35, 47] However, to avoid any potential concern, families with members who are immunocompromised should generally be advised not to keep *Mycobacterium*-infected pets.

Feline Leprosy

Diane T. Lewis and Gail A. Kunkle

ETIOLOGY AND PATHOGENESIS

M. lepraemurium, the agent of rat leprosy, is believed to be the causative agent of feline leprosy. The organism is unable to be cultivated by routine mycobacterial methods but has been cultured on 1% Ogawa egg yolk medium. Disease transmission to cats is thought to occur via bites or contact with infected rats. Occurrence of the disease in cats has been confined to seaport cities of the western United States, New Zealand, Great Britain, Australia, and the Netherlands, with a greater incidence in the winter. It is possible that feline leukemia virus (FeLV)–or feline immunodeficiency virus (FIV)–associated immunosuppression is involved in the pathogenesis.[33, 66]

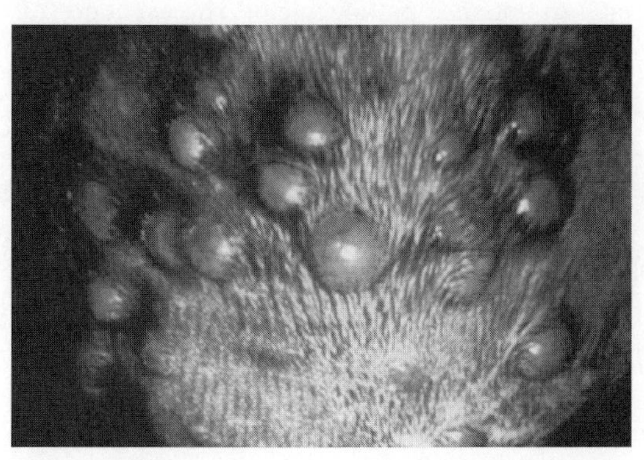

Figure 50–5. Multiple cutaneous nodules on the dorsal neck of a cat with feline leprosy. (Courtesy of Dr. Kirk Haupt, Seattle, WA.)

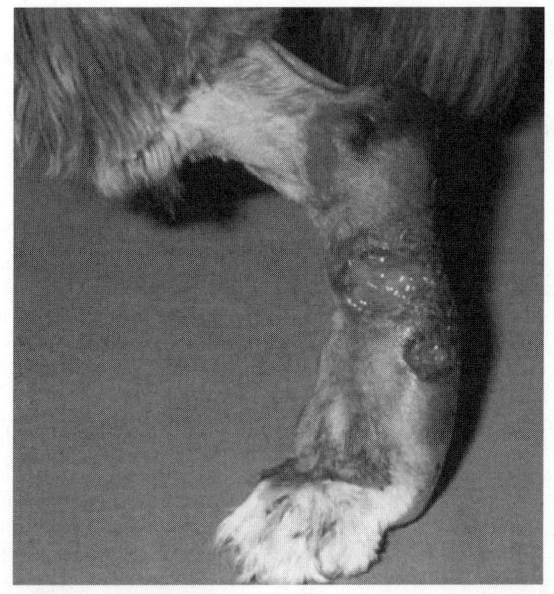

Figure 50–6. Ulcerated nodules of feline leprosy on the limb of a cat. (Courtesy of Dr. Kirk Haupt, Seattle, WA.)

CLINICAL SIGNS

Feline leprosy is primarily a cutaneous disease; cats are in good health otherwise. Nonpainful, frequently ulcerated, soft, fleshy nodules confined to the skin and subcutis are noted on the face, forelimbs, and trunk of young cats (Figs.

50–5 and 50–6). Regional lymph nodes usually are enlarged, although systemic infection is uncommon.

DIAGNOSIS

Diagnosis is made through clinical findings: the presence of very large numbers of acid-fast bacilli in histologic sections (Fig. 50–7) or impression smears from tissue and culture of affected tissue. A diffuse, granulomatous inflammatory infiltrate composed of vacuolated macrophages is present on histologic examination of tissue. With acid-fast stains, such as Ziehl-Neelson, numerous acid-fast bacilli are noted within the macrophages or extracellularly within dermal vacuoles. The organisms are visible with silver stains. Culture results will be negative when conditions are used to grow the tuberculous bacilli and rapidly growing mycobacteria. PCR amplification of 16S rRNA gene sequences has been utilized to substantiate *M. lepraemurium* as the cause of feline leprosy.[28b] In addition, a novel mycobacterium with nucleotide sequence resembling *M. malmoense* was identified in a few cases.

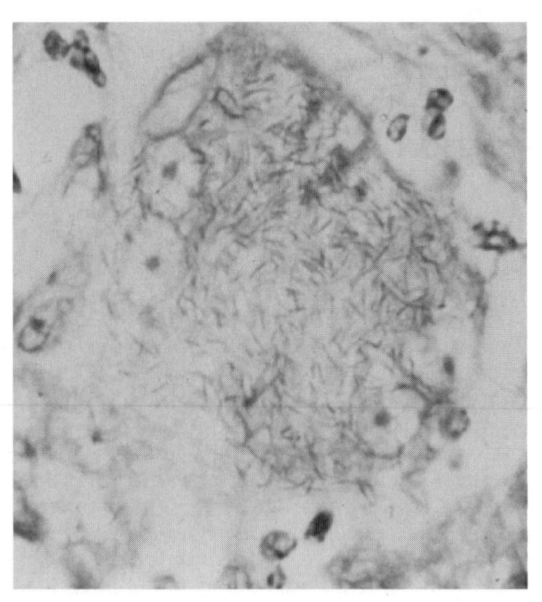

Figure 50–7. Microscopic appearance of nodular lesion from the face of a FeLV-positive cat. Large numbers of organisms are visible (acid-fast stain, × 100). (Courtesy of Dr. Boyd Jones, University College Dublin, Dublin, Ireland.)

TREATMENT

Complete surgical excision of all nodules has proved beneficial in many cats. When this approach is not feasible, clofazimine has been successful in a small number of cases. The drug appears to have minimal toxicity. Dapsone may be another alternative to surgery, although toxicity may occur in some cats.

Because the disease is acquired from rodents, preventing exposure to rodents will likely minimize the possibility of disease in cats.

Opportunistic Rapid-Growing Mycobacterial Infections

Diane T. Lewis and Gail A. Kunkle

ETIOLOGY

There are numerous saprophytic, nontuberculous, nonlepromatous species called opportunistic or atypical mycobacteria. They are divided into the slow-growing and the fast-growing species (see Table 50–1). Although the slow-growing opportunistic mycobacteria are responsible for several well-characterized cutaneous diseases in people, they are less commonly identified as pathogens in the dog and cat, possibly as a result of the lengthy time needed for culture. The exception to this low frequency of isolation is the slow-growing MAC organisms, which belong to the opportunistic group and have been discussed previously with TB. Rapidly growing, opportunistic mycobacteria have been isolated from many cats and several dogs with cutaneous lesions as well as from rare pulmonary infections.

EPIDEMIOLOGY

These opportunistic mycobacteria are ubiquitous in nature, especially in water and wet soil. They are not pathogenic for animals under normal circumstances. Animal-to-animal transmission does not generally occur. Most opportunistic mycobacteria infecting dogs and cats are acquired from the environment after trauma to the skin or soft tissues. Bite or scratch injuries have also been responsible for infection (see Chapter 53). The respiratory or alimentary systems rarely are points of entry for these organisms, and the location of bacilli entry in the body is important in determining the type of resulting disease. Most opportunistic mycobacterial lesions are localized tissue reactions to the presence of acid-fast bacilli in the skin or deeper tissues via puncture or fight wounds. Inoculation of the acid-fast bacilli into adipose tissue seems to enhance pathogenicity. The existence of tissue injury, predisposing disease conditions, or impairment of the host's immunologic defense mechanism has often been identified in people but not commonly in animals.

M. fortuitum, *M. chelonae (M. chelonei)*, and *M. smegmatis* are the species commonly isolated from canine and feline opportunistic mycobacterial infections in the United States. *M. smegmatis*, *M. phlei*, and other similar but as yet unidentified species are most common in Australia. Cats seem more susceptible to infection and exhibit a higher infection rate than do dogs. Abscesses or granulomas are the typical lesions that develop.

CLINICAL FINDINGS

Opportunistic mycobacteriosis in cats most commonly causes multiple fistulous tracts associated with purulent or

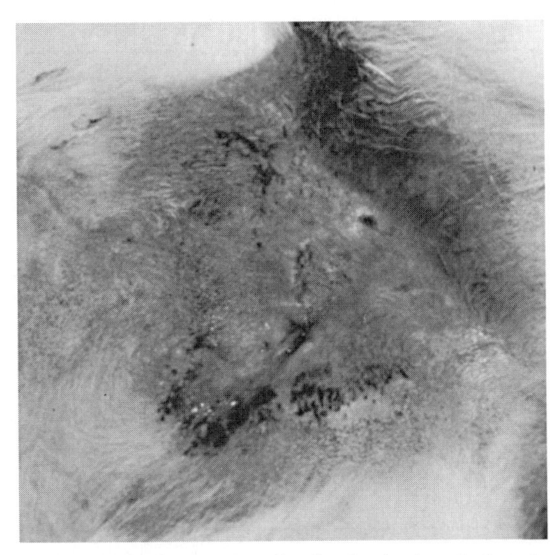

Figure 50–8. Multiple draining fistulas in the inguinal region of a cat caused by chronic infection by *M. fortuitum*.

serosanguineous drainage into the caudal abdominal, inguinal, and lumbar subcutaneous tissues (Fig. 50–8). Cutaneous or subcutaneous nodules that periodically drain develop with or without punctate ulcers and spreading granulomatous proliferation. By use of careful methodology, *M. fortuitum* or *M. smegmatis* can generally be isolated from these lesions. Most cats, even those with extensive cutaneous involvement, remain active and somewhat normal except for serous drainage from the tracts. Fever occasionally occurs, but anorexia, weight loss, and other features of chronic infections usually are absent. Response to antibiotic therapy usually is temporary, and these lesions may wax and wane for years.

Dogs with opportunistic mycobacteriosis usually have a history of bite wounds or trauma followed by granulomatous proliferation of cutaneous tissues with serous or seropurulent drainage (Fig. 50–9). Pulmonary infections with *M. fortuitum*,[65] systemic infection with *M. smegmatis*,[22] and disseminated subcutaneous *M. fortuitum* infection[18] have been reported.

DIAGNOSIS

The diagnosis of opportunistic mycobacteriosis is not always easy, and a diligent search for organisms in tissue biopsy samples is usually required, especially in cats. Tissue biopsy samples will generally reveal extensive granulomatous to pyogranulomatous inflammation of the dermis and panniculus. Application of acid-fast stains (especially Fite's method), followed by extensive searching, may reveal a few organisms within extracellular lipid vacuoles surrounded by neutrophils and macrophages. Frozen-section biopsy specimens have improved staining capacity and demonstration of organisms. The rapid Ziehl-Neelsen method also is useful. The presence of acid-fast bacteria in exudates alone may be suggestive of infection; however, it is not confirmatory, because other acid-fast saprophytes exist.

Organisms may be difficult to detect because of their scarcity, and repeated biopsies may be necessary to confirm their presence. Pyogranulomatous panniculitis can also be seen with nocardiosis, which should be considered more likely than mycobacteriosis if granules are found in the exudate or tissues (see Chapter 49).

Bacterial culture of deep tissue (especially the panniculus) biopsy specimens and identification of the organism are essential for definitive diagnosis. Cultures from multiple tissue samples may be necessary. The mycobacteria begin to grow rapidly within 3 to 5 days of inoculation onto culture media. *Staphylococcus* species or other organisms may be secondarily present on the surface and may overgrow the blood agar plate, preventing identification of the pathogen. For this reason, medium specifically intended for mycobacterial isolation (see Tuberculous Mycobacterial Infections, Bacterial Isolation) should be used, and the plates should be held for 3 weeks. The final identification of acid-fast organisms from culture requires biochemical or genetic methods.

THERAPY

If a rapidly growing mycobacterium has been isolated, species identification should be performed. This approach can be expensive and is not universally available. Currently, the National Jewish Center for Immunology and Respiratory Medicine in Denver, Colorado, performs identification and susceptibility tests for mycobacteria. If antibiotic susceptibility testing is to be done, specific drugs should be requested. *M. fortuitum* and *M. smegmatis* are usually sensitive to high dosages of fluoroquinolones (ciprofloxacin, enrofloxacin, and ofloxacin) and others,[20, 42, 56] whereas *M. chelonae* is not. *M. chelonae* is usually only sensitive to clarithromycin.[62] Those drugs found most useful both in vitro and in vivo are listed in Table 50–5. Antibacterial therapy should be chosen on the basis of susceptibility data and should be maintained for at

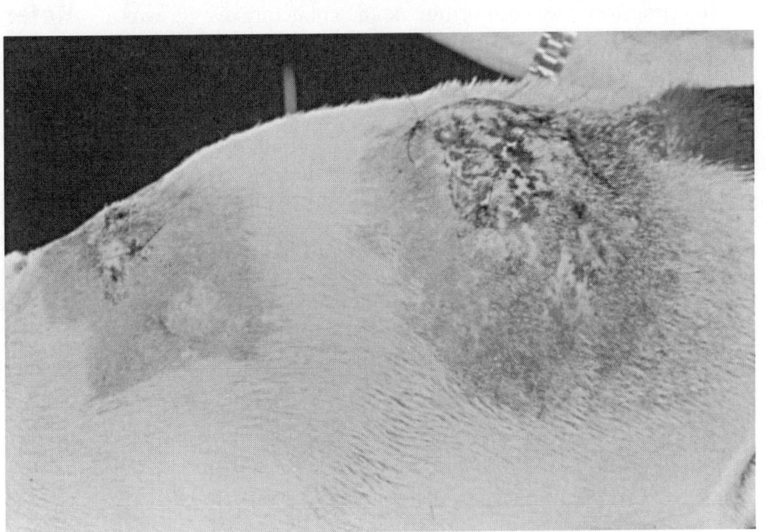

Figure 50–9. Granulomatous draining masses caused by *M. chelonae* infection in a dog.

Table 50–5. Drug Dosages for Lepromatous and Opportunistic Mycobacterial Infections

DRUG	SPECIES	DOSE (mg/kg)[b]	ROUTE	INTERVAL (HOURS)	DURATION (WEEKS)
Lepromatous[c]					
Dapsone	D	1[d]	PO	8	2
	C	50 mg total/cat	PO	12	2
Clofazimine[e]	C	8	PO	24	6[f]
Opportunistic (Slow and Rapid Growing)					
Gentamicin	B	2	SC, IM	8–12	2–4[g]
Amikacin	B	5–10	SC, IM	8–12	2–4
Kanamycin	B	5–7	SC, IM	12	2–4[g]
Doxycycline or minocycline	B	5–12.5	PO, IV	12	4–6
Trimethoprim-sulfonamide	D	15–30	PO	12	4–6
	C	10	PO	12	4[g,h]
Chloramphenicol	D	25–50	PO	8	4–6
	C	15–40	PO	8–12	3–4[h]
Enrofloxacin	B	5–15	PO	12	3–16[i,j]
Clofazimine	B	8	PO	24	3–4[e,f]
Clarithromycin	C	15	PO	12	6–8
Cefuroxime	B	11–22	PO	12	4–16

[a]For specific information about each drug consult Drug Formulary, Appendix 8.
[b]Dose per administration at specified interval. Dose is expressed as mg/kg unless otherwise stated.
[c]Surgical removal is the most effective therapy. An alternative regimen that might work in cases of treatment failures would include doxycycline and a fluoroquinolone, with or without rifampin.
[d]For induction therapy; later switch to 0.3–0.6 mg/kg per dose.
[e]Because of difficulty of fractionating liquid in capsules, cats are usually given one 50-mg capsule per dose.
[f]After 6 weeks, begin twice weekly interval of administration.
[g]Monitor blood urea nitrogen weekly for evidence of nephrotoxicity; often combined with other drugs.
[h]Must check hemogram weekly for evidence of myelosuppression.
[i]For the dosage of other quinolones, see Drug Formulary, Appendix 8.
[j]Avoid in young animals.
D = dog; C = cat; B = dog and cat.

least 6 weeks, because these infections are deep. In some cases clinical cure was achieved only after 6 to 8 months of therapy. Opportunistic mycobacteria are usually resistant to antituberculous drugs. In human infections, increased resistance to the fluoroquinolones has been observed when they are used as monotherapy.[1]

Surgical resection or debulking of large granulomatous masses has been more beneficial in dogs than in cats. Cats may improve with surgical resection of small lesions, but dehiscence, proliferation of the wound margins, and further progression of lesions are common sequelae. However, radical surgical resection with tissue advancement flaps and appropriate antibiotic therapy has been reported successful in some cats.[42]

PROGNOSIS

The prognosis for opportunistic mycobacteriosis in cats and dogs is guarded. Although some cats have been cured with fluoroquinolone therapy alone, others require lifelong treatment. Some cats may show complete resolution of clinical signs with antibiotic therapy, but once it is stopped, lesions recur. After years of chronic cutaneous lesions, a few cats have developed visceral masses containing acid-fast rods. Dogs apparently have a better prognosis for remission on the basis of current reports. In spite of expensive, long-term therapy, an infected pet who has continual serous drainage must occasionally be euthanized.

PUBLIC HEALTH CONSIDERATIONS

Because these organisms are free-living saprophytes, there is little risk of transmission of these infections from animal to animal or animal to human. However, wound disinfection and contact precautions are usually advised, especially if immunosuppressed people are present in the same environment. Sodium hypochlorite (100 ppm available chlorine) rapidly kills these organisms on contaminated surfaces or inanimate objects.

Subcutaneous inoculation of *M. chelonae* organisms into a person reportedly occurred through penetration of dog hair into the owner's Achilles tendon by prolonged and vigorous rubbing of the person's ankle on that person's pet terrier.[44] Tendonitis caused by *M. chelonae* resulted. Cultures of the dog's hair and of tap water from the patient's home were negative for mycobacteria. Human hospital-acquired infections have also occurred. Contamination of multiple-dose–injection syringes, peritoneal dialysis and hemodialysis machines, bronchoscopes, and some surgical equipment has led to severe nosocomial infections. Similar problems have not been reported in veterinary hospitals, but the potential exists.

References

1. Alangaden GJ, Lerner SA. 1997. The clinical use of fluoroquinolones for the treatment of mycobacterial diseases. *Clin Infect Dis* 25:1213–1221.
1a. Aranaz A, Liebana E, Pickering X, et al. 1996. Use of polymerase chain reaction in the diagnosis of tuberculosis in cats and dogs. *Vet Rec* 138:276–280.
2. Barnes PF, Barrows SA. 1993. Tuberculosis in the 1990's. *Ann Intern Med* 119:400–410.
3. Bermudez LE, Petrofsky M, Kolonoski P, et al. 1992. An animal model of *Mycobacterium avium* complex disseminated infection after colonization of the intestinal tract. *J Infect Dis* 165:75–79.
4. Bleck S, Boyer J. 1996. Personal communication. Lexington Veterinary Associates, Lexington, MA.
5. Blunden AS, Smith KC. 1996. A pathological study of a mycobacterial infection in a cat caused by a variant with cultural characteristics between *Mycobacterium tuberculosis* and *M. bovis*. *Vet Rec* 138:87–88.
6. Boireau E, Andre-Fontaine G, Blanchard D, et al. 1994. Serological analysis by A6O antigen ELISA and BCG immunoblotting in domestic carnivores experimentally vaccinated with *Mycobacterium bovis* BCG. *Int J Med Microbiol Virol Parasitol Infect Dis* 281:85–94.
7. Bottger EC, Hirschel B, Coyle MB. 1993. *Mycobacterium genavense* sp. nov. *Int J Syst Bacteriol* 43:841–843.

8. Cammarata G, Caniatti M, Parodi-Cammarata M. 1991. Localizzazioni: e forme poco comuni di tubercolosi nel cane e nel gatto. *Arch Vet Ital* 42:112–129.
8a. Carpentier E, Drovillard B, Dailloux M, et al. 1995. Diagnosis of tuberculosis by amplicor *Mycobacterium tuberculosis* test: a multicenter study. *J Clin Microbiol* 33:3106–3110.
9. Chen ZH, Butler WR, Baumstark BR, et al. 1996. Identification and differentiation of *Mycobacterium avium* and *M. intracellulare* by PCR. *J Clin Microbiol* 34:1267–1269.
10. Clarridge JE, Shawar RM, Shinnick TM, et al. 1993. Large scale use of polymerase chain reaction for detection of *Mycobacterium tuberculosis* in a routine mycobacteriology laboratory. *J Clin Microbiol* 31:2049–2056.
11. Clercx C, Coignoul F, Jakovljevic S, et al. 1992. Tuberculosis in dogs: a case report and review of the literature. *J Am Anim Hosp Assoc* 28:207–211.
12. Collins FM. 1994. The immune response to mycobacterial infection. Development of new vaccines. *Vet Microbiol* 40:95–110.
13. Cousins DV, Francis BR, Gow BL. 1989. Advantages of a new agar medium in the primary isolation of *Mycobacterium bovis. Vet Microbiol* 20:89–95.
14. De Lisle GW. 1993. Mycobacterial infections in cats and dogs. *Surveillance* 20:24–26.
15. De Lisle GW, Collins DM, Loveday AS, et al. 1990. A report of tuberculosis in cats in New Zealand and the examination of strains of *Mycobacterium bovis* by DNA restriction endonuclease analysis. *N Z Vet J* 38:10–13.
15a. Eggers JS, Parker GA, Braaf HA, et al. 1997. Disseminated *Mycobacterium avium* infection in three miniature schnauzer littermates. *J Vet Diagn Invest* 9:424–427.
16. Evans LM. 1995. Mycobacterial lymphadenitis in a cat. *Feline Pract* 23:14–17.
17. Formston C. 1994. Retinal detachment and bovine tuberculosis in cats. *J Small Anim Pract* 35:5–8.
18. Fox LE, Kunkle GA, Homer BL, et al. 1995. Disseminated subcutaneous *Mycobacterium fortuitum* infection in a dog. *J Am Vet Med Assoc* 206:53–55.
19. Frieden TR, Sterling T, Pablos-Mendez A, et al. 1993. The emergence of drug-resistant tuberculosis in New York City. *N Engl J Med* 328:521–526.
20. Garcia-Rodriguez JA, Garcia ACG. 1993. In vitro activities of quinolones against mycobacteria. *J Antimicrobial Chemother* 32:797–808.
21. Greene CE. 1990. Tuberculous mycobacterial infections, pp 558–566. *In* Greene CE (ed), Infectious diseases of the dog and cat. WB Saunders, Philadelphia, PA.
22. Grooters AM, Couto CG, Andrews JM, et al. 1995. Systemic *Mycobacterium smegmatis* infection in a dog. *J Am Vet Med Assoc* 206:200–202.
23. Gunn-Moore DA. 1996. Unpublished observations. University of Bristol, England, UK.
24. Gunn-Moore DA, Jenkins PA. 1994. Tuberculosis in cats. *Vet Rec* 134:336.
25. Gunn-Moore DA, Jenkins JA, Lucke VM. 1996. Feline tuberculosis: a literature review and discussion of 19 cases caused by an unusual mycobacterial variant. *Vet Rec* 138:53–58.
26. Hoop RK, Böttger EC, Pfyffer GE. 1996. Etiological agents of mycobacterioses in pet birds between 1986 and 1995. *J Clin Microbiol* 34:991–992.
27. Hooper DC, Wolfson JS. 1991. Fluoroquinolone antimicrobial agents. *N Engl J Med* 324:384–393.
28. Horsburgh CR. 1991. *Mycobacterium avium* complex infection in the acquired immunodeficiency syndrome. *N Engl J Med* 324:1332–1338.
28a. Hosoe K, Mae T, Yamashita K, et al. 1996. Identification and antimicrobial activity of urinary metabolites of a rifamycin derivative in a dog. *Xenobiotica* 26:321–332.
28b. Hughes MS, Ball NW, Beck L-A, et al. 1997. Determination of the etiology of presumptive feline leprosy. *J Clin Microbiol* 35:2464–2471.
29. Huitema H, van Vloten J. 1960. Murine tuberculosis in a cat. *Antonie Leeuwenhock* 29:235–240.
30. Inderlied CB, Kemper CA, Bermudez LEM. 1993. The *Mycobacterium avium* complex. *Clin Microbiol Rev* 6:266–310.
31. Iseman MD. 1989. *Mycobacterium avium* complex and the normal host. *N Engl J Med* 321:896–898.
32. Jackson R, de Lisle GW, Morris RS. 1995. A study of the environmental survival of *Mycobacterium bovis* on a farm in New Zealand. *N Z Vet J* 43:346–352.
33. Jones B. 1996. Personal communication. Massey University, Palmerston North, NZ.
34. Jordan HL, Cohn LA, Armstrong DJ. 1994. Disseminated *Mycobacterium avium* complex infection in three siamese cats. *J Am Vet Med Assoc* 204:90–93.
35. Kaufman AC, Greene CE, Rakich P, et al. 1995. Treatment of localized *Mycobacterium avium* complex infection in a cat with clofazimine and doxycycline. *J Am Vet Med Assoc* 207:457–459.
36. Kiehn TE, Hoefer H, Böttger EC, et al. 1996. *Mycobacterium genavense* infection in pet animals. *J Clin Microbiol* 34:1840–1842.
37. Kim DY, Cho DY, Newton JC, et al. 1994. Granulomatous myelitis due to *Mycobacterium avium* in a dog. *Vet Pathol* 31:491–493.
38. Kirschner RA, Parker BC, Falkinham JO. 1992. Epidemiology of infection by nontuberculosis mycobacteria. *Am Rev Respir Dis* 145:271–275.
39. Kocagoz T, Yilmaz E, Ozkara S, et al. 1993. Detection of *Mycobacterium tuberculosis* in sputum samples by polymerase chain reaction using a simplified procedure. *J Clin Microbiol* 31:1435–1438.
40. Kulski JK, Khinsoe C, Pryce T, et al. 1995. Use of a multiplex PCR to detect and identify *Mycobacterium avium* and *M. intracellulare* in blood culture fluids of AIDS patients. *J Clin Microbiol* 33:668–674.
41. Kunkle GA. 1990. Lepromatous and atypical mycobacterial infections, pp 567–569. *In* Greene CE (ed), Infectious disease of the dog and cat. WB Saunders, Philadelphia, PA.
42. Malik R, Hunt GB, Goldsmid SE, et al. 1994. Diagnosis and treatment of pyogranulomatous panniculitis due to *Mycobacterium smegmatis* in cats. *J Small Anim Pract* 35:524–530.
43. Mason KV, Wilkinson GT, Blacklock Z. 1989. Some aspects of mycobacterial diseases of the dog and cat, pp 36–37. *In* Proceedings of the 5th Annual AAVD and ACVD Members' Meeting, St. Louis, MO.
44. McKinsey DS, Dykstra M, Smith DL. 1995. The terrier and the tendinitis. *N Engl J Med* 5:332.
45. Michaud AJ. 1994. The use of clofazimine as treatment for *Mycobacterium fortuitum* in a cat. *Feline Pract* 22:7–9.
46. Miller J, Jenny A, Rhyan J, et al. 1996. Diagnosis of tuberculosis in formalin-fixed, paraffin-embedded tissues by polymerase chain reaction (PCR), p 82. *In* Proceedings of the American Association of Veterinary Laboratory Diagnosticians, Little Rock, AR.
47. Miller MA, Greene CE, Brix AE. 1995. Disseminated *Mycobacterium avium-intracellulare* complex infection in a miniature schnauzer. *J Am Anim Hosp Assoc* 31:213–216.
48. Morfitt DC, Matthews JA, Thoen CO, et al. 1989. Disseminated *Mycobacterium avium* serotype 1 infection in a seven month old cat. *J Vet Diagn Invest* 1:354–356.
49. Picardeau M, Vincent V. 1996. Typing of *Mycobacterium avium* isolates by PCR. *J Clin Microbiol* 34:389–392.
50. Ragg JR, Moller H, Waldrup KA. 1995. The prevalence of bovine tuberculosis (*Mycobacterium bovis*) infections in feral populations in cats *(Felis catus)*, ferrets *(Mustela furo)* and stoats *(Mustelae erminea)* in Otago and Southland, New Zeland. *N Z Vet J* 43:328–332.
51. Roccabianca P, Caniatti M, Scanziani E, et al. 1996. Feline leprosy: spontaneous remission in a cat. *J Am Anim Hosp Assoc* 32:189–193.
52. Rupp ME, Schultz AW, Davis JC. 1994. Discordance between tuberculin skin test results with two commercial purified protein derivative preparations. *J Infect Dis* 169:1174–1175.
53. Shackelford C, Reed W. 1989. Disseminated *Mycobacterium avium* infection in a dog. *J Vet Diagn Invest* 2:273–275.
54. Shafran SD, Singer J, Zarowny DP, et al. 1996. A comparison of two regimens for the treatment of *Mycobacterium avium* complex bacteremia in AIDS. *N Engl J Med* 335:377–383.
55. Stewart LJ, White SD, Kennedy FA, et al. 1993. Case report: cutaneous *Mycobacterium avium* infection in a cat. *Vet Dermatol* 4:87–90.
56. Studdert VP, Hughes KL. 1992. Treatment of opportunistic mycobacterial infections with enrofloxacin in cats. *J Am Vet Med Assoc* 201:1388–1390.
56a. Talbot EA, Perkins MD, Fagundes S, et al. 1997. Disseminated Bacille Calmette-Guérin disease after vaccination: case report and review. *Clin Infect Dis* 24:1139–1146.
57. Thoresen OF, Saxegaard F. 1993. Comparative use of DNA probes for *Mycobacterium avium* and *Mycobacterium intracellulare* and serotyping for identification and characterization of animal isolates of the *M. avium* complex. *Vet Microbiol* 34:83–88.
58. Tvedten HW, Walker RD, DiPinto NM. 1990. *Mycobacterium* bacteremia in a dog: diagnosis of septicemia by microscopical evaluation of blood. *J Am Anim Hosp Assoc* 26:359–363.
59. Van Dorssen CA. 1960. *Microbacteria micoti* in a cat. *Tijdschr Diergeneesk* 85:404–412.
60. Van Soolingen D, de Haas PEW, Haagsma J, et al. 1994. Use of various genetic markers in differentiation of *Mycobacterium bovis* strains from animals and humans and for studying epidemiology of bovine tuberculosis. *J Clin Microbiol* 32:2425–2433.
61. Vaneechoutte M, De Beenhouwer H, Claeys G, et al. 1993. Identification of *Mycobacterium* species by using amplified ribosomal RNA restriction analysis. *J Clin Microbiol* 31:2061–2065.
62. Wallace RJ, Brown BA, Onyi GO. 1992. Skin, soft tissue, and bone infections due to *Mycobacterium chelonae chelonae*: importance of prior corticosteroid therapy, frequency of disseminated infections, and resistance to oral antimicrobials other than clarithromycin. *J Infect Dis* 166:405–412.
63. Whitbread TJ. 1993. Mycobacterial infection in cats (letter). *Vet Rec* 132:492.
64. White PD, Kowalski JT. 1991. Enrofloxacin response of cutaneous atypical mycobacterial infection in two cats, p 95. *In* Proceedings of the 7th Meeting of the American Association of Veterinary Dermatologists and the American College of Veterinary Dermatologists, Scottsdale, AZ.
65. Wylie KB, Lewis DD, Pechman RD, et al. 1993. Hypertrophic osteopathy associated with *Mycobacterium fortuitum* pneumonia in a dog. *J Am Vet Med Assoc* 202:1986–1988.
66. Yager JA, Scott DW. 1993. The skin and appendages, pp 531–738. *In* Jubb KVF, Kennedy PC, Palmer U (eds), Pathology of domestic animals, ed 4, vol 1. Academic Press, San Diego, CA.
67. Zeiss CJ, Jardine J, Huchzermeyer H. 1994. A case of disseminated tuberculosis in a dog caused by *Mycobacterium avium-intracellulare. J Am Anim Hosp Assoc* 30:419–424.

Chapter **51**

Dermatophilosis

Craig E. Greene

ETIOLOGY AND EPIDEMIOLOGY

Dermatophilosis (cutaneous streptothrichosis) is an exudative skin disease caused by the actinomycete *Dermatophilus congolensis*. Chronic exposure of the skin to trauma or moisture and immunosuppressive therapy or concurrent debilitating diseases may predispose the patient's skin to overgrowth and colonization by *D. congolensis*. This aerobe or facultative anaerobe is a normal dermal inhabitant of a number of mammalian species, including horses, sheep, goats, and cattle. Although not primary hosts, cats[4, 7–9] and dogs[2, 5] can be naturally infected. Contamination of puncture wounds is presumed to occur in infected cats. Acquisition from the soil, contact with another carrier animal, or latent infection with the organism by the affected animal cannot be excluded in reported cases.

Dermatophilosis has been produced experimentally in dogs after inoculation of the organism onto previously damaged skin[10] and in cats by subcutaneous inoculation.[7]

CLINICAL FINDINGS

Dogs

Spontaneous dermatophilosis in dogs has been confined to the skin. As a primary dermatologic disease, dermatophilosis produces minimal signs of systemic illness, although emaciation and debilitation may be associated with an underlying immunosuppressive disease process. Lesions in dogs, which are frequently found on haired portions of the skin, consist of dry, adherent scabs that become entrapped in surrounding hair (Fig. 51–1). Removal of the crusts reveals underlying erythematous and ulcerated skin.

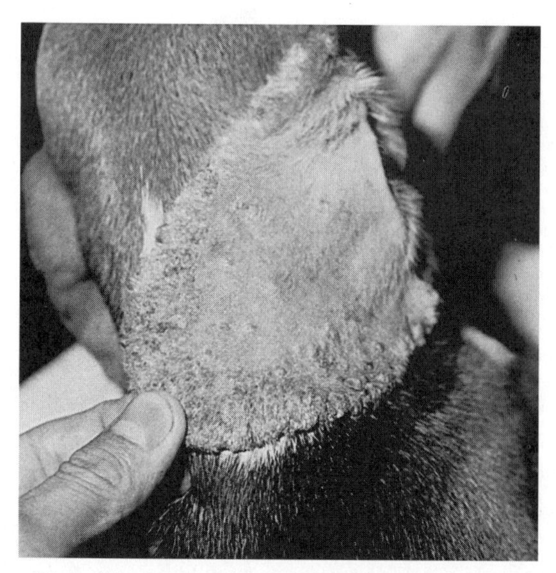

Figure 51–1. Skin lesions of dermatophilosis in a beagle. Note the crusty lesions that surround tufts of hair on the ear margins.

Cats

In affected cats, deeper abscesses in muscle and lymph nodes and in subcutaneous tissues have been more characteristic. The lesions are submucosal or subcutaneous pyogranulomas that may produce chronic draining fistulas. Fever, anorexia, and regional lymphadenomegaly or abscess formation are common. Ulcerative granulomas in cats that involve the tongue or urinary bladder were also described.[1, 9]

DIAGNOSIS

The simplest and most rapid means of establishing a diagnosis involves removing the dried scabs from epidermal lesions or taking biopsy samples of deeper tissues where abscesses are found. Samples are minced in small amounts of sterile saline or nutrient broth. Some of the material is also used to prepare wet mounts or air-dried smears for microscopic examination, and the remainder is submitted for culture. Wet mounts can be stained with new methylene blue; dried specimens are heat fixed and are best stained by Giemsa methods, although Wright's and Gram's stains are suitable. Exudates or minced preparations usually contain large numbers of neutrophils in clusters around gram-posi-

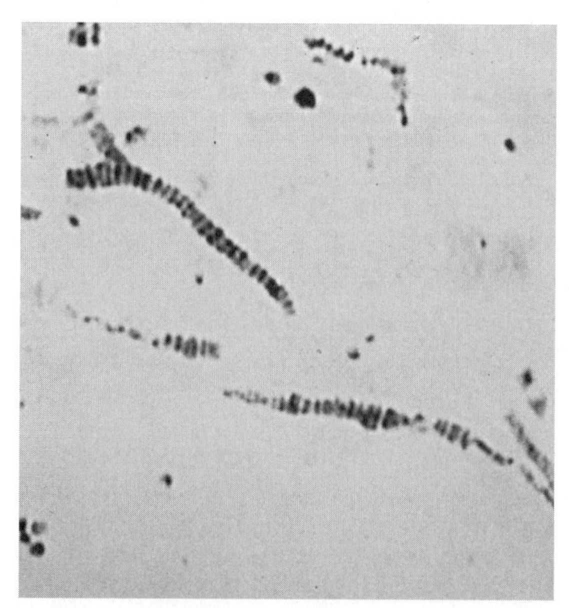

Figure 51–2. Cytologic characteristics of *D. congolensis*. Note the filaments of paired rows of cocci, which give the appearance of "stacked coins" (Gram's stain, × 4300). (Courtesy of Dr. Emmett Shotts, University of Georgia, Athens, GA.)

Table 51–1. Drug Therapy for Dermatophilosis

DRUG	SPECIES	DOSE[a] (mg/kg)	ROUTE	INTERVAL (HOURS)	DURATION (DAYS)
Penicillin V[b]	B	10	PO	8	7–10
Gentamicin	B	2	IM	12	7
Amp(amox)icillin	B	20	PO	8–12	7–10

[a]Dose per administration at specified interval. For additional information, see Drug Formulary, Appendix 8.
[b]Penicillin may be given alone or in combination with gentamicin.
B = dog and cat, PO = oral, IM = intramuscular.

tive branching filamentous organisms. The filaments are recognized by their characteristic transverse and longitudinal divisions that result in three to eight paired rows of coccoid spores arranged in linear fashion (Fig. 51–2). Monoclonal antibodies to *D. congolensis* have been used with indirect FA staining to specifically identify the organism in clinical samples.[6]

Sterile specimens from scabs or biopsy samples may be cultured aerobically at 25°C and aerobically or anaerobically at 37°C on solid nutrient agar, such as blood or brain-heart infusion media. Small, grayish, raised colonies surrounded by a zone of hemolysis are typically produced. The organism can be further identified by its biochemical properties or after experimental inoculation in laboratory animals.

PATHOLOGIC FINDINGS

Histologically, the organism produces an exudative, suppurative dermatitis characterized by epidermal hyperkeratosis and subcorneal abscesses with underlying dermal edema and hemorrhage. Branching hyphae and clusters of coccoid bodies are usually in the parakeratotic layer. There is little involvement of hair follicles. In cats, the lesions consist of pyogranulomas in subcutaneous tissues or lymph nodes. The organism may be identified by H and E–stained preparations in the periphery of necrotic lesions. The banded filamentous nature is best demonstrated by Twart's modified Gram's stain.

THERAPY

Treatment involves keeping the animal's skin dry and hair clipped around the periphery of the lesions or, where lesions are extensive, over the entire body. Clipping the hair and subsequently bathing with 2% lime sulfur or organic iodine preparations facilitate the softening and removal of the impervious, dry, adherent crusts. Bathing and removing crusts should be continued for a minimum of 2 weeks.

The infecting organism is susceptible to a number of antimicrobial agents in vitro; however, on the basis of cost and efficacy, penicillin derivatives are the most practical choice (Table 51–1). Penicillin may be given alone or in combination with an aminoglycoside. Ampicillin has been administered successfully to treat cats with abscesses. Attempts must be made to find and eliminate the causes of dermatophilosis if treatment is to be successful and permanent.

PUBLIC HEALTH CONSIDERATIONS

People are accidental secondary hosts of *D. congolensis*. People handling infected carcasses or tissues can develop exudative pustular dermatitis.[3] The disease in people is extremely rare, and approximately 10 cases have been reported in the literature.[3] Lesions usually consist of multiple white pustules 2 to 5 mm in diameter at the site of contact. These lesions neither spread nor coalesce but resolve within 2 weeks, and more rapidly if the lesions are opened to drain.

References

1. Baker GJ, Breeze RG, Dawson CO. 1972. Oral dermatophilosis in a cat: a case report. *J Small Anim Pract* 13:649–653.
2. Blancou J. 1973. Infection of a dog with *Dermatophilus congolensis. Rev Elev Med Vet Pays Trop* 26:289–291.
3. Bucek J, Pospisil L, Moster M, et al. 1992. Experimental dermatophilosis. *Zentralbl Veterinarmed B* 39:495–502.
4. Carakostas MC, Miller RI, Woodward MG. 1984. Subcutaneous dermatophilosis in a cat. *J Am Vet Med Assoc* 185:675–676.
5. Chastain CB, Carithers RW, Hogle RM, et al. 1976. Dermatophilosis in two dogs. *J Am Vet Med Assoc* 169:1079–1080.
6. How SJ, Lloyd DH. 1988. Use of monoclonal antibody in the diagnosis of infection by *Dermatophilus congolensis. Res Vet Sci* 45:416–417.
7. Jones RT. 1976. Subcutaneous infection with *Dermatophilus congolensis* in a cat. *J Comp Pathol* 86:415–421.
8. Miller RI, Ladds PW, Mudie A, et al. 1983. Probable dermatophilosis in 2 cats. *Aust Vet J* 60:155–156.
9. O'Hara JP, Cordes DO. 1963. Granulomata caused by dermatophilosis in two cats. *N Z Vet J* 11:151–154.
10. Richard JL, Pier AC, Gysewski SJ. 1973. Experimentally induced canine dermatophilosis. *Am J Vet Res* 34:797–799.

Chapter 52

Feline Abscesses

Craig E. Greene

ETIOLOGY AND PATHOGENESIS

Percutaneous abscesses are the most common bacterial infections of feline skin. Abscesses develop more frequently in cats than in dogs owing to the tough, elastic nature of feline skin, which readily seals over contaminated puncture wounds, causing the accumulation of subcutaneous exudates. Sharp teeth and fighting behavior, especially of adult males, are important predisposing factors to abscess formation. The size and degree of abscess formation depend on many factors, including the overlying skin tension, amount of dead space, and gravitation of exudate below the point of penetration. Pus-filled cavities that form above the puncture site drain easily. Cavities that gravitate below the puncture site become overdistended and may repeatedly drain through the puncture site without complete resolution. Abscesses associated with foreign bodies, underlying osteomyelitis, or certain organisms such as *Nocardia* or *Mycobacterium* also tend to recur, persist, or spread in tissues.

Because abscesses usually result from bites and scratches, the most common organisms found within them are resident oral microflora (Table 52–1).[2, 3, 5, 6, 9, 11, 15, 17] Although more difficult to cultivate, anaerobes are more frequently isolated than aerobes. Cats that sustain bite injuries are more likely to become infected with feline immunodeficiency virus (FIV) (see Chapter 13).

CLINICAL FINDINGS

The clinical signs of abscess formation in cats reflect the site and severity of the infection. Abscesses are usually located around the cat's legs, face, back, and base of the tail. Some cats have a noticeable swelling with few other signs of illness, whereas more extensive infection is associated with fever (39.7–40.6°C [103.6–105.2°F]), anorexia, depression, and regional lymphadenomegaly. Pain is usually present at the site of infection, and there may or may not be obvious swelling or warmth. Mature abscesses that are ready to discharge are usually tender with a soft, fluctuant central area. Feline skin easily stretches over distended abscesses. Redness or discoloration is rarely apparent unless the blood vascular supply has been compromised. Drainage of white, creamy, purulent material occurs spontaneously or after surgical lancing. Foul-smelling, red-brown discharges tend to be associated with anaerobic bacterial infections. Systemic signs often abate once the abscess ruptures, and the only evidence of infection may be matted hair at the site of drainage. Careful examination in the area of swelling usually reveals a small puncture wound covered by a crust.

Additional clinical manifestations reflect various sequelae that can occur. Lameness or paralysis will be apparent with myositis, osteomyelitis, septic arthritis, or diskospondylitis. Depression, stiffness, lethargy, nuchal rigidity, or seizures can be seen with meningitis. Osteomyelitis also causes chronic or recurrent draining fistulas that only temporarily respond to antibiotics. Respiratory distress, dyspnea, and stridor are noted with pyothorax, sinusitis, and rhinitis. Vestibular signs can be noted if otitis media or interna develops. Signs of bacteremia and systemic infection include malaise and fever or reflect those of another organ system of hematogenous localization.

Table 52–1. Bacteria Isolated From Feline Abscesses[a]

GENUS	SPECIES	%[b]
Anaerobes		
Porphyromonas[c]	*tectum, heparinolyticus, gingivalis, salivosus, melaninogenicus, corrodens, fragilis,* others	27–45
Fusobacterium	*nucleatum, necrophorum, russii,* others	17–64
Peptostreptococcus	*anaerobius*	11–45
Clostridium	*perfringens, novyi, sordellii, septicum, chauvoei, tetani, villosum*	6.5
Propionibacterium	*acnes, freudenreichii*	4.2
Bifidobacterium	spp.	1.2
Lactobacillus	spp.	1.2
Eubacterium	*lentum*	0.6
Aerobes/Facultative		
Pasteurella	*multocida*[d]	13–27
Actinomyces	*viscosus, odontolyticus*	7–18
Nocardia	spp.	
Staphylococcus	spp.	14
Rhodococcus	*equi*	27
Enterobacteriaceae	other than *E. coli* listed below	13
Streptococcus	spp.	4.8–13
Enterococcus	spp.	12
Lactobacillus	spp.	1.8
Escherichia	*coli*	0.6

[a]Summarized from data in references 2, 3, 5–9, 11, 15–17.
[b]Percentage of those isolates cultured from feline abscesses.
[c]Previously *Bacteroides*.
[d]Has been reclassified, see Etiology, Chapter 53.

DIAGNOSIS

Determining the presence of an abscess is usually based on clinical history and examination. Abscesses should be expected in cats that develop an acute onset of unexplained fever, anorexia, or lameness, even in the absence of an obvious swelling, because abscess formation may be delayed or hidden. The differential leukocyte count can help in determining the extent of infection and the animal's ability to control it. A low count with an inappropriate shift is associated with diffuse infection or cellulitis. A mature neutrophilia is more characteristic of a walled-off or mature abscess. Severe leukopenia (< 4000 cells/m^3), with or without an associated anemia, may be present in cats infected with feline leukemia virus (FeLV) or FIV that develop chronic or recurrent abscesses as a result of immunosuppression. Unlike those in FeLV- or FIV-infected cats, the leukograms usually improve in immunocompetent cats after the abscesses drain.

Causes of recurrent or nonhealing abscesses in cats include retroviral infections as previously discussed, underlying osteomyelitis, neoplasia or foreign body, or infection with organisms such as *Nocardia*, *Mycobacterium*, fungi, or parasites such as *Cuterebra*. Chronic or recurrent draining abscesses should be evaluated by radiography for underlying osteomyelitis, by cytology and culture for possible fungal or unusual bacterial infection, or by surgical exploration for the presence of a foreign body or parasite. Culture of abscess wounds for bacteria is not generally indicated because surgical debridement and empiric antimicrobial therapy are often effective. Anaerobic bacteria are difficult to culture.

THERAPY

Abscesses vary in severity and in the extent of therapeutic intervention required. Small, localized abscesses that drain spontaneously by the time animals are presented for examination require that the hair around the wound be clipped and cleaned with hydrogen peroxide or dilute iodophor solutions. More extensive infections that cause signs of systemic illness may require antibiotic administration, surgical drainage, or supportive care.

Antibiotic Therapy

This has a decided but not absolute role in the management of abscesses in cats. Although mortality and complications resulting from abscesses have been reduced with the use of antibacterials, these agents should not be given indiscriminately or in the absence of other adjunctive measures. Antibiotics alone are ineffective in penetrating walled-off abscesses that require drainage. Empiric antibiotic therapy should be discontinued and extensive diagnostic investigation initiated if abscesses or fever persist longer than 1 to 2 weeks or re-form after repeated surgical drainage.

Penicillin derivatives are antibiotics of choice for treating abscesses because they are bactericidal and have marked activity against the more frequently encountered organisms (Table 52–2). Penicillin V, amoxicillin, or ampicillin may be dispensed in oral forms to be administered by the client. However, amoxicillin or ampicillin may not always be as effective as penicillin in treating anaerobic infections. Because of a similar antibacterial spectrum, chloramphenicol can be substituted for penicillin, but it is bacteriostatic and frequently causes anorexia. It can be hazardous to people. If anaerobes are suspected, penicillin, second- or third-generation cephalosporins, chloramphenicol, clindamycin, and metronidazole have the greatest efficacy. Certain *Fusobacterium* spp. also have been susceptible to erythromycin and doxycycline (see also Therapy, Chapter 41).[16] *Rhodococcus* has been primarily susceptible to aminoglycosides, chloramphenicol, and erythromycin (see also Rhodococcal Infections, Chapter 35).[6] Topical application or direct instillation of antibiotics into the abscess cavity is ineffective because, with the exception of nitrofurans, none work in the presence of pus. Hydrogen peroxide or chlorhexidine solutions and nitrofurazone powder or solution are empirically placed in surgically opened abscess cavities without documented efficacy. Systemic antibiotic therapy may be beneficial in minimizing abscess formation when given immediately after bite wound contamination or with diffuse cellulitis (see also Bite Wound Infections, Chapter 53). Within 24 hours of injury, a single injection of procaine penicillin G can thwart the development of an abscess.[10] Although therapeutic drainage has been advocated for most abscesses, medical therapy alone has proved efficacious in treating affected people.[1a] Antimicrobial treatment of abscesses in cats may be considered when surgical intervention will alter delicate anatomic structures or will involve considerable anesthetic risk. Less favorable outcomes are associated with large (> 5 cm) lesions or with mixed bacterial populations.[1a] Without surgical drainage, medical therapy must be continued for longer periods of at least 14 to 28 days.

***Table 52–2. Drug Therapy for Feline Abscesses*[a]**

DRUG	DOSE[b]	ROUTE	INTERVAL (HOURS)	DURATION (DAYS)[c]
Penicillin G	30,000–50,000 U/kg	SC, IM, IV	12	5–7
Penicillin V	20 mg/kg	PO	12	5–7
Ampicillin (amoxicillin)	20 mg/kg	PO, SC, IV	8–12	5–7
Chloramphenicol	15 mg/kg	PO, SC, IV	8	5–7
Clindamycin	10 mg/kg	PO, IM	12	5–7
Metronidazole	10 mg/kg	PO, IV	8–12	5–7
Doxycycline	5–10 mg/kg	PO, IV	12	5–7

[a]See also Drug Therapy for Anaerobic Infections, Table 41–10, and Rhodococcal Infections, Table 35–6.
[b]Dose per administration at specified interval. See Appendix 8.
[c]Treatment is required for at least 14 to 28 days if surgical drainage is not performed.

Surgery

Surgical intervention is reserved for mature or ruptured abscesses. Diffuse cellulitis or early abscesses should be allowed to mature before surgical drainage is performed. Applying warm compresses daily or soaking affected extremities in warm, saturated Epsom salt solutions may hasten the maturation process. Both have been beneficial in keeping already established drainage sites open until proper healing can occur. Surgical therapy usually involves creating drainage openings at the most ventral portion of an abscess cavity. Controversy exists as to the degree and type of surgical closure indicated. Most veterinarians debride the abscess cavity and remove a small portion of overlying skin to prevent premature closure. Placement of soft rubber tubing that exits at the lowest point of incision with partial closure is frequently used to maintain a drainage opening. A few veterinarians, advocating complete primary closure of the abscess cavity after extensive debridement, argue that more rapid healing and less postoperative drainage are achieved.[4] Systemic antibiotic therapy is probably essential whenever partial or complete surgical closure is performed because the likelihood of organisms remaining in the wound is high, and the risk of systemic spread increases.

Surgical drainage must be established whenever abscess formation occurs within closed cavities. Retrobulbar abscesses must be drained by passing a probe from immediately behind the last upper molar upward into the retrobulbar space. Infraorbital abscesses are usually associated with infection of the upper carnassial tooth, which must be extracted. Sinusal, nasal, and chronic middle-ear abscesses also require surgical drainage with debridement of bone because of the loculation of pus within cavities surrounded by bone. Abscesses associated with underlying osteomyelitis must be treated by surgical debridement of infected bone. Foreign bodies or material must be removed from abscess cavities before they will heal.

Castration is recommended as a preventive measure to abscess formation because it reduces the fighting and roaming behavior of male cats. Progestogens can be given similarly to modify behavior, but the necessity of their continued use induces many undesirable side effects.

References

1. Amato JFR, Grisi L, Neto MP. 1990. Two cases of fistulated abscesses caused by *Lagochilascaris major* in the domestic cat. *Mem Inst Oswaldo Cruz* 85:471–473.

1a. Bamberger DM. 1996. Outcome of medical treatment of bacterial abscesses without therapeutic drainage: a review of cases reported in the literature. *Clin Infect Dis* 23:592–603.
2. Berg JN, Fales WH, Scanlan CM. 1979. Occurrence of anaerobic bacteria in diseases of the dog and cat. *Am J Vet Res* 40:876–881.
3. Biberstein EL, Knight HD, England K. 1968. *Bacteroides melaninogenicus* in diseases of domestic animals. *J Am Vet Med Assoc* 153:1045–1049.
4. Anonymous. 1972. Cat abscesses and suturing controversy. *Feline Pract* 2:22–28.
5. Dobbinson SS, Tannock GW. 1985. A bacteriological investigation of subcutaneous abscesses in cats. *N Z Vet J* 33:27–29.
6. Elliott G, MacKenzie CP, Lawson GHK. 1986. *Rhodococcus equi* infection in cats. *Vet Rec* 118:693–694.
7. Greene CE. 1990. Feline abscesses, pp 595–598. *In* Greene CE (ed), Infectious diseases of the dog and cat. WB Saunders, Philadelphia, PA.
8. Hoshuyama S, Kanoe M, Amimoto A. 1996. Isolation of obligate and facultative anaerobic bacteria from feline subcutaneous abscesses. *J Vet Med Sci* 58:273–274.
9. Jang SS, Lock, Biberstein EL. 1975. A cat with *Corynebacterium equi* lymphadenitis clinically simulating lymphosarcoma. *Cornell Vet* 65:232–239.
10. Joshua JO. 1971. Abscesses and their sequelae in cats. Part 1. *Feline Pract* 1:9–12.
11. Kanoe M, Kido M, Toda M. 1984. Obligate anaerobic bacteria found in canine and feline purulent lesions. *Br Vet J* 140:257–262.
12. Love DN, Bailey M, Johnson RS. 1980. Antimicrobial susceptibility patterns of obligatory bacteria from subcutaneous abscesses and pyothorax in cats. *Aust Vet Pract* 10:168–170.
13. Love DN, Johnson JL, Moore LVH. 1989. *Bacteroides* species from the oral cavity and oral-associated diseases of cats. *Vet Microbiol* 19:275–281.
14. Love DN, Jones RF, Bailey M, et al. 1978. Bacteria isolated from subcutaneous abscesses in cats. *Aust Vet Pract* 8:87–90.
15. Love DN, Jones RF, Bailey M, et al. 1979. Isolation and characterization of bacteria from abscesses in the subcutis of cats. *J Med Microbiol* 12:207–212.
16. Love DN, Jones RF, Bailey M. 1980. Characterization of *Fusobacterium* species isolated from soft tissue infections. *J Appl Bacteriol* 48:325–331.
17. Love DN, Jones FR, Bailey M. 1981. Characteristics of *Bacteroides* species isolated from soft tissue infections of cats. *J Appl Bacteriol* 50:567–575.
18. Malik R, Martin P, Davis PE, et al. 1996. Localized *Corynebacterium pseudotuberculosis* infection in a cat. *Aust Vet Pract* 26:27.

Chapter 53

Bite Wound Infections

Craig E. Greene, Ellie J. C. Goldstein, and John C. Wright

Dog and Cat Bite Infections

EPIDEMIOLOGY

Although it is reported that 2 to 3 million animal bite wounds are inflicted on people in the United States annually,[13a, 64a] less than half are ever reported. Animal bite wounds are fourth among the most commonly reported human illnesses each year in the United States. Bites of family members from their pets are even more drastically underreported. Nearly 1% of emergency visits of humans to hospitals concern bite injuries. Veterinarians and animal health personnel are at greater risk for injury by dogs and cats than the general population.[41] Results of a survey of a group of veterinarians in the United States indicated that approximately 65% had sustained a major animal-related injury. Animal bites and scratches accounted for 34% and 3.8% of the trauma, respectively. Dogs were involved in 24% and cats in 10% of those injuries. In their careers, 92% of the veterinarians surveyed had sustained dog bites, 81% cat bites, and 72% cat scratches. The following epidemiologic discussion focuses on non–veterinary-practice-related bite injuries for which the veterinarian may be consulted concerning the disposition of the dog or cat responsible for causing the bite, although the information can be applicable to injuries that occur within a veterinary practice setting. The principles discussed with respect to treatment of injured people can also be applied to wounds of dogs and cats that are bitten in fighting. The characteristics surrounding dog- and cat-related injuries are discussed next and summarized in Table 53–1.

Dogs

Risk factors for dog bites include the dog's age, breed and size, medical health, sex, and reproductive status.[23, 44, 55, 62, 77] Bites are likely to be delivered by reproductively intact male, large-sized (> 22.7 kg [> 50 lbs]), 6-month to 4-year-old, mixed-breed, German shepherd, or Chow Chow dogs. However, breed-specific statements are potentially inaccurate because of breed popularity, and misidentification, inaccurate estimates of breed's prevalence, and differences in aggressive behavior. Reports citing large dogs as most frequent biters may underestimate bites from smaller dogs.[77] However, serious bites to children are commonly inflicted by large dogs.[12, 23, 44] Dogs cited for causing a high percentage of severe or fatal bites have included pit bulls, Rottweilers, German shepherds, Chow Chows, and huskies.[65] However, in one Florida county, golden retrievers and Cocker spaniels have caused more bites in incidence studies than German shepherds. Despite breed behavior, the most important contributory factor is the degree of responsibility exercised by the animal's owner.

Other aspects of the dog bite event include the victim, dog-person relationship, and the bite-event setting.[79] Approximately 75% of bite injuries are in people younger than 21 years, with peak incidence at 5 to 9 years of age. This information may be biased by more frequent attention given to wounds of children compared with those of adults. Although males constitute approximately 65% of all reported bite victims, boys and girls younger than 6 years account for almost 60% of all fatal bite injuries. *Any* movement in the presence of *some* dogs is likely to lead to dog aggression, especially involving children.[49, 62] Bending over, reaching toward, hugging, or grabbing the collar of a dog are human behaviors that may increase bite likelihood, especially in the context of fear, possessiveness, or dominance. Other *kinds* of dog aggression and their eliciting behaviors are discussed elsewhere.[79, 81]

Table 53–1. Characteristics of Aggressive Dogs and Cats, People Injured, and Injury Event

CHARACTERISTICS OF CATS AND DOGS EXHIBITING AGGRESSION		
	Cats	**Dogs**
Age	ID	< 5 years (49%)
Sex	Female (67%)	Male (70–79%)
Ownership status	Stray (57%)	Owned (a significant number of these owned aggressive dogs live in a household with at least one child)
Reproductive status	ID	Intact (not neutered)
Size	ID	Large dogs (> 50 lbs)
Breed	ID	Total annual number of bites: mixed-breed and German shepherds Bite rates: German shepherds and Chow Chows Highest rate of severe/fatal bites: pit bulls, German shepherds, Chow Chows
CHARACTERISTICS OF PEOPLE INJURED BY CATS AND DOGS		
	Victims of Aggression by Cats	**Victims of Aggression by Dogs**
Age	25–34 years	< 20 years old, with significant occurrence in 5- to 9-year-olds
Sex	Females (59%)	Males (62%)
Relationship to animal	Victim does not usually own cat	Victim is family member or acquaintance of owners Dog owners are most frequently bitten by dogs, not necessarily by their own dogs
CHARACTERISTICS OF THE INJURY EVENT		
	Common Cat Bite Scenario	**Common Dog Bite Scenario**
Kinds of aggression	Fear-related aggression Play aggression Redirected aggression Biting and petting syndrome	Dominance aggression Possessive aggression Fear-related aggression Protective/territorial aggression Punishment induced Pain elicited
Time of year	May through August (warm weather)	May through August (warm weather)
Time of day	9:00 AM to noon	Late afternoon
Other factors	If the cat is owned, 50% of the victims are the owners	Unusually high incidence of bites by chained dogs who are restrained on their own property
Typical wound characteristics	80% of all bites require medical attention 50% of all wounds become infected 29% of all cat bite victims return to doctor after initial visit because of complications Wounds consist of scratches (70%), punctures (27%), and tears (3%) to finger (21%), arm (18%), foot or leg (8%), face or neck (7%), and multiple body location (3%)	20–60% of all bites require medical attention ID 5% of all dog bite victims return to doctor after initial visit because of complications Wounds consist primarily of puncture and tears to extremities (76%) and to face (15%) 70% fatal injuries to children < 9 years old Highest death rate to neonates (< 1 month old) Death rates of neonates 295/100 million; for children 1–11 months old, 47/100 million

ID = insufficient data.

In general, people are more likely to be victimized by dog bites if they own a dog, if the biting *dog* is owned but not by the victim, and if the dog lives in a household with at least one child.[23, 49, 77] Recipients of reported bites are more likely to be neighbors, followed by household members, although bites to household members are probably under-reported.[12, 81]

Other precipitating factors include chaining a dog for long periods of time,[23] geographic location, time of year, time of day, and weather. A majority of dog bite injuries occur between April and September, when warm weather is conducive to outdoor activity.[77] Dog and victim characteristics are summarized in Table 53–1.

Cats

Compared with the dog bite event, much less has been reported about feline aggression (biting and scratching) toward people. Cat bites number approximately 400,000 per year in the United States, and cat-induced wounds have a greater propensity than dog bites for becoming infected. Cat bites constitute 5% to 25% of animal-related injuries to people, whereas other domestic and wild animals account for less than 1% of reported bites.

In general, the most common cat bite events have been reported to involve unowned female cats that bit or scratched adult women. Bite setting characteristics include warm weather (summer) and late afternoon. The proportion of cat-induced wounds have been described as scratches, punctures, or tears.[78] Owned cats bit people on the neck, face, and multiple sites, whereas strays inflicted injuries to the hand. Older people were more likely to be bitten on the hand. Cat and victim characteristics are summarized in Table 53–1.

Wounds

Dog bite wounds may become infected, resulting in functional impairment, although cat bite wounds have the greatest risk of becoming infected.[43] Most bite infections are minor; however, at least 10% require suturing and between 1% and 5% require hospitalization.[75]

The infecting organism in bite or scratch injuries usually corresponds to the normal oral microflora of dogs and cats (compare Table 53–2 with Table 89–1), although organisms from the environment or victim's skin may also contaminate the injury. Bite wounds are usually polymicrobial, with a mean of three to four species involving aerobes and anaerobes.[16, 69] Although greater than 80% of cultures produce pathogens, only 15% to 20% become clinically infected.[26] The

Table 53–2. Organisms Isolated From Infected Human Wounds Caused by Dog or Cat Bites or Scratches

ORGANISM	REPORTED % OF ISOLATES[a] Dog	REPORTED % OF ISOLATES[a] Cat
Viruses		
Rabies virus (Chapter 22)	NA	NA
Motor paralysis agent		R
Bacteria		
Gram-negative Aerobes		
Yersinia pestis (Chapter 47)		NA
Francisella tularensis (Chapter 48)	R	R
Bartonella henselae (Chapter 54)		NA
Pasteurella spp.[b]	25–54	50–78
Pseudomonas spp.	8	NR
Actinobacillus actinomycetemcomitans	6	NR
Capnocytophaga canimorsus (DF-2)	NA	NA
Capnocytophaga cynodegmi (DF-2-like)	NA	NA
Unclassified rods (NO-1, EF-4, VE-2)[c]	4	NR
Weeksella zoohelcum (formerly CDC IIj)	4	NR
Neisseria weaveri (formerly CDC M-5)	4	11
Brucella suis	NA	NR
Acinetobacter calcoaceticus	NR	11
Moraxella spp.[e]	NA	22
Haemophilus aphrophilus	4	NR
Streptobacillus moniliformis	R	NR
Chromobacterium	2	NR
Flavobacterium spp.	NA	NR
Neisseria spp.	2	11–25
Eikenella corrodens	NA	NR
Escherichia coli	2	NR
Spirillum minor	NR	19
Proteus mirabilis	2	NR
Enterobacter cloacae	R	11
Klebsiella	2	NR
Citrobacter freundii	R	R
Mycobacterium fortuitum	R	NR
Gram-positive Aerobes		
Enterococcus	4–9	NR
Streptococcus spp.[d]	40–46	50–52
Staphylococcus (coagulase-positive)[f]	23–36	33
Staphylococcus epidermidis	19	7–70
Corynebacterium spp.	8–20	11–25
Micrococcus spp.	6	NR
Diphtheroids	4	25
Bacillus spp.	4	NR
Nocardia spp. (Chapter 49)	R	R
Anaerobes		
Porphyromonas[g]	32	22
Prevotella[h]	23	22
Propionibacterium spp.	18–21	NR
Bacteroides spp.[h]	11–32	22
Eubacterium plautii	11	NR
Fusobacterium spp.[j]	5–36	30
Clostridium spp.	5	11
Clostridium tetani (Chapter 43)	R	R
Leptotrichia buccalis	5	NR
Peptostreptococcus spp.	5–18	16
Veillonella parvula	5	NR
Actinomyces (see Chapter 49)	R	NR
Fungi		
Blastomyces dermatitidis (Chapter 59)	R	NR

[a]Percentage based on isolates of those wounds of patients who sought medical attention.
[b]*Pasteurella multocida* ss *multocida* C, 52%, D, 14%; *P. multocida* ss *septica* C, 30%, D, 14%; *P. dagmatis* C, 4%, D, 5%; *P. stomatis* C, 4%; *P. canis* D, 27%; *P. multocida* ss *gallicida* D, 5%; *P. pneumotropica* D, 5%; *P. stomatis* D, 5%.
[c]EF-4, VE-2 (*Pasteurella* or *Actinobacillus* like); IIj (*Flavobacterium* like); M-5 (*Moraxella* like). DF-2 now classified as *Capnocytophaga* spp.
[d]*Streptococcus mitis* C, 33%, D, 36%; *S. sanguis* II C, 19%, D, 18%; *S. equinus* C, 11%, D, 5%; *S. pyogenes* D, 9%; *S. constellatus* C, 4%, D, 4%; *S. mutans* D, 4%, C, 4%; *S. agalactiae* C, 4%; *S. sanguis* C, 4%, D, 5%; *S. sanguis* I C, 4%.
[e]*Moraxella cutarrhalis* C, 11%; *M. osloensis* C, 11%; *M. atlantae* C, 7%; *M. nonliquefaciens* C, 4%.
[f]*Staphylococcus epidermidis* C, 7%, D, 23%; *S. wameri* C, 7%, D, 5%; *S. aureus* C, 4%, D, 14%; *S. cohnii* D, 5%; *S. intermedius* D, 9%, C, 4%; *S. coagulase* neg D, 5%; *S. xylosus* D, 4.5%; *S. haemolyticus* C, 4%; *S. hominis* C, 4%; *S. hyicus* C, 4%; *S. sciuri/lentis* C, 4%; *S. simulans* C, 4%.
[g]*Porphyromonas gingivalis* C, 7%, D, 9%; *P. cangingivalis* C, 4%, D, 5%; *P. canoris* C, 4%, D, 4%; *P. salivosa* C, 4%, D, 4%; *P. circumdentaria* C, 4%; *Porphyromonas* spp. D, 5%; *P. cansulci* C, rare; *P. levii*-like D, rare; *P. macacae* C, rare; *Porphyromonas* sp. D, rare, C, rare.
[h]*Prevotella bivia* C, 11%; *P. heparinolytica* C, 7%, D, 14%; *P. intermedia/nigrescens* D, 5%; *P. melaninogenica* D, 5%; *Prevotella* sp. C, 8%; *P. zoogleoformans* D, rare, C, rare.
[i]*Bacteroides tectum* C, 22%, D, 14%; *B. ureolyticus* D, 9%; *B. gracilis* D, 5%; *B. fragilis* D, 5%.
[j]*Fusobacterium nucleatum* C, 26%, D, 18%; *F. russi* C, 15%, D, 5%; *F. gonidiaformans* C, 4%, D, 5%.
Data compiled from Talan D, Goldstein EJC, Emergency Medicine Animal Bite Infection Study Group. 1996. Bacteriology of infected dog and cat bite wounds. Society for Academic Emergency Medicine, Denver, CO; Greene CE, Lockwood R, Goldstein EJC. 1990. Bite infection. In infectious diseases of the dog and cat. WB Saunders, Philadelphia, PA; Citron DM et al. 1996. *Clin Infect Dis* 23(Suppl):S78–S82.
D = dog; C = cat; NA = not available; R = rare or isolated reports; NR = not reported.

risk of infection is highest (approximately 40%) for crush injuries, puncture wounds, wounds in areas of pre-existing edema, and wounds of the hand.[25] Despite the numerous aerobic and anaerobic organisms that contaminate bite wounds, only a few such as *Pasteurella multocida* and *Capnocytophaga canimorsus* consistently cause systemic manifestations. When present, anaerobic bacteria are usually isolated in mixed cultures. *Bacterioides* spp., *Prevotella* spp., and other anaerobic gram-negative bacilli are often involved.[1] About 4% to 20% of dog bite wounds and 20% to 50% of cat bite wounds for which medical attention is sought become clinically infected. Clinical infections usually occur within 8 to 24 hours after injury. An unusual form of motor neuron disease suspected to be caused by a virus occurred after a cat bite.[29]

The public health aspects of rabies, tetanus, and bartonellosis are covered in Chapters 22, 43, and 54, respectively. People who have been bitten may have to be hospitalized for their injury if they develop significant local or systemic infection; are unresponsive to oral antibiotics; have penetrating wounds of tendons, joints, or CNS; have open fractures; develop blood loss or airway injury; require reconstructive surgery; require wound elevation; have head or hand injuries; or are immunocompromised.[75]

Pasteurella Infections

Pasteurella species are small, nonmotile, gram-negative, bipolar-staining bacilli that are clinically significant in many dog and cat bite wounds. These organisms normally inhabit the nasal, gingival, and tonsillar regions of approximately 12% to 92% and 52% to 99% of dogs and cats, respectively, as well as many other animals. *Pasteurella* species have been reclassified based on their DNA homology. *P. multocida* subspecies *multocida* and subspecies *septica* were the most common isolates from clinically healthy cats, whereas *P. canis* was not commonly isolated from healthy dogs.[10, 51] This same distribution is seen with respect to bite-associated infections. Strains isolated from cats were more commonly pathogenic

(71%) than those from dogs (8%). *P. multocida* subspecies *multocida* and subspecies *septica* have been isolated in more serious or systemic infections caused by biting or licking of wounds by dogs or cats.[35] The frequency of isolation is as follows: in cat wounds, *P. multocida*, 50%, and *P. septica*, 30%; in dog bite wounds, *P. canis*, 27%, *P. multocida*, 13%, and *P. septica*, 13%.[27] *P. dagmatis* isolations are rare.[15] Although many cats and dogs harbor *Pasteurella* in their saliva, the risk of infection in people is low in the absence of bite wounds.[63]

Although dog bites account for more than 80% of emergency room visits related to animal bites, cats are responsible for approximately 75% of bites or scratches contaminated with *Pasteurella*. Over 50% of all cat bite wounds and 20% to 30% of all dog bite wounds are contaminated with *Pasteurella*.[43] *Pasteurella* infections also have been reported after bite injuries caused by large exotic Felidae. Scratch injuries produced by dogs are less likely to cause *Pasteurella* infections than cat scratches, unless the scratch is also associated with a bite injury.[50] The fact that cats frequently lick their paws or that, when they scratch, they also hiss, thereby producing aerosolized secretions that contaminate the wounds, is probably related to the increase in *Pasteurella*-infected scratches. A *Pasteurella* throat abscess developed after tonsillectomy in a person that was licked daily on her hands by her dog.[35] *Pasteurella* meningitis developed in a person with extensive dental caries who regularly kissed the family dog. *Pasteurella* has been isolated from the oral cavity of some people who kissed their dogs and cats but not from those who did not.[3, 4] *Pasteurella* acquired from pets may also cause a variety of upper respiratory tract infections, including tonsillitis,[82] sinusitis,[5, 53] and epiglottiditis.[64] Submandibular cellulitis (Ludwig's angina) developed in a previously healthy person 10 days after playing with a dog.[17] *Pasteurella* peritonitis has developed in dialysis patients after a cat scratch or bite that penetrated the tubing of their home dialysis machines.[45] Nontraumatic domestic cat exposure has also been associated with *Pasteurella* peritonitis in people with hepatic cirrhosis.[39] Joint arthroplasties have become infected with *P. multocida* when people have been bitten by cats.[11, 21]

Although a majority of human *P. multocida* infections are related to animal bites, humans also may develop pasteurellosis from nonbite animal exposure. In most of these cases, licking of intact or injured skin and inhalation or ingestion of animal secretions are the most likely sources of entry. Infections associated with inhaled microorganisms or those that disseminate frequently localize in the GI or respiratory tracts or CNS. Patients who are immunosuppressed or who have predisposing underlying illness such as diabetes mellitus and hepatic dysfunction are more likely to develop bacteremia and die. In infants and children, meningitis has been reported following face-licking by family dogs.[73]

Most *Pasteurella* infections occur in people who have frequent contact with farm or pet animals. Presumably, bites in people in urban environments are related to dog, cat, or other small animal or rodent exposure.

Capnocytophaga Infections

C. canimorsus is a slow-growing (3–11 days in culture), thin filamentous, non-spore-forming, nonmotile, pleomorphic, facultative aerobic, gram-negative bacillus previously labeled dysgonic fermenter-2 (DF-2). It causes fatal septicemia predominantly after dog bites and less commonly cat bites or scratches.[47, 73a] It has been isolated from the oral cavity of 16% and 18% of clinically healthy dogs and cats, respectively.[75] Many cases have been reported in the literature with a 30% mortality rate. *C. canimorsus* has an unusual propensity to cause systemic bacteremia, presumably because of its tropism for endothelial surfaces and its inherent resistance to serum complement. The majority of infections with *C. canimorsus* have occurred in immunocompromised individuals older than 40 years. A splenectomized veterinarian died from illness after a dog bite. Most people who developed fatal complications of *C. canimorsus* infection had underlying disorders, such as functional or surgical splenectomy, glucocorticoid therapy, Hodgkin's disease, alcoholism, peptic ulcer, arteriosclerotic heart disease, hemoglobinopathy, immune-mediated thrombocytopenia, granulomatous or other chronic lung disease, chronic arthritis, macroglobulinemia, intestinal malabsorption, or old age (> 65 years). Presumably, these disorders caused defects in the phagocytic immune defenses, and the victims could not eliminate this organism from the blood. As with pasteurellosis, some patients with *C. canimorsus* sepsis have had exposure to dogs, cats, or other carnivores or to outdoor environments but with no known bites.

Ocular keratitis and blepharitis have developed in people with close association of their pet dogs or cats and in other people with no known animal exposure. Corneal scratch injuries from cats have also produced keratitis in people. Results from DNA hybridization and biochemical studies have determined that the more virulent species isolated from people with septicemia were *C. canimorsus* and those from localized (noninvasive) wound infections or keratitis were *C. cynodegmi* (DF-2 like). Other *Capnocytophaga* spp. are part of the normal gingival flora of people and cause problems such as conjunctivitis, periodontitis, gingivitis, abscesses, and body cavity infections.[18] In addition, they can cause bacteremia in immunocompromised individuals.[28] Infections with other *Capnocytophaga* are not associated with animal exposure.

CLINICAL FINDINGS

The type of injury after dog bite wounds varies, including abrasions, punctures, avulsions, and lacerations. Dog bites cause severe crushing injuries and lacerations with ligamentous tearing and tissue necrosis. A majority of lesions of adults are primarily on the upper extremities and trunk. Young children generally receive facial injuries because of their small stature and lack of experience with dogs and because the dogs tend to bite the face and mouth as part of aggressive behavior. Dogs biting other dogs most commonly injure the extremities followed by the head, neck, thorax, and abdomen.[14]

Cat scratches frequently occur on the handler's extremities and usually are associated with attempts to restrain the animal. Cat bites are deep, and the cat's sharp teeth are more likely to produce wounds that become foci for abscess formation and resultant complications such as osteomyelitis.

Signs indicating wound infection include localized swelling or reddening and pain with or without a purulent drainage. The type of organism and site of bite are most important in determining the clinical course of the injury. Infections caused by the two most clinically significant organisms, *C. canimorsus* and *Pasteurella*, are discussed next.

Pasteurella Infections

These infections are more progressive than those produced by many other bacteria. The time from bite until onset of infection has been 12.3 hours, 15.0 hours, and 24.0 hours for *Streptococcus*, *Pasteurella*, and *Staphylococcus*, respectively.[69] Usually within 8 to 48 hours, cellulitis develops at the site of injury with *Pasteurella* spp. Erythema, tenderness, and swelling occur in association with a serosanguineous to purulent, malodorous, dark yellow–colored discharge. Lymphadenomegaly and low-grade fever (> 38°C [100.5°F]) develop in some patients. Cellulitis can lead to extensive infection of deeper tissues or potentially fatal septicemia. Septicemia is characterized by persistent chills, fever, and collapse. Chronic osteomyelitis, septic or post-traumatic arthritis, tenosynovitis, meningitis, and smoldering abscesses also can occur.

Capnocytophaga Infection

Although inconsistent, cellulitis is the most common finding after bite wounds contaminated by *C. canimorsus* and *C. cynodegni*. Bite infections caused by *Eubacterium plautii* can appear to be similar to those of *C. canimorsus*.[22] In some cases, eschariform lesions, characterized by formation of purplish-black necrotic tissue around the bite site, are seen. Splenectomized or immunosuppressed patients, including those with advanced age or hepatic cirrhosis, develop the most severe illness from septicemia, characterized by fever, malaise, myalgia, vomiting, diarrhea, abdominal pain, dyspnea, hypotension, thrombocytopenia with purpura, symmetric peripheral gangrene, oliguria, disseminated intravascular coagulation, and death.[57] Fatality rate has been over 25%, and acute myocardial infarction has been reported in some people. Regardless of the clinical spectrum, most patients are continuously bacteremic. Localization of the septic process without death can occur, and some people develop endocarditis, purulent meningitis, and polyarthritis. The organisms may not be demonstrated on microscopic examination of tissues, although they may be in blood films of some patients with severe bacteremia and in blood culture.

Capnocytophaga isolates may be detected within 72 hours in culture, but up to 7 to 10 days is typical. Growth is enhanced in the presence of carbon dioxide and with serum-enriched media. The laboratory should be advised if *Capnocytophaga* is suspected so that specific tests can be performed to detect these unusual gram-negative organisms. Because identification of these organisms takes a relatively long time, antimicrobial therapy must be instituted immediately without definitive identification.

THERAPY

Judging from the discrepancy between the number of reported versus the number of estimated bite cases, not all affected people seek medical attention. Bites should be reported to public health officials, whose job it is to investigate the incident and to make recommendations concerning the treatment of the bite victim and disposition of the animal. Only a few states have developed formal guidelines for handling these cases. Immunocompromised individuals who are bitten or scratched should *always* be instructed to seek medical attention immediately.

Although not primarily responsible for the treatment of human victims, veterinarians should be aware of the proper protocols for medical care of bite wounds in people. Thorough washing of all bite wounds and scratches with soap and water is essential. Soaking in an aqueous organic iodine solution (1% povidone-iodine) may also be beneficial. Surgical scrub should not be used because it is toxic to tissue. It is important that wounds be irrigated with physiologic solutions such as normal saline or lactated Ringer's solution. Intermittent, pulsating, high-pressure irrigation, which streams isotonic fluids directly into the wound, has been most effective in dislodging contaminating bacteria. Irrigation is usually performed with an 18- to 20-gauge blunted needle or catheter, a 20- to 50-ml syringe, and approximately 150 ml of solution.[43]

The degree of surgical intervention frequently depends on the site and type of bite. Facial injuries bleed profusely and produce highly visible scarring; therefore, they are routinely sutured. Extremity wounds are less visible and often are more contaminated and prone to infection; therefore, they are often treated as open wounds. Puncture wounds that show minimal hemorrhage should be irrigated, although some physicians have cautiously excised the margins of the wound, leaving it open to drain. Any wound that becomes infected should be cultured. The affected extremity should be elevated to prevent swelling.

Antimicrobial therapy with penicillin or ampicillin-amoxicillin for 3 to 7 days has been recommended for all penetrating bite injuries, even though studies have questioned routine prophylaxis. This recommendation is based on the fact that most animal bite wound isolates, with the exception of staphylococci, are susceptible to penicillin G. Early initiation of antimicrobial prophylaxis can reduce the severity of infection, but the difference in overall numbers of infections that develop is not statistically significant when empirical prophylaxis is used. Drugs with a gram-positive and anaerobic spectrum, such as penicillins, are usually effective for this purpose. Amoxicillin-clavulanate has been a first-choice therapy; penicillin V is an alternative for less severe injuries. Doxycycline has been an alternative for penicillin-allergic patients. There is generally little need for culture of clinically uninfected bite wounds. Because of their polymicrobic nature, clinically infected bite wounds should be cultured. Resistant bacteria require use of cephalosporins or penicillinase-resistant antibiotics. Tetracycline is an alternative for patients who are allergic to β-lactam drugs. Use of erythromycin, clindamycin, first-generation cephalosporins, or dicloxacillin is often associated with microbial resistance, especially to *Pasteurella* spp.

For a discussion of therapy of rabies virus–, anaerobic bacteria–, or *Clostridium tetani*–infected wounds, refer to Chapters 22, 41, and 43, respectively.

Pasteurella Infections

Penicillin and its analogs such as ampicillin are the single most effective antibiotics to control this infection in adults. Tetracyclines, chloramphenicol, and some cephalosporins are similarly effective. Bacterial resistance to β-lactamase–resistant penicillins and to cephalosporins has been reported in 18% to 50% of animal isolates. Erythromycin does not control infection, and relapses can occur after it is discontinued.

Capnocytophaga Infections

Many cases of *C. canimorsus* sepsis are fatal in immunocompromised hosts; however, some people may completely recover even without antimicrobial therapy. Physicians and veterinarians should realize the potential risk of dog ownership in immunocompromised people and advise them to seek immediate medical care and antimicrobial treatment after bite injuries. Response to therapy in individuals treated early enough in the course of septicemia has generally been dramatic but not always curative. The organism shows in vitro susceptibility to many antimicrobials, including penicillin, ampicillin, amoxicillin-clavulanate, cephalosporins, tetracycline, carbenicillin, clindamycin, chloramphenicol, erythromycin, imipenem, and quinolone. Isolates have been resistant to the typical drugs, such as colistin, gentamicin, and kanamycin, selected to treat gram-negative infections. Variable susceptibility has been found to trimethoprim-sulfamethoxazole. Penicillin should be used as a first choice. In severely ill people a third-generation cephalosporin has been recommended to be given concurrently with penicillin because penicillin-resistant strains of *Capnocytophaga* and *Pasteurella* have been isolated on occasion.

PREVENTION

Avoidance of actions that precipitate aggression by dogs and cats is key in preventing bite injuries (Table 53–3). With respect to dogs, pet owners can avoid those breeds or predominant breeds with known aggressive tendencies. Male, unneutered, free-roaming dogs of German shepherd, pit bull, or Chow Chow breeding seem to present the greatest risk. Neutering aggressive male dogs is advised. Early experiences and socialization, including proper handling and attention during the neonatal period, are essential for puppies and kittens. People with a high occupational risk, such as animal control officers, postal employees, meter readers, and animal health workers, need education programs to help them interpret canine and feline communicative behavior. Crown reduction, an endodontic method for disarming the canine teeth, has been described to reduce the injury caused by biting dogs and cats[66] but is probably not very effective in dealing with injury from dog bites.[61, 80]

Table 53–3. Recommendations to Limit Dog Bites

ANIMAL HEALTH PROFESSIONALS	DOG OWNERS
1. Use extra caution in handling pit bulls, Rottweilers, wolf hybrids, Chow Chows.	1. Avoid dog breeds with known aggressive tendencies.
2. Separate vicious dogs from each other and handling personnel. Provide leashes and carriers.	2. Do not bother ill animals or animals that are eating.
3. Always muzzle dogs with known or suspected vicious tendencies.	3. Socialize dogs and cats beginning at an early age.
4. Use metal choke collar and a chain leash on vicious dogs.	4. Take dogs to obedience classes beginning as pups.
5. Snap bolt cages or runs containing vicious dogs.	
6. Always have two people in a room when handling or working around vicious dogs.	

Rat Bite Infections

Two commensal organisms of rodents are responsible for a bacterial disease of dogs, cats, and people who have direct or indirect contact with rodent tissues or their secretions. *Streptobacillus moniliformis* is a small (0.25–0.5 μm × 1–3 μm), motile, aerobic, pleomorphic gram-negative bacillus with unipolar flagella. *Spirillum minus* is a gram-negative spiral organism (3–5 μm) that is motile by means of polar flagellar bundles.

These species of bacteria are found as resident nasopharyngeal flora in up to 50% of wild or laboratory rodents. Subclinical infections of rats with *S. moniliformis* are prevalent worldwide, although in some cases rats develop abscess formation and purulent infection. Other rodents such as mice and guinea pigs more commonly develop clinical illness when infected. With *S. minus*, the prevalence of infection in rats is more variable, depending on the geographic location; however, most are inapparently infected.

Dogs and cats contaminate their oral cavities with these bacteria while catching rodents. They can also harbor these agents subclinically and act as mechanical vectors because they can transmit their recently acquired infection to people by biting.[56] Occasionally, abscesses occur in dogs or cats presumably as a result of a rat bite.

Infected people have fever, myalgia, arthralgia, lymphadenitis, and generalized exanthematous eruptions that may develop weeks to months after bites.[6] Epidemic infections have rarely been reported after laboratory or food-borne contamination. Endocarditis and polyarthritis are chronic sequelae. With infections caused by *S. moniliformis*, the site of the original bite usually heals by the time clinical signs are seen. With infections caused by *S. minus*, the healed wound may become reinflamed and later ulcerate during the course of febrile illness. Regional lymphadenitis and lymphangitis are common in the region of the bite.

S. moniliformis can be isolated in culture on serum-enriched media, and a diagnosis requires notifying the laboratory of the suspicion that this organism may be involved. Isolation from blood must not be made in blood culture media because the typical anticoagulant, polyanethol sulfonate, inhibits the organism's growth. *S. moniliformis* has the propensity to convert to pleomorphic, cell wall–deficient, L forms in vivo or in vitro, during unfavorable growth conditions or during β-lactam therapy (see also L-Form Infections, Chapter 32). *S. minus* does not grow on laboratory media; therefore, dark-field examination of exudates or inoculation of mice with blood from affected patients is necessary to confirm the infection.

Penicillin is the drug of choice for infection caused by either organism. Tetracyclines are indicated in the event of resistant or L-form infections (see Appendix 8 for dosages). Oral infections of dogs and cats are usually inapparent, and so treatment is not necessary. In the case of abscess formation, surgical drainage should accompany antimicrobial therapy.

References

1. Alexander CJ, Citron DM, Gerardo SH, et al. 1997. Characterization of saccharolytic *Bacteroides* and *Prevotella* isolates from infected dog and cat bite wounds in humans. *J Clin Microbiol* 35:406–411.
2. Andersen BM, Steigerwalt AG, O'Connor SP, et al. 1993. *Neisseria weaveri* sp. nov., formerly CDC group M-5, a gram-negative bacterium associated with dog bite wounds. *J Clin Microbiol* 31:2456–2466.
3. Arashima Y, Kumasaka K, Okuyama K, et al. 1992. Clinicobacteriological study of *Pasteurella multocida* as a zoonosis (1). *Kansenshogaku Zasshi* 66:221–224.
4. Arashima Y, Kumasaka K, Okuyama K, et al. 1992. Clinicobacteriological study of *Pasteurella multocida* as a zoonosis (2). *Kansenshogaku Zasshi* 66:232–235.
5. Arashima Y, Kumasaka K, Okuyama K, et al. 1992. The first report of human chronic sinusitis by *Pasteurella multocida* subsp *multocida* in Japan. *Kansenshogaku Zasshi* 66:232–235.
6. Azimi P. 1990. Pets can be dangerous. *Pediatr Infect Dis* 9:670–684.
7. Ballard WT, Cooper RR. 1994. An environmental hazard to the diabetic foot—a case report. *Iowa Orthop J* 14:171–173.

8. Barnham M, Holmes B. 1992. The isolation of CDC group M-5 and *Staphylococcus intermedius* from infected dog bites. *J Infect* 25:332–334.
9. Beck AM. 1991. The epidemiology and prevention of animal bites. *Semin Vet Med Surg* 6:186–191.
10. Biberstein EL, Spencer SJ, Kass PH, et al. 1990. Distribution of indole-producing urease-negative pasteurellas in animals. *J Vet Diagn Invest* 3:319–323.
10a. Butt TS, Khan A, Ahmad A, et al. 1997. *Pasteurella multocida* infectious arthritis with acute gout after a cat bite. *J Rheumatol* 24:1649–1652.
11. Braithwaite BD, Giddins G. 1992. *Pasteurella multocida* infection of a total hip arthroplasty. A case report. *J Arthroplasty* 7:309–310.
12. Brogan TV, Bratton SL, Dowd MD, et al. 1995. Severe dog bites in children. *Pediatrics* 96:947–950.
13. Citron DM, Gerardo SH, Claros MC, et al. 1996. Frequency of isolation of *Porphyromonas* species from infected dog and cat bite wounds in humans and their characterization by biochemical tests and arbitrarily primed polymerase chain reaction fingerprinting. *Clin Infect Dis* 23(Suppl):S78–S82.
13a. Cornwell JM. 1997. Dog bite prevention: responsible pet ownership and animal safety. *J Am Vet Med Assoc* 210:1147–1148.
14. Cowell AK, Penwick RC. 1989. Dog bite wounds: a study of 93 cases. *Compend Cont Educ Pract Vet* 11:313–325.
15. David C, Brasme L, Vinsonneau M, et al. 1996. *Pasteurella dagmatis* and dog bite wound. *Med Malad Infect* 26:594–595.
16. Dire DJ. 1992. Emergency management of dog and cat bite wounds. *Emerg Med Clin North Am* 10:719–736.
17. Dryden MS, Dagliesh D. 1996. *Pasteurella multocida* from a dog causing Ludwig's angina. *Lancet* 347:123.
18. Esteban J, Albalate M, Caramelo C, et al. 1995. Peritonitis involving a *capnocytophaga* sp in a patient undergoing continuous ambulatory peritoneal dialysis. *J Clin Microbiol* 33:2471–2472.
19. Fajfar-Whetstone CJ, Coleman L, Biggs DR, et al. 1995. *Pasteurella multocida* septicemia and subsequent *Pasteurella dagmatis* septicemia in a diabetic patient. *J Clin Microbiol* 33:202–204.
19a. Finegold SM, Jousimiessomer H. 1997. Recently described clinically important anerobic bacteria—medical aspects. *Clin Infect Dis* 25:S88–S93.
20. Fox LE, Kunkle GA, Homer BL, et al. 1995. Disseminated subcutaneous *Mycobacterium fortuitum* infection in a dog. *J Am Vet Med Assoc* 206:53–55.
20a. Freud HK, Colomes JL, Sainz CS, et al. 1997. Animal bites—study of 606 cases. *Rev Clin Espan* 197:560–563.
21. Gabuzda GM, Barnett PR. 1992. *Pasteurella* infection in a total knee arthroplasty. *Orthop Rev* 21:601–605.
22. Garre M, Le Hanaff C, Bensonsan TT, et al. 1991. Fulminant *Eubacterium plautii* infection following dog bite in an asplenic man. *Lancet* 338:384–385.
23. Gershman KA, Sacks JJ, Wright JC. 1994. Which dogs bite? A case-control study of risk factors. *Pediatrics* 93:913–917.
24. Goldstein EJ. 1989. Management of human and animal bite wounds. *J Am Acad Dermatol* 21:1275.
25. Goldstein EJ. 1991. Household pets and human infections. *Infect Dis Clin North Am* 5:117–130.
26. Goldstein EJ. 1992. Bite wounds and infection. *Clin Infect Dis* 14:633–638.
27. Goldstein EJ. 1997. Unpublished observations, Alden Research Laboratory, Santa Monica, CA.
28. Gomez-Garces JL. Alos JI, Sanchez J, et al. 1994. Bacteremia by multidrug-resistant *Capnocytophaga sputigena*. *J Clin Microbiol* 32:1067–1069.
29. Greene CE, Lockwood R, Goldstein EJ. 1990. Bite and scratch infections, pp 614–620. *In* Greene CE (ed), Infectious diseases of the dog and cat. WB Saunders, Philadelphia, PA.
30. Greenhalgh C, Cockington RA, Raftos J. 1991. An epidemiological survey of dog bites presenting to the emergency department of a children's hospital. *J Pediatr Child Health* 27:171–174.
31. Hodgin EC, Michaelson F, Howerth EW, et al. 1992. Anaerobic bacterial infections causing osteomyelitis/arthritis in a dog. *J Am Vet Med Assoc* 201:886–888.
32. Hollis DG, Moss CW, Daneshvar MI, et al. 1993. Characterization of Centers for Disease Control group NO-1, a fastidious nonoxidative, gram-negative organism associated with dog and cat bites. *J Clin Microbiol* 31:746–748.
33. Holmes B, Costas M, On SLW, et al. 1993. *Neisseria weaveri* sp. nov. (formerly CDC Group M-5) from dog bite wounds of humans. *Int J Syst Bacteriol* 43:687–693.
34. Holmes B, Costas M, Wood AC. 1990. Numerical analysis of electrophoretic protein patterns of group EF-4 bacteria, predominantly from dog-bite wounds of humans. *J Appl Bacteriol* 68:81–91.
35. Holst E, Rollof J, Larsson L, et al. 1992. Characterization and distribution of *Pasteurella* species recovered from infected humans. *J Clin Microbiol* 30:2984–2987.
36. Howell JM, Woodward GR. 1990. Precipitous hypotension in the emergency department caused by *Capnocytophaga canimorsus* sp nov sepsis. *Am J Emerg Med* 8:312–314.
36a. Hudspeth MK, Gerardo SH, Citron DM, et al. 1997. Growth characteristics and a novel method for identification (the Wee-Tab System) of *Porphyromonas* species isolated from infected dog and cat bite wounds in humans. *J Clin Microbiol* 35:2450–2453.
37. Kelly PJ, Mason PR, Els J, et al. 1992. Pathogens in dog bite wounds in Harare, Zimbabwe. *Vet Rec* 131:464–466.
38. Kneafsey B, Condon KC. 1995. Severe dog bite injuries, introducing the concept of pack attack: a literature review and seven case reports. *Injury* 26:37–41.
39. Koch CA, Mabee CL, Robyn JA, et al. 1996. Exposure to domestic cats risk factor for *Pasteurella multocida* peritonitis in liver cirrhosis. *Am J Gastroenterol* 91:1447–1449.
40. Korbel R. 1990. Epizootiology, clinical aspects and therapy of *Pasteurella multocida* infection in bird patients after cat bite. *Tierarztl Prax* 18:365–376.
41. Landercasper J, Cogbill TH, Strutt PJ, et al. 1988. Trauma and the veterinarian. *J Trauma* 28:1255–1258.
42. Lee J. 1994. *Staphylococcus intermedius* isolated from dog-bite wounds. *J Infect* 29:105.
43. Lewis KT, Stiles M. 1995. Management of cat and dog bites. *Am Fam Physician* 52:479–485, 489–490.
44. Lockwood R. 1994. The ethology and epidemiology of canine aggression. *In* Serpel J (ed), The domestic dog: its evolution, behaviour & interactions with people. Cambridge University Press, Cambridge, England.
45. London RD, Bottone EJ. 1991. *Pasteurella multocida*: zoonotic cause of peritonitis in a patient undergoing peritoneal dialysis. *Am J Med* 91:202–204.
46. Lynch JA. 1989. Comments about public health risks. *Can Vet J* 30:931.
47. Mahrer S, Raik E. 1992. *Capnocytophaga canimorsus* septicemia associated with cat scratch. *Pathology* 24:194–196.
48. Malnick H, Adhami ZN, Galloway A. 1991. Isolation and identification of *Capnocytophaga canimorsus* (DF-2) from blood culture. *Lancet* 338:384.
49. Mathews JR, Lattal KA. 1994. A behavioral analysis of dog bites to children. *J Dev Behav Pediatr* 15:44–52.
50. Matsiu T, Kayashima K, Kito M, et al. 1996. Three cases of *Pasteurella multocida* skin infection from pet cats. *J Dermatol* 23:502–504.
51. Mohan K, Kelly PJ, Hill FW, et al. 1997. Phenotype and serotype of *Pasteurella multocida* isolates from diseases of dogs and cats in Zimbabwe. *Comp Immunol Microbiol Infect Dis* 20:29–34.
51a. Mulligan ME, Citron DM, Kwok RY, et al. 1997. Immunoblot characterization of *Porphyromonas* species from infected dog and cat bite wounds in humans. *Clin Infect Dis* 25:S98–S99.
52. Moore F. 1997. I've just been bitten by a dog: surgical toilet, appropriate antibiotics, and advice to come back if infection develops. *BMJ* 314:88–90.
53. Nakano H, Sekitami T, Ogata Y, et al. 1993. Paranasal sinusitis due to *Pasteurella multocida*. *Nippon Jibiinkoka Gakkai Kaiho* 96:192–196.
54. Ndon JA. 1992. *Capnocytophaga canimorsus* septicemia caused by a dog bite in a hairy cell leukemia patient. *J Clin Microbiol* 30:211–213.
55. Overall KL. 1995. Sex and aggression. *Canine Pract* 20:16–18.
56. Peel M. 1993. Dog-associated bacterial infections submitted to an Australian reference laboratory 1981–1992. *Pathology* 25:379–384.
57. Pers C, Gahrn-Hansen B, Frederiksen W. 1996. *Capnocytophaga canimorsus* septicemia in Denmark 1982–1995: review of 39 cases. *Clin Infect Dis* 23:71–75.
58. Rayan GM, Downard D, Cahill S, et al. 1991. A comparison of human and animal mouth flora. *J Okla State Med Assoc* 84:510–515.
59. Reina J, Borrell N. 1992. Leg abscess caused by *Weeksella zoohelcum* following a dog bite. *Clin Infect Dis* 14:1162.
60. Reisner IR. 1991. The pathophysiologic basis of behavior problems. *Vet Clin North Am Small Anim Pract* 21:207–224.
61. Reisner IR. 1992. Crown reduction for biting pets. *Adv Small Anim Med Surg* 4:3.
62. Reisner IR, Erb HN, Houpt KA. 1994. Risk factors for behavior-related euthanasia among dominant-aggressive dogs: 110 cases (1989–1982). *J Am Vet Med Assoc* 205:855–863.
62a. Rieck D. 1997. Dog bite prevention from animal control's perspective. *J Am Vet Med Assoc* 210:1145–1146.
63. Rollof J, Nordin-Fredriksson G, Holst E. 1989. *Pasteurella multocida* occurs in a high frequency in the saliva of pet dogs. *Scand J Infect Dis* 21:583–584.
64. Ryberg J, White P. 1993. *Pasteurella multocida* as a cause of acute epiglottiditis. *Lancet* 341:381.
64a. Sacks JJ, Kresnow M, Houston B. 1996. Dog bites: how big a problem? *Injury Prev* 2:52–54.
65. Sacks JJ, Lockwood R, Hornreich J, et al. 1996. Fatal dog attacks 1989–1994. *Pediatrics* 97:891–895.
66. Shipp AD. 1991. Crown reduction. Disarming of biting pets. *J Vet Dent* 8:4–6.
67. Sinclair CL, Zhou C. 1995. Descriptive epidemiology of animal bites in Indiana. *Pub Health Rep* 110:64–67.
68. Szpakowski NM, Bonnett BN, Martin SW, et al. 1989. An epidemiological investigation into the reported incidents of dog biting in the city of Guelph. *Can Vet J* 30:937–942.
69. Talan DA, Goldstein EJC. 1996. Bacteriology of infected dog and cat bite wounds. Meeting, *Soc Acad Emerg Med*, Denver, CO.
70. Talan DA, Goldstein EJC, Staatz D, et al. 1989. *Staphylococcus intermedius*: clinical presentation of a new human dog bite pathogen. *Ann Emerg Med* 18:410–413.
71. Talan DA, Staatz D, Staatz A, et al. 1989. Frequency of *Staphylococcus intermedius* as human nasopharyngeal flora. *J Clin Microbiol* 27:2393.
72. Talan DA, Staatz D, Staatz A, et al. 1989. *Staphylococcus intermedius* in canine gingiva and canine-infected human wound infections. *J Clin Microbiol* 27:78–81.

73. Tammemagi M. 1989. Hazards of dogs licking humans' faces. *Can Vet J* 30:929–931.
73a. Valtonen M, Lauhio A, Carlson P, et al. 1995. *Capnocytophagia canimorsus* septicemia: fifth report of a cat-associated infection and five other cases. *Eur J Clin Microbiol Infect Dis* 14:520–523.
74. Walker RD, Walshaw R, Riggs CM, et al. 1995. Recovery of two mycoplasma species from abscesses in a cat following bite wounds from a dog. *J Vet Diagn Invest* 7:154–156.
75. Weber DJ, Hansen AR. 1991. Infections resulting from animal bites. *Infect Dis Clin North Am* 5:663–680.
76. Wolf JS, Turzan C, Cattolica EV, et al. 1993. Dog bites to the male genitalia: characteristics management and comparison with human bites. *J Urol* 149:286–289.
77. Wright JC. 1990. Reported dog bites: are owned and stray dogs different? *Anthrozoos* 4:113–119.
78. Wright JC. 1990. Reported cat bites in Dallas: characteristics of the cats, the victims and the attack events. *Pub Health Rep* 105:420–424.
79. Wright JC. 1991. Canine aggression toward people: bite scenarios and prevention. *Vet Clin North Am* 21:299–314.
80. Wright JC. 1992. Crown reduction for biting pets. *Adv Small Anim Med Surg* 4:4.
81. Wright JC. 1996. Canine aggression: dog bites to people, pp 240–246. *In* Voith VL, Borchelt PL (eds), Reading in companion animal behavior. Veterinary Learning Systems, NJ.
82. Zhao G, Galina L, Hanyanun W, et al. 1993. Human tonsillitis associated with porcine *Pasteurella multocida* infection. *Lancet* 342:491.

Chapter 54

Bartonellosis

Edward B. Breitschwerdt and Craig E. Greene

ETIOLOGY

Species of *Bartonella* are fastidious, arthropod-transmitted, hemotropic, small, curved, gram-negative bacteria. They include organisms that once comprised the genera of *Bartonella*, *Rochalimaea*, and *Grahamella* (Table 54–1).[6, 11, 67] *B. bacilliformis*, the original type species, is the cause of a focally occurring vasculoproliferative and hemolytic disease of people in the Andes Mountains of Peru. *B. (Rochalimaea) quintana*, the cause of trench fever in World War I, has been associated with bacillary angiomatosis, endocarditis, and chronic lymphadenomegaly, predominantly in immunocompromised people.[23, 27, 45] *B. (Rochalimaea) henselae* has been isolated from clinically healthy cats and people with bacillary angiomatosis, visceral bacillary peliosis (extravasation of blood), relapsing fever with bacteremia, meningitis, encephalitis, neuroretinitis, endocarditis, and cat-scratch disease (CSD).[43, 59, 63, 69] A closely related species, *B. clarridgeiae*, comprises approximately 10% of *Bartonella* isolates from clinically healthy cats[8] and has been serologically associated with CSD-like illness in people.[8, 37, 48] *Afipia felis*, a bacterium once thought to be the cause of CSD, has been isolated from people with CSD on rare occasions.[29] *B. (Rochalimaea) elizabethae* was isolated from an HIV-infected human with endocarditis,[25] and *B. (Rochalimaea) vinsonii* has only been isolated from voles. *B. vinsonii* subsp. *berkhoffii* has been isolated from the blood of healthy and diseased dogs.[49] Five species from the former genus *Grahamella*—*B. talpae*, *B. peromysci*, *B. grahamii*, *B. taylorii*, and *B. doshiae*—isolated from small feral animals were unified in the genus *Bartonella*.[6] Additional species or subspecies, for which the pathogenic potential in cats, dogs, or people has yet to be defined, will be added to the genus *Bartonella* in

Table 54–1. Comparison of Recognized Disease-Producing Members of the Genus Bartonella[a]

ORGANISM	CLASSIC DISEASES	GEOGRAPHIC OCCURRENCE	VECTOR[b]	RESERVOIR HOST	INCIDENTAL HOST	CLINICAL FEATURES
B. bacilliformis	Oroya fever	Andes Mountains	Sandfly	Human[d]	Human	Hemolytic anemia, fever, asymptomatic bacteremia, indolent angiomatous skin lesions (verruga peruana)
B.[c] *quintana*	Trench fever	Focal WWI worldwide	Body louse	Human[d]	Human	Bacteremia, localized tissue infection; angiomatosis, peliosis, granulomatous and pyogenic inflammation, lymphadenitis
B.[b] *henselae*	Cat-scratch disease	Worldwide	Cat flea, tick?	Cat	Human	Same as for *B. quintana*
B. clarridgeiae	Cat-scratch disease	Worldwide?	Cat flea?	Cat	Human	Same as for *B. quintana*
B.[c] *vinsonii* subsp. *berkhoffii*	—	?	Brown dog tick	?	Dog	Endocarditis, bacteremia in splenectomized dog
B.[c] *elizabethae*	—	?	?	?	Human	Endocarditis, bacteremia

[a]Also includes other organisms of uncertain pathogenicity—*B. vinsonii* (Canadian vole agent) and former *Grahamella* species (*B. talpae, B. peromysci, B. grahamii, B. taylorii, B. doshiae*)—that infect small mammals, fish, and birds.
[b]Sandfly = *Phlebotomus* spp.; body louse = *Pediculus humanus*; cat flea = *Ctenocephalides felis*; brown dog tick = *Rhipicephalus sanguineus*.
[c]Formerly *Rochalimaea*.
[d]Nonhuman primates have been experimentally infected.
WWI = World War I; ? = unknown.

the future.[43] The following discussion of *Bartonella* in animals focuses on *B. henselae* and *B. clarridgeiae* and on *B. vinsonii* subsp. *berkhoffii*, which have been established as causes of cat and dog infections, respectively. Species of *Bartonella* infecting people and their zoonotic implications are discussed under Public Health Considerations.

EPIDEMIOLOGY

B. henselae and *B. clarridgeiae*

Both serologic and blood culture data indicate that exposure to *Bartonella* spp., most frequently *B. henselae*, is prevalent among cats in the United States and, presumably from preliminary data from other countries, throughout most temperate regions of the world (Table 54–2). A seroepidemiologic survey, incorporating 577 samples from throughout North America, identified an overall prevalence of 28%; rates ranged from a low of 4% to 7% in the Midwest and Great Plains region to 60% in the Southeast (Fig. 54–1).[39] Seroepidemiologic studies in cats generally show a higher prevalence of seroreactivity with age, warmer temperature, and higher humidity and in feral cats and those infested with fleas.[8, 18, 43, 49, 78] Although CSD has been associated historically and epidemiologically with exposure to kittens,[17, 78] of 21 CSD-associated cats, 16 were older than 6 months and the 2 oldest were between 5 and 7 years.[50] *B. henselae* was cultured from 17 of 19 of these asymptomatic cats.

Table 54–2. Geographic Prevalence of Bartonellosis in Cats

GEOGRAPHIC LOCATION	ENVIRONMENT	NUMBER TESTED	% POSITIVE
Serologic Testing FA			
California[20]	Z	114	30.0
Connecticut[75]	BP	48	79.2
	PV	29	37.9
Northern California[18]	IS, VH	205	81.0
Georgia[16]	VH, PV	73	47.9
Kansas[16]	PV	10	50.0
Maine[16]	PV	52	65.4
Baltimore, MD[17]	AS	345	12.2
	IS	195	11.8
	PV	24	12.5
	FT	9	44.0
Maryland[16]	PV, AS	612	13.2
North Carolina[3, 50]	VH	114	40.4
	VH	518	21.0
Texas[16]	VH	567	37.9
North America[39]	PV	628	27.9
Egypt[16]	PV	42	11.9
Israel[3]	VH	114	39.5
The Netherlands[c, 3a]	AS	113	50.0
Portugal[16]	PV	14	6.7
South Africa[41]	PV, AS	52	21.0
Switzerland[30]	PV	700	6.0
Zimbabwe[41]	PV, AS	119	24.0
Blood Culture			
Northern California[15]	IS, VH	205	39.5
San Francisco, CA[43]	PV	37	41.0
	AS	22	41.0
	FT	2	50.0
North Carolina[50]	BP	19	89.0
France[b, 37]	FT	94	53.0
Germany[65]	PH	100	13.0
Japan[54]	PV	24	8.0
	AS	9	11.0
The Netherlands[3a]	AS	113	22.0
	PH	50	56.0
Sydney, Australia[7]	PV, FT	77	35.0

[a]See accompanying maps, Fig. 54–1.
[b]Two strains of *B. henselae* were isolated, and 30% of the cats had *B. clarridgeiae* as their isolate.
[c]An ELISA was used in this study.
Z = exotic cats in zoos; BP = cats of *Bartonella*-infected people; PV = sick cats at private veterinarian; IS = impounded strays; VH = veterinary teaching hospital patients; AS = animal shelter; FT = feral trapped cats; PH = privately owned healthy cats.

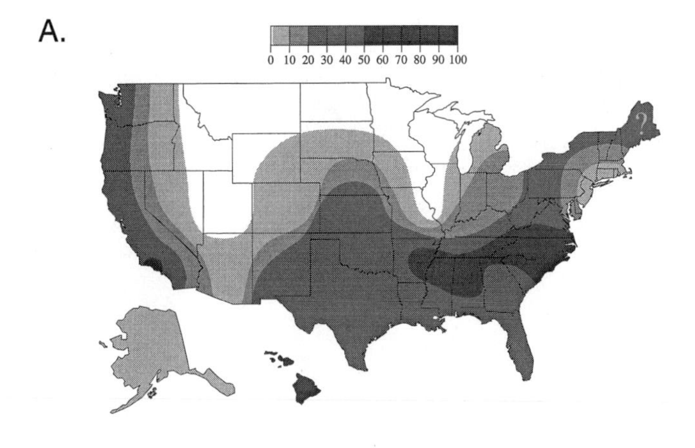

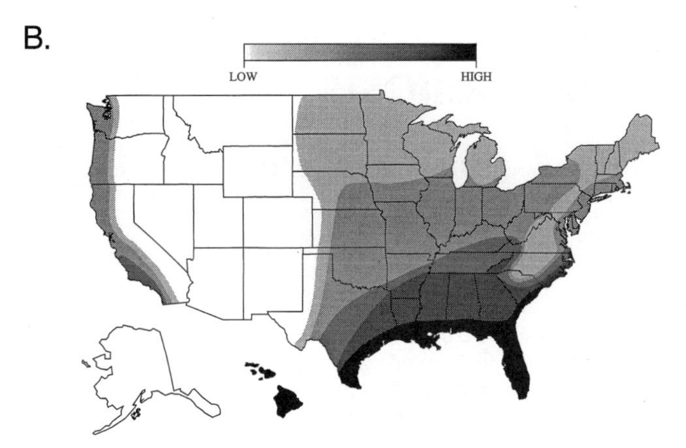

Figure 54–1. *A*, Percentage of pet cats with *Bartonella henselae* antibodies throughout the United States based on samples received from 29 geographic regions. *B*, Estimated cat flea prevalence throughout the United States based on temperature and humidity data. (From Jameson PH, Greene CE, Regnery RL, et al. 1995. *J Clin Microbiol* 33:1879–1883.)

B. henselae is the predominant, but not the only, cause of CSD. *B. quintana* has on occasion been reported to produce lymphadenomegaly similar to CSD,[27] but this agent has not been cultured from cats or associated with cat exposure, as has *B. henselae*. At least one other *Bartonella* spp., *B. clarridgeiae*, infects clinically healthy cats. The role of species other than *B. henselae* in zoonotic transmission is uncertain. *B. clarridgeiae* was isolated from a pet cat that induced an inoculation papule, fever, and CSD (regional lymphadenomegaly) in the owner, who developed antibodies to this organism but not to *B. henselae*.[8, 48] It has also been isolated from a cat whose owner was concurrently infected with *B. henselae*[21] and from a lower proportion of cats during serosurveys.[37] A small percentage of naturally infected cats may be coinfected with both *B. henselae* and *B. clarridgeiae*.[35b] Other *Bartonella* variants have been found in culture of blood from a low proportion of cats during serosurveys.[3a, 35b, 37, 39, 52, 66] Genetic variants may be useful in future epidemiologic studies to determine the involvement of the cat as a reservoir and may help to incriminate vectors responsible for their transmission.[5]

B. vinsonii subspecies *berkhoffii*

On the basis of seroepidemiology data in dogs, *B. vinsonii* subspecies *berkhoffii* appears to be transmitted by the brown dog tick, *Rhipicephalus sanguineus*. Seroreactivity to this organism was detected in only 3.6% (69/1920) serum samples from sick dogs compared with 36% (54/151) of the sera being reactive to *Ehrlichia canis*.[8, 58] Seropositive dogs were more likely to live in rural environments, be free to roam, and have heavy tick exposure. Seroreactivity to *B. vinsonii* correlated with seroreactivity to *Babesia canis* and *E. canis*.

PATHOGENESIS

B. henselae is an intraerythrocytic bacterium.[46] Multiple organisms can be observed within the same erythrocyte by EM (Fig. 54–2). It remains to be determined whether the intracellular presence of the bacteria influences erythrocyte fragility, results in the early removal of erythrocytes by the mononuclear phagocytic system, or allows the parasite continued existence. Experimentally, *B. henselae* can be transmitted to specific pathogen-free (SPF) cats by IV or IM blood transfusion but not by IM inoculation of urine sediment.[47] Transient mild anemia has been observed in *B. henselae* experimentally infected cats during the immediate post-transfusion period. Other consistent hematologic abnormalities have not been detected in experimentally infected cats during periods of at least 21 months duration.[46, 47]

The high prevalence of bacteremia in the healthy cat population indicates that *B. henselae* is frequently and unknowingly transmitted to recipient cats during blood transfusion therapy. *B. henselae* has been cultured and detected by polymerase chain reaction (PCR) from fleas obtaining blood meals from naturally infected cats.[19, 43] Infection has been transmitted via fleas from naturally infected to laboratory-reared SPF cats.[19] Whether fleas serve as a biologic or mechanical vector has not been clearly established. Flea and/or ear mite infestations were found to be associated with seropositivity in exotic cats.[20] Fleas have become infected after ingesting blood via artificial feeding devices.[37a] Ticks have been incriminated in some human infections.[51]

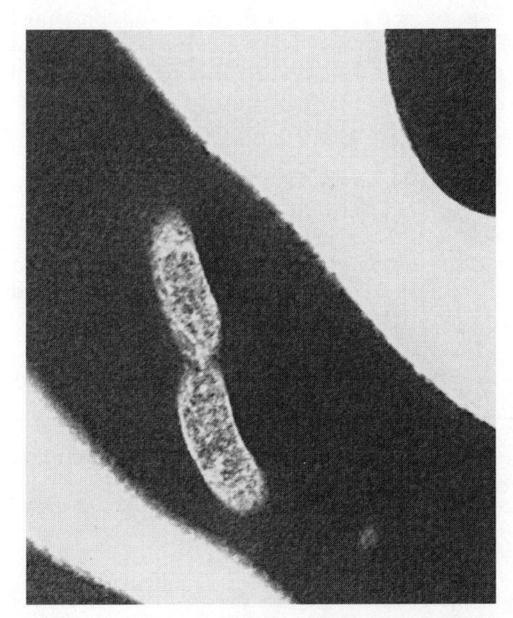

Figure 54–2. Transmission electron photomicrograph of two *B. henselae* organisms inside a feline erythrocyte. Staining was with methanol uranyl acetate and then lead citrate (× 30,420). (Courtesy of KL Kordick and EB Breitschwerdt, North Carolina State University, Raleigh, NC).

Cats are efficient reservoirs for *Bartonella* spp., which can be transmitted by arthropod vectors. Transmission does not occur in cats in the absence of arthropod vectors.[1, 19, 33] Considering the cellular tropisms of *B. henselae* in human beings with CSD or bacillary angiomatosis, it is probable that the organism can infect endothelial cells, macrophages, and potentially other canine or feline cells. *B. bacilliformis* releases an angiogenic factor that is responsible for the vascular proliferation,[24] and the other related species may react similarly. Experimentally infected cats develop an increasing antibody titer to the organism and, despite this titer rise, have variable degrees and duration of bacteremia.[32, 33] High-dose antimicrobial therapy may facilitate the clearance of the bacteremia, and once they have cleared the infection, cats are immune to rechallenge by ID inoculation of cultured organisms. Rechallenge by blood transmission between cats has not shown protection.

CLINICAL FINDINGS

B. henselae

For the clinical features of human infections, see Public Health Considerations. Whether members of the genus *Bartonella* are pathogenic for cats or contribute to previously described instances of argyrophilic bacteria in lymph nodes of cats with persistent lymphadenomegaly[42] or to peliosis hepatis[13] remains to be determined. Self-limiting febrile illness of 48 to 72 hours duration and transient, nonlocalizing neurologic dysfunction, including lethargy, persistent staring into space, unresponsiveness to environmental stimuli, and mild postural reaction deficits in all limbs, developed in a naturally infected cat and two *B. henselae* experimentally infected cats.[47] In other studies,[35a] experimentally IV infected SPF cats developed transient fever, anorexia, generalized peripheral lymphadenomegaly, and inflammatory lesions in multiple organs. Other naturally infected cats have developed brief periods of pronounced fever after routine surgical procedures that resolved without antibiotic therapy.

Most studies of naturally infected cats indicate that the infection, despite the persistent associated bacteremia, is subclinical. If at all pathogenic, *B. henselae* is a subtle pathogen in that clinical signs may develop only in chronically infected cats during periods of stress or potentially in conjunction with concurrent diseases. Although bacteremia can persist for months to years in apparently healthy cats, the causative role of this organism in chronic feline diseases deserves consideration. Owing to the high percentage of chronically bacteremic but healthy cats, establishing a cause-and-effect relationship between bacteremia and specific disease manifestations is difficult.

B. vinsonii subspecies *berkhoffii*

A novel organism, *B. vinsonii* subspecies *berkhoffii* was isolated from the blood and heart valves of a dog with endocarditis, from the blood of a clinically healthy dog,[9, 49] and from five other dogs with endocarditis.[10] This organism is probably responsible for the endocarditis in a number of dogs in which culture results are negative. Clinical signs in affected dogs have been typical of endocarditis, including lethargy, inappetence, shifting leg lameness, and heart murmur.[9] This organism also causes granulomatous lymphadenitis in dogs.[10]

DIAGNOSIS

Testing serum for antibodies to *B. henselae* provides useful epidemiologic information in screening populations of cats for evidence of *B. henselae* infections, but is of limited clinical utility in documenting actively infected cats. The indirect FA procedure is the reference standard but is accurate only to the genus level. Among experimentally infected SPF cats, the pattern of bacteremia and the magnitude and duration of IgM or IgG response to the organism are highly variable.[33, 47] Very high antibody titers (>256) appear to correlate well with obtaining positive blood culture results in both naturally and experimentally infected cats. However, some cats with lower but detectable antibody titers have culture-negative test results, and some seronegative cats are culture positive. These preliminary results indicate a poor correlation between the mere presence of serum antibody and blood culture documentation of bacteremia. In some instances, seropositivity has been statistically associated with kittens that are bacteremic or in CSD-affected households.[18, 78] However, in other studies, cats associated with CSD were mostly older than 6 months; indirect FA titers were highly variable, not always corresponding to findings of blood culture.[50] Some *Bartonella*-infected cats that are seronegative may be infected with the closely related strains or different species that have lesser degrees of serologic cross-reactivity.[3, 21, 32, 50] Other cats that are seropositive but have culture negative results may have intermittent bacteremia or may be reacting to exposure to other closely related species of bacteria.

The most accurate and efficient means of diagnosing infection is by blood or tissue culture. Presumably, because of higher levels of bacteremia in cats, *B. henselae* is easier to isolate from feline blood or tissue specimens compared with those of humans. *B. henselae* bacteremia of up to 1000 organisms/ml can be found in 25% to 41% of healthy cats.[18, 43] *B. henselae* bacteremia can persist in clinically healthy cats for periods of at least 22 months.[50] Some isolates of *B. henselae*, obtained from cats that had induced CSD in their owners, caused a relapsing pattern of bacteremia when blood was inoculated into SPF cats.[47]

After surgical preparation, blood for culture can be taken into sterile EDTA tubes or directly into centrifugation-lysis tubes (Isolator Microtubes, Wampole Labs, Cranbury, NJ). Alternatively, EDTA blood can be frozen and thawed before culture to produce cell lysis. Because *B. henselae* is intraerythrocytic, cell lysis improves the sensitivity and rapidity of colony formation.[12] Colonies are usually detected within 7 to 21 days, but it can take up to 56 days. Primary isolation of *Bartonella* is usually performed on solid media containing sheep, rabbit, or human blood-based agar or chocolate and charcoal yeast extract agar at 37°C at high humidity, in 5% carbon dioxide–enriched atmosphere. Chemically defined liquid media have also been developed.[77] Differentiation of isolated *Bartonella* at the species level usually requires immunocytochemistry or genetic analysis.[40, 56, 64, 65]

On necropsy of experimentally infected SPF cats, lymphoid hyperplasia and inflammatory foci in the spleen and lymph nodes were noted.[3a] Focal neutrophilic inflammation was observed in the livers of some cats.

THERAPY

Antimicrobial efficacy for eliminating *B. henselae* bacteremia in cats has not been clearly established for any antibiotic. Several of the antibiotics considered effective for treating people (see Public Health Considerations) are ineffective for cats, even with a prolonged duration of therapy. Treatment failures occur with amoxicillin, doxycycline, and enrofloxacin in both natural and experimental *B. henselae* bacteremic cats.[8, 62] Some suppressive effect on bacteremia has been found with doxycycline and erythromycin at recommended dosages.[62] On the contrary, when used at higher than recommended dosages for 1 week, doxycycline, amoxicillin, and amoxicillin-clavulanate were effective in suppressing bacteremia in experimentally infected cats.[33] In controlled studies, rifampin has been effective in clearing bacteremia alone and in combination with doxycycline.[32] Enrofloxacin for 14 or 28 days has also been effective.[48a] Recommended dosages are listed in Table 54–3; however, because of the uncertainty of their efficacy, several follow-up cultures performed at 2- to 4-week intervals should always be obtained to ensure effectiveness.[33, 48a, 62] Cultures should be taken at least 3 weeks after the antimicrobial therapy has been discontinued.[33] Perhaps of little consequence to the cat, pharmacologic elimination of *Bartonella* bacteremia has important implications for maintaining the pet in the household of an immunocompromised individual. Because routine treatment of feline bartonellosis may induce resistant strains, recommendations are to treat cats owned by immunocompromised people or when euthanasia is the only alternative to treatment.[48a]

PREVENTION IN CATS

On the basis of our current understanding of zoonotic implications associated with *Bartonella* infection in cats, vaccination seems desirable to decrease potential human exposure to this organism. Cats that are treated and recover from *Bartonella* bacteremia after experimental ID infections with cultured organisms appear to be resistant to reinfections.[1, 33, 62] Similar immunity is not found with IV transfusion of blood from infected cats.[47] Nevertheless, a vaccine might be effective in protecting cats from vector inoculation after exposure and reduce their public health risk, especially for immunodeficient owners. No vaccines are available. Cats in such households should be screened for infection with blood culture. Any cat with positive results should be treated with high levels of antimicrobials as discussed previously and retested to determine whether they are clear.[33, 62] Cats should also be screened for *B. henselae* infection before being used as blood donors.

PUBLIC HEALTH CONSIDERATIONS

Bartonella spp. have become associated with several distinct clinical syndromes in people: bacillary angiomatosis,[23, 45] bacillary peliosis,[43, 59] relapsing fever with bacteremia,[69, 76]

Table 54–3. Suggested Antibiotic Dosage for Bartonellosis of Dogs and Cats[a]

DRUG	DOSE (mg/kg)	ROUTE	INTERVAL (HOURS)	DURATION (WEEKS)
Enrofloxacin	22.7 mg total	PO	12	2–4
Doxycycline	10–22 mg/kg	PO	12	2–4
Rifampin	10 mg/kg	PO	24	2

[a]Data from Kordick, et al: *Antimicrob Agents Chemother* 41:2448–2455; Greene, University of Georgia, unpublished observations. Greene et al: *J Clin Microbiol* 34:1682–1685, 1996. Efficacy of these drugs to treat bacteremic cats is controversial. Giving these drugs for 4 weeks appears to be more efficacious than for 2 weeks. Dosages were based on giving whole tablets for convenience. Rifampin is effective alone or in combination with doxycycline but has to be reformulated so that the dosage given here can be administered. Rifampin should always be given in combination to reduce bacterial resistance. For further information on these drugs, see Drug Formulary, Appendix 8.

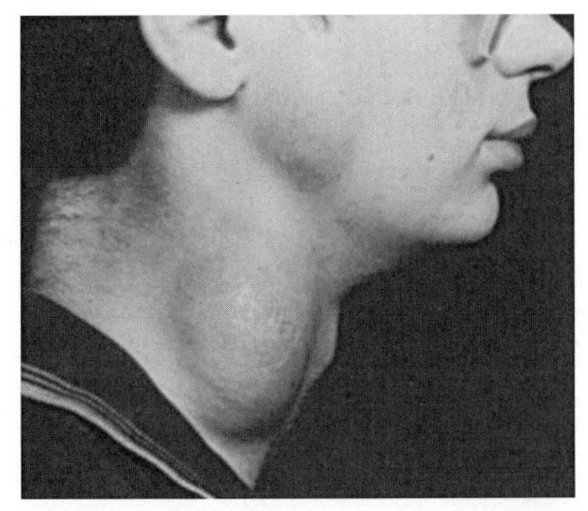

Figure 54–3. Enlarged lymph nodes in a person with CSD.

CSD,[2, 26, 60] endocarditis,[25, 36, 70] granulomatous hepatosplenic syndrome,[31] retinitis and swelling of the optic nerve,[77] arthritis,[36a] osteolytic lesions,[44, 73] and pulmonary granulomas in a chronically ill renal transplant patient.[14] A substantial role for *B. henselae* in the pathogenesis of AIDS encephalopathy has also been proposed.[68] The clinical syndrome in an affected person is highly dependent on their immune status. Immunocompetent individuals tend to contain the infection to regional lymph nodes, and localized or regional pyogranulomatous lymphadenitis ensues (Fig. 54–3). In the immunodeficient host, bacteremia and disseminated lesions develop. Vasculoproliferative lesions are most common in these individuals. In tissues, the organisms have a positive staining reaction to silver.

Bacillary angiomatosis, also called epithelioid angiomatosis, is a vascular proliferative disease of the skin in *Bartonella*-infected patients that is characterized by multiple, blood-filled, cystic tumors.[23, 45] Depending on the visceral parenchymal organs involved, the condition is referred to as bacillary peliosis hepatitis, bacillary splenic peliosis, or systemic bacillary angiomatosis. Vascular lesions have also been detected in the lymph nodes, bone, heart, CNS, oropharynx, larynx, endobronchus, duodenum, and colon.[38] These vascular manifestations can be caused by either *B. henselae* or *B. quintana*, and have been more frequently documented in immunocompromised individuals (particularly AIDS patients), although immunocompetent individuals have been affected.

Persistent or relapsing fever accompanied by malaise, anorexia, and weight loss have been found in immunocompromised[14, 45, 69] or immunocompetent[51, 76] individuals with *B. henselae* infections. Persistent bacteremia of approximately 3 months' duration was identified in an immunocompetent man who was potentially infected by tick exposure.[51] This report suggests that, similar to the situation in cats and potentially dogs, people can experience prolonged illness with persistent bacteremia. Endocarditis and resultant persistent bacteremia have also been features of infections with *B. quintana*, *B. elizabethae*, and *B. vinsonii*.

For nearly a century, CSD, a regional lymphadenomegaly, has been associated with animal contact, particularly cat scratches. In the early 1980s, small silver-stained, gram-negative bacteria were seen in the lymph nodes of CSD patients.[75] In 1988, a bacterium, later designated *Afipia felis*, was cultured from the lymph node and was considered to be the cause of CSD. In studies of immunosuppressed patients with bacillary angiomatosis, an organism later named *B. henselae* was recovered. Seroreactivity linked this organism to patients with CSD,[61, 78] and *B. henselae* was identified from such cases from lymph nodes by genetic and cultural methods.[2] Now there is little doubt that *B. henselae* is the predominant cause of CSD. Unfortunately, even currently, the clinical diagnosis of CSD by some physicians is being made in people having both an unexplained lymphadenomegaly and known association with cats without obtaining definitive testing for bartonellosis. Before eliminating a suspected cat from a household, people thought to have such illnesses should have the sera tested for *Bartonella*-specific antibodies and/or tissues or blood examined for *Bartonella* organisms by various methods.[2a, 55a]

Because of disparate results among studies and an overall lack of microbiologic data in clinical therapeutic trials, numerous issues related to treatment of human *Bartonella* infection remain controversial. In contrast to the apparent lack of response to antimicrobial treatment in human CSD patients,[15, 53] bacillary angiomatosis, parenchymal bacillary peliosis, and acute *Bartonella* bacteremia appear to respond to antimicrobial treatment, particularly in immunocompromised individuals.[35] In people, doxycycline, erythromycin, and rifampin are recommended antibiotics,[55] but clinical improvement has been reported with penicillin, gentamicin, ceftriaxone, ciprofloxacin, and azithromycin. Treatment for 2 weeks in immunocompetent individuals and 6 weeks in immunocompromised individuals is generally recommended. Relapses, associated with bacteremia, have been reported in immunocompromised people despite treatment for 6 weeks.

PREVENTION IN PEOPLE

Although vector transmission data are in the preliminary stages of development, it appears that elimination of fleas and ticks would decrease transmission of *B. henselae* and *B. vinsonii* to cats and dogs, respectively. Factors influencing the transmission of *B. henselae* or *B. clarridgeiae* to humans via a scratch or bite remain largely undetermined. Although perhaps related to inhibitors in saliva, efforts to amplify *B. henselae* DNA from saliva of infected cats using PCR analysis have not been definitively successful.[32] Salivary spread may not be a means of transmission as once suspected. Although not substantiated, cat fleas (*Ctenocephalides* spp.) may be responsible for transmission of disease to people either directly through sucking blood of people or indirectly through contamination of cat scratch or bite wounds with flea excreta from the animal's hair coat or local environment. Although the quantity of serologic or blood culture data in the literature is limited, the zoonotic implications of *Bartonella* infections in cats appear to be substantial for both immunocompromised and immunocompetent people. Cats belonging to individuals infected with HIV should be screened by blood culture for bartonellosis.

References

1. Abbott RC, Chomel BB, Kasten RW. 1997. Experimental and natural infection with *Bartonella henselae* in domestic cats. *Comp Immun Microbiol Infect Dis* 20:41–51.

1a. Anderson B, Lu E, Jones D, et al. 1995. Characterization of a 17-kilodalton antigen of *Bartonella henselae* reactive with sera from patients with cat scratch disease. *J Clin Microbiol* 33:2358–2365.

2. Anderson B, Sims K, Regnery R, et al. 1994. Detection of *Rochalimaea henselae* DNA in specimens from cat scratch disease patients by PCR. *J Clin Microbiol* 32:942–948.

2a. Avidor B, Kletter Y, Abulafia S, et al. 1997. Molecular diagnosis of cat scratch disease: a two-step approach. *J Clin Microbiol* 35:1924–1930.

3. Baneth G, Kordick DL, Hegarty BC, et al. 1996. Comparative seroreactivity

to *Bartonella henselae* and *Bartonella quintana* among cats from Israel and North Carolina. *Vet Microbiol* 50:161–162.
3a. Bergmans AMC, de Jong CMA, van Amerongen G, et al. 1997. Prevalence of *Bartonella* species in domestic cats in the Netherlands. *J Clin Microbiol* 35:2256–2261.
4. Bergmans AMC, Groothedde JW, Schellekens JFP, et al. 1995. Etiology of cat scratch disease: comparison of polymerase chain reaction detection of *Bartonella* (formerly *Rochalimaea)* and *Afipia felis* DNA with serology and skin tests. *J Infect Dis* 171:916–923.
5. Bergmans AMC, Schellekens JFP, van Embden JDA, et al. 1996. Predominance of two *Bartonella henselae* variants among cat-scratch disease patients in the Netherlands. *J Clin Microbiol* 34:254–260.
6. Birtles RJ, Harrison TG, Saunders NA, et al. 1995. Proposals to unify the genera *Grahamella* and *Bartonella*, with descriptions of *Bartonella talrae* comb. nov., *Bartonella peromysci* comb. nov., and three new species, *Bartonella grahamii* sp. nov., *Bartonella taylorii* sp. nov., and *Bartonella doshiae* sp. nov. *Int J Syst Bacteriol* 45:1–8.
7. Branley J, Wolfson C, Waters P, et al. 1996. Prevalence of *Bartonella henselae* bacteremia, the causative agent of cat scratch disease in an Australian cat population. *Pathology* 28:262–265.
8. Breitschwerdt EB. 1996. Unpublished data. North Carolina State University, Releigh, NC.
9. Breitschwerdt EB, Kordick DL, Malarkey DE, et al. 1995. Endocarditis in a dog due to infection with a novel *Bartonella* subspecies. *J Clin Microbiol* 33:154–160.
10. Breitschwerdt EB, Pappalardo BL. 1997. Unpublished data. North Carolina State University, Raleigh, NC.
11. Brenner DJ, O'Connor SP, Winkler HH, et al. 1993. Proposals to unify the genera *Bartonella* and *Rochalimaea*, with descriptions of *Bartonella quintana* comb. nov., *Bartonella vinsonii* comb. nov., *Bartonella henselae* comb. nov., and *Bartonella elizabethae* comb. nov., and to remove the family *Bartonellaceae* from the order Rickettsiales. *Int J Syst Bacteriol* 43:777–786.
12. Brenner SA, Rooney JA, Manzewitsch P, et al. 1997. Isolation of *Bartonella (Rochalimaea) henselae*: effects of methods of blood collection and handling. *J Clin Microbiol* 35:544–547.
13. Brown PJ, Henderson JP, Galloway P, et al. 1994. Peliosis hepatis and telangiectasis in 18 cats. *J Small Anim Pract* 35:7377.
14. Caniza MA, Granger DL, Wilson KH, et al. 1995. *Bartonella henselae*: etiology of pulmonary nodules in a patient with depressed cell-mediated immunity. *Clin Infect Dis* 20:1505–1511.
15. Carithers HA. 1985. Cat-scratch disease: an overview based on a study of 1,200 patients. *Am J Dis Child* 139:1124–1133.
16. Childs JE, Olson JG, Wolf A, et al. 1995. Prevalence of antibodies to *Rochalimaea* species (cat scratch disease agent) in cats. *Vet Rec* 136:519–520.
17. Childs JE, Rooney JA, Cooper JL, et al. 1994. Epidemiologic observations on infection with *Rochalimaea* species among cats living in Baltimore, MD. *J Am Vet Med Assoc* 204:1775–1778.
18. Chomel BB, Abbott RC, Kasten RW, et al. 1995. *Bartonella henselae* prevalence in domestic cats in California: risk factors and association between bacteremia and antibody titers. *J Clin Microbiol* 33:2445–2450.
19. Chomel BB, Kasten RW, Floyd-Hawkins K, et al. 1996. Experimental transmission of *Bartonella henselae* by the cat flea. *J Clin Microbiol* 34:1952–1956.
20. Chomel BB, Yamamoto K, Kasten RW, et al. 1996. *Bartonella* infection in domestic and wild cats in the USA. Association with ectoparasite infestation. Presented at the International Conference on Emerging Zoonoses, Jerusalem, Israel.
21. Clarridge JE, Raich TJ, Pirwani D, et al. 1995. Strategy to detect and identify *Bartonella* species in routine clinical laboratory yields *Bartonella henselae* from human immunodeficiency virus-positive patient and unique *Bartonella* strain from his cat. *J Clin Microbiol* 33:2107–2113.
22. Cockerell CJ, Friedman-Kien AE. 1988. Epithelioid angiomatosis and cat scratch disease bacillus (letter). *Lancet* 1:1334–1335.
23. Cockerell CJ, Tierno PM, Friedman-Kien AE, et al. 1991. Clinical, histologic, microbiologic, and biochemical characterization of the causative agent of bacillary (epithelioid) angiomatosis: a rickettsial illness with features of bartonellosis. *J Invest Dermatol* 97:812–817.
24. Conley T, Slater L, Hamilton K. 1994. *Rochalimaea* species stimulate human endothelial cell proliferation and migration in vitro. *J Lab Clin Med* 124:521–528.
25. Daly S, Worthington MG, Brenner DJ, et al. 1993. *Rochalimaea elizabethae* sp. nov. isolated from a patient with endocarditis. *J Clin Microbiol* 31(4):872–881.
26. Dolan MJ, Wong MT, Regnery RL, et al. 1993. Syndrome of *Rochalimaea henselae* adenitis suggesting cat scratch disease. *Ann Intern Med* 118:331–336.
27. Drancourt M, Moal V, Brunet P, et al. 1996. *Bartonella (Rochalimaea) quintana* infection in a seronegative hemodialyzed patient. *J Clin Microbiol* 34:1158–1160.
28. English CK, Wear DJ, Margileth AM, et al. 1988. Cat-scratch disease. Isolation and culture of the bacterial agent. *JAMA* 259:1347–1352.
29. Giladi M, Avidor B, Kletter Y, et al. 1996. Cat scratch disease. The rare role of *Afipia felis* (abstract 33), p 922. Presented at the 34th Annual Meeting of the Infectious Disease Society of America.
30. Glaus T, Hofmann-Lehmann R, Greene C, et al. 1997. Seroprevalence of *Bartonella henselae* infection and correlation with disease status in cats in Switzerland. *J Clin Microbiol* 35:2883–2885.
31. Golden SE. 1993. Hepatosplenic cat-scratch disease associated with elevated anti-*Rochalimaea* antibody titers. *Pediatr Infect Dis J* 12:868–871.
32. Greene CE. 1997. Unpublished data. University of Georgia, Athens, GA.
33. Greene CE, McDermott M, Jameson PH, et al. 1996. *Bartonella henselae* infection in cats: evaluation during primary infection, treatment, and rechallenge infection. *J Clin Microbiol* 34:1682–1685.
34. Groves MG, Harrington KS. 1993. *Rochalimaea henselae* infections: newly recognized zoonoses transmitted by domestic cats. *J Am Vet Med Assoc* 204:267–271.
35. Guerra LG, Neira CJ, Boman D, et al. 1993. Rapid response of AIDS-related bacillary angiomatosis to azithromycin. *Clin Infect Dis* 17:264–266.
35a. Guptill L, Slater L, Wu Ching-Ching, et al. 1997. Experimental infection of young specific pathogen–free cats with *Bartonella henselae. J Infect Dis* 176:206–216.
35b. Gurfield AN, Boulouis H-J, Chomel BB, et al. 1997. Coinfection with *Bartonella clarridgeiae* and *Bartonella henselae* and with different *Bartonella henselae* strains in domestic cats. *J Clin Microbiol* 35:2120–2123.
36. Hadfield TL, Warren RI, Kass M, et al. 1994. Endocarditis caused by *Rochalimaea henselae. Hum Pathol* 24:1140–1141.
36a. Hayem F, Chacar S, Hayem G, et al. 1996. *Bartonella henselae* infection mimicking systemic onset juvenile chronic arthritis in a 2 1/2-year old girl. *J Rheumatol* 23:1263–1265.
37. Heller R, Artois M, Xemar V, et al. 1997. Prevalence of *Bartonella henselae* and *Bartonella clarridgeiae* in stray cats. *J Clin Microbiol* 35:1327–1331.
37a. Higgins JA, Radulovic S, Jaworski DC, et al. 1996. Acquisition of the cat scratch disease agent *Bartonella henselae* by cat fleas (Siphonaptera: Pulicidae). *J Med Entomol* 33:490–495.
38. Huh YB, Rose S, Schoen RE, et al. 1996. Colonic bacillary angiomatosis. *Ann Intern Med* 124:735–737.
39. Jameson PH, Greene CE, Regnery RL, et al. 1995. Prevalence of *Bartonella henselae* antibodies in pet cats throughout regions of North America. *J Infect Dis* 172:1145–1149.
40. Joblet C, Roux V, Drancourt M, et al. 1995. Identification of *Bartonella (Rochalimaea)* species among fastidious gram-negative bacteria on the basis of the partial sequence of the citrate-synthase gene. *J Clin Microbiol* 33:1879–1883.
41. Kelly PJ, Matthewman LA, Hayter D, et al. 1996. *Bartonella henselae* in southern Africa, evidence for infection in domestic cats and implications for veterinarians. *J S Afr Vet Assoc* 67:182–187.
42. Kirkpatrick CE, Moore FM, Patnaik AK, et al. 1989. Argyrophilic, intracellular bacteria in some cats with idiopathic peripheral lymphadenopathy. *J Comp Pathol* 101:341–349.
43. Koehler JE, Glaser CA, Tappero JW. 1994. *Rochalimaea henselae* infection: a new zoonosis with the domestic cat as a reservoir. *JAMA* 271:531–535.
44. Koehler JE, Quinn FD, Berger TG, et al. 1992. Isolation of *Rochalimaea* species from cutaneous and osseous lesions of bacillary angiomatosis. *N Engl J Med* 327:1625–1631.
45. Koehler JE, Tapero JW. 1993. Bacillary angiomatosis and bacillary peliosis in patients infected with human immunodeficiency virus. *Clin Infect Dis* 17:612–624.
46. Kordick DL, Breitschwerdt EB. 1995. Intraerythrocytic presence of *Bartonella henselae. J Clin Microbiol* 33:1655–1656.
47. Kordick DL, Breitschwerdt EB. 1997. Relapsing bacteremia after blood transmission of *Bartonella henselae* to cats. *Am J Vet Res* 58:492–497.
48. Kordick DL, Hilyard EJ, Hadfield TL, et al. 1997. *Bartonella clarridgeiae,* a newly recognized zoonotic pathogen causing inoculation papules, fever, and lymphadenopathy (cat scratch disease). *J Clin Microbiol* 35:1813–1818.
48a. Kordick DL, Papich MG, Breitschwerdt EB. 1997. Efficacy of enrofloxacin or doxycycline for treatment of *Bartonella henselae* or *Bartonella clarridgeiae* infection in cats. *Antimicrob Agents Chemother* 41:2448–2455.
49. Kordick DL, Swaminathan B, Greene CE, et al. 1996. *Bartonella vinsonii* subsp. *berkhoffii* subsp. nov., isolated from dogs; *Bartonella vinsonii* subsp. *vinsonii*; and emended description of *Bartonella vinsonii. Int J Syst Bacteriol* 46:704–709.
50. Kordick DL, Wilson KH, Sexton DJ, et al. 1995. Prolonged *Bartonella* bacteremia in cats associated with cat-scratch disease patients. *J Clin Microbiol* 33:3245–3251.
50a. Lawson PA, Collins MD. 1996. Description of *Bartonella clarridgeiae* sp. nov. isolated from the cat of a patient with *Bartonella henselae* septicemia. *Med Microbiol Lett* 5:64–73.
51. Lucey D, Dolan KJ, Moss CW, et al. 1992. Relapsing illness due to *Rochalimaea henselae* in immunocompetent hosts: implication of therapy and new epidemiological associations. *Clin Infect Dis* 14:683–688.
52. Marano N, Regnery R, Greene CE, et al. 1998. Examination of *Bartonella henselae* isolates from North American cats and introduction of a unique species. Manuscript in preparation.
53. Margileth AM. 1992. Antibiotic therapy for cat-scratch disease: clinical study of therapeutic outcome in 268 patients and a review of the literature. *Pediatr Infect Dis J* 11:474–478.
54. Maruyama S, Nogami S, Inoue I, et al. 1996. Isolation of *Bartonella henselae* from domestic cats in Japan. *J Vet Med Sci* 58:81–83.
55. Maurin M, Raoult D. 1993. Antimicrobial susceptibility of *Rochalimaea*

quintana, Rochalimaea vinsonii, and the newly recognized *Rochalimaea henselae*. *J Antimicrob Chemother* 32:587–594.
55a. Mouritsen CL, Litwin CM, Maiese RL, et al. 1997. Rapid polymerase chain-reaction based detection of the causative agent of cat-scratch disease (*Bartonella-henselae*) in formalin-fixed, paraffin-embedded samples. *Human Pathol* 28:820–826.
55b. Noah DL, Kramer CM, Verbsky MP, et al. 1997. Survey of veterinary professionals and other veterinary conference attendees for antibodies to *Bartonella-henselae* and *Bartonella-quintana*. *J Am Vet Med Assoc* 210:342–344.
56. Norman AF, Regnery R, Jameson P, et al. 1995. Differentiation of *Bartonella*-like isolates at the species level by PCR-restriction fragment length polymorphism in the citrate synthase gene. *J Clin Microbiol* 33:1797–1803.
57. Pappalardo BL, Correa MT, York CC, et al. 1996. *Rhipcephalus sanguineous*: a probable vector for transmission of *Bartonella vinsonii* to dogs (abstract 12). Presented at the Sesquiannual Meeting of the American Society of Rickettsiology and Rickettsial Diseases, Montery, CA.
58. Pappalardo BL, Correa MT, York CC, et al. 1997. Epidemiologic evaluation of the risk factors associated with exposure and seroreactivity to *Bartonella vinsonii* in dogs. *Am J Vet Res* 58:467–471.
58a. Rath PM, von Recklinghausen G, Ansorg R. 1997. Seroprevalence of immunoglobulin G antibodies to *Bartonella henselae* in cat owners [letter]. *Eur J Clin Microbiol Infect Dis* 16:326–327.
59. Reed JA, Brigati DJ, Flynn SD, et al. 1992. Immunocytochemical identification of *Rochalimaea henselae* in bacillary (epithelioid) angiomatosis, parenchymal bacillary peliosis, and persistent fever with bacteremia. *Am J Surg Pathol* 16:650–657.
60. Regnery RL, Anderson BE, Clarridge JE III, et al. 1992. Characterization of a novel *Rochalimaea* species, *R. henselae* sp. nov., isolated from blood of a febrile, human immunodeficiency virus-positive patient. *J Clin Microbiol* 30:265–274.
61. Regnery RL, Olson JG, Perkins BA, et al. 1992. Serological response to *Rochalimaea henselae* antigen in suspected cat-scratch disease. *Lancet* 339:1443–1445.
62. Regnery RL, Rooney JA, Johnson AM, et al. 1996. Experimentally induced *Bartonella henselae* infections followed by challenge exposure and antimicrobial therapy in cats. *Am J Vet Res* 57:1714–1719.
63. Relman DA, Loutit JS, Schmidt TM, et al. 1990. The agent of bacillary angiomatosis: an approach to the identification of uncultured pathogens. *N Engl J Med* 323:1573–1580.
64. Rodriguez-Barradas MC, Hamill RJ, Houston ED, et al. 1995. Genomic fingerprinting of *Bartonella* species by repetitive element PCR for distinguishing species and isolates. *J Clin Microbiol* 33:1089–1093.
65. Roux V, Raoult D. 1995. Inter- and intraspecies identification of *Bartonella* (*Rochalimaea*) species. *J Clin Microbiol* 33:1573–1579.
66. Sander A, Buhler C, Pelz K, et al. 1997. Detection and identification of two *Bartonella henselae* variants in domestic cats in Germany. *J Clin Microbiol* 35:584–587.
67. Schwartzman WA. 1992. Infections due to *Rochalimaea*: the expanding clinical spectrum. *Clin Infect Dis* 15:893–902.
68. Schwartzman WA, Patnaik M, Barka NE, et al. 1994. *Rochalimaea* antibodies in HIV-associated neurologic disease. *Neurology* 144:1312–1316.
69. Slater LN, Welch DF, Hensel D, et al. 1990. A newly recognized fastidious gram-negative pathogen as a cause of fever and bacteremia. *N Engl J Med* 323:1587–1593.
70. Spach DH, Callis KP, Paauw DS, et al. 1993. Endocarditis caused by *Rochalimaea quintana* in a patient infected with human immunodeficiency virus. *J Clin Microbiol* 31:692–694.
71. Ueno H, Hohdatsu T, Muramatsu Y, et al. 1996. Does coinfection of *Bartonella henselae* and FIV induce clinical disorders in cats. *Microbiol Immunol* 40:617–620.
72. Ueno H, Muramatsu Y, Chomel BB, et al. 1995. Seroepidemiological survey of *Bartonella* (*Rochalimaea*) *henselae* in domestic cats. *Microbiol Immunol* 39:339–341.
73. Waldvogel K, Regnery RL, Anderson BE, et al. 1994. Disseminated cat-scratch disease: detection of *Rochalimaea henselae* in affected tissue. *Eur J Pediatr* 153:23–27.
74. Wear DJ, English CK, Margileth AM. 1990. Cat scratch disease, pp 632–638. *In* Greene CE (ed), Infectious diseases of the dog and cat. WB Saunders, Philadelphia, PA.
75. Wear DJ, Margileth AM, Hadfield TL, et al. 1983. Cat scratch disease. A bacterial infection. *Science* 221:1403–1405.
76. Welch DF, Hensel DM, Pickett DA, et al. 1993. Bacteremia due to *Rochalimaea henselae* in a child: practical identification of isolates in the clinical laboratory. *J Clin Microbiol* 31:2381–2386.
77. Wong MTAI, Dolan MJ, Lattuada CP, et al. 1995. Neuroretinitis, aseptic meningitis, and lymphadenitis associated with *Bartonella (Rochalimaea) henselae* infection in immunocompetent patients and patients infected with human immunodeficiency virus type 1. *J Infect Dis* 21:352–360.
78. Zangwill KM, Hamilton DH, Perkins BA, et al. 1993. Cat scratch disease in Connecticut. Epidemiology, risk factors, and evaluation of a new diagnostic test. *N Engl J Med* 329(1):8–13.

Chapter 55

Surgical and Traumatic Wound Infections

Craig E. Greene

Bacterial infections have been a limiting factor in successful healing of operative wounds since the very beginnings of surgery. The use of aseptic methods and minimization of tissue trauma were major breakthroughs in reducing postoperative infections. Subsequent development of antibiotics and their use in surgery brought further reductions in surgical infections. The prevalence of nosocomial infections has increased again, owing to more invasive and prolonged surgical procedures and synthetic implants.

ETIOLOGY

The major source of bacteria contaminating surgical wounds is the patient's endogenous microflora. Despite disinfection, skin-associated bacteria can be reduced but not eliminated. Bacteria residing in the deeper parts of the skin such as the hair follicles and sebaceous glands are not removed or killed by preparative scrubbing. They may enter deeper tissues during the initial incision. Nosocomial infections can also arise from inadequate sterilization of surgical equipment, operating room air flow, or transfer from the veterinary staff or hospital environment. Microbes indigenous to the hospital environment are most problematic because they are often antimicrobial resistant. A classification of human surgical wound contamination that can be applied to veterinary practice is summarized in Table 55–1. Predictably, the infection risk increases with the wound classification. In a study of 1574 dogs and cats with clean, clean

Table 55–1. Classification of Surgical Wounds and Indications for Prophylaxis

CLEAN	CONTAMINATED
1. Elective surgery	1. Fresh traumatic wound
2. No entry into mucosal surface	2. Spillage from GI surface
3. No break in asepsis	3. Acute inflammation encountered
4. No inflammation or drainage encountered	4. Dental prophylaxis[a]
CLEAN CONTAMINATED	**INFECTED**
1. Entry into GI, GU, RT mucosae	1. Abscessed material present
2. No unusual contamination	2. Viscus perforated
3. Minor break in asepsis	3. Older (> 4 hr) traumatic wound
	4. Suppuration encountered

[a]For dental prophylaxis, see Gingivitis, Chapter 89.
GI = gastrointestinal tract; GU = genitourinary tract; RT = respiratory tract.
From National Research Council: *Ann Surg* 160:1–192, 1964. Used with permission.

contaminated, contaminated, or dirty surgical wounds, infection rates were 4.7%, 5.0%, 12.0%, and 10%, respectively.[4]

Clean surgical wounds involve surgical incision sites where no prior trauma or inflammation is present; no break in sterile technique occurs; and mucosal surfaces such as the respiratory, genitourinary, or alimentary tract are not compromised. *Clean contaminated surgical wounds* involve minor breaks in surgical technique (such as a torn glove) or contact with normal mucosae of the GI tract without spillage of viscus contents or uninfected genitourinary, biliary, or respiratory tracts. It also includes otherwise clean procedures in which drains are placed. *Contaminated surgical wounds* are operative wounds in which there is accidental spillage from the GI tract from penetration of an infected viscus or tissue, foreign bodies, devitalized tissue or pus, or a break in sterile technique. Bacterial contamination is suspected, but purulent discharge is absent. Clean lacerations of the skin or subcutaneous tissue that are not already infected are often categorized in this group. Contaminated surgical wounds have a high risk for postoperative infections. For example, after colonic spillage, isolated pathogens are often mixed; up to five species are present. Aerobic species are usually *Escherichia coli* and enterococci, and anaerobes are *Bacteroides*, anaerobic cocci, and clostridia (see Chapter 89, Intra-Abdominal Infections).[8] *Infected (dirty) surgical or traumatic wound infections* are already infected surgical wounds or nonsurgical defects or breaks in the skin associated with blunt trauma. Devitalized tissues, foreign bodies, or purulent discharges are often observed. Examples of this type of wound are previously perforated viscus, devitalized wounds, compound fractures, foreign bodies, pus pockets, and acute cellulitis. Traumatic wounds are assumed to be contaminated and have a subsequent increased risk of infection because microbes bypass the anatomic and immunologic barriers of the host. Bacteria within these wounds have often already spread systemically. Establishment of tissue infection depends on the type and depth of the injury, damage to the vascular supply, devitalization of the tissue, and delay in the presentation for treatment. For orthopedic injuries, post-traumatic osteomyelitis occurs whenever a broken bone has a contaminated open wound, an avascular fragment, and a milieu of damaged necrotic tissue or hemorrhage.[3] See Musculoskeletal Infections, Chapter 86. After trauma and hospitalization, urinary and IV catheter infections are most common, followed by pneumonia and intra-abdominal and wound infections. Organisms are often staphylococci, *E. coli*, *Enterobacter*, *Pseudomonas*, and *Klebsiella*.

Table 55–2. Sources of Infection Associated With Surgical Manipulations

PREOPERATIVE
Pre-existing infection
Abscess formation
Traumatic wounds
Foreign bodies
Viscus perforation
INTRAOPERATIVE
Air-borne, inadequate air filtration
Operating room personnel
Hands or gloves
Mucosae or skin of patient
Drain placement
Hematogenous dissemination
Opening viscus
Contaminated surgical materials
POSTOPERATIVE
IV catheters
Urinary catheters
Drains
Hematogenous to implants

Contributing Factors

Many factors contribute to the likelihood of developing postoperative infection, which can occur at various times before, during, or after the operative event (Table 55–2). A number of precautions can be taken to reduce the risk for infection (Table 55–3). Preoperative preparation of the surgical site is a critical factor in preventing wound infection (see Chapter 94). Skin trauma produced during surgical preparation greatly increases the local bacterial population. Preoperative clipping time is an important factor in the development

Table 55–3. Methods to Reduce Infection of Surgical Wounds

PREOPERATIVE
Minimize preoperative hospitalization.
Treat with antimicrobial or avoid surgery in animals with concurrent infections.
Treat remote sites of infection before operating.
Widely clip hair around the incision site.
Shave skin just before surgery.
Prepare skin with povidone-iodine or chlorhexidine.
INTRAOPERATIVE
Use prophylactic antimicrobials when:
Manipulating contaminated tissues or intestine
For prolonged surgical procedures (> 3 hr)
With synthetic implants
Keep surgical room free of dust and insects.
Keep surgical field clean and use routine antiseptic technique.
Ensure accurate sharp incision and dissection.
Avoid normal skin or mucosal flora from contacting body cavities or internal tissues.
Minimize drying and exposure of handled tissues.
Debride surgically all tissues to healthy vascular areas.
Remove all foreign bodies, avascular tissue, and dead space.
Irrigate contaminated areas with antimicrobial or disinfectant solutions.
Avoid circulatory compromise.
Use meticulous hemostasis to avoid tissue hemorrhage and blood clots.
Place stab wound drains at other than incision sites.
Delay surgical closure with dead space.
Handle soft tissues and abdominal viscera gently.
POSTOPERATIVE
Use delayed closure of contaminated wounds.
Change IV catheters routinely.
Prevent aspiration pneumonia.
Keep drainage established and irrigate healing wounds.

of postoperative wound infection.[4] Animals with surgical sites clipped before anesthetic induction rather than immediately before surgery were three times likely to develop surgical wound infections. Those clipped hours to days before the surgery, for ultrasonographic studies, had a postoperative infection rate three times greater.[4]

Delayed wound healing, caused by excessive numbers of sutures, foreign implants, or devascularized tissues, serves as a focus for infection after contamination.[1] Dead space between tissues should be avoided, and all surgical wounds should be closely approximated. Although surgically placed drains allow for removal of blood or pus in dead space areas, they may delay closure or allow entry of organisms into wounds. IV catheters and intubation used in surgical or trauma patients also increase the risk of infection. Drains and IV catheters should be removed as soon as possible during the recovery period to minimize the direct or hematogenous colonization of the surgical site.

Surgical technique is perhaps the single most important factor in preventing postoperative infections. The risk of tissue infection is directly proportional to the increased amount of tissue handling and trauma. Vascular compromise to tissue, excessive electrocautery, and bleeding into tissue spaces are the major contributory factors. Foreign material and blood clots allow for adherence and facilitate replication of microorganisms. Experimentally, use of fibrinolytic agents prevents infections, abscesses, and adhesions after surgery. A biofilm composed of polysaccharide glycocalix and bacteria can colonize the surface of prosthetic implants during the surgical procedure.[1] Bacteria that seed surgical sites or implants can remain dormant for months to years, or, less frequently, the sites can be seeded during the healing and recovery phases. In some animals, occult orthopedic infections develop with bacteria remaining at the site of the healed fracture without causing clinical or radiographic evidence of osteomyelitis.[5] The infection may persist locally until such time as any orthopedic implants are removed.

The duration of surgery has a major influence on the overall risk of wound infection. Drying of tissue and airborne contamination are also major factors. Tissue counts of less than 10^5 organisms per gram of tissue are needed to ensure proper incisional healing. Bacterial counts may double for every hour of operative time. Nosocomial infections develop in 1% of patients after procedures less than 30 minutes and in 14% after procedures more than 3.5 hours. In dogs and cats, risk for postoperative infection was twice as high for those undergoing procedures lasting 90 minutes compared with those lasting 60 minutes.[4] Ultraclean surgical rooms have been shown to reduce the prevalence of postoperative infection; however, in most operating rooms with high-volume air exchange and perioperative antimicrobial use in extended procedures, postoperative infections can be minimized.

Localized infections at distant sites can spread to operative wounds hematogenously. Bacterial translocation denotes the spread of viable bacteria from the lumen of the GI tract into the blood stream via the portal circulation. Manipulation of the intestines during surgery may lead to distant postsurgical infection or sepsis. The majority of culturable translocating bacteria in mesenteric lymph nodes and blood are *E. coli*.[9] In corresponding experiments, anesthesia without intestinal manipulation produced minimal bacteremia in itself. Prolonged (>48 hours) fasting before and after surgery caused increased bacteremia in animals with intestinal manipulation, presumably because of intestinal stasis and bacterial overgrowth. Bacterial translocation is also increased with endotoxemia, abdominal irradiation, splenectomy, biliary obstruction, and hemorrhagic shock.

Host immunosuppression by a concurrent disease or an inherent immunodeficiency disorder may increase the risk of postoperative infection. Dogs rendered immune deficient by treatment with glucocorticoid and azathioprine had increased prevalence of infected vascular grafts compared with immunocompetent dogs.[1] Diabetes mellitus, hyperadrenocorticism, obesity, and malnutrition are predisposing factors. A relative immunodeficiency state may occur in traumatized animals as a result of hemorrhage, glucocorticoid therapy, and reduced cell-mediated immunity from cytokine dysregulation. Previous urinary outflow obstruction has been shown to predispose cats to postoperative infection after perineal urethrostomy in comparison to unobstructed cats having the same surgery.[6] Although anesthesia has been associated with in vitro alterations in leukocyte chemotaxis, mobility, and lymphocyte stimulation, actual documentation of impaired host immune responses in vivo has not been confirmed.

Prolonged hospitalization increases the risk from infection with antimicrobial-resistant bacteria. Wet dressings reduce the fibrin seal formation on a wound and may allow for the maceration of tissue and proliferation of bacteria at the incision site. Prophylactic antibiotics should not be used indiscriminately in surgical procedures but only when contamination of tissues is expected (see Antimicrobial Prophylaxis).

CLINICAL SIGNS

The signs of infection are often masked in the traumatized patient, and complicating infection should be considered with any worsening of clinical parameters. Fever and leukocyte changes are not always predictive. Some local inflammation or serous discharges are expected at the incision site of any surgical procedure. A diagnosis of post-traumatic infection can be made from soft tissue swelling, hyperesthesia, fever, and leukocytosis. Additional signs that may be associated with systemic infections are increased respiratory distress, hyperglycemia or hypoglycemia, renal failure, thrombocytopenia, icterus, and severe mental depression.

DIAGNOSIS

Postsurgical infections are characterized locally by heat, swelling, pain, and erythema at the incision site. Unfortunately, these same signs may be present in the initial healing phases after surgery. Systemic manifestations of infection are more easily discernible rectal temperature elevations and leukocytoses or left shifts in the hematologic test findings. Wounds involving intestinal perforation and burns are always contaminated and therefore require immediate attention. For deeper wounds, radiographs of the skeleton or ultrasonograms of the soft tissues may reveal deeper tissue damage, soft tissue swelling, or gas formation. With chronic orthopedic infection, bony lysis, proliferation of bone, or sequestra develop. Cytology of exudates and biopsy or culture of tissues is most definitive. Deep-sample culturing of infected wounds must be performed with surgical entry or needle penetration because surface contaminants are common. Material thus obtained should be sealed in an airtight container and submitted to a laboratory as soon as possible in an attempt to culture anaerobic agents that often are present.

THERAPY

Extensive debridement or surgical drainage of wounds may be required to prevent wound infection and to reduce extensive swelling or abscess formation. Wounds should be covered to prevent extensive drying of devitalized tissues, and drainage should be encouraged by incomplete closure or drain placement. Occlusive dressings containing adequate absorbent material should be changed whenever drainage is present. To encourage formation of sufficient granulation tissue, limbs should be immobilized or supported. Chronic nonhealing scar tissue should be resected from the wound. Prolonged hospitalization and indiscriminate use of topical or systemic antibiotics favor the overgrowth of resistant bacteria. Surgical drains, IV catheters, and intubations of trauma patients also increase the risk of infections. For intra-abdominal infections and suspected or documented ruptured viscus, antimicrobial therapy should be provided against fecal flora, including anaerobes and gram-negative *Enterobacteriaceae* (see Intra-Abdominal Infections, Chapter 89). For orthopedic injuries with mandibular and maxillary or open fractures, penicillins or cephalosporins, respectively, are often administered.

PREVENTION

Surgical Equipment

A review of hospital and equipment disinfection procedures is presented in Chapter 94. The disinfection of surgical tools and facilities is intimately involved with the operative procedure. Surgical equipment should be appropriately sterilized with steam autoclaves or ethylene oxide, rather than by cold disinfection, and should be stored in dust-free enclosed cabinets. Cold disinfection should be avoided when possible because it may be associated with the increased risk of infections from soil saprophytes such as *Clostridium tetani* (see Chapter 43). All surfaces in operating rooms that do not contact the patient should be routinely disinfected with phenolic compounds. Floors can be washed with disinfectants and wet mopped or polished. Wet mops or vacuums with filtered exhaust elements can pick up excess disinfectant and loosening debris. Built-up disinfectant films can be removed with a solution of 0.12 L (one-half cup) of vinegar in 3.8 L (1 gallon) of water. Dry mops and brooms should never be used to clean hospital floors because they disseminate microorganisms in dust. Personnel should wear face masks to minimize aerosol contamination in surgery areas. Handwashing and gloving for surgery are superior to handwashing alone in minimizing the spread of skin microflora to the patient. Antisepsis of the skin at the incision site is similar to that for preparing IV catheter sites, but there is a final application of tincture of iodine or iodophor solution just before the animal is draped. For a discussion of cleanliness and sterility of anesthesia and nebulizer equipment, see Chapter 94.

Lavage

Contaminated wounds should be lavaged with copious amounts of prewarmed saline solution. Pressure is delivered by a 35-ml syringe and 18-gauge needle or similar sized catheter. Lavage without jet irrigation is not effective. Local antibiotic instillation may achieve higher concentrations of drugs in the desired tissue with minimal toxicity. Because antibiotics are readily absorbed, they should not be instilled in body cavities. Chlorhexidine has been used as a successful wound disinfectant.

Antimicrobial Prophylaxis

A majority of nosocomial infections occur in hospitalized animals undergoing surgery. Preoperative and intraoperative antimicrobials have been shown repeatedly to reduce the prevalence of postoperative infection when strict antisepsis cannot be maintained, such as in surgery of the bowel, respiratory and biliary tracts, and oropharyngeal region. For dental procedures, see Chapter 89. Organisms that contaminate relatively avascular subcutaneous tissues, bone fragments, or serosal surfaces are often commensals of skin and mucosal surfaces. There are surgical situations in which antimicrobial therapy administered before the procedure for anticipated infection may be beneficial (Table 55–4). Short-term, clean surgical procedures in dogs and cats have no difference in infection rates when antimicrobial prophylaxis is compared with placebo. Prophylactic antimicrobial therapy is desirable in conjunction with surgical drainage of abscesses.

The success of prophylaxis depends heavily on the chosen antimicrobial. Because of their low toxicity and activity against the commonly infecting staphylococci, cephalosporins have been the mainstay of prophylaxis for surgery. Because of its prolonged duration of activity, cefazolin has been a popular choice among surgeons.

The timing of administration of antibiotics is an important factor in the prevention of surgical wound infections. The success involves timing the administration of the drug slightly before (<2 hours) or during the surgery to achieve maximum concentration during the operative procedure and not continued for longer than 24 hours after surgery. If antimicrobial prophylaxis is considered as an afterthought, it will *not* be effective. In 1574 dogs and cats with clean surgical wounds, animals not receiving antibodies had 30 of 677 (4%) infected wounds.[4] Those receiving only perioperative antibiotics as outlined previously had 3 of 135 (2.2%) infected wounds, whereas animals receiving antibiotics in some other prescribed manner had 21 of 334 (6.3%) infections. When only postoperative antibodies were given, the infection rate was 8.3%.

Oral therapy is given 1 hour before, IM injections one-half hour before, and IV therapy immediately at the beginning of the anesthetic induction as an IV bolus. With the exception of colonic surgery, in which prophylaxis is started earlier, the initial dose of a systemically administered drug should be given parenterally at the time of anesthetic induction. For colonic surgery, systemic antimicrobial therapy, combined with mechanical cleaning of the large bowel to reduce the microflora, is started 48 hours before surgery. Enemas with isotonic lavage fluids and cathartics are often used.

Even with clean surgeries, the operating field is considered to be contaminated if the procedure lasts longer than 3 hours. Another dose of antimicrobials should be given at that time to maintain concentrations for the length of the operation. Redosing the drug at the time of closure may be needed if the procedure takes longer than 3 hours. Antimicrobials penetrate formed tissue exudates and blood clots poorly but will be readily incorporated in the latter if they are present in the plasma during clot formation. The risk of contamination is present until there is a firm fibrin seal forming between the wound edges 3 to 5 hours postoperatively. For this reason a final dose of antimicrobial is recommended for contaminated procedures when the closure is being completed. When contamination is suspected but infection is not documented, antimicrobial therapy should never be given for more than 12 to 24 hours after surgery. Measures should be taken to reduce the risk of infection after antimicrobial prophylaxis, because infection with resistant organism is more likely. Hospitalization, stress, and invasive procedures

Table 55–4. Indications and Drugs for Antimicrobial Prophylaxis or Treatment in Surgery

SURGICAL CLASS	EXAMPLES	ASSOCIATED BACTERIA	RECOMMENDED THERAPY	
			First Choice	Alternative
Prophylaxis				
Clean	Routine surgery	None	None	None
Clean contaminated	Genital surgery	Aerobes: gram-negative Anaerobes	Cefazolin	Fluoroquinolone
	Prolonged (> 3 hrs) surgery, orthopedic prosthesis, amputation, open fracture reduction	*E. coli*, staphylococci, streptococci	Cephalosporins, cefazolin	β-lactamase–resistant penicillin
	Intra-abdominal	Aerobes: gram-negative Anaerobes	Cefoxitin	Gentamicin, metronidazole
	Dentistry	Aerobes: gram-positives and anaerobes	Chloramphenicol	Ampicillin, amoxicillin
Contaminated	Bite wounds	Aerobes and anaerobes	Amoxicillin-clavulanate	Clindamycin
	Enterotomy with leakage	Aerobes: streptococci, enterococci Anaerobes: bifidobacteria, clostridia, fusobacteria, *Bacteroides*	Cefoxitin	Aminoglycoside, metronidazole
	Biliary infection cholecystectomy	Enterobacteriaceae (*E. coli, Klebsiella, Proteus*), *Bacteroides, Clostridium*	Cefazolin	Gentamicin
	Colonic resection[a]	*E. coli, Bacteroides*	Gentamicin, clindamycin	Cefoxitin
Treatment				
Infected	Abscesses	Aerobes	Gentamicin	Aminoglycoside, clindamycin
	Ruptured bowel, colonic leakage	Anaerobes	Metronidazole	
	Pyometra	Aerobes and anaerobes	Cefazolin	Fluoroquinolone

[a]Oral therapy starting 48 hr before surgery and before anesthesia includes neomycin and metronidazole, enemas for cleaning. Routine prophylaxis not recommended with soft tissue (cyst removal, laparotomy not involving a viscus, inguinal hernia repair, mastectomy, tonsillectomy, simple lacerations); neurologic (laminectomy, fenestration); ophthalmic (lens extraction); orthopedic (rhinotomy or rhinoplasty).

should be avoided in immunosuppressed patients. If perioperative antibiotics are used, they should be bactericidal drugs in which the effectiveness is limited as much as possible to the suspected contaminant (see Table 55–4). Systemic antibiotics are thought to enter host tissues at the time of surgery and should be maintained at high concentrations during the entire procedure. A full course of antibiotics at the proper dosage should be provided; anything less is often ineffective in the absence of an adequate immune system. If results of susceptibility testing are conflicting or indicate that organisms are not susceptible to the particular drug, antibiotics should not be changed if the patient appears to be responding.

There are several disadvantages of antimicrobial chemoprophylaxis, some so serious that the risk of therapy might outweigh the benefits. Bacterial resistance or drug toxicities may occur. Chloramphenicol may interfere with barbiturate metabolism; some cephalosporins (cefamandole, cefoperazone, and cefotetan) may cause hypoprothrombinemia; and aminoglycosides may cause neuromuscular blockade or nephrotoxicity. Prophylaxis with antimicrobials may suppress normal microflora and increase the risk of infection with resistant microorganisms (superinfection). Multiple antibiotic-resistant bacteria such as enterococci, staphylococci, and *Klebsiella* have been isolated with increasing resistance. See Antimicrobial Chemotherapy (Chapter 34) and the Drug Formulary (Appendix 8) for additional information on drugs and their dosages.

References

1. Bandyk DF, Kinney EV, Riefsnyder TI, et al. 1993. Treatment of bacteria-biofilm graft infection by in situ replacement in normal and immune-deficient states. *J Vasc Surg* 18:398–406.
2. Boothe HW, Slater MR, Hobson HP, et al. 1992. Exploratory celiotomy in 200 nontraumatized dogs and cats. *Vet Surg* 21:452–457.
3. Braden TD. 1991. Posttraumatic osteomyelitis. *Vet Clin North Am Small Anim Pract* 21:781–811.
4. Brown DC, Conzemius MG, Shofer F, et al. 1997. Epidemiologic evaluation of postoperative wound infections in dogs and cats. *J Am Vet Med Assoc* 210:1302–1306.
5. Doherty MA, Smith MM. 1995. Contamination and infection of fractures resulting from gunshot trauma in dogs: 20 cases (1987–1992). *J Am Vet Med Assoc* 206:203–205.
6. Griffin DW, Gregory CR. 1992. Prevalence of bacterial infections after perineal urethrostomy in cats. *J Am Vet Med Assoc* 200:681–684.
7. Houston KA, McRitchie DI, Rotstein OD. 1990. Tissue plasminogen activator reverses the deleterious effect of infection on colonic wound healing. *Ann Surg* 211:130–135.
8. Nord CE. 1990. Incidence and significance of intraperitoneal aerobic and anaerobic bacteria. *Clin Ther* 12(Suppl B):9–20.
9. Salman FT, Buyruk MN, Gurler N, et al. 1992. The effect of surgical trauma on the bacterial translocation from the gut. *J Pediatr Surg* 27:802–804.
10. Sanchez IR, Swaim SF, Nusbam KE, et al. 1988. Effects of chlorhexidine diacetate and povidone-iodine on wound healing in dogs. *Vet Surg* 17:291–295.
11. Vasseur PB, Levy J, Dowd E, et al. 1988. Surgical wound infection rates in dogs and cats. *Vet Surg* 17:60–64.
12. Wendelburg K. 1993. Surgical wound infection, pp 54–56. *In* Bojrab M (ed), Disease mechanisms in small animal surgery. Lea & Febiger, Philadelphia, PA.
13. Wittmann DH, Bergstein JM, Frantzides C. 1991. Calculated empiric antimicrobial therapy for mixed surgical infections. *Infection* 19:5345–5350.

Section III

FUNGAL DISEASES

Chapter 56

Laboratory Diagnosis of Fungal and Algal Infections

Spencer S. Jang and Ernst L. Biberstein

Specific diagnosis of fungal and algal infections in animals requires laboratory procedures that include direct microscopic examination and culture, frequently supported by serologic tests. Many such direct examinations and primary cultures and some serologic tests are now well within the scope of in-office diagnostic procedures for veterinary practice. The development of improved methods for mycologic diagnosis is directed at rapid procedures using prepackaged identification sets and reagents,[4] serologic kits, automated systems, and molecular techniques.[15] In a high proportion of such cases, confirmation by a specialty laboratory will still be necessary to establish a definitive diagnosis.

SPECIMENS FOR LABORATORY DIAGNOSIS

A satisfactory sample should be representative of the focus of infection and of an adequate size to permit direct examination and culture. Except in systemic infections suggesting fungemia and requiring blood culture, samples should be obtained from the site of infection as indicated by lesions, signs, or symptoms. Because systemic mycoses are usually acquired via the respiratory tract, lung tissue or airway exudates are preferred samples.[12] In certain disseminated mycotic infections, urine may also be an appropriate specimen to culture.

SAMPLE COLLECTION

When collecting skin scrapings for dermatophyte culture,[18] briefly clean the lesion, particularly the periphery, with 70% alcohol; iodine is harmful to dermatophytes. Surface antisepsis, when feasible, aids in the collection of uncontaminated samples and thereby ensures a significant result. Before venipuncture, the skin must be disinfected by swabbing with 70% alcohol followed by 2% iodine.

Swabs are of limited value in fungal isolation and their use is discouraged. If no alternative collection method is available, specimens received on swabs in a suitable transport medium (see Chapter 33) should be cultured without delay.[12] Swabs for direct smears preferably should not consist of cotton because recovery rates are poor and inexperienced observers may mistake cotton fibers for hyphae. Blood for cultures can be collected directly by IV catheter (see Chapter 87) or syringe into conventional and biphasic blood culture bottles, automated blood systems, and lysis-centrifugation systems (see Isolation).[19] A fresh needle is used for transfer of blood, 1 ml per 10 ml of culture medium, from syringe to the culture bottle.

Urine is best taken by percutaneous cystocentesis, which ensures a sample uncontaminated by bacterial or fungal flora in the lower genitourinary tract (see Chapter 91).

Stool specimen cultures for diagnosis of fungal infections of the GI tract are generally misleading.[12] It is best to take biopsy specimens for histologic examination.

Scrapings for dermatophyte culture are best obtained with a scalpel blade or the edge of a glass microscope slide from the marginal, most active portion of the ringworm lesion. Use of a Wood's lamp may identify hairs infected with certain dermatophyte species. The hair roots are then plucked with forceps for culture. Nails are collected by clipping. The surface of heavily keratinized structures is scraped away for access to deeper portions. Claw surfaces are disinfected with alcohol.

The surface of skin pustules, nodules, vesicles, and so forth is disinfected, and aspiration is done with sterile needle and syringe. A biopsy may be required if fungi fail to grow from the aspirate, scraping, or swab. Normal tissue, along with portions from all zones of the lesion, should be taken.[8] Opened skin lesions are not disinfected or cleaned because such procedures may remove or kill the organisms.

Fluids and contents of abscesses are collected through aspiration by needle and syringe. Large volumes, adequate for centrifugation, are best. Any granules should be included and characterized. Bone marrow is likewise sampled by needle and syringe or core needle biopsy. At least 3 ml of CSF is desirable via lumbar or cisternal puncture. For lung sampling, a transtracheal or bronchial wash or bronchial brushing is done (see Chapter 88).[3a]

Necrotic material or curettings and other surgically collected material should be handled aseptically pending examination and culture. Corneal lesions are sampled by scraping several times with a sterile Kimura spatula or nylon brush (see Fig. 93–6). Slide preparation and culture are done at the site and time of collection.

TRANSPORTATION AND PRESERVATION

For referral to a diagnostic laboratory, tissue and fluid samples should be shipped by the most expeditious route in secure, sturdy, leakproof containers. Accompanying information on the type of sample submitted and any clinical information and other circumstances will assist the laboratory in selecting appropriate methods of processing the submittal, including media, incubation conditions, and safety precautions.

Specimens that cannot be promptly processed can be held in a suitable bacterial transport medium (see Chapter 33). They are refrigerated at 4°C but not frozen for periods up to 12 to 15 hours.[12] Refrigeration may delay proliferation of slow-growing fungi for 1 to 2 days. *Aspergillus* and zygomycetes are sensitive to refrigeration.[12] If a specimen suspected of harboring a zygomycete cannot be promptly cultured, overnight storage at room temperature in a bacteriologic transport medium is permissible.[12] Some fungi have been recovered from specimens up to 2 weeks in transit, but this type of delay is not recommended.[12]

Urine specimens may be kept under refrigeration up to 12 hours before culture.[12] Most bacteria and yeasts will multiply in urine kept at room temperature. The Urine C & S Transport Kit (Becton Dickinson, Rutherford, NJ) delays growth of bacteria and *Candida albicans* for up to 48 hours at room temperature. Vaginal swabs in transport medium or aspirates may be held under refrigeration before processing.

Blood culture bottles or lysis-centrifugation tubes (see Isolation), if subject to delay in processing, can be held at room temperature up to 16 hours. CSF and fluids from serous cavities and joints should be processed as soon as possible. The presence of proteins and carbohydrates in CSF contributes to its qualities as a maintenance medium. CSF should be held at room temperature if not cultured immediately.

Nasal curettings and excised polyps may be divided between sterile containers for culturing and jars of 10% buffered formalin for histologic preparation aimed at detection of rhinosporidiosis (Fig. 56–1). Impression smears of nasal tissue should be made before fixation of specimens (see Fig. 64–2). Tissue and bone marrow may be moistened with a small amount of sterile saline if transport is delayed.

Skin scrapings, nails, and hairs can be collected in a clean envelope or a sterile culture dish for mailing. Skin scrapings also can be held in place between glass slides taped at both ends. Such samples should not be kept in tightly sealed containers because resulting accumulation of moisture can lead to overgrowth by saprophytes.[18] Storage is best at room temperature; refrigeration can be harmful for some dermatophytes.[12]

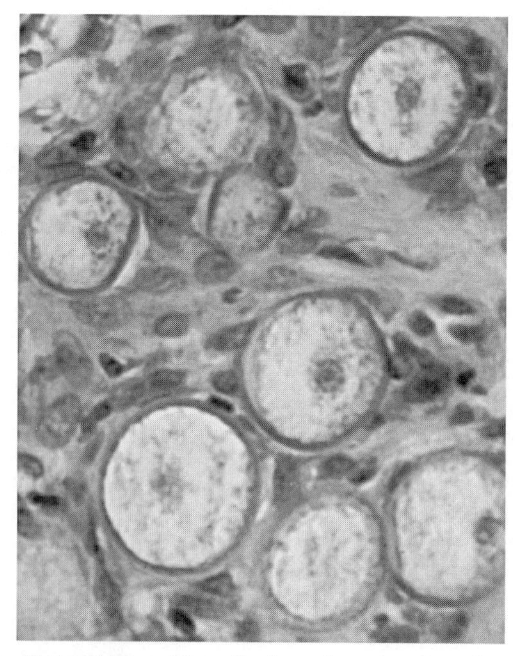

Figure 56–1. *Rhinosporidium.* Section of nasal polyp, dog. Thick-walled proliferating spherules (H and E ×500).

PROCESSING OF SPECIMENS

The complete processing of specimens involves direct microscopic examination, isolation, identification, and serology. In the following sections, some of the procedures are considered, with particular reference to their feasibility as in-office tests. No special equipment, beyond that required for basic clinical bacteriology, is needed for fungal diagnosis. For incubation purposes, an undisturbed area where room temperature (about 25°C) remains fairly constant is adequate. A hand lens (8–10×) or a dissecting microscope is helpful in the early recognition of fungal colonies.

Direct Microscopic Examination

The search for diagnostically significant fungal structures[2] may involve preparation of stained or unstained wet mounts, fixed stained smears, and histologic sections.[1] Some of these techniques are simple and rapid and may provide the clinician with a presumptive or even definitive diagnosis and a time-saving guide to therapy (Table 56–1).

Wet Mounts. Specimen material may be suspended on a slide in saline, water, or, preferably, 10% potassium hydroxide (KOH), which clears the preparation of tissue admixtures, leaving fungal elements intact. Examination should begin under low power (100×) and with subdued light, with the condenser racked down to achieve maximum contrast. When structures suggestive of fungal elements are seen, higher magnification (400×) is needed for confirmation.

The KOH digestion method is employed universally in preparation of cutaneous samples suspected of harboring dermatophytes (see Chapter 58). The hair or skin scraping to be examined is placed into a drop of 10% KOH on a clean slide (Fig. 56–2*A*). The crusty material is teased apart with forceps or dissecting needles and covered with a coverslip. Gently press the coverslip down to expel any bubbles. This preparation is passed over an open flame several times, but care must be taken not to boil the mixture. This slide is examined immediately for the presence of arthroconidia or fungal chains embedded in the material (Fig. 56–2*B* and *C*). If no organisms are initially observed, the slide is re-examined in 30 minutes. A mixture of 20% KOH and 36% dimethyl sulfoxide[8, 18] or 25% KOH or NaOH with 5% glycerol increases penetration and clarity of specimens.[12, 18] Nails may require up to 2 hours for better clearing.

India ink (Pelikan) or nigrosin (1% aqueous), when mixed on a slide with fluids or exudates containing *Cryptococcus neoformans*, provides a dark background outlining the large capsules surrounding the yeast cells (see Fig. 61–6*B*). Less than 50% of culture-positive human CSF samples are proved to be infected by this method.[1]

Less generally available but useful methods of unstained wet mount study include phase microscopy, in which the visibility of fungal structures against a background of tissue debris is improved, and fluorescent microscopy, in which a specimen is prepared by mixing with an equal volume of 10% to 20% KOH and 0.5% calcofluor white[1, 7] (Difco, Detroit, MI) on a slide. The specimen is examined on a fluorescent

Table 56–1. Direct Examination of Fungi in Clinical Specimens

STAIN OR REAGENT	USAGE	TEXT FIGURES/DISADVANTAGES
Gram's	Stains bacteria, yeasts, and other fungi	*Cryptococcus neoformans* (Fig. 56–3); *Malassezia pachydermatis* (Fig. 56–4); *Sporothrix schenckii* (Fig. 56–5); some fungi stain variably or not at all
Potassium hydroxide	Clearing tissue and cellular debris from variety of specimens to provide greater visibility of fungal elements	Dermatophytes (Fig. 56–2); artifacts develop after preparation time; experience required
India ink	Observation for presence or absence of capsules of fungal cells against a dark background	*C. neoformans* (Fig. 61–6); problems of artifacts can occur in the stain, poor sensitivity
Calcofluor white	A fluorescent brightener binding to polysaccharide such as cellulose and chitin	Detects variety of fungal elements; requires fluorescent microscope
Wright's	Stain for cytologic exam of peripheral blood, bone marrow, and body fluids, organ impressions	*Histoplasma capsulatum* (Fig. 60–7); *Aspergillus* (Fig. 65–7); *Candida* (Fig. 66–3B), *Prototheca* (Fig. 79–4); limited use
Gomori's methenamine silver	Detection of fungal elements in histologic section	*Candida albicans* (Fig. 66–2); not readily available to most clinical laboratories
Hematoxylin and eosin	Cytologic stain used for detection of fungal elements	*Rhinosporidium* (Fig. 56–1); *Coccidioides immitis* (Fig. 62–8); *Prototheca* (Fig. 79–1); usually requires large numbers of fungi to be detected with this stain

microscope equipped with a 365-nm exciter filter and a barrier filter that will transmit light at 410 nm. The fungal wall will fluoresce brilliantly.

Fixed Smears. Gram's stain is commonly done on most routine clinical specimens and will detect most fungi. It is of limited use in differentiating fungi because most will stain gram positive or unpredictably, and it produces distortion in cell morphology. Yeasts often can be detected because they retain the primary crystal violet stain (Fig. 56–3). Fungal cell

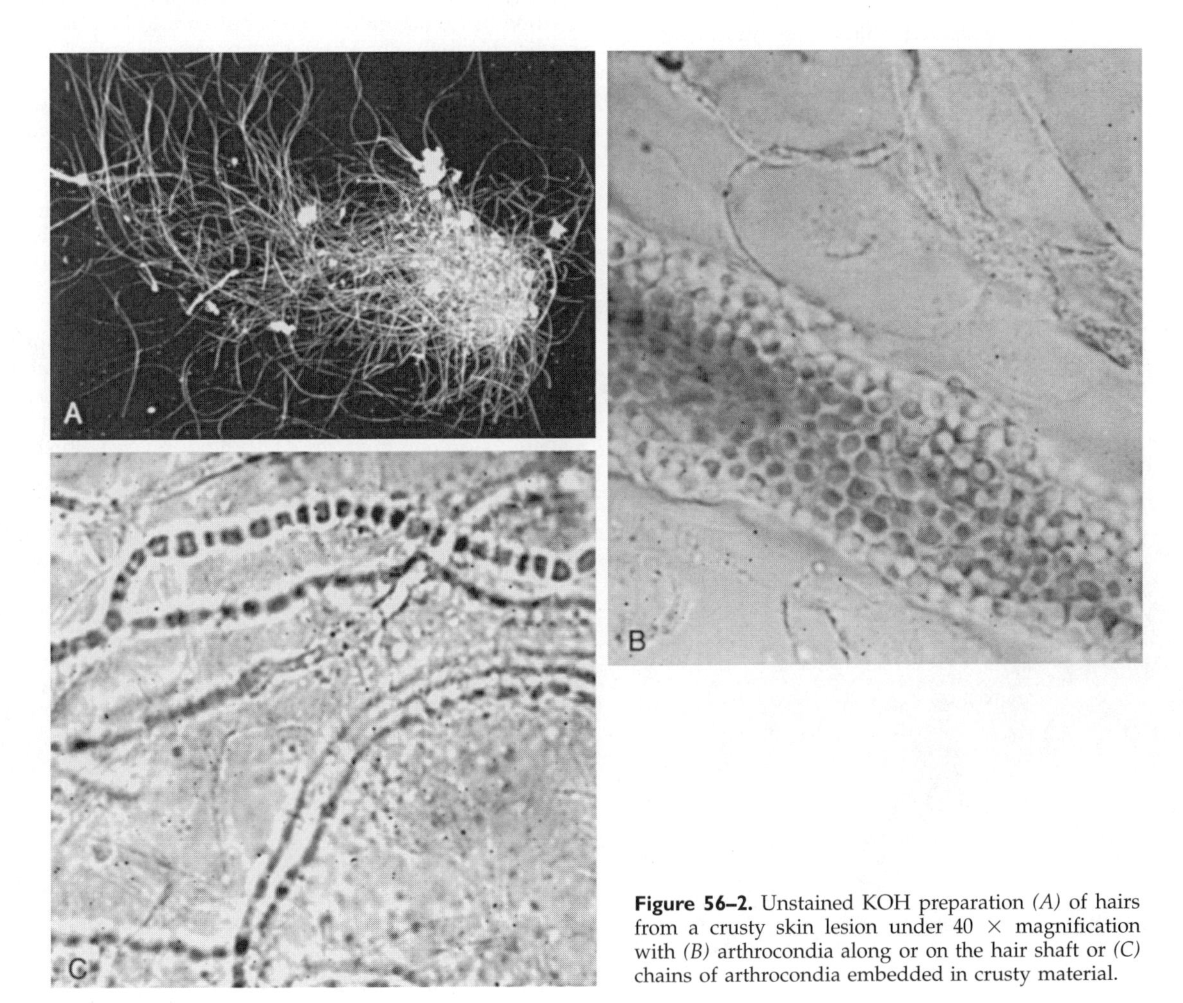

Figure 56–2. Unstained KOH preparation *(A)* of hairs from a crusty skin lesion under 40 × magnification with *(B)* arthrocondia along or on the hair shaft or *(C)* chains of arthrocondia embedded in crusty material.

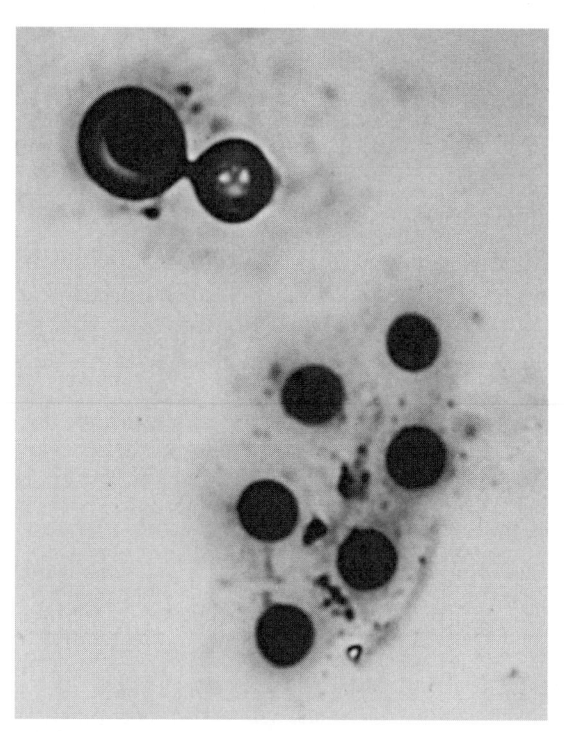

Figure 56–3. *Cryptococcus neoformans.* Nasal granuloma of a cat. Budding forms, *top center;* hazy zone around the six cells below represent capsules (Gram's stain, ×5000).

walls often appear as unstained halos. The usefulness of Gram's stain is generally limited to smears in which *Candida, Malassezia* (Fig. 56–4), *Geotrichum, Trichosporum,* or the yeast form of *Sporothrix* spp. (Fig. 56–5) is suspected.

Romanowsky-type stains, such as Wright's, Giemsa Leishman's, and Diff-Quik, will stain many fungi, especially yeasts, and are the stains of choice for the tissue phase of *Histoplasma capsulatum* (see Fig. 60–7). As with Gram's stain, fungal cell walls remain unstained by these procedures.

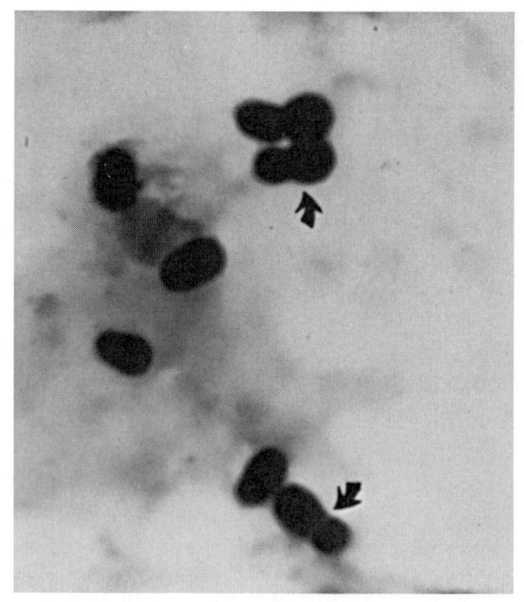

Figure 56–4. *Malassezia pachydermatis.* Ear exudate, dog. Budding yeast cells *(arrows)* have "shoe print" appearance (Gram's stain, ×5000).

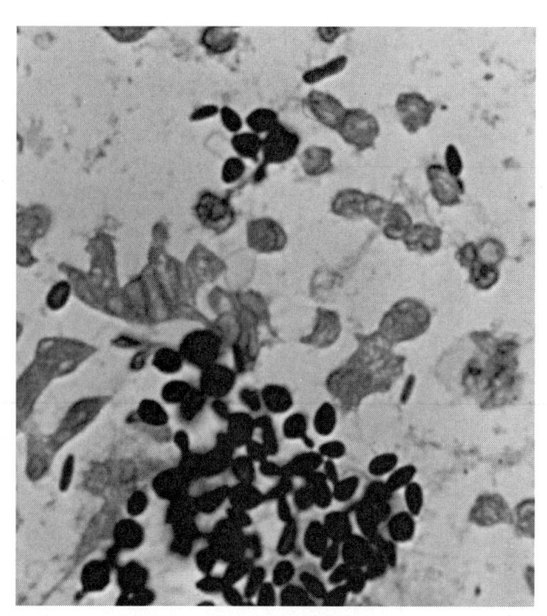

Figure 56–5. *Sporothrix schenckii.* Cutaneous exudate of a cat. Note budding yeasts, oval, rod, and cigar-shaped forms (Gram's stain, ×2000).

A special fungal stain applicable to direct smears is a modified periodic acid–Schiff (PAS), which colors mycotic structures and some other extraneous and tissue components selectively red. This application is beyond the scope of most routine office laboratory work but should be obtainable as a service through any histology laboratory.

Fluorescent microscopy has had some limited application in mycologic diagnosis. Currently, no fluorescent diagnostic reagents are available commercially and no diagnostic services use this approach.

Advances in molecular techniques such as the polymerase chain reaction (PCR) are currently being tested and utilized for special fungi detections. PCR has been especially demonstrated to detect the presence of fungal DNA in laboratory and clinical samples.[6, 9–11, 14, 16, 17]

Histology. Stained sections from biopsy and necropsy specimens often provide critical diagnostic information about mycotic infections. Routine hematoxylin and eosin (H and E) stain permits detection of the tissue phase of dimorphic fungi causing systemic mycoses (coccidioidomycosis, histoplasmosis, blastomycosis, cryptococcosis). With filamentous fungi, it may demonstrate hyphae in tissues, often providing an indication as to their septate or nonseptate nature and thereby helping with their classification. More specific for fungi is the preferred Gomori's methenamine silver,[1] which stains fungal structures brownish-black against a pale green background, and a number of PAS stains, which make mycotic elements appear dark red against a contrasting background, depending on the counterstain. Many laboratories utilize H and E as a counterstain, which permits better pathologic characterization of the lesion than do other procedures.

Isolation

Inoculation of a suitably prepared specimen on any appropriate medium is required. Preparation of specimens may include centrifugation of fluid samples, grinding of biopsy and other tissues, surface sterilization of necropsy specimens by searing, repeated washing of granules from mycetomas

Table 56–2. Isolation Media for Fungi

MEDIUM (COMMERCIAL SOURCE)	SELECTIVE FEATURES	PRINCIPAL USE/LIMITATION IN MYCOLOGIC DIAGNOSIS
Blood agar (Remel Labs, Lenexa, KS)	Highly nutritious for most fungi	General purpose, converts some dimorphic fungi to yeast form; noninhibitory, nonselective, easily overgrown
Potato flake agar (Remel Labs, Lenexa, KS)	Low pH, highly nutritious for most fungi	To induce sporulation of fungi
Inhibitory mold agar (Remel Labs, Lenexa, KS)	Gentamicin and chloramphenicol for bacterial suppression	General purpose; not for dermatophytes
Sabouraud's dextrose agar (Remel Labs, Lenexa, KS; marketed as SAB DUET with DTM in a two-compartment plate by Bacti-lab, Mountain View, CA)	Low pH, modest nutritional quality; addition of chloramphenicol and cycloheximide inhibits bacteria and some fungi	General purpose; added antibiotics for isolation from contaminated environment such as recovery of dermatophytes; cycloheximide inhibits *Cryptococcus, Aspergillus, Scedosporium apiospermum* (*Pseudallescheria boydii*), some *Candida* spp; chloramphenicol inhibits some yeasts
DTM (Remel Labs, Lenexa, KS; Bacti-lab, Mountain View, CA)	Gentamicin, tetracycline, and cycloheximide are inhibitors; glucose and phenol red are indicators	Isolation of dermatophytes, which turn yellow medium to red in 48 hours; not for sporulation; may produce atypical colonial growth; natural pigmentation obscured; nondermatophytes turn yellow medium to red eventually
RSM (marketed as DERM DUET with DTM in a two-compartment plate by Bacti-lab, Mountain View, CA)	Cycloheximide and chloramphenicol are inhibitors; glucose and bromothymol blue are indicators	For dermatophytes, which turn blue medium green early; prompt conidial and pigment development permits identification; color change of RSM not as intense as of DTM with some dermatophytes

DTM = dermatophyte test medium; RSM = rapid sporulation medium.

with saline, or filtration of CSF and blood. Scrapings, swabs, and blood may be inoculated directly without further preparation.

Because many pathogenic fungi, when propagated on agar media, constitute air-borne health hazards, laboratories often prefer tubes and bottles over Petri plates for isolation purposes. If plates are used, they should be secured with oxygen-permeable tape. All examinations of cultures producing aerial mycelium should be carried out in biologic safety cabinets. Most fungi grow on media used routinely in microbiologic diagnosis (Table 56–2). These media should be utilized when the sample is obtained from an uncontaminated site, that is, one that has no resident flora and is not exposed to the external environment such as CNS, internal organ, or joints. Samples originating from cutaneous sources or mucous membranes that harbor such flora are cultured on selective media that may contain broad-spectrum antibacterial and antimycotic agents (see Table 56–2) for the suppression of bacteria and nonpathogenic fungi, respectively. A low pH (≤6.0) of the medium may further limit bacterial overgrowth. Yeasts can be selectively recovered from specimens heavily contaminated with bacteria by propagation on a medium of pH 3.5 to 4.0. Fungal cultures are optimally incubated at 25° to 30°C. Incubation at 37°C allows bacterial overgrowth and causes failure of some fungal pathogens to grow. An atmosphere of 40% to 50% humidity is favorable for most fungi.[7]

The Isolator system (Wampole Laboratories, Cranbury, NJ) has improved the number and rate of fungal isolations from blood.[19] It involves lysis and centrifugation of 10 ml of blood. The supernatant is removed from the upper stopper, and the concentrate is removed from the bottom stopper and plated. The isolation rates of *H. capsulatum* and *C. neoformans* have improved with the Isolator.[19] Broth bottles used for bacterial blood cultures should not be expected to detect fungi other than certain yeasts. Biphasic bottles contain 50 ml of brain-heart infusion broth and brain-heart infusion agar. A biphasic bottle is inoculated with 10 ml of blood, vented, and incubated in an upright position. After daily examination, it is tilted so that the broth floods the agar surface.

Identification

Microscopic morphology of fungal reproductive structures is the most helpful criterion for identification. Other criteria are macroscopic colonial features under different conditions of incubation, nutritional and metabolic properties, antigenic characteristics, and pathogenicity for experimental animals.

Agar cultures are examined daily during the first 2 weeks of incubation and twice weekly thereafter. Allow 4 to 6 weeks for slow-growing fungi. Some common zygomycetes (*Mucor, Rhizopus* spp.) grow rapidly and abundantly, filling a tube or Petri dish within 2 or 3 days. Fruiting bodies may be visible as black specks in the colorless mycelium (Fig. 56–6). Aerial mycelium is grossly less prominent but more intensely pigmented by the presence of fruiting structures with *Aspergillus* (Fig. 56–7) and *Penicillium* spp. (Fig. 56–8). Some fungi produce soluble pigment that diffuses through the medium (e.g., *Microsporum canis*). In others, pigment is confined to parts of the organism and may be best observed either on the surface or on the reverse side of the colony. The colony surface varies according to mycelial growth patterns from smooth ("glabrous") to powdery, velvety, and cottony. Yeasts, which form no or little pseudomycelium, produce mucoid, creamy, pasty, or waxy colonies.

Low-power (25–50×) microscopy helps in early detection of mycelial growth and such diagnostic features as macroconidia and microconidia of dermatophytes (Figs. 56–9, 56–10, 56–11). Once colonial growth is established, identification is based largely on microscopic examination for hyphal charac-

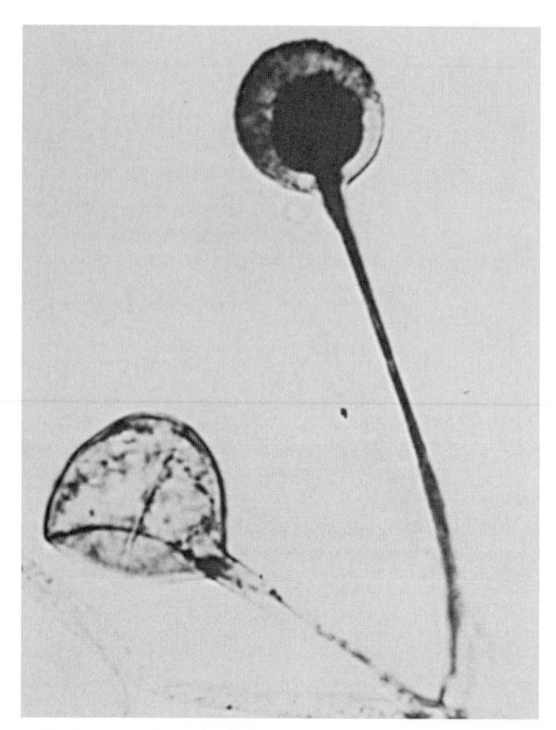

Figure 56–6. *Mucor* in culture. Sporangia form on sporangiophores; note nonseptate, broad hyphae (LPAB, ×2000).

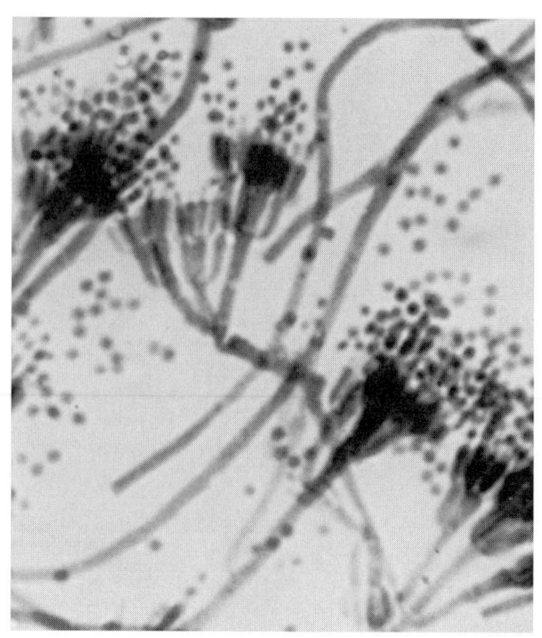

Figure 56–8. *Penicillium.* Fruiting heads give brushlike appearance (LPAB, ×500).

teristics: septate versus nonseptate, pigmented (dematiaceous) (Fig. 56–12) versus nonpigmented (hyaline), and conidia and their supporting structures. This step obviously involves opening of a culture vessel and should be done only by trained, experienced personnel and under conditions in which exposure to people and animals and contamination of the environment can be avoided.

At the in-office laboratory level, it is feasible to make "teased preparations" or transparent adhesive (Scotch) tape lactophenol aniline blue mounts (LPAB, Remel Labs, Lenexa, KS) from mold cultures by using appropriate precautions. Diagnostic features are usually better preserved in their natural interrelationships in Scotch tape mounts (Figs. 56–13 and 56–14). In the absence of a laminar flow hood, such attempts should be restricted to macroscopically positive dermatophyte cultures.

The slide culture procedure probably exceeds the capabilities of most veterinary practices and should be left to clinical laboratories. This procedure permits study of undisturbed fungal structures by using LPAB (Figs. 56–15 and 56–16).

The germ tube test allows rapid differentiation of *C. albicans* (see Chapter 66) from most of the other, usually nonpathogenic, *Candida* spp. Serum, 0.5 to 1 ml, is inoculated lightly with suspect growth and incubated at 35°C for 2 to 3 hours. A drop of the suspension is then examined microscopically (100× and 400×) for the presence of germ tubes

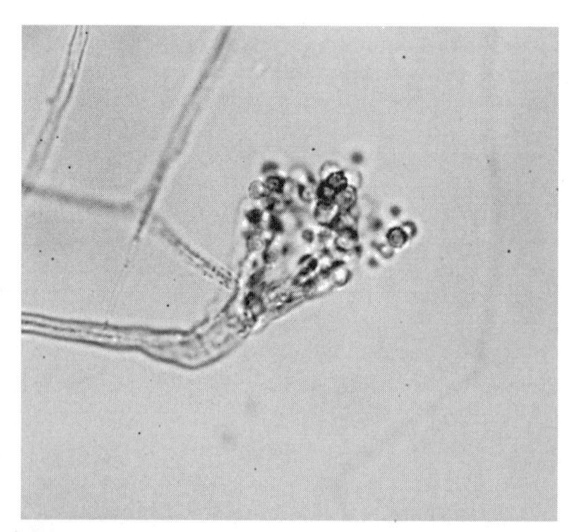

Figure 56–7. *Aspergillus deflectus.* Columnar conidial head resembling a briar pipe and biseriate arrangement of phialides (LPAB, ×500).

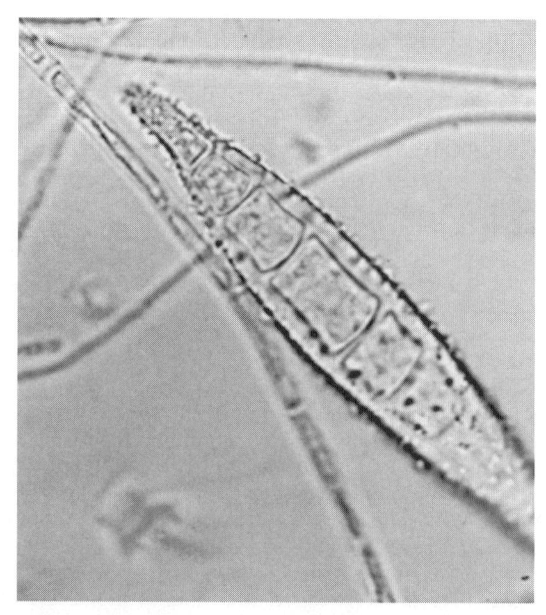

Figure 56–9. *Microsporum canis* in culture. Rough and thick-walled multicellular spindle-shaped macroconidia. Note curved, pointed ends (LPAB, ×2000).

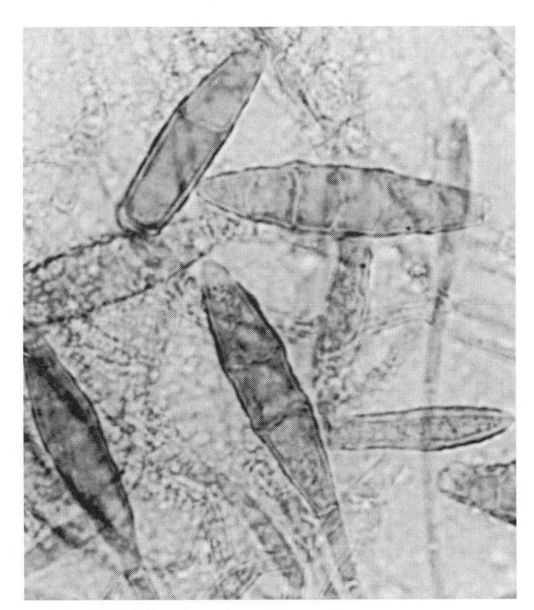

Figure 56–10. *Microsporum gypseum* in culture. Numerous multicellular, fairly thin-walled macroconidia with rounded ends (LPAB, ×2000).

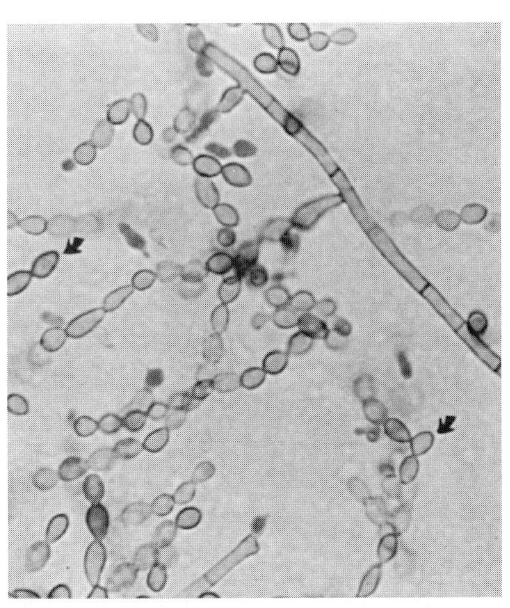

Figure 56–12. *Cladophialophora bantiana* in culture. Oval conidia occurring in chains. Note dematiaceous (dark-pigmented) appearance of some conidia and mycelium *(arrows)* (LPAB, ×2000).

sprouting from yeast cells (blastoconidia) of *C. albicans* (Fig. 56–17).

Commonly used differential media include Czapek agar (Difco, Detroit, MI) for the differentiation of *Aspergillus* spp.; cornmeal agar for the demonstration of chlamydospores in *C. albicans* and their absence in most other *Candida* spp.; Trichophyton agars (Remel Labs, Lenexa, KS) for the identification of *Trichophyton* species by their growth factor needs[8, 18]; Christensen's urea agar (Difco, Detroit, MI) for production of urease by *Cryptococcus, Rhodotorula, Trichophyton,*[8, 18] and *Trichosporon* spp.; and CHROMagar Candida (Hardy Diagnostics, Santa Maria, CA) for culture and identification of *C. albicans, C. krusei, C. tropicalis,* and *Trichosporon* spp.[13]

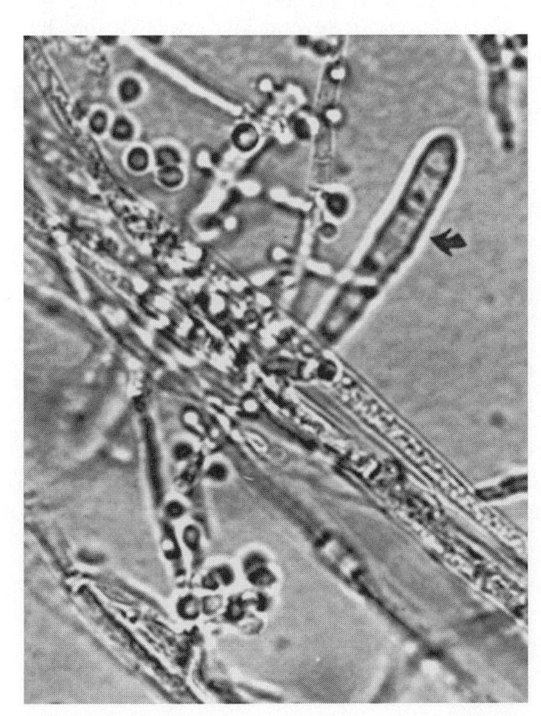

Figure 56–11. *Trichophyton mentagrophytes* in culture. Spherical microconidia and one thin-walled, multicellular, cigar-shaped macroconidium *(arrow)* (LPAB, ×2000).

For definitive identification of the dimorphic fungi *Coccidioides immitis, H. capsulatum,* and *Blastomyces dermatitidis,* antisera are commercially available (ImmunoMycologics, Norman, OK) for use in agar immunodiffusion exoantigen test. The antigen is prepared from an extract of mycelial growth.[12]

Much more rapid and sensitive assays are possible with labeled, single-stranded, species-specific DNA probes to hybridize with DNA or RNA of the target organism.[7] Probes are commercially available (AccuProbe, Gen-Probe Inc., San Diego, CA) for identification of specific dimorphic fungi as identified by the exoantigen method.

Among miniaturized prepackaged identification sets for

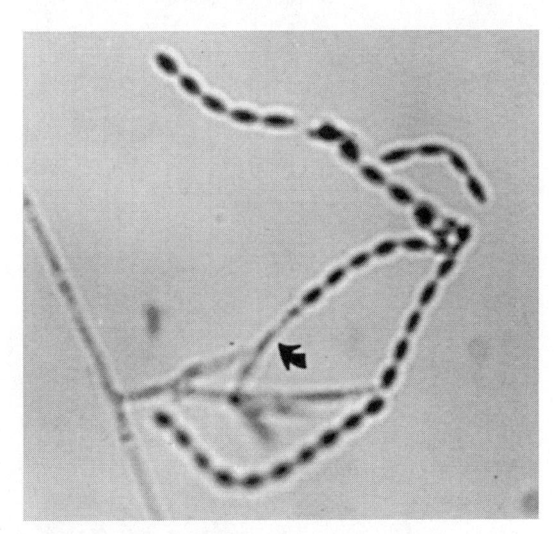

Figure 56–13. *Paecilomyces* in culture. Ovoid chains of conidia attached to a phialide *(arrow)* that is usually tapered (not visible) (LPAB, ×2000).

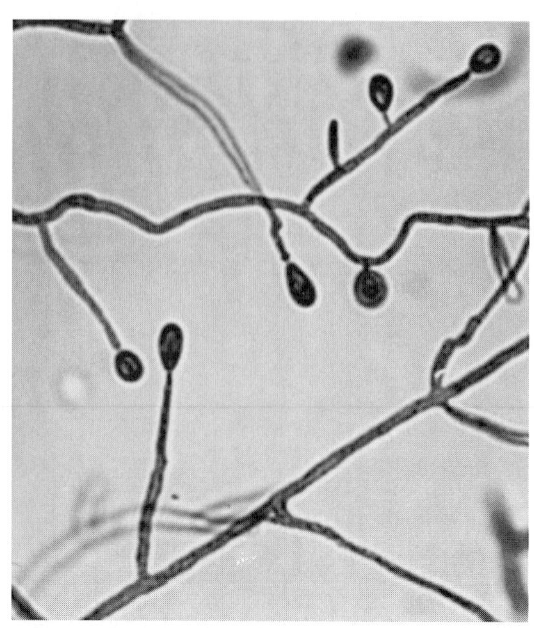

Figure 56–14. *Scedosporium apiospermum* (= asexual stage of *Pseudallescheria boydii*). Single elliptical conidia attached to tips of conidiophores arising along the hyphae (LPAB, ×2000).

yeast and *Prototheca* spp. isolates the API 20C (bioMerieux Vitex, Inc, Hazlewood, MO) and the Uni-yeast-tek system (Remel Labs, Lenexa, KS) are utilized.[3] All rely on tests that are scored to yield a single number, which is listed in a code book and translates into a yeast species. Identification can be completed within 4 hours to several days and more conveniently and generally more rapidly than by conventional methods. Rapid multiple biochemical test systems lack the data base for the more unusual yeasts. Automated systems such as Vitex Yeast biochemical card (bioMerieux Vitex, Inc,

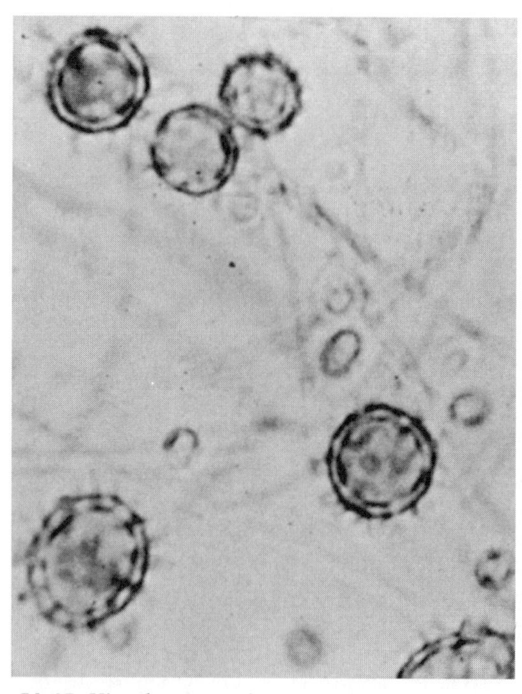

Figure 56–15. *Histoplasma capsulatum* in culture. Tuberculate macroconidia (LPAB, ×2000).

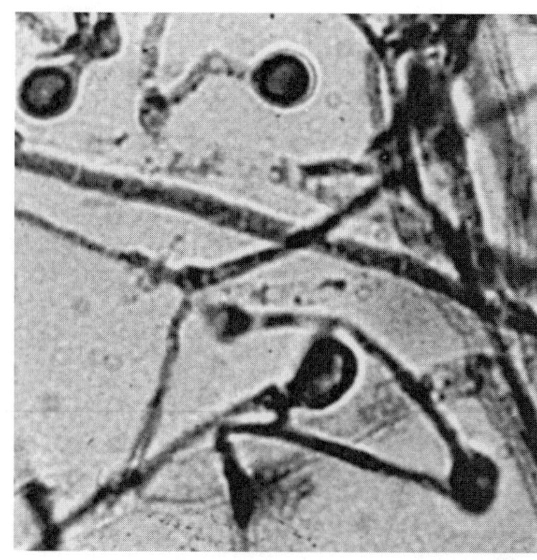

Figure 56–16. *Blastomyces dermatitidis* in culture. One-celled conidia on short conidiophores, "lollypop" appearance (LPAB, ×2000).

Hazlewood, MO) and Microbial Identification System (MIS) (Hewlett-Packard Co., Palo Alto, CA, and Microbial ID, Inc. [MIDI], Newark, DE) require continued expansion and updating of the veterinary data base for improved quality.

Serologic Testing

Reagents designed to detect antigens and antibodies in body fluids are becoming commercially available in increasing numbers. An antigen detection kit, the *Cryptococcus neoformans* latex agglutination test (Meridian Diagnostics, Cincinnati, OH),[1] is one of several kits available that has been adapted for use in office laboratories (see Chapter 61, Table 61–3, and Appendix 6). For a discussion of antibody testing of particular fungal infections, see the respective chapters.

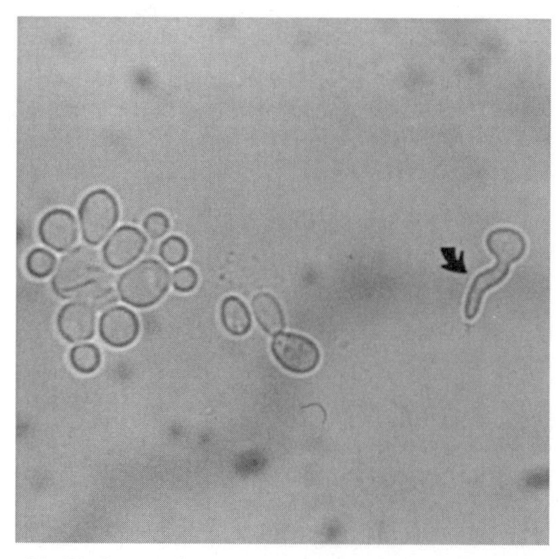

Figure 56–17. Germ tube test. Formation of germ tube *(arrow)* characteristic of *Candida albicans*. Blastoconidia on left. (Wet mount, ×2000.)

References

1. Aslanzadeh J, Roberts GD. 1991. Direct microscopic examination of clinical specimens for the laboratory diagnosis of fungal infections. *Clin Microbiol Newslett* 13(24):185–188.
2. Barenfanger J. 1990. Identification of yeast and other fungi from direct microscopic examination of clinical specimens. *Clin Microbiol Newslett* 12(2):9–15.
3. Fenn JP, Segal H, Barland B, et al. 1994. Comparison of updated Vitek yeast biochemical card and API 20C yeast identification systems. *J Clin Microbiol* 32(5):1184–1187.

3a. Hawkins EC, DeNicola DB. 1990. Cytologic analysis of tracheal wash specimens and bronchoalveolar lavage fluid in the diagnosis of mycotic infections in dogs. *J Am Vet Med Assoc* 197:79–83.

4. Hazen KC. 1995. New and emerging yeast pathogens. *Clin Microbiol Rev* 8(4):462–478.
5. Jang SS, Biberstein EL. 1990. Laboratory diagnosis of fungal and algal infections, pp 639–648. *In* Greene CE (ed), Infectious diseases of the dog and cat. WB Saunders, Philadelphia, PA.
6. Jordan JA. 1994. PCR identification of four medically important *Candida* species using a single primer pair. *J Clin Microbiol* 32(12):2962–2967.
7. Kwon-Chun KJ, Bennett JE. 1992. Laboratory diagnosis medical mycology. Lea & Febiger, Malvern, PA.
8. Larone DH. 1996. Culture and identification of dermatophytes. *Clin Microbiol Newslett* 18(5):33–38.
9. Maiwald M, Kappe R, Sonntag HG. 1994. Rapid presumptive identification of medically relevant yeasts to the species level by polymerase chain reaction and restriction enzyme analysis. *J Med Vet Mycol* 32:115–122.
10. Melchers WJG, Verweij PE, van DenHurk P, et al. 1994. General primer-mediated PCR for detection of *Aspergillus* species. *J Clin Microbiol* 32(7):1710–1717.
11. Mitchell TG, Freedman EZ, White TD, et al. 1994. Unique oligonucleotide primers in PCR identification of *Cryptococcus neoformans*. *J Clin Microbiol* 32(1):253–255.
12. Murray PR, Baron EJ, Pfaller MA, et al. 1995. Manual of clinical microbiology, ed 6. American Society for Microbiology Press, Washington, DC.
13. Odds FC, Bernaerts R. 1994. CHROMagar *Candida*, a new differential isolation medium for presumptive identification of clinically important *Candida* species. *J Clin Microbiol* 32(8):1923–1928.
14. Rath PM, Marggraf G, Dermoumi H, et al. 1995. Use of phenotypic and genotypic fingerprinting methods in the strain identification of *Aspergillus fumigatus*. *Mycoses* 38:429–434.
15. Roberts GD, Pfaller MA, Gueho E, et al. 1992. Developments in the diagnostic mycology laboratory. *J Med Vet Mycol* 30(1):241–248.
16. Spreadbury C, Holden D, Aufauvre-Brown A. 1993. Detection of *Aspergillus fumigatus* by polymerase chain reaction. *J Clin Microbiol* 31(3):615–621.
17. Walsh TJ, Francesconi A, Kasai M, et al. 1995. PCR and single stranded conformational polymorphism for recognition of medically important opportunistic fungi. *J Clin Microbiol* 33(12):3216–3220.
18. Weitzman I, Summerbell RC. 1995. The dermatophytes. *Clin Microbiol Rev* 8(2):240–259.
19. Witebsky FG, Gill VJ. 1995. Fungal blood culture systems: which ones and when to use them. *Clin Microbiol Newslett* 17(21):161–164.

Chapter 57

Antifungal Chemotherapy

Craig E. Greene and A. D. J. Watson

SYSTEMIC ANTIFUNGALS

Table 57–1 lists various systemic antifungal drugs and the circumstances for their use. Chapters 58 to 69 provide information on their applications in specific diseases and details on the dosage and usage are given in the Drug Formulary (Appendix 8).

Griseofulvin

This orally administered antifungal drug is produced by *Penicillium griseofulvum*. Absorption from the GI tract is facilitated by addition of fat to the diet. The drug has also been improved by production of microsized and ultramicrosized formulations. Griseofulvin is effective against infections caused by dermatophytes but not yeasts.

Griseofulvin is deposited in the epidermal layers of the skin and dermal appendages as they are formed. Several weeks of therapy are required for complete drug distribution throughout cell layers and for inhibition of fungal growth. Resistance rarely develops during therapy.

Iodides

A solution of 20% sodium iodide or 100% potassium iodide has been given orally to treat cutaneous sporotrichosis (Chapter 63). The mechanism of action of the iodides is uncertain because they are not directly toxic to *Sporothrix* in vitro. Iodides are all less toxic than amphotericin B (AMB), which should be reserved for second choice or for disseminated disease. Iodism, manifested clinically as dermal eruption with hair loss, may occur as a result of therapy.

Amphotericin B and Other Polyenes

AMB is a lipophilic polyene isolated from *Streptomyces nodosus* that binds to sterols in cell membranes of eukaryotic organisms and causes increased permeability and leakage of nutrients and electrolytes. Nystatin is another polyene applied topically (see Topical Antifungals). AMB has greater binding affinity for ergosterol, the major sterol of fungal cell membranes, than for cholesterol, which is present in mammalian host cells. Because it is poorly absorbed across the GI mucosa or skin, AMB must be given parenterally (usually IV) for the treatment of systemic mycoses. Most of the drug is metabolized locally at tissue sites, and lesser amounts are excreted in the urine. Standard IV preparations contain lyophilized AMB combined with deoxycholate and buffer in a colloidal state (ABD). ABD has been diluted and given SC, which appears to delay its absorption and reduce its nephrotoxicity, allowing larger amounts of the drug to be given.[31] Lipid-based formulations are now available with lower toxicity (Table 57–2); however, merely giving ABD in

Table 57–1. Systemically Used Antifungal Drugs[a]

GENERIC NAME (TRADE NAME)	ROUTE OF ADMINISTRATION	CLINICAL FORMULATION	INDICATIONS	
			First	Alternate
Griseofulvin (Fulvicin, Grisactin)	PO	Capsules, tablets, suspension	Dermatophytosis	None
Sodium or potassium iodide	PO	Solution (20% NaI–100% KI)	Sporotrichosis	None
Amphotericin B[b] (Fungizone, AmBisome, Amphocil, Abelcet)	IV, SC	See Table 57–2	Rapidly progressive or severe systemic mycosis, systemic aspergillosis, or sporotrichosis mucormycosis	Imidazole-resistant cryptococcosis or other systemic mycosis
Flucytosine (Ancobon)	PO	Capsules (250, 500 mg)	Cryptococcosis in combination with amphotericin B	Systemic candidiasis
Miconazole (Monistat i.v.)	IV	Ampules (10 mg/ml in 20 ml)	Systemic mycosis	None
Ketoconazole (Nizoral)	PO	Tablets (200 mg)	Systemic mycosis in dogs, systemic aspergillosis, miscellaneous fungal infections	Adjunctive with enilconazole in resistant aspergillosis, systemic mycosis in cats, dermatophytosis
Itraconazole (Sporanox)	PO	Capsules (100 mg) Oral suspension (100 mg/10 ml)	Cutaneous sporotrichosis, systemic mycosis in cats and small dogs, miscellaneous fungal infections, malasseziosis	Adjunct with nasal aspergillosis, systemic mycoses if funds available, dermatophytosis
Fluconazole (Diflucan)	PO, IV	Capsules (50, 100, 150, 200 mg) Oral suspension (10 or 40 mg/ml in 35 ml) IV solution (2 mg/ml in 50 or 100 ml)	CNS, meningeal or ocular systemic mycosis	Systemic mycosis in cats, candidiasis

[a]For additional information on drugs and dosages, see Drug Formulary, Appendix 8.
[b]See Table 57–2.

a fat emulsion did not alter nephrotoxicity.[42] In contrast, commercially prepared lipid-encapsulated formulations are taken up well into organs of the mononuclear phagocyte system where the organism resides; they have relatively low accumulation in the kidneys.[25] Lipid-based formulations can be given at a higher dose and may be effective in treating resistant or unresponsive mycoses. Occasionally, the drug is used for topical therapy of mycotic disease. See the Drug Formulary (Appendix 8) about the various preparations and for specific information regarding its use.

The fungal organisms affected by AMB are listed in Table 57–1. Zygomycetes (Mucoraceae) are variably susceptible, and *Aspergillus* is usually resistant. Lipid-based formulations are more effective against zygomycosis and fusariosis, and they should be the first choice for these diseases.[19a]

AMB had been the first line of therapy for rapidly progressive or disseminated deep mycotic infections. Resistance rarely, if ever, develops during treatment, but relapses may occur when the drug is discontinued. Oral azoles such as ketoconazole (KTZ), itraconazole (ITZ), and fluconazole (FCZ) have become alternatives for treatment of uncomplicated systemic mycoses.

Hamycin is another polyene that has efficacy against *Candida*, *Cryptococcus*, *Histoplasma*, *Blastomyces*, and *Aspergillus*. It has been given orally, topically, and intraperitoneally to treat various mycotic conditions although with toxicity. A dog

Table 57–2. Comparison of Clinical Formulations of Amphotericin B (AMB)[a]

ABBREVIATION	FORMULATION	BRAND NAME: MANUFACTURER	DIAMETER	COMPOSITION	RATIO	LD_{50} (MURINE)
ABD	Deoxycholate	Fungizone: Squibb	≥ 300 nm	Detergent deoxycholate/buffer/AMB	0.8/0.5/1	3
L-AMB[1]	Liposome encapsulated	AmBisome: Nexstar, San Dimas, CA	55–75 nm	Hydrogenated soy phosphatidylcholine/cholesterol/distearoylphosphatidylglycerol/AMB	2/1/0.8/0.4	175
ABCD[11, 13]	Colloidal dispersion, lipid disk particle	Amphocil: Sequus, Menlo Park, CA	~115 nm	Cholesterylsulfate/AMB	1/1	38
ABLC[21]	Lipid complex, ribbon shape	Abelcet: Liposome Co., Princeton, NJ	2000–11,000 nm	Dimyristoylphosphatidylcholine/dimyristoylphosphatidylglycerol/AMB	7/3/10	40

[a]For additional information, see Drug Formulary, Appendix 8.

with disseminated aspergillosis was treated with some success.[24] Liposomal encapsulation of this drug has been associated with increased efficacy and reduced toxicity.[37]

Flucytosine

Flucytosine or 5-fluorocytosine (FCY) is a fluorinated pyrimidine originally synthesized as an antineoplastic agent. It interferes with pyrimidine metabolism and resultant DNA synthesis in yeasts.

FCY is effective against *Cryptococcus*, *Candida*, and other yeasts but has little or no effect on other deep mycotic agents or on *Aspergillus*. Localized candidiasis or cryptococcal infections respond best, but resistance to FCY frequently develops during therapy. For this reason, the drug is always given in combination with AMB. Skin eruption, similar to that with azoles, has been observed in treated dogs.[33]

Azole Derivatives

Synthetic imidazole derivatives were originally produced as broad-spectrum anthelmintics with activity against some gram-positive bacteria and protozoa. Like AMB, they inhibit sterol synthesis as one of their main effects, but they are generally less toxic. They also inhibit nucleic acid, triglyceride, and fatty acid synthesis and alter oxidative enzyme biochemistry. At low concentrations they are fungistatic, and at higher concentrations, which cannot be achieved systemically, they are fungicidal. Thiabendazole was initially recognized as being effective in treating human dermatophytoses. Miconazole, clotrimazole, and enilconazole are available in creams and lotions and can be formulated into solutions for the topical treatment of fungal infections of the skin, such as dermatophytosis and candidiasis (see Topical Antifungals and Drug Formulary, Appendix 8). However, oral therapy with an azole, griseofulvin or terbinafine, is needed for nail infections. The orally administered azoles are becoming widely used in human and veterinary medicine to treat systemic and opportunistic fungal infections. In vitro susceptibility testing of the drugs shows variable efficacy against different fungi, but in vitro does not always parallel in vivo efficacy. Azole derivatives are discussed here under systemic therapy or under topical antifungal therapy on the basis of their respective uses.

Miconazole. It is partially absorbed after oral administration and is effective when given parenterally; thus, it is more valuable than clotrimazole for treating systemic fungal infections. The drug penetrates joint and ocular fluids and CSF at variable rates. It is primarily metabolized by the liver and, with metabolites, excreted in the urine. It is rarely administered systemically now because less toxic and more potent oral azoles are available. Miconazole is now used topically to treat dermatophyte and yeast infections.

Ketoconazole. This drug is less active than miconazole but better absorbed from the GI tract, making it convenient for the treatment of systemic mycoses and chronic mucocutaneous candidiasis. Absorption is improved in acid media; therefore, antacids and H_2-receptor antihistamine antagonists should not be given concurrently. The drug is predominantly bound to plasma albumin, entering all tissues and body fluids in therapeutic concentrations with the exception of seminal, CNS, and ocular locations. The drug is distributed throughout the skin and subcutaneous tissues. Owing to this observed beneficial effect, it has been used in treating superficial fungal infections of the skin and hair. Metabolites of the drug, produced in the liver, lack antifungal activity.

Occasional nausea, partial anorexia, and vomiting in dogs can be overcome if the drug is given with meals and by dividing the daily dose into three or four administrations. Additional side effects of KTZ are similar to those of other azoles. Frequently, reversible subclinical increases in activities of hepatic transaminases and alkaline phosphatase (ALP) in blood occur as manifestations of hepatotoxicity. Less commonly, clinical hepatitis develops, and if treatment continues or dosages are high enough, it may be fatal. Histologic findings in affected animals include enlarged portal tracts, bile duct proliferation, and infiltration with mononuclear cells. KTZ may produce endocrine dysfunction by suppressing testosterone and cortisol synthesis.

KTZ is most effective in vitro against yeast and dimorphic fungi, such as *Candida*, *Malassezia*, *Coccidioides*, *Histoplasma*, and *Blastomyces*, and is less effective against *Cryptococcus*, *Sporothrix*, and *Aspergillus*. Evidence suggests that in rapidly progressing systemic mycoses, such as many cases of blastomycosis, patients should first be treated with AMB and then maintained on KTZ (see Amphotericin B and Other Polyenes). The action of KTZ alone often occurs so slowly (5–10 days) that the disease progresses before the drug has a chance to take effect. In contrast, KTZ has been given alone in dogs and cats to successfully treat coccidioidomycosis and some cases of histoplasmosis and cryptococcosis, although relapses are common when host defenses are inadequate. Preference for more active and generally less toxic ITZ or FCZ has been apparent for treatment of these infections. Where underlying immunosuppression is thought to be responsible for the fungal disease, concurrent treatment with AMB is recommended. There is no evidence that KTZ provides synergistic effects with other antifungals except AMB, and even that evidence is inconclusive. For dosing and detailed information on administration, see Drug Formulary, Appendix 8, and Chapters 58 to 69.

Unfortunately, as noted with many of the other antifungal drugs, eradication of systemic fungi with azole drugs is often incomplete. Relapses can occur when maintenance therapy is discontinued. Infections in areas where the drug cannot easily reach, such as bone and CNS, are especially difficult to treat. Therapy should always continue at least 4 weeks after disease is no longer detectable clinically.

ITZ. This broad-spectrum azole has more potent activity than KTZ against *Candida*, *Aspergillus*, and dermatophytes. It can be given orally or parenterally; it is widely distributed in body tissues with the exception of the CNS. The best success in treating human patients has been with (in decreasing order) paracoccidioidomycosis, blastomycosis, sporotrichosis, noninvasive aspergillosis, meningeal cryptococcosis, and aspergilloma. Some patients with zygomycosis or other fungal infections also respond to ITZ treatment. In small animal practice, it has been most effective in treating blastomycosis (Chapter 59), histoplasmosis (Chapter 60), cryptococcosis (Chapter 61), and coccidioidomycosis (Chapter 62). Toxicity appears less than that with KTZ, probably because ITZ more selectively inhibits fungal rather than mammalian enzymes. Higher dosages should be expected to cause similar side effects as those of KTZ. Dosage adjustments do not appear to be necessary in the presence of renal dysfunction. Bioavailability after oral administration is erratic; however, it can be maximized by giving ITZ with a full meal. An oral solution improves absorption (see Drug Formulary, Appendix 8).[3a]

FCZ. This orally active agent has been used to treat systemic mycoses, including cryptococcal meningitis, blastomycosis, and histoplasmosis and for superficial infections, including candidiasis and dermatophytosis. FCZ crosses the blood-brain and blood-CSF barriers better than the other azole derivatives. It also is water soluble, is well absorbed orally, and has a long half-life, making it potentially valuable for treating susceptible fungal infections. Toxicity appears to be less than that of KTZ. It has poor activity against *Aspergillus* species.

Other azoles. Vibunazole is a derivative with oral and topical activity. Its activity is most impressive in treating aspergillosis after oral administration. ICI 195,739 is an investigational compound with more potent activity than any of the currently available drugs. It readily penetrates fungal cell walls. In animal experiments it has been effective in treating superficial and systemic mycotic and some protozoal infections.

Terbinafine

An antifungal allylamine derivative has been extremely effective for treating people with chronic dermatophytosis of the nails. A dosage of 250 mg daily has been used for 6 and 12 months for finger and toe nail infections, respectively. Improvement or resolution usually occurs by 3 to 6 months of therapy. Side effects have been minimal. This drug would have potential value for the treatment of canine and feline onychomycosis.

Chitin Synthesis Inhibitors

Newer compounds that are being investigated as systemic antifungals are the polyoxins and nikkomycins. These are inhibitors of chitin synthesis in the fungal cell walls. In vitro studies have shown marked efficacy against *Coccidioides* and *Blastomyces* with lesser activity against *Candida* and *Cryptococcus*. Filamentous fungi seem more resistant. Lufenuron, a chitin synthesis inhibitor used to control fleas, has been effective in the treatment of coccidioidomycosis (see Chapter 62 and Drug Formulary, Appendix 8).[2] Inhibitors of fungal glucan synthesis, including aculeacins, echinocandins, and papulacandins are also being investigated.[57] One promising fungal cell wall inhibitor is cilofungin, a lipopeptide derivative effective against systemic candidiasis and *Aspergillus* in laboratory animals when given by continuous IV infusions. The benanomicins and pradimicins damage the mannan component of fungal cell wall by calcium chelation, but their present limitation is poor oral bioavailability.

Table 57–3. Agents Commonly Used Topically Against Fungi and Yeasts

GENERIC NAME	CLINICAL FORMULATION (% ACTIVITY)	SUSCEPTIBLE ORGANISMS (MOST TO LEAST)	COMMENTS AND RECOMMENDATIONS FOR VETERINARY USAGE
Miscellaneous			
Mercaptans	Captan Technical grade powder (45%)	Dermatophytes	Not recommended, toxic, carcinogenic, ineffective
Chlorhexidine	Nolvasan[a], Chlorhexiderm[a, b] Solution (1%), shampoo (0.5%)	Dermatophytes	Poor efficacy
Tolnaftate	Tinactin[c] Cream, powder, solution, aerosol liquid (1%)	Dermatophytes	Spot treatment: animals can ingest, bitter taste
Undecylenic acid and salts	Powder, ointment, cream, 2–10% soap, liquid, foam[c]	Dermatophytes	Spot treatment: animals can ingest, bitter taste
Halprogin	Halotex[d] Cream, solution (1%)	Dermatophytes, *Malassezia*	Spot treatment, ear medicant
Lime sulfur	Lymdyp[b]	Dermatophytes	Odor, stains hair, good for dermatophytosis, very safe in puppies and kittens, stains jewelry
Ciclopirox olamine	Loprox[e] Cream, lotion (1%)	*Malassezia*, dermatophytes, *Candida*	Spot treatment only
Naftifine hydrochloride	Naftin[f] Cream, gel (1%)	Dermatophytes	Spot treatment
Polyenes			
Amphotericin B	Fungizone[h] Cream, lotion, ointment (3%)	*Candida*	Limited use as irrigant for affected mucosal tissues
Nystatin	Mycostatin[c] Ointment, cream, or powder (10^5 μg); suspension (10^5 U/ml); tablets 5×10^5 U	*Candida*, dermatophytes, variable *Aspergillus*	Limited as irrigant for affected mucosal tissues
Imidazoles			
Thiabendazole	Solution (13%)	Dermatophytes, *Candida*, *Aspergillus*	Third choice for nasal aspergillosis
Ketoconazole	Nizoral[i] Cream, shampoo, solution (2%)	Dermatophytes, *Malassezia*	Poor efficacy in dermatophytosis
Econazole nitrate	Spectazole[j] Cream, spray, powder (1%)	Dermatophytes, *Candida*	Spot treatment, may need to treat whole animal
Miconazole nitrate	Micatin[j] Powder, shampoo, cream, lotion (2%)	Dermatophytes, *Candida*, *Malassezia*, *Leishmania*	Spot treatment, shampoo efficacy undocumented
Clotrimazole	Lotrimin, Mycelex[c] Cream, lotion, solution (1%)	Dermatophytes, *Candida*, *Aspergillus*	First choice for nasal aspergillosis
Enilconazole	Imaverol[i] Solution (10%)	Dermatophytes, *Aspergillus*	Second choice for canine nasal aspergillosis, toxic to cats

[a] Fort Dodge. [b] DVM Pharmaceuticals. [c] Various, over the counter. [d] Westwood Squibb. [e] Hoechst. [f] Allergan. [g] Herbert. [h] E-R Squibb. [i] Janssen. [j] Ortho.

Combination Therapy

Simultaneous administration of antifungal agents is indicated under selected circumstances. Combined use of AMB and FCY is beneficial in treating cryptococcal infections; presumably AMB facilitates penetration of FCY into the fungal cell. Synergism has also been subjectively assessed in the treatment of blastomycosis, coccidioidomycosis, and histoplasmosis by combining AMB and azole derivatives.

TOPICAL ANTIFUNGALS

Many formulations are used in the treatment of dermatophytosis and superficial yeast infections (Table 57–3). See also Dermatophytosis, Chapter 58. Undecylenic acid is an unsaturated fatty acid given in combination with zinc to treat dermatophytosis. Its mechanism of action is unknown. Mercaptans, organic mercurial compounds, have been utilized as plant fungicides and can be applied as a dilute dip for affected animals at low cost. Tolnaftate, a synthetic lipid-soluble compound, has also been used; hyperkeratotic plaques must be removed before its application to ensure its effectiveness. Topical cuprimyxin, a copper-containing compound, is highly effective against *Malassezia*. Iodochlorhydroxyquin is a halogenated oxyquinoline that has been given orally as an antifungal, antiprotozoal, and antibacterial agent in dogs. Overdosages have caused CNS toxicity. Chlorhexidine solution (0.5%) has been recommended as a daily dip or shampoo for persistent dermatophyte infections, although its efficacy is poor.[10, 56] Haloprogin is a broad-spectrum topical antifungal drug that may be more helpful against dermatophyte and *Candida* infections.

Nystatin is a polyene antibiotic, closely related to AMB, that is produced by *Streptomyces noursei*. It is poorly absorbed after oral administration or topical application to skin or mucous membranes. Because it is very toxic to internal tissues, parenteral administration must be avoided. Although nystatin is somewhat effective against dermatophytes and *Aspergillus*, its primary use has been to treat candidiasis.

The azole derivatives are discussed with the systemic antifungal drugs. Thiabendazole (13%) has been used as a three-times-weekly dip for 3 weeks to treat cats with dermatophytosis. Clotrimazole is very effective against yeasts, dermatophytes, and *Aspergillus*. Because of its limited absorption, severe GI irritative effect, and systemic toxicity, it has been confined to topical application (see Chapter 65 and Drug Formulary, Appendix 8).[6] It was more effective than miconazole in treating dermatophytosis in dogs and cats when applied as a 1% solution twice daily for 2 weeks. Enilconazole is a topically applied derivative that has been valuable in the treatment of nasal aspergillosis (see Chapter 65 and Drug Formulary, Appendix 8). Several other topical azole preparations from human medicine are listed in Table 57–3.

References

1. Adler-Moore JP, Proffitt RT. 1993. Development, characterization, efficacy, and mode of action of AmBioSome, a unilamellar liposomal-formulation of amphotericin B. *J Lipsome Res* 3:376–381.
2. Bartsch R, Greene R. 1997. New treatment of coccidioidomycosis. *Vet Forum* April 25:50–52.
3. Bekersky I, Puhl RJ, Hanson G, et al. 1994. The pharmacokinetics of DMP lactate, a new agent against opportunistic infections in male beagle dogs. *Drug Metab Dispos* 22:233–236.

3a. Bernard EM, Armstrong D. 1997. Treatment of opportunistic fungal infections: Clinical overview and perspective. *Int J Infect Dis* 1(suppl 1):528–531.

3b. Boothe DA, Herring I, Calvin J, et al. 1997. Itraconazole disposition after single oral and intravenous and multiple dosing in healthy cats. *Am J Vet Res* 58:872–877.

4. Brooks DE, Legendre AM, Gum GG, et al. 1991. The treatment of canine ocular blastomycosis with systemically administered itraconazole. *Prog Vet Comp Ophthalmol* 1:263–268.
5. Cohn MS. 1992. Superficial fungal infections. *Postgrad Med* 91:239–252.
6. Conte L, Ramis J, Mis R, et al. 1992. Pharmacokinetic study of [14C] flutrimazole after oral and intravenous administration in dogs. *Arzneimforsch/Drug Res* 42:854–858.
7. Craig AJ, Ramzan I, Malik R. 1994. Pharmacokinetics of fluconazole in cats after intravenous and oral administration. *Res Vet Sci* 57:372–376.
8. Davies C, Troy GC. 1996. Deep mycotic infections in cat. *J Am Anim Hosp Assoc* 32:380–391.
9. DeBoer DJ, Moriella KA. 1995. Inability of two topical treatments to influence the course of experimentally induced dermatophytosis in cats. *J Am Vet Med Assoc* 207:52–57.
10. DeBoer DJ, Moriello KA, Cairns R. 1995. Clinical update on feline dermatophytosis: part II. *Compend Cont Educ Pract Vet* 17:1471–1480.
11. Fielding RM, Singer AW, Wang LH. 1992. Relationship of pharmacokinetics and drug distribution in tissue to increased safety of amphotericin B colloidal dispersion in dogs. *Antimicrob Agents Chemother* 36:299–307.
12. Fielding RM, Smith PC, Wang LH, et al. 1991. Comparative pharmacokinetics of amphotericin B after administration of a novel colloidal delivery system, ABCD, and a conventional formulation to rats. *Antimicrob Agents Chemother* 35:1208–1213.
13. Goulden V, Goodfield MJD. 1995. Treatment of childhood dermatophyte infections with oral terbinafine. *Pediatr Dermatol* 12:53–54.
14. Graybill JR, Stevens DA, Galgani N, et al. 1990. Itraconazole treatment of coccidioidomycosis. *Am J Med* 89:282–290.
15. Greene CE. 1990. Antifungal chemotherapy, pp 649–658. *In* Greene CE (ed), Infectious diseases of the dog and cat. WB Saunders, Philadelphia, PA.
16. Greene RT, Troy GC. 1995. Coccidioidomycosis in 48 cats: a retrospective study (1984–1993). *J Vet Intern Med* 9:86–91.

16a. Guillot J, Chermette R. 1997. The treatment of mycoses in carnivores. *Point Veterinaire* 28:51–61.

17. Guo LS, Fielding RM, Mufson D. 1991. Pharmacokinetic study of a novel amphotericin B colloidal dispersion with improved therapeutic index. *Ann N Y Acad Sci* 618:586–588.
18. Heit MC, Riviere JE. 1995. Antifungal therapy: ketoconazole and other azole derivatives. *Compend Cont Educ Pract Vet* 17:21–31.
19. Herbrecht R. 1996. The changing epidemiology of fungal infections: are the lipid-based forms of amphotericin B an advance? *Eur J Haematol* 56:12–17.

19a. Herbrecht R, Letscher V, Kurtz JE, et al. 1997. Amphotericin B lipid complex in the management of emerging fungal pathogens. *Int J Infect Dis* 1(suppl 1):542–546.

20. Hodges RD, Legendre AM, Adams LG, et al. 1994. Itraconazole for the treatment of histoplasmosis in cats. *J Vet Intern Med* 8:409–413.

20a. Jankegt R, deMarie S, Bakker-Woudenberg I, et al. 1992. Liposomal and lipid formulations of amphotericin B. *Clin Pharmacokinet* 23:279–291.

21. Janoff AS, Perkins WR, Saletan SL, et al. 1993. Amphotericin B lipid complex (ABLC) a molecular rationale for the attenuation of amphotericin B related toxicities. *J Liposome Res* 3:451–471.
22. Jezequel SG. 1994. Fluconazole: interspecies scaling and allometric relationships of pharmacokinetic properties. *J Pharm Pharmacol* 46:196–199.
23. Jones TC. 1995. Overview of the use of terbinafine (Lamisil®) in children. *Br J Dermatol* 132:683–689.
24. Kaufman AC, Greene CE, Selcer BA, et al. 1994. Systemic aspergillosis in a dog and treatment with hamycin. *J Am Anim Hosp Assoc* 30:132–136.
25. Krawiec DR, McKiernan BC, Twardock AR, et al. 1996. Use of amphotericin B lipid complex for treatment of blastomycosis in dogs. *J Am Vet Med Assoc* 209:2073–2075.
26. Kumar B, Kaur I, Chakrabarti A, et al. 1991. Treatment of deep mycoses with itraconazole. *Mycopathologia* 115:169–174.
27. Lanthier T, Chaliforex A. 1991. Enilconazole as an adjunct to the treatment of four cases of canine nasal aspergillosis. *Can Vet J* 32:110–112.
28. Leenders AC, de Marie S. 1996. The use of lipid formulations of amphotericin B for systemic fungal infections. *Leukemia* 10:1570–1575.
29. Leitner MI, Meingassner JG. 1994. The efficacy of orally applied terbinafine, itraconazole and fluconazole in models of experimental trichophytoses. *J Med Vet Mycol* 32:181–188.
30. Levy JK. 1991. Ataxia in a kitten treated with griseofulvin. *J Am Vet Med Assoc* 198:105–106.
31. Malik R, Craig AJ, Wigney DI, et al. 1996. Combination chemotherapy of canine and feline cryptococcosis using subcutaneously administered amphotericin B. *Aust Vet J* 73:124–128.
32. Malik R, Dill-Macky E, Martin P, et al. 1995. Cryptococcosis in dogs: a retrospective study of 20 consecutive cases. *J Med Vet Mycol* 33:291–297.
33. Malik R, Medeiros C, Wigney DI. 1996. Suspected drug eruption in 7 dogs during administration of flucytosine. *Aust Vet J* 74:285–288.
34. Malik R, Wigney DI, Muir DB, et al. 1992. Cryptococcosis in cats: clinical and mycological assessment of 29 cases and evaluation of treatment using orally administered fluconazole. *J Med Vet Mycol* 30:133–134.
35. Medleau L, Greene CE, Rakich PM. 1990. Evaluation of ketoconazole and

itraconazole for treatment of disseminated cryptococcosis in cats. *Am J Vet Res* 51:1454–1458.
36. Medleau L, Jacobs GJ, Marks MA. 1995. Itraconazole for the treatment of cryptococcosis in cats. *J Vet Intern Med* 9:39–42.
37. Mehta RT, McQueen TJ, Keyhani A, et al. 1991. Liposomal hamycin: reduced toxicity and improved antifungal efficacy in vitro and in vivo. *J Infect Dis* 164:1003–1006.
38. Moriello KA, DeBoer DJ. 1995. Efficacy griseofulvin and itraconazole in the treatment of experimentally induced dermatophytosis in cats. *J Am Vet Med Assoc* 207:439–444.
39. Nichols AJ, Koster PF, Brooks DP, et al. 1992. Effect of fenoldopam on the acute and subacute nephrotoxicity produced by amphotericin B in the dog. *J Pharmacol Exp Ther* 260:269–274.
39a. Oliva G, Gradoni L, Ciaramella P, et al. 1995. Activity of liposomal amphotericin B (AmBiosome) in dogs naturally infected with *Leishmania infantum*. *J Antimicrob Chemother* 36:1013–1019.
40. Oppenheim BA, Herbrecht R, Kusne S. 1995. The safety and efficacy of amphotericin B colloidal dispersion in the treatment of invasive mycoses. *Clin Infect Dis* 21:1145–1153.
41. Plotnick AN, Boshoven EW, Rosychuk RA, et al. 1997. Primary cutaneous coccidioidomycosis and subsequent drug eruption to itraconazole in a dog. *J Am Anim Hosp Assoc* 33:139–143.
42. Randall SR, Adams LG, White MR, et al. 1996. Nephrotoxicity of amphotericin B administered to dogs in a fat emulsion versus five percent dextrose solution. *Am J Vet Res* 57:1054–1058.
43. Rubin SI, Krawiec DR, Gelberg H, et al. 1989. Nephrotoxicity of amphotericin B in dogs, a comparison of two methods of administration. *Can J Vet Res* 53:23–28.
44. Sharkey PK, Rinaldi MG, Dunn JF, et al. 1991. High dose itraconazole in the treatment of severe mycoses. *Antimicrob Agents Chemother* 35:707–713.
45. Sharp NJH, Harvey CE, O'Brien JA. 1991. Treatment of canine nasal aspergillosis/penicilliosis with fluconazole (UK-49,858). *J Small Anim Pract* 32:513–516.
46. Sharp NJH, Sullivan M. 1989. Use of ketoconazole in the treatment of canine nasal aspergillosis. *J Am Vet Med Assoc* 194:782–786.
47. Sharp NJH, Sullivan M, Harvey CE, et al. 1993. Treatment of canine nasal aspergillosis with enilconazole. *J Vet Intern Med* 7:40–43.
48. Shelton GH, Grant CK, Lineberger ML, et al. 1990. Severe neutropenia associated with griseofulvin therapy in cats with feline immunodeficiency virus. *J Vet Intern Med* 4:317–320.
49. Szoka FC Jr, Tang M. 1993. Amphotericin B formulated in liposomes and lipid-based systems: a review. *J Liposome Res* 3:363–375.
50. Thorpe JE, Baker N, Bromet-Petit M. 1990. Effect of oral antacid administration on the pharmacokinetics of oral fluconazole. *Antimicrob Agents Chemother* 34:2032–2033.
51. Van Oosterhoust ICAM, Venker-van-Haagen AJ. 1991. Aspergillosis: report on diagnosis and treatment. *Tijdschr Diergeneeskd* 116(Suppl):37–38.
52. Wali JP, Aggarwal P, Gupta V, et al. 1992. Ketoconazole in the treatment of antimony- and pentamidine-resistant kala-azar. *J Infect Dis* 166:215–216.
53. Wang LH, Smith PC, Anderson KL, et al. 1992. High performance liquid chromatographic analysis of amphotericin B in plasma, blood, urine and tissues for pharmacokinetic and tissue distribution studies. *J Chromatogr* 579:259–268.
53a. Ward H. 1994. Itraconazole for the treatment of histoplasmosis in cats. *J Vet Intern Med* 9:39–42.
54. Werner AH, Werner BE. 1993. Feline sporotrichosis. *Compend Cont Educ Pract Vet* 15:1189–1225.
55. White MH, Anaissie EJ, Kusne S, et al. 1997. Amphotericin B colloidal dispersion vs amphotericin B as therapy for invasive aspergillosis. *Clin Infect Dis* 24:635–642.
56. White-Weithers N, Medleau L. 1995. Evaluation of topical therapies for the treatment of dermatophyte infected hairs from dogs and cats. *J Am Anim Hosp Assoc* 31:250–253.
57. Zornes LL, Stratford RE. 1997. Development of a plasma high-performance liquid chromatographic assay for LY303366, a lipopeptide antifungal agent, and its application in a dog pharmacokinetic study. *J Chromatograph B* 695:381–387.

Chapter **58**

Dermatophytosis

Carol S. Foil

ETIOLOGY

Transient Fungal Microflora

Dogs and cats harbor many saprophytic molds and yeasts on their hair coats and probably on dermatitic skin as well. The most common fungi isolated from the hair coats of clinically healthy cats are *Alternaria*, *Aspergillus*, *Cladosporium*, *Penicillium*, *Rhizopus*, and *Trichoderma*.[61, 62, 67] From dogs, the same fungi are isolated with somewhat different frequencies.

Dermatophytes (*Microsporum canis*, *M. gypseum*, *M. vanbreuseghemi*, *Trichophyton verrucosum*, *T. mentagrophytes*, *T. rubrum*, *Epidermophyton*) have also been isolated from the hair coats of normal dogs and cats.[67, 79] Whether these isolations represent subclinical infections or transient flora is uncertain. *M. canis* causes a persistent nonsymptomatic infection in some long-haired cats, but the prevalence in cats varies markedly among reports, depending on the geography as well as the circumstances of the survey, illustrating the difficulty in distinguishing subclinical infection from transient carriage. Two surveys of pet cats from temperate climates found a very low incidence of carriage of *M. canis* on asymptomatic cats.[61, 92] Most isolations from asymptomatic cats are from animals in multiple-cat households or catteries,[62, 92] from cats at shows, or from stray and free-roaming cats in tropical urban environments. Where animals are congregated in a potentially contaminated facility, it is not possible to distinguish true infection from transient carriage by means of brush culturing. Illustrating this feature of dermatophyte surveys, a study of catteries in the northern United States showed that, within a facility, cats were either not culture positive or, in *M. canis*–affected catteries, virtually all cats were positive.[62] It is also not uncommon to isolate geophilic dermatophytes from the feet of animals that are allowed outdoors.

Pathogenic Dermatophytes

Dermatophytosis is a cutaneous infection with one of a number of keratinophilic species of fungi. The great majority of canine and feline dermatophytosis cases worldwide are caused by *M. canis*, *T. mentagrophytes*, or the geophilic species *M. gypseum*,[9, 40] although the list of species of dermatophytes that have been reported occasionally or rarely from symptomatic or asymptomatic dogs and cats is extensive (Table

Table 58–1. Dermatophyte Species Reported From Specimens From Dogs and Cats

SPECIES	HOSTS	GEOGRAPHIC RANGE
Zoophilic		
M. canis[a] (includes *M. distortum*)	B	Worldwide
M. equinum (horses; resembles *M. canis*)	D	?; rare
M. nanum (pigs)	B	Worldwide
M. gallinae	B	Worldwide
T. equinum (horses)	B	Worldwide
T. verrucosum (cattle, sheep)	B	Worldwide
Sylvatic		
T. mentagrophytes, includes *T. m. erinacei* (hedgehogs) and	B	Worldwide
T. m. quinckeanum (mice)	B	
M. persicolor (voles)	B; not in hair	Europe and Canada
Geophilic		
M. cookei	B	Worldwide
M. fulvum (resembles *M. gypseum*)	B	Worldwide
M. vanbreuseghemi[a]	B	Eurasia and North America
T. simii	B	India; frequently infects monkeys and poultry
M. gypseum	B	Worldwide, especially warm climates
T. terrestre	B; not in hair	Not very pathogenic
T. ajelloi	B; not in hair	Worldwide, not very pathogenic
Anthropophilic		
E. floccosum	B	Worldwide
M. audouinii[a]	B	Worldwide
T. megninii	B	Africa, Europe
T. rubrum	B	Worldwide
T. schoenleinii	B	Africa, Asia; rare in Americas
T. tonsurans	B	Worldwide, especially Latin America
T. violaceum	B	Worldwide; rare in North America

[a]This species fluoresces when illuminated with ultraviolet light.
B = both dog and cat; D = dog; ? = uncertain.

58–1). The prevalence of infections caused by each of the three common etiologic agents varies geographically (Table 58–2). In cats, over 90% of cases are caused by *M. canis* worldwide. There is morphologic and biochemical variability among isolates from cats, however.[56] The incidence of *M. gypseum*, which is most common in tropical and subtropical humid areas, varies seasonally, being more common in summer and autumn.[40]

Simultaneous infection of dogs with more than one dermatophyte species may occur. Of combined infections, those caused by *M. gypseum* and *T. mentagrophytes* have been the most common.

EPIDEMIOLOGY

Prevalence

Fungal skin disease is overdiagnosed in veterinary medicine, especially in the dog. In all studies of skin diseases of dogs and cats in which fungal cultures have been performed, the prevalence of dermatophyte infections seems to be about 2% of all dermatologic cases. The percentage of positive culture results among specimens submitted from suspected ringworm cases has ranged from less than 4% to 50%.[5, 40, 46, 86] In the United Kingdom, a survey showed that culture results were positive from only 16% of 8349 specimens from dogs or cats suspected of having dermatophytosis,[86] whereas in Turin, Italy, the figure was 40% of cases examined.[46] These figures may reflect not only geographic variation but also differences in the types of cases chosen for dermatophyte culture.

Transmission

Dermatophytes are spread between animals or to persons from animals by direct contact or by contact with infected hair and scale in the environment or on fomites. Transmission to a child from the interior of a used car was reported.[94] The incubation period is 1 to 3 weeks. The source of *M. canis* is often an infected cat or fomites contaminated by cats. In most *Trichophyton* infections, dogs and cats are suspected of being exposed by contact with rodents or their nests. *M. gypseum* is a geophilic organism that inhabits rich soil. Dogs and cats are exposed by digging and rooting in contaminated areas.

Table 58–2. Relative Frequency (%) of Dermatophytes Species Isolated From Dogs and Cats in Surveys From Various Geographic Locations

	M. CANIS		*M. GYPSEUM*		*T. MENTAGROPHYTES*	
LOCATION	Cats	Dogs	Cats	Dogs	Cats	Dogs
Austria	91	58	—	—	5	19
Indiana[24]	93	63	0	5	7	32
Louisiana[40]	92	43	7	44	2	11
Norway[92a]	96	84	0	0	4	5
New Zealand[24]	90	74	4	9	2	11
Spain[5a]	97	71	3	14	0	14
United Kingdom[86]	92	65	<1	<1	6	24

Table 58–3. Clinical Features of Canine and Feline Dermatophytosis

PRESENTATION	HOST	FUNGAL SPECIES	COMMENTS
Classic	B	Mc, Mg	Circular patch of alopecia, scale, central healing
Alopecia	B	Mc, Tm	Irregular to widespread, long-haired cats, Yorkshire terriers
Miliary dermatitis	C	Mc	Always consider dermatophytosis
Folliculitis, furunculosis	D	Mc, Mg, Tm	May be localized, regional (facial), or generalized
Onychomycosis	B	Mc, Mg, Tm	Rare; often with paronychia
Kerion	D	Mg, Tm	Highly inflamed, single or multiple
Granulomas	B	Mc, Mg, Tm	Rare—most often in Persians or Himalayans with generalized *M. canis*
Asymptomatic	B	Mc	Especially long-haired cats; also Yorkshire terriers

B = both dog and cat; C = cat; D = dog; Mc = *Microsporum canis*; Mg = *M. gypseum*; Tm = *Trichophyton mentagrophytes*.

Infections with anthropophilic species are acquired as reverse zoonoses by direct contact with infected persons.

Dermatophyte infections of dogs and cats involve the hair shaft and follicle. Infected hair shafts are fragile, and dislodged hair fragments containing infectious arthrospores are the most efficient means of transmission to other hosts. Such material may remain infectious in the environment for many months. One study found that samples of hair stored for 18 months could yield positive culture results.[92]

Host Factors

Susceptibility to infection is poorly understood, but the ability to mount an inflammatory response plays a crucial role in terminating an infection. As with many infectious diseases, young animals are predisposed to acquiring symptomatic dermatophyte infections. This finding is partly due to a delay in development of adequate host immunity. Dermatophyte infections in healthy dogs are usually self-limiting.

Humoral and cellular immune responses develop after recovery from dermatophyte infections in immunocompetent cats, making them immune to reinfections.[87] Immunodeficient hosts will be at greater risk for acquiring infections, and their infections may be more serious, more widespread, or more prolonged. Glucocorticoid therapy is particularly likely to increase susceptibility to dermatophytosis by means of inhibiting local inflammation. In cats, increased frequency of isolation of *M. canis* is reported in feline immunodeficiency virus–infected animals.[43] Widespread and recalcitrant *M. canis* dermatophytosis was reported in a cat after bone marrow transplantation for acute myeloid leukemia.[28] Other more subtle aberrations in the immune response may influence the likelihood of acquiring and retaining a dermatophyte infection. For example, atopic people are at increased risk for dermatophytosis as a result of local inhibition of T-lymphocyte function and inflammation.

CLINICAL FINDINGS

It is dangerous to diagnose dermatophytosis on the basis of clinical signs alone, not only because of the protean nature of the dermatologic findings but also because there are several other skin diseases, such as demodicosis and staphylococcal folliculitis as well as allergy and pruritus in cats, that mimic the classic ringworm lesion. Because the infection is follicular in dogs and usually so in cats, the most consistent clinical sign is one or more patches of alopecia with variable scaling and crusting. Some patients may develop a classic ring lesion with central healing and fine follicular papules on the periphery. Generally, however, signs and symptoms are highly variable and depend on the degree of inflammation and hair shaft destruction. Some of the clinical presentations of dermatophytosis are characterized in Table 58–3.

Cat

Feline dermatophytosis often appears as irregular patchy alopecia (Fig. 58–1) or patches of scale with minor alopecia or hair breakage; this is the most common presentation in long-haired cats. Other syndromes include classic circular patches of alopecia with scaling, miliary dermatitis, focal or multifocal pruritic dermatitis, onychomycosis, and granulomatous dermatitis. Rarely diffuse alopecia with hyperpigmented patches of long hair has been observed.[78]

Granulomatous dermatitis, in the form of well-circumscribed, ulcerated dermal nodules, is infrequently recognized in cats (Fig. 58–2). The lesions occur on cats afflicted with more generalized typical *M. canis* infections. Interestingly, a report described different strains of *M. canis* isolated from the granulomatous lesions and from the surface infections of the same cat.[56] These lesions have been called mycetomas, pseudomycetomas, and Majocchi's granulomas. This form of disease carries a poor prognosis for resolution, and one case description[79] and a cat seen by the author show that the disease can have a fatal outcome, with deep ulceration leading to sepsis.

Dog

Dogs often develop classic foci of alopecia with follicular papules, scales, and crusts. Dermatophytosis should be considered in any papular or pustular eruption. Facial folliculitis

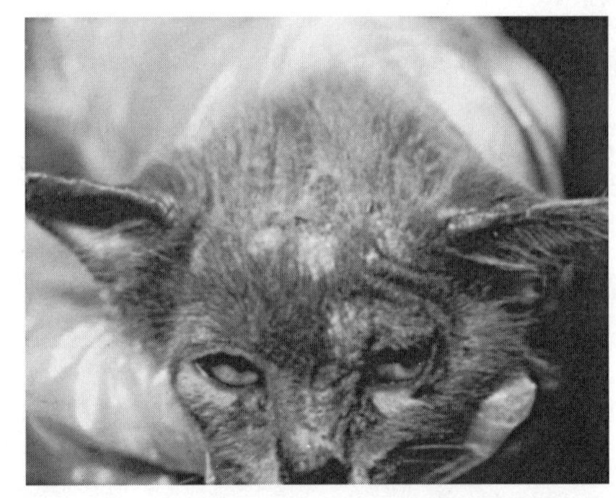

Figure 58–1. Dermatophytosis in this kitten with *Microsporum canis* is characterized by patchy alopecia with marked scaling and hyperkeratosis.

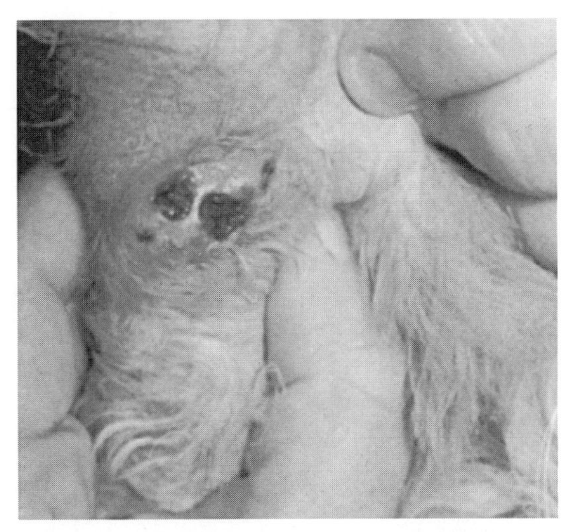

Figure 58–2. Granulomatous dermatitis has developed in this cat with generalized dermatophyte infection caused by *Microsporum canis*. Microscopically, this lesion resembled a mycetoma. (Courtesy of Dr. Gail Kunkle, University of Florida, Gainesville, FL.)

and furunculosis, superficially mimicking an autoimmune skin disease, can develop (Fig. 58–3). Nodular skin lesions (kerion) may also be caused by dermatophytosis (Fig. 58–4). Kerion is a common presenting sign of *M. gypseum* infection. Onychomycosis may be manifest by chronic ungual fold inflammation, with or without footpad involvement, or the claw alone may be infected, which causes claw deformity and fragility.

Demodicosis and dermatophytosis can be clinically indistinguishable but can be reliably differentiated by a skin scraping. Superficial folliculitis, especially when accompanied by the spreading rings of erythema and exfoliation that have been characterized as "staphylococcal hypersensitivity" or "superficial spreading pyoderma," is more often mistaken for dermatophytosis. Staphylococcal skin lesions of seborrheic spaniels are also often misdiagnosed as ringworm.

DIAGNOSIS

Although there has been research focused on cellular and humoral responses to dermatophytes infections,[13, 18, 88, 90] only

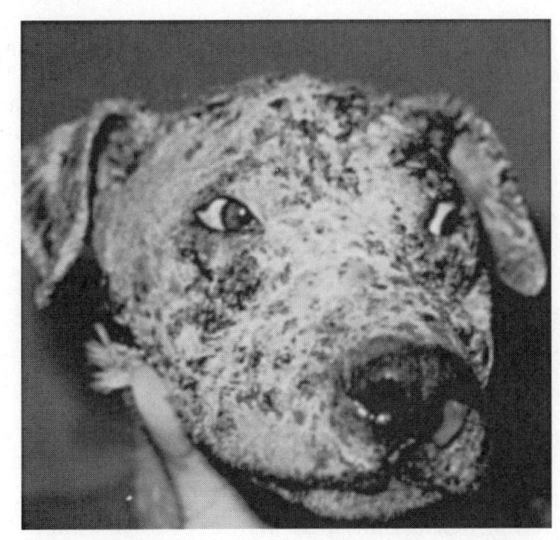

Figure 58–3. Facial folliculitis and furunculosis in this dog was caused by *Trichophyton mentagrophytes*. This dog was referred as a suspected pemphigus foliaceus case.

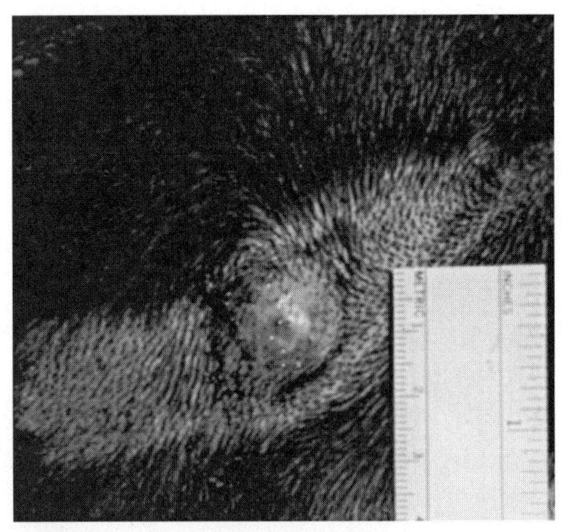

Figure 58–4. This nodular skin lesion on a dog is a kerion caused by *Microsporum gypseum*.

preliminary work has been reported in serologic diagnosis in canine dermatophytosis.[74] Follow-up studies examining cross-reacting antibodies and experimental and naturally occurring feline ringworm are needed, because serology could be a useful tool for protecting cat breeders from importing infected animals to their facilities. It may soon become possible, also, to investigate the appropriateness of the immune response to infection in groups of persistently infected animals.[89] Other new developments in diagnosis include the production of polymerase chain reaction probes and immunohistochemical stains for the various species of dermatophytes.[3, 73] These have yet to be developed for commercial use. Calcofluor white has been mentioned to improve the diagnostic accuracy of direct microscopic examination of hairs (see following discussion).[91] Improvements in commercial in vitro fungal susceptibility testing continue to be reported.[95]

Direct Microscopic Examination

Hair and scales may be mounted in 10% to 20% potassium hydroxide (KOH) overnight or heated gently for 10 minutes for clearing of keratin and visualization of fungal elements. It is useful to try to examine Wood's light–positive hairs in this manner. Even in experienced hands, this technique is time consuming and may be diagnostic in only a few cases. It may lead to misinterpretation if saprophytic fungal spores are present in the specimen (Fig. 58–5). Dermatophytes never form macroconidia in tissue (see Figs. 56–9, 56–10, and 56–11), but rather form hyphae and arthroconidia on hair and scale (see Fig. 56–2). One investigation has recommended hair examination with a solution of calcofluor white and Evans blue (1:9) in equal volume of 20% KOH for superior visualization of fungal elements.[91]

Wood's Light Examination

M. canis infections may show fluorescence on Wood's light examination. The use of a screening examination with a Wood's lamp can be very valuable in the hands of an experienced diagnostician. However, a negative result should not be used to rule out dermatophytosis, because not all infections exhibit fluorescence. The specificity of the Wood's lamp examination was tested against culture and found once again

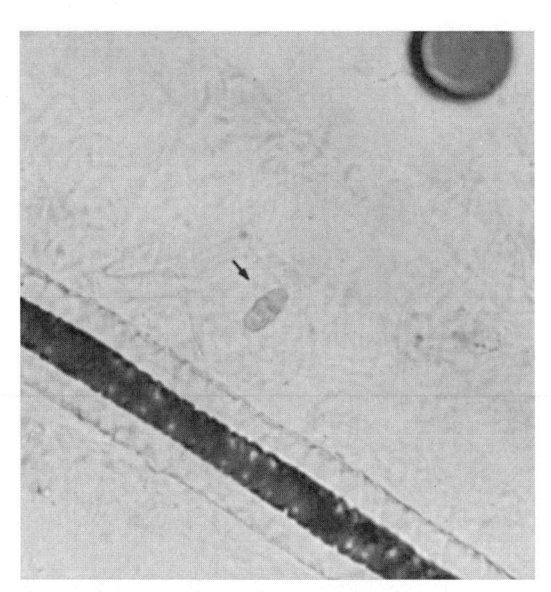

Figure 58–5. This KOH-digested microscopic preparation of hair and scale from a dog contains a multiloculated fungal spore that may be mistaken for a dermatophyte macroconidium. It is an *Alternaria* spore. Dermatophytes never produce macroconidia in tissue.

to have a sensitivity of about 50% for *M. canis* infection.[86] The specificity was found to be high in the same study, but it is not difficult for the less experienced clinician to mistake scale and medication for a positive result. True fluorescence is quite bright, apple-green, and should be only within the shafts of infected hairs. Moriello and DeBoer[65] have emphasized some technical features for improved accuracy in the use of the Wood's lamp. They advised that the lamp should be turned on and warm (3–5 minutes) before the examination. The suspect lesion should be held under the lamp for a similar amount of time. The Wood's lamp can also be utilized to examine a contaminated environment for fluorescing hairs.[60]

Fungal Culture

Definitive diagnosis of dermatophytosis is made by culture, although it is neither perfectly sensitive nor always specific for the diagnosis.[86] Several important principles should be followed to ensure accurate specimen collection.

Specimen Collection

If done properly, clipping and cleaning the lesions to be cultured will reduce contaminant growth. The hair should be clipped to 0.5-cm length and the area patted clean with an alcohol-moistened gauze and then allowed to dry. The hair stubble should be collected from several suspect sites with hemostats by grasping the hair shafts close to the skin and rolling the hairs from the follicles. Hairs that are broken and near active inflammation should be selected. Scales should be included in the sample. Exudates or antiseptics should not be transferred to the medium.

If surgical biopsy is performed on nodular lesions, aseptically collected and transported tissue should be submitted for cultural as well as histologic examination.

Media and Incubation

Culture can readily be performed as an in-office procedure employing dermatophyte test medium (DTM) (see also Table 56–2). DTM consists of Sabouraud's dextrose agar, phenol red as pH indicator, and antimicrobials to inhibit bacterial and saprophytic mold growth. For incubation, DTM containers should be loosely capped at room temperature and protected from UV light and desiccation. They should be inspected daily for a color change of the medium to red and simultaneous growth of a cottony mycelium. If the color change occurs later, which may be caused by saprophyte growth exhausting the carbohydrate in the medium, the result will be a false-positive reading.

After 7 to 10 days of growth, most colonies will begin to produce spores, which will allow specific identification. A suspect colony that fails to produce spores or is difficult to identify, as is often the case in *Trichophyton* species, should be sent to a qualified diagnostic laboratory. Dysgonic varieties of *M. canis* (sometimes called *M. canis* var *distortum*) may occasionally be isolated, particularly from cat colonies.[70, 81] These varieties grow under the surface of the agar, giving a feathery or snowflake-like appearance. They do not produce conidia or a red color change on DTM.[65] These can be converted to more typical forms by a diagnostic laboratory for identification.[47]

Zoophilic dermatophyte colonies are white to buff-colored on DTM (or yellowish to pinkish below on Sabouraud's dextrose agar). If blue, green, dark brown, or black fungal contaminants have overgrown a colony suspected of being a dermatophyte, subculturing will be necessary.

Culturing Asymptomatic Animals

Brush culturing is the preferred method of obtaining such specimens. A sterilized toothbrush or a surgical scrub brush is satisfactory for this technique. The animal's hair coat is brushed thoroughly and extensively. The bristles are then impressed directly onto the culture medium in several sites.

Onychomycosis

When dermatophytosis is suspected as a cause of chronic paronychia, special culture techniques may be needed. In many cases the hair surrounding the ungual fold may be infected and may be cultured as done elsewhere on the body, taking special care to clip and clean to reduce contaminant growth. However, in dogs, geophilic fungi may contaminate pre-existing foot lesions, so it may be necessary to correlate cultural findings with histologic demonstrations of fungi in hair or claw. Otherwise, repeated isolation of fungus from the lesions may be regarded as evidence of causation. If the claws alone are affected, a scalpel blade may be used to shave fine pieces from the proximal end of clipped or surgically excised specimens for culture. In this case, untreated Sabouraud's dextrose agar as well as DTM should be used.

Histopathology

Biopsy examination is not as sensitive as culture in the diagnosis of dermatophytosis. When the significance of culture results is questioned, demonstration of the organism in biopsy specimens is more definitive. Histologic examination is most helpful in detecting the nodular forms of dermatophytosis (the kerion and granulomatous ringworm), especially because these lesions are often culture negative. Shaved, clipped, or surgically excised specimens of claws may be submitted for histologic examination in cases of paronychia, onychorrhexis, or onychomadesis. If fungal organisms are present, they will be readily visible within the substance of the claw.

THERAPY

Topical Therapy

It is still my opinion that all animals with dermatomycosis should receive topical therapy; however, this recommendation has become controversial in light of new investigations that have shown little antifungal efficacy with common topical agents.[16, 65, 97] Furthermore, it has been shown that clipping of the hair along with topical therapy can spread and exacerbate existing ringworm lesions.[59, 63] However, there is no more efficient way to loosen and discard infectious hair and scale from affected pets, so the recommendation of topical treatment is made to decrease ongoing environmental contamination and human exposure. Clipping and topical therapy can also shorten the length of systemic treatment before mycologic cure. In short-haired cats with limited visible lesions, only infected hairs around the periphery of the lesions should be removed with scissors. Clipping of the entire hair coat with a number 10 blade is recommended in animals with generalized lesions.

See Table 58–4 for comments about the efficacy of commonly prescribed topical therapies. Currently, lime sulfur dips (4–8 oz/gal), miconazole (MCZ) and ketoconazole (KTZ) shampoos, and enilconazole rinse are currently recommended as most likely to be effective. The latter is available in Europe and Canada as a rinse for dogs only. It is widely used to treat cats in Europe,[7] and, although the safety in cats has been questioned,[65] a reported study in 14 Persian cats using 0.2% whole body rinses produced no adverse reactions.[20] A combination 2% chlorhexidine/2% MCZ shampoo was shown to significantly decrease the time to mycologic cure in combination with systemic therapy.[69] Creams, ointments, and lotions are not formulated to penetrate infected hair shafts and follicles. In some cases in cats with ringworm, there is significant fungal growth in the stratum corneum as well as within hairs and follicles. In extremely scaly infections and localized lesions in cats, these products could theoretically be helpful. To apply topical therapies such as lime sulfur, gauze sponges can be used to press the dip into the skin without rubbing, which can spread infection. An Elizabethan collar can be worn by the animal after treatment to allow the solution to dry. Vomiting and mental depression have been observed in cats that lick the freshly applied solution.[59]

Kerions and granulomatous lesions do not require specific antifungal therapy unless more widespread disease is also present. The kerion should be cleansed gently to remove exudate and avoid the potential for scarring. Feline dermatophyte granulomas should be surgically excised. Systemic antibiotics may be required if extensive purulent exudation has developed.

Systemic Therapy

Topical treatment removes spores from the hair shafts, and systemic treatment acts at hair follicles. Not every patient requires systemic therapy. In dogs, localized lesions and even generalized *M. canis* or *M. gypseum* infections can resolve without treatment.[48] Cats and kittens with seemingly localized disease can also self-cure, but infection can be prolonged (>60–100 days). It can be more widespread than clinically suspected, so treatment is recommended in infected cats. Systemic treatment is also recommended in dogs with *Trichophyton* infection or with any immunocompromised state. Drugs and dosage regimens are summarized in Table 58–5.

There have been several reports of sensitivity testing of *M. canis* isolates from cats and dogs.[42, 68, 77] In vitro, griseofulvin (GFV), KTZ, and itraconazole (ITZ) appear to be almost uniformly efficacious. In practice, GFV and ITZ are currently the systemic treatments of choice. See Drug Formulary, Appendix 8, for additional information on each drug.

GFV. This fungistatic drug is expensive, and long-term side effects are not uncommon. It should be used only when diagnosis is certain. Fortunately, dermatophytosis is rare in adult dogs, which would require the largest dosages. Like many antifungal agents, GFV is poorly water soluble; thus, GI absorption after oral dosing is variable and incomplete. Absorption is enhanced by administration with a fat-containing meal or by formulations containing polyethylene glycol. Particle size (micronization) also greatly affects oral absorption and bioavailability.

Dosages recommended for dogs and cats are not based on modern pharmacologic studies. Dosages that have proved to be effective in the largest numbers of cases are higher than manufacturer's recommendations, and significant toxicities may be encountered. The most common side effects are vomiting, diarrhea, and anorexia. These can be partially avoided by dividing the daily dose into two administrations. Bone marrow suppression and neurologic signs have occurred, probably as idiosyncratic reactions. GFV is teratogenic and

Table 58–4. Recent Information About the Efficacy of Various Topical Agents Recommended for Treatment of Dermatophytosis in Dogs and Cats

TOPICAL AGENT	AVAILABLE FORMULATIONS	COMMENTS ON EFFICACY[a]
Captan	Shampoo, rinse	Poor performance in vitro
Chlorhexidine	Shampoo, rinse	No advantage over control treatment in experimental clinical infection; inferior in in vitro tests
Clotrimazole	Cream, lotion	Creams and lotions not formulated to penetrate infected hair
Enilconazole	Rinse, fogger	Superior in in vitro tests
Ketoconazole	Shampoo, cream	Tested in animal models, fair efficacy; creams not formulated to penetrate infected hair
Lime sulfur	Rinse	Superior at 1:16 dilution in in vitro tests
Miconazole	Shampoo, cream	Superior in in vitro tests
Povidone-iodine	Shampoo, rinse, ointment	Poor performance in vitro
Sodium hypochlorite	Rinse	Inferior (1:10 dilution) in in vitro tests

[a]In vitro tests performed with infected hair.

Table 58–5. Drugs for Systemic Therapy of Dermatophytosis in Dogs and Cats [a]

DRUG	DOSE[b] (mg/kg)	ROUTE	INTERVAL (HOURS)	DURATION[c] (WEEKS)
Griseofulvin				
Microsized[d]	25–50	PO	12	4–8
Ultramicrosized[e]	5–10	PO	24	4–8
Ketoconazole[f]	10	PO	24	3–4
Itraconazole[g]	5–10	PO	24	3–4

[a]See Drug Formulary, Appendix 8, for additional information on each drug.
[b]Dose per administration at specified interval.
[c]Follow-up brush culture should be negative before discontinuing therapy.
[d]Trade names: Grifulvin V, Fulvicin U/F, Grisactin. For small kittens, usually culture negative at 8 weeks and cured at 10 weeks.
[e]Dose is approximately two thirds that of microsized preparation. Some preparations contain polyethylene glycol to facilitate absorption. Trade names: Fulvicin P/G, Grisactin Ultra, Gris-PEG.
[f]Trade name: Nizoral; cats often receive 50 mg total dose daily; with side effects, every other day treatment is used.
[g]Trade name: Sporanox. Capsules may be opened and contents divided to administer recommended doses.

must never be given during the first two thirds of pregnancy. For a further discussion of toxicity, see Griseofulvin, Chapter 57.

KTZ. This has been shown to be a moderately effective fungistatic drug against *M. canis* and *T. mentagrophytes*. It has been used successfully to treat canine and feline[49] dermatophytosis. Less favorable results were reported in long-haired animals. KTZ should be reserved for cases in which intolerance of GFV is a problem and in which ITZ cannot be substituted because of greater expense. Side effects of KTZ are GI and hepatotoxic and inhibition of steroidal hormone synthesis (see Ketoconazole, Chapter 57).

ITZ. This is better tolerated by cats and dogs than either KTZ or GFV and is comparable or superior to GFV in its efficacy for *M. canis*.[41, 64] In human medicine, ITZ has proved helpful in chronic, recalcitrant dermatophytosis, including onychomycosis.[19, 31, 32, 82] Signs of hepatotoxicity have been reported uncommonly in cats, and cutaneous vasculitis is reported in dogs. Most patients, however, tolerate the drug well at the dosages recommended for treatment of dermatophytosis. ITZ is not recommended in pregnancy. The drug is available in 100-mg capsules that can be opened and dispensed to small animals in butter or food in the appropriate dosages (see Drug Formulary, Appendix 8). I have used it in kittens as young as 8 weeks. The drawback is the lack of licensing for use in animals and the high expense of the medication. A liquid suspension for oral use, with higher bioavailability than capsules, is licensed.

Duration. Cats should be treated systemically until the fungus cannot be cultured from three sequential weekly cultures. Monitoring should begin at 3 weeks after treatment is instituted. Cats can appear clinically normal before their skin and hair are cleared of fungal organisms. Although a Wood's light can help to screen for dermatophytes, positive fluorescence may occur in some hair shafts in which fungus has been inactivated.[59]

Vaccination. A killed *Microsporum* vaccine for prophylactic and therapeutic use in cats and kittens has been introduced in the United States (Fel-O-Vax MC-K, Fort Dodge Laboratories, Fort Dodge, IO). In field trials conducted by the manufacturer, vaccine reduced the size of clinical lesions after several weeks. However, there are no controlled studies to demonstrate vaccine efficacy against natural or challenge exposure.[59] The product is labeled for both treatment and prevention of lesion development but not for prevention of infection. Three doses are recommended for either treatment or prevention. Testing of another vaccine that is commercially available has shown questionable efficacy for protection against infection in cats when they were placed in contact with asymptomatically infected cats.[17, 59] Furthermore, mycologic cure was difficult to demonstrate. Concern is focused on the possibility that the use of this product in breeding situations may lead to the selling and distributing of inapparently affected kittens and an increase in the number of cases in exposed persons and new multiple cat household contaminations.[96] Local reactions may occur at the site of vaccination of some cats. Nevertheless, interest in a vaccination program in multiple-cat households remains high. A killed vaccine has been demonstrated in the guinea pig model to protect vaccinates from lesion development after natural exposure.[71] A modified live vaccine protocol has been very successful in control of *T. verrucosum* infections in calves in northern Europe.[30]

ENVIRONMENTAL CONTROL

In each confirmed case of dermatophytosis in dogs and cats, there is an environmental cleanup problem to be handled. The environment is particularly likely to be heavily contaminated in multiple-cat households, even with good daily cleaning practices.[65] Investigations have shown that many previously recommended environmental decontamination procedures are ineffective.[65] Although 1% formalin and undiluted bleach are effective in killing all spores,[59] they are too caustic. None are effective in an environment heavily contaminated with hair. Current recommendations included very thorough vacuuming and cleaning so that no visible hair contamination is present. This is followed by triple cleansing and disinfecting with stabilized chlorine dioxide disinfectants or 1:10 household bleach solutions.[60] Any materials or fomites that cannot be thoroughly treated in this manner should be discarded. Enilconazole in the form of a spray (Clinafarm Spray, Janssen Pharmaceuticals, Belgium) or fogger (Clinafarm Smoke) is available in some countries, and some data are available to indicate decent efficacy in an *M. canis*–contaminated environment.

PUBLIC HEALTH CONSIDERATIONS

Pet Owners

Transmission to people of *M. canis* infection by nonsymptomatic cats, and even occasionally by dogs[36] and fomites,[94] continues to be reported. Immunocompromised persons may be at increased risk for infections and for more serious infections.[37] Moriello and DeBoer[65] listed the circumstances in which risk of transmission from cats is thought to warrant special consideration: adoption of kittens from animal shelters or catteries with any known history of dermatophytosis, exposure of pet cats to large numbers of other animals (e.g., at shows or for breeding), and age (e.g., kittens and young persons are both at increased risk for infection). Almost half of people exposed to infected cats do acquire the infection. The majority of persons living in households with an infected cat become infected. Worldwide, the reported number of cases of human infection with *M. canis* continues to increase.[79]

Animal Health Workers

For handlers of small animals, the occupational risk of acquiring dermatophytosis is not as great as for those working with cattle, for whom ringworm is the most commonly reported zoonosis. Not surprisingly, *M. canis* is most often implicated in cases involving small animal practitioners and their employees. An investigation of veterinary clinics in Italy revealed that, in 15 of 50 clinics, *M. canis* could be isolated from the floors of waiting rooms, examination rooms, radiology rooms, and wards.[44] Veterinary practitioners must be vigilant in protecting themselves and their employees from this very unpleasant zoonosis.[38]

Person-to-Animal Transmission

This is illustrated in the isolation of the anthropophilic dermatophyte species that are listed in Table 58–1. *M. canis* may be transmitted from people to household pets as well.

Transmission to Other Domestic Animals

M. canis–infected cats have been implicated as the source of infection in farm animals, including pigs, lambs, and rabbits.[29, 33]

References

1. Aly R. 1994. Ecology and epidemiology of dermatophyte infections. *J Am Acad Dermatol* 31:S21–S25.
2. Biberstein EL. 1990. Dermatophytes, pp 272–285. *In* Biberstein EL, Zee YC (eds), Review of veterinary microbiology. Blackwell Scientific Publications, Boston, MA.
3. Bock M, Maiwald M, Kappe R, et al. 1994. Polymerase chain reaction-based detection of dermatophyte DNA with a fungus-specific primer system. *Mycoses* 37:79–84.
4. Bond R, Middleton DJ, Scarff DH, et al. 1992. Chronic dermatophytosis due to *Microsporum persicolor* infection in three dogs. *J Small Anim Pract* 33:571–576.
5. Breuer-Strosberg R. 1993. Nachweishäufigkeit von Dermatophyten bei Katzen und Hunden in Österreich. *DTW Dtsch Tierarztl Wochenschr* 100:483–485.

5a. Cabanes FJ, Abarca ML, Bragulat MR. 1997. Dermatophytes isolated from domestic animals in Barcelona, Spain. *Mycopathologica* 137:107–113.

6. Caretta G, Mancianti F, Ajello L. 1989. Dermatophytes and keratinophilic fungi in cats and dogs. *Mycoses* 32:620–626.
7. Carlotti D-N. 1996. Personal communication. St. Eulaly, France.
8. Carlotti D-N, Couprie B. 1988. Dermatophyties du chien et du chat: actualités. *Pract Méd Chir Animal Compagnie* 23:450–457.
9. Casillas del Collado M. 1991. Estudio etiológico de las dermatofitosis en perros y gatos. *Rev Iberoam Micol* 8:13–15.
10. Connole MD. 1990. Review of animal mycoses in Australia. *Mycopathologia* 11:133–164.
11. DeBoer DJ, Moriello KA. 1994. Development of an experimental model of *Microsporum canis* infection in cats. *Vet Microbiol* 42:289–295.
12. DeBoer DJ, Moriello KA. 1993. Humoral and cellular immune responses to *Microsporum canis* in naturally occurring feline dermatophytosis. *J Med Vet Mycol* 31:121–131.
13. DeBoer DJ, Moriello KA. 1994. The immune response to *Microsporum canis* induced by a fungal cell wall vaccine. *Vet Dermatol* 5:47–55.
14. DeBoer DJ, Moriello KA. 1995. Clinical update on feline dermatophytosis—part I. *Compend Cont Educ Pract Vet* 17:1197–1265.
15. DeBoer DJ, Moriello KA. 1995. Clinical update on feline dermatophytosis—part II. *Compend Cont Educ Pract Vet* 17:1471–1481.
16. DeBoer DJ, Moriello KA. 1995. Inability of two topical treatments to influence the course of experimentally induced dermatophytosis in cats. *J Am Vet Med Assoc* 207:52–56.
17. DeBoer DJ, Moriello KA. 1995. Investigations of a killed dermatophyte cell-wall vaccine against infection with *Microsporum canis* in cats. *Res Vet Sci* 59:110–113.
18. DeBoer DJ, Moriello KA, Cooley AJ. 1991. Immunological reactivity to intradermal dermatophyte antigens in cats with dermatophytosis. *Vet Dermatol* 2:59–67.
19. De Doncker P, Decroix J, Piérard GE, et al. 1996. Antifungal pulse therapy for onychomycosis. A pharmacokinetic and pharmacodynamic investigation of monthly cycles of 1-week pulse therapy with itraconazole. *Arch Dermatol* 132:34–41.
20. DeJaham C, Pagé N, Lambert AJ, et al. 1996. Toxicity study of enilconazole emulsion in the treatment of dermatophytosis in Persian cats, p 38. Presented at the Third World Congress of Veterinary Dermatology, Edinburgh, Scotland.
21. Elliot C, Plant JD. 1995. A comparison of the performance of five growth media used to culture and identify *Microsporum canis*, pp 28–29. Presented at the meeting of AAVD/ACVD, Las Vegas, NV.
22. Euzeby J. 1992. Mycologie medicale compareé. Les mycoses des animaux et leur relations avec les mycoses de l'homme, Vol 1. Foundation Merieux, Lyon, France.
23. Ferreiro L, Polack B, Larcher G, et al. 1996. Relations between canine and feline dermatophytosis and enzymatic activity of *Microsporum canis* strains, p 148. Presented at the Third World Congress of Veterinary Dermatology, Edinburgh, Scotland.
24. Foil CS. 1990. Dermatophytosis, pp 659–668. *In* Greene CE (ed), Infectious diseases of the dog and cat. WB Saunders, Philadelphia, PA.
25. Foil CS. 1993. Dermatophytosis, pp 22–33. *In* Griffin CE, Kwochka KW, MacDonald JM (eds), Current veterinary dermatology. The science and art of therapy. Mosby Year Book, St Louis, MO.
26. Foil CS. 1994. Fungal Diseases. *Clin Dermatol* 12:529–542.
27. Gambale W, Larsson CE, Moritami MM, et al. 1993. Dermatophytes and other fungi of the haircoat of cats without dermatophytosis in the city of Sao Paulo, Brazil. *Feline Pract* 21:29–33.
28. Gasper PW, Rosen DK, Fulton R. 1996. Allogeneic marrow transplantation in a cat with acute myeloid leukemia. *J Am Vet Med Assoc* 208:1280–1284.
29. Gonzales Cabo JF, Bárcena Asensio MC, Gómez Rodriguez F, et al. 1995. An outbreak of dermatophytosis in pigs caused by *Microsporum canis*. *Mycopathologia* 129:79–80.
30. Gordon PJ, Bond R. 1996. Efficacy of a live attenuated *Trichophyton verrucosum* vaccine for control of bovine dermatophytosis. *Vet Rec* 139:395–396.
31. Hanifen JM, Tofte SJ. 1988. Itraconazole therapy for recalcitrant dermatophyte infections. *J Am Acad Dermatol* 18:1077–1080.
32. Hay RJ, Clayton YM, Moore MK, et al. 1990. Itraconazole in the management of chronic dermatophytosis. *J Am Acad Dermatol* 23:561–564.
33. Hormansdorfer S, Heinritzi K, Bauer J. 1995. *Microsporum canis* Als Ursache Einer Bestandsenzootie Beim Schwein. Ein Fallbericht. *Tierarztl Prax* 23:465–468.
34. Ikesyoji R, Takahashi M, Igami N, et al. 1992. Distribution of dermatophyte carriers in cats. *J Jpn Vet Med Assoc* 45:430–431.
35. Jand SK, Gupta MP. 1989. Dermatomycosis in dogs. *Mycoses* 32:104–105.
36. Katoh T, Maruyama R, Nishioka K, et al. 1991. Tinea corporis due to *Microsporum canis* from an asymptomatic dog. *J Dermatol* 18:356–359.
37. King D, Cheever LW, Hood A, et al. 1996. Primary invasive cutaneous *Microsporum canis* infections in immunocompromised patients. *J Clin Microbiol* 34:460–462.
38. Korting HC, Zienicke H. 1990. Dermatophytoses as occupational dermatoses in industrialized countries. Report on two cases from Munich. *Mycoses* 33:86–89.
39. Kwon-Chung KJ, Bennett JE. 1992. Medical mycology. Lea & Febiger, Philadelphia, PA.
40. Lewis DT, Foil CS, Hosgood G. 1991. Epidemiology and clinical features of dermatophytosis in dogs and cats at Louisiana State University: 1981–1990. *Vet Dermatol* 2:53–58.
41. López-Gómez S, Del Palacio A, Van Cutsem J, et al. 1994. Itraconazole versus griseofulvin in the treatment of tinea capitis: a double-blind randomized study in children. *J Dermatol* 33:743–747.
42. Macura AB. 1993. In vitro susceptibility of dermatophytes to antifungal drugs: a comparison of two methods. *Int J Dermatol* 32:533–536.
43. Mancianti F, Giannelli C, Bendinelli M, et al. 1992. Mycological findings in feline immunodeficiency virus-infected cats. *J Med Vet Mycol* 30:257–259.
44. Mancianti F, Papini R. 1996. Isolation of keratinophilic fungi from the floor of private veterinary clinics in Italy. *Vet Res Commun* 20:161–166.
45. Mansfield PD, Stringfellow JS. 1990. Isolation of *Microsporum vanbreuseghemi* from skin lesions of a dog. *J Am Vet Med Assoc* 197:875–876.
46. Marchisio VF, Gallo, MG, Tullio V, et al. 1995. Dermatophytes from cases of skin disease in cats and dogs in Turin, Italy. *Mycoses* 38:239–244.
47. Mavroudeas D, Velegraki A, Leonardopoulos J, et al. 1996. Effect of glucose and thiamine concentrations on the formation of macroconidia in dermato-

phytes. Occurrence of dysgonic *Microsporum canis* strains in Athens, Greece. *Mycoses* 39:61–66.
48. Medleau L, Chalmers SA. 1992. Resolution of generalized dermatophytosis without treatment in dogs. *J Am Vet Med Assoc* 201:1891–1892.
49. Medleau L, Chalmers SA. 1993. Ketoconazole for the treatment of dermatophytosis in cats. *J Am Vet Med Assoc* 200:77–78.
50. Medleau L, Kuhl KA. 1992. Dealing with chronic recurring dermatophytosis. *Vet Med* 87:1101–1104.
51. Medleau L, Moriello KA. 1992. Feline dermatophytosis, pp 547–551. *In* Kirk RW, Bonagura JD (eds), Current veterinary therapy: XI. Small animal practice. WB Saunders, Philadelphia, PA.
52. Medleau L, Rakich PM. 1994. *Microsporum canis* pseudomycetomas in a cat. *J Am Anim Hosp Assoc* 30:573–576.
53. Medleau L, Ristic Z. 1992. Diagnosing dermatophytosis in dogs and cats. *Vet Med* 87:1086–1091.
54. Medleau L, White-Weithers NE. 1991. Dermatophytosis in cats. *Compend Cont Educ Pract Vet* 13:557–561.
55. Medleau L, White-Weithers NE. 1992. Treating and preventing the various forms of dermatophytosis. *Vet Med* 87:1096–1100.
55a. Mignon BR, Losson B. 1997. Prevalence and characterization of *Microsporum canis* carriage in cats. *J Med Vet Mycol* 35:249–256.
56. Morganti L, Tampieri MP, Galuppi R, et al. 1992. Morphological and biochemical variability of *Microsporum canis* strains. *Eur J Epidemiol* 8:340–345.
57. Moriello KA. 1990. Management of dermatophyte infections in catteries and multiple-cat households. *Vet Clin North Am Small Animal Pract* 20:1457–1474.
58. Moriello KA. 1992. Management of dermatophytosis in catteries, pp 89–94. *In* August J (ed), Consultations in feline internal medicine. WB Saunders, Philadelphia, PA.
59. Moriello KA. 1996. Treatment of feline dermatophytosis: revised recommendations. *Feline Pract* 24:32–36.
60. Moriello KA. 1997. Personal Communication. University of Wisconsin, Madison, WI.
61. Moriello KA, DeBoer DJ. 1991. Fungal flora of the coat of pet cats. *Am J Vet Res* 52:602–606.
62. Moriello KA, DeBoer DJ. 1991. Fungal flora of the haircoat of cats with and without dermatophytosis. *J Med Vet Mycol* 29:285–292.
63. Moriello KA, DeBoer DJ. 1994. Dermatophytosis, pp 219–226. *In* August J (ed), Consultations in feline internal medicine 2. WB Saunders, Philadelphia, PA.
64. Moriello KA, DeBoer DJ. 1994. Efficacy of griseofulvin and itraconazole in the treatment of experimental feline dermatophytosis. *J Am Vet Med Assoc* 207:439–444.
65. Moriello KA, DeBoer DJ. 1995. Feline dermatophytosis: recent advances and recommendations for therapy. *Vet Clin North Am Small Animal Pract* 25:901–921.
66. Moriello KA, DeBoer DJ. 1996. Environmental decontamination of *Microsporum canis*: in vitro studies on the efficacy of disinfectants, p 39. Presented at the Third World Congress of Veterinary Dermatology, Edinburgh, Scotland.
67. Moriello KA, Kunkle GA, DeBoer DJ. 1994. Isolation of dermatophytes from the haircoats of stray cats from selected animal shelters in two different geographic regions in the United States. *Vet Dermatol* 5:57–62.
68. Okamoto K, Yoshimori K, Akuzawa M, et al. 1994. Drug sensitivity of *Microsporum canis* isolates from dogs and cats. *J Jpn Vet Med Assoc* 47:118–122.
69. Paterson S, Pott JM, Jones A. 1996. The use of a 2% chlorhexidine/2% miconazole shampoo in the treatment of dermatophytosis, p 72. Presented at the Third World Congress of Veterinary Dermatology, Edinburgh.
70. Philpot CM, Newman MJ. 1992. Preliminary report on the isolation of a dysgonic variety of *Microsporum canis* together with the normal variety from a cattery. *Mycopathologia* 120:73–77.
71. Pier AC, Hodges AB, Lauze JM, et al. 1995. Experimental immunity to *Microsporum canis* and cross reactions with other dermatophytes of veterinary importance. *J Med Vet Mycol* 33:93–97.
72. Pier AC, Smith JMB, Alexiou H, et al. 1994. Animal ringworm—its etiology, public health significance and control. *J Vet Med Mycol* 32(Suppl):133–150.
73. Piérard GE, Arrese JE, De Doncker P, et al. 1996. Present and potential diagnostic techniques in onychomycosis. *J Am Acad Dermatol* 34:273–277.
74. Pinter L, Noble WC, Ellis J, et al. 1992. The value of enzyme-linked immunosorbent assay (ELISA) in the sero-diagnosis of canine dermatophytosis due to *Microsporum canis*. *Vet Dermatol* 3:65–70.
75. Piontelli LE, Toro SM. 1987. Domestic animals (dogs and cats) as fungus reservoirs. *Boletin Micologico* 3:149–158.
76. Product Information. Fel-o-vax Mc-K, Fort Dodge Laboratory, Fort Dodge, IA.
77. Puccini S, Valdré A, Papini R, et al. 1992. In vitro susceptibility to antimycotics of *Microsporum canis* isolates from cats. *J Am Vet Med Assoc* 201:1375–1377.
78. Reedy LM. 1995. An unusual presentation of feline dermatophytosis. *Feline Pract* 23:25–27.
79. Richard JL, Debey MC, Chermette R, et al. 1994. Advances in veterinary mycology. *J Med Vet Mycol* 32(Suppl):168–187.
80. Rycroft AN, McLay C. 1991. Disinfectants in the control of small animal ringworm due to *Microsporum canis*. *Vet Rec* 129:239–241.
81. Sanchez J, Velasco P, Quindos G. 1989. Isolation of dysgonic strains of *Microsporum canis* in Bilbao (Spain). *J Med Vet Mycol* 27:391–395.
82. Saul A, Bonifaz A. 1990. Itraconazole in common dermatophyte infections of the skin: fixed treatment schedules. *J Am Acad Dermatol* 23:554–558.
83. Scott DW, Miller WH Jr, Griffin CE. 1995. Fungal skin diseases, pp 329–391. *In* Scott DW, Miller WH, Griffin CE (eds), Muller & Kirk's small animal dermatology, ed 5. WB Saunders, Philadelphia, PA.
84. Scott DW, Paradis M. 1990. A survey of canine and feline skin disorders seen in a university practice: Small Animal Clinic, University of Montreal, Saint-Hyacinthe, Quebec (1987-1988). *Can Vet J* 31:830–835.
85. Shelton GH, Grant CK, Linenberger ML, et al. 1990. Severe neutropenia associated with griseofulvin therapy in cats with feline immunodeficiency virus. *J Vet Intern Med* 4:317–319.
86. Sparkes AH, Gruffydd-Jones TJ, Shaw SE, et al. 1993. Epidemiological and diagnostic features of canine and feline dermatophytosis in the United Kingdom from 1956 to 1991. *Vet Rec* 133:57–61.
87. Sparkes AH, Gruffydd-Jones TJ, Stokes CR. 1996. Acquired immunity in experimental feline *Microsporum canis* infection. *Res Vet Sci* 61:165–168.
88. Sparkes AH, Stokes CR, Gruffydd-Jones TJ. 1993. Humoral immune responses in cats with dermatophytosis. *Am J Vet Res* 54:1869–1873.
89. Sparkes AH, Stokes CR, Gruffydd-Jones TJ. 1994. SDS-PAGE separation of dermatophyte antigens, and Western immunoblotting in feline dermatophytosis. *Mycopathologia* 128:91–98.
90. Sparkes AH, Stokes CR, Gruffydd-Jones TJ. 1995. Experimental *Microsporum canis* infection in cats: correlation between immunological and clinical observations. *J Med Vet Mycol* 33:177–184.
91. Sparkes AH, Werrett G, Stokes CR, et al. 1994. Improved sensitivity in the diagnosis of dermatophytosis by fluorescence microscopy with calcofluor white. *Vet Rec* 134:307–308.
92. Sparkes AH, Werrett G, Stokes CR, et al. 1994. *Microsporum canis*: inapparent carriage by cats and the viability of arthrospores. *J Small Anim Pract* 35:397–401.
92a. Stenwig H. 1985. Isolation of dermatophytes from domestic animals in Norway. *Nord Vet Med* 37:161–169.
93. Symoens F, Fauvel E, Nolard N. 1989. Évolution de la contamination de l'air et des surfaces par *Microsporum canis* dans une habitation. *Bull Soc Fr Mycol Med* 18:293–298.
94. Thomas P, Kurting HC Strassl W, et al. 1994. *Microsporum canis* infection in a 5-year-old boy: transmission from the interior of a second-hand car. *Mycoses* 37:141–142.
95. Van Cutsem J, Kurata H, Matsuoka H, et al. 1994. Antifungal drug susceptibility testing. *J Vet Med Mycol* 32(Suppl):267–276.
96. Wenrick CJ. 1994. *Microsporum canis* vaccine (letter). *J Am Vet Med Assoc* 205:969.
97. White-Weithers N, Medleau L. 1995. Evaluation of topical therapies for the treatment of dermatophytosis in dogs and cats. *J Am Anim Hosp Assoc* 31:250–253.

Chapter 59

Blastomycosis

Alfred M. Legendre

ETIOLOGY

Blastomycosis is a systemic mycotic infection caused by the dimorphic fungus *Blastomyces dermatitidis*. In nature, *Blastomyces* grows as a saprophytic mycelial form that produces infective spores. At body temperatures, the organism transforms into the yeast form in tissues. A gene, *bys-1*, controls the change of the fungus from a mycelial to a yeast phase.[8] Budding yeasts are 5 to 20 μm in diameter and have a thick, refractile, double-contoured cell wall. Dogs and people most commonly are infected with *Blastomyces*, but cats, horses, sea lions, lions, wolves, ferrets, and polar bears have developed systemic blastomycosis.

EPIDEMIOLOGY

Natural Reservoir

The reservoir for *Blastomyces* is thought to be the soil; however, recovery of the organism from sites of suspected exposure is uncommon. Growth of the organism in the environment appears to require sandy, acid soil and proximity to water. Environmental survival of *Blastomyces* is further restricted because normal soil organisms in most areas will destroy *Blastomyces* inoculated into the soil. A special set of environmental conditions, "an ecologic niche," is required for proliferation of the organism. Organisms have been recovered from a beaver dam where a number of schoolchildren became exposed to the organism.[15] Living near a waterway is a risk factor for infection with blastomycosis. In a Wisconsin study, 95% of dogs with blastomycosis lived within 400 m of water.[3] Rain or heavy dew appears to facilitate the release of infectious spores. Access to sites that have been excavated also increases the risk for infection with blastomycosis because of exposure to organisms deep in the soil.[3] Even within endemic regions, *Blastomyces* is not widely distributed. Most people and dogs that live in such areas show no serologic or skin test evidence of exposure. A "point source" where exposure occurs within an enzootic area is more likely. For example, it is not unusual to find neighborhoods in which a number of dogs with blastomycosis are identified over a short period of time. Some owners have had a number of dogs develop blastomycosis, suggesting a foci in their immediate environment. Suspected common-source exposure of dogs and people while duck and raccoon hunting has been reported.[17]

In other systemic fungal infections such as histoplasmosis, aspergillosis, and coccidioidomycosis, many animals are exposed but few develop significant disease. However, in canine blastomycosis, subclinical infection is uncommon or rarely recognized. When tissues from pound dogs in endemic areas were cultured for fungal organisms, *Blastomyces* was found in 2% and *Histoplasma* in 50%.[17]

Geographic Distribution

Blastomycosis, caused by *B. dermatitidis*, is principally a disease of North America, but it has been identified in Africa and Central America. South American blastomycosis in people is caused by a different organism, *Paracoccidioides brasiliensis*, which has never been isolated from dogs or cats. Blastomycosis has a well-defined endemic distribution that includes the Mississippi, Missouri, and Ohio River valleys, the mid-Atlantic states, and the Canadian provinces of Quebec, Manitoba, and Ontario (Fig. 59–1)[26]; however, the distribution may be enlarging. Blastomycosis also occurs sporadically in New York.[9] Pets visiting or hunting in enzootic areas may become infected. A history of travel to an endemic area should increase the clinician's index of suspicion for blastomycosis.

Mode of Infection

Most cases of blastomycosis are acquired by inhalation of the spores from mycelial growth in the environment. The spores enter the terminal airway and establish a primary infection in the lungs. The size of the yeast when it grows at body temperature precludes its entering the terminal airway in an aerosol. Inoculation of *Blastomyces* into a wound from soil appears to be uncommon in the dog, but in solitary skin infections without systemic disease the possibility of direct inoculation cannot be excluded.[21] Because of the rarity of focal skin disease, cutaneous blastomycosis in the dog should be considered a manifestation of disseminated disease.

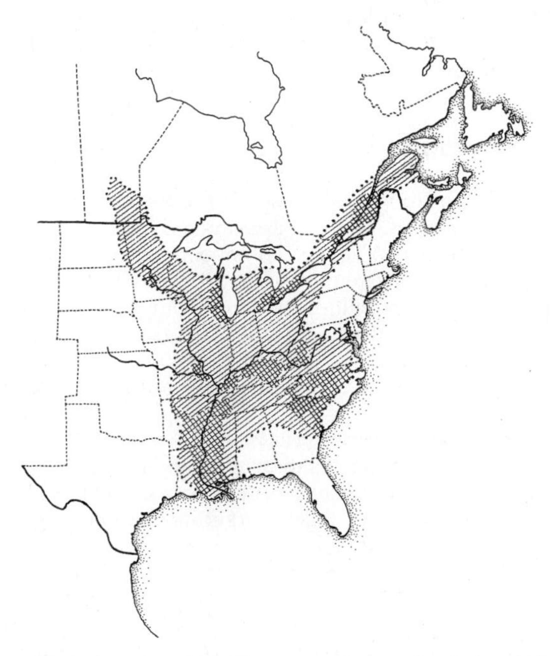

Figure 59–1. Area in which blastomycosis is endemic is within the dotted lines. Areas of highest incidence are cross-hatched. (From Rippon JW: Medical Mycology, ed 3. WB Saunders, 1988, pp 474–505. Reprinted with permission.)

PATHOGENESIS

Host Signalment

There does not seem to be a breed, age, or sex predisposition in the cat.[18] Sex and breed differences in the development of disease have been noted in dogs. Male dogs are more frequently infected than female dogs, and in dogs with equally severe blastomycosis, a greater percentage of females survive treatment.[17] In people, there is a 9:1 male–female ratio, which has, in part, been attributed to the increased exposure of males while hunting. An epidemiologic study using the Veterinary Medical Data Base (Purdue University, West Lafayette, IN) identified sporting dogs and hounds to be at greater risk.[27] This finding was attributed to outdoor activity as a risk factor for developing blastomycosis. Many of these breeds are brought to high-risk areas to hunt. Certain nonsporting breeds such as Doberman pinschers were also at increased risk.[17, 27] Large-breed dogs, in general, are more commonly infected than small-breed dogs. This finding also may reflect increased exposure from outdoor activities and roaming in larger dogs. The highest prevalence is in 2-year-old dogs; most cases occur in dogs 1 to 5 years of age. There does not appear to be a seasonal occurrence in the southeastern United States, but a greater number of cases have been found from late spring through late fall in Wisconsin.[17]

Dissemination of Organisms

After *Blastomyces* becomes established in the lungs, it disseminates throughout the body. The preferred sites in the dog are the skin, eyes, bones, lymph nodes, subcutaneous tissues, external nares, brain, and testes. Less commonly affected sites are mouth, nasal passages, prostate, liver, mammary gland, vulva, and heart. Dissemination is thought to occur via blood and lymphatic routes. Although lung entry occurs in almost all cases, lung lesions may resolve by the time the sites of disseminated infection become apparent. Occasionally, a focal lesion occurs from a puncture wound,[21] but generally a solitary lesion should be considered part of a systemic process.

Host Response

There appear to be distinct species differences in susceptibility to *Blastomyces*. The dog appears to be more susceptible to infection than people, and in enzootic areas of Arkansas, the incidence of blastomycosis is 10 times higher in dogs than in people. Epidemiologic studies in an endemic area of Wisconsin also identified a 10-fold greater incidence of blastomycosis in dogs compared with people.[1, 3] Among dogs in the highly endemic area, young age and close proximity to shoreline were risk factors.[4] The incidence in dogs was 1420 per 100,000 dogs per year.[3]

Dogs appear to have a shorter prepatent period and tend to develop the disease before people do when exposed at the same time.[17] Dogs may inhale a larger inoculum of organisms than people because they are closer to the ground. The larger the dose of inoculum, the earlier are the progression of the disease and death of the host.[17] Considerable variation in pathogenicity of isolated strains has also been demonstrated.[23] Cats have uncommonly been infected with *Blastomyces*. A 5-year survey of the Veterinary Medical Data Program identified 3 cats compared with 324 dogs with blastomycosis.[17]

Many factors in innate resistance of the host to blastomycosis are still unclear. A majority of dogs experimentally infected by exposure to contaminated soil recover from blastomycosis without treatment.[17] It is likely that under natural circumstances many infected dogs become mildly symptomatic and that the respiratory disease resolves spontaneously. However, nearly all dogs with clinical signs that have warranted veterinary attention have disseminated disease and should be aggressively treated. Recovery from symptomatic blastomycosis without treatment rarely occurs in dogs, but it has occurred in people.[17]

Dogs with disseminated disease are probably immunosuppressed, which further hinders their immune response. Forty percent of dogs with blastomycosis are lymphopenic. There is also a significant reduction in lymphocyte reactivity to mitogens when lymphocytes are cultured in autologous sera, suggesting a circulating factor that suppresses immune response.[17] Whether this reduced lymphocyte response is a cause or effect is uncertain. Recovery from mycotic diseases is attributed to cell-mediated immunity. Although antibody production occurs in most cases, it is not protective. Dogs with severe disseminated disease appear to have the greatest concentration of antibodies.

CLINICAL FINDINGS

Dogs

Dogs with blastomycosis usually have clinical signs that include anorexia, weight loss, cough, dyspnea, ocular disease, lameness, or skin lesions. Signs of disease usually have been present for a few days to a week but may have been apparent for up to a year. In some dogs, the disease process seems to stabilize; animals may show minimal signs for weeks to months, and then the disease suddenly progresses with worsening of signs. In many cases, there has been a history of antibiotic therapy with minimal or temporary improvement.

The physical findings in blastomycosis vary greatly. Mental depression is frequent but inconsistently noted. About 40% of dogs have a fever of 39.4°C (103°F) or greater. Dogs with chronic lung disease are often severely emaciated. Lymphadenomegaly of one or more nodes is a frequent finding.

A majority (85%) of dogs with blastomycosis have lung lesions with characteristic dry, harsh lung sounds. Dogs with mild lung disease show exercise intolerance, and severely affected dogs have dyspnea at rest. Coughing is a variable finding. Thoracic radiographs are indicated for dogs suspected of having blastomycosis because some dogs have lung changes without respiratory signs. Diffuse, nodular interstitial and bronchointerstitial lung changes are most commonly seen (Fig. 59–2). Other less common manifestations include well-marginated solitary to multiple cystic or solid nodules to masses. Tracheobronchial lymphadenomegaly occurs in some dogs. Pleural effusion, pneumomediastinum, and cavitary lung lesions are also observed. Chylothorax and solid fibrous masses are uncommon manifestations of thoracic blastomycosis. Solid fibrous masses may partially occlude the great vessels.

Up to 40% of dogs with blastomycosis have ocular lesions, the most common of which is uveitis. Early signs of uveitis are aqueous flare, miosis, blepharospasm, and photophobia (Fig. 59–3). Retinal separation with detachment (see Fig. 93–13), retinal granulomas, and vitreal hemorrhage are also seen (Fig. 59–4). Severe corneal edema may prevent good visualization of the internal ocular structures. Glaucoma secondary to angle closure occurs in blastomycosis.[5] Periorbital cellulitis

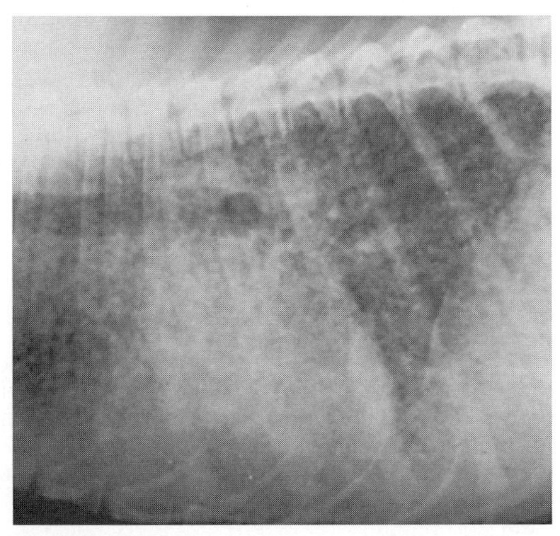

Figure 59–2. Severe, diffuse miliary to nodular interstitial pulmonary infiltrate. (Courtesy of Dr. Bill Adams, University of Tennessee, Knoxville, TN.)

and involvement of the nictitating membrane also occur. Uveitis in conjunction with signs of respiratory or skin disease should alert the clinician to consider blastomycosis. Early diagnosis and appropriate treatment are essential to preservation of vision in blastomycosis (see also Chapter 93).

Skin lesions, found in 20% to 40% of dogs with blastomycosis, may be ulcerated with drainage of a serosanguineous or purulent fluid (Fig. 59–5). Other lesions may be granulomatous, proliferative, and meaty (Fig. 59–6). There may be well-defined subcutaneous abscesses. Although the skin lesions may be found anywhere, the planum nasale, the face, and the nail beds appear to be preferred sites.

Bone involvement occurs in up to 30% of infected dogs. Lameness is the primary sign in affected animals and may be the only sign of disease. Special procedures, such as bone scans, may identify a greater percentage of dogs with bone involvement. Lesions usually involve the appendicular skeleton or vertebrae; they are usually osteolytic with periosteal proliferation and soft tissue swelling (Fig. 59–7). A majority of the bone lesions are solitary and occur distal to the stifle and elbow. Fungal osteomyelitis must be differentiated from primary and metastatic bone tumors and bacterial osteomyelitis.

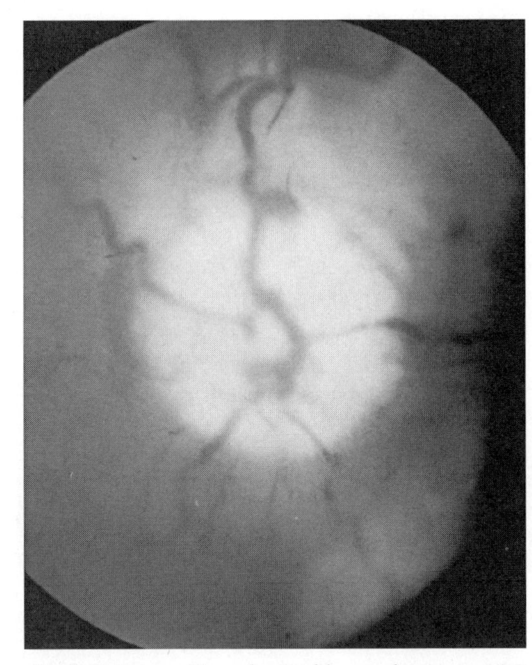

Figure 59–4. Optic neuritis and retinal hemorrhages associated with blastomycosis of the eye and central nervous system. (Courtesy of Dr. Dennis Brooks, University of Tennessee, Knoxville, TN.)

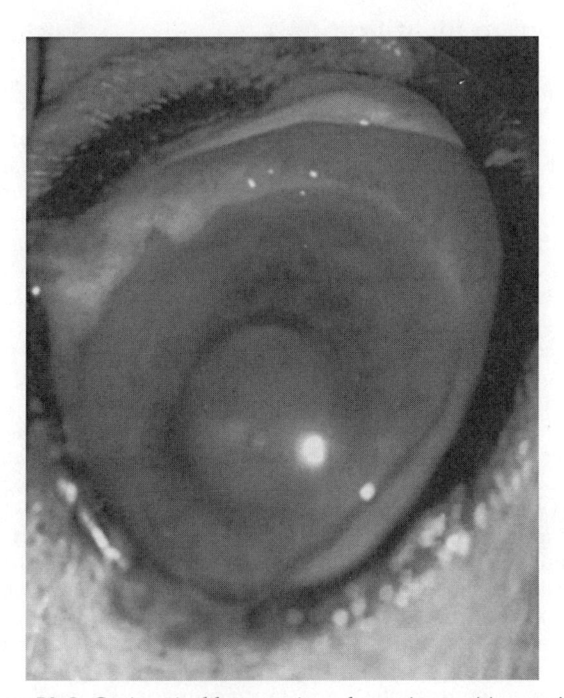

Figure 59–3. Conjunctival hyperemia and anterior uveitis associated with blastomycosis. (Courtesy of Dr. Dennis Brooks, University of Tennessee, Knoxville, TN.)

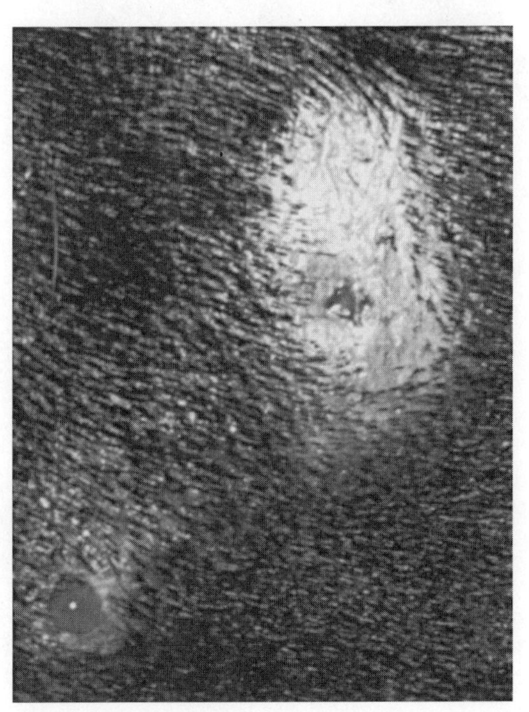

Figure 59–5. Draining tract from subcutaneous abscess producing a serosanguineous discharge. (Courtesy of Dr. Lynn Schmeitzel, University of Tennessee, Knoxville, TN.)

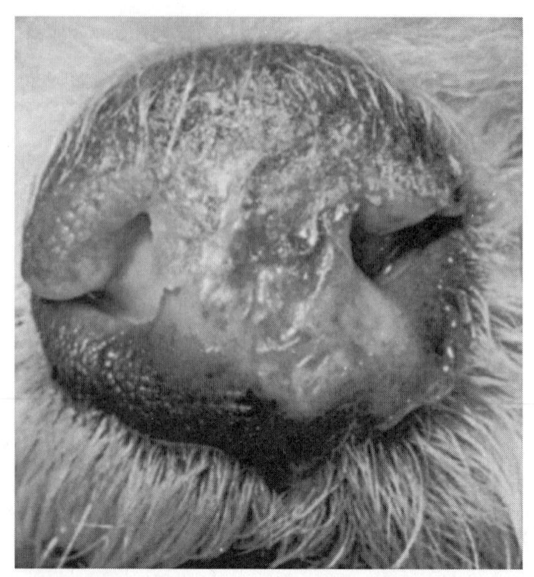

Figure 59–6. Proliferative granulomatous blastomycosis lesion of the nose causing distortion. (Courtesy of Dr. Lynn Schmeitzel, University of Tennessee, Knoxville, TN.)

A variety of other tissues may be less commonly infected, including testes, prostate, kidney, bladder, brain, and nasal passages. The testes and epididymis may be greatly enlarged and painful. Involvement of the prostate gland produces swelling and pain. Dogs with involvement of the kidneys, bladder, or prostate may have organisms in the urine. Meningeal and secondary brain involvement usually develops with widely disseminated disease but may develop without multisystemic manifestations. Depression, seizures, and neurologic deficits are noted with CNS infections. Nasal discharge and obstruction of airflow through the nose occur when blastomycosis involves the nasal passages. Lesions have been found in most organs of infected dogs except the stomach and intestinal tract.

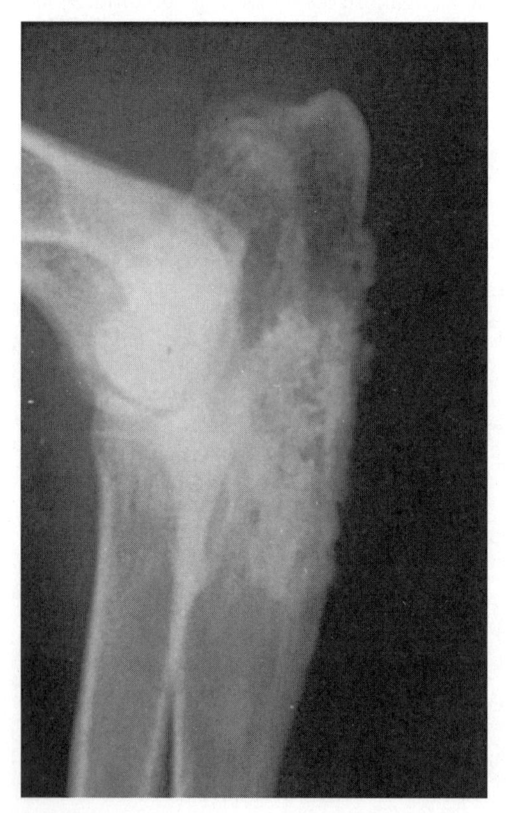

Figure 59–7. Semiaggressive bone lesion characterized by osteolysis and amorphous bone production of the proximal ulna. (Courtesy of Dr. Bill Adams, University of Tennessee, Knoxville, TN.)

Cats

Cats have lesions similar to those of dogs, but too few cats have been evaluated to derive a reliable characterization of predominant signs. Dyspnea, visual impairment, draining skin lesions, and weight loss have been the most frequent findings. Intracranial CNS disease and posterior paralysis also have been reported.[22] Clinical signs reflect the involved tissues: lung, lymph node, kidney, eye, CNS, skin, GI tract, pleura, and peritoneum.[22]

DIAGNOSIS

Clinical Laboratory Testing

Preliminary laboratory evaluation shows a mild normocytic, normochromic anemia attributed to chronic inflammation. Most dogs have a moderate leukocytosis (17,000–30,000 WBC/μl) with a mild left shift, and lymphopenia is common. Serum biochemical profiles show hyperglobulinemia and hypoalbuminemia. The greater globulin concentrations are due to an increase in α_2-globulin and a polyclonal increase in immunoglobulin. The only other biochemical change that may be seen is hypercalcemia of granulomatous disease (12.5–17.5 mg/dl), which may occur without bone lesions.[11] Elevated serum calcium concentrations return to normal after treatment of the blastomycosis. Hypercalcemia may be associated with renal failure.

Organism Identification

Diagnosis should be made by identification of the organism by cytologic or histologic evaluation. Any of the common cytologic stains can be used. Because of the cost of therapy, a definitive cytologic rather than a serologic diagnosis is preferred. The combination of aspirates of enlarged lymph nodes and impression smears of skin lesions or cytology of draining exudates will yield organisms in more than half the cases (Fig. 59–8). The cytologic reaction is characteristically pyogranulomatous including nondegenerate neutrophils and macrophages (which may be epithelioid in appearance) with occasional multinucleated giant cells. Plasma cells, lymphocytes, and fibroblasts are also seen. Occasionally, a suppurative reaction can predominate.[13] Organisms are usually plentiful in fulminating disease. When the disease is primarily ocular and less invasive diagnostic procedures have failed, vitreous aspirates or histologic examination of enucleated blind eyes will identify the disease as blastomycosis. In dogs with productive coughs, a tracheal wash may contain the organism but this test is less reliable than other procedures, probably because of the primarily interstitial site of infection. Lung aspirates can be used when the lung is the only affected site and the results of the tracheal wash are negative. Pneumothorax is a potential complication of lung aspiration, although severe complications are uncommon. Premedication with atropine is recommended before lung aspiration to prevent excessive vagal stimulation. In dogs with urinary tract

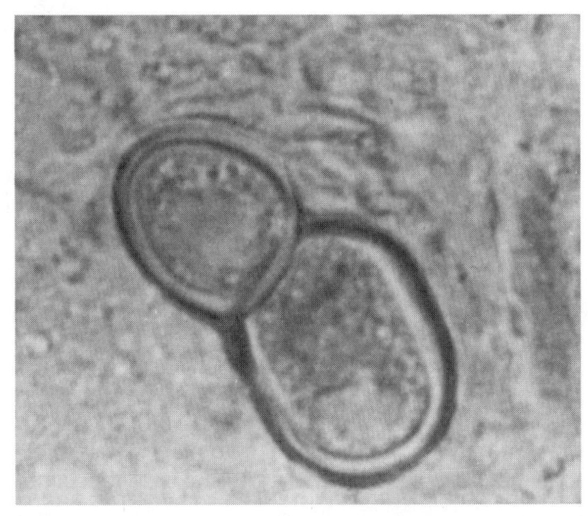

Figure 59–8. Budding yeast form of *Blastomyces* (new methylene blue, ×1260).

or prostatic blastomycosis, the organism may be found on urinalysis. In dogs with brain involvement, organisms rarely may be found on examination of the CSF. Culture of cytologic specimens is not recommended for in-clinic laboratories because of the danger to personnel of infection from the mycelial form of the organism (see Fig. 56–16).[10]

Atypical pulmonary fibrous masses containing organisms in small inflammatory foci may develop in lieu of the usual granulomatous reaction. These fibrous masses have few organisms and cytology of aspirates is usually unrewarding. Surgical biopsies are required, and multiple histologic sections with fungal staining are needed to find the organisms.

Serologic Testing

Only after a search for organisms has been made should serologic testing be done to help establish a diagnosis. Although serologic testing alone is not definitive, a combination of compatible history, clinical signs, and suggestive radiographs in conjunction with positive serology may be substituted for identification of the organism.

The agar-gel immunodiffusion test (AGID), which has replaced the complement fixation test, is currently the most commonly utilized serologic test available for diagnosis of blastomycosis. It has a sensitivity and specificity in the dog of greater than 90%.[19, 24] The AGID test has been used in only a few infected cats, and results have been positive in only one of three cats tested.[22] AGID test results in dogs may be negative early in the development of infections. Although the intensity and the number of bands seen on the AGID tend to decrease after successful treatment, the persistence of antibodies in cured animals precludes AGID for evaluating response to therapy or relapse afterwards. A number of ELISAs have been evaluated, but these tests are not commercially available at this time. They may be more sensitive in identifying dogs with early disease or infected cats. Purification of the antigens in ELISA testing improves the test specificity and discrimination between fungal infections.[12]

PATHOLOGIC FINDINGS

Blastomycosis produces purulent to pyogranulomatous lesions in infected tissues of dogs and cats. The yeasts are admixed with neutrophils, macrophages, and multinucleated giant cells. Lymph nodes are hyperplastic with increased numbers of plasma cells and macrophages. In tissue, the broad-based, budding yeasts are best demonstrated by special stains (periodic acid–Schiff, Gridley's fungal, or Gomori's methenamine silver stain). Filamentous forms in lieu of the yeast form have been found in the tissue of people and dogs.[17]

THERAPY

For a summary of the dosage regimens discussed next, see Table 59–1.

Amphotericin B

Amphotericin B (AMB) is an effective, rapidly acting, fungicidal drug for the treatment of a variety of systemic fungal infections, including blastomycosis. Because AMB is nephrotoxic and has been given IV, it has been replaced as the drug of choice for blastomycosis by itraconazole (ITZ), which is equally effective and safer.[20] For further information on AMB and its precautions, see Drug Formulary, Appendix 8.

In dogs that cannot absorb oral medications or that have not responded to ITZ treatment, AMB can be a life-saving drug. AMB deoxycholate should be given at a dose of 0.5 mg/kg every other day. The blood urea nitrogen (BUN) concentration should be monitored closely and the AMB discontinued when the BUN approaches 50 mg/dl. A cumulative dose of 8 to 10 mg/kg will be required for cure of

Table 59–1. Drug Therapy for Blastomycosis[a]

DRUG	SPECIES	DOSE (mg/kg)[b]	ROUTE	INTERVAL (HOURS)	DURATION[c] (DAYS)
Itraconazole	D[d]	5	PO	24	60
	C	5	PO	12	60
Fluconazole	D	5	PO	12	60
AMB lipid complex[e]	D	1	IV	3 times weekly	[f]
AMB	D	0.5	IV	3 times weekly	[g]
	C	0.25	IV	3 times weekly	[h]

[a]See text and Drug Formulary, Appendix 8, for additional information concerning administration of each drug.
[b]Dose per administration at specified interval.
[c]This is the minimum duration of therapy, which should continue for at least 1 month beyond the last detection of clinical illness or infection.
[d]Preferred drug and dosage therapy; when expense is a factor, other regimens may be considered; should be given every 12 hours for the first 5 days; see text.
[e]There are three lipid formulations available (see Drug Formulary, Appendix 8). Efficacy at this dose has been established for ABLC (Abelcet, Liposome Co., Princeton, NJ).
[f]Stop when cumulative dose reaches 12 mg/kg.
[g]Stop when azotemic or cumulative dose reaches 4–6 mg/kg, then start azole; or when cumulative dose is 8–10 mg/kg when given alone.
[h]Stop when azotemic or cumulative dose reaches 4 mg/kg.
D = dog; C = cat; B = both dog and cat; AMB = amphotericin B.

blastomycosis. Cats should be given no more than 0.25 mg/kg every other day.

AMB lipid complex (see Drug Formulary, Appendix 8) has been less toxic when given to treat dogs with systemic blastomycosis.[16] The effective dose is similar to or slightly higher than that of AMB deoxycholate, but the drug is much less nephrotoxic although considerably more expensive.

Itraconazole

Dogs. ITZ is an azole drug of the triazole group (for additional information, see Drug Formulary, Appendix 8). Dogs with blastomycosis respond to treatment with ITZ as rapidly as with AMB and more rapidly than with ketoconazole (KTZ). Compared with AMB, ITZ is easier to administer and has fewer side effects. Because ITZ is given PO, dogs can be treated at home. Although the cost of ITZ is greater, the cost of treatment is similar to that for AMB when the expense of IV administration and frequent monitoring of renal function is considered.

Fifty-four percent of dogs treated with 5 mg/kg/day of ITZ were cured compared with 57% in a historical control group treated with AMB.[20] The relapse rates and the mortality rates between ITZ and AMB treated dogs were very similar. The 5 mg/kg/day dose of ITZ was better than the 10 mg/kg/day dose. The cure and relapse rates were similar, but the lower dose group had fewer adverse effects. ITZ appears to penetrate into the eye in dogs with active disease, because the dogs with ocular blastomycosis of the posterior chamber often respond to ITZ treatment.[7] ITZ is not excreted in the urine so it cannot be used in urinary tract disease. The ease of administration, the decreased likelihood of toxicity, and the efficacy of ITZ make it the drug of choice for the treatment of blastomycosis. The only disadvantage to ITZ treatment is its high cost.

For dogs, ITZ should be started at a dosage of 5 mg/kg every 12 hours for 5 days to maximize blood concentrations rapidly. The dosage is reduced to 5 mg/kg/day for the remainder of the treatment. ITZ treatment should be continued for at least 60 days and for at least 1 month after all signs of disease have resolved. Most dogs with mild to moderate lung involvement can be cured with a 60-day course of treatment. Dogs with severe lung involvement should be treated for at least 90 days. Dogs treated with ITZ for 60 to 90 days had a recurrence rate of 20%, which is identical to the experience with AMB.[20] Recurrence usually occurs within 1 year of completion of treatment. Occasionally a dog may have a recurrence 1 to 2 years after treatment. For additional information on itraconazole, see Drug Formulary, Appendix 8.

Cats. Cats with blastomycosis have been treated with 5 mg/kg given every 12 hours. This is an effective, safe treatment for most cats. There are no studies on the efficacy of lower drug dosages.

Adverse Effects. The most common adverse effect of ITZ treatment is anorexia associated with hepatotoxicity. Ninety-two percent of dogs receiving 5 mg/kg/day had no clinical signs of toxicity.[20] Only 1 of 24 dogs studied had serum alanine aminotransferase activities above 200 U/L. Increases in liver enzymes correlate to serum concentrations of ITZ. Serum concentrations of ITZ can vary tremendously in dogs receiving the same dose of drug. If toxicity occurs, medication should be stopped until the appetite returns and the serum liver enzyme activities return to below 100 U/L. The medication is reinstituted at half the former dose with monitoring of serum liver enzymes every 2 weeks.

Ulcerative dermatitis occurred in 7.5% of dogs receiving 10 mg/kg/day of ITZ, but it did not occur in any dog receiving 5 mg/kg/day[20] (Fig. 59–9). Ulcers were usually focal, 1 to 2.5 cm in diameter, and circular, with ischemic dermis from an underlying vasculitis. The lesions healed quickly after ITZ was stopped. Lesions did not recur when ITZ was restarted at a decreased dose. This reaction must not be interpreted as a recurrence of blastomycosis.

Serum concentration of ITZ can be measured to ensure that the dog is receiving enough drug.[20] Serum ITZ concentrations of 2 μg/ml or greater appear to be adequate. Serum samples can be sent to The Fungus Testing Lab, University of Texas Health Science Center, 7703 Floyd Curl Drive, San Antonio, Texas 78284; (210) 567-4131.

Prognosis

The prognosis for dogs and cats with blastomycosis is good. The two prognostic factors for survival are brain involvement and severity of lung disease. Dogs with brain involvement usually die, but occasionally such a dog can be successfully treated. A 10-mg/kg/day dose should be used in dogs with brain disease. The severity of lung infiltrates may worsen in the first 2 to 3 days of treatment and the worsening of signs has been attributed to an inflammatory response to the killing of organisms in the lungs. Death usually results from respiratory failure and occurs in 50% of the dogs with severe lung disease during the first 7 days of treatment. Improved survival rates can be achieved only with earlier diagnosis of the condition before severe lung disease occurs. For ocular lesions, dogs with mild posterior segment disease, without complete retinal separation, have good prognoses for retaining vision.[5] Dogs with severely affected eyes, with endophthalmitis and/or glaucoma, have poor prognoses for improvement in vision.

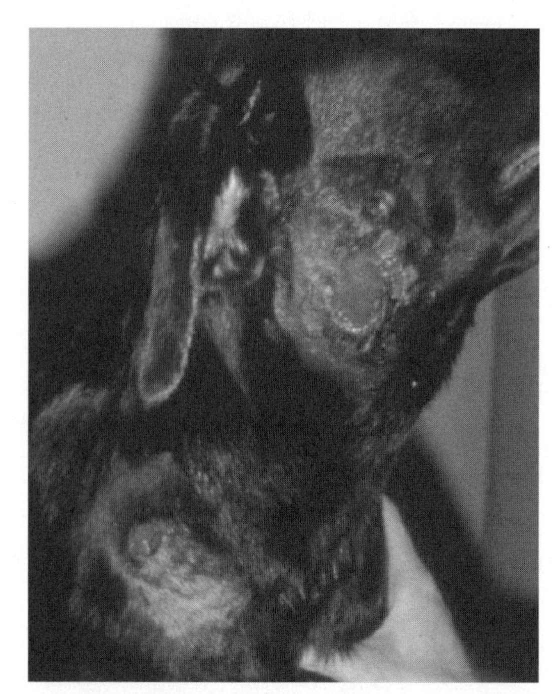

Figure 59–9. Ulcerative dermatitis may occur in some dogs treated with 10 mg/kg/day of itraconazole. (Reprinted with permission from Legendre AM, Rohrbach BW, Toal RL, et al. *J Vet Intern Med* 10:365–371, 1996.)

Treatment of Relapse

Approximately 20% of the dogs will relapse after treatment with AMB alone, or AMB plus KTZ treatment.[20] Relapse after apparently successful treatment usually occurs in the first 6 months after completion of therapy, but recurrences can occur up to 15 months after completion of therapy.[17, 20] Likelihood of relapse is related to severity of the initial lung disease. Reinfection after successful treatment does not appear to occur, and the recurrence of infection is probably due to reactivation of a residual site of infection. Recurrence of disease can be effectively treated with another 60- to 90-day course of ITZ. The *Blastomyces* organisms do not appear to develop resistance to the ITZ. Retreatment has an 80% or greater chance of producing a cure.

PREVENTION

The ecologic niche for growth of *Blastomyces* has not been identified; therefore, preventive measures are not possible. Even if the site were identified, sterilization of the soil is impossible. Restriction of the animals from lakes and creeks in areas where other dogs have become infected may be helpful. Dogs should be kept away from construction sites where there has been digging. Dogs kenneled in a heavily shaded area where the soil remains moist may be at increased risk. Removal of some tree branches to allow sunshine into the kennel area may be helpful in reducing the risk of infection. No vaccine is available for prevention of blastomycosis.

PUBLIC HEALTH CONSIDERATIONS

There is no danger from aerosol transmission of the yeast phase of the organism from animals to people or from people to people. Penetrating wounds contaminated by the organism have produced infections in people. Care should be taken to avoid getting bitten when handling a dog with blastomycosis.[17] Accidental inoculation of organisms by contaminated knives or needles should be avoided at necropsy or during fine-needle aspiration.[17, 25] Culturing of the organism should be restricted to laboratories with proper facilities. Primary pulmonary blastomycosis has readily occurred in laboratory workers exposed to cultures of the mycelial form of *Blastomyces dermatitidis*.[10, 17]

References

1. Baumgardner DJ, Buggy BP, Mattson BJ, et al. 1992. Epidemiology of blastomycosis in a region of high endemicity in north central Wisconsin. *Clin Infect Dis* 15:629–635.
2. Baumgardner DJ, Burdick JS. 1991. An outbreak of humans and canine blastomycosis. *Rev Infect Dis* 13:898–905.
3. Baumgardner DJ, Paretsky DP, Yopp AC. 1995. The epidemiology of blastomycosis in dogs: north central Wisconsin, USA. *J Med Vet Mycol* 33:171–176.
4. Baumgardner DJ, Turkal NW, Paretsky DP. 1996. Blastomycosis in dogs. A 15 year survey in a very highly endemic area near Eagle River, Wisconsin. *Wild Environ Med* 7:1–8.
5. Bloom JD, Hamor RE, Gerding PA. 1996. Ocular blastomycosis in dogs: 73 cases, 108 eyes (1985–1993). *J Am Vet Med Assoc* 209:1271–1274.
6. Bono JL, Legendre AM, Scalarone GM, et al. 1995. Detection of antibodies and delayed hypersensitivity with Rotofor preparative IEF fractions of *Blastomyces dermatitidis* yeast phase lysate antigen. *J Med Vet Mycol* 33:209–214.
7. Brooks DE, Legendre AM, Gum GG, et al. 1991. The treatment of ocular blastomycosis with systemically administered itraconazole. *Prog Vet Comp Ophthalmol* 4:263–268.
8. Burg EF III, Smith LH Jr. 1994. Cloning and characterization of bys1, a temperature-dependent cDNA specific to the yeast phase of the pathogenic dimorphic fungus *Blastomyces dermatitidis*. *Infect Immun* 62:2521–2528.
9. Ĉoté E, Barr SC, Allen C, et al. 1997. Blastomycosis in six dogs in New York State. *J Am Vet Med Assoc* 210:502–504.
10. Ĉoté E, Barr SC, Allen C, et al. 1997. Possible transmission of *Blastomyces dermatitidis* via culture specimen. *J Am Vet Med Assoc* 210:479–480.
11. Dow SW, Legendre AM, Stiff M, et al. 1986. Hypercalcemia associated with blastomycosis in dogs. *J Am Vet Med Assoc* 188:706–709.
12. Fisher MA, Bono JL, Abuodeh RO, et al. 1995. Sensitivity and specificity of an isoelectric focusing fraction of *Blastomyces dermatitidis* yeast lysate antigen for the detection of canine blastomycosis. *Mycoses* 38:177–182.
13. Garma-Avina A. 1995. Cytologic findings in 43 cases of blastomycosis diagnosed ante-mortem in naturally-infected dogs. *Mycopathologia* 131:87–91.
14. Hurst SF, Kaufman L. 1992. Western immunoblot analysis and serologic characterization of *Blastomyces dermatitidis* yeast from extracellular antigens. *J Clin Microbiol* 30:3043–3049.
15. Klein BS, Vergeront JM, Weeks RJ, et al. 1986. Isolation of *Blastomyces dermatitidis* in soil associated with a large outbreak of blastomycosis in Wisconsin. *N Engl J Med* 314:529–534.
16. Krawiec DR, McKiernan BC, Twardock AR, et al. 1996. Use of an amphotericin B lipid complex for treatment of blastomycosis in dogs. *J Am Vet Med Assoc* 209:2073–2075.
17. Legendre AM. 1990. Blastomycosis, pp 669–678. *In* Greene CE (ed), Infectious diseases of the dog and cat. WB Saunders, Philadelphia, PA.
18. Legendre AM. 1994. Systemic mycotic infections, pp 553–564. *In* Sherding R (ed), Diseases of the cat. Churchill Livingstone, New York, NY.
19. Legendre AM, Becker RU. 1980. Evaluation of the agar-gel immunodiffusion test in the diagnosis of canine blastomycosis. *Am J Vet Res* 41:2109–2111.
20. Legendre AM, Rohrbach BW, Toal RL, et al. 1996. Treatment of blastomycosis with intraconazole in 112 dogs. *J Vet Intern Med* 10:365–371.
21. Marcellin-Little DJ, Sellon RK, Kyles AE, et al. 1996. Chronic localized osteomyelitis caused by atypical infection with *Blastomyces dermatitidis* in a dog. *J Am Vet Med Assoc* 209:1877–1879.
22. Miller PE, Miller LM, Schoster JV. 1990. Feline blastomycosis: a report of three cases and literature review (1961 to 1988). *J Am Anim Hosp Assoc* 26:417–424.
23. Moser SA, Koker PJ, Williams JE. 1988. Fungal-strain dependent alterations in the time course and mortality of chronic murine pulmonary blastomycosis. *Infect Immun* 56:34–39.
24. Phillips WE, Kaufman L. 1980. Cultural and histopathologic confirmation of canine blastomycosis diagnosed by an agar-gel immunodiffusion test. *Am J Vet Res* 41:1263–1265.
25. Ramsey DT. 1994. Blastomycosis in a veterinarian. *J Am Vet Med Assoc* 205:968.
26. Rippon JW. 1988. Medical mycology, ed 3, pp 474–505. WB Saunders, Philadelphia, PA.
27. Rudmann DG, Coolman BR, Perez CM, Glickman LT. 1992. Evaluation of risk factors for blastomycosis in dogs: 857 cases (1980–1990). *J Am Vet Med Assoc* 201:1754–1759.
28. Scalarone GM, Legendre AM, Clark KA, et al. 1992. Evaluation of a commercial DNA probe assay for the identification of *Blastomyces dermatitidis* from dogs. *J Med Vet Mycol* 30:43–49.
29. Seawell BW, Legendre AM, Scalarone GM. 1990. Enzyme immunoassay detection of antibodies in canine blastomycosis using *Blastomyces dermatitidis* lysate antigens. *Mycoses* 33:483–489.
30. Seawell BW, Scalarone GM. 1990. Comparison of enzyme immunoassay and immunodiffusion for the detection of canine blastomycosis. *Mycoses* 33:375–381.

Chapter 60

Histoplasmosis

Alice M. Wolf

ETIOLOGY

The etiologic agent of American histoplasmosis is the soil-borne, dimorphic fungus *Histoplasma capsulatum*. This organism can survive wide fluctuations in environmental temperature and prefers areas with moist, humid conditions. *H. capsulatum* grows best in soil containing nitrogen-rich organic matter such as bird and bat excrement. Although most affected animals have exposure to the outdoor environment, some affected cats have been exclusively housed indoors. This finding suggests that even accumulations of household dust or soil-containing house plants may be potential sources of infection.

EPIDEMIOLOGY

H. capsulatum is endemic throughout large areas of the temperate and subtropical regions of the world (Fig. 60–1). The fungus has been isolated from soil in 31 of the continental United States. Most clinical cases occur in the central United States in the region of the Ohio, Missouri, and Mississippi Rivers. Histoplasmosis can appear in traditionally non-endemic regions if local environmental conditions are altered to favor fungal growth. Obtaining a detailed travel history is important to identify patients that may have acquired infection while in endemic regions.[10]

It is difficult to determine true rates for histoplasmosis in companion animals because most infections are subclinical. The prevalence of infection probably parallels that in the human population in endemic regions.

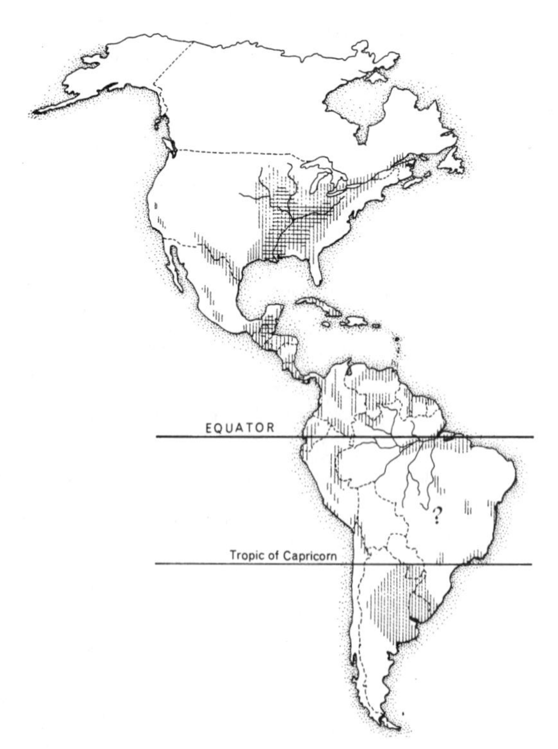

Figure 60–1. The incidence and prevalence of histoplasmosis in North and South America based on skin testing surveys. The darker-shaded areas indicate zones of very high endemicity. (From Rippon JW: Medical Mycology, ed 3. WB Saunders, Philadelphia, 1988. Reprinted with permission.)

PATHOGENESIS

The life cycle of *H. capsulatum* is similar to that of other dimorphic fungi. The free-living, mycelial stage in soil produces macroconidia (5–18 μm) (see Fig. 56–15) and microconidia (2–5 μm) that are the source of infection for mammals. Histoplasmosis is probably acquired by inhalation of microconidia that are small enough to reach the lower respiratory tract. The incubation period after exposure is approximately 12 to 16 days.[8] The microconidia convert to the yeast phase in the lung and reproduce by budding. The yeast organisms are phagocytized by cells of the host's mononuclear phagocyte system and undergo further intracellular replication. Infection may be grossly limited to the pulmonary tree; however, lymphatic and hematogenous dissemination of *H. capsulatum* can occur early in the course of the disease because of the intracellular location of the fungus. Severe clinical disease can result if the dose of infective spores is large or if the immune system of the host is compromised. The cellular immune system will rapidly bring the infection under control in most patients. T-cell immunity is critical for clearance of the organism. In some hosts, *H. capsulatum* may establish a dormant phase and may not be totally eliminated from the mononuclear phagocyte system.[8a] With subsequent immunosuppression, reactivation of infection can occur.

The occurrence of GI histoplasmosis without respiratory tract involvement suggests that the GI tract may also be a primary site of infection. However, experimental studies have failed to reliably produce GI disease after oral administration of *H. capsulatum* spores.

CLINICAL FINDINGS

Cats

Cats are very susceptible hosts and are at least as likely as dogs to develop clinical histoplasmosis. The age range of cats affected with histoplasmosis is 4 months to 14 years; the majority of cases occur in young cats (< 4 years).[12] There is no apparent breed predilection; females appear to be more commonly affected than males.[12]

Most infected cats have disseminated disease and exhibit a wide range of nonspecific clinical signs, including depression, weight loss, fever, anorexia, and pale mucous membranes.[5] Coughing is uncommon, but dyspnea, tachypnea, and abnormal lung sounds are found in more than half of affected cats. Other frequent findings include peripheral or visceral lymphadenomegaly, splenomegaly, and hepatomegaly. Occasionally, *Histoplasma* infects the eye, causing conjunctivitis, granulomatous blepharitis, granulomatous chorioretinitis, retinal detachment, and optic neuritis.[12, 13, 17] Some cats have had osseous lesions, causing soft tissue swelling and lameness. The skin is infrequently affected with nodular or ulcerated lesions.[20] Rare clinical findings include oral ulcers, nasal polyps, vomiting, and diarrhea.

Dogs

Histoplasmosis has been reported in dogs ranging in age from 2 months to 14 years. Most affected dogs are young (< 4 years), and there is no apparent sex predilection. Pointers, Weimaraners, and Brittany spaniels are overrepresented in some published reports.[26]

Inappetence, weight loss, and fever unresponsive to antibiotic therapy occur in most cases of canine histoplasmosis. In some dogs, the clinical signs may be limited to the respiratory tree and include dyspnea, coughing, and abnormal lung sounds. However, in most dogs, clinical signs result from disseminated histoplasmosis with GI involvement.[6, 16] Signs of large-bowel diarrhea with tenesmus, mucus, and fresh blood in the stool are the most common clinical findings (Fig. 60–2). Pale mucous membranes often are found in patients with bone marrow involvement or GI blood loss. Extensive *Histoplasma* infiltration of the small bowel can cause a voluminous, watery stool with an accompanying protein-losing enteropathy. Hepatomegaly, visceral lymphadenomegaly, splenomegaly, icterus, and ascites are frequent associated findings. Unusual signs include vomiting, peripheral lymphadenomegaly, and lameness as a result of osseous infection. Ocular lesions and skin lesions as described for cats have also been reported in the dog. Neurologic involvement, recognized with dissemination of infection in dogs, is rare.[19]

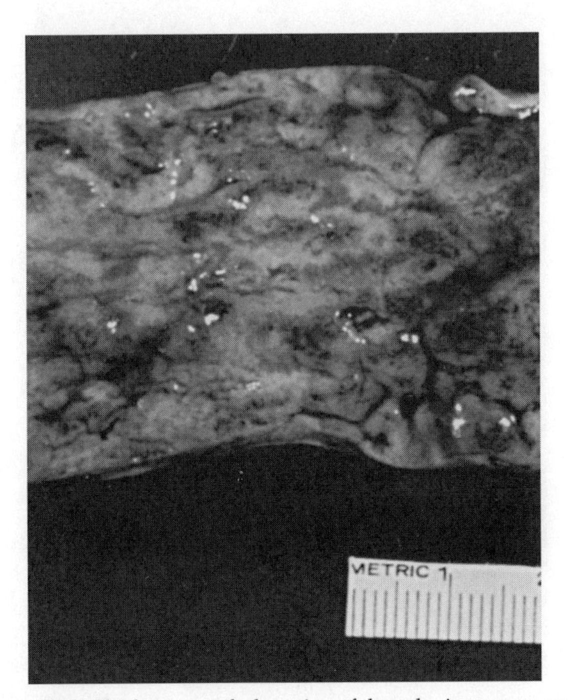

Figure 60–2. Thickening and ulceration of the colonic mucosa caused by histoplasmosis results in large bowel diarrhea containing mucus and fresh blood.

DIAGNOSIS

Clinical Laboratory Testing

The most common hematologic abnormality in both dogs and cats with disseminated histoplasmosis is normocytic, normochromic, nonregenerative anemia. The anemia probably results from both chronic inflammatory disease, *Histoplasma* infection of the bone marrow, and intestinal blood loss in GI disease. Leukocyte counts are variable. Neutrophilic leukocytosis with monocytosis and eosinopenia is found most frequently. Leukopenia and thrombocytopenia have also been reported. Severe pancytopenia has been observed in some cats. *Histoplasma* organisms may be found during routine blood film examination in circulating monocytes, neutrophils, and, rarely, eosinophils. Performing 1000-cell differential counts or examining buffy coat smears will enhance detection of infected cells.

Abnormal coagulation function tests have been found in some thrombocytopenic dogs with disseminated histoplasmosis, suggesting the presence of microangiopathic hemolysis. Disseminated intravascular coagulation (DIC) in these dogs may occur as a result of extensive *Histoplasma* infiltration of the liver. Hemolysis and an increased bleeding tendency associated with DIC may enhance the severity of the anemia in these patients.

Biochemical profiles are usually unremarkable in dogs with pulmonary histoplasmosis. Hypoalbuminemia is a fairly consistent finding in cats with disseminated histoplasmosis. Some cats have had hyperproteinemia, hyperglobulinemia, and mild elevations of serum glucose and alanine aminotransferase (ALT) activities. Dogs with disseminated disease may have hypoproteinemia and severe hypoalbuminemia as a result of intestinal blood loss or protein-losing enteropathy. Liver dysfunction in affected dogs may cause hypoalbuminemia, hyperbilirubinemia, elevated serum alkaline phosphatase and ALT values, and abnormal results on liver function tests.[3] Hypercalcemia (probably associated with granulomatous disease) has been reported in several cats.[12]

Urinalyses are usually normal in dogs and cats with histoplasmosis. Most cats have tested negative for feline leukemia virus and feline immunodeficiency virus infections.

Radiography–Ultrasonography

Thoracic radiographs of dogs and cats with active pulmonary histoplasmosis usually exhibit a linear or diffuse pulmonary interstitial pattern associated with granulomatous fungal pneumonia (Fig. 60–3). The infiltrates often are coalescing and may appear miliary or grossly nodular (Fig. 60–4). True alveolar involvement in pulmonary histoplasmosis is rare. Hilar lymphadenomegaly is common in dogs but rare in cats. Pleural effusion occurs infrequently in the dog. Pulmonary calcification, indicative of inactive pulmonary histoplasmosis, is occasionally seen in dogs.

The interpretation of abdominal radiographs in dogs with GI histoplasmosis may be difficult because of the emaciated condition of the patient or the presence of abdominal fluid. Noncontrast studies may demonstrate hepatomegaly, splenomegaly, or ascites (Fig. 60–5). Barium contrast examination may reveal irregularities of the intestinal mucosa and thickening of the intestinal walls.

Ultrasound examination of dogs with liver involvement reveals hyperechoic liver parenchyma.[3] Nodular and infarctive lesions have also been observed.

Osseous involvement with histoplasmosis is rare in the cat and even less common in the dog. The typical radiographic

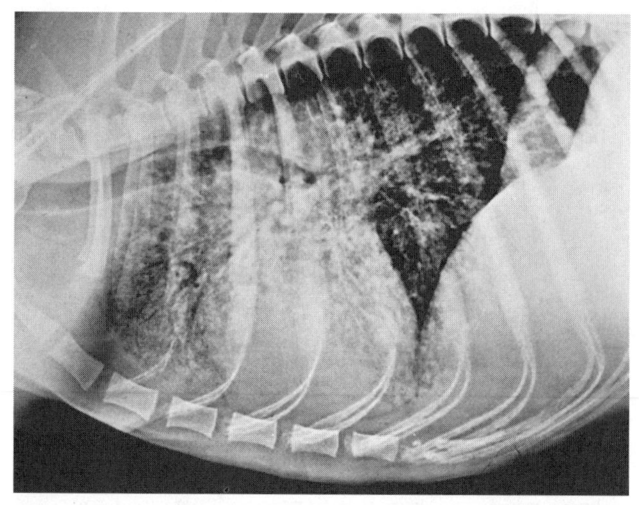

Figure 60–3. Lateral thoracic radiograph of a 3-year-old mixed breed dog with pulmonary histoplasmosis showing a mixed pattern of coalescing interstitial, nodular, and peribronchial infiltrates throughout the lungs. Minimal alveolar involvement is seen in the periphery of the lung.

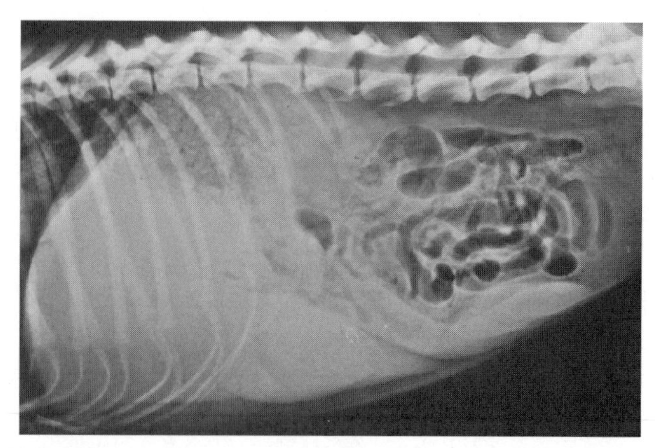

Figure 60–5. Lateral radiograph of the abdomen of a 5-year-old male English setter with disseminated histoplasmosis and resultant severe hepatomegaly and splenomegaly. (From Clinkenbeard KD, et al: *Comp Cont Educ Pract Vet* 11:1355, 1989. Reprinted with permission.)

appearance of bony lesions is a mixed pattern of osteolysis, subperiosteal bone proliferation, and periosteal new bone formation (Fig. 60–6). Intra-articular infection has been observed in both dogs and cats but is rare.[13] In the cat, *Histoplasma* most frequently infects the metaphyses of long bones with a predilection for the bones of and adjacent to the carpal and tarsal joints.

Endoscopy

Endoscopic examination of dogs with colonic histoplasmosis reveals mucosal thickening, granularity, friability, and ulceration.[16] Cytologic or histologic examination of rectal scrapings and biopsy samples usually reveals large numbers of *Histoplasma* organisms.

Transtracheal Wash–Bronchoalveolar Lavage

Transtracheal wash (TTW) and bronchoalveolar lavage (BAL) have been suggested as methods by which to evaluate patients with suspected pulmonary mycotic infections in which organisms were not recovered by other noninvasive methods.[11] Generally, BAL is superior to TTW because the collected cells are more representative of the interstitial and distal portions of the airway. BAL requires anesthesia and causes more respiratory compromise than TTW; therefore, patients must be evaluated carefully before undergoing this procedure. Fungal organisms may not be numerous in specimens recovered with either procedure, and the sensitivity of these tests has not been thoroughly evaluated.

Cytologic and Histologic Findings

Histoplasma organisms are usually numerous in infected tissues. A definitive diagnosis can often be made by fine-

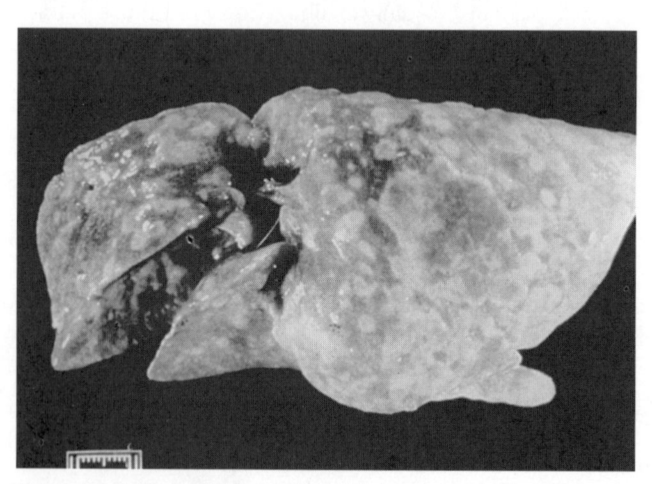

Figure 60–4. Lungs from a 2-year-old domestic shorthaired cat that died from widespread, fulminating, granulomatous pneumonia caused by *H. capsulatum*.

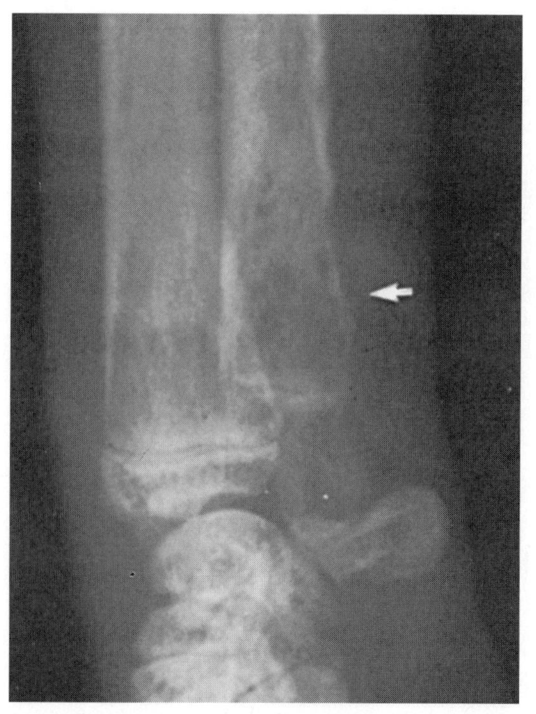

Figure 60–6. Lateral radiograph of the distal radius and ulna of a 5-year-old cat showing diffuse osteolysis and new reactive bone formation *(arrow)* characteristic of osseous histoplasmosis.

needle aspiration and exfoliative cytology.[20] The organisms are usually contained within cells of the mononuclear phagocyte system; single or multiple yeast cells may be present within each phagocytic cell. Routine Wright's or Giemsa's hematologic stains demonstrate the organism as a small (2–4 μm) round body with a basophilic center and lighter halo caused by shrinkage of the yeast during staining (Fig. 60–7*A* and 7*B*). In the cat, *Histoplasma* organisms are most easily recovered from bone marrow, lung, and lymph node aspirates. Rectal scrapings; imprints of colonic biopsy specimens; and aspirates of liver, lung, spleen, and bone marrow are most productive in the dog. *Histoplasma* organisms have been found in macrophages in peritoneal and pleural effusions, and these and other tissues should be examined as warranted by the clinical signs in each case.[15]

Tissue biopsy may be required if exfoliative cytology is not diagnostic. Affected tissues demonstrate granulomatous inflammation, but *Histoplasma* organisms are difficult to detect with routine H and E stain. Special fungal stains (periodic acid–Schiff, Gomori's methenamine silver, Gridley's fungal stain) should be used to enhance detection of the organisms if histoplasmosis is suspected.

CSF

CNS involvement is rare in dogs or cats with histoplasmosis. CSF specimens from affected dogs demonstrate increased protein and cellularity.[19] The granulomatous cellular response consists of nondegenerate neutrophils, macrophages, monocytes, and occasional lymphocytes. *Histoplasma* organisms have been identified in CSF macrophages in some patients.

Fungal Isolation

Attempts to culture *H. capsulatum* in a routine practice setting are *not* recommended because of the pathogenic potential of this organism. *H. capsulatum* can be cultured from tissue specimens, fine-needle aspirates, and body fluids. The yeast phase produces white, moist colonies when inoculated on blood agar and incubated at 30°C or 37°C (see Chapter 56 and Fig. 56–15). The mycelial phase will develop within 7 to 10 days on routine fungal culture media incubated at room temperature. Microconidia produced by the mycelial phase are infectious, and cultures exhibiting fluffy white or buff-brown mycelial growth should be handled with caution.

Immunodiagnosis

ID skin tests for reactivity to histoplasmin are unreliable in companion animals and cannot be used to confirm the diagnosis of histoplasmosis. Serologic tests (agar-gel immunodiffusion, complement fixation) for antibodies directed against *Histoplasma* antigens are often falsely negative in animals with active naturally occurring disease.[12, 15] Test results may be false positive in an animal with prior exposure that has recovered from infection. Even in human infections, cross-reactivity of the urine test for *Histoplasma* antigens occurs in people with blastomycosis and penicilliosis.[23a] Currently, no consistently reliable immunodiagnostic test is available for identification of histoplasmosis in companion animals.

THERAPY

Pulmonary histoplasmosis in the dog may be self-limiting and can resolve without treatment.[8] However, antifungal che-

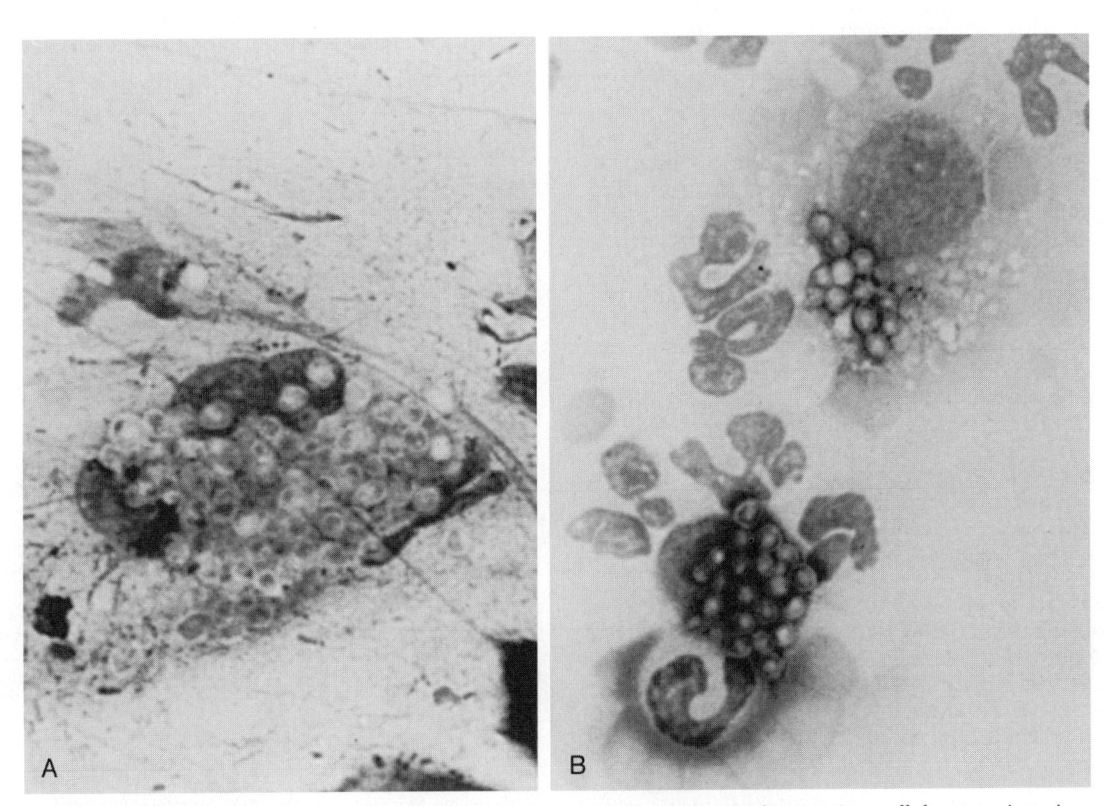

Figure 60–7. *A*, Cytologic preparation of a rectal scraping from a dog with histoplasmosis showing intracellular organisms in a macrophage. (Wright's stain, × 800). This is one of the best and most common ways to confirm a diagnosis of histoplasmosis in dogs with GI disease. *B*, *H. capsulatum* in circulating blood monocytes. This organism can also be found in neutrophils and, rarely, in eosinophils (Wright's stain, × 1000). (Courtesy of Dr. Ken Latimer, University of Georgia, Athens, GA.)

Table 60–1. Therapy for Histoplasmosis[a]

DRUG	SPECIES	DOSE[b] (mg/kg)	ROUTE	INTERVAL (HOURS)	DURATION (MONTHS)
Itraconazole	B	10	PO	12–24	4–6[c]
Fluconazole	B	2.5–5	PO	12–24	4–6[c]
AMB[d]	B	0.25–0.5	IV	48[e]	[f]

[a]See Drug Formulary (Appendix 8) for further information.
[b]Dose per administration at specified interval.
[c]Minimum time; each case must be evaluated independently; see text. Treat for at least 2 months after resolution of clinical signs.
[d]Given in conjunction with a concurrently administered oral azole. See Table 57–2 and Drug Formulary, Appendix 8, for alternate formulations and dosages of AMB.
[e]Monday-Wednesday-Friday schedule usually used.
[f]Continue until cumulative dose of 5–10 mg/kg is reached in dogs and 4–8 mg/kg in cats.
B = both dog and cat; AMB = amphotericin B.

motherapy is recommended because dissemination can occur early in the course of infection (Table 60–1). Itraconazole (ITZ) is currently the drug of choice for the treatment of histoplasmosis in animals. Treatment is usually initiated once daily; however, pharmacokinetic studies in cats indicate significant variability among cats in the PO absorption of ITZ, and twice daily dosing (at 10 mg/kg) may be required in some to achieve the desired therapeutic effect.[2] The oral solution is more consistently absorbed than capsules, allowing for 10 mg/kg once daily dosing. See Drug Formulary, Appendix 8, for detailed information on the use of ITZ.

Despite the reportedly poor penetration of ITZ into the CNS and eye, several cats with *Histoplasma*-induced ocular lesions had complete resolution of disease with a standard course of ITZ therapy.[12, 27]

In dogs or cats with severe or fulminating pulmonary or GI histoplasmosis with dissemination, combination therapy with amphotericin B (AMB) and ITZ or high loading doses of ITZ may provide more rapid control of the fungal infection (see Table 60–1). See the Drug Formulary, Appendix 8, for further information on AMB. ITZ treatment is initiated at the same time as AMB administration and is continued after termination of the AMB regimen.

The duration of antifungal treatment required for each patient is variable and is determined by the severity of infection and the patient's clinical response. The response to therapy should be evaluated by monitoring the resolution of clinical signs, hematologic and biochemical abnormalities, and radiographic lesions. Generally, most patients are treated with oral antifungal drugs for at least 4 to 6 months.

Another orally administered triazole, fluconazole (FCZ), has better penetration into the CNS and eye than ITZ (see Drug Formulary, Appendix 8). FCZ is preferred for patients with neurologic involvement or ocular lesions that are refractory to AMB or ITZ treatment. FCZ may also be used for animals that do not tolerate ITZ therapy. It is not as effective as ITZ in treatment of people with histoplasmosis.[18]

KTZ, the first licensed oral azole antifungal agent, has lower potency against *Histoplasma* and increased relative toxicity compared with ITZ and FCZ. For these reasons, it is not recommended as a first-choice treatment unless expense becomes a limiting factor. See Drug Formulary (Appendix 8) for further information.

The ability to treat animals with histoplasmosis effectively has improved significantly because of the availability of safe and efficacious oral azole antifungal drugs. Dogs and cats with pulmonary histoplasmosis have a fair to excellent prognosis. The prognosis for animals with disseminated histoplasmosis is fair to good depending on the severity of fungal involvement.

PREVENTION

Effective immunoprophylaxis is not clinically available for histoplasmosis. In laboratory experiments, several constituents extracted from the cell wall and cell membrane of *H. capsulatum* protect mice against infection.[8a] A genetic recombinant–produced version of one of these extracts, heat shock protein 60, protects mice against challenge with yeast cells.[10a] Prevention consists of avoiding exposure to *Histoplasma*-infected soil in endemic areas. Soil containing bird or bat excrement enhances the growth of *Histoplasma* and is particularly dangerous. Formalin (3%) or formaldehyde solution may be used for soil decontamination if small, focal sources of infection can be identified.

PUBLIC HEALTH CONSIDERATIONS

Both companion animals and humans residing in or traveling through endemic regions of the country are at risk of exposure to *H. capsulatum*. Concurrent common-source infection of humans and animals has been observed; however, as with the other systemic mycoses, direct transmission of histoplasmosis from animal to animal or animal to human has not been reported.[8, 24] Fungal cultures containing mycelial growth of *H. capsulatum* are highly infectious and should be handled with extreme caution.

References

1. Blischok D, Bender H. 1996. What is your diagnosis—15-year-old male domestic shorthair cat. *Vet Clin Pathol* 25:114.
2. Boothe DM, Herrig I, Calvin J, et al. 1997. Itraconazole disposition following single oral, intravenous, and multiple oral dosing in healthy cats. *Am J Vet Res* 58:872–877.
3. Chapman BL, Hendrick MJ, Washabau RJ. 1993. Granulomatous hepatitis in dogs: nine cases (1987–1990). *J Am Vet Med Assoc* 203:680–684.
4. Clinkenbeard KD, Wolf AM, Cowell RL, et al. 1989. Canine disseminated histoplasmosis. *Compend Cont Educ Pract Vet* 11:1347–1360.
5. Clinkenbeard KD, Wolf AM, Cowell RL, et al. 1989. Feline disseminated histoplasmosis. *Compend Cont Educ Pract Vet* 11:1223–1233.
6. Como JA, Dismukes WE. 1994. Oral azole drugs as systemic antifungal therapy. *N Engl J Med* 330:263–272.
7. Costa EO, Diniz LSM, Netto CF, et al. 1994. Epidemiological study of sporotrichosis and histoplasmosis in captive Latin American wild mammals, Sao Paulo, Brazil. *Mycopathologica* 125:19–22.
8. Davies SF, Colbert RL. 1990. Concurrent human and canine histoplasmosis from cutting decayed wood. *Ann Intern Med* 113:252–253.
8a. Deepe GS. 1997. *Histoplasma capsulatum:* darling of the river valleys. *ASM News* 63:599–604.
9. Dismukes WE, Bradsher RW Jr, Cloud GC, et al. 1992. Itraconazole therapy for blastomycosis and histoplasmosis. *Am J Med* 93:489–497.
10. Eilert D, Hoskinson JJ. 1993. What is your diagnosis? Diffuse nodular interstitial-to-alveolar pattern throughout the lungs. *J Am Vet Med Assoc* 202:456–457.
10a. Gomez FJ, Allendoerfer R, Deepe GS. 1995. Vaccination with recombinant heat shock protein 60 from *Histoplasma capsulatum* protects mice against pulmonary histoplasmosis. *Infect Immun* 63:2587–2595.
11. Hawkins EC, DeNicola DB. 1990. Cytologic analysis of tracheal wash specimens and bronchoalveolar lavage fluid in the diagnosis of mycotic infections in dogs. *J Am Vet Med Assoc* 197:79–83.
12. Hodges RD, Legendre AM, Adams LG, et al. 1994. Itraconazole for the treatment of histoplasmosis in cats. *J Vet Intern Med* 8:409–413.

13. Huss BT, Collier LL, Collins BK, et al. 1994. Polyarthropathy and chorioretinitis with retinal detachment in a dog with systemic histoplasmosis. *J Am Anim Hosp Assoc* 30:217–224.
14. Kauffman CA. 1994. Newer developments in therapy for endemic mycoses. *Clin Infect Dis* 19(Suppl 1):s28–32.
15. Kowalewich N, Hawkins EC, Skrowronek AJ, et al. 1993. Identification of *Histoplasma capsulatum* organisms in the pleural and peritoneal effusions of a dog. *J Am Vet Med Assoc* 202:423–426.
16. Leib MS, Codner EC, Monroe WE. 1991. Common colonoscopic findings in dogs with chronic large bowel diarrhea. *Vet Med* 86:913–921.
17. McCalla T, Collier L, Wigton D, et al. 1992. Ocular histoplasmosis in the cat (abstract). *Vet Pathol* 29:470.
18. McKinsey DS, Kauffman CA, Pappas PG, et al. 1996. Fluconazole therapy for histoplasmosis. *Clin Infect Dis* 23:996–1001.
19. Meadows RL, MacWilliams PS, Dzata G, et al. 1992. Diagnosis of histoplasmosis in a dog by cytologic examination of CSF. *Vet Clin Pathol* 21:122–125.
20. Rosychuk RA, White SD. 1991. Systemic infectious diseases and infestations that cause cutaneous lesions. *Vet Med* 86:164–181.
21. Sanford SE. 1991. Disseminated histoplasmosis in a young dog. *Can Vet J* 32:692.
22. Sarosi GA, Davies SF. 1994. Therapy for fungal infections. *Mayo Clin Proc* 69:1111–1117.
23. Van Cauteren H, Heykants J, De Coster R, et al. 1987. Itraconazole: pharmacokinetic studies in animals and humans. *Rev Infect Dis* 9(Suppl 1):s43–s46.
23a. Wheat J, Wheat H, Connolly P, et al. 1997. Cross reactivity in *Histoplasma capsulatum* variety *capsulatum* antigen assays of urine samples from patients with endemic mycoses. *Clin Infect Dis* 24:1169–1171.
24. Wolf AM. 1989. Systemic mycoses. *J Am Vet Med Assoc* 194:1192–1196.
25. Wolf AM. 1990. Diagnosing and treating the four most common pulmonary mycoses in cats. *Vet Med* 85:994–1001.
26. Wolf AM. 1990. Histoplasmosis, pp 679–686. *In* Greene CE (ed), Infectious diseases of the dog and cat. WB Saunders, Philadelphia, PA.
27. Zuckerman JM, Tunkel AR. 1994. Itraconazole: a new triazole antifungal agent. *Infect Control Hosp Epidemiol* 15:397–410.

Chapter **61**

Cryptococcosis

Gilbert J. Jacobs and Linda Medleau

ETIOLOGY

Several different species of the genus *Cryptococcus* exist in the environment. *C. neoformans* is primarily responsible for disease in people and animals. Sporadic reports have been made of human infection from *C. laurentii* and *C. albidus*, which are commonly isolated from normal skin and indoor and outdoor air. The ability of *C. neoformans* to grow at 37°C may explain its pathogenicity in mammals because other cryptococcal species grow poorly at this temperature. The growth of the organism is inhibited at temperatures above 39°C. *C. neoformans* is a saprophytic, round, yeastlike fungus (3.5–7 μm in diameter) with the ability to form a large (1–30 μm thick) heteropolysaccharide capsule (Fig. 61–1). The capsule confers its virulence and resistance to desiccation. The organism may or may not produce the capsule when growing on artificial media or when growing naturally in the environment, but it always produces the capsule in tissues.[31] *C. neoformans* reproduces by forming one or two buds (blastoconidia) that are connected to the parent cell by a narrow isthmus (see Fig. 61–1). The buds may break off when small; as a result, the yeast population varies in size. Unlike other dimorphic fungi, the yeast phase of *C. neoformans* is always found under normal laboratory conditions and in infected tissues. The sexual reproductive phase can be demonstrated only under controlled laboratory conditions.

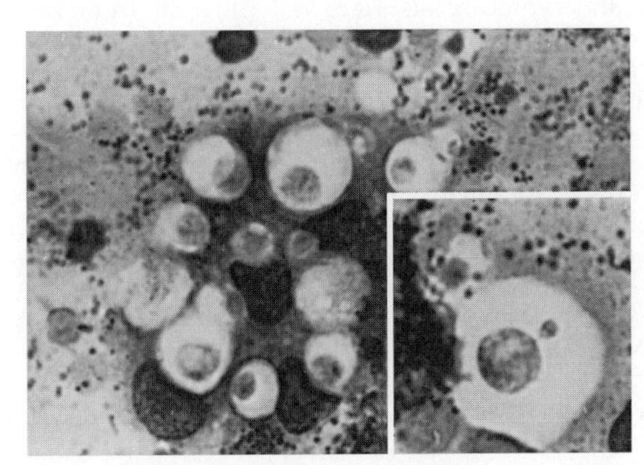

Figure 61–1. Numerous cryptococcal organisms in an impression smear of the nasal exudate from a cat. The thick nonstaining capsule is visible (Wright's stain, × 1000). *Inset* (has been enlarged): typical budding appearance of *Cryptococcus*.

EPIDEMIOLOGY

C. neoformans is worldwide in distribution and, in addition to people, infects a variety of domestic and wild mammals, including the cat and the dog. In contrast to the other systemic mycoses, the prevalence of cryptococcosis in cats is equal to or greater than that in dogs.

Two variants (var. *neoformans* and *gattii*) and five serotypes (A, B, C, D, AD) of *C. neoformans* have been identified on the basis of antigenic differences in glucuronoxylomannan, the main component of *C. neoformans* capsular polysaccharide.[43] Because cryptococcal infection has emerged as a serious health problem in HIV-infected persons with AIDS, subtyping *C. neoformans* in people has become more important to identify cluster cases and environmental sources of infection.

C. neoformans var. *neoformans,* which contains serotypes A, D, and AD, has been isolated from several environmental sources, such as soil and foods (fruits), and the oropharynx, GI tract, and skin of healthy people. Avian (particularly pigeon) excreta is the chief reservoir.[11] The organism passes through the gut of pigeons, but spontaneous avian cryptococcosis is extremely rare. Presumably the pigeon's high body temperature (42°C [107.6°F]) protects it from infection. In pigeon droppings, cryptococci may remain viable for at least

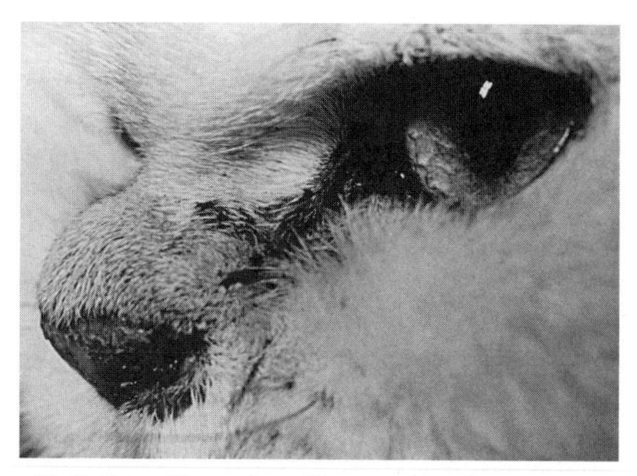

Figure 61–2. Cat with nasal swelling resulting from cryptococcosis.

2 years unless exposed to drying or sunlight.[31] The high concentration of creatinine in pigeon droppings may favor cryptococcal growth. However, pigeon feces provide an alkaline, hyperosmolar environment that is rich in many nitrogen-containing compounds besides creatinine.

C. neoformans var. *neoformans* is the variety that most often causes clinical disease in temperate regions of the world. *C. neoformans* var. *gattii* contains serotypes B and C. It seems to occupy a specific ecologic niche, having been isolated only from the bark and leaf litter of Eucalyptus trees. No other environmental source of the fungus has been detected so far.[11] *C. neoformans* var. *gattii* has been reported as a cause of cryptococcosis in people and dogs in tropic and subtropic regions of the world where Eucalyptus trees are found.[24]

PATHOGENESIS

The exact mode of infection is unknown, but the most likely route is through inhalation of air-borne organisms. In the environment, *Cryptococcus* is unencapsulated and thus reduced in size, increasing the chances of aerosolization and inhalation. After inhalation, the organism may deposit in the upper respiratory tract, inducing nasal granulomas (Fig. 61–2), or lodge in the alveoli, inducing pulmonary granulomas (Fig. 61–3). Studies in random-source dogs and cats have asymptomatic colonization of the nasal passages of 14% and 7% of the animals, respectively.[28] Once in the respiratory tract, cryptococci regenerate their capsules. The production of a thick capsule and abundant release of a glycoprotein into the circulation are hallmarks of virulence. The capsule interferes with antigen presentation, subsequent immune response, and elimination of the organism. In addition, intravascular cryptococcal antigens prevent leukocytes from migrating into acute or delayed hypersensitivity reaction sites.[10] Increased virulence has also been found in those strains that produce phospholipases.[7]

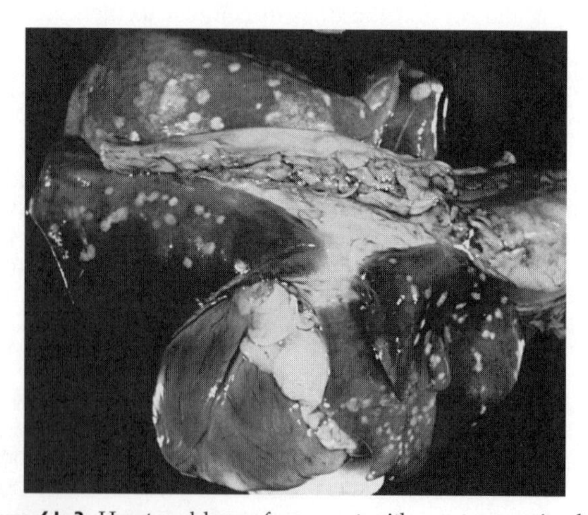

Figure 61–3. Heart and lungs from a cat with cryptococcosis, showing multiple white pulmonary nodules.

Cryptococcal infection can disseminate hematogenously, often to the CNS, from the respiratory system or extend locally from the nasal cavity. When CNS signs eventually appear, there may be no evidence of respiratory infection. Encapsulated organisms in tissues are too large (5–20 μm) to enter terminal airways, so that spread from the upper to lower airways is unlikely. However, shrunken, unencapsulated cryptococci that are small enough for alveolar deposition have been isolated from pigeon feces and soil.[31] It is theoretically possible to inhale the basidiospores of the sexual (mold) stage directly into the alveoli, but it is uncertain whether this mode of infection occurs naturally.

Cryptococcosis has been experimentally induced in cats by intranasal and intrathecal administration of organisms.[32] Under natural circumstances, primary GI infection is unlikely. Drinking unpasteurized milk from cattle with cryptococcal mastitis did not induce disease. However, under certain circumstances, direct inoculation of the organisms could result in disease in animals (see also Public Health Considerations).

The establishment and spread of infection in the host are highly dependent on immunity. As with most fungal infections, cell-mediated immunity is an important mechanism of resistance to cryptococcal infection. The natural resistance of people to cryptococcosis is so strong that the presence of the disease is a signal to look for predisposing immunosuppression. Most humans with cryptococcal meningitis have other conditions that have inhibitory effects on lymphocyte number or function, such as lymphoreticular malignancy, glucocorticoid or other immunosuppressive therapy, sarcoidosis, or AIDS. Reports show that 5% to 10% of all patients with AIDS develop cryptococcosis.[8] As in people, both experimental and natural cases of cryptococcal infection in dogs and cats have been accelerated or worsened by glucocorticoid therapy.[31] In cats, infections with feline leukemia virus (FeLV) or feline immunodeficiency virus (FIV) have been speculated to be predisposing factors for cryptococcosis.[31] However, in one study, the prevalence of FeLV and FIV infections in cats with cryptococcosis was the same as or less than that for the population as a whole.[12, 44] Furthermore, leukocyte and lymphocyte subset numbers in FIV-positive and FIV-negative cats with cryptococcosis were not different from those in healthy cats,[44] and seropositivity for FIV did not impart an unfavorable prognosis.[27] Thus, underlying diseases are often not detected in cats with cryptococcosis, and factors predisposing to infections remain elusive.[12] In dogs, immunosuppressive diseases such as ehrlichiosis have been associated with fatal disseminated cryptococcosis,[31] but in one study immunosuppressive factors could be identified in less than 6% of affected dogs.[3]

CLINICAL FINDINGS

Cats

Cryptococcosis is the most common of the systemic mycoses in the cat. *C. neoformans* var. *neoformans* and var. *gattii* have been isolated in cats with cryptococcosis.[27] There is no sex predisposition, and the age range of affected cats is broad

Table 61–1. Frequency of Clinical Signs Reported in 110 Cats with Cryptococcosis[12, 31]

CLINICAL SIGNS	NUMBER AFFECTED
Sneezing, snuffling, nasal discharge	58
Skin lesions	48
Nasal mass	40
Abnormal ocular signs	15
Abnormal CNS signs	15

(1–13 years, average 5.0 years). In some studies, Siamese cats are overrepresented.[27] Cats with cryptococcosis usually have one or more of the following sites affected: respiratory, cutaneous, CNS, and ocular (Table 61–1). The nasal cavity is affected in more than 80% of cases. Upper respiratory tract signs are most common and include sneezing; snuffling; and mucopurulent, serous or hemorrhagic, unilateral or bilateral, chronic nasal discharge. In some cases, a flesh-colored, polyp-like mass is evident in the nostril, or a firm, hard, subcutaneous swelling over the bridge of the nose is evident (see Fig. 61–2). Often there is submandibular lymphadenomegaly. Ulcerated or proliferative lesions in the oral cavity are occasionally seen in conjunction with upper respiratory tract infections.[24a, 31] Lower respiratory tract signs are rare in cats. Radiographs of the nasal passages may show increased opacity and possible destruction of the nasal turbinates. Thoracic radiographs are usually normal, although small nodular lesions may be present. Rarely, a secondary bronchopneumonia or pulmonary nodules may be found.

Cutaneous lesions are also common in cats with cryptococcosis. The skin or subcutaneous tissues have been affected in approximately 40% to 50% of reported cases. In most cats with dermal lesions, multiple lesions have been present or other organ systems affected. This finding suggests that the skin lesions are the result of dissemination from another site rather than direct infection of the skin caused by trauma. Cutaneous lesions other than over the nose are usually papules and nodules that are fluctuant to firm and range from 1 to 10 mm in diameter (Fig. 61–4). Larger lesions tend to ulcerate, leaving a raw surface with a serous exudate. Pruritus is usually nonexistent to mild, and peripheral lymphadenomegaly is common.

Neurologic signs associated with cryptococcosis in cats are variable, depending on lesion location in the CNS, and include depression, changes in temperament, seizures, circling, head pressing, ataxia, paresis, apparent loss of smell, and blindness. These signs may occur alone or in association with other clinical signs and may result from the presence of a mass (granuloma) or from meningoencephalitis or meningomyelitis. In people, CNS cryptococcal infection is associated with high intracranial pressure, which contributes to the pathogenesis of neurologic signs. The pathogenesis of the increase in intracranial pressure is obscure but, in addition to inflammation, may be due to increased CSF osmolality caused by the presence of high-molecular-weight cryptococcal polysaccharide or the production of D-mannitol by the cryptococcal organism.[35] Cranial nerve involvement is common. Upper motor neuron limb deficits are usually present owing to brain involvement, although lower motor neuron spinal cord or nerve root lesions also have been described.

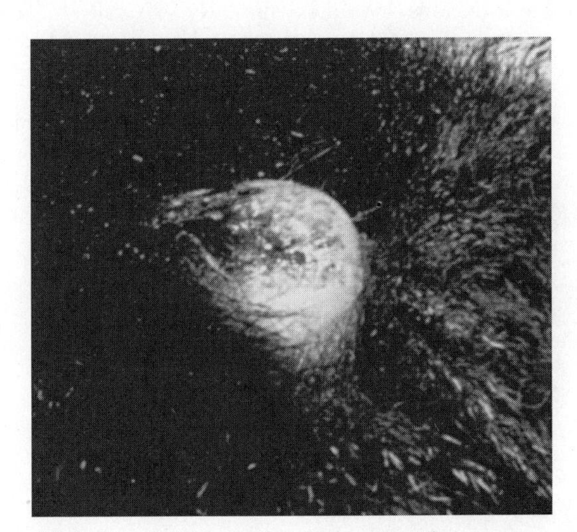

Figure 61–4. A nodule on the head of a cat with cutaneous cryptococcosis.

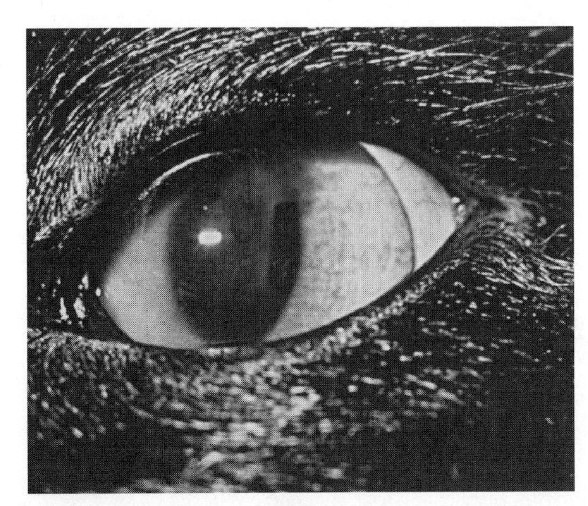

Figure 61–5. Anterior uveitis with aqueous flare in a cat with disseminated cryptococcosis.

Ocular abnormalities occur in some affected cats, especially those with CNS signs. The most common ocular signs are dilated, unresponsive pupils and blindness due to exudative retinal detachment, granulomatous chorioretinitis, panophthalmitis, and optic neuritis (see Systemic Fungal Infections, Chapter 93). The fundus also can be affected without apparent visual loss. Chorioretinitis is probably a consequence of hematogenous spread and suggests multisystemic involvement, whereas optic neuritis usually is associated with CNS inflammation.[31] An anterior uveitis is also present in some cats (Fig. 61–5). A case of mediastinal infection and chylous effusion in a cat associated with cryptococcosis has been reported,[30] as has ocular adnexal infection as the only clinical lesion.[29]

Fever is uncommon in affected cats and, when present, is mild, usually less than 39.5°C (103°F). Cryptococcosis is often chronic, causing listlessness and anorexia with resultant weight loss. Other reported signs are peripheral lymphadenomegaly unassociated with skin lesions, bone lysis associated with subcutaneous infection, chronic cough, and, rarely, renal failure due to kidney involvement.

Dogs

The average age of affected dogs has been 3.5 years, primarily young adult dogs (< 4 years, 80% between 1 and 7 years) with no gender predisposition.[24] Doberman pinschers and Great Danes in Australia and the American cocker spaniel in North America are breeds overrepresented for crypto-

Table 61–2. Frequency of Clinical Signs Reported in 28 Dogs with Cryptococcosis

CLINICAL SIGNS	NUMBER AFFECTED
Abnormal CNS signs	21
Abnormal ocular signs	18
Anorexia-emaciation	12
Skin lesions	6
Fever	5
Peripheral lymphadenomegaly	5
Nasal discharge	4
Dry cough	3
Vomiting	3
Lytic bone lesions	3
Vaginal discharge	1

coccal infections.[3, 24] Most cases are due to *C. neoformans* var. *neoformans* but var. *gattii* has also been isolated.[24]

Weight loss and lethargy are common nonspecific findings. Major organ systems affected by canine cryptococcosis are the CNS and the eyes (Table 61–2). CNS signs are typically multifocal and attributable to meningitis alone or accompanying encephalomyelitis and include head tilt, nystagmus, facial paralysis, paresis to paraplegia or tetraplegia (usually upper motor neuron), ataxia, circling, seizure, and cervical hyperesthesia. Most dogs with CNS cryptococcal infections have intraneural sites.[4] The most common ocular abnormalities are exudative granulomatous chorioretinitis, retinal hemorrhage, papilledema, and optic neuritis associated with dilated pupils and blindness. Anterior uveitis is occasionally present. A retrobulbar abscess with lysis of the bone of the orbit has been reported in one dog. One study found a high incidence of nasal cavity involvement; thus, associated rhinosinusitis from cryptococcosis may be subclinical and underestimated in dogs.[24]

Cutaneous involvement may also be seen in association with systemic disease. Skin lesions are usually characterized by ulcers that may involve the nose, tongue, gums, hard palate, lips, or nail beds. Other rarely reported lesions have included pharyngeal abscess formations[24a] and skin wounds with multiple draining sinuses.

Fever (39.4–40.5°C [103–105°F]) is noted in about 25% of cases of natural infections. Less common clinical signs include lameness caused by lytic bone lesions and peripheral lymphadenomegaly.

DIAGNOSIS

Cytologic Examination

The most rapid method of diagnosis is cytologic evaluation of nasal and skin exudates, CSF, tissue aspirates, and samples obtained by paracentesis of the aqueous or vitreous chambers of the eye. Although Wright's stain has been used most often in the diagnosis of cryptococcosis, it can cause the organism to shrink and the capsule to become distorted. New methylene blue (Fig. 61–6*A*) and Gram's (see Fig. 56–3) stain are considered to be better than Wright's stain for this reason. With Gram's stain the organism retains crystal violet, whereas the capsule stains lightly red with safranin. The organism can be seen with low (× 100) power. India ink may also help to visualize the organism, which appears unstained and silhouetted against a black background (Fig. 61–6*B*). Ink is not as helpful as the other stains unless budding is seen, because lymphocytes, fat droplets, and aggregated India ink particles may be confused with the organism. Cytologic examination can also be performed on tissue biopsy samples. Impression smears may be made directly, or part of the biopsy can be macerated with a scalpel, mixed with 1 ml of 15% potassium hydroxide (KOH), incubated at 37°C for 30 minutes, and examined microscopically for budding organisms. The KOH will digest all other cells and debris.

Cytologic examination of nasal or cutaneous exudates, masses, CSF, or ocular fluid has revealed organisms in a majority of cases.[4] Urine sediment should be evaluated because many dogs have subclinical renal infection from cryptococcosis.[4] It is suspected that *C. neoformans* can be mistaken for fat droplets in urine sediment.[13] Although cytologic examination is a rapid test, negative results do not eliminate the possibility of cryptococcosis from consideration. Unencapsulated organisms may be overlooked unless a large number are present.

Serologic Testing

The detection of cryptococcal capsular antigen by the latex agglutination procedure is the most widely utilized and is a clinically helpful serologic test. Current methods use agglutination with anticryptococcal globulin–sensitized latex beads or particles or ELISA with polyclonal antibody capture and monoclonal detection. Current tests detect all known serotypes and can be used for serum, urine, or CSF. They provide a rapid diagnostic method in suspected cases in which the organism has not been visualized or cultured (Table 61–3). In people, commercial kits typically demonstrate 90% to 100% sensitivity and 97% to 100% specificity.[41, 45] Results have been similar for cats.[12, 34] Although not documented, its use in canine infections should be similarly valuable. In people, false-negative titers can be seen when the disease is localized or when there are prozone effects in cases of antigen excess.[4, 34] False-positive titers have been seen in people with *Klebsiella* infections. They also occur when rheumatoid factors

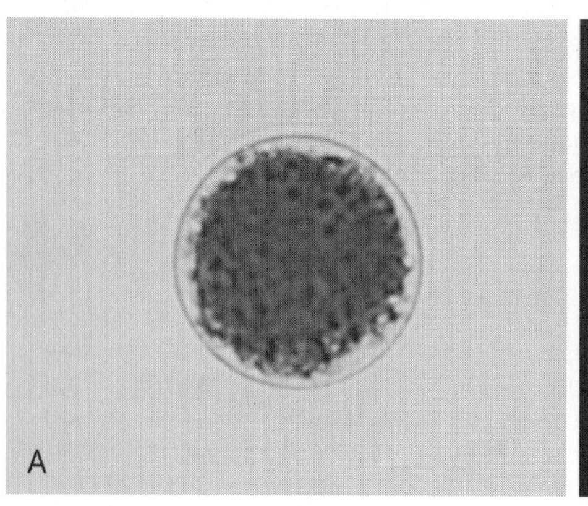

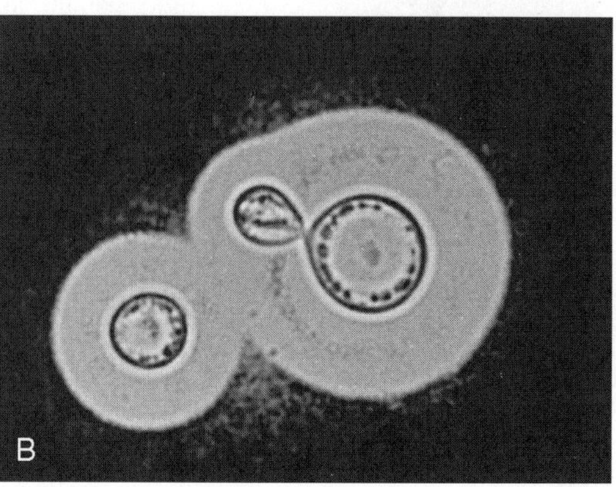

Figure 61–6. New methylene blue *(A)* and India ink *(B)* preparations of CSF from a dog with cryptococcal meningoencephalitis. Budding is evident in the India ink preparation.

Table 61–3. Immunodiagnostic Kits for Detection of Cryptococcal Antigen in Clinical Specimens [a]

NAME	MANUFACTURER
Latex Agglutination Tests	
Crypto-LA	Wampole Laboratories, Cranbury, NJ
CALAS	Meridian Diagnostics, Cincinnati, OH
Crypto-Lex	Trinity Laboratories, Raleigh, NC
Myco-Immune	American MicroScan, Rahway, NJ
Immy Latex-Crypto Antigen	Immunomycologics Inc, Norman, OK
ELISA	
Premier EIA	Meridian Diagnostics, Cincinnati, OH

[a] See Appendix 6 for more information on manufacturers and available kits.

or other macroglobulins in serum are present or when the sample is obtained from a patient receiving low-molecular-weight hydroxyethyl starches in place of albumin for vascular filling.[31, 37, 45] False-positive reactions can also be seen artifactually by introduction of talc from latex gloves during CSF collection or by various soaps used to clean ring slides for testing.[5] The specificity of this test has been improved by modification in which the serum to be tested is pretreated with a protease (pronase).[25, 31, 41] Infections with the closely related yeast *Trichosporon* may cause some cross-reactivity (see Chapter 67).

Titers can be quite high (10,000) in affected cats, although even a titer of 1 is considered to be a positive result. Titration of antigen in serum and CSF has been utilized to determine prognosis and to evaluate response to treatment. However, titer results using different kits can vary considerably, and methods should not be altered when monitoring response to treatment.[16] When monitored in a consistent fashion, titers have been useful in evaluating the progress of cats during therapy.[31] A good prognosis is indicated by a decrease in antigen titer, whereas a persistent titer after treatment suggests continued infection. Titer reductions may actually lag behind clinical improvement.[25]

CSF serology may be more sensitive for CNS cryptococcosis than cytology or CSF culture and is preferred to serum serology in animals with neurologic signs. Cryptococcal antigen can be detected in other body fluids such as pleural fluid or bronchoalveolar lavage fluid. When there is a high clinical suspicion for cryptococcal infection but cytologic and serum results are negative, testing for cryptococcal antigen from tissue aspirates can be diagnostic.[22]

Tissue Biopsy

Because of the rapidity of cytologic evaluation, impression smears or KOH preparations should always be made from biopsy samples. If no organisms are seen, part of the sample can be used for culture, and the rest can be processed for routine histologic examination. On H and E staining, the organism stains as a faint, eosinophilic, round-to-oval body surrounded by a clear halo, which is the unstained capsule (Fig. 61–7). The organism is more easily visualized with periodic acid–Schiff, methenamine silver, or Masson-Fontana stain, but the capsule still does not stain. Mayer's mucicarmine is the definitive stain, because the cryptococcal capsule appears as a rose-red color and the organism appears pink against a blue background. Other fungi that have similar morphologic characteristics do not stain with this method. The large capsule and the thin cell wall of *Cryptococcus* differentiate it from *Blastomyces*. Its budding and lack of endospores distinguish it from *Coccidioides immitis*.

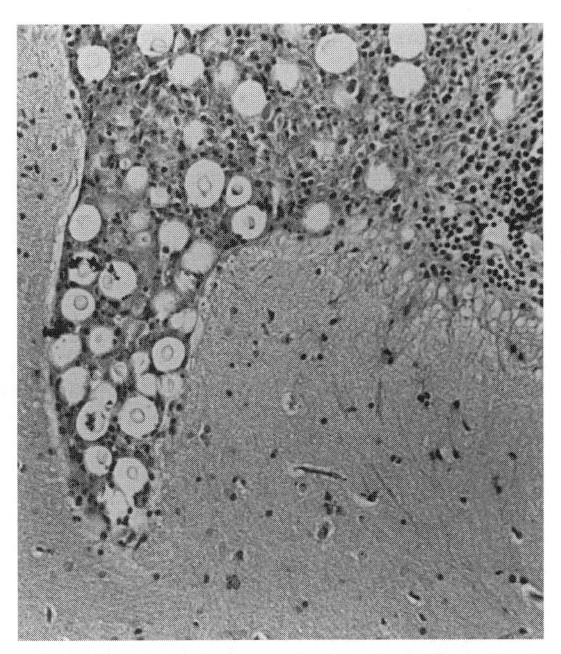

Figure 61–7. Histologic section of brain and meninges from a dog with cryptococcal meningoencephalitis showing numerous organisms and an inflammatory response (H and E, × 400).

Fungal Isolation

The organism can be cultured from exudate, CSF, urine, joint fluid, and tissue samples fairly easily if a large enough sample volume is obtained. Sabouraud's agar with antibiotics is used when bacterial contamination is likely. *Cryptococcus* is sensitive to media that contain cycloheximide. The organism should be cultured at both 25° and 37°C; growth will occur in 48 hours to 6 weeks, depending on the amount of inoculum. The organism forms white, creamy colonies that yellow with age, are mucoid when the organism forms its capsule, and are dry when it is unencapsulated. Characteristics employed to identify the organism are its morphology (i.e., presence of the capsule), growth at 37°C, urea hydrolysis, response to various assimilation tests, and virulence for mice. Cultures of CSF are often positive in CNS cryptococcosis, and fungal culture of CSF is always recommended in suspected cases when the organism cannot be demonstrated cytologically or serologically. Obtaining a positive culture is enhanced by sediment of 15 to 20 ml of CSF, although this amount cannot be safely obtained from dogs or cats.[4] Relative to cytologic examination or serologic testing, fungal isolation has limited immediate clinical utility because a positive culture finding may take several weeks. Polymerase chain reaction has been used to detect *C. neoformans* in human clinical specimens.[40]

PATHOLOGIC FINDINGS

A lesion associated with cryptococcosis can vary from a gelatinous mass, consisting of numerous organisms with minimal inflammation, to a granuloma formation. In people, the degree of granuloma formation has been directly related to the lesion duration. The granuloma is composed of aggregates of encapsulated organisms within a connective tissue reticulum (see Fig. 61–7). The primary cellular response is composed of macrophages and giant cells with a few plasma cells and lymphocytes. Epithelioid and giant cells and areas of caseation are less common than those with the other systemic mycoses.

Cats

In cats that die or are euthanized, the respiratory system is usually affected. Typically, the nasal cavity contains a granulomatous lesion, and in some instances the lungs are affected (see Fig. 61–3). Lesions of the CNS are usually meningitis, peripheral neuritis, frequently involving the optic nerve, and granulomatous chorioretinitis. Occasionally, a granulomatous mass rather than a diffuse meningoencephalitis is found. Other affected organs are skin and subcutaneous tissues, kidneys, and lymph nodes that drain infected areas. Renal granulomas have been found in approximately 30% of cases. Granulomas have also been found occasionally in the spleen, adrenal glands, thyroid glands, and liver.

Dogs

In contrast to cats, dogs that die or are euthanized because of cryptococcosis infection usually have severe disseminated disease, and most have CNS or ocular involvement. The lesions are usually meningoencephalitis; peripheral neuritis of the optic, facial, or vestibular nerves; and granulomatous chorioretinitis. Approximately 50% of dogs in reported cases had lesions in the respiratory tract, usually in the lungs and nasal cavities, or sinuses.[24] Other affected organs include kidneys, lymph nodes, spleen, liver, thyroid gland, adrenal glands, pancreas, bone, GI tract, muscle, myocardium, prostate gland, heart valves, and tonsils. In one instance, a dog had acute eosinophilic periportal hepatitis associated with cryptococcal organisms.

THERAPY

When large masses are protruding from the external nares into the nasopharynx or from the skin surface, surgical removal or debulking is indicated. This can offer immediate relief from obstruction or physical injury and reduce the amount of granulomatous tissue and organisms, facilitating systemic antifungal chemotherapy. Drugs used to treat cryptococcosis are the polyenes, azoles, and flucytosine (FCY).

Amphotericin B and Flucytosine

Amphotericin B (AMB) inhibits the formation of fungal cell membranes and has been given alone to successfully treat cats with cryptococcosis (Table 61–4). Lower dose rates should be given initially and then gradually increased when it is determined that the cat has not become azotemic (see also Chapter 57). Because cats require such a small amount per dose, a bottle of AMB can be reconstituted in sterile water, divided into small aliquots, and frozen. Each week an aliquot can be thawed, with a portion diluted for treatment, and the remainder refrigerated for later that week. For each treatment, the AMB is diluted in a small volume of 5% dextrose solution and administered by bolus IV infusion rather than by IV drip.

There are several disadvantages of utilizing AMB in treating cryptococcosis when given IV. There is a high frequency of adverse reactions, particularly nephrotoxicity. Long-term hospitalization and constant monitoring are often necessary during treatment. Even cats successfully treated with AMB have developed transient renal failure that necessitated parenteral fluid administration and delayed further treatment. Treatment failures can be associated with resistance, poor tissue penetration, and poor response in neutropenic patients.

A study described a simple, less expensive, and less toxic method of administering AMB as a SC infusion for treating infected dogs and cats[23] (see Table 61–4 and Drug Formulary, Appendix 8). Three different AMB derivatives are currently under investigation. These are lipid formulations such as combining AMB with lipid bilayers (i.e., liposomes), which may reduce toxicity and increase tissue concentration. AMB lipid complex has been used in the treatment of blastomycosis in dogs and might be tried in cryptococcosis (see Drug Formulary, Appendix 8).[17, 21]

FCY can be administered alone or in combination with AMB (see Table 61–4).[31] When FCY is used alone, however, the development of drug resistance may occur. Combination

Table 61–4. Therapy for Cryptococcosis

DRUG	SPECIES	DOSE (mg/kg)[a]	ROUTE	INTERVAL[c]	DURATION (MONTHS)
Flucytosine	C	30	PO	6 hr	1–9
		50	PO	8 hr	1–9
and/or		75	PO	12 hr	1–9
	D	50–75	PO	8 hr	1–12
Amphotericin B (deoxycholate)	C	0.1–0.5	IV	3 times/week	[b]
	D	0.25–0.5	IV	3 times/week	[b]
	C	0.5–0.8	SC	3 times/week	[c]
Amphotericin B (lipid complex)	D	1.0	IV	3 times/week	[d]
Ketoconazole	C	5–10[e]	PO	12 hr	6–10[f]
		10–20[e, g]	PO	24 hr	6–10[f]
	D	5–15	PO	12 hr	6–10
		30	PO	24 hr	6–10
Itraconazole	C	5–10	PO	12 hr	6–10[f]
		20	PO	24 hr	6–10[f]
Fluconazole	B	5–15	PO	12–24 hr	6–10

[a]Dose per administration at specified interval.
[b]Until a cumulative dosage of 4–10 mg/kg is reached.
[c]Add each dose to 400 ml of 0.45% saline, 2.5% dextrose to a total cumulative dosage of 8 to 26 mg/kg.[23] See Drug Formulary, Appendix 8.
[d]With lipid-complex drug, dose per administration and cumulative dosage may be slightly increased; has been effective for blastomycosis (see Chapter 59); until a cumulative dosage of 8–12 mg/kg has been reached; for various formulations of amphotericin B see Table 57–2 and Drug Formulary, Appendix 8.
[e]If toxicity develops, the dose should be changed to 50 mg/kg cat every other day.
[f]Range may vary from 6 to 10 months.
[g]If lack of response to therapy or toxicity is noted at these dosages, then ITZ, FCZ, or AMB lipid preparations should be used.
C = cat; D = dog; B = both dog and cat.

therapy with AMB and FCY, therefore, is recommended. There have also been reports of successful treatment in cats utilizing FCY in combination with ketoconazole (KTZ).[36, 39] Drug eruptions have also occurred.

There are few reports of treatment of infected dogs with AMB with or without FCY.[26] The meningoencephalitis frequently observed in dogs is more like the disease in humans and carries a more guarded prognosis than does the disease in cats. Neurologic signs in dogs have progressed during treatment or after AMB has been discontinued.[31] The inability of AMB or FCY to cross the blood-brain and blood-CNS barriers explains the limited efficacy of these drugs in cases of cryptococcal meningoencephalitis; thus, they must be combined with other antifungal agents such as itraconazole (ITZ) or fluconazole (FCZ) for CNS infection. Intrathecal AMB has been provided in severe cases of cryptococcal meningitis in humans. Persistence of cryptococci in the prostate gland and urine after AMB treatment has been reported in people, particularly those with AIDS.[2, 6]

Ketoconazole

KTZ, an imidazole derivative, has been administered successfully as an oral treatment for cats and dogs with cryptococcosis.[4, 31, 32] In general, the dose is given once or twice daily but may have to be given less frequently in cats that develop toxicity (see Table 61–4). Because KTZ is fungistatic and, therefore, slow acting, treatment may be needed for several months. Treatment should be continued until serum cryptococcal antigen titer findings are negative or for 1 month past resolution of all clinical signs.

KTZ absorption from the GI tract is greatly enhanced by giving it with food. Side effects of KTZ in cats include anorexia, vomiting, diarrhea, elevated serum liver enzyme activities, and icterus.[31] Giving KTZ with food and dividing the daily dose may help alleviate signs of anorexia or vomiting. If anorexia persists, KTZ therapy should be stopped until the cat is eating normally. It is then reinstituted at a lower dose or on an alternate-day basis. Cats with CNS manifestations do not respond to treatment with KTZ.[13]

KTZ has been used less commonly to treat infected dogs, but the response has not been as consistent as in cats.[31] Presumably, this occurrence is related to the tendency for dogs to have disseminated or neurologic manifestations that are difficult to treat. Dogs with disseminated cryptococcosis have not improved or have relapsed, whereas those with primarily cutaneous manifestations recovered after 3 months of treatment. KTZ penetrates poorly into the CNS; thus, in general, KTZ should not be given alone to treat CNS cryptococcosis.

Itraconazole

ITZ is a triazole antifungal agent (see Table 61–4 and Drug Formulary, Appendix 8). Its basic principles of activity are similar to those of KTZ. ITZ is also administered orally but appears to have fewer side effects than KTZ in cats.[32] ITZ has been successful in the treatment of experimental cryptococcosis in mice, rabbits, and cats,[31, 32] and in clinical cases in which KTZ treatment was unsuccessful.

Treatment duration is long; the mean is about 8.5 months.[33] Adverse effects of ITZ are primarily GI (anorexia, vomiting), but hepatic disease with elevation of alanine aminotransferase (ALT) activity can develop. Rarely, vasculitis with severe cutaneous ulceration can develop. If adverse effects develop, ITZ should be discontinued for about 2 weeks and then readministered at half the original dose. ALT activity should be monitored every 2 weeks for the first month of treatment and then once monthly thereafter. ITZ is well absorbed, but bioavailability is improved by concurrent administration of food. ITZ is metabolized by the liver and extensively distributed to lipophilic tissues. Its concentration in kidney, liver, and skin is 2 to 20 times greater than in plasma.[33] Although it is not well distributed into the CNS, ITZ still has been given successfully to treat humans and cats with cryptococcal meningitis.[9, 27] Newer triazoles such as FCZ may have better efficacy in penetrating the blood-CSF barrier.

Fluconazole

FCZ is a triazole antifungal agent similar to ITZ (see Drug Formulary, Appendix 8). It seems to result in fewer toxic side effects than KTZ or ITZ. Mild transient anorexia has been observed in cats.[27] Bioavailability exceeds that for ITZ. FCZ is widely distributed, including the CNS with good CSF penetration (CSF:serum ratio is 60%–80%).[27, 38] FCZ is eliminated primarily by renal excretion; thus, the dose should be adjusted in patients with renal failure. FCZ has been provided successfully to treat cryptococcosis in cats.[27] There are anecdotal reports of successful treatment in dogs with CNS cryptococcosis. In people, FCZ at high doses has been successful in suppressing relapses from sequestered cryptococcal infection of the prostate gland in about 50% of cases.[2] Development of fungal resistance to FCZ has been observed with long-term suppressive treatment of cryptococcosis in AIDS patients.[1]

Immunologic Therapy

Immunization has never been an important strategy for the prevention of mycosis.[17] However, it has been demonstrated in mice that some monoclonal antibodies of the IgG_3 subclass may protect against cryptococcal infection, and immunization with cryptococcal capsular antigen may also confer protection.[17] Cryptococcal meningitis in people has been successfully treated with inoculation of rabbit antibody to *C. neoformans* in combination with AMB.[15] In addition, diethylcarbamazine has been effective in vitro and in cryptococcal meningitis in mice in reducing the number of organisms.[20]

Treatment Outcomes

A study in cats showed that treatment outcome was not influenced by gender or magnitude of pretreatment serum antigen titer but was influenced adversely by seropositivity for FeLV or FIV.[19] Furthermore, serial titers were valuable in the ongoing assessment of patients' progress and prognosis and optimal duration of treatment. A favorable prognosis was associated with a progressive decrease in serum antigen titers of at least 10-fold at the end of 2 months. Recommendations were to continue treatment for 1 month after resolution of clinical signs and after decrease of the cryptococcal titer by at least two orders of magnitude, but preferably until the titer was undetectable.[19] Cryptococcosis in people who are immunocompromised is more likely to be disseminated and relapse rates are higher; thus, maintenance treatment for those individuals is recommended.[6, 8, 38] Similarly, FeLV- or FIV-infected cats may require maintenance treatment.[19, 27]

PREVENTION

The major means of prevention is restricting animal contact with areas of high concentrations of pigeon droppings, especially those inside shaded, damp buildings. The number of organisms can be greatly reduced by repeated cleaning of pigeon habitats with hydrated lime diluted in water 40 g/L (1 lb/3 gal) plus 1.5 g/L sodium hydroxide. This solution should be applied at a rate of 1.36 L/m^2 (1 gal/30 ft^2).[31]

PUBLIC HEALTH CONSIDERATIONS

Unlike culture of other systemic fungi, culture of *Cryptococcus* is not a public health hazard, because only the yeast form is routinely grown, and this form does not aerosolize from media. Contact with infected pets is also not a risk, because the organism does not aerosolize from sites of tissue infection. The organism from tissues or body fluids does not spread between people or animals. Although infection can be produced by experimental inoculation of animals, this has not been reported spontaneously. The major public health significance of infected pets is that their source of exposure is also a potential source of exposure for associated humans.

References

1. Armengou A, Porcar C, Mascaro J, et al. 1996. Possible development of resistance to fluconazole during suppressive therapy for AIDS-associated cryptococcal meningitis. *Clin Infect Dis* 23:1337–1338.
2. Bailly MP, Boibieux A, Biron F, et al. 1991. Persistance of *Cryptococcus neoformans* in the prostate: failure of fluconazole despite high doses. *J Infect Dis* 164:435–436.
3. Berthelin CF, Bailey CS, Kass PH, et al. 1994. Cryptococcosis of the nervous system in dogs: part 1. Epidemiologic, clinical, and neuropathologic features. *Prog Vet Neurol* 5:88–97.
4. Berthelin CF, Legendre AM, Bailey CS, et al. 1994. Cryptococcosis of the nervous system in dogs: part 2. Diagnosis, treatment, monitoring, and prognosis. *Prog Vet Neurol* 5:136–146.
5. Blevins LB, Fenn J, Segal H, et al. 1995. False-positive cryptococcal antigen latex agglutination caused by disinfectants and soaps. *J Clin Microbiol* 33:1674–1675.
6. Bozzette SA, Larsen RA, Chiu J, et al. 1991. Fluconazole treatment of persistent *Cryptococcus neoformans* prostatic infection in AIDs. *Ann Intern Med* 115:285–286.
6a. Brocklebank J. 1997. British Columbia: canine *Cryptococcus neoformans. Can Vet J* 38:724.
7. Chen SCA, Muller M, Zhou JZ, et al. 1997. Phospholipase activity in *Cryptococcus neoformans*: a new virulence factor? *J Infect Dis* 175:414–420.
8. Chuck SL, Sande MA. 1989. Infections with *Cryptococcus neoformans* in the acquired immunodeficiency syndrome. *N Engl J Med* 321:794–799.
9. Denning DW, Tucker RM, Hanson LH, et al. 1989. Itraconazole therapy for cryptococcal meningitis and cryptococcosis. *Arch Intern Med* 149:2301–2308.
10. Dong ZM, Murphy JW. 1995. Intravascular cryptococcal culture filtrate (cneF) and its major component glucuronoxylomannan (Gxm) are potent inhibitors of leukocyte accumulation. *Infect Immun* 63:770–778.
11. Ellis DH, Pfeiffer TJ. 1990. Natural habitat of *Cryptococcus neoformans* var. *gattii. J Clin Microbiol* 28:1642–1644.
12. Flatland B, Greene RT, Lappin MR. 1996. Clinical and serologic evaluation of cats with cryptococcosis. *J Am Vet Med Assoc* 209:1110–1113.
13. Gerds-Grogan S, Dayrell-Hart B. 1997. Feline cryptococcosis, a retrospective evaluation. *J Am Anim Hosp Assoc* 33:118–122.
14. Glass E, De Lahunta A, Kent M. 1996. A cryptococcal granuloma in the brain of a cat causing focal signs. *Prog Vet Neurol* 7:141–144.
15. Gordon MA, Casadevall A. 1995. Serum therapy for cryptococcal meningitis. *Clin Infect Dis* 21:1477–1479.
16. Hamilton JR, Noble A, Denning DW, et al. 1991. Performance of *Cryptococcus* antigen latex agglutination kits on serum and cerebrospinal fluid specimens of AIDS patients before and after pronase treatment. *J Clin Microbiol* 29:333–339.
17. Hay RJ. 1994. Antifungal drugs on the horizon. *J Am Acad Dermatol* 31:582–585.
18. Hofmann S, Heider HJ, Hinrichs V, et al. 1997. Systemic cryptosporidiosis in a dog. Case report. *Tierarztl Umschau* 52:100–106.
19. Jacobs GJ, Medleau L, Calvert CC, et al. 1997. Cryptococcal infection in cats: factors influencing treatment outcome, and results of sequential serum antigen titers in 35 cats. *J Vet Intern Med* 11:1–4.
20. Kitchen LW. 1996. Adjunctive immunologic therapy for *Cryptococcus neoformans* infections. *Clin Infect Dis* 23:209.
21. Krawiec DR, McKiernan BC, Twardock AR, et al. 1996. Use of amphotericin B lipid complex for treatment of blastomycosis in dogs. *J Am Vet Med Assoc* 209:2073–2075.
22. Liaw Y-S, Yang P-C, Yu C-J, et al. 1995. Direct determination of cryptococcal antigen in transthoracic needle aspirate for diagnosis of pulmonary cryptococcosis. *J Clin Microbiol* 33:1588–1591.
23. Malik R, Craig AJ, Wigney D, et al. 1996. Combination chemotherapy of canine and feline cryptococcosis using subcutaneously administered amphotericin B. *Aust Vet J* 73:124–128.
24. Malik R, Dill-Macky E, Martin P, et al. 1995. Cryptococcosis in dogs: a retrospective study of 20 consecutive cases. *J Vet Med Mycol* 33:291–297.
24a. Malik R, Martin P, Wigney DI, et al. 1997. Nasopharyngeal cryptococcosis. *Aust Vet J* 75:483–488.
25. Malik R, McPetrie R, Wigney D. 1996. A latex cryptococcal antigen agglutination test for diagnosis and monitoring of therapy for cryptococcosis. *Aust Vet J* 74:358–364.
26. Malik R, Medeiros C, Wigney D, et al. 1996. Suspected drug eruption in dogs during administration of flucytosine. *Aust Vet J* 74:285–288.
27. Malik R, Wigney DI, Muir DB, et al. 1992. Cryptococcosis in cats: clinical and mycological assessment of 29 cases and evaluation of treatment using orally-administered fluconazole. *J Med Vet Mycol* 30:133–144.
28. Malik R, Wigney DI, Muir DB, et al. 1997. Asymptomatic carriage of *Cryptococcus neoformans* in the nasal cavity of dogs and cats. *J Med Vet Mycol* 35:27–31.
29. Martin CL, Stiles J, Willis M. 1996. Ocular adnexal cryptococcosis in a cat. *Vet Comp Ophthalmol* 6:225–229.
30. Meadows RL, MacWilliams PS, Dzata G, et al. 1993. Chylothorax associated with cryptococcal mediastinal granuloma in a cat. *Vet Clin Pathol* 22:109–116.
31. Medleau L, Barsanti JB. 1990. Cryptococcosis, pp 687–695. *In* Greene CE (ed), Infectious diseases of the dog and cat. WB Saunders, Philadelphia, PA.
32. Medleau L, Greene CE, Rakich PM. 1990. Evaluation of ketoconazole and itraconazole for treatment of disseminated cryptococcosis in cats. *Am J Vet Res* 51:1454–1458.
33. Medleau L, Jacobs GJ, Marks MA. 1995. Itraconazole for the treatment of cryptococcosis in cats. *J Vet Intern Med* 9:39–42.
34. Medleau L, Marks MA, Brown J, et al. 1990. Clinical evaluation of a cryptococcal antigen latex agglutination test for diagnosis of cryptococcosis in cats. *J Am Vet Med Assoc* 196:1470–1473.
35. Megson GM, Stevens DA, Hamilton JR, et al. 1996. D-Mannitol in cerebrospinal fluid of patients with AIDs and cryptococcal meningitis. *J Clin Microbiol* 34:218–221.
36. Mikiciuk MG, Fales WH, Schmidt DA. 1990. Successful treatment of feline cryptococcosis with ketoconazole and flucytosine. *J Am Anim Hosp Assoc* 26:199–201.
37. Millon L, Barale T, Julliot M-C, et al. 1995. Interference by hydroxyethyl starch used for vascular filling in latex agglutination test for cryptococcal antigen. *J Clin Microbiol* 33:1912–1919.
38. Moncino MD, Gutman LT. 1990. Severe systemic cryptococcal disease in a child: review of prognostic indicators predicting treatment failure and an approach to maintenance therapy with oral fluconazole. *Pediatr Infect Dis J* 9:363–368.
39. Shaw SE. 1988. Successful treatment of 11 cases of feline cryptococcosis. *Aust Vet Pract* 18:135–139.
40. Tanaka K, Miyazaki T, Maesaki S, et al. 1996. Detection of *Cryptococcus neoformans* gene in patients with pulmonary *Cryptococcus. J Clin Microbiol* 34:2826–2828.
41. Tanner DC, Weinstein MP, Fedorciw B, et al. 1994. Comparison of commercial kits for detection of cryptococcal antigen. *J Clin Microbiol* 32:1680–1684.
42. Tjalsma EJ. 1997. Two cases of cryptococcosis in the cat. *Tijdschrift Diergeneesk* 122:128–132.
43. Turner SH, Cherniak R. 1991. Multiplicity in the structure of the glucuronoxylomannan of *Cryptococcus neoformans*, pp 123–142. *In* Latge JP, Boucias D (eds), Fungal cell wall and immune response. Springer-Verlag, Heidelberg, Germany.
44. Walker C, Malik R, Canfield PJ. 1995. Analysis of leucocytes and lymphocyte subsets in cats with naturally occurring cryptococcosis but differing feline immunodeficiency virus status. *Aust Vet J* 72:93–97.
45. Warren RJ, Perceval A, Dwyer BW. 1993. Comparative evaluation of cryptococcal latex tests. *Pathology* 25:76–80.

Chapter 62

Coccidioidomycosis

Russell T. Greene

ETIOLOGY

Coccidioides immitis is a soil-borne fungus restricted to certain geographic regions. It grows in soil and culture medium as a mycelium. It forms thick-walled, barrel-shaped, rectangular, multinucleate arthroconidia, 2 to 4 μm wide and 3 to 10 μm long (Fig. 62–1). These arthroconidia alternate with smaller, thin-walled, nonviable cells. The latter degenerate, releasing the arthroconidia to be dispersed by wind. The arthroconidia can germinate to yield new hyphae or serve as the infecting form for animals and humans (Fig. 62–2). When inhaled, the arthroconidia, in the presence of the phagocytic cells and increased carbon dioxide, convert into a different morphologic form. They shed all but one nucleus, round up, and enlarge to produce an immature spherule. The nucleus undergoes division, which is followed by inward partitioning of the cytoplasm, resulting in a mature spherule with endospores in the center. The spherule, gradually enlarging to 20 to 200 μm in diameter, eventually breaks open to release endospores, which form new spherules at 37°C or mycelia at room temperature. Transformation from arthroconidia to immature spherules can be completed within 2 to 3 days. Intact spherules are poorly chemotactic for neutrophils. Those neutrophils that do attach cannot penetrate the wall of the spherule (Fig. 62–3). The endospores are the vulnerable stage of *C. immitis* in the body. They attract large numbers of neutrophils and are small enough to be phagocytized.

EPIDEMIOLOGY

The mycelial phase of *C. immitis* has been found in nature only in a specific ecologic region, the Lower Sonoran life zone. Geographically, the Lower Sonoran life zone is within the southwestern United States, Mexico, and Central and South America (Guatemala, Honduras, Colombia, Venezuela, Paraguay, Argentina) (Fig. 62–4). This zone is characterized by sandy, alkaline soils, high environmental temperature (summer mean >26.6°C [79.9°F]; winter mean 4–12°C [39.2–53.6°F]), low annual rainfall (3–20″), and low elevation (sea level to a few hundred feet). During prolonged periods of high temperature and low soil moisture, *C. immitis* survives below the soil surface at depths as great as 20 cm, where competitive organisms are few. After a period of rainfall, *C. immitis* returns to the soil surface, sporulates, and releases large numbers of arthroconidia to be disseminated by the wind. Epidemics in people have occurred after dust storms, following the rainy season, or after earthquakes.[14] Endemically, the incidence of disease is highest in the late summer and early fall, when the soil is dry and crops are being harvested. Occupational and recreational exposure of people and animals in the outdoors leads to a greater risk of infection. In the United States, the disease is often referred to as Valley Fever after the occurrence of an epidemic in the San Joaquin Valley of California, but it is also prevalent in Arizona and southwestern Texas. The disease is less common in New Mexico, Nevada, and Utah. A few endemic areas are found in Central and South America, particularly Venezuela.

Although the majority of cases in animals and people are diagnosed within the southwestern United States, an occasional case may be identified outside this area. Usually, these "stray" cases have a history of residence or travel within an endemic area. Serologic surveys indicate that most human and canine inhabitants in endemic areas become infected; however, most infections are subclinical or cause only mild, transient respiratory signs. It is estimated that only 40% of people infected develop respiratory symptoms and very few develop systemic manifestations. In the remaining 60%, the only evidence of infection is seroconversion. Although not proven, it is thought that the same statistics concerning infections and clinical signs in domestic animals are similar.

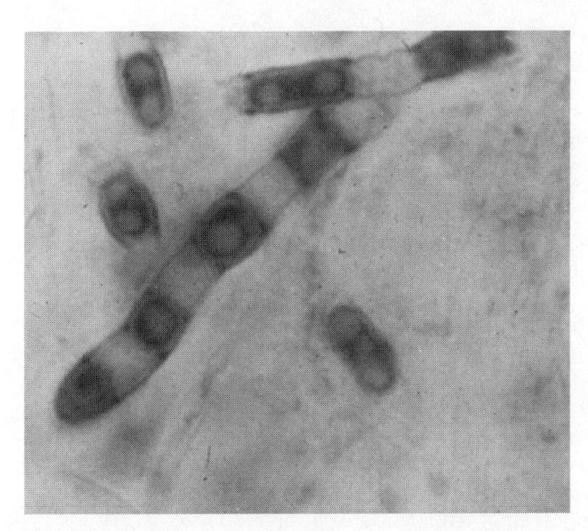

Figure 62–1. Lactophenol cotton blue preparation from a *C. immitis* colony. The arrangement of the barrel-shaped arthroconidia of *C. immitis* is a characteristic alternating pattern of live and dead arthroconidia. These arthroconidia are extremely dangerous, and mycelial cultures should only be handled within a biosafety hood (× 100).

PATHOGENESIS

The major route of infection is by inhalation. Very few (<10) arthroconidia must be inhaled to produce disease. The incubation period from inhalation to onset of abnormal respiratory signs is 1 to 3 weeks. Primary localized infection of the skin lesions from penetrating wounds has rarely been reported. Experimentally, ID inoculation or skin scarification produces only localized infection in a small percentage of animals.

After inhalation, the conidia first enter the bronchioles and alveoli and then extend into the peribronchiolar tissue, eventually causing subpleural lesions. The first cellular response is neutrophilic, followed by monocytes, lymphocytes, and plasma cells. As with all fungal infections, cell-mediated immunity is more important than humoral immunity in elim-

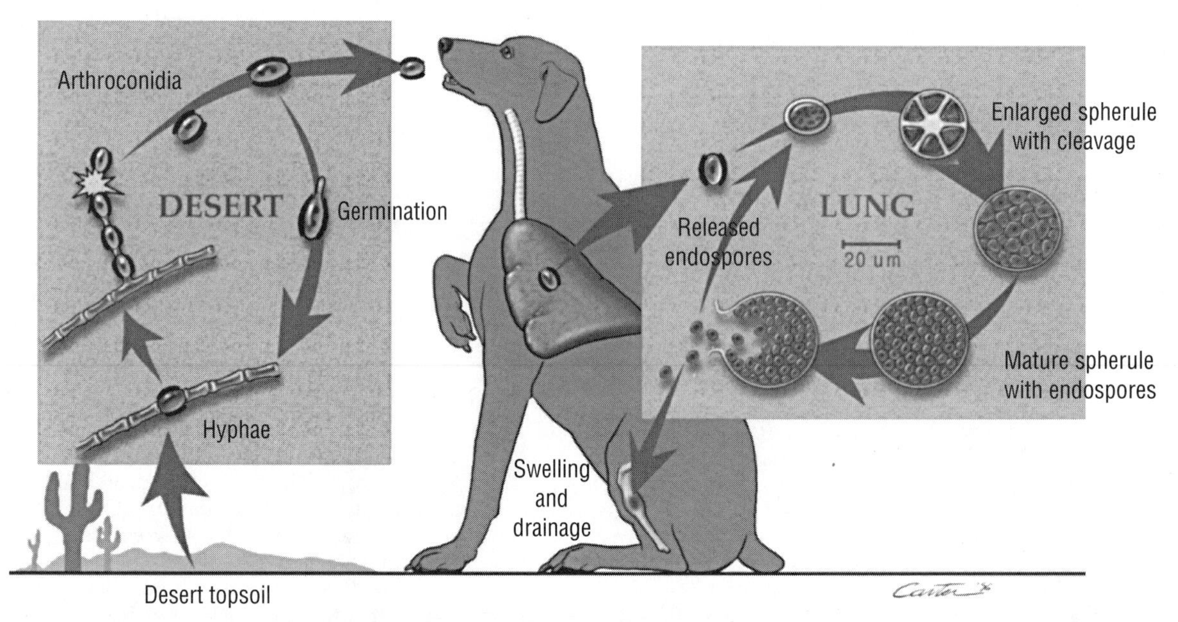

Figure 62–2. Life cycle of *C. immitis*. In the soil (an arthroconidium) or in culture of infected tissues (an endospore), the single cell germinates to become hyphae, which eventually form arthroconidia that can break off to form new hyphae. Once inhaled, these arthroconidia enter the lung, change morphologically to a round spherule that undergoes repeated internal divisions until it is filled with thousands of endospores. Each endospore has the capacity to become a new spherule. They also disseminate to infect distant tissues. Swelling and drainage occur at lesion sites close to skin surfaces.

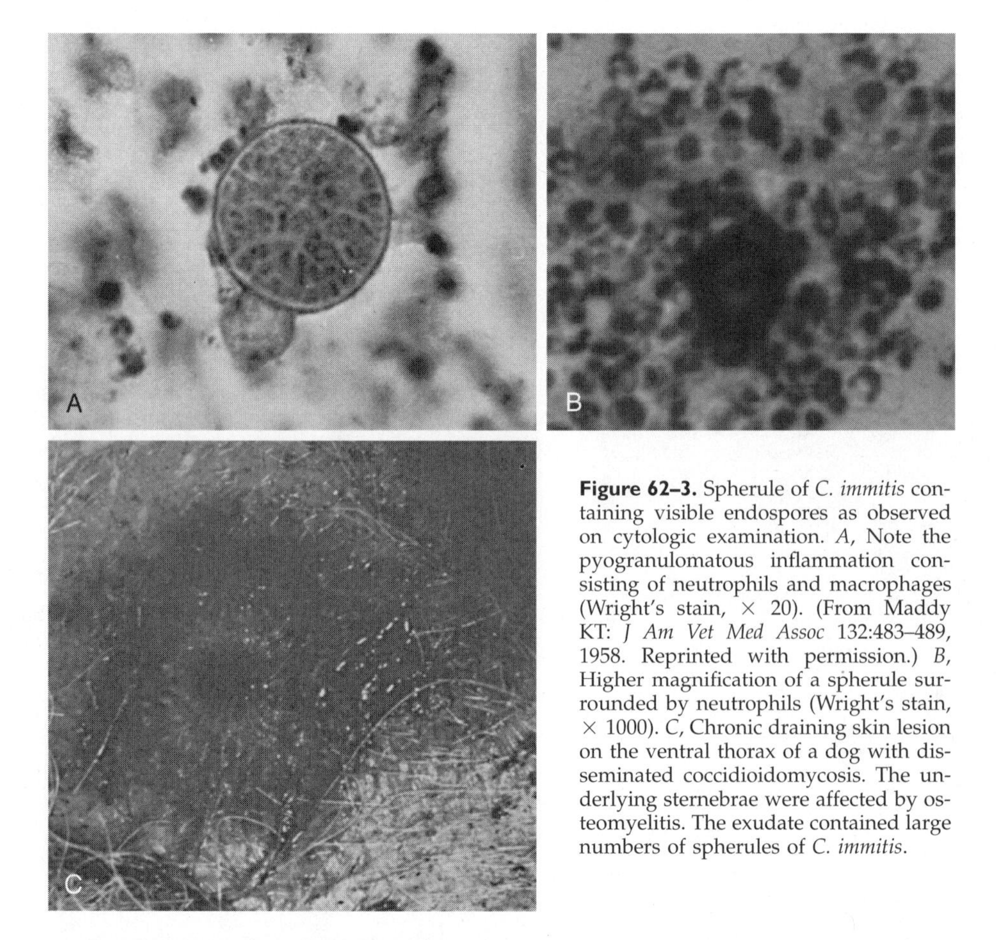

Figure 62–3. Spherule of *C. immitis* containing visible endospores as observed on cytologic examination. *A*, Note the pyogranulomatous inflammation consisting of neutrophils and macrophages (Wright's stain, × 20). (From Maddy KT: *J Am Vet Med Assoc* 132:483–489, 1958. Reprinted with permission.) *B*, Higher magnification of a spherule surrounded by neutrophils (Wright's stain, × 1000). *C*, Chronic draining skin lesion on the ventral thorax of a dog with disseminated coccidioidomycosis. The underlying sternebrae were affected by osteomyelitis. The exudate contained large numbers of spherules of *C. immitis*.

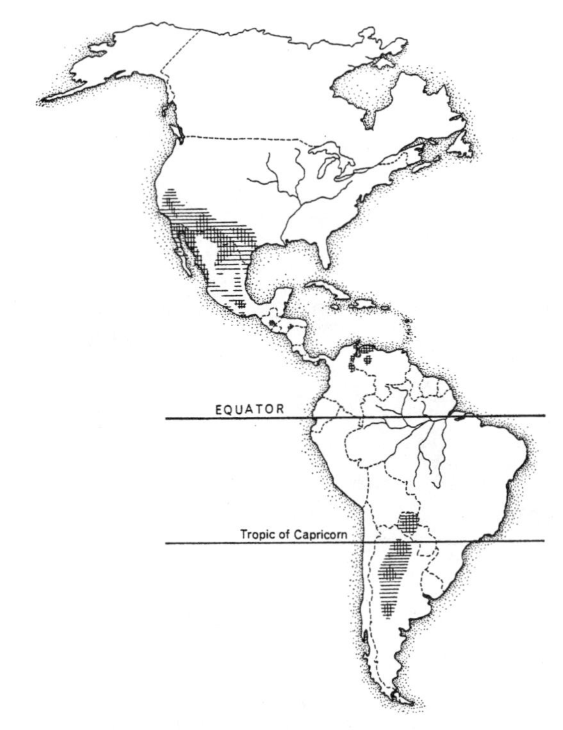

Figure 62–4. Worldwide distribution of incidence and prevalence of coccidioidomycosis. The areas marked by horizontal lines indicate incidence; the cross-hatched areas indicate regions of high endemicity. From Rippon JW (ed): Medical Mycology, 3rd ed. WB Saunders, 1988, p 436. Reprinted with permission.

ination of infection. Antibody response to two different antigens of the fungus has been used to detect infection (see Diagnosis).

Recovery from initial infection in people results in lifelong immunity, but resistance to reinfection in animals is uncertain. With massive exposure or depressed cellular immunity, pulmonary infection can become more extensive, and the organism can invade the hilar lymph nodes and distant tissues. If disease progresses beyond the hilar lymph nodes, which it can do within 10 days of exposure, it is considered to have disseminated. Dissemination involves the reproductive cycle from spherules to endospores to new spherules. If the disease disseminates, the organs that are usually affected are, in decreasing order of frequency, bones, eyes, heart and pericardium, testicles, brain, spinal cord, and visceral organs (primarily spleen, liver, kidney). Ocular lesions begin as a chorioretinitis and extend into the anterior chamber. The intestinal mucosa and endocardium are rarely affected. Virtually all other tissues can be affected. Signs referable to dissemination usually occur about 4 months after pulmonary signs develop, but this period is variable, and the respiratory infection may have never been noticed. Disseminated cases usually have a chronic course of months to years.

CLINICAL FINDINGS

Dogs

The high prevalence of positive skin test reactions in epidemiologic surveys of healthy dogs indicates that the most common form of coccidioidomycosis is an asymptomatic or mild, undiagnosed respiratory tract infection. When clinical respiratory disease develops, it can be characterized by either a dry, harsh cough similar to that associated with tracheobronchitis or a wet, moist, productive cough. The dry cough is usually a result of a hilar lymphadenomegaly or diffuse pulmonary interstitial disease, and the productive one is usually a result of alveolar involvement. Fever, partial anorexia, and weight loss are commonly present in both situations. The pulmonary disease can resolve or worsen. The latter course leads to severe generalized pneumonia with a worsening of respiratory signs.

Clinical signs most commonly associated with disseminated disease include, in decreasing order of frequency, persistent or fluctuating fever, anorexia, weight loss, depression and weakness, lameness, localized peripheral lymphadenomegaly, draining skin lesions, keratitis, uveitis, and acute blindness. GI signs as well as generalized peripheral lymphadenomegaly are extremely uncommon. Signs of right- or left-sided congestive heart failure can also occur. Cardiac dysfunction arises from disturbances in blood flow, conduction, and myocardial contractility, resulting from lesions in the myocardium, conduction system, and pericardium. The latter lesion often results in constrictive pericarditis. Seizures, ataxia, behavioral changes, and coma have been associated with lesions in the CNS.

Lameness usually is accompanied by painful bone swellings (Fig. 62–5). Bone lesions usually are initially localized to one bone but may progress to involve multiple sites. The lesions generally occur in the long bones in the distal diaphysis, metaphysis, and epiphysis and typically there is a combination of lysis and production. Lesions occur in the axial skeleton but only at a 10% prevalence compared with the appendicular skeleton. Joint infection is not typical, although secondary immune-mediated polyarthritis has developed in infected dogs.

Skin lesions that begin as small bumps and progress to abscesses, ulcers, or draining tracts are almost always found over sites of infected bone (see Fig. 62–5). Most cutaneous involvement results from systemic spread of the organism. Naturally occurring primary cutaneous infection from penetrating injury is extremely rare in dogs.[12]

Cats

Signs associated with *C. immitis* infection in cats are similar to those described in dogs; however, skin lesions are the most frequent type of infection found in cats. It is very common to have skin infections without underlying bone involvement. Fever, inappetence, and weight loss are commonly found concurrently with skin lesions. Coughing, wheezing, and respiratory difficulties are only occasionally recognized with feline *C. immitis* infections possibly because

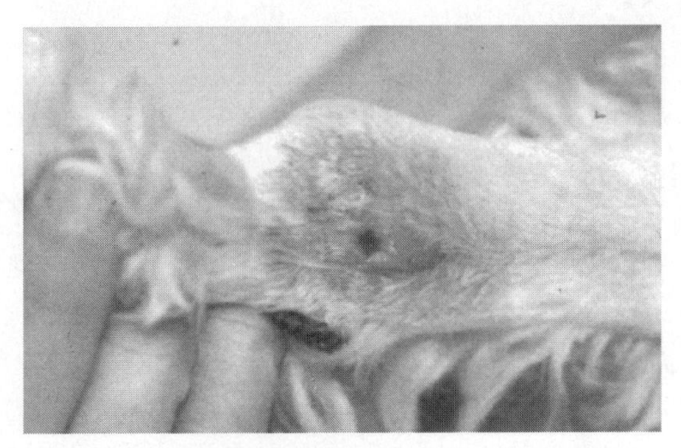

Figure 62–5. Left carpal swelling with a draining fistula in a dog with disseminated coccidioidomycosis. The underlying bone had evidence of an osteomyelitis.

cats limit their physical activity. Appendicular bone lesions, like lung lesions, are recognized seldomly in feline infections compared with canine infections. When bone lesions are present in cats, the radiographic changes are similar to those observed in dogs. Ocular lesions of chorioretinitis and anterior uveitis occur with about the same frequency in cats as they do in dogs.

DIAGNOSIS

Clinical Laboratory Findings

Hematologic changes may include mild nonregenerative anemia and moderate neutrophilic leukocytosis, often with a left shift. Eosinophilia of blood and CSF, common in human coccidioidomycosis, is quite variable in animals. Hyperglobulinemia and hypoalbuminemia are common, reflecting a chronic persistent inflammatory disease. Hypercalcemia unassociated with bone lesions has not yet been described in affected dogs or cats, but has been found with other systemic mycoses and in some human patients. An osteotrophic factor similar to humoral hypercalcemia of malignancy has been postulated.

Radiography

Thoracic radiographic findings vary with the severity of the disease. A diffuse interstitial pattern is most common but is often mixed with a localized alveolar pattern (Fig. 62–6). Miliary to nodular interstitial densities may be found. Pulmonary abscess formation, fibrosis, and bronchiectasis (rarely calcification) may be sequelae to severe pulmonary infection. Hilar lymphadenomegaly is quite common, affecting most dogs with chronic illness, but calcification of the hilar lymph nodes or sternal lymphadenomegaly is rare. Pericardial and pleural effusion may occur secondary to right-sided myocardial failure or, more frequently, to pericarditis. Radiographic findings of osteomyelitis are typically a mixture of both lysis and production (Fig. 62–7).

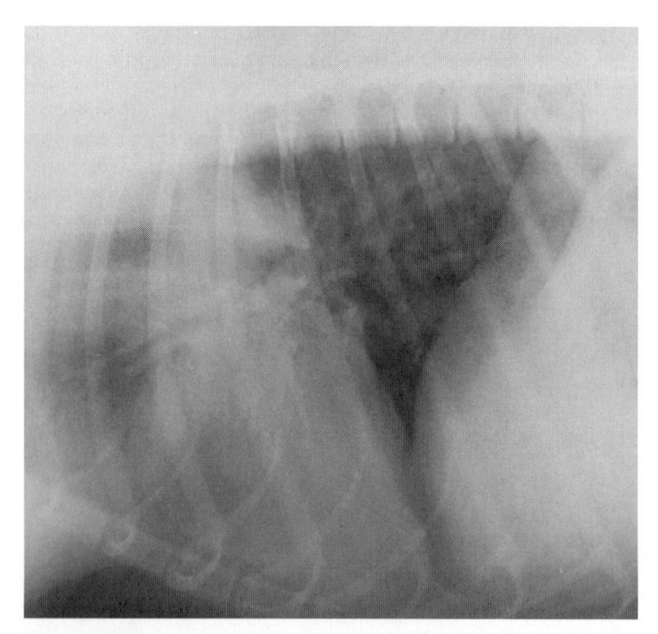

Figure 62–6. Lateral thoracic radiograph of a dog with pulmonary coccidioidomycosis, showing a hilar lymphadenopathy and diffuse interstitial pattern.

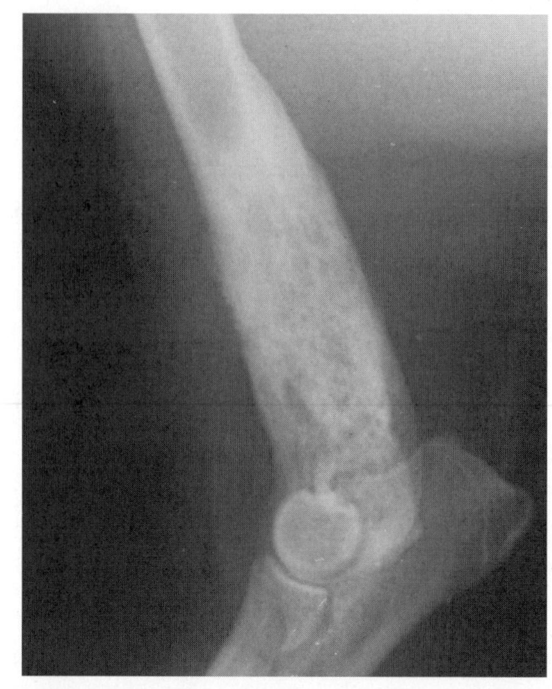

Figure 62–7. Radiograph of the distal humerus of a dog with disseminated coccidioidomycosis. Lesions are classically a mixture of lysis and production.

Cytology

Coccidioidomycosis is conclusively diagnosed by cytologic or histologic visualization of the organism. However, because of lesion localization or cost associated with invasive procedures, demonstration of the organism is often not possible. In such cases, a diagnosis is based on history, clinical findings, and serologic test results.

As with other nodular interstitial diseases, false-negative results are common with transtracheal or bronchial washings. The chance of a positive yield increases if alveolar disease is present. Spherules are frequently found in aspirates of enlarged nodes or in impression smears of draining lesions (Fig. 62–8).

The organism can be seen in unstained preparations under

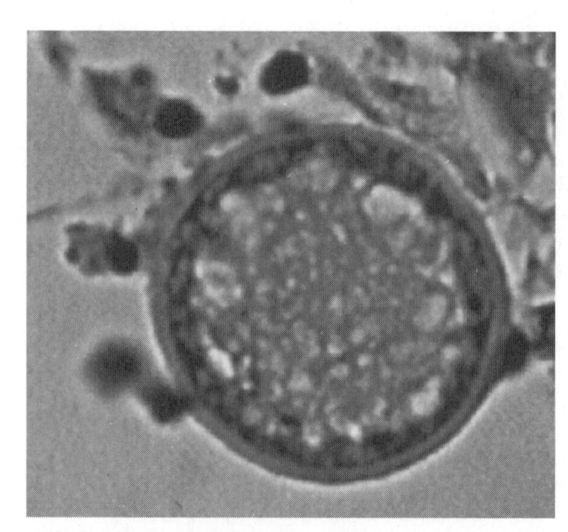

Figure 62–8. Histopathology of *C. immitis*–induced lesion with a large *C. immitis* spherule surrounded by pyogranulomatous inflammation (H and E, × 100).

reduced light as a large (10–80 μm), round, double-walled structure with endospores. Ten percent potassium hydroxide can clear an unstained specimen, although stained preparations are more typical. The organism is readily recognized with standard Wright's stain, but to specifically stain the fungal structures, the best stains are Papanicolaou's (PAP) and periodic acid–Schiff (PAS). With PAP stain, the capsular wall is refractile and purple-black, the cytoplasm yellow, and the endospores red-brown. Not all spherules will contain recognizable endospores. Smaller spherules may have a crumpled, transparent wall. With PAS stain, the wall is deep red to purple and the endospores are bright red. Large numbers of neutrophils may surround the spherules, making them difficult to visualize.

Biopsy

In histopathology specimens, the organism usually can best be found in microabscesses. Spherules are detected employing routine H and E stains, but for optimal visualization special stains such as PAS or Grocott-Gomori's methenamine silver should be used. Spherules may be difficult to find in bone biopsy samples because of the reactive bone that forms within lesions. Repeated biopsies may be necessary to find the organism. Pathologists recommend that several biopsy samples be taken from the same lesion. Often redirecting the biopsy needle through the same insertion site to obtain several core samples is most successful. Immunofluorescence techniques can also be utilized to identify *C. immitis* spherules in tissues or cytologic preparations, but false-negative results can occur and rarely are these techniques needed.

Fungal Isolation

C. immitis grows on a wide range of common fungal culture media and blood agar. Attempts should *not* be made to culture and identify this organism within veterinary practices. Instead, samples should be sent to laboratories familiar with biosafety precautions. The mycelial phase grows best at 25°C to 30°C. It usually grows within 3 days but may require more time if the number of organisms in the sample is low. The characteristic pattern of alternating live and dead arthroconidia associated with the appearance of the fungal colony allows for presumptive identification, but additional in vitro and in vivo methods can further definitively identify the organism. Veterinarians, technicians, and laboratory personnel must recognize that arthroconidia from mycelial growth are highly infectious.

Serologic Testing

Dogs. When the organism cannot be demonstrated by cytology or biopsy, detection of antibodies to the organism is commonly used as a presumptive test. The two classic antigens for serotesting are the tube precipitin (TP) and complement fixation (CF). The names for these differently prepared antigens were based on the types of tests that were initially utilized to detect antibodies. The antibody response to the TP antigen has been shown to be primarily IgM, whereas the antibody response to the CF antigen is associated more with IgG. For interpretation of TP and CF antibody titers in naturally infected dogs refer to Table 62–1.

Advances in molecular diagnostics have brought new methods of antibody detection. Clinicians should always check with the laboratory performing the serologic tests to determine which method is being used. Instead of the TP and CF methods, some laboratories employ the latex agglutination, AGID, or ELISA methods for detection of these same antibodies. See Table 62–2 for a comparison of these methods. TP and CF antigens are still used in AGID tests. Because the antigens and the antibody responses were named well before these newer techniques, it makes the serologic terminology confusing. Even more confusing is the fact that many of these new assays have not been fully evaluated utilizing animal serum. Assumptions have often been made concerning their accuracy based on limited research in humans. Because of the nature of the disease and the studies that have been completed to date, it is usually difficult to determine which of the tests are correct versus incorrect when discrepancies are noted. Further serologic studies with corresponding histologic, cytologic, or mycologic confirmation are needed. Advantages of the AGID and the ELISA methods over the classic CF test are that these newer methods are less complicated to perform and interference by anticomplementary factors, which can be found in 15% to 25% of normal dog sera, does not occur.

Tests to detect antigenemia in people have been developed and used on an investigational basis. Antigen detection would be helpful in early cases before seroconversion or in immunodeficiencies when seroreactivity does not develop. Interference by various components in serum has been a major problem with antigen tests; however, newer techniques are being evaluated. Appendix 5 should be consulted for information concerning the submission of samples for serologic testing of coccidioidomycosis.

Cats. Early publications suggest that serologic tests were not useful diagnostic aids. However, a review of 48 feline cases indicated that both TP and CF antibodies were routinely

Table 62–1. Interpretation of Serologic Testing for Coccidioidomycosis in Dogs and Cats

VARIABLE	TP ANTIBODY: NEGATIVE	TP ANTIBODY: POSITIVE
CF ANTIBODY: NEGATIVE	1. No infection 2. Early infection; if disease suspected, repeat test in 4–6 weeks to detect positive TP or CF test results 3. Rapidly fatal, fulminating infection in severely immunocompromised animal	1. Early or mild infection: TP test results become positive 2 weeks postexposure and may become negative after 4–6 weeks
CF ANTIBODY: POSITIVE	1. Past exposure or disease, healing or localized lesions, or long-standing residual titer (especially if weak CF titer, 1:4 or less) 2. Chronic infection: TP antibody frequently disappears after 4–6 weeks; the higher the CF titer, the more likely is severe or disseminated disease 3. Higher CF titers $\geq$ 1:64 most frequently seen with severe pulmonary or disseminated lesions	1. Early or active infection: the greater the CF titer, the more likely that disease is severe or disseminated 2. Chronic infection: positive TP tests occur later in infections or at the time of dissemination or recrudescence

CF = complement fixation, primarily IgG; TP = tube precipitin, primarily IgM.

Table 62–2. Comparison of Serologic Tests for Coccidioidomycosis[a]

TEST (ABBREVIATION)	MEASURED IMMUNOGLOBULIN	COMMENTS
TP	IgM	Positive results early in disease. Titer may increase with reactivation or dissemination.
CF	IgG	Good test for quantitative titers. Considered reference test for IgG. Positive results occur later in infection and rise with dissemination. Titer remains elevated months after successful treatment or if arrested. Titer gradually decreases with successful treatment. False-negative results occur in some immunosuppressed or anergic animals.
Latex agglutination	IgM	Some false-positive results occur in canine sera. Detects acute (< 1 mo) infections.
Immunodiffusion (AGID)		
TP antigen (IDTP)	IgM	More sensitive than TP in detecting recent (< 1 mo) infections.
CF antigen (IDCF)	IgG	Good correlation with ELISA IgG with quantitative immunodiffusion. Most sensitive screening test for IgG.
ELISA		
IgM	IgM	Some (~15%) false-positive results compared with IDTP; also cross-reacts with some blastomycosis sera.
IgG	IgG	Good correlation with CF and IDCF: OD readings do not always correlate directly with CF titers. Cross-reacts with some blastomycosis sera.

[a]Based on data from Greene RT: unpublished observations, 1996; Pappagianis D, Zimmer BL: *Clin Microb Rev* 3:247–268, 1990.
TP = tube precipitin; CF = complement fixation; IDTP = immunodiffusion tube precipitin; IDCF = immunodiffusion complement fixation; OD = optical density.

detected in feline infections.[6] Both antibodies appear to persist for long periods in cats, even when therapy is initiated and maintained.

Skin Testing

Skin testing is used for epidemiologic surveys and evaluation of immunocompetence to *C. immitis* rather than as a diagnostic tool. The accuracy of ID testing with coccidioidin is subject to antigen variability. A positive reaction is an induration of 5 mm or greater area 24 to 36 hours after injection. A positive test indicates past or present infection. In people, the test result becomes positive within 1 week, after development of respiratory signs, whereas in dogs a positive test result has been found within 3 to 8 weeks of natural exposure. In healthy people, a positive skin test result indicates past exposure and resistance to infection and remains positive for years. About 5% of people and 10% of dogs with disseminated disease have a negative skin test owing to severe immunosuppression. Skin testing is not especially specific because cross-reactions with histoplasmin and blastomycin can occur. Use of an antigen from the spherule phase, spherulin, has not proven diagnostically superior to coccidioidin in people.

PATHOLOGIC FINDINGS

The lesion induced by *C. immitis* in dogs and cats is usually pyogranulomatous and is most often seen in the lungs. On gross inspection, lesions may vary from miliary to massive, from red to gray to white, from nodular to diffuse, and from firm to caseous or liquefactive (Fig 62–9). Tracheobronchial lymph nodes are often increased in size and firm. Bone enlargement is found in dogs with coccidioidal osteomyelitis. At the time bone lesions are observed, lung lesions may have resolved. With CNS involvement, granulomas have been found in the cerebrum and midbrain. A granulomatous uveitis, retinitis, and keratitis may be present. In dogs with granulomatous pericarditis, the organism can be found in pericardial fluid. In dogs, right-sided heart failure is more commonly caused by coccidioidal pericarditis than myocarditis.

THERAPY

Proper therapy of coccidioidomycosis in dogs and cats typically involves long-term antifungal drug treatment (Table 62–3); however, success is unpredictable. Mildly affected animals do not require treatment. There is controversy as to whether animals with primary pulmonary disease should be treated, because many cases may resolve spontaneously. In humans with initial mild primary pulmonary involvement, therapy is avoided unless there is chronic (6-week) debilitation. In dogs and cats, therapy has generally been instituted earlier for fear of dissemination. Animals with severe pulmonary infections, those with increasing reciprocal titers of CF antibody (especially ≥16), and those with fever, weakness, lameness, or worsening clinical signs are candidates for therapy. All animals with disseminated disease should also be treated.

Because of the cost and potential toxicity of treatment, caution should be exercised when a diagnosis is based on serologic data alone. Positive CF titers of 8 or less are suspect for infection in animals. Those patients with clinical illness may be treated, and serotesting should be repeated in 3 to 4 weeks to determine whether the titer is rising. Many dogs in enzootic areas have reciprocal titers of 4 or less from prior

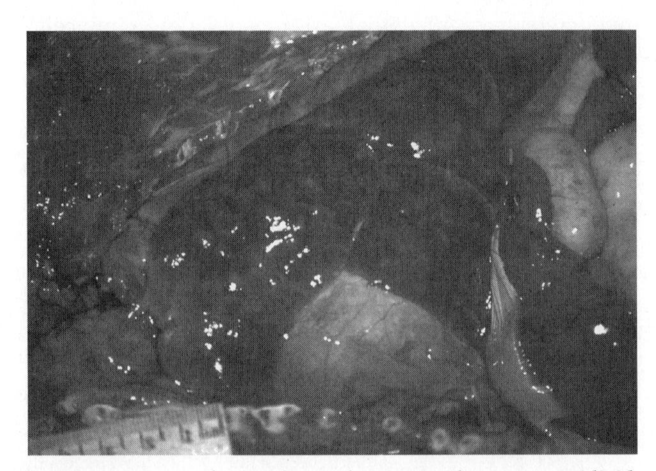

Figure 62–9. Lungs from a dog with severe pulmonary coccidioidomycosis showing multiple light-colored granulomas throughout the lung lobes.

Table 62–3. Antifungal Therapy of Coccidioidomycosis

DRUG	SPECIES	DOSE[a]	ROUTE	INTERVAL (HOURS)	DURATION (MONTHS)
Ketoconazole	D	5–10 mg/kg	PO	12	8–12[b]
	C	50 mg (total)	PO	12–24	[b]
Itraconazole	D	5 mg/kg	PO	12	[b]
	C	25–50 mg (total)	PO	12–24	[b]
Fluconazole	D	5 mg/kg	PO	12	[b]
	C	25–50 mg (total)	PO	12–24	[b]
Amphotericin B[c]	D	0.4–0.5 mg/kg	IV	48–72[d]	[e]
Lufenuron	D	5 mg/kg	PO	24	4[f]

[a]Dose per administration at specified interval. For additional information, see Drug Formulary, Appendix 8.
[b]Not based on controlled studies, but typical duration with dissemination generally 12 months. Primary respiratory diseases often require shorter therapy.
[c]Amphotericin is rarely used because of its nephrotoxicity. It can be used alone or in combination with an azole. If used in combination, the recommended cumulative dose is often half.
[d]Given Monday and Thursday or Monday, Wednesday, and Friday.
[e]Until cumulative dose is 8–11 mg/kg.
[f]Efficacy of therapy and minimum dosage regimen has not been established. Maintenance therapy may be needed for longer periods. This treatment is still experimental.
D = dog; C = cat.

exposure. Symptomatic animals with these low titers should have additional diagnostic procedures performed rather than be treated. Although animals can be infected and seronegative, this situation appears to be rare.

Deciding whether to terminate therapy is based on resolution of the clinical disease, radiographic appearance of bone and lung lesions, and serologic titers. Serologic titers alone may not be helpful to determine whether the disease is in remission because CF titers may stabilize or decrease only slightly. However, long-term monitoring of serologic response is beneficial to determine whether the titer is rising. Rising titers suggest poor absorption of drug or poor therapeutic response. If blood levels of the drug suggest adequate absorption, an alternate therapy should be considered.

If uveitis is the only sign of active infection and it is not improving with antifungal therapy, enucleation should be performed. It has been curative, without further treatment, in at least one cat.[6]

The three azole drugs, ketoconazole (KTZ), itraconazole (ITZ), and fluconazole (FCZ), are most commonly prescribed in this order of frequency. For many years, amphotericin B (AMB) was the only drug available; however, because of its adverse effects and need for IV administration, it is less commonly administered. The newer route of SC administration has not been evaluated in this disease (see Drug Formulary, Appendix 8).

Ketoconazole

The drug of choice to initially treat coccidioidomycosis has been KTZ. It has been used to treat coccidioidomycosis in a large number of dogs and cats in the southwestern United States. See the Drug Formulary (Appendix 8) for detailed information about this drug.

The recommended dosages for KTZ are listed in Table 62–3. The duration of therapy has been variable, depending on the site and extent of disease. Relapses are common if the drug is not administered on a daily basis for an adequate period of time. Treatment of animals with bone or disseminated coccidioidomycosis typically requires a minimum of 1 year. Because GI absorption of the drug is variable, it is helpful to measure a 2- to 4-hour postpill KTZ blood level after 2 to 3 weeks of treatment.

Poor response and relapses occur with KTZ. Serologic tests should be repeated after 4 to 6 weeks of therapy. If the CF titer has continued to rise or clinical signs are deteriorating, an alternative azole or, rarely, AMB should be considered (see Table 62–3).

In people with nonmeningeal coccidioidomycosis, KTZ appears to be fungistatic; most patients improve, but relapses are common even at higher than recommended dosages, and cures occur in only approximately 30%. For meningeal disease, KTZ has been considered a poor choice for treatment because of its decreased penetration into the CSF and CNS. In the past, intrathecal AMB was given for CNS coccidioidomycosis, but the drug is very irritating by this route. Because of its excellent pharmacokinetics and CNS penetration, FCZ is recommended for these cases (see Fluconazole, Chapter 57, and Drug Formulary, Appendix 8).

Itraconazole and Fluconazole

The newer azoles, ITZ and FCZ, are thought to be more efficacious in treating coccidioidomycosis in humans; however, there are no controlled studies in dogs or cats demonstrating similar efficacy. In some cases, these drugs are more effective, resolving the clinical signs with fewer side effects. In others, the newer azole has failed when it was tried first, only to have the infection controlled with KTZ. As with KTZ, some of the animals treated with ITZ or FCZ develop relapses. These drugs may be an alternative but not a panacea. Side effects of hepatic dysfunction, GI upsets, and skin reactions[12] can also occur as they do with KTZ.

Amphotericin B

AMB, previously the drug of choice for treating canine coccidioidomycosis, is still indicated in animals that are unable to tolerate an azole compound. The toxicities and difficulties of administering AMB make it less desirable than KTZ for dogs (see Chapter 57). Lipid formulations of AMB are available and are thought to have less toxicity but have not been clinically tested in dogs or cats (see Drug Formulary, Appendix 8). The dose of AMB to induce remission when used alone or in combination is listed in Table 62–3. Periodic, once-monthly maintenance injections of AMB, given at the same daily dose, may be required over extended periods to prevent relapses.

Chitin Synthesis Inhibitors

Chitin synthesis inhibitors are newer antifungal agents that also interfere with formation of the cell wall of fungi. One drug, Nikkomycin-Z (Shaman Pharmaceuticals, Inc., San

Francisco, CA), is near the stage of clinical trials. These compounds are cidal, rather than static as are the azoles, and, in comparison, require relatively low doses for shorter time periods. Lufenuron, a chitin synthesis inhibitor, is licensed for control of flea infestation in dogs and cats. Instead of once-monthly treatment, the drug was given daily for 16 weeks.[2] Clinical improvement began after 1 week, and resolution of radiographic lesions in the lungs (if present) occurred after 10 weeks. For further information, see Drug Formulary, Appendix 8.

PROGNOSIS

The prognosis for localized respiratory coccidioidomycosis without treatment is good; however, many dogs have been routinely treated to decrease the chance of dissemination. Without treatment, dogs with disseminated disease will usually die or have to be euthanized shortly after the disease is discovered. In more than 90% of these dogs, signs resolve with KTZ therapy; however, complete recovery rates in animals that require no further maintenance therapy are much lower. Complete recovery rates vary with the severity of the disease and dissemination, ranging from 90% with only pulmonary involvement to 0% with multiple bone involvement. An overall recovery rate of approximately 60% has been noted. Many infected cats show clinical improvement with KTZ therapy; however, relapses have been common, especially when medication was discontinued.[6] Some cats have a relapse each time treatment is stopped (i.e., multiple relapses).

PREVENTION

No vaccine is available to prevent infections, although a killed spherule vaccine was found to be highly protective against coccidioidal infection in mice. A similar vaccine in people failed to demonstrate protection. Current studies are examining the use of purified antigens as vaccines.

Immunotherapy has been tried with little or variable success in people utilizing a variety of drugs and cytokine inducers. Similarly, levamisole and acemannan have been empirically given to infected dogs with little success. All immunosuppressive drugs, including glucocorticoids, should be avoided or withdrawn before and during therapy. Synthetic immunomodulators or those produced by recombinant DNA techniques may offer an approach in the future.

PUBLIC HEALTH CONSIDERATIONS

Coccidioidomycosis is generally accepted as being noncontagious because the infectious arthroconidial form of the agent is not produced in tissues. Except for one unusual case, in which disseminated meningeal coccidioidomycosis developed in a veterinarian who performed a necropsy on a horse with disseminated disease,[8] there is no known direct spread from animal to person. This veterinarian may have been exposed to arthroconidia growing in improperly preserved infected tissue or, less likely, directly to aerosolized or inoculated spherules from fresh tissues or discharges. In general, infected animals are not considered public health hazards. However, veterinarians should be cognizant of the potential problem of placing bandages over draining lesions. The tissue drainage may contaminate the bandage material and provide a suitable environment for arthroconidia development.

In contrast, handling of mycelial cultures of the organism in the laboratory is extremely dangerous, and precautions must be taken to prevent arthroconidia release into the air. Laboratory technicians have also developed primary cutaneous lesions while working with the mycelial phase or while injecting suspected cultures into laboratory rodents.

References

1. Barsanti JA, Jeffery KL. 1990. Coccidioidomycosis, pp 687–695. *In* Greene CE (ed), Infectious diseases of the dog and cat. WB Saunders, Philadelphia, PA.
2. Bartsch R, Greene R. 1997. New treatment of coccidioidomycosis. *Vet Forum*, April, 50–52.
3. Catanzaro A, Galgiani JN, Levine BE, et al. 1995. Fluconazole in the treatment of chronic pulmonary and nonmeningeal disseminated coccidioidomycosis. *Am J Med* 98:249–256.
4. Gade W, Ledman DW, Wethington R, et al. 1992. Serological responses to various *Coccidioides* antigen preparations in a new enzyme immunoassay. *J Clin Microbiol* 30:1907–1912.
5. Graybill JR, Stevens DA, Galgiani JN, et al. 1990. Itraconazole treatment of coccidioidomycosis. *Am J Med* 89:282–290.
6. Greene RT, Troy GC. 1995. Coccidioidomycosis in 48 cats: a retrospective study (1984–1993). *J Vet Intern Med* 9:86–91.
7. Kirkland TN, Fierer J. 1996. Coccidioidomycosis: a reemerging infectious disease. *Emerging Infect Dis* 2:192–199.
8. Kohn GJ, Linné SR, Smith CM, et al. 1992. Acquisition of coccidioidomycosis at necropsy by inhalation of coccidioidal endospores. *Diagn Microbiol Infect Dis* 15:527–530.
9. Martins TB, Jaskowski TD, Mouritsen CL, et al. 1995. Comparison of commercially available enzyme immunoassay with traditional serological tests for detection of antibodies to *Coccidioides immitis*. *J Clin Microbiol* 33:940–943.
10. Mirels LF, Stevens DA. 1997. Update on treatment of coccidioidomycosis. *West J Med* 166:58–59.
11. Pappagianis D, Zimmer BL. 1990. Serology of coccidioidomycosis. *Clin Microbiol Rev* 3:247–268.
12. Plotnick AN, Boshoven EW, Rosychuk RA. 1997. Primary cutaneous coccidioidomycosis and subsequent drug eruption to itraconazole in a dog. *J Am Anim Hosp Assoc* 33:139–143.
13. Rippon JW (ed). 1988. Medical mycology: the pathogenic fungi and the pathogenic Actinomycetes, ed 3. WB Saunders, Philadelphia, PA.
14. Schneider E, Hajjeh RA, Spiegel RA, et al. 1997. A coccidioidomycosis outbreak following the Northridge California earthquake. *J Am Med Assoc* 277:904–908.
15. Sekhon AS, Issac-Renton J, Dixon JM, et al. 1991. Review of human and animal cases of coccidioidomycosis diagnosed in Canada. *Mycopathologia* 113:1–10.
16. Sinke JD, Sjollema BE. 1994. Coccidioidomycosis in a dog. *Vet Q* 16(Suppl 1):64S.
17. Stevens DA. 1995. Coccidioidomycosis. *N Engl J Med* 332:1077–1082.

Chapter **63**

Sporotrichosis

Edmund J. Rosser, Jr., and Robert W. Dunstan

ETIOLOGY AND EPIDEMIOLOGY

Sporotrichosis is a mycotic disease caused by the dimorphic fungus *Sporothrix schenckii*. *S. schenckii* exists in a mycelial form at environmental temperatures (25–30°C) and in a yeast form at body tissue temperature (37°C). The organism is distributed worldwide and can be found preferentially in soils that are rich in decaying organic matter. It has also been isolated from barberry and rose bush thorns, sphagnum moss, tree bark, and mine timbers.[11, 15, 17] Sphagnum moss has been associated with sporadic outbreaks of sporotrichosis,[3a] including a multistate outbreak in forestry workers and seedling handlers.[2] The sphagnum moss was harvested in Wisconsin and used as a packing for conifer seedlings.[1] *S. schenckii* does not grow on the living sphagnum moss in bogs, but grows and sporulates well on moist, dead sphagnum moss after harvest.[22] The handling of stored hay bales has also been associated with outbreaks.[1a]

The usual means of acquiring sporotrichosis is via the inoculation of the infectious organism into tissues.[15, 17] The disease in dogs is often associated with a puncture wound caused by a thorn or wood splinter and, therefore, is most frequently observed in hunting dogs. In cats, sporotrichosis is most commonly identified in intact male cats that are allowed to roam outdoors. Infection presumably occurs via the inoculation of the organism from a puncture wound caused by the contaminated claw of another cat.[15] Although contamination of a puncture wound by organisms in the environment is considered an important mechanism in acquiring the disease in people, contact exposure of people to cats infected with *S. schenckii* is now considered a significant means by which a zoonotic infection can be established[13] (see Public Health Considerations).

CLINICAL FINDINGS

Sporotrichosis can occur in three clinical forms: cutaneous, cutaneolymphatic, and disseminated. In many instances more than one of these forms may be present concurrently. In addition to the cutaneous manifestations, dogs and cats may have a history of lethargy and anorexia, and on physical examination may be depressed and febrile which suggests the potential for *disseminated* disease. This finding should alert the clinician to the possibility of an immunocompromised animal. In general, the clinical presentations of this disease are different in dogs and cats.

Dogs

Sporotrichosis in dogs usually develops in the cutaneous or cutaneolymphatic form; the disseminated form of the disease is extremely rare.[15] The *cutaneous* form is a multinodular condition, typically occurring on the trunk or head (Fig. 63–1), with the nodules in the dermal and subcutaneous layers. The nodules may or may not be ulcerated. Ulcerated nodules are associated with purulent exudate and crust formation. Dogs with the *cutaneolymphatic* form usually develop nodules on the distal aspect of one limb. The infection then ascends proximally following lymphatic vessels, and secondary nodules develop, which may also ulcerate and drain a purulent exudate. The cutaneolymphatic form is usually associated with regional lymphadenomegaly.

Cats

Lesions usually occur on the distal aspects of the limbs, head, or tail base region. Draining puncture wounds that first appear are similar to fight wound abscesses or cellulitis. Previous treatment with soaks and systemic antibiotics for bacterial infection results in poor or partial improvement. Subsequently, the affected areas become ulcerated, drain a purulent exudate, and form large crusted lesions (Fig. 63–2). Extensive areas of necrosis may develop, exposing muscle and bone. The disease process may be further complicated by autoinoculation, occurring when the cat licks and scratches the lesions and then continues with normal grooming behavior, which results in multiple lesions on the extremities, face, and ears. The involvement of the lymphatic system may or may not be apparent during the physical examination of affected cats. However, with necropsy or biopsy of internal organs, most cats have evidence of disseminated disease with lymph node and lymphatic vessel involvement. *Sporothrix* organisms are commonly present.

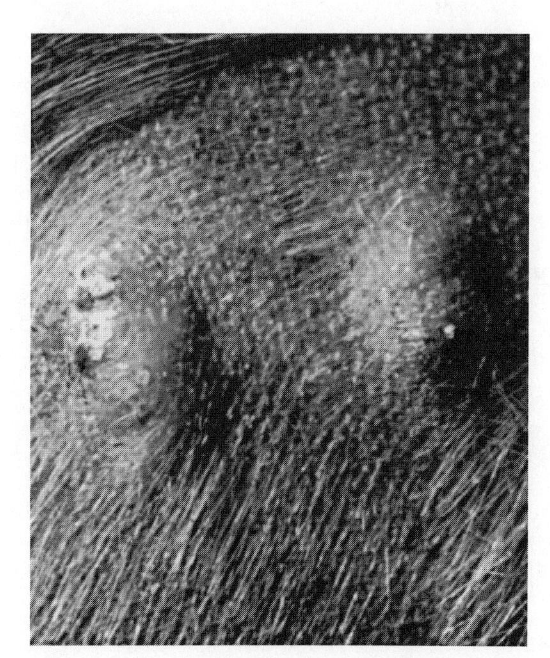

Figure 63–1. Canine sporotrichosis with multiple nodules in the abdominal region.

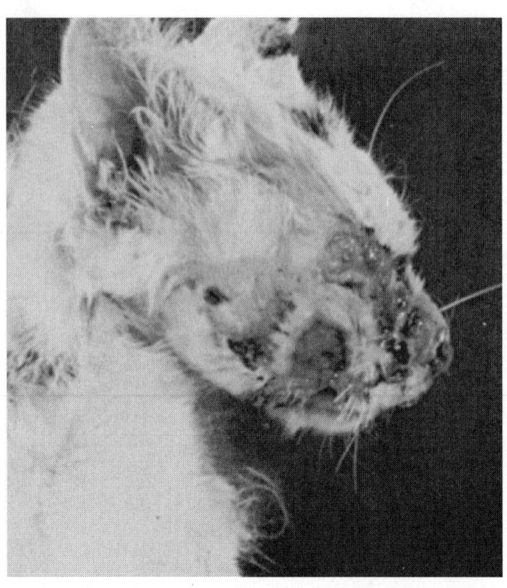

Figure 63–2. Feline sporotrichosis with multiple nodules, ulceration, and draining tracts. (From Dunstan RW et al: *J Am Acad Dermatol* 15:37–45, 1986. Reprinted with permission.)

DIAGNOSIS

The initial presentation of dogs or cats with sporotrichosis is similar to that of an animal with a deep cutaneous bacterial infection. The clinician should become suspicious of the possibility of sporotrichosis if the appropriate use of systemic antibiotics for a deep pyoderma results in minimal or partial improvement. When bacterial cultures have been performed, the ulcerative and exudative lesions of sporotrichosis are often secondarily infected with bacterial organisms, especially *Staphylococcus intermedius*.

Cytology

Exudates from draining lesions should first be examined cytologically and stained for the presence of fungal organisms using either the periodic acid–Schiff (PAS) or Gomori's methenamine silver (GMS) stain. The organism is often difficult to find in the exudates from dogs, and sporotrichosis should not be ruled out on the basis of negative cytologic findings. In contrast, *S. schenckii* is often easily identified in the exudates from cats. However, one case report[5] and our own experience have indicated that the organism can be difficult to find on cytologic examination of exudates from cats as well as dogs. When present, *S. schenckii* appears as a pleomorphic yeast that is round, oval, or cigar-shaped and may be found within macrophages and inflammatory cells or found extracellularly (Figs. 63–3 and 56–5).

Fungal Isolation

When culturing for the presence of *S. schenckii*, samples of the exudate from deep within a draining tract and a piece of tissue surgically removed for a macerated tissue culture should be submitted. This approach is especially important in the dog, in which there usually are very few organisms present in the lesion. It is also advisable to alert the laboratory to which samples have been submitted that a diagnosis of sporotrichosis is being considered.

Histopathologic Findings

Whenever possible, the best specimens to submit for histologic examination are biopsy samples of early-forming, intact nodules. The histologic pattern observed in sporotrichosis of the dog and cat is a nodular to diffuse pyogranulomatous inflammatory reaction. It is primarily located in the dermal and subcutaneous tissues and may extend to involve the underlying skeletal muscle. As with cytologic examination, it is easier to find the organism in lesions of cats compared with those of dogs. In the feline lesions, organisms are frequently so numerous that they are readily demonstrated within the pyogranulomatous reaction, even on H and E–stained sections. However, experience has indicated that the organism can occasionally be difficult to demonstrate on histopathologic examination of tissues in cases of feline sporotrichosis. Because there are usually only a few organisms in canine tissues, slides should be counterstained with a fungal stain such as PAS or GMS, and even then, each section of tissue should be carefully examined.

Immunofluorescence Testing

Specific fluorescent antibody detection of the organism is most useful in establishing the diagnosis in dogs when the results of the just-mentioned procedures have been negative or when attempts at culturing the organism have failed.[15] This diagnostic procedure can be performed by the Centers for Disease Control and Prevention, Atlanta, Georgia, on a sample of exudate or preferably on affected tissue from a patient suspected of having the disease (see Appendix 5). Serologic testing for antibodies to the organism is available, but a positive result indicates exposure and not necessarily active infection.

THERAPY

In the management of sporotrichosis in dogs and cats, the use of glucocorticoids or any immunosuppressive drug is contraindicated both during and after the treatment of the disease. Immunosuppressive doses of glucocorticoids have

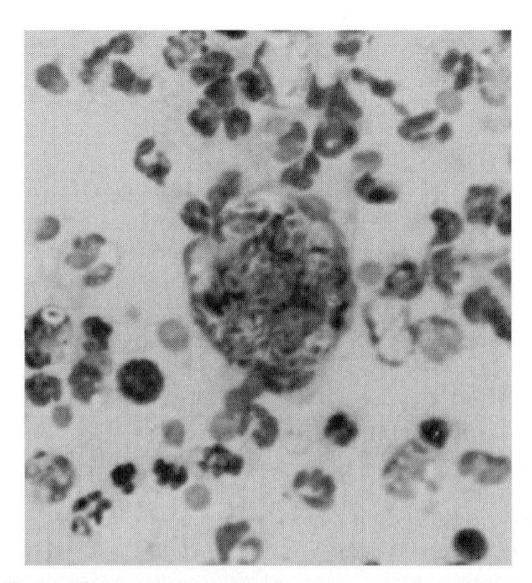

Figure 63–3. Photomicrograph of an impression smear from an ulcerated nodule in a cat with sporotrichosis. Notice the numerous fungal organisms within a macrophage (Wright-Giemsa stain, × 27). (Courtesy of Dr. Patricia White, Charlotte, MI.)

Table 63–1. Drug Therapy for Sporotrichosis[a]

DRUG	SPECIES	DOSE (mg/kg)[b]	ROUTE	INTERVAL (HOURS)	DURATION (MONTHS)
SSKI[c]	D	40	PO	8	≥2
	C	20	PO	12	
Ketoconazole[d]	D	5–15	PO	12	≥2
	C	5–10	PO	12	
Itraconazole[e]	D	5–10	PO	12–24	≥2
	C	5–10	PO	12–24	

[a]Continue treatment at least 30 days beyond resolution of all clinical signs, usually involving 2 or more months of treatment.
[b]Dose per administration at the specified interval. See Drug Formulary, Appendix 8, for additional information.
[c]See iodide, Drug Formulary; treatment of choice for dogs.
[d]Preferred therapy for dogs; toxicity more likely in cats on higher dosages.
[e]Preferred therapy for cats; toxicity more likely in dogs on higher dosages.
SSKI = supersaturated solution of potassium iodide; D = dog; C = cat.

been shown to cause a recurrence of the clinical disease after it has apparently resolved.[15] Any concurrent bacterial infection should be simultaneously treated for 4 to 8 weeks with an appropriate antibiotic on the basis of the results of culture and sensitivity.[14]

Dogs

The treatment of choice for dogs is the oral administration of a supersaturated solution of potassium iodide (SSKI) with food for 30 days beyond apparent clinical cure (Table 63–1). When sporotrichosis is not treated for an adequate period of time, it can often recur. Care should be taken to observe the dog for any signs of iodism (ocular and nasal discharge, dry hair coat with excessive scaling, vomiting, depression, and collapse). If iodism is observed, the medication should be discontinued for 1 week. If the side effects were mild, they may not recur, and therapy should then be reinstituted. If the side effects recur or if the initial reactions were severe, an alternative treatment should be considered. Ketoconazole (KTZ) can be provided in dogs that do not tolerate SSKI as well as those that are refractory to iodide therapy (see Table 63–1). We have successfully treated a dog with sporotrichosis using KTZ at 15 mg/kg, given every 12 hours for 1 month beyond the apparent clinical cure (which required 3.5 months of treatment). KTZ is usually well tolerated by dogs, but the potential for hepatotoxicity should be monitored during therapy (see Drug Formulary, Appendix 8). [14, 18] Itraconazole has also been shown to be a relatively safe and effective drug in the treatment of sporotrichosis in people.[7, 12, 19, 20] However, in dogs, hepatotoxicity was reported to occur in about 10% of the cases when itraconazole was given at a dosage of 5 mg/kg twice daily.[6] (See Drug Formulary, Appendix 8.)

Cats

Treatment of sporotrichosis in the cat is more difficult than in the dog because of the cat's greater sensitivity for the development of toxic side effects from iodides (vomiting, anorexia, depression, twitching, hypothermia, and cardiovascular failure) and KTZ (anorexia, depression, vomiting, diarrhea, fever, neurologic signs, and jaundice).[6, 15] We recommend itraconazole as the treatment of choice for sporotrichosis in cats (see Table 63–1). The treatment should be continued for 30 days beyond the apparent clinical cure. Itraconazole has been shown to be effective in the treatment of systemic or disseminated sporotrichosis in people and is becoming the recommended treatment of choice.[4, 7, 9, 19, 20] Because disseminated sporotrichosis commonly occurs in cats, the use of itraconazole seems most rational. Preliminary observations indicate that itraconazole is an effective alternative for the treatment of feline sporotrichosis and is better tolerated by cats than either iodides or KTZ.[6, 8, 18] The potential for hepatotoxicity exists, and it is recommended that serum liver enzymes be monitored monthly during therapy. The most common side effect of itraconazole in cats is anorexia; other reported side effects include vomiting, weight loss, and depression.[8] The triazole derivative saperconazole is undergoing clinical trials and appears to be well tolerated and more effective than itraconazole in the treatment of sporotrichosis in people.[3, 12]

PUBLIC HEALTH CONSIDERATIONS

Traditionally, sporotrichosis has been considered to have minimal zoonotic potential. However, several reports have documented the transmission of sporotrichosis to people by contact with an infected wound or exudate from an infected cat.[13, 15] The ready transmission of sporotrichosis from animals to people appears to be a feature limited to feline sporotrichosis, presumably because of the copious numbers of organisms found in tissues, exudates, and feces of infected cats. Theoretically, transmission from infected dogs or people seems less likely because it is often difficult to demonstrate the presence of the organism.

The population that is potentially at greatest risk for acquiring sporotrichosis from an infected cat includes veterinarians, their assistants, and anyone exposed during treatment. In some instances, infection has occurred after nontraumatic exposure to an infected cat, when there had been no known pre-existing injury or penetrating wound on the person before contracting the disease. With these considerations in mind, it is advisable that people handling cats suspected of having sporotrichosis wear disposable gloves. Afterward, they should remove the gloves carefully and wash their forearms, wrists, and hands with either a chlorhexidine or povidone-iodine scrub.

References

1. Dixon DM, Salkin IF, Duncan RA, et al. 1991. Isolation and characterization of *Sporothrix schenckii* from clinical and environmental sources associated with the largest U.S. epidemic of sporotrichosis. *J Clin Microbiol* 29:1106–1113.

1a. Dooley DP, Bostic PS, Beckius ML. 1997. Spook house sporotrichosis—a point-source outbreak of sporotrichosis associated with hay bale props in a Halloween haunted house. *Arch Intern Med* 157:1885–1887.

2. England T, Kasten MJ, Martin R, et al. 1989. Multistate outbreak of sporotrichosis in seedling handlers, 1988. *Arch Dermatol* 125:170.

3. Franco L, Gomez I, Restrepo A. 1992. Saperconazole in the treatment of systemic and subcutaneous mycoses. *Int J Dermatol* 31:725–729.

3a. Hajjeh R, McDonnell S, Reef S, et al. 1997. Outbreak of sporotrichosis among tree nursery workers. *J Infect Dis* 176:499–504.
4. Kaufman CA. 1994. Newer developments in therapy for endemic mycoses. *Clin Infect Dis* 19(Suppl 1):S28–S32.
5. Kennis RA, Rosser EJ, Dunstan RW. 1994. Difficult dermatologic diagnosis. *J Am Vet Med Assoc* 204:51–52.
6. Legendre AM. 1995. Antimycotic drug therapy, pp 327–331. *In* Bonagura JD (ed), Kirk's current veterinary therapy XII. WB Saunders, Philadelphia, PA.
7. Mercurio MG, Elewski BE. 1993. Therapy of sporotrichosis. *Semin Dermatol* 12:285–289.
8. Messinger LM. 1995. Therapy for feline dermatoses. *Vet Clin North Am* 25:986–987.
9. Odds FC. 1993. Itraconazole: a new oral antifungal agent with a very broad spectrum of activity in superficial and systemic mycoses. *J Dermatol Sci* 5:65–72.
10. Peaston A. 1993. Sporotrichosis, a clinical vignette. *J Vet Intern Med* 7:44–45.
11. Rafal ES, Rasmussen JE. 1991. An unusual presentation of fixed sporotrichosis: a case report and review of the literature. *J Am Acad Dermatol* 25:928–932.
12. Restrepo A. 1994. Treatment of tropical mycoses. *J Am Acad Dermatol* 31:S91–S102.
13. Rosser EJ. 1990. Sporotrichosis and public health, pp 633–634. *In* Kirk RW (ed), Current veterinary therapy X. WB Saunders, Philadelphia, PA.
14. Rosser EJ. 1993. Sporotrichosis, pp 49–53. *In* Griffin CE, Kwochka KW, MacDonald JM (eds), Current veterinary dermatology: the science and art of therapy. Mosby–Year Book, St. Louis, MO.
15. Rosser EJ, Dunstan RW. 1990. Sporotrichosis, pp 707–710. *In* Greene CE (ed), Infectious diseases of the dog and cat. WB Saunders, Philadelphia, PA.
16. Sanford SE. 1992. Persistent sporotrichosis in a dog. *Can Vet J* 33:826.
17. Shadomy HJ, Utz JP. 1993. Sporotrichosis, pp 2492–2494. *In* Fitzpatrick TB, Eisen AZ, Wolff K, et al (eds), Dermatology in general medicine. McGraw-Hill, Inc, New York, NY.
18. Sherding RG, Johnson SE. 1992. Intestinal histoplasmosis, pp 610–611. *In* Kirk RW, Bonagura JD (eds), Current veterinary therapy XI. WB Saunders, Philadelphia, PA.
19. Van Cutsem J. 1992. In vitro antifungal spectrum of itraconazole and treatment of systemic mycoses with old and new antimycotic agents. *Chemotherapy* 38(Suppl 1):3–11.
20. Winn RE, Anderson J, Piper J, et al. 1993. Systemic sporotrichosis treated with itraconazole. *Clin Infect Dis* 17:210–217.
21. Zamri-Saad M, Salmiyah TS, Jasni S, et al. 1990. Feline sporotrichosis: an increasingly important zoonotic disease in Malaysia. *Vet Rec* 127:480.
22. Zhang X, Andrews JH. 1993. Evidence for growth of *Sporothrix schenckii* on dead but not on living sphagnum moss. *Mycopathologia* 123:87–94.

Chapter **64**

Rhinosporidiosis

Edward B. Breitschwerdt and M. Cecilia Castellano

ETIOLOGY AND EPIDEMIOLOGY

Rhinosporidiosis, a mycotic disease caused by *Rhinosporidium seeberi*, induces tumor-like growths of epithelial tissues in domestic animals, birds, and people.[5, 7] The disease is endemic in India, Sri Lanka, and Argentina and is reported sporadically from other parts of the world, including the United States. Infection most frequently involves mucous membranes of the nasal cavity, but infrequently, infection can involve the ear, pharynx, larynx, trachea, esophagus, genital and urinary mucosae, and skin. Reported cases of canine rhinosporidiosis have involved only the nasal cavity. Rhinosporidiosis has not been reported in cats.

R. seeberi is a fungal organism of uncertain classification.[5] The infectious fungal nature of the disease has been questioned.[1] Although earlier attempts to culture the organism using conventional fungal culture media were not successful, modification of the culture parameters has resulted in the successful isolation of *R. seeberi* from human patients in India.[6] The organism has also been grown in tissue culture, utilizing an epithelioid rectal tumor cell line.[8] Complete development of *R. seeberi* appears to require interaction with epithelial cells. The organism appears to induce in vitro cellular proliferation.

The infective unit is a small (8 μm), round spore that proliferates in epithelial tissue to produce sporangia (or nodular bodies, 300–400 μm), which are grossly visible on the superficial surface of the polyp. Sporangia undergo a maturation process, resulting in the production of 16,000 to 20,000 spores that are expelled, leaving an empty sporangial case.

PATHOGENESIS

The pathogenesis of canine rhinosporidiosis has not been characterized in detail owing to the difficulties associated with propagation of the organism. In contrast to the human disease, in which dissemination can develop, reported canine cases have been limited to nasal involvement.

Reports from endemic regions suggest that infection is acquired by mucosal contact with stagnant water. Mucous membrane trauma is a predisposing factor. In arid countries, most human infections are ocular, and dust is postulated to be a fomite. In the United States, canine rhinosporidiosis has been reported only in the southern states; however, occurrence of the disease in a dog native to Ontario suggests the possibility of more widespread distribution in North America. The disease occurs in large-breed dogs; many are exposed to flowing or impounded fresh water. In the dog, there appears to be a sex predilection for males, as is true of infections in people and horses. Behavioral as well as biologic factors may be responsible for this apparent predilection.

CLINICAL FINDINGS

Clinical findings include wheezing, sneezing, unilateral seropurulent nasal discharge, and epistaxis. Polyps may be visible in the nares or may be visualized by rhinoscopy in the rostral nasal cavity (Fig. 64–1). Single or multiple polyps ranging in size from a few millimeters up to 3 cm are pink, red, or pale gray and are covered with numerous pinpoint, white sporangia. Polyps may be sessile or pedunculated, and

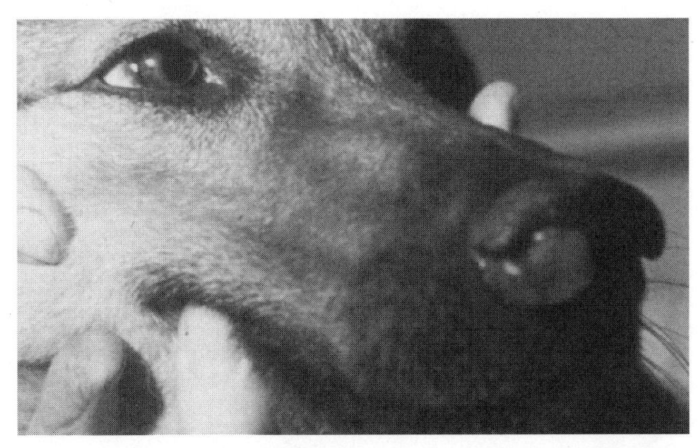

Figure 64–1. A 2-year-old male dog of mixed German shepherd breeding from Argentina, with a bright red sessile growth in the right nostril. Rhinosporidiosis was diagnosed on histologic examination.

the superficial surface is irregular and glistening and may be ulcerated.

DIAGNOSIS

The organism can be demonstrated by H and E, Gridley's toluidine blue, periodic acid–Schiff, or Grocott's stains. Cytologic examination of nasal exudate or histologic examination of the polyp should allow diagnosis by visualization of *R. seeberi* spores (Fig. 64–2).

PATHOLOGIC FINDINGS

Microscopically, polyps are composed of fibrovascular tissue lined by squamous or columnar epithelium that is frequently ulcerated.[2] Sporangia are visualized and may be releasing spores through the epithelium to the superficial surface (see Fig. 56–1). A superficial exudate, most prominent in areas of spore extrusion, is composed of spores, neutrophils, epithelia, and erythrocytes. A mixed inflammatory response, consisting predominantly of plasma cells and lymphocytes and, to a lesser extent, macrophages, is scattered throughout the tissue.

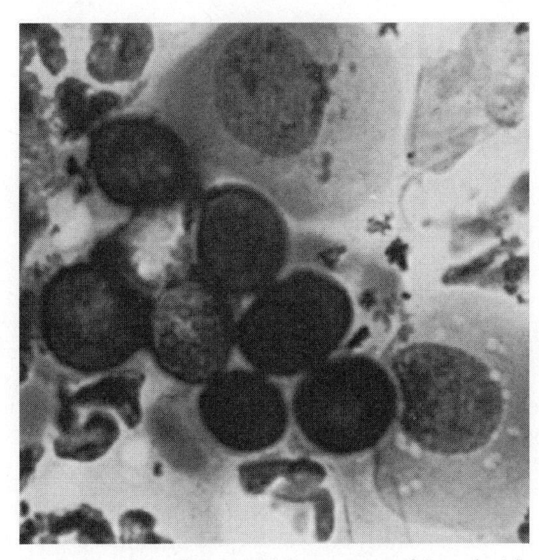

Figure 64–2. Nasal exudate containing spores of *R. seeberi* (× 1000). (Courtesy of Drs. Roger Easley and Donald Meuten, North Carolina State University, Raleigh, NC.)

THERAPY

Surgical excision remains the treatment of choice and may be curative when a single polyp is excised. Because of the frequent rostral location of the polyps, surgical excision through the nares or by an anterolateral approach to the nares generally is possible, negating the necessity for the more invasive dorsonasal flap procedure. Recurrence has been reported after surgery in dogs with single or multiple polyps. Dapsone (1 mg/kg every 8 hours for 2 weeks, followed by 1 mg/kg every 12 hours for 4 months) was likely curative in a dog that had recurrence of polyps after surgical extirpation.[9] Dapsone has been used to treat human rhinosporidiosis with variable success.[4,7] Ketoconazole (8.7 mg/kg every 8 hours for 21 days) eliminated nasal discharge in a dog after 4 days, and visual and cytologic resolution of the polyps occurred after 21 days of therapy.[2] The dog was treated with ketoconazole (8.7 mg/kg every 8 hours) for an additional 21 days; however, recurrence 6 months later necessitated surgical excision of a large polyp (Fig. 64–3). Interestingly, this dog again developed nasal rhinosporidiosis several years after moving from the United States to England. The utility of medical therapy in canine rhinosporidiosis requires additional evaluation.

PUBLIC HEALTH CONSIDERATIONS

There is no evidence to support the possibility of direct transmission of *R. seeberi* from animals to people. Dogs and people appear to be infected from common environmental sources.

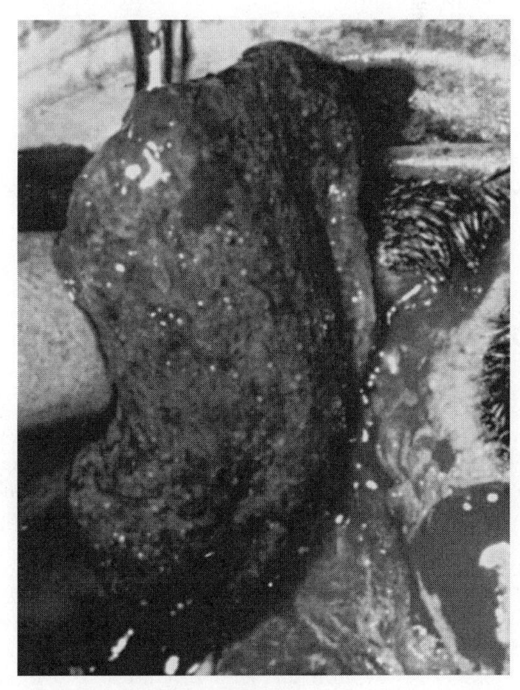

Figure 64–3. Surgically excised nasal polyp. Miliary white foci on the surface are sporangia of *R. seeberi*.

References

1. Ahluwalia KB. 1992. New interpretations in rhinosporidiosis, enigmatic disease of the last nine decades. *J Submicrosc Cytol Pathol* 24:109–114.
2. Breitschwerdt EB. 1986. Unpublished observations. North Carolina State University, Raleigh, NC.
3. Breitschwerdt EB. 1990. Rhinosporidiosis, pp 711–713. *In* Greene CE (ed), Infectious diseases of the dog and cat. WB Saunders, Philadelphia, PA.
4. Job A, Venkateswaran S, Mathan M, et al. 1993. Medical therapy of rhinosporidiosis with dapsone. *J Laryngol Otol* 107:809–812.
5. Kennedy FA, Buggage RR, Ajello L. 1995. Rhinosporidiosis—a description of an unprecedented outbreak in captive swans (*Cygnus* spp.) and a proposal for revision of ontogenic nomenclature of *Rhinosporidium seeberi*. *J Vet Med Mycol* 33:157–165.
6. Kishnamoorthy S, Sreedharan VP, Koshy P, et al. 1989. Culture of *Rhinosporidium seeberi*: preliminary report. *J Laryngol Otol* 103:178–180.
7. Kwon-Chung KJ. 1994. Phylogenetic spectrum of fungi that are pathogenic to humans. *Clin Infect Dis* 19(Suppl 1):S1–S7.
8. Levy MG, Meuten DJ, Breitschwerdt EB. 1986. Cultivation of *Rhinosporidium seeberi* in vitro: interaction with epithelial cells. *Science* 234:474–476.
9. Mahakrisnan A, Rajasekaram V, Pandian PI. 1981. Disseminated cutaneous rhinosporidiosis treated with dapsone. *Trop Geogr Med* 33:189–192.
10. Radovanovic Z, Vukovic Z, Jankovic S. 1997. Attitude of involved epidemiologists toward the first European outbreak of rhinosporidiosis. *Eur J Epidemiol* 13:157–160.

Chapter 65

Aspergillosis and Penicilliosis

Aspergillus and *Penicillium* are saprophytic fungi, ubiquitous in the environment, that generally cause either nasal or pulmonary and disseminated infections in dogs and cats. *Penicillium* are often confused with *Aspergillus* on gross or histologic appearance, and culture is required to distinguish the two. Cats may have GI mucosal localization. Rarely do solitary lesions occur outside the nasal passages; nasal infections have not been suspected to disseminate.[21]

Nasal infection has been most commonly associated with *A. fumigatus* and dissemination with *A. terreus*. *Aspergillus* and *Penicillium* are common contaminants of body or mucosal surfaces and the respiratory tract, so that culture without histologic or cytologic evidence of associated inflammation can be misleading. Host immunocompetence is an important determinant in the development of these opportunistic fungal infections. Pre-existing nasal disease, prolonged antimicrobial therapies, or secretory IgA immune deficiencies may be important in the development of nasal infections. Cell-mediated immunity is a major factor in limiting systemic spread of infection.

Immunosuppressive conditions, such as diabetes mellitus, persistent granulocytopenia, cytotoxic chemotherapy, glucocorticoid therapy, concurrent infection, and hereditary cell-mediated immunodeficiency, are often associated with disseminated disease. German shepherd dogs are as predisposed to opportunistic infections (especially aspergillosis and hyalohyphomycosis) as they are to rickettsial diseases (see Chapters 28 and 29). For a discussion of infection with other opportunistic saprophytic fungi, see Chapter 68.

Canine Nasal Aspergillosis–Penicilliosis

Nick J. H. Sharp

ETIOLOGY

Nasal aspergillosis is a relatively common disease in dogs. It is encountered much more frequently than is nasal penicilliosis. The two conditions are indistinguishable other than by culture and subsequent differentiation using the appearance of the conidial heads (Figs. 65–1, 56–7, and 56–8). *A. fumigatus* is the most common species encountered, although *A. niger*, *A. nidulans*, and *A. flavus* are occasionally involved. The species of *Penicillium* causing nasal penicilliosis have not been defined. These organisms all branch dichotomously at 45-degree angles and form septate, nonpigmented hyphae of approximately 5 to 7 mm diameter in culture and in tissue specimens. Both groups of fungi are ubiquitous saprophytes and are regarded as opportunistic pathogens.

PATHOGENESIS

In humans, paranasal aspergillosis has been classified into allergic, noninvasive, invasive, and fulminant forms, which probably reflect a continuous spectrum of disease. The first two forms have been considered to represent extramucosal disease, whereas the latter two are variants of the tissue-invasive disease.[15, 17a, 46] Extramucosal disease usually occurs in immunocompetent individuals, whereas tissue-invasive disease is more common in immunocompromised patients,[2] although it can occur in otherwise healthy people.[22, 45] The fulminant form, which only occurs in immunocompromised patients, is a rapidly progressive gangrenous mucoperiostitis, which advances to destruction of the nasal cavity and paranasal sinuses within a few days.[33]

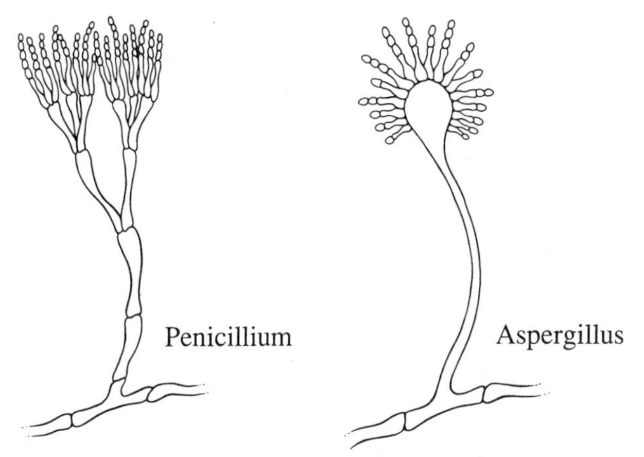

Figure 65–1. Conidial heads of *Aspergillus* species (right) and *Penicillium* species (left). In the former, phialides arise in two series from a terminal vesicle; in the latter conidiophores have primary branches and phialides that bear chains of conidia.

Nasal aspergillosis in dogs spans the noninvasive and invasive forms of the disease spectrum in humans. Only one instance of a completely noninvasive process or "fungal ball" has been reported in dogs.[47] The canine disease usually remains confined to the nasal cavity or paranasal sinus, but marked destruction of turbinate mucosa and bone is nearly always seen, probably as a result of vasculitis and vascular necrosis of submucosal vessels.[47] An obviously invasive form of the disease does occur in dogs in which the organism erodes through the medial wall of the orbit into periorbital soft tissue structures.[54] Invasion of the cranial vault has also been documented in canine nasal aspergillosis.[39] The fulminant form has not been recognized in dogs. Dogs with disseminated aspergillosis do not generally have any nasal involvement (see next section).

Canine nasal aspergillosis usually occurs without concomitant malignant or immunosuppressive disease, and affected dogs are in otherwise excellent health.[51] Immunologic studies performed before and after treatment have, however, revealed both T- and B-cell dysfunction, which can persist long after the organism has been eliminated.[47, 51] It is unclear whether these results reflect the cause or the consequence of infection.[51] Products of *A. fumigatus* have been shown to inhibit lymphocyte transformation of both B and T cells in vitro.[47] *A. fumigatus* has also been shown to produce an endotoxin that is both hemolytic and dermonecrotic.[59] This toxin presumably causes the turbinate necrosis and erosion of the rhinarium, which occur in canine nasal aspergillosis.

CLINICAL FINDINGS

This disease is usually seen in dolichocephalic and mesocephalic dogs and is very rare in brachycephalic breeds. Dogs of any age may be affected, but approximately 40% are 3 years or younger and 80% are 7 years or younger.[51] The main clinical features are shown in Table 65–1. The three hallmarks of canine nasal aspergillosis–penicilliosis are a profuse sanguinopurulent discharge that may alternate with periods of epistaxis; an ulceration of the external nares (Fig. 65–2); and a pain or discomfort in the facial region. Some dogs with infections restricted to the frontal sinus do not show nasal discharges or nasal ulcerations.

Table 65–1. Clinical Features of 35 Dogs With Nasal Aspergillosis–Penicilliosis

CLINICAL FEATURES	% AFFECTED
Profuse nasal discharge	91
Nasal pain	85
Ulceration of the external nares	77
Sanguinopurulent discharge	76
Frontal sinus infection	65
Epistaxis	63
Mucopurulent discharge	24
Sparse nasal discharge	9

DIAGNOSIS

Several techniques can be applied to the diagnosis of this disease, but no single test is accurate enough when considered in isolation. False-positive and false-negative results occur with cytologic, histopathologic, mycologic, and serologic testing. Blind cytologic examination or culture of discharge is often unrewarding and can erroneously suggest the disease to be a simple bacterial rhinitis. Cytologic examination may also reveal *Aspergillus* or *Penicillium* as contaminants (see Figs. 56–7 and 56–8). *Pseudomonas* spp. or other Enterobacteriaceae are common secondary infections of necrotic tissue within the nasal chamber. Caution should also be taken in interpreting a positive fungal culture result. After culture of nasal swabs taken blindly from normal dogs or from dogs with nasal neoplasia, 30% to 40% cultured positive for either *Aspergillus* or *Penicillium* spp. Histologic examination performed on tissues obtained by blind biopsy through the nares may also result in a diagnosis of nonspecific rhinitis if fungal colonies are missed.[47] The most informative diagnostic tests are radiographic, rhinoscopic, and serologic examinations.

The radiologic features of nasal aspergillosis are summarized in Figure 65–3. In a review of 71 dogs with nasal aspergillosis, all showed destruction of turbinate bones, 57 dogs (80%) showed associated areas of increased radiolucency, and only 1 (1.4%) dog showed an overall increase in radiopacity. Frontal sinus osteomyelitis, demonstrated in the rostrocaudal or "skyline" frontal sinus projection, occurred in 23 (80%) of 29 dogs evaluated.[47] These findings are in contrast to those seen with nasal neoplasia, in which an increase in radiolucency is very unusual, and most dogs

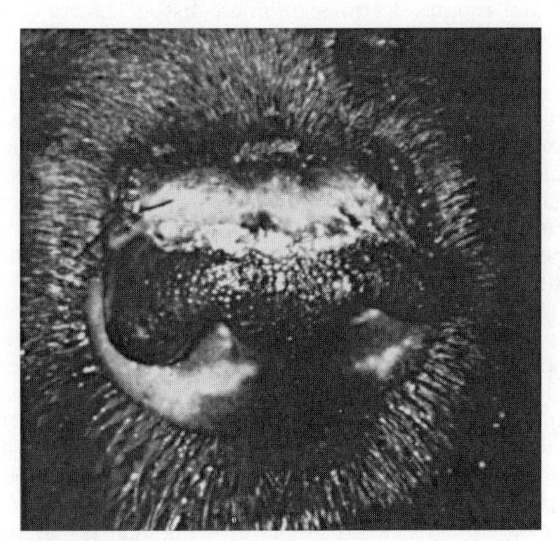

Figure 65–2. Ulceration of the external nares in association with *A. fumigatus* infection.

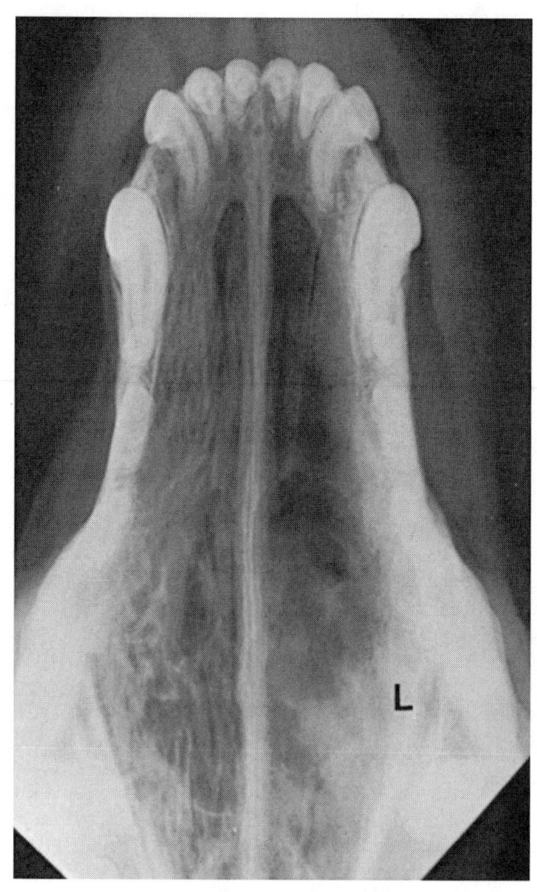

Figure 65–3. Intraoral dorsoventral radiograph of the nasal cavity of a dog with aspergillosis, showing typical turbinate destruction and an increase in radiolucency in the left (L) nasal chamber.

show either an increase in radiopacity or a mixed density.[51] Computed tomographic (CT) features of nasal neoplasia and aspergillosis have been reported but not compared.[4, 32, 38, 58] In human paranasal aspergillosis, the CT density of paranasal concretions was found to be a very useful predictor of fungal disease,[28] but attenuation measurement was not useful in the one dog studied to date.[8]

Rhinoscopy is a particularly valuable diagnostic tool because the fungus destroys turbinate tissue leaving a large airspace within the nasal cavity, which in turn affords good visualization of fungal plaques. An otoscope with a bright light source can sometimes be used as the sole means of directing a fungal plaque biopsy. An arthroscope is better, but probably the best instrument is a 3- to 5-mm diameter flexible pediatric bronchoscope. A working channel to the bronchoscope greatly facilitates the biopsy of plaques. Fungal plaques appear as a white, yellow, or light-green mold lying on the mucosa. Plaques within the frontal sinus can also be identified by introducing an arthroscope or a bronchoscope through a small trephine hole in the frontal bone; the tip of the instrument may be kept free of blood if the animal is placed on its back. Biopsy of fungal plaques under direct visualization is the best (and probably the only) way to obtain meaningful samples for mycologic examination. Mycologic confirmation is possible by cytologic (Fig. 65–4) or histologic examination or by culture on a fungal medium such as Sabouraud's dextrose agar.

Serologic diagnosis is possible utilizing agar gel immunodiffusion (AGID), counter immunoelectrophoresis (CIE), and ELISA techniques to detect fungi-specific serum antibodies.

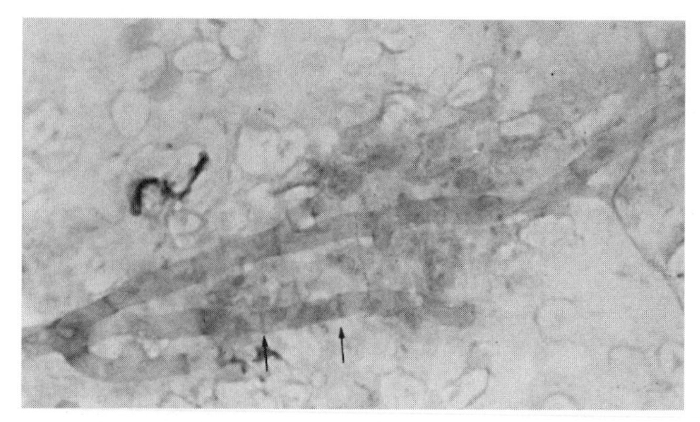

Figure 65–4. Cytologic preparation of nasal exudate from a dog to show *Aspergillus* with septate hyphae *(arrows)*. (From Sharp NJH, Sullivan M, Harvey CE: *In Practice* 14:27–31, 1992. Reprinted with permission.)

The AGID test has been performed for many years but can have a 6% false-positive rate. Fifteen percent false-positive results were found using CIE, although others have reported no false-positive or false-negative results with this technique. Corresponding data are unavailable for ELISA, but this test has given reliable results over the past 10 years. It is advisable to use antigens that identify both *Aspergillus* and *Penicillium* spp. for any of the serologic tests.[47] For further information on laboratories and test kits available for performing these assays, see Appendices 5 and 6, respectively.

Several criteria have been suggested to allow a definitive diagnosis of nasal aspergillosis–penicilliosis before the institution of therapy.[47, 51] The most simple scheme requires that the dog be positive for at least two, and preferably three, diagnostic criteria (Table 65–2).[48]

The most important differential diagnosis for nasal aspergillosis is nasal neoplasia. Rhinoscopic examination is often very frustrating for the examiner in nasal neoplasia, and false-positive results (30–40%) are a problem with serologic testing. Clinically, it is unusual for dogs with nasal neoplasia to show marked nasal pain or ulceration at the external nares. Differentiation is best made by radiographic examination followed by tissue biopsy through the nostril.[36, 52] Although both nasal neoplasia and aspergillosis cause consistent turbinate destruction, the soft tissue mass of nasal neoplasia causes a marked increase in radiopacity and rarely causes the increased radiolucency typical of fungal rhinitis. Furthermore, the earliest signs of turbinate destruction in nasal neoplasia predominate in the caudal nasal chamber, whereas the rostral chamber is initially affected in aspergillosis. A good tissue biopsy specimen clearly differentiates the two conditions, but it is not unusual for several attempts to be required before neoplastic tissue is recovered, even in large tumors. Other causes of nasal disease such as foreign bodies, dental disease, and chronic rhinitis do not usually produce the degree of turbinate destruction seen in aspergillosis or neopla-

Table 65–2. Diagnostic Criteria for Nasal Aspergillosis

VARIABLE	CRITERIA
Radiology	Features typical of fungal rhinitis
Rhinoscopy	Fungal plaques on nasal or sinus mucosa
Mycology	*Aspergillus* or *Penicillium* on culture, cytology, or histology
Serology	Positive AGID, CIE, or ELISA result

AGID = agar gel immunodiffusion; CIE = counter immunoelectrophoresis.

sia. An idiopathic destructive rhinitis has been reported in dogs with clinical features that are identical to aspergillosis–penicilliosis, but no fungal organisms could be found on rhinoscopic, mycologic, or serologic examination.[47]

THERAPY

Systemic Therapy

Several antifungal drugs have been used to treat nasal aspergillosis–penicilliosis in the past (Table 65–3).[47] Of these, the newer azole derivatives fluconazole and itraconazole have shown the best results, but success rates do not exceed 60% to 70%. Fluconazole should be used at 2.5 mg/kg PO BID and itraconazole at 5 mg/kg PO BID—both for a minimum of 10 weeks.[30, 50] Five percent of dogs on itraconazole have to have the medication stopped because of hepatic injury; therefore, liver enzymes should be monitored with this drug.[30] Systemic therapy is indicated as part of the treatment regimen if the fungus has invaded extranasal structures (see following discussion). The results obtained for systemic therapy are not as good as those obtained for topical agents.

Topical Therapy

For several years, the standard treatment for this disease was an enilconazole emulsion delivered via tubes surgically implanted into the nasal chambers and frontal sinuses.[53] Although this approach resulted in the elimination of the fungus in more than 90% of affected dogs, it had several disadvantages. The twice-daily irrigation of drug for 7 days was labor intensive, often very messy, not always well tolerated by the dog, and was considerably complicated if the dog removed one or both tubes. Enilconazole has only lately become available in the United States, and therefore efforts were made to find a substitute.

Dogs were treated with clotrimazole, used as the commercially available solution in polyethylene glycol (Lotrimin, Schering Corp., Kenilworth, NJ).[10] Furthermore, topical therapy was revolutionized by administering the clotrimazole not as a flush but instead as an infusion using general anesthesia.[11] This regimen eliminated many of the aforementioned disadvantages of enilconazole but caused no loss of efficacy. The distribution of topical agents after noninvasive infusion via the external nares has been studied in both normal dog skulls and in dogs with fungal rhinitis.[32, 44] Each frontal sinus has several noncommunicating compartments, and the method of delivery significantly influences final drug distribution.[44] The best drug distribution is obtained by noninvasive, IN delivery utilizing a 1-hour soak under anesthesia. This method also has the advantage of preserving the nasofrontal ostia.[11, 44] Foley catheters (24-French diameter) occlude the nasopharynx (along with gauze sponges) to deliver drug through the external nares into the dorsal nasal meatus (10 French) and to occlude the external nares (12 French) (Fig. 65–5). A 1% solution of clotrimazole is introduced under pressure (60 ml per side for middle to large breeds, to a pressure of 15 cm H_2O) to enhance drug distribution. Furthermore, by placing the dog on its back and then rotating the head, very good distribution is obtained, even into diseased frontal sinuses. Care must be taken after the procedure is completed to allow the solution to drain out with the dog in sternal recumbency and its head tilted ventrally and to remove all gauze sponges and suction the pharynx.[32] Inflammation and edema of the pharynx with postoperative airway obstruction were observed as complications in one dog receiving a second treatment.[6a] Propylene glycol and isopropyl alcohol in a commercial clotrimazole preparation were the suspected irritants. Mixing the powdered drug or crushed tablets of drug in polyethylene glycol to a 1% formulation may be a safer alternate (see Drug Formulary, Appendix 8). In addition, prolonged recovery from pentobarbital anesthesia was noted in this dog, presumably as a result of hepatic microsomal enzyme inhibition by clotrimazole.[6a, 10a] Anesthetic agents that rely on hepatic elimination for recovery might be avoided. Another potential contraindication to this technique is extension of drug to the brain across a damaged cribriform plate. The risks of this appear to be low, but a CT study should be performed when it is a potential concern. The results in dogs treated by the intranasal delivery and 1-hour clotrimazole soak are excellent; 17 of 18 dogs (94%) were considered to be cured.[31] In a comparison study between invasive (surgical) and noninvasive (intranasal) administration of clotrimazole to 11 dogs, the noninvasive method was more effective.[3a]

In the few cases in which clotrimazole therapy fails, enilconazole irrigation could be considered as a follow-up treatment. Enilconazole is ideal as a topical agent because it is also active in the vapor phase, which enhances its distribution throughout the nasal chamber.[54] Enilconazole has become available for poultry in the United States as Clinafarm-EC (Sterwin Labs, Inc, Millsboro, DE). Clinafarm-EC contains alcohol and has a slightly different formulation from the one used previously (Imaverol, Janssen). I have administered the drug for irrigation of the nasal chambers and frontal sinuses in two dogs with no ill effects. Clinifarm-EC has also been used as an infusion, but irritant effects were observed[6a, 32a] similar to those with alcohol-containing preparations of clotrimazole. The drug was administered after endoscopic placement of lavage tubes in the caudal portion of the nasal cavity and frontal sinuses.[32a] Enilconazole (Clinifarm-EC) in a final concentration of 5% and 50 to 200 ml–volume was used in the treatment, during general anesthesia, of six dogs with nasal aspergillosis. The dogs received two or three treatments with each one lasting 45 to 60 minutes. All the dogs showed

Table 65–3. Therapy for Nasal Aspergillosis

DRUG	SPECIES	DOSE[a]	ROUTE	INTERVAL (HOURS)	DURATION (WEEKS)	EFFICACY (%)
Clotrimazole	D	60 ml each side	IN[b]	Once	prn	90
Enilconazole	D	10 mg/kg	IN[c]	12–24	1	80–90
Itraconazole	D	5 mg/kg	PO	12	10	60–70
	C	10 mg/kg	PO	24	10	?
Fluconazole	D	2.5–5 mg/kg	PO	12	10	60

[a]Dose per administration at the specified interval. See Drug Formulary, Appendix 8, for further information.
[b]See text and Figure 65–5 for a description of the administration technique. A 1-hour infusion under anesthesia is recommended.
[c]Should only be used as a daily infusion of small volumes. The 1-hour infusion method is effective in only 50% of cases. Available as Imaverol or Clinifarm-EC, see text.
D = dog; C = cat; IN = intranasal; prn = as needed; ? = unknown.

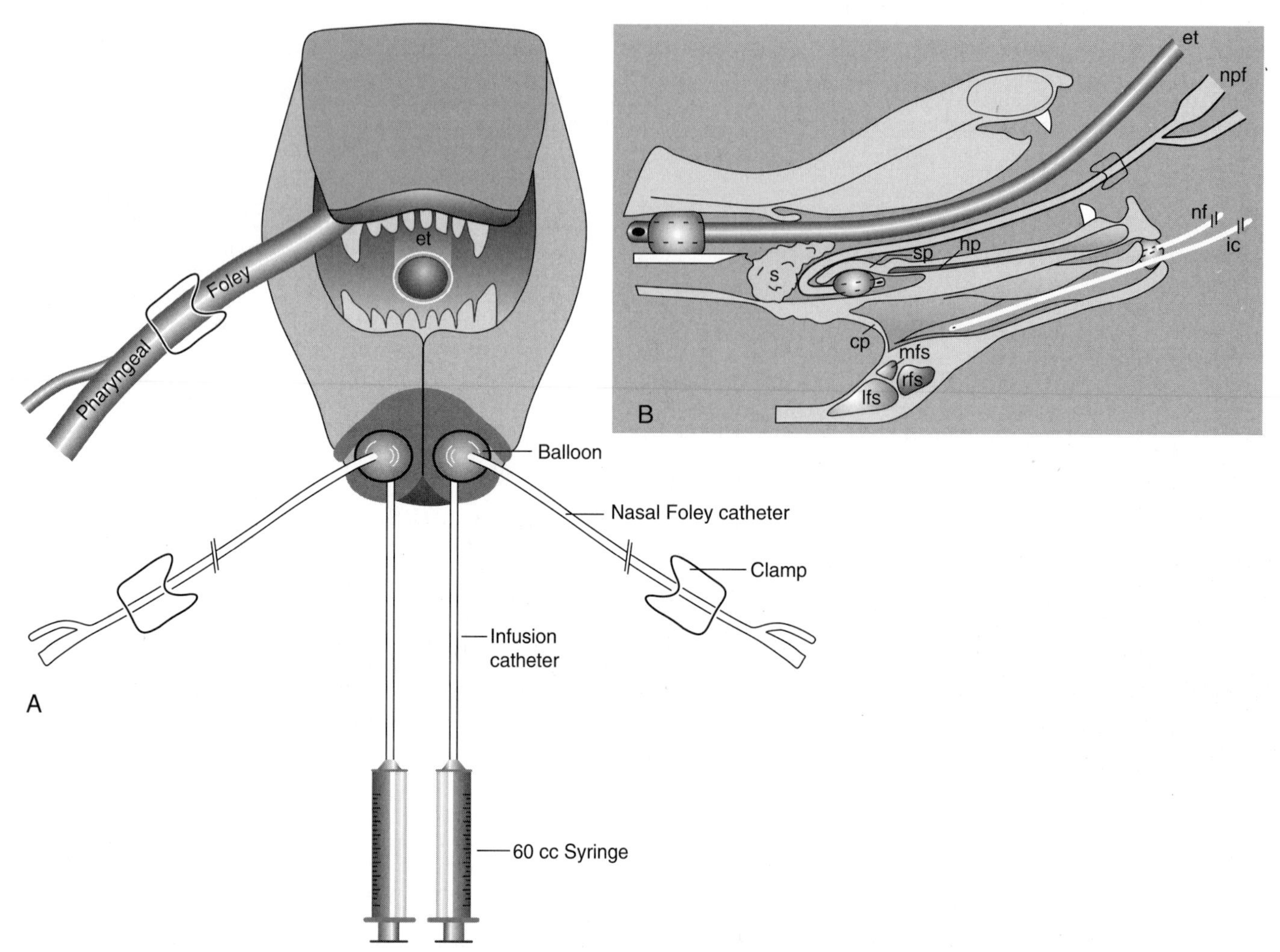

Figure 65–5. *A,* Catheter position with the dog in dorsal recumbency. A Foley catheter with the balloon inflated in the nasopharynx and pharyngeal gauze sponges (not shown) minimize leakage of infusate caudally. A cuffed endotracheal tube (et) further diminishes the risk of aspiration. Sixty-milliliter syringes are used to inject infusate into the dorsal nasal meatus via polypropylene infusion catheters. Infusion catheters are attached to water manometers via three-way stopcocks, so that intranasal pressures can be monitored. Inflated Foley catheter balloons obstruct the nares to diminish leakage of infusate rostrally. Tubing clamps on Foley catheters are closed when fluid is observed within the catheter lumen. *B,* Sagittal section showing the position of the endotracheal tube (et), nasopharyngeal Foley catheter (npf), pharyngeal sponges (s), infusion catheter (ic), and rostral nasal Foley catheter (nf) in relation to the hard palate (hp), soft palate (sp), cribriform plate (cp), rostral frontal sinus (rfs), medial frontal sinus (mfs), and lateral frontal sinus (lfs). (From Mathews KG, Koblik PD, Richardson EF, et al: *Vet Surg* 25:309–319, 1996. Reprinted with permission.)

favorable clinical response soon after treatment. Three dogs that were followed for a mean of 16.5 months had marked clinical improvement.

Imaverol has been utilized as a 1-hour infusion but has produced very disappointing results. In one study involving four dogs, none were cured by the 1-hour infusion and three even appeared to be made worse. Two of these dogs did respond to subsequent twice daily irrigation with the drug. Three other dogs were randomly assigned to a 1-hour infusion with clotrimazole during the same study period, and all were cured.[3] In another study of 10 dogs treated with a 1-hour Imaverol infusion, 5 were cured and 5 failed treatment.[20] In both of these studies, fairly high concentrations of enilconazole were given (5–10%). These are probably much higher than necessary to kill the fungus and may result in exposure of the nasal mucosa to excessive levels of the detergent base in Imaverol, which may well be toxic.[3]

A 1-hour infusion with clotrimazole should now be considered the treatment of choice for nasal aspergillosis–penicilliosis. The one possible exception is when the cribriform plate is damaged. I have used Imaverol flush in two such cases with no complications. Any clotrimazole or enilconazole solution should preferably not contain alcohol or other irritants. Topical therapy with either enilconazole or clotrimazole will fail when the organism invades soft tissue structures outside the nasal cavity, such as the orbit or cranial vault. These cases require a combination of topical therapy with a systemically active agent such as itraconazole.[31, 46, 54]

Surgery

Rhinotomy and turbinectomy have no roles in the treatment of fungal rhinitis. It is my opinion that rhinotomy should be performed only if all other attempts to obtain a cure have been unsuccessful. Even then, if the rhinotomy reveals fungal plaques, the tendency to continue with a turbinectomy should be strongly resisted. Experience suggests that turbinectomy is of no benefit in controlling the nasal discharges and is often detrimental.[29, 47, 54, 64] Rather than curetting turbinate tissue, the surgeon should view the procedure as diagnostic only; large fungal mats can be removed, but care must be taken to cause as little damage as possible to nasal and turbinate mucosa and to the nasofrontal ostia.[32] Open nasal cavity treatment of nasal aspergillosis with povidone-iodine solution is also not recommended as a first-line therapy for nasal aspergillosis–penicilliosis.[42] Treatment should be delivered as described under Topical Therapy.

PROGNOSIS

The best indication of successful therapy is the rapid resolution of nasal pain, sanguineous discharge or epistaxis, and ulcerated nares. In some dogs, a mild mucopurulent, crusty discharge may persist at one or both nostrils, presumably as a result of the reorganized nasal architecture. Serology is of only limited value in assessing the response to treatment. Although both AGID and ELISA titers tend to decline within 1 to 2 years of successful therapy, this occurrence is not a reliable indicator. Positive titers may persist for more than 2 years (ELISA) or 5 years (AGID) in dogs that remain free of disease.[51]

Relapse of fungal disease does not appear to be a common problem with canine nasal aspergillosis–penicilliosis. Of 43 dogs that had shown resolution of clinical signs after treatment with a variety of systemic and topical antifungal drugs, only one suffered a relapse of fungal rhinitis during follow-up periods ranging from 6 months to 5.5 years.[51] Recurrence of fungal disease is usually signified by a return of facial pain and ulceration of the nares. A bacterial rhinitis may develop in up to 25% of dogs after successful resolution of the primary fungal disease. Bacterial rhinitis is characterized by a return of the profuse nasal discharge, usually without blood or facial pain. Fungal plaques are absent in these cases, and the discharge responds to antibiotic therapy based on culture and sensitivity results.[29, 54, 63]

PUBLIC HEALTH CONSIDERATIONS

There are no documented instances of infection in humans arising from dogs or cats. Infection in all species occurs from common environmental sources. It seems prudent, however, for the clinician to inform an owner that immunosuppressed individuals should not be exposed to affected animals that may be discharging large quantities of fungal hyphae and spores. In addition, both clinicians and owners who wear contact lenses should remember that *Aspergillus* species can cause a potentially devastating ocular disease.[67]

Feline Nasal Aspergillosis–Penicilliosis

Nick J. H. Sharp

Although rare diseases, both *Aspergillus* and *Penicillium* spp. have been incriminated in frontal sinus infections in cats. The infections extended into the soft tissues of the orbit and caused proptosis in two animals; one cat also demonstrated *Penicillium* pneumonitis. The immune status of these animals was not evaluated. A third cat with aspergillosis of the nasal cavity and frontal sinus was feline leukemia virus (FeLV) positive.[47] This cat had a positive result on AGID testing and was successfully treated by rhinotomy and turbinectomy. Itraconazole is preferable to ketoconazole for systemic therapy in cats and should be given at a dosage of 10 mg/kg once daily.[30, 34] There is no information on the topical application of enilconazole or clotrimazole in the cat.

Canine Disseminated Aspergillosis

Michael J. Day

ETIOLOGY AND PATHOGENESIS

Most cases of canine disseminated aspergillosis have occurred in German shepherd dogs (age range, 2–8 years) and have been reported from Australia[12, 27, 65] and California.[12, 23] The disease has also been documented in Spain,[40, 43] Belgium,[7] the United Kingdom,[5] and the eastern United States.[5, 9, 18, 26] It is probably more ubiquitous than the reports suggest. In those cases in which the species has been identified, infection has involved, in decreasing frequency, *A. terreus*, *A. deflectus*, *A. flavipes*, and *A. fumigatus*. This finding contrasts with nasal aspergillosis (see previous discussion), in which *A. fumigatus* is most common. The portal of entry of *Aspergillus* is thought to be via the respiratory tract with subsequent hematogenous spread. As with any blood-borne pathogen, common sites of embolic dissemination of fungal organisms are the intervertebral discs, renal glomeruli, and uveal tracts. Other parenchymatous organs or muscles and long bones may be affected sites. Disseminated aspergillosis in people is usually secondary to immunodeficiency or immune suppression, although invasive *Aspergillus* has been described in immunocompetent individuals.[25] Predisposing factors for canine aspergillosis may include a combination of optimum climatic conditions, an access to particular strains of *Aspergillus*, and a subtle defect in mucosal immunity that may have a genetic basis.[13] German shepherd dogs are also susceptible to infection with a range of other opportunistic fungi.[64] Glucocorticoids should never be administered to dogs with aspergillosis, and their

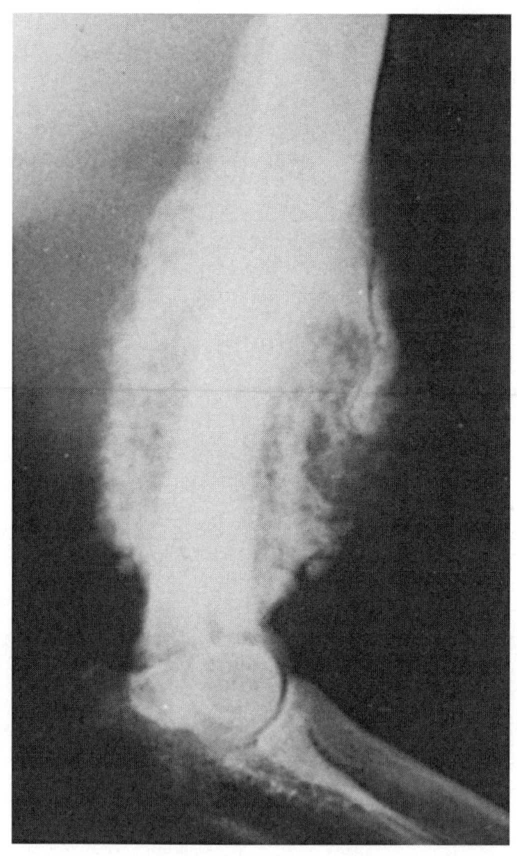

Figure 65–6. Canine disseminated aspergillosis. Radiograph of humeral lesion. Note extensive cortical destruction and new bone formation.

inadvertent use has precipitated dissemination of the infection in some cases.

CLINICAL FINDINGS

Disease involves multiple organ systems and develops over several months, but most dogs are terminally ill when first examined. The most consistent clinical features are vertebral pain progressing to paraparesis, paraplegia, or limb lameness with pronounced swelling and discharging sinus tracts. A sudden onset of paraplegia may result from rupture of an infected intervertebral disc or subluxation from an instability.

Other nonspecific clinical signs include anorexia, weight loss, muscle wasting, pyrexia, weakness, lethargy, and vomiting. Occasionally, dogs have clinical evidence of CNS involvement, lymphadenomegaly with cutaneous edema, and pyometra. Uveitis or endophthalmitis may be clinically apparent some months before generalized illness develops and thus may be important in early diagnosis.

DIAGNOSIS

The most consistent hematologic abnormality is the presence of mature neutrophilia. Eosinophilia or monocytosis may be apparent. Biochemical analysis may reveal elevations in total protein concentration, blood urea nitrogen, and serum alkaline phosphatase, alanine aminotransferase, and amylase activities. Radiography of affected long bones reveals areas of lysis and cortical destruction, with similar changes in sternebrae and vertebral bodies associated with diskospondylitis (Fig. 65–6). In the few cases with bronchopulmonary involvement, interstitial alveolar or consolidated alveolar patterns have been observed.[7]

Methods to diagnose aspergillosis include cytology, culture, serology, and histopathology. An effective and simple diagnostic test involves examination of a sterile-collected urine sample for the presence of hyphal elements (Fig. 65–7). Fungal elements may also be observed on cytologic examination of blood, synovial fluid, lymph node, bone, or intervertebral disc material. Confirmation of fungal involvement by culture on Sabouraud's dextrose agar requires at least 5 to 7 days. Several methodologies are available to measure *Aspergillus*-specific antibodies in serum. The AGID, CIE, ELISA, and FA may provide rapid serologic confirmation, but not all dogs with disseminated infection have detectable *Aspergillus* antibodies. For example, kits utilizing *A. fumigatus* as an antigen may not detect antibodies to those dogs with disseminated infection caused by *A. terreus*.[56] For further information on laboratories and test kits for antibody assays, see Appendices 5 and 6, respectively. In humans with invasive aspergillosis, efforts to detect *Aspergillus* antigens in body fluids have focused on detection of galactomannan or other carbohydrates in serum or urine by latex agglutination (Pastorex *Aspergillus* latex agglutination test; Sandofi Diagnostics Pasteur, Marnes-La-Coquette, France) or ELISA methods.[41, 46a, 62] False-negative results in serum correspond to low test sensitivity, whereas false-positive results in urine correspond to reaction to other fungi and organisms causing urinary tract infections.[24, 57, 66] Polymerase chain reaction has also been utilized on a limited experimental and clinical basis to improve the sensitivity and specificity of *Aspergillus* detection.[35, 55]

PATHOLOGIC FINDINGS

Gross changes include focal osteomyelitis and multiple, pale granulomas in kidneys and spleen that also may be seen in lymph nodes, myocardium, pancreas, and liver. Occasionally, pulmonary congestion or GI mucosal reddening or ero-

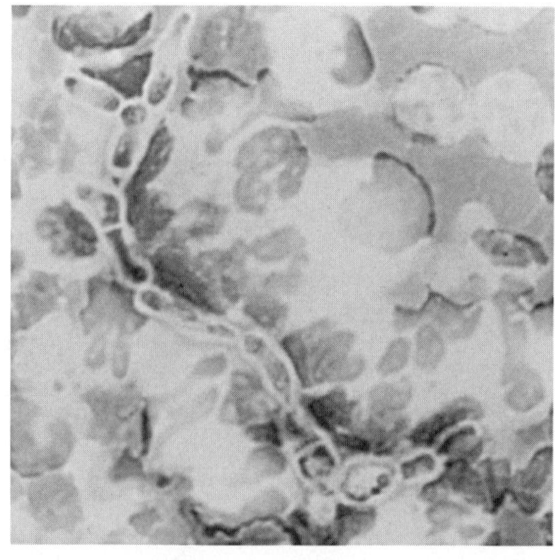

Figure 65–7. Microscopic appearance of stained urine sediment from a dog with disseminated aspergillosis. Branching hyphal elements amid leukocytes and erythrocytes (Wright's stain, × 1000). (Courtesy of Drs. E. Mahaffey and A. Kaufman, University of Georgia, Athens, GA.)

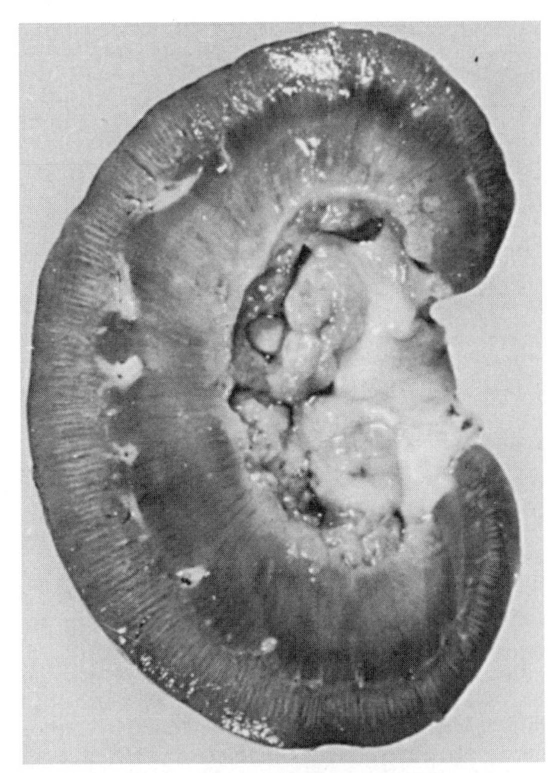

Figure 65–8. Canine disseminated aspergillosis. Sagittal section of kidney with fungal mass in renal pelvis and scattered fungal granulomata *(A. terreus)*.

sions may be found. Microscopic granulomas may be associated with areas of slow vascular flow in liver, lungs, eyes, and pancreas and occasionally in prostate, thyroid, uterine submucosa, and brain. Infarcted areas secondary to thrombi containing fungal elements have been found in spleen, kidneys (Fig. 65–8), and liver. Lesions contain varying numbers of septate, branching hyphae that may have characteristic lateral branching aleuriospores (Fig. 65–9*A*). Intralesional hyphae are best visualized by periodic acid–Schiff or Gomori's methenamine silver stain, and they have been identified by immunostaining with specific antisera (Fig. 65–9*B*).[5, 43] The cellular infiltrates may be predominantly neutrophilic or may also include macrophages, giant cells, lymphocytes, and plasma cells.[14, 43]

THERAPY AND PROGNOSIS

Severely ill dogs have poor prognoses. Treatments, including supportive therapy of fluids and antibiotics, together with thiabendazole or ketoconazole with and without concurrent 5-fluorocytosine, have been unsuccessful. Hamycin, an experimental polyene related to amphotericin B (AMB), showed partial effectiveness in treating one dog.[26] Only two systemic antifungals are effective: AMB and itraconazole (Table 65–4). Response to amphotericin B has been most promising, but response has been suboptimal and requires hospitalization with IV therapy. Some human patients who fail to respond to AMB do so to lipid-associated AMB or itraconazole.[16] AMB generally is contraindicated by pre-existing renal damage. In one dog, intrarenal perfusion of AMB was performed utilizing indwelling nephrostomy catheters.[56] The induction of long-term clinical remission has been achieved in four dogs with oral itraconazole (5 to 10 mg/kg daily for up to 1095 days).[27, 64] In one dog the infection was eliminated; others had resolution of clinical illness but eventually died from disseminated aspergillosis after therapy was discontinued. One dog was euthanized while improving clinically during treatment because of radiographic evidence of additional spondylitic lesions. The surviving dog was not a German shepherd.

In people with disseminated aspergillosis, itraconazole is a useful drug in treatment, but similar failures or relapses are common in the most immunocompromised patients.[17]

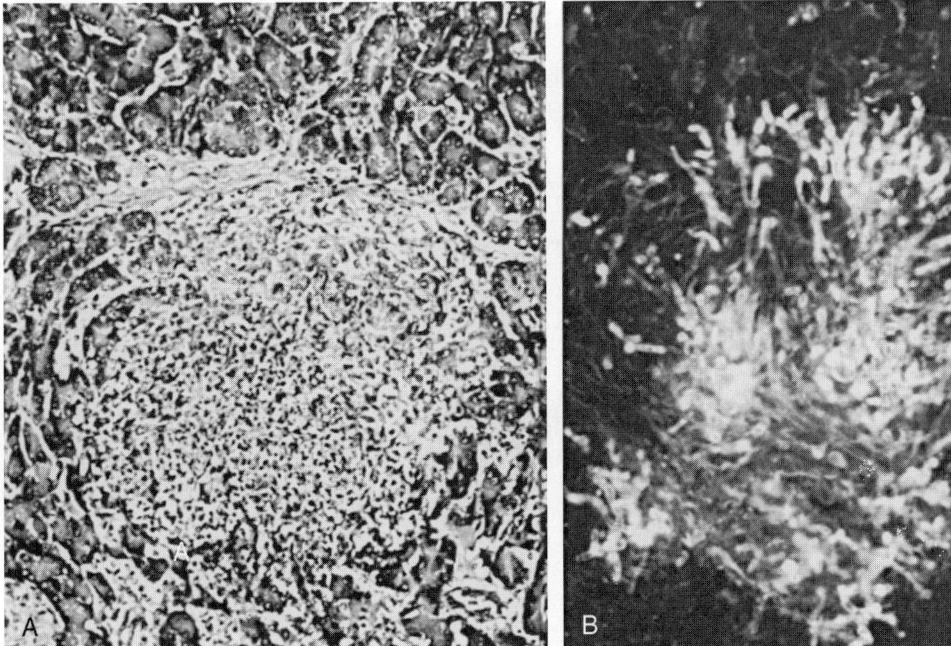

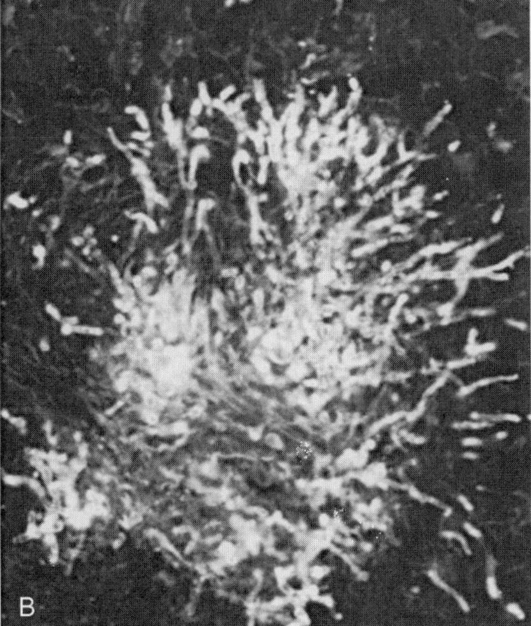

Figure 65–9. Canine disseminated aspergillosis. *A*, Fungal granuloma in pancreas (H and E, × 140). *B*, Fungal hyphae within a granuloma marked with antiserum to *A. terreus* (FA, × 320).

Table 65–4. Therapy for Disseminated Aspergillosis

DRUG	SPECIES	DOSE (mg/kg)	ROUTE	INTERVAL (HOURS)	DURATION
Amphotericin B (deoxycholate)	D	0.25	IV	48	[a]
Itraconazole	B	2.5–5	PO	12	prn[b]
Amphotericin B (lipid based)	B	3–5	IV	48	[c]

[a]Until a cumulative dose of 4–8 mg/kg is reached for cats and 8–12 mg/kg for dogs.
[b]Therapy to control infection may require months to years, although clinical remissions may be achieved; the infection may reactivate in a variable time period after discontinuing treatment.
[c]Until a cumulative dose of 12 mg/kg is reached.
See Drug Formulary, Appendix 8, for further information.
D = dog; B = dog and cat; prn = as needed.

Feline Disseminated Aspergillosis

Michael J. Day

Feline aspergillosis largely occurs in cats up to 2 years of age that often are terminally ill. Unlike dogs with aspergillosis, most affected cats have concurrent immunosuppressive diseases such as panleukopenia, feline infectious peritonitis, FeLV infection, or multiple diseases, or they have had dystocia or have been receiving glucocorticoid or antibiotic therapy.[37] Aspergillosis has not been reported in cats with feline immunodeficiency virus infection, although such cats may have other opportunistic mycoses.[6] Clinical signs are referable to GI or pulmonary involvement, with nonspecific findings similar to those in dogs. Hematologic findings are variable and may reflect other underlying diseases.

Necropsy findings may include pulmonary granulomata, GI ulcers, or pseudomembranes and involvement of urinary system or CNS. The lesions are characterized by hemorrhage and necrosis, with variable numbers of inflammatory cells and fungal hyphae that may invade blood vessels, leading to thrombosis.

References

1. Berry WL, Leisewitz AL. 1996. Multifocal *Aspergillus terreus* discospondylitis in two German shepherd dogs. *Tydskr S Afr Vet Ver* 67:222–228.
2. Blaugrund SM, Sarti EJ, Lin PT, et al. 1988. Paranasal sinus disease with intracranial extension: aspergillosis versus malignancy. *Larygnoscope* 98:632–635.
3. Bray JP, White RAS, Duncan B et al. 1998. Treatment of canine nasal aspergillosis with a new non-invasive technique: failure with enilconazole. In press.
3a. Burbidge HM, Clark WT, Read R, et al. 1997. Canine nasal aspergillosis. Results of treatment using clotrimazole as a topical agent. *Aust Vet Pract* 27:79.
4. Burk RL. 1992. Computed tomographic imaging of nasal disease in 100 dogs. *Vet Radiol Ultrasound* 33:177–180.
5. Butterworth SJ, Barr FJ, Pearson GR, et al. 1995. Multiple discospondylitis associated with *Aspergillus* species infection in a dog. *Vet Rec* 136:38–41.
6. Callanan JJ. 1995. Feline immunodeficiency virus infection, pp 111–130. *In* Willett BJ, Jarrett O (eds), Feline immunology and immunodeficiency. Oxford University Press, Oxford, England.
6a. Caulkett N, Lew L, Fries C. 1997. Upper airway obstruction and prolonged recovery from anesthesia following intranasal clotrimazole administration. *J Am Anim Hosp Assoc* 33:264–267.
6b. Caulkett NA, Lew L, Shmon (Fries) C. 1997. Nasal aspergillosis: Treatment with clotrimazole. *J Am Anim Hosp Assoc* 33:476–477.
7. Clercx C, McEntee K, Snaps F, et al. 1996. Bronchopulmonary and disseminated granulomatous disease associated with *Aspergillus fumigatus* and *Candida* species infection in a golden retriever. *J Am Anim Hosp Assoc* 32:139–145.
8. Codner EC, Lurus AG, Miller JB, et al. 1993. Comparison of computed tomography with radiography as a non-invasive diagnostic technique for chronic nasal discharge in dogs. *J Am Vet Med Assoc* 202:1106–1110.
9. Dallman MJ, Dew TL, Tobias L, et al. 1992. Disseminated aspergillosis in a dog with diskospondylitis and neurologic deficits. *J Am Vet Med Assoc* 200:511–513.
10. Davidson A, Komtebedde J, Pappagianis D, et al. 1992. Treatment of nasal aspergillosis with topical clotrimazole, p 807. Presented at the 10th ACVIM Forum, San Diego, CA.
10a. Davidson A, Mathews KG. 1997. Nasal aspergillosis: treatment with clotrimazole. *J Am Anim Hosp Assoc* 33:475–476.
11. Davidson A, Pappagianis D. 1995. Treatment of nasal aspergillosis with topical clotrimazole, pp 899–901. *In* Bonagura JD and Kirk RW (eds), Kirk's current veterinary therapy XII. WB Saunders, Philadelphia, PA.
11a. Davies C, Troy GC. 1996. Deep mycotic infections in cats. *J Am Anim Hosp Assoc* 32:380–391.
12. Day MJ. 1990. Aspergillosis and penicilliosis, pp 719–722. *In* Greene CE (ed), Infectious diseases of the dog and cat. WB Saunders, Philadelphia, PA.
13. Day MJ. 1996. Low IgA concentration in the tears of German shepherd dogs. *Aust Vet J* 74:433–434.
14. Day MJ, Penhale WJ. 1991. An immunohistochemical study of canine disseminated aspergillosis. *Aust Vet J* 68:383–386.
15. deCarpentier JP, Ramamurthy L, Denning DW, et al. 1994. An algorithmic approach to *Aspergillus* sinusitis. *J Laryngol Otol* 108:314–318.
16. Denning DW. 1996. Therapeutic outcome in invasive aspergillosis. *Clin Infect Dis* 23:608–615.
17. Denning DW, Lee JY, Hostetler JS, et al. 1994. NIAID mycoses study group multicenter trial of oral itraconazole therapy for invasive aspergillosis. *Am J Med* 97:135–144.
17a. de Shazo RD, Chapin K, Swain RE. 1997. Fungal sinusitis. *N Engl J Med* 337:254–259.
18. Gelatt KN, Chrisman CL, Samuelson DA, et al. 1991. Ocular and systemic aspergillosis in a dog. *J Am Anim Hosp Assoc* 27:427–431.
19. Guerin SR, Walker MC, Kelly DF. 1993. Cavitating mycotic pulmonary infection in a German shepherd dog. *J Small Anim Pract* 34:36–39.
20. Holt D. 1996. Personal communication. Veterinary Hospital of the University of Pennsylvania, Philadelphia, PA.
21. Houston A, Moore A, Hanna FY. 1995. Mycotic osteomyelitis in a dog following nasal aspergillosis. *Vet Rec* 137:349–350.
22. Jahrsdoerfer RA, Ejercito VS, Johns MME, et al. 1979. Aspergillosis of the nose and paranasal sinuses. *Am J Otolaryngol* 1:6–14.
23. Kahler JS, Leach MW, Jang S, et al. 1990. Disseminated aspergillosis attributable to *Aspergillus deflectus* in a Springer Spaniel. *J Am Vet Med Assoc* 197:871–874.
24. Kappe R, Schulze-Berge A. 1994. New cause for false-positive results with the pastorex *Aspergillus* antigen latex agglutination test. *J Clin Microbiol* 31:2489–2490.
25. Karim M, Alam M, Shah AA, et al. 1996. Chronic invasive aspergillosis in apparently immunocompetent hosts. *Clin Infect Dis* 24:723–733.
26. Kaufman AC, Greene CE, Selcer BA, et al. 1994. Systemic aspergillosis in a dog and treatment with hamycin. *J Am Anim Hosp Assoc* 30:132–136.
27. Kelly SE, Shaw SE, Clark WT. 1995. Long-term survival of four dogs with disseminated *Aspergillus terreus* infection treated with itraconazole. *Aust Vet J* 72:311–313.
28. Krennmair G, Lenglinger F, Muller-Schelken H. 1994. Computed tomography (CT) in the diagnosis of sinus aspergillosis. *J Craniomaxillofacial Surg* 22:120–125.
29. Lanthier T, Chalifoux A. 1991. Enilconazole as an adjunct to the treatment of four cases of canine nasal aspergillosis. *Can Vet J* 32:110–112.

30. Legendre AM. 1995. Treatment of nasal aspergillosis with topical clotrimazole, pp 327–331. *In* Bonagura JD, Kirk RW (eds), Kirk's current veterinary therapy XII. WB Saunders, Philadelphia, PA.
31. Mathews KG, Davidson AP, Richardson EF, et al. 1998. Topical clotrimazole therapy in dogs with nasal aspergillosis—comparison of intranasal vs surgical infusions: 59 cases (1990–1996). *J Am Vet Med Assoc*. In press.
32. Mathews KG, Koblik PD, Richardson EF, et al. 1995. Computed tomographic assessment of noninvasive intranasal infusions in dogs with fungal rhinitis. *Vet Surg* 25:309–319.
32a. McCullough SM, McKiernan BC, Grodsky BS. 1998. Endoscopically placed tubes for administration of enilconazole for treatment of nasal aspergillosis in dogs. *J Am Vet Med Assoc* 212:67–69.
33. McGill TJ, Simpson G, Healy GB. 1980. Fulminant aspergillosis of the nose and paranasal sinuses: a new clinical entity. *Laryngoscope* 90:748–754.
34. Medleau L, Greene CE, Rakich PM. 1990. Evaluation of ketoconazole and itraconazole for treatment of disseminated cryptococcosis in cats. *Am J Vet Res* 51:1454–1458.
35. Melchers WJG, Verweij PE, van den Hurk P, et al. 1994. General primer-mediated PCR for detection of *Aspergillus* species. *J Clin Microbiol* 32:1710–1717.
36. Morrison T, Read R, Eger C. 1989. A retrospective study of nasal tumors in 37 dogs. *Aust Vet Pract* 19:130–134.
37. Ossent P. 1987. Systemic aspergillosis and mucormycosis in 23 cats. *Vet Rec* 120:330–333.
38. Park RD, Beck ER, LeCouteur RA. 1992. Comparison of computed tomography and radiography for detecting changes induced by malignant nasal neoplasia in dogs. *J Am Vet Med Assoc* 201:1720–1724.
39. Parker AJ, Cunningham JG. 1971. Successful removal of an epileptogenic focus in a dog. *J Small Anim Pract* 12:513–521.
40. Pastor J, Pumarola M, Cuenca R, et al. 1993. Systemic aspergillosis in a dog. *Vet Rec* 132:412–413.
41. Patterson TF, Miniter P, Patterson JE, et al. 1995. *Aspergillus* antigen detection in the diagnosis of invasive aspergillosis. *J Infect Dis* 171:1553–1558.
42. Pavletic MM, Clark GN. 1991. Open nasal cavity and frontal sinus treatment of chronic canine aspergillosis. *Vet Surg* 20:43–48.
43. Perez J, Mozos E, Chacon-M. de Lara F, et al. 1996. Disseminated aspergillosis in a dog: an immunohistochemical study. *J Comp Pathol* 115:191–196.
44. Richardson EF, Mathews KG. 1995. Distribution of topical agents in the frontal sinuses and nasal cavity of dogs: comparison between current protocols for treatment of nasal aspergillosis and a new non-invasive technique. *Vet Surg* 24:476–483.
45. Romett JL, Newman RK. 1982. Aspergillosis of the nose and paranasal sinuses. *Laryngoscope* 92:764–766.
46. Rowe-Jones JM, Freedman AR. 1994. Adjuvant itraconazole in the treatment of destructive sphenoid aspergillosis. *Rhinology* 32:203–207.
46a. Severens JL, Donnelly JP, Meis JFGM, et al. 1997. Two strategies for managing invasive aspergillosis: a decision analysis. *Clin Infect Dis* 25:1148–1154.
47. Sharp NJH. 1990. Aspergillosis and penicilliosis, pp 714–719. *In* Greene CE, (ed), Infectious diseases of the dog and cat. WB Saunders, Philadelphia, PA.
48. Sharp NJH. 1998. Aspergillosis/Penicilliosis. *In* Gorman N (ed), Canine medicine and therapeutics. Blackwell Science, New York, NY.
49. Sharp NJ, Harvey CE. 1991. Aspergillosis: report on diagnosis and treatment. *Tijdschr Diergeneeskd* 116(Suppl 1):35S–37S.
50. Sharp NJH, Harvey CE, O'Brien JA. 1991. Treatment of canine nasal aspergillosis with fluconazole (UK-49,858). *J Small Anim Pract* 32:513–516.
51. Sharp NJH, Harvey CE, Sullivan M. 1991. Canine nasal aspergillosis/penicilliosis. *Compend Cont Educ Pract Vet* 13:41–49.
52. Sharp NJH, McEntee M, Gilson SD, et al. 1991. Nasal cavity and frontal sinuses. *Prob Vet Med* 3:170–187.
53. Sharp NJH, Sullivan M, Harvey CE. 1992. Treatment of canine nasal aspergillosis. *In Practice* 14:27–31.
54. Sharp NJH, Sullivan M, Harvey CE, et al. 1993. Treatment of canine nasal aspergillosis with enilconazole. *J Vet Intern Med* 7:40–43.
55. Spreadbury C, Holden D, Aufauvre-Brown A, et al. 1993. Detection of *Aspergillus fumigatus* by polymerase chain reaction. *J Clin Microbiol* 31:615–621.
56. Starkley RJ, McLoughlin MA. 1996. Treatment of renal aspergillosis in a dog using nephrostomy tubes. *J Vet Intern Med* 10:336–338.
57. Swanik CMA, Meis JFGM, Rijs AJMM, et al. 1997. Specificity of a sandwich enzyme linked immunosorbent assay for detecting *Aspergillus* galactomannan. *J Clin Microbiol* 35:257–260.
58. Thrall DE, Robertson ID, McLeod DA, et al. 1989. A comparison of radiographic and computed tomographic findings in 31 dogs with malignant nasal cavity tumors. *Vet Rad* 30:59–66.
59. Tilden EB, Hatton EH, Freeman S, et al. 1961. Preparation and properties of the endotoxins of *Aspergillus fumigatus* and *Aspergillus flavus*. *Mycopathol Mycolog Appl* 14:325–346.
60. Van Cutsem J. 1991. Aspergillosis in pet animals and treatment of experimental infection in laboratory animals. *Tijdschr Diergeneeskd* 116(Suppl 1):38S–39S.
61. Van Oosterhout IC, Venker van Haagen AJ. 1991. Aspergillosis: report on diagnosis and treatment. *Tijdschr Diergeneeskd* 116(Suppl 1):37S–38S.
62. Verweij PE, Stynen D, Rijs JMM, et al. 1995. Sandwich enzyme-linked immunosorbent assay compared with pastorex latex agglutination test for diagnosing invasive aspergillosis in immunocompromised patients. *J Clin Microbiol* 33:1912–1914.
63. Watt PR. 1994. Diagnosis and treatment of nasal aspergillosis in a Doberman pinscher. *Aust Vet Pract* 24:182–185.
64. Watt PR, Robins GM, Galloway AM, et al. 1995. Disseminated opportunistic fungal disease in dogs: 10 cases (1982–1990). *J Am Vet Med Assoc* 207:67–70.
65. Wigney DL, Allan GS, Hay LE, et al. 1990. Osteomyelitis associated with *Penicillium* verruculosum in a German shepherd dog. *J Small Anim Pract* 31:449–452.
66. Wijnands LM, van Leusden FM, Puyk RJT, et al. 1994. Pitfalls in immunoblot detection of *Aspergillus* antigens associated with invasive infection. *J Clin Microbiol* 32:2339–2340.
67. Wilhelmus KR, Robinson NM, Font RA, et al. 1988. Fungal keratitis in contact lens wearers. *Am J Ophthalmol* 106:708–714.
68. Wilson SM, Odeon A. 1992. Disseminated *Aspergillus terreus* infection in a dog. *J Am Anim Hosp Assoc* 28:447–458.

Chapter 66

Candidiasis, Torulopsosis, and Rhodotorulosis

Craig E. Greene and Francis W. Chandler

Candidiasis

ETIOLOGY

Members of the genus *Candida* are dimorphic fungi in the family Cryptococcaceae. In the yeast phase, *Candida* spp. normally inhabit the alimentary, upper respiratory, and genital mucosae of mammals. A sexual stage has not been identified, and the small (2–6 μm), thin-walled, ovoid, yeastlike cells reproduce by budding. *Candida* spp., especially *C. albicans* and *C. parapsilosis*, have been the most commonly isolated fungal organisms cultured from the ears, nose, oral cavity, and anus of clinically normal dogs. Occasionally, *C. tropicalis, C. pseudotropicalis, C. guilliermondii*, and *C. krusei* have been found on human and animal body surfaces. Only rarely are *Candida* spp. isolated from soil or as laboratory contaminants.

EPIDEMIOLOGY

Candida spp., first acquired by the neonate as it passes through the birth canal, colonize the oral, GI, upper respiratory, and genital mucosae for the life of the animal, but their presence normally evokes no reaction. The intact skin is an abnormal site for *C. albicans* except at mucocutaneous junctions of body orifices. Opportunistic infections may result if the skin becomes chronically traumatized or moistened. Under certain circumstances, *Candida* spp. also can invade deeper host tissues and proliferate as blastoconidia, pseudohyphae, and branched, septate hyphae (Fig. 66–1). In other instances, they may disseminate via the blood stream to many tissues (Fig. 66–2*A* and *B*).

PATHOGENESIS

Local proliferation of *Candida* spp. in wounds or on mucosal surfaces is the first step in spread of infection. Overgrowth of *Candida* is probably inhibited under most circumstances by a variety of factors, including intestinal, genital, and cutaneous microflora. Factors that upset the normal endogenous microflora, such as prolonged broad-spectrum antibiotic therapy, may allow *Candida* to proliferate, especially in the external auditory meatus, oropharynx, and GI tract.[8, 12] Similarly, disruption of cutaneous or mucosal barriers by burns, surgery, cytotoxic agents, trauma, or indwelling vascular or urinary catheters allows a pathway for *Candida* to enter the body from the body surfaces or the environment. Once in the body, cell-mediated immunity appears to be an important determinant of further spread of infection. There also is evidence that *Candida* cell wall mannan, a glycoprotein, has immunosuppressive properties that facilitate persistent infection.[10] Prolonged immunosuppression, cytotoxic chemotherapy causing persistent neutropenia, diabetes mellitus, long-term glucocorticoid therapy, and prolonged antibiotic therapy have resulted in an increased incidence of both localized and disseminated candidiasis. Circulating neutrophils appear to be a major defense against candidiasis; candidiasis has occurred in neutropenic persons and in dogs with experimentally induced and spontaneous neutropenia. A similar predisposition has not been substantiated for the occurrence of disseminated candidiasis in cats. One cat with disseminated infection, however, had concurrent toxoplasmosis, diabetes mellitus, and suspected hyperadrenocorticism.[4]

In disseminated candidiasis, the microcirculation of tissues, such as lung, skin, kidneys, liver, brain, myocardium, eyes, intervertebral disc, and skeletal muscle, acts to filter and clear the blood of yeasts. This activity results in embolic colonization and microabscess formation at these sites.

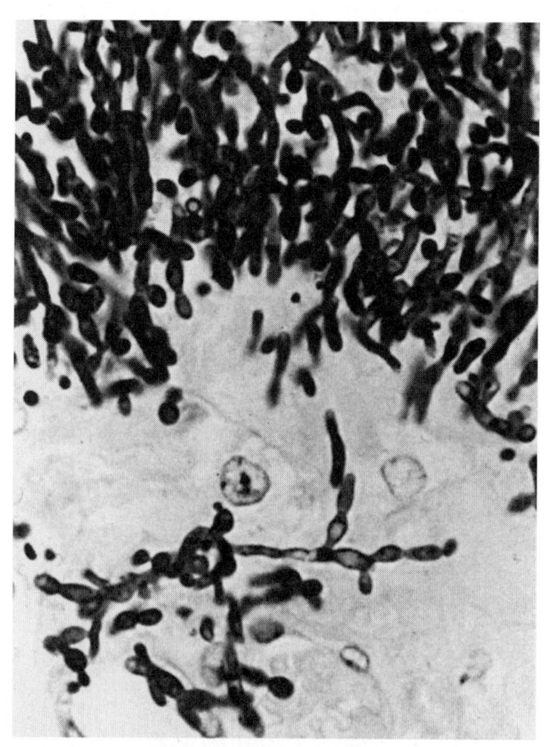

Figure 66–1. Invasive candidiasis. Budding yeast-like cells (blastoconidia) and segmentally constricted pseudohyphae of *C. albicans* invade the esophageal mucosa (PAS, × 700).

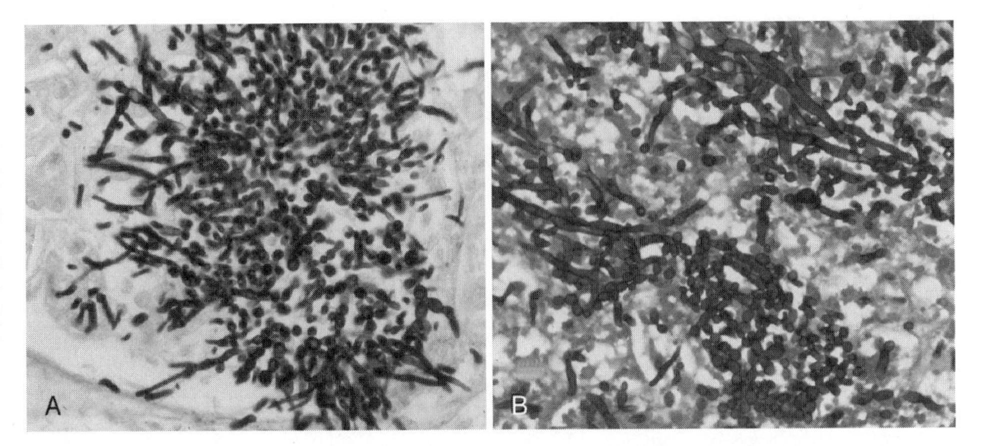

Figure 66–2. Hematogenous renal candidiasis caused by *C. albicans*. *A*, A glomerulus contains spherical to oval blastoconidia and peripheral, radially oriented pseudohyphae (Gomori's methenamine silver stain, × 300). *B*, Blastoconidia and branched, septate hyphae with parallel contours proliferate within a necrotic renal papilla (Gomori's methenamine silver with H and E counterstain, × 300).

CLINICAL FINDINGS

Localized candidiasis is found in chronically immunosuppressed dogs and cats and in those with nonhealing ulcers of the oral, upper respiratory, GI, or genitourinary mucosae. Lesions are characterized by nonhealing ulcers covered by whitish-gray plaques with hyperemic margins (Fig. 66–3*A* and *B*). A white vaginal or preputial discharge may be seen in candidiasis of the genital mucosa. Dysuria and hematuria are features of *Candida* urocystitis.[3] Chronic lesions of the skin or nail beds may appear as nonhealing, erythematous, moist, exuding, and crusting. Superficial ocular infections appear as conjunctival congestion and corneal ulceration.[4]

Disseminated candidiasis has been recognized in dogs and cats. Although clinical signs frequently reflect involvement of particular organ systems, lesions in dogs and cats with multisystemic infection are often widespread. Fever and the sudden appearance of multiple raised erythematous to hemorrhagic skin lesions have been described in canine systemic candidiasis. The lesions begin as small wheals or macules that eventually ulcerate (Fig. 66–4*A* and *B*). Pain and reluctance to move are common manifestations of myositis. Dogs with systemic candidiasis also have peripheral lymphadenomegaly and fistulous drainage resulting from underlying osteomyelitis. Cats with systemic infection have developed uveitis, chorioretinitis, neurologic deficits, and pleural effusions.[4]

DIAGNOSIS

Hematologic findings usually are normal in localized infections; however, leukopenia and thrombocytopenia may be associated with disseminated disease. Muscle and liver enzyme concentrations may be increased, depending on the tissues affected.

Isolation methods, which first involve lysis centrifugation, release fungi from leukocytes, increasing the ability to grow *Candida* spp. and decreasing the time between inoculation and growth of the organism. *Candida* spp. grow well on blood agar; therefore, they are often isolated from specimens submitted for bacterial culture. *Candida* grow rapidly at room temperature or 37°C, producing smooth or wrinkled, creamy white, yeastlike colonies. Colonies are composed of spheroidal to oval yeastlike cells 5 to 7 μm in diameter, pseudohyphae, and septate hyphae 3 to 5 μm in width. Pseudohyphae are composed of elongated yeastlike cells that remain attached end to end in chains. They can be distinguished from true hyphae by having prominent constrictions at points of attachment between adjacent cells. Septate hyphae are tubular with parallel contours. The thick-walled chlamydoconidia, 8 to 12 μm diameter, are spheroidal. *C. albicans* is further identified by a positive germ tube test (see Fig. 56–17 and associated text) and patterns of carbohydrate metabolism.

Antemortem blood samples for culture are best obtained

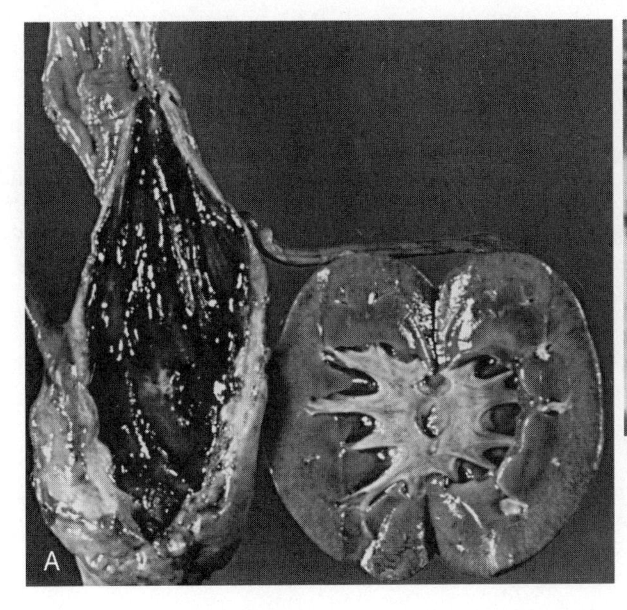

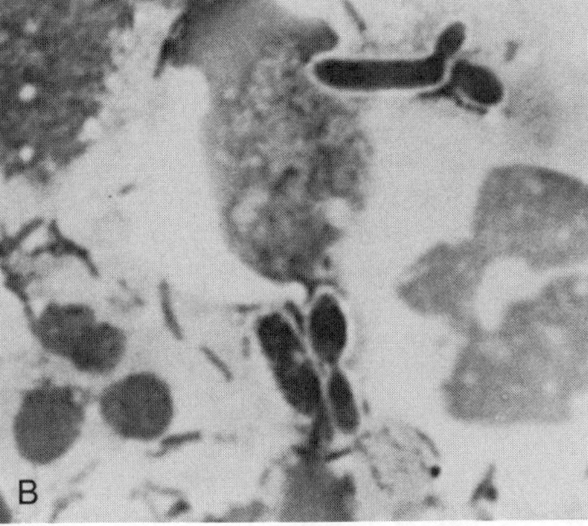

Figure 66–3. *A*, Bladder from a dog with secondary *Candida* cystitis as a result of long-term cyclophosphamide therapy. *B*, Stained urinary sediment contains blastoconidia with leukocytes.

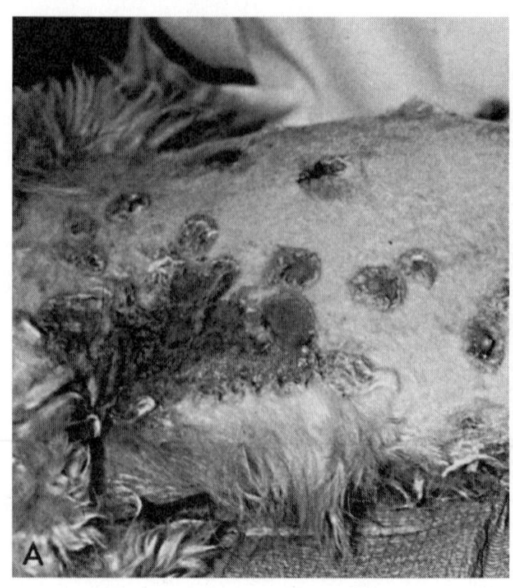

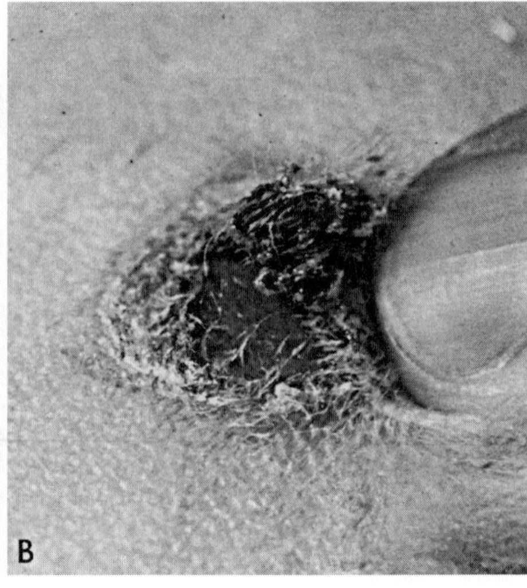

Figure 66–4. *A*, Ulcerative dermatitis in a dog with concurrent polymyositis. *Candida* was cultured from the lesions, and the disease responded to therapy with ketoconazole. *B*, Closer view of a skin lesion.

from peripheral arteries, because most of the organisms, effectively filtered out by tissues, never reach the systemic venous circulation. Because consistent renal embolization occurs with disseminated infection, *Candida* spp. are more easily isolated from urine than from the blood. Candiduria in patients without lower urinary tract signs or indwelling urinary catheters usually reflects hematogenous spread to the kidneys. Recovery of *Candida* spp. from a normally sterile fluid such as CSF or joint fluid is indicative of invasive candidiasis. Organisms may sometimes be cultured from many tissues at surgery or necropsy, but such results should be interpreted with caution. Culture of *Candida* spp. from cutaneous or mucosal surfaces or exudates alone should not be considered an absolute indicator of infection. Histologic confirmation of invasion and host reaction are essential. Cutaneous or mucosal tissue biopsy samples should be submitted for histologic and cultural examinations simultaneously. Biopsies of liver, spleen, lung, and kidney may be needed to document hematogenous spread. A definitive histologic diagnosis can sometimes be made in the presence of negative culture results.

A number of nonculture methods have been developed for the diagnosis of disseminated candidiasis in serum, whole blood, or urine specimens.[11] D-Arabinitol, a low-molecular weight metabolite, has been increased in serum of humans with disseminated candidiasis. Artifactual increases of D-arabinitol that occur in renal failure are distinguished by comparing its concentration with that of serum creatinine.

As a more rapid alternative to culture methods, polymerase chain reaction has been used to detect *Candida* spp. in blood and urine.[9] A number of tests also have been developed on an experimental basis to detect soluble antigens of *Candida* spp. such as mannan in blood and urine using ELISA and latex agglutination (LA) immunoassays.[6] Two LA tests are commercially available for clinical detection of *Candida* antigens in body fluids: Pastorex *Candida* (Sanofi Diagnostics Pasteur, Marres-la Coquette, France) and Cand-Tec (Ramco Laboratories, Inc., Houston, TX)].

PATHOLOGIC FINDINGS

Animals that die of disseminated candidiasis have gross lesions consisting of multiple white foci in the heart, liver, spleen, lymph nodes, CNS, kidneys, or other organs. Microscopic evaluation reveals multifocal abscesses or areas of necroses that contain abundant blastoconidia, pseudohyphae, and true hyphae surrounded by mixed inflammatory (budding yeastlike) cells (see Figs. 66–1, Fig. 66–2*A*, and Fig. 66–2*B*). Infiltrates are usually minimal in profoundly immunosuppressed or leukopenic animals. Occasionally, hyphal angioinvasion or occlusion of small and medium-size arteries by systemic candidal emboli results in nodular, hemorrhagic infarcts. Caution must be exercised in diagnosing localized, superficial candidal infections on the basis of cytologic or histologic study of mucocutaneous lesions unless hyphal elements and numerous inflammatory cells are present (see Fig. 66–3*B*). The different *Candida* spp. are morphologically and tinctorially indistinguishable in clinical specimens. Culture is needed for definitive species identification. Test kits are available to confirm genus identity in clinical or culture specimens (see Appendix 6).

THERAPY

Treatment of superficial candidiasis involves drying of nonmucosal lesions. Antifungal susceptibility testing is unreliable. Mucosal lesions can be treated with topical nystatin, gentian violet (1:10,000), miconazole creams, or topical amphotericin B (AMB) lotions (Table 66–1). Systemic candidiasis can be treated with IV AMB, but the drug's nephrotoxicity in otherwise compromised hosts can be fatal. Ketoconazole and other related benzimidazoles are currently the drugs of choice for treating infected dogs (Table 66–2). Liposome-encapsulated AMB has been relatively effective and nontoxic in preliminary studies. Supplemental administration of oral vitamin A might be recommended because it has been shown to increase resistance to infection by *Candida*.

Table 66–1. Recommended Drugs for Topical Treatment of Candidiasis and Trichosporonosis

GENERIC (BRAND) DRUG	FORMULATION	INTERVAL (HOURS)	DURATION (WEEKS)
Nystatin (Nilstat)	100,000 U/g	8–12	1–2
Miconazole (Conofite)	2%	12–24	2–4
Clotrimazole (Lotrimin)	1%	6–8	1
Amphotericin B (Fungizone)	3%	6–8	1

Table 66–2. Recommended Drugs for Systemic Treatment of Candidiasis and Trichosporonosis

SYSTEMIC DRUG	SPECIES	DOSE[a]	ROUTE	INTERVAL (HOURS)	DURATION[b] (WEEKS)
Ketoconazole	D	5–11 mg/kg	PO	12	5
	C	50 mg total	PO	12–24	4
Itraconazole	B	5–10 mg/kg	PO	12–24	4
Fluconazole	B	5 mg/kg	PO	12	4

[a]Dose per administration at specified interval. For additional information on these drugs, see Drug Formulary, Appendix 8.
[b]May have to extend therapy based on response.
D = dog; C = cat; B = dog and cat.

Torulopsosis

Torulopsis glabrata, which had been tentatively merged with the genus *Candida* as *C. glabrata,* is now considered to be taxonomically distinct. *T. glabrata* has been rarely associated with urinary tract infection (UTI) in immunocompromised dogs and cats.[4a] Disseminated infections have not yet been recognized in these animals. *T. glabrata* is part of the microbial flora of the skin and mucosal surfaces of human and animals and is an environmental saprophyte.

This yeast gains access to the genitourinary tract from local contamination and ascending infection or from embolic spread to the kidneys in disseminated infection. Immunosuppression or chronic antimicrobial therapy contributes to colonization. Infection may be subclinical, although signs of lower UTI, hematuria, and dysuria have been noted. In smears and sections of infected tissue, *T. glabrata* closely resembles *Histoplasma capsulatum.* In comparison, in H and E–stained tissues, *T. glabrata* shows no pseudocapsule or "halo" effect as does *H. capsulatum.* With Gomori's methenamine silver (GMS) stain, *T. glabrata* are larger, bud more frequently, and are more often extracellular and not in clusters. Unlike *Candida, T. glabrata* reproduces only by budding and is always a yeast form in tissue or culture. Treatment of lower UTI would involve local infusion of antifungal solutions, although systemic antifungal therapy, as outlined for candidiasis, would be more convenient and appropriate should disseminated infections be recognized.

Rhodotorulosis

Yeasts of the genus *Rhodotorula* are saprophytes, found in the domestic environment on shower curtains and in bathtub grout and as commensals of moist skin. They can be isolated as contaminants and are rarely isolated from clinical specimens of the urinary tract. Granulomatous epididymitis was associated with this infection in a dog,[7] and disseminated infections have occurred in immunocompromised people.

This yeast may gain access to the genitourinary tract through local contamination. The yeast has caused septicemia and meningitis in people on long-term IV therapy. Contamination of IV catheter sites is the presumed route of these infections. As with candidiasis, immunocompromised states are associated with disseminated infections.

Rhodotorula can be isolated on routine mycologic media at room temperature after 3 to 4 days incubation. Colonies are smooth and salmon-pink and contain 10 μm-diameter encapsulated yeasts. Biochemical characteristics have been described.[7]

In the dog with granulomatous epididymitis, severe swelling of the scrotum was observed. Treatment with antibiotics was ineffective, and the scrotum became firm. Surgical removal of the testes and epididymides was performed. The epididymides were swollen and, when sectioned, contained firm connective tissues, multifocal hemorrhages, and abscesses. On histopathologic examination, marked infiltration of neutrophils and macrophages with fibrosis was found in the dilated and partially ruptured ductus deferens. In surrounding stroma, focal collections of macrophages contained eosinophilic, spherical, 5- to 8-μm diameter, yeastlike structures. The intracellular yeasts stained positive by periodic acid-Schiff and GMS procedures. Removal of the affected testes and epididymides was curative. In case of disseminated infections, systemic antifungal therapy, as for candidiasis, is indicated.

References

1. Beco L, Heimann M, Heyneman M, et al. 1996. Cutaneous candidiasis associated with hypersensitivity and a post injection nodular granulomatous panniculitis in a cat. *Ann Med Vet* 140:451.
2. Brain PH. 1993. Urinary tract candidiasis in a diabetic dog. *Aust Vet Pract* 23:88.
3. Fulton RB, Walker RD. 1992. *Candida albicans* urocystitis in a cat. *J Am Vet Med Assoc* 200:524–526.
4. Gerding PA, Morton LD, Dye JA. 1994. Ocular and disseminated candidiasis in an immunosuppressed cat. *J Am Vet Med Assoc* 204:1635–1638.

4a. Greene CE. 1996. Unpublished information. University of Georgia, Athens, GA.

5. Greene CE, Chandler FW. 1990. Candidiasis, pp 723–727. *In* Greene CE (ed), Infectious diseases of the dog and cat. WB Saunders, Philadelphia, PA.
6. Herent P, Stynen D, Fernando H, et al. 1992. Retrospective evaluation of two latex agglutination tests for detection of circulating antigens during invasive candidosis. *J Clin Microbiol* 30:2158–2164.
7. Kadota K, Uchida K, Nagatomo T, et al. 1995. Granulomatous epididymitis related to *Rhodotorula glutinis* infection in a dog. *Vet Pathol* 32:716–718.
8. McKellar QA, Rycroft A, Anderson L, et al. 1990. Otitis externa in a Foxhound pack associated with *Candida albicans. Vet Rec* 127:72.
9. Miyakawa Y, Mabuchi T, Fukazawa Y. 1993. New method for detection of *Candida albicans* in human blood by polymerase chain reaction. *J Clin Microbiol* 31:3344–3347.
10. Nelson RD, Shibata N, Podzorski RP, et al. 1991. *Candida* mannan: chemistry, suppression of cell-mediated immunity, and possible mechanisms of action. *Clin Microbiol Rev* 4:1–19.
11. Reiss E, Morrison CJ. 1993. Nonculture methods for diagnosis of disseminated candidiasis. *Clin Microbiol Rev* 6:311–323.
12. Sparks TA, Kemp DT, Wooley RE, et al. 1994. Antimicrobial effect of combinations of EDTA-Tris and amikacin or neomycin on the microorganisms associated with otitis externa in dogs. *Vet Res Commun* 18:241–249.

Chapter **67**

Trichosporonosis

Craig E. Greene and Francis W. Chandler

ETIOLOGY

Trichosporon spp., yeastlike fungi that exist in nature as soil saprophytes, are members of the family Cryptococcaceae. In culture they form hyaline yeastlike cells, mycelia, and characteristic arthroconidia. *Trichosporon* spp. are not considered to be primary pathogens because they are distributed in the environment worldwide and form a minor component of normal skin and mucosal flora of people and animals.

T. beigelii (=T. cutaneum), a transient skin commensal, is recognized as the agent of white piedra, a nodular mycosis of hair shafts affecting people, monkeys, and horses in temperate to tropical climates. It has been linked to the syndrome of human seasonal hypersensitivity pneumonitis in Japan[12, 14] and catheter-associated infections. *T. capitatum (= Blastoschizomyces capitatus, Geotrichum capitatum)* has been incriminated as causing abortion in a cow and horse. Both *T. beigelii* and *T. capitatum* have caused systemic infections in people, especially in patients being treated for hematologic malignancies and in recipients of renal and bone marrow transplants. *T. pullulans* and *T. beigelii* have caused infections in three cats. Biochemical and genetic studies indicate that cutaneous skin, mucosal, and environmental isolates differ from those that cause disseminated illness.[8, 9, 15]

PATHOGENESIS

Most cases of trichosporonosis in people have been disseminated and fatal, and they have occurred in patients with severe immunosuppression who were also neutropenic. Many had received multiple or broad-spectrum antibiotics for documented or presumed bacterial infections, whereas others had neoplastic diseases or organ transplants. Presumably, the fungus invades mucosal surfaces of the respiratory, GI, or urogenital tracts of immunosuppressed hosts, with subsequent dissemination. A few cases of valvular endocarditis caused by *Trichosporon* spp. have been reported.[1, 7]

Feline infections have been characterized by mixed suppurative and granulomatous inflammation of the mucosal and submucosal or subcutaneous tissues. Evidence for immunosuppression has not been apparent in all affected cats, but one had multicentric lymphosarcoma.

CLINICAL FINDINGS

One cat was reported to have a fever, an inspiratory stertor, and a protruding unilateral nasal mass (Fig. 67–1) similar to that caused by *Cryptococcus neoformans*.[5] Later spread to regional lymph nodes and pulmonary tissues was suspected. Another cat had a chronic ulcerative subcutaneous lesion at the site of a bite wound.[2] A third cat suffered from chronic hematuria and dysuria as a result of chronic cystitis complicated by the yeast infection.[2] In people, clinical findings are usually those of fungal sepsis, with fever that is unresponsive to antibiotic therapy. Cutaneous lesions, chorioretinitis, and signs referable to renal glomerular and pulmonary vascular localization are most frequent.

DIAGNOSIS

Mere culture of *Trichosporon* spp. from cutaneous or mucosal surfaces can be misleading because the organism is a normal constituent of the endogenous microflora in these areas. Biopsy with histologic confirmation of host reaction and invasion of the deeper tissues by characteristic fungal elements is more specific for documentation of pathogenicity.

Trichosporon spp. can be grown on Sabouraud's or Mycosel agar (Becton Dickinson Microbiology Systems, Cockeysville, MD) at 25°C, and after several days, spreading cream-colored yeastlike colonies are formed. Wet-mount lactophenol blue-stained preparations show hyaline, septate hyphae, arthroconidia (10.4×2.5 μm), and pleomorphic blastoconidia (2.5 to 8 μm in diameter). The characteristic arthroconidia are produced by segmentation and fragmentation of hyphae. Unlike those of *C. neoformans*, blastoconidia of the *Trichosporon* spp. do not show a capsule when stained with mucin stains or India ink. The species are distinguished from each other by differences in various carbon and nitrogen sources for growth.

T. beigelii produces a heat-stable, cell wall antigen that is antigenically similar to the capsular polysaccharide of *C. neoformans*. The latex agglutination test, used to detect cryptococcal capsular polysaccharide antigen (see Chapter 61), has been used to diagnose disseminated *T. beigelii* infection in people and in experimentally infected rabbits.[11, 16] Pretreatment of sera with pronase, which presumably disrupts immune complexes and nonspecific protein binding to the fungal capsule, increased the sensitivity of the antigen detection test.[16] In a case of nasal infection caused by *T. pullulans* in a cat,[5] cryptococcal antigen test findings of serum were negative before clinical evidence of dissemination.

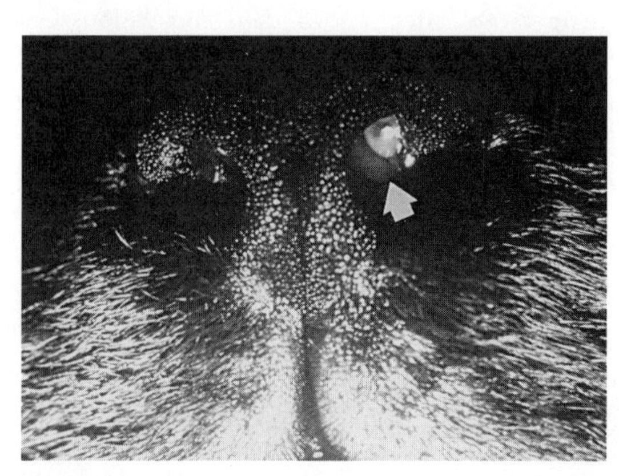

Figure 67–1. Mass *(arrow)* protruding from the nostril of the cat with nasal trichosporonosis. (From Greene CE et al: *J Am Vet Med Assoc* 187:946–948, 1985. Reprinted with permission.)

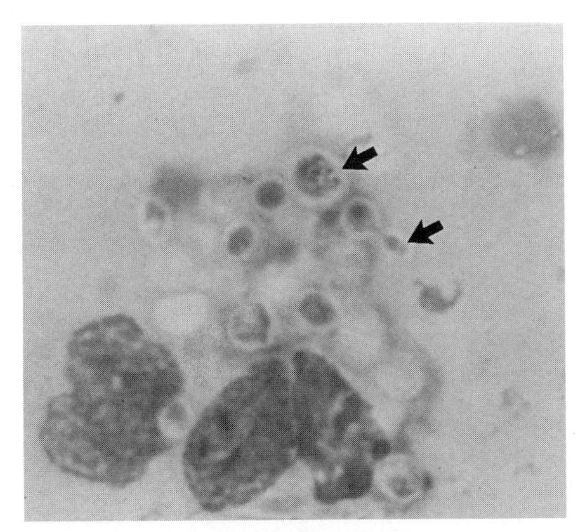

Figure 67–2. Macrophage with multiple intracytoplasmic yeasts *(arrows)* in an impression smear of the mass on which a biopsy was done shown in Figure 67–1 (Wright's stain, × 800). (From Greene CE et al: *J Am Vet Med Assoc* 187:946–948, 1985. Reprinted with permission.)

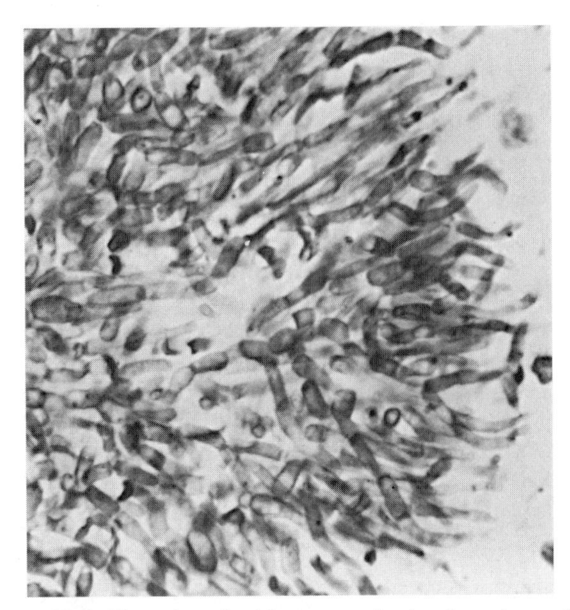

Figure 67–4. Disseminated trichosporonosis. A microcolony of *Trichosporon beigelii* consists of yeast-like cells, true hyphae, and arthroconidia formed by septal disarticulation of hyphae (Gomori's methenamine silver stain, × 850).

PATHOLOGIC FINDINGS

Histologic findings in trichosporonosis are similar to those of disseminated aspergillosis and consist of abscesses and nodular infarcts, with mycotic vascular invasion, thrombosis, and infiltration of neutrophils and macrophages. Spherical to oval yeastlike organisms (blastoconidia), 3 to 8 μm in diameter, arthroconidia, and septate hyphae can be seen in tissue sections or in impression smears (Figs. 67–2 and 67–3). In disseminated lesions, fungal elements often proliferate from a central nidus to produce a radial or sunburst pattern of growth (Fig. 67–4). All fungal elements stain positively with periodic acid–Schiff and Gomori's methenamine silver stains as a result of polysaccharides in the fungal cell walls. The arthroconidia, formed by hyperseptation and disarticulation of hyphal segments, are sometimes difficult to demonstrate. When this problem occurs, *Trichosporon* spp. and *Candida* spp. can be mistaken for each other and must be distinguished by immunohistologic or cultural studies.

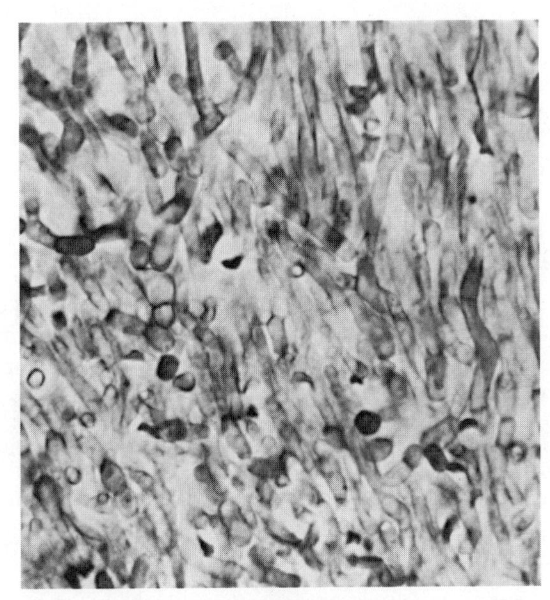

Figure 67–3. Disseminated trichosporonosis. Pleomorphic blastocoidia and branched, septate hyphae of *Trichosporon beigelii* occupy a nodular splenic infarct (Gomori's methenamine silver stain, × 850).

THERAPY

Trichosporon spp. are more susceptible in vitro to benzimidazole compounds than to amphotericin B (AMB) or flucytosine. Resistance to AMB often has been demonstrated when treating infected people,[18] but itraconazole (ITZ) has been effective.[1] Cats should be treated orally with ITZ (see Table 66–2). Cats that develop anorexia, vomiting, or diarrhea may need to have the dosage reduced to 50 mg total on alternate days. ITZ is not as hepatotoxic in cats as ketoconazole. Reduction of the dosage has been associated with relapse of disease. Surgical removal of a nasal granuloma in one cat was incomplete, and the infection later disseminated.

References

1. Chaumentin G, Boibieux A, Piens MA, et al. 1996. *Trichosporon inkin* endocarditis: short term evolution and clinical report. *Clin Infect Dis* 23:396–397.
2. Doster AR, Erickson ED, Chandler FW. 1987. Feline trichosporomosis. *J Am Vet Med Assoc* 190:1184–1186.
3. Ellner K, McBride ME, Rosen T, et al. 1991. Prevalence of *Trichosporon beigelii*. Colonization of normal paragenital skin. *J Med Vet Mycol* 29:99–103.
4. Greene CE, Chandler FW. 1990. Trichosporosis, pp 728–730. *In* Greene CE (ed), Infectious diseases of the dog and cat. WB Saunders, Philadelphia, PA.
5. Greene CE, Miller DM, Blue JL. 1985. *Trichosporon* infection in a cat. *J Am Vet Med Assoc* 187:946–948.
6. Gueho E, Faergemann J, Lyman C, et al. 1994. *Malassezia* and *Trichosporon*: two emerging pathogenic basidiomycetous yeast-like fungi. *J Med Vet Mycol* 32:367–378.
7. Keay S, Denning DW, Stevens DA. 1991. Endocarditis due to *Trichosporon beigelii*: in vitro susceptibility of isolates and review. *Rev Infect Dis* 13:383–386.
8. Kemker BJ, Lehmann PF, Lee JW, et al. 1991. Distinction of deep versus superficial clinical and nonclinical isolates of *Trichosporon beigelii* by isoenzymes and restriction fragment length polymorphisms of rDNA generated by polymerase chain reaction. *J Clin Microbiol* 29:1677–1683.

9. Lee JW, Melcher GA, Rinaldi MG, et al. 1990. Patterns of morphologic variation among isolates of *Trichosporon beigelii*. *J Clin Microbiol* 28:2823–2827.
10. Lopes JO, Alves SH, Benevenga JP, et al. 1994. *Trichosporon beigelii* peritonitis associated with continuous ambulatory peritoneal dialysis. *Rev Inst Med Trop Sao Paulo* 36:121–123.
11. Melcher GP, Reed KD, Rinaldi MG, et al. 1991. Demonstration of a cell wall antigen cross-reacting with cryptococcal polysaccharide in experimental disseminated trichosporonosis. *J Clin Microbiol* 29:192–195.
12. Mizobe T, Yamasaki H, Doi K, et al. 1993. Analysis of serotype-specific antibodies to *Trichosporon cutaneum* types I and II in patients with summer-type hypersensitivity pneumonitis with monoclonal antibodies to serotype-related polysaccharide antigens. *J Clin Microbiol* 31:1949–1951.
13. Nahass GT, Rosenberg SP, Leonardi CL, et al. 1993. Disseminated infection with *Trichosporon beigelii*: report of a case and review of the cutaneous and histologic manifestations. *Arch Dermatol* 129:1020–1023.
14. Nishiura Y, Nakagawayoshida K, Suga M, et al. 1997. Assignment and serotyping of *Trichosporon* species—the causative agents of summer-type hypersensitivity pneumonitis. *J Med Vet Mycol* 35:45–52.
15. Sugita T, Nishikawa A, Shinoda T, et al. 1995. Taxonomic position of deep-seated, mucosa associated, and superficial isolates of *Trichosporon cutaneum* from trichosporonosis patients. *J Clin Microbiol* 33:1368–1370.
16. Walsh TJ, Lee JW, Melcher GP, et al. 1992. Experimental *Trichosporon* infection in persistently granulocytopenic rabbits: implications for pathogenesis, diagnosis and treatment of an emerging opportunistic mycosis. *J Infect Dis* 166:121–133.
17. Walsh TJ, Melcher GP, Lee JW, et al. 1993. Infections due to *Trichosporon* species: new concepts in mycology, pathogenesis, diagnosis and treatment. *Curr Top Med Mycol* 5:79–113.
18. Walsh TJ, Melcher GP, Rinaldi MG, et al. 1990. *Trichosporon beigelii*, an emerging pathogen resistant to amphotericin B. *J Clin Microbiol* 28:1616–1622.

Chapter 68

Miscellaneous Fungal Infections

Carol S. Foil

This chapter discusses pythiosis, a common but not easily classified mycosis, and several opportunistic fungal infections that infect dogs and cats sporadically. The diseases and agents are summarized in Table 68–1. Diagnosis of any infection by a saprophytic fungus must be made on the basis of isolation of the organism from tissue (not exudate) and tissue invasion by a morphologically compatible organism. Several agents, belonging to diverse taxonomic groups, produce granulomas containing similar, wide, nonseptate hyphae. "Phycomycoses," as these infections have been termed, are more properly classified as either pythioses or zygomycoses. Uncultured lesions should not be classified by pathologic features without the aid of immunohistochemistry, because the epidemiology, treatment, and prognosis of pythiosis and zygomycosis are dissimilar.

Pythiosis

Pythiosis is a cutaneous, GI, or multisystemic granulomatous disease that affects dogs, cats, horses, cattle, and people worldwide in wet, tropical, and subtropical climates. The dog and horse are most commonly affected.

ETIOLOGY

Pythiosis is caused by an aquatic pathogen, *Pythium insidiosum*[4, 43] (synonyms: "*Hyphomyces destruens*," *P. destruens*, and *P. gracile*). This water mold is a member of the protoctistid class Oomycetes. Water molds differ from true fungi in producing motile, flagellate zoospores; having cell walls with cellulose and β-glucan but without chitin; and having fundamentally different nuclear division and mitochondrial and Golgi structures. Their plasma membranes typically lack sterols such as ergosterol, which is the target of action of most classic antifungal drugs. The only member of this class currently recognized to cause disease in mammals is *P. insidiosum*. Other members of the genus *Pythium* are plant pathogens of some economic importance. The pathogens most closely related according to molecular studies are the *Prototheca* species (see Chapter 69).[32]

The infective stage is the biflagellate aquatic zoospore. Zoospore release is seasonal and associated with warm weather. Water lilies and other aquatic plants and submerged grasses, including rice plants, are thought to be the normal hosts.

EPIDEMIOLOGY

Pythiosis has been reported in Australia, Brazil, Burma, Colombia, Costa Rica, Indonesia, Japan, New Guinea, Thailand, and the United States. In the United States, most cases are from states bordering the Gulf of Mexico. However, reports of cases in dogs from as far north as Kentucky[42] and North Carolina show that pythiosis is not as geographically restricted as previously assumed.

Large-breed male dogs are affected most frequently, although a reported series of cases had females predominate.[15] Many develop infection in autumn but are presented for medical evaluation between August and December. Animals are probably exposed by standing in or drinking warm, stagnant fresh water containing newly emerged zoospores. The zoospores in water move toward damaged plant or animal

Table 68–1. Miscellaneous Fungal Infections of Dogs and Cats

DISEASE	AGENT	FUNGAL CHARACTERISTICS	SPECIES	PRIMARY ORGAN SYSTEM OR TISSUE AFFECTED
Pythiosis	*Pythium insidiosum*[a]	Broad, poorly septate hyphae	Dog, cat rarely	GI, subcutaneous, disseminated rarely
Zygomycosis				
Mucormycosis	*Mucor, Rhizopus, Rhizomucor, Absidia*	Broad, poorly septate hyphae	Dog, cat	CNS, GI, disseminated
Entomophthoromycosis	*Conidiobolus*	Broad, poorly septate hyphae with eosinophilic sleeves	Dog	Nasal, pharyngeal, subcutaneous
	Basidiobolus		Dog	Subcutaneous, pulmonary
Adiaspiromycosis	*Emmonsia (Chrysosporium) parva*	Adiaspores	Dog	Lung
Hyalohyphomycosis	*Acremonium (Cephalosporium)*	Branching septate hyphae with chlamydospores	Dog	Cutaneous nodules, disseminated, keratomycosis
	Chrysosporium	Swollen hyphae and yeastlike bodies	Dog	Diskospondylitis
	Fusarium	Branching, septate hyphae with ballooning ends	Dog, cat	Pyelonephritis, cutaneous, disseminated, keratomycosis
	Geotrichum	Short, septate hyphae and yeastlike bodies	Dog	Cutaneous, disseminated
	Paecilomyces	Branching septate hyphae, dilated hyphae, and yeastlike bodies	Dog, cat	Nasal granuloma, CNS, disseminated
	Pseudallescheria[b] (= *Scedosporium*)	Septate, branching hyphae and racket hyphae	Dog	Osteomyelitis, respiratory, keratomycosis
Phaeohyphomycosis	*Alternaria*	Darkly pigmented septate hyphae with swollen bodies	Dog, cat	Nasal, subcutaneous, keratomycosis
	Bipolaris[c]	Branching, septate, lightly pigmented hyphae with globose elements	Dog, cat	Subcutaneous, paranasal sinusitis, rarely disseminated
	Cladosporium[d]	Lightly pigmented septate hyphae, bizarre forms, yeastlike cells	Cat, dog	CNS, keratomycosis, cutaneous, disseminated
	Curvularia	Moderately pigmented hyphae with swollen forms and yeastlike bodies	Dog, cat	Subcutaneous, sporotrichoid, keratomycosis
	Exophiala	Pale pigmented hyphae and yeastlike bodies	Cat	Subcutaneous, on face and feet, rhinitis
	Moniliella	Darkly pigmented pseudohyphae and yeastlike cell	Cat	Subcutaneous
	Ochroconis	Pigmented hyphae?	Cat	Disseminated
	Phialemonium	Pleomorphic with darkly pigmented hyphae and swollen yeastlike elements	Dog	Osteomyelitis, cutaneous nodules, tracts
	Phialophora	Pigmented pseudohyphae with globose yeastlike bodies	Cat	Subcutaneous
	Pseudomicrodochium	Pigmented hyphae with bizarre forms	Dog	Cutaneous
	Scolecobasidium	Septate pigmented hyphae with globose swellings	Cat	Subcutaneous
	Stemphyllium	Pigmented hyphae	Cat	Subcutaneous
Eumycotic mycetoma (white grain)	*Acremonium*	Unpigmented tissue grains with hyphae and chlamydospores	Dog?	Intra-abdominal and disseminated
	Pseudallescheria		Dog	Intra-abdominal
Eumycotic mycetoma (black grain)	*Curvularia*	Pigmented tissue grains with hyphae and chlamydospores	Dog, cat	Subcutaneous on extremities
	Madurella		Dog	Intra-abdominal
	Phaeococcus		Cat	Subcutaneous, tail head

[a] Synonyms: *Hyphomyces destruens, P. destrans, P. gracile.* An oomycete in the kingdom Chromista or Protoctista depending on systematics.
[b] Synonyms: *Petriellidum, Allescheria;* saprophytic stage = *Scedosporium apiospermum.*
[c] Synonym: *Drechslera.*
[d] Synonyms: *Cladosporium bantianum, Xylohypha bantiana, Torula bantiana, Cladosporium trichoides.*

tissues. Interestingly, some cases are observed in small dogs in the suburbs with no known history of access to a standing body of water. This occurrence raises the possibility that the organism proliferates in temporary stands of water or even on wet turf grass.

Intact skin is probably resistant to invasion. It is not known whether zoospores can penetrate intact oropharyngeal or GI mucosa. Immune suppression is not an apparent prerequisite for infection.

CLINICAL FINDINGS

The **GI form** of the disease predominates in the dog. Affected dogs have a history suggestive of an upper GI obstruction with palpable abdominal mass or, less often, chronic diarrhea and weight loss. Any part of the GI tract may be affected with a markedly infiltrative granulomatous enteritis (Fig. 68–1); the stomach and duodenum are the most common sites. Diarrhea may be present if the distal small intestine is affected, and hematochezia is seen in cases of colonic involvement. Oropharyngeal infection is less common, and chronic esophagitis has been reported, associated with hypersalivation.[55] Signs of systemic illness develop only after intestinal obstruction, infarction, or perforation; therefore, in most cases the disease is far advanced before diagnosis is made.

The **subcutaneous** and **nasopharyngeal forms** of pythiosis are seen less frequently in dogs[22] and occur rarely in cats[5, 13] (Fig. 68–2). German shepherd dogs may be predisposed to the subcutaneous form, and this form seems to be more common in the southeastern United States than in the rest of the geographic range. Cutaneous trauma or abrasion often precedes infection. Large spongy and proliferative lesions with ulceration and draining tracts may develop from dermal

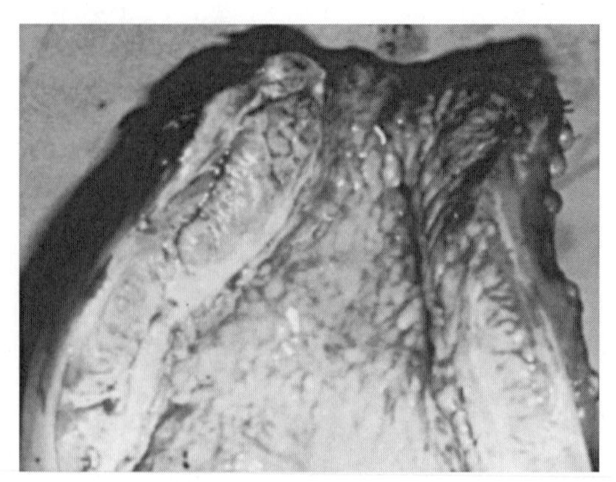

Figure 68–1. A surgically resected gastric pylorus demonstrating marked infiltration of the wall caused by gastric pythiosis.

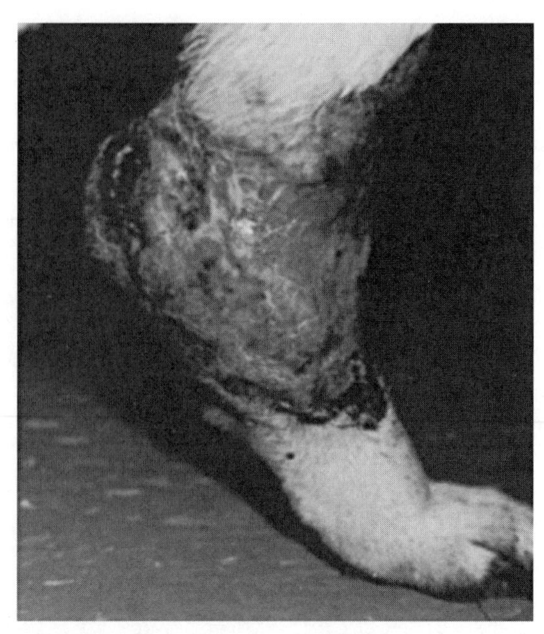

Figure 68–3. Canine subcutaneous pythiosis is the cause of this lesion on the hock of a German shepherd. The swelling and ulceration surround the limb. The lesion is infarcted in several sites.

nodules. Lesions may enlarge rapidly and become quite destructive; some animals develop necrosis. The most common sites are on the extremities and the tail head or perineum. Occasionally, the nodules are pruritic; early lesions on the limbs may resemble lick granulomas. Some limb lesions will progress to involve the entire circumference of the limb (Fig. 68–3). The face may become involved as an extension of oropharyngeal disease. Most patients show no symptoms of systemic illness, although severe cutaneous infarction and sepsis develop in a small percentage of advanced cases in the dog.

Rarely, disseminated disease develops in dogs with either the cutaneous or GI form. Granulomatous foci and infarctions affect various internal organs. The use of glucocorticoids, either locally or systemically, may be associated with rapid dissemination. Other host factors associated with dissemination are not known.

DIAGNOSIS AND PATHOLOGIC FINDINGS

Diagnosis can occasionally be established cytologically if lesions are accessible. Macerated tissue fixed in 10% potassium hydroxide (KOH) may be examined by direct microscopic inspection for the presence of typical wide, poorly septate, and branching hyphal elements. In GI disease, exploratory laparotomy reveals diffuse to irregular transmural thickening of a discrete segment of the tract, with variable irregular mucosal ulceration. Occasionally, only mesenteric lymph nodes are affected. Histologically, the disease shows granulomatous inflammation with fibrosis. In some specimens, large, irregular areas of liquefaction necrosis with eosinophils, neutrophils, plasma cells, and hyphal elements are surrounded by macrophages, epithelioid cells, and giant cells. The organisms typically are found in areas of liquefaction necrosis but are rare in the centers of discrete granulomas and are never found in the intervening connective tissue. *Pythium* does not stain well on hematoxylin and eosin sections but may be observed as clear spaces delineated by a narrow band of eosinophilic material intimately associated with the hyphal wall. When pythiosis is suspected, Gridley-stained or Gomori's methenamine silver–stained sections should be examined. Hyphae have thick, almost parallel walls ranging in diameter from 2.5 to 8.9 μm. A highly specific and sensitive indirect immunoperoxidase technique has been developed for use on tissue with hyphal elements and may be applied to canine as well as equine lesions.[7] Because the organism in tissue is quite similar to zygomycetes, when this test is not applied it is necessary to have cultural as well as histologic information to establish the diagnosis.

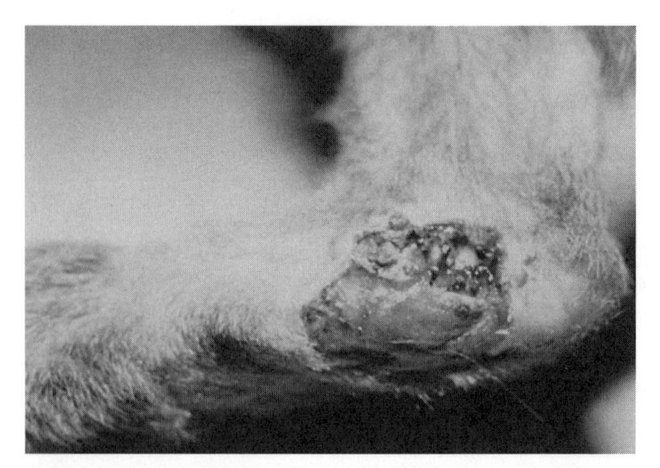

Figure 68–2. Feline cutaneous pythiosis demonstrating the less destructive ulcerative lesion typical of the feline disease (compare with canine lesion in Figure 68–3).

Pythium grows rapidly on blood agar, brain-heart infusion broth, and Sabouraud's dextrose when bits of aseptically obtained tissue are inoculated at 35°C to 37°C. Most of the plate is covered within 24 hours. Growth is poor and sparse at 20°C. The colony is typically dull yellow to white or colorless, growing with a finely radiate pattern into a flat, submerged mat with very short aerial growth. Incubation in water agar with sterile grass blades at 35°C to 37°C is necessary for production of the diagnostic zoosporangia and biflagellate zoospores.[44] FA tests and immunodiffusion exoantigen tests have been developed for identification of isolates at the Centers for Disease Control (CDC) in Atlanta, Georgia but are not commercially available.[57] These tests have been evaluated for specificity in comparison with other *Pythium* species as well as zygomycetes.[26, 27]

Failure to grow the organism from infected tissue is usually related to sample handling. The tissue should not be ground with mortar and pestle before being placed on the agar. It is advisable to submit specimens to veterinary diagnostic laboratories, where the microbiologist is more likely to be familiar with *Pythium* and its characteristic growth patterns. *Pythium* is sensitive to temperature stress and dehydration. Bacterial contamination may also be detrimental to organism isolation. When samples must be shipped or when delay between sample collection and plate inoculation is likely, tissue specimens should be washed thoroughly with sterile saline. The sample is then transported at room temperature via an overnight express delivery service in a sterile saline–ampicillin (100 μg/ml) solution. An immunodiffusion test for the serologic identification of anti-*Pythium* antibody production in horses is now available commercially (Spectrum Laboratories, Mesa, AZ).

THERAPY

The prognosis in the patient with pythiosis is poor unless the affected tissue can be completely excised. In the GI tract, this approach often requires radical resection, but complete resection can be curative.[11] When lesions are on an extremity, amputation can be curative. Wide and deep excision of skin lesions followed by skin grafting may be successful, but if excision is not complete the graft may become reinfected (Fig. 68–4). Unfortunately, many animals are not presented until complete excision is not feasible.

Attempts to treat canine pythiosis with antifungal medical therapy in conjunction with surgery have generally been frustrating. Metalaxyl (Ridomil; Ciba Geigy Corp., Summit, NJ), a fungicide used to treat plant diseases caused by Oomycetes, has been used in dogs and in a rabbit model, but the results have been disappointing owing in part to the systemic toxicity of the compound. Streptomycin has been given to control Oomycetes causing hop downy mildew disease of plants. No clinical investigation of this drug in pythiosis has been carried out. Although both topically and parenterally administered amphotericin B (AMB) and sodium or potassium iodide have been used with limited success in the horse, amphotericin B (AMB) and ketoconazole (KTZ) treatment of subcutaneous disease in dogs have been unsuccessful. *P. insidiosum* has been studied for in vitro response to a number of traditional antifungal agents, and miconazole (MCZ) showed the most consistently low minimum inhibitory concentrations (MICs).[63] Fluconazole, KTZ, and itraconazole (ITZ) gave inconsistent but encouraging results. ITZ has been used to treat several dogs and one cat diagnosed with cutaneous or GI pythiosis.[68] No response was observed in the cat.

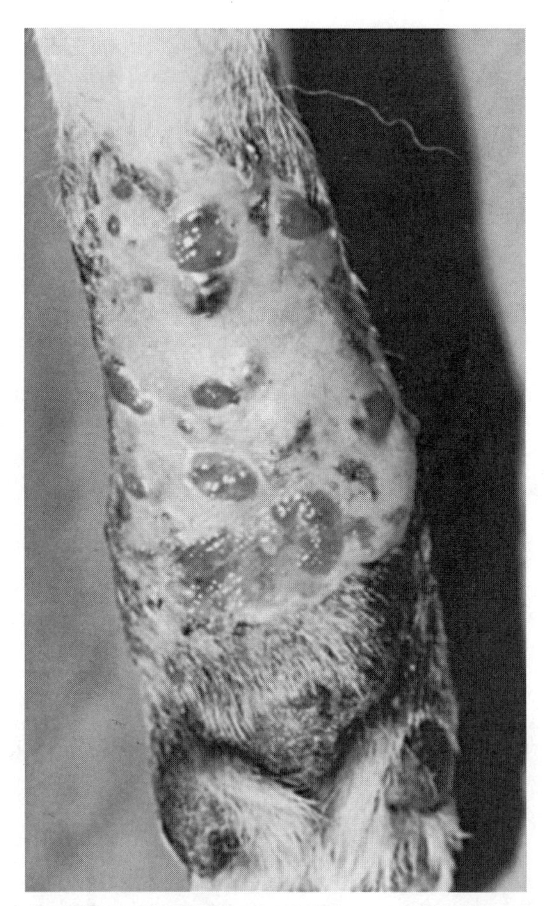

Figure 68–4. The split-thickness graft that was done after a resection of a subcutaneous pythiosis lesion has become infiltrated with new granulomatous nodules. The leg was amputated, resolving the disease.

Some improvement has been observed in all the canine cases, and some have been apparently cured of GI disease that was incompletely resectable at the time of presentation.[68] Lipid-complexed AMB has effected an apparent long-term remission in one dog with unresectable GI disease.[68]

A vaccine derived from ultrasonicated hyphae of *P. insidiosum* has been utilized with good success in the treatment of cutaneous disease in the horse.[45] Response in the dog has not been documented, although this approach has been taken in few cases and newer vaccine formulations may improve efficacy.

Zygomycosis

ETIOLOGY

Fungi in the class Zygomycetes that cause disease in animals and humans belong to two orders that cause diverse types of disease. The order Mucorales includes the genera *Rhizopus, Mucor, Rhizomucor, Mortierella,* and *Absidia,* among others. The term *mucormycosis* has been applied to this group of infections. The order Entomophthorales contains the genera *Conidiobolus* and *Basidiobolus,* and *entomophthoromycosis* is the term sometimes applied to their infections of animals and people. Of the three species of *Conidiobolus (C. coronatus, C. incongruus, C. lamprauges),* only the first has been specifically identified in dog or cat disease.

Only one confirmed report exists of disseminated *Basidiobolus ranarum (haptosporus)* infection in a dog. Disseminated disease with any entomophthoromycete in any species is rarely reported. There are two reports of localized canine conidiobolomycosis *(C. coronatus).*[21, 35] GI and pharyngeal entomophthoromycosis caused by undetermined species has been defined on the basis of fungal morphology in tissue by a skilled investigator in two additional dogs.

A chronically infected cervical bite wound in a dog has

been culturally confirmed as caused by *Absidia corymbifera*. In another report of canine zygomycosis of the pancreas, however, the diagnosis was based on morphologic description of the pathology and organism without confirmation by fungal culture findings. Other cases of systemic "phycomycosis" reported in dogs from western Europe and the northeastern United States in some older reports are likely to have been zygomycosis, but these were not cultured nor differentiated from pythiosis. Lesions in the affected animals involved the kidney, GI tract, heart muscle, or disseminated tissues. Some reports have been made of "mucormycosis" in cats with diabetes or with immunosuppressive diseases such as feline leukemia virus infection and panleukopenia.[51] *Mortierella parasitica* has been isolated from a tracheal lesion, and *Rhizomucor pusillus*, from a cerebral zygomycosis in cats.

EPIDEMIOLOGY

Zygomycetes are widely distributed in nature, and the Mucorales are common contaminants in cultures. Entomophthorales are soil saprophytes and insect pathogens that are most commonly restricted to tropical and subtropical climates. The portal of entry may be via the GI or respiratory tracts or via wound inoculation. In people and animals, a compromised immune system or pre-existing local tissue damage is usually necessary for invasion by Mucorales. In a report of systemic mycoses in cats, of which 12 were identified as mucormycoses, 70% had what were considered to be predisposing conditions, including 17% with panleukopenia.[51] However, in most confirmed and suspected cases in dogs and in infections with the Entomophthorales, such factors have not been documented. Mucormycosis has been recognized with increasing frequency in cats[51] and is associated with the use of deferoxamine (iron chelator) in people.[67] The latter is of interest because this agent is being used in some veterinary plastic surgical procedures. The natural distribution of *Basidiobolus* in northern Australia have been studied.[76] It was recovered from the feces of amphibians, reptiles, and wallabies, and from wood lice and leaf litter. Inoculation by biting insects has been suspected in cutaneous disease in the horse, and the organism can be isolated from the mouth parts of biting flies. *Conidiobolus* lesions are invariably nasal or facial, and presumably inspiration is the route of infection.

CLINICAL FINDINGS

Entomophthoromycosis

A young German shepherd dog developed nasal infection that was reminiscent of the most common form of conidiobolomycosis in farm animals, with nasal discharge and stertorous breathing.[2a, 35] These signs were associated with a ragged and extensive palatal ulcer (Fig. 68–5). In a second case, a young golden retriever had a subcutaneous mass that had developed from initially small nodules on the chest wall and hind limb.[21] Whereas the chest wall lesion seemed to regress over the course of the dog's illness, the lesion on the limb showed relentless enlargement and worsening with ulceration and limb edema, despite treatment.[21] This dog was vomiting. It had granulomas on the pleura and peritoneum and in the lungs, liver, and spleen at necropsy.

Mucormycosis

The disease is poorly defined in dogs and cats, and most diagnoses have been obtained by necropsy examination. It is difficult to draw conclusions about typical clinical findings; most reported cases have involved the GI or respiratory tract and have had acute to subacute courses. Many patients have vomited and have had palpable abdominal masses. Some of these cases may have actually been misdiagnosed with abdominal pythiosis. In disseminated disease, the clinical presentations include GI erosion, lymphadenomegaly with calcification, encephalitis, pneumonia, and cutaneous nodules and ulcers.[67] A series of cases reported in cats included animals with icterus,[51] and most had nonspecific signs of serious systemic illness. The rhinocerebral form of zygomycosis seen in immunocompromised people does not appear to occur in dogs and cats.

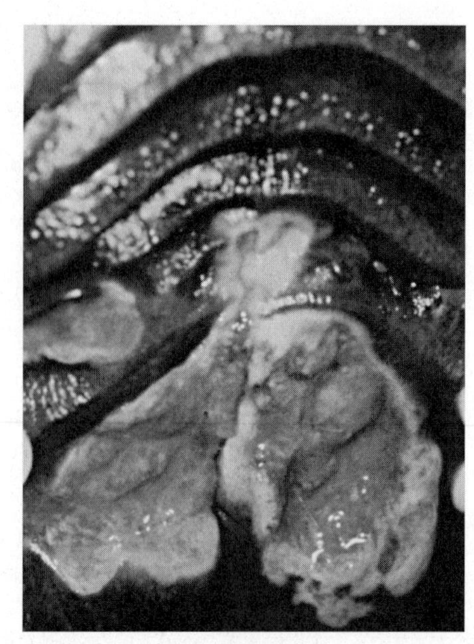

Figure 68–5. Irregular and deep palatal ulcer in a dog with conidiobolomycosis and nasal discharge. This lesion resolved with itraconazole treatment, and there was no recurrence.

DIAGNOSIS AND PATHOLOGIC FINDINGS

Rapid analysis of impression smears or tissue macerated in 10% KOH may provide a tentative diagnosis of zygomycotic disease. In most reported cases, fungal elements are abundant within necrotic centers of tissue masses. The hyphae are broad (> 5μ) and poorly septate. Histologically, special stains are useful, although hyphae are surrounded with eosinophilic granular material (Splendore-Hoeppli) and are found within eosinophilic granulomas. The only problematic differential diagnosis histologically is pythiosis.

Zygomycetes are, for the most part, readily cultured from properly obtained surgical specimens or even from uncontaminated swabs (see Fig. 56–6). However, not all microbiology laboratories have the capability of specific identification of isolates, so referral to reference laboratories may be required.[67]

For publishable cases and on individual requests, there are experimentally available ELISA[28] and immunodiffusion assays[23, 26] for serologic testing in people with either mucormycosis or subcutaneous entomophthoromycosis, and there are immunohistochemical techniques for use on tissue specimens.[25]

THERAPY

For disseminated and abdominal mucormycosis, the patient's prognosis is grave. When GI lesions can be completely excised, there is some hope of a cure. The susceptibility of most of the Mucorales to antimycotic agents is quite variable, and in vitro susceptibility testing is recommended. Seriously ill dogs or cats should be treated with initial AMB therapy while results are awaited. All of the imidazoles and triazoles were not effective in experimental guinea pig *Rhizopus* infection, but AMB was effective in 75%.[71] Disseminated zygomycosis in neutropenic people has been almost uniformly fatal; however, AMB-lipid complex and granulocyte–colony-stimulating factor followed by suppressive AMB maintenance therapy has been effective in one person.[20] For therapeutic dosages in an animal, see Drug Formulary, Appendix 8.

In horses and in humans, subcutaneous entomophthoromycoses have been treated successfully with a variety of modalities, including hyperthermia, SC administration of AMB, systemic and local MCZ and systemic KTZ,[70] and potassium and sodium iodides. Unfortunately, none of these treatments are consistently useful. Susceptibility testing for several isolates of *Basidiobolus* and *Conidiobolus* has been reported.[69, 75] MCZ and KTZ showed most consistent activity. AMB is active against some isolates. Most reports of cures in human cases have been achieved with surgery and long-term ITZ. When these infections are confined to the skin, surgical resection may be curative with or without follow-up chemotherapy. Because antifungal chemotherapy is long term, it should ideally be based on results of in vitro susceptibility tests.

Adiaspiromycosis

Adiaspiromycosis affects the lungs of humans, foxes, and rodents. It is caused by an enlarging but nongerminating spore of the fungus *Emmonsia (Chrysosporium) parva*, a soil inhabitant. Invasive infections with *Emmonsia* are occasionally described in dogs,[72] but only one pathologically well-documented case of adiaspiromycosis is available.[30] Fungal pneumonia and incidental findings at necropsy are the expected clinical correlates. The spores tend to mineralize in other species with adiaspiromycosis. In pathologic specimens, the spores must be distinguished from the spherules of *Coccidioides* and *Rhinosporidium*; however, the adiaspores are exceedingly thick walled and generally devoid of contents. *Emmonsia* spp. are regularly isolated in surveys of mycologic flora of dog and cat hair coats.

Hyalohyphomycosis

Hyalohyphomycoses are opportunistic infections caused by nondematiaceous fungi that form hyphal elements in tissue. Aspergillosis and penicilliosis (see Chapter 65) are, by convention, not included. Cases of hyalohyphomycosis described in dogs or cats are summarized in Table 68–1.

ETIOLOGY

In animals and humans, 47 species of fungus, classified in 23 genera in 3 phyla (Deuteromycota, Ascomycota, and Basidiomycota) have been implicated as agents in hyalohyphomycosis.[40] An unidentified species of *Acremonium* has been associated with disseminated disease[66] and with multifocal subcutaneous disease,[19] *A. "hyalinum"* with osteomyelitis and nephritis, and *A. kilense* with keratoconjunctivitis in dogs. *Fusarium* sp. was the cause of an interesting unilateral pyelonephritis and an undocumented case of disseminated disease in Australian dogs. *F. solani* was isolated from an ear lesion of a cat.[10] *Geotrichum candidum* infection has been reported in disseminated diseases[59] and in infections after bite wounds; it has also been reported as a cause of cutaneous nodules and superficial dermatitis[65] in dogs and as a cause of disease in cats.

Paecilomyces fumosoroseus, P. varioti, P. lilacinus, and other *Paecilomyces* sp.[49] have been associated with cutaneous and disseminated lesions in dogs and cats.[38, 54] *Pseudallescheria* (synonyms: *Allescheria, Petriellidium, Scedosporium apiospermum*) *boydii* has been isolated from dogs with pneumonia and from dogs with osteomyelitis and with disseminated disease.[61] Hypercalcemia, as noted with other granulomatous diseases, was found in a dog with disseminated infection.[38]

The fungi associated with hyalohyphomycosis are generally ubiquitous soil saprophytic molds and are common contaminants of laboratory cultures. *Paecilomyces lilacinus* is found in tap water and contaminates "sterile" solutions. *Geotrichum*, which is difficult to distinguish mycologically from *Trichosporon*, may also be considered a normal part of the oral and GI flora.[33] Kwon-Chung and Bennett[33] considered many of the reported cases of invasive *Geotrichum* infection in animals and humans to have questionable identifications of the agent. *P. boydii* causes disease in human beings much more commonly than the other agents of hyalohyphomycosis and causes disparate syndromes, especially in immunocompromised persons, including sinusitis, keratitis, brain abscess, arthritis, fungal ball, endocarditis, cutaneous disease, and disseminated disease.

Although saprophytic fungi are considered opportunistic infectious agents, in local or disseminated disease in dogs and cats, rarely is an associated predisposing condition identified. *Fusarium* infections, in particular, are associated with neutropenia in humans, and *P. boydii* is associated with neutropenia and with HIV infection,[40] but these types of associations have not yet been made for companion animals. However, a tendency to affect the German shepherd breed[72] and a dissemination after treatment with glucocorticoids[59] have been noted.

CLINICAL FINDINGS

Altogether, too few cases of any individual type of infection in this category exist to draw conclusions about any propensity of a particular fungal species to cause a particular clinical syndrome. *Geotrichum*, in particular, and *Paecilomyces* may colonize epithelial surfaces and thus may be more likely to begin as local disease after wounding or to remain confined to skin or mucosae. For each species, however, there are reports of disseminated disease, which can result from immunosuppression caused by terminal illness, immunosuppressive drugs, or long-term antibiotic usage. Dissemination is apparently hematogenous. Signs vary with the organ system affected, which includes the nasal passages, sinuses, lungs, CNS, myocardium, bone and bone marrow, lymph nodes, spleen, kidneys, liver, peritoneum, and pleura. Pneumonia has been prominent in dogs with disseminated geotrichosis.[59] One case of unilateral pyelonephritis with local extension into the retroperitoneal space was associated with *Fusarium*.[12] There are cases of cutaneous and subcutaneous nodules, localized or widespread. *Acremonium*, *Fusarium*, and *Pseudallescheria* (and *Scedosporium*) are reported as causes of canine keratomycosis.[39]

DIAGNOSIS AND PATHOLOGIC FINDINGS

Many potentially pathogenic fungi in this group of agents are common laboratory contaminants. Furthermore, most can frequently be isolated from the skin and hair coats of normal animals.[8, 18, 47, 48] Documentation of invasive disease involves cultural and histopathologic correlation. Histopathologically, tissue invasion and morphologic characteristics compatible with a fungus from culturing properly obtained clinical specimens renders the most definitive diagnosis (see Figs. 56–13 and 56–14). Specimens should not be contaminated with epithelial flora or obtained from open wounds. When appropriate specimens were not obtained for fungal culture or when histopathologic specimens are the only material available, most pathogenic fungal species can be tentatively identified with immunohistochemical techniques. In the United States, this type of testing is generally obtainable only by referral of the specimens to the CDC in Atlanta, GA, however.

THERAPY

Animals with disseminated or CNS disease carry a grave prognosis. In many reported cases, treatment has been attempted with AMB or imidazole. Many reports have described treatment with ITZ in particular. In a report of disseminated paecilomycosis in a dog, initial apparent response to combined flucytosine and fluconazole therapy was followed by recurrence and death.[49] In some cases, treatment seems to prolong the survival of dogs with disseminated disease,[38, 66, 72] but few dogs have been reported to survive disseminated hyalohyphomycosis. If treatment is to be attempted, the isolate should be subjected to in vitro susceptibility testing to formulate a rational therapeutic plan. In keratitis or deep infection with *P. boydii* in humans, combination therapy with amphotericin and antifungal azoles is recommended.[40] When disease is localized, surgical removal is the treatment of choice, although dissemination might be expected. Keratitis is often treated with topical natamycin or MCZ. A special note should be made regarding the treatment of *Paecilomyces* infection, because the various species in the genus have apparently very different drug susceptibilities. *P. varioti* is reportedly sensitive to AMB and flucytosine, whereas *P. lilacinus* is resistant to these and sensitive to imidazoles and even to griseofulvin.[9]

Phaeohyphomycosis

ETIOLOGY AND EPIDEMIOLOGY

Phaeohyphomycoses are uncommon opportunistic infections caused by a number of ubiquitous saprophytic and plant pathogenic molds with the characteristic of forming pigmented (dematiaceous) hyphal elements in tissue. The pigment is melanin; the fungus may be very pale to very dark and will generally stain with Masson-Fontana melanin in histopathologic sections. Taxonomy of the commonly implicated agents is confusing, and generic names are changed frequently. A review stated that 101 species, belonging to 57 genera, classified as Deuteromycetes, have been described as agents of phaeohyphomycosis in animals or humans.[40] These fungi are thought to be one of the major emerging groups of pathogenic fungi in laboratory diagnosis.[41]

In phaeohyphomycosis, hyphae differ from those associated with most hyalohyphomycoses by having thick walls, varying diameters, and yeastlike swellings. Phaeohyphomycosis differs from the human disease *chromoblastomycosis* in that the spherical yeastlike bodies lack septa in two perpendicular planes, as is seen in the sclerotic bodies of the chromoblastomycosis infection. Phaeohyphomycosis should also be distinguished from dark-grain mycetomas, which are discussed in the following section. All of these infections caused by pigmented fungi are often called "chromomycoses."

The organisms that have been isolated from canine and feline phaeohyphomycotic infections include *Alternaria alternata*,[52] *A. infectoria*,[60] *Bipolaris (Drechslera) spicifera*,[73] *Cladosporium (Xylohypha) bantianum (= X. emmonsii?)*,[36] *Cladosporium trichoides*, *Curvularia geniculatu*, *Curvularia lunata*, *Exophiala jeanselmei*,[44, 46] (=*Phialophora gougerotti*),[37] *E. spinifer*,[9a, 29] *Moniliella suaveolens*, *Ochroconis (Dactylaria) gallopavum*,[53] *Phialemonium obovatum*, *Phialophora verrucosa*, *Pseudomicrodochium suttonii*, *Scolecobasidium humicola*, and *Stemphyllium* sp.

Alternaria, *Xylohypha*, *Bipolaris*, *Exophiala*, *Phialemonium*, *Phialophora*, and *Stemphyllium* are ubiquitous wood and soil saprophytes. *Moniliella* has been recovered from cheese, butter, and margarine. *Scolecobasidium* is usually a cause of phaeohyphomycosis in cold-blooded vertebrates. Several of the potentially pathogenic species have been cultured from the skin of clinically healthy people, cats, and dogs.[8, 18, 47, 48] Animals and people presumably are exposed to infection with dematiaceous fungi by wound contamination, especially through wood slivers, although initial respiratory tract colonization cannot be ruled out in systemic cases. The route of exposure in cerebral phaeohyphomycosis is not understood, and extension from sinus infection, orbital injury, and middle ear infection has been postulated for human cases. *Bipolaris* species are usually associated with paranasal sinus infections in humans,[40] and rhinitis has been described in a cat.[46] Some species of *Cladosporium* demonstrate neurotropism. Only rarely are cases of phaeohyphomycosis in animals associated with other systemic disorders. These infections are not associated with HIV-induced immunosuppression in humans. Intact granulocyte function is the important defense mecha-

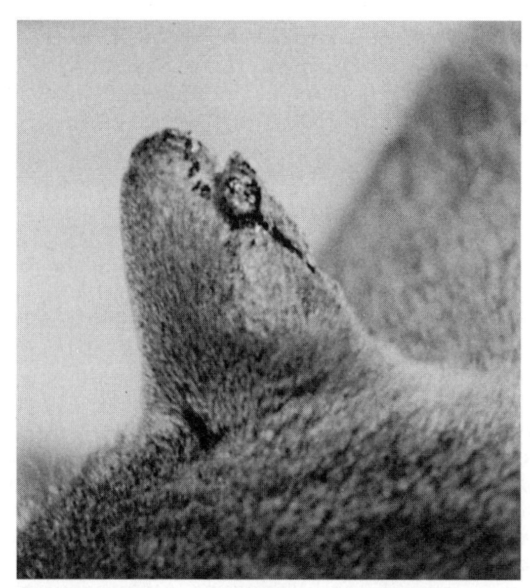

Figure 68–6. Cutaneous phaeohyphomycosis on the pinna of a cat showing ulcerated and crusted nodule. This lesion was pigmented clinically and on cut surface. The disease was resolved by routine excisional biopsy.

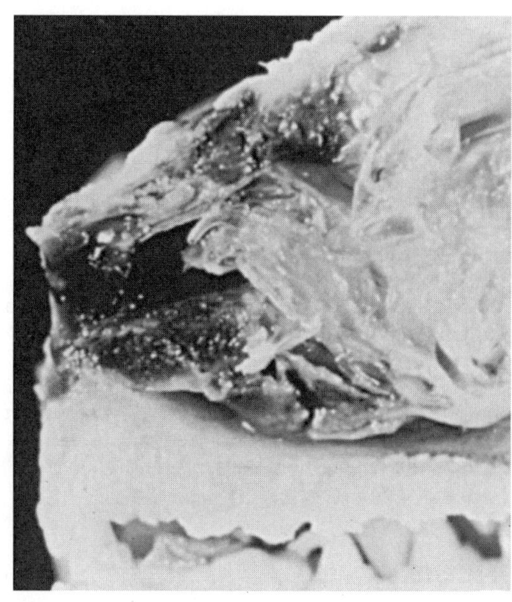

Figure 68–8. This necropsy specimen of a cat with nasal phaeohyphomycosis illustrates the darkly pigmented nature of the infiltrate. The pigment is imparted by fungal melanin. (Courtesy of Dr. Richard I. Miller, Australia.)

nism against these infectious agents.[40] Persistent lymphopenia has been either a cause or an effect of infection in dogs with systemic infections.[36] Hyperglobulinemia can occur as a result of a persistent but ineffective humoral response to eliminate the infection. Of the reported cases, one dog had been treated with long courses of glucocorticoids, one dog had ehrlichiosis, and one cat had leukemia. All of these patients had disseminated phaeohyphomycosis.

CLINICAL FINDINGS

Subcutaneous Phaeohyphomycosis

Singular or multifocal, poorly circumscribed, and ulcerating or fistulizing nodules and plaques characterize this infection (Figs. 68–6 and 68–7). The fungal pigmentation is often apparent in the tissue. In cats, the lesions may resemble chronic bacterial abscesses or thick-walled "cysts." The disease may evolve over weeks to months, and in dogs, cutaneous lesions have been associated with osteomyelitis. In a report of phaeohyphomycosis in a dog caused by *Curvularia geniculatum*, the lesions had a sporotrichoid appearance, with involvement of lymphatics and lymph nodes on the affected limb.[3] Most cases have been described in cats, and lesions in this species most often occur on the face or distal extremities (Fig. 68–8). *Bipolaris spicifera*, *Exophiala jeanselmei*, and *Phialophora verrucosa* are the most common isolates.

Cerebral (Encephalitic or Brain Abscess) Phaeohyphomycosis

The agents involved are almost always *Cladosporium (Xylohypha)* species. Dogs and cats are both affected. CNS disease can also develop as a manifestation of disseminated phaeohy-

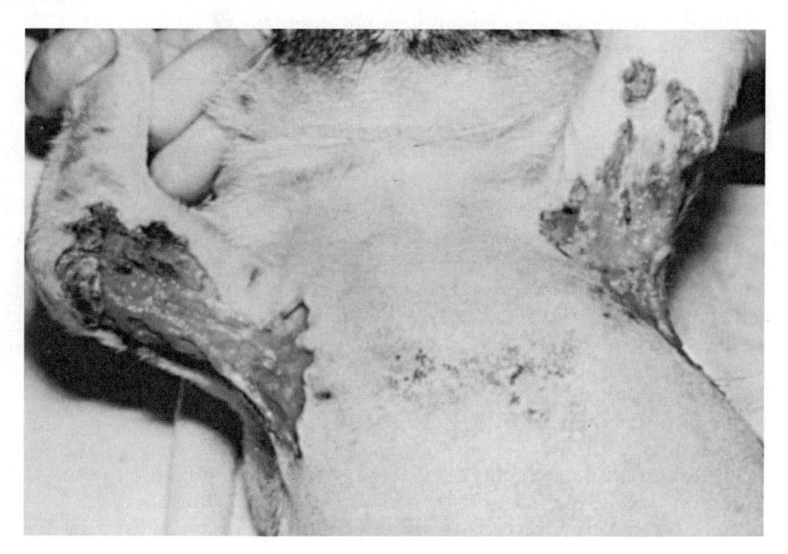

Figure 68–7. This extensive cutaneous ulceration is caused by subcutaneous phaeohyphomycosis due to *Bipolaris spicifera*. (Courtesy of Dr. Kenneth Kwochka, The Ohio State University.)

phomycosis. Neurologic dysfunction varies with the site of disease, because most cases are localized brain abscess.

Keratomycosis in a cat has been associated with *Cladosporium (Xylohypha)* and in dogs with *Alternaria* and *Curvularia*.

Disseminated Phaeohyphomycosis

Systemic disease usually has an acute to subacute course, with symptoms referable to the organ system involved. As noted, CNS disease is prominent and is invariably fatal, and some patients have potentially immunosuppressive conditions. One report may serve as an example.[62] An 8-year-old Maltese cross dog with ehrlichiosis demonstrated CNS signs and hepatomegaly from infection with *Cladosporium bantianum*. Necropsy revealed pigmented fungal granulomas in the liver parenchyma, spleen, renal cortices, adrenal glands, and gray and white matter of the CNS.

DIAGNOSIS

Direct examination of exudate or macerated tissue mounted in KOH may reveal the pigmented fungal elements. As with other opportunistic mycoses, confirmation of the diagnosis is based on the concomitant demonstration of hyphae in tissue and culture of a morphologically compatible organism from properly obtained tissue specimens. These organisms grow readily on Sabouraud's dextrose agar, although specialized agar may be required to encourage production of the identifying fruiting bodies (see Fig. 56–12). In any case, some expertise is required for specific mycologic identification, and referral to specialized laboratories may be required.[67] When culture cannot be obtained, specific identification of the most commonly pathogenic species may be performed with experimental immunohistochemical techniques, available at the CDC.

THERAPY

The animal's prognosis in disseminated CNS disease or in widespread cutaneous disease is grave. In the localized cutaneous forms often seen in cats, successful treatment has been described. When the lesions are excisable, surgery may be curative, but recurrence at the same or at new sites is common.

In unexcisable or recurrent cases, antifungal chemotherapy may be helpful but response is unpredictable. Drugs should be chosen on the basis of in vitro susceptibility testing; the imidazoles show variable in vitro activity against saprophytic organisms. A cat apparently has been cured after multiple excisions and treatment with KTZ. Yet another has been treated successfully with AMB. In other feline cases, treatment with both KTZ and flucytosine was unsuccessful. In a published report, a dog with disseminated cutaneous infection with *Phialemonium curvatum* was cured long term with KTZ (5 mg/kg/day).[6] Surprisingly, there are as yet few reported cases in veterinary medicine concerning the usefulness of the triazoles for these disease syndromes. ITZ treatment of human subcutaneous and musculoskeletal phaeohyphomycosis has been reviewed[64]; of 17 patients assessed, only 3 were cured, although another 6 improved. In all cases the fungal isolates were reported as susceptible to ITZ on in vitro testing. A cat with granulomatous rhinitis caused by *Exophiala jeanselmei* was successfully treated with oral ITZ given for 30 days.[46]

Eumycotic Mycetoma

Mycetomas are pyogranulomatous nodules that contain tissue grains or granules. Within the grains are dense colonies of organisms along with host-derived matter, usually necrotic debris.

ETIOLOGY

When mycetomas are caused by fungi, they are known as eumycotic mycetomas to distinguish them from actinomycotic lesions (see Chapter 49) and botryomycosis. Eumycotic mycetomas must also be differentiated from the pseudomycetomas seen in generalized dermatophytosis in long-haired cats. (See Chapter 58.)

Eumycotic mycetomas may be caused by fungi that impart their pigmented appearance to the grains in tissue. These are called black- or dark-grain mycetomas. Black-grain mycetomas have been associated with infections by *Curvularia* spp. and *Madurella* spp. When the agents are unpigmented, they cause white-grain mycetomas. White-grain mycetomas have been caused by *Acremonium* and *Pseudallescheria*. Most eumycotic mycetomas are confined to the subcutaneous tissues, but white-grain mycetomas on the body wall may be extensions of abdominal cavity disease. Fungal isolation from affected dogs and cats has not been done in all cases. Of the black-grain mycetomas, *Curvularia geniculata* is the most common isolate, and cases caused by *C. spicifera*, *C. lunata*,[14] and *C. senegalensis*[10] have been reported. In abdominal and body wall white-grain mycetoma of the dog, *P. boydii* and *Acremonium hyalinum* have been isolated. Disseminated infection was caused by *Acremonium* sp. in a dog.[66] *Madurella grisea* has been isolated from a cat with mycetoma, and *M. mycetomatis* from a dog.[34]

CLINICAL FINDINGS

In white-grain mycetomas, most infections have involved abdominal cavity organs. Dogs have developed peritonitis or abdominal masses after contamination from unrelated surgical wound dehiscence. As with aspergillosis, German shepherd dogs have the greatest prevalence rate of infection. Peritonitis and intra-abdominal granulomas accompanied by symptoms typical of septic peritonitis are noted. Lesions within the abdomen have tissue grains and are usually caused by *P. boydii*. Systemic infection caused by *Acremonium* was characterized by signs of neurologic dysfunction, uveitis, and visceral granulomas.[66] A black-grain mycetoma caused by *M. mycetomatis* developed at the site of a uterine stump, subsequent to wound dehiscence following ovariohysterectomy.[34]

Cutaneous mycetoma has been the typical finding of black-grain infection. Infection probably develops at the site of a superficial wound, possibly contaminated by a plant foreign body. Such cases are more often reported in dogs than in cats and are most often caused by *Curvularia* spp. In one cat, a black mycetoma developed after a bite wound. Lesions are cutaneous nodules, relatively poorly circumscribed, usually on the extremities or the face. They do not often ulcerate widely, but fistulas may form within the nodule. Most become surmounted by alopecic and hyperkeratotic epidermis. Cycles of healing and ulceration may lead to firm swelling and scarring. Black tissue grains may be visible within the exudate, or the exudate or the tissue itself may appear black. Some nodules are so heavily pigmented that they are mistaken for cutaneous melanomas. On the limbs and feet, the infectious process may involve underlying bone.

DIAGNOSIS AND PATHOLOGIC FINDINGS

A presumptive diagnosis of mycetoma may be made if there are grains within exudate from any draining tract. Cytologic investigation must be directed at the tissue grains, because the organism is often scant or absent elsewhere within exudate or tissue. Grains may be crushed and smeared on a slide for staining in some cases. Black grains are often gritty and may require digestion in 10% KOH before they can be mounted for microscopic study. The fungal elements are usually quite evident in thinly smeared or flattened grains. Serum may be tested for specific antibodies by agar gel immunodiffusion. In histopathologic specimens, common fungi may be identified by immunohistochemical techniques.

Investigation by culture technique is otherwise necessary to confirm cytologic findings and to identify the causative organism. Tissue grains may be collected from exudate and washed in sterile saline for culturing. Alternatively, surgically excised tissue, if it contains grains, may be cultured. Fungal isolates should be retained for possible in vitro susceptibility testing. The agents associated with mycetomas in dogs and cats are readily cultured on standard media.

THERAPY

The prognosis in abdominal mycetoma is guarded, because patients described to date have had extensive involvement of abdominal organs and have not responded to debridement and/or chemotherapy. Cutaneous mycetoma is not a life-threatening disease but is difficult to resolve. Radical surgical excision has been the treatment most often used in human cases. Amputation of affected limbs may be necessary; spontaneous resolution does not occur. Any attempt at antifungal chemotherapy should be based on in vitro susceptibility testing of the isolate. Even if an antifungal chemotherapeutic agent that may be helpful is identified, it is apparently difficult to attain effective levels within the tissue grains where the organism resides. Successful outcomes have been reported in human cases with local hyperthermia treatments and improvement with high-dose ITZ.[58]

References

1. Allison N, McDonald RK, Guist SR, et al. 1989. Eumycotic mycetoma caused by *Pseudallescheria boydii* in a dog. *J Am Vet Med Assoc* 194:797–799.
2. Barboza-Quintana A, Guiris-Andrade DM, Ramirez-Romero R, et al. 1990. Zygomycotic enteritis in the dog: case report. *Vet Mex* 21:425–428.

2a. Bauer RW, LeMarie SL, Roy AF. 1997. Oral conidiobolomycosis in a dog. *Vet Derm* 8:115–120.

3. Beale KM, Pinson D. 1990. Phaeohyphomycosis caused by two different species of *Curvularia* in two animals from the same household. *J Am Anim Hosp Assoc* 26:67–70.
4. Bentinck-Smith J, Padhye AA, Maslin WR, et al. 1989. Canine pythiosis—isolation and identification of *Pythium insidiosum*. *J Vet Diagn Invest* 1:295–298.
5. Bissonnette KW, Sharp NJH, Dykstra MH, et al. 1991. Nasal and retrobulbar mass in a cat caused by *Pythium insidiosum*. *J Med Vet Mycol* 29:39–44.
6. Bourdeau P, Daix B, Martel AF, et al. 1996. Pyogranulomatous panniculitis due to *Phialemonium curvatum* in the dog, p 129. In Proceedings of the Third World Congress of Veterinary Dermatology, Edinburgh.
7. Brown CC, McClure JJ, Triche P, Crowder C. 1988. Use of immunohistochemical methods for diagnosis of equine pythiosis. *Am J Vet Res* 49:1866–1868.
8. Caretta G, Mancianti F, Ajello L. 1989. Dermatophytes and keratinophilic fungi in cats and dogs. *Mycoses* 32:620–626.
9. Castro LGM, Salebian A, Sotto MN. 1990. Hyalohyphomycosis by *Paecilomyces lilacinus* in a renal transplant patient and a review of human *Paecilomyces* species infections. *J Med Vet Mycol* 28:15–26.

9a. Chermette R, Ferreiro L, Debievre C, et al. 1997. *Exophiala spinifera* nasal infection in a cat and a literature review of feline phaeohyphomycoses. *J Mycol Med* 7:149–158.

10. Connole MD. 1990. Review of animal mycoses in Australia. *Mycopathologia* 11:133–164.
11. Cooper RC Jr, Allison N, Boring JG. 1991. Apparent successful treatment of intestinal pythiosis with vascular invasion in a dog. *Canine Pract* 16:9–12.
12. Day MJ, Holt PE. 1994. Unilateral fungal pyelonephritis in a dog. *Vet Pathol* 31:250–252.
13. Duncan D, Hodgin C, Bauer R, Brignac M. 1992. Cutaneous pythiosis in four cats (abstract). *Vet Pathol* 29:5.
14. Elad D, Orgad U, Yakogson B, et al. 1991. Eumycetoma caused by *Curvularia lunata* in a dog. *Mycopathologia* 116:113–118.
15. Fischer JR, Pace LW, Turk JR, et al. 1994. Gastrointestinal pythiosis in Missouri dogs: eleven cases. *J Vet Diagn Invest* 6:380–382.
16. Foil CS. 1990. Miscellaneoous fungal infections, pp 731–741. *In* Greene CE (ed), Infectious diseases of the dog and cat. WB Saunders, Philadelphia, PA.
17. Foil CS. 1994. Fungal Diseases. *Clin Dermatol* 12:529–542.

17a. Fuchs A, Brever R, Axman H, et al. 1996. Subcutaneous mycosis in a cat due to *Staphylotrichum coccosporum*. *Mycosis* 39:381.

18. Gambale W, Larsson CE, Moritami MM, et al. 1993. Dermatophytes and other fungi of the haircoat of cats without dermatophytosis in the city of Sao Paulo, Brazil. *Feline Pract* 21:29–33.
19. Gonzales-Cabo JF, Latre-Cequiel MV, Solans-Aisa C, et al. 1987. Aislamiento de *Acremonium* sp. En un caso de dermatitis canina. *Med Vet* 4:93–96.
20. Gonzalez CE, Couriel DR, Walsh TJ. 1997. Disseminated zygomycosis in a neutropenic patient: successful treatment with amphotericin B lipid complex and granulocyte colony-stimulating factor. *Clin Infect Dis* 24:192–196.
21. Hillier A, Kunkle GA, Ginn PE, et al. 1994. Canine subcutaneous zygomycosis caused by *Conidiobolus* sp.: a case report and review of *Conidiobolus* infections in other species. *Vet Dermatol* 5:205–213.
22. Howerth EW, Brown CC, Crowder C. 1989. Subcutaneous pythiosis in a dog. *J Vet Diagn Invest* 1:81–83.
23. Imwidthaya P, Srimuang S. 1992. Immunodiffusion test for diagnosing basidiobolomycosis. *Mycopathologia* 118:127–131.
24. Jand SK, Gupta MP. 1989. Dermatomycosis in dogs. *Mycoses* 32:104–105.
25. Jensen HE, Aalbaek B, Lind P, et al. 1996. Immunohistochemical diagnosis of systemic bovine zygomycosis by murine monoclonal antibodies. *Vet Pathol* 33:176–183.
26. Kaufman L, Mendoza L, Standard PG. 1990. Immunodiffusion test for serodiagnosing subcutaneous zygomycosis. *J Clin Microbiol* 28:1887–1890.
27. Kaufman L, Standard PG. 1987. Specific and rapid identification of medically important fungi by exoantigen detection. *Ann Rev Microbiol* 41:209–225.
28. Kaufman L, Turner LF, McLaughlin DW. 1989. Indirect enzyme-linked immunosorbent assay for zygomycosis. *J Clin Microbiol* 27:1979–1982.
29. Kettlewell P, McGinnis MR, Wilkinson GT. 1989. Phaeohyphomycosis caused by *Exophiala spinifera* in two cats. *J Med Vet Mycol* 27:257–264.
30. Koller LD, Patton NM, Whitsett DK. 1976. Adiaspiromycosis in the lungs of a dog. *J Am Vet Med Assoc* 169:1316–1317.
31. Kumar B, Kaur I, Chakrabati A, et al. 1991. Treatment of deep mycoses with itraconazole. *Mycopathologia* 115:169–174.
32. Kwon-Chung KJ. 1994. Phylogenetic spectrum of fungi that are pathogenic to humans. *Clin Infect Dis* 19(Suppl 1):S1–S7.
33. Kwon-Chung KJ, Bennett JE. 1992. Medical mycology. Lea & Febiger, Philadelphia, PA.
34. Lambrechts N, Collett MG, Henton M. 1991. Black grain eumycetoma (*Madurella mycetomatis*) in the abdominal cavity of a dog. *J Med Vet Mycol* 29:211–214.
35. LeMarie SL, Bauer RW, Foil CS, et al. 1994. Conidiobolomycosis in a dog (abstract). *Vet Dermatol* 5:144.
36. Lobetti RG. 1996. Leukogram and serum globulin values in two dogs with systemic *Xylohypha bantiana* infection. *J S Afr Vet Assoc* 67:91–92.
37. Malik R, Wigney D, Muir D. 1994. Phaeohyphomycosis caused by *Exophiala jeanselmei* in a cat. *Aust Vet Pract* 24:27–31.
38. March PA, Knowles K, Dillavou CL, et al. 1996. Diagnosis, treatment, and temporary remission of disseminated paecilomycosis in a Vizsla. *J Am Anim Hosp Assoc* 32:509–514.
39. Marlar AB, Miller PE, Canton DD, et al. 1994. Canine keratomycosis: a

report of eight cases and literature review. *J Am Anim Hosp Assoc* 30:331–340.
40. Matsumoto T, Ajello L, Matsuda T, et al. 1994. Developments in hyalohyphomycosis and phaeohyphomycosis. *J Med Vet Mycol* 32(Suppl):329–349.
41. Matsumoto T, Padhye AA, Ajello L. 1987. Medical significance of the so-called black yeasts. *Eur J Epidemiol* 3:87–95.
42. McLaughlin BG, Ayer AA. 1995. Gastrointestinal pythiosis in a dog from Kentucky. *Can Pract* 20:17–19.
43. Mendoza L, Hernandez F, Ajello L. 1993. Life cycle of the human and animal Oomycete pathogen *Pythium insidiosum*. *J Clin Microbiol* 31:2967–2973.
44. Mendoza L, Prendas J. 1988. A method to obtain rapid zoosporogenesis of *Pythium insidiosum*. *Mycopathologia* 104:59–62.
45. Mendoza L, Villalobos J, Calleje CE, et al. 1992. Evaluation of two vaccines for the treatment of pythiosis insidiosi in horses. *Mycopathologia* 119:89–95.
46. Michaud AJ. 1993. Phaeohyphomycotic rhinitis due to *Exophiala jeanselmei* in a domestic cat. *Feline Pract* 21:19–23.
47. Moriello KA, DeBoer DJ. 1991. Fungal flora of the coat of pet cats. *Am J Vet Res* 52:602–606.
48. Moriello KA, DeBoer DJ. 1991. Fungal flora of the haircoat of cats with and without dermatophytosis. *J Med Vet Mycol* 29:285–292.
49. Nakagawa Y, Mochizuki R, Iwasaki K, et al. 1996. A canine case of profound granulomatosis due to *Paecilomyces* fungus. *J Vet Med Sci* 58:157–159.
50. Nuttall W, Woodgyer A, Butler S. 1990. Phaeohyphomycosis caused by *Exophiala jeanselmei* in a domestic cat. *N Z Vet J* 38:123.
51. Ossent P. 1987. Systemic aspergillosis and mucormycosis in 23 cats. *Vet Rec* 120:330–333.
52. Outerbridge CA, Myers SL, Summerbell RC. 1995. Phaeohyphomycosis in a cat. *Can Vet J* 36:629–630.
53. Padhye AA, Amster RL, Browning M, et al. 1994. Fatal encephalitis caused by *Ochroconis gallopavum* in a domestic cat (*Felis domesticus*). *J Med Vet Mycol* 32:141–145.
54. Patterson JM, Rosendal S, Humphry J, et al. 1983. A case of disseminated paecilomycosis in the dog. *J Am Anim Hosp Assoc* 19:569–574.
55. Patton CS, Hake R, Newton J. 1996. Esophagitis due to *Pythium insidiosum* infection in two dogs. *J Vet Intern Med* 10:139–142.
56. Piontelli LE, Toro SM. 1987. Domestic animals (dogs and cats) as fungus reservoirs. *Bol Micol* 3:149–158.
57. Pracharktam R, Changtrakool P, Sathapatayavongs B, et al. 1991. Immunodiffusion test for diagnosis and monitoring of human pythiosis insidiosi. *J Clin Microbiol* 29:2661–2662.
58. Resnik BI, Burdick AE. 1995. Improvement of eumycetoma with itraconazole. *J Am Acad Dermatol* 33:917–919.
59. Rhyan JC, Stackhouse LL, Davis EG. 1990. Disseminated geotrichosis in two dogs. *J Am Vet Med Assoc* 197:358–360.
60. Roosje PJ, de Hoog GS, Koeman JP, et al. 1993. Phaeohyphomycosis in a cat caused by *Alternaria infectoria* EG Simmons. *Mycoses* 36:11–12.
61. Salkin IF, Cooper CR, Bartges JW, et al. 1992. *Scedosporium inflatum* osteomyelitis in a dog. *J Clin Microbiol* 30:2797–2800.
62. Schroeder H, Jardine JE, Davis V. 1994. Systemic phaeohyphomycosis caused by *Xylohypha bantiana* in a dog. *J S Afr Vet Assoc* 65:175–178.
63. Sekon AS, Padhye AA, Garg AK. 1992. In vitro sensitivity of *Penicillium marneffei* and *Pythium insidiosum* to various antifungal agents. *Eur J Epidemiol* 8:427–432.
64. Sharkey PK, Graybill JR, Rinaldi MG, et al. 1990. Itraconazole treatment of phaeohyphomycosis. *J Am Acad Dermatol* 23:577–586.
65. Sidhu RK, Singh KB, Jand SK, et al. 1993. Cutaneous geotrichosis in a dog and its handler—a case report. *Indian J Anim Health* 32:1.
66. Simpson KW, Khan KNM, Podell M, et al. 1993. Systemic mycosis caused by *Acremonium* sp in a dog. *J Am Vet Med Assoc* 203:1296–1299.
67. Smith JMB. 1989. Opportunistic mycoses of man and other animals. CAB International, Exeter, England.
68. Taboada J. 1992. Oomycosis (pythiosis): biology, clinical disease and therapeutic implications, pp 715–718. In Proceedings of the 10th Annual Meeting of the American College of Veterinary Internal Medicine, San Diego, CA.
69. Taylor GD, Sekhon AS, Tyrell DLJ, et al. 1987. Rhinofacial zygomycosis caused by *Conidiobolus coronatus*: a case report including in vitro sensitivity to antimycotic agents. *Am J Trop Med Hyg* 36:398–401.
70. Towersey L, Wanke B, Ribeiro Estrella R, et al. 1988. *Conidiobolus coronatus* infection treated with ketoconazole. *Arch Dermatol* 124:1392–1396.
71. Van Cutsem J, van Gerven F, Fransen J, et al. 1989. Treatment of experimental zygomycosis in guinea pigs with azoles and with amphotericin B. *Chemotherapy* 35:267–272.
72. Watt PR, Robins GM, Galloway AM, et al. 1995. Disseminated opportunistic fungal disease in dogs: 10 cases (1982–1990). *J Am Vet Med Assoc* 207:67–70.
73. Waurzyniak BJ, Hoover JP, Clinkenbeard KD, et al. 1992. Dual systemic mycosis caused by *Bipolaris spicifera* and *Torulopsis glabrata* in a dog. *Vet Pathol* 29:566–569.
74. Wolf AM. 1995. Opportunistic algal and fungal infections, pp 324–327. *In* Bonagura JD, Kirk RW (eds), Kirk's current veterinary therapy XII: small animal practice. WB Saunders, Philadelphia, PA.
75. Yangco BG, Okafor JI, TeStrake D. 1984. In vitro susceptibilities of human and wild-type isolates of *Basidiobolus* and *Conidiobolus* species. *Antimicrob Agents Chemother* 25:413–416.
76. Zahari P, Hirst RG, Shipton WA, et al. 1990. The origin and pathogenicity of *Basidiobolus* species in northern Australia. *J Med Vet Mycol* 28:461–468.

Chapter **69**

Protothecosis

Craig E. Greene

ETIOLOGY

Protothecosis is caused by *Prototheca* (a saprophytic achlorophyllous alga that is closely related to the green algae of the genus *Chlorella*). In culture or in tissue, the cells are spherical to oval and range from 1.3 to 13.4 μm in diameter and 1.3 to 16.1 μm in length. The size varies with the stage of development, the species, and the medium used for culture. Organisms have a hyaline cell wall approximately 0.5 μm thick; a granular, basophilic cytoplasm; and a small, centrally located nucleus. In smaller, immature forms, a nucleus may not be evident. Reproduction is by endosporulation, with irregular nuclear and cytoplasmic cleavage resulting in 2 to 20 or more endospores. The mother cell ruptures, discharging tiny replicas that enlarge, mature, and repeat the life cycle. Empty cell casings scattered among intact algal cells may be seen in lesions. Typical *Prototheca* in tissue are seen in Figure 69–1.

Of the three recognized species of *Prototheca*, *P. stagnora*, *P. zopfii*, and *P. wickerhamii*, the last two have been incriminated as pathogens. The species can be differentiated by sugar and alcohol assimilation tests or by FA methods.

EPIDEMIOLOGY AND PATHOGENESIS

The disease has been identified in people and animals of Europe, Asia, Oceania, and North America; a preponderance of cases in the latter region are restricted to the southeastern United States.[6] Ecologically, *Prototheca* are primarily found in

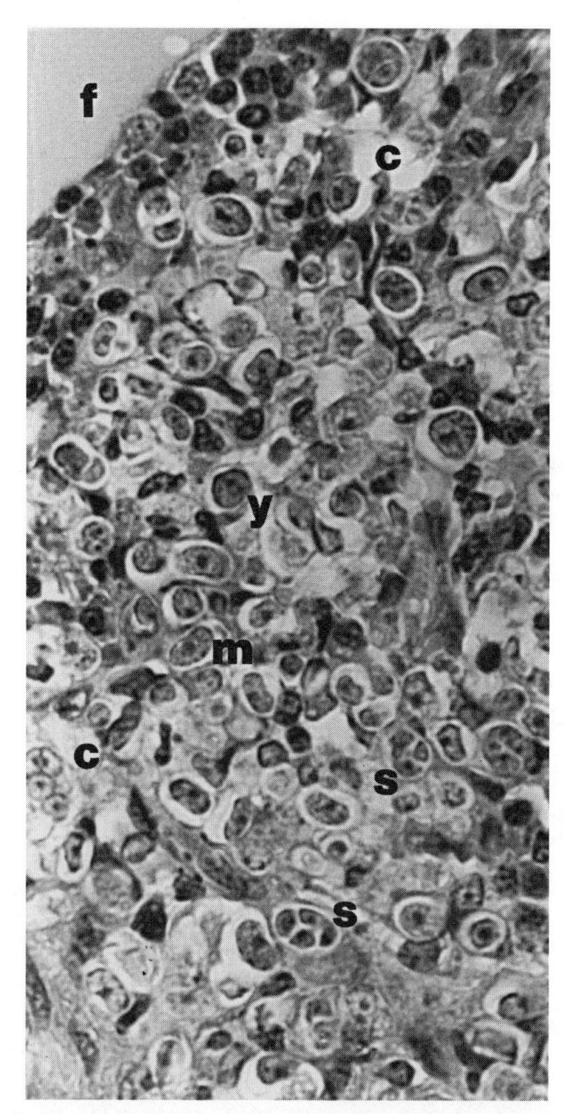

Figure 69–1. *Prototheca* in various stages of development. The lesion is in the thyroid gland. (y = young spherical cell; m = more mature oval cell; s = sporulating cells; c = empty casings of cells that have discharged their spores; f = follicle) (H and E, × 400).

raw and treated sewage, slime flux of trees, and animal wastes. From these sources, *Prototheca* secondarily contaminate water systems, soil, and food, from which they may be ingested by, or come into contact with injured skin or mucosa of, people and animals. Although *Prototheca* can be isolated from freshly voided human and animal feces, the algae are regarded as transient contaminants and only rarely cause diseases. Protothecosis is a sporadic illness that primarily occurs when the host's immune resistance is suppressed or altered, often by pre-existing or concurrent disease. Lack of cell-mediated immunity seems to be a more important factor than decreased humoral responses in allowing entrance of *Prototheca* into tissues and establishment of infection. An association has been made between the develop of protothecosis in people with AIDS.[9, 18] Cases have also occurred in people at sites of prolonged endotracheal intubation or peritoneal catheterization.[4, 7] Another pathogenetic mechanism noted in some infected people is a deficiency in the ability of the host's neutrophils to specifically destroy *Prototheca* after phagocytosis. There has been no evidence of failure of either humoral immunity or cell-mediated immunity in such patients. Evaluation of immune function in one dog with disseminated protothecosis revealed depressed T-lymphocyte function and neutrophil inhibition. A serum inhibitory factor may have been responsible for both findings.

In people, infection is usually cutaneous or SC or bursal, although mucosal, catheter-related, and disseminated infections occur. Cutaneous and localized infections are frequently seen in cats. In contrast, in nearly all canine cases, evidence of protracted colitis with multisystemic dissemination is reported. This finding suggests that, after ingestion by dogs, the colon may be the common site of replication with subsequent spread to other organs by blood and lymph.

Virulence of the organism may differ between species of *Prototheca*. In cutaneous cases in both dogs and cats, only *P. wickerhamii* has been isolated. In contrast, *P. zopfii* is nearly always isolated from disseminated cases in dogs. Breed susceptibility may also be a factor in dogs because a disproportionate number of cases have occurred in collies.[15] There is no age predilection, but a majority of the cases have been in female dogs.

CLINICAL FINDINGS

Dogs

Protothecosis in dogs is generally a widely disseminated disease with clinical signs varying in kind and severity, depending on the tissues involved. The kidney, liver, heart, intestine, brain, and eye are the most common sites of localization. The most frequently reported clinical observation is bloody diarrhea, which is usually intermittent and protracted. Melena or hematochezia may be observed. Weight loss and debility become more pronounced over the course of the disease. Clinical signs attributed directly to involvement of the CNS have been reported in about 40% of the dogs and have included marked depression, ataxia, circling, incoordination, and paresis. Deafness has been observed as have signs of renal failure. Only a few cases of the cutaneous manifestation of the disease have been reported in dogs. Skin lesions are chronic, of many months duration, and characterized by nodules, draining ulcers, and crusty exudates of the trunk and extremities and mucosal surfaces (Fig. 69–2). Even in cutaneous cases, lesions may be disseminated, involving other organs such as the joints, lymph nodes, heart, and lungs.

The eyes are involved in two thirds of the cases, and in some dogs blindness may be the presenting complaint. Leukokoria resulting from vitreous clouding is seen frequently when dogs are first presented for examination. Generally, ophthalmoscopic examination reveals exudative clouding of the fluid in one or both chambers and multiple white, raised foci or streaks in the retina (Fig. 69–3), often accompanied by small hemorrhages. Retinal detachment is usually evident.

Cats

Only the cutaneous form of protothecosis has been reported in cats. Lesions usually occur as large, firm cutaneous nodules on the limbs or feet. They have also been reported on the nose, forehead, pinna, and base of the tail. All cats have been in good health otherwise.

DIAGNOSIS

Whenever a dog with a history of protracted bloody diarrhea coupled with ocular lesions is presented, protothecosis

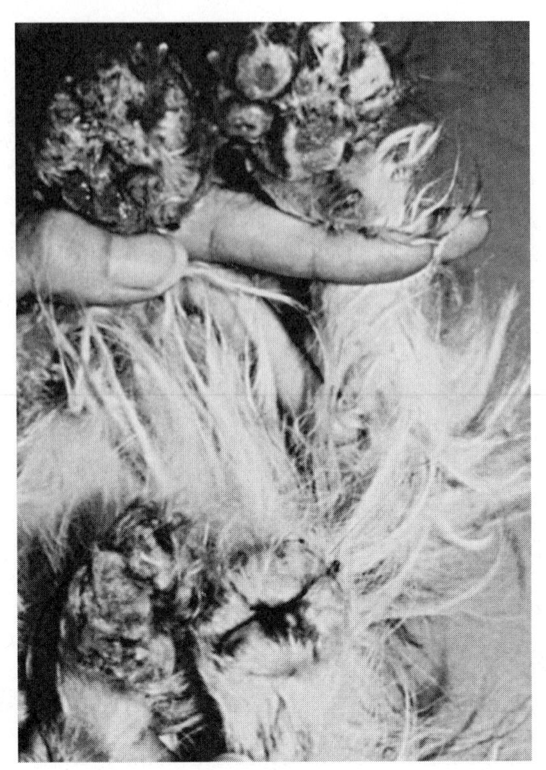

Figure 69–2. Heavy crusts on the footpads of all four feet of a dog with a rare cutaneous form of protothecosis.

should be suspected. Similar suspicion is warranted for cats that develop nodular and ulcerative skin lesions.

Clinical Laboratory Findings

Laboratory data have not been well characterized in the cases of canine and feline protothecosis. Generally, the results of the CBC are within reference ranges, and serum hepatic enzymes rarely are slightly elevated. If present, abnormalities in the CSF may include marked pleocytosis (>100 cells/μl), with granulocytes and lymphocytes being the predominant nucleated cell types, and increased protein (>100 mg/dl).

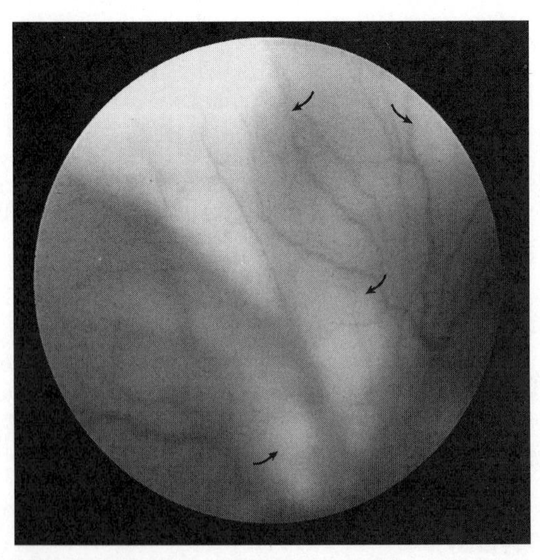

Figure 69–3. Ophthalmoscopic appearance of the ocular fundus from a dog with protothecosis. The retina contains multiple white foci *(arrows)*. (Courtesy of Dr. Susan M. Winston, Marietta, GA.)

Algal Identification and Isolation

Clinically, organisms have been found by culture of fluid obtained by vitreous centesis or CSF, examination of Wright's-stained rectal scrapings (Fig. 69–4), and histologic evaluation of lesion biopsy specimens or enlarged lymph nodes. Because *Prototheca* commonly invades Bowman's space and renal tubules after embolization, finding the organism in the urinary sediment is an accurate way to determine that dissemination of infection has occurred.

Because *Prototheca* and *Chlorella* species are morphologically indistinguishable and because organisms in tissues stained with H and E show variability in staining, Gomori's methenamine silver or periodic acid–Schiff stain is preferred. With these stains, large starch granules are readily seen in *Chlorella* sp. but not in *Prototheca* sp. The presence of chloroplasts is characteristic of *Chlorella*. *Chlorella* has not been reported to infect the dog or cat; however, it has been observed in several other animal species and frequently has been improperly identified as *Prototheca*.

Prototheca grows readily on a variety of laboratory media, such as Sabouraud's cycloheximide-free dextrose agar at 25°C to 37°C, forming white to light tan colonies within 2 to 7 days. Characteristic organisms, in all stages of development, can be recognized by staining a smear from the colony with Gram's iodine stain (Fig. 69–5).

Ribostamycin-impregnated discs have been used to grossly differentiate *Candida* and *Prototheca* colonies on Sabouraud's glucose agar. *Prototheca* shows a halo of inhibition around the discs, whereas *Candida* does not. *Prototheca* species have been separated by the use of clotrimazole-impregnated discs, because *P. wickerhamii* is susceptible to clotrimazole, whereas *P. zopfii* is resistant.

There may be sufficient morphologic differences between

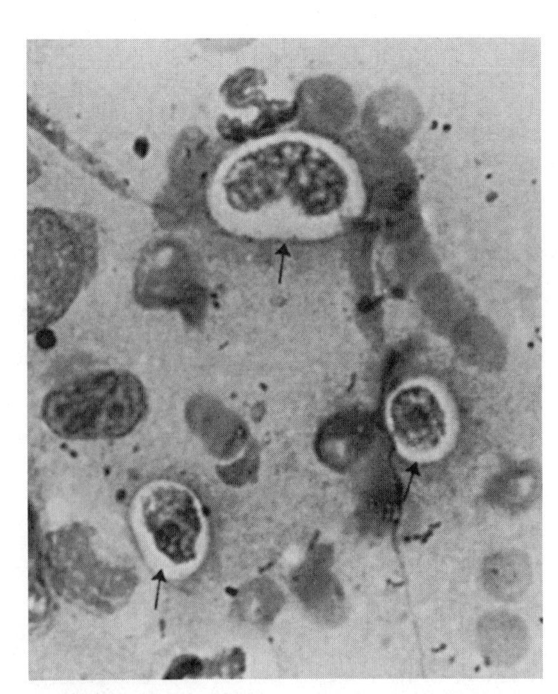

Figure 69–4. Protothecal cells *(arrows)* in a smear of a rectal scraping from a dog with disseminated protothecosis (Wright's stain, × 1008). (Courtesy of Dr. Ken Latimer, University of Georgia, Athens, GA.)

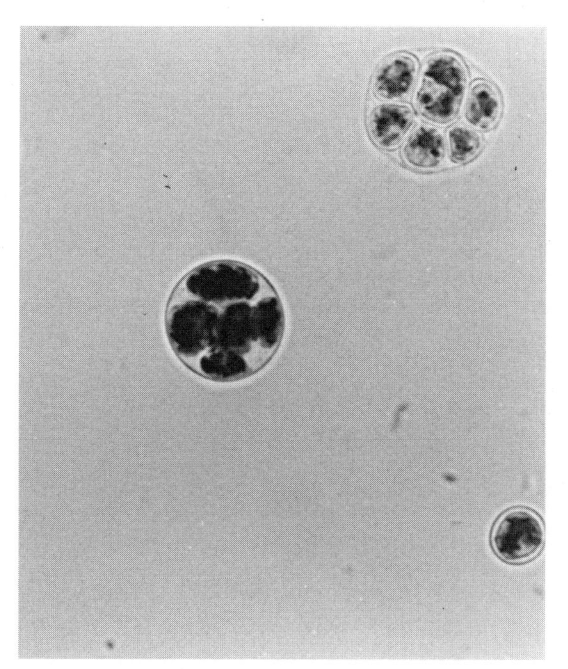

Figure 69–5. Sporulating and nonsporulating forms of *P. zopfii* isolated from canine CSF (Gram's iodine stain, × 1000). (From Tyler DE et al: *J Am Vet Med Assoc* 176:987–993, 1980. Reprinted with permission.)

P. zopfii and *P. wickerhamii* to establish histologic identification of species; however, these are too subtle for pathologists who see these organisms infrequently to appreciate. When species identification is required, preserved biopsy and necropsy tissues and unstained histologic sections can be examined at specialized laboratories by the indirect FA technique (see Appendix 5). The slower but more routine method of culturing followed by sugar and alcohol assimilation testing can be done in most diagnostic laboratories.

PATHOLOGIC FINDINGS

Dogs

Protothecosis occurs predominantly as a disseminated disease, producing lesions in a wide variety of tissues. Lesions in parenchymatous organs and on serosal surfaces are diffusely scattered throughout the tissues and are seen as white to tan granular foci measuring 0.5 to 2 mm in diameter or as streaks measuring 0.5 × 2 to 3 mm in length. This pattern especially is seen in the myocardium, skeletal muscle, intestinal muscularis, lymph nodes, thyroid, liver, and loose connective tissue. In the kidney, lesions tend to be larger, often measuring up to several centimeters in size and surrounded by a peripheral ring of hemorrhage. They also have a radiating linear pattern and may appear in either the cortex or medulla. Gross lesions have been reported throughout the intestinal tract, but the colon is most commonly affected. The lesions in the mucosa may vary from diffuse reddening to marked nodular thickening with scattered ulcerations, which are often hemorrhagic. Tiny white foci, as just described, are frequently seen in the muscularis and serosa. Gross sectioning of the eye reveals a gray-white cloudy exudate, often with red streaks in one or both chambers and beneath the retina, which is detached.

Microscopically, a variety of host reactions may be seen. Usually, there is little evidence of necrosis and only a minimal mixed inflammatory cell infiltration at the periphery of *Prototheca* cell clusters. The infiltrate consists mostly of macrophages, lymphocytes, neutrophils, and plasma cells, the last of which may be present in inordinately large numbers. Infrequently, the inflammatory reaction is more pronounced and may be granulomatous or pyogranulomatous. In such lesions, many *Prototheca* cells are contained within macrophages and multinucleate giant cells. Hemorrhage and necrosis more commonly are seen in the kidneys, heart, and intestines.

In the colon, lesions consist of masses of organisms often arranged in cords or nodules, replacing most of the mucosa and extending into and filling the submucosa (Fig. 69–6). Small focal colonies of organisms are seen throughout the muscularis and serosa. Inflammatory cell response is mixed but usually is minimal. Focal ulcerations of the mucosal surface and hemorrhage are frequently encountered. When there has been a history of prolonged diarrhea, granulation tissue may be seen intermingled with organisms in the mucosa and submucosa (see Fig. 69–6). In the kidney, multiple focal aggregates of *Prototheca* cells are seen in the interstitium of the cortex, medulla, and occasionally the papillae. Minimal to marked necrosis and inflammatory cell infiltrate occur at the periphery of the organism cluster. The cellular infiltrate consists of plasma cells (which often predominate), lymphocytes, macrophages, and occasionally granulocytes. Lesions in the brain and spinal cord usually occur as widely scattered, small foci of necrosis with an infiltration of mixed inflammatory cells. Numbers of *Prototheca* cells in these foci vary from none to large aggregates. Similar findings may be present in the inner ear. Focal to diffuse granulomatous chorioretinitis with retinal detachment and severe retinal degeneration are the most common ocular lesions seen microscopically. Masses of organisms are seen within the vitreous and between the retina and choroid. Lesser numbers occur focally in the choroid. The inflammatory infiltrate is mixed and may be pyogranulomatous.

In cutaneous lesions, masses of *Prototheca* cells occur in the dermis, subcutis, and subjacent skeletal muscles. The epidermis has zones of hyperkeratosis, ulceration, and atrophy with the typical inflammatory cell response. Ulcerated surfaces are necrotic and secondarily infected with bacteria.

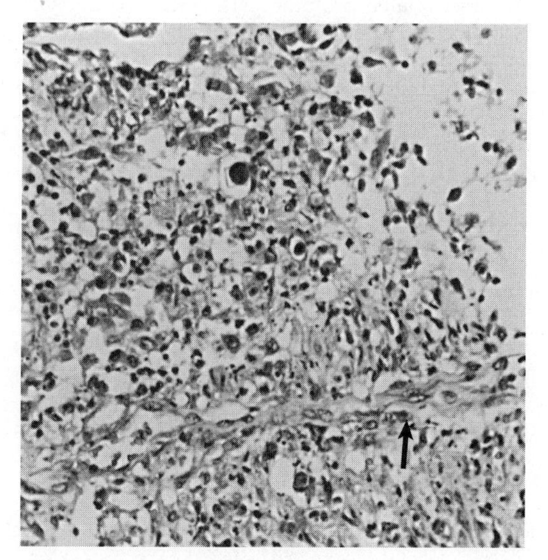

Figure 69–6. The mucosa of the colon from a dog has been replaced by masses of *Prototheca* cells. Only a few mixed mononuclear inflammatory cells are scattered throughout the lesion. A wisp of granulation tissue is seen at the arrow (H and E, × 100).

When cutaneous lesions extend into the nasal mucosa, necrosis, ulceration, hemorrhage, and infiltration of neutrophils and plasma cells mixed with large masses of proliferating *Prototheca* are seen. Regional lymph nodes commonly are invaded secondarily. In one dog with cutaneous protothecosis, the amount of inflammatory cell infiltrates before treatment was scanty but increased during treatment, whereas the number of organisms was reduced.[12a] These findings suggested that viable organisms inhibited the immune response or were less immunoreactive in tissues than dead ones.

Cats

Localized cutaneous lesions in cats are gray-white subcutaneous or dermal masses of variable consistency that extend deeply into the underlying tissue and intermesh with tendons, nerves, and blood vessels. Histologically, they are granulomas characterized by densely packed epithelioid cells and sparse, multinucleated giant cells. Neutrophils and plasma cells may be prominent in some lesions. Masses of *Prototheca* in all stages of reproduction constitute the bulk of the lesion.

THERAPY

Because protothecosis usually occurs as a single focal cutaneous lesion in people and cats, wide excision has been successful and the preferred therapeutic approach. A variety of antimicrobials have been tried therapeutically in infected people and animals. However, in most instances, treatment has failed. These have included systemic administration of various antibacterial drugs, amphotericin B (AMB), griseofulvin, potassium iodide, and pentamidine isethionate and topical application of antibiotics, copper sulfate, AMB lotion, gentian violet, brilliant green, and chlorinated lime. Treatment of human cutaneous protothecosis with AMB alone in combination with oral tetracycline or with ketoconazole (KTZ) or fluconazole has been successful.[8] With localized cutaneous lesions, surgery is recommended to remove the lesions in conjunction with systemic antifungal chemotherapy. However, in one of the few successfully treated human cases of disseminated protothecosis, AMB and transfer factor were used. In vitro studies on *P. wickerhamii* have shown a synergistic effect between AMB and tetracycline, and one person with cutaneous protothecosis was effectively treated with this combination. Treatment with AMB alone was successful in alleviating the progression of clinical signs for 1 year in a dog with cutaneous and systemic infection with *P. wickerhamii*.[17] See Table 69–1 for appropriate dosages.

An immunocompetent person having disseminated infection with *P. wickerhamii* was successfully treated with AMB for several weeks in conjunction with 3 months of KTZ.[2] Cutaneous *P. wickerhamii* infection in a human with AIDS did not respond to itraconazole but did resolve with AMB therapy.[1a] Susceptibility testing was predictive in this case and may be indicated owing to the variable responses achieved between these two antifungal agents in human and animal infections. An immunocompetent person who developed a localized granuloma was successfully treated with itraconazole.[13] In a human, successful treatment of a *P. wickerhamii*–infected wrist wound with orally administered KTZ has been reported. Hepatotoxicity, which developed in response to the treatment, spontaneously resolved after cessation of the treatment.

KTZ was effective in causing regression of multifocal cutaneous abscesses caused by infection with *Prototheca* species in a dog.[10] Treatment was continued for 4 months, although long-term follow-up is not available. The organism showed marked in vitro susceptibility to KTZ. In another dog with cutaneous manifestations of *P. wickerhamii* infection, oral KTZ therapy for 6 months resolved the lesions except for scrotal granuloma, which necessitated surgical removal.[4a] Unfortunately, a clinical relapse occurred 5 months later.

AMB was not effective in the treatment of ocular protothecosis (*P. zopfii*) in a dog.[11] Initial treatment reduced the lesion in the eye, and blood culture results became negative, but, because of the development of renal toxicity, the therapy was discontinued. Subsequently, lower doses failed to stop the progression of the lesions. In the same dog simazine, an algicidal drug used to clean fish tanks, gentamicin, and KTZ also were tried without success.

In vitro, clotrimazole (CTZ) has no activity against *P. zopfii* but is highly efficacious against *P. wickerhamii*. Because *P. zopfii* is the most common species infecting dogs, CTZ probably might not be of value in treating canine protothecosis. In contrast, because cutaneous protothecosis in both dogs and cats is caused by *P. wickerhamii*, topically applied CTZ might be the drug of choice for this form of protothecosis. Topical CTZ did not appear to alter the course of successful therapy with systemic KTZ in one dog.[4a]

Aminoglycosides such as gentamicin have in vitro activity against *Prototheca*, but their clinical usefulness has not been well substantiated. Ribostamycin, an aminoglycoside antibiotic closely related to kanamycin, is an effective in vitro agent against all species of *Prototheca*, especially *P. zopfii*. Although not commercially available, ribostamycin was used on an

Table 69–1. Proposed Drug Therapy for Protothecosis[a]

DRUG	SPECIES	DOSE (mg/kg)[b]	ROUTE	INTERVAL (HOURS)	DURATION (DAYS)
Amphotericin B	D	0.25–0.5	IV	3 times weekly	[c] [d]
	C	0.25	IV	3 times weekly	[d]
and					
Tetracycline	B	22	PO	8	[e]
Ketoconazole[f]	B	10–15	PO	12–24	28–42
Itraconazole[f]	B	5–10	PO	12	28–42
Fluconazole	B	2.5–5	PO, IV	12	28–42
Clotrimazole	B		Topical		

[a]Although these regimens have been used to treat people and experimental animals, none has yet been extensively used in treating affected dogs and cats; see text.
[b]Dose per administration at specified interval. See Drug Formulary, Appendix 8, for additional information on each drug.
[c]Until cumulative dose = 8 mg/kg. Higher doses of lipid formulations are used, see Drug Formulary, Appendix 8.
[d]Until cumulative dose = 4 mg/kg. Higher doses of lipid formulations are used, see Drug Formulary, Appendix 8.
[e]Continued while receiving amphotericin B. The synergistic effect of tetracycline has not been well substantiated.
[f]Effective against *P. wickerhamii* but not against *P. zopfii*.
D = dog; C = cat; B = dog and cat.

experimental basis to treat a dog with chorioretinitis as the primary manifestation of the disease caused by *P. zopfii*.[14] The drug was administered at a dose of 12.5 mg/kg given IM twice daily. Ocular manifestations improved, but later the dog died with disseminated lesions.

PUBLIC HEALTH CONSIDERATIONS

Protothecosis is considered to be acquired from environmental exposure and is not transmissible between hosts. Humans, dogs, and cats are continually being exposed to this ubiquitous organism, but the disease is infrequent. Immunocompetent people and animals have less risk of developing clinical disease or dissemination. Handling of wastes or exudates from infected pets would carry no greater risk than environmental exposure. However, as a general recommendation, immunocompromised people should be advised against close contact with these animals. Hospitalized people receiving immunosuppressive or surgical therapy or those with IV, endotracheal, or peritoneal catheters have been at greatest risk.

References

1. Blogg JR, Sykes JE. 1995. Sudden blindness associated with protothecosis in a dog. *Aust Vet J* 72:147–149.

1a. Carey WP, Kaykova Y, Bandres JC, et al. 1997. Cutaneous protothecosis in a patient with AIDS and a severe functional neutrophil deficit: successful therapy with amphotericin B. *Clin Infect Dis* 25:1265–1266.

2. Chan JC, Jeffers LJ, Gould EW, et al. 1990. Visceral protothecosis mimicking sclerosing cholangitis in an immunocompetent host: successful antifungal therapy. *Rev Infect Dis* 12:802–807.

3. Fuchs A, Fidler G, Meissel H. 1996. Protothecosis in a dog. *Wiener Tierarztl Monatsschr* 83:60–63.

4. Gibb AP, Aggarwal R, Swainson CP. 1991. Successful treatment of *Prototheca* peritonitis complicating continuous ambulatory peritoneal dialysis. *J Infect* 22:183–185.

4a. Ginel PJ, Perez J, Molleda JM, et al. 1997. Cutaneous protothecosis in a dog. *Vet Rec* 140:651–653.

5. Hasegawa PM, Ono K, Lee CW. 1990. A new staining solution for the morphological studies of fungi and prototheca. *Jpn J Vet Sci* 50:527–531.

6. Huerre M, Ravisse P, Solomon H, et al. 1993. Human protothecosis and environment. *Bull Soc Pathol Exot* 86:484–488.

7. Iacoviello VR, DeGirolami PC, Lucarini J, et al. 1992. Protothecosis complicating prolonged endotracheal intubation: case report and literature review. *Clin Infect Dis* 15:959–967.

8. Kim ST, Suh KS, Chae YS, et al. 1996. Successful treatment with fluconazole of protothecosis developing at the site of an intralesional corticosteroid injection. *Br J Dermatol* 135:803–806.

9. Laeng RH, Egger C, Schaffner T, et al. 1994. Protothecosis in an HIV-positive patient. *Am J Surg Pathol* 18:1261–1264.

10. Macartney L, Rycroft AN, Hammil J. 1988. Cutaneous protothecosis in the dog: first confirmed case in Britain. *Vet Rec* 123:494–496.

11. Moore FM, Schmidt GM, Desai D, et al. 1985. Unsuccessful treatment of disseminated protothecosis in a dog. *J Am Vet Med Assoc* 186:705–708.

12. Pal M, Hasegawa A, Ono K, et al. 1990. A new staining solution for the morphological studies of fungi and *Prototheca*. *Jpn J Vet Sci* 52:527–531.

12a. Perez J, Ginel PJ, Lucena R, et al. 1997. Canine cutaneous protothecosis: an immunohistochemical analysis of the inflammatory cell infiltrate. *J Comp Pathol* 117:83–89.

13. Pierard GE, Rurangirwa A, Arrese-Estrada J, et al. 1990. Cutaneous protothecosis treated with itraconazole. *Ann Soc Belg Med Trop* 70:105–112.

14. Scagliotti RH. 1989. Personal communication. Sacramento, CA.

15. Thomas JB, Preston N. 1990. Generalized protothecosis in a collie dog. *Aust Vet J* 67:25–27.

16. Tyler DE. 1990. Protothecosis, pp 742–750. *In* Greene CE (ed), Infectious diseases of the dog and cat. WB Saunders, Philadelphia, PA.

17. Wilkinson GT, Leong G. 1988. Protothecosis in a dog. *Aust Vet Practit* 18:47–49.

18. Woolrich A, Koestenblatt E, Don P, et al. 1994. Cutaneous protothecosis and AIDS. *J Am Acad Dermatol* 31:920–924.

Section
IV

PROTOZOAL DISEASES

Chapter 70

Laboratory Diagnosis of Protozoal Infections

Michael R. Lappin and Janet P. Calpin

Successful diagnosis of a protozoal infection is dependent on the careful choice of procedures. For example, saturated sodium nitrate fecal flotation is not useful for many enteric protozoal infections because the specific gravity of most protozoal cysts is greater than that of this solution. Trophozoites, in contrast, are killed by the sodium nitrate solution. Furthermore, accurate diagnosis of a protozoal infection, whether it is caused by an enteric, a systemic, or a blood-borne organism, also depends on the proper collection and preservation of the clinical sample. Radiographic techniques involving barium sulfate may hinder detection of intestinal protozoa for a week or more.[2] Antibiotics and other medications also may affect the recovery of protozoa from stool and blood samples. In addition, many enteric organisms are shed intermittently, requiring examination of multiple samples.

Formulas and detailed procedures for the diagnostic tests described in this chapter can easily be performed in the veterinary office.[2, 3] The collection and preservation of clinical samples to be sent to specialized testing laboratories are discussed. The reader is referred to the chapters on specific protozoal diseases and Appendix 5 for discussion of specific specialized tests and lists of the commercial, state, and federal laboratories that perform them.

FECES

Sample Collection and Storage

At least 5 g of fresh feces should be collected and placed in a clean, dry container that is sealed with a tight-fitting lid. The sample should be free of contaminants such as urine and litter. If blood or mucus is present in the stool, it should be included in the sample.

Microscopic examination of the sample should be done as soon as possible, especially if the feces are diarrheic. Diarrheic stool samples should be maintained at room temperature and examined within 30 minutes of collection because they may contain fragile trophozoite stages of the infectious agent, which cannot survive refrigeration. If immediate examination is impossible, the sample should be mixed with a preservative (see Preservation of Feces). Formed stools, which do not usually contain trophozoites, should be refrigerated if there is any delay in examination. If the container is tightly sealed to prevent desiccation, the sample may be usable for up to 1 week.

Examination of Feces

Table 70–1 lists the recommended microscopic procedures for the diagnosis of GI protozoal infections.

Direct Smear. The direct smear technique is usually reserved for diarrheic samples or for examination of mucus in the sample. The substage condenser of the microscope must be adjusted to maximum contrast, because the unstained organisms appear transparent. When available, the phase-contrast or dark-field microscope may aid in the demonstration of motile trophozoites.

Fresh Saline Smear. The saline smear is made by placing a drop of physiologic saline on a clean microscope slide. The amount of feces that adheres to the end of an applicator stick is mixed evenly with the saline so that the smear is thin. A coverslip is applied, and the slide is systematically scanned using low power (10× objective). It may be necessary to warm the smear to enhance the motility of *Entamoeba histolyt-*

Table 70–1. Recommended Procedures for the Diagnosis of Gastrointestinal Protozoans of the Dog and Cat

ORGANISM	STAGE	PROCEDURE
Entamoeba histolytica	Trophozoites Cysts	Direct smear Direct smear
Giardia	Trophozoites Cysts	Direct smear Zinc sulfate centrifugation flotation technique or formalin-ether sedimentation
Pentatrichomonas *Balantidium coli*	Trophozoites Trophozoites Cysts	Direct smear Direct smear Zinc sulfate centrifugation flotation technique
Coccidia (*Toxoplasma, Isospora, Sarcocystis, Hammondia, Besnoitia,* and *Cryptosporidium*)	Oocysts	Sheather's sugar centrifugation flotation technique

ica. Motility and structural features of protozoa are best examined using the high-dry objective (40 or 43×). Generally, use of the oil immersion objective is not recommended for examining fresh wet mounts. After motility has been observed, stain may be added to the saline smear to aid in the specific identification of the organism.

Stained Smear. Adding stain to the wet mount through the edge of the coverslip will aid in visualizing internal structures of protozoa. Because staining the preparation kills the organism, the examination for motility must be done first. Table 70–2 describes the trophozoites found on direct smears from dogs and cats.

Iodine stains have traditionally been utilized to reveal the internal structural detail of protozoans. D'Antoni's iodine and Lugol's solution are the most popular.[2, 3] When employed correctly, iodine stains the cytoplasm of cysts yellow-gold, whereas the nuclei are paler and refractile. Methylene blue in acetate buffer (pH 3.6) has been used to stain trophozoite stages, especially those of *E. histolytica.*[2] An aqueous solution of eosin will stain fecal debris bright red, but trophozoites and cysts will remain colorless. Acid methyl green is recommended for staining the macronucleus of *Balantidium coli.*[1, 3]

Fecal Flotation. Fecal concentration methods help to confirm the presence of protozoal cysts or oocysts. Protozoal cysts are more frequently found in formed stools, whereas coccidian oocysts, especially *Cryptosporidium,* are more frequently found in diarrheic feces.

Sheather's sugar or zinc sulfate centrifugation technique for intestinal parasites is recommended as a routine diagnostic procedure that can be performed in the veterinary clinic. The solution is inexpensive, and the technique is effective in revealing *Toxoplasma, Cryptosporidium,* and other coccidia.[2, 3] The hypertonicity of the solution will distort the cysts of *Giardia;* however, the distortion itself may be diagnostic. Most *Giardia* cysts are oval, and the cytoplasm is pulled to one side so that a half- or quarter-moon shape is presented.

The zinc sulfate centrifugation technique reveals protozoal and helminthic parasites in feces.[2, 3] Although it causes some distortion of protozoans, it distorts *Giardia* cysts less than the sugar solution. For this reason, zinc sulfate can be applied to verify the identity of *Giardia*-like cysts revealed by sugar flotation. *Giardia* cysts also take up iodine, which helps to distinguish them from coccidian oocysts, which do not stain.

Fecal sedimentation will recover protozoal and helminthic parasites present in the feces; however, the resultant sample will also contain debris. The formalin-ether and formalin-ethyl acetate sedimentation techniques are recommended for concentrating *Giardia* cysts.[3] The sedimentation procedure is similar for the two techniques; the only difference is whether ethyl acetate or ether is used. Although ether is extremely flammable and explosive, it is especially effective in concentrating cysts from stools that have a high fat content.[4]

Fecal Culture

Fecal protozoal culture is rarely performed in small animal practice, and specialized diagnostic laboratories that perform the procedure have to be identified before sample submission. The sample should be fresh and sent by the most rapid means available. For this reason, a presumptive diagnosis of most enteric protozoan infections is made on morphologic appearance of the organism. However, specific media have been developed that will support the growth of *E. histolytica, B. coli,* and *Pentatrichomonas* species.

Preservation of Feces

If there is a delay in examining a fecal sample for protozoa or if the sample is to be sent to a diagnostic laboratory for further analysis, a preservative must be added to it. It is important that the fecal sample be broken up and thoroughly mixed with the preservative before shipment to the laboratory.

Polyvinyl Alcohol (PVA) Preservation. The greatest advantage of the PVA technique is that permanent-stained slides may be made at a later date from a stool sample that has been fixed in PVA. Another advantage is that the formalin-ether sedimentation technique can be performed on PVA-fixed specimens. The fixative remains stable for years; however, it contains mercury, and care must be exercised in handling and storing the solution. PVA can be employed to fix large volumes of feces or individual smears on microscope slides.[2, 3]

Merthiolate-Iodine-Formalin (MIF) Preservation. The MIF preservation procedure has the advantage of both preserving the sample and staining any protozoans that may be present. This technique involves mixing two stock solutions immediately before use. The Lugol's solution (iodine) can also be utilized to stain direct smears (see Direct Smear). The disadvantages of this method are that the iodine solution does not have a long shelf-life and permanent-stained slides cannot be made from MIF-preserved material.[2, 3]

Table 70–2. Protozoal Trophozoite Identification by Direct Fecal Smear

		DISTINGUISHING MORPHOLOGY	
ORGANISM	SIZE (μm)	FRESH SMEAR	STAINED SMEAR
Entamoeba histolytica	12–50	Constantly changes shape when active; moves by means of finger-like projections of cytoplasm; one nucleus that is difficult to see; may contain erythrocytes	Nucleus usually has evenly distributed peripheral chromatin and centrally located, compact karyosome
Giardia	9–21 × 5–15 × 2–4	Bilaterally symmetric; pear shaped on dorsoventral view; crescentic on lateral view; rolling movement by means of flagella; contains two nuclei	Two large nuclei, each with prominent karyosomes and axonemes and median bodies, give monkey-faced appearance
Pentatrichomonas	5–20 × 3–14	Oval to pear shaped; wobbly, jerky, rapid movement by means of flagella; undulating membrane visible	Oval nucleus in anterior half of body; axostyle protruding from posterior end
Balantidium coli	50–150	Oval shape; revolving movement by means of cilia; macronucleus may be visible	Large kidney bean-shaped macronucleus is prominent; occasionally micronucleus may be seen

Ten Percent Formalin Preservation. This technique is effective in preserving protozoal cysts; however, it is not recommended for trophozoites. Several grams of feces are mixed with 10% formalin that has been warmed to 60°C. As with the MIF procedure, the major disadvantage is that permanent-stained smears cannot be prepared from formalin-fixed specimens.[2, 3]

Permanent Staining of Fecal Smears. Frequently, positive identification of intestinal protozoa can be made only by specialized laboratories using a permanent staining method. Samples that have been fixed in PVA can be submitted to a diagnostic laboratory, where trichrome or iron-hematoxylin stains can be utilized.[2, 3]

Organism Confirmation

Animal inoculation can be utilized to differentiate some coccidian parasites. Oocysts of *Toxoplasma gondii* cannot be distinguished from those of *Hammondia hammondi* or *Besnoitia darlingi* morphologically; only *T. gondii* is infectious for human beings. These coccidians are passed from cats as unsporulated oocysts, which are not infectious. If it should be necessary to submit feces to a laboratory for coccidial identification, a simple procedure enhances oocyst sporulation. The stool is mixed with 2.5% potassium dichromate and strained through cheesecloth to remove large debris. The suspension is sporulated at room temperature in an open container, but the dichromate solution should not be allowed to decrease in volume. Sporulation takes 3 to 5 days or longer, after which the specimen should be refrigerated until identification is completed. Sporulated oocysts of *T. gondii* are highly infectious; therefore, great caution should be taken during sporulation and subsequent handling of this material. If *T. gondii* is suspected, the diagnostic laboratory should be contacted before sporulation for instructions regarding shipment of material, because it is not recommended that infectious material be sent via parcel post. Several weeks are generally required for the organisms to mature in the host animal.

Fecal Immunodiagnostic Tests

ELISA and FA procedures for detection of *Giardia* spp. and *Cryptosporidium* spp. antigens or cysts and oocysts, respectively, in feces are commercially available (see Appendix 6). Minimal information is available about sensitivity and specificity of these assays for dogs and cats. If used, the results of these assays should be interpreted with the results from fecal examination techniques. Polymerase chain reaction (PCR) for demonstration of some enteric protozoans in feces is being studied. Predictive values of coproantibodies against *Cryptosporidium* spp. and *T. gondii* are being evaluated.

WHOLE BLOOD

Collection

Films to be studied for the diagnosis of blood-borne protozoal infections may be made from either fresh blood or blood that has been collected into edetate acid (EDTA). Table 70–3 lists the protozoans that may be seen on blood films or tissue smears. Care should be taken in handling the sample, because hemolysis of the erythrocytes and destruction of the parasites will hinder positive identification. If fresh blood is used, the film must be made before the blood clots. Some blood-borne protozoans, especially *Babesia*, are more readily demonstrated if blood from microcapillary beds (ear margin, toenail) is collected to make films. If blood culture is to be performed, the blood collection site, preferably the jugular vein, should be prepared aseptically.

Table 70–3. Practical Techniques for the Diagnosis of Blood-Borne and Systemic Protozoal Infections

ORGANISM	BLOOD FILMS	ASPIRATE IMPRESSIONS	TISSUE IMPRESSIONS
Toxoplasma	+[a]	+	+
Neospora	?	+	+
Trypanosoma	+	+	+
Leishmania	−	+	+
Hepatozoon	+	−	+
Encephalitozoon	−	+[b]	−
Cytauxzoon	+	−	+
Babesia	+	−	−
Entamoeba histolytica	−	+	−
Pneumocystis	−	+	+

[a] Rare.
[b] May give negative results in seropositive animals.
+ = useful or indicated; − = not used; ? = uncertain.

Preparation of Blood Films

When diagnostic blood films are made, the microscope slide must be completely clean. If slides are to be sent to a diagnostic laboratory for protozoal identification, both thick and thin films (at least two of each) should be prepared.

Thick Films. A larger amount of blood is examined with a thick film, thereby increasing the chances of detecting parasites, especially when the parasitemia is mild. However, organisms may be distorted in thick films; therefore, thin films should be made for proper identification.

Two to three small drops of blood are placed on a clean microscope slide and spread in a circular motion over a 2-cm area with the corner of another slide. When fresh blood is used, it should be stirred on the slide for 30 seconds to prevent formation of fibrin strands. If EDTA-anticoagulated blood is used, additional stirring is unnecessary. The film should be air dried at room temperature with the slide kept on a flat surface. The choice of stain will determine whether the film will have to be laked (i.e., immersed in distilled water to rupture and remove the erythrocytes) (see Staining of Blood Films). Thick films to be stored for later examination or shipped to a diagnostic laboratory should be laked. Films should be stored in a cool (20°C), dry, clean place.

Thin Films. A small drop of blood is placed at one end of a clean microscope slide. The short edge of another clean slide (the spreader slide) is placed in the middle of the slide at a 30-degree angle and pulled back toward the blood. The blood is allowed to spread along the width of the spreader slide; then, in a fairly rapid, even motion, the spreader slide is pushed across the length of the slide, dragging the blood along. The blood should not be pushed across the slide, because this will rupture many cells and parasites. The blood film should be air dried at room temperature. As with thick films, the staining method will determine the need for prior fixation (see Staining of Blood Films). If the films are not stained within 48 hours, they should be fixed in 100% methyl alcohol (methanol). Slides should be stored as for thick films.

Staining Blood Films

Both Giemsa stain and Wright's stain are available commercially in ready-to-use form. The choice of stain is a matter of personal preference. Generally, however, Giemsa stain is chosen for differentiation of blood protozoans and Wright's stain for differential leukocyte counts.

When treated properly with Giemsa stain, erythrocytes should be pale gray-blue; leukocyte cytoplasm should stain blue, and the nucleus should be purple; eosinophilic granules should be a bright pink, and neutrophilic granules should stain a deep blue, whereas the nucleus should be red. Giemsa stain is a permanent stain, and slides can be kept for years when properly stored.

With Wright's stain, erythrocytes are light-tan; the nuclei of leukocytes are bright blue, and the cytoplasm is lighter. Eosinophilic granules are red, and neutrophilic granules are pink. Protozoal cytoplasm stains a light blue, whereas the nucleus is a deeper blue. Wright's stain has a tendency to fade with time.

Examination of Blood Films

Thin blood films can be examined with or without coverslips. If a coverslip is utilized, only the number 1 size is thin enough to allow proper focusing with a microscope. A neutral mounting medium prevents the stain from bleaching. The mounting medium will also aid in viewing the cells with low- and high-dry objectives and will prevent the coverslip from moving when the oil immersion objective is in place. If a coverslip is not used with the thin blood film, a small drop of oil may be placed on the slide and thinly spread over the blood film. This procedure eliminates the diffraction of light around blood cells during scanning with the low- and high-dry objectives. After scanning, another drop of oil should be added, and with the oil immersion objective the film should be systematically examined for blood parasites, which usually are located and best visualized at the feathered end and edges of the film.

Thick films may be examined with or without coverslips. After the microscope is focused and the slide scanned with low power, oil may be applied and the film examined for parasites.

Blood Culture and Laboratory Animal Inoculation

Blood culture or animal inoculation with whole blood can be employed to identify some protozoan parasites. Specific media have been developed to support the growth of trypanosomes and *Leishmania*. See individual chapters for specific discussion of these techniques.

Xenodiagnosis

Xenodiagnosis uses a laboratory-reared, parasite-free arthropod vector of the disease in question. The vector is allowed to feed on a suspected infected host. After feeding, the vector must be maintained until the parasite has had sufficient time to develop (which may be 6 weeks). Then it is examined for the parasitic stage of the organism. Historically, xenodiagnosis has been employed in the detection of trypanosomiasis.

SEROLOGIC TESTING

Serodiagnosis of protozoal diseases involves the testing of serum for the presence of antibodies against the parasite, antigens of the parasite, or immune complexes containing parasite antigens. Parasite-specific serum antibody testing has been utilized as a diagnostic aid in most blood-borne and systemic protozoal diseases. The major advantages of antibody testing include ease of sample collection, low cost of most procedures, and wide availability of most assays.

Sample Handling

Blood should be collected for serologic testing as described earlier in this chapter, except that blood is dispensed into a clean tube that does not contain an anticoagulant. It should be processed to prevent hemolysis. Separated serum samples may be frozen before testing. Thawing during shipment to a diagnostic laboratory should not affect the outcome of most serologic tests as long as bacterial growth is minimized. Sodium azide should be added to the tube if transport will take more than a few days.

Antibody Detection. IgG class antibody responses have been studied most extensively. Unfortunately, IgG develops to detectable levels well after clinical disease has begun and then remains elevated for months to years with most protozoal infections. Diagnosis of recent or active infection through IgG measurement necessitates demonstration of a fourfold rising titer. IgM and IgA serologic responses have been studied with some protozoal infections, particularly *T. gondii* and *Cryptosporidium* spp. In general, IgM is the first antibody produced after an antigenic exposure in dogs and cats. The major problem associated with measurement of any antibody class is that the presence of antibodies in serum does not correlate directly with the presence of clinical illness. Sensitivity and specificity also vary with different assays. If immunosuppression is present concurrently with protozoal infection, parasite-specific antibody responses may be diminished.

Antigen Detection. The detection of parasite-specific circulating serum antigens has been used in the diagnosis of *Pneumocystis* and *Toxoplasma* infections. Antigen detection can be beneficial for the diagnosis of protozoal infection, especially in cases with concurrent immunosuppression and poor specific antibody production. Problems include the presence of antigen in clinically normal individuals and the potential presence of cross-reactive antigens. *T. gondii*–containing IgM and IgG class immune complexes have been detected in serum from healthy and clinically ill cats.

OTHER BODY FLUIDS

Protozoans are occasionally identified in aqueous humor, CSF, pleural and/or peritoneal effusions, urine, duodenal fluids, and transtracheal washings or bronchoalveolar lavages. Fluids should be examined immediately with the direct smear technique to reveal motile protozoans that may be present (see Table 70–3). *Giardia* trophozoites are commonly detected in duodenal fluids collected from dogs by endoscopy. Aqueous humor, CSF, urine, and airway washings should be concentrated by centrifugation at $2000 \times g$ for 5 minutes before making impressions or smears. Stained smears should be made utilizing the technique described for staining thin blood films.

An aliquot of collected material should be placed in an EDTA tube and in a sterile tube and stored at room temperature while cytologic evaluation is completed. Further specialized procedures including antibody measurement, antigen measurement, PCR, culture, or animal inoculation can then be performed from these specimens as indicated.

Protozoans like *Neospora caninum* or *T. gondii* are rarely demonstrated cytologically in aqueous humor or CSF. However, *T. gondii* is detected in some clinically ill cats by PCR (see Chapter 80). Demonstration of *T. gondii*–specific local production of antibody or antigen in aqueous humor or CSF can help to support the diagnosis of toxoplasmosis. Samples for antibody detection, antigen detection, or organism detection by PCR should be frozen immediately and transported to the laboratory frozen. Samples for culture or laboratory animal inoculation should be transported immediately without freezing or preservatives.

TISSUE SPECIMENS

Tissue Aspirates

Fine-needle aspirates from lymph nodes, spleen, liver, and bone marrow will occasionally demonstrate protozoans. Aspirated material should be examined for motile protozoans by the direct methods. If aspirated material is compressed between two slides, the impression that results when the slides are pulled apart can be stained as described for thin blood films and examined for the internal morphology of protozoa. Alternatively, a small amount of aspirated material is placed on a microscope slide and then spread by repeatedly passing the tip of a 22-gauge needle through the material, drawing it along the slide. This technique may lessen the destruction of cells.

Tissue Biopsy

A tissue impression should be made from any biopsy material. The cut edge of the tissue should be blotted on a paper towel to remove the excess blood, and the specimen should be touched to a clean microscope slide. The resulting impression is one cell layer thick and, when stained as for thin blood films, should reveal parasitized cells (see Table 70–3).

If possible, a biopsy specimen should be examined as a fresh preparation (by frozen sectioning and staining) so that a rapid diagnosis can be made. However, the accessibility of the diagnostic laboratory will influence the usefulness of this technique. If there will be a delay in the examination of biopsy material, it should be preserved in 10% buffered formalin; then, on arrival at the diagnostic laboratory, the tissue can be handled as for routine histologic processing. Immunofluorescent or immunoperoxidase staining techniques can be performed at some diagnostic and research laboratories. These procedures can aid in the specific identification of tissue forms of protozoans. Although many of these techniques are effective utilizing formalin-fixed tissue, fresh-frozen tissue gives superior results in some, especially PCR. Tissue for culture or laboratory animal inoculation should be submitted without freezing. Glutaraldehyde-based fixatives are superior to formalin for EM.

References

1. Adam KMG, Paul J, Zaman V. 1971. Medical and veterinary protozoology. Churchill Livingstone, London.
2. Ash LR, Orihel TC. 1987. Parasites: a guide to laboratory procedures and identification. ASC Press, Chicago, IL.
3. Greene CE. 1990. Appendix 12: Some preservation, staining, and microscopy techniques for infectious disease agents, pp 916–920. *In* Greene CE (ed), Infectious diseases of the dog and cat. WB Saunders, Philadelphia, PA.
4. Traunt AL, Elliot SH, Kelly MT, et al. 1981. Comparison of formalin-ethyl ether sedimentation, formalin-ethyl acetate sedimentation, and zinc sulfate flotation techniques for detection of intestinal parasites. *J Clin Microbiol* 13:882–884.

Chapter 71

Antiprotozoal Chemotherapy

Craig E. Greene and A. D. J. Watson

Table 71–1 summarizes the indications for current antiprotozoal drugs. Chapters 72 to 83 should be consulted for details concerning chemotherapy of specific diseases. Dosages of various drugs are available in the Drug Formulary (Appendix 8).

AZO-NAPHTHALENE DRUGS

Trypan blue was one of the first compounds used to treat babesiosis. Because local irritation and abscesses develop after SC injection, it is administered IV. Trypan blue does not completely eliminate *Babesia*, but infected animals recover from illness and remain in a state of premunition. They must be treated with aromatic diamidines (see later discussion) within 1 month to effect a cure. A disadvantage of trypan blue is that it stains all body tissues and secretions for several weeks.

ACRIDINE DYES

Quinacrine, developed as a human antimalarial drug, has been administered to dogs as an alternative treatment to nitroimidazoles for giardiasis. It becomes incorporated into the DNA of the organism and inhibits nucleic acid synthesis. Evidence of toxicity includes vomiting, fever, pruritus, neurologic signs, yellow discoloration of urine or tissues, and hepatic dysfunction. It is no longer available in the United States.

QUINOLINE DERIVATIVES

Diiodohydroxyquin and iodochlorhydroxyquin are halogenated oxyquinolines that have been provided as topical antifungal drugs. They are also amebicidal when administered

Table 71–1. Properties of Antiprotozoal Drugs

GENERIC NAME (TRADE NAME)	INFECTIONS INDICATED	
	First Choice	Alternate Choice
Azo-Naphthalene Dyes		
Trypan blue	None	*Babesia*
Acridine Dyes		
Quinacrine hydrochloride (Atabrine, Keybrin)	None	*Giardia*
Quinoline Derivatives		
Diiodohydroxyquin (iodoquinol; Diodoquin, Yodoxin)	*Balantidium*	*Entamoeba*
Iodochlorhydroxyquin (clioquinol; Vioform)	*Balantidium*	*Entamoeba*
Hydroxynaphthoquinones		
Atovaquone (Mepron)	None	*Pneumocystis, Toxoplasma, Babesia*
Aromatic Diamidines		
Pentamidine isethionate (Lomidine, Pentam, NebuPent) (also phenamidine)	*Babesia, Acanthamoeba*	*Leishmania Pneumocystis*
Diminazene aceturate (Berenil, Ganaseg)	*Cytauxzoon, Babesia,* African *Trypanosoma*	*Hepatozoon*
Imidocarb dipropionate (Imizol)	*Babesia, Hepatozoon, Cytauxzoon*	*Ehrlichia*
Amicarbalide (Diamipron)	*Ehrlichia*	None
Nitroimidazoles		
Metronidazole (Flagyl, Stomorgyl[a])	*Giardia, Pentatrichomonas*	*Entamoeba, Balantidium*
Dimetridazole (Emtryl)	*Entamoeba, Balantidium*	None
Tinidazole (Fasigyn)	*Pentatrichomonas*	*Babesia*
Benzimidazoles		
Fenbendazole (Panacur)	Helminths	*Giardia*
Albendazole (Valbazan)	*Giardia, Encephalitozoon*	None
Ionophores		
Monensin (Rumensin, Coban)	Coccidia	*Toxoplasma*
Lasalocid (Bovatec)	Coccidia	None
Salinomycin (Bio-cox)	Coccidia	None
Antimonials		
Sodium stibogluconate (Pentostam)	*Leishmania*	None
Meglumine antimonate (Glucantime)	*Leishmania*	None
Antibacterials		
Paromomycin (Humatin, Aminosidine)	*Cryptosporidium, Pentatrichomonas*	*Entamoeba, Giardia, Leishmania*
Furazolidone (Furoxone)	Coccidia	*Giardia*
Nifurtimox (Lampit)	*Trypanosoma cruzi*	*Leishmania*
Tetracycline (many)	*Balantidium*	None
Trimethoprim-sulfonamide (Tribrissen, Ditrim, Bactrim, Septra)	*Pneumocystis,* coccidia, *Cyclospora, Neospora*	*Acanthamoeba*
Pyrimethamine (Daraprim)	*Toxoplasma, Neospora*	*Pneumocystis*
Spiramycin (Rovamycin, Stomorgyl[a])	*Cryptosporidium*	*Toxoplasma*
Clindamycin (Antirobe, Cleocin)	*Toxoplasma, Neospora*	*Babesia*
Azithromycin (Zithromax)	*Toxoplasma*	*Babesia, Cryptosporidium*
Miscellaneous		
Bismuth-N-glycollylarsanilate (Milibis-V)	None	*Entamoeba, Giardia*
Amprolium (Amprol, Corid)	None	Coccidia
Amphotericin B (Fungizone, Albecet[b])	*Acanthamoeba*	*Leishmania*
Toltrazuril (Baycox)	Coccidia, *Hepatozoon*	*Toxoplasma*
Ketoconazole	*Leishmania*	None
Allopurinol (Zyloprim[c])	*Leishmania*	*Trypanosoma cruzi*
Interferon-γ[c]	*Leishmania* (experimental)	None

See Drug Formulary, Appendix 8, for further information on these drugs.
[a] Combination of metronidazole (25, 125, 250 mg) with spiramycin (46.9, 234, 469 mg) in tablets.
[b] Lipid formulations preferred.
[c] Used in combination with antimonials for leishmaniasis.

orally. They are not absorbed systemically and have relatively low toxicity. Signs of toxicity are abdominal pain, diarrhea, and neurologic signs, all of which have been reported in dogs. Atovaquone is a closely related hydroxynaphthoquinone derivative licensed to treat *Pneumocystis* infections.

AROMATIC DIAMIDINES

Phenamidine, pentamidine, diminazene, amicarbalide, and imidocarb, which are diamidine derivatives, are the drugs of choice for treating *Babesia*, *Cytauxzoon*, and African *Trypanosoma* infections in dogs and cats. They are also effective against some other protozoa (see Table 71–1) and act by interfering with nucleic acid metabolism. These drugs are formulated as salts to reduce irritation after parenteral (IM or SC) injection.

Diamidines are rapidly effective and usually resolve clinical signs and parasitemia within 24 hours. They do not completely eradicate the organisms but have residual activity after a single injection. These drugs are avidly concentrated in parenchymal organs such as the liver and brain and are slowly metabolized or excreted unchanged. The slow metabolism and elimination of diamidines contribute to their prophylactic effects for many weeks after a single injection. Subtherapeutic dosages may allow organisms to develop resistance to these drugs.

NITROIMIDAZOLES

These drugs are effective against anaerobic enteric protozoa that cause trichomoniasis, amebiasis, giardiasis, and balantidiasis. They affect both the intraintestinal and the invasive parasites. Within anaerobic protozoa and bacteria, the nitrogroup undergoes reduction to produce various unstable metabolites, some of which have antimicrobial activity. The drugs are generally much less effective against microaerophilic or aerobic microorganisms. Metronidazole, tinidazole, nimorazole, dimetridazole, and ornidazole are close structural analogs marketed in various regions of the world. Metronidazole is the most widely used of these compounds. In addition to protozoa, it is active against obligate spore-forming anaerobes such as *Clostridium*, some non-spore-forming anaerobes such as *Campylobacter*, and microaerophilic organisms such as Enterobacteriaceae.

Metronidazole is almost completely absorbed after oral administration. Food does not reduce the extent of absorption but may delay its rate. IV administration of metronidazole may be preferable in severely ill patients but is expensive. The drug distributes widely and penetrates body tissues, extracellular fluids, and even pus-filled cavities. Metronidazole achieves good concentrations in the CNS even in the absence of inflammation. It is extensively metabolized in the liver, but there is also renal excretion of active drug.

Metronidazole has been administered alone and with spiramycin to treat periodontal disease and stomatitis and in combination with aminoglycosides to treat mixed infections associated with bowel perforation and intra-abdominal sepsis (see Chapter 89). In people, the drug is effective in the treatment of intra-abdominal, pelvic, pleuropulmonary, CNS, and bone and joint infections.

Side effects of metronidazole include GI irritation with signs of vomiting and anorexia, glossitis, and stomatitis. Neurologic signs may be seen after 7 to 10 days of treatment with high ($\geq$66 mg/kg/day) dosages and may be resolved when therapy is discontinued, but some dogs have developed fatal encephalopathy, persistent seizures, or cerebellar and central vestibular ataxia.

BENZIMIDAZOLES

Fenbendazole and albendazole are broad-spectrum drugs of this class that are used to treat a wide range of infections with helminths and selected protozoa by affecting microtubule synthesis in their cytoskeletons. Both drugs have been effective and relatively safe in the treatment of intestinal giardiasis. Myelotoxicity has been observed in dogs and cats,[33a] but can be reversed after treatment is discontinued.

IONOPHORES

These compounds form lipid-soluble complexes with cations, which facilitate transport of these ions across biologic membranes. They are antibiotics isolated from *Streptomyces* spp. and are provided primarily as coccidiostats. Monensin, lasalocid, and salinomycin, the compounds of veterinary interest, cause accumulation of intracellular ions within the parasite, interfering with its metabolism. Their use has primarily been as growth promoters in food animal practice, although monensin has been provided experimentally to reduce shedding of *Toxoplasma* oocysts by cats. The ionophores also have antibacterial activity and have been used experimentally to treat endotoxic shock in dogs. Because of their stimulatory effects on cardiac contractility and myocardial perfusion, their toxicity may be increased by concurrent administration of cardiac glycosides.

ANTIMONIALS

Sodium stibogluconate and meglumine antimonate, which are pentavalent antimony compounds, are two of the main agents in the treatment of leishmaniasis.[10, 31, 35, 36, 36a] The dosage is based on the amount of antimony compound administered. Treatment with these drugs is not curative, and two or three courses may be necessary. Side effects include anorexia, vomiting, nausea, myalgia, and lethargy. ECG abnormalities and nephrotoxicity can develop at higher dosages.

ANTIBACTERIALS

Paromomycin and furazolidone are nonabsorbable antibacterials, previously discussed under antibacterial therapy (Chapter 34). They are effective in treating some intestinal protozoal infections. Because of potential intestinal absorption and nephrotoxicity, paromomycin, an aminoglycoside, must be administered with caution in treating amebiasis when bowel lesions are extensive. Furazolidone and sulfonamides are effective in treating intestinal coccidial infections. Nifurtimox, a nitrofuran derivative, is suppressive but not curative for *Trypanosoma cruzi* infections. Nausea, vomiting, and convulsions may be side effects.

Trimethoprim, a previously discussed antibacterial diaminopyrimidine compound that inhibits folic acid synthesis, has broad-spectrum antimicrobial activity. Combined with sulfonamides, it has been provided to treat *Pneumocystis* and coccidial infections. Pyrimethamine is closely related but is more effective against protozoa than trimethoprim. It has been used in combination with sulfonamides to treat infections with *Neospora* and *Toxoplasma*.

Several newer antifolate drugs (see Chapter 80) under development may also be active against these two protozoa. Clindamycin, a lincosamide antimicrobial drug, and certain macrolides (azithromycin, clarithromycin) are also active against *Toxoplasma* and possibly *Neospora*.

Spiramycin, a macrolide antibiotic, has an antibacterial spectrum similar to that of erythromycin but is less effective. Absorption after PO administration is adequate for therapeutic purposes, and it is widely distributed and reaches high concentrations in tissues from which it is slowly eliminated in the bile and urine. It has had limited use for bacterial infections in veterinary medicine but is now marketed in combination with metronidazole, primarily to treat periodontal and oral infections. Spiramycin has been found to be somewhat effective for treating intestinal cryptosporidiosis and has been given to treat acute toxoplasmosis in people.

MISCELLANEOUS DRUGS

Bismuth-*N*-glycollylarsanilate is an anthelmintic drug that is a second choice in treating giardiasis. Amprolium is a thiamine inhibitor that is commonly chosen to treat coccidiosis in dogs, although not approved by the Food and Drug Administration for this purpose (see Chapter 81). Overdoses may produce neurologic signs. Toltrazuril is a new anticoccidial agent that is unrelated to the others. It appears to be very effective in eliminating coccidia in most species without interfering with a persistent host immune response. Toltrazuril has been provided to control oocyst shedding by cats acutely infected with *Toxoplasma*. The drug can be given PO in water or food, systemically by SC injection, or by topical application. Allopurinol is a pyrazolopyrimidine that interferes with nucleic acid synthesis in *Leishmania* and *T. cruzi*. It has been licensed to treat hyperuricemia and gout in people but is now being utilized to treat American trypanosomiasis and leishmaniasis in endemic areas (see Chapters 72 and 73).[13, 17, 19, 21]

References

1. Armitage K, Flanigan T, Carey J, et al. 1992. Treatment of cryptosporidiosis with paromomycin. *Arch Intern Med* 152:2497–2499.
2. Barr SC, Bowman DD, Heller RL. 1994. Efficacy of fenbendazole against giardiasis in dogs. *Am J Vet Res* 55:988–990.
3. Barr SC, Bowman DD, Heller RL, et al. 1993. Efficacy of albendazole against giardiasis in dogs. *Am J Vet Res* 54:926–928.
4. Barr SC, Jamrosz GF, Hornbuckle WE, et al. 1994. Use of paromomycin for treatment of cryptosporidiosis in a cat. *J Am Vet Med Assoc* 205:1742–1743.
5. Berman JD. 1997. Human leishmaniasis: clinical, diagnostic, and therapeutic developments in the last 10 years. *Clin Infect Dis* 24:684–703.
6. Chang HR, Comte R, Pechere JC. 1990. In vitro and in vivo effects of doxycycline of *Toxoplasma gondii*. *Antimicrob Agents Chemother* 34:775–780.
7. Dow SW, LeCouteur RA, Poss ML, et al. 1989. Central nervous system toxicosis associated with metronidazole treatment of dogs. Five cases (1984–1987). *J Am Vet Med Assoc* 195:365–368.
8. Egbe-Nwiyi TN, Antia RE. 1993. The effect of trypanocidal drug treatment on the haematological changes in *Trypanosoma brucei brucei* infected splenectomized dogs. *Vet Parasitol* 50:23–33.
9. Font A, Roura X, Fondevila D, et al. 1996. Canine mucosal leishmaniasis. *J Am Anim Hosp Assoc* 32:131–137.
10. Gramiccia M, Gradoni L, Orsini S. 1992. Decreased sensitivity to meglumine antimoniate (Glucantime) of *Leishmania infantum* isolated from dogs after several causes of drug treatment. *Ann Trop Med Parasitol* 86:613–620.
11. Greene CE. 1990. Antiprotozoal chemotherapy, pp 758–762. *In* Greene CE (ed), Infectious diseases of the dog and cat. WB Saunders, Philadelphia, PA.
12. Hay WH, Shell LG, Lindsay DS, et al. 1990. Diagnosis and treatment of *Neospora caninum* infection in a dog. *J Am Vet Med Assoc* 197:87–89.
13. Herwaldt BL, Neva FA, Berman JD. 1992. Allopurinol in the treatment of American cutaneous leishmaniasis. *N Engl J Med* 327:498.
14. Hiles RA, Mong S, Bekersky I, et al. 1994. Inhalation toxicity of aerosolized pentamidine isethionate in rats and dogs. *Fundam Appl Toxicol* 23:382–390.
15. Hughes WT. 1995. The role of atovaquone tablets in treating *Pneumocystis carinii* pneumonia. *J Acquir Immune Defic Syndr Hum Retrovirol* 8:247–252.
16. Kock N, Kelly P. 1991. Massive hepatic necrosis associated with accidental imidocarb dipropionate toxicosis in a dog. *J Comp Pathol* 104:113–116.

16a. Lamothe J. 1997. A new prospect on canine leishmaniasis: treatment with amphotericin B. *Prat Med Chir Comp* 32:133–141.

17. Lester SJ, Kenyon JE. 1996. Use of allopurinol to treat visceral leishmaniasis in a dog. *J Am Vet Med Assoc* 209:615–617.
18. Lindsay DS, Blagburn BL. 1991. Coccidial parasites of cats and dogs. *Compend Cont Educ Pract Vet* 13:759–765.

18a. Ling GV, Ruby AL, Harrold DR, et al. 1991. Xanthene-containing urinary calculi in dogs given allopurinol. *J Am Vet Med Assoc* 198:1935–1940.

19. Liste F, Gascon M. 1995. Allopurinol in the treatment of canine visceral leishmaniasis. *Vet Rec* 137:23–24.
20. Lynen L, Van Damme W. 1992. Local application of diminazene aceturate: an effective treatment for cutaneous leishmaniasis. *Ann Soc Belge Med Trop* 72:13–19.
21. Marr JJ. 1991. Purine analogs as chemotherapeutic agents in leishmaniasis and American trypanosomiasis. *J Lab Clin Med* 118:111–119.
22. Martinez S, Marr JJ. 1992. Allopurinol in the treatment of American cutaneous leishmaniasis. *N Engl J Med* 326:741–744.
23. Matthewmann LA, Kelly PJ, Brouqui P, et al. 1994. Further evidence for the efficacy of imidocarb dipropionate in the treatment of *Ehrlichia canis* infection. *J S Afr Vet Assoc* 65:104–107.
24. Mayhew IG, Smith KC, Dubey JP, et al. 1991. Treatment of encephalomyelitis due to *Neospora caninum* in a litter of puppies. *J Small Anim Pract* 32:609–612.
25. Motzel SL, Wagner JE. 1990. Treatment of experimentally induced cytauxzoonosis in cats with parvaquone and buparvaquone. *Vet Parasitol* 35:131–138.

25a. Oliva G, Gradoni, Ciaramella P, et al. 1995. Activity of liposomal amphotericin B (AmBiosome) in dogs naturally infected with *Leishmania infantum*. *J Antimicrob Chemother* 36:1013–1019.

26. Onyeyili PA, Anika SM. 1990. Effects of the combination of DL-α-difluoromethylornithine and diminazene aceturate in *Trypanosoma congolense* infection of dogs. *Vet Parasitol* 37:9–19.
27. Onyeyili PA, Anika SM. 1991. Diminazene aceturate residues in the tissues of healthy, *Trypanosoma congolense* and *Trypanosoma brucei brucei* infected dogs. *Br Vet J* 147:155–158.
28. Penzhorn BL, Lewis BD, DeWaal DT, et al. 1995. Sterilization of *Babesia canis* infections by imidocarb alone or in combination with diminazene. *J S Afr Vet Assoc* 66:157–159.
29. Peregrine AS, Mamman M. 1993. Pharmacology of diminazene: a review. *Acta Trop* 54:185–203.

29a. Poli A, Sozzi S, Guidi G, et al. 1997. Comparison of aminosidine (paromomycin) and sodium stilbogluconate for treatment of canine leishmaniasis. *Vet Parasitol* 71:263–271.

30. Rehg JE, Hancock ML, Woodmansee DB. 1988. Anticryptosporidial activity of sulfadimethoxine. *Antimicrob Agents Chemother* 12:1907–1908.
31. Slappendel RJ, Teske E. 1997. The effect of intravenous or subcutaneous administration of meglumine antimonate (Glucantime) in dogs with leishmaniasis. A randomized clinical trial. *Vet Q* 19:10–13.
32. Slater CA, Sickel JZ, Visvesvara GS, et al. 1994. Brief report: successful treatment of disseminated *Acanthamoeba* infection in an immunocompromised patient. *N Engl J Med* 331:85–87.
33. Sobottka I, Albrecht H, Schaefer H, et al. 1995. Disseminated encephalitozoon (septata) intestinalis infection in a patient with AIDS: novel diagnostic approaches and autopsy-confirmed parasitological cure following treatment with albendazole. *J Clin Microbiol* 33:2948–2952.

33a. Stokol T, Randolph JF, Nachbar S, et al. 1997. Development of bone marrow toxicosis after albendazole administration in a dog and a cat. *J Am Vet Med Assoc* 210:1753–1756.

34. St. Omer VV. 1978. Efficacy and toxicity of furazolidone in veterinary medicine. *Vet Med Small Anim Clin* 73:1125–1132.
35. Sundar S, Rosenkaimer F, Murray HW. 1994. Successful treatment of refractory visceral leishmaniasis in India using antimony plus interferon-γ. *J Infect Dis* 170:659–662.
36. Valladares JE, Alberola J, Estebam M, et al. 1996. Disposition of antimony after the administration of N-methylglucamine antimonate to dogs. *Vet Rec* 138:181–183.

36a. Valladares JE, Freixas J, Franquelo JA, et al. 1997. Pharmacokinetics of liposone encapsulated meglumine antimonate after intramuscular and subcutaneous administration in dogs. *Am J Trop Med Hyg* 57:403–406.

37. Wong BK, Woolf TF, Chang T, et al. 1990. Metabolic disposition of trimetrexate, a nonclassical dihydrofolate reductase inhibitor in rat and dog. *Drug Metab Dispos* 18:980–986.

Chapter **72**

Trypanosomiasis

American Trypanosomiasis

Stephen C. Barr

ETIOLOGY AND LIFE CYCLE

Trypanosoma cruzi, the etiologic agent of American trypanosomiasis or Chagas' disease, is a hemoflagellate protozoan of the class Zoomastigophorea and family Trypanosomatidae. The organism exists in three morphologic forms. The trypomastigote or blood form is 15 to 20 μm long, with a flattened spindle-shaped body and a centrally placed vesicular nucleus. A single free flagellum originates from a basal body near the large subterminal kinetoplast (situated posterior to the nucleus) and passes along the body to project anteriorly (Fig. 72–1). The intracellular or amastigote form is approximately 1.5 to 4.0 μm in diameter and ovoid, and it contains a large, round nucleus and rodlike kinetoplast. The flagellum is small and not always obvious under light microscopy. Epimastigotes, the third morphologic form, are found in the reduviid vector (subfamily Triatomae), commonly known as the kissing bug. This flagellated and spindle-shaped form has a kinetoplast situated anterior to the nucleus.

Infection usually occurs when trypomastigotes are deposited in the insect vector's feces at the bite site (Fig. 72–2). Oral ingestion of infected insects will cause infection in opossums and might be a possible route of infection in dogs. Other less common routes include blood transfusions, congenital factors, or ingestion of meat or milk from infected lactating animals.[13] Trypomastigotes usually enter macrophages and myocytes, either locally or systemically, after hematogenous spread. Once intracellular, trypomastigotes transform into amastigotes, which multiply by binary fission. These transform into trypomastigotes before rupture of and release from the cell. Rapid intracellular multiplication cycles ensure a rapid rise in parasitemia before effective immunity develops. The vector becomes infected by ingesting circulating trypomastigotes, which transform to epimastigotes and multiply by binary fission. Transformation of the epimastigotes back into trypomastigotes occurs in the vector's hindgut before the trypomastigotes are passed in the feces (see Fig. 72–2).

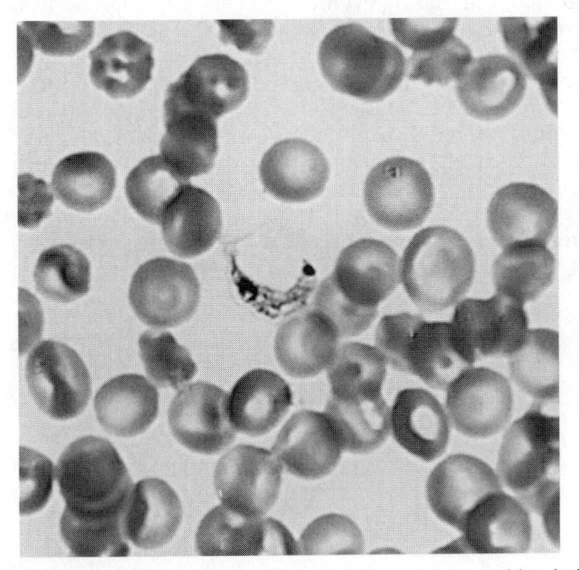

Figure 72–1. Trypomastigote form of *T. cruzi* in a blood film (Wright's stain, × 1000).

EPIDEMIOLOGY

T. cruzi infects humans and a wide range of domestic and wild animal species in the Americas. It is a major human health problem in South America (especially Brazil, Venezuela, Argentina) and Central America and is gaining importance in Mexico. Few human cases involving transmission by vectors have been reported in the United States. However, large numbers of people have emigrated to the United States from endemic regions, and an estimated 50,000 to 100,000 *T. cruzi*–infected people now reside here. Consequently, the number of cases associated with transfusion transmission have steadily risen.[25, 32] Most canine cases in the United States occur in Texas, especially in areas close to the Mexican border.[2] Isolated canine cases occur in other southern states,[2, 12, 33, 36] although the infection was found to be endemic in a group of Walker hounds in Virginia (Fig. 72–3).[13] The mother and a majority of her pups were found to be infected, suggesting transplacental or transmammary infection.

Usual transmission of *T. cruzi* depends on the confluence of reservoirs, vectors, parasites, and hosts (people or animals) in a single habitat. There are two extremes of vector behavior: those that are habitually domiciliated and those that are habitually sylvan; many species are intermediate in behavior. Because of this variation, vectors tend to have either domestic or sylvan cycles, with cross-over between the two occasionally. Of the many Triatomae species that can feed on people in South America, only three, *Triatoma infestans, T. dimidiata,* and *Rhodnius prolixus*, are related to the epidemiology of human infections. They are efficient human vectors because they feed on blood from both people and domestic reservoir mammals (dog, cat, guinea pigs), reproduce prolifically while cohabiting close to people, and defecate soon after taking a blood meal. Infection rates in these vectors can be as high as 100% south of the equator. In comparison, infection rates of the two principal vectors in the United States, *T. protracta* and *T. sanguisuga*, are 20%. These two vectors are peridomestic, and their inability to adapt to living in human dwellings, their different feeding and defecation habits, and their lack of access to people with a higher standard of housing are some reasons for low infection rates in the United States.

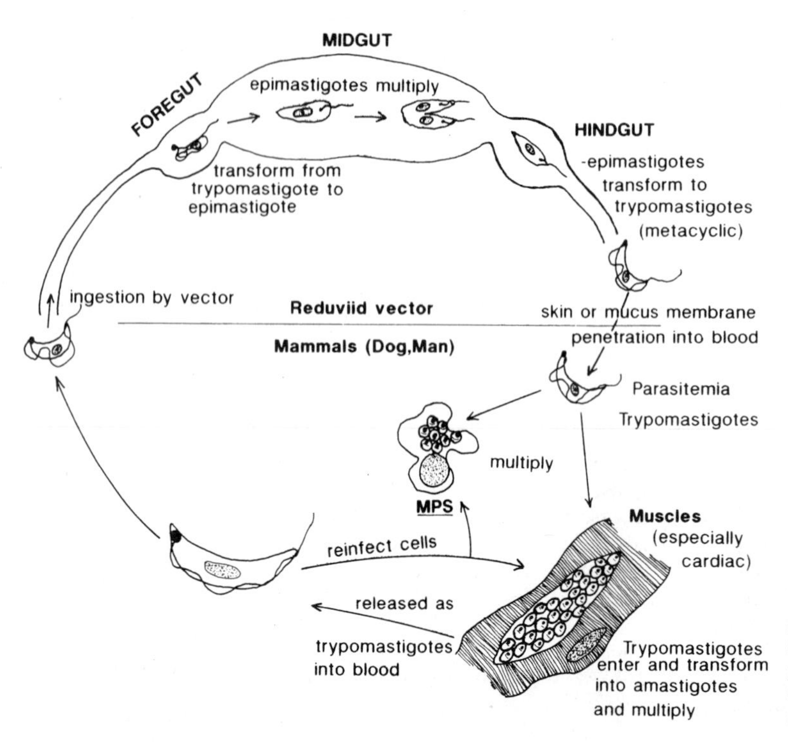

Figure 72–2. Life cycle of *T. cruzi*. Replication by epimastigotes occurs in the vector. Trypomastigotes in the vector's feces infect the host and divide intracellularly as amastigotes. Host cells rupture, releasing trypomastigotes, which enter other cells or the blood stream. Vectors become infected by ingesting blood containing trypomastigotes.

The principal sylvan reservoir hosts of *T. cruzi* in the southern United States are opossums, raccoons, and armadillos.[2, 5, 15, 24] Similarly, in Maryland,[38] Oklahoma,[23] North Carolina,[24] and Georgia,[30] raccoons and opossums are the main reservoir hosts. In California and New Mexico, the main sylvan hosts are various mouse, squirrel, and rat species.[2] Although *T. cruzi* isolates from infected vectors, animal reservoirs, and people in North America show similar in vitro characteristics to those of isolates from South America,[6] these isolates tend to be less pathogenic in mice than South American isolates.[5] Because inoculation of *T. cruzi* isolates from opossums and armadillos into dogs experimentally produces a similar disease described in naturally acquired cases of acute and chronic canine trypanosomiasis, it is likely that dogs in nature are infected with the same isolates as these sylvan hosts.[9–11]

PATHOGENESIS

T. cruzi trypomastigotes enter host cells soon after infection, multiply unhindered, escape the immune response, and are transported throughout the body primarily within macrophages. Parasitemia develops within a few days and peaks 2 to 3 weeks PI, coinciding with acute clinical disease.[9] The pathogenesis of the acute phase is thought to result from cell damage as trypomastigotes rupture from host cells, especially cardiac myocytes, and, in some cases, neurologic tissue. Most clinical signs during the acute stage are referable to this cell destruction. The period from infection to development of acute disease is variable with puppies showing severe disease 2 weeks PI. Dogs infected after 6 months of age may show no signs of acute disease other than slight depression and low-rising parasitemia.

By 4 weeks PI, parasitemias have dropped to undetectable levels probably owing to a rising specific immune response to the parasite, and signs of acute disease diminish. Dogs tend to remain asymptomatic for months or years. During this time, there is a progressive development of myocardial degeneration, leading eventually to biventricular dilative cardiomyopathy of unknown pathogenesis.[1a]

There are many theories concerning the cause of the cardiomyopathy, including damage by toxic parasite products and autoimmune-mediated mechanisms leading to autonomic nervous system disruption.[22] Further studies suggest that local spasm of the coronary microvasculature, eventually leading to myocardial ischemia, may lead to progressive cardiac myocyte destruction. Cardiac dilatation occurs when fibrosis no longer permits efficient compensatory hypertrophy.[1, 35]

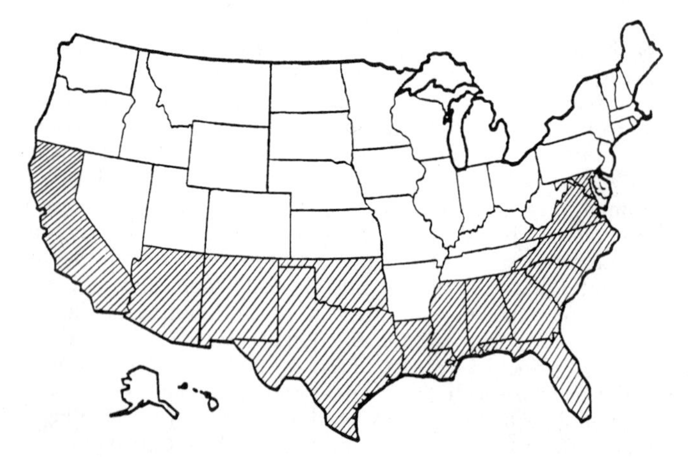

Figure 72–3. Distribution of *T. cruzi* in dogs, vectors, and reservoir hosts in the United States.

CLINICAL FINDINGS

Dogs

Clinically affected dogs develop either acute or chronic disease. Acute disease occurs mainly in dogs younger than 1 year and is sudden in onset, with signs referable to right-sided heart failure. Generalized lymphadenomegaly may precede and is invariably present during acute illness. Signs referable to acute myocarditis, such as sudden collapse and death of a previously normal young dog, have been reported most frequently. Pale mucous membranes, slowed capillary refill time, weak pulse with deficits, tachyarrhythmia, and terminal hypothermia and respiratory distress are common. Most infected dogs that do not die suddenly develop ascites, hepatomegaly, and splenomegaly owing to right-sided heart failure. Anorexia and diarrhea are also common during acute disease. Neurologic signs referable to meningoencephalitis, including pelvic limb ataxia, profound weakness, and hyperreflexive spinal reflexes suggestive of distemper, have been found in naturally and experimentally infected dogs.[2, 9, 14] During acute disease, dogs, like experimentally infected mice, probably suffer a profound immunosuppression because of altered interleukin-2 activity.[35] Such immunosuppression has been proposed as the cause of the development of distemper in pups with acute canine trypanosomiasis after they received modified live distemper vaccine.[13] ECG changes during acute disease are highly variable and include alteration in ST-T segments, T-wave inversion, low-amplitude QRS complexes, positive polyphasic ventricular premature contractions, and first- and second-degree heart block.[10]

Survivors of acute myocarditis will become aparasitemic and asymptomatic, and they develop chronic myocarditis with cardiac dilatation over the next 8 to 36 months.[9, 10] During the long asymptomatic period between acute and chronic disease in the dog, the ECG may be normal except for the intermittent occurrence of ventricular arrhythmias, which can be exacerbated by exercise or excitement.[3] Sudden death during this stage can occur and is thought to be caused by fatal cardiac arrhythmias. As cardiac dilatation occurs, ECG abnormalities become more prevalent and clinical signs referable to right-sided and eventually left-sided chamber failure occur. These cases are indistinguishable from chronic dilative cardiomyopathy seen in large breeds of dogs and often are diagnosed as such until histology or immunohistochemistry findings are available.[11–13] Trypanosomiasis should be considered in any dog with signs of myocarditis or cardiomyopathy.

Megaesophagus and other megaviscus syndromes described in humans with chronic Chagas' disease have not been described in dogs spontaneously or experimentally infected with *T. cruzi*.

Cats

Cats are reported to be susceptible to South American isolates of *T. cruzi*, but little information is available regarding clinical disease. There are no reports of domestic feline trypanosomiasis from North America.

DIAGNOSIS

Radiographic and Clinical Laboratory Findings

Thoracic radiography is of value in the diagnosis of pleural effusion, pulmonary edema, and chamber dilation in both acute and chronic myocarditis. ECG is valuable in the diagnosis of the dilative cardiomyopathy of chronic disease. Thinning of ventricular walls, large end-diastolic volumes, and low shortening fractions (usually <20%) are often present.[10]

Hematology is of little specific diagnostic value. A lymphocytosis may occur in the acute phase in a small number of cases. Alanine aminotransferase activity may be elevated as a result of hepatic hypoxia. Creatine kinase (CK) and lactate dehydrogenase activities are rarely elevated during acute disease. Elevations of serum CK (isoenzyme MB) do occur but are too variable and transient to be of any diagnostic value in the dog.[9] The abdominal effusion is typically a modified transudate from cardiac causes.

Cytology

Trypomastigotes can be identified in the blood just before and during acute disease (see Fig. 72–1). Although organisms are identified in most cases of acute trypanosomiasis, rarely are they found in chronic cases. Parasitemias are often so low, however, that organisms can be missed during routine examination of Wright's-stained blood films. Trypomastigotes may be pelleted for examination from plasma (obtained by centrifugation of 50 ml of heparinized blood at 800 *g* for 10 minutes) by further centrifugation (8000 *g* for 15 minutes). High-power (400 ×) examination of the buffy coat–plasma interface of a centrifuged microhematocrit tube may reveal characteristically motile parasites. A thick-film buffy coat smear, stained with Wright's or Giemsa stain or examined as a wet preparation for trypomastigote movement, is also an effective means of concentrating trypomastigotes. Lymph node aspirates or impression smears may be positive even when parasitemias are very low. Abdominal effusions may contain organisms that can be identified cytologically. Polymerase chain reaction has been shown to have higher sensitivity than microscopic methods in detecting parasitemia.[26]

Isolation

Isolation of organisms into germ-free hosts or cell culture systems is a sensitive but time-consuming practice. Blood agar slants overlaid with liver infusion tryptose (LIT) medium or LIT alone are effective for isolating trypomastigotes from blood of an infected animal but can take from 2 to 20 weeks to become positive for epimastigotes.[2] Direct inoculation of blood into a Vero cell monolayer will usually result in the development of intracellular amastigote forms and trypomastigotes in media after 2 to 4 weeks.

Weanling laboratory inbred mice (C3H) inoculated IP or SC with the patient's blood will usually develop detectable parasitemias 10 to 30 days later. The sensitivity can be increased by treating mice with glucocorticoids before and after inoculation.

Serologic Testing

The indirect FA, direct hemagglutination, and complement fixation tests are most commonly used.[2] These tests confirm the presence of antibodies to *T. cruzi* and, although most cross-react with antibodies to *Leishmania* and *T. rangeli* in South America, they are sensitive and specific for North American isolates. A central laboratory is available on a limited research basis in North America for *T. cruzi* serologic assays (Appendix 5). Titers usually become positive by 3 weeks PI at the time when parasitemias are declining.[7]

PATHOLOGIC FINDINGS

In acute disease, lesions usually are confined to the heart, especially the right side. Subendocardial and subepicardial hemorrhages as well as multiple yellow to white myocardial spots and streaks mainly involve the coronary groove.[2, 11] Hepatic, splenic, and renal congestion as well as pulmonary edema may be present secondary to cardiac failure. Micro-

Table 72–1. Therapy for American and African Trypanosomiasis[a]

DISEASE	DOSE (mg/kg)[b]	ROUTE	INTERVAL (HOURS)	DURATION (MONTHS)
American Trypanosomiasis				
Nifurtimox[c]	2–7	PO	6	3–5
Benznidazole	5	PO	24	2
African Trypanosomiasis				
Diminazene aceturate[d]	3.6–7	IM	2 weeks[16]	[e]

[a]See Drug Formulary, Appendix 8, for additional information on each drug.
[b]Dose per administration at specified interval.
[c]Lampit (Bayer) is an investigational drug in the United States. Available only from the Centers for Disease Control, Atlanta, GA, for treatment of human infections.
[d]Available for use in endemic areas.
[e]Repeat therapy as needed to control relapse or reinfection.

scopically, a diffuse granulomatous inflammation, hydropic degeneration and necrosis of myofibrils, and a mononuclear cellular infiltrate typify acute cases. Numerous pseudocysts containing amastigotes are often associated with the inflammatory response. Mild granulomatous myositis and organisms can be found in other organs, including the smooth muscle of the stomach, small intestine, bladder, and skeletal muscle. A nonsuppurative encephalitis has also been found.

Chronic disease is characterized by a bilaterally enlarged flaccid heart with areas of thinning of the ventricular walls owing to fibrous plaques. Histologically, there are multifocal coalescing areas of lymphoplasmacytic inflammation and mild necrosis with extensive loss of myocardial fibers and replacement by fibrous tissue. Organisms are seldom found in tissues. The apex of the heart is one of the more likely areas to find them.[11]

THERAPY

The investigational drug nifurtimox (Bayer 2502 or Lampit, Bayer Ag, Leverkusen-Bayerwerk, Germany), available in the United States from the Centers for Disease Control, Atlanta, Georgia, has been reported to be successful in treating experimental and natural cases of canine trypanosomiasis (Table 72–1).[2] Improved survival has been shown to occur in dogs treated concurrently with anti-inflammatory doses of glucocorticoids.[2] Benznidazole has been shown to produce cures in acute Chagas' disease in people. Benznidazole and nifurtimox are considered the recommended therapies for Chagas' disease.[37] Ketoconazole, gossypol, and allopurinol have been investigated, but the results of these studies are less than convincing.[19, 27, 31] For further information on nifurtimox, see Drug Formulary, Appendix 8.

Supportive therapy, including furosemide and theophylline, is indicated in cases of dilatational myocarditis. Cardiac arrhythmias may require specific therapy, depending on the source and severity of the disturbance. If the disease is diagnosed and treated early enough, the mortality rate of acute disease can be decreased. However, dogs surviving acute disease invariably develop chronic cardiac disease in 8 to 30 months. Their prognoses must be guarded because the outcome is usually fatal.

PREVENTION

Preventing contact between dogs and infected vectors by upgrading housing of the dogs will do much to limit infection. Residual insecticides should be sprayed monthly in peridomiciliary structures (woodpiles, chicken houses) and dog kennels. Oral cythioate (Proban, Bayer, Shawnee, KS; 3 mg/kg every other day) given to dogs housed outdoors will reduce vector numbers; once reduced, the dose can be given twice a week. Limiting contact between dogs and infected reservoir hosts (opossums, raccoons, armadillos) and their vectors is virtually impossible but would limit infection. Most cases in the United States have been reported in hunting dogs, which do have an increased risk of exposure.[8] Dogs should not be fed raw meat of reservoir hosts. Blood donors in endemic areas should be screened serologically to determine previous exposure to *T. cruzi*.

PUBLIC HEALTH CONSIDERATIONS

An estimated 20 million Latin Americans are infected with Chagas' disease, but only 3 naturally acquired cases have been reported in the United States.[2] Several factors are probably responsible for this low prevalence of Chagas' disease. First, the North American species of *Triatoma* have usually left the host when they defecate, unlike the South American insect, which defecates while still on the host. Because contact with infected feces is the usual mode of transmission, this behavior limits the chance of contact. Second, the density of infected *Triatoma* in human dwellings is much less in the United States than it is in endemic areas of South America. Third, more cases of human Chagas' disease may have occurred in the United States but have gone unrecognized because of a low index of suspicion. Because it is estimated that 50,000 to 100,000 infected people now reside in the United States, there is probably more risk of catching *T. cruzi* from blood transfusion than from infected vectors.

Chagas' disease in dogs and wild hosts is of considerable public health significance because of the severity of and difficulty in treating the disease in people. Veterinarians should take particular care in treating such cases and make owners aware of the potential zoonotic risk. Blood samples taken from infected dogs are potentially infective, and laboratory staff should be appropriately instructed in their handling.

African Trypanosomiasis

Craig E. Greene

ETIOLOGY AND EPIDEMIOLOGY

Trypanosomiasis is an important hemoparasitic disease of animals and people in Africa (i.e., sleeping sickness). *T. brucei* comprises a group of indistinguishable flagellated hemoparasites in the subgenus *Trypanozoon*. Some of the subspecies cause human sleeping sickness. *T. brucei brucei* and *T. congolense*, a species in the subgenus *Nannomonas*, are parasites of wild and domestic animals, but do not infect people. Host species differ in their susceptibility to infection, and dogs are particularly susceptible to *T. congolense* and *T. brucei brucei*.[28]

These parasites are transmitted by tsetse flies of the genus *Glossina*, which are widespread in Africa. Mechanical transmission by other vectors and congenital transmission does not occur. Rare laboratory inoculations have developed. Flies become infected after ingesting blood containing short trypomastigotes. The organism has a developmental cycle in the insect vector. It transforms into slender trypomastigotes, which enter the salivary glands, becoming epimastigotes. Transmission occurs when these are inoculated by the fly during feeding on a new host.

PATHOGENESIS

Once in the mammalian host, these parasites can replicate unimpeded by immune defenses. Unlike *T. cruzi*, they undergo continual antigenic variation of their outer glycoprotein coat.

Replication in the host results in widespread hemolymphatic dissemination. From the site of inoculation, inflammation spreads to the lymph nodes and spleen. Pericarditis and myocarditis, anemia, thrombocytopenia leukocytosis, and disseminated intravascular coagulation can occur. Invasion of the CNS occurs in final stages of the disease with a diffuse meningoencephalitis.

The spleen is important in the production of antibodies and immune response to these hemoprotozoans. Splenectomy delays the onset of anemia and increases parasitemia and febrile responses.[17]

CLINICAL FINDINGS

Clinical signs in acutely infected dogs consist of anorexia and fever; edema of the face, genitalia, and SC tissues; purulent ocular and nasal discharges; orchitis in males; and pale mucosae and weakness. Petechial hemorrhage and mucosal bleeding, lymphadenomegaly, and splenomegaly also occur.

DIAGNOSIS AND PATHOLOGIC FINDINGS

Hematologic changes during the course of infection include a decline in hematocrit with reticulocytosis and elevated mean corpuscular volume. The WBC count often decreases with neutropenia, lymphopenia, and eosinopenia and thrombocytopenia. In other cases, leukocytosis with neutrophilia has been noted.

Immunodiagnostic methods include detection of an antibody response using indirect FA and ELISA methods, of which the latter is more sensitive. Trypanosome species–specific monoclonal antibodies have been utilized to detect circulating antigen in infected dogs.[18]

At necropsy, edema and subcutaneous hemorrhages may be visible in many organs. Hepatosplenomegaly and lymphadenomegaly may be apparent. Lymphoplasmacytic infiltrates are found in many organs.

TREATMENT

Few drugs exist in the treatment of African trypanosomiasis (see Table 72–1). Isometamidium chloride was the first used. Arsenicals such as cymelarsan (RM 110, Merial, Iselin, NJ) and an enzyme inhibitor, difluoromethylornithine (DFMO; Hoechst Marion-Roussel, Somerville, NJ), have shown efficacy in experimental studies.[28, 34] DFMO has been combined with diminazene in treating infected dogs. Although relapses have occurred with this combination, they were lower than those that developed with either drug alone. Trypanosomes may cross the blood-brain barrier, evading the effective drugs, which are molecularly too large to cross.[16] Diminazene appears to be the most effective drug against relapses. It is available for treatment of affected cattle. Appropriate dosages are listed in Table 73–1. Further information on its use appears in the Drug Formulary, Appendix 8. Concentrations of diminazene are higher in brain tissue of infected dogs compared with healthy dogs,[28, 29] presumably as a result of inflammation of the blood-brain barrier. Melarsoprol is effective in penetrating the nervous system but is available only on an experimental basis.

References

1. Andrade ZA, Andrade SG, Correa R, et al. 1994. Myocardial changes in acute *Trypanosoma cruzi* infection: ultrastructural evidence of immune damage and the role of microangiopathy. *Am J Pathol* 144:1403–1411.

1a. Andrade ZA, Andrade SG, Sadigursky M, et al. 1997. The indeterminate phase of Chagas disease: ultrastructural characterization of cardiac changes in the canine model. *Am J Trop Med Hyg* 57:328–336.

2. Barr SC. 1990. American trypanosomiasis, pp 763–768. *In* Greene CE (ed), Infectious diseases of the dog and cat. WB Saunders, Philadelphia, PA.

3. Barr SC. 1991. Canine American Trypanosomiasis. *Compend Cont Educ Pract Vet* 13:745–755.

4. Barr SC, Brown C, Dennis VA, et al. 1990. Infections of inbred mice with three *Trypanosoma cruzi* isolates from Louisiana mammals. *J Parasitol* 76:918–921.

5. Barr SC, Brown C, Dennis VA, et al. 1991. The lesions and prevalence of *Trypanosoma cruzi* in opossums and armadillos from southern Louisiana. *J Parasitol* 77:624–627.

6. Barr SC, Dennis VA, Klei TR. 1990. Growth parameters in axenic and cell cultures, protein profiles, and zymodeme typing of three *Trypanosoma cruzi* isolates from Louisiana mammals. *J Parasitol* 76:631–638.

7. Barr SC, Dennis VA, Klei TR, et al. 1991. Antibody and lymphoblastogenic responses of dogs experimentally infected with *Trypanosoma cruzi* isolates from North American mammals. *Vet Immunol Immunopathol* 29:267–283.

8. Barr SC, Dennis VA, Klei TR. 1991. Serologic and blood culture survey of *Trypanosoma cruzi* for infection in four canine populations of southern Louisiana. *Am J Vet Res* 52:570–573.

9. Barr SC, Gossett KA, Klei TR. 1991. Clinical, clinicopathologic, and parasitologic observations of trypanosomiasis in dogs infected with North American *Trypanosoma cruzi* isolates. *Am J Vet Res* 52:954–960.

10. Barr SC, Holmes RA, Klei TR. 1992. Electrocardiographic and echocardiographic features of trypanosomiasis in dogs inoculated with North American *Trypanosoma cruzi* isolates. *Am J Vet Res* 53:521–527.

11. Barr SC, Schmidt SP, Brown CC, et al. 1991. Pathologic features of dogs

inoculated with North American *Trypanosoma cruzi* isolates. *Am J Vet Res* 52:2033–2039.
12. Barr SC, Simpson RM, Schmidt SP, et al. 1989. Chronic dilatative myocarditis caused by *Trypanosoma cruzi* in two dogs. *J Am Vet Med Assoc* 195:1237–1241.
13. Barr SC, van Beek O, Carlisle-Nowak MS, et al. 1995. *Trypanosoma cruzi* infection in Walker Hounds from Virginia. *Am J Vet Res* 56:1037–1044.
14. Berger SL, Palmer RH, Hodges CC, et al. 1991. Neurologic manifestations of trypanosomiasis in a dog. *J Am Vet Med Assoc* 198:132–134.
15. Burkholder JE, Allison TC, Kelly VP. 1980. *Trypanosoma cruzi* (Chagas) (protozoa: Kinetoplastida) in invertebrate, reservoir and human hosts of the lower Rio Grande Valley of Texas. *J Parasitol* 66:305–311.
16. Chukwu CC, Anene BM, Onuekwusi KO, et al. 1990. Relapse infection after chemotherapy in dogs experimentally infected with *Trypanosoma brucei brucei*. *J Small Anim Pract* 31:141–144.
17. Egbe-Nwiyi TN, Anita RE. 1993. The effect of trypanocidal drug treatment on the haematological changes in *Trypanosoma brucei brucei* infected splenectomised dogs. *Vet Parasitol* 50:23–33.
18. Egbe-Nwiyi TN, Anita RE. 1995. Use of monoclonal antibodies for detecting *T. brucei brucei* infection in splenectomised dogs. *J Small Anim Pract* 36:229–232.
19. Gallerano RH, Marr JJ, Sosa RR. 1990. Therapeutic efficacy of allopurinol in patients with chronic Chagas' disease. *Am J Trop Med Hyg* 43:159–166.
20. Gürtler RE, Cécere MC, Rubel DN, et al. 1991. Chagas disease in northwest Argentina: infected dogs as a risk factor for the domestic transmission of *Trypanosoma cruzi*. *Trans R Soc Trop Med Hyg* 85:741–745.
21. Harrus S, Harmelin A, Presenty B. 1995. *Trypanosoma congolense* infection in two dogs. *J Small Anim Pract* 36:83–86.
22. Hudson L. 1981. Immunobiology of *Trypanosoma cruzi* infection and Chagas' disease. *Trans R Soc Trop Med Hyg* 75:493–498.
23. John DT, Hoppe KL. 1986. *Trypanosoma cruzi* from wild raccoons in Oklahoma. *Am J Vet Res* 47:1056–1059.
24. Karsten V, Davis C, Kuhn R. 1992. *Trypanosoma cruzi* in wild raccoons and opossums in North Carolina. *J Parasitol* 78:547–549.
25. Kirchhoff LV. 1993. American trypanosomiasis (Chagas' disease)—a tropical disease now in the United States. *N Engl J Med* 329:639–644.
26. Kirchhoff LV, Votava JR, Ochs DE, et al. 1996. Comparison of PCR and microscopic methods for detecting *Trypanosoma cruzi*. *J Clin Microbiol* 34:1171–1175.
27. Marr JJ, Docampo R. 1986. Chemotherapy for Chagas' disease: a perspective of current therapy and considerations for future research. *Rev Infect Dis* 8:884–903.
28. Onyeyili PA, Anika SM. 1990. Effects of the combination of DL-α-difluoromethylornithine and diminazene aceturate in *Trypanosoma congolense* infection of dogs. *Vet Parasitol* 37:9–19.
29. Onyeyili PA, Anika SM. 1991. Diminazene aceturate residues in the tissues of healthy *Trypanosoma congolense* and *Trypanosoma brucei brucei* infected dogs. *Br Vet J* 147:155–162.
30. Pung OJ, Banks CW, Jones DN, et al. 1995. *Trypanosoma cruzi* in wild raccoons, opossums, and Triatomine bugs in southeast Georgia, USA. *J Parasitol* 81:324–326.
31. Rovai LE, Aoki A, Gerez de Burgos NM, et al. 1990. Effect of gossypol on trypomastigotes and amastigotes of *Trypanosoma cruzi*. *J Protozool* 37:280–286.
32. Schmunis GA. 1991. *Trypanosoma cruzi*, the etiologic agent of Chagas' disease: status in the blood supply in endemic and nonendemic countries. *Transfusion* 31:547–557.
33. Snider TG, Yaeger RG, Dellucky J. 1992. Myocarditis caused by *Trypanosoma cruzi* in a native Louisiana dog. *J Am Vet Med Assoc* 177:247–249.
34. Syakalima M, Yasuda J, Hashimoto A. 1995. Preliminary efficacy trial of cymelarsan in mice artificially infected with *Trypanosoma brucei brucei* isolated from a dog in Zambia. *Jpn Vet Res* 43:93–97.
35. Tanowitz HB, Kirchhoff LV, Simon D, et al. 1992. Chagas' disease. *Clin Microbiol Rev* 5:400–419.
36. Tippit TS. 1978. Canine Trypanosomiasis (Chagas' disease). *Southwest Vet* 2:97–104.
37. Viotti R, Vigliano C, Armenti H, et al. 1994. Treatment of chronic Chagas' disease with benznidazole: clinical and serologic evolution of patients with long-term follow-up. *Am Heart J* 127:151–162.
38. Walton BC, Bauman PM, Diamond LS, et al. 1958. The isolation and identification of *Trypanosoma cruzi* from raccoons in Maryland. *Am J Trop Med Hyg* 7:603–610.

Chapter 73

Leishmaniasis

Robbert J. Slappendel and Luis Ferrer

Leishmaniasis is a worldwide infectious disease of people and wild and domestic animals that is caused by diphasic protozoans of the genus *Leishmania*. It is a frequent cause of clinical disease in dogs and is less common in cats. Infected dogs serve as reservoirs of the disease for people in many countries where leishmaniasis is endemic. Interest in the disease has also increased in nonendemic countries because of the ever-increasing international traffic of tourists and immigrants accompanied by pets. Dogs easily carry this chronic insidious disease unnoticed.

Different leishmanial species occur in various parts of the Old World and the New World and are responsible for a wide spectrum of clinical illness in people (Fig. 73–1). Rough estimates suggest that some 350 million people are at risk of acquiring the infection and that 12 million are currently infected. Depending on the leishmanial species involved, dogs may or may not frequently or sporadically be involved in sylvan and urban cycles.[59]

ETIOLOGY

On the basis of the difference in development in sandflies, the genus *Leishmania* is divided into the subgenera *Leishmania* and *Viannia*. Within these subgenera, many species and subspecies have been recognized. Currently, classification is mainly based on discrimination by biochemical methods, including DNA peptide mapping, immunologic reactivity to monoclonal antibodies and membrane-shed antigens, and especially isoenzyme patterns (so-called zymodemes). A number of different *Leishmania* species sharing major characters have been grouped into so-called "complexes."

On the basis of clinical signs in humans, the disease may be divided into cutaneous leishmaniasis (CL), mucocutaneous leishmaniasis (MCL), and visceral leishmaniasis (VL). These forms are caused by various leishmanial species (Table 73–1).

Canine leishmaniasis is often classified as VL because it is associated with the *Leishmania* species that cause VL in humans, but in dogs there is usually both visceral and cutaneous involvement.

EPIDEMIOLOGY

The natural cycle of infection is usually a zoonosis with blood-sucking sandflies serving as vectors, transmitting the

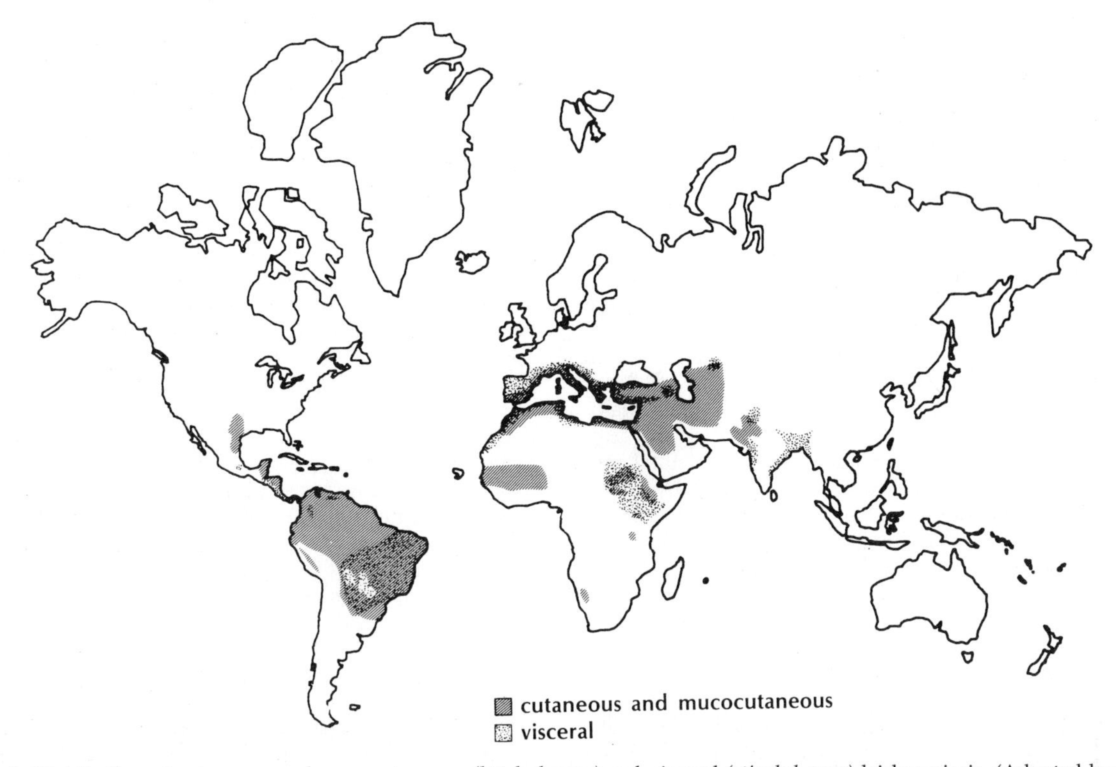

Figure 73–1. Distribution of cutaneous and mucocutaneous *(hatched areas)* and visceral *(stippled areas)* leishmaniasis. (Adapted by permission from *The Leishmaniases*. The WHO Expert Committee. WHO Technical Report Series No. 701. Geneva, WHO, 1984.)

parasite among wild or domestic animals and humans. Sandflies of the genus *Phlebotomus* in the Old World and *Lutzomyia* in the New World are the primary vectors. Most species of sandflies are active mainly at sunset, rarely at night, from early spring to late autumn. They do not roam more than approximately 1500 m from their breeding places.

Wild and domestic dogs are the main reservoirs for VL in people, but even in countries with a high infection rate among dogs, the incidence of VL in native human inhabitants is generally low.[59] In some regions in the Far East and East Africa, humans themselves appear to be the reservoir. The main reservoir hosts for CL and MCL are rodents and other wild animals, but dogs may play a role in its epidemiology in some regions. Cats are only rarely infected with *Leishmania*. See Public Health Considerations for further information regarding animals as reservoirs for infections.

In the vertebrate host, *Leishmania* is found in macrophages only as a nonflagellate form, the amastigote, which is ovoid or round, 2.5 to 5.0 μm long × 1.5 to 2.0 μm wide. In addition to a reddish nucleus, a characteristic purple, rod-shaped kinetoplast is generally visible after Wright's or Giemsa staining (Fig. 73–2).

Amastigotes multiply by binary fission, rupture out of the macrophage, and infect new cells. Sandflies can ingest the amastigotes when they suck blood from an infected host. In the sandfly, the organisms multiply and undergo a series

Table 73–1. Leishmanial Species and the Diseases They Cause in Humans Worldwide

CLINICAL DISEASE	OLD WORLD	NEW WORLD
Cutaneous	*L. aethiopica* complex	*L. mexicana* complex
	L. aethiopica	*L. mexicana*
	L. major complex	*L. venezuelensis*
	L. major	*L. amazonensis*
	L. tropica complex	*L. pifanoi*
	L. tropica	*L. garnhami*
	L. killicki	*L. braziliensis* complex (*Viannia*)
		L. braziliensis[a]
		L. panamensis[a]
		L. guyanensis[a]
		L. peruviana
		L. lainsoni[b]
Visceral	*L. donovani* complex	
	L. donovani	*L. chagasi*[a]
	L. infantum[c]	

[a]May also cause mucocutaneous leishmaniasis.
[b]Not definitively assigned.
[c]Main causative agents of canine leishmaniasis.

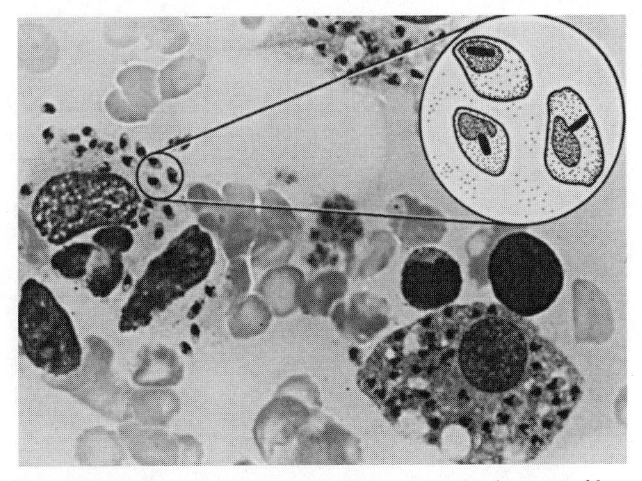

Figure 73–2. Amastigotes in macrophages in stained smear of bone marrow aspirate (May-Grünwald-Giemsa stain). *Inset*: schematic drawing of amastigotes. (From Slappendel RJ: *Vet Q* 10:1–16, 1988. Reprinted with permission.)

of morphologic alterations, including transformation into a flagellate form, the promastigote. Promastigotes may be injected into the skin of a vertebrate host when the fly feeds again. After inoculation into the host, they lose their flagella and again change into amastigotes (Fig. 73–3).

Old World

Clinical information about leishmaniasis in small animals has been almost exclusively based on studies in dogs from countries around the Mediterranean basin and from Portugal. Sporadic autochthonous cases have also been reported in other European countries in which no sandflies exist.[10b] These may have resulted from the bite of a sandfly incidentally imported by means of rapid modern transportation, because the life span of a sandfly is about 2 weeks. Horizontal mechanical transmission, directly from dog to dog or by a vector, such as the brown dog tick,[36] are other rare possibilities. Usually, however, canine leishmaniasis in nonendemic regions is found in imported dogs and dogs that have visited endemic areas. The latter type of case has been reported in the United States, Canada, and many European countries.

The inciting organism in dogs in the Old World is almost exclusively *L. infantum,* although *L. tropica* may be involved incidentally. Both species occur in the Mediterranean area, and they are morphologically indistinguishable. Dogs infected with *L. tropica* seem to be asymptomatic or may have only small cutaneous lesions that are not readily detected. Parasites with *L. tropica*–specific zymodemes have been isolated in dogs in Egypt, Israel, and Morocco,[10] but dogs are probably rarely involved in the epidemiology of CL.

The frequency of canine infections may vary greatly according to differences in environmental conditions and vectors. High prevalences of canine leishmaniasis as have been reported in the past are now rarely observed and may have been due to biased calculations. Even in regions with high infection rates, the prevalence rarely exceeds 10%.[13, 43]

In the Old World, infection of dogs occurs mostly in arid zones of rural areas and at the periphery of certain towns. Dogs may attract sandflies into houses, facilitating transmission to people. The geographic distribution of VL in people (see Fig. 73–1) is caused mainly by parasites of the *L. donovani* complex (see Table 73–1) and generally coincides with the distribution of leishmaniasis in dogs. In northwestern India, Bangladesh, Nepal, and parts of East Africa, VL is an anthropozoonosis caused by *L. donovani,* which does not occur in dogs. In Senegal, canine leishmaniasis is well known, but human infection seems to be extremely rare.[10a, 59]

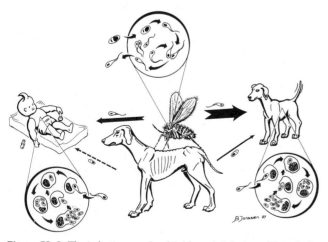

Figure 73–3. The infectious cycle of *Leishmania infantum.* (The relative incidence of contamination is indicated by the boldness of the *arrows.*)

New World

The distribution of leishmaniasis in the New World is shown in Figure 73–1. The endemic region is extending northward, probably up into Mexico.[59] In humans in South and Central America, VL is clinically similar to that of Old World VL caused by *L. infantum,* but the etiologic agent is *L. chagasi.* Domestic and wild dogs are considered reservoir hosts, and the epidemiology resembles that of VL in the Mediterranean basin. In addition, hen houses close to habitations attract wild, carnivorous animals, which are considered to be the sylvan reservoirs. Chickens may also constitute a major feeding host for sandflies.[59]

Autochthonous foci of VL in dogs in the United States have been reported in Ohio, Oklahoma, and Texas.[9, 49] These states may represent newly established endemic foci in which diseased hosts from other areas have infected native sandfly populations. *L. infantum* was involved in the infection in Oklahoma. Antileishmania antibodies were detected in asymptomatic dogs in Michigan and Alabama after the diagnosis of VL in one dog.[9]

CL in humans is caused by parasites of the *L. mexicana* complex and the *L. braziliensis* complex (see Table 73–1). It is associated with a wide variety of clinical manifestations but is usually limited to single or multiple skin lesions. MCL or "espundia," which may be caused by *L. braziliensis* and *L. panamensis,* has a propensity to disseminate to mucous tissues. Rodents rather than Canidae are involved in the epidemiology of New World CL and MCL, but parasites of the *L. braziliensis* and *L. mexicana* complexes have been demonstrated in canine specimens.[59] In Texas, antileishmania antibodies were detected in five dogs from a household in which *L. mexicana*–associated CL occurred in people. *L. mexicana* has been isolated also in Texas from cutaneous nodules in cats.[4, 50] Equines may also be involved in the epidemiology of CL.[1, 59]

PATHOGENESIS

Not every dog experimentally or naturally infected with *Leishmania* develops disease.[28, 44] Studies indicate that protective immunity to leishmaniasis in dogs is mediated by T cells and the cytokines they produce.[44] Resistance to experimental infection with *L. infantum* in dogs is associated with proliferation of peripheral blood lymphocytes, which produce interleukin-2, tumor necrosis factor, and interferon-γ (IFN-γ) on parasite antigen–specific stimulation. In addition, *L. infantum*–infected macrophages are lysed in a histocompatibility complex–restricted manner by $CD8^+$ and/or $CD4^+$ cytotoxic T cells. These phenomena are lacking in symptomatic (i.e., nonresistant) dogs, in which local infection of the skin[31e] is usually followed by multiplication of the parasite in macrophages and dissemination throughout the body. T-cell response to leishmanial antigen is suppressed in infected dogs, and a marked IgG response to the parasite ensues.[34, 45] Intracellular killing of the parasite by neutrophils and monocytes is also impaired.[8]

Clinical signs may develop in a period of 3 months to 7 years after infection. T-lymphocyte regions in the lymphoid organs become depleted, but antibody-producing B-cell regions proliferate. The proliferation of B lymphocytes, plasma cells, histiocytes, and macrophages in concert with the attraction of eosinophils results in generalized lymphadenomegaly, sometimes hepatosplenomegaly, and consistent hyperglobulinemia. The immunoglobulin response is usually enormous; however, it is nonprotective and eventually detrimental. Specific antibodies probably opsonize amastigotes, thus enhancing their phagocytosis by macrophages, within which the parasite continues to survive and to multiply. Numerous coincidental antibodies are also produced, including autoantibodies that may be associated with the development of pathologic phenomena such as immune-mediated thrombocytopenia and anemia.

A potential hazard of impaired T-cell regulation with exuberant B-cell activity is the generation of large amounts of circulating immune complexes (CICs).[31b] CIC deposition in the walls of blood vessels may cause vasculitis, polyarthritis, uveitis, and glomerulonephritis. In dogs, CIC deposition in the kidneys eventually results in renal failure, which is the main cause of death of dogs with leishmaniasis. CIC may also include cryoglobulins. These proteins may precipitate in the blood vessels of the extremities when exposed to cold, thus causing ischemic necrosis.[50]

Canine leishmaniasis is most often associated with a variety of skin lesions, which are generalized rather than local because *L. infantum* disseminates all over the body.[46] Generalized nodular lesions probably indicate a less effective immune response than that with generalized alopecia.[17a] Rarely are skin lesions restricted to a few ulcerations or nodules.

Dogs with leishmaniasis may show signs of a hemorrhagic diathesis, chiefly epistaxis. Apart from nasal ulcers, possible causes include paraglobulinemia, which may interfere with fibrin polymerization and which, in concert with uremia, may inhibit thrombocyte function. In addition, thrombocytopenia may develop as a result of CIC, autoantibodies, splenic pooling, or bone marrow failure. Anemia usually develops as a sequel to the decreased erythropoiesis of chronic disease but may be aggravated by blood loss and/or an antibody-related decrease in red blood cell survival.

CLINICAL FINDINGS

Dogs

In dogs, *Leishmania* infection usually causes chronic systemic disease. The incubation period varies from 3 months to as long as 7 years. Signs are highly variable and often begin with slight but progressive dullness and insidious exercise intolerance. The clinical findings in canine leishmaniasis are presented in Table 73–2.

Table 73–2. Clinical Findings in 80 Dogs With Leishmaniasis

HISTORY EXAM FINDINGS	% OF DOGS	PHYSICAL EXAM ABNORMALITIES	% OF DOGS
Decreased endurance	67.5	Lymphadenomegaly	90.0
Weight loss	64.0	Skin involvement	89.0
Somnolence	60.0	Cachexia	47.5
Increased fluid intake	40.0	Abnormal locomotion	37.5
Anorexia	32.5	Hyperthermia	36.0
Diarrhea	30.0	Conjunctivitis	32.5
Vomiting	26.0	Palpable spleen	32.5
Polyphagia	15.0	Abnormal nails	20.0
Epistaxis	15.0	Rhinitis	10.0
Melena	12.5	Keratitis	7.5
Sneezing	10.0	Pneumonia	2.5
Coughing	6.0	Icterus	2.5
Fainting	6.0	Uveitis	1.3
		Panophthalmitis	1.3

Modified from Slappendel RJ: *Vet Q* 10:1–16, 1988. Used with permission.

Almost 90% of dogs with overt leishmaniasis have cutaneous involvement (Fig. 73–4). Dermatologic abnormalities may occur in the absence of other signs of disease, but any animal with dermal manifestations of leishmaniasis should be presumed to have visceral involvement, because the parasites are usually disseminated throughout the body before skin lesions develop. The skin problems vary in character and extent but are rarely pruritic. Most dogs develop a progressive and symmetric alopecia with intense, dry desquamation, usually commencing on the head and extending to the rest of the body. In addition, some animals develop ulcerations, which are particularly located on the nose and the pinna, or chapping of the muzzle or the footpads. Less frequently, there are mucocutaneous ulcers, cutaneous nodules, or pustular eruptions.[21, 29, 30] Some dogs develop ocular lesions, including keratoconjunctivitis and lymphoplasmacytic or granulomatous uveitis.[21a] Abnormally long or brittle nails (onychogryphosis), a rather specific finding, occur in a small proportion of the patients.

Weight loss and muscle atrophy are the most common signs of visceral involvement. Some dogs lose weight despite having a ravenous appetite, but serious loss of condition is usually associated with anorexia and other signs of renal failure, including mental depression, polyuria, polydipsia, and vomiting. Transient diarrhea may occur.

In cases of overt disease, decreased physical activity is obvious and related to somnolence, decreased endurance, and locomotion disturbances. The last may be due to neuralgia, polyarthritis, polymyositis, footpad clefts, interdigital ulcers, or even osteolytic lesions or proliferative periostitis. Body temperature may fluctuate but is usually normal or subfebrile. Immunosuppression may promote the occurrence of concomitant infections; hence, the clinical picture may be complicated by demodicosis, pyoderma, GI disease, pneumonia, and so on. Combined infections with *Ehrlichia*, *Babesia*, and *Dirofilaria* are quite common if *Leishmania* infection occurs in regions where these organisms are also endemic. Other less common manifestations have been reported, including pericardial tamponade,[19] chronic colitis,[15] pemphigus,[22] and polyarthritis.[52] Thrombosis has also occurred as a result of the nephrotic syndrome caused by glomerulonephritis.[17a, 18] An increased association between leishmaniasis in dogs and lymphoid neoplasia or hemangiosarcoma has been suggested.[32] Signs caused by, or complications of, disseminated intravascular coagulation may occur.[20] Many dogs visiting or living in endemic areas contract visceral leishmaniasis. Some of the less common manifestations may actually be caused by other coincidental diseases.

Cats

Cats are rarely clinically affected,[7a, 42b] even when they have been seropositive. Nodular lesions on the nose and ears have been observed in cats in an endemic region of Venezuela.[7a] CL caused by *L. mexicana* was diagnosed in one cat from south Texas.[4, 50] Nodules on the pinna were the only clinical finding initially after amputation, but 2 years later the cat developed lesions at the surgical site, muzzle, and nasal mucosa. Cats were refractory to experimental infection with a Kenyan strain of *L. donovani*.[1a]

DIAGNOSIS

Clinical Laboratory Testing

The abnormalities (and percentages) reported in 1988 in 80 untreated dogs are shown in Table 73–3. Clinical signs were

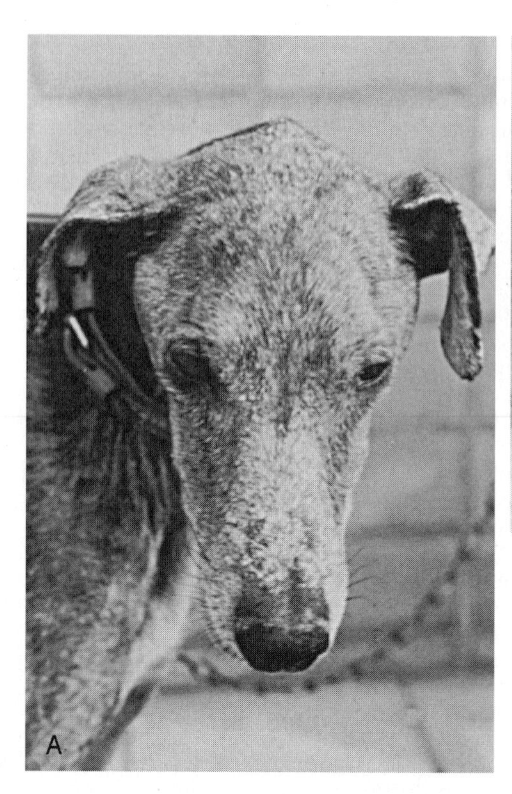

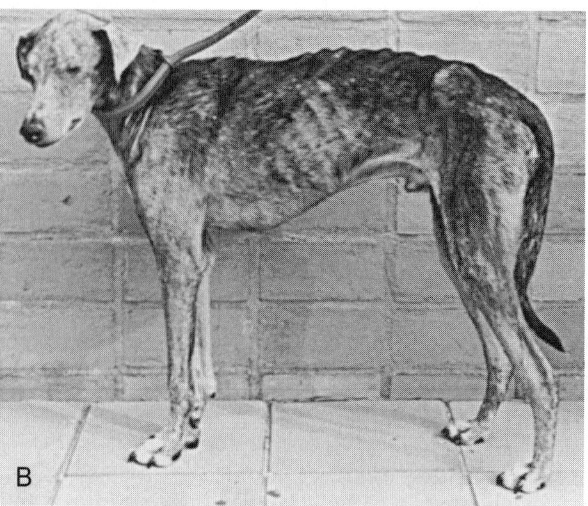

Figure 73–4. *A* and *B*, Dog with characteristic features of leishmaniasis. Notice the thin haircoat, excessive scaling, cachexia, and muscle atrophy. (From Slappendel RJ: *Vet Q* 10:1–16, 1988. Reprinted with permission.)

obvious in the great majority of these cases. With the present refinement of diagnostic methods and increased knowledge of the disease, diagnosis is more often made in an earlier stage, when proteinuria, thrombocytopenia, azotemia, and hypercreatinemia are still absent. Urinary protein-creatinine ratio and enzymuria have been proposed as tests for assessing renal damage in affected animals.[42, 42a]

Serologic Testing

A wide range of immunodiagnostic tests has been developed using complement fixation, indirect FA, and ELISA methods.[31d, 51a, 56a] Very high specificity and sensitivity have been achieved with a commercially available direct agglutination test containing stabilized purified parasite proteins (Dog-DAT, Lyopharma, Bilthoven, The Netherlands)[17, 24, 41] (see Appendix 6).

Serologic tests may verify the presence of antibodies but do not prove or disprove active disease. However, in an animal with compatible clinical illness, a positive titer strongly supports the preliminary diagnosis. Depending on the sensitivity and specificity of the test methods, false-positive or false-negative results may be obtained. Antibodies may be absent in some dogs harboring *Leishmania,* although rarely in those with clinical signs of the disease. In addition, spontaneous elimination of the parasite without development of clinical disease may occur in approximately 10% to 20% of apparently healthy seropositive dogs.[43]

Decreasing titers detected by indirect FA, DAT, or ELISA have been utilized to monitor therapy.[2, 9a, 14, 58] Results are not consistent and relapses can occur frequently despite a negative test result.

Table 73–3. Clinical Laboratory Abnormalities in 80 Dogs With Leishmaniasis

ABNORMALITY	% OF DOGS
Hyperglobulinemia	100
Hypoalbuminemia	94
High total serum protein	91
Proteinuria	85
Positive Coombs' test result (mostly weak)	84
High alanine aminotransferase activity	61
High serum alkaline phosphatase activity	51
Thrombocytopenia	50
Azotemia	45
Hypercreatinemia	38
Positive results for antinuclear antibody	31
Leukopenia, associated with low normal or decreased lymphocyte count	22
Positive results for lupus erythematosus cells	13
Leukocytosis with left shift	8

Modified from Slappendel RJ: *Vet Q* 10:1–16, 1988. Used with permission.

Organism Identification

Definitive diagnosis is usually based on cytologic or histologic identification of amastigotes, free or in macrophages, in routinely stained smears from lymph nodes or bone marrow. The specificity of these methods is virtually 100%, but, depending on the time spent searching for parasites, the sensitivity is maximally ±80% in dogs with clinical signs of the disease and lower in seropositive dogs without signs. The detection of amastigotes in tissues such as spleen and liver is less practical. Identification of amastigotes in skin lesion biopsies may be facilitated by immunoperoxidase staining.[16] The diagnosis may also be established by the culture of parasites from tissues in Novy-MacNeal-Nicolle medium or Schneider's Drosophila medium or by the inoculation of hamsters.

A very sensitive and specific diagnostic method used in dogs, which may be used routinely in the near future, is the

Table 73–4. Antimicrobial Therapy for Canine Leishmaniasis

DRUG	DOSE (mg/kg)[a]	ROUTE	INTERVAL (HOURS)	DURATION[b] (WEEKS)
Meglumine antimonate (Glucantime)	100	IV, SC	24	3–4
Sodium stibogluconate[c] (Pentostam)	30–50	IV, SC	24	3–4
Allopurinol[d]	6–8	PO	8	26
	15	PO	12	26

[a]Dose per administration at specified interval. For further information on use of these drugs, see Drug Formulary, Appendix 8.
[b]All long-term survivors will have to be treated on multiple occasions because of relapses.
[c]Available in the United States for treatment of human infections by special request from the Centers for Disease Control, Atlanta, GA.
[d]Some studies suggest combined therapy with allopurinol and antimony compounds is superior for treating *L. infantum* infections.

demonstration of leishmanial DNA in bone marrow and other tissue biopsy specimens by polymerase chain reaction.[2, 35]

PATHOLOGIC FINDINGS

Severely affected patients are cachectic. The organs mainly affected are the skin and elements of the mononuclear-phagocyte system in diverse sites. Generalized enlargement of lymph nodes is usually present. Hepatosplenomegaly may be present but is less common. These organs and tissues enlarge from increased numbers of cells consisting of histiocytes, macrophages (which may be parasitized), eosinophils, lymphocytes, and plasma cells. Small, light-colored nodular foci, which are granulomas, may occur in various organs, including the skin and the kidneys. Mucosal ulcerations in the stomach, intestine, and colon have been seen occasionally. Petechiae and ecchymotic bleeding in mucosal and serosal membranes are rare. Kidney lesions include CIC-induced glomerulonephritis, interstitial nephritis, and occasionally amyloidosis.[38] Amyloid deposits may also be present in other organs. The bone marrow is usually red and abundant, but erythropoiesis is ineffective. Osteolytic or proliferative periosteal processes may be found in various parts of the skeleton in some patients. In the nervous system, organisms may be found in inflammatory cells in the choroid plexus.[40]

THERAPY

Leishmaniasis is more resistant to therapy in dogs than in people, and *Leishmania* organisms are rarely completely eliminated with available drugs. Relapses necessitating retreatment are the rule rather than the exception, although some dogs may eventually become free of clinical disease.

Traditionally, treatment consists of pentavalent antimonials (Sb^{5+}), which selectively inhibit the protozoal enzymes required for glycolytic and fatty acid oxidation. Two Sb^{5+}-containing agents have been administered to dogs: meglumine antimonate (Glucantime, Rhône-Mérieux, Lyon, France) and sodium stibogluconate (Pentostam, Wellcome, Beckenham, United Kingdom) (see Drug Formulary, Appendix 8). Both agents are expensive, require daily injections, and may cause serious adverse effects. Meglumine should produce fewer side effects than stibogluconate but is not available in the United States. Dosage regimens vary widely. We recommend the dosage schedule in Table 73–4. There is no justification for alternate-day administration, which is often advocated. Sb^{5+} is quickly excreted with the urine. Only a small part is reduced to the toxic Sb^{3+}, which may accumulate in the body. However, normal doses of the drug rarely cause signs of toxicity unless administered daily for longer than 2 months or administered to a patient with serious renal, cardiac, or hepatic failure. Antimonials may be injected IM, SC, or IV. IM injections in the thigh have resulted in severe lameness as a result of muscle fibrosis. Possible local complications of SC administration are less serious but include local inflammation. IV injections may cause thrombophlebitis and hence thrombosis. Results of pharmacokinetic studies of Sb^{5+} compounds in dogs are controversial,[54, 56] but the clinical effect and parasitologic clearance is the same when 100 mg meglumine antimonate/kg is given IV once daily or SC divided in two daily doses.[51]

In some dogs, treatment with meglumine antimonate seems to alter the immunopathologic status of the patient without accomplishing a definite cure, a situation comparable to that of people with so-called post-kala-azar dermal lesions (PKDL). In dogs, this immune alteration may result in the development of granulomatous dermal nodules and iridocyclitis (Fig. 73–5), as described in African PKDL in humans.[43] In people and experimental animals, combined Sb^{5+} and interferon-γ has been effective in treating Sb^{5+}-resistant infections.[3, 37, 53]

A new alternative to injection of Sb^{5+} is the administration of allopurinol (see Drug Formulary, Appendix 8). In *Leishmania* species, allopurinol is aminated to analogues of adenosine and incorporated into RNA, which inhibits multiplication of the parasite. This drug is cheaper than Sb^{5+} compounds; can be administered orally; is readily available, even in the United States; and has few adverse effects. Consumption of allopurinol causes hyperxanthinuria, which may

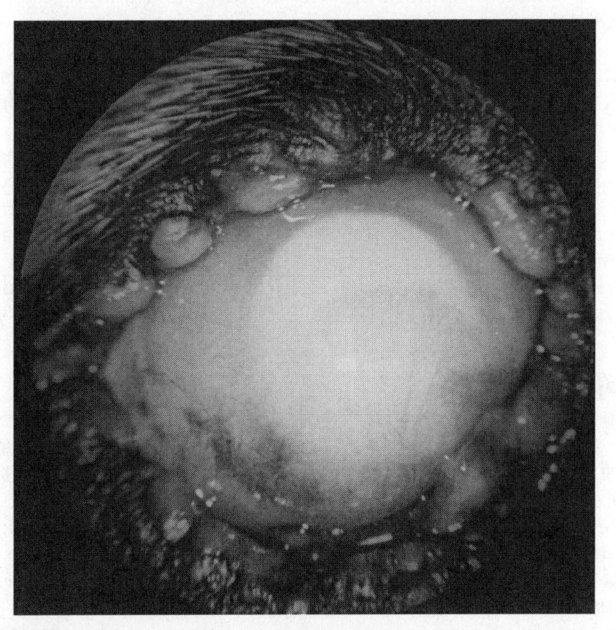

Figure 73–5. Iridocyclitis, keratoconjunctivitis, and nodular blepharitis in a dog with chronic leishmaniasis after multiple courses of injections with meglumine antimonate. (Courtesy of Dr. F. C. Stades, Utrecht, The Netherlands.)

incidentally produce urolithiasis. This may be prevented by concurrent administration of a low protein diet.[4a] It is used with increasing frequency by veterinarians in the Mediterranean area, especially in combination with Sb^{5+}.[1, 14, 55] In treating infected people, allopurinol and Sb^{5++} therapy is more effective than stibogluconate alone.[33] As with meglumine, dosage schedules vary widely and the optimal dose has not been defined. Results of a retrospective inquiry among 52 practices in and around Madrid suggest that remission of canine leishmaniasis is obtained more frequently and that relapses are postponed longer with a combination of meglumine and allopurinol than with meglumine alone.[55] Clinical remission may also be obtained by treating with allopurinol alone. I (RJS) found that a dose of 7 mg/kg TID nearly always results in dramatic clinical improvement within 3 weeks and reduction of parasites to undetectable numbers. However, relapses are consistent once therapy has been discontinued. Even after conscientious administration of the drug for 6 months, complete recovery is rare.[31] Relapses develop more insidiously and are less serious than with meglumine.

Antifungal agents, especially amphotericin B (AMB), ketoconazole, and itraconazole, or other antiprotozoal drugs such as diminazene have also been utilized with variable success,[30a, 40a, 45a] but reports of their effects are anecdotal. Drugs that are coupled to liposomes or other lipid-carrier substances specifically taken up by macrophages have been effective in the treatment of experimental leishmaniasis but have not yet been successful in the treatment of spontaneous leishmaniasis in dogs. Lipid-associated AMB has been effective in the treatment of people with visceral leishmaniasis that is resistant to antimonials.[6] Treated dogs showed clinical improvement without eliminating infection.[40a]

The aminoglycoside aminosidine (paromomycin) has shown some preliminary evidence of effectiveness when compared with antimonials in treating dogs with *L. infantum* infection.[45a] Since many dogs with leishmaniasis have renal dysfunction, this drug is contraindicated for such animals. Kidney function must be closely monitored as in AMB.

If dogs are seriously ill, and especially if they are in severe renal failure, it may be necessary to restore fluid and acid-base balances before antimicrobial drugs are administered. Antimicrobial treatment should be started at a lower dose and anti-inflammatory, but not immunosuppressive, doses of glucocorticoids should be given during the first few days. Because of its lower toxicity, allopurinol is preferred over an Sb^{5+} compound in these cases.

The prognosis mainly depends on renal function at the start of treatment. In dogs with serious renal insufficiency, the prognosis is very poor. In dogs with leishmaniasis without renal insufficiency, there is a 75% probability of survival for more than 4 years with good quality of life after treatment with meglumine for 3 to 6 weeks, with additional treatment when relapses occur.[51]

PREVENTION

Currently, no prophylactic drugs or vaccines are effective against leishmaniasis. Prevention of the disease in endemic areas is difficult and depends on control of the insect vectors, detection and extermination of the animal reservoirs, and early detection and treatment of the infected pets. Eradication of the breeding places of sandflies has resulted in limited control of the disease.

Measures to protect the individual dog include keeping the animal indoors as much as possible from 1 hour before sunset to 1 hour after dawn during the vector season and the use of repellents, insecticides, and fine mesh screens to keep kennels and houses free of sandflies. Deltamethrin collars may effectively protect dogs from bites of sandflies.[27a] Owners who live in *Leishmania*-free countries should leave their pets at home when visiting endemic areas.

PUBLIC HEALTH CONSIDERATIONS

Leishmania species described in dogs with clinical signs of leishmaniasis have almost exclusively been parasites of the *L. donovani* complex, which causes VL. VL is a serious disease that may be fatal when untreated. Traditionally, VL affected mainly young children and infants, but now it is also often a complicating factor in adults infected with HIV or receiving cytostatic or immunosuppressive drugs.[23, 27, 47, 58, 59]

In the Old World, sandflies pass *L. infantum* from dogs to people. Considering the low incidence of *L. infantum*–associated VL in native inhabitants in endemic regions in Europe,[13] the risk of such an infection in healthy people is very low. By consequence, the risk of infection of people in areas without sandflies is remote, even when they live in close contact with infected dogs. However, rare infections by direct contact from animals to people have been reported. Direct contact with contaminated injection needles or with open wounds or exudates from dogs with leishmaniasis, therefore, should be strictly avoided. The risk of direct transmission seems to be greater between dogs than from dogs to people.[25]

In regions of the New World where *L. chagasi* causes endemic American visceral leishmaniasis, the spread and maintenance of human infection have been attributed to canine reservoirs. However, in a controlled study in three isolated valleys in Brazil, no difference in human seroconversion rate occurred between populations where infected dogs were or were not eliminated.[10c] This finding suggests, in the New World, that dogs are not the principal reservoirs and that human-sandfly-human transmission may be important in the spread and maintenance of infection.

In the United States, treatment of dogs infected with *Leishmania* presents a dilemma to veterinarians and public health officials because of the potential of establishing new zoonotic foci.[48] For pet owners, this outlook is probably rarely a convincing argument to euthanize their infected dogs. Even owners in zoonotic regions rarely cooperate in that respect, despite the fact that the presence of sandflies makes possible the risk, however remote, of transmission of the disease from their pets to members of their own family.

References

1. Alvar J, Molina R, San Andres M, et al. 1994. Canine leishmaniasis, parasitological and entomological follow-up after chemotherapy. *Ann Trop Med Parasitol* 88:371–378.

1a. Anjili CO, Githure JI. 1993. Refractioness of domestic cats to infection with a Kenyan strain of *Leishmania donovani*. *East Afr Med J* 70:322.

1b. Aquilar CM, Rangel EF, Garcia L, et al. 1998. Zoonotic cutaneous leishmaniasis due to *Leishmania (Viannia) braziliensis* associated with domestic animals in Venezuela and Brazil. *Mem Inst Oswaldo Cruz* 84:19–28.

2. Ashford DA, Bozza M, Freire M, et al. 1995. Comparison of the polymerase chain reaction and serology for the detection of canine visceral leishmaniasis. *Am J Trop Med Hyg* 50:251–255.

3. Badaro R, Falcoff E, Badaro FS, et al. 1990. Treatment of visceral leishmaniasis with pentavalent antimony and interferon gamma. *N Engl J Med* 322:16–21.

4. Barnes JC, Stanley O, Craig TM. 1993. Diffuse cutaneous leishmaniasis in a cat. *J Am Vet Med Assoc* 202:416–418.

4a. Bartges JW, Osborne CA, Felice LJ, et al. 1995. Influence of allopurinol and two diets on 24-hour urinary excretions of uric acid, xanthine, and ammonia by healthy dogs. *Am J Vet Res* 56:595–601.

5. Belazzoug S. 1992. Leishmaniasis in Mediterranean countries. *Vet Parasitol* 44:15–19.
6. Berman JD. 1997. Human leishmaniasis: clinical, diagnostic and chemotherapeutic developments in the last 10 years. *Clin Infect Dis* 24:684–703.
7. Binhazim AA, Chapman WL, Latimer KS, et al. 1992. Canine leishmaniasis caused by *Leishmania leishmania infantum* in two labrador retrievers. *J Vet Diagn Invest* 4:299–305.
7a. Bonfante-Garrido R, Urdaneta I, Urdaneta R, et al. 1991. Natural infection of cats with *Leishmania* in Barquisimeto, Venezuela. *Trans R Soc Trop Med Hyg* 85:53.
8. Brandonisio O, Panunzio M, Faliero SM, et al. 1996. Evaluation of polymorphonuclear cell and monocyte functions in *Leishmania infantum*-infected dogs. *Vet Immunol Immunopathol* 53:95–103.
9. Bravo L, Frank LA, Brenneman KA. 1993. Canine leishmaniasis in the United States. *Compend Cont Educ Pract Vet* 15:699–708.
9a. Ciaramella P, Oliva G, De Luna R, et al. 1997. A retrospective clinical study of canine leishmaniasis in 150 dogs naturally infected with *L. infantum*. *Vet Rec* 141:539–543.
9b. Deplazes P, Arnold P, Skaggs J, et al. 1992. Parasitological and immunological progress control during and after chemotherapy of leishmaniasis in dogs. *Schweiz Arch Tiercheilkd* 134:85–93.
10. Dereure J, Rioux JA, Gallego M, et al. 1991. *Leishmania tropica* in Morocco: infection in dogs. *Trans R Soc Trop Med Hyg* 85:595.
10a. Desjeux P, Bray RS, Dedet JP, et al. 1982. Differentiation of canine and cutaneous leishmaniasis strains in Senegal. *Trans R Soc Trop Med Hyg* 76:163–168.
10b. Diaz-Espineria MM, Slappendel RJ. 1997. A case autochthonous canine leishmaniasis in the Netherlands. *Vet Q* 19:69–71.
10c. Dietze R, Barros GB, Teixeira L, et al. 1997. Effect of eliminating seropositive canines on the transmission of visceral leishmaniasis in Brazil. *Clin Infect Dis* 25:1240–1242.
11. Dye C, Killick-Kendrick R, Vitutia MM, et al. 1992. Epidemiology of canine leishmaniasis prevalence, incidence and basic reproduction number calculated from a cross sectional serological survey on the island of Goza Malta. *Parasitology* 105:35–41.
12. Evans TG, Vasconcelos IAB, Lima JW, et al. 1990. Canine visceral leishmaniasis in Northeast Brazil: assessment of serodiagnostic methods. *Am J Trop Med Hyg* 42:118–123.
13. Ferrer L. 1992. Leishmaniasis, pp 266–270. *In* Kirk RW, Bonagura JD (eds), Current veterinary therapy XI. WB Saunders, Philadelphia, PA.
14. Ferrer L, Aisa MJ, Roura X. 1995. Serological diagnosis and treatment of canine leishmaniasis. *Vet Rec* 136:514–516.
15. Ferrer L, Jvanola B, Ramos JA, et al. 1991. Chronic colitis due to *Leishmania* infection in two dogs. *Vet Pathol* 28:342–343.
16. Ferrer L, Rabanal R, Domingo M, et al. 1988. Identification of *Leishmania* amastigotes in canine tissues by immunoperoxidase staining. *Res Vet Sci* 44:194.
17. Fisa R, Gallego M, Riera C, et al. 1997. Serologic diagnosis of canine leishmaniasis by dot ELISA. *J Vet Diagn Invest* 9:50–55.
17a. Fondevila D, Vilafranca M, Ferrer L. 1997. Epidermal immunocompetence in canine leishmaniasis. *Vet Immunol Immunopathol* 56:319–327.
17b. Font A, Closa JM. 1997. Ultrasonographic localization of a caudal vena cava thrombus in a dog with leishmaniasis. *Vet Radiol Ultrasound* 38:394–396.
18. Font A, Closa JM, Molina A, et al. 1993. Thrombosis and nephrotic syndrome in a dog with visceral leishmaniasis. *J Small Anim Pract* 34:466–470.
19. Font A, Durall N, Domingo M, et al. 1993. Cardiac tamponade in a dog with visceral leishmaniasis. *J Am Anim Hosp Assoc* 29:95–121.
20. Font A, Gines C, Closa JM, et al. 1994. Visceral leishmaniasis and disseminated intravascular coagulation in a dog. *J Am Vet Med Assoc* 204:1043–1044.
21. Font A, Roura X, Fondevila D, et al. 1996. Canine mucosal leishmaniasis. *J Am Anim Hosp Assoc* 32:131–138.
21a. Garcia-Alonso M, Blanco A, Reina D, et al. 1996. Immunopathology of the uveitis in canine leishmaniasis. *Parasite Immunol* 18:617–623.
22. Ginel PJ, Mozos E, Fernandez A, et al. 1993. Canine pemphigus foliaceus associated with leishmaniasis. *Vet Rec* 133:526–527.
22a. Gothe R, Nolte I, Kraft W. 1997. Leishmaniasis in dogs in Germany: epidemiological case analysis and alternatives to conventional causal therapy. *Tierarztl Prax* 25:68–73.
23. Gramiccia M, Gradoni L, Troiana M. 1995. Heterogeneity among zymodemes of *Leishmania infantum* from HIV-positive patients with visceral leishmaniasis in south Italy. *FEMS Microbiol Lett* 128:33–38.
24. Harith AE, Slappendel RJ, Reiter I, et al. 1989. Application of a direct agglutination test for detection of specific anti-*Leishmania* antibodies in the canine reservoir. *J Clin Microbiol* 27:2252–2257.
25. Harris MP. 1994. Suspected transmission of leishmaniasis. *Vet Rec* 135:339.
26. Huss BT, Ettinger SJ. 1992. Visceral leishmaniasis, Rocky Mountain Spotted Fever, and von Willebrand's disease in a giant schnauzer. *J Am Anim Hosp Assoc* 28:221–225.
27. Jimenez MI, Laguna F, de la Torre F, et al. 1995. New *Leishmania infantum* zymodemes responsible for visceral leishmaniasis in patients co-infected with HIV in Spain. *Trans R Soc Trop Med Hyg* 89:33.
27a. Killick-Kendrick R, Killick-Kendrick M, Focheux C, et al. 1997. Protection of dogs from bites of phlebotomine sandflies by deltamethrin collars for control of canine leishmaniasis. *Med Vet Entomol* 11:105–111.
28. Killick-Kendrick R, Killick-Kendrick M, Pinelli E, et al. 1994. A laboratory model of canine leishmaniasis: the inoculation of dogs with *Leishmania infantum* promastigotes from midguts of experimentally infected phlebotomine sandflies. *Parasite* 1:311–318.
29. Kontas VJ, Koutinas AF. 1993. Old world canine leishmaniasis. *Compend Cont Educ Pract Vet* 15:949–960.
30. Koutinas AF, Scott DW, Kantos V, et al. 1992. Skin lesions in canine leishmaniasis (kala-azar): a clinical and histopathological study of 22 spontaneous cases in Greece. *Vet Dermatol* 3:121–130.
30a. Lamothe J. 1997. A new prospect on canine leishmaniasis: treatment with amphotericin B. *Prat Med Churg Anim Comp* 32:133–141.
31. Lester SJ, Kenyon JE. 1996. Use of allopurinol to treat visceral leishmaniosis in a dog. *J Am Vet Med Assoc* 209:615–617.
31a. Liste F, Gascon M. 1995. Allopurinol in the treatment of canine visceral leishmaniasis. *Vet Rec* 137:23–24.
31b. Lopez R, Lucena R, Novales M, et al. 1996. Circulating immune complexes and renal function in canine leishmaniasis. *Zentralbl Veterinarmed [B]* 43:469–474.
31c. Lucena R, Ginel PJ, Lopez R, et al. 1996. Antinuclear antibodies in dogs with leishmaniasis. *Zbl Vet Med* 43:255–259.
31d. Mancianti F, Pedonese F, Poli A. 1996. Evaluation of dot enzyme-linked immunosorbent assay (DOT-ELISA) for the serodiagnosis of canine leishmaniasis as compared with indirect immunofluorescence assay. *Vet Parasitol* 65:1–9.
31e. Marchal IS, Marchal T, Moore PF, et al. 1997. Infection of canine Langerhans cell and interdigitating dendritic cell by *Leishmania infantum* in spontaneous canine leishmaniasis. *Rev Med Vet* 148:29.
32. Margarito JM, Ginel PJ, Molleda JM, et al. 1994. Haemangiosarcoma associated with leishmaniasis in three dogs. *Vet Rec* 134:66–67.
33. Martinez S, Gonzales M, Vernaza ME. 1997. Treatment of cutaneous leishmaniasis with allopurinol and stibogluconate. *Clin Infect Dis* 24:165–169.
34. Martinez-Moreno A, Moreno T, Martinez-Moreno FJ, et al. 1995. Humoral and cell-mediated immunity in natural and experimental canine leishmaniasis. *Vet Immunol Immunopathol* 48:209–220.
35. Mathis A, DePlazes P. 1995. PCR and in vitro cultivation for detection of *Leishmania* spp in diagnostic samples from humans and dogs. *J Clin Microbiol* 33:1145–1149.
36. McKenzie KK. 1984. A study of the transmission of canine leishmaniasis by the tick, *Rhipicephalus sanguineus*, and an ultrastructural comparison of the promastigote. Doctoral dissertation (0664), Oklahoma State University, Stillwater, OK.
37. Murray HW. 1990. Effect of continuous administration of interferon-γ in experimental visceral leishmaniasis. *J Infect Dis* 161:992–994.
38. Nieto CG, Navarrete I, Habela MA, et al. 1992. Pathological changes in kidneys of dogs with natural *Leishmania* infection. *Vet Parasitol* 45:33–47.
39. Nieto CG, Navarrete I, Habela MA, et al. 1992. Seroprevalence of canine leishmaniasis around Cáceres, Spain. *Prevent Vet Med* 13:173–178.
40. Nieto CG, Viñuelas J, Blanco A, et al. 1996. Detection of *Leishmania infantum* amastigotes in canine choroid plexus. *Vet Rec* 139:346–347.
40a. Oliva G, Gradoni L, Ciaramella P, et al. 1995. Activity of liposomal amphotericin B (AmBisome) in dogs naturally infected with *L. infantum*. *J Antimicrob Chemother* 36:1013–1019.
41. Oskam L, Slappendel RJ, Beijer EGM, et al. 1996. Dog-DAT: a direct agglutination test using stabilized, freeze-dried antigen for the serodiagnosis of canine visceral leishmaniasis. *J Clin Microbiol FEMS Immunol Med Microbiol* 16:235–239.
42. Palacio J, Liste F, Gascon M. 1995. Urinary protein/creatinine ratio in the evaluation of renal failure in canine leishmaniasis. *Vet Rec* 137:567–568.
42a. Palacio J, Liste F, Gascon M. 1997. Enzymuria as an index of renal damage in canine leishmaniasis. *Vet Rec* 140:477–480.
42b. Passos VMA, Lasmar EB, Gontijo CMF, et al. 1996. Natural infection of a domestic cat *(Felis domesticus)* with *Leishmania* (Viannia) in the metropolitan region of Belo Horizonte, State of Minas Cerais, Brazil. *Mem Inst Oswald Cruz* 91:19–20.
43. Peters W, Killick-Kendrick R (eds). 1987. The leishmaniasis in biology and medicine. Academic Press, London.
44. Pinelli E, Gonzalo RM, Boog CJP, et al. 1995. *Leishmania infantum*-specific T cell lines derived from asymptomatic dogs that lyse infected macrophages in a major histocompatibility complex-restricted manner. *Eur J Immunol* 25:1594–1600.
45. Pinelli E, Killick-Kendrick R, Nagenaar J, et al. 1994. Cellular and humoral immune responses in dogs experimentally and naturally infected with *Leishmania infantum*. *Infect Immun* 62:229–235.
45a. Poli A, Sozzi S, Guidi G, et al. 1997. Comparison of aminosidine (paromomycin) and sodium stibogluconate for treatment of canine leishmaniasis. *Vet Parasitol* 71:263–271.
46. Pratts N, Ferrer L. 1994. A possible mechanism in the pathogenesis of cutaneous lesions in canine leishmaniasis. *Vet Rec* 137:103–104.
47. Rosenthal E, Marty P, Poizot-Martin I, et al. 1995. Visceral leishmaniasis and HIV-1 co-infection in southern France. *Trans R Trop Med Hyg* 89:159–162.
48. Sellon R. 1992. Leishmaniasis in the United States, pp 271. *In* Kirk RW, Bonagura JD (eds), Current veterinary therapy XI. WB Saunders, Philadelphia, PA.

49. Sellon RK, Menard MM, Meuten DJ, et al. 1993. Endemic visceral leishmaniasis in a dog from Texas. *J Vet Intern Med* 7:16–19.
50. Slappendel RJ, Greene CE. 1990. Leishmaniasis, pp 769–777. *In* Greene CE (ed), Infectious diseases of the dog and cat. WB Saunders, Philadelphia, PA.
51. Slappendel RJ, Teske E. 1997. The effect of intravenous or subcutaneous administration of meglumine antimonate (Glucantime) in dogs with leishmaniasis. A randomized clinical trial. *Vet Q* 19:10–13.
51a. Soto M, Requena JM, Quijada L, et al. 1998. Multicomponent chimeric antigen for serodiagnosis of canine visceral leishmaniasis. *J Clin Microbiol* 36:58–63.
52. Spreng D. 1993. Leishmanial polyarthritis in two dogs. *J Small Anim Pract* 34:559–563.
53. Sundar S, Rosenkaimer F, Murray HW. 1994. Successful treatment of refractory visceral leishmaniasis in India using antimony plus interferon-γ. *J Infect Dis* 170:6559–6562.
54. Tassi P, Ormas P, Madonna M, et al. 1994. Pharmacokinetics of N-methylglucamine antimonate after intravenous, intramuscular and subcutaneous administration in the dog. *Res Vet Sci* 56:144–150.
55. Tesouro MA, Amusategui I, Mazzucchelli F, et al. 1995. Tratamiento de la leishmaniosis canina. *Ilustre Col Oficial Vet Madrid M-24629.*
56. Valladares JE, Alberola J, Esteban M, et al. 1996. Disposition of antimony after the administration of N-methylglucamine antimonate to dogs. *Vet Rec* 138:181–183.
56a. Vercammen F, Berkvens D, Leray D, et al. 1997. Development of a slide ELISA for canine leishmaniasis and comparison with 4 serological tests. *Vet Rec* 141:328–330.
57. Vercammen F, de Deken R. 1995. Treatment of canine leishmaniasis with allopurinol. *Vet Rec* 137:252.
58. Vercammen F, de Deken R. 1996. Antibody kinetics during allopurinol treatment in canine leishmaniasis. *Vet Rec* 139:264.
59. WHO Expert Committee on the Control of the Leishmaniases. 1990. Control of the leishmaniases. *WHO Tech Rep Ser* 793.

Chapter **74**

Hepatozoonosis

Thomas M. Craig

ETIOLOGY AND EPIDEMIOLOGY

Hepatozoonosis is a tick-borne disease caused by *Hepatozoon*, which are classified in the family Haemogregarinidae order Eucoccidiorida class Sporozoea in the phylum Apicomplexa. Although some workers consider each host to have a separate species of *Hepatozoon*, others describe infections in nondomestic Felidae and other carnivores as being caused by *H. canis*. It is uncertain whether infections in wild and domestic cats are caused by the same or another species. The host range *H. canis* in mammalian carnivores includes domestic dogs, jackals, coyotes, foxes, hyenas, genet, palm civet, and African cats (lion, leopard, and cheetah).[5, 7] Undetermined *Hepatozoon* spp. have been isolated from other feline hosts, including domestic cats and native American cats (ocelots and bobcats).[2, 5] The unique features of infected North American dogs suggest that a different strain or species is causing disease (Table 74–1). Rodents are the most commonly infected order of mammals, although infection is reported in marsupials, insectivores, and ungulates. The relationships among carnivorous hosts of *Hepatozoon* and their common arthropod vectors are uncertain.

H. canis occurs throughout Africa, southern Europe, Asia (including the Middle East), and islands of the Pacific and Indian Oceans, where the tick vector *Rhipicephalus sanguineus* is found. In the United States, hepatozoonosis was first described in the Texas Gulf Coast[5]; however, infected dogs have now been reported from Texas to Georgia.[15] In Brazil, neutrophilic inclusions were found in a wild crab-eating fox *(Cerdocyon thous)*.[1] The relationship of this parasite to North American strains is uncertain since leucocyte inclusions are more typical of non-American strains.

The life cycle of *H. canis*, as it is currently understood, is similar to that of other *Hepatozoon* species (Fig. 74–1). The vector tick ingests isogamonts in monocytes or neutrophils as part of its blood meal. Syngamy occurs in the gut of the tick. The ookinete (zygote) penetrates the gut wall, and sporogony occurs in the haemocoel of the tick. The oocyst that is formed consists of the numerous sporocysts, each containing 12 to 24 sporozoites.[5] There is no evidence that the sporozoites migrate to the salivary gland or mouth parts of the tick, so, to become infected, the dog must ingest the tick. After the tick is ingested, the sporozoites are released; penetrate the dog's intestinal wall; and are carried by blood or lymph to mononuclear phagocyte or endothelial cells of the spleen, bone marrow, lungs, liver, or muscle where merogony occurs.

Schizonts have been found in a number of tissues, predominantly the lung, myocardium, and skeletal muscle, and have been detected in the liver, spleen, and lymph nodes. A cyst is a thick-walled structure containing a schizont, which develops into merozoites. Macroschizonts and microschizonts have been described, although the relationship of the various stages of meront development is uncertain. Macroschizonts may produce a few large merozoites, which become schizonts. Microschizonts may, in turn, produce a large number of micromerozoites, giving rise to gamonts in leukocytes. Schizont and cystic stages described in the North American strain of *H. canis* vary from those reported elsewhere (see Table 74–1).[5, 15]

Although transmission of *H. canis* to the dog usually occurs via ingestion of the vector tick, there may be other means. Experimentally, infection did not result from parenteral inoculation of tissues or blood from infected dogs, but from inoculation of emulsified tick tissues.[5] Vertical transmission of *H. canis* was reported in puppies reared in a tick-free environment. Both meronts and gamonts were seen in puppies—meronts on the 16th day of life and gamonts beginning from day 21 to 31.[20]

Two types of vertebrate hosts are recognized. In one type (predator host), all stages of the organism (schizonts, gamonts, and cysts) are formed. In the other type (prey host), only cysts are formed.[5] When sporozoites enter the predacious host, schizonts are formed. These schizonts give rise to

Table 74–1. Comparative Features of* H. canis *or Related Species Infecting Dogs and Cats

VARIABLE	NORTH AMERICAN	NON-AMERICAN
Host	Domestic dogs, coyotes, fox Domestic cats, bobcats, ocelots Other: raccoon	Domestic dogs, foxes, hyenas, jackals Domestic cats, lions, cheetah, leopards Other: impala, genet, marten
States or Countries	Dogs: Texas, Oklahoma, Louisiana, Alabama, Georgia Cats: California	Dogs: Africa, Southern Europe, Israel, Japan, Malaysia, islands of the Pacific and Indian Oceans, Brazil (?) Cats: India, Nigeria, South Africa, Israel
Clinical signs	Gait dysfunction: stiffness, hyperesthesia, muscle atrophy, and weakness; mucopurulent, oculonasal discharges; recurrent fever; weight loss; polydipsia, polyuria; bloody diarrhea	Subclinical infections, lethargy, fever, anorexia, depression, weight loss, pale mucosae, weakness, petechiae, ecchymoses, epistaxis (some combined infections)
Laboratory findings	Leukocytosis with hypersegmented neutrophils, normocytic normochromic anemia, mildly elevated SAP activity, hypoglycemia, low urea nitrogen, variable hyperglobulinemia Gametocytes rare (0.1%) in blood smears	Neutrophilic leukocytosis variable, anemia, hyperglobulinemia, hypoalbuminemia, elevated CK and SAP activities, thrombocytopenia, proteinuria Gametocytes frequent (60–90%) in blood smears
Radiography	Periosteal proliferation	No bony changes (except 1 dog in Japan)
Tissue biopsy	Large lamellar cysts, pyogranulomas and myositis of skeletal, cardiac, and intestinal smooth muscle. Pyogranulomas in pancreas, tongue, lymph nodes, kidney, spleen, and lung	Wheel-spoke pattern schizonts found in the liver, lymph nodes, spleen, kidneys, lungs, pancreas, and bone marrow. Pyogranulomas not noted. Hepatitis, pneumonia, glomerulonephritis.
Treatment	Trimethoprim-sulfonamide, nonsteroidal anti-inflammatory drugs, toltrazuril	Imidocarb, diminazene

SAP = serum alkaline phosphatase; CK = creatine kinase.

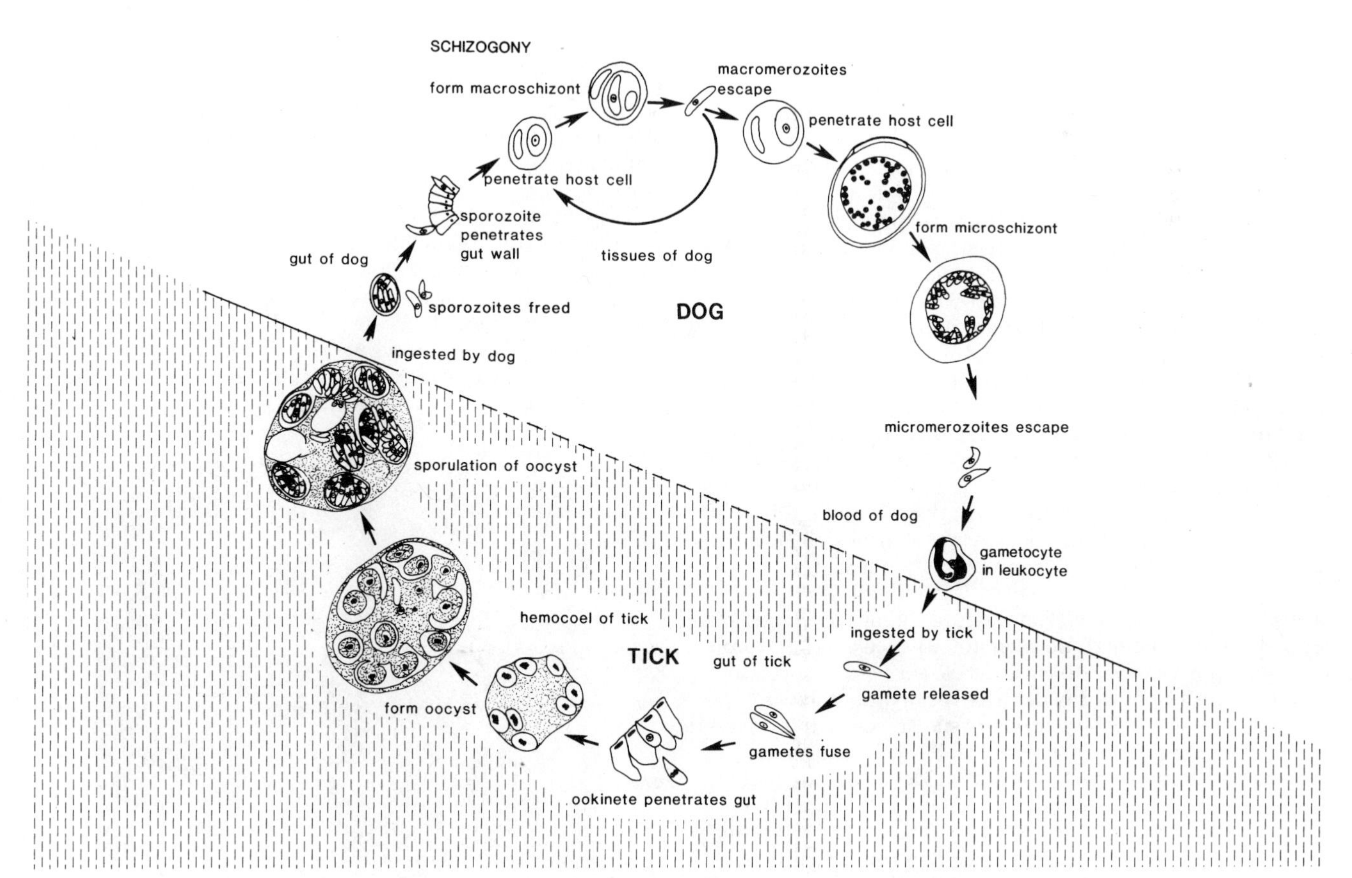

Figure 74–1. Life cycle of *Hepatozoon canis* in the dog and tick *Rhipicephalus sanguineus*.

either gamonts, which in turn infect arthropods, or long-lived cysts, which can be freed from the host only if it is eaten. The host with only the cyst forms cannot infect arthropods but may serve as a source of infection for an animal that preys on it. Transmission via ingestion of infected tissues has not yet been recognized for *H. canis*, although it would seem to be an efficient method of spread. Numerous vectors have been incriminated in the transmission of *Hepatozoon* species in other hosts. If vectors that normally feed on one host are eaten by another host, the second host may become infected by a *Hepatozoon*.

The geographic distribution of *H. canis* in dogs is essentially that of *R. sanguineus*. However, in some localities other vectors have been implicated in transmission. In areas of Japan where *H. canis* is extant, *R. sanguineus* is not an important ectoparasite.[17, 18] Oocysts, presumably those of *H. canis*, were found in *Amblyomma maculatum*, *Haemaphysalis longicornis*, and *H. flava* collected from infected dogs.[19, 29a]

The onset of clinical cases of hepatozoonosis is apparently seasonal in the warmer months, as is a rise and fall in the circulating parasitemia.[5, 15, 22] Epidemiologic features of infection with *Hepatozoon* spp., which are similar to those of other hemoprotozoa in endemic localities, were described in *H. erhardovae* of tropical rat fleas *(Xenopsylla cheopis)* and bank voles *(Clethrionomys glareolus)*. Generally, the parasitemia occurred in waves, and the interval between peaks of parasitemia became longer. There was a progressive reduction in the height of each succeeding parasitemic wave. Reinfection, even with a different geographic strain, did not cause a new rise in parasitemia.[5]

PATHOGENESIS

Observations of naturally and experimentally infected dogs indicate that the hepatozoonosis syndrome is complex and factors other than the presence of the organism are necessary to induce the clinical syndrome. *H. canis* has been identified in leukocytes of clinically normal dogs in Africa, Japan, and Israel.[3, 23] Lack of illness may reflect either differences in strains or host factors. Immunosuppression or concurrent infections with canine distemper virus, canine parvovirus, *Toxoplasma*, *Leishmania*, *Babesia*, or *Ehrlichia* appears to be important.[1b, 2, 9] Experimentally infected dogs have been given glucocorticoids or were from a litter of puppies having congenital defects in their neutrophil function.[5] The age of the dog at the time of infection apparently influences clinical manifestations, especially that of periosteal bone proliferation. Susceptibility may also be related to age, because dogs older than 4 to 6 months were resistant to experimental infection.[5]

The progression of the infection in dogs from ingestion of sporozoites in the tick until the onset of clinical signs has not been well studied. In dogs experimentally infected, a bloody diarrhea beginning 2 or 3 days PI lasted for 2 days to 2 weeks. An elevated rectal temperature initially occurred on day 7 PI and remained elevated for 24 weeks. The lymph nodes became visibly swollen 3 weeks PI. Leukocytosis occurred 4 weeks PI as did ocular discharge and cachexia.[5]

The progression of the various tissue stages of the organism is not known. The first recognizable schizonts, seen approximately 2 months PI, were well developed. Amyloid deposits have occurred in multiple organs, and vasculitis and glomerulonephritis have developed in fatal cases, suggesting that immune complexes may be important in the pathogenesis of disease.[5] Humoral immunity is stimulated by *H. canis*,[27] but there is no evidence that antibodies are protective; instead they may predispose patients to immune complex formation.

The role of immunologic insufficiency from age, genetics, or concurrent infections in hepatozoonosis has not been established. However, it may be an explanation for the sporadic nature of the disease. Additional investigations are necessary to determine the cause of periosteal bone proliferation, leukemoid response, and apparent susceptibility to disease by some infected dogs.

CLINICAL FINDINGS

Dogs

Fever and emaciation are the two most frequently reported clinical signs.[5, 8, 12, 13, 15, 23] Other signs such as anemia, diarrhea, anorexia, and paraparesis have been noted in some reports. The syndrome associated with the North American strain of *H. canis* seems to be clinically distinct, even if other infections are concurrently seen in the affected dogs (see Table 74–1). Within regions, there may be strain differences, because in North American cases, the sign of bloody diarrhea has only been noted in Texas.[15]

Antibiotic unresponsive fever (39.3 to 40.9°C [102.7–105.6°F]), cachexia, depression, generalized muscle atrophy and hyperesthesia (especially noticeable over the paraspinal regions), purulent ocular and nasal discharges, and mild anemia are seen in most dogs.[5, 13, 15, 16, 23, 26]

Hyperesthesia was manifest by stiffness and reluctance to move and cervical and/or trunk rigidity, which probably resulted from periosteal reaction and muscle inflammation. The dogs assumed a "master's voice" stance (Fig. 74–2). Pain, particularly in the lumbar region, may resemble traumatic or degenerative disease of the spine. Because of fever, lumbar pain, and leukocytosis, a few cases were initially suspected of having pyelonephritis. Ocular abnormalities, present in some dogs, have included low tear production, focal retinal scarring, hyperpigmentation and hyperreflectivity, mild papilledema, and uveitis with active inflammatory fundic lesions.[15]

The course of the disease is often prolonged, with periods of apparent remission interspersed with episodes of fever and pain. In responding cases, the periods of remission were longer and the painful episodes less often. In fatal cases, the reverse seemed to be true. Perhaps the most unusual observation of this chronic febrile disease was the normal appetite exhibited by many dogs until near the time of death, although other dogs were anorexic.

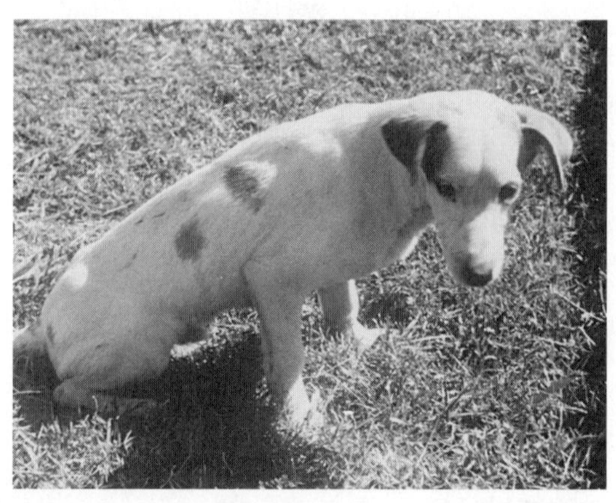

Figure 74–2. Six-month-old terrier mix with hepatozoonosis. Notice the extreme emaciation and "master's voice" posture.

In dogs that appeared to be in a state of remission, the use of glucocorticoids or allowing noninfected *R. sanguineus* to feed on the dog usually resulted in recurrence of a febrile episode within a few days. Then a few days after cessation of glucocorticoids or removal of ticks, the dog would again experience remission. Dogs apparently overcame the clinical disease spontaneously even though organisms were found in the tissues later.[15]

Cats

Schizonts are found in tissues of domestic cats at necropsy more frequently than are clinical signs earlier. In a parasitemic cat from Israel, weakness, hypersalivation, lingual mucosal ulceration, and lymphadenomegaly were observed.[2] The cat was treated with doxycycline and recovered. A cat from Hawaii had weight loss, ulcerative glossitis, pyrexia, progressive anemia, serous ocular discharge, and icterus.[5] Laboratory abnormalities were similar to those in dogs infected with North American strains.

DIAGNOSIS

Clinical Laboratory Findings

An elevated leukocyte count is typical of the naturally occurring disease, with the count ranging from 20,000 to 200,000 cells/μl.[1b, 5, 12, 15] Infection with the North American strain is usually associated with a neutrophilia with an occasional left shift.[5, 15] In other cases, a normal leukocyte count, with an increase in eosinophils of up to 20% of the total leukocyte count, was found.[5] A mild normocytic, normochromic, regenerative anemia has been a consistent finding with reported cases of hepatozoonosis. Thrombocytosis (422,000–916,000 platelets/μl) has been evident in some dogs.[15] Thrombocytopenia would only be expected with concurrent *Ehrlichia* infection.

Abnormalities of serum chemistry during hepatozoonosis include lowered glucose and albumin concentrations, occasional hyperglobulinemia, and increased alkaline phosphatase activity and inorganic phosphorus concentration.[1, 5, 15] Slight alterations in other serum constituents, such as elevated blood urea nitrogen concentrations, have been encountered. One striking abnormality is low serum glucose concentration. The extremely low glucose concentration, 10 to 15 mg/dl, is considered to be an artifact of the extreme neutrophilia and its effect on in vitro glucose catabolism from the time of blood collection until the time of serum separation. This artifact may be overcome by collection of blood in sodium fluoride. Protein-losing nephropathy with high urine protein-creatinine ratios from glomerulopathy is evident in some dogs[15] and may progress to more severe renal tubular failure. Generalized polymyopathy may be found with electromyography. CSF cytology may be within reference limits, or there may be lymphocytic pleocytosis.[15] Lymph node aspirates are characterized by hyperplasia with cytologic examination. Results of synoviocentesis analysis are those of nonseptic inflammation.[15] Bone marrow cytologic findings are granulocytic hyperplasia and erythroid hypoplasia with a high myeloid-erythroid ratio.

Radiography

Radiographic findings may range from spectacular to nonexistent. Periosteal bone proliferation was associated with the attachment of muscle on most bones of the body except the skull (Figs. 74–3 and 74–4).[5, 15, 23] Bony changes have been noted in the vertebrae, pelvis, radius, ulna, humerus, femur, fibula, and tibia. Not all infected dogs develop this unique

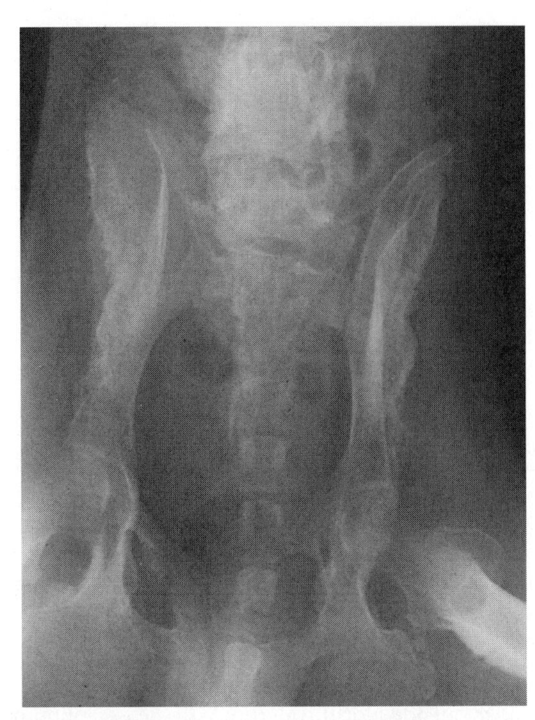

Figure 74–3. Radiograph of the pelvis and lumbar vertebrae of a dog with periosteal new bone proliferation associated with *Hepatozoon canis*.

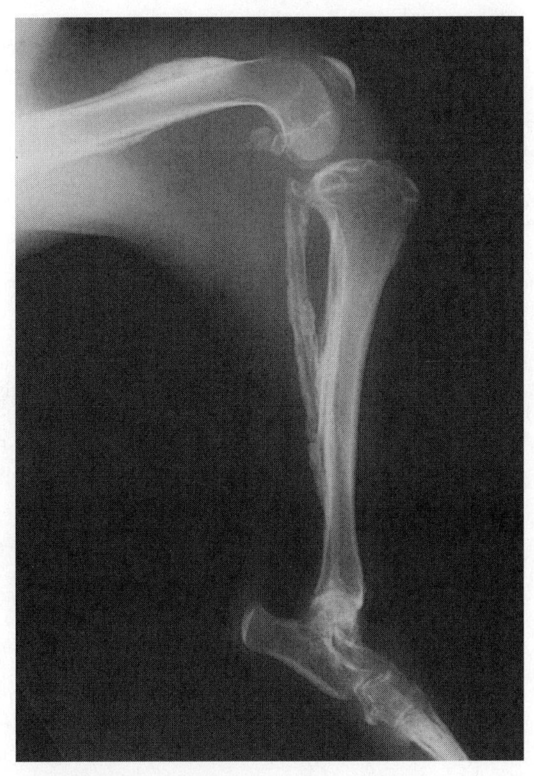

Figure 74–4. Radiograph of femur, tibia, and fibula of dog infected with *Hepatozoon canis*.

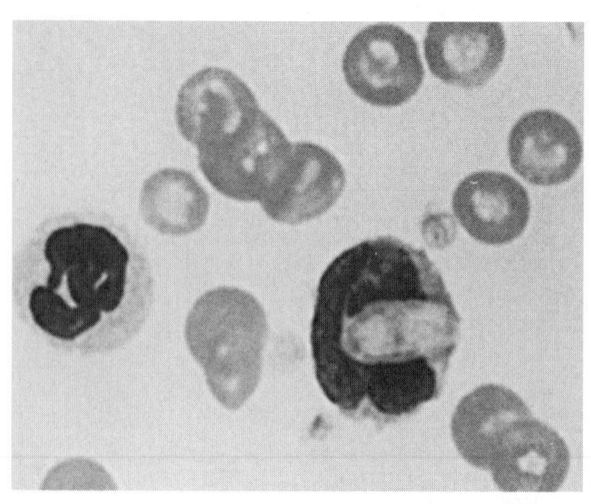

Figure 74–5. Gamont of *Hepatozoon canis* in neutrophilic leukocyte on a peripheral blood smear (Giemsa, × 1200).

lesion. The radiographic lesions are more common in younger dogs (<1 year) than in older dogs. It is not known whether the radiographic changes are associated with rapid skeletal growth or are indicative of a more severe infection in the young. Bony lesions have not been described in infected dogs outside North America with the exception of one case in Japan.[23]

Organism Identification

A definitive diagnosis of *H. canis* infection is made by finding the organism in Romanovsky's-stained blood films. The gamonts, found in both neutrophils and monocytes, stain an ice-blue color with Giemsa or Leishman's stain (Fig. 74–5). Especially in low concentrations, parasites can be better identified with special staining, which can be time consuming.[5] If films are not made shortly after blood collection, many gamonts appear to leave host cells, and nonstaining capsules are all that remains. Unless the capsules are present in great numbers, they can be easily overlooked. Although infected animals outside the United States have high parasitemias (60–90% of peripheral neutrophils),[1b, 5, 8, 13] the gamonts of the North American strain are very difficult to find (0.1% of peripheral neutrophils) (see Table 74–1).[5, 15] When a dog does have a detectable parasitemia, only 1 or 2 cells per 1000 leukocytes are infected. Gamont-infected leukocytes appear to be enzymatically inactive, although nonparasitized neutrophils have normal activity.[11, 19, 24]

Muscle biopsy is a convenient and more consistent means of establishing a diagnosis of hepatozoonosis in animals infected with the North American strain (see Pathologic Findings).[5, 15] Multiple or sequential biopsy specimens may need to be examined to facilitate detection of the organism in some dogs.[15]

Serologic Testing

H. canis infection incites antibody response. A survey in Israel using gamonts as antigens in an indirect FA test indicated a 33% prevalence of seropositivity, whereas only 1% of dogs tested had circulating gamonts detected.[3] In the United States, a serologic test might be of more value in clinical or epidemiologic studies because gamonts are infrequent in blood specimens.

PATHOLOGIC FINDINGS

The consistent gross lesion of dogs infected with *H. canis* is cachexia. Muscle atrophy is especially evident in the temporal region. Dogs are often anemic and may have an enlarged liver and spleen. There may be pulmonary congestion, lymphadenomegaly, gastric mucosa congestion, polyarthritis, and pale kidneys.[5] Grossly, the pyogranulomas may be visualized as 1- to 2-mm in diameter, white to tan foci scattered throughout the cardiac, skeletal, and intestinal smooth muscles; tongue; liver; skin lymph nodes; pancreas; lymph node; lung; and kidney.[29]

Schizonts are named for the size of the merozoites that they contain; the microschizont, which contains micromerozoites, is larger than a macroschizont. Microschizonts with a characteristic wheel spoke–like pattern can be found in spleen, liver, lymph nodes, kidneys, lungs, pancreas, and bone marrow of infected dogs outside North America (Fig. 74–6). This pattern has not been seen in schizonts from dogs in the Texas Gulf Coast or other areas in the United States.

Microscopically, schizonts have been found in the skeletal cardiac and intestinal smooth muscles, lymph nodes, spleen, liver, kidneys, and skin of infected dogs in the United States. Muscle from dogs infected with the North American strain contain unique cystlike microschizonts (250–500 μm diameter), which have also been described in native Felidae (Fig. 74–7).[6, 15] This structure contains a nucleus (15–60 × 30–90 μm) surrounded by bluish, mucinous, or often granular material and fine laminar membranes.

Occasionally, accumulations of small structures are seen, which may represent developing macroschizonts (Fig. 74–8). The individual structures are approximately 10 μm in diameter, with the total grouping about the size of a cyst. Whether a cyst always gives rise to multiple macroschizonts is unknown.

Pyogranulomas composed of macrophages and neutrophils are seen in the muscle, but there is no evidence of encapsulation. Inflammatory cells are often seen in fascial planes away from the organism (Fig. 74–9). The granulomas are similar to those in Chagas' disease (see American Trypanosomiasis, Chapter 72), from which hepatozoonosis must be differentiated. During the growth and maturation of the

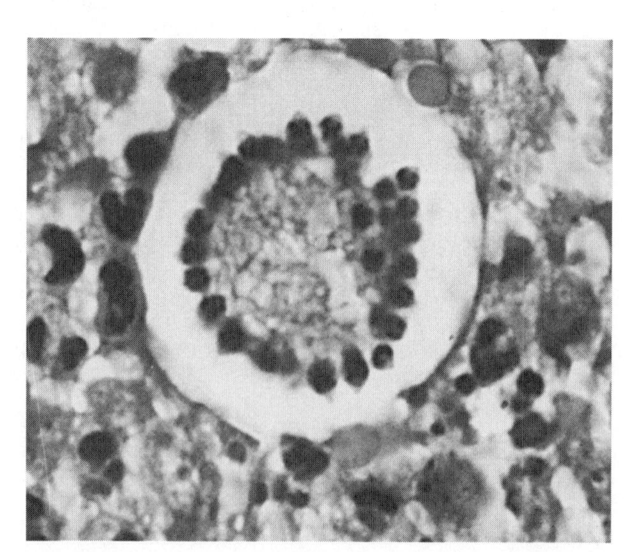

Figure 74–6. Schizont of *H. canis* in the spleen of a dog from Israel. The wheel-spoke pattern is typical of schizonts in the spleen and other organs of dogs with disseminated hepatozoonosis outside the U.S. (H and E, × 400. Courtesy of Dr. Gad Baneth, The Hebrew University of Jerusalem.)

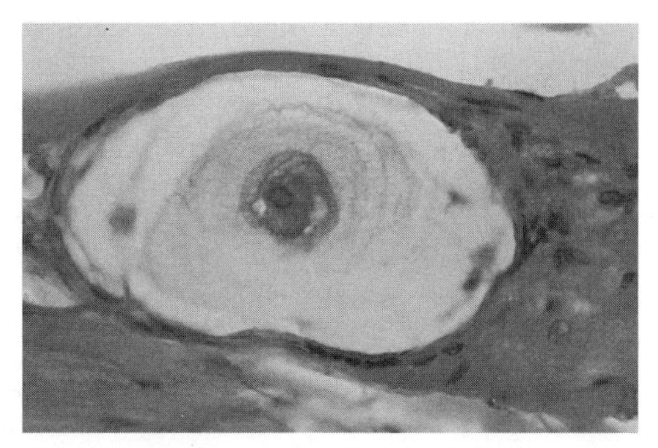

Figure 74–7. Cyst with central nucleus in skeletal muscle. The nucleus is surrounded by fine laminar membranes (H and E, × 1200).

meront, there is no inflammatory response. However, on release of merozoites, an intense granulomatous response composed of equal numbers of macrophages and neutrophils with varying numbers of eosinophils is observed. Pyogranulomatous vasculitis is characterized by fibrinoid and mineralization changes in blood vessel walls.[29] Few lymphocytes or plasma cells are associated with the lesions, and giant cells have not been found. In tissues, especially the muscles, there are large accumulations of neutrophils, which may account for the pain, fever, and stimulation of periosteal bone proliferation (see Fig. 74–3).

The North American strain has a predilection for cardiac muscles; however, organisms are numerous in skeletal muscle and, occasionally, the smooth muscle of the intestine. The organisms have not been observed in the liver or kidneys and only rarely in spleen, lymph nodes, or skin of dogs infected with this strain. The granulomatous response to this strain of *H. canis* appears to be more striking than that ascribed to others.

The cause of death has not always been established in fatal cases of hepatozoonosis. As previously noted, amyloidosis and immune complex disorders may develop. Concomitant disease or chronic progressing debilitation leads to cachexia and death.

THERAPY

Several antiprotozoal agents have been administered in an effort to control hepatozoonosis, although none are known to consistently cause an improvement in the clinical outcome of the infection, even though parasitemias may be reduced (Table 74–2). Recovery occurs in few dogs; most, however, have temporary improvement with relapses and death within 2 years of clinical diagnosis. Most dogs experience relapse 3 to 6 months after treatment. Clearance of blood forms has been reported with imidocarb dipropionate.[5] The effect of imidocarb therapy has been inconsistent, apparently depending on severity of signs, geographic locality, and criteria for clinical response.[1b, 5, 15] Treatment with diminazene aceturate apparently had little effect on the course of disease.[5] Treatment of hepatozoonosis with a combination of oxytetracycline and primaquine resulted in recovery of a cat.[5] A combination of tetracycline and imidocarb was reported to cause a clinical remission and clearance of a parasitemia; however, at least some of the dogs so treated were concurrently infected with *Ehrlichia canis*.[12] Whether the response was a direct effect of the drug on *Hepatozoon* or an indirect effect on *Ehrlichia* is unknown.

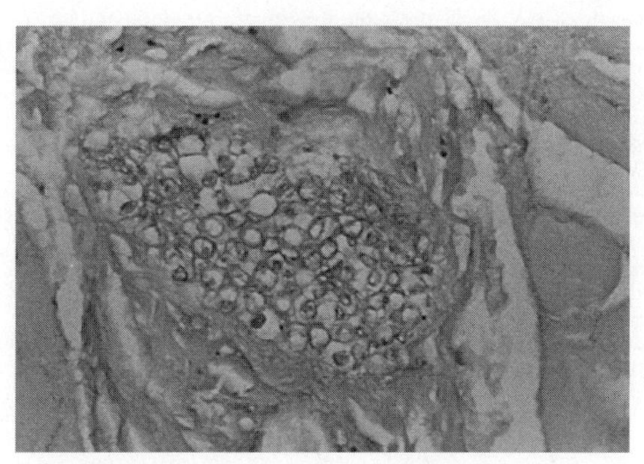

Figure 74–8. Skeletal muscle with developing macroschizonts (H and E, × 400).

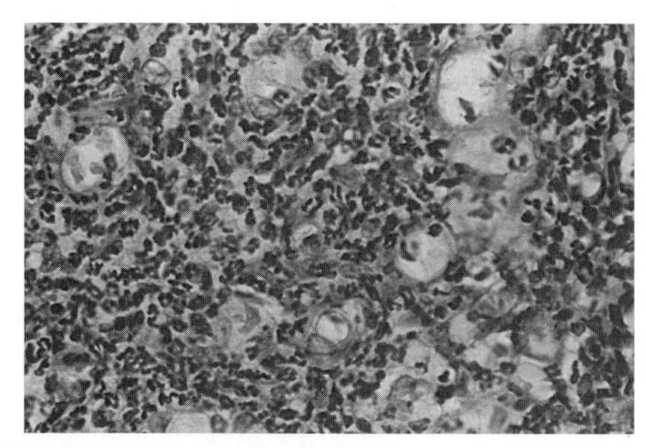

Figure 74–9. Pyogranuloma, thought to be associated with the invasion of a group of macroschizonts of *Hepatozoon canis*. Several schizonts, each containing one to three macromerozoites, are incorporated within the granuloma (H and E, × 1200).

Toltrazuril, a coccidiostat, has been administered to voles, and it protected them from experimental hepatozoonosis but did not clear them of infection.[5] Excellent clinical response was seen in dogs treated with oral toltrazuril at 5 mg/kg BID for 5 days. However, relapse occurred, and there was no evidence of clearing the cyst forms from the muscle.[15] Clindamycin was also used as a chemotherapeutic agent with either toltrazuril or trimethoprim-sulfonamide and pyrimethamine. With the clindamycin, trimethoprim-sulfonamide, pyramethamine combination, the clinical response was favorable, but relapse of signs occurred in 3 to 4 months.[15]

The criteria for effectiveness of a drug in a disease like hepatozoonosis are difficult to ascertain because of the complex nature of the disease and the chronicity of the bone and muscle lesions. None of the criteria utilized by various authors seem to be consistently valid in determining the value of treatment.

Symptomatic palliative treatment with nonsteroidal anti-inflammatory agents seems to be the most important aspect of therapy at this time. Drugs such as aspirin, phenylbutazone, and flunixin seem to be of value in relieving discomfort in clinical cases. In many instances, administration of these drugs will provide temporary clinical relief, and the owner can adjust the frequency of administration to the reappearance of clinical signs.[5] Each individual dog seems to respond to palliative treatment uniquely, and the ideal treatment must be adjusted depending on the degree of pain and extent of side effects. Glucocorticoids may give temporary clinical relief but should probably be avoided for long-term therapy because they apparently exacerbate the disease.[5]

Table 74–2. Antiprotozoal Therapy for Hepatozoonosis

DRUG	WHERE TREATED	SPECIES	DOSE (mg/kg)[a]	ROUTE	INTERVAL (HOURS)	DURATION (DAYS)
Diminazene aceturate	Texas[5]	D[b]	3.5	IM	Once	1
Imidocarb dipropionate	Nigeria[8]	D[c]	5	SC	Once	1
Imidocarb dipropionate	Nigeria[8]	D[c]	6	SC	14 days	14
and						
tetracycline			22	PO	8	14
Imidocarb dipropionate	Spain[5]	D[c]	5	SC	14 days	14
and						
doxycycline			10	PO	Daily	14
Trimethoprim sulfadiazine	India[26]	D[c]	30	IV	24	5
and						
dexamethasone						
Trimethoprim-sulfonamide	Alabama[15]	D	15	PO	12	14
and						
pyrimethamine			0.25	PO	24	14
and						
clindamycin			10	PO	8	14
Primaquine phosphate	South Africa[5]	C	2	PO	Once	
and						
oxytetracycline			50	PO	12	7
Toltrazuril	Alabama[15]	D[d]	5	PO	12	5

[a] Dose per administration at specified interval.
[b] Apparent clinical response, no change in parasitemia.
[c] Drugs may clear parasitemia but do not always reverse clinical signs of infection. Supportive anti-inflammatory therapy or anticholinergic may be needed. See text and Drug Formulary, Appendix 8.
[d] Initial clinical response followed by relapse.
D = dog; C = cat.

PREVENTION

Control of ticks by routine dipping of dogs from infested premises is important to limit the spread of disease. The transmission of *H. canis* only occurs transtadially or by male ticks; transovarial transmission is unknown. Environmental control of the vector by preventing it from feeding on infected dogs, therefore, will help prevent spread. Home or kennel environments should be sprayed on a routine basis. Regular dipping of dogs from infested premises will kill any ticks feeding at that time.

If vectors other than *R. sanguineus* are involved, they will have to be identified in order for control programs to be instituted. In a few instances in which the disease was recognized, careful scrutiny of the dog's home environment failed to reveal *R. sanguineus*. Kissing bugs (family Reduviidae) were found, but no oocysts of *H. canis* have been recovered from these insects. Large numbers of *Dermacentor variabilis*, American dog ticks, were associated with bobcats and ocelots infected with *Hepatozoon* species.[5] Structures resembling *H. canis* oocysts have been identified in an *Amblyomma* tick removed from an infected dog in Alabama.[15, 29] Infected *Haemaphysalis* ticks were found with *Hepatozoon*-infected dogs in Japan.[19]

Until the development of an effective antiprotozoal agent and a serologic test that is sensitive enough to identify inapparent carriers, the prevention of hepatozoonosis will be largely a matter of controlling known vectors. The importance of transplacental transmission in maintaining the infection is unknown at this time. Direct transmission via predation seems unlikely in infected house pets; however, it may have a role in the spread of infection in wildlife hosts. Control of wildlife reservoir hosts is unlikely to be successful.

PUBLIC HEALTH CONSIDERATIONS

Infection with *Hepatozoon* sp. was described in a human patient with occasional chills, anemia, and jaundice in the Philippines.[4] Hypersegmentation of the nucleus of unparasitized neutrophils, as is seen in many canine infections, was noted in this case. Morphologically, the gamonts resembled *H. canis*, but the identification was far from certain. Whether the scarcity of reports of infection in humans is due to the rarity of instances in which they ingest suitable vectors or to natural resistance is unknown. Attempts to experimentally infect primates are not known.

References

1. Alencar NX, Kohayagawa A, Santarem VA. 1997. *Hepatozoon canis* infection of wild carnivores in Brazil. *Vet Parasitol* 70:279–282.
1a. Baneth G, Aroch I. Presentey B. 1997. *Hepatozoon canis* infection in a litter of Dalmation dogs. *Vet Parasitol* 70:201–206.
1b. Baneth G, Harmelin A, Presentey B-Z. 1995. *Hepatozoon canis* infection in two dogs. *J Am Vet Med Assoc* 206:1891–1894.
2. Baneth G, Lavy E, Presentey B-Z, Shkap V. 1995. *Hepatozoon* sp. parasitemia in a domestic cat. *Feline Pract* 23(2):10–12.
3. Baneth G, Shkap V, Presentey B-Z, Pipano E. 1996. *Hepatozoon canis*: the prevalence of antibodies and gametocytes in dogs in Israel. *Vet Res Commun* 20:41–46.
3a. Baneth G, Weigler B. 1997. Retrospective case-control study of Hepatozoonosis in dogs in Israel. *J Vet Intern Med* 11:365–370.
4. Carlos ET, Cruz FB, Cabiles CC, et al. 1971. *Hepatozoon* sp. in the WBC of a human patient. *Univ Philipp Vet* 15:5–7.
5. Craig TM. 1990. Hepatozoonosis, pp 778–785. *In* Greene CE (ed), Infectious diseases of the dog and cat. WB Saunders, Philadelphia, PA.
5a. Deinert M, Kraft W, Gothe R. 1997. *Hepatozoon canis* infection of dogs in Germany: case report and epidemiology. *Tierarztl Prax* 25:254–256.
6. Droleskey RE, Mercer SH, DeLoach JR, Craig TM. 1993. Ultrastructure of *Hepatozoon canis* in the dog. *Vet Parasitol* 50:83–99.
7. Dubey JP, Bwangamoi O. 1994. *Microbesnoitia leoni* Bwangamoi 1989, from the African lion (Panthera leo) redetermined as a junior synonym of *Hepatozoon canis* (James 1905) Wenyon 1926. *J Parasitol* 80:333–334.
8. Ezeokoli CD, Ogunkoya AB, Abdullahi R, et al. 1983. Clinical and epidemiological studies on canine hepatozoonosis in Zaria, Nigeria. *J Small Anim Pract* 24:455–460.
9. Harmelin A, Dubey JP, Yakobson B, et al. 1992. Concurrent *Hepatozoon canis* and *Toxoplasma gondii* infections in a dog. *Vet Parasitol* 43:131–136.
10. Hervas J, Carrasco L, Gomez-Villamandos JC, et al. 1995. Acute fatal hepatozoonosis in a puppy: histopathological and ultrastructural study. *Vet Rec* 137:518–519.

10a. Hervas J, Carrasco L, Sierra MA, et al. 1997. Ultrastructural findings in natural canine hepatozoonosis. *Zentralbl Vet Med B* 44:119–125.
11. Ibrahim NDG, Rahamathulla PM, Njoku CO. 1989. Neutrophil myeloperoxidase deficiency associated with canine hepatozoonosis. *Int J Parasitol* 19:915–918.
12. Jaurequi Latorre E, Lopez Giron M. 1995. Canine hepatozoonosis. *Vet Int* 7(1):30–38.
13. Kontos V, Koutinas A. 1991. Canine hepatozoonosis: a review of 11 naturally occurring cases. *Eur J Comp Anim Proct* 2:26–30.
14. Latorie EJ, Giron ML. 1995. Canine hepatozoonosis. *Vet International* 7:30–38.
15. Macintire DK, Vincent-Johnson N, Dillon AR, et al. 1997. Canine hepatozoonosis: in dogs of 22 cases (1989–1994). *J Am Vet Med Assoc* 210:916–922.
16. Mundim AV, Jacomini JO, Mundim MJS, et al. 1992. *Hepatozoon canis* (James, 1905) Em caes de Uberlandia, Minas Gorais. Relato de dois Casos. *Braz J Vet Res Anim Sci* 29:359–361.
17. Murata T, Animoto A, Shiramizu K, et al. 1993. Survey on canine *Hepatozoon canis* infection in the western area of Yamaguchi Prefecture. *Jpn Vet Med Assoc* 46:395–397.
18. Murata T, Inoue M, Abe H, et al. 1998. Ticks collected from the *Hepatozoon canis* infected dogs. *J Vet Med Sci*. In press.
19. Murata T, Inoue M, Kanoe M, et al. 1993. Ultrastructure and cytochemical characteristics of leukocyte infected with *Hepatozoon canis*. *J Vet Med Sci* 55:1043–1045.
20. Murata T, Inoue M, Tateyama S, et al. 1993. Vertical transmission of *Hepatozoon canis* in dogs. *J Vet Med Sci* 55:867–868.
21. Murata T, Inoue M, Taura Y, et al. 1995. Detection of *Hepatozoon canis* oocyst from ticks collected from the infected dogs. *J Vet Med Sci* 57:111-112.
22. Murata T, Shinoda K, Inoue M, et al. 1993. Seasonal periodical appearance of *Hepatozoon canis* gamont in the peripheral blood. *J Vet Med Sci* 55:877–879.
23. Murata T, Shiramizu K, Hara Y, et al. 1991. First case of *Hepatozoon canis* infection of a dog in Japan. *J Vet Med Sci* 53:1097–1099.
24. Murata T, Taqani R, Inoue M, et al. 1994. Investigation of the nitroblue tetrazolium reduction of neutrophils in the dog infected with *Hepatozoon canis*. *Exp Anim* 43:101–103.
25. Panciera RJ, Gatto NJ, Crystal MA, et al. 1997. Canine hepatozoonosis in Oklahoma. *J Am Anim Hosp Assoc* 33:221–225.
26. Prathaban S, Jayathangaraj MG, Rasheed MA. 1992. Canine cerebral hepatozoonosis—a case report. *Indian Vet J* 69:67–68.
27. Shkap V, Baneth G, Pipano E. 1994. Circulating antibodies to *Hepatozoon canis* demonstrated by immunofluorescence. *J Vet Diagn Invest* 6:121–123.
28. Smith TG. 1996. The genus *Hepatozoon*. *J Parasitol* 82:565–585.
29. Vincent-Johnson N, Macintire DK, Baneth G. 1997. Canine hepatozoonosis: pathophysiology, diagnosis, and treatment. *Compend Cont Educ Pract Vet* 19:51–65.
29a. Vincent-Johnson N, Macintire DK, Linsay DS. 1996. Preliminary studies in the transmission of *Hepatozoon canis*. *Proc Am Coll Vet Intern Med* 14:761.
30. Waner T, Baneth G, Zuckerman A, et al. 1994. *Hepatozoon canis* size measurement of gametocyte using image analysis technology. *Comp Haematol Int* 4:1–3.

Chapter 75

Encephalitozoonosis

Peter J. Didier, Elizabeth S. Didier, Karen Snowden, and John A. Shadduck

ETIOLOGY

Encephalitozoonosis in dogs and cats is caused by the obligate, intracellular protozoan *Encephalitozoon cuniculi*, which is a member of the Phylum Microspora. More than 1000 species of microsporidia exist, classified into approximately 100 genera, which infect insects and members of all classes of vertebrates.[4] To date, three species of the genus *Encephalitozoon* have been described: *E. hellem*, *E. intestinalis* (previously named *Septata intestinalis*), and three strains of *E. cuniculi*.[3, 12, 16, 19] Mature spores of *E. cuniculi* are small and oval shaped measuring approximately 1.5 μm × 2.5 μm and contain the distinctive coiled polar tubule or filament and extrusion apparatus that distinguish microsporidia from all other protozoans (Fig. 75–1). The polar tubule is used for propelling the sporoplasm (containing the microsporidian nucleus) into the host cell. Spores also contain a posterior vacuole, and the spore coat contains an outer glycoprotein coat, a middle layer containing chitin, and an internal plasma membrane.

Infection of most mammalian hosts with *E. cuniculi* occurs by ingestion or inhalation of spores from contaminated urine or feces that are shed by infected hosts.[4] Infection by transplacental transmission and traumatic inoculation have been reported as well.[30] Once internalized, infectious spores invade host cells by propelling the sporoplasm through the everting polar tubule by a process called "germination." In the case of *E. cuniculi*, the sporoplasm develops within a host cell–derived membrane-bound parasitiferous vacuole (Fig. 75–2). The organisms undergo schizogony (also termed merogony), which is an asexual process of cell division or binary fission. During sporogony and maturation, organisms develop the spore coat and organelles (the polar tubule, endoplasmic reticulum, polar cap). The host cells eventually rupture to release organisms that infect new cells or environmentally resistant spore forms, which are shed with the urine or feces.[4] Typical organs of localized infection in dogs and cats include the kidney, liver, and brain.[30]

EPIDEMIOLOGY

Natural infections of *E. cuniculi* have been described in a wide range of hosts, including rabbits, mice, cats, dogs, foxes, and humans.[4, 30] Of the three strains of *E. cuniculi*, strain I has been primarily isolated from rabbits. Strain II has only been isolated from mice, and strain III has been isolated from dogs and humans.[7, 11, 12, 24] Differences in these isolates have been confirmed by protein electrophoresis, Western blot immunodetection, and small subunit ribosomal RNA gene sequence analysis. No epidemiologic information exists about the relationship between the human and canine isolates of *E. cuniculi*. However, strain I (primarily from rabbits) can infect mice, cats, and sheep in experimental situations.[25, 30] A comparison of isolates from humans and rabbits suggests that this is a zoonotic strain.[8] A strain of *E. cuniculi* from a dog produced a subclinical infection in immunocompetent monkeys.[33] Relatively few isolates of *E. cuniculi* have been avail-

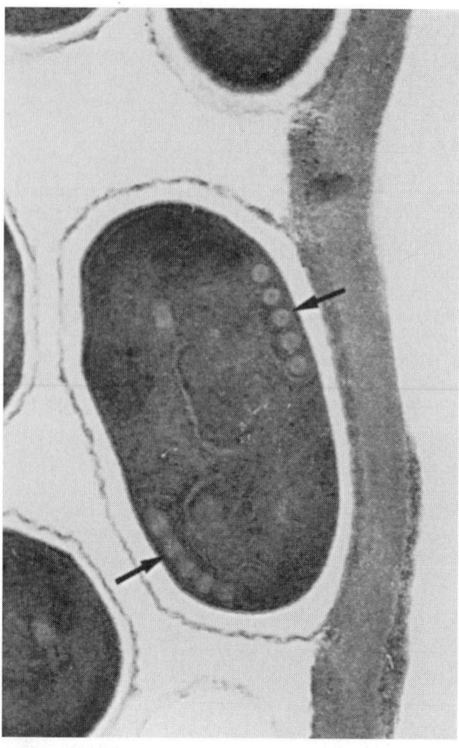

Figure 75–1. Cross-section of a mature spore of *E. cuniculi.* Polar filaments *(arrows)* and electron-lucent spore wall are demonstrated. The sporoplasm is contained within the electron-dense material (lead citrate/uranyl acetate; × 35,000). (From Shadduck JA et al: *Vet Pathol* 15:449–460, 1978. Reprinted with permission.)

able for comparison, so that the host specificity of the *E. cuniculi* strains is still unclear.

Few studies have been published on the prevalence rates of naturally acquired *E. cuniculi* infections. In a group of stray dogs that were housed three per cage in a kennel in London, 13.3% of the dogs were found to express specific antibodies to *E. cuniculi.*[17] In South Africa, a serologic study of 220 serum samples submitted for clinical evaluation suggested a prevalence of 18% in domestic dogs.[29] Among 52 dogs with renal failure, 12 (23%) expressed specific antibodies for *E. cuniculi* compared with the presence of specific antibodies in 2 of 42 (5%) control dogs.[28] Based on the presence of specific antibodies, a prevalence of 70% was also reported in 50 dogs housed in kennels. This high prevalence was perhaps due to confinement and closer contact to contaminated urine or feces.[29] In an urban animal shelter, 6 of 20 dogs were found to be excreting microsporidial spores in the stools.[18] Natural infections of cats with *E. cuniculi* are rare, and no prevalence data have been published.[30]

Clinically significant infections of *E. cuniculi* generally occur in neonatal and young puppies, acquired by transplacental transmission and ingestion or inhalation of spores shed from the mother.[30] Older dogs may become infected with microsporidia by inhalation or ingestion of spores from contaminated urine or feces or by ingestion of tissues from rabbits or mice infected with *E. cuniculi.*[23, 30] Experimental canine infections also may be transmitted by IP inoculation, whereas kittens may be infected experimentally by intracerebral, IP, or oral inoculation. Cats and older dogs generally show few or no clinical signs of disease, but do sporadically shed organisms in the urine. Younger dogs infected with microsporidia have clinical signs associated with renal disease.[28, 30] In experimental studies, microsporidiosis is chronic, asymptomatic in healthy immunocompetent animals, but becomes severe and lethal in T cell–depleted animals.

CLINICAL FINDINGS

Dogs

Clinical signs in neonatal dogs appear within a few weeks post partum, and several pups in a litter may be affected with stunted growth and general unthriftiness. As infection progresses, animals show signs of renal failure and neurologic abnormalities such as depression, ataxia, convulsions,

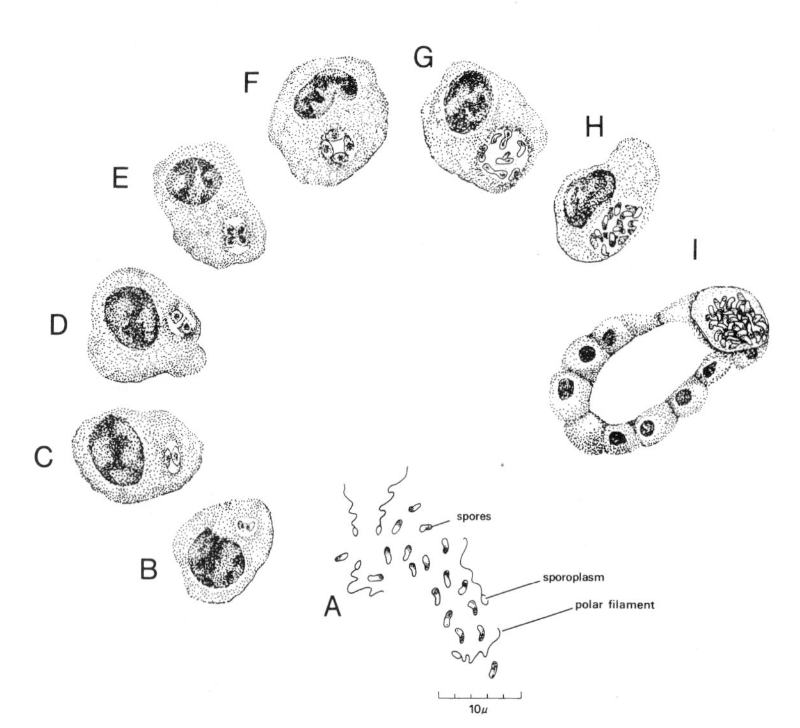

Figure 75–2. Diagram of the intracellular life cycle of *E. cuniculi* in a renal tubular epithelial cell. The diagram is based on light and electron microscopic examination of parasites. *A,* Mature spores, some with sporoplasm extruded by means of the polar tubule. *B–G,* Proliferative forms of the parasite (schizonts) in the parasitophorous vacuole. Binary fission occurs in contact with the membrane of the vacuole. As maturation progresses, spores collect in the center of the vacuole. *H–I,* Parasitophorous vacuole containing spores and proliferative forms. These stages are visible under the light microscope. The vacuole *(I)* ruptures and releases its spores *(A)* into the renal tubule lumen.

and blindness.[5, 22, 23, 30] Animals may develop signs of aggressive behavior, consisting of viciousness, biting, and abnormal vocalization. The high frequency of anti–*E. cuniculi* antibodies in dogs with azotemia suggests that *E. cuniculi* may contribute to chronic renal disease in dogs.[28, 30]

Clinical laboratory findings are available only for experimentally infected dogs.[30, 31] A normochromic, normocytic anemia is a consistent finding and may result from severe renal lesions with depression of erythropoietin production. In contrast, leukocytes, especially lymphocytes and monocytes, are increased. Bone marrow is hypercellular, with a preponderance of large mononuclear cells. Serum biochemical findings include increased alanine aminotransferase and alkaline phosphatase (in the high normal to slightly elevated range), variable blood urea nitrogen and creatinine, and increased total serum protein. CSF may have increased protein and cells in animals that display behavioral and neurologic signs and higher anti–*E. cuniculi* IgG levels in the CSF than in serum. Urinalysis may demonstrate hematuria and pyuria.

Cats

Clinical signs in feline encephalitozoonosis are variable. Severe muscle spasms, superficial corneal infection with blepharospasm, depression, paralysis, and death have been found in those with natural infections but could not be repeated in experimental trials.[30] Clinical laboratory findings specifically for cats have not been reported.

DIAGNOSIS

Immunologically competent hosts produce specific antibodies to *E. cuniculi*, which can be detected by methods such as indirect FA staining and ELISA.[30] An FA titer greater than 1:20 or an ELISA titer of 1:800 or greater is considered to be positive for the presence of antibodies to *E. cuniculi*.[17, 29, 30] Serologic tests, however, are not commercially available, and there is concern about the diagnostic reliability of serologic tests in immunologically immature puppies or in casually exposed hosts. Diagnostic methods, therefore, have been directed toward detection of the microsporidian spores in urine, stool, and tissue specimens.

The small size and poor staining qualities have made *Encephalitozoon* difficult to visualize with routine parasitologic and histologic techniques. They are easily missed with hematoxylin and eosin staining, especially when organisms are present in low numbers.

Transmission EM is still considered the standard for the specific diagnosis of microsporidiosis. Observation of the polar tubule distinguishes microsporidia from other organisms (see Fig. 75–1).[4, 30] However, it is relatively insensitive, costly, and time consuming and requires technical expertise.[9]

Cytologic examination of body fluids is of prime importance in making a clinical diagnosis in disseminated infections. Spores shed into the urine from parasitized renal tubular epithelial cells are readily identifiable in the sediment with either Gram's or Ziehl-Neelsen staining.[30] Stained spores are gram positive, whereas the proliferative stages are gram negative. Microsporidia are also difficult to distinguish from other gram-positive bacteria in stool specimens. When viewed with cross-polarizing filters, *Encephalitozoon* and other microsporidia are birefringent in appearance, unlike the coccidians, *Toxoplasma gondii* and *Isospora* species. Microsporidia are easily stained with the modified trichrome stains (using 10-fold higher concentrations of chromotrope 2R) and appear bright pink with a diagonal pink band and a clear posterior vacuole, whereas bacteria stain with the counterstain.[6, 9, 15, 20, 38] Yeasts also stain bright pink but lack a posterior vacuole, and they are usually larger and more round than oval compared with microsporidia. Chitin-staining fluorochromes (e.g., Calcofluor White 2MR, American Cyanamid, Princeton, NJ) are useful for detecting the microsporidia, which stain as white to turquoise oval halos when viewed under UV microscopy.[6, 9, 21, 34, 35] These staining methods, however, do not discriminate between species of microsporidia. FA methods using monoclonal antibodies or hyperimmune polyclonal antisera specifically identify microsporidia (Fig. 75–3). These reagents are not yet commercially available.[1, 9, 24, 26, 36, 40, 42] Development of a polymerase chain reaction method should provide a sensitive, specific, and reliable diagnostic procedure for microsporidiosis. This method is not yet commercially available.[7, 11, 12, 16, 24, 36, 37, 39, 41]

PATHOLOGIC FINDINGS

Gross lesions of canine encephalitozoonosis, based on experimental infections, include hepatomegaly, petechiae on multiple organs, patchy consolidation and edema of lung, fibrinous pericarditis, regional enteritis, focal myocardial degeneration, swollen kidneys, hemorrhagic cystitis, and splenomegaly.[30] The kidney may contain mild petechiae to severe cortical cysts and infarcts (Fig. 75–4). Brain may contain thrombosis of meningeal blood vessels, focal encephalomalacia, and cystic spaces within the parenchyma. In naturally infected blue foxes, nodular thickening of the extramural coronary arteries and lymphadenomegaly have been seen.[30]

Histologically, dogs and blue foxes with encephalitozoonosis consistently have nonsuppurative meningoencephalitis (Fig. 75–5).[22, 30] Fibrinoid necrosis of small and medium-sized arteries of the brain can result in thrombosis and encephalomalacia. Parasitophorous vacuoles occur in glial cells. Kidneys of dogs, cats, and foxes have multifocal nonsuppurative interstitial nephritis. Parasitophorous vacuoles with organisms are present in the renal tubular epithelia. In the heart, focal myocardial necrosis, vasculitis, and fibrinoid

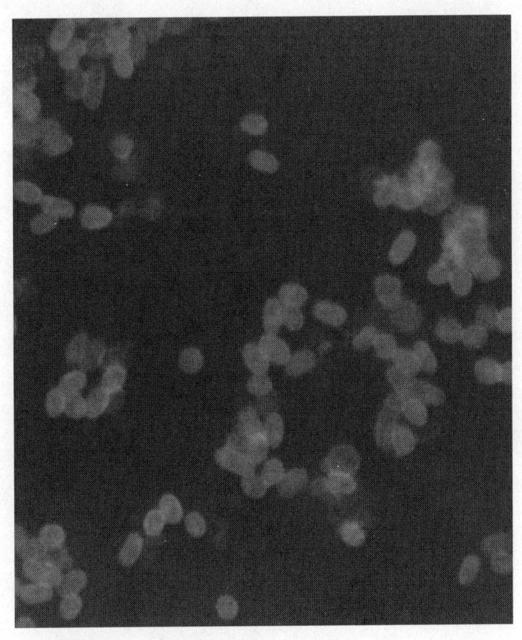

Figure 75–3. Indirect FA test of *E. cuniculi* spores in urine sediment (fluorescein isothiocyanate, × 2400).

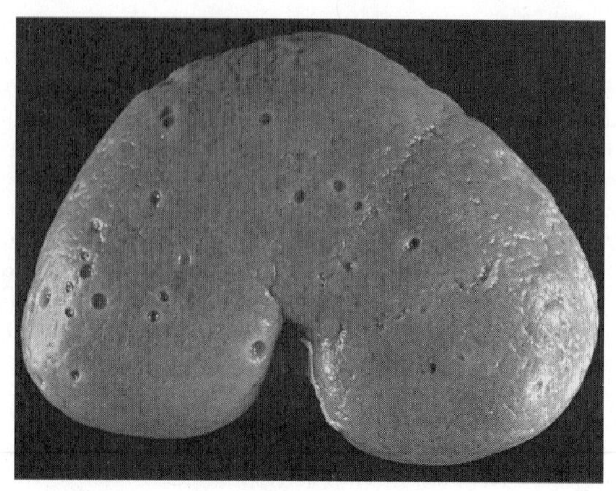

Figure 75–4. Kidney with pale, firm cortex that has an irregular subcapsular surface and numerous projecting cysts filled with clear fluid. (From Shadduck JA et al: *Vet Pathol* 15:449–460, 1978. Reprinted with permission.)

necrosis of small and medium-sized arteries are associated with *E. cuniculi* in endothelial cells and smooth muscle cells. In experimental infections, livers of dogs and cats contain vascular fibrinoid necrosis, focal hepatic necrosis, and lymphoplasmacytic infiltration associated with *E. cuniculi* in hepatocytes, Kupffer's cells, and endothelial cells. In blue foxes, ocular lesions are attributable to arterial lesions of the short and long ciliary arteries and retinal vessels. Other nonspecific lesions include pulmonary edema, nonsuppurative interstitial pneumonia and enteritis, lymphadenomegaly, reticuloendothelial hyperplasia of the spleen, and hyperplasia of the bone marrow.[30]

THERAPY

No treatment has been reported for either canine or feline encephalitozoonosis. In vitro experiments demonstrate that the antibiotic fumagillin inhibits the replicative ability of the organism without damaging the host cell, but the drug in its present formulation is toxic for systemic use in mammals.[30] Topical fumagillin has been administered to successfully treat microsporidial keratitis in persons infected with HIV. Its use in dogs and cats with microsporidiosis has not been reported.[10, 13] The benzimidazole albendazole has been successful for the treatment of *E. intestinalis* and *E. cuniculi* in AIDS patients.[2, 7, 10, 34] Its use for treating dogs and cats with microsporidiosis has not been published. In adult humans, the dose is 400 mg given twice daily for 4 weeks or longer. In vitro and in vivo studies suggest that the parasite is inhibited by antifolate drugs. Trimethoprim or pyrimethamine and sulfonamides, alone or in combination with albendazole, have been effective in treating humans with disseminated infections.[14] Should these drugs be given to dogs, the dosages can be found in the Drug Formulary (Appendix 8).

PREVENTION AND PUBLIC HEALTH CONSIDERATION

Microsporidia are increasingly recognized as causing opportunistic infections in persons with AIDS and those with

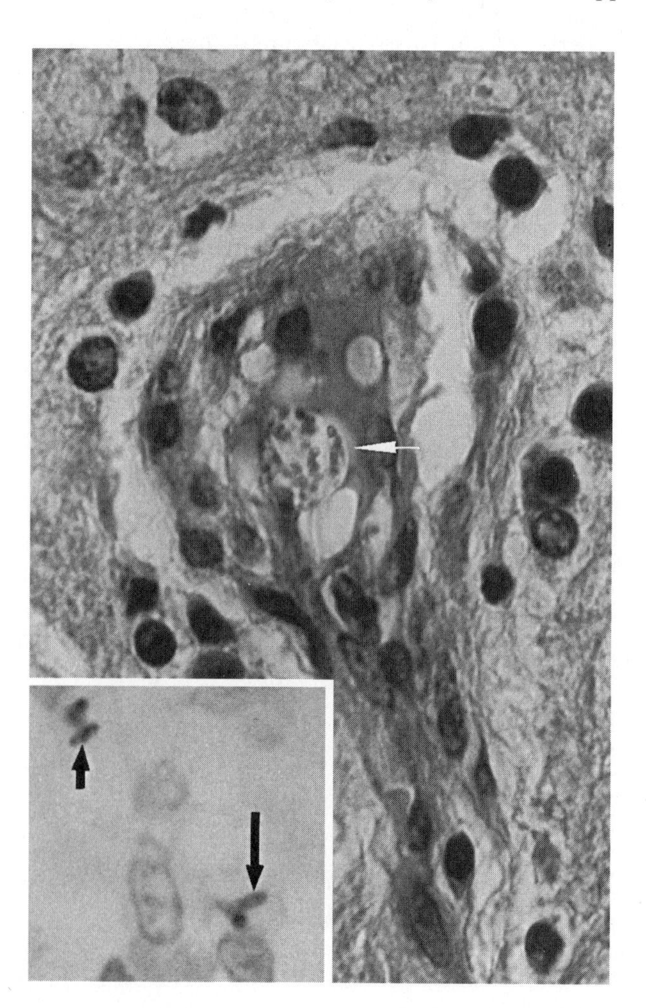

Figure 75–5. Parasitophorous vacuole *(arrow)* in endothelial cells of cerebral vessel with mononuclear perivascular cuff from a dog (H and E, × 1300). *Inset, E. cuniculi* spores *(arrows)* free in brain parenchyma of an experimentally infected kitten. Note the lack of an inflammatory response (Gram's stain, × 2000). (From Shadduck JA et al: *Vet Pathol* 15:449–460, 1978. Reprinted with permission.)

Table 75–1. Species of Microsporidia Infecting People and Animals

MICROSPORIDIA	HUMAN SYNDROME	NATURALLY INFECTED ANIMALS
Encephalitozoon cuniculi	Peritonitis, hepatitis, rhinosinusitis, seizures, nephritis	Rabbit (strain I) Mouse (strain II) Dog (strain III) Cats, foxes, rodents, primates, birds
Encephalitozoon hellem	Conjunctivitis, keratoconjunctivitis, rhinosinusitis, bronchiolitis, pneumonia, disseminated infection	Budgerigars
Encephalitozoon intestinalis	Diarrhea, disseminated infection	?
Enterocytozoon bieneusi	Diarrhea, malabsorption, weight loss, rhinitis, bronchitis, pneumonia, cholecystitis, cholangitis	Primates, swine
Pleistophora spp.	Myositis	Australian terrestrial mammals, insects, neon tetra fish
Nosema cannoir	Disseminated infection	Invertebrates
Nosema ocularum	Keratitis	Invertebrates
Vittaforma corneae	Keratitis	?
Trachipleistophora hominis	Myositis, keratitis, rhinosinusitis	?
Microsporidium spp.[a]	Keratitis	?

[a]Collective term for unclassified microsporidia.
? = unknown animals.

the immunosuppression of organ transplantation. The high seroprevalence in immunocompetent hosts suggests that most infections are subclinical.[34a] In persons with AIDS, *E. intestinalis* and *E. hellem* are the most frequent causes of disease and probably result from opportunistic spread of endogenous microflora. At least 10 species of microsporidia are known to infect humans, including *E. cuniculi* strain III, which infects dogs (Table 75–1).[11, 12] In one report, however, a 10-year-old girl underwent seroconversion to *E. cuniculi* after close contact with an infected puppy.[23] However, it is unknown whether dogs infect humans or whether humans infect dogs with microsporidia.

Sanitation is important in suspected cases of encephalitozoonosis, because environmentally resistant spores may be shed in urine or feces. Spores can readily be rendered uninfective by a variety of disinfectants; the most commonly available are 2% phenol, 10% formalin, and 70% ethyl alcohol. Infectivity is unaffected by sonication, freezing and thawing, and pH ranging from 4 to 9. Infectivity of spores stored in neutral buffer at 4°C and 20°C is maintained beyond 24 days, indicating that spore survival is possible in a humid environment at ambient temperatures.[30]

References

1. Aldras AM, Orenstein JM, Kotler DP, et al. 1993. Detection of microsporidia by indirect immunofluorescence antibody test using polyclonal and monoclonal antibodies. *J Clin Microbiol* 32:608–612.
2. Blanshard C, Ellis DS, Tovey DG, et al. 1992. Treatment of intestinal microsporidiosis with albendazole in patients with AIDS. *AIDS* 6:311–313.
3. Cali A, Kotler DP, Orenstein JM. 1993. *Septata intestinalis*, n.g., n. sp., an intestinal microsporidian associated with chronic diarrhea and dissemination in AIDS patients. *J Protozool* 40:101–112.
4. Canning EU, Lom J. 1986. The microsporidia of vertebrates. Academic Press, New York, NY.
5. Cole JR, Sangster LT, Sulzer CR, et al. 1982. Infections with *Encephalitozoon cuniculi* and *Leptospira interrogans*, serovars grippotyphosa and ballus, in a kennel of foxhounds. *J Am Vet Med Assoc* 180:435–437.
6. DeGirolami PC, Ezratty CR, Desai G, et al. 1995. Diagnosis of intestinal microsporidiosis by examination of stool and duodenal aspirate with Weber's modified trichrome and Uvitex 2B stains. *J Clin Microbiol* 33:805–810.
7. DeGroote MA, Visvesvara GS, Wilson ML, et al. 1995. Polymerase chain reaction and culture confirmation of disseminated *Encephalitozoon cuniculi* in a patient with AIDS: successful therapy with albendazole. *J Infect Dis* 171:1375–1378.
8. Deplazes P, Mathis A, Baumgartner R, et al. 1996. Immunologic and molecular characteristics of *Encephalitozoon*-like microsporidia isolated from humans and rabbits indicate that *Encephalitozoon cuniculi* is a zoonotic parasite. *Clin Infect Dis* 22:557–559.
9. Didier ES, Orenstein JM, Aldras AM, et al. 1995. Comparison of three staining methods for detecting microsporidia in fluids. *J Clin Microbiol* 33:3138–3145.
10. Didier ES, Rogers LB, Brush AD, et al. 1996. Diagnosis of disseminated microsporidian *Encephalitozoon hellem* infection by PCR-southern analysis and successful treatment with albendazole and fumagillin. *J Clin Microbiol* 34:947–952.
11. Didier ES, Visvesvara GS, Baker MD, et al. 1996. A microsporidian isolated from an AIDS patient corresponds to the *Encephalitozoon cuniculi* strain III, originally isolated from domestic dogs. *J Clin Microbiol* 24:2835–2837.
12. Didier ES, Vossbrinck CR, Baker MD, et al. 1995. Identification and characterization of three *Encephalitozoon cuniculi* strains. *Parasitology* 111:411–421.
13. Diesenhouse MC, Wilson LA, Corrent GC, et al. 1993. Treatment of microsporidial keratoconjunctivitis with topical fumagillin. *Am J Ophthalmol* 115:293–298.
14. Field AS, Marriott DJ, Milliken ST, et al. 1996. Myositis associated with a newly described microsporidian, *Trachipleistophora hominis*, in a patient with AIDS. *J Clin Microbiol* 34:2803–2811.
15. Garcia LS, Bruckner DA. 1993. Diagnostic medical parasitology, ed 2. American Society for Microbiology, Washington, DC.
16. Hartskeerl RA, van Gool T, Schuitema ARJ, et al. 1995. Genetic and immunological characterization of the microsporidian *Septata intestinalis* Cali, Kotler, and Orenstein, 1993: reclassification to *Encephalitozoon intestinalis*. *Parasitology* 110:277–285.
17. Hollister WS, Canning EU, Viney M. 1989. Prevalence of antibodies to *Encephalitozoon cuniculi* in stray dogs as determined by an ELISA. *Vet Rec* 124:332–336.
18. Jafri HS, Reedy T, Moorhead AR, et al. 1993. Detection of pathogenic protozoa in fecal specimens from urban dwelling dogs (abstract 361). Presented at the 42nd Annual Meeting of the American Society of Tropical Medicine and Hygiene, Atlanta, GA.
19. Katiyar SK, Visvesvara G, Edlind TD. 1995. Comparisons of ribosomal RNA sequences from amitochondrial protozoa: implications for processing, mRNA binding and paromomycin susceptibility. *Gene* 152:27–33.
20. Kokoskin E, Gyorkos TW, Camus A, et al. 1994. Modified technique for efficient detection of microsporidia. *J Clin Microbiol* 32:1074–1075.
21. Luna VA, Stewart BK, Bergeron DL, et al. 1995. Use of the fluorochrome calcofluor white in the screening of stool specimens for spores of microsporidia. *Am J Clin Pathol* 103:656–659.
22. McCully RM, van Dellen AD, Basson PA, et al. 1978. Observations on the pathology of canine microsporidiosis. *Onderstepoort J Vet Res* 45:75–92.
23. McInnes EF, Stewart CG. 1991. The pathology of subclinical infection of *Encephalitozoon cuniculi* in canine dams producing pups with overt encephalitozoonosis. *J S Afr Vet Assoc* 62:51–54.
24. Mertens RB, Didier ES, Fishbein MC, et al. 1997. Disseminated *Encephalitozoon cuniculi* microsporidiosis: infection of the brain, heart, kidneys, trachea, adrenals, urinary bladder, spleen, and lymph nodes in an AIDS patient. *Mod Pathol* 10:68–77.
25. Schmidt EC, Shadduck JA. 1983. Murine encephalitozoonosis model for studying the host-parasite relationship of a chronic infection. *Infect Immun* 40:936–942.
26. Schwartz DA, Visvesvara GS, Diesenhouse MC, et al. 1993. Pathologic features and immunofluorescent antibody demonstration of ocular mi-

crosporidiosis (*Encephalitozoon hellem*) in seven patients with acquired immunodeficiency syndrome. *Am J Ophthalmol* 115:285–292.
27. Stewart CG, Collett MG, Snyman H. 1986. The immune response in a dog to *Encephalitozoon cuniculi* infection. *Onderstepoort J Vet Res* 53:35–37.
28. Stewart CG, Reyers F, Snyman H. 1988. The relationship between primary renal disease in dogs and antibodies to *Encephalitozoon cuniculi. J S Afr Vet Assoc* 59:19–21.
29. Stewart CG, van Dellen AF, Botha WS. 1979. Canine encephalitozoonosis in kennels and the isolation of *Encephalitozoon* in tissue culture. *J S Afr Vet Assoc* 50:165–168.
30. Szabo JR, Pang V, Shadduck JA. 1990. Encephalitozoonosis, p 786–791. *In* Greene CE (ed), Infectious diseases of the dog and cat. WB Saunders Co, Philadelphia, PA.
31. Szabo JR, Shadduck JA. 1987. Experimental encephalitozoonosis in neonatal dogs. *Vet Pathol* 24:99–108.
32. Van Dellen AF, Botha WS, Boomker J, et al. 1978. Light and electron microscopical studies on canine encephalitozoonosis: cerebral vasculitis. *Onderstepoort J Vet Res* 45:165–186.
33. Van Dellen AF, Stewart CG, Botha WS. 1989. Studies of *Encephalitozoonosis* in vervet monkeys *(Cercopithecus pygerythrus)* orally inoculated with spores of *Encephalitozoon cuniculi* isolated from dogs (*Canis familiaris*). *Onderstepoort J Vet Res* 56:1–22.
34. Van Gool T, Snijders F, Reiss P, et al. 1993. Diagnosis of intestinal and disseminated microsporidial infections in patients with HIV by a new rapid fluorescence technique. *J Clin Pathol* 46:694–699.
34a. Van Gool T, Vetter JCM, Weinmayr B, et al. 1997. High seroprevalence of *Encephalitozoon* species in immunocompetent subjects. *J Infect Dis* 175:1020–1024.
35. Vavra J, Chalupsky J. 1982. Fluorescence staining of microsporidian spores with the brightener Calcofluor White M2R. *J Protozool* 29(Suppl):503.
36. Visvesvara GS, Leitch GJ, da Silva AJ, et al. 1994. Polyclonal and monoclonal antibody and PCR-amplified small-subunit rRNA identification of a microsporidian, *Encephalitozoon hellem*, isolated from an AIDS patient with disseminated infection. *J Clin Microbiol* 32:2760–2768.
37. Vossbrinck CR, Baker M, Didier ES, et al. 1992. rDNA sequences of *Encephalitozoon hellem* and *Encephalitozoon cuniculi*: species identification and phylogenetic construction. *J Eukaryot Microbiol* 40(3):354–362.
38. Weber R, Bryan RT, Owen RL, et al. 1992. Improved light-microscopical detection of microsporidia spores in stool and duodenal aspirates. *N Engl J Med* 326:161–166.
39. Weiss LM, Cali A, Levee E, et al. 1992. Diagnosis of *Encephalitozoon cuniculi* infection by western blot and the use of cross-reactive antigens for the possible detection of microsporidiosis in humans. *Am J Trop Med Hyg* 47:456–462.
40. Weiss LM, Zhu X, Cali A, et al. 1994. Utility of microsporidian rRNA in diagnosis and phylogeny: a review. *Folia Parasitol* 41:81–90.
41. Zhu X, Wittner M, Tanowitz HB, et al. 1993. Small subunit rRNA sequence of *Enterocytozoon bieneusi* and its potential diagnostic role with use of the polymerase chain reaction. *J Infect Dis* 168:1570–1575.
42. Zierdt CH, Gill VJ, Zierdt WS. 1993. Detection of microsporidian spores in clinical samples by indirect fluorescent antibody assay using whole-cell antisera to *Encephalitozoon cuniculi* and *Encephalitozoon hellem*. *J Clin Microbiol* 31:3071–3074.

Chapter **76**

Cytauxzoonosis

Ann B. Kier and Craig E. Greene

ETIOLOGY AND EPIDEMIOLOGY

Cytauxzoon felis causes a usually fatal tick-borne blood protozoal disease of domestic cats *(Felis domesticus)* and exotic Felidae from several south central and southeastern states in the United States. The natural reservoir host appears to be the North American bobcat *(Lynx rufus)*. Fatal cytauxzoonosis was reported in a captive-reared white tiger *(Panthera tigris)* at a private breeding facility in northern Florida.[8] Florida panthers *(Felis concolor coryi)* and a Texas cougar *(Felis concolor)* at this facility were also suspected to be infected. The organism has previously been recognized in the erythrocytes of cheetahs *(Acinonyx jubatus)*.[12] Iatrogenic transmission from a Florida panther to a domestic cat has been reported.[3] Cytauxzoonosis, caused by similar organisms as evaluated by light microscopy, was first described in Africa, affecting ungulates. EM of a natural, fatal case of African cytauxzoonosis in a tsessebe calf *(Damaliscus lunatus)* reported the size and appearance similar to those described for *C. felis*.[11]

Cytauxzoon has been classified in the order Piroplasmida and family Theileriidae. This family has both an erythrocytic and a leukocytic, or tissue, phase. In the case of *C. felis*, the tissue phase consists of large schizonts that develop within macrophages, whereas *Theileria*, a more familiar genus of this family, has its exoerythrocytic phase primarily within lymphocytes. The Babesiidae, a related family, is characterized by having only or primarily an erythrocytic (piriform) phase in the mammalian host, that is indistinguishable from the erythrocytic form in *Cytauxzoon*. Although no serologic cross-reactivity has been reported between *C. felis* and the South African parasites *T. taurotragi* and *B. felis*, RNA gene sequence analysis links *C. felis*, *B. equi*, and *B. rodhaini* to both the theilerias and babesias, with some suggestion that these three organisms be reclassified within a separate family.[1, 5]

In the life cycle of *C. felis*, schizonts develop primarily within mononuclear phagocytes, first as indistinct vesicular structures within the cytoplasm of infected cells and later as large, distinct, nucleated schizonts that actively undergo division by schizogony and binary fission. The phagocytes line the lumens of the veins within almost every organ and become huge and numerous, often occluding the vessel like a thrombus. Multiplication of schizonts within host cells is observed ultrastructurally to be true schizogony, without host cell division. Later in the course of the disease, schizonts develop buds (merozoites) that separate and eventually fill the entire host cell. The host cell probably ruptures, releasing the merozoites into the blood or tissue fluid. Merozoites appear in macrophages 1 to 3 days before they are observed in erythrocytes. These organisms, which then invade uninfected erythrocytes, produce late-stage parasitemias that are detected on examination of blood films, usually 1 to 3 days before death.[13]

The apparently sporadic occurrence, short course of illness, and usually fatal nature of the disease indicate that the domestic cat is likely an incidental dead-end host. However, at least two cats with naturally occurring cases and two experimentally inoculated, untreated cats have survived.[9, 16, 18] Blood from naturally parasitemic bobcats was inoculated into the two domestic cats, causing persistent asymptomatic erythroparasitemias. In contrast, bobcats usually develop a nonfatal form of the disease and serve as potential carriers. Infection of erythrocytes as high as 60% in clinically healthy bobcats has been reported. However, transmission of one isolate in an experimentally inoculated domestic cat back to a bobcat was fatal.[14]

Ticks likely are the natural vector for *Cytauxzoon*, because most cases have been associated with the presence of ticks on the hosts. Tick *(Dermacentor variabilis)* transmission from wild-caught, splenectomized bobcats with parasitemia to two splenectomized domestic cats resulted in the fatal form of the disease. Subinoculation of blood from bobcats to cats appeared to transmit only the erythrocytic piroplasm stage.[2] The fatal form of the disease with extraerythrocytic stages develops only, or primarily, after tick transmission of the organism or inoculation of tissues from fatally infected cats. In the white tiger that developed naturally occurring fatal disease in Florida, two female Lone Star ticks *(Amblyomma americanum)* were present on the inguinal skin.[8]

PATHOGENESIS

Rapid multiplication of the tissue phase of the parasite may cause mechanical obstruction of blood flow, especially through the lungs. By-products of tissue parasites may be toxic, pyrogenic, and vasoactive, whereas the blood phase may induce destruction and phagocytosis of erythrocytes. Disseminated intravascular coagulation (DIC) has been a complication based on laboratory findings in naturally infected cats.[8, 9] Infected cats appear to die from a shocklike state.

CLINICAL FINDINGS

In the naturally occurring disease, affected cats develop nonspecific clinical signs that lead to a rapid course of illness and death, usually in fewer than 5 days. Most cats are presented from May through September, and geographic clusters of infection may be observed. Access to an outdoor, wooded environment or tick exposure is typically noted. Anorexia, dyspnea, lethargy, dark urine, dehydration, depression, icterus and pallor, anemic heart murmur, capillary refill time greater than 2 seconds, and fever (39.4–41.6°C [103–107°F]) have been observed. Hypothermia, recumbency, and coma are clinical findings in terminally ill cats.

Clinical signs in experimentally induced cytauxzoonosis have been similar to those in naturally occurring cases. Incubation periods have varied from 5 to 20 days, probably attributable to type and dose of inoculum, method of cryopreservation, and individual cat response. After a febrile period (39.9–40.1°C [103.8–104.2°F]), the temperature may become subnormal, and the cat may have difficulty breathing. Parasitized erythrocytes are observed late in the disease, during the febrile episode. Cats usually die 2 or 3 days after the temperature peak, and the entire course of clinical illness usually takes less than a week.

Normocytic normochromic anemia; variable leukocyte counts but often leukopenia; thrombocytopenia; high serum concentrations of total bilirubin and glucose; low serum concentrations of albumin, cholesterol, and potassium; high serum glucose and alanine aminotransferase activity; and bilirubinuria are common abnormalities in clinical cases.[10] The percentage of parasitized erythrocytes during illness ranges from 0.5% to 4%. The number of nucleated erythrocytes may increase slightly. Although blood urea nitrogen and ammonia concentrations and hepatic enzyme activities may be elevated in febrile or comatose animals, they may not be elevated earlier in the course of disease. Along with thrombocytopenia; prolonged activated coagulation, activated partial thromboplastin time, and prothrombin time tests; and increased fibrin split products will be present in cats with DIC.[8, 9]

DIAGNOSIS

Cytauxzoonosis should be considered in the differential diagnosis when a cat that is allowed access to tick-infested wooded areas becomes depressed and develops high temperature and possibly anemia and jaundice. Diagnosis is made by demonstrating the erythrocyte phase (piroplasms) in Wright's- or Giemsa-stained thin blood films. The piroplasms within erythrocytes appear as round "signet ring"–shaped bodies, 1 to 1.5 μm in diameter; bipolar oval "safety-pin" forms, 1 × 2 μm; tetrad forms; or anaplasmoid round "dots," less than 0.5 μm in diameter (Fig. 76–1). All forms may occur in a single blood film. The cytoplasm of the piroplasm stains light blue and the nucleus dark red or purple. The number of parasitized cells varies from cat to cat and with the stage of the disease. A single cell usually contains only one parasite, but pairs and tetrads (Maltese crosses) are observed occasionally. The erythrocytic stage of *Cytauxzoon* may appear similar to the ring form of *Haemobartonella* and to piriforms of *Babesia*. If the parasitemia is low, the schizogenous tissue phase is usually found in Wright's- or Giemsa-stained aspirates or impression smears of bone marrow, spleen, or lymph node.[7] Phagocytes containing tissue phase schizonts are sometimes found on the feathered edge of a peripheral blood smear.

In cats that die, histologic confirmation should be made from standard formalin-fixed tissues (lung, lymph node, spleen, liver, heart, brain) that are sent to a veterinary pathology laboratory for parasite evaluation, because haemobartonellosis and babesiosis do not have a tissue stage. A direct FA test for the detection of the tissue phase[17] and a microfluorometric immunoassay system for the detection of the se-

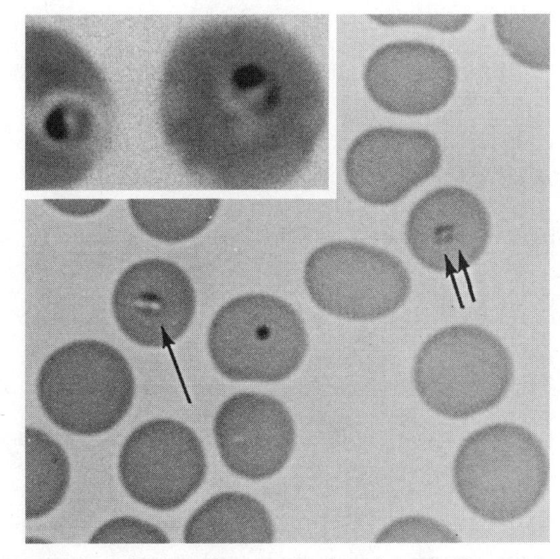

Figure 76–1. Feline erythrocytes infected with *Cytauxzoon* piroplasms: ring *(single arrow)* and dividing forms *(double arrows)*. The Howell-Jolly body is included for comparison of size and structure (Giemsa-Triton stain, × 1000). *Inset*, Enlarged view of ring forms in parasitized erythrocytes.

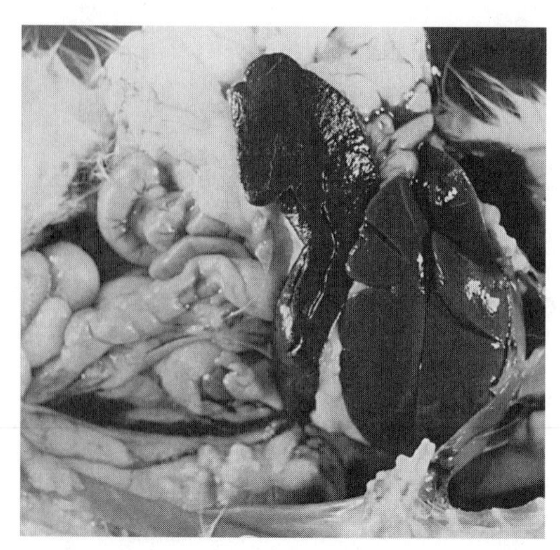

Figure 76–2. Gross lesions in a cat experimentally infected with *C. felis* include a greatly enlarged spleen and a slightly enlarged liver with rounded edges and distended veins.

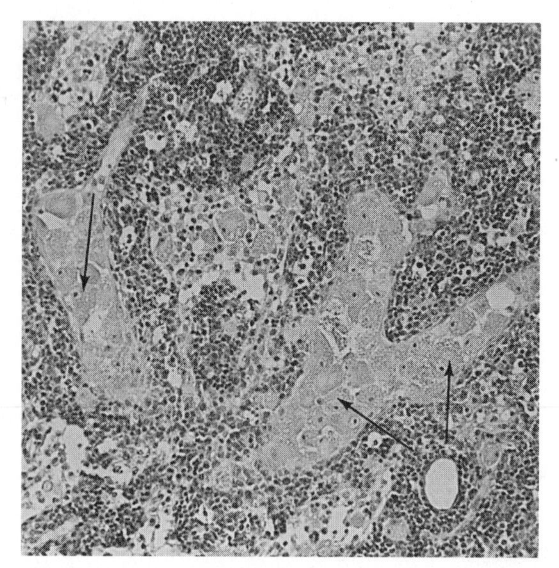

Figure 76–3. Numerous infected mononuclear phagocytes filling the lumina and lining the walls of veins *(arrows)* within a lymph node from a cat experimentally infected with *C. felis* (H and E, × 400).

rum antibody to *C. felis*[4] have been developed; however, neither is commercially available.

PATHOLOGIC FINDINGS

Gross findings in domestic cats include dehydration; pallor; icterus; hydropericardium; hydrothorax; enlarged, edematous, and hemorrhagic lymph nodes; accentuated hepatic lobular pattern; intra-abdominal venous distention; splenomegaly; and petechial and ecchymotic hemorrhages on the serosal surfaces of abdominal organs and lungs. The lungs are frequently congested and edematous, often with petechiae throughout (Fig. 76–2).

The characteristic lesion on histologic examination of feline cytauxzoonosis is the accumulation of large numbers of parasitized mononuclear phagocytes containing schizonts in various stages of development. These cells are particularly prevalent within the lumens of veins of the lungs, liver, lymph nodes, and spleen, making these vessels appear partially or completely occluded (Fig. 76–3). Minimal inflammatory reaction is present in affected tissues. Spleen and lymph node should be used for tissue impression films, which should be stained with Wright's or Giemsa stain.

THERAPY

Preliminary attempts to treat cats that have either naturally or experimentally induced disease have had very limited success. In approximately 500 naturally and experimentally infected cats known to us, 8 cats have recovered, and of these, 4 were experimentally infected cats that appeared to be immune to reinfection. A number of cats have been treated, but even with the most effective drugs, the mortality rate approaches 50%. Of the recovered cats, supportive fluid therapy is essential. Parvaquone, sodium thiacetarsamide, buparvaquone, and tetracycline do not appear to be effective. One cat treated with fluids, enrofloxacin, and tetracycline survived with a reduction and final elimination of blood parasites.[18] Most success in treatment has been with the carbanilide compounds diminazene or imidocarb. One cat with DIC that was treated with fluids, SC heparin, enrofloxacin, and diminazene aceturate (see Drug Formulary, Appendix 8), had an immediate improvement in its clinical state and elimination of the parasitemia by 4 days after treatment was instituted.[9] Morphologic examination of the organisms in blood smears showed a degenerating appearance within 48 hours after the drug therapy was instituted. Two sequential injections of diminazene are most efficacious.[9] Although enrofloxacin was administered in treating both of these surviving cats, its efficacy on protozoa has not been determined. Two other affected housemate cats and a cat from a different household were successfully treated with diminazene alone.[9] Furthermore, a much larger number (approximately 100) of cats has been treated successfully (50% survival) with imidocarb dipropionate alone (see Drug Formulary, Appendix 8).[6] In addition to fluid therapy, imidocarb is given in two injections with a 2-week interval. Concurrent first-generation cephalosporins have been given to cats that are severely

Table 76–1. Therapy for Cytauxzoonosis[a]

DRUG	DOSE[b] (mg/kg)	ROUTE	INTERVAL[c] (HOURS)	DURATION (DAYS)
Heparin	100–150 U/kg	SC	8	As needed
Enrofloxacin[d]	5.0 mg/kg	PO, SC	8–12	7–10
Imidocarb dipropionate	5.0 mg/kg	IM	14 days	14[e]
Diminazene aceturate	2.0 mg/kg	IM	7 days	7[e]

[a]See Drug Formulary, Appendix 8, for specific information on each drug.
[b]Dose per administration at specified interval.
[c]Interval in hours unless otherwise specified.
[d]The efficacy of this drug alone is uncertain. Use of imidocarb or diminazene is recommended instead or in combination.
[e]Two injections will be given at the specified interval with this regimen.

leukopenic for the first 7 to 10 days.[6] Recommended dosages for these drugs are listed in Table 76–1.

PREVENTION

A conscientiously applied ectoparasite control program and confinement indoors during tick season could be beneficial in preventing cytauxzoonosis, because all naturally occurring cases known to us have involved cats that were free to roam in wooded, tick-infested areas.

References

1. Allsopp MTEP, Cavalier-Smith T, DeWall DT, et al. 1994. Phylogeny and evolution of the piroplasms. *Parasitology* 108(2):147–152.
2. Blouin EF, Kocan AA, Glen BL, et al. 1984. Transmission of *Cytauxzoon felis* (Kier, 1979) from bobcats, *Felis rufus* (Schreber), to domestic cats by *Dermacentor variabilis* (Say). *J Wildl Dis* 20:241–242.
3. Butt MT, Bowman D, Barr MC, et al. 1991. Iatrogenic transmission of *Cytauxzoon felis* from a Florida panther (*Felis concolor coryi*) to a domestic cat. *J Wildl Dis* 27(2):342–347.
4. Cowell RL, Fox JC, Panciera RJ, et al. 1988. Detection of anticytauxzoon antibodies in cats infected with a *Cytauxzoon* organism from bobcats. *Vet Parasitol* 28:43–52.
5. Escalante AA, Ayala FJ. 1995. Evolutionary origin of *Plasmodium* and other Apicomplexa based on rRNA genes. *Proc Natl Acad Sci U S A* 92:5793–5797.
6. Fly BR, Fly BA. 1997. Personal communication. Nolensville, TN.
7. Franks PT, Harvey JW, Shields RP, et al. 1988. Hematological findings in experimental feline cytauxzoonosis. *J Am Anim Hosp Assoc* 24:395–401.
8. Garner MM, Lung NP, Citino S, et al. 1996. Fatal cytauxzoonosis in a captive-reared white tiger (*Panthera tigris*). *Vet Pathol* 33:82–86.
9. Greene CE. 1996. Unpublished observations. University of Georgia, Athens, GA.
10. Hoover JP, Walker DB, Hedges JD. 1994. Cytauxzoonosis in cats: eight cases (1985–1992). *J Am Vet Med Assoc* 205(3):455–460.
11. Jardine JE. 1992. The pathology of cytauxzoonosis in a tsessebe (*Damaliscus lunatus*). *J S Afr Vet Assoc* 63(1):49–51.
12. Kier AB. 1990. Cytauxzoonosis, pp 792–795. *In* Greene CE (ed), Infectious diseases of the dog and cat. WB Saunders, Philadelphia, PA.
13. Kier AB, Wagner JE, Kinden DA. 1987. The pathology of experimental cytauxzoonosis. *J Comp Pathol* 97:415–432.
14. Kier AB, Wightman SF, Wagner JE. 1982. Interspecies transmission of *Cytauxzoon felis*. *Am J Vet Res* 43:102–105.
15. Kocan AA, Kocan KM, Blovin EF, et al. 1992. A redescription of schizogony of *Cytauxzoon felis* in the domestic cat. *Trop Vet Med Curr Issues Perspect* 653:161–167.
16. Motzel SL, Wagner JE. 1990. Treatment of experimentally induced cytauxzoonosis in cats with parvaquone and buparvaquone. *Vet Parasitol* 35:131–138.
17. Shindel N, Dardiri AH, Ferris DH. 1978. An indirect fluorescent antibody test for the detection of *Cytauxzoon*-like organisms in experimentally infected cats. *Can J Comp Med* 42:460–465.
18. Walker DB, Cowell RL. 1995. Survival of a domestic cat with naturally acquired cytauxzoonosis. *J Am Vet Med Assoc* 206(9):1363–1365.

Chapter 77

Babesiosis

Joseph Taboada

ETIOLOGY

Babesiosis is a disease of worldwide significance caused by tick-borne hematozoan organisms of the genus *Babesia* (Table 77–1).[29, 55, 58] *B. canis* and *B. gibsoni* are the two species capable of natural infection in the dog, whereas *B. felis*, *B. cati*, *B. herpailuri*, and *B. pantherae* have been reported in cats.[29, 58]

Dogs

B. canis is the more important of the two organisms that affect dogs. It is a large (2.4 μm × 5.0 μm), piriform-shaped organism that may occur singly or paired within erythrocytes (Fig. 77–1*A*). Its range is greater, covering most of southern Europe; Africa; Asia; and North, Central, and South America. Vector ticks include *R. sanguineus*, *Dermacentor reticulatus*, *D. marginatus*, and *H. leachi* in natural conditions and *D. andersoni* and *Hyalomma marginatum* in experimental ones.[13, 29] *B. gibsoni* is a small, pleomorphic (1.0 μm × 3.2 μm) organism usually observed singly within erythrocytes (Fig. 77–1*B*). It is found primarily in northern Africa and the southern parts of Asia but is endemic in the southwestern United States. It is sporadically noted in areas near military bases, where military working dogs that have been transported around the world are housed.[10] *B. gibsoni*'s potential geographic range correlates with that of the vector ticks, *Haemaphysalis bispinosa* and *R. sanguineus*.[29] The existence of a third species, *B. vogeli*, has been proposed, but it is probably a strain of *B. canis*.[63]

On the basis of serologic and cross-immunity studies as well as differences in pathogenicity and vectors, a trinomial nomenclature system for *B. canis* has been proposed.[63] *B. canis vogeli* is the proposed name for the strain that occurs in tropical and subtropical regions of most continents and is transmitted by the brown dog tick, *R. sanguineus*. It is the least pathogenic of the three strains and is the one found in the United States. *B. canis canis* is the name proposed for the strain in Europe and parts of Asia. It is intermediate in pathogenicity and is transmitted by ticks of the *Dermacentor* genus. *B. canis rossi* is the proposed name given to the highly pathogenic strain transmitted by *H. leachi* that is found in southern Africa.

Cats

Feline babesiosis has not been studied as extensively as the disease in dogs. *B. felis* is a highly pathogenic species found in southern Africa and the Sudan. *B. cati* is less pathogenic and found primarily in India. There have been no cases of feline babesiosis reported in the United States. *B. herpailuri*

Table 77–1. Common Babesias, Vectors, and Distribution

SPECIES	TYPICAL MORPHOLOGY	RECOGNIZED TICK VECTORS	GEOGRAPHIC DISTRIBUTION
Canine			
Babesia canis vogeli, Babesia canis canis, Babesia canis rossi	Large (2.4 × 5.0 μm), paired piriform bodies	*Rhipicephalus sanguineus, Dermacentor reticulatus, Haemaphysalis leachi, Hyaloma plumbeum* (?)	Africa, Asia, Australia, Europe, and Central, South, and North America
Babesia gibsoni	Small (1.0 × 3.2 μm), usually singular annular bodies	*Rhipicephalus sanguineus, Haemaphysalis bispinosa*	Predominantly Far East, Asia Less important: United States, southern Europe
Feline			
Babesia felis	Small (0.9 × 0.7 μm), single or paired annular bodies	Unknown	Africa, southern Asia
Babesia herpailuri	Large (2.7 × 2.2 μm), single or paired piriform bodies	Unknown	Africa
Babesia cati	Small (1.0 × 2.5 μm), single or paired annular bodies	Unknown	India
Human[a]			
Babesia microti	Small, pleomorphic bodies	*Ixodes scapularis (dammini), Ixodes ricinus, Ixodes trianguliceps*	North America: northeastern, Great Lakes region, Europe (rare)
Babesia divergens	Small, pleomorphic bodies	*Ixodes ricinus*	Northern Europe, Missouri?[16]
Babesia bovis	Large, piriform bodies	*Boophilus* spp.	Southern Europe
Babesia spp. (*B. gibsoni*–like, WA-1)	Ring forms and tetrads	*Dermacentor*?	Washington State,[49] northern California

[a]Humans are thought to be accidental hosts for babesias of other species: *Babesia microti* (rodent); *Babesia divergens, Babesia bovis* (cattle); *Babesia equi* (horse).
Modified from Taboada J, Merchant SR. *Vet Clin North Am Small Anim Pract* 21:103–123, 1991. Used with permission.

and *B. pantherae* are large organisms of wild Felidae in Africa that have been transmitted experimentally to the domestic cat.[29]

EPIDEMIOLOGY

In the United States, canine babesiosis occurs most commonly along the Gulf Coast and in the south, central, and southwestern states. Arkansas, Arizona, Florida, and Oklahoma seem to be states where cases are most common. Reported prevalence has ranged from 3.8% to 59%.[57] The seroprevalence is higher in adult dogs than in dogs younger than 1 year.[7] In a serosurvey of dogs in Florida, 46% of 393 greyhounds were seropositive. The prevalence within kennels ranged from 17% to 100%; the lower prevalence was noted in kennels where more intensive tick control was performed. None of 50 adult non-greyhound pet dogs surveyed were seropositive, implicating both environment and breed susceptibility as factors in determining seroprevalence in endemic areas.[57] Outbreaks may occur and are often localized to a relatively small area or to a kennel. Veterinarians in one practice may see affected dogs commonly, while neighboring practices in the same area may not see any at all.[55]

Although the seroprevalence is highest in adult dogs, dogs younger than 1 year are most susceptible to infection.[22] Dogs younger than 2 months may be protected by maternally derived antibody. Age may be a less significant factor in the pathogenesis of clinical disease caused by *B. gibsoni* and the more virulent strains of *B. canis*, however.

PATHOGENESIS

Transmission of babesias is by the bite of infected ixodid ticks. The adult female tick is most important in transmission, but all stages of the tick are likely to be infected.[13] Once in the host, *Babesia* spp. attach to the erythrocyte membrane and are engulfed by endocytosis (Fig. 77–2).[19] Once in the erythrocyte, the red blood cell membrane that surrounds the

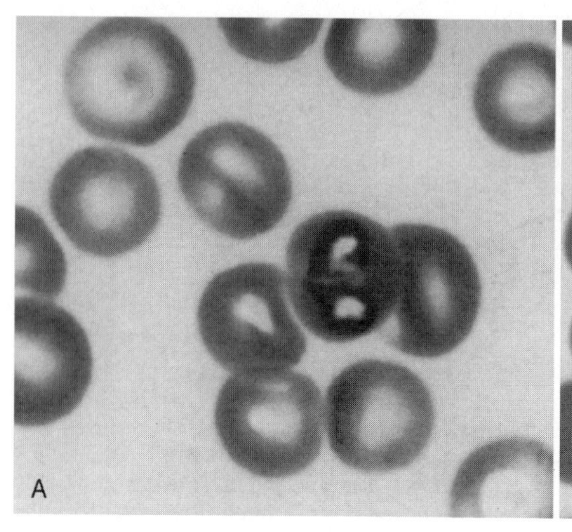

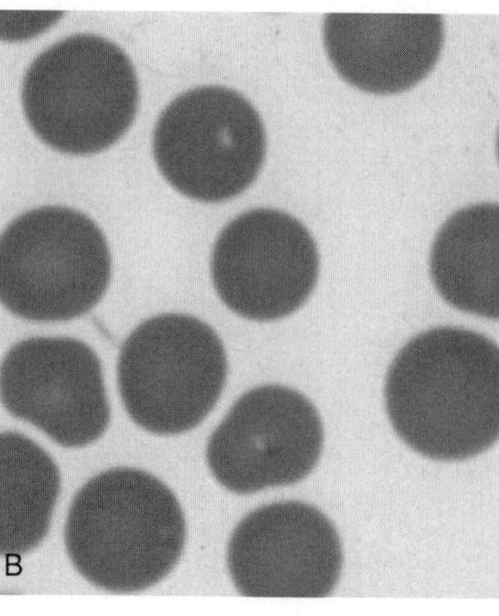

Figure 77–1. *A,* A pair of large piriform-shaped merozoites of *Babesia canis* within an erythrocyte from a 3-week-old Neopolitan mastiff puppy with acute babesiosis. From Taboada J: *In* Bonagura J (ed): Current Veterinary Therapy XII. WB Saunders, 1995, p 317. Reprinted with permission. *B,* Individual merozoites of *B. gibsoni* in two erythrocytes from a military dog. (Courtesy of Dr. George Moore, U.S. Army.)

parasite disintegrates, and all subsequent stages are in direct contact with the host cell cytoplasm. *Babesia* multiply within the erythrocytes by repeated binary fission, resulting in merozoites. As many as 16 merozoites of *B. canis* may be seen in a single red blood cell, but they most commonly occur singly or paired. Ticks are infected by merozoites during feeding. A complex life cycle involving both transtadial and transovarial transmission ensues that results in sporozoite formation in cells of the tick's salivary glands.[13, 19] When infected ticks feed, the sporozoites are passed with saliva into the circulation of the host. The tick must feed a minimum of 2 to 3 days for transmission of *B. canis* to occur.[36] After infection, there is usually a significant host immune response generated. The immune system does not appear able to completely clear infection, and recovered animals are usually chronic carriers of the parasite. Poor humoral immune response is common in pups younger than 8 months.

Transplacental transmission probably occurs and may result in fading puppies. I have diagnosed *B. canis* infection in a 36-hour-old greyhound pup that was born to a seropositive bitch. The pup's packed cell volume (PCV) was decreased compared with its four littermates.[56]

The pathogenicity of *Babesia* organisms is determined primarily by the species and strain involved.[51, 63, 71] Host factors, such as the age of the host and the immunologic response generated against the parasite or vector tick, are also important.

Two syndromes, one characterized by hemolytic anemia and the other by hypotensive shock and/or multiple-organ dysfunction, account for most of the clinical signs observed in animals with babesiosis (Fig. 77–3).[21, 22] Parasitemia results in increased osmotic fragility of erythrocytes, hemolysis (often of an intravascular nature), and subsequent anemia.[34] However, the severity of anemia is not proportional to the low degree of parasitemia usually observed. Direct parasitic damage contributes to the anemia. However, induction of serum hemolytic factors, increased erythrophagocytic activity of macrophages, and secondary immune system–induced damage after formation of antierythrocyte membrane antibodies are also important to the pathogenesis.[3–5, 42, 43, 46, 47] Oxidative stress is another possible reason for damage to erythrocytes that results in increased susceptibility to phagocytosis.[44] Increased urinary methemoglobinemia has been found in dogs with naturally occurring *B. canis* infections.[32] Lipid peroxidation occurring during babesiosis infection increases rigidity of both parasitized and nonparasitized erythrocytes and slows their passage through capillary beds. Soluble parasite proteases activate the kallikrein system and induce fibrinogen-like protein (FLP) formation. These FLPs increase erythrocyte "stickiness," leading to further sludging of erythrocytes in the capillaries. Vascular stasis from sludging of parasitized cells within capillary beds is thought to contribute to the acute anemia as well as to many of the other potential clinical signs. The most severe sludging appears to occur in the CNS and muscles.[71] Rhabdomyolysis and acute renal failure have been complications of babesiosis.[23, 33]

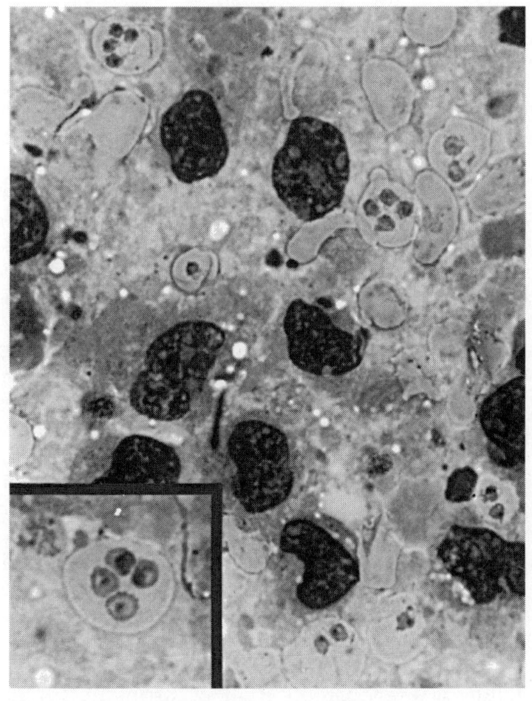

Figure 77–2. Impression smear of the spleen obtained at necropsy from a naturally infected dog. Numerous erythrocytes contain one or more *B. canis* organisms (Wright's-Giemsa stain, × 1100). (Courtesy of Peter MacWilliams, DVM, PhD, and Charles W. Qualls, Jr, DVM, PhD.)

Disseminated intravascular coagulation (DIC) can be a devastating complication of canine babesiosis. *Babesia* proteases may induce increases in plasma kallikrein levels, which can activate the intrinsic cascade at factor XII. Thrombocytopenia is common, especially in dogs infected with *B. gibsoni*. This finding can be a result of DIC but is also likely a result of immune-mediated platelet destruction. Membranoproliferative glomerulonephritis is seen in some infected dogs and may have an immune-mediated pathogenesis.

Tissue hypoxia is an important contributor to many of the clinical signs caused by the most pathogenic *Babesia* strains. Causes of hypoxia include anemia, shock, vascular stasis, excessive endogenous production of carbon monoxide, parasitic damage to hemoglobin, and decreased ability of hemoglobin from *Babesia*-infected dogs to off-load oxygen.[22, 32, 50–61, 71] The resultant tissue damage probably results in the release of cytokines, which would be expected to support widespread inflammation and further damage to multiple-organ systems.[22] Hypoxia appears to be more important than hemoglobinuria in producing damage to the kidneys of experimentally infected dogs.[33]

CLINICAL FINDINGS

Dogs

Babesiosis may follow hyperacute, acute, chronic, or subclinical courses (Table 77–2). Most infected dogs in the United States are subclinical carriers.[57] Acute disease characterized by fever, lethargy, and acute anemia is the most common clinical syndrome, whereas the hyperacute presentation characterized by shock and extensive tissue damage is rare.[10, 12] Acute signs of infection are typical of *B. gibsoni* and the more virulent strains of *B. canis*.[9, 10] Chronic manifestations of *B. canis* infection are poorly characterized and have not been reported in the United States.[22]

The hyperacute presentation, although uncommon, can have devastating consequences. It is characterized by hypotensive shock, hypoxia, extensive tissue damage, and vascular stasis. A high percentage of dogs with this form of babesiosis die despite therapy. In the United States, this form of the disease is most common in puppies and has been reported in one adult Doberman pinscher after surgical stress and blood transfusion from an infected greyhound blood donor.[12] Shock, coma, or death after less than a 1-day history of anorexia, lethargy, and hematuria may be seen. Dogs with hyperacute babesiosis are usually heavily parasitized and have a history of heavy tick infestation.

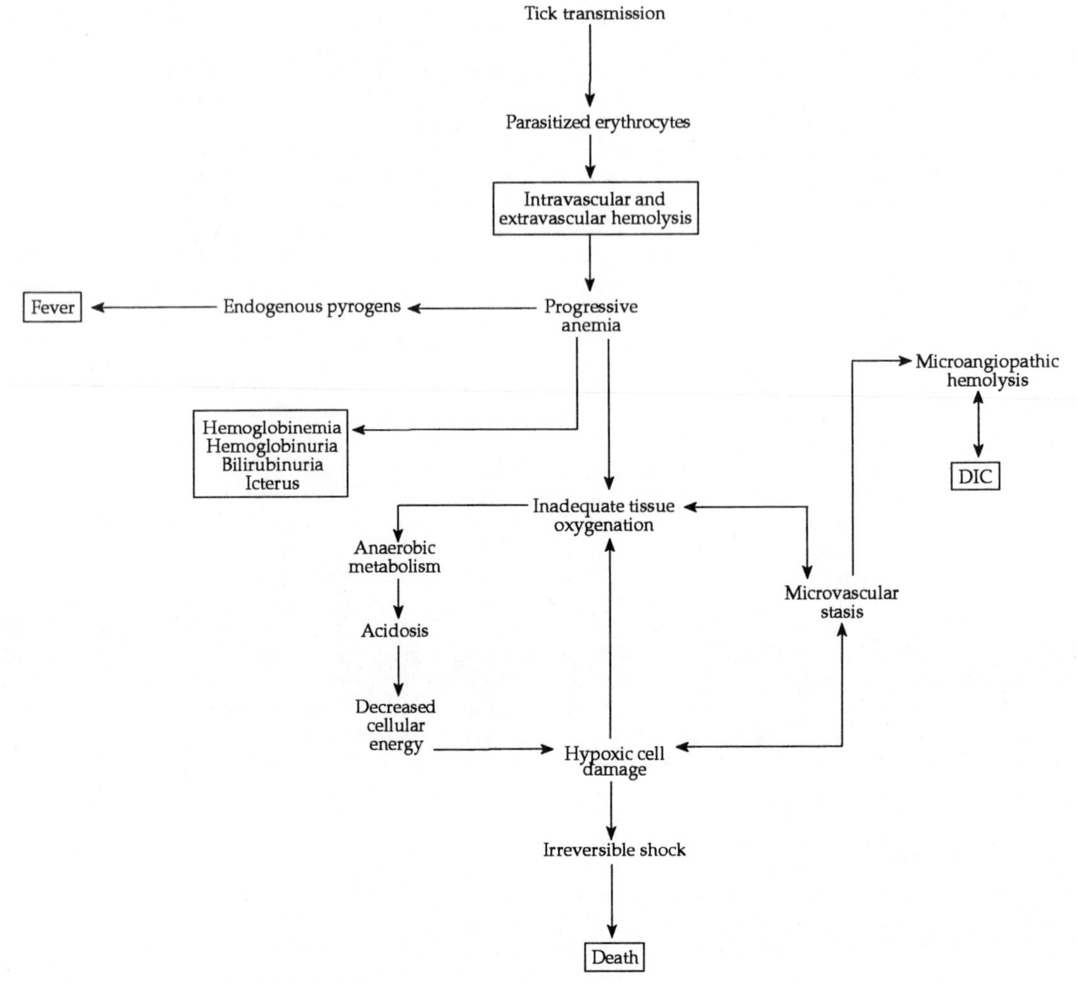

Figure 77–3. Proposed pathogenesis of canine babesiosis.

Acute disease is characterized by anorexia, hemolytic anemia, thrombocytopenia, lymphadenomegaly, and splenomegaly.[2, 20, 22] Anorexia, lethargy, fever, and vomiting are also common. Fatalities may occur, especially in puppies or *B. gibsoni*–infected adults, but most animals with acute disease recover with treatment. Hematuria and icterus may be noted, especially in *B. canis*–infected dogs. The acute presentation is most typical of *B. gibsoni* infections encountered in Asia and the southwestern United States and *B. canis* infections encountered in Africa, Australia, and southern Europe. Immune-mediated hemolytic anemia and systemic lupus erythematosus are the primary diseases that must be differentiated from this form of babesiosis.

A paradoxic phenomenon of intravascular hemolysis with hemoconcentration despite normal plasma proteins is occasionally seen in dogs infected with severely pathogenic strains of *B. canis*. This finding has been termed "red biliary" and is typified by mucous membrane congestion and grossly visible hemoglobinemia and/or hemoglobinuria.[22] The hemoconcentration is characterized by a slightly increased PCV and has been associated with neurologic signs, acute renal failure, DIC, and pulmonary edema.

Chronic infections are primarily reported in *B. canis*–infected dogs in southern Africa and are characterized by intermittent fever, decreased appetite, and marked loss of body condition. The chronic form of the disease may occur in *B. gibsoni*–infected dogs in the United States but has not been well documented after *B. canis* infection.[10]

A wide variety of "atypical signs" and complications of *Babesia* infection have been reported.[22] These signs are less common than the hyperacute and acute presentations described previously. Unfortunately, it is difficult to state whether many of the atypical signs are induced by *Babesia* alone or by concurrent disease. Respiratory manifestations are usually self-limiting and range from mild upper respiratory tract signs to dyspnea. GI signs may include vomiting, constipation, diarrhea, and ulcerative stomatitis. Ascites and edema, especially periorbital, peripheral limb, and scrotal edema, may be seen. Pulmonary edema is often a fatal complication that may be caused by increased capillary permeability similar to that in adult respiratory distress syndrome.[8, 17, 22] Rarely, hemorrhages, varying from petechiae to ecchymotic patches, occur secondary to thrombocytopenia and DIC. Musculoskeletal manifestations include a *Babesia*-associated masticatory myositis, joint swelling, and back pain. With severe rhabdomyolysis, dogs show muscle discomfort, dark-colored urine, muscle tremors, and abnormal gait.[23] Acute renal failure is a rare complication, occurring in less than 3% of cases in one report.[22, 33] CNS manifestations are referred to as "cerebral babesiosis."[21] Signs may include seizures, weak-

Table 77–2. Clinical Findings in Dogs with Babesiosis

SPECTRUM	DURATION
Nonspecific Clinical Signs	**Hyperacute Presentation**
Anorexia	Hypothermia
Lethargy	Shock
Weakness	Coma
Pyrexia	Disseminated intravascular coagulation
Weight loss	Metabolic acidosis
	Death
Atypical Clinical Signs	**Acute Presentation**
Ascites	Hemolytic anemia
Edema	Icterus
Constipation	Splenomegaly
Diarrhea	Lymphadenopathy
Ulcerative stomatitis	Vomiting
Hemorrhage	
Congested mucous membranes	**Chronic Presentation**
Polycythemia	
Ocular and nasal discharge	Intermittent pyrexia
Respiratory distress	Partial anorexia
Masticatory myositis	Loss of body condition
Temporomandibular joint pain	Lymphadenopathy
Back pain	
Central nervous system signs	
Seizures	
Ataxia	
Paresis	

Modified from Taboada J. *In* Bonagura JD (ed), Kirk's current veterinary therapy: XII. Small animal practice. WB Saunders, 1995. Used with permission.

ness, ataxia, and vestibular or cerebellar signs. The neurologic manifestations are thought to be caused by sludging of parasitized erythrocytes within capillaries of the CNS with subsequent tissue hypoxia (Fig. 77–4). Many of the other atypical manifestations may have a similar cause. Dual infections with *Babesia* spp. and *Ehrlichia canis* may contribute to the diversity of clinical signs described, because the vector ticks for both *E. canis* and *B. canis* are the same in some areas and both organisms may be present in the same tick population.

Subclinically infected dogs are common in certain populations. Greyhounds in the United States have a very high seroprevalence, but adult dogs rarely show clinical signs. Parasites will rarely be found on blood smears from asymptomatic carriers, making identification of this group of dogs difficult without performing serologic screening tests. The primary importance of this group of dogs may be in their role as a potential source of infection to susceptible puppies in breeding colonies or as a source of infection through blood transfusion.[12, 57] Babesiosis can be a significant and underdiagnosed cause of morbidity and mortality of puppies from breeding colonies located in endemic areas. The seroprevalence among adults in affected kennels will often reveal a seroprevalence of over 75% and can serve as a serologic marker for the disease. This finding is compared with seroprevalences typically less than 20% in well-managed kennels from endemic areas where anemic puppies are less likely to be encountered.[57] Most subclinical carriers will never show clinical signs of babesiosis; however, they may rarely show signs when subjected to stress or to treatment with glucocorticoids.[9, 37]

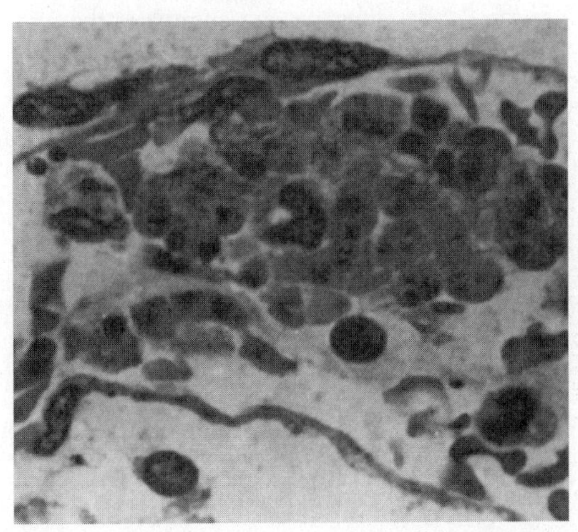

Figure 77–4. Cerebral vessel filled with numerous erythrocytes parasitized by *B. canis* (H and E, × 1200). (Courtesy of Dr. Charles W. Qualls, Jr, Oklahoma State University, Stillwater, OK.)

Cats

Those with naturally occurring babesiosis usually are younger than 2 years and may show lethargy, anorexia, weakness, rough hair coat, or diarrhea. Fever and icterus are rarely observed. Chronic anemia can be severe and is the underlying reason for the clinical signs. Cats usually adapt to the anemia and may have only mild clinical signs until they experience the stress of a physical examination or diagnostic evaluation.

DIAGNOSIS

The primary differential diagnoses for acute uncomplicated babesiosis are immune-mediated hemolytic anemia, zinc or onion toxicity, clostridial septicemia, and GI hemorrhage mimicking a hemolytic anemia. The clinical pathologic changes are nonspecific; the primary hematologic abnormalities are anemia and thrombocytopenia.[2, 20, 38, 45] The prevalence of thrombocytopenia is higher than that in dogs with ehrlichiosis. A mild, normocytic, normochromic anemia is generally noted in the first few days PI, and the anemia then becomes macrocytic, hypochromic, and regenerative as the disease progresses. The reticulocytosis is proportional to the severity of the anemia. Uncommonly, a relative polycythemia with normal plasma protein concentration may be noted.[22] Leukocyte abnormalities are inconsistently observed but may include leukocytosis, neutrophilia, neutropenia, lymphocytosis, and eosinophilia.[20, 45] A leukemoid response similar to that in cases of immune-mediated hemolytic anemia is occasionally seen.[31] Autoagglutination of erythrocytes in saline was noted in 21% of 134 dogs with babesiosis in one study, and nearly 85% of infected dogs were positive on direct antiglobulin (Coombs') test in another, making it difficult to differentiate the disease from immune-mediated hemolytic anemia if organisms are not apparent.[22]

Serum chemistry values are usually normal. Hypokalemia may be found in severely affected animals but is probably nonspecific because of decreased potassium intake. Hyperkalemia and hypoglycemia were noted in severely affected animals in one study.[20] Serum proteins are typically normal, but hyperglobulinemia is found in some dogs with *B. canis* infection.[56] A study of dual infections with *B. canis* and *E. canis* showed that the prevalence of hyperglobulinemia was higher in dogs with dual infections than in dogs infected singly with either organism.[38] Azotemia and metabolic acidosis are common and appear to contribute to morbidity and mortality. Hyperbilirubinemia is a consistent finding during acute disease caused by *B. canis* but not that caused by *B. gibsoni*.[20, 68a] Liver enzyme activities may be increased during severe disease. Bilirubinuria, hemoglobinuria, proteinuria, and granular casts may be observed on urinalysis.

Cats infected with *B. felis* have similar but less severe clinicopathologic findings. The anemia is usually macrocytic; hyperbilirubinemia is common. Serum chemistry abnormalities are usually restricted to mild increases in liver enzyme activity.

The definitive diagnosis of babesiosis is dependent on demonstration of organisms within infected erythrocytes or on positive serology. *B. canis* are large piriform-shaped organisms, usually present singly or in pairs (see Fig. 77–1*A*), whereas smaller singular intracellular organisms are likely to be *B. gibsoni* (see Fig. 77–1*B*). Parasitemias are often low, especially in *B. canis*–infected dogs, making thorough examination of thin blood smears necessary. Blood collected from the peripheral capillary beds in the ear tip or nail bed may yield higher numbers of parasitized cells.[20] Erythrocytes adjacent to the buffy coat are also more likely to be infected. Occasionally, phagocytized organisms and erythrocyte fragments are seen in neutrophils. Although the organisms within erythrocytes may be numerous in some acutely infected animals, they are rarely evident in chronically infected or asymptomatic carriers. Evaluation of stained slides can be tedious and requires a significant time commitment on the part of the laboratory technician. Flow cytometric techniques correlate closely with conventional light microscopic techniques for identification of *Babesia*-parasitized erythrocytes and degree of reticulocytosis.[14, 62] In addition, the methods of concentrating and staining of buffy coat improve the sensitivity of parasite detection.[39]

Because of the difficulties in detecting *Babesia* parasites, especially in chronic carriers, immunodiagnostics are often essential to recognize infected hosts. Serodiagnostics have proved reliable as a method of indirect parasite detection in either patent or occult infections that have been present long enough for an immune response to be generated.[50, 69] For canine babesiosis, the indirect FA test is probably the most reliable and most commonly used test for detection of babesial antibody.[50] Although laboratory methods differ, generally titers greater than or equal to 80 to *B. canis* on a single sample are sufficient for diagnosis. A cut-off titer of 320 or greater has been determined for incriminating *B. gibsoni* infection.[72] Very young dogs or dogs seen early in the disease course may be serologically negative, however, making it necessary to evaluate convalescing serum in some cases.[7] Antibodies were not detected in 36% of dogs with *B. canis* parasitemia in one study.[7] Cross-reactivity between *B. canis* and *B. gibsoni* make parasite identification necessary to differentiate between the two species. This test is especially important in areas like the southwestern United States, where both species are endemic. ELISA and dot-ELISA techniques for antibody detection have been developed. These tests are most often utilized for seroepidemiologic studies rather than clinical diagnosis.[7, 50] Dogs infected with *B. gibsoni* may have false-positive serologic test results for *Toxoplasma gondii* and *Neospora caninum* as well as for *B. canis*.[72]

PATHOLOGIC FINDINGS

Pathologic findings include staining of tissues with hemoglobin or bilirubin, hepatosplenomegaly, lymphadenopathy, and dark-reddish kidneys.[64] Edema and hemorrhage, which may indicate vascular injury and poor tissue oxygenation in severely affected dogs, are often most severe in the lungs. Large numbers of parasitized erythrocytes may be noted in capillary beds, especially in the brain. Nonparasitized cells often line the endothelial surface with parasitized cells sludged in the lumen. Microthrombi of many tissues may be evident in animals exhibiting signs of DIC. Large numbers of parasitized cells are often evident in the spleen. Impression smears of the spleen may substantiate the diagnosis of babesiosis at necropsy (see Fig. 77–4). Nonspecific findings include erythroid hyperplasia in the bone marrow, extramedullary hematopoiesis of the liver and spleen, mononuclear phagocyte system hyperplasia, and centrolobular necrosis of the liver. Vasculitis, associated with multifocal deposits of IgM in inflamed arteries and renal glomeruli, has been observed in *B. gibsoni* infections.[70a] In chronic cases of canine babesiosis and cases of feline babesiosis, the only gross finding may be splenomegaly.

THERAPY

Dogs generally show clinical improvement within 24 hours of treatment with antibabesial drugs (Table 77–3).[28] The Drug Formulary, Appendix 8, should be consulted for further information on all drugs used. Unfortunately, of the most effective of the babesiacidal drugs, diminazene aceturate and phenamidine isethionate are not approved for use in the United States. Diminazene aceturate is the most commonly used drug worldwide.[27] It is an aromatic diamidine derivative in the same class of drugs as phenamidine isethionate and pentamidine isethionate. Diminazene aceturate is effective when given IM, although clearance of infection is inconsistent even at higher doses. *B. gibsoni* infections are less responsive to diminazene than *B. canis* infections. Dogs are more susceptible to the toxic effects of the drug than other species. Side effects include pain and swelling at the injection site, GI irritation, and neurologic manifestations. Phenamidine isethionate is available in many countries as a licensed drug for treatment of canine babesiosis. Pentamidine isethionate (Pentam 300, Abbott Labs, Abbott Park, IL) has been approved for use in the United States by the Food and Drug Administration as an orphan drug for treatment of *Pneumocystis* pneumonia in people. The drug has been effective against *B. canis* and *B. gibsoni*.[28] The drug has not been as extensively studied as the other diaminidines. Side effects include injection site pain, hypotension, tachycardia, and vomiting.

A carbanilide member of the diaminidine family, imidocarb dipropionate, is a very effective drug against *B. canis* with few side effects.[6, 28] It is available in the United States (see Drug Formulary, Appendix 8.) It is less effective against *B. gibsoni*. At the suggested dose (see Table 77–3), imidocarb eliminates the *Babesia* infection and eliminates the infectivity of ticks engorging on treated animals for up to 4 weeks after treatment. A single dose of 7.5 mg/kg or a single dose of 6 mg/kg the day following a dose of diminazene at 3.5 mg/kg has also been shown to clear infections.[48] Imidocarb is also effective against *E. canis* and is, therefore, the drug of choice in dual infections.[6] It has a protective prophylactic activity of up to 6 weeks after a single injection.[66] Side effects are uncommon and are thought to be related to an anticholinesterase effect of the drug. They include transient salivation, lacrimation, vomiting, diarrhea, muscle tremor, restlessness, tachycardia, and dyspnea.[1] An overdose of 10 times resulted in hepatic necrosis and death in one dog.[26]

Quinuronium sulfate has been effective in treatment of dogs with *B. canis* infection.[26a] Dogs showed clinical improvement within 24 to 48 hours of treatment.

Trypan blue (1% solution) is effective in treating dogs with mild to moderate signs of infection with *B. canis* (see Table 77–3).[24, 53] It has also been recommended for patients with severe infections because it lacks the anticholinergic properties of imidocarb and the CNS toxicity of the other diami-

Table 77–3. Selected Babesiacidal Compounds Used in the Treatment of Canine and Feline Babesiosis[a]

GENERIC (BRAND)	DOSE (mg/kg)[b]	ROUTE	INTERVAL (HOURS)	DURATION (DAYS)	*BABESIA CANIS*	*BABESIA GIBSONI*	*BABESIA FELIS*
Imidocarb dipropionate (Imizol)[c]	5.0–6.6	IM	14 days	14	+ + +	?	–
	7.5	IM	Once	NA			
Diminazene aceturate (Berenil, Ganaseg)[c]	3.5	IM	Once[d]	NA	+ + +	+ +	+
Phenamidine isethionate (Lomadine, Phenamidine)[c]	15.0	SC	24	2	+ + +	+ +	–
Pentamidine isethionate (Pentam 300)[e]	16.5	IM	24	2	+ +	+ +	?
Trypan blue	10.0	IV	Once	NA	+ +	–	–
Primaquine phosphate (Primaquine)	0.5	IM	Once	NA	?	–	+ + +
Metronidazole (Flagyl, Protostat)	25–65	PO	24	5–7	–	+	?
Clindamycin (Antirobe, Cleocin)[f]	12.5–25	PO	12	7–10	?	?	?
Doxycycline (Vibramycin)[g]	10.0	PO	12	7–10	+	?	?
Azithromycin (Zithromax)[h]	5–10	PO	12	7–10	?	?	?
Atovaquone (Mepron)[h]	13.3	PO	8	5–7	?	?	?
Quinuronium sulfate (Acaprin)	0.25	SC	48	2	+ +	?	?

[a]For specific information on each drug, see Drug Formulary, Appendix 8.
[b]Dose per administration at specified interval.
[c]Drugs not approved for use in the United States. Available in other countries as oxopirvedine (Merial), where it is combined with an antihistamine, oxomemazine.
[d]For *B. canis*, this dose is sufficient; for *B. gibsoni* repeat dose in 24 hours. These total dosages of 7.0 mg/kg or higher are associated with an increased risk of neurotoxicity.
[e]Orphan drugs.
[f]Anecdotal evidence for effectiveness against *Babesia canis*.
[g]Only shown to reduce or prevent parasitemia while dogs were infected during treatment.
[h]Effective against *Babesia microti* in a hamster model.
+ + + = very good; + + = good; + = fair to poor; – = not effective; ? = unknown; NA = not applicable.

dines; thus, it is less likely to aggravate shock or hypotension.[28] Trypan blue does not clear infections and results in bluish discoloration of tissues and plasma. Metronidazole has been utilized with limited success in treating *B. gibsoni*.

Clindamycin is the treatment of choice for *B. microti* in people, and there have been numerous anecdotal reports of success in treating canine babesiosis at 25 to 50 mg/kg per day. However, many infected dogs will recover completely without specific babesiacidal therapy if adequate supportive measures are taken, making interpretation of uncontrolled treatment observations difficult. I currently recommend that infected dogs be treated with aggressive supportive care and clindamycin if the specific antibabesial drugs are not available. Controlled trials evaluating the efficacy of clindamycin in dogs are needed. Azithromycin and atovaquone are newer drugs that are effective against *B. microti* in hamster models.[18, 70] Doxycycline has been effective in preventing or reducing parasitemia when dogs were being treated at the time of infection.[68]

Treatment of feline babesiosis has not been as critically evaluated as its canine counterpart.[28] Most babesiacidal drugs appear to be ineffective. Primaquine phosphate, an antimalarial compound, administered PO or as an IM injection, is effective and is currently the drug of choice (see Table 77–3). However, the effective dose, 0.5 mg/kg, is very close to the lethal dose of 1.0 mg/kg.

Supportive therapy is very important in the management of animals with babesiosis.[25] Many animals will recover without specific babesiacidal therapy. IV fluids should be administered to animals that are dehydrated or in shock. Whole blood or packed erythrocytes should be transfused to patients that are severely anemic. Transfusion may normalize acid-base as well as arterial oxygen status.[30] In severely acidemic animals, sodium bicarbonate infusion may need to be given. Acidosis is a poor prognostic factor if left untreated. Treatment of concurrent stressors, especially GI parasitism, is also important.

Whether glucocorticoids are indicated is controversial. The immune system is implicated in many of the clinical manifestations of canine babesiosis, especially the hemolytic anemia. In one study, 20% of dogs with *B. canis* infection had hemolytic anemias that were not responsive to antibabesial therapy alone.[22] Treatment with immunosuppressive doses of glucocorticoids is sometimes necessary. Long-term use is probably not indicated, however, and in most dogs the glucocorticoid dosage can be tapered over 2 to 3 weeks. This therapy may predispose the animals to other infections and has the potential to induce babesial relapse.[37] The monocyte-macrophage system is important in control of *Babesia* parasitemia. Reduction in this system's function will often result in more severe parasitemia shortly after glucocorticoids are initiated.

PREVENTION

The difficulty in obtaining specific therapeutic compounds for treatment of *Babesia* makes prevention of paramount importance. Preventive measures alone may be sufficient to control *B. canis* outbreaks in kennels in the southeastern United States. The primary means of prevention is the control of the vector tick.[54] Frequent inspection of the skin and hair coat for ticks is important because it takes a minimum of 2 to 3 days of feeding for transmission of the parasite to occur. New animals should be serologically tested, treated, and quarantined before being introduced into a colony. Flea and tick collars, although not very effective for flea control, are reasonably effective for tick control when used in conjunction with inspection, topical ascaricide application, and environmental control. Fipronil (TopSpot, Frontline; Merial, Iselin, NJ) appears to be effective as a topical product for tick control.

Premunition (subclinical infection) is important in controlling clinical signs of disease in areas where more virulent strains of *Babesia* are endemic.[48] In these areas, completely clearing infections may not be desirable. The role premunition plays in immunity in areas where less virulent strains are endemic is not known.

Duration of protective immunity against canine babesiosis is limited. Antibody titers gradually decline between 3 and 5 months after infection.[63, 67] Dogs are protected against homologous infection within 5 to 8 months after infection.[67] Cross-protection between strains does not occur, and seropositivity is no guarantee of protection against heterologous challenge.

A vaccine produced from cell culture–derived exoantigens of *B. canis* is available in Europe.[41] An efficacy of 70% to 100% has been reported, with the disease occasionally seen in the vaccinates generally being mild.[40] Other field studies have been less impressive. Vaccination does not prevent infection but appears to block the initiation of many of the pathologic processes involved in disease pathogenesis (see Fig. 77–2).[51, 51a] Vaccines may limit the parasitemia, reduction in hematocrit, and development of splenomegaly.[51a] Differences in strain antigenicity substantially limit the usefulness of the commercial vaccine in other areas.

Babesia organisms can be transmitted by transfusion, making control in a blood donor colony especially important.[12] All prospective canine blood donors should be serologically tested for babesiosis. Positive animals should be identified and culled from the program. Splenectomy increases the likelihood of finding parasites in animals with occult infection and is, therefore, indicated. Blood smears should be examined for *Babesia* daily for 2 weeks after splenectomy and then periodically thereafter.

Babesiosis in Greyhounds

There is a high prevalence of babesiosis among greyhounds in the United States.[57] This finding is likely due to both breed susceptibility and environmental factors that lead to extensive exposure to vector ticks. The likely organism involved is the Gulf Coast strain of *B. canis vogeli*, which rarely causes clinical disease in adults. Of the 16,000 greyhounds that were adopted through rescue leagues in 1995, 20% to 60% were likely to test positive for *Babesia*. This concern is commonly voiced by adopting owners, greyhound rescue organizations, and veterinarians. The question of what to do with these animals is not an easy one to answer. The likelihood of the adopted greyhound developing clinical babesiosis is low, as is the likelihood of the dog serving as an epidemiologic significant source of spread of the disease. However, the risk to other dogs is great if the positive animal is placed in a breeding kennel in which dogs are housed together and tick control is not adequate or if the animal is used as a canine blood donor. A single IM dose of imidocarb dipropionate at 7.5 mg/kg will apparently clear the carrier state. This approach should be considered in situations in which risk of spread is likely. In other situations, the owner should be aware of the seropositive status so that, should clinical signs consistent with babesiosis arise, their attending veterinarian can be alerted to the possibility of the disease.

PUBLIC HEALTH CONSIDERATIONS

Babesiosis is a significant tick-borne zoonosis of humans throughout Europe and in the Northeast and upper Midwest of the United States. Cases have been described in Missouri, northern California, and the state of Washington. The majority of infections are mild or nonsymptomatic; some, however, result in severe illness and death. People with AIDS are especially at risk.[11, 49] There does not appear to be a *Babesia* that is host specific for humans. As for other tick-borne zoonoses, people serve as accidental hosts for babesias of animals when they are bitten by infected ticks. *B. microti* is the primary parasite affecting humans in the Northeast and upper Midwest of the United States (see Table 77–1). The vector tick is *Ixodes scapularis (dammini)*, the vector tick of Lyme borreliosis. The disease is usually mild and self-limiting or easily managed with clindamycin and quinine. Severe disease only occasionally occurs. A more severe form of human babesiosis is caused by *B. bovis* and *B. divergens* in Europe and *B. equi* in the United States. This form of the disease usually occurs in splenectomized people and is often fatal. A closely related organism to *B. divergens* was isolated from a splenectomized person in Missouri who was suffering from a fatal illness.[15] A similar syndrome of more severe disease in splenectomized people occurs in the western United States. Genetic analysis has shown that this northern California and Washington strain was most closely related to, but distinct from, the theilerial species and the canine pathogen *B. gibsoni* than to other *Babesia*.[49] Human babesiosis caused by companion animal babesias has only been reported once; acute renal failure was reported in association with *B. canis*.[35] However, companion animals are a source of exposure to the ticks that may harbor other organisms more likely to affect humans.

References

1. Abdullah AS, Sheikh-Omar AR, Baggot AR, et al. 1984. Adverse effects of imidocarb dipropionate (*Imizol®*) in a dog. *Vet Res Commun* 8:55–59.
2. Abdullahi SU, Mohammed AA, Trimnell AR, et al. 1990. Clinical and haematological findings in 70 naturally occurring cases of canine babesiosis. *J Small Anim Pract* 31:145–147.
3. Adachi K, Tateishi M, Horii Y, et al. 1994. Reactivity of serum anti-erythrocyte membrane antibody in *Babesia gibsoni*–infected dogs. *J Vet Med Sci* 56:997–999.
4. Adachi K, Tateishi M, Horii Y, et al. 1995. Immunologic characteristics of anti-erythrocyte membrane antibody produced in dogs during *Babesia gibsoni* infection. *J Vet Med Sci* 57:121–123.
5. Adachi K, Yoshimoto A, Hasegawa T, et al. 1992. Anti-erythrocyte membrane antibodies detected in sera of dogs naturally infected with *Babesia gibsoni*. *J Vet Med Sci* 54:1081–1084.
6. Adeyanju BJ, Aliu YO. 1982. Chemotherapy of canine ehrlichiosis and babesiosis with imidocarb dipropionate. *J Am Anim Hosp Assoc* 18:827–830.
7. Bobade PA, Oduye OO, Aghomo HO. 1989. Prevalence of antibodies against *Babesia canis* in dogs in an endemic area. *Rev Elev Med Vet Pays Trop* 42:211–217.
8. Boustani MR, Lepore TJ, Gelfand JA, et al. 1994. Acute respiratory failure in patients treated for babesiosis. *Am J Respir Crit Care Med* 149:1689–1691.
9. Breitschwerdt EB. 1990. Babesiosis, pp 796–803. *In* Greene CE (ed), Infectious diseases of the dog and cat. WB Saunders, Philadelphia, PA.
10. Conrad P, Thomford J, Yamane I, et al. 1991. Hemolytic anemia caused by *Babesia gibsoni* infection in dogs. *J Am Vet Med Assoc* 199:601–605.
11. Falagas ME, Klempner MS. 1996. Babesiosis in patients with AIDS: a chronic infection presenting as fever of unknown origin. *Clin Infect Dis* 22:809–812.
12. Freeman MJ, Kirby BM, Panciera DL, et al. 1994. Hypotensive shock syndrome associated with acute *Babesia canis* infection in a dog. *J Am Vet Med Assoc* 204:94–96.
13. Friedhoff KT. 1988. Transmission of *Babesia*, pp 23–52. *In* Ristic M (ed), Babesiosis of domestic animals and man. CRC Press, Boca Raton, FL.
14. Fukata T, Ohnishi T, Okuda S, et al. 1996. Detection of canine erythrocyte infected with *Babesia gibsoni* by flow cytometry. *J Parasitol* 82:641–642.
15. Herwaldt BL, Persing DH, Precigout EA, et al. 1996. A fatal case of babesiosis in Missouri: identification of another piroplasm that infects humans. *Ann Intern Med* 124:643–650.
16. Herwaldt BL, Springs FE, Roberts PP, et al. 1995. Babesiosis in Wisconsin: a potentially fatal disease. *Am J Trop Med Hyg* 53:146–151.
17. Horowitz ML, Coletta F, Fein AM. 1994. Delayed onset adult respiratory distress syndrome in babesiosis. *Chest* 106:1299–1301.
18. Hughes WT, Helieh SO. 1995. Successful prevention and treatment of babesiosis with atovaquone. *J Infect Dis* 172:1042–1046.
19. Igarashi I, Aikawa M, Kreier JP. 1988. Host cell–parasite interaction in babesiosis, pp 53–69. *In* Ristic M (ed), Babesiosis of domestic animals and man. CRC Press, Boca Raton, FL.
20. Irwin PJ, Hutchinson GW. 1991. Clinical and pathological findings of *Babesia* infection in dogs. *Aust Vet J* 68:204–209.

21. Jacobson LS. 1994. Cerebellar ataxia as a possible complication of babesiosis in two dogs. *J S Afr Vet Assoc* 65:130–131.
22. Jacobson LS, Clark IA. 1994. The pathophysiology of canine babesiosis: new approaches to an old puzzle. *J S Afr Vet Assoc* 65:134–145.
23. Jacobson LS, Lobetti RG. 1996. Rhabdomyolysis as a complication of canine babesiosis. *J Small Anim Pract* 37:286–297.
24. Jacobson LS, Reyers F, Berry WL, et al. 1996. Changes in haematocrit after treatment of uncomplicated canine babesiosis: a comparison between diminazene and trypan blue, and an evaluation of the influence of parasitaemia. *J S Afr Vet Assoc* 67:77–82.
25. Jacobson LS, Swan GE. 1995. Supportive treatment of canine babesiosis. *J S Afr Vet Assoc* 66:95–105.
26. Kock N, Kelly P. 1991. Massive hepatic necrosis associated with accidental imidocarb dipropionate toxicosis in a dog. *J Comp Pathol* 104:113–116.
26a. Kontos VJ, Koutinas AF. 1997. Clinical observations in 15 spontaneous cases of canine babesiosis. *Canine Pract* 22:30–34.
27. Kuttler KL. 1980. Pharmacotherapeutics of drugs used in treatment of anaplasmosis and babesiosis. *J Am Vet Med Assoc* 176:1103–1108.
28. Kuttler KL. 1988. Chemotherapy of babesiosis, pp 227–242. *In* Ristic M (ed), Babesiosis of domestic animals and man. CRC Press, Boca Raton, FL.
29. Kuttler KL. 1988. World-wide impact of babesiosis, pp 1–22. *In* Ristic M (ed), Babesiosis of domestic animals and man. CRC Press, Boca Raton, FL.
30. Leisewitz AL, Guthrie AJ, Berry WL. 1996. Evaluation of the effect of whole-blood transfusion on the oxygen status and acid-base balance of *Babesia canis* infected dogs using oxygen status algorithm. *J S Afr Vet Assoc* 67:20–26.
30a. Littman MP. 1991. Clinical babesiosis in 26 dogs from Pennsylvania and New Jersey (abstract 95). Presented at the Meeting of the American College of Veterinary and Internal Medicine, Ninth Annual Veterinary Medical Forum, New Orleans, LA.
31. Lobetti RG. 1995. Leukaemoid response in two dogs with *Babesia canis* infection. *J S Afr Vet Assoc* 66:182–184.
32. Lobetti RG, Reyers F. 1996. Methaemoglobinuria in naturally occurring *Babesia canis* infection. *J S Afr Vet Assoc* 67:88–90.
33. Lobetti RG, Reyers F, Nesbit JW. 1996. The comparative role of hemoglobinemia and hypoxia in the development of canine babesial nephropathy. *J S Afr Vet Assoc* 67:188–198.
34. Makinde MO, Bobade PA. 1994. Osmotic fragility of erythrocytes in clinically normal dogs and dogs with parasites. *Res Vet Sci* 57:343–348.
35. Marsaudon E, Camenen J, Testou D, et al. 1995. *Babesia canis* human babesiosis causing a 40-day anuria. *Ann Med Intern* 146:451–452.
36. Martinod S, Brossard M, Moreau Y. 1985. Immunity of dogs against *Babesia canis*, its vector tick *Dermacentor reticulatus*, and *Ixodes ricinus* in endemic area. *J Parasitol* 71:269–273.
37. Masuda T, Baba E, Arakawa A. 1983. Relapse of canine babesiosis after prednisolone treatment. *Mod Vet Pract* 64:931–932.
38. Matthewman LA, Kelly PJ, Bobade PA, et al. 1993. Infections with *Babesia canis* and *Ehrlichia canis* in dogs in Zimbabwe. *Vet Rec* 133:344–346.
39. Mattia AR, Waldron MA, Sierra LS. 1993. Use of the quantitative buffy coat system for detection of parasitemia in patients with babesiosis. *J Clin Microbiol* 31:2816–2818.
40. Moreau Y, Martinod S, Fayet G. 1988. Epidemiologic and immunoprophylactic aspects of canine babesiosis in France, pp 191–196. *In* Ristic M (ed), Babesiosis of domestic animals and man. CRC Press, Boca Raton, FL.
41. Moreau Y, Vidor E, Bissuel G, et al. 1989. Vaccination against canine babesiosis: an overview of field observations. *Trans R Soc Trop Med Hyg* 83(Suppl):95–96.
42. Morita T, Saeki H, Imai S, et al. 1995. Reactivity of anti-erythrocyte antibody induced by *Babesia gibsoni* infection against aged erythrocytes. *Vet Parasitol* 58:291–299.
43. Murase T, Naede Y. 1990. Increased erythrophagocytic activity of macrophages in dogs with *Babesia gibsoni* infection. *Nippon Juigaku Zasshi* 52:321–327.
44. Murase T, Ueda T, Yamato O, et al. 1996. Oxidative damage and enhanced erythrophagocytosis in canine erythrocytes infected with *Babesia gibsoni*. *J Vet Med Sci* 58:259–261.
45. Omamegbe JO, Uche UE. 1985. Haemogram studies in Nigerian local dogs suffering from ancylostomiasis, babesiosis, and trypanosomiasis. *Bull Anim Health Prod Afr* 33:335–338.
46. Ohnishi T, Suzuki S. 1994. Changes of serum hemolytic activity and the number of reticulocytes in canine *Babesia gibsoni* infection. *J Vet Med Sci* 56:611–612.
47. Ohnishi T, Ueda K, Horie M, et al. 1990. Serum hemolytic activity in dogs with *Babesia gibsoni*. *J Parasitol* 76:564–567.
48. Penzhorn BL, Lewis BD, de Waal DT, et al. 1995. Sterilisation of *Babesia canis* infections by imidocarb alone or in combination with diminazene. *J S Afr Vet Assoc* 66:157–159.
49. Persing DH, Herwaldt BL, Glaser C, et al. 1995. Infection with a *Babesia*-like organism in northern California. *N Engl J Med* 332:298–303.
50. Reiter I, Weiland G. 1989. Recently developed methods for the detection of babesial infections. *Trans R Soc Trop Med Hyg* 83(Suppl):21–23.
51. Schetters TH, Kleuskens J, Scholtes N, et al. 1995. Strain variation limits protective activity of vaccines based on soluble *Babesia canis* antigens. *Parasite Immunol* 17:215–218.
51a. Schetters TH, Kleuskens J, Scholtes NC, et al. 1997. Vaccination of dogs against *Babesia canis* infection. *Vet Parasitol* 73:35–41.
52. Shakespeare AS. 1995. The incidence of canine babesiosis amongst sick dogs presented to the Onderstepoort veterinary academic hospital. *J S Afr Vet Assoc* 66:247–250.
53. Sinha BP, Ghosh P. 1986. Treatment of clinical cases of canine babesiosis. *Indian J Vet Med* 6:94–97.
54. Smith RD, Kakoma I. 1989. A reappraisal of vector control strategies for babesiosis. *Trans R Soc Trop Med Hyg* 83(Suppl):43–52.
55. Taboada J. 1995. Canine babesiosis, pp 315–319. *In* Bonagura JD (ed), Kirk's current veterinary therapy: XII. Small animal practice. WB Saunders, Philadelphia, PA.
56. Taboada J. 1997. Unpublished data. Louisiana State University, Baton Rouge, LA.
57. Taboada J, Harvey JW, Levy MG, et al. 1992. Seroprevalence of babesiosis in greyhounds in Florida. *J Am Vet Med Assoc* 200:47–50.
58. Taboada J, Merchant SR. 1991. Babesiosis of companion animals and man. *Vet Clin North Am Small Anim Pract* 21:103–123.
59. Taylor JH, Guthrie AJ, Leisewitz A. 1991. The effect of endogenously produced carbon monoxide on the oxygen status of dogs infected with *Babesia canis*. *J S Afr Vet Assoc* 62:153–155.
60. Taylor JH, Guthrie AJ, van der Walt JG, et al. 1993. The effect of *Babesia canis* induced haemolysis on the canine haemoglobin oxygen dissociation curve. *J S Afr Vet Assoc* 64:141–143.
61. Taylor JH, Janse Van Renburg J. 1995. Electrophoretic separation of canine haemoglobin in dogs with babesiosis. *J S Afr Vet Assoc* 66:219–221.
62. Uemura T, Suzuki S, Ohnishi T. 1990. Flow cytometric enumeration of reticulocytes in the peripheral blood from canine infected with *Babesia gibsoni*. *Zentralbl Veterinarmed* 37:468–472.
63. Uilenberg G, Franssen FFJ, Perie NM, et al. 1989. Three groups of *Babesia canis* distinguished and a proposal for nomenclature. *Vet Q* 11:33–40.
64. Valli VEO. 1993. The hematopoietic system, pp 101–265. *In* Jubb KVF, Kennedy PC, Palmer N (eds), Pathology of domestic animals, ed 4. Academic Press, San Diego, CA.
65. Vercammen F, DeDeken R, Maes L. 1995. Clinical and serological observations on experimental infections with *Babesia canis* and its diagnosis using the IFAT. *Parasite* 2:407–410.
66. Vercammen F, DeDeken R, Maes L. 1996. Prophylactic activity of imidocarb against experimental infection with *Babesia canis*. *Vet Parasitol* 63:195–198.
67. Vercammen F, DeDeken R, Maes L, et al. 1996. Prophylactic treatment of experimental canine babesiosis (*Babesia canis*) with doxycycline. *Vet Parasitol* 66:251–255.
68. Vercammen F, DeDeken R, Maes L. 1997. Duration of protective immunity in experimental canine babesiosis after homologous and heterologous challenge. *Vet Parasitol* 68:51–55.
68a. Vercammen F, DeDeken R, Maes L. 1997. Hematological and biochemical profiles in experimental canine babesiosis (*Babesia canis*). *Vlaams Diergeneesk Tijdsch* 66:174–178.
69. Weiland G, Reiter I. 1988. Methods for the measurement of the serological response to *Babesia*, pp 143–162. *In* Ristic M (ed), Babesiosis of domestic animals and man. CRC Press, Boca Raton, FL.
70. Weiss LM, Wittner M, Wasserman S, et al. 1993. Efficacy of azithromycin for treating *Babesia microti* infection in the hamster model. *J Infect Dis* 168:1289–1292.
70a. Wozniak EJ, Barr BC, Thomford JW, et al. 1997. Clinical, anatomic, and immunopathologic characterization of *Babesia gibsoni* infection in the domestic dog (*Canis familiaris*). *J Parasitol* 83:692–699.
71. Wright IG, Goodger BV. 1988. Pathogenesis of babesiosis, pp 99–118. *In* Ristic M (ed), Babesiosis of domestic animals and man. CRC Press, Boca Raton, FL.
72. Yamane I, Thomford JW, Gardner IA. 1993. Evaluation of the indirect fluorescent antibody test for diagnosis of *Babesia gibsoni* infections in dogs. *Am J Vet Res* 54:1579–1584.

Chapter **78**

Enteric Protozoal Infections

Stephen C. Barr

The enteric protozoa covered in this chapter are limited to four protozoan genera: *Giardia*, *Pentatrichomonas*, and *Entamoeba* in the phylum Sarcomastigophora and *Balantidium* in the phylum Ciliophora. Salient characteristics of these organisms and the diseases they may cause are presented in Table 78–1. Enteric protozoa of the phylum Apicomplexa are discussed in Chapters 80 (Toxoplasmosis), 81 (Enteric Coccidiosis), and 82 (Cryptosporidiosis). Detailed coverage of laboratory methods for diagnosis of enteric protozoan infections is presented in Chapter 70.

Giardiasis

ETIOLOGY AND EPIDEMIOLOGY

Giardia, a protozoan parasite found in the intestinal tract of human beings and most domestic animals throughout the world, has two morphologic forms. The intestinal lumen-dwelling motile form, the trophozoite, is approximately 15 μm long and 8 μm wide. Under light microscopy, the trophozoite is easily identified by its "smiling face" appearance formed by the two nuclei in the anterior third (forming the eyes), the axonemes passing longitudinally between the nuclei (forming the nose), and the median bodies (forming the mouth) situated transversely in the posterior third (Fig. 78–1). Four pairs of flagella complete the rather comical appearance of this form. The second form, the cyst, is responsible for transmission and environmental survival. It is approximately 12 μm long and 7 μm wide. Because the cyst contains two incompletely separated but formed trophozoites, the axonemes, fragments of the ventral discs, and up to four nuclei can be seen within (Fig. 78–2). The cyst is susceptible to desiccation under dry, hot conditions but can survive for several months outside the host in wet, cold conditions.

The life cycle is direct (Fig. 78–3). After ingestion, cysts (trophozoites are noninfective) excyst in the duodenum on exposure to gastric acids and pancreatic enzymes. The two released trophozoites separate, mature, and attach to the brush border of the villous epithelium. The distribution of trophozoites within the intestinal tract varies with host and diet. In dogs, the organism seems to prefer the duodenum and jejunum[45] but has been found from the ileum to the duodenum.[14] Circumstantial evidence indicates that trophozoites occupy the upper intestinal tract (duodenum) in infected symptomatic dogs[29] and the lower tract (jejunum) in infected nonsymptomatic dogs.[3, 48] In cats, trophozoites have been found throughout the intestinal tract.[25, 29] In dogs, a high-carbohydrate diet rather than a high-protein diet[45] may favor trophozoite habitation of the upper tract. In humans, *Giardia* is often found in chronic atrophic gastritis (often associated with *Helicobacter pylori* infection or gastric adenocarcinoma) when there is a decrease in gastric acidity.[13, 39] Trophozoites adhere (using a ventral adhesive disc) to the brush border of the intestinal mucosa and move from one attachment site to another using flagella. Encystation of trophozoites is stimulated by bile salts and fatty acids at slightly alkaline pH[29]; however, the site and mechanism are unknown. Trophozoites may be passed in diarrheic stools, but cysts are more routinely shed. Whereas cysts may survive for days to weeks in cool, moist conditions, trophozoites do not survive long outside the host. On excretion, the relatively resistant, ellipsoidal cysts are immediately infective to another host.

Table 78–1. Comparison of Some Enteric Protozoa in Dogs and Cats

ORGANISM	STAGE	AVERAGE SIZE (μm)	NATURAL HOSTS	ORGAN PARASITIZED	PATHOGENIC MECHANISMS	CLINICAL SIGNS
Giardia[a]	Tr Cy	15 × 10 × 3 10 × 8	D, C, H, other mammals	Small intestine	Damage to glycocalyx and microvilli on intestinal epithelium; inhibition of some digestive enzymes; host elicits inflammatory response	None to chronic diarrhea, continuous or intermittent; malabsorption
Pentatrichomonas hominis	Tr	8 × 5	D, C, H, other mammals	Large intestine	Probably none; considered harmless commensal but may be opportunistic pathogen	None to diarrhea
Entamoeba histolytica	Tr Cy	25 (diam.) 12 (diam.)	D, C, H, NHP	Large intestine	Invades colonic wall, producing ulcers; may metastasize to extraintestinal sites	None to diarrhea; dysentery
Balantidium coli	Tr Cy	60 × 35 50 (diam.)	D, P, H, NHP	Large intestine	Invades colonic wall, producing ulcers (metastases rare)	None to diarrhea; dysentery

[a] Some *Giardia* species may be identical.
Tr = trophozoite; Cy = cyst; D = dog; C = cat; H = human being; NHP = nonhuman primate; P = pig.

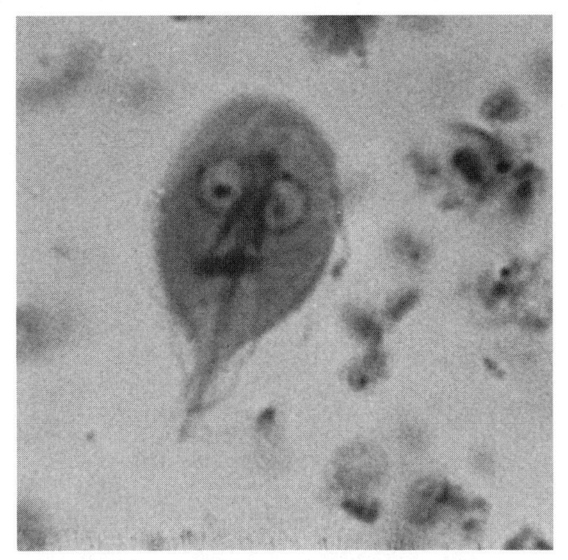

Figure 78–1. *Giardia* trophozoite in a fecal smear stained to enhance the characteristic organelles (iron hematoxylin, × 2000).

The prepatent period of *Giardia* infection ranges from 5 to 12 days (mean, about 8 days) in dogs and from 5 to 16 days (mean, about 10 days) in cats. The onset of disease, when it occurs, may precede cyst shedding by 1 to 2 days.

The prevalence of *Giardia* is approximately 10% in well-cared-for dogs, 36% to 50% in puppies, and even 100% in breeding kennels.[29] The prevalence in cats ranges from 1.4% to 11%.[29] Overall, in the general population of both species, the overall incidence averages approximately 2.5%.[31, 35, 44] Although the prevalence of giardiasis is high in cats and dogs, obvious clinical disease is rare. Immunodeficient adults, the young, and group-housed animals (breeding kennels, catteries, and laboratory animal colonies) have a high prevalence of *Giardia* infection. Glucocorticoid therapy at anti-inflammatory dosages (1 mg/kg/day of prednisolone) for 10 days, allowed replication and reshedding of *Giardia*.[48]

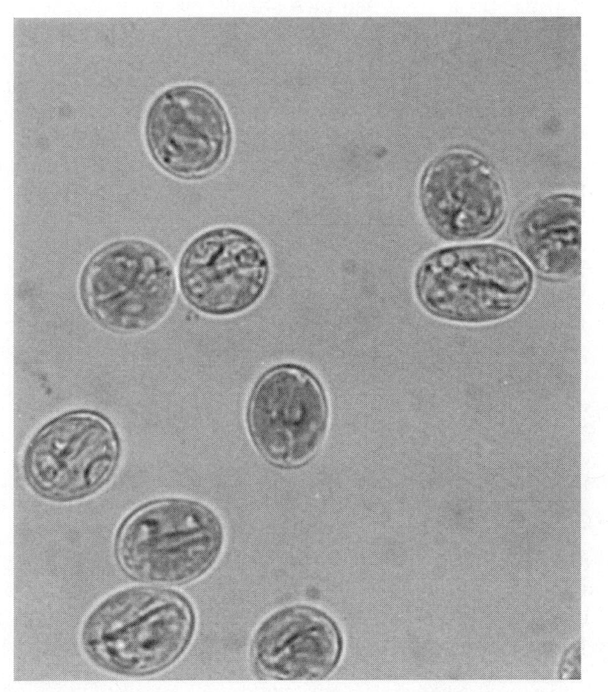

Figure 78–2. *Giardia* cysts concentrated from the feces of a cat by the zinc sulfate centrifugal flotation technique. Cyst wall, nuclei, axonemes, and median bodies are apparent in several of the cysts (iodine, × 1100).

PATHOGENESIS

Because there are virtually no studies of how *Giardia* causes clinical disease in dogs and cats, most of the following information is extrapolated from human studies. In humans, infection can cause malabsorption of vitamin B_{12}, folate, iron (leading to anemia),[23] triglycerides, lactose, and, less commonly, sucrose.[21] Specific histologic changes have not been identified in the small-bowel mucosa[36]; however, parasite-related pathogenic factors have been implicated in abnormally rapid sloughing of intestinal epithelial cells, leading to failure of new epithelial cells arising in the crypts to differentiate fully into columnar cells with microvilli. Blunting of intestinal villi and microvilli results in decreased absorptive surface area.[1]

Putative differences in virulence of *Giardia* strains, as well as host genetics and immune status, probably determine the outcome of an infection. Not only do morphologically identical human *Giardia* isolates vary in respect to their surface antigens,[32] susceptibility to proteases,[33] and genetic profiles,[8] they vary in their virulence.[9, 10] An intact cellular and humoral[28] immune system is important for overcoming infection and developing protective immunity.[19] Absence of an S-IgA response to one of *Giardia* heat shock proteins is associated with persistent infection despite an IgG response to this protein and IgA responses to other *Giardia* polypeptides.[11] Few studies involve dogs or cats; the prevalence of *Giardia* infection in a colony of IgA-deficient beagles was higher than that of normal animals.[29] Administration of immunosuppressive amounts of glucocorticoids will lead to recrudescence of *Giardia* infections in dogs.[48]

CLINICAL FINDINGS

Most infections (where cysts are being passed in the feces) are nonsymptomatic. Acute diarrhea tends to occur in very young puppies and kittens shortly after infection. In older cats and dogs, diarrhea may be acute and short lived, intermittent, or chronic. Feces are often malodorous, pale, and steatorrheic. Affected animals may experience weight loss secondary to diarrhea, but rarely will they become inappetent.[29] Although *Giardia* cysts and trophozoites can be seen in the stool of dogs with small- or large-bowel diarrhea with weight loss,[16] the organism is unlikely to be the sole cause of the diarrhea. Giardiasis does not in itself produce fever or emesis.

DIAGNOSIS

Finding cysts or trophozoites in the feces or samples taken from the intestinal tract is the most definitive means of diagnosing giardiasis, because clinical signs and laboratory test results (hemogram, serum biochemistry, radiology) are not pathognomonic. The prevalence of *Giardia* is high, even when giardiasis often goes undetected.[29] Reasons for this occurrence may include failure to consider it in the differential diagnosis, failure to recognize the organisms, use of inappropriate methods for fecal analysis, and intermittent excretion of organisms in feces of infected individuals.

A fecal smear, especially in symptomatic patients, may

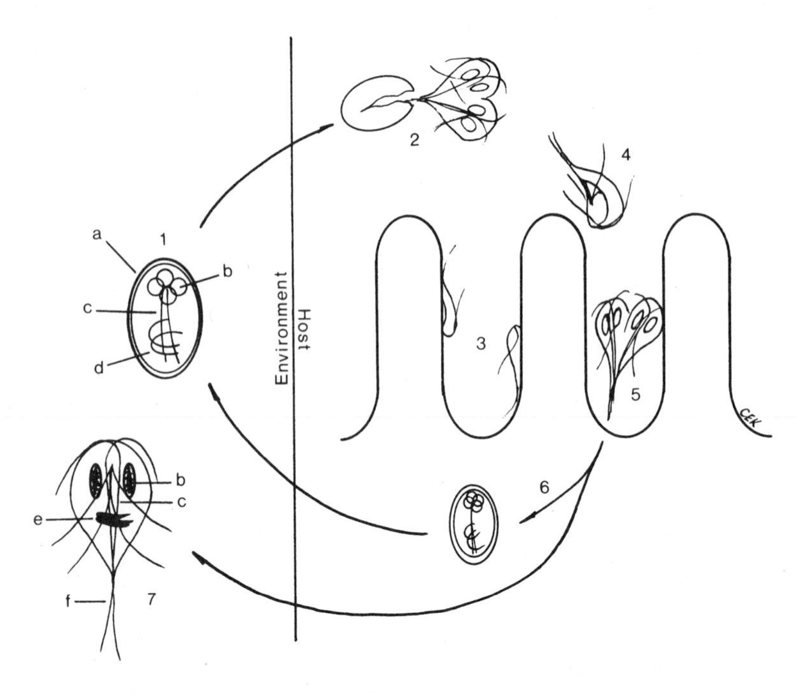

Figure 78–3. Diagram of *Giardia* life cycle, indicating organelles of cyst and trophozoite visible by light microscopy. After cyst (1) is ingested by the host, excystation (2) occurs in the small intestine. Trophozoites (3–5) attach to the mucosa or swim freely in the lumen, where they divide asexually. Following encystment, cysts are excreted (6) in the feces, completing the cycle. Excreted trophozoites (7) do not survive. Key to structural features: a, cyst wall; b, nuclei; c, axonemes (recurrent flagella); d, adhesive disk fragments; e, median bodies; f, flagella. (From Kirkpatrick CE: *Vet Clin North Am [Small Anim Pract]* 17:1377–1387, 1987. Reprinted with permission.)

reveal trophozoites distinctive by their erratic tumbling motion and concave ventral disc. *Giardia* trophozoites can be distinguished from those of *Pentatrichomonas hominis* (the only other organism that resembles *Giardia*) because the latter have a smoother rolling motion, no concave ventral disc, a single nucleus, and an undulating membrane (Fig. 78–4). A drop of feces is mixed with a drop of normal saline on a glass slide, a coverslip is applied, and the specimen is examined immediately under 40× with the condenser in its lowest position. Morphology of the organisms can be better appreciated by adding a drop of Lugol's iodine (which kills the parasite, thereby rendering it immobile) to a drop of feces. Finding organisms in a fecal smear provides a definitive diagnosis of *Giardia* infection, but a negative result does not rule it out.

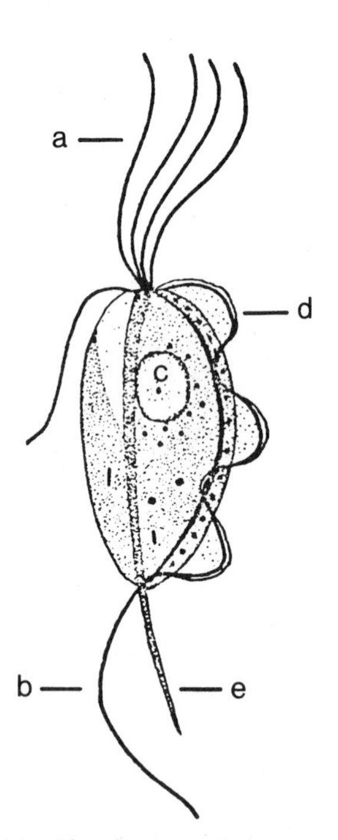

Figure 78–4. Drawing of *P. hominis* trophozoite indicating some of the characteristic organelles. Key: a, anterior flagella; b, posterior flagellum; c, nucleus; d, undulating membrane; e, axostyle. (Modified from Wenrich SH: *J Parasitol* 33:177–188, 1947, with permission.)

If a direct smear provides a negative result, the zinc sulfate concentration technique (ZSCT) should be performed.[29, 48] This method is also effective in demonstrating nematode eggs in the feces of cats and dogs and is superior to sucrose (of equal density) flotation because it is less likely to distort the organisms. Because cats and dogs shed *Giardia* organisms intermittently,[24, 29] and the presence of organisms in feces does not necessarily parallel the severity of clinical signs, at least three fresh fecal samples should be examined over a period of 3 to 5 days to maximize the chance of ruling out infection. Approximately 70% and 93% of *Giardia*-positive dogs can be identified with one and two ZSCTs, respectively.[29, 48] For shipping, fecal samples should be refrigerated at 4°C to ensure survival for at least 2 days; cysts will not survive in 10% formalin. Slides prepared by the ZSCT should be examined within 10 minutes of preparation because the cysts shrink with time and lose the internal morphologic characteristic appearance that differentiates them from other organisms. Cysts may be distinguished from coccidian oocysts and sporocysts by internal structure and by observing that *Giardia* cysts will take up iodine, whereas the former organisms will not. Yeasts also will stain with iodine; however, yeasts are oval, not ellipsoidal, and are about half the size of *Giardia* cysts. Further, close observation of yeast cells may reveal budding. If steatorrhea frustrates attempts at flotation, the formalin–ethyl acetate sedimentation method to concentrate *Giardia* cysts from a fecal specimen is usually successful.

Commercial ELISA kits to detect fecal *Giardia* antigens (see Appendix 6) have over 97% sensitivity and over 96% specificity in humans.[42, 50] In dogs, the ProSpecT/Giardia ELISA kit (Alexon Inc, Mountain View, CA) was found to be slightly less sensitive and have a slightly lower relative specificity than the ZSCT.[3] The test may be slightly more effective than a single ZSCT in diagnosing *Giardia* infections in dogs.[49] Frozen fecal samples or samples preserved in formalin fixative can be used. Given that the ELISA kits are technically more difficult to perform and more expensive than the ZSCT, they do not seem to offer any advantages over performing three ZSCTs for the diagnosis of giardiasis in dogs. The ELISA test has not been adequately evaluated in the cat, although it will detect infected fecal samples.

Like the ELISA kits, the direct immunofluorescent test (using fluorescent-labeled monoclonal antibodies to detect *Giardia* cysts in feces) is highly sensitive (100%) and specific (99.8%) in people.[50] Although not extensively evaluated in cats and dogs, one such test (Merifluor Cryptosporidium/ Giardia Direct Immunofluorescence Assay, Meridian Diagnostics, Cincinnati, OH) is more sensitive than the sucrose gradient flotation and ZSCT at identifying infected feces from cattle and sheep, especially when the cyst concentration in the feces is low.[47] One would expect a similar finding for feces from small animals. Because the test requires a fluorescent microscope, it is more likely to be used in diagnostic laboratories. Feces should be collected fresh and preserved as soon as possible in 10% formalin or sodium acetate–acetic acid formalin.

Two techniques used to collect a sample from the duodenum for the microscopic examination of trophozoites have reportedly had disparate findings. In one study, examination for trophozoites of duodenal aspirates collected during gastroduodenoscopy or exploratory laparotomy has been shown to be more efficacious than a ZSCT on a single fecal sample from the same dogs suffering from clinical giardiasis.[38] However, in another study performed in nonsymptomatic dogs, a single sample was found to be as effective as a duodenal aspirate for the diagnosis of giardiasis.[48] The disparity between these findings may be explained by the fact that, in subclinical dogs, the organism colonizes various levels (not always including the duodenum) anywhere along the small intestine.[14] Duodenal aspiration to specifically rule out *Giardia* infection is clinically impractical but could be performed if the dog was undergoing gastroduodenoscopy for other reasons.

The second technique utilized to sample duodenal contents, a commercially available peroral nylon string test (Entero-test, HDC Corp., San Jose, CA), has been found to be both safe and accurate for the diagnosis of giardiasis in people.[41] The test is not safe or effective in diagnosing infection in nonsymptomatic dogs,[3] although it has been effective in detecting trophozoites in two symptomatic dogs. The test has not been evaluated in cats. See Appendix 6 for information on this product.

THERAPY

In the United States, no drug used to treat giardiasis in small animals is officially approved for that purpose. However, a number of licensed drugs have been employed commonly in human patients and small animals to treat giardiasis. Some of the reportedly effective treatment regimens in dogs and cats are shown in Table 78–2.[4–6, 29] Fenbendazole (Panacur granules 22.2%, Hoechst-Roussel Agri-Vet Co, Somerville, NJ), at the dose approved in dogs for the control and removal of roundworms, hookworms, and whipworms, and the tapeworm *Taenia pisiformis*, was effective in removing *Giardia* cysts from feces in 100% of dogs (6 of 6 dogs treated) in a controlled trial,[6] and in 9 of 10 dogs in another study.[47a] No side effects were seen at this dose regimen, nor is fenbendazole (like some other benzimidazoles) thought to be teratogenic. It is safe to treat puppies as young as 6 weeks at these doses. Mild diarrhea has been the only side effect noted. These results suggest that fenbendazole alone could be used to treat giardiasis or to rule out (by therapeutic trial) *Giardia* and whipworm infections as a cause of chronic diarrhea in the dog. Fenbendazole has not been evaluated in cats. Albendazole given to dogs for 2 days was 90% efficacious in clearing *Giardia* cysts from feces[4]; however, a longer regimen (5 days) is needed in cats.[5] No side effects were seen in cats at doses provided, nor in beagles treated at 30 mg/kg body weight orally once a day for 13 weeks.[43] However, albendazole is potentially more toxic, causing myelosuppression. Albendazole, but not fenbendazole, is suspected of being teratogenic[12] and, therefore, should not be given to pregnant animals.

Metronidazole (a nitroimidazole) has been administered extensively in dogs and cats for the treatment of giardiasis. It is less effective than albendazole or fenbendazole against *Giardia* in vitro and in vivo. The drug is only 67% effective in eliminating *Giardia* from infected dogs and has been associated with the acute development of neurologic signs, including anorexia and vomiting, with deterioration to pronounced generalized ataxia and vertical positional nystagmus. This situation has resulted in euthanasia in some animals.[15, 20] Cats often resent the administration of metronidazole because of the very bitter taste of the tablets. Drug resistance to metronidazole by various isolates of *Giardia* is a serious concern in people and the drug has been described as "obsolete" for the treatment of *Giardia*.[18, 46] At high doses (see Table 78–2), quinacrine is 100% effective but is associated

Table 78–2. Drug Therapy for Enteric Protozoal Infections[a]

DRUG	SPECIES	DOSE[b]	ROUTE	INTERVAL (HOURS)	DURATION (DAYS)	INFECTION
Fenbendazole	D	50 mg/kg	PO	24	3	G
Albendazole	D	25 mg/kg	PO	12	2	G
	C	25 mg/kg	PO	12	5	G
Metronidazole	D	15–30 mg/kg[c]	PO	12–24	5–7	G, T, A, B
	C	10–25 mg/kg	PO	12–24	5–7	G, T, A, B
Tinidazole	D	44 mg/kg	PO	24	6	G, T?, A?, B?
Ipronidazole	D	126 mg/L[d]	PO	Ad libitum	7	G
Quinacrine	D	9 mg/kg	PO	24	6	G
	D	6.6 mg/kg	PO	12	5	G
Furazolidone	C	4 mg/kg[e]	PO	12	7–10	G
Tetracycline	D	22 mg/kg	PO	8	7–10	B
Paromomycin	C	125–160 mg/kg	PO	12	5	T, A

[a] For additional information on each drug, see Drug Formulary, Appendix 8. For coccidial infections, see Chapter 81; for Cryptosporidiosis, Chapter 82.
[b] Dose per administration at specified interval.
[c] Neurotoxicity has been noted with higher doses previously recommended; see Nitroimidazoles, Chapter 77. To facilitate the dosage to smaller animals, the 250- or 500-mg tablets may be ground, or smaller tablet size (50 or 100 mg) may be used. This may be placed in a palatable base (see Drug Formulary, Appendix 8).
[d] In drinking water.
[e] In suspension, 200 mg/day maximum.
D = dog; C = cat; G = giardiasis; T = trichomoniasis; A = amebiasis; B = balantidiasis.

with a 50% rate of side effects (lethargy and fevers) toward the end of the therapeutic regimen.[29] These side effects regress spontaneously within 2 to 3 days after stopping drug administration. Like albendazole and metronidazole, quinacrine should not be given to pregnant animals. Quinacrine has not been demonstrated to be effective in cats.

Ipronidazole, a feed-water additive for the treatment of blackhead in turkeys and *Trichomonas foetus* in cattle, has been provided effectively in drinking water to treat giardiasis in two greyhounds. Unfortunately, the drug has not been more extensively tested. Tinidazole, another nitroimidazole, has an efficacy against giardiasis similar to metronidazole,[29] but it is unavailable in the United States. Furazolidone is effective in treating giardiasis in cats, but side effects of diarrhea and vomiting can occur.[29] Furazolidone has not been well evaluated in dogs. Like many of the other anti-*Giardia* compounds, furazolidone is suspected of being teratogenic and should not be used in pregnant queens.[29] See the Drug Formulary, Appendix 8, for more information on these drugs.

CONTROL

To date, no drug has been convincingly proved to be 100% effective against *Giardia*. Trials testing the efficacy of drugs against *Giardia* are based on clearing cysts from feces, not removing organisms from the intestinal tract. Thus, because it is possible that these compounds do not clear organisms but only inhibit cyst production for a time, it is unknown whether treated animals may be a source of infection in the future. Certainly, autoinfection occurs by virtue of viable cysts present in fecal material adherent to the external hair coat or present in a cold, moist environment. Because the prepatent period can be extremely short for *Giardia*, it is possible for an animal to become reinfected and start excreting cysts again within 5 days after the last treatment. Owing to these factors, it is virtually impossible to prevent reinfection of household pets or animals held in uncontrolled environments. Preliminary trials in kittens, using a killed trophozoite vaccine (Langford/Cyanamid, Guelph, Ontario, Canada), have shown protection against diarrhea, weight loss, and cyst shedding.[37] Lesser numbers or no cysts and reduced cyst viability were found in vaccinates compared with unvaccinated kittens.

In controlled environments (cattery or kennel situation), four main approaches should be employed to control *Giardia*: (1) decontaminating environment, (2) using drugs to treat animals, (3) cleaning cysts from coats, and (4) preventing reintroduction of infection.[2]

In a cattery or kennel, it is first necessary to establish a "clean area." In a small facility, all the animals should be moved out of the facility while it is being cleaned. In a large facility, clean areas can be created over time by setting up a few cages or runs on a rotation basis once animals are moved out to a holding facility. Before moving animals to the holding facility, they should be treated (preferably with fenbendazole or albendazole) and moved to the holding facility on the last day of treatment. Once moved, the cages or runs should be steam or chemically cleaned after all fecal material has been picked up. Quaternary ammonium (QUAT)–containing disinfectants (Roccal, Winthrop Labs, New York, NY; Totil, Calgon Corp., St. Louis, MO), when used at the manufacturers' recommended concentrations, are very effective in inactivating *Giardia* cysts (1 minute at room temperature).[29] QUATs lose considerable activity when used in the presence of organic matter. The kennel should be allowed to dry thoroughly after cleaning (cysts are extremely susceptible to drying) and preferably left dry and empty for several days before being repopulated. Before repopulating the clean area, the animals should be bathed to remove all fecal material from their coats with a general pet shampoo and thoroughly rinsed. The animals should be bathed again (especially the perianal area) with a QUAT compound. QUAT compounds can irritate skin and mucous membranes with repeated or prolonged exposure but appear to produce no ill effects when applied for 3 to 5 minutes followed by thorough rinsing. The coat is allowed to dry thoroughly before returning the animal to the clean area. Animals should then be treated again, preferably with a different compound than initially used, once back in the clean facility. Theoretically, the only way *Giardia* can be reintroduced into a clean area is by an infected animal or by fomite transmission. New animals introduced into the kennel or cattery should be treated and their coats cleaned as discussed regardless of whether they are *Giardia* negative on fecal examination. Fomite transmission can be avoided by donning shoe covers before entering the facility or cleaning boots with a QUAT foot bath. Fecal samples should be periodically checked using the ZSCT, which should detect whether the process has been effective.

PUBLIC HEALTH CONSIDERATIONS

Giardia is the most common intestinal parasite affecting people in North America. Many infections are acquired by drinking unfiltered municipal water originating from *Giardia*-contaminated streams, rivers, or lakes.[26] Infants and children in day care facilities appear to have a particularly high risk for infection. Although scant direct evidence links zoonotic infections from dogs and cats, molecular and immunologic analyses of *Giardia* isolates from animals (including dogs) and human beings suggest that *Giardia* isolates are not highly host specific.[7, 17, 22] However, attempts to induce giardiasis in dogs and cats by administering *Giardia* organisms obtained from people have yielded equivocal results.[29] Genotyping of isolates by PCR methods in an isolated community of cohabitating people and dogs could not document cross infection.[25a] In one instance, a human volunteer was experimentally infected with *Giardia* from an animal.[30] It seems prudent to regard *Giardia*-infected pets as a potential source of human infection and treat infected animals as long as uncertainty remains.

Chlorine disinfection of public drinking water is not effective in controlling *Giardia* contamination, and filtration must be used. Organic chlorine compounds such as *N*-halamines are stable in water and have shown marked efficacy in inactivating *Giardia* cysts within 2 minutes at 22°C.

Trichomoniasis

ETIOLOGY AND EPIDEMIOLOGY

Pentatrichomonas hominis is a piriform flagellate inhabiting the large intestines (particularly the cecum) of people, dogs, cats, and some other mammals. Transmission is direct via the fecal-oral route. The organisms exist only in the trophozoite stage. Trophozoites bear five anteriorly directed flagella and a single, posteriorly directed flagellum that arises at the anterior end and courses along the body of the trophozoite attached to the undulating membrane, a characteristic feature of trichomonads. A rigid, rod-shaped organelle, the axostyle, runs through the trophozoite and protrudes from the posterior end (see Fig. 78–4).

CLINICAL FINDINGS

It is widely thought that *P. hominis* does not cause disease in dogs and cats, although it is possible that it is an opportunistic pathogen. There is no doubt that large numbers of trophozoites may be seen in diarrheic feces of dogs, yet an unambiguous, causal relationship remains to be established. Large-bowel diarrhea characterized by fresh blood and mucus has been observed in cats.[20a, 40]

DIAGNOSIS AND THERAPY

Microscopic examination of fecal smears, as described previously for *Giardia* trophozoites, will reveal the tiny, motile trophozoites (see Table 78–1). The trophozoites of *P. hominis* must be distinguished from those of *Giardia* because intercurrent infections can occur. If desired, trichomoniasis may be eliminated with metronidazole at the dosages given for *Giardia* (see Table 78–2). In some cats, treatment with metronidazole, tylosin, fenbendazole, and enrofloxacin has been ineffective.[20a] Paromomycin appears to be the most effective therapy.[10a, 20a]

Amebiasis

ETIOLOGY AND EPIDEMIOLOGY

Entamoeba histolytica is a facultatively parasitic ameba that predominantly infects people and nonhuman primates. Although the prevalence of amebiasis in the United States has declined considerably over the last several decades, *E. histolytica* remains an important parasite in many tropical areas around the world.

Trophozoites either inhabit the colonic lumen as commensals or invade the colonic wall. Rarely do they disseminate to other organs such as the liver, lungs, brain, perianal skin, and genitalia (Figs. 78–5 and 78–6). Various strains of *E. histolytica* differ in virulence. Cysts, passed in human feces, are the infective stages. Because encystment of trophozoites rarely occurs in dogs and cats, amebiasis is among those unusual diseases that are transmissible from humans to pets but seldom vice versa.

Willaertia is a genus of free-living saprophytic amebas

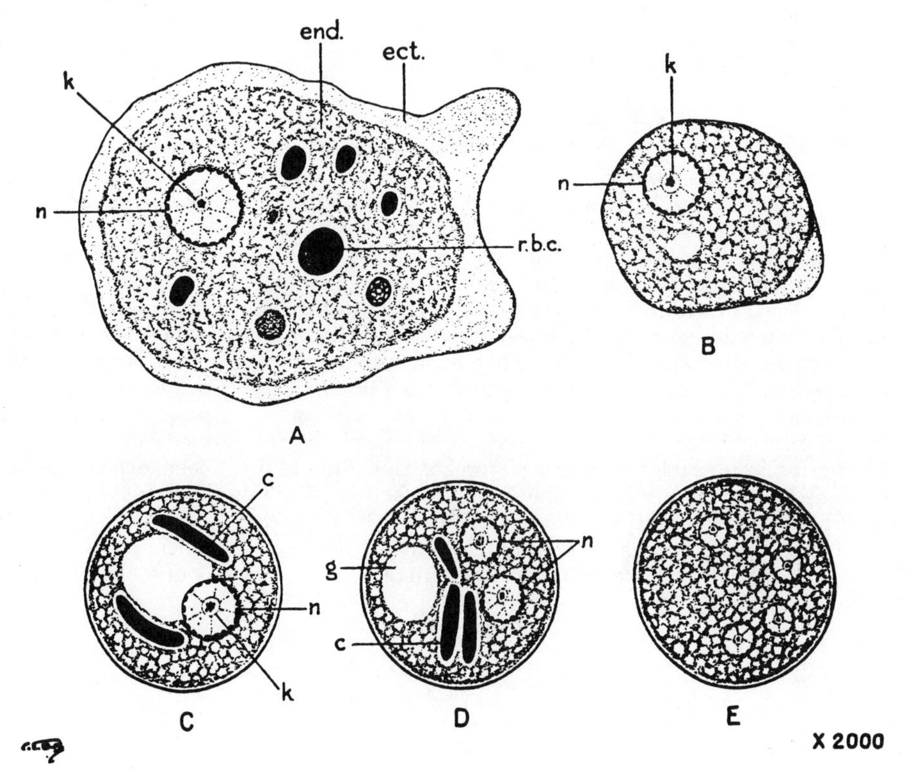

Figure 78–5. Schematic depiction of *E. histolytica* trophozoite *(A)* and various stages of cyst development *(B–E)*. Key: c, chromatoid bodies; g, glycogen vacuole; k, karyosome; n, nucleus; r.b.c., red blood cell; end., endoplasm; ect., ectoplasm. (From Brown HW, Neva FA: *Basic Clinical Parasitology*, ed 5. Copyright Appleton-Century-Crofts, 1983. Reprinted with permission.)

closely related to *Naegleria*. The latter species has been identified in human infections in which trophozoites are found in tissues. This finding contrasts with *Acanthamoeba* (see Chapter 79) that produces tissue cysts.

PATHOGENESIS AND PATHOLOGIC FINDINGS

E. histolytica trophozoites damage the intestine by attaching to and lysing host cells and secreting enzymes that disrupt intercellular connections. The presence of certain bacteria and a host with deficient protein intake contribute to parasite virulence. The host's own cellular immune response to tissue-invading amebas can exacerbate the damage. Secretory diarrhea may be induced by serotonin and other factors secreted by the trophozoites.

Invasive amebiasis results in erosion or ulceration of the colonic mucosa. Microscopic examination of infected colonic tissue may reveal the classic flask-shaped ulcer of amebiasis, which is the result of mucosal undermining by trophozoites in the submucosa. Trophozoites may be seen in sections stained with H and E, iron hematoxylin, or periodic acid–Schiff reaction (see Fig. 78–6).

CLINICAL FINDINGS

E. histolytica infections are usually nonsymptomatic but can lead to signs of severe ulcerative colitis, including dysentery. Fulminant, untreated amebiasis may prove fatal. Extraintestinal amebiasis, a serious complication, is rare in dogs and unknown in cats. In such cases, signs would be referable to the parasitized tissue (e.g., lung). Vulval swelling and bloody vaginal discharge have been reported in a dog with uterine, cervical, and vaginal invasion with trophozoites.

A gastric infection with *Willaertia* was described in a dog with gastric ulceration and adenocarcinoma.[42a] The dog had been receiving glucocorticoids for paraparesis and was vomiting and had melena.

DIAGNOSIS AND THERAPY

Definitive diagnosis of amebiasis in dogs and cats requires finding *E. histolytica* trophozoites in feces or tissues (see Table 78–1). Trophozoites are difficult to detect in fecal specimens. Direct smears of fresh feces reveal the sluggish, ameboid motility of the trophozoites. In invasive amebiasis, trophozoites may contain erythrocytes. Macrophages in feces may be confused with trophozoites. Methylene blue staining of a wet mount may be helpful in revealing amebas. Trichrome- or iron-hematoxylin–stained fecal smears are ideal for diagnosis, but these techniques are best left to a reference laboratory (Appendix 5). Fecal concentration methods (i.e., flotation or sedimentation) are unsuitable for *E. histolytica* trophozoites. In clinically affected animals, a more reliable means of detecting the trophozoites is the microscopic examination of a sectioned biopsy specimen of colonic mucosa (see Fig. 78–6). An ELISA-based antigen test has been shown to be parasite specific in dogs[34] but its clinical application has not been evaluated. For available test kits, see Appendix 6.

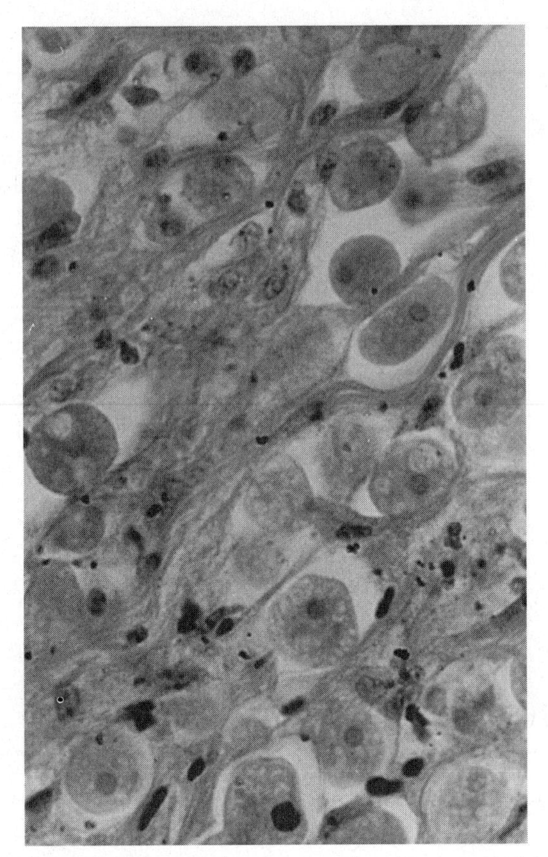

Figure 78–6. Numerous *E. histolytica* trophozoites in a section from the wall of a human colon. Each organism contains a single darkly stained nucleus; in some of the trophozoites, pale vacuoles are apparent (H and E, × 540).

Colitis caused by *E. histolytica* rapidly responds to metronidazole at doses recommended for treatment of giardiasis (see Table 78–2), but dogs can continue to shed organisms.[1, 27]

Diagnosis of free-living amebiasis is best achieved by tissue biopsy. Trophozoites, rather than cysts, are identified in tissue margins of the ulcer and in the serosal exudate. Immunostaining can be used to determine the species of ameba present.[42a]

PUBLIC HEALTH CONSIDERATIONS

Although amebiasis is a potentially serious human disease, it is unlikely that dogs and cats are significant reservoirs of these parasites for people. It is more likely that dogs and cats acquire their infections from human feces or from food or water contaminated by human feces. Although amebiasis is not a zoonosis, the finding of *E. histolytica* in a pet should prompt the veterinarian to suggest that the owners seek medical advice. The owners could have infected the pet or been exposed to a common source of *E. histolytica* cysts. With free-living amebiasis, people and animals are at risk for exposure to the same environmental sources. Immunocompetency is important in determining whether infection becomes established.

Balantidiasis

ETIOLOGY AND EPIDEMIOLOGY

Balantidium coli is a relatively large (see Table 78–1), ciliated protozoan found throughout the world. Although the pig is the most frequently infected animal, dogs and people sometimes become infected with *B. coli*. Infection in the cat has not been reported. Like *E. histolytica*, *B. coli* trophozoites inhabit the colon, either as commensals or invasive parasites, and cysts are passed in the feces. Cysts are infective when ingested by a susceptible host.

PATHOGENESIS AND PATHOLOGIC FINDINGS

Why normally commensal *B. coli* trophozoites may become virulent in some instances remains an unanswered question. Certain colonic bacteria and concurrent *Trichuris vulpis* (whipworm) infections may contribute to *B. coli* invasiveness.

The gross and microscopic features of balantidiasis closely resemble those of amebiasis in the colon. Unlike amebiasis, extraintestinal metastases of *B. coli* trophozoites is very rare. Routinely processed sections of affected colonic tissue will reveal the trophozoites with their characteristic cilia and bean-shaped macronucleus (Figs. 78–7 and 78–8).

CLINICAL FINDINGS

Balantidiasis is clinically indistinguishable from some other causes of hemorrhagic colitis, including amebiasis and trichuriasis. There may be a history of contact with swine, although pigs are usually nonsymptomatic.

DIAGNOSIS AND THERAPY

B. coli cysts and, occasionally, trophozoites may be detected on fecal flotation, using the ZSCT. Fresh fecal smears in an isotonic solution are preferred to demonstrate the motile trophozoites. The distinctive macronucleus of both cyst and trophozoite (Figs. 78–7, 78–8, and 78–9) is invisible unless stained. A drop of acidic methyl green solution (1 g methyl green, 1 ml glacial acetic acid, 100 ml water) added to the preparation will reveal the macronucleus in most of the organisms after a few minutes of contact.

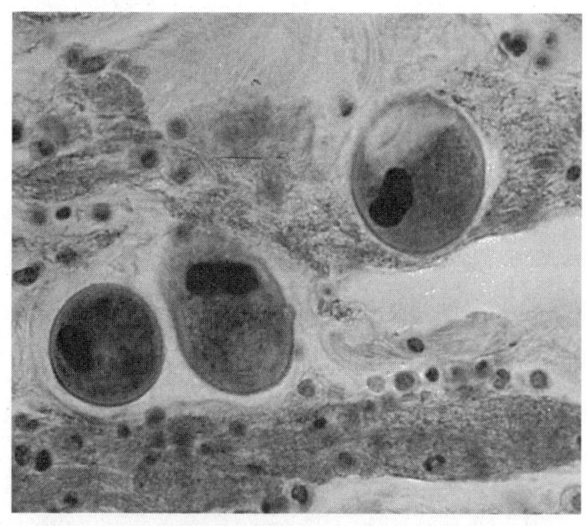

Figure 78–8. *B. coli* trophozoites in a section from the wall of a human colon. Note the prominent parasite macronuclei and the surrounding inflammatory response (H and E, × 250).

Reports of therapy of canine balantidiasis are lacking. However, on the basis of human clinical studies, oral metronidazole (see Table 78–2) or tetracyclines should prove effective in the dog.

PUBLIC HEALTH CONSIDERATIONS

Because *B. coli*–infected dogs may excrete cysts in their feces, the potential for transmission of the parasite from dog to people exists. Compared with swine, however, dogs are

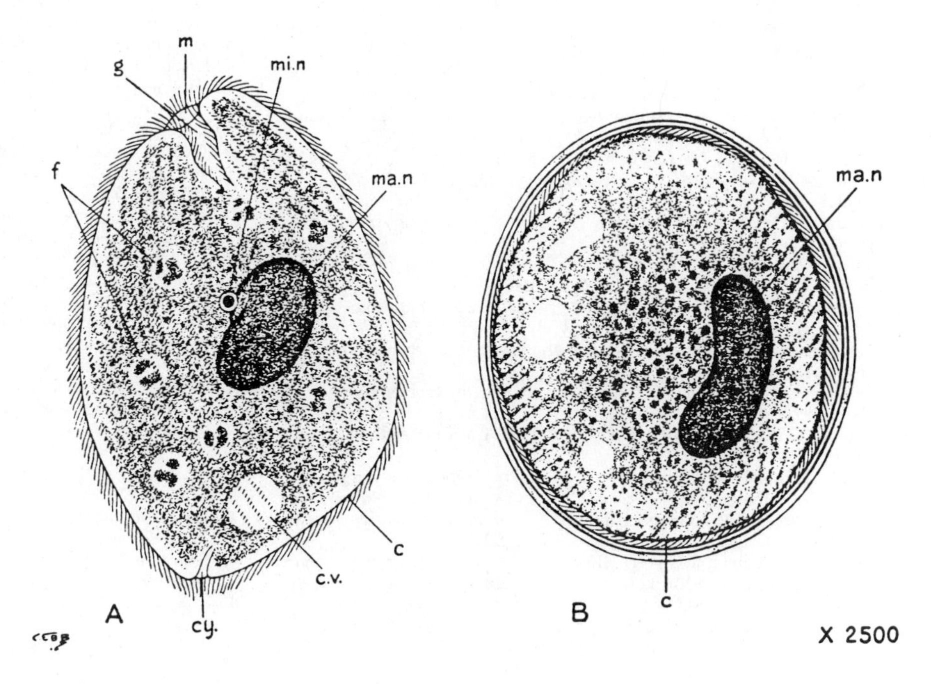

Figure 78–7. Schematic diagram of a *B. coli* trophozoite *(A)* and cyst *(B)*. Key: c, cilia; c.v., contractile vacuole; cy., cytopyge; f, food vacuole; g, gullet; m, mouth; ma.n, macronucleus; mi.n, micronucleus. (From Brown HW, Neva FA: *Basic Clinical Parasitology*, ed 5. Copyright Appleton-Century-Crofts, 1983. Reprinted with permission.)

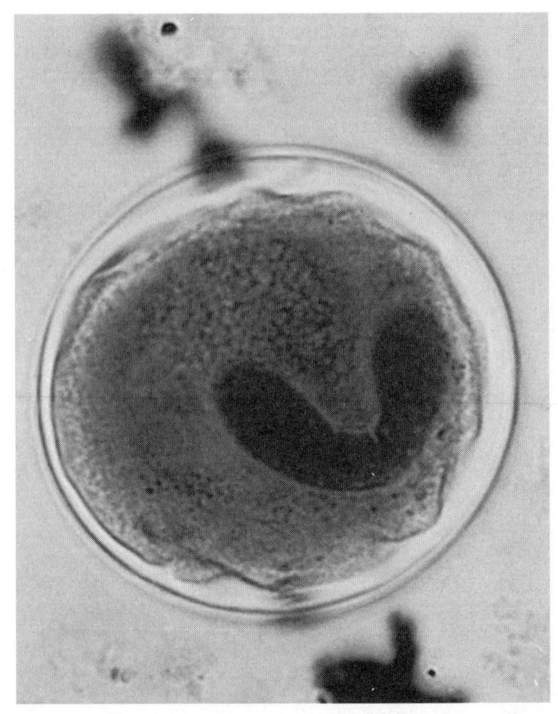

Figure 78–9. *B. coli* cyst in a fixed and stained fecal smear. The hyaline cyst wall and macronucleus are conspicuous. (Giemsa stain, × 1200.)

so uncommonly infected that they cannot be considered significant reservoirs of *B. coli* for people.

References

1. Ajuwape ATP, Nottidge HO. 1993. Amoebiasis in a four-month-old puppy: a case report. *Trop Vet* 11:69–73.
2. Barr SC, Bowman DD. 1994. Giardiasis in dogs and cats. *Compend Cont Educ Pract Vet* 16:603–611.
3. Barr SC, Bowman DD, Erb HN. 1992. Evaluation of two test procedures for diagnosis of giardiasis in dogs. *Am J Vet Res* 53:2028–2031.
4. Barr SC, Bowman DD, Heller RL, et al. 1993. Efficacy of albendazole against giardiasis in dogs. *Am J Vet Res* 54:926–928.
5. Barr SC, Bowman DD, Heller RL, et al. 1993. Efficacy of albendazole against *Giardia* sp in dogs and cats. *Proc Am Assoc Vet Parasitol* 83:56.
6. Barr SC, Bowman DD, Heller RL. 1994. Efficacy of fenbendazole against giardiasis in dogs. *Am J Vet Res* 55:988–990.
7. Baruch AC, Isaac-Renton J, Adam RD. 1996. The molecular epidemiology of *Giardia lamblia*: a sequence-based approach. *J Infect Dis* 174:233–236.
8. Carnaby S, McHugh TD, Katelaris PH, et al. 1991. DNA fingerprinting of *Giardia lamblia* with the M13 bacteriophage genome. *Gut* 32:596–597.
9. Cevallos AM, Carnaby S, James M, et al. 1992. Small intestinal injury in a neonatal rat model of giardiasis is strain dependent. *Gastroenterology* 109:766–773.
10. Cevallos AM, Farthing MJG. 1992. Differences in functional mucosal damage between *Giardia lamblia* isolates. *Gut* 33:176.

10a. Chamberlin T. 1998. Williamsburg, VA. Personal communication.

11. Char S, Cevallos AM, Yamson P, et al. 1993. Impaired IgA response to *Giardia* heat shock antigen in children with persistent diarrhoea and giardiasis. *Gut* 34:38–40.
12. Davidson RA. 1984. Issues in clinical parasitology: the treatment of giardiasis. *Am J Gastroenterol* 79:256–261.
13. Doglioni C, De Boni M, Cielo R, et al. 1992. Gastric giardiasis. *J Clin Pathol* 45:964–967.
14. Douglas H, Reiner DS, Gault MJ, et al. 1988. Location of *Giardia* trophozoites in the small intestine of naturally infected dogs in San Diego, pp 65–69. *In* Wallis PM, Hammond BR (eds), Advances in *Giardia* research. University of Calgary Press, Calgary, Alberta, Canada.
15. Dow SW, LeCouteur RA, Poss ML, et al. 1989. Central nervous system toxicosis associated with metronidazole treatment of dogs: five cases (1984–1987). *J Am Vet Med Assoc* 195:365–368.
16. Ewing GO, Aldrete A. 1973. Canine giardiasis presenting as chronic ulcerative colitis: a case report. *J Am Anim Hosp Assoc* 9:52–55.
17. Ey PL, Bruderer T, Wehrlic C, et al. 1996. Comparison of genetic groups determined by molecular and immunological analyses of *Giardia* isolated from animals and humans in Switzerland and Australia. *Parasitol Res* 82:52–60.
18. Farbey MD, Reynoldson JA, Thompson RCA. 1995. In vitro drug susceptibility of 29 isolates of *Giardia duodenalis* from humans as assessed by an adhesion assay. *Int J Parasitol* 25:593–599.
19. Farthing MJG. 1990. Immunopathology of giardiasis. *Springer Semin Immunopathol* 12:269–282.
20. Fitch R, Moore M, Roen D. 1992. Metronidazole neurotoxicity in a dog. *Prog Vet Neurol* 2:307–309.

20a. Gookin J. North Carolina State University. Personal communication.

21. Hartong WA, Gourley WK, Arvanitakis C. 1979. Giardiasis: clinical spectrum and functional-structural abnormalities of the small intestinal mucosa. *Gastroenterology* 77:61–69.
22. Hay DC, Savva D, Nowell F. 1990. Characterization of *Giardia* species of canine and human origin using RFLPs. *Vet Rec* 126:274.
23. Heazlewood VJ. 1987. Giardiasis and vitamin B12 deficiency. *Aust N Z J Med* 17:261.
24. Hewlett EL, Andrews JS, Ruffier J, et al. 1982. Experimental infection of mongrel dogs with *Giardia lamblia* cysts and cultured trophozoites. *J Infect Dis* 145:89–93.
25. Hitchcock DJ, Malewitz TD. 1956. Habitat of *Giardia* in the kitten. *J Parasitol* 42:286.

25a. Hopkins RM, Meloni BP, Groth DM, et al. 1997. Ribosomal RNA sequencing reveals differences between the genotypes of *Giardia* isolates recovered from humans and dogs living in the same locality. *J Parasitol* 83:44–51.

26. Isaac-Renton J, Moorehead W, Ross A. 1996. Longitudinal studies of *Giardia* contamination in two community drinking water supplies: cyst levels, parasite viability, and health impact. *Appl Environ Microbiol* 62:47–54.
27. Jani RG, Dave MR. 1992. A case study of amoebic dysentery in a pup. *Indian Vet J* 69:852–853.
28. Janoff EN, Smith PD. 1994. The role of immunity in *Giardia* infections, pp 215–233. *In* Meyer EA (ed), Giardiasis. Elsevier, New York, NY.
29. Kirkpatrick CE. 1990. Enteric protozoal infections, pp 804–814. *In* Greene CE (ed), Infectious diseases of the dog and cat. WB Saunders, Philadelphia, PA.
30. Majewska AC. 1994. Successful experimental infections of a human volunteer and Mongolian gerbils with *Giardia* of animal origin. *Trans R Soc Trop Med Hyg* 88:360–362.
31. Milstein TC, Goldsmid JM. 1995. The presence of *Giardia* and other zoonotic parasites of urban dogs in Hobart, Tasmania. *Aust Vet J* 72:154–155.
32. Nash TE, Herrington DA, Levine MM, et al. 1990. Antigenic variation of *Giardia lamblia* in experimental human infections. *J Immunol* 144:4362–4369.
33. Nash TE, Merritt JW, Conrad JT. 1991. Isolate and epitope variability in susceptibility of *Giardia lamblia* to intestinal proteases. *Infect Immun* 59:1334–1340.
34. Nogami S, Inove I, Araki K, et al. 1991. Specificity of commercially available *Entamoeba histolytica* antigen in enzyme-linked immunosorbent assay (ELISA) to sera from dogs with various parasitic infections. *J Vet Med Sci* 53:729–731.
35. Nolan TJ, Smith G. 1995. Time series analysis of the prevalence of endoparasitic infections in cats and dogs presented to a veterinary teaching hospital. *Vet Parasitol* 59:87–96.
36. Oberhuber G, Stolte M. 1990. Giardiasis: analysis of histological changes in biopsy specimens of 80 patients. *J Clin Pathol* 43:641–643.
37. Olson ME, Morck DW, Ceri H. 1995. The efficacy of a *Giardia lamblia* vaccine in kittens. *Can J Vet Res* 60:249–256.

37a. Ortega YR, Adam RD. 1997. *Giardia*: overview and update. *Clin Infect Dis* 25:545–550.

38. Pitts RP, Twedt DC, Mallie KA. 1983. Comparison of duodenal aspiration with fecal flotation for diagnosis of giardiasis in dogs. *J Am Vet Med Assoc* 182:1210–1211.
39. Quincey C, James PD, Steele RJC. 1992. Chronic giardiasis of the stomach. *J Clin Pathol* 45:1039–1041.
40. Romatowski J. 1996. An uncommon protozoan parasite (*Pentatrichomonas hominis*) associated with colitis in three cats. *Feline Pract* 24:10–14.
41. Rosenthal P, Liebman WM. 1980. Comparative study of stool examinations, duodenal aspiration, and pediatric Entero-Test for giardiasis in children. *J Pediatr* 96:278–279.
42. Rosoff JD, Sanders CA, Sonnad SS, et al. 1989. Stool diagnosis of giardiasis using a commercially available enzyme immunoassay to detect *Giardia*-specific antigen 65 (GSA 65). *J Clin Microbiol* 27:1997–2002.

42a. Steele KE, Visvesvara GS, Bradley GA, et al. 1997. Amebiasis in a dog with gastric ulcers and adenocarcinoma. *J Vet Diagn Invest* 9:91–93.

43. Theodorides VJ, Daly IW, Kraeer P, et al. 1989. Human safety studies with albendazole. *Proc Am Assoc Vet Parasitol* 55:41.
44. Tonks MC, Brown TJ, Ionas G. 1991. *Giardia* infection of cats and dogs in New Zealand. *N Z Vet J* 39:33–34.
45. Tsuchiya H. 1931. The localization of *Giardia canis* (Hegner, 1922) as affected by diet. *J Parasitol* 18:232–246.
46. Upcroft JA, Upcroft P. 1993. Drug resistance and *Giardia*. *Parasitol Today* 9:187–190.
47. Xiao L, Herd RP. 1993. Quantitation of *Giardia* cysts and *Cryptosporidium*

oocysts in fecal samples by direct immunofluorescence assay. *J Clin Microbiol* 31:2944–2946.
47a. Zajac AM, LaBranche TP, Donoghue AR, et al. 1998. Efficacy of fenbendazole in the treatment of experimental *Giardia* infection in dogs. *Am J Vet Res* 59:61–63.
48. Zajac AM, Leib MS, Burkholder WJ. 1992. *Giardia* infection in a group of experimental dogs. *J Small Anim Pract* 33:257–260.
49. Zajac AM, Leib MS, Saunders G, et al. 1992. Experimental infection of dogs with *Giardia*. *Proc Am Assoc Vet Parasitol* 82:55.
50. Zimmerman SK, Needham CA. 1995. Comparison of conventional stool concentration and preserved-smear methods with Merifluor *Cryptosporidium/Giardia* direct immunofluorescence assay and ProSpecT *Giardia* EZ microplate assay for detection of *Giardia lamblia*. *J Clin Microbiol* 33:1942–1943.

Chapter 79

Acanthamebiasis

Craig E. Greene

ETIOLOGY

Acanthamoeba is a genus of ubiquitous free-living amebas found in fresh and salt water, soil, and sewage. Organisms of this genus cause pneumonia and encephalitis in people and animals and disseminated dermatitis and chronic keratitis in people. Acanthamebiasis has been reported in dogs mostly as solitary cases, except possibly in a greyhound kennel where multiple dogs have been infected. Acanthamebiasis has not been described in cats.

Acanthamoeba has a relatively simple life cycle with two stages in the environment and host tissues. A vegetative replicating trophozoite feeds mostly on bacteria in nature and host cells in vivo. A cyst phase is often able to resist adverse environmental conditions, including desiccation and possibly host immune responses. Several *Acanthamoeba* species are pathogenic for animals and people. *A. castellanii* and *A. culbertsoni* have been found in canine infections. Two related organisms, *Naegleria fowleri* and *Leptomyxida amebae*, also cause meningoencephalitis in people but are not known to infect dogs or cats.

EPIDEMIOLOGY

In dogs, epizootics of acanthamebiasis have been observed in greyhounds, whereas singular cases have been described in a German shepherd dog and an immunosuppressed Akita. Young dogs appear to be most susceptible. Affected greyhounds varied from 4 to 13 months of age. In outbreaks, organisms are thought to be acquired from a common environmental source rather than from other animals. The source of infection and the incubation period in dogs are unknown.

Immunosuppressed persons such as organ transplant patients, AIDS patients, alcoholics, diabetics, or otherwise debilitated individuals are at high risk and are particularly susceptible to acanthamebiasis. In critically ill or debilitated people, *Acanthamoeba* species typically cause a chronic granulomatous meningoencephalitis, which may last for more than a week to months before death occurs. Amebic keratitis has been seen in otherwise healthy people who wear contact lenses or who have minor corneal trauma. Tap water, used to make saline solutions, has been incriminated.[6]

In people, routes of infection may include inhalation of organisms from contaminated air or water during breathing or swimming. The organisms can replicate in the upper or lower respiratory tract after inhalation or in skin or other tissues after penetrating injuries. They then spread to the CNS by hematogenous means. Alternatively, infection of the cornea and nasal passage might lead to a retrograde spread to the nervous system via optic and olfactory nerves, respectively.

CLINICAL FINDINGS

Clinical manifestations of canine acanthamebiasis and canine distemper are remarkably similar. Initial signs include mild oculonasal discharge, anorexia, and lethargy. Rectal temperature varies from normal to as high as 40.5°C (105°F). Respiratory distress and neurologic signs follow. Most dogs eventually show neurologic dysfunction. Coughing and dyspnea may be observed after a few days. Neurologic signs include incoordination, head tilt, stumbling, dysmetria, and seizures. Severely affected dogs are tetraplegic, in lateral recumbency, and unable to right themselves. Less severely affected greyhounds are permanently disabled for performance racing.

DIAGNOSIS

The clinical laboratory abnormalities in acanthamebiasis are nonspecific. Leukopenia is due to marked lymphopenia in greyhounds and reduction in all types of blood leukocytes in other breeds. The cause of the leukopenia is unknown but may be concurrent infectious disease, stress, or specific factor(s) produced by the *Acanthamoeba*.

Premortem diagnosis of acanthamebiasis in dogs has been rare. Culture or biopsy of affected tissues would be the most specific means of confirmation. Although lung and CNS tissues are not readily accessible, the possibility of finding organisms in CSF and tracheal washings has not been evaluated.

Amebas can be cultured from lesions by special methods that are not done in most laboratories because biocontainment facilities are needed.[1] Organisms grow sparingly on potato dextrose agar, where amebas grow as individual colonies with many cysts, or on non-nutrient agar seeded with bacteria, where they grow more rapidly as a confluent expanding ringlike mass of trophozoites with cysts at the central portion. Organisms can also be isolated in cell culture, where they cause cytopathic effects. Mouse inoculation can be used to test the pathogenicity of isolated strains.

PATHOLOGIC FINDINGS

Lung and brain lesions have been observed grossly in all cases. Lung lesions vary from light-tan to deep-red, raised, semisolid nodules distributed uniformly throughout all lobes. The nodules show a tendency to coalesce, and intralesional cavitations have been noted. Brain lesions may be large, multifocal, and visible on the meningeal surfaces of the cerebrum and cerebellum and vary from red to tannish-brown as the result of recent hemorrhage or necrosis.

Microscopically, lung and brain lesions are generally circumscribed to coalescing areas of granulomatous inflammation; however, focally diffuse meningeal inflammatory infiltrates have been seen. Thrombi, hemorrhage, necrosis, and mixed inflammatory cell infiltrates are present in the subarachnoid space of the meninges. Perivascular inflammation in the neuropil is composed of a mixture of macrophages, some neutrophils, and plasma cells. Trophozoites and occasional cyst forms of *Acanthamoeba* are seen within alveolar spaces and terminal bronchioles (Fig. 79–1). In brain lesions, the amebas are best visualized in perivascular and subarachnoid spaces, because in the neural parenchyma they are often masked by the presence of infiltrating inflammatory cells. Lesions in other tissues are not consistent, but granulomatous foci in the glomeruli of some dogs have been observed associated with trophozoites.

Histologic and FA methods are utilized to demonstrate and identify the organism in tissues. Free-living pathogenic amebas are difficult to differentiate microscopically from certain mammalian cells, especially macrophages. The diagnostic feature of *Acanthamoeba* in histologic sections is the centrally located nucleolus ("targetoid karyosome") and

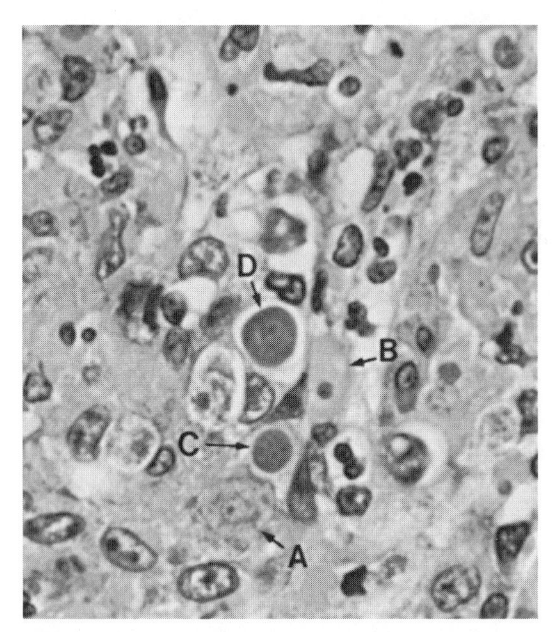

Figure 79–1. Lung of greyhound, pneumonia. Several *Acanthamoeba* are clustered together. Note the morphologic progression from trophozoite to cyst form (*arrows* A–D) (H and E, × 400).

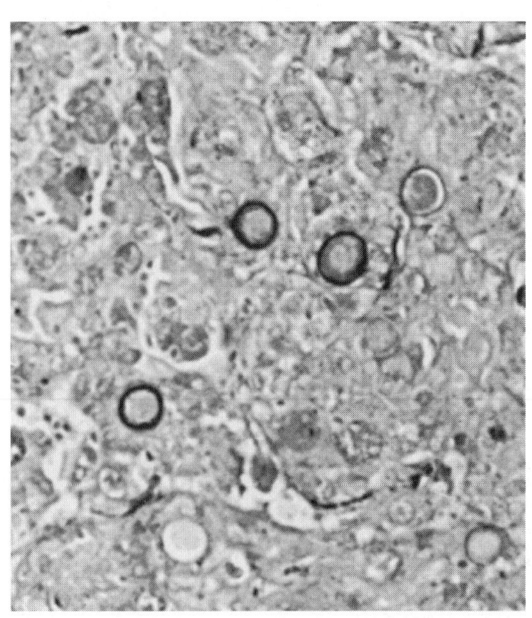

Figure 79–2. Lung of greyhound, pneumonia; same case as Figure 79–1. Only the cell wall of the cyst form is stained. The body of the *Acanthamoeba* apart from the cell wall takes up the background stain (Gomori's methenamine silver stain, × 320).

vacuolated cytoplasm. No histochemical stain has been found to be specific for *Acanthamoeba*. Periodic acid–Schiff and Gomori's methenamine silver methods stain only the cyst wall (Fig. 79–2). Direct FA staining is specific and reliable on deparaffinized sections of formalin-fixed tissue and, with specific conjugates, can distinguish between various species of *Acanthamoeba*.

THERAPY AND PREVENTION

There is no well-established therapeutic regimen for systemic acanthamebiasis and no consistent susceptibility. Drugs active against *Acanthamoeba* in vitro include polyene antifungals (amphotericin B) and imidazoles (ketoconazole) and the antitubercular drug rifampicin, among others.[4] Rifampicin was effective in treating mice with meningitis.[4] In one immunocompromised person with disseminated skin lesions from *A. rhysodes* infection, treatment was successful with topical chlorhexidine gluconate and ketoconazole cream and systemic treatment with pentamidine followed by itraconazole.[11] Combination therapy with IV pentamidine, oral fluconazole, flucytosine, and sulfadiazine is recommended in people with disseminated and CNS infections.[7] Sulfadiazine has been beneficial in treating experimental infection in mice, and trimethoprim-sulfonamide was effective in curing a child with meningoencephalitis after 8 weeks of therapy.[9] Should a dog be identified as being infected, one or more of these drugs should be used. The dosage of trimethoprim-sulfonamide is 30 mg/kg given every 12 hours.

Dogs may be exposed to low numbers of *Acanthamoeba* throughout their lifetimes. Because these are free-living amebas, prevention is accomplished by avoiding access to contaminated water. Pathogenic free-living amebas are found more frequently in thermally enriched and polluted discharge water from industrial plants, lakes, and swimming pools. Nonthermally enriched water contains fewer amebas. A 0.5% solution of sodium hypochlorite is a satisfactory aqueous disinfectant. Because *Acanthamoeba* feed on bacteria, water sources can be initially screened for amebas by testing for coliforms.

PUBLIC HEALTH CONSIDERATIONS

There is no known transmission of infection between hosts, and infections are thought to originate solely from environmental sources. The dog, however, serves as sentinel for human infection because of a common environmental exposure.

References

1. Bauer RW, Harrison LR, Watson CW, et al. 1993. Isolation of *Acanthamoeba* sp. from a greyhound with pneumonia and granulomatous amebic encephalitis. *J Vet Diagn Invest* 5:386–391.
2. Brasseur G, Favenneck L, Perrine D, et al. 1994. Successful treatment of *Acanthamoeba* keratitis by hexamidine. *Cornea* 13:459–462.
3. Buergelt CD, Harrison LR, Bauer RW. 1991. Diagnostic exercise: pneumonia and CNS disturbances in young greyhound dogs. *Lab Anim Sci* 41:76–77.
4. Das SR, Asiri AS, El-Soofi A. 1991. Protective and curative effects of rifampicin in *Acanthamoeba* meningitis of the mouse. *J Infect Dis* 163:916–917.
5. Harrison LR, Bauer RW. 1990. Acanthamebiasis, pp 815–817. *In* Greene CE (ed), Infectious diseases of the dog and cat. WB Saunders, Philadelphia, PA.
6. Kilvington S, Larkin DFP, White DG, et al. 1990. Laboratory investigation of *Acanthamoeba* keratitis. *J Clin Microbiol* 28:2722–2725.
7. Murakawa GJ, McCalmont T, Altman J, et al. 1995. Disseminated acanthamebiasis in patients with AIDS. A report of five cases and a review of the literature. *Arch Dermatol* 131:1291–1296.
8. Niederkorn JY, Ubelaker JE, McCulley JP, et al. 1992. Susceptibility of corneas from various animal species to in vitro binding and invasion by *Acanthamoeba castellanii*. *Invest Ophthalmol Vis Sci* 33:104–112.
9. Sharma PP, Gupta P, Murali MV, et al. 1993. Primary amebic meningoencephalitis caused by *Acanthamoeba*: successfully treated with cotrimoxazole. *Indian Pediatr* 30:1219–1222.
10. Sison JP, Kemper CA, Loveless M, et al. 1995. Disseminated *Acanthamoeba* infection in patients with AIDS: case reports and review. *Clin Infect Dis* 20:1207–1216.
11. Slater CA, Sickel JZ, Visvesvara GS, et al. 1994. Brief report: successful treatment of disseminated *Acanthamoeba* infection in an immunocompromised patient. *N Engl J Med* 331:85–87.

Chapter **80**

Toxoplasmosis and Neosporosis

J. P. Dubey and Michael R. Lappin

Toxoplasmosis

ETIOLOGY

Toxoplasma gondii is an obligate intracellular coccidian parasite that infects virtually all species of warm-blooded animals, including people. Domestic cats and other Felidae are the definitive hosts. All nonfeline hosts are intermediate hosts. There are three infectious stages: sporozoites in oocysts, tachyzoites (actively multiplying stage), and bradyzoites (slowly multiplying stage) enclosed in tissue cysts. Oocysts are excreted in feces, whereas tachyzoites and bradyzoites are found in tissues.

EPIDEMIOLOGY

The three major modes of transmission are congenital infection, ingestion of infected tissues, and ingestion of oocyst-contaminated food or water (Fig. 80–1). Other minor modes of transmission include transfusion of fluids or transplantation of organs.[33]

Enteroepithelial Life Cycle

This cycle is found only in the definitive feline host. Most cats are thought to become infected by ingesting intermediate hosts infected with tissue cysts. Bradyzoites are released in the stomach and intestine from the tissue cysts when the cyst wall is dissolved by digestive enzymes. Bradyzoites penetrate the epithelial cells of small intestine and initiate the five types (A–E) of predetermined asexual stages (Fig. 80–2). These types, A to E, are equivalent to schizonts of other intestinal coccidia. After an undetermined number of generations, merozoites released from type D or E form male (micro) or female (macro) gamonts. The microgamont divides and forms several biflagellate microgametes, which are released and swim to and penetrate macrogamonts. A wall is formed around the fertilized macrogamont to form an oocyst. Oocysts are round to oval, 10×12 μm, and are unsporulated (uninfective) when passed in feces. After exposure to air and moisture for 1 to 5 days, oocysts sporulate and contain two sporocysts, each with four sporozoites. Sporozoites are banana shaped, approximately 8×2 μm, and can survive in the oocyst for many months, even under harsh environmental conditions.

The entire enteroepithelial (coccidian) cycle of *T. gondii* can be completed within 3 to 10 days after ingestion of tissue cysts and occurs in up to 97% of naive cats. However, after ingestion of oocysts or tachyzoites, the formation of oocysts is delayed until 18 days or more, and only 20% of cats fed oocysts will develop patency.[31] The differences in the life cycle that account for this delay and resistance are uncertain,

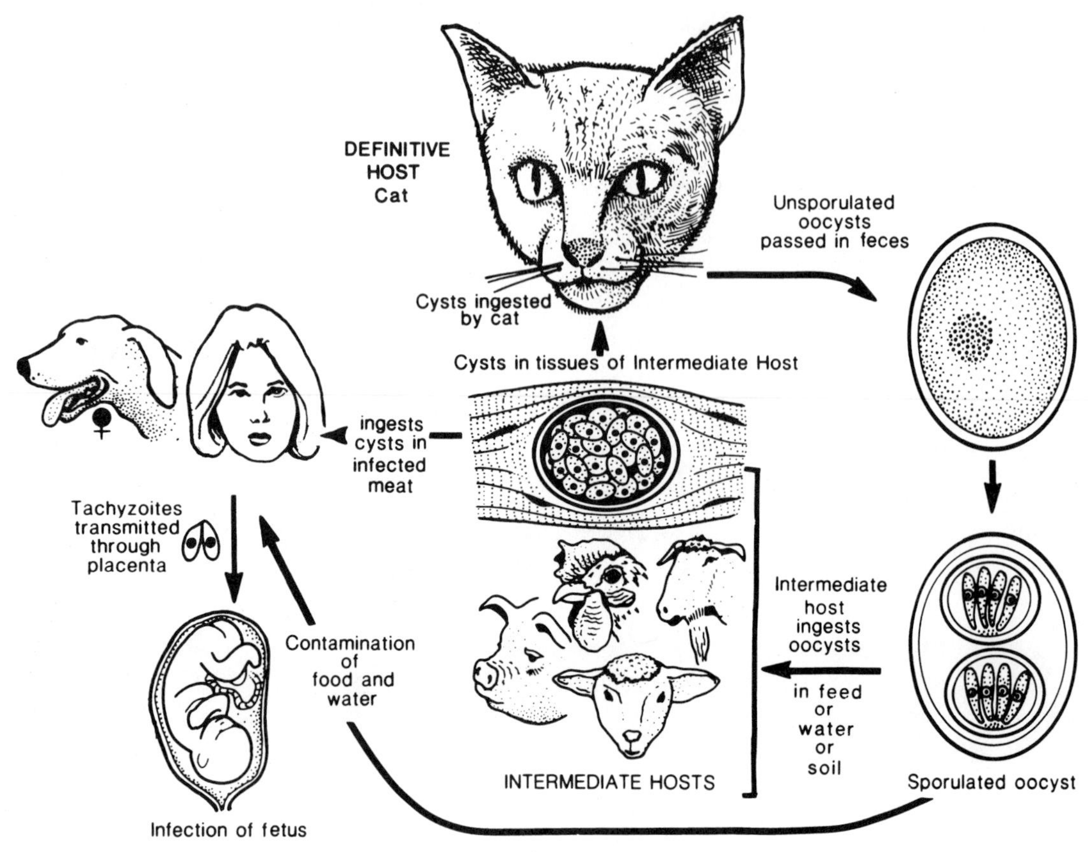

Figure 80–1. Life cycle of *T. gondii.*

but bradyzoites are probably precursors of enteroepithelial replication.

Experimentally, dogs have been fed sporulated oocysts from cat feces, which passed through into their feces for 2 days PI.[103a] Although these dogs seroconverted, no clinical signs of infection or enteroepithelial replication occurred. Dogs ingesting cat litter would serve only as potential mechanical vectors for transmission to people.

Extraintestinal Life Cycle

The extraintestinal development of *T. gondii* is the same for all hosts, including dogs, cats, and people, and is not dependent on whether tissue cysts or oocysts are ingested. After the ingestion of oocysts, sporozoites excyst in the lumen of the small intestine and penetrate intestinal cells, including the cells in the lamina propria. Sporozoites divide into two by an asexual process known as endodyogeny and thus become tachyzoites. Tachyzoites are lunate in shape, approximately 6 × 2 μm (Figs. 80–3 and 80–4), and multiply in almost any cell of the body. If the cell ruptures, they infect new cells. Otherwise, tachyzoites multiply intracellularly for an undetermined period and eventually encyst. Tissue cysts grow intracellularly and contain numerous bradyzoites (Figs. 80–5 and 80–6). Bradyzoites resemble tachyzoites in structure except that they are thinner and the nucleus is located at the posterior end of the parasite. Biologically, bradyzoites differ from tachyzoites in that they can survive the digestive process in the stomach, whereas tachyzoites are usually killed. Tissue cysts vary in size from 15 to 60 μm and usually conform to the shape of the parasitized cell. Tissue cysts are

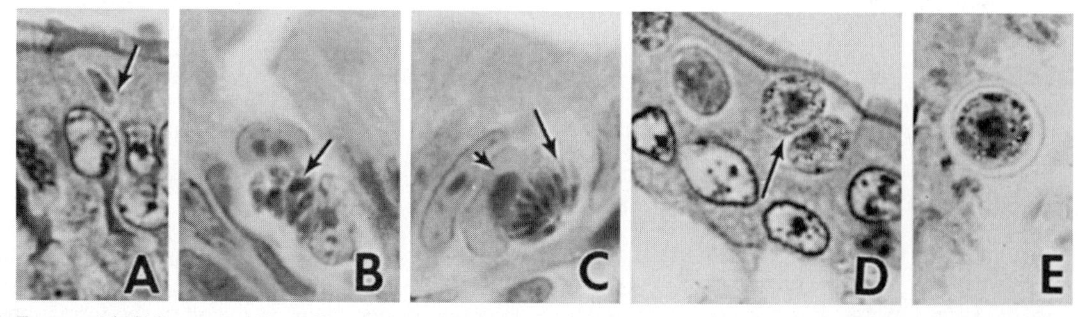

Figure 80–2. Enteroepithelial stages of *T. gondii* in the small intestine of cats (H and E, × 1000). *A*, Merozoite *(arrow)* above the epithelial cell nucleus. *B*, Type B meront *(arrow)*. *C*, Type C meront *(arrow)* in banana-shaped merozoites. The epithelial cell nucleus *(arrowhead)* is hypertrophied. *D*, Two female gamonts on right *(arrow)*, each with one nucleus, and a male gamont on left. *E*, Unsporulated oocyst in intestinal lumen.

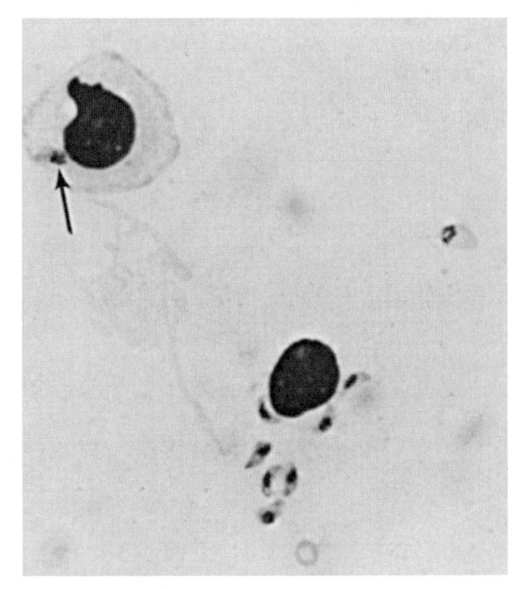

Figure 80–3. Tachyzoites of *T. gondii* in impression smear from lung. One tachyzoite is within a macrophage *(arrow)*, and others are being liberated from the host cell (Giemsa, × 1250). (From Dubey JP: *In* Kreier JP (ed): *Parasitic Protozoa*, Vol 3. Academic Press, 1977, pp 101–237. Reprinted with permission.)

separated from the host cell by a thin (<0.5 μm) elastic wall (see Fig. 80–6). Tissue cysts are formed in the CNS, muscles, and visceral organs and probably persist for the life of the host. Some variation in tissue tropism for cyst formation has been observed.[32a]

Congenital Transmission

Parasitemia during pregnancy can cause placentitis followed by spread of tachyzoites to the fetus. In people or sheep, congenital transmission occurs usually when the woman or ewe becomes infected during pregnancy. Little is known of transplacental toxoplasmosis in dogs, although its prevalence is thought to be less common than that in sheep and goats. Many kittens born to queens infected with *T. gondii* during gestation became infected transplacentally or via suckling.[16, 35, 42, 130] Clinical illness was common, varying with the stage of gestation at the time of infection, and some newborn kittens shed oocysts.[42]

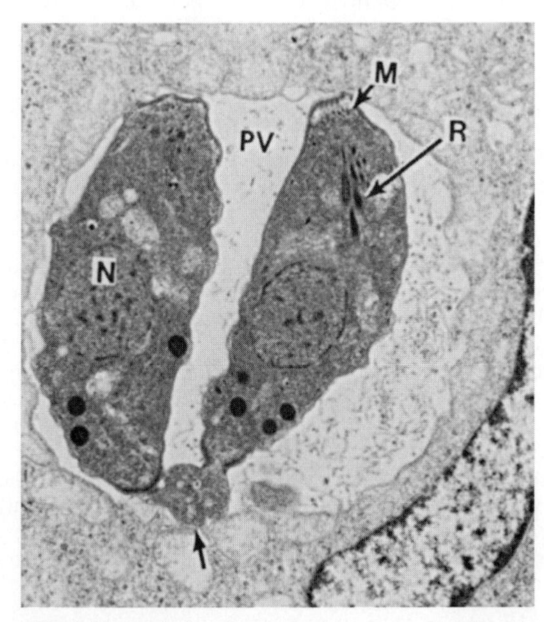

Figure 80–4. Transmission electron micrograph of tachyzoites of *T. gondii.* Tachyzoites are separated from the host cell cytoplasm by a parasitophorous vacuole (PV). One tachyzoite has divided into two progeny that are still attached at the posterior end. Note central nucleus (N), rhoptries (R), and micronemes (M) anterior to the nucleus (× 10,000). (Courtesy of Dr. C. A. Speer, Montana State University, Bozeman, MT.)

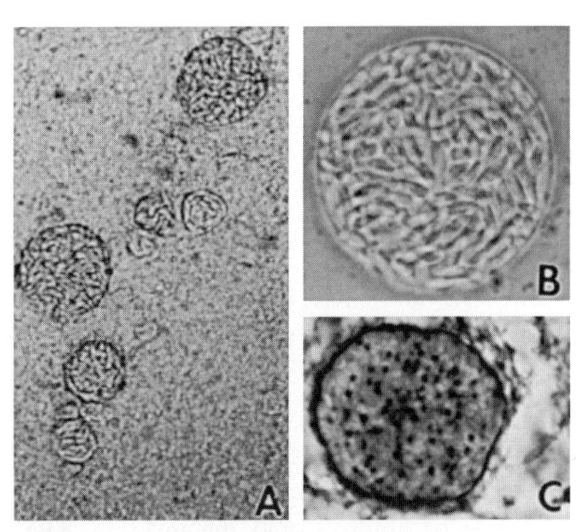

Figure 80–5. *T. gondii* tissue cysts from brain of experimentally infected mice. *A*, Different-size tissue cysts (unstained smear, × 300). *B*, High magnification to show a thin cyst wall and banana-shaped bradyzoites (unstained smear, × 1000). *C*, Tissue cyst in section. The cyst wall is argyrophilic (silver stain, × 1000).

PATHOGENESIS

The type and severity of clinical illness with *T. gondii* infections are dependent on the degree and localization of tissue injury. Tachyzoites are the invasive asexual forms of the parasite that require intracellular existence for replication and survival. All cell types appear susceptible. Cell necrosis is due to the intracellular growth of *Toxoplasma*. *T. gondii* does

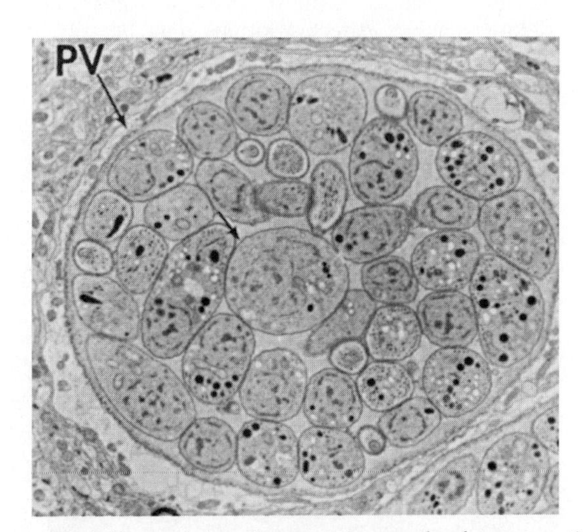

Figure 80–6. Transmission electron micrograph of a young tissue cyst of *T. gondii* in the brain of a mouse, 21 days PI. The tissue cyst is separated from the cytoplasm of the neuron by a parasitophorous vacuole (PV). One bradyzoite *(shorter arrow)* is dividing (× 6500). (Courtesy of Dr. D. J. P. Ferguson, Oxford University, England.)

not produce a toxin. In infections acquired after the ingestion of tissue cysts or oocysts, initial clinical signs are due to the necrosis of intestine and associated lymphoid organs caused by tachyzoites. *T. gondii* then spreads to extraintestinal organs via blood or lymph and focal necrosis may develop in many organs (Fig. 80–7). The brain, liver, lungs, skeletal muscle, and eyes are common sites of initial replication and chronic persistence of infection. The clinical outcome is determined by the extent of injury to these organs, especially vital organs such as the heart, lung, liver, and adrenal glands. Although acute disseminated infections can be fatal, the host often recovers.

By about the third week after infection, tachyzoites begin to disappear from visceral tissues and may localize as tissue cysts (as bradyzoites). These cysts may persist in the host for life. Tissue cysts may rupture, and released bradyzoites may initiate a clinical relapse during immunosuppression, such as with antitumor or glucocorticoid therapy (Fig. 80–8). The mechanism of reactivation is not known.

Why some infected dogs or cats develop clinical toxoplasmosis whereas others remain well is not fully understood. Age, sex, host species, strain of *T. gondii*, number of organisms, and stage of the parasite ingested may account for some of the differences. Postnatally acquired toxoplasmosis is generally less serious than prenatally acquired infection. Stress may also aggravate *T. gondii* infection. Concomitant illness or immunosuppression may make a host more susceptible because *T. gondii* proliferates as an opportunistic pathogen. Clinical toxoplasmosis in dogs is often associated with canine distemper or other infections, such as ehrlichiosis, or with glucocorticoid therapy. In some cases, however, predisposing disorders cannot be found. Historically, the prevalence of canine toxoplasmosis has decreased with the routine use of distemper vaccines.[37] Some cases of clinical feline toxoplasmosis have been observed concomitantly with glucocorticoid therapy, haemobartonellosis, feline leukemia virus (FeLV) and immunodeficiency virus (FIV) infections, and feline infectious peritonitis.[25, 34, 35, 69, 99, 121, 135] In contrast, experimental FIV and FeLV infections in cats were not documented to produce reactivated or more severe acute infections.[89, 91, 122]

CLINICAL FINDINGS

Cats

Clinical toxoplasmosis is most severe in transplacentally infected kittens.[35, 42, 48] Affected kittens may be stillborn or may die before weaning. Kittens may continue to suckle until death. Clinical signs reflect inflammation of the liver, lungs, and CNS. Affected kittens may have an enlarged abdomen because of enlarged liver and ascites. Encephalitic kittens may sleep most of the time or cry continuously.

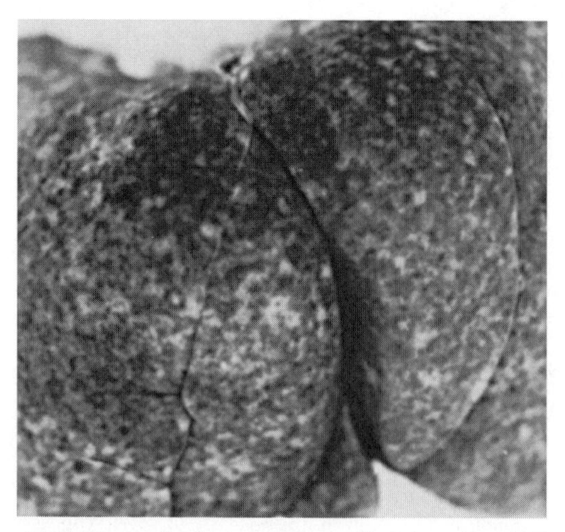

Figure 80–7. Liver of a kitten congenitally infected with *T. gondii*. Numerous white-yellowish areas of discoloration are due to necrosis produced by tachyzoites.

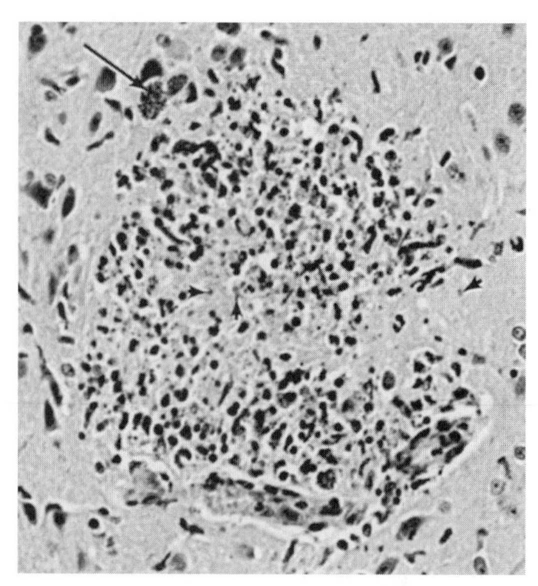

Figure 80–8. A focus of reactivation of toxoplasmosis in the cerebrum of a chronically infected cat medicated with glucocorticoids. Tissue cysts *(arrow)* are present at the periphery of the lesion. Numerous tachyzoites *(arrowheads)* are present in the necrotic area but are not visible at this magnification (H and E, × 400). (From Dubey JP, Frenkel JK: *Vet Pathol* 11:350–379, 1974. Reprinted with permission.)

Anorexia, lethargy, and dyspnea due to pneumonia have been commonly recognized features of postnatal toxoplasmosis (Table 80–1). Other clinical signs include persistent or intermittent fever, anorexia, weight loss, icterus due to hepatitis or cholangiohepatitis, vomiting, diarrhea, abdominal effusion, hyperesthesia on muscle palpation, stiffness of gait, shifting leg lameness, and neurologic deficits.[34, 93] In 100 cats with histologically confirmed toxoplasmosis, clinical syndromes were diverse but infection of pulmonary (97.7%), CNS (96.4%), hepatic (93.3%), pancreatic (84.4%), cardiac (86.4%), and ocular (81.5%) tissues were most common.[34] Clinical signs may be sudden or may have a slow onset. The disease may be rapidly fatal in some cats with severe respiratory or CNS signs. Anterior or posterior uveitis involving one or both eyes is common.[34, 88, 93, 96] Iritis, iridocyclitis, or chorioretinitis can occur alone or concomitantly. Aqueous flare, keratic precipitate, lens luxation, glaucoma, and retinal detachment are common manifestations of uveitis. Chorioretinitis may occur in both tapetal and nontapetal areas (see Toxoplasmosis, Chapter 93). Ocular toxoplasmosis occurs in some cats without polysystemic clinical signs of disease. In experimental *T. gondii* in cats, those infected concurrently with FIV developed severe pneumonitis and hepatitis, whereas those not infected with FIV developed multifocal chorioretinitis and anterior uveitis.[23, 25] Neurologic and ocular manifestations that occur in the absence of other systemic signs are more common with reactivated than acute infection.

Dogs

Clinical signs may be localized in respiratory, neuromuscular, or GI systems or may be caused by generalized infection.

Table 80–1. Clinical Findings in Feline Toxoplasmosis

Fever
Anorexia, lethargy
Weight loss
Muscle pain, hyperesthesia
Respiratory tract disease
  Conjunctivitis
  Rhinitis
  Coughing
  Dyspnea, tachypnea
  Diffuse harsh bronchovesicular sounds
Vomiting, diarrhea
Abdominal discomfort
Icterus
Abdominal effusion
Arthritis, joint pain, shifting lameness
Cardiac arrhythmias, sudden death
Splenomegaly
Lymphadenomegaly
Neurologic signs
  Ataxia
  Circling
  Behavioral changes
  Seizures
  Twitching
  Tremors
Ocular signs
  Retinochoroiditis, retinal hemorrhages
  Optic neuritis
  Optic nerve atrophy
  Anisocoria
  Blindness
  Anterior uveitis, aqueous flare, hyphema, velvety iris
  Glaucoma
  Lens luxation
  Retinal detachment
Neonatal (transplacental infection)
  Stillbirth
  Fading kittens
  Organ dysfunction (liver: hepatomegaly, icterus, ascites; lung: dyspnea; CNS: sleeping, crying)

The neurologic form of toxoplasmosis may last for several weeks without involvement of other systems, whereas severe disease involving the lungs and liver may kill dogs within a week.[33] Generalized toxoplasmosis is seen mostly in dogs younger than 1 year and is characterized by fever, tonsillitis, dyspnea, diarrhea, and vomiting. Icterus usually results from extensive hepatic necrosis. Myocardial involvement is usually subclinical, although arrhythmias and heart failure may develop as predominant findings in some older dogs.

The most dramatic clinical signs in older dogs have been associated with neural and muscular systems. Neurologic signs depend on the site of lesion in the cerebrum, cerebellum, or spinal cord. Seizures, cranial nerve deficits, tremors, ataxia, and paresis or paralysis may be seen. Dogs with myositis may initially show abnormal gait, muscle wasting, or stiffness. Paraparesis and tetraparesis may rapidly progress to lower motor neuron paralysis. Canine toxoplasmosis is clinically similar to *Neospora caninum* infection, which was previously confused with toxoplasmosis (see Neosporosis later). Although these diseases are similar, toxoplasmosis appears to be more prevalent in cats and neosporosis in dogs.

There are only a few reports of ocular lesions associated with toxoplasmosis in dogs. Retinitis, anterior uveitis, iridocyclitis, ciliary epithelium hyperplasia, and optic nerve neuritis have been noted (see Toxoplasmosis, in Chapter 93).

DIAGNOSIS

Clinical Laboratory Findings

Routine hematologic and biochemical parameters may be abnormal in cats and dogs with acute systemic toxoplasmoses. Nonregenerative anemia, neutrophilic leukocytosis, lymphocytosis, monocytosis, and eosinophilia are most commonly observed. Leukopenia of severely affected cats may persist until death and is usually characterized by an absolute lymphopenia and neutropenia with an inappropriate left shift, eosinopenia, and monocytopenia. In experimentally infected cats, neutropenia and lymphopenia persist for 5 to 12 days. Leukocytosis was seen in the recovery phase of illness.[91] Lymphocyte counts greater than 7000 cells/μl were common from 28 to 154 days after primary inoculation.[91] Secondary exposure of cats to *T. gondii* did not result in significant changes in leukocyte numbers.[91]

Biochemical abnormalities during the acute phase of illness include hypoproteinemia and hypoalbuminemia. Hyperglobulinemia has been detected in some cats with chronic toxoplasmosis.[93] Marked increases in serum alanine aminotransferase (ALT) and aspartate aminotransferase (AST) have been noted in animals with acute hepatic and muscle necrosis. Dogs generally have increased serum alkaline phosphatase (ALP) activity with hepatic necrosis, but this occurs less frequently in cats. Serum creatine kinase activity is also increased in cases of muscle necrosis. Serum bilirubin levels have been increased in animals with acute hepatic necrosis, especially cats that develop cholangiohepatitis or hepatic lipidosis. Cats or dogs that develop pancreatitis may show increased serum amylase and lipase activities. Cats often show proteinuria and bilirubinuria. Cats with pancreatitis may have reduced serum total calcium with normal serum albumin concentrations.[34]

Cytology

Tachyzoites may be detected in various tissues and body fluids by cytology during acute illness (see Fig. 80–3). They are rarely found in blood, CSF, fine-needle aspirates, and transtracheal or bronchoalveolar washings[53, 67] but are more common in the peritoneal and thoracic fluids of animals' developing thoracic effusions or ascites.

Inflammatory changes are usually noted in body fluids. In suspected feline toxoplasmosis of the nervous system, CSF protein levels were within reference ranges to a maximum of 149 mg/dl, and nucleated cells were a maximum of 28 cells/ml.[93] Lymphocytes predominate, but a mixture of cells may be found.

Radiology

Thoracic radiographic findings, especially in cats with acute disease, consist of a diffuse interstitial to alveolar pattern with a mottled lobar distribution.[129] Diffuse symmetric homogeneous increased density due to alveolar coalescence has been noted in severely affected animals. Mild pleural effusion can be present. Abdominal radiographic findings may consist of masses in the intestines or mesenteric lymph nodes or homogeneous increased density as a result of effusion. Loss of contrast in the right abdominal quadrant can indicate pancreatitis.

Fecal Examination

Despite the high prevalence of serum antibodies in cats worldwide, the prevalence of *T. gondii* oocysts in feces is low. In the United States, less than 1% of cats shed oocysts on any given day.[33] Because cats usually shed *T. gondii* oocysts for only 1 to 2 weeks after their first exposure, oocysts are rarely found in routine fecal examination. Moreover, cats usually are not clinically ill and do not have diarrhea during the period of oocyst shedding. Although cats are considered immune to reshedding of oocysts, they may shed a few oocysts after rechallenge with different strains more than 6 years later.[30] Cats that are immune have partial asexual development of *T. gondii* in their intestines compared with complete development cycle in naive cats.[26] Immunosuppression with high dose (10–80 mg/kg daily PO or weekly IM) of prednisolone will cause chronically infected cats to reexcrete oocysts, whereas a lower dose (5 mg/kg IM for 4 weeks) will not.[86]

T. gondii oocysts in feline feces are morphometrically indistinguishable from oocysts of *Hammondia hammondi* and *Besnoitia darlingi*, which also occur in cats (see Chapter 81). Oocysts of these coccidians can be differentiated only by sporulation and subsequent animal inoculation. If 10-μm–sized oocysts are found, they should be considered to be *T. gondii* until proved otherwise. Further inoculations should be attempted only in a diagnostic laboratory with competence in this procedure because of the infectious nature of the organism.

Because of their small size, oocysts of *T. gondii* are best demonstrated by centrifugation using Sheather's sugar solution. Five to 10 g of feces are mixed with water to a liquid consistency, and the mixture is strained with gauze. Two parts Sheather's sugar solution (500 g sugar, 300 ml water, and 6.5 g melted phenol crystals) are added to one part fecal suspension and centrifuged in a capped centrifuge tube. Care should be taken not to fill the tube to the top to prevent spills or aerosols. After centrifugation at 1000 *g* for 10 minutes, remove 1 to 2 drops from the meniscus by a dropper, place on a microscope slide, cover with a coverslip, and examine at low-power (× 100) magnification. *T. gondii* oocysts are about one fourth the size of *Isospora felis* and one eighth the size of *Toxocara cati* (the common roundworm of the cat) (Fig. 80–9).

Serologic Testing

Once infected, animals harbor toxoplasmic tissue cysts for life. IgG in kittens born to chronically infected queens is transferred in colostrum and persists for 8 to 12 weeks after birth.[120] Serologic surveys indicate that *T. gondii* infections are prevalent worldwide. Approximately 30% of cats and dogs in the United States have *T. gondii* antibodies. The prevalence

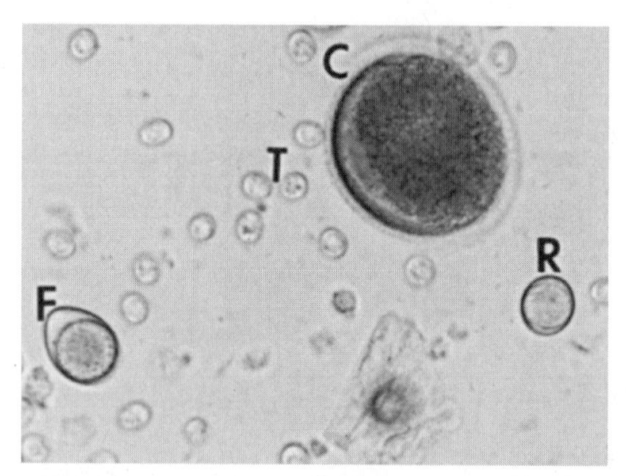

Figure 80–9. Unsporulated oocysts of *T. gondii* (T), *Isospora felis* (F), and *I. rivolta* (R) and an egg of the roundworm *Toxocara cati* (C) in a flotation of feline feces (unstained, × 410). (From Dubey JP: *J Am Vet Med Assoc* 169:1061–1078, 1976. Reprinted with permission.)

of seropositivity increases with age of the cat or dog because of the chance of exposure rather than susceptibility.

Multiple serologic tests for the detection of antibodies have been used in the diagnosis of toxoplasmosis (Table 80–2). The use of these tests in cats has been reviewed.[80] No single serologic assay exists that can definitively confirm toxoplasmosis. The Sabin-Feldman dye test is highly sensitive and specific for human toxoplasmosis but not necessarily for cats. Moreover, the test is too technical to perform in diagnostic laboratories and uses live *T. gondii*.

The indirect FA technique is comparable to the dye test but does not require live antigen. Some false-positive, polar staining that can occur with the indirect FA test has been attributed to Fc receptors on the surface of *T. gondii* tachyzoites that nonspecifically bind immunoglobulin. The indirect FA can be adapted to detect IgM, IgG, or IgA antibodies, using whole or immunoblotted antigen (see later).

Agglutination tests have the advantage of being species independent and are available in commercial kits that have been developed for use in people. The indirect hemagglutination (IHA) test (TMP-test, Wampole Labs, Carter Wallace Inc., Cranbury, NJ) does not require live antigen but is less sensitive than the dye test and indirect FA test.[95] Its main drawback is that it primarily measures IgG and is usually not positive during acute infection.

The latex agglutination test (LAT) (Toxo-test, Eiken Chemical Co., Tokyo, Japan; Synkit Inc., Chatsworth, CA) is somewhat more sensitive for serologic screening; however, it cannot be used to distinguish immunoglobulin classes. The modified agglutination test (MAT; Toxo-Screen DA, Biomerieux, Marcy-l'Etoile, France) detects only IgG antibodies but is extremely sensitive compared with the other available assays.[107] The MAT has been improved in its sensitivity and specificity in distinguishing acute and chronic *Toxoplasma* infections in people and cats by using acetone-fixed and formalin-fixed trophozoites, respectively.[43] Antibodies to acetone-fixed antigen are elevated only during acute (<3 months) infection, whereas antibodies to formalin-fixed antigen may remain high for several years.[52] For additional information on commercial laboratory testing and test kits, see Appendices 5 and 6, respectively.

ELISA, with and without immunoblotting, has been adapted for the detection of IgM, IgG, and IgA class antibodies against *T. gondii* in feline sera.[16, 80, 84, 91] ELISA methods are as sensitive as indirect FA and more sensitive than LAT or IHA. Immunoblots of separated antigens, reacted with an animal's sera and ELISA, can be used to identify specific target antigens. Comparison of antigen recognition patterns by serum from infected queens and their kittens by immunoblot aids in the diagnosis of neonatal toxoplasmosis.[16]

The kinetics of *T. gondii*–specific IgM, IgG, and IgA serum immune responses in experimentally inoculated cats are shown in Figure 80–10. Approximately 80% of experimentally inoculated cats develop detectable IgM titers; 100% develop detectable IgA and IgG titers. Chronic persistence of high IgG titers merely reflects continued presence of *Toxoplasma* antigen. Documentation of a positive IgM titer or an increasing IgG or IgA titer (fourfold) can verify recent infection but not necessarily oocyst shedding.[118] Some cats do not develop detectable IgM titers, and positive IgM titers can persist for months to years after infection. Thus, this antibody class does not accurately predict the oocyst shedding period. Some cats may not develop IgG titers to *T. gondii* for 4 to 6 weeks, well after the completion of the oocyst shedding period. Following the initial detection of IgG or IgA antibodies in serum, maximal titers are often reached in 2 to 3 weeks, leaving a narrow window for the documentation of an increasing titer.[48] Optimally, both serum samples should be

Table 80–2. Serologic Tests for Feline Toxoplasmosis

TEST	EARLIEST DETECTION (WEEKS)	ANTIBODY CLASS	TITER (LEAST SIGNIFICANT LEVEL OF REACTIVITY[a])	GUIDELINES FOR ACTIVE INFECTION
Sabin-Feldman	1–2	IgG, IgM	16	Fourfold rise over 2–3 wk
Indirect FA				
IgM	1–2	IgM	64	Positive with IgG negative
IgG	2	IgG	64	Fourfold rise over 2–5 wk
Indirect hemagglutination	2	IgG	64	Fourfold rise over 2–3 wk; insensitive
Latex agglutination	2	IgG	64	Fourfold rise over 2–3 wk
Modified agglutination test				
Acetone-fixed antigen	1–2	IgG	100	Fourfold rise over 2–3 wk or high titer with low formalin-fixed; titers remain high for 3 mo
Formalin-fixed	2	IgG	—	Fourfold rise over 2–3 wk; titers remain high for years
ELISA				
IgM	1–2	IgM	64	Titer > 256 and negative; IgG indicates active infection
IgG	2	IgG	64	Fourfold rise over 2–3 wk

[a] Titers may vary between laboratories on the basis of individual methodologies. Whenever comparisons are being made, both samples should be processed at the same time by the same lab.
For additional information on test availability, see Laboratory Listings, Appendix 5.
Modified from Lindsay DS, Dubey JD: *Compend Cont Educ Pract Vet* 19:448–461, 1997. Used with permission.

assessed at the same time in the assay to avoid interassay variation. After experimental inoculation of cats, IgG titers greater than 30,000 are commonly detected by MAT 6 years after inoculation; thus, high IgG titers do not prove recent or active infection.[43] Some seropositive cats will shed lower numbers of oocysts after oral inoculation with *T. gondii*, and so the presence of serum antibodies does not prove intestinal immunity.[30] Because of these findings, the measurement of serum antibodies in healthy cats cannot accurately predict the oocyst shedding period. In general, for *assessing human health risk*, serologic test results from healthy cats can be interpreted as follows:

1. A seronegative cat is not likely currently shedding oocysts but will likely shed oocysts if exposed; this cat poses the greatest public health risk.
2. A seropositive cat is probably not currently shedding oocysts and is less likely to shed oocysts if re-exposed or immunosuppressed. It is still recommended that potential exposure to oocysts be minimized.

Because antibodies occur in the serum of both healthy and diseased cats, results of these serologic tests do not independently prove clinical toxoplasmosis. Antibodies of the IgM class are commonly detected in the serum or aqueous humor of clinically ill or FIV-infected cats, but not healthy cats, and they may be a better marker of clinical disease than IgG or IgA.[91, 93, 94, 96] *T. gondii*–specific IgM is occasionally detected in the serum of cats with chronic or reactivated infection and does not always correlate with recent exposure. A *tentative antemortem diagnosis* of clinical toxoplasmosis in dogs or cats can be based on the following combination of serology and clinical parameters:

1. Serologic evidence of recent or active infection consisting of high IgM titers, or fourfold or greater, increasing or decreasing, IgG or other antibody titers (after treatment and/or recovery)
2. Exclusion of other causes of the clinical syndrome
3. Beneficial clinical response to an anti-*Toxoplasma* drug.

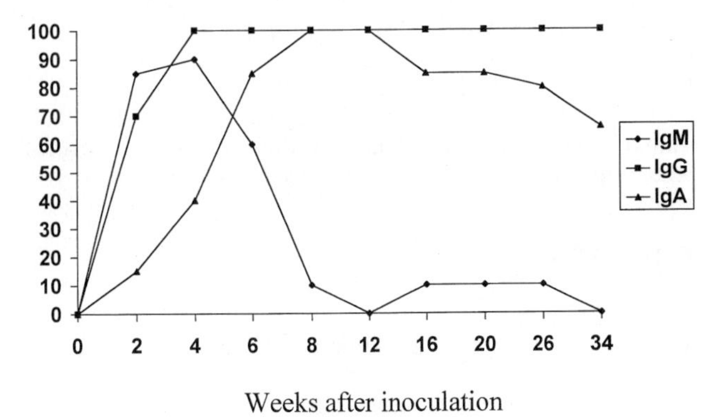

Figure 80–10. IgM, IgG, and IgA serum antibodies in cats experimentally inoculated with *T. gondii*.

Aqueous Humor and CSF Assessment

In dogs and cats with toxoplasmic encephalitis or uveitis, both protein and leukocytes may be increased in CSF or aqueous humor.[96] Cells are usually a mixed population of large and small mononuclear cells and neutrophils; the organism is rarely seen.

When assessing specific antibodies in aqueous humor or CSF, one must differentiate those produced locally from those passively diffusing across a damaged vascular barrier. As with serologic testing for other CNS or ocular infections, a comparison of antibody in CSF or aqueous humor can be made with that of serum for *Toxoplasma* and another nonocular infectious agent such as calicivirus[71] (see also Immunologic Testing, Canine Distemper, Chapter 3). This coefficient is calculated by the following:

$$\text{Antibody coefficient} = \frac{\textit{Toxoplasma}\text{-specific antibody aqueous (or CSF)}}{\textit{Toxoplasma}\text{-specific antibody serum}} \times \frac{\text{Other agent-specific antibody serum}}{\text{Other agent-specific antibody aqueous (or CSF)}}$$

Titers or equivalent numerical values from ELISA or other assays are substituted in the formula.

Antibody coefficient values greater than 1, and especially greater than 8, are considered stronger evidence for local production of *Toxoplasma* antibody and associated infection than for nonselective leakage from inflammation.[96] Ideally, to avoid variables inherent in test sensitivity, the same methodologies (e.g., ELISA, FA, agglutination) should be employed in the assays for both infectious agents. For examination of

CSF and CNS infection, the other agent should be a pathogen that is likely to have a serum titer such as a vaccine antigen, but does not cause CNS infection. Calicivirus is also suitable for this purpose in cats. In some experimentally infected cats, high *T. gondii*–specific IgG antibody coefficients can be detected for 3 to 4 months after inoculation. Caution must be exercised in assuming that this increased value always correlates with CNS or ocular replication of organisms. In some cats previously exposed to *T. gondii*, nonspecific immune stimulation resulted in an increased antibody coefficient (>1) on CSF or aqueous humor.[85] Analysis of IgM in aqueous humor shows better discrimination in cats with uveitis.[96]

Transient local production of *T. gondii*–specific antibodies in the eyes (IgG and IgA) and CNS (IgG) of cats has been documented after primary and secondary experimental inoculation.[18, 83, 99, 114] Local production of *T. gondii*–specific IgM has only been detected in client-owned, naturally exposed cats with uveitis or clinical signs of encephalitis, suggesting that this antibody class in CSF or aqueous humor may be a marker of clinical disease.[96] *T. gondii*–specific antigens can be detected in the aqueous humor of some cats with uveitis.[85, 96]

Organism Detection

The presence of *T. gondii* can be confirmed by animal or cell culture inoculation. Laboratory mice are the most susceptible animals. Homogenized suspensions of tissues or body fluids obtained at necropsy or biopsy may be used to infect laboratory mice or tissue culture. Cleaned, sporulated oocysts obtained from feces similarly may be used to infect mice. Generally mice are inoculated SC or IP. Beginning 4 to 6 days PI, peritoneal exudates of mice are examined for tachyzoites of *T. gondii* in intraperitoneally inoculated mice. Tissue cysts are present 4 to 6 weeks PI mostly in neural tissue. *Toxoplasma* antibodies in mice have developed by 6 weeks PI and can be demonstrated by any one of the serologic tests mentioned. Lack of parasite demonstration does not mean that the mice are not infected with *T. gondii*, and serologic verification is necessary.

ELISAs detecting *T. gondii* antigen, free and immune complexed, have been studied in naturally and experimentally infected cats.[92] Clinically ill cats and those with ocular involvement were more likely to have immune complexes in serum. Although this finding may have a role in disease development, the detection of circulating antigen does not confirm that *T. gondii* is responsible for clinical illness in a given animal.

Polymerase chain reaction (PCR) can be used to verify the presence of *T. gondii* in biologic specimens.[74, 109, 133] PCR has been performed to detect *T. gondii* in the blood of people with acute toxoplasmosis.[64] False-negative results occur, and chronically infected people may not be identified. PCR followed by restriction analysis can also be used to determine genotypes of infecting strains.[73a] *T. gondii* can be detected transiently in the aqueous humor by PCR after primary and secondary inoculation of cats.[15] The organism was commonly identified before the detection of antibody production by the eye. In client-owned, naturally exposed cats, the organism was detected in the aqueous humor from 8 of 43 cats with uveitis and 2 of 23 healthy cats.[15] Because *T. gondii* can be detected without the clinical signs of uveitis, positive PCR results in aqueous humor do not prove that the ocular signs are from toxoplasmosis.

PATHOLOGIC FINDINGS

Dogs

Grossly, necrosis is the predominant lesion, particularly in the brain, lung, liver, and mesenteric lymph nodes. Pulmonic lesions consist of gray-white nodular foci up to 5 mm in diameter and are found in the subpleura and in the parenchyma. The bronchial lymph nodes are often enlarged and necrotic. Grossly visible necrotic foci are also seen in pancreas, liver, kidneys, and spleen. Multiple ulcers up to 10 mm in diameter are observed in the stomach and small intestines. In the CNS, areas of discoloration and necroses up to 12 mm in diameter and cerebellar atrophy have been observed.

Myositis involving the muscles of the limbs has been observed in dogs with *T. gondii* infections. The affected muscles are pale and reduced in mass and, in severe, chronic cases, are grossly replaced by connective tissue. Fibrosis and scarring are usually not as prominent as those occurring with neosporosis (see later).

Microscopically, pulmonic lesions consist of fibrinous exudation and necrosis involving alveolar walls, blood vessels, and bronchioles. The alveolar lumina are filled with fibrin and occasionally with lymphocytes, neutrophils, and eosinophils. The alveolar lining and terminal epithelial cells are hypoplastic and infiltrated with lymphocytes, plasma cells, and multinucleated giant cells. Necrosis, the predominant muscular lesion, involves myofibers, small blood vessels, and surrounding connective tissues. Necrotic myofibers are replaced by fibrosis. Neural lesions consist of necrosis, gliosis, and vasculitis and are characteristic of multifocal nonsuppurative meningoencephalomyelitis. Lesions seen early in blood vessels consist of endothelial cell proliferation, necrosis, and perivascular cuffing. Neuronal necrosis, mild malacia, and some astrocytosis may be seen. Multifocal leptomeningeal infiltrates of macrophages, plasma cells, and some lymphocytes and neutrophils are found. In dogs with *T. gondii* polymyositis, noninflammatory degenerative changes are observed in peripheral nerves and nerve roots. Immunoperoxidase staining can be used to demonstrate *T. gondii* definitively in tissues to distinguish it from *N. caninum*.

Cats

The gross and microscopic findings may be similar to those seen in dogs; however, in feline toxoplasmosis, necrosis is predominantly in the liver (see Fig. 80–7), mesenteric lymph nodes, pancreas, and lungs.[34, 48] CNS lesions are similar to those found in dogs. Granulomas may be present in intestines and mesenteric lymph nodes. Tissue cysts in naturally infected cats have always been identified as *Toxoplasma* and not *Neospora*. Cholangiohepatitis, found in cats infected with *Toxoplasma*, has not been reported in any other host. The bile ducts are hyperplastic and plugged with desquamated bile duct epithelium and exudate. *T. gondii* schizonts (not tachyzoites) were seen in the biliary epithelium in both naturally occurring and experimentally induced disease.

THERAPY

Available drugs usually suppress replication of *T. gondii* and are not completely effective in killing the parasite. Dosages for these drugs are summarized in Table 80–3.

Clindamycin is the drug of choice for treating clinical toxoplasmosis in dogs and cats. Because of its good intestinal absorption, oral and parenteral dosages are similar. Clinda-

Table 80–3. Therapy for Toxoplasmosis

DRUG	SPECIES	DOSAGE (mg/kg)[a]	ROUTE	INTERVAL (HOURS)	DURATION (WEEKS)
Extraintestinal Cycle (Systemic Infection)					
Clindamycin	D	3–13[b]	PO, IM	8	2
	D	10–20	PO, IM	12	2
	C	8–17	PO, IM	8	2–4
	C	10–12.5	PO, IM	12	2–4
Sulfonamides[c] and	B	30	PO	12	2
Pyrimethamine[d]		0.25–0.5	PO	12	2
Trimethoprim-sulfonamide	C	15	PO	12	2–4
Enteroepithelial Cycle (Oocyst Shedding by Cats)					
Clindamycin	C	50	PO, IM	24	1–2
	C	12.5–25	PO, IM	12	1–2
Sulfonamides[c] and	C	100	PO	24	1–2
Pyrimethamine[e]		2.0	PO	24	1–2
Monensin	C	[e]	PO	24	1–2
Toltrazuril	C	5–10	PO	24	2

[a]Dose per administration at specified interval. See Therapy, in text, for other drugs being investigated to treat systemic infections.
[b]Use proportionally higher doses per kilogram in small (< 5 kg) dogs.
[c]Twice this dosage is used if sulfonamides are used alone.
[d]Available only in 25-mg tablets. For proper dosing of cats, must be divided. More effective than trimethoprim.
[e]Mixed as 0.02% (w/w) concentration in dry weight of food.
D = dog; C = cat; B = dog and cat.

mycin dosages for treating toxoplasmosis are greater than those for treating anaerobic infections for which the drug is marketed.

Clinical signs of systemic illness usually begin to resolve within 24 to 48 hours after institution of therapy. Appetite improves, hyperesthesia disappears, and fever usually subsides. Lower motor neuron deficits and muscle atrophy may take weeks to resolve in animals with polymyositis. Clindamycin has been effective in crossing the blood-brain and blood-vascular barriers in *Toxoplasma*-infected animals and people. Neurologic deficits improve, but signs may not totally resolve because of permanent damage caused by CNS inflammation. Active chorioretinitis generally subsides within 1 week. Some cases of anterior segment inflammation thought to be from toxoplasmosis have resolved with the administration of clindamycin alone.[93] However, because intraocular inflammation commonly leads to lens luxation and glaucoma, cats with anterior segment inflammation should be treated with topical, oral, or injectable glucocorticoids (see Toxoplasmosis, in Chapter 93). Clinical doses of glucocorticoids are not likely to exacerbate systemic disease.[86] Cats with concurrent FIV infections do not respond as well as FIV-naive cats to therapy. Clindamycin, given early in the course of acute experimental infection of cats, caused increased inflammatory reaction and tumor necrosis factor-α levels.[24] These effects have not been substantiated in naturally infected cats and may be related to the increased killing of actively replicating parasites, decreased IgM titer development, or decreased phagocytic activity caused by the drug.

Oral clindamycin can cause anorexia, vomiting, and diarrhea in dogs and cats, especially at higher dosages.[62] These side effects appear to be related to local GI irritation, because parenteral therapy at similar dosages does not cause them in the same animals. The side effects stop soon after the dosage is reduced or therapy is discontinued. *Clostridium difficile* overgrowth has not been documented in dogs and cats as it has been in people treated with clindamycin (see Drug Formulary, Appendix 8 and Clindamycin, Chapter 34).

Although less suitable than clindamycin, the combination of rapid-acting sulfonamides, such as sulfadiazine, sulfamethazine, sulfamerazine, and triple sulfas, and pyrimethamine is synergistic in the therapy of systemic toxoplasmosis. Pyrimethamine has greater efficacy than trimethoprim when used in combination. Because mental depression, anemia, leukopenia, and thrombocytopenia from bone marrow suppression develop rapidly in antifolate-treated cats compared with dogs, frequent hematologic monitoring is required, especially if therapy lasts longer than 2 weeks. Although trimethoprim-sulfonamide crosses the blood-brain barrier well, it has been reported to be ineffective in treating a dog with severe uveitis and optic neuritis.[39]

Bone marrow suppression can often be corrected with the addition of folinic acid (5.0 mg/day) or brewer's yeast (100 mg/kg/day) to the animal's diet. Baker's yeast, which contains folic acid, is inexpensive and as effective as folinic acid. The parasite uses preformed folic acid better than folinic acid. Nevertheless, pyrimethamine and sulfonamides inhibit folic–folinic acid metabolism in *T. gondii* to a greater extent than in the mammalian cell, so that supplementation with folic acid does not completely reverse therapeutic efficacy when used in combination with pyrimethamine and sulfonamides.

Doxycycline and minocycline have been shown to be effective in vitro and in vivo on experimental infections in mice and on cerebral toxoplasmosis in humans.[113] It might be considered when side effects are noted with clindamycin or antifolates.

Several new drugs, such as trimetrexate and piritrexim, which are antifolates; roxithromycin, a macrolide; atovaquone, a hydroxynaphthoquinone; and arprinocid, a purine analog and an anticoccidial drug, have been effective in treating experimental toxoplasmosis in mice, but they are not available for clinical use in cats or dogs. Azithromycin and clarithromycin are newer macrolides that are licensed for human use and show in vitro and in vivo activity against *T. gondii* (see Drug Formulary, Appendix 8). Trioxane derivatives have been shown to be effective against *T. gondii* in vitro. Spiramycin, used in Europe for prevention of transplacental transmission of *Toxoplasma*, has not been as effective in treating postnatally infected people.

In addition to pyrimethamine-sulfonamide combinations, pyrimethamine has been administered in combination with clindamycin and dapsone. Limited clinical and experimental studies have shown synergy with azithromycin-pyrimethamine, clarithromycin-minocycline, clarithromycin or azithromycin and sulfonamides, and atovaquone with pyrimethamine or sulfonamides.[2, 142] Biologic response modifiers such as interferon-γ have been given synergistically in combination therapy with antimicrobials.[3]

Oocyst Shedding in Cats

This has been partially controlled only when high doses of pyrimethamine and sulfonamide have been provided (see Table 80–3). Oocyst excretion also has been reduced by the dosages of clindamycin recommended for systemic chemotherapy.

Monensin, an anticoccidial drug used in poultry and cattle feeds, is effective in suppressing oocyst shedding when placed in dry cat food within 1 to 2 days PI. It did not prevent infected cats from developing immunity against shedding of oocysts in subsequent exposure to *Toxoplasma*. Toxicity was not noted when the drug was fed for extended periods, despite its known tendency to produce a myopathy in dogs and horses. Toltrazuril has been highly effective when given on a daily basis in preventing oocyst shedding after infection or reshedding after glucocorticoid-induced immunosuppression. These drugs may be beneficial in treating cats owned by pregnant women to reduce the risk of potential exposure of the fetuses to oocysts.

PREVENTION

Preventing toxoplasmosis in dogs and cats involves measures intended to reduce the incidence of feline infections and subsequent shedding of oocysts into the environment (see also Chapter 99). Kittens raised outdoors usually become infected shortly after they are weaned and begin to hunt. Cats should preferably be fed only dry or canned, commercially processed cat food. The prevalence of canine and feline toxoplasmosis has been higher in countries where raw meat products are fed to pets. Freezing or γ-ray irradiation can kill tissue cysts without affecting meat quality.[29, 51] Household pets should be restricted from hunting and eating potential intermediate hosts or mechanical vectors, such as cockroaches, earthworms, and rodents. If meat is provided, it should always be thoroughly cooked, even if frozen before feeding. Cats should be prevented from entering buildings where food-producing animals are housed or where feed storage areas are located.

The development of protective immunity in toxoplasmosis appears to be strain and/or stage specific.[117] An oral vaccine containing live bradyzoites of a mutant strain (T-263) is being developed in the hope of reducing oocyst shedding by cats.[32, 58] The vaccine strain itself does not produce oocyst shedding.[58] Although not commercially available, the value of a vaccine for cats would be to reduce the environmental contamination in areas of human habitation.

PUBLIC HEALTH CONSIDERATIONS

Worldwide, nearly 500 million people have *T. gondii* antibodies. The seroprevalence of *T. gondii* is highest (approaching 100%) in warm, moist, or tropical climates and lowest in the arid and the frigid regions of the world.[33] The rate of congenital infection varies among countries, being higher in continental Europe and South America than in North America.[33] In the United States, prevalence is highest in the East and in the Appalachian Mountain regions and is lowest in the southwestern arid regions and northwestern mountain regions. Approximately 25% to 50% of people tested in the United States have antibodies to *Toxoplasma*.

Clinical disease in people is similar to that in infected intermediate hosts, such as dogs. Transplacental infection can develop when previously noninfected people become infected during pregnancy. In immunocompromised or HIV-infected women, the fetus can become infected from a chronically infected mother. The fetus is affected most severely when infection takes place during the first half of gestation. Retinochoroiditis is the primary clinical disease in congenitally infected children. Prenatal detection of fetal infection and treatment of the pregnant mother have greatly reduced the morbidity of disease in newborn infants.

Postnatally acquired infections are generally nonsymptomatic and self-limiting, usually persisting for 1 to 12 weeks. Such infections with persistent or recurrent lymphadenomegaly may resemble infectious mononucleosis or Hodgkin's disease and usually are not fatal unless the host is severely immunosuppressed and the infection becomes disseminated. Reactivation of chronic latent (encysted) infection also is possible. It has been seen in AIDS patients when *Toxoplasma* encephalitis is the predominant illness.

Oocyst survival is an important determinant of the distribution and maintenance of the disease in nature.[50a] Oocysts, which are shed by cats, contaminate the environment and are ingested by herbivorous animals, who subsequently infect carnivorous animals higher in the food chain, such as humans. Oocysts can survive up to 18 months during unfavorable environmental conditions and are resistant to most disinfectants. People become infected by ingesting bradyzoite-infected meat (usually pork, goat, or lamb).[18a] Ingestion of raw goat's milk may be an additional source of human toxoplasmosis. Laboratory accidents, blood transfusions, and organ transplants are additional sources of infection.

Although oocysts are key in the epidemiology of toxoplasmosis, there is no correlation between toxoplasmosis in adults and cat ownership (see Chapter 99). Most cats become infected from carnivorousness soon after weaning and shed oocysts for only short periods (<3 weeks) thereafter. Cats found to be shedding *T. gondii* oocysts should be hospitalized for this period and treated to eliminate shedding, particularly when a pregnant woman is present in the household. To prevent inadvertent environmental contamination, cat owners should practice proper hygienic measures on a routine basis. Because infected cats rarely have diarrhea, and they groom themselves regularly, direct fecal exposure from handling infected cats is unlikely. Oocysts were not detected in fur of cats that had shed large numbers of *T. gondii* oocysts.[30]

Litter boxes should be changed daily, because usually at least 24 hours are necessary for oocysts to reach the infective stage. Oocyst sporulation depends on environmental temperature (Table 80–4). Unsporulated oocysts are more susceptible

Table 80–4. Effects of Temperature on* Toxoplasma *Oocyst Sporulation

TEMPERATURE	DAYS
23.8°C (75.8°F)	1–3
15°C (59°F)	5–8
11°C (51.8°F)	21

to disinfection and environmental destruction; therefore, control efforts should be directed at this stage. Litter pans should be disinfected with scalding water. Cat feces should be disposed of in the septic system, incinerated, or sealed tightly in a plastic bag before placing in a sanitary landfill. Only organic litters that are biodegradable should be placed in the septic system. High-temperature composting to kill oocysts remains to be proved. Under no circumstances should litter boxes be dumped into the environment.

Oocysts survive best in warm, moist soil, a factor that helps to explain the high prevalence of disease in temperate and tropical climates. They also withstand exposure to constant freezing temperature, drying, and high environmental temperature up to 18 months or more, especially if they are covered and out of direct sunlight. A cat's natural instinct to bury or hide its feces provides the protected environment for oocyst survival. Children's sandboxes should be covered to prevent cats from defecating in them. Mechanical vectors, such as sowbugs, earthworms, and houseflies, have been shown to contain oocysts, and cockroaches and snails are additional mechanical vectors. Control of these invertebrates will help reduce the spread of infection. Dogs that commonly roll in foreign feces were examined for their potential to act as mechanical vectors for oocysts. Oocyst sporulation did not occur when cat feces were placed on the skin and fur of dogs kept at 19° to 22°C and 40% to 100% relative humidity.[103a]

Sporulated oocysts resist most disinfectants, and only 10% ammonia is effective when it is in contact with contaminated surfaces for 10 minutes. Because of the time required for chemical disinfection and the fumes produced by ammonia, immersing litter pans in boiling or scalding water usually is the easiest means of disinfection. Steam cleaning can decontaminate hard impervious surfaces.

Outbreaks of human infections have been reported when oocyst-contaminated dust particles were inhaled or ingested. Dispersion of oocysts can also occur by earth-moving or cultivating equipment, shoes, animal feet, wind, rain, and fomites. Streams can become contaminated via water run-off. Stray and wild cats have been known to contaminate streams.

***Table 80–5. Survival of* Toxoplasma**

CONDITIONS	MAXIMAL SURVIVAL TIME
Bradyzoites	
−3°C (26.6°F)	3 weeks
−6°C (21.2°F)	11 days
50°C (122°F)	20 min
58°C (136°F)	10 min
61°C (142°F)	4 min
64°C (147.2°F)	1 min
Oocysts	
Unsporulated	
−21°C (−5.8°F)	1 day
4°C (39°F)	months
37°C (98.6°F)	1 day
50°C (122°F)	10 min
Sporulated	
−20°C (−4°F)	28 days
50°C (122°F)	30 min
55°C (122°F)	1 min
5% Ammonia	60 min

A report of military recruits infected by drinking oocyst-contaminated stream water in a jungle has been made.[33] Water from streams or ponds should always be boiled before drinking. Heating utensils to 70°C for at least 10 minutes will kill oocysts.

Prevention of human toxoplasmosis involves avoiding exposure of susceptible hosts, which includes the unborn fetus and immunosuppressed adult. Risk of exposure by contact with infected meat can be avoided by cooking all meat to an internal temperature greater than 67°C (Table 80–5). Microwaving does not kill all *T. gondii* because of uneven heating.[108] γ-Ray irradiation at doses of 5 centigray has been effective.[51] Freezing of meat in home freezers (−12°C) for at least 24 hours is an effective method for killing organisms. Good personal hygiene dictates that hands be washed well after handling raw meat. Animal care technicians cleaning cat cages should wear masks and protective clothing.

T. gondii–*like Infection of Cats*

T. gondii is thought to be a single species despite its widespread host range. An unidentified, structurally different, *Toxoplasma*-like parasite has been found in five cats with systemic and/or neurologic manifestations that could be confused with toxoplasmosis.[36, 38, 50] Fever and multisystemic signs had been present in some cats, and some had predominant signs of cervical spinal cord injury, which are unusual for toxoplasmosis. Some reactivity was noted to *T. gondii* in serologic testing. In one cat in which CSF was examined, an elevated WBC count (117/μl) and protein level (186 mg/μl) were present, and the cells were predominantly lymphocytes. Histologically, nonsuppurative inflammation was observed in many organs, including the CNS. As distinct from *T. gondii*, there were many tissue cysts and free bradyzoites; tachyzoites in inflammatory lesions were lacking. The tissue cysts were larger than those of *T. gondii*, they had thinner walls, and ultrastructurally they had micronemes arranged in rows. Although not evaluated, treatment of this organism would likely be similar to that of toxoplasmosis. The significance of this parasite awaits elucidation of its life cycle and host range.

Neosporosis

ETIOLOGY

Neospora caninum is a recognized protozoan of the phylum Apicomplexa; before 1988 it had been confused with *T. gondii*. Its tachyzoites and tissue cysts resemble those of *T. gondii* under light microscope. The complete life cycle of this organism is unknown, but a carnivorous definitive host is suspected. As with other coccidia, herbivores likely become infected from ingesting oocysts shed by the definitive host and by subclinical congenital infection from transplacental

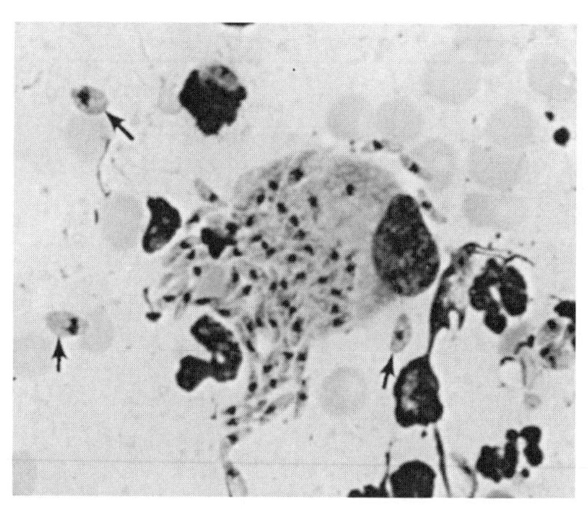

Figure 80–11. Numerous tachyzoites of *N. caninum* in a smear of an ulcer in the skin of a dog. Dividing tachyzoites *(arrows)* are thicker than nondividing tachyzoites (Giemsa, × 750).

transmission.[1] Tachyzoites are 5 to 7 μm × 1 to 5 μm, depending on the stage of division (Fig. 80–11). They divide into two zoites by endodyogeny. In infected carnivores, tachyzoites are found within macrophages, polymorphonuclear cells, spinal fluid, and neural and other cells of the body. Individual organisms are ovoid, lunate, or globular. They contain one or two nuclei and are arranged singly, in pairs, or in groups of four or more. Cell necrosis occurs after rapid intracellular replication of tachyzoites. Widespread dissemination of tachyzoites to many organs may occur in the acute phases, with subsequent restriction to neural and muscular tissues in more chronically affected dogs.[6]

Nonseptate tissue cysts (up to 100 μm in diameter) are found only in neural cells (brain, spinal cord, peripheral nerves, and retina) (Fig. 80–12). They may be round or elongated. The cyst wall is 1 to 4 μm thick and encloses slender periodic acid–Schiff-positive bradyzoites. Rupture of tissue cysts is associated with a granulomatous inflammatory reaction in the involved tissue.

EPIDEMIOLOGY

Naturally occurring infections in dogs have been found throughout the world. Seroprevalence of clinically healthy dogs is usually much less than 20% but much greater than the prevalence of clinical illness, suggesting subclinical infections.[104, 136] Purebred dogs, especially German shorthaired pointers, Labrador retrievers, boxers, golden retrievers, basset hounds, and greyhounds have been noticeably prevalent in published case reports.[128] Experimental transmission in dogs can occur after oral (carnivorousness) and parenteral (experimental) administration, but transplacental transmission may be the predominant route in natural infections. Suppositions are that the chronically infected bitch develops parasitemia during gestation, which spreads transplacentally to the fetus. Successive litters from the same subclinically infected dam may be born infected, and the majority of, but not all, puppies in a litter have clinical manifestations.[41] Other pups may carry the infection subclinically with reactivation in later life with immunosuppressive illnesses or administration of MLV vaccines or glucocorticoids. Postnatal acquisition of infection is thought to be uncommon.[136] In contrast to toxoplasmosis, underlying immunodeficiencies or concurrent illnesses are not consistently detected in canine neosporosis.

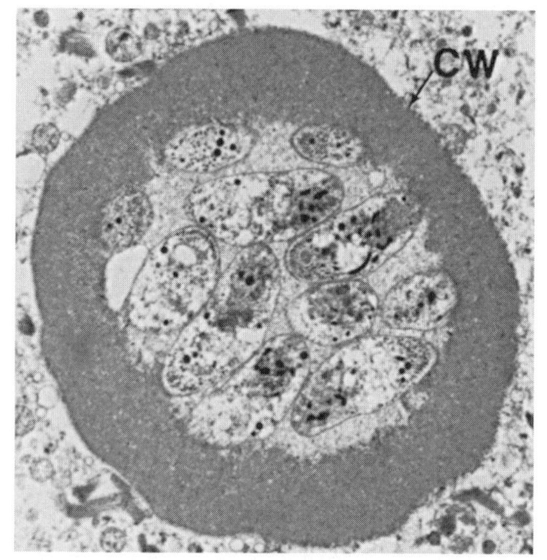

Figure 80–12. Transmission electron micrograph of a tissue cyst of *N. caninum* in the brain of a dog. Note the thick cyst wall (CW) and bradyzoites (× 9939).

CLINICAL FINDINGS

Naturally occurring infections have been reported worldwide in dogs, cattle, sheep, goats, horses, and deer but, experimentally, mice, rats, and domestic cats are also susceptible and show illness.[45] A predominant manifestation in herbivores is abortion. Neonatal death and in utero mortality

Table 80–6. Clinical Features of Canine Neosporosis

Clinical Features
PUPS (< 6 MONTHS)
Ascending LMN Rigid Paralysis to Tetraparesis (polymyositis, radiculitis, encephalomyelitis)[4, 7, 19, 22, 55, 68, 76, 78, 125, 137, 138, 139a]
Variable CNS signs
Monoparesis or paraparesis to tetraparesis
Can progress to paralysis
Muscle atrophy
Rigid hyperextension
Hyperesthesia
Incontinence
Respiratory muscle paralysis
Cranial muscle paralysis (cranial myositis)
Dysphagia
Trismus
Glossal paralysis
DOGS (> 6 MONTHS)
LMN Flaccid Paralysis (regional or generalized myositis older dogs)[61, 138]
Lameness and focal hyperesthesia
Acute flaccid LMN signs
Paraparesis to tetraparesis
Diffuse hyperesthesia
Muscle hypotonia
CNS Manifestations (meningitis, encephalomyelitis, cerebellitis)[7, 40, 138]
Paraparesis, tetraparesis, ataxia
Tremors and ataxia (cerebellitis)[75]
Head tilt
Seizures
Behavior changes
Altered thirst
Blindness, anisocoria (retinitis, choroiditis, optic neuritis)
Systemic Signs
Fever, dyspnea, cough (pneumonia)[63]
Cardiac arrhythmias, sudden death (myocarditis)[7, 78, 116, 139a]
Ulcerative, pruritic skin lesions (pyogranulomatous dermatitis)[49, 59a]
Regurgitation, megaesophagus (esophagitis, esophagomyositis)
Fever, vomiting, icterus (pancreatitis, hepatitis)

LMN = lower motor neuron.

may result depending on the time of infection during pregnancy. *N. caninum* has also been identified as a less common cause of equine protozoal myelitis than is *Sarcocystis neurona*.[110]

Dogs

It is likely that many dogs diagnosed with toxoplasmosis before 1988 actually had neosporosis. In general, clinical findings in dogs are similar to those of toxoplasmosis, but neurologic deficits and muscular abnormalities predominate (Table 80–6). Clinical signs may also include those of hepatic, pulmonary, and myocardial involvement, but any tissue can become involved. Both pups and older dogs are clinically affected, and the infections can be transmitted congenitally. The most severe and frequent infections have been in young (<6 months) dogs that presented with ascending paralysis of the limbs. In the youngest pups, signs are often noticed beginning at 3 to 6 weeks of age. Features that distinguish neosporosis from other forms of paralysis are gradual muscle atrophy and stiffness, usually as an ascending paralysis; the pelvic limbs are more severely affected than the thoracic limbs. Paralysis progresses to rigid contracture of the muscles of the affected limb (Fig. 80–13). This arthrogryposis is a result of the scar formation in the muscles from lower motor neuron damage and myositis. In some pups, joint deformation and genu recurvatum may develop. Cervical weakness, dysphagia, and ultimately death occur. In some dogs, the progression may become static. Dogs do not develop severe intracranial manifestations and maintain alert attitudes. They can survive for months with hand feeding and care but remain paralyzed with associated complications. Older dogs, which are less commonly affected, often have signs of multifocal CNS involvement or polymyositis; less common manifestations result from myocarditis, dermatitis, pneumonia, or multifocal dissemination. Death can occur in dogs of any age.

Experimental studies suggest that *N. caninum* can cause early fetal death, mummification, resorption, and birth of weak pups.[45] Although abortion is a major feature of the disease in cattle, there are no reports of abortion in dogs.

Cats

N. caninum can induce a fatal infection in experimentally inoculated cats.[47] It is most severe in prenatally and neonatally infected kittens. Subclinical disease was found in adult cats. These cases were more severe and acute when immunosuppressed with glucocorticoids. As in dogs, encephalomyelitis, polymyositis, and hepatitis are the predominant lesions. Natural infections have not been documented.

DIAGNOSIS

Hematologic and biochemical findings have been variable, depending on the organ system of involvement. With muscle disease, creatine kinase and AST activities have been in-

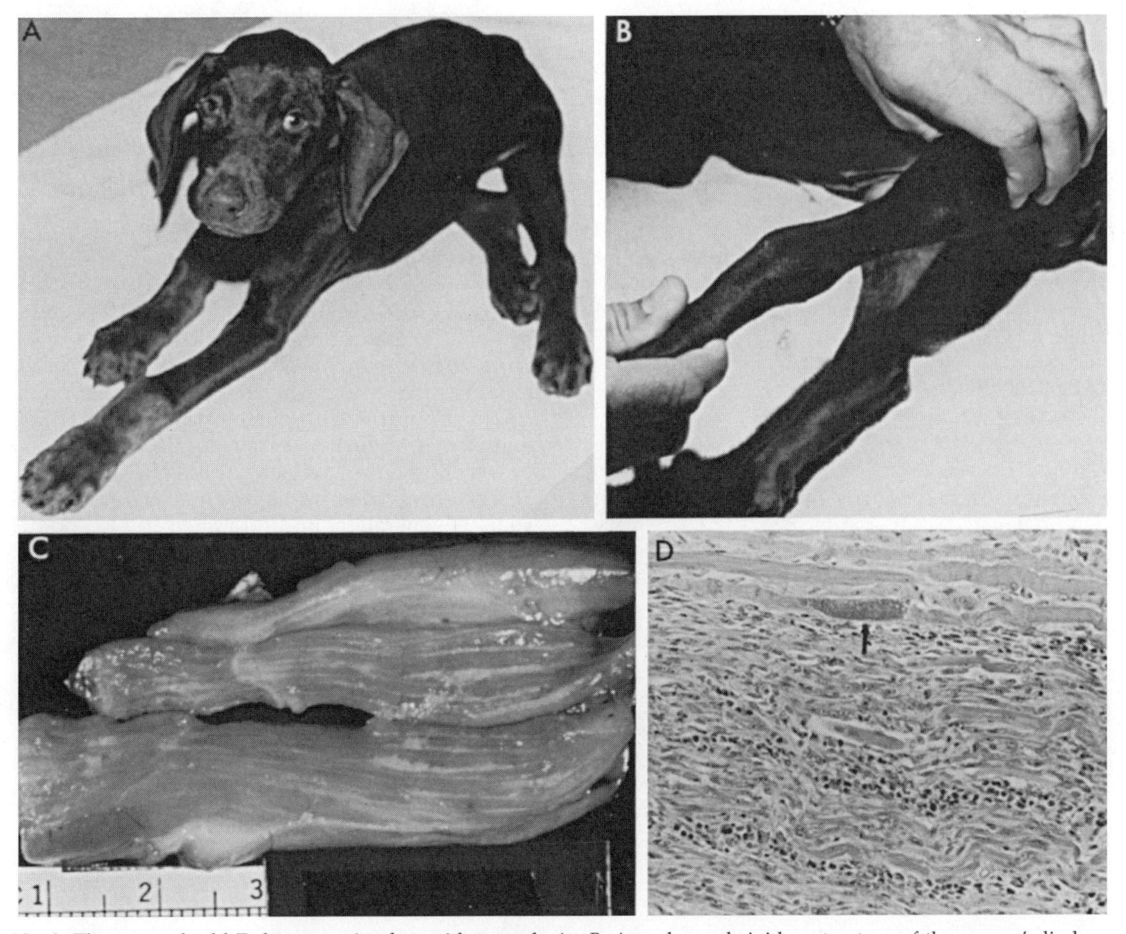

Figure 80–13. *A*, Three-month-old Doberman pinscher with tetraplegia. *B*, Atrophy and rigid contracture of the puppy's limbs are apparent. *C*, Gross and *D*, microscopic appearances of muscle fibers in chronic myositis. A group of organisms *(arrow)* is shown in *D* (H and E, × 40).

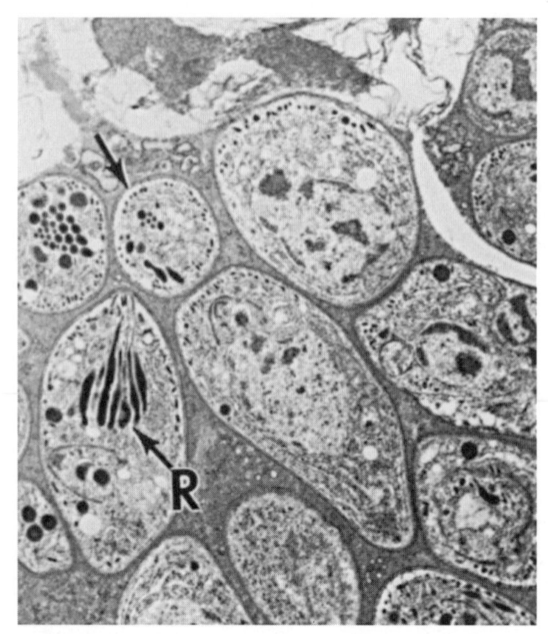

Figure 80–14. Several tachyzoites of *N. caninum* directly in the cytoplasm of a myelinated cell *(arrow)* in the spinal cord of a dog. Several tachyzoites are dividing into two by endodyogeny. Numerous electron-dense rhoptries (R) in tachyzoites distinguish *N. caninum* from *T. gondii* (× 10,425).

creased. Serum ALT and alkaline phosphatase activities are increased in dogs that develop hepatic inflammation. CSF abnormalities have included mild increases in protein (>20 but <150 mg/dl) and nucleated cell (>10 but <100 cells/dl) concentrations. Differential leukocyte counts included lymphocytes, monocytes and macrophages, neutrophils, and eosinophils in decreasing numbers.[22, 121a] CSF results can be within reference limits in some dogs.[68] Electromyographic abnormalities have consisted of spontaneous activity of fibrillation potentials, positive sharp waves, and occasional repetitive discharges. Nerve conduction velocities may be reduced in the most severely affected limbs, especially proximally, but they are often within reference range. Low evoked action potentials may be found with myositis.

Serologic Testing

Demonstrating serum antibodies to *N. caninum* can help confirm the diagnosis of neosporosis. Serum is reacted with cell-cultured *N. caninum*. Serum indirect FA titers can vary between laboratories; however, in one reference laboratory, values of 200 or greater are considered positive and values are often greater than 800.[102] CSF can be tested, but titers are of lesser magnitude (50–800).[7] Some false-positive titers exist in previously exposed dogs that may be infected, but they remain nonsymptomatic with values of 800 or greater. Indirect FA IgG titers in most species increase 1 to 2 weeks after infection.[46] Higher indirect FA have been found in clinically versus subclinically affected dogs and in those with the longest duration of illness.[6] ELISA methods are comparable but more sensitive than the indirect FA procedures.[12] A direct agglutination test measuring IgG was as sensitive and specific as an indirect FA test with the advantage of being useful in a variety of host species.[126a] Antibodies to *T. gondii* do not cross-react with *N. caninum*, at dilutions of 1:50 or less, so that serum or CSF antibody titers to *T. gondii* in *Neospora*-infected dogs are negative. Slight cross-reactivity with sera from dogs infected with *Babesia gibsoni* but not *B. canis* has been observed.[143] Some cross-reactivity has been observed with ELISA testing when crude extracts are used as antigens.[45] Western blots show four major antigens (17, 29, 30, and 37 kD) that appear to be specific for *Neospora*.[12]

Organism Detection

N. caninum may be found in CSF or tissue aspirates and biopsies of some dogs and may be detected with any material used to stain blood films. Biopsy of affected muscle may yield a definitive diagnosis when organisms are detected. *N. caninum* tachyzoites are similar to *T. gondii* tachyzoites by light microscopy (Fig. 80–14). Tissue cysts of *N. caninum* have thicker walls than those of *T. gondii* (Fig. 80–15). *N. caninum* can be grown in cell culture and in mice. *N. caninum* must be distinguished from *T. gondii* in sections by immunochemical stains.[21] Structural differences can also be detected with transmission EM. *T. gondii* has a thinner cyst wall and fewer micronemes and rhoptries. The use of molecular genetics and PCR to distinguish *Neospora* from other related parasites has been reviewed.[45]

PATHOLOGIC FINDINGS

Gross lesions include multifocal streaks of necrosis, fibrosis, and mineralization of striated muscles, especially the diaphragm. Hepatomegaly, pneumonia, and discoloration of brain or spinal cord tissues may be apparent on cut section.

Nonsuppurative encephalomyelitis, polyradiculoneuritis, ganglionitis, myositis (of all striated muscles), and myofibrosis are the predominant histologic findings (see Fig. 80–13). The encephalomyelitis is characterized by inflammation, axonal degeneration, and formation of glial nodules in gray and white matter. Parasites are most consistently found in the cerebrum regardless of the clinical presentation.[6] Tissue

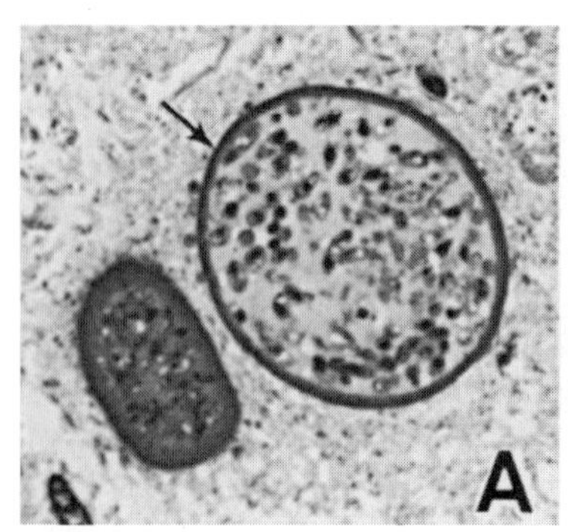

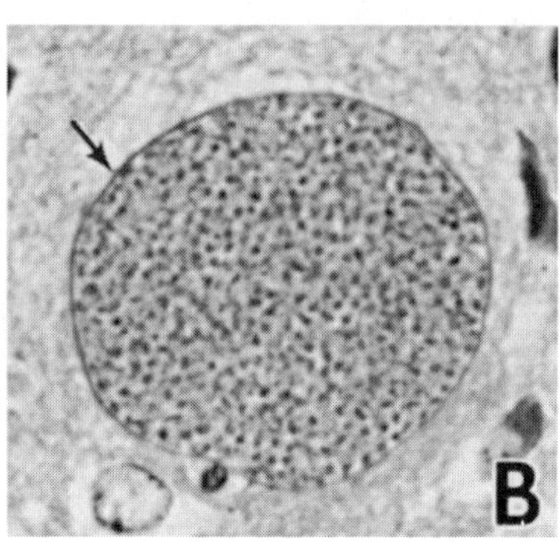

Figure 80–15. Comparison of tissue cysts of *N. caninum (A)* and *T. gondii (B)* in the brain (H and E, × 750). The cyst wall *(arrows)* of *N. caninum* is thicker than that of *T. gondii*.

Table 80–7. Drug Therapy for Neosporosis [a]

DRUG	SPECIES	DOSE (mg/kg)	ROUTE	FREQUENCY (HOURS)	DURATION (WEEKS)
Trimethoprim-sulfonamide	D	15–20	PO	12	4–8
		10–15	PO	8	4–8
Clindamycin [b]	D	7.5–15	PO, SC	8	4–8
		15–22	PO, SC	12	4–8
Pyrimethamine *and*	D	1	PO	24	2–4
sulfonamide [c]	D	15–30	PO	12	

[a]For additional information on listed drugs, see Appendix 8.
[b]Also been used in combination with trimethoprim-sulfonamide or pyrimethamine.
[c]Can be substituted with trimethoprim-sulfonamide.
D = dog.

cysts are present only in central or peripheral neural tissues, whereas tachyzoites are present in many tissues. Tissue cysts are often present, even in treated animals. A radiculoneuritis is often present in young dogs. Muscle lesions can range from focal necrosis to generalized inflammation of all skeletal muscles and esophageal and cardiac muscles. Inflammation and necrosis of other tissues also occur. Tachyzoites are frequently found in the lung, liver, adrenal and thyroid glands, and uterus but usually with no clinical significance.[6] *N. caninum* appears to induce more inflammation than *T. gondii* and has been found to cause severe phlebitis and dermatitis. Nonsuppurative myocarditis, pneumonia, and hepatitis are commonly present as subclinical lesions. Lesions caused by *N. caninum* are similar to those by *T. gondii* or to granulomatous meningoencephalitis. Confirmation, therefore, requires serologic or immunohistochemical methods.

THERAPY

Information on effective therapy for this disease is limited. However, drugs used for therapy of toxoplasmosis should be tried early in the course of illness. In vitro assays have shown activity of dihydrofolate reductase inhibitors (trimethoprim), ionophone antibiotics (monensin and salinomycin), macrolides (azithromycin, clarithromycin, and erythromycin), tetracyclines (doxycycline and minocycline), and lincosamides (clindamycin).[101] Clindamycin, sulfadiazine, and pyrimethamine alone or in combination have been administered to treat canine neosporosis (Table 80–7).[45] However, clinical improvement is not likely in the presence of muscle contracture or rapidly advancing paralysis.[45] To reduce the chance of illness, all dogs in an affected litter should be treated as soon as the diagnosis is made in one littermate. Older (>16 weeks) puppies and adult dogs respond better to treatment.[7] In adult dogs with acute lower motor neuron paralysis from myositis, dysfunction is often more amenable to early treatment because scar contracture is less common.[61] There is no known therapy to prevent a bitch from transmitting infection to her pups.

PREVENTION

In dogs, *N. caninum* can be transmitted repeatedly through successive litters and litters of their progeny. This should be considered when planning the breeding of *Neospora*-infected bitches.[41] Until the definitive host is known, specific control measures will not be known. There is no vaccine to combat neosporosis.

PUBLIC HEALTH CONSIDERATIONS

The zoonotic potential of *N. caninum* is unknown. Nonhuman primates can be experimentally infected.[71a]

References

1. Anderson ML, Reynolds JP, Rowe JD, et al. 1997. Evidence of vertical transmission of *Neospora* sp infection in dairy cattle. *J Am Vet Med Assoc* 210:1169–1172.
2. Araujo FG, Prokocimer P, Remington JS. 1992. Clarithromycin-minocycline is synergistic in a murine model of toxoplasmosis. *J Infect Dis* 165:788.
3. Araujo FG, Remington JS. 1991. Synergistic activity of azithromycin and γ-interferon in murine toxoplasmosis. *Antimicrob Agents Chemother* 35:1672–1673.
4. Barber J, Trees AJ, Owen M. 1993. Isolation of *Neospora caninum* from a British dog. *Vet Rec* 129:531–532.
5. Barber JS, Holmdahl OJ, Owen MR, et al. 1995. Characterization of the first European isolate of *Neospora caninum*. *Parasitol* 111:563–568.
6. Barber JS, Payne-Johnson CE, Trees AJ. 1996. Distribution of *Neospora caninum* within the central nervous system and other tissues of six dogs with clinical neosporosis. *J Small Anim Pract* 37:568–574.
7. Barber JS, Trees AJ. 1996. Clinical aspects of 27 cases of canine neosporosis. *Vet Rec* 139:439–443.
8. Barber JS, van Ham L, Polis I, et al. 1997. Seroprevalence of antibodies to *Neospora caninum* in Belgian dogs. *J Small Anim Pract* 38:15–16.
9. Bjerkas I, Dubey JP. 1991. Evidence that *Neospora caninum* is identical to the *Toxoplasma*-like parasite of Norwegian dogs. *Acta Vet Scand* 32:407–410.
10. Bjerkas I, Jenkins MC, Dubey JP. 1994. Identification and characterization of *Neospora caninum* tachyzoite antigens useful for diagnosis of neosporosis. *Clin Diagn Lab Immunol* 1:214–221.
11. Bjorkman C. 1994. Prevalence of antibodies to *Neospora caninum* and *Toxoplasma gondii* in Swedish dogs. *Acta Vet Scand* 35:445–447.
12. Bjorkman C, Lunden A, Holmdahl J, et al. 1994. *Neospora caninum* in dogs: detection of antibodies by ELISA using an iscom antigen. *Parasite Immunol* 16:643–648.
13. Burkhardt E, Dubey JP, Korte G, et al. 1992. Zwei erkrankungen Infolge einer Infection mit *Neospora caninum* bei Hundewelpen in Deutschland. *Kleintierpraxis* 37:701–706.
14. Burney DP, Lappin MR, Cooper CM. 1995. Demonstration of *Toxoplasma gondii*-specific IgA in the serum of cats. *Am J Vet Res* 56:769–773.
15. Burney DP, Lappin MR, Dow SW, et al. 1996. Detection of *Toxoplasma gondii* in aqueous humor from experimentally inoculated cats. *J Vet Intern Med* 10:178.
15a. Buxton D, Maley SW, Pastoret PP, et al. 1997. Examination of red foxes (*Vulpes vulpes*) from Belgium for antibody to *Neospora caninum* and *Toxoplasma gondii*. *Vet Rec* 141:308–309.
16. Cannizzo K, Lappin MR, Cooper CM, et al. 1996. *Toxoplasma gondii* antigen recognition by serum IgM, IgG and IgA of queens and their neonatally infected kittens. *Am J Vet Res* 57:1327–1330.
17. Chavkin MJ, Lappin MR, Powell CC, et al. 1992. Seroepidemiologic and clinical observations of 93 cases of uveitis in cats. *Prog Vet Comp Ophthalmol* 12:29–36.
18. Chavkin MJ, Lappin MR, Powell CC, et al. 1994. *Toxoplasma gondii*-specific antibodies in the aqueous humor of cats with toxoplasmosis. *Am J Vet Res* 55:1244–1249.
18a. Choi WY, Nam HW, Kwak NH, et al. 1997. Foodborne outbreaks of human toxoplasmosis. *J Infect Dis* 175:1280–1282.
19. Cochrane SM, Dubey JP. 1993. Neosporosis in a Golden retriever dog from Ontario. *Can Vet J* 34:232–233.

20. Cole RA, Lindsay DS, Blagburn BL, et al. 1995. Vertical transmission of *Neospora caninum* in dogs. *J Parasitol* 81:208–211.
21. Cole RA, Lindsay DS, Dubey JP, et al. 1993. Detection of *Neospora caninum* in tissue sections using murine monoclonal antibody. *J Vet Diagn Invest* 5:579–584.
22. Cuddon P, Lin DS, Bowman DD, et al. 1992. *Neospora caninum* infection in English Springer Spaniel littermates. *J Vet Intern Med* 6:325–332.
22a. D'Amore E, Falcone E, Busani L, et al. 1997. A serological survey of feline immunodeficiency virus and *Toxoplasma gondii* in stray cats. *Vet Res Commun* 21:355–359.
23. Davidson MG, Lappin MR, English RV, et al. 1993. A feline model of ocular toxoplasmosis. *Invest Ophthalmol Vis Sci* 34:3653–3659.
24. Davidson MG, Lappin MR, Rottman JR, et al. 1996. Paradoxical effect of clindamycin in experimental acute toxoplasmosis in cats. *Antimicrob Agent Chemother* 40:1352–1359.
25. Davidson MG, Rottman JB, English RV, et al. 1993. Feline immunodeficiency virus predisposes cats to acute generalized toxoplasmosis. *Am J Pathol* 143:1486–1497.
26. Davis SW, Dubey JP. 1995. Mediation of immunity to *Toxoplasma gondii* oocyst shedding in cats. *J Parasitol* 81:882–886.
27. Dubey JP. 1990. *Neospora caninum*: a look at a new *Toxoplasma*-like parasite of dogs and other animals. *Compend Cont Educ Pract Vet* 12:653–664.
28. Dubey JP. 1992. A review of *Neospora caninum* and *Neospora*-like infections in animals. *J Protozool Res* 2:40–52.
29. Dubey JP. 1994. Toxoplasmosis. *J Am Vet Med Assoc* 205:1593–1598.
30. Dubey JP. 1995. Duration of immunity to shedding of *Toxoplasma gondii* oocysts in cats. *J Parasitol* 81:410–415.
31. Dubey JP. 1996. Infectivity and pathogenicity of *Toxoplasma gondii* oocysts for cats. *J Parasitol* 82:957–961.
32. Dubey JP. 1996. Strategies to reduce transmission of *Toxoplasma gondii* to animals and humans. *Vet Parasitol* 64:65–70.
32a. Dubey JP. 1997. Tissue cyst tropism in *Toxoplasma gondii*: a comparison of tissue cyst formation in organs of cats, and rodents fed oocysts. *Parasitology* 115:15–20.
33. Dubey JP, Beattie CP. 1988. Toxoplasmosis of animals and man, pp 1-220. CRC Press, Boca Raton, FL.
34. Dubey JP, Carpenter JL. 1993. Histologically confirmed clinical toxoplasmosis in cats: 100 cases (1952–1990). *J Am Vet Med Assoc* 203:1556–1566.
35. Dubey JP, Carpenter JL. 1993. Neonatal toxoplasmosis in littermate cats. *J Am Vet Med Assoc* 203:1546–1549.
36. Dubey JP, Carpenter JL. 1993. Unidentified *Toxoplasma*-like tissue cysts in the brain of three cats. *Vet Parasitol* 45:319–321.
37. Dubey JP, Carpenter JL, Topper MJ, et al. 1989. Fatal toxoplasmosis in dogs. *J Am Anim Hosp Assoc* 25:659–664.
38. Dubey JP, Fenner WR. 1993. Clinical segmental myelitis associated with an unidentified *Toxoplasma*-like parasite in a cat. *J Vet Diagn Invest* 5:472–480.
39. Dubey JP, Greene CE, Lappin MR. 1990. Toxoplasmosis and neosporosis, pp 818–834. *In* Greene CE (ed), Infectious diseases of the dog and cat. WB Saunders, Philadelphia, PA.
40. Dubey JP, Higgins RJ, Smith JH, et al. 1990. *Neospora caninum* encephalomyelitis in a British dog. *Vet Rec* 126:193–194.
41. Dubey JP, Koestner A, Piper RC. 1990. Repeated transplacental transmission of *Neospora caninum* in dogs. *J Am Vet Med Assoc* 197:857–860.
42. Dubey JP, Lappin MR, Thulliez P. 1995. Diagnosis of induced toxoplasmosis in neonatal cats. *J Am Vet Med Assoc* 207:179–185.
43. Dubey JP, Lappin MR, Thulliez P. 1995. Long-term antibody response of cats fed *Toxoplasma gondii* tissue cysts. *J Parasitol* 81:887–893.
44. Dubey JP, Lindsay DS. 1993. Neosporosis. *Parasitol Today* 9:452–458.
45. Dubey JP, Lindsay DS. 1996. A review of *Neospora caninum* and neosporosis. *Vet Parasitol* 67:1–59.
46. Dubey JP, Lindsay DS, Adams DS, et al. 1996. Serologic responses of cattle and other animals infected with *Neospora caninum*. *Am J Vet Res* 57:329–336.
47. Dubey JP, Lindsay DS, Lipscomb TP. 1990. Neosporosis in cats. *Vet Pathol* 27:335–339.
48. Dubey JP, Mattix ME, Lipscomb TP. 1996. Lesions of neonatally induced toxoplasmosis in cats. *Vet Pathol* 33:290–295.
49. Dubey JP, Metzger FL, Hattel AL. 1995. Canine cutaneous neosporosis: clinical improvement with clindamycin. *Vet Derm* 6:37–43.
50. Dubey JP, Peters D, Brown C. 1992. Unidentified *Toxoplasma*-like tissue cyst–forming coccidium in a cat (*Felis catus*). *Parasitol Res* 78:39–42.
50a. Dubey JP, Rollor EA, Smith K, et al. 1997. Low seroprevalence of *Toxoplasma gondii* in feral pigs from a remote island lacking cats. *J Parasitol* 83:839–840.
51. Dubey JP, Thayer DW. 1994. Killing of different strains of *Toxoplasma gondii* tissue cysts by irradiation under defined conditions. *J Parasitol* 80:764–767.
52. Dubey JP, Thulliez P. 1989. Serologic diagnosis of toxoplasmosis in cats fed *Toxoplasma gondii* tissue cysts. *J Am Vet Med Assoc* 194:1297–1299.
53. Eddlestone SM, Hoskins JD, Hosgood G, et al. 1996. Case presentation. *Compend Cont Edu Pract Vet* 18:774–779.
54. Ellis J, Luton K, Baverstock PR, et al. 1994. The phylogeny of *Neospora caninum*. *Mol Biochem Parasitol* 64:303–311.
55. Flagstad A, Jensen HE, Bjerkas I, et al. 1995. *Neospora caninum* infection in a litter of Labrador retriever dogs in Denmark. *Acta Vet Scand* 36:387–391.
56. Frenkel JK. 1990. Toxoplasmosis in human beings. *J Am Vet Med Assoc* 196:240–248.
57. Frenkel JK. 1990. Transmission of toxoplasmosis and the role of immunity in limiting transmission of illness. *J Am Vet Med Assoc* 196:233–240.
58. Frenkel JK, Pfefferkorn ER, Smith DD, et al. 1991. Prospective vaccine prepared from a new mutant of *Toxoplasma gondii* for use in cats. *Am J Vet Res* 52:759–763.
59. Freyre A, Choromanski L, Fishback JL, et al. 1993. Immunization of cats with tissue cysts, bradyzoites, and tachyzoites of the T-263 strain of *Toxoplasma gondii*. *J Parasitol* 79:716–719.
59a. Fritz D, George C, Dubey JP, et al. 1997. *Neospora caninum*: associated nodular dermatitis in a middle-aged dog. *Canine Pract* 22:21–24.
60. Gasser RB, Edwards G, Cole R. 1993. Neosporosis in a dog. *Aust Vet Pract* 23:190–193.
61. Greene CE, Cook JR, Mahaffey EA. 1985. Clindamycin for treatment of *Toxoplasma* polymyositis in a dog. *J Am Vet Med Assoc* 187:631–633.
62. Greene CE, Lappin MR, Marks A. 1993. Effect of clindamycin on clinical, hematologic, and biochemical parameters in healthy cats. *J Am Anim Hosp Assoc* 28:323–326.
63. Greig B, Rossow KD, Collins JE, et al. 1995. *Neospora caninum* pneumonia in an adult dog. *J Am Vet Med Assoc* 206:1000–1001.
64. Guy EC, Joynson HM. 1995. Potential of the polymerase chain reaction in the diagnosis of active *Toxoplasma* infection by detection of parasite in blood. *J Infect Dis* 173:319–322.
65. Harmelin A, Dubey JP, Yakobson B, et al. 1992. Concurrent *Hepatozoon canis* and *Toxoplasma gondii* infections in a dog. *Vet Parasitol* 43:131–136.
66. Hass JA, Shell L, Sanders G. 1989. Neurological manifestations of toxoplasmosis: a literature review and case summary. *J Am Anim Hosp Assoc* 25:253–260.
67. Hawkins EC, Davidson MG, Meuten DJ, et al. 1997. Cytologic identification of *Toxoplasma gondii* in bronchoalveolar lavage fluid of experimentally infected cats. *J Am Vet Med Assoc* 210:648–650.
68. Hay WH, Shell LG, Lindsay DS, et al. 1990. Diagnosis and treatment of *Neospora caninum* infection in a dog. *J Am Vet Med Assoc* 197:87–89.
69. Heidel JR, Dubey JP, Blythe LL, et al. 1990. Myelitis in a cat infected with *Toxoplasma gondii* and feline immunodeficiency virus. *J Am Vet Med Assoc* 196:316–318.
70. Henriksen P, Dietz HH, Henriksen SA. 1994. Fatal toxoplasmosis in five cats. *Vet Parasitol* 55:15–20.
71. Hill SL, Lappin MR, Carman J, et al. 1995. Comparison of methods for estimation of *Toxoplasma gondii*-specific antibody production in the aqueous humor of cats. *Am J Vet Res* 56:1181–1187.
71a. Ho MSY, Barr BC, Tarantal AF, et al. 1997. Detection of *Neospora* from tissues of experimentally infected rhesus macques by PCR and specific DNA probe hybridization. *J Clin Microbiol* 35:1740–1745.
72. Holmdahl JM, Mattsson JG, Uggla A. 1994. The phylogeny of *Neospora caninum* and *Toxoplasma gondii* based upon ribosomal RNA sequences. *FEMS Microbiol Lett* 119:187–192.
73. Hoskins JD, Bunge MM, Dubey JP, et al. 1991. Disseminated infection with *Neospora caninum* in a ten-year-old dog. *Cornell Vet* 81:329–334.
73a. Howe DK, Honore S, Derouin F, et al. 1997. Determination of genotypes of *Toxoplasma gondii* strains isolated from patients with toxoplasmosis. *J Clin Microbiol* 35:1411–1414.
74. Hyman JA, Johnson LK, Tsai MM, et al. 1995. Specificity of polymerase chain reaction identification of *Toxoplasma gondii* infection in paraffin-embedded animal tissues. *J Vet Diagn Invest* 7:275–278.
74a. Innes EA. 1997. Toxoplasmosis: comparative species susceptibility and host immune response. *Comp Immunol Microbiol Infect Dis* 20:131–138.
75. Jackson W, de Lahunta A, Adaska J, et al. 1995. *Neospora caninum* in an adult dog with progressive cerebellar signs. *Prog Vet Neurol* 6:124–127.
76. Jacobson LS, Jardine JE. 1993. *Neospora caninum* infection in three Labrador littermates. *J S Afr Vet Assoc* 64:47–51.
77. Jardine JE. 1996. The ultrastructure of bradyzoites and tissue cysts of *Neospora caninum* in dogs: absence of distinguishing morphological features between parasites of canine and bovine origin. *Vet Parasitol* 62:231–240.
78. Jardine JE, Dubey JP. 1992. Canine neosporosis in South Africa. *Vet Parasitol* 44:291–294.
79. Knowler C, Wheeler SJ. 1995. *Neospora caninum* infection in three dogs. *J Small Anim Pract* 36:172–177.
79a. Kornberg M, Kosfeld HU. 1997. *Neospora caninum* in a dog. *Kleintierpraxis* 42:235–236.
80. Lappin MR. 1996. Feline toxoplasmosis: interpretation of diagnostic test results. *Semin Vet Med Surg* 11:154–160.
81. Lappin MR, Burney DP, Dow SW, et al. 1996. Detection of *Toxoplasma gondii* in aqueous humor from client-owned cats. *J Vet Intern Med* 10:179.
82. Lappin MR, Burney DP, Dow SW, et al. 1996. Polymerase chain reaction for the detection of *Toxoplasma gondii* in aqueous humor of cats. *Am J Vet Res* 37:1589–1593.
83. Lappin MR, Burney DP, Hill SA, et al. 1995. Demonstration of *Toxoplasma gondii*-specific IgA in the aqueous humor of cats. *Am J Vet Res* 56:774–778.
84. Lappin MR, Bush DJ, Reduker DW. 1994. Feline serum antibody responses to *Toxoplasma gondii* and characterization of target antigens. *J Parasitol* 80:73–80.
85. Lappin MR, Chavkin MJ, Mununa KR, et al. 1996. Feline ocular and cerebrospinal fluid *Toxoplasma gondii*-specific humoral immune responses

following specific and nonspecific immune stimulation. *Vet Immunol Immunopathol* 55:23–31.
86. Lappin MR, Dawe DL, Lindl P, et al. 1992. The effect of glucocorticoid administration on oocyst shedding, serology, and cell-mediated immune responses of cats with acute or chronic toxoplasmosis. *J Am Anim Hosp Assoc* 27:625–632.
87. Lappin MR, Dawe DL, Lindl P, et al. 1992. Mitogen and antigen-specific induction of lymphoblast transformation in cats with subclinical toxoplasmosis. *Vet Immunol Immunopathol* 30:207–210.
88. Lappin MR, Dow SW, Reif JS, et al. 1997. Elevated interleukin 6 activity in aqueous humor of cats with uveitis. *Vet Immunol Immunopathol* 58:17–26.
89. Lappin MR, Gasper PW, Rose BJ, et al. 1992. Effect of primary phase feline immunodeficiency virus infection on cats with chronic toxoplasmosis. *Vet Immunol Immunopathol* 35:121–131.
90. Lappin MR, George JW, Pedersen NC, et al. 1995. Experimental induction of toxoplasmosis in cats chronically infected with feline immunodeficiency virus. *J Clin Microbiol* 82:733–742.
91. Lappin MR, George JW, Pedersen NC, et al. 1996. Primary and secondary *Toxoplasma gondii* infection in normal and feline immunodeficiency virus infected cats. *J Parasitol* 82:733–742.
92. Lappin MR, Gigliotti A, Cayatte S, et al. 1993. Demonstration of *Toxoplasma gondii*-antigen containing immune complexes in the serum of cats. *Am J Vet Res* 54:415–419.
93. Lappin MR, Greene CE, Winston S, et al. 1989. Clinical feline toxoplasmosis: serologic diagnosis and therapeutic management of 15 cases. *J Vet Intern Med* 3:139–143.
94. Lappin MR, Marks A, Greene CE, et al. 1993. Effect of feline immunodeficiency virus infection on *Toxoplasma gondii*-specific humoral and cell-mediated immune responses of cats with serologic evidence of toxoplasmosis. *J Vet Intern Med* 7:95–100.
95. Lappin MR, Powell CC. 1991. Comparison of latex agglutination, indirect hemagglutination, and ELISA techniques for the detection of *Toxoplasma gondii*-specific antibodies in the serum of cats. *J Vet Intern Med* 5:299–301.
96. Lappin MR, Roberts SM, Davidson MG, et al. 1992. Enzyme-linked immunosorbent assays for the detection of *Toxoplasma gondii*-specific antibodies and antigens in the aqueous humor of cats. *J Am Vet Med Assoc* 201:1010–1016.
97. Lathe CL. 1994. *Neospora caninum* in British dogs. *Vet Rec* 134:532.
98. Lin DS, Bowman DD. 1991. Cellular responses of cats with primary toxoplasmosis. *J Parasitol* 77:272–279.
99. Lin DS, Bowman DD, Jacobson RH. 1992. Immunological changes in cats with concurrent *Toxoplasma gondii* and feline immunodeficiency virus infections. *J Clin Microbiol* 30:17–24.
100. Lindsay DS, Blagburn BL, Dubey JP. 1997. Feline toxoplasmosis and the importance of the *Toxoplasma gondii* oocyst. *Comp Cont Educ Pract Vet* 19:448–461.
101. Lindsay DS, Butler JM, Rippey NS, et al. 1996. Demonstration of synergistic effects of sulfonamides and dihydrofolate reductase/thymidine synthase inhibitors against *Neospora caninum* tachyzoites in cultured cells, and characterization of mutants resistant to pyrimethamine. *Am J Vet Res* 57:68–72.
102. Lindsay DS, Dubey JP, Blagburn BL. 1996. Canine neosporosis. *Small Anim Med Diag* 2:7–12.
103. Lindsay DS, Dubey JP, Butler JM, et al. 1996. Experimental tissue cyst induced *Toxoplasma gondii* infections in dogs. *J Eukaryot Microbiol* 43:5113.
103a. Lindsay DS, Dubey JP, Butler JM, et al. 1997. Mechanical transmission of *Toxoplasma gondii* oocysts by dogs. *Vet Parasitol* 73:27–33.
104. Lindsay DS, Dubey JP, Upton SJ, et al. 1990. Serological prevalence of *Neospora caninum* and *Toxoplasma gondii* in dogs from Kansas. *J Helminthol Soc Wash* 57:86–87.
105. Lindsay DS, Mitschler RR, Toivio-Kinnucan, et al. 1993. Association of host cell mitochondria with developing *Toxoplasma gondii* tissue cysts. *Am J Vet Res* 54:1663–1667.
106. Lindsay DS, Rippey NS, Cole RA, et al. 1994. Examination of the activities of 43 chemotherapeutic agents against *Neospora caninum* tachyzoites in cultured cells. *Am J Vet Res* 55:976–981.
107. Ljungstrom B-L, Lunden A, Hoglund J, et al. 1994. Evaluation of a direct agglutination test for detection of antibodies against *Toxoplasma gondii* in cat, pig, and sheep sera. *Acta Vet Scand* 35:213–216.
108. Lunden A, Uggla A. 1992. Infectivity of *Toxoplasma gondii* in mutton following curing, smoking, freezing or microwave cooking. *Int J Food Microbiol* 15:357–363.
109. MacPherson JM, Gajadhar AA. 1993. Sensitive and specific polymerase chain reaction detection of *Toxoplasma gondii* for veterinary and medical diagnosis. *Can J Vet Res* 57:45–48.
110. Marsh AE, Barr BC, Madigan J, et al. 1996. Neosporosis as a cause of equine protozoal myeloencephalitis. *J Am Vet Med Assoc* 209:1907–1913.
111. Mayhew IG, Smith KC, Dubey JP, et al. 1991. Treatment of encephalomyelitis due to *Neospora caninum* in a litter of puppies. *J Small Anim Pract* 32:609–612.
112. McGlennon NJ, Jeffries AR, Casas C. 1990. Polyradiculoneuritis and polymyositis due to a *Toxoplasma*-like protozoan: diagnosis and treatment. *J Small Anim Pract* 31:102–104.
113. Morris JT, Kelly JW. 1992. Effective treatment of cerebral toxoplasmosis with doxycycline. *Am J Med* 93:107–108.
114. Munana KR, Lappin MR, Powell CC, et al. 1995. Sequential measurement of *Toxoplasma gondii*-specific antibodies in the cerebrospinal fluid of cats with experimentally induced toxoplasmosis. *Prog Vet Neurol* 6:627–631.
115. Munday BL, Dubey JP, Mason RW. 1990. *Neospora caninum* infection in dogs. *Aust Vet J* 67:76.
116. Odin M, Dubey JP. 1993. Sudden death associated with *Neospora caninum* myocarditis in a dog. *J Am Vet Med Assoc* 203:831–833.
117. Omata Y, Aihara Y, Kanda M, et al. 1996. *Toxoplasma gondii* experimental infection in cats vaccinated with ^{60}Co-irradiated tachyzoites. *Vet Parasitol* 65:173–183.
118. Omata Y, Oikawa H, Kanda M, et al. 1990. Experimental feline toxoplasmosis: humoral immune responses of cats inoculated orally with *Toxoplasma gondii* cysts and oocysts. *Jpn J Vet Sci* 52:865–867.
119. Omata Y, Oikawa H, Kanda M, et al. 1991. Enhancement of humoral immune responses of cats after inoculation with *Toxoplasma gondii*. *J Vet Med Sci* 53:163–165.
120. Omata Y, Oikawa H, Kanda M, et al. 1994. Transfer of antibodies to kittens from mother cats chronically infected with *Toxoplasma gondii*. *Vet Parasitol* 52:211–218.
120a. Omata Y, Taka A, Terada K, et al. 1997. Isolation of coccidian enteroepithelial stages of *Toxoplasma gondii* from the intestinal mucosa of cats by Percoll density-gradient centrifugation. *Parasitol Res* 83:574–577.
121. O'Neil SA, Lappin MR, Reif JS, et al. 1991. Clinical and epidemiological aspects of feline immunodeficiency virus and *Toxoplasma gondii* coinfections in cats. *J Am Anim Hosp Assoc* 27:211–220.
121a. Patitucci AN, Alley MR, Jones BR, et al. 1997. Protozoal encephalomyelitis of dogs involving *Neospora caninum* and *Toxoplasma gondii* in New Zealand. *NZ Vet J* 45:231–235.
122. Patton S, Legendre AM, McGavin MD, et al. 1991. Concurrent infection with *Toxoplasma gondii* and feline leukemia virus. *J Vet Intern Med* 5:199–201.
123. Pimenta AL, Piza ET, Cardoso RB, et al. 1993. Visceral toxoplasmosis in dogs from Brazil. *Vet Parasitol* 45:323–326.
124. Poncelet L, Bjerkas I, Charlier G, et al. 1990. Confirmation of the presence of *Neospora caninum* in Belgium. *Ann Med Vet* 134:501–503.
125. Pumarola M, Anor S, Ramis AJ, et al. 1996. *Neospora caninum* infection in a Napolitan mastiff dog from Spain. *Vet Parasitol* 64:315–317.
126. Rhyan JC, Dubey JP. 1992. Toxoplasmosis in an adult dog with hepatic necrosis and associated tissue cysts and tachyzoites. *Canine Pract* 17:6–10.
126a. Romand S, Thulliez P, Dubey JP. 1998. Direct agglutination test for serologic diagnosis of *Neospora caninum* infection. *Parasitol Res* 84:50–53.
127. Rudback E, Mannonen J, Nikander S, et al. 1991. *Neospora caninum:* a new parasite in Finland? *Fin Vet J* 97:526–529.
128. Ruehlmann D, Podell M, Oglesbee M, et al. 1995. Canine neosporosis: case report and literature review. *J Am Anim Hosp Assoc* 31:174–183.
129. Sardinas JC, Chastain CB, Collins BK, et al. 1994. *Toxoplasma* pneumonia in a cat with incongruous serological test results. *J Small Anim Pract* 351:104–107.
130. Sato K, Iwamoto I, Yoshiki K. 1993. Experimental toxoplasmosis in pregnant cats. *J Vet Med Sci* 55:1005–1009.
131. Sheahan BJ, Caffrey JF, Dubey JP, et al. 1993. *Neospora caninum* encephalomyelitis in seven dogs. *Ir Vet J* 46:3–7.
132. Sreter T, Sebestyen P, Dubey JP. 1992. Neosporosis in a dog in Hungary. *Parasitol Hung* 25:5–8.
133. Stiles J, Prade R, Greene CE. 1996. Detection of *Toxoplasma gondii* in feline and canine biological samples by use of the polymerase chain reaction. *Am J Vet Res* 57:264–267.
134. Tenter AM, Vietmeyer C, Johnson AM, et al. 1994. ELISAs based on recombinant antigens for seroepidemiological studies on *Toxoplasma gondii* infection in cats. *Parasitology* 109:29–36.
135. Toomey JM, Carlisle-Nowak MM, Barr SC, et al. 1995. Concurrent toxoplasmosis and feline infectious peritonitis in a cat. *J Am Anim Hosp Assoc* 31:425–428.
136. Trees AJ, Guy F, Tennant BJ, et al. 1993. Prevalence of antibodies to *Neospora caninum* in a population of urban dogs in England. *Vet Rec* 132:125–126.
137. Umemura T, Shiraki K, Morita T, et al. 1992. Neosporosis in a dog: the first case report in Japan. *J Vet Med Sci* 54:157–159.
138. Vanham LM, Thoonen H, Barber JS, et al. 1996. *Neospora caninum* infection in the dog. Typical and atypical cases. *Vlaams Diergeneesk Tijdschr* 65:326–335.
139. Wallace MR, Rossetti RJ, Olson PE. 1993. Cats and toxoplasmosis risk in HIV-infected adults. *JAMA* 269:76–77.
139a. Weissenbock H, Dubey JP, Suchy A, et al. 1997. Neosporosis causing encephalomalacia and myocarditis in young dogs. *Wien Tierarztl Monatsschr* 84:233–237.
140. Wilson M, Ware DA, Juranek DD. 1990. Serologic aspects of toxoplasmosis. *J Am Vet Med Assoc* 196:277–281.
141. Wolf M, Cachin M, Vandevelde M, et al. 1991. Clinical diagnosis of protozoal myositis-encephalitis syndrome *(Neospora caninum)* in puppies. *Tierarztl Prax* 19:302–306.
142. Wong SY, Remington JS. 1993. Biology of toxoplasmosis. *AIDS* 7:299–316.
143. Yamane I, Thomford JW, Gardner IA, et al. 1993. Evaluation of the indirect fluorescent antibody test for diagnosis of *Babesia gibsoni* infections in dogs. *Am J Vet Res* 54:1579–1584.

Chapter **81**

Enteric Coccidiosis

J. P. Dubey and Craig E. Greene

Coccidia are obligate intracellular parasites normally found in the intestinal tract. They belong to phylum Apicomplexa, class Sporozoasida, order Eucoccidiorida, and, depending on the species, family Eimeriidae, Cryptosporidiidae, or Sarcocystidae. Coccidian genera that infect cats and dogs are *Isospora* (also called *Cystoisospora*), *Hammondia, Besnoitia, Sarcocystis, Toxoplasma, Neospora* (see Chapter 80), *Cryptosporidium*, and *Cyclospora* (see Chapter 82).[2] A *Caryospora* infection is also discussed in this section. Another coccidian genus, *Eimeria*, found commonly in herbivores, birds, lagomorphs, and rodents, is found only in feces of dogs and cats after they ingest intestinal contents or feces from these animals. The oocysts pass unchanged through the feline or canine intestine. Some coccidians of dogs remain unclassified.

INTESTINAL COCCIDIOSIS

All coccidians have an asexual and a sexual cycle. In some genera, such as *Sarcocystis*, the asexual and sexual cycles occur in different hosts, whereas in *Isospora* both cycles may occur in the same host (Table 81–1 and Fig. 81–1). The oocyst is the environmentally resistant stage in the life cycle of all coccidia and is excreted in feces of the definitive host.

A representative coccidian life cycle is best described as follows. Oocysts are passed unsporulated in feces and contain a single nucleated mass called a sporont, which almost fills the oocyst (Fig. 81–2). After exposure to warm (20–37°C) environmental temperatures and moisture, oocysts sporulate, forming two sporocysts. Within each sporocyst are four sporozoites (Fig. 81–3). The sporozoites are banana shaped and are the infective stage (Fig. 81–4). They can survive environmental exposure inside the oocysts for many months. After the ingestion of sporulated oocysts by cats or dogs, sporozoites excyst in the intestinal lumens, and the sporozoites initiate the formation of schizonts or meronts. During schizogony or merogony, the sporozoite nucleus divides into two, three, or more nuclei, depending on the parasite and the stage of the cycle. After nuclear division, each nucleus is surrounded by cytoplasm, forming a merozoite. The number of merozoites within a schizont varies from two to several hundred, depending on the stage of the cycle and the species of coccidia. Merozoites are released from the schizont when the host cell ruptures. The number of schizogonic cycles varies with the parasitic species. First-generation merozoites repeat the asexual cycle and form second-generation schizonts or transform into male (micro) and female (macro) gamonts. The microgamont divides into many tiny microgametes. A microgamete fertilizes a macrogamete, and an oocyst wall is formed around the zygote. The life cycle is completed when unsporulated oocysts are excreted in feces.

Isospora

Members of the genus *Isospora*, the most commonly recognized coccidians infecting dogs or cats, are species specific for the definitive host. At least four species, *I. canis, I. ohioensis, I. burrowsi*, and *I. neorivolta*, infect dogs, and two species, *I. felis* and *I. rivolta*, infect cats.

Epidemiology. The life cycle of *Isospora* infecting dogs and cats is similar to the basic coccidian intestinal cycle, except an asexual cycle can also occur in the definitive or intermediate host. On ingestion by definitive or suitable paratenic (intermediate) hosts, oocysts excyst in the presence of bile, and free sporozoites invade the intestine. Some sporozoites penetrate the intestinal wall and enter mesenteric lymph nodes or other extraintestinal tissues, where they form enlarging unicellular cysts (Fig. 81–5). If no replication occurs, the term paratenic, rather than intermediate, host is used. Monozoic cysts of *Isospora* may remain in extraintestinal tissues of definitive and paratenic hosts for the life of the host. In dogs and cats, these cysts may serve as a source of intestinal reinfection and relapse of enteric coccidiosis. Ingestion of monozoic cysts in paratenic hosts leads to intestinal infection in the definitive dog and cat host. The life cycle after the

Table 81–1. Comparison of Some Coccidial Genera That Infect Dogs and Cats

	SEXUAL CYCLE: INTESTINAL REPLICATION		MEANS OF TRANSMISSION	ASEXUAL CYCLE: EXTRAINTESTINAL REPLICATION	
	Definitive Host	Form of Oocyst Passed	Direct Transmission Possible	Intermediate or Paratenic Hosts	Location of Tissue Cysts
Isospora	B	U	Yes	Dog, cat, many other mammals	Extraintestinal or lymphoid tissues (monozoic)
Besnoitia	C	U	No	Many vertebrates	Fibroblasts
Hammondia	B	U	No	Herbivores, rodents	Skeletal muscle
Sarcocystis	B	S[a]	No	Many vertebrates	Cardiac and skeletal muscle
Cryptosporidium	B	S[b]	Yes	None	None
Toxoplasma	C	U	Yes	Many vertebrates	Many tissues

[a]Free sporocysts.
[b]Naked sporozoites.
B = both dog and cat; C = cat; U = unsporulated; S = sporulated.

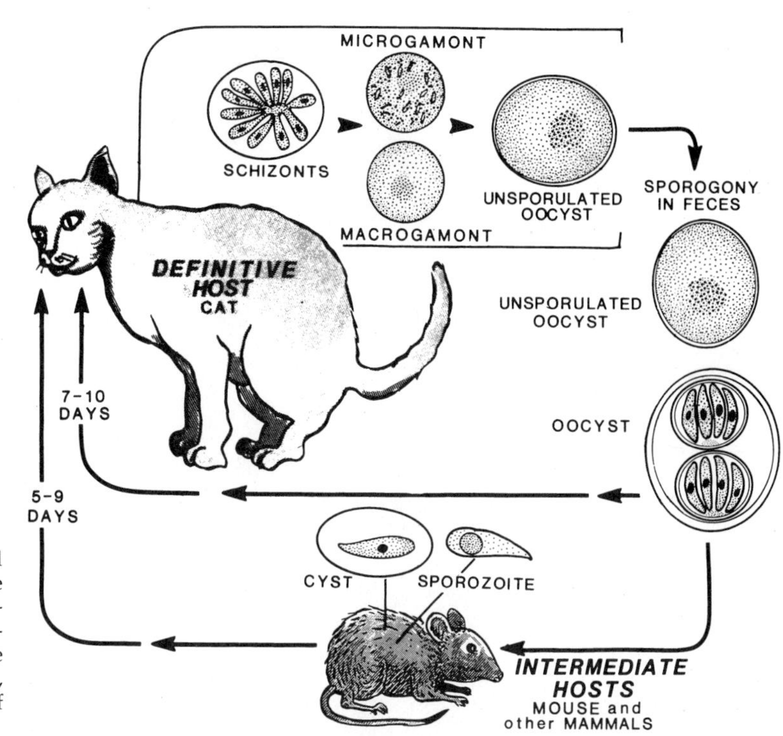

Figure 81–1. Life cycle of *Isospora felis*, which is typical of the *Isospora* spp. The mode of transmission may be direct, via ingestion of sporulated oocysts from the environment, or indirect, via ingestion of cysts in prey animals. Sexual and asexual reproduction of the parasite occurs in the intestines of the definitive host (in this case, a cat), and unsporulated oocysts are shed in the feces of definitive hosts.

ingestion of paratenic host is the same as after the ingestion of sporulated oocysts from feces.

Clinical Findings. Diarrhea with coccidiosis in immunocompetent animals probably represents incidental or concurrent infections with coccidia and other infectious agents because coccidial infection can be present in the absence of clinical illness. Enzootic infections are frequently found in catteries or kennels where animals are congregated. Clinical signs are most apparent in neonates. Experimental studies have shown that clinical signs of intestinal disease are uncommon unless large numbers of oocysts are fed to very young (<1 month) or immunosuppressed animals. Clinically, severe diarrhea has been associated with naturally occurring coccidiosis in immunosuppressed dogs and cats. Diarrhea with weight loss and dehydration and, rarely, hemorrhage is the primary sign attributed to coccidiosis in dogs and cats. Anorexia, vomiting, mental depression, and ultimately death may be seen in severely affected animals. Severely immunosuppressed dogs and cats may have extraintestinal stages in macrophages of the lymphocyte-depleted mesenteric lymph nodes or extraintestinal tissues.

Intestinal coccidiosis may be manifest clinically when dogs or cats are shipped or weaned or experience a change in ownership. Diarrhea might result from the extraintestinal stages of *Isospora* returning to the intestines. Monozoic cysts do not cause clinical disease in paratenic hosts.

Diagnosis. Intestinal coccidial infection in dogs and cats is diagnosed by identification of the oocysts with any of the fecal flotation methods commonly used to diagnose parasitic infections (see Fecal Examination, Chapter 70). In dogs, only *I. canis* can be identified with certainty by oocyst size and shape (see Fig. 81–2). The two species of *Isospora* occurring in cats can be readily distinguished by oocyst size (see Fig. 80–9). Oocysts of *I. felis* in cats and *I. canis* in dogs are large

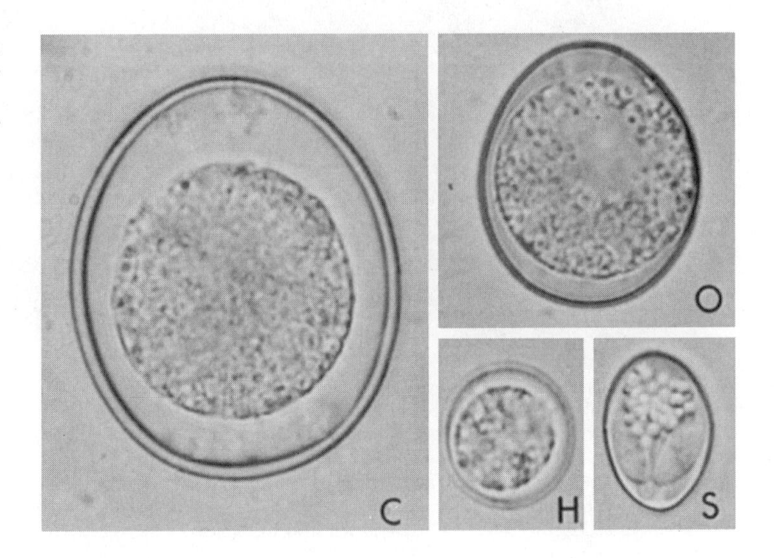

Figure 81–2. Unsporulated oocysts of *Isospora canis (C), I. ohioensis (O),* and *Hammondia heydorni (H)* and sporulated sporocyst of *Sarcocystis* sp. *(S)* from canine feces (unstained, × 1700). (From Dubey JP: *J Am Vet Med Assoc* 169:1061–1078, 1976, with permission.)

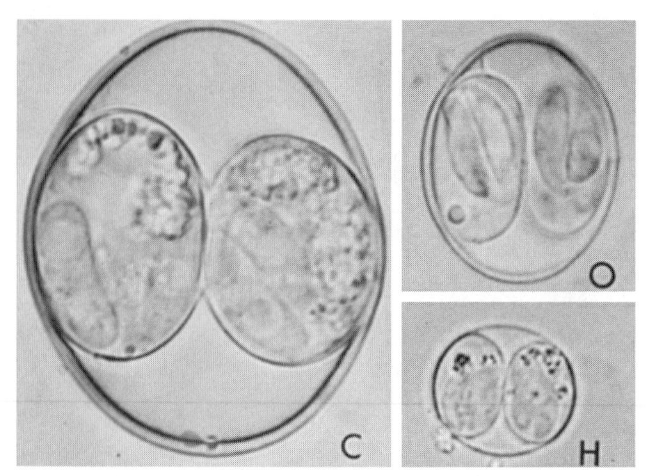

Figure 81–3. Sporulated oocysts of *Isospora canis (C), I. ohioensis (O),* and *Hammondia heydorni (H).* Compare with Figure 81–2 (unstained, × 1700). (From Dubey JP: *J Am Vet Med Assoc* 169:1061–1078, 1976, with permission.)

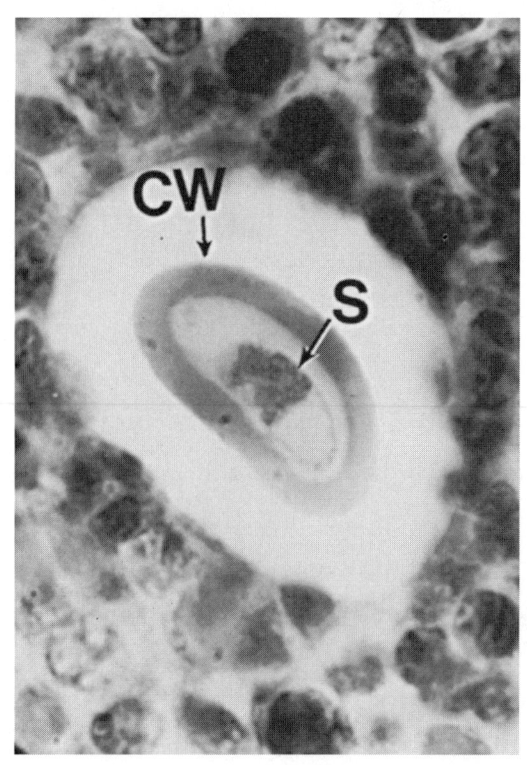

Figure 81–5. Tissue cyst of *Isospora felis* in smear of mesenteric lymph node of an experimentally infected mouse. The sporozoite *(S)* is surrounded by a thick cyst wall *(CW).* The vacuole around the cyst wall is a fixation artifact (periodic acid–Schiff, × 1250).

and easily distinguished from small oocysts, whereas it is almost impossible to distinguish *I. rivolta, I. burrowsi,* and *I. ohioensis* morphologically (Fig. 81–6; see also Fig. 80–9). Although *I. felis–, I. rivolta–, I. canis–,* and *I. ohioensis*–like oocysts are passed unsporulated in freshly excreted feces, they sporulate partially by the time fecal examination is made. Partially sporulated oocysts contain two sporocysts without sporozoites. *Isospora* species may sporulate within 8 hours of excretion, and these *Isospora* are highly infectious.

Therapy. The presence of underlying disease or host immunosuppression should be suspected whenever coccidial infections persist for extended periods in older animals or whenever associated with chronic diarrhea. Treatment is often indicated in bitches and their newborn puppies because of the severity of clinical signs at this age. If diarrhea or dehydration is severe, parenteral fluid therapy must be considered as a supportive measure. Blood transfusion may be required when severe intestinal hemorrhage results in anemia.

Specific therapy involves the use of drugs that are coccidiostatic rather than curative (Table 81–2). However, as with many protozoal diseases, the presence of low-level infection may lead to premunition.

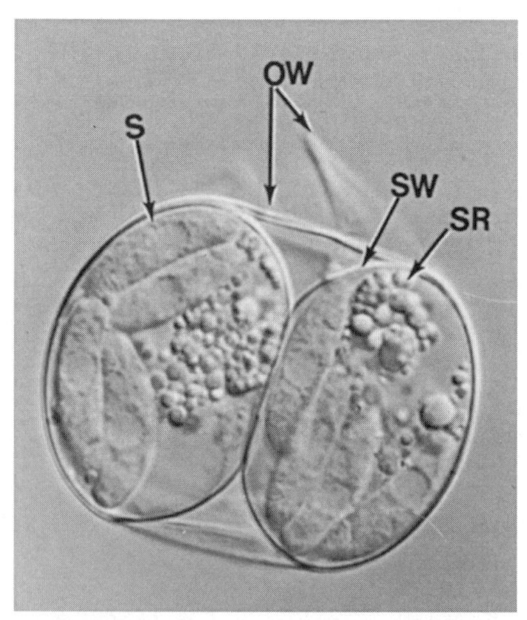

Figure 81–4. *Isospora canis* sporulated oocyst treated with 5.25% sodium hypochlorite solution to dissolve part of the oocyst wall *(OW).* Two sporocysts occupy most of the oocyst. Each sporocyst has a thin sporocyst wall *(SW),* four banana-shaped sporozoites *(S),* and a sporocystic residual body *(SR).* The SR may be compact or dispersed (unstained, × 1600). (From Kirkpatrick CE, Dubey JP: *Vet Clin North Am Small Anim Pract* 17:1405–1420, 1987, with permission.)

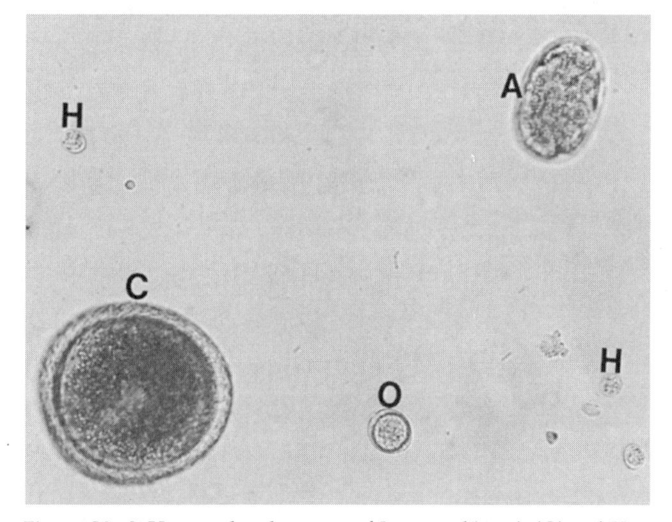

Figure 81–6. Unsporulated oocysts of *Isospora ohioensis (O)* and *Hammondia heydorni (H)* compared with eggs of the nematodes *Toxocara canis (C)* and *Ancylostoma caninum (A)* in a flotation of canine feces (unstained, × 385). (From Dubey JP: *J Am Vet Med Assoc* 169:1061–1078, 1976, with permission.)

Table 81–2. Anticoccidial Drugs for Dogs and Cats

DRUG	SPECIES	DOSE (mg/kg)[a]	ROUTE	INTERVAL (HOURS)	DURATION (DAYS)
Sulfamethoxine[b]	B	50–60	PO	24	5–20
Sulfaguanidine	B	100–200	PO	8	5
Trimethoprim-sulfonamide	D	30–60[c]	PO, SC	24	5
	B	15–30[d]	PO, SC	12–24	5
Ormetoprim-sulfadimethoxine	D	66[e]	PO	24	7–23
Furazolidone[f]	B	8–20	PO	12–24	5
Amprolium	D	300–400 (total)[g]	PO	24	5
	D	110–200 (total)[h]	PO	24	7–12
	C	60–100 (total)	PO	24	7
Quinacrine	B	10	PO	24	5
Spiramycin	H	50–100 (total)[i]	PO	24	5
Toltrazuril	D	10	PO	Medicated feed	2–6
Roxithromycin	H	2.5	PO	12	15

[a]Dose per administration at specified interval.
[b]Other sulfonamides, such as sulfadimidine and sulfaguanidine, can be used, but sulfaquinoxaline should be avoided owing to its interference with vitamin K synthesis with potential hemorrhagic complications.
[c]Greater than 4 kg body weight.
[d]Less than 4 kg body weight.
[e]Consists of 11 mg ormetoprim and 55 mg sulfadimethoxine.
[f]When furazolidone is combined with sulfonamides, 50% of this dose is used.
[g]Total dose/day. Lower dosage recommended for puppies and maximum of 300 mg total/day (see Drug Formulary, Appendix 8).
[h]Total dose/day. Combine 150 mg amprolium and 25 mg sulfadimethoxine/kg/day for 14 days.
[i]Total dose/day. Dose on a milligram per kilogram basis is listed in Drug Formulary, Appendix 8.
B = dog and cat; D = dog; C = cat; H = human.

Sulfonamides have long been the drugs of choice for the treatment of coccidiosis. Rapid-acting sulfonamides, such as sulfadimethoxine or sulfaguanidine, can be given alone or in combination with other antifolate drugs such as trimethoprim. Trimethoprim-sulfonamide offers the advantages of being readily available and of having lower toxicity compared with other drugs. It should be considered a drug of first choice. Nitrofurazone can be administered alone or in combination with sulfonamides. Nitrofurazone is also available as a 4.59% soluble powder that can be added to drinking water (up to 1 g/2 L) for 7 days.

Amprolium is considered an effective preventive and treatment for coccidiosis in kenneled puppies. Although it is not currently approved for use in dogs, it can be administered as an undiluted liquid and a paste, but it is unpalatable in these forms (see Drug Formulary, Appendix 8).

Quinacrine, spiramycin, toltrazuril, tetracycline, and roxithromycin have been provided on a limited basis to treat canine and feline coccidiosis. Their use might be considered if more established treatment regimens fail or protozoal resistance develops.

Prevention. Coccidiosis tends to be a problem in areas of poor sanitation. The fecal shedding of large numbers of environmentally resistant oocysts makes infection likely under such conditions. Animals should be housed so as to prevent contamination of food and water bowls by oocyst-laden soil or infected feces. Feces should be removed daily and incinerated. Oocysts survive freezing temperatures. Runs, cages, food utensils, and other implements should be disinfected by steam cleaning or immersion in boiling water or by 10% ammonia solution. Animals should have limited access to intermediate hosts and should not be fed uncooked meat. Insect control is essential in animal quarters and food storage areas because cockroaches and flies may serve as mechanical vectors of oocysts. Coccidiostatic drugs can be given to infected bitches before or soon after whelping to control the spread of infection to puppies.

Hammondia

Two species of *Hammondia* exist in domestic animals: *H. hammondi*, with cats as definitive hosts, and *H. heydorni*, with dogs and coyotes as definitive hosts.[2] Unlike *Isospora* spp., *H. hammondi* and *H. heydorni* have obligatory two-host life cycles similar to *T. gondii* (see Chapter 80 and Table 81–1). For *H. hammondi*, goats and rats are natural intermediate hosts, and the domestic cat *(Felis catus)* and the European wild cat *(Felis sylvestris)* are the definitive hosts. *H. hammondi* does not invade extraintestinal tissues of the cat, and cats are infected only by eating tissue cysts. Experimentally, many warm-blooded animals, including monkeys, cattle, sheep, goats, pigs, rabbits, guinea pigs, and mice, can serve as intermediate hosts. Intermediate hosts become infected by ingesting sporulated oocysts, which resemble those of *T. gondii.* Sporozoites excyst in the intestinal lumen, invade the intestinal wall, and multiply as tachyzoites in the intestines, mesenteric lymph nodes, and other tissues. The parasite eventually encysts principally in muscles (Fig. 81–7).

H. heydorni's life cycle is similar to that of *H. hammondi* except that dogs and coyotes are definitive hosts. Cattle, sheep, goats, buffaloes, camels, moose, and deer serve as intermediate hosts. The structure of the parasite in the intermediate hosts is not known. Both *H. hammondi* and *H. heydorni* are nonpathogenic. Therefore, no treatment is necessary.

Besnoitia

Cats, but not dogs, are definitive hosts for two species of *Besnoitia* in the United States: *B. wallacei* of rats and mice and *B. darlingi* of opossums and, possibly, lizards.

The life cycle of *Besnoitia* is similar to those of *H. hammondi* and *T. gondii* (see Table 81–1). Cats become infected by ingesting tissue cysts (Fig. 81–8), and schizonts and gamonts are formed in intestinal goblet cells. Unsporulated oocysts are shed in feces, and they are difficult to distinguish from those of *H. hammondi*. Intermediate hosts become infected by ingesting sporulated oocysts. The parasite develops in connective tissue, and cysts may become macroscopic. *Besnoitia* is considered nonpathogenic for cats, and no treatment is necessary.

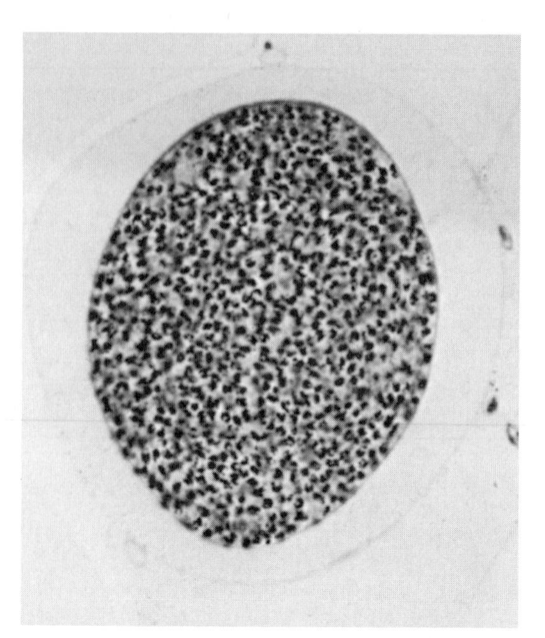

Figure 81-7. *Hammondia hammondi* tissue cyst in section of abdominal muscle of an experimentally infected mouse. Note the thin cyst wall enclosing hundreds of periodic acid–Schiff–positive bradyzoites (× 750).

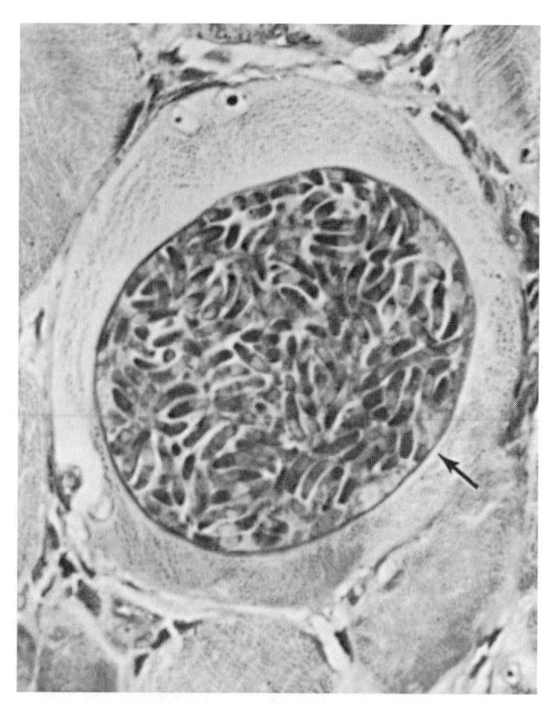

Figure 81-9. Cross-section of sarcocyst of *Sarcocystis muris* in a myocyte. The sarcocyst wall *(arrow)* is thin and encloses numerous banana-shaped bradyzoites. There is no host reaction around the sarcocyst (Giemsa stain, × 750).

Sarcocystis

Infections resulting from *Sarcocystis* are ubiquitous in reptiles, birds, and warm-blooded animals.[2] Virtually all cattle and sheep are infected with this parasite. There are more than 90 species of *Sarcocystis*. *Sarcocystis* spp. have an obligatory two-host life cycle (see Table 81–1). Carnivores (predators) are definitive hosts, and herbivores (prey) are intermediate hosts. As the name implies, the parasite forms tissue cysts (called sarcocysts) in muscles and neural tissues (Fig. 81–9). Sarcocysts are thin or thick walled, and the zoites are usually separated from each other by septa. Cats and dogs become infected by ingesting sarcocysts. The life cycle of *Sarcocystis* is distinct from other coccidians of domestic animals in that oocysts sporulate within the definitive host and are excreted in the feces in an infective form (Fig. 81–10). The intermediate hosts become infected by ingesting sporocysts or oocysts. One to three generations of schizogony occur in blood vessels or in hepatocytes (depending on the species of intermediate hosts), and merozoites then invade skeletal muscles and nerve cells, where they form sarcocysts (Figs. 81–10 and 81–11). Certain species of *Sarcocystis*, transmissible via dogs, are pathogenic in cattle, sheep, goats, pigs, and mule deer, whereas species transmissible via cats are generally nonpathogenic.

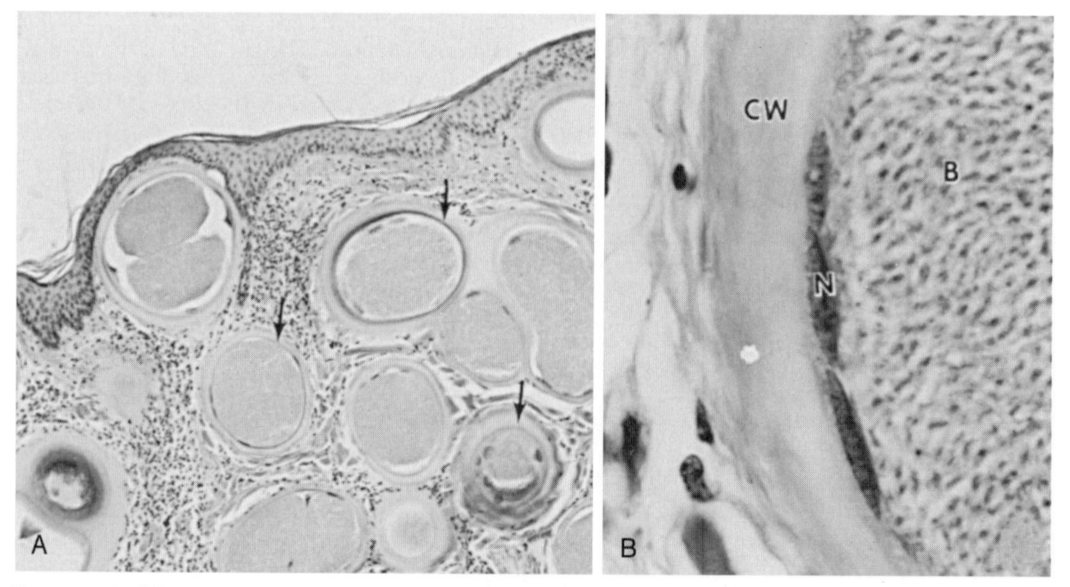

Figure 81-8. Tissue cysts of *Besnoitia besnoiti* in skin of a naturally infected cow (H and E). *A*, Arrows point to thick cyst walls (× 150). *B*, Note thick cyst wall *(CW)* incorporating host cell nuclei *(N)* and numerous bradyzoites *(B)* (× 750).

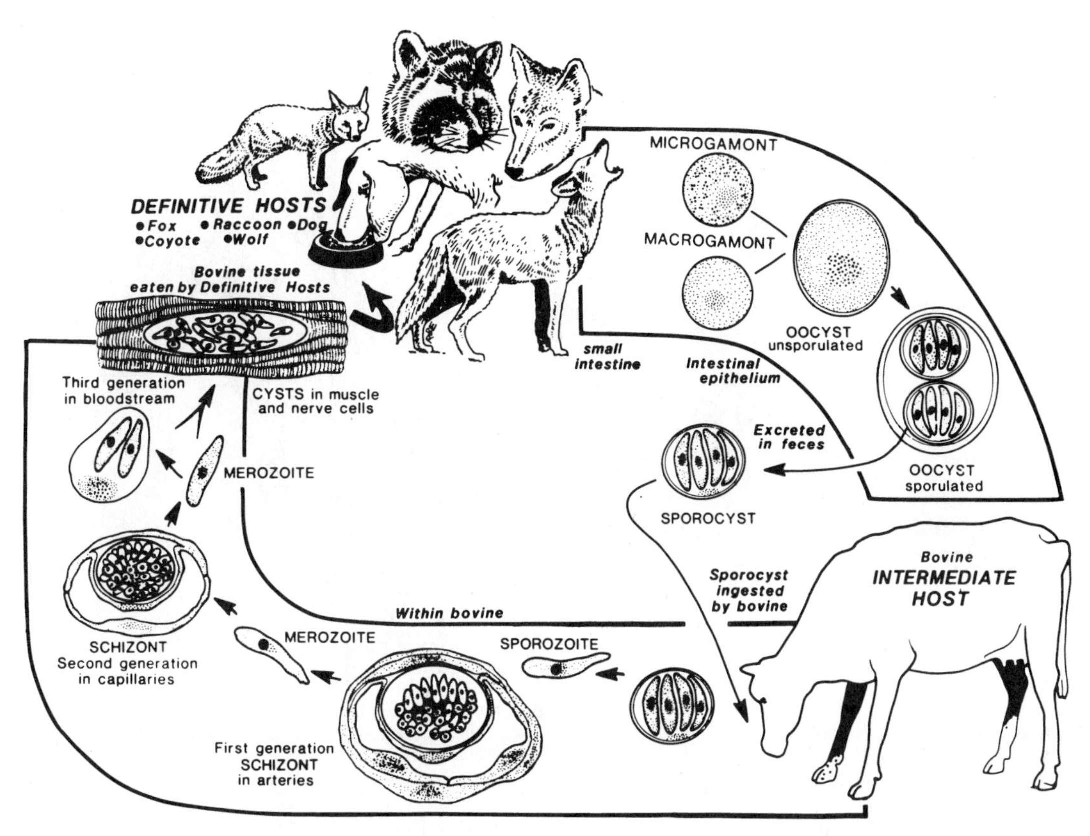

Figure 81–10. Life cycle of *Sarcocystis cruzi*, which is typical of *Sarcocystis* spp. Carnivores are definitive hosts, supporting the sexually replicating stages of the parasite, and herbivores are intermediate hosts, supporting the asexually replicating stages of the parasite. Sporulated oocysts or, more commonly, sporocysts are excreted in the feces of carnivores. (Modified from Dubey JP, Fayer R: *Br Vet J* 139:371–377, 1983, with permission.)

More than 20 species of *Sarcocystis* infect both cats and dogs. It is not possible to differentiate species on the basis of measurement of sporocysts. *Sarcocystis* is excreted in feces fully sporulated, often as free sporocysts when examined microscopically (Fig. 81–12). They are small and, because of low density, lie at a different plane of focus than other parasites.

Sarcocystis spp. are not pathogenic for the intestinal tract of dogs or cats, and no treatment is necessary. Infections can be prevented by feeding only cooked meat. Occasionally, sarcocysts are found in skeletal muscles of immunosuppressed or wild cats and dogs, but their life cycle is unknown.[4, 7]

VISCERAL AND CUTANEOUS SARCOCYSTOSIS

Another group of *Sarcocystis*-like parasites has been identified in tissues as schizonts, which cause fatal encephalomyelitis in horses, dogs, raccoons, minks, and cats. The parasite in horses has been called *Sarcocystis neurona* and is a principal cause of equine protozoal myelitis (see also Neosporosis, Chapter 80). One of these *Sarcocystis*-like parasites (*Sarcocystis canis*) has been described as occurring in Rottweiler dogs in the United States.[9–11] Only asexual stages (schizonts) were seen in various cells, including neurons, hepatocytes, and dermal cells (Figs. 81–13 and 81–14). Affected dogs were 2-day-old to adult dogs and were presented clinically with neurologic and hepatic signs and dermatitis. Schizonts were 5 to 25 × 4 to 20 μm in size and contained 6 to 40 merozoites. Merozoites were arranged occasionally around a residual body. The parasite was named *S. canis* because it differed from other species of *Sarcocystis*. Its life cycle is unknown.

Sarcocystis-associated meningoencephalomyelitis was

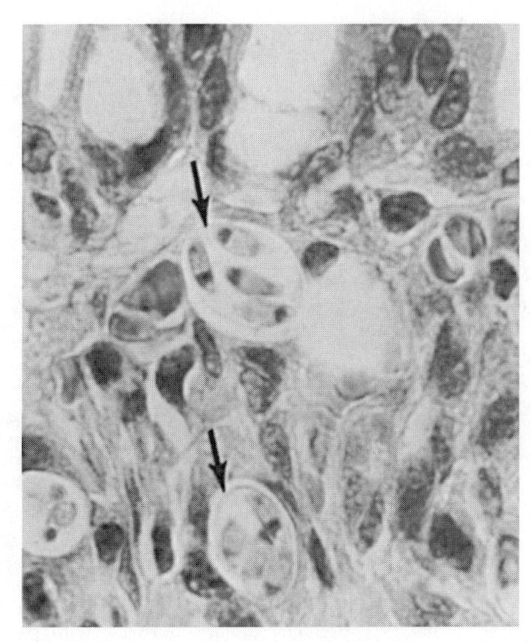

Figure 81–11. Sporocysts (*arrows*) in the lamina propria of small intestine of dog fed *S. cruzi*–infected beef (H and E, × 1250).

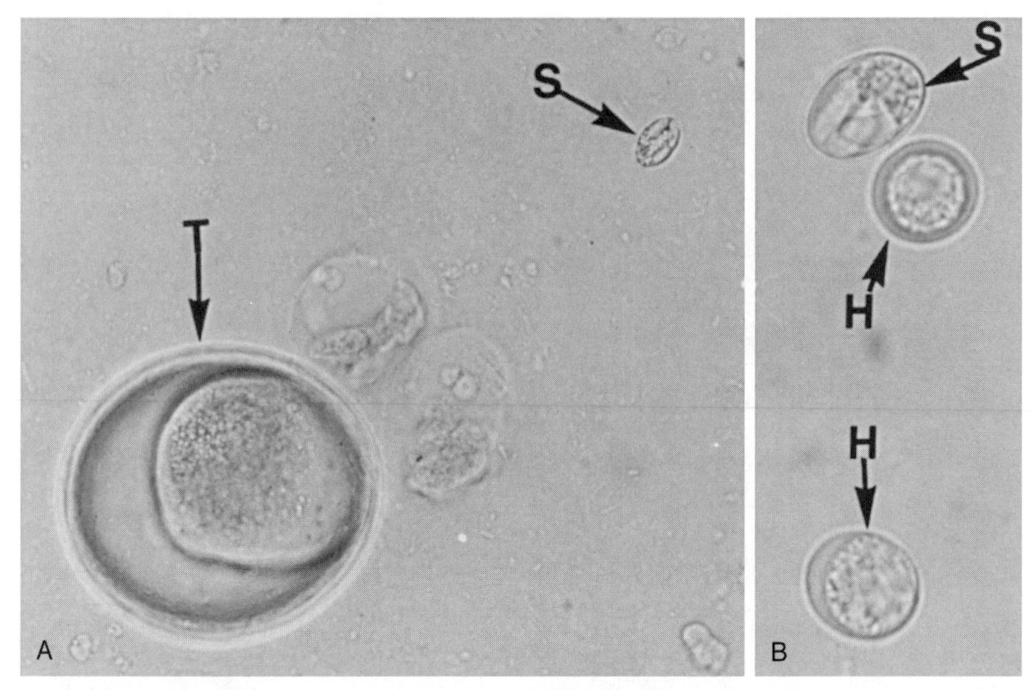

Figure 81–12. Sporulated *Sarcocystis cruzi* sporocysts *(S)*, unsporulated *Hammondia hammondi (H)*, and *Toxascaris leonina* egg *(T)* in fecal flotation of canine feces (unstained, *A*, × 430; *B*, × 1250). (From Dubey JP: *J Am Vet Med Assoc* 169:1061–1078, 1976, with permission.)

described in a 13-week-old Burmese kitten with lethargy, depression and crying, and upper motor neuron hemiparesis.[8]

VISCERAL AND CUTANEOUS CARYOSPOROSIS

A *Caryospora bigenetica*–like organism has been isolated from cutaneous nodules in five dogs ranging in age from 2 to 6 months. The dogs were thought to be concurrently affected with distemper virus–like infection.[3]

The skin nodules were up to 2 cm in diameter, and some had a central ulcerated area through which serohemorrhagic exudate could be expressed. Microscopically, the dermatitis was characterized by edema and infiltrations by polymorphonuclear cells, eosinophils, and macrophages (Fig. 81–15). Schizonts, male and female gamonts, unsporulated and sporulated oocysts, and caryocysts were seen in macrophages. In one dog, infection had spread to the lymph nodes.

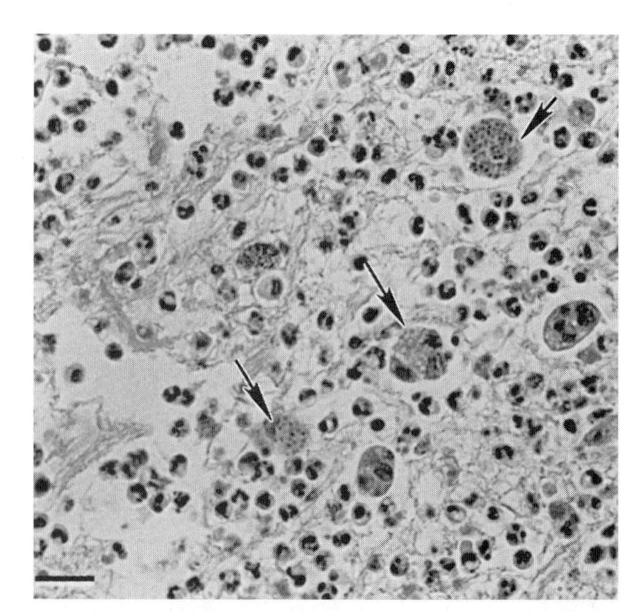

Figure 81–13. *Sarcocystis canis* schizonts in section of a dermal ulcer from a dog. Note distended macrophages *(arrows)* with parasites among inflammatory exudate, mainly neutrophils (H and E, × 750; bar = 10 μm).

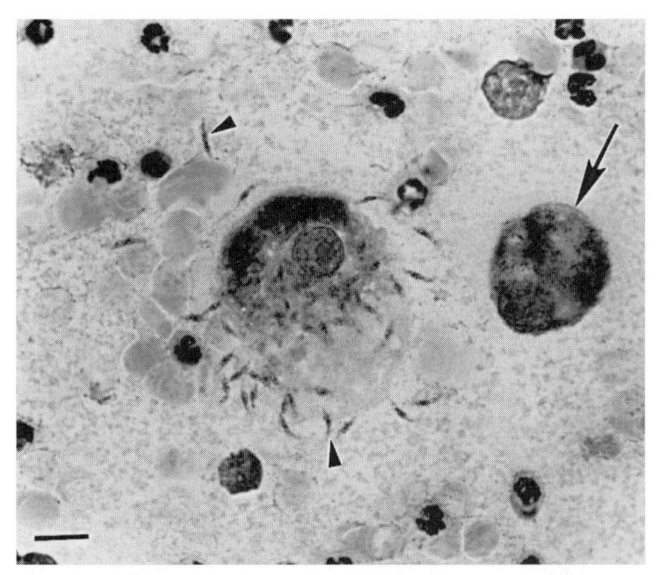

Figure 81–14. An intact *Sarcocystis canis* schizont *(arrow)* and several merozoites *(arrowheads)* released from a ruptured schizont in a smear of exudate from dermal ulcer of a dog (Giemsa stain, × 750; bar = 10 μm).

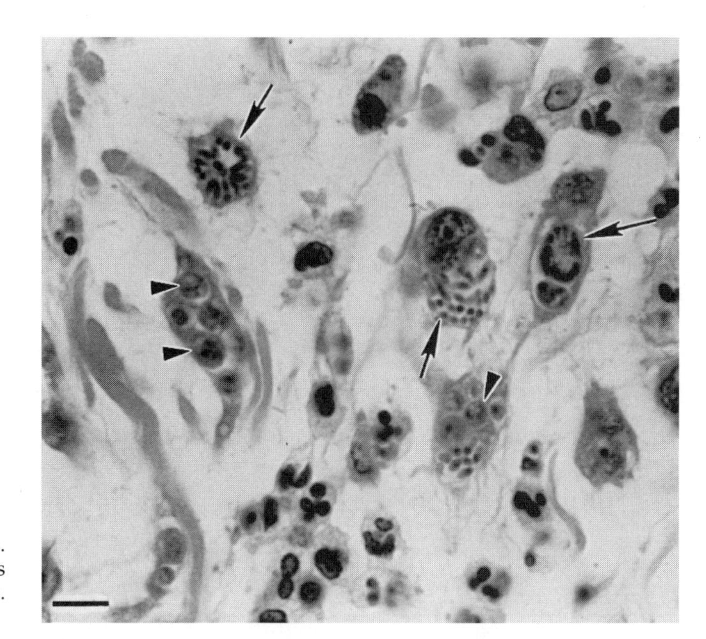

Figure 81–15. Section from skin of a dog with *Caryospora* dermatitis. Note numerous *Caryospora* stages in dermal cells including gamonts *(arrowheads)* and schizonts *(arrows)* (H and E, × 750; bar = 10 μm). (From Dubey et al: *J Parasitol* 76:552–556, 1990, with permission.)

Members of the genus *Caryospora* have an oocyst with one sporocyst that contains eight sporozoites, and they typically parasitize mostly reptiles and raptors. At least two species, *C. bigenetica* and *C. simplex* are parasitic in rodents and snakes. *Caryospora* spp. have a complicated life cycle involving asexual and sexual multiplication both in the prey (rodent) and the predator (snake). In addition to usual schizonts and gamonts, sporulated oocysts and monozoic cysts (called caryocysts) are formed in connective tissue cells of the prey. The caryocysts (unlike sporocysts and oocysts) have a thin cyst wall enclosing the host cell nucleus. Two unusual features of *Caryospora* stages are noted in histologic sections of dog tissue: 1) the small size (<15 μm) of all developmental stages, and 2) the presence of gamonts, schizonts, and oocysts in a single macrophage.

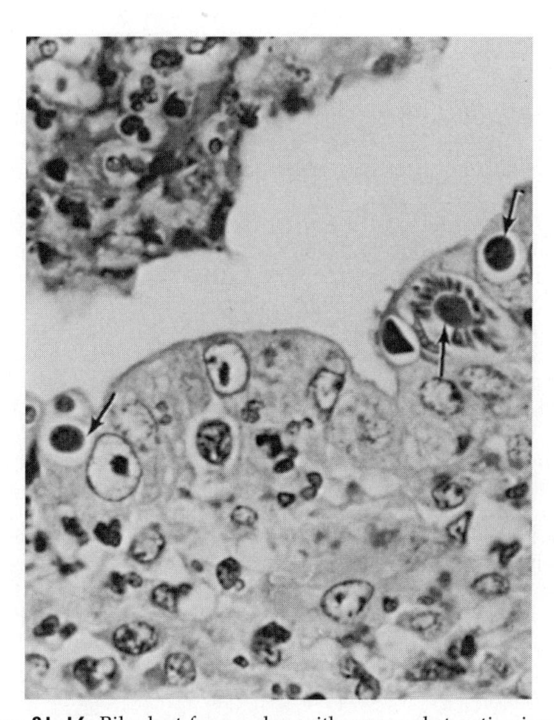

Figure 81–16. Bile duct from a dog with severe obstructive jaundice reported by Lipscomb and colleagues (1989). Parasites *(arrows)* are present in epithelial cells of bile duct. One schizont has merozoites radiating from a residual body. Inflammatory cells are present in bile duct lumen (H and E, × 750).

INTRAHEPATIC BILIARY COCCIDIOSIS IN DOGS

Intrahepatic biliary coccidiosis is a rare condition in dogs.[13] Clinical signs are those associated with hepatic disease: icterus, weight loss, and vomiting. Small and large bile ducts are enlarged because of inflammation and desquamation of epithelial cells. Lesions may extend into hepatic parenchyma. Asexual stages (schizonts) of an unidentified coccidium are found in biliary epithelial cells (Fig. 81–16). This coccidium is different from *Toxoplasma*, *Sarcocystis*, *Hammondia*, *Cryptosporidium*, and any other known coccidium of the dog.

INTRAPULMONARY COCCIDIOSIS IN DOGS

An adult dog with clinical signs of weakness, fever, diarrhea, dehydration, weight loss, and harsh lung sounds was found to have canine distemper complicated by pulmonary infection with coccidia-like organisms.[14] Asexual stages of coccidia were observed in cytoplasmic vacuoles of many bronchiolar epithelial cells.

References

1. Bwangamoi O, Ngatia TA, Richardson JD. 1993. *Sarcocystis*-like organisms in musculature of a domestic dog *(Canis familiaris)* and wild dogs *(Lycaon pictus)* in Kenya. *Vet Parasitol* 49:201–205.
2. Dubey JP. 1993. *Toxoplasma, Neospora, Sarcocystis*, and other tissue cyst-forming coccidia of humans and animals, pp 1–158. *In* Kreir JP (ed), Parasitic protozoa, vol 6. Academic Press, New York, NY.
3. Dubey JP, Black SS, Sangster LT, et al. 1990. *Caryospora*-associated dermatitis in dogs. *J Parasitol* 76:552–556.
4. Dubey JP, Bwangamoi O. 1994. *Sarcocystis felis* (Protozoa: sarcocystidae) from the African lion *(Panthera leo)*. *J Helminthol Soc Wash* 61:113–114.
5. Dubey JP, Cosenza SF, Lipscomb TP, et al. 1991. Acute *Sarcocystis*-like disease in a dog. *J Am Vet Med Assoc* 198:439–444.

6. Dubey JP, Greene CE. 1990. Enteric coccidiosis, pp 835–846. *In* Greene CE (ed), Infectious diseases of the dog and cat. WB Saunders, Philadelphia, PA.
7. Dubey JP, Hamir AN, Kirkpatrick CE, et al. 1992. *Sarcocystis felis* sp. n. (Protozoa: Sarcocystidae) from bobcats *(Felis rufus)*. *J Helminthol Soc Wash* 59:227–229.
8. Dubey JP, Higgins RJ, Barr BC, et al. 1994. *Sarcocystis*-associated meningoencephalomyelitis in a cat. *J Vet Diagn Invest* 6:118–120.
9. Dubey JP, Slife LN. 1990. Fatal encephalitis in a dog associated with an unidentified coccidian parasite. *J Vet Diagn Invest* 2:233–236.
10. Dubey JP, Slife LN, Speer CA, et al. 1991. Fatal cutaneous and visceral infection in a Rottweiler dog associated with a *Sarcocystis*-like protozoon. *J Vet Diagn Invest* 3:72–75.
11. Dubey JP, Speer CA. 1991. *Sarcocystis canis* n. sp. (Apicomplexa: Sarcocystidae), the etiologic agent of generalized coccidiosis in dogs. *J Parasitol* 77:522–527.
12. Dubey JP, Speer CA, Fayer R. 1989. Sarcocystosis of animals and man, pp 1–215. CRC Press, Boca Raton, FL.
13. Lipscomb TJ, Dubey JP, Pletcher JM, et al. 1989. Intrahepatic biliary coccidiosis in a dog. *Vet Pathol* 26:343–345.
14. Neu S, Dubey JP. 1992. Pulmonary coccidiosis in a dog. *J Vet Diagn Invest* 4:490–492.
15. Omata Y, Oikawa H, Kanda M, et al. 1991. Humoral immune response to *Isospora felis* and *Toxoplasma gondii* in cats experimentally inoculated with *Isospora felis*. *J Vet Med Sci* 53:1071–1073.
16. Omata Y, Oikawa H, Mikazuki M, et al. 1990. *Isospora felis*: possible evidence for transmission of parasites from chronically infected mother cats to kittens. *Jpn J Vet Sci* 52:665–666.
17. Saito M, Shibata Y, Kobayashi T, et al. 1996. Ultrastructure of the cyst wall of *Sarcocystis* species with canine final host in Japan. *J Vet Med Sci* 58:861–867.

Chapter **82**

Cryptosporidiosis and Cyclosporiasis

Stephen C. Barr

Cryptosporidiosis

ETIOLOGY AND EPIDEMIOLOGY

Cryptosporidium is a ubiquitous coccidian genus in the suborder Eimeria, family Cryptosporidiidae, phylum Apicomplexa that inhabits the epithelium of the respiratory and digestive systems of reptiles, birds, and mammals. Infections of the ileum are most common, but gastric, respiratory, and conjunctival infections have been observed in immunosuppressed hosts. Many species have been described. Most species may be relatively host specific. Those found in reptiles and birds apparently do not infect mammals. Only two species are recognized in mammals on the basis of the very small oocyst size, namely *C. parvum* (4–5 μm in diameter) and *Cryptosporidium* sp. (6–8 μm in diameter a.k.a. *C. muris*). Oocysts are often difficult to demonstrate in the feces without special techniques. The biology of *Cryptosporidium* sp. is not well known and its host range is limited,[2] and it will not be considered further. In contrast, *C. parvum* is by far the most commonly occurring species in mammals and, similar to *Toxoplasma*, has a wide mammalian host range.[48] It has been reported in rodents, domestic livestock, cats, dogs, people, and numerous wild mammals. Ruminants, especially calves, are considered reservoir hosts. Cross-infection between various mammalian hosts occurs.[46] Despite their host specificity, experimentally, *C. parvum* from calves can induce respiratory signs in chickens,[52] although most such attempts have failed.[48] A high prevalence of serum antibodies to cryptosporidia in most species tested, including cats, suggests that exposure to the parasite is common.[45] In a clinical and postmortem study in metropolitan domestic and feral cats, the prevalence of infection was 5.1% and 12.1%, respectively.[43] In rural cats from the surrounding area, the prevalence was 12.3%.[47] One study of stray dogs in California, in which only 2% of dogs were excreting oocysts, suggested that the numbers of dogs excreting oocysts at any one time may be low.[13]

The life cycle of cryptosporidians differs from most other coccidians (Fig. 82–1). All stages of development (asexual and sexual) of cryptosporidia occur within one host.[48] After ingestion, oocysts excyst in the GI tract, releasing infective sporozoites, which become enclosed as trophozoites within parasitiferous vacuoles of the microvillous surface of enterocytes rather than in the cytoplasm (Fig. 82–2). The trophozoites proliferate (asexually) by merogony to produce, sequentially, two types of meronts. Within 24 hours, type I meronts (containing eight merozoites) leave the parasitiferous vacuole to invade other epithelial cells where they develop into more type I meronts or type II meronts (containing four merozoites). The type II meronts do not undergo merogony but produce sexual reproductive stages (gamonts). The zygotes formed by sexual reproduction (gametogony between male microgamonts and female macrogamonts) form either thick-walled (excreted in the feces) or thin-walled (autogenous reinfection) oocysts each containing four sporozoites.

Oocysts of cryptosporidia are spread via the fecal-oral route. Fecal contamination of food or drinking water is a common source of infection. The organism is extremely infective; as few as 100 oocysts are necessary to precipitate disease in people.[37]

PATHOGENESIS

Cryptosporidia are either primary pathogens or secondary invaders in a variety of immunosuppressive diseases of ani-

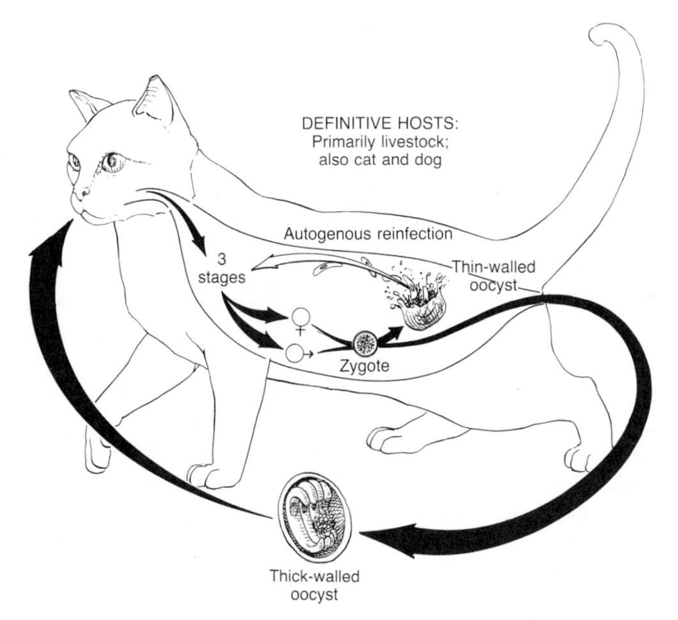

Figure 82–1. Life cycle of *Cryptosporidium*.

mals and people. Crowding and unsanitary practices increase the risk of exposure. Cryptosporidial diarrhea is common among calves in intensive raising units and among children in day care centers.

Cryptosporidiosis may cause malabsorption or secretory diarrhea, but the underlying mechanisms are unknown. Functional impairment (glucose-stimulated sodium and water absorption) and morphologic changes (villous atrophy, crypt hyperplasia, and cell infiltration) have been reported in pigs experimentally infected with *C. parvum*.[1, 42] Although secretory toxins have been implicated in the electrogenic chloride secretory stimulation,[20] the mechanism of action is unclear.[37] Lymphocytic duodenitis and intestinal bacterial overgrowth have been documented in a young cat with cryptosporidiosis; however, it is unknown whether *Cryptosporidium* species caused the lesion.[22]

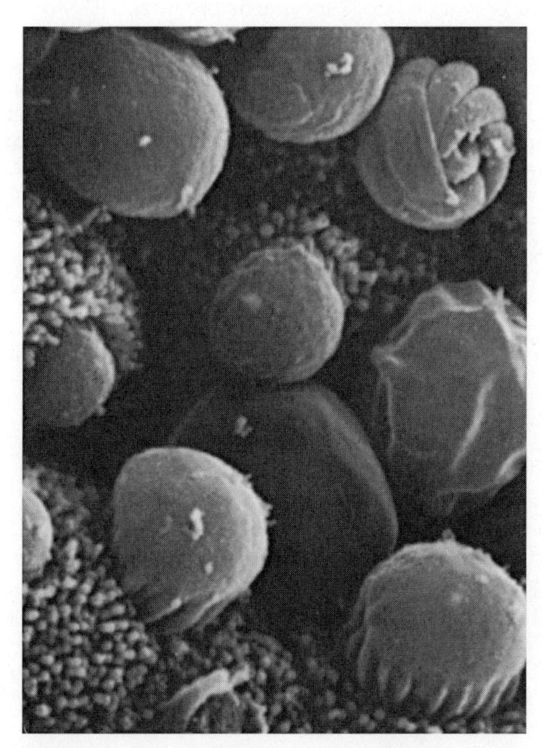

Figure 82–2. Scanning electron microphotograph of various stages of *Cryptosporidium* on the epithelial cell microvillous surface of the cloaca of a young chicken (× 5000). (Courtesy of Sandy L. White, Lilly Research Labs, Greenfield, IN. From Current WL: *ASM News* 54:605–612, 1988, with permission.)

Both humoral and cell-mediated immunity participate in the host response to infection with *C. parvum*. Although cryptosporidial cysts are excreted by nonsymptomatic cats or dogs, most case reports document a potential cause of systemic (feline leukemia virus [FeLV], feline immunodeficiency virus, canine distemper, parvovirus) or local (GI lymphoma, coronavirus, *Campylobacter, Isospora* spp., *Toxocara cati*) immunosuppression in infected symptomatic animals.[18, 31, 57] Concurrent infections with various organisms (*Capillaria* spp., *T. cati, Isospora felis, Pharyngostomum cordatum*) were detected in normal cats excreting cryptosporidial oocysts in the feces. Cryptosporidiosis was found to be more common among nonsymptomatic young and newborn kittens as compared with older (>6 months) cats.[43]

CLINICAL FINDINGS

Cats

Because experimental inoculations of *C. parvum* of healthy adult cats or healthy 6-week-old kittens resulted in nonsymptomatic infections, it is questionable whether cryptosporidia infections can cause diarrhea in healthy animals. Diarrhea can be self-limiting or absent in naturally infected immunocompetent cats. Pathogenicity undoubtedly is greater in immunodeficient cats. Intestinal cryptosporidiosis in other FeLV-negative or FeLV-positive cats has also been associated with chronic anorexia, weight loss, and persistent diarrhea.[57] The diarrhea is usually of a small-bowel nature, characterized by high-volume, low-frequency stools with significant weight loss. Tenesmus, fresh blood, swelling, and discomfort may be seen with chronicity.

Dogs

Experimental infection of healthy pups resulted in oocyst shedding without accompanying disease.[57] Naturally occurring cryptosporidiosis has been reported in a 1-week-old pup that died after an episode of diarrhea and dyspnea,[48] whereas other pups infected with cryptosporidia did not show clinical signs suggestive of infection.[57] As in cats, signs of diarrhea are most severe in immunosuppressed dogs. Cryptosporidiosis has been described in immunosuppressed pups with distemper[57] and in dogs with GI lymphoma.[4] Cryptosporidial infection has been diagnosed in an adult dog with persistent diarrhea and malabsorption syndrome and no obvious cause for immunosuppression.[19]

Calves and Other Animals

Although cryptosporidial infection in calves without clinical signs of diarrhea is common, it is an important cause of diarrhea of varying severity (from mild intermittent to profuse watery with dehydration) among calves younger than 3 weeks.[49] The organism has also been identified in the bronchial epithelium of a calf.[38] Cryptosporidial diarrhea also is an important disease among young ruminants found in zoos. Less severe infections have been reported in young swine, lambs, and foals. The coccidian is fairly common in birds, infecting the digestive and respiratory tracts and the bursa of Fabricius, and may be a primary pathogen. In captive snakes, cryptosporidia causes gastritis and subsequent vomiting because it parasitizes the stomachs of these reptiles.[48]

People

People of all ages may become infected with cryptosporidia, and the severity of disease depends on the immunocompetence of the host. Most people develop transient clinical signs and recover. Cryptosporidiosis is an increasingly common cause of death in people with AIDS.[61] Individuals with congenital immunodeficiency disease may survive for years with cryptosporidiosis when fed parenterally. Immunocompetent persons may be infected readily with *Cryptosporidium* as demonstrated when more than 400,000 people in Milwaukee developed diarrhea as a result of contracting the organism via the public water supply.[34] Enzootic infections by this means are very common.[7, 17, 35] Infection among veterinary students is common after contact with infected calves and has been documented after contact with infected lambs,[15] a dog,[19] and cats.[12, 29, 33] Severe stress or concurrent infection by viruses or bacteria serves to exacerbate the diarrheal syndrome.

In people, there has been a causal connection between oocysts being shed in the stool and GI signs.[26] The typical prepatent period is 5 to 7 days. Clinical signs, which may last from 2 to 26 days in immunocompetent people, may include nausea, abdominal cramps, low-grade fever, and anorexia. Occasionally, episodes last longer. Diarrhea may be profuse, and dehydration is a common sequela. Nonsymptomatic infections do occur, especially in recovery phases of the illness. Conversely, symptomatic patients can have intermittently negative stools.[26]

DIAGNOSIS

Fecal Examination

Fecal oocyst excretion directly coincides with the onset and duration of clinical signs. Because cryptosporidial oocysts are directly infective when shed in the feces, caution must be used to avoid accidental infection. To destroy the oocyst, 1 part 100% formalin (38% formaldehyde) should be mixed with 9 parts fluid feces before performing fecal examination procedures. Sodium acetate–acetic acid–formalin is another acceptable fixative, but polyvinyl alcohol fixatives are not compatible with most staining procedures. Samples should also be formalinized before shipment to a diagnostic laboratory and should be placed in a nonbreakable container. The outside of the container should be disinfected to avoid accidental infection of laboratory personnel. Oocysts may be seen microscopically on direct smears of feces, but concentration techniques, such as Sheather's sugar solution, can be used (see Fecal Examination, Chapter 80). Because oocysts are slightly smaller than erythrocytes and because of transparency, unstained preparations utilizing conventional light microscopy do not permit accurate identification.[57] When searching for cryptosporidial oocysts on unstained preparations, phase-contrast microscopy is often recommended; however, bright-field microscopy can be used (Fig. 82–3). A wet preparation with crystal violet is applied on fluid stools, and oocysts can readily be seen because they do not stain (Fig. 82–4). Because the small and refractile oocysts cling to the coverslip on Sheather's flotation, focusing immediately

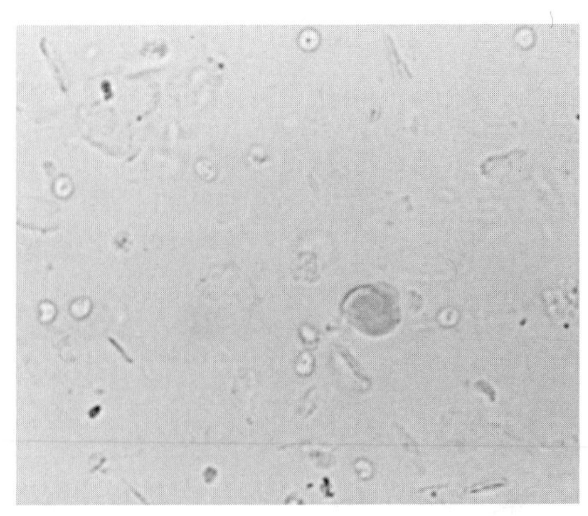

Figure 82–3. Cryptosporidial oocyst as seen with bright-field microscopy using Sheather's sugar flotation (× 160).

beneath the coverslip is imperative. Oocysts appear as circular, sometimes concave, discs that are refractile and pink with bright-field microscopy. Dark shadows of sporozoites may be seen within the oocysts.

Beagle pups experimentally infected with *C. parvum* of calf origin commenced shedding oocysts 3 to 5 days PI with a peak shedding at 7 to 9 days PI. Shedding lasted for at least 80 days at a low or intermittent level.

Other procedures, used by diagnostic laboratories to demonstrate cryptosporidial oocysts in fluid stools, include formalin-ethyl acetate (FEA) sedimentation technique or examination of direct smears of feces or intestinal contents with negative stains, such as Kinyoun's modified carbolfuchsin and crystal violet.[25, 33a, 36, 44] Using the FEA concentration method on watery stool specimens provided 100% detection with direct FA or acid-fast staining when 10^4 oocysts/g or more were present.[65] For formed stools, 5×10^4 or more was needed for indirect FA and 5×10^5 oocysts/g or more for acid-fast staining. A modification of the acid-fast technique utilizing dimethyl sulfoxide has simplified the procedure and has stained the internal structure of the organism. Newer but more expensive auramine-rhodamine staining techniques are very sensitive.[36] Staining methods allow for easier detection of the oocysts and their differentiation from yeasts, which stain darker and are slightly smaller than cryptosporidia, are

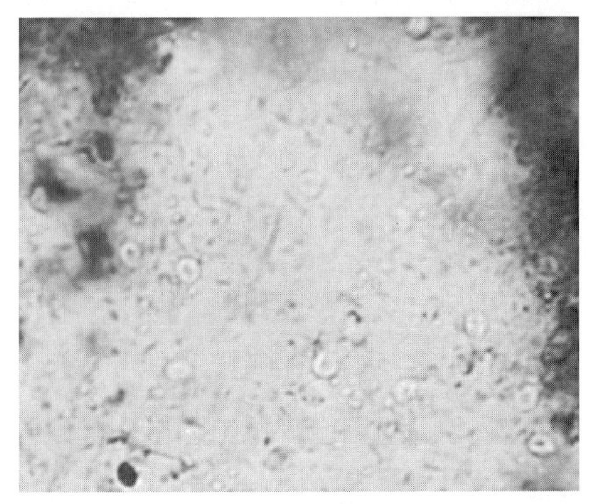

Figure 82–4. Wet preparation of cryptosporidial oocysts. Their appearance is accentuated by lack of internal staining (crystal violet, × 125).

oval, appear in clumps, and may show budding. Commercial kit staining methods are available.[48] A direct FA kit for staining cryptosporidial oocysts (and *Giardia* cysts) in feces is commercially available (Merifluor, Meridian Diagnostics, Cincinnati, OH); although extensive evaluations have not been reported in dogs and cats, the test is effective for oocyst detection in fecal samples from calves and sheep.[68] Several ELISA tests (ProSpecT and ProSpecTR, *Cryptosporidium* Microtiter Assay, Alexon, Sunnyvale, CA; Color-Vue *Cryptosporidium*, Seradyn, Indianapolis, IN) for the detection of cryptosporidial antigen in feces are also available but not yet evaluated for dog and cat feces. Nested polymerase chain reaction (PCR) has been used to detect *C. parvum* DNA in feces of symptomatic people with 500 oocysts/g of feces, some of whom had negative results with acid-fast staining.[3] Similar high sensitivity has been reported for PCR detection in calf feces.[65] Flow cytometry has also been used to increase the sensitivity of oocyst detection.[63a] See Appendix 5 for the laboratories that perform diagnostic tests and Appendix 6 for further information on test kits available for diagnosis of this disease.

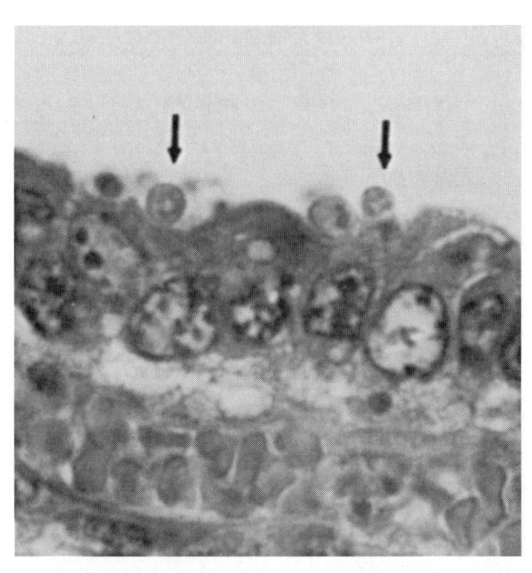

Figure 82–5. *Cryptosporidium (arrows)* in intestine from an infected calf is characteristically located at the microvillous border (H and E, × 250).

Serologic Testing

An ELISA was developed to measure *Cryptosporidium*-specific IgG in feline sera.[29c] Positive antibody titers were correlated with exposure, but not necessarily active infection or oocyst shedding. This test might be used as an epidemiologic surveillance tool.

Animal Inoculation

Oocysts for animal inoculation may be harvested by sugar centrifugation and stored in a refrigerator in 2.5% potassium dichromate for up to 6 months without appreciable loss of viability. Neonatal mice are inoculated per os, and the intestinal tissues are examined microscopically 1 week later.

Intestinal Biopsy

Gross lesions consist of enlarged, congested mesenteric lymph nodes, and changes are most severe in the distal ileum. The mucosa is hyperemic and may contain watery, yellow contents. Giemsa and routine H and E stains are effective as most parasite stages are basophilic (Fig. 82–5). As a routine method of diagnosis, biopsy is costly and time consuming and lacks sensitivity because only small amounts of tissue can be examined.

Specimens may be fixed in Bouin's or formalin solutions. Samples must be fixed within hours of biopsy or death because autolysis causes rapid loss of the intestinal surface that contains the organisms. Microscopic lesions vary in degree of villous atrophy; reactive lymphoid tissue; and inflammatory infiltrates in the lamina propria, consisting of neutrophils, macrophages, and lymphocytes. Parasites may be found throughout the intestines but are usually most numerous in the distal small intestine. EM readily identifies organisms by their unique ultrastructural characteristics and location within distinctive parasitiferous vacuoles.[48] EM shows that the organism is covered by the host cell microvillous membrane and, therefore, is intracellular but extracytoplasmic in location.

THERAPY

Infections in immunocompetent animals or persons are usually self-limiting, and full recovery soon ensues. To date, there have been few drugs used successfully for treating cryptosporidiosis, although more than 100 have been screened.[28] Spiramycin showed early promise, but subsequent studies did not corroborate its efficacy.[54] Eflornithine,[60] oral bovine dialyzable extract,[40] and hyperimmune bovine colostrum[56] have shown clinical benefit. The aminoglycoside antibiotic, paromomycin (Humatin, Parke-Davis, Morris Plains, NJ) is effective in treating acute intestinal cases of cryptosporidiosis in humans,[10] calves,[14] mice,[21] and rats.[64] Clinical signs of disease and oocyst shedding were eliminated in cats and dogs after paromomycin was administered for 5 days (Table 82–1).[4, 5] Although paromomycin seems effective against ileal infections, it was ineffective against cecal and biliary tract infections in immunosuppressed rats.[59] Tylosin (11 mg/kg PO BID for 28 days) was helpful in relieving diarrhea in a cat with cryptosporidiosis and lymphocytic duodenitis,[22, 29b] and this finding may be related to its antibacterial effects. Neither prior clindamycin nor metronidazole were effective in treating this cat. Azithromycin, a macrolide antibiotic, was more effective than paromomycin when used at identical regimens against cryptosporidial infection involving the ileum, cecum, or biliary tract of immunosuppressed rats.[59] Azithromycin has been effective in treating an immunocompetent man with cryptosporidiosis acquired from a calf[6] and is currently being tested in human trials. For additional information on this drug, see Chapter 34, and the Drug Formulary, Appendix 8.

Parenteral fluid replacement is usually indicated if dehydration is severe. Antibiotic therapy for eliminating secondary bacterial invaders may be necessary.

PUBLIC HEALTH CONSIDERATIONS

Cryptosporidial infections in people were not recognized until 1976. Since that time, it has been diagnosed with increasing frequency. Animal handlers, medical personnel, people living or traveling in developing countries, and children in day care facilities have the highest risk of exposure. Be-

Table 82–1. Drug Therapy for Cryptosporidiosis[a]

DRUG	SPECIES	DOSE[b] (mg/kg)	ROUTE	INTERVAL (HOURS)	DURATION (DAYS)
Paromomycin	B	125–165	PO	12	5[4, 5]
Azithromycin[c]	D	5–10	PO	12	5–7
	C	7–15	PO	12	5–7

[a]See Drug Formulary, Appendix 8, for specific information on drugs.
[b]Dose per administration at specified interval.
[c]Dose for systemic infections; effective level for this disease has not been established.
B = dog and cat; D = dog; C = cat.

tween 4% and 7% of human patients admitted to hospitals for gastroenteritis have cryptosporidiosis, and infections are more common during the warm, humid months. Aquatic transmission via drinking water, the source of infection for more than 400,000 people in Milwaukee in 1993,[34] and swimming pools[35, 39] have been major sources of infection. One outbreak in the United States has also been associated with a recreational lake.[29a] Food contamination with feces from infected people or animals is less common.[28] Although there are only weak epidemiologic data implicating household pets as sources of cryptosporidiosis in humans, there are several reports of human infection after contact with infected cats[29] and a dog.[19] There are numerous reports of transmission from calves to humans.[30, 32, 41] Genetic analyses of human and bovine isolates have shown that two types of *C. parvum* exist.[53a] One is involved with calf-to-human, human-to-human, human-to-calf, and other interspecies transmissions. The other is an exclusive anthroponotic cycle with people being both the reservoir and affected population. Because cryptosporidiosis can be fatal in immunocompromised people, especially those with AIDS, it is essential that owners of infected animals be made aware of the zoonotic risks.

In immunocompetent people, GI signs include profuse watery diarrhea, low-grade fever, vomiting, and abdominal discomfort in decreasing frequency. Diarrhea usually lasts 3 to 12 days. Infants, children, and the elderly have more chronic persistent diarrhea and dehydration. In immunodeficient persons, especially those with AIDS, the diarrhea becomes chronic (usually 20 or longer weeks), debilitating, and potentially fatal. In addition, respiratory tree, biliary, and pancreatic duct colonization has been reported in immunodeficient people with associated clinical signs.[9]

Cryptosporidia are resistant to commercial bleach (5.25% sodium hypochlorite); routine chlorination of drinking water does not affect oocyst viability.[58] Of the common disinfectants, only formol saline (10% solution) and ammonia (5% solution) were effective in destroying the viability of cryptosporidial oocysts. However, oocysts had to be in contact with the disinfectants for 18 hours. More concentrated (50%) ammonia solutions have been effective after 30 minutes. Moist heat (steam or pasteurization [>55°C]), freezing and thawing, or thorough drying are more practical means of disinfection. Swimming pools can be disinfected by using high chlorine concentrations for long periods (3 mg/L of water for 53 hours or 8 mg/L for 20 hours).[27] Excellent sanitation and liberal use of boiling water for scalding food and water bowls should minimize contamination in a clinical environment.

Cyclosporiasis

Cyclospora cayetanensis is a member of subclass Coccidia in the phylum Apicomplexa that infects people in tropical climates worldwide. For many years it was considered to be a cyanobacterium, a blue-green alga, or a large (8–10 μ) strain of *Cryptosporidium*. Phylogenetically, it is most closely related to *Eimeria*.[54a] Veterinarians should be aware that this parasite may be mistaken for *Cryptosporidium*. Both *Cyclospora* and *Cryptosporidium* have similar appearing unsporulated oocysts in feces and produce similar GI signs.[67] The morphology and features of *Cyclospora* that distinguish it from other coccidial oocysts are listed in Table 82–2. The life cycle of *Cyclospora* is unknown, but transmission occurs through contaminated water. The oocyst dies immediately when desiccated. At least 2 weeks are required for sporulation of oocysts to be infectious. Outbreaks correspond to the time of the rainy season in endemic countries. Drinking contaminated water or eating unwashed berries imported from some countries in South America have been implicated as risk factors in the United States,[8] where the prevalence in stool specimens submitted to diagnostic laboratories is generally less than 0.5%.[24, 62] Carriage rates of up to 20% of diarrheic people are found in endemic tropical countries. Animals or insects may act as reservoir hosts maintaining the organism in nature. Although other animals, including dogs or cats, might be infected, this has been currently identified only as a human pathogen. In Mexico, feces of cats were examined to no avail; however, large numbers of oocysts morphologically and biologically resembling *C. cayetanensis* were found in poultry feces.[16] Fowl feces may be involved in contamination of poultry meat, water supplies, and/or vegetables or fruits. Animal-to-human or person-to-person transmission is not yet documented. The upper small intestine is the site of replication in immunocompetent hosts, and more diffuse intestinal involvement occurs in the immunosuppressed hosts.[53] Malabsorption is caused by inflammation, villous atrophy, and crypt hyperplasia.

Cyclosporiasis has relapsing watery diarrhea, fatigue, systemic flulike manifestations, and weight loss in susceptible humans such as those infected with HIV, those receiving organ transplants or immunosuppressants, and those traveling to different geographic areas. Clinical signs are infrequent or transient in immunocompetent hosts, who usually recover within several weeks.[50a]

Diagnosis is made by microscopic detection of oocysts in fecal specimens. These can be confused with *Cryptosporidium* and *Isospora*, which also stain acid fast in stool specimens. However, *Cyclospora* has a variable staining intensity on an individual preparation. Although PCR has been used for

Table 82–2. Comparison of Coccidial Oocysts and Transmission

VARIABLE	*CYCLOSPORA*	*CRYPTOSPORIDIUM*	*ISOSPORA*	*TOXOPLASMA*
Definitive host	Human Animal?	Human, dog, cat Other animals	Human, dog, cat Other animals	Cat
Intestinal biopsy				
Intracellular stages	T, S, M	T, S, M, G	T, S, M, G	T, S, M, G
Intracellular location	Deep seated	Intramembranous, extracytoplasmic	Deep seated	Deep seated
Size in tissue (μm)	4–16	2–5	3–15	3–15
Feces				
Oocyst size (μm)	8–10	4–6	10–19 × 20–30 Varies with species	12 × 10
Sporulated oocyst				
Number sporocysts	2	0	2	2
Number sporozoites per sporocyst	2	Four per oocyst	4	4
Acid-fast staining	Variable	Yes	Yes	Yes
UV autofluorescence 365-nm filter	Blue-green Circles	None	None	None
Auramine fluorescence	Weak	Bright	Variable	Variable
Zoonotic transmission	Unknown	Many animals	None, host specific	Cat
Host-to-like-host transmission	Unknown	Yes	Yes	Yes, uncommon via oocyst

T = trophozoite; S = schizont; M = merozoite; G = gametocyte.

Modified from Soave R: *Clin Infect Dis* 23:429–437, 1996, with permission of the University of Chicago Press; Sun et al: *Am J Clin Pathol* 105:216–220, 1996, copyright © 1996, by the American Society of Clinical Pathologists. Reprinted with permission.

specific detection of the organism in fecal specimens, cross-amplification with other coccidia has not been determined.[55] Organisms can also be detected on jejunal aspiration or biopsy. Unlike cryptosporidiosis, cyclosporiasis responds to 7 days of treatment with trimethoprim-sulfonamides with rapid cessation of diarrhea and shedding of oocysts.[23]

References

1. Argenzio RA, Liacos JA, Levy ML, et al. 1990. Villous atrophy, crypt hyperplasia, cellular infiltration and impaired glucose sodium absorption in enteric cryptosporidiosis of pigs. *Gastroenterology* 98:1129–1140.
2. Aydin Y, Ozkul IA. 1996. Infectivity of *Cryptosporidium muris* directly isolated from the murine stomach for various laboratory animals. *Vet Parasitol* 66:257–262.
3. Balatbat AB, Jordan GW, Tang YJ, et al. 1996. Detection of *Cryptosporidium parvum* DNA in human feces by nested PCR. *J Clin Microbiol* 34:1769–1772.
4. Barr SC, Guilford WG, Jamrosz GJ, et al. 1994. Paromomycin for the treatment of *Cryptosporidium* in dogs and cats (abstract). *Am Coll Vet Int Med* 12:138.
5. Barr SC, Jamrosz GJ, Hornbuckle WE, et al. 1994. Use of paromomycin for treatment of cryptosporidiosis in a cat. *J Am Vet Med Assoc* 205:1742–1743.
6. Bessette RE, Amsden GW. 1995. Treatment of non-HIV cryptosporidial diarrhea with azithromycin. *Ann Pharmacother* 29:991–993.
7. Bridgman SA, Robertson RMP, Syed Q, et al. 1995. Outbreak of cryptosporidiosis associated with a disinfected groundwater supply. *Epidemiol Infect* 115:555–566.
8. Colley DG. 1996. Widespread foodborne cyclosporiasis outbreaks present major challenges. *Emerging Infect Dis* 2:354–356.
9. Current WL, Garcia LS. 1991. Cryptosporidiosis. *Clin Microbiol Rev* 4:325–358.
10. Danziger LH, Kanyok TP, Novak RM. 1993. Treatment of cryptosporidial diarrhea in an AIDS patient with paromomycin. *Ann Pharmacother* 27:1460–1462.
11. Dubey JP, Speer CA, Fayer R. 1990. Cryptosporidiosis of man and animals. CRC Press, Boca Raton, FL.
12. Egger M, Nguyen X, Schaad UB, et al. 1990. Intestinal cryptosporidiosis acquired from a cat. *Infection* 18:177–178.
13. El-Ahraf A, Tacal JV, Sobin M, et al. 1991. Prevalence of cryptosporidiosis in dogs and human beings in San Bernardino county, California, USA. *J Am Vet Med Assoc* 198:631–634.
14. Fayer R, Ellis W. 1993. Paromomycin is effective as prophylaxis for cryptosporidiosis in dairy calves. *J Parasitol* 79:771–774.
15. Fleta-Zaragozano J, Clavel A, Quilez J, et al. 1994. Human cryptosporidiosis acquired from a pet lamb. *Pediatr Infect Dis J* 13:935.
16. Garcia-Lopez HL, Rodriguez-Tovar LE, Medina-Dela Garza, CE. 1996. Identification of *Cyclospora* in poultry. *Emerging Infect Dis* 2:356–357.
17. Goldstein ST, Juranek DD, Ravenholt O, et al. 1996. Cryptosporidiosis: an outbreak associated with drinking water despite state-of-the-art water treatment. *Ann Intern Med* 124:459–468.
18. Goodwin MA, Barsanti JA. 1990. Intractable diarrhea associated with intestinal cryptosporidiosis in a domestic cat also infected with feline leukemia virus. *J Am Anim Hosp Assoc* 26:365–368.
19. Greene CE, Jacobs GJ, Prickett D. 1990. Intestinal malabsorption and cryptosporidiosis in an adult dog. *J Am Vet Med Assoc* 197:365–369.
20. Guarino A, Canani RB, Casola A, et al. 1995. Human intestinal cryptosporidiosis: secretory diarrhea and enterotoxic activity in Caco-2 cells. *J Infect Dis* 171:976–983.
21. Healey MC, Yang S, Rasmussen KR, et al. 1995. Therapeutic efficacy of paromomycin in immunosuppressed adult mice infected with *Cryptosporidium parvum*. *J Parasitol* 81:114–116.
22. Hill LS, Lappin MR. 1995. Cryptosporidiosis in the dog and cat, pp 728–731. *In* Bonagura JD (ed), Kirk's current veterinary therapy, ed 12. WB Saunders, Philadelphia, PA.
23. Hoge CW, Shlim DR, Ghimire M, et al. 1995. Placebo-controlled trial of co-trimoxazole for *Cyclospora* infections. *Lancet* 345:691–693.
24. Huang P, Weber JT, Sosin DM, et al. 1995. The first reported outbreak of diarrheal illness associated with *Cyclospora* in the United States. *Ann Intern Med* 123:409–414.
25. Ignatius R, Lehman M, Miksits K, et al. 1997. A new acid-fast trichrome stain for simultaneous detection of *Cryptosporidium parvum* and microsporidial species in stool specimens. *J Clin Microbiol* 35:446–449.
26. Jokipii L, Jokipii A. 1986. Timing of symptoms and oocyst excretion in human cryptosporidiosis. *N Engl J Med* 315:1643–1647.
27. Juranek DD. 1995. Cryptosporidiosis: sources of infection and guidelines for prevention. *Clin Infect Dis* 21:S57–S61.
28. Khaw M, Panosian CB. 1995. Human antiprotozoal therapy: past, present, and future. *Clin Microbiol Rev* 8:427–439.
29. Koch KL, Shankey TV, Weinstein GS, et al. 1983. Cryptosporidiosis in a patient with hemophilia, common variable hypogammaglobulinemia, and the acquired immunodeficiency syndrome. *Ann Intern Med* 99:337–340.

29a. Kramer MH, Sorhage FE, Goldstein ST, et al. 1998. First reported outbreak in the United States of cryptosporidiosis associated with a recreational lake. *Clin Infect Dis* 26:27–33.

29b. Lappin MR, Dowers K, Edsell D, et al. 1997. Cryptosporidiosis and inflammatory bowel disease in a cat. *Feline Pract* 25:10–13.

29c. Lappin MR, Ungar B, Brownhahn B, et al. 1997. Enzyme-linked immunosorbent assay for the detection of *Cryptosporidium parvum* IgG in the serum of cats. *J Parasitol* 83:957–960.

30. Lengerich EJ, Addiss DG, Marx JJ, et al. 1993. Increased exposure to cryptosporidia among dairy farmers in Wisconsin. *J Infect Dis* 167:1252–1255.
31. Lent SF, Burkhardt JE, Bolka D. 1993. Coincident enteric cryptosporidiosis and lymphosarcoma in a cat with diarrhea. *J Am Anim Hosp Assoc* 29:492–496.
32. Levine JF, Levy MG, Walker RL, et al. 1988. Cryptosporidiosis in veterinary students. *J Am Vet Med Assoc* 193:1413–1414.
33. Lewis IJ, Hart CA, Baxby D. 1985. Diarrhoea due to *Cryptosporidium* in acute lymphoblastic leukemia. *Arch Dis Child* 60:60–62.

33a. Lloyd S, Smith J. 1997. Pattern of *Cryptosporidium parvum* oocyst excretion by experimentally infected dogs. *Int J Parasitol* 27:799–801.

34. MacKenzie WR, Hoxie NJ, Proctor ME, et al. 1994. A massive outbreak in Milwaukee of *Cryptosporidium* infection transmitted through the public water supply. *N Engl J Med* 331:161–173.

35. MacKenzie WR, Kazmierczak JJ, Davis JP. 1995. An outbreak of cryptosporidiosis associated with a resort swimming pool. *Epidemiol Infect* 115:545–553.
36. MacPherson DW, McQueen R. 1993. Cryptosporidiosis: multiattribute evaluation of six diagnostic methods. *J Clin Microbiol* 31:198–202.
37. Martins CAP, Guerrant RL. 1995. *Cryptosporidium* and cryptosporidiosis. *Parasitol Today* 11:434–436.
38. Mascaro C, Arnedo T, Rosales MJ. 1994. Respiratory cryptosporidiosis in a bovine. *J Parasitol* 80:334–336.
39. McAnulty JM, Fleming DW, Gonzalez AH. 1994. A community-wide outbreak of cryptosporidiosis associated with swimming at a wave pool. *JAMA* 272:1597–1600.
40. McMeeking A, Borkowsky W, Klesius PH, et al. 1990. A controlled trial of bovine dialyzable leukocyte extract for cryptosporidiosis in patients with AIDS. *J Infect Dis* 161:108–112.
41. Miron D, Kenes J, Dagan R. 1991. Calves as a source of an outbreak of cryptosporidiosis among young children in an agricultural closed community. *Pediatr Infect Dis J* 10:438–441.
42. Moore R, Tzipori S, Griffiths JK, et al. 1995. Temporal changes in permeability and structure of piglet ileum after site-specific infection by *Cryptosporidium parvum*. *Gastroenterology* 108:1030–1039.
43. Mtambo MMA, Nash AS, Blewett DA, et al. 1991. *Cryptosporidium* infection in cats: prevalence of infection in domestic and feral cats in the Glasgow area. *Vet Rec* 129:502–504.
44. Mtambo MMA, Nash AS, Blewett DA, et al. 1992. Comparison of staining and concentration techniques for detection of *Cryptosporidium* oocysts in cat fecal specimens. *Vet Parasitol* 45:49–57.
45. Mtambo MMA, Nash AS, Wright SE, et al. 1995. Prevalence of specific anti-*Cryptosporidium* IgG, IgM and IgA antibodies in cat sera using an indirect immunofluorescence antibody test. *Vet Parasitol* 60:37–43.
46. Mtambo MMA, Wright SE, Nash AS, et al. 1996. Infectivity of a *Cryptosporidium* species isolated from a domestic cat (*Felis domestica*) in lambs and mice. *Res Vet Sci* 60:61–63.
47. Nash AS, Mtambo MMA, Gibbs HA. 1993. *Cryptosporidium* infection in farm cats in the Glasgow area. *Vet Rec* 133:576–577.
48. O'Donoghue PJ. 1995. *Cryptosporidium* and cryptosporidiosis in man and animals. *Int J Parasitol* 25:139–195.
49. Ongerth J, Stibbs H. 1989. Prevalence of *Cryptosporidium* infection in dairy calves in western Washington. *Am J Vet Res* 50:1069–1070.
50. Ortega YR, Gilman RH, Sterling CR. 1994. A new coccidian parasite (Ampicomplexa: Eimeriidae) from humans. *J Parasitol* 80:625–629.
50a. Ortega YR, Nagle R, Gilman RH, et al. 1997. Pathologic and clinical findings in patients with cyclosporiasis and a description of intracellular parasite life-cycle stages. *J Infect Dis* 176:1584–1589.
51. Ortega YR, Sterling CR, Gilman RH, et al. 1993. *Cyclospora* species: a new protozoan pathogen of humans. *N Engl J Med* 328:1308–1312.
52. Palkovic L, Marousek V. 1989. The pathogenicity of *Cryptosporidium parvum* Tyzzer, 1912 and *C. baileyi* current, Upton et Haynes, 1986 for chickens. *Folia Parasitol* 36:209–217.
53. Pape JW, Verdier RI, Boncy M, et al. 1994. *Cyclospora* infection in adults infected with HIV: clinical manifestations, treatment, and prophylaxis. *Ann Intern Med* 121:654–657.
53a. Peng MM, Xiao L, Freeman AR, et al. 1997. Genetic polymorphism among *Cryptosporidium parvum* isolates: evidence of two distinct human transmission cycles. *Emerg Infect Dis* 3:567–573.
54. Peterson C. 1992. Cryptosporidiosis in patients infected with the human immunodeficiency virus. *Clin Infect Dis* 15:903–909.
54a. Pieniazek NJ, Herwaldt BL. 1997. Reevaluating the molecular taxonomy: Is human-associated *Cyclospora* a mammalian *Eimeria* species? *Emerg Infect Dis* 31:381–383.
55. Pieniazek NJ, Slemenda SB, da Silva AJ, et al. 1996. PCR confirmation of infection with *Cyclospora cayetanensis*. *Emerging Infect Dis* 2:357–358.
56. Plettenberg A, Stoehr A, Stellbrink HJ, et al. 1993. A preparation from bovine colostrum in the treatment of HIV-positive patients with chronic diarrhea. *Clin Invest* 71:42–45.
57. Prestwood AK. 1990. Cryptosporidiosis, pp 847–853. *In* Greene CE (ed), Infectious diseases of the dog and cat. WB Saunders, Philadelphia, PA.
58. Quinn CM, Betts WB. 1993. Longer term viability status of chlorine-treated *Cryptosporidium* oocysts in tap water. *Biomed Lett* 48:315–318.
59. Rehg JE. 1994. A comparison of anticryptosporidial activity of paromomycin with that of other aminoglycosides and azithromycin in immunosuppressed mice. *J Infect Dis* 170:934–938.
60. Rolston KVI, Fainstain V, Bodey GP. 1989. Intestinal cryptosporidiosis treated with eflornithine: a prospective study among patients with AIDS. *J Acquir Immune Defic Syndr* 2:426–430.
61. Selik RM, Chu SY, Ward JW. 1995. Trends in infectious diseases and cancers among persons dying of HIV infection in the United States from 1987 to 1992. *Ann Intern Med* 123:933–936.
62. Soave R. 1996. *Cyclospora*: an overview. *Clin Infect Dis* 23:429–437.
63. Sun T, Ilardi CF, Asnis D, et al. 1996. Light and electron microscopic identification of *Cyclospora* species in the small intestine: evidence of the presence of asexual life cycle in human host. *Am J Clin Pathol* 105:216–220.
63a. Valdez LM, Dang H, Okhuysen PC, et al. 1997. Flow cytometric detection of *Cryptosporidium* oocysts in human stool samples. *J Clin Microbiol* 35:2013–2017.
64. Verdon R, Polianski J, Gaudebout C, et al. 1994. Evaluation of curative anticryptosporidial activity of paromomycin in a dexamethasone-treated rat model. *Antimicrob Agents Chemother* 38:1681–1682.
65. Weber R, Bryan RT, Bishop HS, et al. 1991. Threshold of detection of *Cryptosporidium* oocysts in human stool specimens: evidence for low sensitivity of current diagnostic methods. *J Clin Microbiol* 29:1323–1327.
66. Webster KA, Pow JDE, Giles M, et al. 1993. Detection of *Cryptosporidium parvum* using a specific polymerase chain reaction. *Vet Parasitol* 50:35–44.
67. Wurtz R. 1994. *Cyclospora*: a newly identified intestinal pathogen of humans. *Clin Infect Dis* 18:620–623.
68. Xiao L, Herd RP. 1993. Quantitation of *Giardia* cysts and *Cryptosporidium* oocysts in fecal samples by direct immunofluorescence assay. *J Clin Microbiol* 31:2944–2946.

Chapter **83**

Pneumocystosis

Craig E. Greene and Francis W. Chandler

ETIOLOGY

Pneumocystis carinii, the etiologic agent of pneumocystosis, occurs worldwide and infects several animal species, including people. A saprophyte of low virulence, it exists in temperate and tropical climates at altitudes up to 5000 feet. Its primary habitat is the mammalian respiratory tract. Estimates of latent human infections range from 1% to 10% of the population. Subclinical or latent infections also are common in rats, mice, guinea pigs, rabbits, cats, sheep, and various wild animals. Clinical pneumonia has been reported to occur spontaneously in dogs, pigs, horses, goats, nonhuman primates, and people. Air-borne transmission is suspected because healthy animals become infected when they are housed with infected animals.[4] It is presumed that the organism may have a yet undiscovered dormant life stage in the environment. Most reports of clinical pneumonia are linked with documented or suspected immunodeficiency in the host. The greater prevalence of pneumocystosis is due not only to a greater awareness of it but also to the increased use of immunosuppressive therapy.

The taxonomy of *P. carinii* is uncertain. It has been classified utilizing freeze-fracture techniques as a unicellular protozoan belonging to the phylum Sarcomastigophora, subphylum Sarcodina. Ultrastructurally, however, its reproductive behavior is similar to the ascospore formation of yeast cells, and its organelles and staining properties for light microscopy resemble those of most pathogenic fungi. Phylogenetic classification based on 16S-like rRNA sequences indicates that *P. carinii* is most closely related to the fungi of the class Ascomycetes, especially *Saccharomyces cerevisiae*. Biologically, however, it behaves like a protozoan and is sensitive to drugs used to treat sporozoan infections. The morphology of the organism and the histopathology of the lesions produced by human and animal isolates throughout the world are similar. Only a single species name has been assigned to the genus *Pneumocystis*, but antigenic differences suggest that several strains may exist. Biologic differences between isolates from different hosts are suggested by the relative difficulty of experimental interspecies transmission.

EPIDEMIOLOGY

P. carinii appears to be maintained in nature by transmission from infected to susceptible animals within a species. The primary mode of spread is thought to be air-borne droplet transmission between hosts. The contagious nature of pneumocystosis is suggested by the epidemic spread that has occurred in institutionalized humans. Sporadic case reports may represent an activation of latent infection by stress, crowding, and immunosuppressive therapy during hospitalization of latent carriers. Clinical disease also has been experimentally activated after glucocorticoid therapy, cytotoxic chemotherapy, and irradiation of laboratory rodents. A higher prevalence of infection has been found in dogs with canine distemper compared with a corresponding control population.[21a]

The entire life cycle of *P. carinii* is completed within the alveolar spaces, where organisms adhere in clusters to the lining cells. Ultrastructural studies have contributed a large body of information concerning the life cycle of *P. carinii* (Fig. 83–1). Two main forms, the trophozoite and cyst, are found. *Pneumocystis* infections are usually limited to the lung; however, organisms have occasionally been reported in extrapulmonary sites in humans. There is one similar report in a dog. Severe immunodeficiency states in people, such as AIDS, can be associated with lymphatic or hematogenous dissemination of the organisms from the lungs to other tissues. Transmission of infection to an offspring may occur via aspiration of amniotic fluid contaminated by placental infection.[16]

PATHOGENESIS

Pneumocystis may be inhaled from the environment and colonize the lower respiratory tract of clinically healthy mammals. *Pneumocystis* organisms rarely multiply to large numbers in the lungs of clinically healthy hosts. Instead, impaired host resistance (especially reduced CD4 T-lymphocyte counts) or pre-existing pulmonary disease allows them to proliferate. The overgrowth and clustering of *P. carinii* within alveolar spaces may lead to alveolocapillary blockage and decreased gaseous exchange. Intra-alveolar organisms are often accompanied by thickening of alveolar septa, but they seldom invade the pulmonary parenchyma and are rarely found in alveolar macrophages. With an adequate immune response, the body may eliminate the infection, although the removal of large amounts of alveolar exudate and cellular debris may take up to 8 weeks. The organism and the inflammatory response it provokes contribute to the pulmonary alveolar damage.

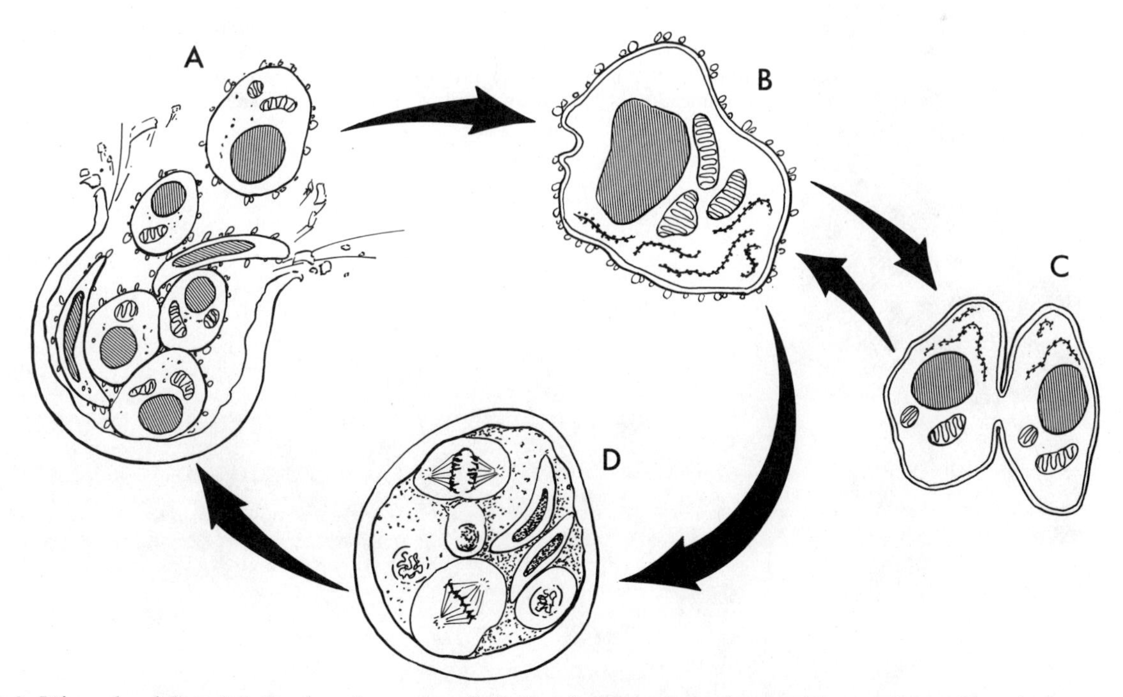

Figure 83–1. Life cycle of *P. carinii.* Trophozoites are small (2–5 μm), thin-walled, pleomorphic organisms with reticular cytoplasm and eccentric nuclei *(A).* They increase in size to form larger (4–7 μm) trophozoites *(B),* which reproduce either by binary fission, dividing into two identical but smaller trophozoites *(C),* or by forming a thick-walled cyst *(D).* The cyst undergoes a process similar to ascospore formation in yeasts whereby nuclear division results in separate chromatin masses in the cytoplasm. Cytoplasmic and nuclear membranes form multiple thin-walled ovoid or crescent-shaped intracystic sporozoites, which are released after rupture of the cyst wall *(A).*

CLINICAL FINDINGS

Cats

In general, pneumocystic infections of cats are latent or subclinical, as they are in people. The organism has been found in the lungs of cats, but clinical disease was not reported. Lung specimens examined from cats suffering from feline leukemia virus infection, interstitial pneumonia, or both have not had evidence of pneumocystosis. Cats that were experimentally infected with *P. carinii* isolated from mice developed cough, tachypnea, and typical pneumonia if they were immunosuppressed with concurrent glucocorticoids.[22] In contrast, subclinical infections occurred in cats that did not receive immunosuppressive therapy.

Dogs

Most canine cases have been in miniature dachshunds younger than 1 year with suspected congenital immunodeficiency,[13] although one case of disseminated pneumocystosis in a Shetland sheepdog also has been reported. Adult Cavalier King Charles spaniels also predominate in clinical reports.[5a, 6, 18a, 21b]

The clinical features of pneumocystic pneumonia are similar to those caused by other pulmonary pathogens except for dry lung sounds, nonproductive cough, and low-grade or absent fever. The typical clinical history in dogs is that of gradual weight loss and respiratory difficulty progressing over 1 to 4 weeks. The weight loss, which occurs in spite of a good appetite in most dogs, may be associated with diarrhea and occasional vomiting. Coughing is not always reported, but reduced exercise tolerance is uniform. Infected animals have responded minimally or temporarily to antibiotic or glucocorticoid therapy.

Abnormalities on physical examination include dyspnea, tachycardia, and increased dry respiratory sounds on thoracic auscultation. Animals are usually in poor condition and cachectic. Although the mucous membranes are generally of normal color, they may be cyanotic in severely affected animals. Affected dogs remain relatively alert and afebrile, although slight (1–2°C [1.8–3.6°F]) elevations of rectal temperature have been reported. Fluid may be present in the thoracic

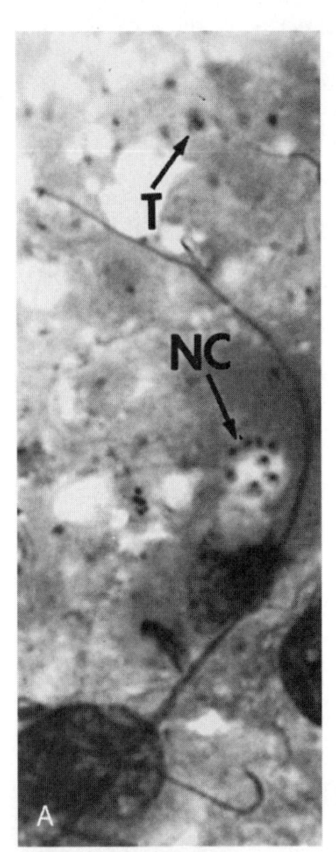

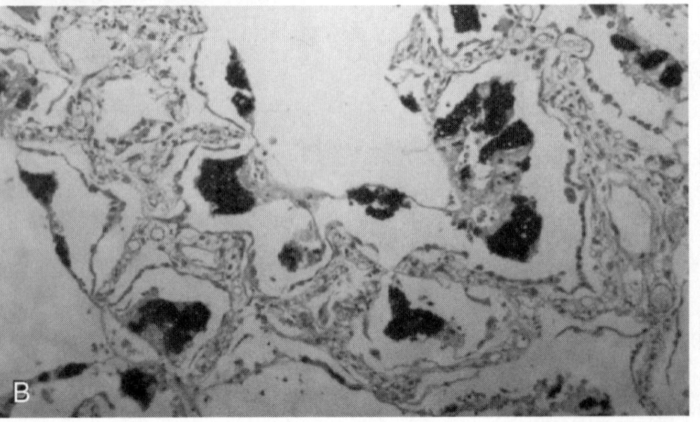

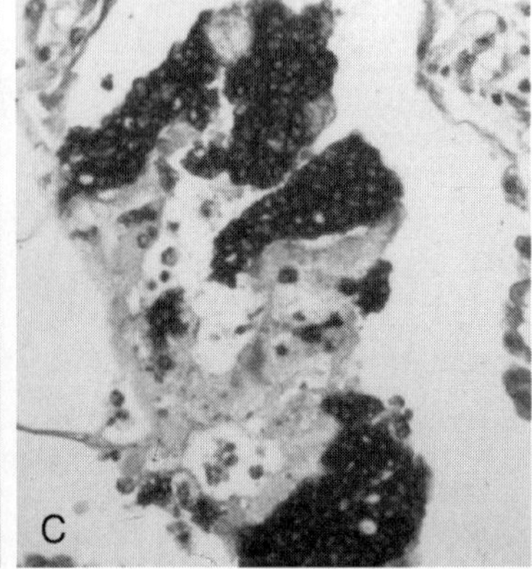

Figure 83–2. *A*, Impression smear of lung tissue from a rat infected with *P. carinii*. Nucleated cysts (NC) and trophozoites (T) are readily demonstrated with Giemsa stain (× 1500). *B*, Immunoperoxidase staining of intra-alveolar cysts and trophozoites of *P. carinii* in a human AIDS patient using monoclonal antibody 2G2 in a routinely prepared biopsy specimen (× 25). *C*, Higher magnification of *B* showing detail of organisms (× 1000).

and peritoneal cavities of some dogs. Ocular fundic lesions known as "cotton wool spots" rarely occur in humans with pneumocystosis, and they represent infarction of the nerve fiber layer. They have not been reported in animal infections.

DIAGNOSIS

Hematologic abnormalities are usually nonspecific, and a neutrophilic leukocytosis with a shift suggesting inflammation is seen most consistently. Less frequently, eosinophilia and monocytosis are found. Polycythemia may occur secondarily to arterial hypoxemia from impaired gaseous exchange. Thrombocytopenia, which can be significant enough to cause bleeding, has been a complication in humans. Biochemical alterations are usually nonspecific. Low globulin levels and decreased lymphocyte stimulation have been found in miniature dachshunds.[13] Low levels of IgA, IgG, and IgM have been apparent. Arterial hypoxemia (oxygen tension [Po_2] ≤ 80), hypocapnia (carbon dioxide tension ≤ 35), and increased arterial blood pH indicate an uncompensated respiratory alkalosis. The Po_2 is often lower than would be expected from the clinical signs and thoracic radiographs.

Findings on thoracic radiography include diffuse, bilaterally symmetric, alveolar to interstitial lung disease, with compensatory emphysema in severely infected animals. Solitary lesion, unilateral involvement, cavitary lesion, spontaneous pneumothorax, or lobar infiltrate occasionally may be present. Tracheal elevation, right-sided heart enlargement, and pulmonary arterial enlargement reflect cor pulmonale secondary to diffuse pulmonary disease.

Serologic tests have been developed for use in people with pneumocystosis, but their diagnostic value is uncertain. Unfortunately, many immunodeficient patients who develop pneumocystosis fail to produce antibody titers, and healthy contacts of these patients frequently have higher titers than the patients themselves. Increased antibody titers to *P. carinii* persist for long periods, offering a valuable index of exposure in epidemiologic studies. However, they are of limited use for an immediate diagnosis. An increase in titer over 2 to 3 weeks is needed to confirm active infection. Circulating *Pneumocystis* antigen has been detected in human serum by counterimmunoelectrophoresis and ELISA methods. However, antigenemia also is found in up to 15% of clinically normal humans who have been tested.

P. carinii has been successfully propagated in cell cultures but not on a continuous basis. Immunosuppressed rodents have been utilized to propagate organisms for serologic and experimental testing. Because of the difficulty of isolation of organisms, diagnosis requires direct demonstration of *P. carinii* in biopsy specimens, respiratory fluids, or occasional extrapulmonary sites. Sputum, transtracheal or endotracheal washings, gastric contents, and oropharyngeal secretions may contain organisms. Transtracheal aspirates have been effective in identifying organisms in dogs.[13] Percutaneous transthoracic needle aspiration is a rapid and simple diagnostic procedure. A 1-inch, 22-gauge needle is inserted through the right thoracic wall into the pulmonary parenchyma, and tissue is rapidly aspirated into 0.2 ml of sterile saline. Samples for cytology may be obtained by endobronchial brushing and transbronchoscopic biopsy, but these procedures require special endoscopic equipment and involve the risks of general anesthesia. Transtracheal or endotracheal lavage is more available to practitioners and has good correlation with transbronchoscopic biopsy findings in confirming a diagnosis. None of the cytologic techniques is as reliable or as definitive as lung biopsy for documenting active pneumocystosis. Unfortunately, endoscopic or percutaneous lung biopsy has the greatest risk of complications. Hemorrhage, secondary infection, pneumothorax, and death from anesthesia have been reported after biopsy in dogs. Open surgical biopsy is the preferred method. Antimicrobial therapy can begin 24 to 48 hours before specimen collection in a patient suspected of having pneumocystosis, without masking the presence of organisms in the sample.

Impression smears for cytologic study should be made from all tissues before fixation for histologic evaluation to facilitate early diagnosis and treatment, because smears can be prepared and stained more rapidly than tissue sections. The cytologic material obtained is placed on a glass microscope slide to dry, after which it is selectively stained with methenamine silver for cysts or with Giemsa for nuclei of intracystic sporozoites and trophozoites (Fig. 83–2*A*). Diff-Quik (a modified Giemsa stain) can be used as a fast and inexpensive screening stain after which negative results can be confirmed with more sensitive staining.[7] Direct or indirect FA testing has been effective in detecting organisms in sputum and tracheal aspirates.[17] Immunoperoxidase techniques have been used to identify *P. carinii* in impression smears and formalin-fixed, paraffin-embedded lung sections (Fig. 83–2*B*). Polymerase chain reaction has been effective in the detection of *P. carinii* in bronchoalveolar lavage specimens from people[12, 14, 19] and lung tissue from dogs.[21b]

PATHOLOGIC FINDINGS

Pathologic findings in pneumocystosis are primarily confined to the lungs, although dissemination to regional lymph nodes and other organs has been reported. On gross examination, the lungs are firm, consolidated, and pale brown or gray (Fig. 83–3). They do not collapse when the chest cavity is opened. Unlike in many pneumonic processes, fluid is not expressed from cut surfaces of the lung. The pulmonary and mediastinal lymph nodes are often enlarged. Despite the apparent lack of pleural inflammation, small amounts of fluid may be found in the pleural cavity. Cardiac enlargement, when present, has been right sided in all cases.

Appropriate histologic staining is essential to ensure detection of *P. carinii* organisms (Table 83–1). The routine H and E stain does not readily demonstrate individual organisms, which may explain why the disease is not recognized more frequently. With this stain, only the hematoxylinophilic nuclei of intracystic sporozoites and trophozoites are demonstrated.

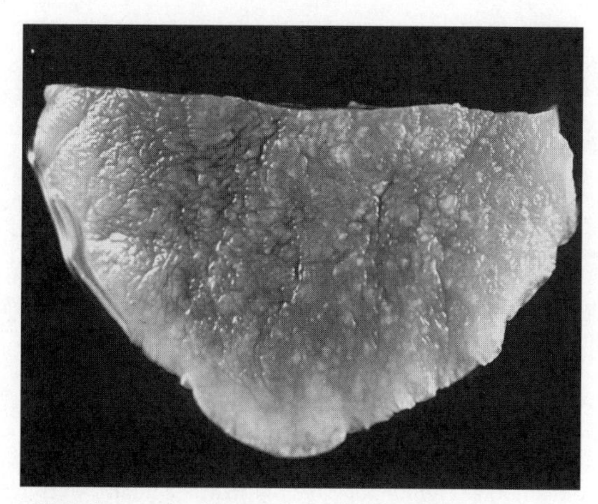

Figure 83–3. Lung of a rhesus monkey with *Pneumocystis* pneumonia in an early stage. The surface of the lung is covered with scattered, pinpoint, grayish-white lesions. These lesions were found throughout the lung when it was sectioned (× 3).

Table 83–1. Comparison of Staining Methods for Demonstrating Pneumocystis in Clinical Specimens

STAIN	REACTION OF		
	Trophozoite	Cyst Wall	Internal Structures
H and E	Unstained	Unstained	Weakly basophilic
Methenamine silver	Unstained	Brownish-black	Unstained
Toluidine blue	Unstained	Purplish-violet	Unstained
Periodic acid–Schiff	Unstained	Red	Unstained
Giemsa	Unstained	Unstained	Magenta
Gram's	Unstained	Positive	Positive

Various modifications of methenamine silver staining can be employed to stain the cyst walls brownish-black, but trophozoites will not be detected (Fig. 83–4). Overstaining with Gomori's methenamine silver (GMS) may cause blackened erythrocytes in alveolar spaces to be mistaken for cyst forms of *Pneumocystis*. Polychrome stains, such as Wright's, Gram's, Giemsa, and methylene blue, will demonstrate nuclei of trophozoites and intracystic sporozoites in cytologic specimens, but the thick walls of cyst forms will not be apparent (see Fig. 83–2*A*).

On histologic examination, alveolar spaces are found to be filled with amorphous, foamy, eosinophilic material that has a honeycomb-like pattern. A few macrophages and desquamated alveolar lining cells also may be present, but polymorphonuclear leukocytes are absent. Special staining methods are needed to identify pneumocysts (see Fig. 83–2*B*). There is little or no phagocytosis of intact *Pneumocystis* organisms. However, nonviable organisms, such as those seen after treatment, are often phagocytosed, and macrophages may contain GMS-positive granular material that represents the residuum of cyst wall degradation. In some instances, alveolar septa are markedly thickened by dense accumulations of plasma cells, lymphocytes, and macrophages. The septa may be widened by fibrosis in chronic infections, especially after treatment. With GMS stain, cyst forms appear as spherical, ovoid, or crescent-shaped structures that range from 4 to 7 μm in diameter and have dotlike, argyrophilic, focal, cyst wall thickenings (Figs. 83–4 and 83–5). Cyst walls also can be demonstrated with other stains (see Table 83–1), and they will fluoresce when stained with orange G of a Papanicolaou stain. Trophozoites in tissue sections and smears are best demonstrated with Giemsa stain, especially using Wolbach's procedure. On ultrastructural examination, intact alveoli appear crowded with trophozoite and cyst stages that totally fill the existing airspaces. Trophozoites commonly line alveoli.

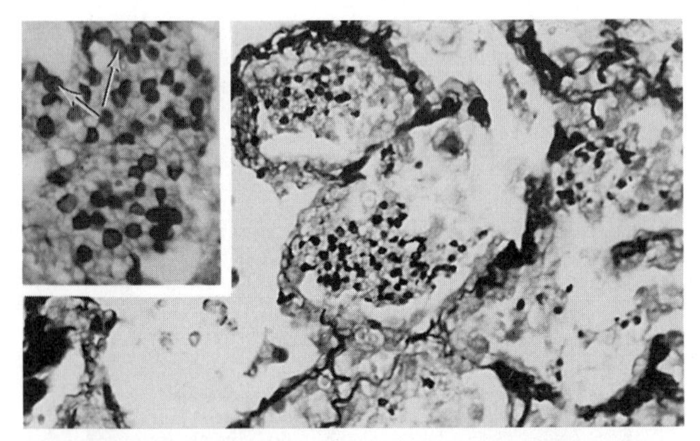

Figure 83–4. *P. carinii* within alveolar spaces in a dog with *Pneumocystis* pneumonia. Light, honeycombed matrix contains trophozoites and cellular debris. Darker ovoid, irregular, and crescent-shaped structures are cysts (× 300). *Inset,* Details of cysts that commonly show darker oval focus of cyst wall *(arrows)* (Gomori's methenamine silver stain, × 600).

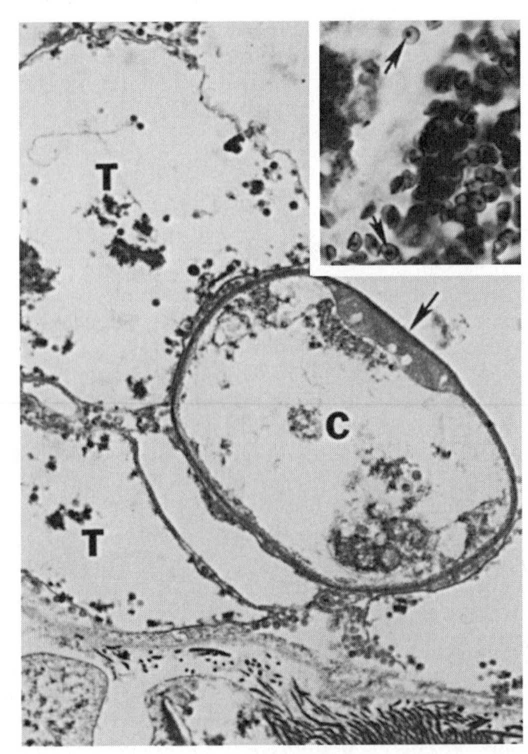

Figure 83–5. Pulmonary pneumocystosis. Alveolar space contains thin-walled trophozoites (T) and a cyst form (C) of *P. carinii.* Segmental, lamellated thickening of cyst wall *(arrow)* corresponds to darkly stained "intracystic" foci seen by light microscopy (uranyl acetate and lead citrate stain, × 22,000). *Inset, P. carinii* cysts in touch imprint contain spherical to oval foci of enhanced staining *(arrows)* that in profile are contiguous with cyst wall (Gomori's methenamine silver stain, × 560).

THERAPY

Supportive care is essential for any patient with pneumocystic pneumonia because of disturbed alveolar gaseous exchange. Oxygen therapy administered by cage, mask, or intubation is needed, and ventilatory assistance also may be required. Aerosol nebulization with mucolytics has been recommended to assist in the dissolution of alveolar debris. Bronchodilators may help reduce airway resistance. Immunosuppressive agents should be temporarily discontinued whenever pneumocystosis is diagnosed in an animal that is receiving such therapy; however, anti-inflammatory doses may be indicated. Antimicrobial chemotherapy of pulmonary pneumocystosis results in a decline in arterial oxygen related to the inflammatory reaction to dying organisms. Administration of anti-inflammatory doses of glucocorticoids has been shown to improve pulmonary function and survival in people.[1, 5, 15]

Specific chemotherapy is most beneficial in cases in which the disease is suspected or diagnosed during its early stages (Table 83–2). Two major chemotherapeutic agents have been used to treat pneumocystosis successfully. Pentamidine isethionate is an aromatic diamidine that has been provided to reduce fatalities from the disease in humans. Its major side effects include impaired renal function, hepatic dysfunction, hypoglycemia, hypotension, hypocalcemia, urticaria, and he-

Table 83–2. Therapy for Pneumocystosis

GENERIC NAME	DOSE[a]	ROUTE	INTERVAL (HOURS)	DURATION (WEEKS)
Specific Agents				
Trimethoprim-sulfonamide	15–20 mg/kg	PO	8	3
	30 mg/kg	PO	12	3
Pentamidine isethionate	4 mg/kg	IV, IM	24	3
Trimetrexate	45 mg/m^2	IV	24	3
Clindamycin and primaquine	3–13 mg/kg	PO	8	3
Atovaquone	15 mg/kg	PO	24	3
Adjunctive Agents				
Aminophylline	10–20 mg/kg	PO	8	3
Prednisone	1 mg/kg	PO	12–24	1
Cimetidine	5 mg/kg	PO	12	3
Levamisole	5 mg/kg	PO	48	3

[a]Dose per administration at specified interval. See Drug Formulary, Appendix 8, for additional information on each drug.

matologic disorders (see Chapter 71). Blood urea nitrogen and glucose are monitored daily during treatment, and the drug is discontinued or dosage is reduced if complications or azotemia occur. IM and IV administration of pentamidine is associated with local inflammation and systemic hypotension, respectively, in people such that aerosolized delivery has been the preferred route of administration. IM administration of this drug has been successful in treating a dog with pneumocystosis. The only side effect is localized pain at the site of injection. Pentamidine also has been successful, at a reduced dosage, in combination with sulfonamides to lower its toxic side effects.

The combination of trimethoprim and sulfamethoxazole has been found more effective and less toxic than pentamidine in treating and preventing *Pneumocystis* pneumonia in immunosuppressed humans. A relatively high oral dosage of 30 mg/kg given every 6 hours for 2 weeks has been recommended in humans so that the drug reaches therapeutically effective serum concentrations. Long-term (up to 2 years) prophylactic therapy for pneumocystosis at this dosage has not caused bone marrow toxicity in children, although changes in oral and fecal microflora have been noted. An increased incidence of mucocutaneous candidiasis was found. Half this dose might be used to treat dogs (see Table 83–2). IV trimethoprim-sulfamethoxazole therapy has been shown to be as or more effective than oral therapy and has the advantage of ease of administration in severely depressed or comatose patients. Folic acid supplementation should be given if side effects such as leukopenia and anemia are observed or if long-term therapy is required. Atovaquone, a hydroxynaphthoquinone, is licensed for the treatment of people with pneumocystosis.[11, 21] This drug is not as effective as pentamidine or trimethoprim-sulfamethoxazole but has lower toxicity. Bioavailability is increased when the drug is given with food with a high fat content.

Combination therapy using clindamycin and primaquine has been effective in vivo and in vitro, but neither drug is effective alone. Further investigation on the naturally occurring disease is needed. Aromatic diamidines, such as diminazene, imidocarb, and amicarbalide, have been more effective than pentamidine in treating experimental *P. carinii* pneumonia (see Chapter 71). Dapsone and trimethoprim, in combination, have been effective in experimental animals and clinical trials in immunosuppressed people with pneumocystosis. Trimetrexate, a lipid-soluble antifolate, has been given concomitantly with leucovorin in people with *Pneumocystis* pneumonia and AIDS. As with most of the other drugs, neutropenia with or without thrombocytopenia has been the main side effect. In experimentally infected animals, *P. carinii* is resistant to imidazole antifungal drugs,[3] but the anthelmintics benzimidazole and albendazole have been effective.[2]

Pneumocystosis in humans and animals is prima facie evidence of immunodeficiency. For this reason, prophylactic treatment with trimethoprim-sulfamethoxazole drugs has been used in hospitalized humans who are receiving irradiation or immunosuppressive agents or who have immunodeficiencies and debilitating diseases. Nonspecific immunostimulants such as cimetidine and levamisole (see Immunotherapy, Chapter 100) have been given adjunctively to treat affected miniature dachshunds. Similar precautions are not warranted in pets because pneumocystosis has not been recognized with similar frequency in such instances.

References

1. Anonymous. 1990. Consensus statement on the use of corticosteroids as adjunctive therapy for *Pneumocystis* pneumonia in the acquired immunodeficiency syndrome. *N Engl J Med* 323:1500–1504.
2. Bartlett MS, Edlind TD, Lee CH, et al. 1994. Albendazole inhibits *Pneumocystis carinii* proliferation in inoculated immunosuppressed mice. *Antimicrob Agents Chemother* 38:1834–1837.
3. Bartlett MS, Queener SF, Shaw MM, et al. 1994. *Pneumocystis carinii* is resistant to imidazole antifungal agents. *Antimicrob Agents Chemother* 38:1859–1861.
4. Bartlett MS, Smith JWM. 1991. *Pneumocystis carinii*, an opportunist in immunocompromised patients. *Clin Microbiol Rev* 4:137–149.
5. Bozzette SA, Finkelstein DM, Spector SA, et al. 1995. A randomized trial of three antipneumocystis agents in patients with advanced human immunodeficiency virus infection. *N Engl J Med* 332:693–699.
5a. Brownlie SE. 1990. A retrospective study of diagnosis in 109 cases of canine lower respiratory disease. *J Small Anim Pract* 31:371–376.
6. Canfield PJ, Church DB, Malik R. 1993. *Pneumocystis* pneumonia in a dog. *Aust Vet Pract* 23:150–154.
7. Cregan P, Yamamoto A, Lum A, et al. 1990. Comparison of four methods for rapid detection of *Pneumocystis carinii* in respiratory specimens. *J Clin Microbiol* 28:2432–2436.
8. Furuta T, Nogami S, Kojima S, et al. 1994. Spontaneous *Pneumocystis carinii* infection in the dog with naturally acquired demodicosis. *Vet Rec* 134:423–424.
9. Greene CG, Chandler FW. 1990. Pneumocystosis, pp 854–861. *In* Greene CE (ed), Infectious diseases of the dog and cat. WB Saunders, Philadelphia, PA.
10. Hong ST, Park KH, Lee SH. 1992. Susceptibility of various animals to *Pneumocystis carinii* infection. *Korean J Parasitol* 30:277–281.
11. Hughes WT. 1995. The role of atovaquone tablets in treating *Pneumocystis carinii* pneumonia. *J Acquir Immune Defic Syndr Hum Retrovirol* 8:247–252.
12. Kitada K, Oka S, Kimura S, et al. 1991. Detection of *Pneumocystis carinii* sequences by polymerase chain reaction: animal models and clinical application to noninvasive specimens. *J Clin Microbiol* 29:1985–1990.
13. Lobetti RG, Leisewitz AL, Spencer JA. 1996. *Pneumocystis carinii* in the miniature dachshund: case report and literature review. *J Small Anim Pract* 37:280–285.

14. Lu JJ, Chen CH, Bartlett S, et al. 1995. Comparison of six different PCR methods for detection of *Pneumocystis carinii*. *J Clin Microbiol* 33:2785–2788.
15. Masur H. 1992. Prevention and treatment of *Pneumocystis* pneumonia. *N Engl J Med* 327:1853–1860.
16. Mortier E, Pouchot J, Bossi P, et al. 1995. Maternal-fetal transmission of *Pneumocystis carinii* in human immunodeficiency virus infection. *N Engl J Med* 332:825.
17. Ng VL, Virani NA, Chaisson RE, et al. 1990. Rapid detection of *Pneumocystis carinii* using a direct fluorescent monoclonal antibody stain. *J Clin Microbiol* 28:2228–2233.
18. Palca J. 1995. A storm over steroid therapy. *Science* 250:1196–1198.
18a. Ramsey IK, Foster A, McKay J, et al. 1997. *Pneumocystis carinii* pneumonia in two Cavalier King Charles spaniels. *Vet Rec* 140:372–373.
19. Roux P, Lavrard I, Porrot JL, et al. 1994. Usefulness of PCR for detection of *Pneumocystis carinii* DNA. *J Clin Microbiol* 32:2324–2326.
20. Settnes OP, Henriksen SA. 1989. *Pneumocystis carinii* in large domestic animals in Denmark. A preliminary report. *Acta Vet Scand* 30:437–440.
21. Stoeckle M, Tennenberg A. 1995. Atovaquone for *Pneumocystis carinii* pneumonia. *Ann Intern Med* 122:314–315.
21a. Sukura A, Laakkonen J, Rudback E. 1997. Occurrence of *Pneumocystis carinii* in canine distemper. *Acta Vet Scand* 38:201–205.
21b. Sukura A, Saari S, Jarvinen A. 1996. *Pneumocystis carinii* pneumonia in dogs. A diagnostic challenge. *J Vet Diagn Invest* 8:124–130.
22. Yuezhong Y, Li Z, Baoping T. 1996. Pneumonia in cats caused by *Pneumocystis carinii* purified from mouse lungs. *Vet Parasitol* 61:171–175.

Chapter **84**

Neurologic Diseases of Suspected Infectious Origin

Marc Vandevelde

Granulomatous Meningoencephalitis Versus Primary Reticulosis

Granulomatous meningoencephalitis (GME) has been reported to occur in dogs in the United States, Australia, New Zealand, and several European countries. It is characterized by disseminated inflammatory lesions in the CNS with perivascular granuloma formation.[46]

The term *primary reticulosis of the CNS* encompasses a range of morphologically different lesions that are thought to be essentially proliferative reactions of the reticulohistiocytic elements originating from the adventitia of the blood vessels, the leptomeninges, and the so-called microglia. With the exception of the rare diffusely growing microgliomatosis, reticulosis is characterized by perivascular mononuclear cuffs containing many histiocytic elements. Adjacent cuffs may merge, leading to the formation of tumor-like lesions. On the basis of cytologic criteria, some lesions have been classified as inflammatory and others as neoplastic reticuloses in addition to transitional forms.[13, 46]

GME was recognized as a disease entity distinct from reticulosis on the basis of clinical and pathologic studies. Retrospective morphologic and immunocytochemical studies demonstrating lymphocytic and histiocytic cell markers have shown that many cases previously classified as reticulosis, especially those with multifocal lesions, have been GME cases.[46] In fact, GME can be associated with the formation of tumor-like mass lesions that usually coexist with characteristic disseminated lesions in other areas of the brain.[6] When such typical disseminated lesions are lacking, other diseases have to be considered.

Immunocytochemistry, demonstrating various immunoglobulin classes, reveals that some of these focal mass lesions are in fact primary lymphosarcomas.[48] GME accounts for the majority of lesions previously called reticulosis. The remaining cases are mostly lymphosarcomas, and, in a few mass lesions, some suspicion remains that they are true histiocytic tumors.[46]

ETIOLOGY

There is little doubt that GME is an infectious disease. However, experimental attempts to transmit the agent in dogs using GME brain tissue have been unsuccessful. Bacteria and fungi can cause granulomatous lesions in the CNS of small animals, but it is unlikely that such agents would have escaped detection on light microscopic examination of GME. It is possible the periodic acid–Schiff–positive and acidophilic inclusions in macrophages in lesions in some cases may be an unidentified infectious agent.[46] Other investigators have searched unsuccessfully for an infectious organism by EM examination of the tissues. Serologic tests for toxoplasmosis have been carried out in a few cases, but the results have been negative.[46] The possibility of rickettsial infection as an underlying cause should also be considered. Certain viral infections such as equine infectious anemia, feline infectious peritonitis, and visna are also associated with granulomatous lesions of the CNS. I believe that the most likely cause of GME is a virus. Canine distemper virus (CDV), which is responsible for a variety of CNS lesions, can be excluded as a cause of GME because systematic immunocytochemical studies in a large number of GME cases failed to find CDV antigen in the lesions.[46] The presence of anti-CDV antibody titers in the CSF of seven dogs with GME is difficult to

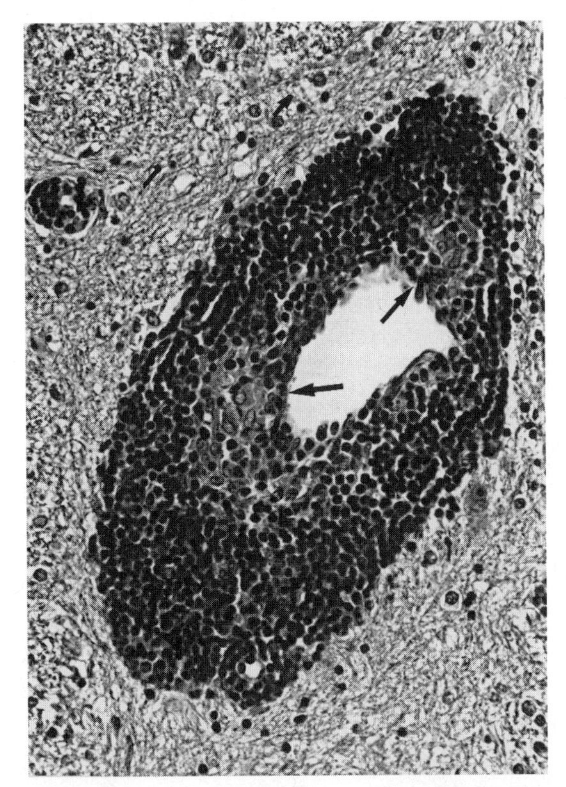

Figure 84–1. Histologic section from a dog with granulomatous meningoencephalitis showing perivascular mononuclear cuffing with eccentrically situated nodular foci of macrophages *(arrows)* (H and E, × 250).

explain in view of the negative immunocytochemical findings. Sophisticated culturing techniques are necessary to identify the agent. Simultaneous onset of the clinical signs in two related Afghan hounds suggests that the disease may be associated with common exposure or genetic predisposition.[18] Lesions consist of infiltrates of major histocompatibility complex class II, antigen-positive macrophages and predominantly CD3 antigen-positive lymphocytes. This finding suggests possible delayed-type hypersensitivity of an organ-specific autoimmune disease.[23b]

CLINICAL FINDINGS

The disease occurs in young to middle-aged dogs. Females are more often affected than males, and there is a higher prevalence for smaller breeds, especially poodles.[6] In dogs with disseminated lesions, there is usually an acute onset, and the disease is always progressive. Death generally occurs within 1 to 8 weeks. Definitive neurologic signs cannot be expected because the lesions are disseminated in the CNS. Signs are associated with the site of most extensive damage and may involve disturbances in gait and postural reactions, with ataxia, dysmetria, paresis, and paralysis; changes in mental status, with confusion, lethargy, and coma; and deficits in cranial nerve function. In the acute stage of the disease, more than half of the animals have fever, and many exhibit paraspinal discomfort or cervical pain.[39] Chronic disease (several months) is possible in the focal form of GME. Large tumor-like masses may develop into focal GME; clinical signs are suggestive of a space-occupying mass. Presenting signs refer to a single site of involvement, most frequently to the posterior fossa, with brain stem and cerebellar signs, and sometimes to the cerebrum. A particular localization of GME, previously called ocular reticulosis, occurs with acute unilateral or bilateral blindness and ophthalmoscopic evidence of optic neuritis.[6]

DIAGNOSIS

Typical hematologic and biochemical findings are lacking. Neutrophilia may be present in the acute disease.[39] The CSF is abnormal, with a marked pleocytosis; cell counts of 100 to more than 1000 WBC/μl are usual. Mononuclear cells predominate, but some neutrophils also are present in most cases.[2] Cytologic examination of the CSF may reveal large anaplastic mononuclear cells with abundant lacy cytoplasm.[6] Electrophoretic examination of the CSF may suggest blood-brain barrier disruption and intrathecal immunoglobulin synthesis.[39] Such changes are not specific for GME. In focal GME, the tumor-like lesions can be detected with diagnostic imaging.[6] EEG patterns studied in some dogs with GME were found to be abnormal.[46]

PATHOLOGIC FINDINGS

Lesions are found in the meninges, brain, and spinal cord, especially in the cervical segments. White matter is generally more severely affected than gray matter. Although the lesions are disseminated, the cerebral hemispheres, the midbrain, and the region around the fourth ventricle are most frequently involved. The lesions, which are strictly associated with the vasculature, consist of perivascular cuffing of monocytes, lymphocytes, plasma cells, and sometimes a few neutrophils. The formation of eccentrically situated nodular foci of macrophages within these cuffs is a characteristic finding in GME (Fig. 84–1). The cuffs can become very large and merge with adjacent cuffs, leading to the formation of tumor-like granulomas.

THERAPY

There is no specific therapy for GME, although improvement frequently has been observed after glucocorticoid administration. However, all known patients have eventually died of the disease despite steroid treatment.

Encephalitis in Pug and Maltese Dogs

This disease was initially described only in the Pug dog breed. It has been known for several years in the United States.[8] The prevalence of this disease outside the United States is uncertain. This breed is relatively uncommon in Europe. Three histologically confirmed cases have been observed in Switzerland, and one clinically suspected case each has been observed in southern Italy, Germany, and Japan.[19c, 24, 47] A necrotizing meningoencephalitis, clinically and pathologically indistinguishable from Pug dog encephalitis, has been reported in five Maltese dogs in the United States.[40]

Stalis and co-workers[40] indicated that the disease may also occur in other miniature breeds.

ETIOLOGY

The cause of Pug and Maltese dog encephalitis is unknown. The distribution and morphology of the lesions are unique for this disease and totally different from the histologic findings in other known CNS infections in small animals. The pathologic findings are, nevertheless, strongly suggestive of an infectious process. Bacterial, fungal, and protozoal organisms may probably be ruled out as potential causes because they would have been detected on histologic examination. The predominantly mononuclear inflammation suggests a viral cause. Viral isolation attempts in two cases, however, were unsuccessful.[10] The restriction of this disease to a few breeds is highly unusual for infections of small animals and strongly suggests predisposing genetic factors. It could be speculated that these breeds may have a breed-specific tissue antigen that could act as a receptor for a hitherto unknown virus or may have a breed-specific composition of the immune response genes leading to an atypical immunologic reaction toward a known pathogen. The predilection of the cerebral hemispheres for involvement with a necrotic inflammatory process is similar to that with α-herpesvirus encephalitides of other species.[8, 40]

CLINICAL FINDINGS

The disease may occur at any age and affects both sexes. The course of the disease is usually 1 to 6 months, but occasionally dogs may die a few days after the onset of signs. The most consistent sign is the occurrence of partial or generalized seizures. Other cerebral signs include decreased consciousness, abnormal behavior, compulsive circling, blindness, generalized ataxia and paresis, and deficient postural reactions.

A few animals may exhibit brain stem signs. The disease is always progressive, and many animals die as a result of severe seizures.[10]

DIAGNOSIS

There are no typical hematologic and biochemical findings. CSF analysis is abnormal in most dogs, with a predominantly mononuclear pleocytosis (usually 90–600 cells/μl) and an increased protein concentration (usually 50–200 mg/dl)[8]; however, these are not specific because other encephalitides are associated with similar CSF changes. The massive necrotizing lesions in the cerebrum can be detected with computed tomography or magnetic resonance imaging.[40]

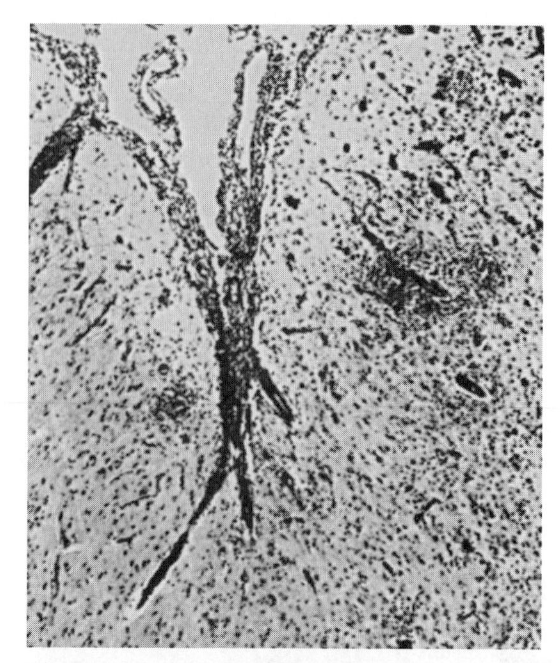

Figure 84–2. Histologic section from a case of Pug dog encephalitis. Severe perivascular and meningeal inflammation as well as necrosis of large areas of the cerebral cortex are evident (H and E, × 100).

PATHOLOGIC FINDINGS

Necrotizing lesions in the cerebrum may be visible on macroscopic examination. The histologic findings are unusual and highly typical for this disease—a disseminated meningitis, choroiditis, and encephalitis with greatest involvement in the cerebrum. The perivascular and meningeal inflammatory infiltrates consisting of lymphocytes, plasma cells, histiocytes, and macrophages have a strong tendency to invade the parenchyma. There are extensive compact subpial and subventricular lesions that may extend deep into the underlying brain tissue, with unusually intense microglial proliferation and total destruction of the original tissue elements. In some areas, there is frank cerebrocortical necrosis. The cerebral white matter also is severely affected, with intense perivascular cuffing and gliosis. In some areas there is leukomalacia with liquefaction and cavitation of the tissue (Fig. 84–2).

THERAPY

There is no treatment for this disease. Glucocorticoids do not alter the course of this necrotizing encephalitis, and antiepileptic drugs are often ineffective in controlling seizures.[10]

Encephalitis in Yorkshire Terriers

This condition appears to be restricted to Yorkshire terriers. The disease was originally reported in Switzerland[43] but also occurs in other western European countries,[49] North America,[23a, 37] and Japan.[11] I believe that the disease is a relatively new entity because retrospective examination of neuropathologic collections did not reveal cases before 1985. Both clinical and pathologic features of this disease differ considerably from the encephalitis in Pug and Maltese dogs.

ETIOLOGY

The cause of Yorkshire terrier encephalitis remains unknown. There is little doubt that an infectious organism is involved. Bacteria, fungi, and parasites can probably be excluded on the basis of microscopic examination of the lesions using appropriate special stains. The appearance of the lesions suggests a viral cause. CDV was excluded by immunocytochemistry and in situ hybridization for CDV antigen and CDV mRNA. The rabies virus and the central European tick-borne encephalitis virus were excluded utilizing similar techniques. To my knowledge, isolation studies have not been attempted.

CLINICAL SIGNS

The total number of documented cases is small, and generalizations are not possible. However, it appears to be predominantly a disease of adult dogs affecting both sexes. Although animals can be presented with acute signs, there is a clear tendency for the disease to become protracted for months or even years. There are no extraneural signs. Neurologic signs refer to the cerebrum with compulsive pacing, seizures, and visual deficits as well as to the brain stem with central vestibular signs (head tilt, vestibular ataxia), anisocoria, and other cranial nerve deficits.

DIAGNOSIS

No specific diagnostic test exists for this disease. Obviously, neurologic signs are not diagnostic per se. Lesions are quite large and, therefore, detectable by imaging techniques.[37] In chronic cases, they appear cystic. CSF changes are marked but not specific for the disease. The differential diagnosis includes chronic distemper encephalitis and GME.

PATHOLOGIC FINDINGS

There are multifocal, destructive inflammatory lesions in the cerebral white matter and in the brain stem. They can be visualized grossly as brownish discoloration on cut section. These lesions have a characteristic appearance, consisting of a malacic center surrounded by a rim of extremely intense perivascular infiltration. Older lesions become cystic with intense astrocytic sclerosis.

Hydrocephalus With Periventricular Encephalitis in Dogs

Hydrocephalus is probably the most common developmental abnormality of the CNS in dogs and may be the result of congenital or acquired stenosis of the mesencephalic aqueduct. Acquired hydrocephalus usually is a result of infectious or neoplastic diseases that lead to obstruction of the CSF drainage pathways. A particular form of acquired hydrocephalus in young dogs is associated with severe periventricular inflammation.[52]

ETIOLOGY

Because of the severe inflammatory changes seen with hydrocephalus, an infectious cause has been suspected. On bacteriologic examination of brain tissue and CSF in two dogs with this disease, three different bacteria were isolated; however, these were thought to be contaminants. It is possible that the disease is caused by a virus, although no infectious agent was found on EM study of the periventricular tissues of two dogs.[52] Canine parainfluenza virus has caused hydrocephalus in dogs after experimental inoculation (see Chapter 7).[3] However, the clinical and pathologic findings in experimental parainfluenza–induced hydrocephalus are totally different from those of the condition described herein. Serum neutralizing antibodies against canine parvovirus were absent.

CLINICAL FINDINGS

This disease occurs in puppies between 2 and 6 months of age. There is no predilection for miniature breeds as occurs with congenital hydrocephalus. The animals are normal at birth and exhibit normal development for the first 2 months of life. At 2 or 3 months of age, acute neurologic signs occur, together with rapidly progressing skull enlargement. Neurologic signs include behavioral changes such as depression, dullness, and hyperactivity. There is progressive incoordination in all limbs, and most animals develop neurologic blindness. Less consistent findings are cranial nerve deficits, which may include deafness, abnormal eye motility, head tilt, and dysphagia. The course of the disease is usually progressive over several days to a few weeks. In some animals, the clinical condition may stabilize.

DIAGNOSIS

No consistent hematologic or biochemical findings are associated with this form of hydrocephalus. CSF abnormalities consist of xanthochromia, increased protein concentration, and pleocytosis, including erythrocytes, mononuclear cells, and macrophages containing erythrocytes. Radiographic examination of the skull reveals abnormalities such as thinning of the cranial vault and homogeneous appearance of the intracranial contents. However, these findings are indicative of hydrocephalus, regardless of its cause. The same can be said for the EEG findings typical of hydrocephalus.

PATHOLOGIC FINDINGS

There is massive enlargement of the cerebral ventricles, which are filled with cloudy, hemorrhagic CSF. The internal surface of the ventricles is focally roughened, with a brownish discoloration. A typical finding is the presence of large dissecting cavities, also called false diverticula, in the cerebral mantle (Fig. 84–3*A*). These communicate with the lateral ventricles. Histologically, there is a severe inflammation with necrosis of the ependymal and subependymal tissues. The lesions are always hemorrhagic. Hemosiderin-laden macrophages are found in old lesions. There is perivascular cuffing with inflammatory cells and, in acute lesions, diffuse infiltration with neutrophils and macrophages (Fig. 84–3*B* and 3*C*). Glial mesenchymal repair tissue is formed later in the course of the disease.

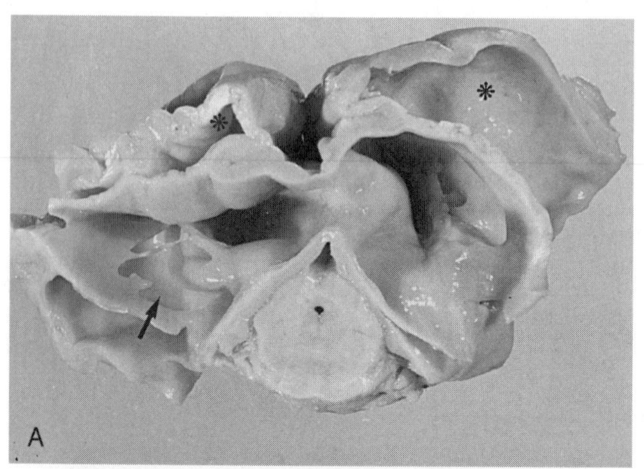

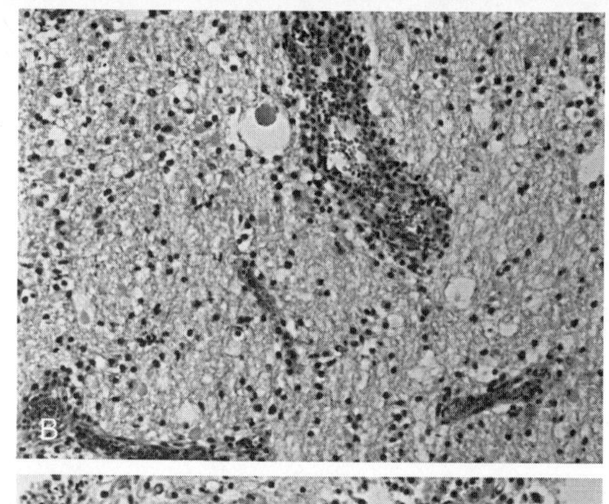

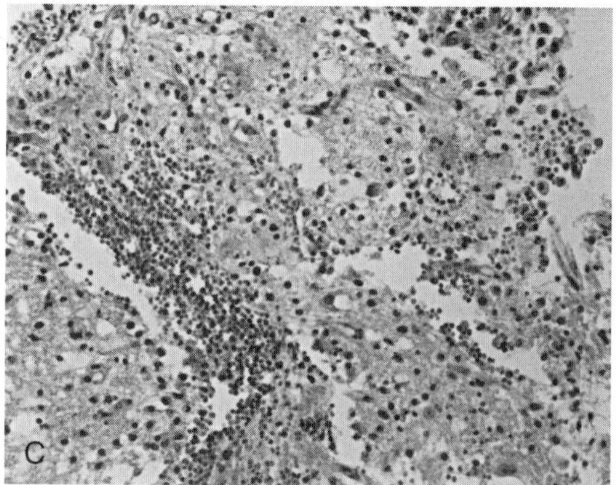

Figure 84–3. Gross and histologic specimens from a dog with periventricular encephalitis. *A,* Occipital area at the level of the midbrain showing greatly enlarged ventricles. False diverticulum *(asterisk)* communicates with the lateral ventricle through a defect *(arrow)* in the ventricular wall. (From Wouda W, et al: *Zentralbl Veterinarmed A* 28:481–493, 1981, with permission.) *B,* Inflammatory changes (cuffing) in the periventricular tissue (H and E, × 100). *C,* Hemorrhage and malacia in periventricular tissue (H and E, × 100).

THERAPY

By the time the condition becomes evident to the owner, severe damage has already taken place. In most cases, the disease is rapidly progressive, leading to severe neurologic impairment. However, in those cases in which the condition stabilizes, conservative therapy with glucocorticoids or surgical treatment may be considered.

Feline Poliomyelitis

Poliomyelitis in domestic cats was first reported in North Africa and Ceylon in the 1950s. Later, additional cases were described in North America and Europe.[21, 25, 46] A clinically and pathologically similar condition occurs in large Felidae (lions and tigers) held in captivity.[15]

ETIOLOGY

Pathologic findings indicate that poliomyelitis in cats is almost certainly caused by a virus. However, ultrastructural studies to demonstrate a specific causal virus in domestic cats have not yet been performed, and the considerable efforts to identify such a virus in lions and tigers, including tissue culture studies, animal inoculation, and serologic studies for known viruses, have been unsuccessful.[46] Comparative pathologic studies suggest that several known spontaneously occurring or experimentally induced viral infections of cats are unlikely to cause poliomyelitis; however, the role of togaviruses should be investigated further.[21] Nonsuppurative encephalitides in cats have been associated with Borna virus infection in some European countries such as Austria, Switzerland, and Sweden (see Chapter 26). Borna disease in cats has been named "staggering disease." However, as far as I can determine, Borna disease in cats is morphologically and clinically distinct from feline poliomyelitis.

CLINICAL FINDINGS

Feline poliomyelitis is an insidious disease; its onset is slow, and it progresses over weeks to months. In many instances, the neurologic signs may stabilize, and some animals may recover. Immature as well as adult cats appear to be susceptible. In cats, the disease is sporadic; to my knowledge, no outbreaks have been recorded in catteries. However, outbreaks in which several lions and tigers were simultaneously affected have occurred in zoologic gardens.[15] The predominant signs are problems in locomotion, including paresis, ataxia, and depressed postural reactions in the pelvic and thoracic limbs. Lower motor neuron involvement is characterized by muscle atrophy and decreased tendon reflexes. Hyperesthesia in the thoracic and lumbar areas is apparent is some cases. Additional neurologic findings, which occur rarely, include epilepsy, cerebellar signs, and pupillary abnormalities.

PATHOLOGIC FINDINGS

Disseminated inflammatory lesions are found in the brain and spinal cord (Fig. 84–4). The spinal cord and medulla oblongata are most severely affected. The lesions consist of perivascular mononuclear cuffing, gliosis, and neuronal degeneration, the last being most obvious in the ventral horns of the spinal cord. In chronic cases very little inflammation may be seen, but neuronal loss and intense astrogliosis in the cord are striking. As a result of neuronal damage, there also is marked diffuse wallerian degeneration of the lateral and ventral columns, resembling a primary degenerative disorder. There are no consistent lesions in other organ systems.

THERAPY

There is no curative treatment for the suspected viral infection. Contact between unaffected cats and those suspected to have the disease should be avoided. The prognosis is not always unfavorable, because large Felidae suspected of having the infection have been known to recover.[15]

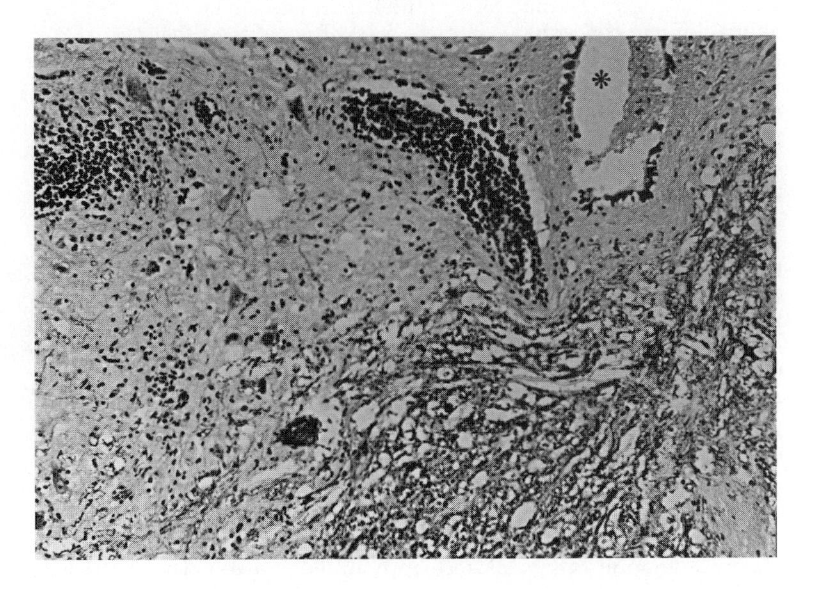

Figure 84–4. Histologic section from the spinal cord of a cat with poliomyelitis showing perivascular cuffing and nodular gliosis in the gray matter. Asterisk indicates central canal (H and E, × 250).

Feline Spongiform Encephalopathy

Feline spongiform encephalopathy (FSE) was first recognized during the bovine spongiform encephalopathy (BSE) epidemic in Great Britain. The first cases were diagnosed in the early 1990s,[26, 54] and approximately 70 cases had been reported by the end of 1995.[4] One case has been described in Norway; it is unknown whether a relation exists; however, the cat was fed commercial dry cat foods imported from Great Britain.[5] Captive wild species of Felidae such as the cheetah (*Acinonyx jubatus*) and puma (*Felis concolor*) that were fed bovine tissues have also been affected.[2a, 23c] The number of cats being reported annually in Great Britain appears to be decreasing,[4] which is expected because measures have been taken to prevent further spreading of the bovine disease. Spongiform change in the CNS of other species, such as that reported in Rottweilers,[24a] may have other causes, but will be scrutinized in the future because of lessons learned in this outbreak.

ETIOLOGY

FSE belongs to the spongiform encephalopathies (SEs), a group of diseases in humans and animals characterized by a very long incubation time and degeneration of the CNS with vacuolation of the neuropil and nerve cells. The SEs are transmissible to other animals, at least under experimental conditions.[9] The exact cause is still unknown; however, accumulation of amyloid fibrils is central in the pathogenesis of these diseases. The protein of which these fibrils consist is called the prion protein (PrP). It is normally a product of nerve cells, but under disease states is modified in such a way that it becomes protease resistant and hence accumulates in the tissue. This disease-inducing modification of the PrP can occur spontaneously; indeed, certain mutations in the PrP gene lead to an SE. Once formed, the modified, abnormal PrP is thought to induce additional copies of itself by interacting with normal PrP. Thus, it is believed that this modified protein becomes itself an infectious agent, the prion.[36] The prion theory is a revolutionary concept in biology, and many questions remain. Scrapie, the classic SE of small ruminants, has been recognized for many years in veterinary medicine. However, this group of diseases became notorious in the late 1980s as a result of the BSE outbreak in Great Britain,[50] where scrapie has been endemic for centuries. BSE was spread by animal protein concentrates in cattle feed. It is believed that the scrapie agent in so-called meat and bone meal derived from abattoir offal and fallen livestock (including scrapie-infected sheep) was no longer properly inactivated because of changes in the production procedures of the rendering industry. As a result, the scrapie agent probably established SE in bovines.

Animals with BSE were undoubtedly also recycled by the rendering industry until the epidemiology of the disease became understood, thus leading to a considerable enrichment of the agent in meat and bone meal before the protein-feeding ban came into effect. By 1996, the outbreak in British cattle involved more than 160,000 confirmed cases. On the basis of strain-typing experiments, there is little doubt that FSE is derived from BSE.[7] It is probable that cats were infected by ingesting BSE-contaminated feed.[54]

CLINICAL FINDINGS

Because of the very long incubation time of SE, the disease affects only adult cats (peak incidence at age 5 years). The neurologic signs develop progressively over several weeks to months and are characterized by behavioral changes and gait abnormalities. There is no focalization of the neurologic signs. The disease is invariably progressive and fatal.

DIAGNOSIS

There are no typical laboratory findings. The suspicion of FSE is based on the age of the animal and the clinical signs. A variety of neurologic conditions have to be considered.

PATHOLOGIC FINDINGS

As in all other SEs, the pathologic findings in FSE are highly characteristic. The changes consist of vacuolation in the neuropil and neurons in a bilaterally symmetric distribution, especially in the thalamus, basal ganglia, and cerebral cortex (Fig. 84–5). In advanced cases, there is neuronal loss and gliosis. There is no inflammation.

THERAPY

All SEs are fatal diseases. Prevention of exposure is the most important measure. Although it is generally very difficult to transmit an SE from one species to another orally, nine other species were found to be infected with BSE in Great Britain.[7] There is little doubt that BSE in these other species resulted from oral exposure. The BSE agent also induced a new variant of Creutzfeldt-Jakob disease in people.[7a, 19a, 29a, 36a] Because of the enormous resistance of the infectious agent to physical and chemical inactivation procedures, high titers of infectivity remain, even in extensively processed contaminated feedstuffs. To prevent exposure to other species, including people, the authorities in endemic countries confiscated all tissues (CNS, lymphoid tissues, intestine) in which the infectious agent could be theoretically present from all bovines at the time of slaughter. This measure came

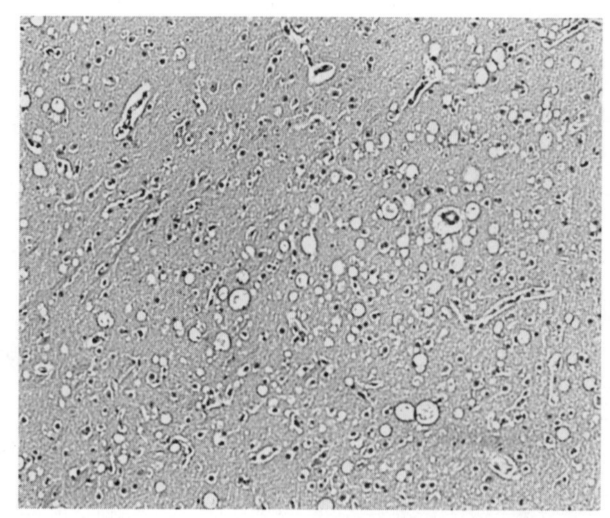

Figure 84–5. Feline spongiform encephalopathy showing small and large vacuoles in the neuropil at the level of the caudate nucleus (H and E, × 100).

into effect in the fourth year of the BSE epidemic and took several years to become completely effective. Thus, most likely, the exposure of other species had taken place before that time. Considering an average incubation period of about 5 years, the peak of the epidemic in cats has certainly been passed.[4] Further spread in the bovine population was prevented by banning the feeding of animal proteins to ruminant species. The BSE epidemic is expected to reach its end by the end of the century.[50] FSE should therefore soon disappear.

Steroid-Responsive Meningitis-Arteritis

Steroid (glucocorticoid)-responsive meningitis-arteritis (SRMA) has been described numerous times in the veterinary literature. Caution must be exercised in assuming that the cases described constitute a homogeneous entity because a variety of inflammatory processes exist, potentially incited by infectious agents and perpetuated by immunopathologic disturbances that can be ameliorated by anti-inflammatory therapy. A syndrome of SRMA has been described in which immune-mediated reactions appear to be primarily directed against the arteries and meninges of the CNS and involve Bernese mountain dogs,[30, 35, 42] boxers,[20, 34, 42] and other middle- to large-breed dogs, usually young adults.[20, 34]

Juvenile polyarteritis, a systemic vasculitis involving medium- to small-sized muscular arteries, predominantly involving the coronary and meningeal vessels, has been commonly reported in laboratory bred and raised beagles 6 to 9 months of age. It is also called the beagle pain syndrome and has been better characterized than the similar-appearing arteritis of the other breeds.[14, 38] Although the syndrome in beagles may be of a more systemic nature, it seems to be the same disease entity as SRMA reported in other breeds.

PATHOGENESIS

Although it resembles immune complex injury, arteritis-vasculitis of beagles and other breeds has not been associated with immune complex deposits in the vascular lesions. Nevertheless, immunoglobulin-producing plasma cells are associated with the lesions. In beagles, increased amounts of circulating immune complexes in one dog, increased rheumatoid factors in two dogs, and decreased C3 in one dog have been found.[19]

Other findings are markedly increased IgA levels in serum, increased percentages of peripheral B cells, decreased percentage of total peripheral T cells, suppressed blastogenic response to mitogens and inability to generate immunoglobulin-secreting plasma cells after activation, and presence of antineutrophil cytoplasmic antibodies. A large portion of the T cells are activated, suggesting the presence of a superantigen.[14, 44a] Elevated interleukin-6 levels in serum have been found in affected beagles, and levels paralleled clinical illness and decreased with glucocorticoid therapy and remission.[22] The uncontrolled IgA synthesis may be the result of immune dysregulation, perhaps induced by an infectious agent. Excessive IgA is likely to play a central role in the pathogenesis of the lesion.

CLINICAL SIGNS

The classic clinical presentation is episodic and recurrent and includes reluctance to move, cervical pain, stiff gait, resistance to neck manipulation, paraspinal hyperesthesia, and high rectal temperature. Chronically affected animals develop neurologic deficits.

DIAGNOSIS

Hematologic findings include a predominantly neutrophilic leukocytosis, and beagles show thrombocytosis.[14] CSF may be blood tinged or xanthochromic from the large amount of protein or blood breakdown. Neutrophilic pleocytosis and erythrophagocytosis are apparent. The highest protein concentrations are usually found in this condition compared with other inflammatory conditions.[42] All dogs synthesize IgG in high concentrations in the CNS.[45]

High IgA concentrations are found in the CSF; it is likely that IgA is also synthesized intrathecally.[42] Simultaneous

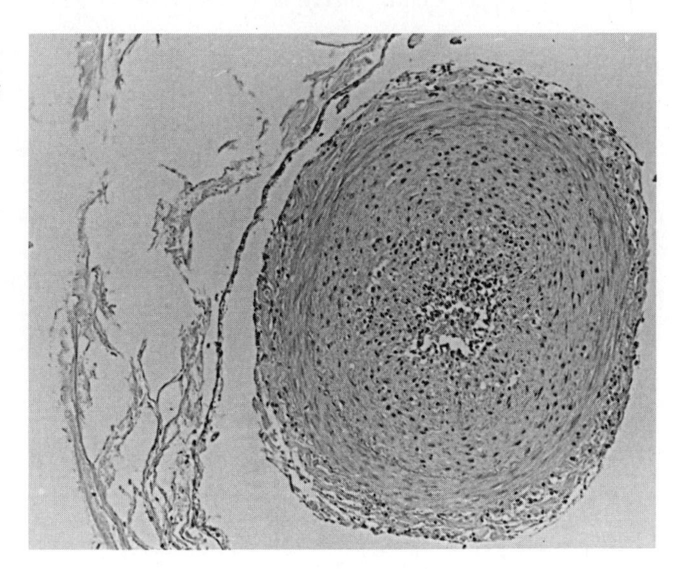

Figure 84–6. Stenosis of spinal meningeal artery from subintimal proliferation in a 3-year-old dog with steroid-responsive meningitis-arteritis. Periluminal inflammatory cell infiltrate and fibrosis of adjacent arachnoidea are also apparent (H and E, × 100).

demonstration of high IgA levels in serum and CSF is highly significant for the diagnosis. Large numbers of neutrophils are predominant in the CSF in acute cases; in chronic cases, mononuclear cells predominate. Mild to moderate hydrocephalus has been documented in some chronic cases with cisternography and neurosonographic techniques.

PATHOLOGIC FINDINGS

At necropsy, subarachnoid hemorrhages extending over the entire length of the meninges of the spinal cord and brain stem have been found in a few cases in which the vascular lesions had led to rupture of major blood vessels. In chronic cases, fibrous thickening of the spinal meninges may be noted. Lesions outside the CNS are relatively rare in affected dogs. Extraneural arteritis is more frequently noted in affected beagles, in which extramural coronary artery vasculitis and myocarditis have been most frequent.

Histologic changes are found in the meninges of the spinal cord and to a much lesser degree in the brain stem. They consist of necrotizing arteritis of medium- and small-sized arteries and associated leptomeningitis (Fig. 84–6). Chronic lesions include proliferative changes of the intima with vascular stenosis and arachnoidal fibrosis. The intramedullary arteries and neural parenchyma can be mildly affected in chronic cases. Occasional vessels may be thrombosed. The meningeal infiltrate contains hemosiderin-laden macrophages in cases in which hemorrhage had occurred. There is no evidence of immune complex deposition, but IgA deposits have been found in the vascular walls of some animals.[45]

TREATMENT

Dogs are unresponsive to antibiotics. If response to antibiotics occurs, it may be coincidental because relapses and intermittent episodes occur. Initial response to glucocorticoid therapy is dramatic. This occurrence contrasts this syndrome with that of granulomatous meningoencephalitis, which has a more rapidly progressive course of illness with deterioration, despite treatment.

Of 32 treated dogs with meningitis-arteritis (long-term glucocorticoid therapy), 13 were euthanized, 7 because of frequent relapses; 12 dogs were free of signs for at least 6 months of treatment, and for up to 4 years after treatment was discontinued; 5 dogs improved but still require therapy; 2 dogs were lost to follow-up.[42]

Conclusions

It is to be expected that additional CNS diseases of suspected infectious origin will be recognized in dogs and cats. The ability to characterize infectious agents in these diseases is limited when formalin-fixed tissues are used. Fresh material for culture should be collected when clinical findings are compatible with one of these disorders. In addition to brain tissue taken for isolation procedures, serum and CSF should be collected and screened for antibody activity against a wide variety of known infectious agents. The advent of widely available, extremely powerful molecular biologic techniques also extends the range of etiologic studies considerably. In addition, it is possible that more systematic ultrastructural studies of appropriately fixed tissues taken from lesions and sites indicated by the clinical examination may be helpful in detecting infectious agents. For a discussion of meningitis of suspected infectious or immune-mediated causes, see Bacterial Infections of the Central Nervous System, Chapter 92.

References

1. Aldhous P. 1990. BSE: spongiform encephalopathy found in cat. *Nature* 345:194.
2. Bailey CS, Higgins RJ. 1986. Characteristics of cerebrospinal fluid associated with canine granulomatous meningoencephalomyelitis: a retrospective study. *J Am Vet Med Assoc* 188:418–421.
2a. Baron T, Belli P, Madec FJY, et al. 1997. Spongiform encephalopathy in an imported cheetah in France. *Vet Rec* 141:270–271.
3. Baumgärtner WK, Krakowka S, Koestner A, et al. 1982. Acute encephalitis and hydrocephalus in dogs caused by canine parainfluenza virus. *Vet Pathol* 19:79–92.
4. Bradley R. 1996. Personal communication. Central Veterinary Laboratory, Weybridge, England.
5. Bratberg B, Ueland K, Wells AH. 1995. Feline spongiform encephalopathy in a cat in Norway. *Vet Rec* 136:444.
6. Braund KG. 1985. Granulomatous meningoencephalomyelitis. *J Am Vet Med Assoc* 186:138–141.
7. Bruce M, Chree A, McDonell I, et al. 1994. Transmission of bovine spongiform encephalopathy and scrapie to mice: strain variation and the species barrier. *Philos Trans R Soc Lond B Bio Sci* 343:405–411.
7a. Collinge J, Sidle KCL, Meads J, et al. 1996. Molecular analysis of prion strain variation and the etiology of new variant CJD. *Nature* 383:685–690.
8. Cordy DR, Holliday TA. 1989. A necrotizing meningoencephalitis of pug dogs. *Vet Pathol* 26:191–194.
9. DeArmond SJ, Prusiner SB. 1995. Etiology and pathogenesis of prion diseases. *Am J Pathol* 146:785–811.
10. De Lahunta A. 1983. Veterinary neuroanatomy and clinical neurology. WB Saunders, Philadelphia, PA.
11. De Lahunta A. 1994. Personal communication. Cornell University, Ithaca, NY.
12. Detweiler DK. 1989. Spontaneous and induced arterial disease in the dog: pathology and pathogenesis. *Toxicol Pathol* 17:94–108.
13. Fankhauser R, Fatzer R, Luginbühl H, et al. 1972. Reticulosis of the central nervous system in dogs. *Adv Vet Sci Comp Med* 16:35–71.
14. Felsburg PJ, Hogenesch H, Somberg RL, et al. 1992. Immunologic abnormalities in canine juvenile polyarteritis syndrome. A naturally occurring animal model of Kawasaki disease. *Clin Immunol Immunopathol* 65:110–128.
15. Flir K. 1973. Encephalomyelitis in the big cats. *DTW Dtsch Tierarztl Wochenschr* 80:401–404.
16. Fraser H, Pearson GR, McConnell I, et al. 1994. Transmission of feline spongiform encephalopathy to mice. *Vet Rec* 134:449.
17. Gruffydd-Jones TJ, Galloway PE, Pearson GE. 1992. Feline spongiform encephalopathy. *J Small Anim Pract* 33:471–476.
18. Harris CW, Didier PJ, Parker AJ. 1988. Simultaneous central nervous system reticulosis in two related Afghan hounds. *Compend Cont Educ Pract Vet* 10:304–310.
19. Hayes TJ, Roberts GKS, Halliwell WH. 1989. An idiopathic febrile necrotizing arteritis syndrome in the dog: Beagle pain. *Toxicol Pathol* 17:129–137.
19a. Haywood AM. 1997. Mechanisms of disease: transmissible spongiform encephalopathies. *N Engl J Med* 337:1821–1828.
19b. Hess PR, Sellon RK. 1997. Steroid-responsive, cervical, pyogranulomatous pachymeningitis in a dog. *J Am Anim Hosp Assoc* 33:461–468.
19c. Hinrichs U, Tobias R, Baumgartner W. 1996. A case of necrotizing meningoencephalitis in a pug dog. *Tierarztl Prax* 24:489–492.
20. Hoff EJ, Vandevelde M. 1981. Necrotizing vasculitis in the central nervous system of two dogs. *Vet Pathol* 18:219–223.
21. Hoff EJ, Vandevelde M. 1981. Non-suppurative encephalomyelitis in cats suggestive of a viral origin. *Vet Pathol* 18:170–180.
22. Hogenesch H, Snyder PW, Scott-Montcrieff JC, et al. 1995. Interleukin-6 activity in dogs with juvenile polyarteritis syndrome: effect of corticosteroids. *Clin Immunol Immunopathol* 77:107–110.
23. Irving G, Chrisman C. 1990. Long term outcome of five cases of corticosteroid-responsive meningomyelitis. *J Am Anim Hosp Assoc* 26:324–328.
23a. Jull BA, Merryman JI, Thomas WB, et al. 1997. Necrotizing encephalitis in a yorkshire terrier. *J Am Vet Med Assoc* 211:1005–1007.
23b. Kipar A, Baumgartner W, Vogi C, et al. 1998. Immunohistochemical characterization of inflammatory cells in brains of dogs with granulomatous meningoencephalitis. *Vet Pathol* 35:43–52.
23c. Kirkwood JK, Cunningham AA, Flach EJ, et al. 1995. Spongiform enceph-

alopathy in another captive cheetah (*Acinonyx jubatus*): evidence for variation in susceptibility or incubation periods between species? *J Zoo Wildl Med* 26:577–582.
24. Kobayashi Y, Ochiai K, Umemura T, et al. 1994. Necrotizing meningoencephalitis in Pug dogs in Japan. *J Comp Pathol* 110:129–136.
24a. Kortz GD, Meier WA, Higgins RJ, et al. 1997. Neuronal vacuolation and spinocerebellar degeneration in young Rottweiler dogs. *Vet Pathol* 34:296–302.
25. Kronevi T, Nordström M, Moreno W, et al. 1974. Feline ataxia due to nonsuppurative meningoencephalomyelitis of unknown etiology. *Nord Vet Med* 26:720–725.
26. Legett MM, Dukes J, Pirie HM. 1990. A spongiform encephalopathy in a cat. *Vet Rec* 127:586–588.
27. Lundgren AL, Czech G, Bode L, et al. 1993. Natural Borna disease in domestic animals other than horses and sheep. *Zentralbl Veterinarmed* 40:298–303.
28. Maeda H, Ozaki K, Horikiri K, et al. 1993. Granulomatous leptomeningitis in Beagle dogs. *Vet Pathol* 30:566–573.
29. Maeda H, Ozaki K, Horikiri K, et al. 1994. Histological and topographical characteristics of canine granulomatous leptomeningitis. *J Comp Pathol* 111:55–63.
29a. Masters CL, Beyreuther K. 1997. Spongiform encephalopathies. Tracking turncoat proteins. *Nature* 388:228–229.
30. Meric SM, Child G, Higgins RJ. 1986. Necrotizing vasculitis of the spinal pachyleptomeningeal arteries in three Bernese mountain dog littermates. *J Am Anim Hosp Assoc* 22:459-465.
31. Meric SM, Perman V, Hardy RM. 1985. Corticosteroid-responsive meningitis in ten dogs. *J Am Anim Hosp Assoc* 21:677–684.
32. Pearson GR, Wyatt JM, Gruffydd-Jones TJ, et al. 1991. Feline spongiform encephalopathy. *Vet Rec* 128:532.
33. Pearson GR, Wyatt JM, Gruffydd-Jones TJ, et al. 1992. Feline spongiform encephalopathy febrile and PrP studies. *Vet Rec* 131:307–310.
34. Poncelet L, Balligand M. 1993. Steroid responsive meningitis in three Boxer dogs. *Vet Rec* 132:361–362.
35. Presthus J. 1991. Aseptic suppurative meningitis in Bernese mountain dogs. *Eur J Comp Anim Pract* 1:24–28.
36. Prusiner SB. 1993. Genetic and infectious prion diseases. *Arch Virol* 50:1129–1153.
36a. Raymond GJ, Hope J, Kocisko DA, et al. 1997. Molecular assessment of the potential transmissibilities of BSE and scrapie to humans. *Nature* 388:285–288.
37. Sawashima Y, Sawashima K, Taura Y, et al. 1996. Clinical and pathological findings of a Yorkshire terrier affected with necrotizing encephalitis. *J Vet Med Sci* 58:659–661.
38. Scott-Moncrieff JC, Snyder PW, Glickman LT, et al. 1992. Systemic necrotizing vasculitis in nine young Beagles. *J Am Vet Med Assoc* 201:1553–1558.
39. Sorjonen DC. 1990. Clinical and histopathological features of granulomatous meningoencephalomyelitis in dogs. *J Am Anim Hosp Assoc* 26:141–147.
40. Stalis IH, Chadwick B, Dayrell-Hart B, et al. 1995. Necrotizing meningoencephalitis of Maltese dogs. *Vet Pathol* 32:230–235.
41. Synge BA, Waters JW. 1992. Spongiform encephalopathy in a Scottish cat. *Vet Rec* 129:320.
42. Tipold A. 1995. Diagnosis of inflammatory and infectious diseases of the central nervous system in dogs. *J Vet Intern Med* 9:304–314.
43. Tipold A, Fatzer R, Jaggy A, et al. 1993. Necrotizing encephalitis in Yorkshire terriers. *J Small Anim Pract* 34:623–628.
44. Tipold A, Jaggy A. 1994. Steroid responsive meningitis-arteritis in dogs. A long-term study of 32 cases. *J Small Anim Pract* 35:311–316.
44a. Tipold A, Somberg R, Felsburg P. 1996. Is there a superantigen effect on steroid-responsive meningitis-arteritis in dogs? *Tierarztl Prax* 24:514–518.
45. Tipold A, Vandevelde M, Zurbriggen A. 1995. Neuroimmunological studies in steroid-responsive meningitis-arteritis in dogs. *Res Vet Sci* 58:103–108.
46. Vandevelde M. 1990. Neurologic diseases of suspected infectious origin, pp 862–865. *In* Greene CE (ed), Infectious diseases of the dog and cat. WB Saunders, Philadelphia, PA.
47. Vandevelde M. 1996. Unpublished observation. University of Bern, Bern, Switzerland.
48. Vandevelde M, Fatzer R, Fankhauser R. 1981. Immunohistologic studies on primary reticulosis of the canine brain. *Vet Pathol* 18:577–588.
49. Van Ham L. 1995. Personal communication. University of Ghent, Belgium.
50. Wells GA, Wilesmith JW. 1995. The neuropathology and epidemiology of bovine spongiform encephalopathy. *Brain Pathol* 5:91–103.
51. Willoughby K, Kelly DF, Lyon DG, et al. 1992. Spongiform encephalopathy in a captive puma (Felis concolor). *Vet Rec* 131:431–434.
52. Wouda W, Vandevelde M, Kihm U. 1981. Internal hydrocephalus of suspected infectious origin in young dogs. *Zentralbl Veterinarmed A* 28:481–493.
53. Wyatt JM, Pearson GR, Smerdon TN, et al. 1990. Spongiform encephalopathy in a cat. *Vet Rec* 126:513.
54. Wyatt JM, Pearson GR, Smerdon TN, et al. 1991. Naturally occurring scrapie-like spongiform encephalopathy in five domestic cats. *Vet Rec* 129:233–236.

Section V

CLINICAL PROBLEMS

Chapter 85

Integumentary Infections

Bacterial Infections of the Skin

Peter J. Ihrke

Pyoderma is defined as a pyogenic or pus-producing bacterial infection of the skin. The diversity of clinical syndromes seen with canine pyoderma is enormous; the effects of lesions vary from minor annoyances to those with life-threatening potential.[24, 25, 38, 54] Pyoderma may be superficial, involving only the epidermis, or deeper, compromising structures in the dermis and the deep, subjacent fatty tissue. This tremendous diversity may be partially responsible for the magnitude of difficulty during diagnosis and management. Misdiagnosis also may result from markedly variable clinical characteristics among pyoderma, among dogs, among different anatomic sites, and between acute and chronic disease. The presence of pus cannot be used as a defining diagnostic characteristic because pus may not be visible grossly. Rapid rupture of pustules leads to less diagnostic crusting. In addition, in deep pyoderma, accumulations of pus in the middermis may not appear on the surface.

Globally, pyoderma is one of the most common causes of canine skin disease. Pyoderma was second only to flea allergy dermatitis in frequency of diagnosis in a study from North American veterinary colleges.[56] In another epidemiologic study performed in a relatively flea-free environment in Canada, bacterial folliculitis and furunculosis ranked first among canine skin diseases, comprising more than one quarter of the dermatology case load.[55] Conversely, pyoderma is an uncommon cause of skin disease in cats, other domestic animals, and humans. Bacterial skin disease in the cat is rare, with the exception of subcutaneous bite wound abscesses (see Chapter 52).

Reasons for the markedly increased frequency of bacterial skin disease in the dog in comparison with other mammalian species are unknown. Various host factors that may result in enhanced susceptibility include the comparatively thin, compact canine stratum corneum, the relative lack of intercellular lipids in the canine stratum corneum, the lack of a lipid-squamous epithelial plug in the entrance of canine hair follicles, and the relatively high pH of canine skin.[25, 35, 40]

ETIOLOGY AND PATHOGENESIS

Normal Microflora of the Skin and Hair

Skin microbial flora is composed of resident and transient bacteria. Resident bacteria are harmless commensals that are able to multiply on both the skin surface and in hair follicles and maintain a static, consistent population. Transient bacteria cannot compete with the established resident flora and may be seeded to the skin from either the mucous membranes or the environment. The total number of resident bacteria found on normal canine skin is not large and may be as little as 350 organisms/cm^2 or less.[25] Studies examining the bacterial flora of normal dogs have documented aerobic organisms, including *Micrococcus* spp., α-hemolytic streptococci, and *Acinetobacter* spp., and anaerobic organisms, among them *Clostridium perfringens* and *Propionibacterium acnes*.[19, 21, 24, 25, 34, 54]

Combined data published over the past decade have clarified the role of *Staphylococcus intermedius*.[2, 4, 5, 19, 21, 25, 34, 39] This organism is probably not a true dermal resident but a contaminant on normal canine hair and either a contaminant or a transient, restricted, local colonist on normal canine skin. Mucous membranes such as those of the anus and nares probably play an important role as sources of this potential skin pathogen. Normal grooming in all dogs and excessive licking in pruritic dogs may seed the skin from the anus and nares.[2–5, 34]

S. intermedius and Other Canine Cutaneous Pathogens

S. intermedius is the primary canine cutaneous pathogen. This organism has been shown to be a species separate and distinct from the human pathogen, *S. aureus*.[17, 25] Pure cultures of this bacterium are grown from most pustules or draining tracts in dogs with pyoderma.

Pathogenicity of staphylococci in humans correlates with various proteins and toxins considered to be virulence factors. Similar data are not available for the dog. The role of various virulence factors such as protein A, leukocidin, hemolysins, epidermolytic toxin, and other soluble products is not known in the dog. When potential virulence factors have been examined comparing *S. intermedius* isolates from normal dogs and dogs with pyoderma, clear differences in toxin profiles, gel electrophoresis of exoproteins, and immunoblotting of concentrated extracellular proteins were not elucidated.[1, 3, 16, 17, 25] Evidently, host factors rather than virulence factors appear to be most important in determining the outcome in canine staphylococcal pyoderma.[1, 3, 17, 25]

Secondary gram-negative invaders such as *Proteus* sp., *Pseudomonas* sp., or *Escherichia coli* may be isolated in conjunction with *S. intermedius*, usually from deep pyodermas. However, if gram-negative bacteria are isolated from a pyoderma without concomitant isolation of *S. intermedius*, the technique used and the results obtained should be questioned. Infection with *S. intermedius* creates a tissue milieu that is conducive to secondary gram-negative bacterial invasion.[24, 25]

Microbial Alterations With Skin Disease

Although the factors that promote the proliferation of *S. intermedius* on skin leading to pyoderma are poorly understood, it is well established that dogs with other skin diseases are more likely to develop secondary pyoderma. Dogs with defects in cornification have a shift in the balance of bacterial species colonizing the skin such that coagulase-positive staphylococci predominate. Clinically, this correlates with an increased frequency of pyoderma in seborrheic dogs. A shift in both the frequency and intensity of staphylococcal colonization has been noted in dogs with atopic dermatitis and contact dermatitis as well as seborrheic dermatitis.[25]

Zoonotic Potential of Skin Pathogens

Because *S. intermedius* is a separate and distinct species from *S. aureus*, this partially explains why humans with a normally functioning immune system are not at great risk for skin or wound infections contaminated with *S. intermedius*. Healthy owners of dogs with staphylococcal pyoderma are not at risk for zoonotic bacterial infection. However, up to 21% of dog bite lesions in people may be infected with *S. intermedius*.[60] These data indicate that a dog with suppurative pyoderma would be of concern if a household member were immunocompromised and bitten or exposed to suppurative discharges. Nevertheless, the pathogenicity of other organisms unassociated with pyoderma would be greater (see Bite Wound Infections, Chapter 53).

Susceptibility and Host Response to Infection

Because *S. intermedius* does not possess the requisite virulence factors to be a potent pathogen for the normal dog, the majority of canine pyoderma are probably associated with underlying disease or other host factors. Diseases such as ectoparasitism, cornification defects (seborrhea), allergy (atopic dermatitis, food allergy, flea allergy dermatitis), and endocrinopathies such as hypothyroidism and Cushing's disease frequently predispose the dog to pyoderma.[14, 25, 30, 54] Pyoderma secondary to cornification defects and allergic diseases are best documented. More broadly, pruritus from any underlying disease, inflammation from any cause, injudicious use of glucocorticoids, and poor grooming contribute to the likelihood of secondary infection.

Infection of the hair follicle is responsible for the majority of canine pyoderma cases. Follicular inflammation, obstruction, atrophy, dysplasia, or degeneration predispose the animal to secondary pyoderma. After pyoderma has been initiated, immunologic incompetence, coexisting disease, pruritus, inflammation, scar tissue formation, and improper initial therapy are negative prognostic factors.[25]

The initiation of a staphylococcal pyoderma requires both invasion and colonization of host tissues and evasion of host immunity. Host defense mechanisms mobilized to prevent this invasion include both immunologic and nonimmunologic processes. Nonimmunologic mechanisms include the desquamation of the stratum corneum (surface and follicular), the lipid intercellular barrier, the epithelial proliferation in response to injury, and the antibacterial effect of inorganic salts found in sebum and sweat. Additionally, resident bacterial competition is a nonimmunologic, "nonhost" defense mechanism. Immunologic host defense mechanisms of the skin include proteins within the intercellular matrix; immunoglobulins within the basement membrane zone; and immunologically active cells such as Langerhans' cells, dermal dendrocytes, lymphocytes, mast cells, and venular endothelial cells present in either the epidermis or dermis.[25]

Host immunologic response may be deleterious as well as beneficial. Some dogs with chronic or recurrent pyoderma exhibit depression of lymphocyte blastogenesis. Exceptionally potent bacterial antigens, termed *superantigens*, may explain the troublesome nature of pyoderma secondary to canine atopic dermatitis and the marked inflammation and pruritus of some canine pyoderma.[25]

Bacterial hypersensitivity has long been hypothesized as a complicating feature of recurrent canine pyoderma. The potential importance of bacterial hypersensitivity has been underscored by work indicating that mast cell degranulation can initiate enhanced epidermal permeability to bacterial antigens in atopic dogs.[39] Another study substantiated a link between antistaphylococcic antibodies and various subgroups of canine pyoderma.[45]

Classification of Pyoderma

Classification based on depth of bacterial involvement is most useful clinically because it provides information on diagnosis, likelihood of underlying disease, prognosis, and response to therapy. In general, the deeper the infection, the more likely it is that underlying causes are present. Deeper infections also require that the clinician be more aggressive both diagnostically and therapeutically. Using depth of bacterial involvement, canine pyoderma may be described as surface, superficial, and deep (Table 85–1).[25]

Surface Pyoderma

This term is used for very superficial erosions of the skin. Although pathogenic bacteria can be cultured from these lesions and contribute to inflammation, bacterial involvement is secondary. Pyotraumatic dermatitis (acute moist dermatitis, hot spots) and intertrigo (skinfold pyoderma) are classified as surface pyoderma. Mucocutaneous pyoderma currently is classified as a surface pyoderma for convenience. Pyotraumatic dermatitis usually develops secondary to flea allergy dermatitis. Intertrigo occurs in skinfolds and is seen in conjunction with friction, poor drainage, and maceration. Mucocutaneous pyoderma is a surface disease of unknown cause that predominantly involves the lips and perioral skin.[26] Surface pyoderma rarely is a diagnostic or therapeutic challenge.

Superficial Pyoderma

Superficial pyodermas are the most common canine bacterial skin diseases. Impetigo is characterized by nonfollicular pustules involving the superficial layers of the epidermis. Superficial folliculitis affects the ostial portion of the hair

Table 85–1. Classification of Canine Pyoderma Based on Depth of Infection

SURFACE PYODERMA
Pyotraumatic dermatitis (acute moist dermatitis, hot spots)
Intertrigo (skinfold pyoderma): lip-fold intertrigo, facial-fold intertrigo, vulvar-fold intertrigo, tail-fold intertrigo, obesity-fold intertrigo
Mucocutaneous pyoderma
SUPERFICIAL PYODERMA
Impetigo (puppy pyoderma)
Superficial bacterial folliculitis[a]
Superficial spreading pyoderma[a]
DEEP PYODERMA
Deep bacterial folliculitis and furunculosis
Muzzle folliculitis and furunculosis (canine acne)
Pyotraumatic folliculitis[a]
Pedal folliculitis and furunculosis[a]
Callus pyoderma (pressure-point pyoderma)
German shepherd dog pyoderma[a]
Cellulitis (secondary to demodicosis or immunologic incompetence)
DISEASES FORMERLY CLASSIFIED AS PYODERMA
Juvenile sterile granulomatous dermatitis and lymphadenitis (juvenile cellulitis, puppy strangles, juvenile "pyoderma")
Hidradenitis suppurativa[b]

[a]Subgroups of superficial and deep pyoderma in which recurrence or recrudescence is more common.
[b]Most were probably bullous pemphigoid or ulcerative dermatosis of the Shetland sheepdog and collie.

follicle and is the most common subgrouping of canine pyoderma. Impetigo and superficial folliculitis are diagnostic challenges because pustules rupture easily, giving rise to crusted papules that are not as easily diagnosed. A third clinical subset of superficial pyoderma, termed *superficial spreading pyoderma,* is characterized by centrifugally expanding erythema and peripheral epidermal collarettes. Superficial spreading pyoderma may be seen alone or in conjunction with superficial folliculitis.

Deep Pyoderma

Infection proceeds deeper in the follicle, and follicular rupture can lead to a granulomatous foreign body tissue response. Deep pyoderma is much less common than superficial pyoderma. Diagnosis of deep pyoderma usually is not difficult, but therapy is often problematic.

CLINICAL FINDINGS

Dermatology has a singular advantage over most other specialty areas in medicine in that skin lesions are visible and available for careful inspection. Excellent lighting is essential for a proper physical examination. A lighted hand lens is beneficial. Frequently, clinical findings can be clarified by clipping the overlying hair from an affected area.

Primary Skin Lesions

An erythematous papule is the most common primary skin lesion seen in most superficial and some deep pyoderma. Papules are circumscribed, solid elevations of the skin and usually are formed in groups. As infection proceeds, pus accumulates in an intraepidermal or follicular location to form a pustule. Small pustules may appear as papules to the naked eye. Intact pustules are often transient in canine skin. If surface rupture of pustules occurs, the resultant lesions are crusted papules. In deep pyoderma, follicular rupture exacerbates inflammation in the adjacent dermis, resulting in a nodule or furuncle. Surface rupture of these deeper lesions may lead to fistulous tracts. Peripheral collarettes are composed of detaching stratum corneum at the margins of inflammation. In deep pyoderma, host response is more intense, producing more obvious inflammation and swelling, thereby creating nodules.

Secondary Skin Lesions

Pustules can rupture spontaneously or can be obliterated by self-trauma. Consequently, ruptured pustules become crusted papules. These crusted papules are less diagnostically based and may be indistinguishable from papules seen with other skin diseases. If crusted papules are grouped, crusts composed of dried pus, exudate, and keratin debris may form and mimic disorders of cornification. Because many canine pyoderma are pruritic, self-traumatic excoriations may obliterate more diagnostic primary lesions and other secondary lesions such as crusted papules.

Alopecia can be seen secondary to pyoderma. Hair fragments are shed from infected follicles. Transient patchy alopecia probably results from premature telogenization and possibly telogen arrest in a normally mosaic, asynchronous hair replacement pattern. Permanent, scarring alopecia secondary to folliculitis is uncommon, in contrast with the condition in people.

Follicular rupture in deep pyoderma leads to nodule formation. Rupture of these nodules leads to draining fistulous tracts. Dermal hemorrhage resulting from follicular rupture and intense inflammation may result in hemorrhagic bullae.

Distribution of Lesions

Acute moist dermatitis, usually secondary to flea allergy, is seen most commonly in the dorsal lumbosacral region. Intertrigo, or skinfold pyoderma, is observed at the specific site of the anatomic defect according to breed. Mucocutaneous pyoderma occurs predominantly on and around the lips but may affect other mucocutaneous junctions.

Uncomplicated superficial pyoderma occurs predominantly in the moist, intertriginous zones of the groin and axilla and, to a lesser extent, the interdigital webs. Impetigo occurs primarily in the groin of prepubescent dogs. Superficial folliculitis and superficial spreading pyoderma are most commonly found in the groin and axilla. Lesions may generalize on the thorax. The attendant patchy, partial alopecia is more distinctive in short-coated dogs. Improper use of glucocorticoids may contribute to the spread of any superficial pyoderma while paradoxically decreasing visible inflammation.

Deep pyoderma usually develop as an extension of superficial pyoderma. A characteristic self-explanatory pattern is seen with interdigital, pressure point, and nasal pyoderma. Because cellulitis is most common secondary to generalized demodicosis, the distribution follows that of the primary disease.

DIAGNOSIS

Differential Diagnoses

Many other skin diseases may mimic canine pyoderma. The differential diagnoses of canine pyoderma have been reviewed.[25] Differential diagnoses are listed in an approximate order of importance in Table 85–2. For additional information, the reader is referred to other sources.[25, 54]

A variety of ancillary procedures may be helpful in diagnosing pyoderma and in determining the presence of underlying diseases or other predisposing factors. Skin scrapings, cytologic examination, and skin biopsy usually are the most useful diagnostic procedures for the evaluation of suspected pyoderma.[25] Conversely, bacterial culture and identification and antibiotic susceptibility testing are overutilized procedures. Bacterial species and susceptibility to antimicrobial therapy can usually be predicted.

Skin Scrapings

Because demodicosis can initiate lesions that mimic uncomplicated pyoderma, skin scrapings should be taken in all suspected cases of canine pyoderma. It is especially important to scrape any pustular or papular lesion with a follicular orientation. In addition to mimicking pyoderma, demodicosis can become secondarily infected. However, lesions will follow the distribution pattern of demodicosis. Skin scrapings are more likely to yield a positive result in suspected cases of lip-fold intertrigo, superficial folliculitis, deep folliculitis, and furunculosis (canine acne, pedal folliculitis), and cellulitis.

Table 85–2. Differential Diagnosis of Canine Pyoderma

SURFACE

Pyotraumatic dermatitis (acute moist dermatitis, hot spots): pyotraumatic folliculitis, demodicosis, neoplasia (especially sweat gland adenocarcinoma), cutaneous metastasis, fixed drug eruption, early necrotizing form of idiopathic nodular panniculitis, early localized vasculitis, focal *Malassezia* dermatitis, candidiasis

Intertrigo (skinfold pyoderma)

Lip-fold intertrigo: localized demodicosis, fixed drug eruption, superficial necrolytic dermatitis ± *Malassezia* dermatitis or candidiasis, zinc-responsive dermatosis, muzzle folliculitis and furunculosis (canine acne), localized pemphigus foliaceus, early pemphigus vulgaris, early bullous pemphigoid

Facial-fold intertrigo: localized demodicosis, *Malassezia* dermatitis, dermatophytosis

Vulvar-fold intertrigo: urinary tract infection with self-trauma, ulcerative dermatosis of the Shetland sheepdog and collie, drug eruption, canine familial dermatomyositis, pemphigus vulgaris, bullous pemphigoid

Tail-fold intertrigo: flea allergy dermatitis

Obesity-fold intertrigo: *Malassezia* dermatitis

Mucocutaneous pyoderma: lip-fold intertrigo, localized demodicosis, early discoid lupus erythematosus, zinc-responsive dermatosis, generic dog food skin disease, muzzle folliculitis and furunculosis (canine acne)

SUPERFICIAL

Impetigo (puppy pyoderma): early flea allergy dermatitis, superficial folliculitis

Superficial bacterial folliculitis: superficial spreading pyoderma, flea allergy dermatitis, demodicosis, pemphigus foliaceus, sarcoptic acariasis, severe impetigo, drug eruption, erythema multiforme, seborrheic dermatitis, sterile eosinophilic pustulosis

DEEP

Deep folliculitis and furunculosis: demodicosis, subcutaneous and deep mycoses, severe maladapted dermatophytosis, sterile granuloma-pyogranuloma, histiocytosis, idiopathic nodular panniculitis, juvenile sterile granulomatous dermatitis and lymphadenitis, vasculitis

Pyotraumatic folliculitis: pyotraumatic dermatitis, demodicosis, neoplasia (especially sweat gland adenocarcinoma), cutaneous metastasis, fixed drug eruption, early necrotizing form of idiopathic nodular panniculitis, early localized vasculitis, focal *Malassezia* dermatitis, candidiasis

Muzzle folliculitis and furunculosis (canine acne): localized demodicosis, early juvenile sterile granulomatous dermatitis and lymphadenitis

Pedal folliculitis and furunculosis: demodicosis, dermatophytosis, subcutaneous and deep mycoses, opportunistic fungal diseases, pelodera dermatitis

Callus pyoderma (pressure-point pyoderma): acral lick dermatitis, generic dog food skin disease, focal actinic comedones

German shepherd dog pyoderma: demodicosis with secondary deep pyoderma, subcutaneous and deep mycoses, opportunistic fungal diseases

Cellulitis (± demodicosis): juvenile sterile granulomatous dermatitis and lymphadenitis (juvenile cellulitis), subcutaneous and deep mycoses, German shepherd dog pyoderma, sterile granuloma-pyogranuloma, idiopathic liquefying panniculitis

Reprinted by permission: Ihrke PJ: Bacterial Skin Disease in the Dog: A Guide to Canine Pyoderma. Veterinary Learning Systems, Princeton, NJ, 1996.

Cytologic Examination

This is a simple, cost-effective, and frequently beneficial diagnostic test for the documentation of canine pyoderma. Material from either direct smears of pustules or draining tracts often yields as much or more useful information than bacterial cultures and is more rapid and cost effective. Specimens should be air dried and stained with either a modified Romanovsky-type Wright's stain *(Diff-Quik)* or new methylene blue. Modified Wright's stain is beneficial both for documenting organisms and for identifying inflammatory cells. The identification of cocci almost always indicates the presence of *S. intermedius*. The presence of degenerating neutrophils supports the diagnosis of pyoderma, especially if cocci are intracellular.

Skin Biopsy

Skin biopsy is a valuable tool that is often neglected in the diagnosis of canine pyoderma. More frequent skin biopsy has led to the more frequent diagnosis of pyoderma. The benefit of skin biopsy can be maximized if basic principles are followed involving timing, lesion selection, method selection, technique, preparation of supportive material, and submission to a dermatopathologist.

Bacterial Culture, Bacterial Identification, and Antibiotic Susceptibility

Bacterial culture is overused in the evaluation and management of canine pyoderma. Bacterial culture and identification and antibiotic susceptibility tests are indicated if mixed infection is suspected (as determined by cytologic examination) and if appropriate empiric antibiotic therapy has not been effective. Cultures of intact pustules, furuncles, and nodules are more likely to yield helpful information. Bacterial cultures are less likely to yield good results from open lesions.

Evaluation for Immunocompetence

Reliable diagnostic tests to determine immunocompetence in the dog still are not available.[13] Gross information can be derived from a CBC and serum electrophoresis. An absolute neutrophilia with a lymphocyte count of at least 1000 to 1500 cells/ml should be observed in normal dogs with ongoing or recurrent pyoderma. A broad-based elevation in the serum electrophoretic pattern in the β and γ ranges should be present.[24, 25] Assays such as in vitro lymphocyte stimulation and bactericidal tests currently are still primarily research tools because of the prohibitive expense and lack of availability. The lack of ability to correct any defects that are documented further detracts from the clinical usefulness of these tests.[14]

THERAPY

Systemic antibiotics usually are not needed in the treatment of most surface pyoderma; topical antibacterial therapy usually is sufficient. In contrast, successful management of most superficial and deep pyoderma requires systemic antibiotic therapy. Topical antibacterial shampoo therapy commonly is applied as an adjunct in the management of most superficial and deep pyoderma to speed recovery, improve patient well-being, and potentially prevent recurrence. Immunomodulatory therapy is used less frequently and usually is an attempt to prevent or diminish the frequency of recurrent infection. Extended regimens of antibiotics are predominantly a last resort in the management of chronic, recurrent pyoderma.

Antibiotic Therapy

The basic principles of systemic antibiotic therapy include the selection of an appropriate antibiotic, the establishment of an optimal dosage, and the maintenance of that dosage for enough time to ensure cure rather than transient remission. Although sequestered foci of infection may not be visible, surface lesions in deep pyoderma commonly heal before deeper lesions have resolved. Antibiotic selection can either be empiric or based on bacterial culture and susceptibility testing. An antibiotic chosen empirically should have a known spectrum of activity directed against *S. intermedius* and, ideally, should not be inactivated by β-lactamases, although most β-lactamase–resistant antibiotics are more expensive. Antibiotic therapy should be maintained for at least 1 week beyond clinical cure for superficial pyoderma and a minimum of 2 weeks beyond clinical cure for all deep pyoderma.

An ideal empiric antibiotic should have a narrow spectrum of activity, minimal side effects, and reasonable cost. It should have been shown to be an effective agent in the management of canine pyoderma. Little clinical evidence exists that bactericidal agents are more effective than bacteriostatic agents in the management of uncomplicated superficial pyoderma. Bactericidal antibiotics are recommended in most deep pyoderma cases and when immunosuppression is confirmed or suspected. Pustules or fistulous tracts should be recultured if *S. intermedius* has not been isolated as the primary pathogen. If multiple isolates are not sensitive to a single oral antibiotic, an antibiotic that is effective against *S. intermedius* should be instituted because staphylococci create a tissue milieu favorable to the replication of secondary bacteria invaders. Results of culture and susceptibility studies and detailed information on individual antibiotics are discussed in greater detail in the Drug Formulary, Appendix 8.[25, 54]

Antibiotics effective in the management of pyoderma are listed in Table 85–3. Penicillin, ampicillin, amoxicillin, and tetracycline are poor choices for the treatment of canine pyoderma. Previous usage may alter antibiotic susceptibility. One study confirmed that more resistant *S. intermedius* and gram-negative isolates were seen more commonly in referral practices than in general practice, and resistant bacterial populations were identified most frequently in deep pyoderma.[46] Many clinical trials have shown various antibiotics to be effective in managing canine pyoderma. These data have been reviewed.[25] Erythromycin, tylosin, lincomycin, clindamycin, chloramphenicol, trimethoprim and ormetoprim-potentiated sulfonamides, oxacillin, cephalexin, cefadroxil, fluoroquinolones, clavulanate-potentiated amoxicillin, and rifampin have been successful in the treatment of various canine pyoderma cases.

Previously, it had been predicted that antibiotic-resistant *S. intermedius* would preclude the administration of many antibiotics common in dermatology. An examination of similarities and differences in antibiotic susceptibility patterns published over the past two decades indicates remarkably little change.[25] *S. intermedius* strains cultured from canine pyoderma apparently are no more resistant to commonly used antibiotics than they were 20 years ago. Many of the antibiotics just mentioned are still effective for the management of canine pyoderma. My preferred narrow-spectrum antibiotics include erythromycin, lincomycin, and oxacillin, and my preferred broad-spectrum antibiotics include cephalexin, cefadroxil, ormetroprim-potentiated sulfonamides, and enrofloxacin.

Owner compliance using different dosing schedule regimens is not well studied in veterinary medicine. Differences in efficacy may correlate with differences in compliance. Antibiotics that need to be given only once or twice daily probably have advantages over those that need to be given three times daily. Ormetoprim-potentiated sulfadimethoxine and enrofloxacin are the only two antibiotics useful in canine pyoderma that can be administered once daily. Cephalexin, cefadroxil, and lincomycin require twice-daily dosing. All other recommended antibiotics require dosing three times daily.

Various "tiered systems" for antibiotic usage have been popularized during the past 5 years or so.[14, 25, 30, 54] The following recommendations comprise the "tiered system" that I recommend. Erythromycin, lincomycin, and ormetoprim-potentiated sulfadimethoxine are recommended for the management of uncomplicated, first-occurrence superficial pyoderma. The advantages and disadvantages of these drugs are listed in Table 85–3. Clindamycin and trimethoprim sulfonamides are other possible candidates for uncomplicated, first-occurrence pyoderma. However, the expense of clindamycin and the potential side effects of trimethoprim sulfonamides are of concern.[29]

First-generation cephalosporins (cephalexin and cefadroxil), enrofloxacin, and oxacillin are recommended for pyoderma refractory to initial antibiotic therapy or recurrent pyoderma. Some veterinary dermatologists have had success with amoxicillin-clavulanate. Chronic, deep pyoderma requires antibiotics with better penetrating ability because sequestered foci of infection and scarring prevent antibiotic access to the site of infection. Cephalexin and enrofloxacin offer better penetrating ability. In the rare circumstances when efficacy is not achieved with these drugs alone, rifampin (in conjunction with cephalexin or oxacillin) may be considered.

Enrofloxacin and other fluoroquinolones have the advantages of once-daily dosing, good tissue penetration, activity against both *S. intermedius* and gram-negative secondary invaders, and less likely development of resistance. Once-daily dosing is recommended because the bactericidal effect is concentration rather than time dependent.[44] Uptake of the drug by macrophages leads to potent tissue-penetrating abilities.

Oxacillin is a β-lactamase–resistant, narrow-spectrum, synthetic penicillin. Advantages include consistent efficacy in pyoderma and few side effects. Price is the primary disadvantage, even as a generic. Oxacillin must be administered three times daily and should be administered at least 1 hour before feeding, because food interferes with absorption.

Topical Therapy

This approach is important in the management of pyoderma. Shampoos are the most commonly used delivery

Table 85–3. Oral Antibiotics Useful for Treating Canine Pyoderma[a]

DRUG NAME (DOSE)	ADVANTAGES	DISADVANTAGES	ASSESSMENT
Erythomycin (10–15 mg/kg TID)	Inexpensive, narrow spectrum	Cross-resistance with lincomycin, vomiting, diarrhea common, TID dosing	Good first empiric choice
Lincomycin (22 mg/kg BID)	Twice-daily dosing, narrow spectrum, low side effects	Cross-resistance with erythromycin, relatively expensive	Good first empiric choice, especially if need BID drug
Ormetoprim-sulfadimethoxine (27.5 mg/kg once daily)	Once-daily dosing, broad spectrum	Relatively expensive, side effects less than with TS?	Good first empiric choice, especially if need once daily drug
Cephalexin or cefadroxil (22 mg/kg BID)	Twice-daily dosing, broad spectrum, resistance is rare, good tissue penetration	Cefadroxil: expensive, generics moderately expensive	Excellent choice refractory-recurrent deep pyoderma, BID drug
Enrofloxacin (5 mg/kg once daily)	Once-daily dosing, broad spectrum, rapidly absorbed, good tissue penetration	Expensive, cannot use in growing dogs	Excellent choice for refractory-recurrent deep pyoderma, once daily drug
Oxacillin (22 mg/kg TID)	Narrow spectrum, resistance is rare, side effects rare	Expensive, TID dosing, food interferes with absorption	Good choice refractory-recurrent deep pyoderma
Amoxicillin-clavulanate (12.5–20 mg/kg BID or TID)	Broad spectrum, side effects rare	Expensive, moisture sensitive; in vivo effect not as good as would be predicted?	Efficacy low, somewhat expensive, for deep pyoderma
TS (22 mg/kg BID)	Inexpensive, BID dosing, broad spectrum	Side effects; keratoconjunctivitis sicca, severe cutaneous drug reactions, hepatic necrosis	Good empiric choice, concern for drug reactions

[a]For additional information on listed drugs, see Drug Formulary, Appendix 8.
TS = trimethoprim-sulfonamide.
Reprinted by permission: Ihrke PJ: Bacterial Skin Disease in the Dog: A Guide to Canine Pyoderma. Veterinary Learning Systems, Princeton, NJ, 1996.

system. Antibacterial shampoos may be effective without concurrent antibiotics in some surface pyodermas and are frequently used as adjunctive therapy in the management of superficial and deep pyodermas. Antibacterial shampoos aid in debridement, encourage drainage, and decrease pain and pruritus. Their desired mechanisms of action are to decrease surface bacterial counts and to limit recolonizing organisms, thereby diminishing the likelihood of recurrent infections. Improvement in patient attitude and owner encouragement are additional benefits.

Available antibacterial shampoos contain benzoyl peroxide, benzoyl peroxide and sulfur, chlorhexidine, ethyl lactate, or triclosan. Twice-weekly antibacterial shampoos are the most common topical therapy. Benzoyl peroxide shampoos may decrease recrudescence in susceptible dogs.

Dogs with deep pyoderma require more aggressive topical therapy. After clipping, dogs benefit from daily antibacterial shampoos or twice-daily whirlpools or soaks. Chlorhexidine or povidone-iodine are added to warm water in whirlpools or soaks. Whirlpools remain a seldomly employed but very beneficial modality of topical therapy for deep pyoderma.

Antibacterial gels, creams, and ointments may be applied in the treatment of limited areas of skin. Cost, messiness, and time required for application limit their usefulness. Benzoyl peroxide is available in a gel vehicle. Mupirocin is a potent antibacterial agent with superior penetrating ability. Mupirocin is formulated for skin surfaces but not mucosal surfaces. It should not be used when absorption of large amounts of the polyethylene glycol vehicle is likely because of the potential for nephrotoxicity.[25]

Immunomodulatory Therapy

This form of treatment for canine pyoderma remains controversial owing to widely varying perceptions of efficacy. If immunomodulation is used, it should be an adjunct to antibiotic and topical therapy with the goal of diminishing the frequency or severity of infection. Immunomodulatory therapy is most efficacious in dogs with idiopathic recurrent superficial pyoderma that respond completely to appropriate therapy, but recurrence follows within weeks after therapy has been discontinued. Most comments in the literature referable to immunomodulatory therapy have been either highly subjective or anecdotal, because it is often given in conjunction with systemic and topical antibacterials. Controlled trials are difficult to perform because immunomodulatory therapy rarely is the sole therapy.

Immunomodulators can be either bacterial or nonbacterial preparations. Commercial products contain either killed *Staphylococcus* or *Propionibacterium (Corynebacterium)* as the antigen. Nonbacterial immunomodulatory drugs include levamisole and cimetidine. (See also Immunostimulants, Chapter 100.)

Staphage Lysate (Delmont Laboratories, Swarthmore, PA) is the most common commercial bacterin in the United States and contains bacterial antigens of *S. aureus* isolated from humans. Staphage Lysate is the only product for which efficacy has been documented (approximately 40% of cases using 0.5 ml twice weekly[15]) by double-blinded, placebo-controlled studies. Autogenous bacterins occasionally are made from the specific staphylococcal organisms isolated from a dog with pyoderma for use in that dog. Inactivation methodology is crucial because the process must kill the organism without disrupting antigenic determinants.

Nonbacterial immunomodulatory therapy is controversial because most reports are anecdotal. Levamisole, a levo-isomer of tetramisole sold as a vermifuge for large animals, may alter lymphocyte and phagocyte immune function. The recommended dosage of the sheep boluses is 2.2 mg/kg given every other day orally. Cimetidine, an H_2-histamine receptor blocker developed for treating gastric ulcers, theoretically could reduce immunosuppression by down-regulating suppressor T lymphocytes, thereby modulating cytokine production. The suggested dosage is 3 to 4 mg/kg orally given twice daily for at least 10 weeks. Controlled studies of efficacy have not been performed with either product.[25]

Factors Complicating Management

Treatment failure and disease recurrence commonly are associated with lack of recognition of factors that can complicate management and influence prognosis. The most common complicating factors include inappropriate initial therapy, unidentified coexisting problems, sequestered foci of infection in deep pyoderma, and external environmental factors such as poor compliance that may not be known to the veterinarian.

Most antibiotic dosages for treatment of pyoderma are largely empiric, because little research has been done in this area. In deep pyoderma, sequestered foci of infection impede antibiotic penetration, and keratin debris from ruptured hair follicles encourages foreign body granulomatous response. Antibiotics that require microbial replication for activity, such as penicillins, are less effective when necrotic tissue and obstructed drainage routes create conditions that are no longer favorable for bacterial multiplication. Consequently, higher dosages are warranted in the management of chronic deep pyoderma.

Concomitant problems such as demodicosis, keratinization defects, hypothyroidism, and steroid abuse may hinder successful management. Pruritus, associated with either a pyoderma or an underlying pruritic disease, is an additional complicating factor.

Assessment of Therapy

All dogs receiving systemic antibiotics for pyoderma should be re-evaluated within 7 to 14 days. If substantial improvement is not noted, the clinician should consider other factors that can complicate management. The clinician should consider owner compliance to the appropriate dosage and drug loss through vomiting, inactivation by food, or malabsorption. The possibility of referral to a veterinary dermatologist should be considered each time that clinical failure occurs.

Recurrent Pyoderma

The small percentage of cases characterized by frequent recurrences is one of the most frustrating aspects of veterinary dermatology. Recurrent pyoderma can be defined as bacterial skin infections that respond completely to appropriate therapy, leaving the dog free of the clinical signs of pyoderma between episodes of infection. Recurrent superficial pyoderma is the most common subgroup. Underlying skin disease or internal medical abnormalities are the most common causes of recurrent canine pyoderma.[14, 25, 30, 54] Causes of recurrent pyoderma have been subdivided into persistent underlying skin disease, bacterial hypersensitivity, immunodeficiency, resistant strains of *S. intermedius*, and nonstaphylococcal pyoderma.[14] Recurrent pyoderma is termed *idiopathic* only if all appropriate diagnostic procedures have failed to reveal a predisposing cause.

Recurrent pyoderma secondary to continuing underlying skin disease may alter the clinical appearance of the predisposing condition, making its identification difficult. Diagnosis of the underlying disease may be facilitated by an appropriate course of antibiotics.

Pruritus can be an important discriminating feature in evaluating recurrent pyoderma. If pruritus is totally ameliorated by antibiotic therapy, the pruritus probably was caused by the bacterial infection. If pruritus is still present after clinical cure, the pruritus is most likely due to an as yet undiagnosed underlying disease.

Recurrent pyoderma commonly is a lifetime disease requiring extensive client communication and counseling. An informed client is more likely to undertake the necessary commitment. Curing underlying diseases may completely prevent recurrent pyoderma. Hypothyroidism is an example of an underlying disease in which pyoderma may be completely eliminated. In contrast, therapy for underlying flea allergy dermatitis seldom completely eliminates secondary pyoderma and requires constant flea control. Many skin diseases that act as triggers for recurrent pyoderma can be controlled but not cured, requiring continuous management. Atopic dermatitis and defects in cornification are examples of skin diseases that rarely respond completely to appropriate aggressive therapy.[25]

Choices in the management of recurrent pyoderma in which successful management of an underlying disease is not possible, or the pyoderma is idiopathic, include long-term topical antibacterial shampoos, immunomodulatory therapy, and extended regimens of systemic antibiotics. Antibacterial shampoo therapy performed once or twice weekly should be attempted initially. If this therapy prevents recurrence, it can be maintained indefinitely. Adjunctive immunomodulatory therapy should be considered as the next option if shampoo therapy alone is unsuccessful.

Extended regimens of antibiotics using subtherapeutic doses to prevent recurrence are viewed as a last resort in the long-term management of recurrent canine pyoderma and should be used only after the current episode of the pyoderma has been brought under complete control. Antibiotics most useful for extended regimens include cephalexin, enrofloxacin, oxacillin, and clavulanate-potentiated amoxicillin.

Risks inherent in the extended administration of systemic antibiotics at subtherapeutic doses include undesirable effects in the patient, induction of antibiotic resistance, and formation and possible dissemination of resistant strains of bacteria in the environment. Relatively high cost is an additional drawback. I prefer every-other-week dosing at therapeutic levels followed by extending the duration of time off antibiotics in gradual increments (2 weeks, 3 weeks). Two days per week dosing at full daily dosage is an additional option. Therapy must be monitored carefully long term to avoid inherent risks.

Malassezia Dermatitis

Craig E. Greene

ETIOLOGY

Malassezia spp. (previously *Pityrosporum*) are saprophytic monopolar yeasts that colonize the skin and mucocutaneous regions of clinically healthy mammals. The genus is divided into two groups based on their lipid dependency in growth media. The lipid-independent form, the species *M. pachydermatis*, contains several genotypes (sequevars).[17c] These have been isolated predominantly from animals, especially domestic carnivores. The lipid-dependent species, which include *M. furfur, M. sympodialis, M. globosa, M. obtusa, M. restricta*, and *M. slooffiae*, have been the predominant isolates from people.[17b] *M. sympodialis* and *M. globosa* have also been isolated from the skin of clinically healthy cats.[5c] Even in dogs, in which *M. pachydermatis* is the main isolate, a single genotype predominates in a given animal. However, multiple genotypes may be found in different skin locations in the same dog and, in some instances, in the same site.[17c] Sequevar type Ia was the most prevalent isolate from various animals and the main one from people. Although *M. pachydermatis* can be readily cultured (or found on histologic examination of skin) from clinically healthy dogs and cats, cytologic detection is more difficult. In clinically healthy skin, the highest numbers on dogs are found on the chin and labial areas, the perianal area, and the dorsal interdigital spaces. Lesser numbers are found in other intertriginal areas, such as the inguinal and axillary regions.[5f, 27a] The organism is a frequent colonizer of the external ear canal. For a discussion of *M. pachydermatis* in otitis externa, see later.

A change in host immunity, altered skin microclimate, or disruption in the epithelial barrier may predispose animals to develop clinical diseases. Chronic inflammatory skin disease is associated with sebaceous gland hyperplasia and increased epithelial cell proliferation. This seborrheic reaction allows the lipophilic yeast to proliferate. The yeast metabolizes surface lipids, resulting in odoriferous byproducts. Atopic dermatitis, endocrinopathy, and pre-existing bacterial pyoderma may be contributing factors to the development of this yeast dermatitis.[5b] Recent antimicrobial therapy, seborrhea, and certain breeds are frequently associated findings.[48] The breeds so involved are basset hound, cocker spaniel, dachshund, West Highland white terrier, silky terrier, Australian terrier, Maltese terrier, Jack Russell terrier, chihuahua, toy and miniature poodles, Shetland sheepdog, collie, German shepherd, golden retriever, and springer spaniel.[5b, 9a]

Despite the apparent proliferation of organisms on the skin of some dogs, clinical signs may be absent. In other animals with severe generalized disease, yeast numbers may be comparatively low. In clinically affected animals, inflammatory reactions are characteristic and have been attributed to byproducts produced by the proliferating fungus. The reason that certain dogs are affected has been attributed to hypersensitivity to extracellular proteins produced by the yeasts.[45a, 45b]

CLINICAL FINDINGS

Primary skin lesions are not typical, although pruritus is a consistent manifestation. Various seborrheic syndromes have been described. The disease is more prevalent in the warmer months with increased humidity. Alopecia, excoriation with erythema, seborrhea, lichenification, and hyperpigmentation are noted.[27a] The appearance of the skin in affected areas has been likened to that of an armadillo or elephant. A noticeable sour odor may also be noted emanating from affected animals. Although some animals develop generalized disease, regional is more common. The most common area is interdigital, causing pododermatitis between the foot pads. Other affected areas are the neck, perianal region, face and lips, axillae, and leg folds. The areas involved in atopic dogs are commonly those that are licked or rubbed, such as the face or feet. In some animals with paronychia, a dark brown discharge may emanate from swollen nail beds. In cats, the disease is less frequent and is usually manifest as alopecia. However, chin acne, or multifocal to generalized erythema and seborrhea, has been described. Typically, there is a poor response to glucocorticoid therapy.

DIAGNOSIS

Cytologic examination is the most common and rapid means of determining infection. Impression smears can be made directly onto glass slides, or by rubbing dry cotton swabs or scalpel blades over surface debris to collect material to be stained. For fixation, slides can be heated or immersed in alcohol as part of the staining process. Wright's or Gram's stains can be used.

In quantitative culture, highest yields can be obtained by use of clear cellophane tape as compared with direct impression, swabbing, detergent scrubs, or skin scrapings.[5a, 5d, 5e, 27a] For culture, the tape is pressed onto the affected skin and then briefly onto the culture medium. For microscopy, the tape used to make the impression is stained directly and then mounted on a clear glass slide for observation. Generally, culture isolation should not exceed 2 colonies/0.5 square inch on a tape/culture preparation or 2 yeasts per field at 1000× of a smear or tape cytologic preparation. The disease is suspected if the organisms exceed this concentration and if clinical signs of compatible lesions are present.

Malassezia can be isolated using modified Dixon's agar, Leeming's medium, or Sabouraud's agar, with optimal growth on the Sabouraud's medium between 32°C and 37°C in a CO_2-enriched environment. These media have the advantage of growing lipid-dependent strains that are occasionally isolated.[5d]

THEARPY

Identifying the underlying factors and correcting them, if possible, offer the most permanent success with treatment. Relapses will occur when topical and systemic therapy are discontinued if the underlying problem has not been remedied. In one cat with generalized *M. pachydermatis* dermatitis, the skin condition resolved once a thymoma was surgically removed.[15a]

The next step in therapy involves reduction in the quantity of surface lipids in the skin. Shampoos containing benzoyl peroxide with sulfur are safest and most effective for this purpose. Selenium sulfide preparations, as used by affected people, are usually too irritating for animals.

Topical medications, in the forms of cremes, shampoos, or rinses, may be used concurrently. They are not very effective alone unless the lesions are very localized.[9a] Shampoos containing azole derivatives, such as ketoconazole (KTZ) 2% or miconazole 2%, cover large areas but become too diluted during application to be effective.

Griseofulvin, the medication used to treat dermatophyte infections, is not effective in *Malassezia* infections. The most effective is systemic antifungal therapy with KTZ at 10 mg/kg, PO, twice daily for 3 to 4 weeks. Itraconazole can be given at 5 to 10 mg/kg, PO, once daily for 2 to 4 weeks. Some animals respond to lower doses. Ingestion of food or lipid improves the absorption of these drugs and can help reduce the amounts needed. For additional information on these drugs, see Drug Formulary, Appendix 8.

A favorable response to treatment usually occurs within 1 to 2 weeks. Pruritus, odor, and erythema usually subside. Treatment may extend up to 4 to 6 weeks in the most severely affected animals. Lower or intermittent maintenance therapy may be tried in animals that experience relapse.

Otitis Externa

Craig E. Greene

ETIOLOGY

Otitis externa is inflammation of the external ear canal. The following discussion focuses on microbial factors. Reviews should be consulted concerning other causes of this condition. For a discussion of otitis media-interna, see Musculoskeletal Infections, Chapter 86. Numerous causative agents have been associated with otitis externa (Table 85–4), and failure to identify and eliminate the underlying cause will result in ineffective treatment. Most microbial infections of the external ear canal are secondary to another disease or factor, making it susceptible to colonization by normal or opportunistic microflora. Bacteria, yeasts, parasites, and viruses have all been incriminated as causing otitis externa. In many cases, an underlying disease can be found, and the role of the infectious organism as the primary cause of otitis externa cannot be substantiated.

The normal ear canal is colonized by a variety of microorganisms that can proliferate with damage or inflammation from the primary factors (Table 85–5). Microfloral overgrowth can exacerbate or perpetuate inflammatory reactions. Coagulase-positive *S. intermedius* is the most common isolate in normal ears and in acute otitis externa, in which it is even more prevalent. β-Hemolytic streptococci are found with equal frequency in normal and diseased ears, so that their pathogenic status is uncertain. Other common organisms rarely found in clinically healthy ears, but rather isolated predominantly in cases of chronic otitis externa, are *Pseudomonas* sp. and *Proteus mirabilis*. Mixed infections usually are composed of *S. intermedius* in conjunction with a gram-negative rod. In cats, *Pasteurella multocida* may also be isolated.

Bacteria or the broad-based budding yeast *M. pachydermatis* may proliferate in an ear canal of an animal predisposed to infection because of other underlying diseases or prolonged antibacterial therapy. *M. canis* is considered to be a secondary invader contributing to or perpetuating and exacerbating inflammation in an already diseased ear canal. In cats, the relative importance of *M. pachydermatis* in disease is less certain because it is found with equal frequency in clinically healthy cats and in those with otitis externa.

The ear mite *Otodectes cyanotis* is believed to be responsible for a majority of feline cases of otitis externa; dogs have a much lower prevalence of infection. Most animals develop a hypersensitivity reaction to the mite that causes the inflammation seen clinically; however, some are nonsymptomatic carriers. In others, the inflammation may lead to a secondary bacterial or yeast infection that can eventually result in the destruction of the mites.

Table 85–4. Predisposing Factors for Otitis Externa

HOST	
Anatomic	
Breed	German shepherd
Conformation	Long droopy ears (cocker, bassett), stenotic canals (English bulldog, Shar pei, chow chow), hair in canals (poodle, schnauzer, bichon, Airedale, wirehaired and fox terriers)
Otitis media-interna	Causing self-inflicted trauma or act as nidus
Masses	Polyps, squamous cell carcinoma, ceruminous gland tumors, papilloma, sebaceous adenoma, ceruminous adenoma, fibroma squamous cell carcinoma, basal cell carcinoma, fibrosarcoma
Hyperkeratosis	Seborrheic diseases (German and Belgian shepherds), sebaceous gland infection (standard poodles, Akitas, Samoyeds), inflammatory polyp (cats)
Immunologic	
Hypersensitivities	Atopic dermatitis, juvenile cellulitis (puppy strangles, golden and Labrador retrievers, dachshund, pointer, Lhasa apso), contact allergies (propylene glycol), food allergy, drug eruption
Immunodeficiency	Debilitation
Autoimmune	Systemic lupus erythematosus, pemphigus foliaceus
Endocrinopathic	Male-feminizing syndrome, hypothyroidism, Sertoli cell tumor, ovarian imbalance
ENVIRONMENT	
Moisture	Swimming (Labrador retrievers), high environmental temperature and humidity
Foreign material	Plant material, excessive otic medicants, soil, exudates, dried wax
Medicants	Yeast infections with chronic antibiotic and glucocorticoid therapy
Astringents	Alcohol, cleansing agents
Trauma	Iatrogenic or self-induced, lacerations of aural mucosa, excessive cleaning or medicants, cotton swabs
AGENT	
Parasites	*Otodectes cynotis* (ear mite), biting flies, chiggers, ticks, *Demodex canis, Sarcoptes, Notoedres,* flea allergy
Bacteria	*S. intermedius,* β-hemolytic streptococci, *Proteus, Pseudomonas*
Fungi	Malassezia canis, Microsporum canis, Candida

CLINICAL FINDINGS

A complete history, especially with regard to the animal's environment and exposure to vegetation and water, is helpful. Pruritus, a major problem with otitis externa, is manifest by head shaking, scratching, or rubbing the ears along the floor or other objects. On physical examination, pinnal or caudal auricular alopecia, matted hair, broken hairs, excoriations, and occasional areas of acute moist dermatitis will be apparent. The external auditory meatus may be erythematous and swollen. In many uncomplicated cases of otitis externa, the clinical findings will be limited to erythema and possibly slight increase in ear wax (ceruminous otitis). When otitis externa is complicated by secondary bacterial or yeast infections, the character and amount of discharge may become more purulent and moist and may have a foul odor (suppurative otitis). Inflammation may be severe, the ear canals may become painful, and self-inflicted trauma may be apparent. Some animals become head shy; others will show evidence of pain only when the canal is palpated. Chronic otitis is characterized by epidermal hyperplasia with thickening of the pinna and narrowing and/or calcification of the ear canal. A thorough examination of the ear, using an otoscope, is needed to determine the presence of secondary changes and the extent of the inflammation and discharge as

Table 85–5. Organisms Isolated From External Ear Canal of Dogs and Cats

ORGANISM	HOST	FREQUENCY OF ISOLATION (%) Clinically Healthy	Otitis Externa	PHYSICAL DESCRIPTION
Gram-Positive Bacteria				
Staphylococci (coagulase positive) includes *S. intermedius*	Dog	9–20	22–40	Light brown or pale yellow exudates
Streptococci (β-hemolytic)	Dog	16	10	Light yellow to light brown exudates
Gram-Negative Bacteria				
Pseudomonas	Dog	0.4	20	Painful, copious light yellow to green exudates, often ulcerated epithelium
Proteus	Dog	0	11	Light yellow exudates ulcerated with chronicity
Escherichia coli	Dog	0	14	Light yellow exudates
Fungi				
Malassezia	Dog	15–49	50–83	Light brown to dark (chocolate) brown exudates
	Cat	23	19	
Metazoans				
Otodectes cyanotis	Dog	0	5–10	Dark brown exudates
	Cat	0	50	

well as the condition of the tympanic membrane. If the canal is very swollen and stenotic, treatment should proceed with a broad-spectrum topical preparation for up to 1 week before performing the otoscopic examination.

DIAGNOSIS

After a complete history and physical otoscopic examination, smears of the ear canal contents should be made. To prevent cross-contamination, a separate, clean otoscope cone must be used for each ear. The canal should be examined for its diameter, amount and type of exudate, foreign bodies, neoplasms, parasites, condition of the tympanic membrane, and integrity of the epithelium. Swabs should be inserted into the horizontal canal of each ear through an otoscope cone to recover material for microscopic examination. One swab should be placed in a drop of mineral oil on a slide and be examined for ear or *Demodex* mites. The swabs are rolled onto microscope slides, and a fast stain based on Giemsa's or Wright's methods is often utilized. Before staining, the slide should be heat fixed by passing it over an open flame two or three times. Heat fixing melts some wax and debris, which causes them to adhere better to the glass slide. Without heat fixing, much of the wax, lipid, and associated yeasts may wash away in the staining process. More than 10 yeasts per high-power field are suggestive of their overgrowth.

Cytologic examination of exudate is needed to evaluate the type of inflammatory response and potential underlying cause. Numbers and morphology of leukocytes, neoplastic cells, and bacteria or fungi should be recorded. Because commensals will be cultured from normal ears, cytologic enumeration of bacteria provides a means of determining their overgrowth and a hint as to their type before culture results become available. When secondary bacterial infections are contributing to the disease, leukocytes and phagocytized bacteria are usually present. When primarily wax and keratin are present, the bacteria observed are most likely incidental but can still contribute to the odor and inflammation by their lipolytic action on waxy debris.

Occasionally, *O. cynotis* or *Demodex* can be identified in examination of a smear. Failure to find mites, especially if secondary infection is present, does not rule out their existence.

Bacterial culture and susceptibility testing offer little additional information compared with good basic cytologic evaluation and are costly. Antimicrobial susceptibility can usually be determined on the basis of organism morphology (Table 85–6). Furthermore, the levels achieved by topical application are much higher than the serum levels of sensitivity disks. Bacterial isolation is of more benefit if the tympanic membrane is ruptured with otitis media or interna and the clinician is contemplating systemic antibiotic therapy. Culture and susceptibility testing also are indicated in chronic otitis externa when primarily bacterial rods are found on a smear or when microorganisms persist in spite of apparent appropriate topical medication. *Malassezia* is better identified by cytology than by culture (see Fig. 56–4). Repeating cytologic examination on subsequent visits will help to evaluate drug resistance or owner compliance. Persistent inflammation in the absence of abundant microorganisms suggests an allergic or ceruminous otitis. Radiographs of bulla should be done with chronic or recurrent otitis when there are associated neurologic signs or when the tympanic membrane is perforated or covered by debris.

THERAPY

Effective treatment and management of otitis externa are best achieved by combining several principles. If possible, predisposing causes should be identified and eliminated. Predisposing factors should be eliminated or prophylactically treated. Topical therapy is especially beneficial because drugs attain their highest concentrations with the fewest systemic effects. To obtain owner compliance, the treatment should be specific and simple. Systemic antibacterial or antifungal therapy may be needed if the external canal is occluded or if otitis media is present. Systemic therapy can be selected on the basis of culture and susceptibility results. For empiric systemic bacterial therapy, drugs used to treat staphylococcal pyoderma such as erythromycin, first-generation cephalosporins, lincomycin, clindamycin, amoxicillin-clavulanate, ormetoprim or trimethoprim-sulfonamides, or fluoroquinolones are most effective. Treatment usually lasts a minimum of 3 to 4 weeks (see Table 85–6).

Cleaning

Depending on the animal's temperament, sedation or anesthesia may be needed for cleaning the ears, which should be dried before initiating therapy. Initial cleaning and drying of the ear canals are essential to complete the otoscopic examination, determine the integrity of the tympanic membrane, and facilitate the penetration of topically administered drugs. Thorough cleansing of the ear canals will remove small secondary foreign bodies as well as degenerated inflammatory cells, free fatty acids, bacterial toxins, wax, and debris. Ear cleaning with physical flushing of the canal may be repeated as needed, but it should not be performed more than two times weekly because it produces mucosal ulceration. Ear-cleaning solutions may be applied more frequently by an owner instilling a few drops just before an otic antimicrobial drug is given. The animal should be allowed to shake its head to disperse the solution, and the excess is removed before instilling the desired medication. Cleaning and flushing solutions are generally disinfectants and are listed in Table 85–7. They are used for initial removal of debris or as ceruminolytics. Ceruminolytics are selected when excessive waxy accumulation is present. In most cases, ceruminolytic agents, such as carbamide peroxide and dioctyl sodium sulfosuccinate, are most effective in emulsifying and facilitating the cleaning procedures and are water soluble. Carbamide peroxide has a foaming action that breaks down debris. Ceruminolytic oils such as squalene, lanolin, and mineral oil are more difficult to clean up. Many combination ceruminolytic and drying products contain organic acids with a ceruminolytic agent or alcohol added. They are easier to clean up and can be used as a one-step procedure. These products must be applied with great caution if the tympanum is ruptured. In a study of several ceruminolytic agents, only a solution containing squalene and isopropyl myristate with liquid petrolatum base (Cerumene, Evsco Pharm., Buena, NJ) was nonirritating to the middle ear in the presence of a ruptured tympanum.[36a] If ceruminolytics are used before the discovery of a ruptured membrane, thorough rinsing with pure water or saline is preferred. Other rinse solutions should not contain detergents or disinfectants because they are ototoxic and are contraindicated with a ruptured tympanic membrane.

Rubber bulb ear syringes are a very efficient way to flush the ear. After the initial flushing, loops can be utilized to remove any remaining material. Cotton swabs should be avoided because they pack exudate and debris down in the ear and may injure the tympanum or epithelial lining. In other cases, especially those with a ruptured tympanum, a feeding tube attached to a 12-ml syringe may be employed for the final flushing as well as cleaning out the bulla. In addition, by applying negative pressure, this is a rapid, atraumatic way of removing residual water. Head tilt and/or ataxia may develop after cleaning as a result of otitis media or interna.

Topical Medicants

Once the ears are clean and dried, topical therapy can be effective in the treatment plan. In general, most ear products contain various combinations of glucocorticoids and antibacterial, antiyeast, and parasiticidal agents in aqueous solution or oil vehicles (Table 85–8). The most appropriate topical drug can be prescribed on the basis of clinical findings, cytology, and diagnosis. Oil vehicles are best applied when the ears are dry, because they will tend to moisturize the skin. In moist exudative ears, water-soluble vehicles are preferred because they are less occlusive. Water-soluble aqueous preparations are most desirable when the tympanic membrane is ruptured. Besides selecting the most appropriate vehicle, the clinician must decide what active ingredients are most appropriate for each case. There is no single perfect topical ear product.

Topical glucocorticoids are most effective when there is early acute inflammation, and high-potency fluocinolone, betamethasone, and dexamethasone are recommended. Al-

Table 85–6. Antimicrobial Selection for Otitis Externa

ACUTE OTITIS	
Cytologic exam: gram-positive cocci, culture; staphylococci, streptococci	
Topical:	Neomycin (Panolog, Forte, Tresaderm, Neopredef), chloramphenicol (Liquichlor) Povidone-iodine (Betadine) dilute 1:50 (intact tympanum); dilute 1:100 (perforated tympanum) Chlorhexidine (Nolvasan) dilute 1:40 in water Acetic acid (white vinegar 5%) dilute 1:3 in water; concentrations of 2–5% are irritating
Cytologic exam: gram-negative bacilli; culture; *Proteus, Escherichia coli*	
Topical:	Neomycin (Panolog), polymyxins (Forte), gentamicin (Gentocin otic) Acetic acid (white vinegar 5%) dilute 1:3 in water Povidone-iodine (Betadine); see above for dilution
Cytologic Exam: yeasts	
Topical:	Nystatin (Panolog), thiabendazole (Tresaderm), miconazole (Surolam, Conofite), clotrimazole (Otomax, Lotrimin)
CHRONIC OR RESISTANT OTITIS	
Yeasts	
Topical:	Clotrimazole (Otomax), miconazole (Surolam, Conofite), clotrimazole (Lotrimin), Silvadene
Systemic:	Ketoconazole 5 mg/kg BID for 2–4 wks, itraconazole 5–10 mg/kg once daily for 2–4 wks
Gram negatives, usually *Pseudomonas*	
Topical:	Gentamicin (Gentocin otic, otomax), polymyxin B, colistin or polymyxin E (Coly-Mycin), polymyxin B (Cortisporin) Polyhydroxidine iodine (Xenodyne, Solvay) dilute 1:3 to 1:5 in water and apply BID
Systemic:	Ormetoprim-sulfadimethoxine, trimethoprim-sulfonamide, first-generation cephalosporin
Culture Pseudomonas	
Topical:	Ticarcillin (Ticar suspension) add 4 g to 4-oz bottle of Oti-clens Tobramycin (Tobrex ophthalmic) Enrofloxacin (Baytril injectable) dilute 50% in water, 3–5 drops BID Amikacin sulfate (Amiglyde-V injectable) undiluted (50 mg/ml) 5–6 drops BID Silver sulfadiazine (Silvadene) dilute 1:1 in water, 4–12 drops BID Tris-EDTA-gentamicin solution (Wooley's solution); see Chapter 34, Table 34–12.
Systemic:	Enrofloxacin, marbofloxacin, orbofloxacin, gentamicin

EDTA = edetic acid.

Table 85–7. Solutions for Management of Otitis Externa

CLASS: INDICATIONS	INGREDIENTS	PRODUCTS
Flushing Solutions		
Primary cleaning of canal with weak antibacterial activity	Cleaning and disinfecting solutions	Betadine, povidone-iodine 10% (dilute 1:10 to 1:50); Xenodyne, polyhydroxidine iodine 0.5% (dilute 1:1 to 1:15); Nolvasan chlorhexidine 2% (dilute 1:40); vinegar, acetic acid 5% (dilute 1:3)
Ceruminolytics		
Permeate and solubilize waxy debris	Squalenes, surfactants, carbamide peroxide, chlorhexidine, DSS, propylene glycol	Cerumene, Clear X, Veterinary Surfactant, Sebo-o-sol, Otic Chlor-7, Otic Clear, Nolvasan Otic, Adams Pan Otic
Ceruminolytic and Drying Agent		
Combinations dissolve wax and dry out canal	As for ceruminolytics but includes acids such as lactic, salicylic, malic, benzoic and acetic, and alcohols	Cerbin-otic, Oti-clens, Epi-otic, Chlorhexiderm Otic, Adams Ear Dessicant, Fresh Ear, VPL Otic Cleanser, Chlor-otic-L, Otic-clear
Drying Agents		
Mild antibacterial activity and dry ear canal acts as astringent on exuding lesions	Organic acids, alcohols, silicone dioxide, as listed for above combinations	Dermal Dry, Otic Domeboro, Panodry, Otic Calm, acetic acid 5% and isopropyl alcohol in a 3:1 ratio

DSS = dioctyl sodium sulfosuccinate.

though they are generally contraindicated in infectious processes, they do reduce the inflammation in the ear canal, which controls pruritus, swelling, exudation, wax build-up, and tissue proliferation and hyperplasia. It is difficult to find a commercial otic medication that is not formulated with glucocorticoids. Because they may predispose the patient to secondary yeast infections and hyperadrenocorticism, the lowest required potency (e.g., hydrocortisone) and frequency are recommended for long-term (>3 mo) treatment. Otic preparations with dexamethasone and triamcinolone have systemic effects and result in signs of hyperadrenalism with iatrogenic pituitary-adrenal suppression. With severely painful or inflamed ears or stenotic canals, systemic prednisone is recommended at a dose of 0.25 to 0.5 mg/kg twice daily for 1 to 2 weeks in dogs, and twice that dose for cats.

Bacterial infections should be treated with topical antibiotics or disinfectants. In general, the aminoglycosides (neomycin, polymyxin, gentamicin) and chloramphenicol are frequently effective. Although the aminoglycosides are potentially ototoxic, especially when topically applied to an ear with a ruptured eardrum, this has not been shown to be a problem (see Aminoglycoside Toxicity, Chapter 34). Optimally, drugs that may later be needed for systemic therapy should not be used topically in acute cases because resistance may develop. Disinfectants are an effective alternative to antibiotics. Iodine and chlorhexidine are good choices against bacteria and yeasts, respectively, but are ototoxic when put into the middle ear. Acetic acid at 2% is effective against *Pseudomonas* species and at 5% is cidal against most bacterial pathogens involved in otitis externa. For *Pseudomonas* infections, otic or ophthalmic medicants containing gentamicin, tobramycin, or polymyxins can be applied, and as a last resort, parenteral enrofloxacin or amikacin solutions can be diluted and instilled twice daily. TRIS–edetic acid (EDTA) preparations are also effective against *Pseudomonas* (see Topical Buffered EDTA Solution, Chapter 34, and Table 34–12).

Secondary yeast infection may occur when systemic or topical antibacterial therapy is prolonged. Cytologic examination should be performed at repeat visits to check for this complication.

When *Malassezia* is present, the topically applied antiyeast agents such as nystatin and thiabendazole contained in many ear medicants are frequently effective. Thiabendazole can be a contact irritant in some dogs. In more difficult cases, 1% miconazole or clotrimazole lotions will usually work. A mixture of 2% boric acid and 2% acetic acid instilled in the ear once daily for 7 weeks was reported to be effective in treating *Malassezia* otitis.[15b] If a *Malassezia* otitis media is diagnosed,

Table 85–8. Broad-Spectrum Veterinary Otic Antimicrobial Preparations

PRODUCT (MANUFACTURER)	FORMULATION/VEHICLE	ANTIBACTERIAL	ANTI-INFLAMMATORY	ANTIYEAST	INDICATIONS
Derma 4 (Pfizer)	Polyethylene	Thiostrepton			
Forte Topical (Upjohn)	Suspension; mineral oil	Penicillin, neomycin, polymyxin	Hydrocortisone	—	Bacteria
Gentocin Otic (Schering)	Solution; propylene glycol, alcohol, glycerine (aqueous)	Gentamicin	Betamethasone	—	Bacteria
Liquichlor (Evsco)	Ointment; mineral oil, squalene, tetracaine	Chloramphenicol	Prednisolone	—	Bacteria
Neo-Predef (Upjohn)	Ointment; lanolin, petrolatum, mineral oil	Neomycin	Isoflupredone	—	Bacteria
Oterna (Coopers)	Ointment; mineral oil	Neomycin	Betamethasone	Monosulfiram	Bacteria, yeasts
Otomax (Schering)	Ointment; mineral oil	Gentamicin	Betamethasone	Clotrimazole	Bacteria, yeasts
Panolog (Solvay)	Ointment; mineral oil	Neomycin	Triamcinolone	Nystatin	Bacteria, yeasts
Surolan (Janssen)	Ointment; petrolatum, mineral oil	Polymyxin B	Prednisolone	Miconazole	Bacteria, yeasts
Tresaderm (MSD-Agvet)	Solution; glycerine, alcohol, propylene glycol (aqueous)	Neomycin	Dexamethasone	Thiabendazole	Bacteria, yeast, mites

then the systemic antifungal ketoconazole given 5 mg/kg every 12 hours, or itraconazole given 5 mg/kg every 24 hours, for 4 to 6 weeks is the preferred treatment (see Chapter 57).

O. cynotis is relatively sensitive to most insecticides, including pyrethrins, rotenone, and thiabendazole. In addition to treating the ears, the whole body and other in-contact animals should be treated. Ivermectin at 250 μg/kg, given PO once weekly for 3 to 4 weeks or SC once every 10 days for two treatments, is effective against *Otodectes*. It also has the advantage of eliminating mites from other areas. However, ivermectin is not approved for use in cats or dogs at this dosage. It is absolutely contraindicated in collies.

Prognosis

The prognosis is generally good in acute (<4 weeks duration) cases of otitis externa when the tympanic membrane is intact. Early control of the disease is important in preventing secondary changes. A guarded-to-good prognosis is indicated in chronic cases unless surgical intervention is advised. Whenever the tympanic membrane is ruptured, otitis media will be present, and the prognosis for complete recovery becomes guarded with medical therapy alone. When secondary changes have progressed to marked fibrosis with narrowing of the ear canal or osteomyelitis of the bulla, surgical intervention may be required. In animals with calcified ear canals, surgery will also be necessary to achieve good results. Lateral (horizontal) ear resection is indicated to facilitate drainage and administer medicants, but it is usually only palliative because diseased tissue often remains. Total (vertical) canal ablation is needed with tissue proliferation and calcification of the ear canal. When clinical signs of middle or inner ear disease occur and fluid density is apparent within the bulla or thickening of the bulla is seen radiographically, bulla osteotomy is the treatment of choice (see also Otitis Media/Interna, Chapter 86).[61] Total canal ablation and lateral bulla osteotomy can be done simultaneously.[28] Although these procedures may resolve the otitis externa and media, postoperative complications are hearing impairment, Horner's syndrome, facial nerve paralysis, and vestibular dysfunction.

References

1. Allaker RP, Garrett N, Kent L, et al. 1993. Characterization of *Staphylococcus intermedius* isolates from canine pyoderma and from healthy carriers by SDS-PAGE of exoproteins, immunoblotting and restriction endonuclease digest analysis. *J Med Microbiol* 39:429–433.
2. Allaker RP, Jensen L, Lloyd DH, et al. 1992. Colonization of neonatal puppies by staphylococci. *Br Vet J* 148:523–528.
3. Allaker RP, Lamport AI, Lloyd DH, et al. 1991. Production of "virulence factors" by *Staphylococcus intermedius* from cases of canine pyoderma and healthy carriers. *Micro Ecol Health Dis* 4:169–173.
4. Allaker RP, Lloyd DH, Bailey RM. 1992. Population sizes and frequency of staphylococci at mucocutaneous sites on healthy dogs. *Vet Rec* 130:303–304.
5. Allaker RP, Lloyd DH, Simpson AI. 1992. Occurrence of *Staphylococcus intermedius* on the hair and skin of normal dogs. *Res Vet Sci* 52:174–176.

5a. Bond R, Collin NS, Lloyd DH. 1994. Use of contact plates for the quantitative culture of *Malassezia pachydermatis* from canine skin. *J Small Anim Pract* 35:68–72.

5b. Bond R, Ferguson EA, Curtis CF, et al. 1996. Factors associated with elevated cutaneous *Malassezia pachydermatis* populations in dogs with pruritic skin disease. *J Small Anim Pract* 37:103–107.

5c. Bond R, Howell SA, Haygood PJ, et al. 1997. Isolation of *Malassezia sympodialis* and *Malassezia globosa* from healthy pet cats. *Vet Rec* 141:200–201.

5d. Bond R, Lloyd DH. 1996. Comparison of media and conditions of incubation for the quantitative culture of *Malassezia pachydermatis* from canine skin. *Res Vet Sci* 61:273–274.

5e. Bond R, Lloyd DH, Plummer JM. 1995. Evaluation of a detergent scrub technique for the quantitative culture of *Malassezia pachydermatis* from canine skin. *Res Vet Sci* 58:133–137.

5f. Bond R, Saijonmaa-Koulumies LEM, Lloyd DH. 1995. Population sizes and frequency of *Malassezia pachydermatis* at skin and mucosal sites of healthy dogs. *J Small Anim Pract* 36:147–150.

5g. Breitwieser F. 1997. Results of bacteriologic and mycologic investigations of otitis media in dogs. *Tierarztl Prax* 25:257–260.

6. Bruyette DS, Lorenz MD. 1993. Otitis externa and otitis media: diagnostic and medical aspects. *Semin Vet Med Surg (Small Anim)* 8:3–9.
7. Burkhard MJ, Meyer DJ, Rosychuck RA, et al. 1995. Monoclonal gammopathy in a dog with chronic pyoderma. *J Vet Intern Med* 9:357–360.
8. Carlotti DN. 1991. Diagnosis and medical treatment of otitis externa in dogs and cats. *J Small Anim Pract* 32:394–400.
9. Chabanne L, Marchal T, Denerolle P, et al. 1995. Lymphocyte subset abnormalities in German shepherd dog pyoderma. *Vet Immunol Immunopathol* 49:189–198.

9a. Charach M. 1997. *Malassezia* dermatitis. *Can Vet J* 38:311–314.

10. Cox CL, Slack RW, Cox GJ. 1989. Insertion of a transtympanic ventilation tube for the treatment of otitis media with effusion. *J Small Anim Pract* 30:517–519.
11. Day MJ. 1994. An immunopathological study of deep pyoderma in the dog. *Res Vet Sci* 56:18–23.
12. Day MJ, Mazza G. 1995. Tissue immunoglobulin G subclasses observed in immune-mediated dermatopathy, deep pyoderma and hypersensitivity dermatitis in dogs. *Res Vet Sci* 58:82–89.
13. DeBoer DJ. 1990. Strategies for management of recurrent pyoderma in dogs. *Vet Clin North Am* 20:1509–1524.
14. DeBoer DJ. 1995. Management of chronic and recurrent pyoderma in the dog, pp 611–617. *In* Bonagura JD (ed), Kirk's current veterinary therapy XII. WB Saunders, Philadelphia, PA.
15. DeBoer DJ, Moriello KA, Thomes CB, et al. 1990. Evaluation of a commercial staphylococcal bacterin for management of idiopathic recurrent superficial pyoderma in dogs. *Am J Vet Res* 51:636–639.

15a. Forster van Hijfte MA, Curtis CF, White RN. 1997. Resolution of exfoliative dermatitis and *Malassezia pachydermatis* overgrowth in a cat after surgical thymoma resection. *J Small Anim Pract* 38:451–454.

15b. Gotthelf LN, Young SE. 1997. New treatment of *Malassezia* otitis externa in dogs. *Vet Forum.* August 46–53.

16. Greene RT, Lammler CH. 1992. Isolation and characterization of immunoglobulin binding proteins from *Staphylococcus intermedius* and *Staphylococcus hyicus*. *J Vet Med B* 39:519–525.
17. Greene RT, Lammler CH. 1993. *Staphylococcus intermedius*: current knowledge on a pathogen of veterinary importance. *J Vet Med B* 40:206–214.

17a. Guedejamarron J, Blanco JL, Garcia ME. 1997. Antimicrobial sensitivity in microorganisms isolated from canine otitis externa. *Zbl Vet Med B* 44:341–346.

17b. Gueho E, Midgley G, Guillot J. 1996. The genus *Malassezia* with description of four new species. *Antonie van Leeuwenhoek* 69:337–355.

17c. Guillot J, Gueho E, Chevrier G, et al. 1997. Epidemiological analysis of *Malasseza pachydermatis* isolates by partial sequencing of the large subunit ribosomal RNA. *Res Vet Sci* 62:22–25.

18. Hallu RE, Gentilini E, Rebuelto M, et al. 1996. The combination of norfloxacin and ketoconazole in the treatment of canine otitis. *Canine Pract* 21:26–28.
19. Harvey RG, Noble WC. 1994. A temporal study comparing the carriage of *Staphylococcus intermedius* on normal dogs with atopic dogs in clinical remission. *Vet Dermatol* 5:1:21–25.
20. Harvey RG, Noble WC, Ferguson EA. 1993. A comparison of lincomycin hydrochloride and clindamycin hydrochloride in the treatment of superficial pyoderma in dogs. *Vet Rec* 132:351–353.
21. Harvey RG, Noble WC, Lloyd DH. 1993. Distribution of propionibacteria on dogs: a preliminary report of the findings on 11 dogs. *J Small Anim Pract* 34:80–84.
22. Hesselbarth J, Witte W, Cuny C, et al. 1994. Characterization of *Staphylococcus intermedius* from healthy dogs and cases of superficial pyoderma by DNA restriction endonuclease patterns. *Vet Microbiol* 41:259–266.
23. Hill PB, Moriello KA. 1994. Canine pyoderma. *J Am Vet Med Assoc* 204:334–340.
24. Ihrke PJ. 1990. Bacterial infections of the skin, pp 72–79. *In* Greene CE (ed), Infectious diseases of the dog and cat. WB Saunders, Philadelphia, PA.
25. Ihrke PJ. 1996. Bacterial skin disease in the dog: a guide to canine pyoderma. Veterinary Learning Systems, Princeton, NJ, pp 1–91.
26. Ihrke PJ, Gross TL. 1995. Canine mucocutaneous pyoderma, pp 618–619. *In* Bonagura JD (ed), Kirk's current veterinary therapy XII. WB Saunders, Philadelphia, PA.
27. Keane KA, Taylor DJ. 1992. Slime producing species in canine pyoderma. *Vet Rec* 130:75.

27a. Kennis RA, Rosser EJ, Olivier NB, et al. 1996. Quantity and distribution of *Malassezia* organisms on the skin of clinically normal dogs. *J Am Vet Med Assoc* 208:1048–1051.

27b. Kiss G, Radvanyi S, Szigeti G. 1996. Characteristics of *Malassezia pachydermatis* strains isolated from canine otitis externa. *Mycoses* 39:313–321.

27c. Kiss G, Radvanyi S, Szigeti G. 1997. New combination for the therapy of canine otitis externa. 1. Microbiology of otitis externa. *J Small Anim Pract* 38:51–56.

28. Krahwinkel DJ, Pardo AD, Sims MH, et al. 1993. Effect of total ablation of the external acoustic meatus and bulla osteotomy on auditory function in dogs. *J Am Vet Med Assoc* 202:949–952.
29. Kunkle GA, Sundlof S, Deisling K. 1995. Adverse side effects of oral antibacterial therapy in dogs and cats: an epidemiologic study of pet owners' observations. *J Am Anim Hosp Assoc* 31:46–55.
30. Kwochka KW. 1993. Recurrent pyoderma, pp 3–21. *In* Griffin CE, Kwochka KW, MacDonald JM (eds), Current veterinary dermatology. Mosby Yearbook, St. Louis, MO.
31. Lane JG. 1990. Surgery of the external and middle ear. *Vet Rep* 3:4–8.
32. Layton CE. 1993. The role of lateral ear resection in managing chronic otitis externa. *Semin Vet Med Surg (Small Anim)* 8:24–29.
33. Little CJL, Lane JG, Pearson GR. 1991. Inflammatory middle ear disease of the dog: the clinical and pathological features of cholesteatoma, a complication of otitis media. *Vet Rec* 128:319–322.
34. Lloyd DH, Allaker RP, Pattinson A. 1991. Carriage of *Staphylococcus intermedius* on the ventral abdomen of clinically normal dogs and those with pyoderma. *Vet Dermatol* 2 (3/4):161–164.
35. Lloyd DH, Garthwaite G. 1982. Epidermal structure and surface topography of canine skin. *Res Vet Sci* 33:99–104.
36. Mansfield PD, Boosinger TR, Attleberger MH. 1990. Infectivity of *Malassezia pachydermatis* in the external ear canal of dogs. *J Am Vet Med Assoc* 16:97–100.
36a. Mansfield PD, Steiss JE, Boosinger TR, et al. 1997. The effects of four commercial ceruminolytic agents on the middle ear. *J Am Anim Hosp Assoc* 33:479–486.
37. Mason I, Moriello K. 1995. Management of infectious disorders, pp 287–294. *In* Moriello K, Mason I (ed), Handbook of small animal dermatology. Pergamon Press, New York, NY.
38. Mason IS. 1991. Canine pyoderma. *J Small Anim Pract* 32:381–386.
39. Mason IS, Lloyd DH. 1989. The role of allergy in the development of canine pyoderma. *J Small Anim Pract* 30:216–218.
40. Mason IS, Lloyd DH. 1993. Scanning electron microscopical studies of the living epidermis and stratum corneum of dogs, pp 131–139. *In* Ihrke PJ, Mason IS, White SD (eds), Advances in veterinary dermatology, ed 2. Pergamon Press, Oxford, England.
41. Mason KV, Evans EG. 1991. Dermatitis associated with *Malassezia pachydermatitis* in eleven dogs. *J Am Anim Hosp Assoc* 27:13–20.
42. McCarthy RT, Caywood DD. 1992. Vertical ear canal resection for end-stage otitis externa in dogs. *J Am Anim Hosp Assoc* 28:545–552.
43. McKellar QA, Rycroft A, Anderson L, et al. 1990. Otitis externa in a Foxhound pack associated with *Candida albicans*. *Vet Rec* 127:15–16.
44. Meinen JB, McClure JT, Rosen E. 1995. Pharmacokinetics of enrofloxacin in clinically normal dogs and mice and drug pharmacodynamics in neutropenic mice with *Escherichia coli* and staphylococcal infections. *Am J Vet Res* 56:1219–1224.
45. Morales CA, Schultz KT, DeBoer DJ. 1994. Antistaphylococcal antibodies in dogs with recurrent staphylococcal pyoderma. *Vet Immmunol Immunopathol* 42:137–147.
45a. Morris DO, Rosser EJ. 1995. Immunologic aspects of *Malassezia* dermatitis in patients with canine atopic dermatitis. In Proceedings of the Annual Meeting of the American Academy/College of Veterinary Dermatology 11:16–17.
45b. Nagata M, Ishida T. 1995. Cutaneous reactivity to *Malassezia pachydermatis* in dogs with seborrheic dermatitis. In 11th proceedings of the AAVD/AAVX meeting, San Diego CA, p 11.
46. Noble WC, Kent LE. 1992. Antibiotic resistance in *Staphylococcus intermedius* isolated from cases of pyoderma in the dog. *Vet Dermatol* 3:71–74.
47. Pedersen K, Wegener HC. 1995. Antimicrobial susceptibility and rRNA gene restriction patterns among *Staphylococcus intermedius* from healthy dogs and from dogs suffering from pyoderma or otitis externa. *Acta Vet Scand* 36:335–342.
48. Plant JD, Rosenkrantz WS, Griffin CE. 1992. Factors associated with and prevalence of high *Malassezia pachydermatitis* numbers on dog skin. *J Am Vet Med Assoc* 201:879–882.
49. Price PM. 1991. Pyoderma caused by *Peptostreptococcus tetradius* in a pup. *J Am Vet Med Assoc* 198:1649–1650.
50. Remidios AM, Fowler DJ, Pharr JW, et al. 1991. A comparison of radiographic versus surgical diagnosis of otitis media. *J Am Anim Hosp Assoc* 27:183.
51. Rosychuck RAW. 1994. Management of otitis externa. *Vet Clin North Am* 24:921–952.
52. Schwarz S, Werckenthin C, Pinter L, et al. 1995. Chloramphenicol resistance in *Staphylococcus intermedius* from a single veterinary centre: evidence for plasmid and chromosomal location of the resistance genes. *Vet Microbiol* 43:151–159.
52a. Scott DW. 1992. Bacteria and yeast on the surface and within non-inflamed hair follicles of skin biopsies from cats with non-neoplastic dermatoses. *Cornell Vet* 82:371–377.
52b. Scott DW. 1992. Bacteria and yeast on the surface and within non-inflamed hair follicles of skin biopsies from dogs with non-neoplastic dermatoses. *Cornell Vet* 82:379–386.
53. Scott DW, Miller WH, Cayatte SM, et al. 1995. Efficacy of tylosin tablets for the treatment of pyoderma due to *Staphylococcus intermedius* infection in dogs. *Can Vet J* 35:617–621.
54. Scott DW, Miller WH, Griffin CE. 1995. Muller and Kirk's small animal dermatology, pp 218–221, 279–328, ed 5. WB Saunders, Philadelphia, PA.
55. Scott DW, Paradis M. 1990. A survey of canine and feline skin disorders seen in a university practice: Small Animal Clinic, University of Montreal, Saint-Hyacinthe, Quebec (1987–1988). *Can Vet J* 31:830–834.
56. Sisco WM, Ihrke PJ, Franti CE. 1989. Regional distribution of the common skin diseases in dogs. *J Am Vet Med Assoc* 195:752–756.
57. Smeak DD, Kerpsack ST. 1993. Total ear canal ablation and lateral bulla osteotomy for management of end-stage otitis. *Semin Vet Med Surg (Small Anim)* 8:30–41.
58. Steiss JE, Boosinger TR, Wright JC, et al. 1992. Healing of experimentally perforated tympanic membranes demonstrated by electrodiagnostic testing and histopathology. *J Am Anim Hosp Assoc* 28:308–310.
59. Studdert VP, Hughes RL. 1991. A clinical trial for a topical preparation of miconazole, polymyxin and prednisolone in the treatment of otitis externa in dogs. *Aust Vet J* 68:193–195.
60. Talan DA, Staatz D, Staatz A, et al. 1989. *Staphylococcus intermedius* in canine gingiva and canine-inflicted human wound infections: laboratory characterizations of a newly recognized zoonotic pathogen. *J Clin Microbiol* 27:1:78–81.
61. Trevor PB, Martin RA. 1993. Tympanic bulla osteotomy for treatment of middle ear disease in cats. 19 cases (1984–1991). *J Am Vet Med Assoc* 202:123–128.
62. Uchida Y, Nakade T, Kitazawa K. 1990. Activity of 5 antifungal agents against *Malassezia pachydermatitis*. *Jpn J Vet Sci* 52:851–853.
63. Uchida Y, Nakade T, Kitazawa K. 1990. Clinico-microbiological study of the normal and otitic external ear canals in dogs and cats. *Jpn J Vet Sci* 52:415–417.
64. Wegener HC, Pedersen K. 1992. Variations in antibiograms and plasmid profiles among multiple isolates of *Staphylococcus intermedius* from pyoderma in dogs. *Acta Vet Scand* 33:391–394.
65. Wisselink MA, Koeman JP, van den Ingh TS, et al. 1990. Investigations on the role of staphylococci in the pathogenesis of German shepherd dog pyoderma. *Vet Q* 12:29–34.

Chapter **86**

Musculoskeletal Infections

Steven C. Budsberg

Musculoskeletal infections involve bones, joints, and muscles. Osteomyelitis is classically defined as inflammation of the cortical bone, medullary cavity, and periosteum.[6, 19] Most cases involve infectious agents, including bacteria, fungi, and viruses. Other potential causes include irritants, such as radiation therapy, or surgical implants; however, these causes are much less common.[6, 19, 23] Bone infections can be divided into skeletal (including the skull and pelvis) and vertebral (including intervertebral disks and vertebral bodies). Diskospondylitis with secondary osteomyelitis developing in the opposing vertebrae is more common in dogs and cats compared with people. In humans, vertebral osteomyelitis often occurs without disk space infection. In animals, vertebral osteomyelitis usually arises from penetrating injuries (see Actinomycosis, Chapter 49) rather than blood-borne infections that cause diskospondylitis.

To understand osteomyelitis, the disease process is best divided into hematogenous and post-traumatic causes. Post-traumatic osteomyelitis can be either acute or chronic.[6, 19, 23] Owing to differences in causes, clinical findings, and treatments, skeletal osteomyelitis and diskospondylitis are discussed separately. Additionally, otitis media is covered in this chapter as it involves the bony structures of the middle and inner ear. Joint and muscle infections that concern soft tissues adjacent to bone are each covered separately. Table 86–1 lists microorganisms commonly associated with musculoskeletal infections.

Table 86–1. Microorganisms Associated With Musculoskeletal Infections[a]

INFECTION	MICROORGANISMS
OSTEOMYELITIS	Bacterial: many Viral: canine distemper virus (3, 100) Fungal: *Blastomyces* (59), *Histoplasma* (60); *Cryptococcus* (61), *Coccidioides* (62), *Aspergillus* (65), *Candida* (66)
DISKOSPONDYLITIS	Dogs: Bacterial–*Staphylococcus intermedius* (36), *Brucella canis* (40), *Nocardia* (49), *Actinomyces* (49), *Streptococcus canis* (35), *Escherichia coli* (37), *Alcaligenes, Micrococcus, Proteus* (35), Mycobacterium (50), *Corynebacterium* Fungal: *Aspergillus terreus* (65), *Paecilomyces varioti* (68), *Fusarium* (68), *Mucor* (68) Cats: *Streptococcus canis* (35), *Actinomyces* (49), *E. coli* (37)
OTITIS MEDIA/INTERNA	*Pasteurella multocida* (53)
JOINT INFECTIONS	Polyarthritis (hematogenous seeding or immune complex deposition) Viral: feline syncytium-forming virus (17), feline calicivirus (16), effusive FIP (11) Rickettsial: granulocytic *Ehrlichia* (28), *Rickettsia rickettsii* (29), *Chlamydia* (31) Mycoplasmal: *Mycoplasma* (32), bacterial L-forms (32) Bacterial: *Staphylococcus* (36), hemolytic *Streptococcus* (35), *E. coli* (37), anaerobes (41), *Pasteurella* (53, 88), *Nocardia* (49), *Proteus* (35), *Pseudomonas* (35), *Yersinia* (39), *Borrelia* (45), *Salmonella* (39), *Erysipelothrix* (35), *Mycobacterium* (50), *Brucella* (40), *Corynebacterium* Fungal: *Histoplasma* (60), *Cryptococcus* (61), *Blastomyces* (59), *Coccidioides* (62), *Aspergillus* (65), *Candida* (66) Protozoal: *Leishmania* (73) Suspected infectious: Akita arthritis (100), Shar pei fever (95)
MYOSITIS	Polymyositis: *Hepatozoon* (74), *Toxoplasma gondii* (80), *Neospora caninum* (80), *Leptospira* (44), *Borrelia* (45) Local myositis: numerous bacteria, toxigenic *Streptococcus canis* (35)

[a]Chapters, for reference, are cited in parentheses.
FIP = feline infectious peritonitis.

Osteomyelitis

ETIOLOGY

Bacterial infections cause most cases of osteomyelitis in clinical practice. *Staphylococcus* accounts for 50% to 60% of cases,[19, 27] and *S. intermedius* is the primary organism. Other gram-positive organisms found less frequently include *Streptococcus*. Gram-negative organisms include *Pasteurella, Escherichia coli, Pseudomonas, Proteus*, and *Klebsiella*. Anaerobic bacteria include *Peptostreptococcus, Bacteroides, Fusobacterium, Actinomyces, Nocardia*, and *Clostridium*.[35] Anaerobic bacteria have been isolated with greater frequency as sample collection, transportation, and incubation techniques have improved.[27, 35] Anaerobic bacteria are rarely isolated alone, and usually other anaerobes and microaerophilic or aerobic bacteria make the environment conducive for anaerobic growth. Polymicrobial infections are becoming more common, presumably because of overuse of antimicrobial agents, which enables resistant bacterial populations to flourish, or because of better bacterial collection and detection methods.

A variety of fungi have been identified in osteomyelitis from regions where the organisms are endemic. In the United States, the most common isolates are *Blastomyces, Coccidioides, Histoplasma*, and *Cryptococcus*.[23, 47] Other organisms reported include *Aspergillus* and *Phialoconidium*. German shepherd dogs have the highest prevalence rate for hematogenous fungal osteomyelitis, making a hereditary immune deficiency a likely contributing factor (see also Disseminated Aspergillosis, Chapter 65).

Although viral agents have been incriminated as causing inflammatory bone diseases, factual data have been limited. However, virulent and vaccine strain canine distemper virus has been suspected as a cause of hypertrophic metaphyseal osteodystrophy and juvenile cellulitis in dogs (see Chapters 3 and 100).[28, 32, 46]

PATHOGENESIS

Hematogenous

Spread of infection via the blood stream from a distant site is rare in dogs and cats. When it occurs, immature animals are usually affected.[20, 23] The animal's predisposition of the metaphyseal region to hematogenous embolization is likely a result, in part, of the microvascular architecture of the region in growing bone. Capillaries that extend into the growth plate have both variable continuous and discontinuous epithelia.[18, 20] Terminally growing capillary buds lack a basement membrane and have discontinuous endothelium.[18, 20] Discontinuities allow circulating microorganisms to escape into the extravascular tissue space during a bacteremic phase. Blood flow through these capillary beds is slow, creating an ideal environment for bacterial lodgment and proliferation. Furthermore, in contrast to secondary spongiosa, leukocytes appear to be absent around primary spongiosa.[18] Bacterial invasion in the region of developing bone may be opposed by only tissue-based macrophages. Unrestricted infection in the metaphyses may spread to the epiphyses, periostea, soft tissues, and adjacent joints. In dogs and cats, unlike other species, transphyseal vessels are absent at birth; thus, infection is usually restricted to the metaphyseal side of the growth plate.[14]

Post-traumatic

Normal bone is resistant to infection. Osteomyelitis is unlikely to develop in the absence of complicating factors, which include tissue ischemia, bacterial contamination, bone necrosis and sequestration, fracture instability, foreign material implantation, and systemic or local alteration in immune response or tissue metabolism.[6, 19, 21, 23] Tissue trauma and subsequent vascular compromise are important factors when discussing post-traumatic osteomyelitis. Soft tissues provide the first blood supply to the ischemic bone during the initial phases of healing. Inoculation of bacteria can occur from direct penetration of a missile or other foreign body, a bite wound, an exposure of the bone via an open fracture, or a surgical intervention. Avascular bone fragments provide an ideal ecologic niche for bacteria to colonize and proliferate. Fracture instability perpetuates the persistence of infection in the bone. Instability may occur when initial stabilization was inadequate or when initial fixation fails. In either case, disruption of the blood supply is caused by damage to proliferating capillaries, promoting tissue and bone necroses and bacterial colonization and growth.

Implantation of foreign material has been associated with increased infection rates.[15, 42] The primary mechanism in biomaterial-centered sepsis is microbial colonization of these materials and adjacent damaged tissues.[21] Tissue necrosis and inflammation along the biomaterial's surface, associated with failure of implant integration into host tissues, serve as a glycoprotein-conditioned substratum for which bacteria have specific receptors.[21] Adherent bacteria produce a matrix of condensed exopolysaccharides known as a glycocalyx.[31] Embedded in the biofilm mixture of glycocalyx, host-derived serum proteins, and cellular debris, bacteria often form into microcolonies (Fig. 86–1). Within biofilm, bacteria are protected from antibodies, phagocytes, and even antibiotics.[21, 23, 31] Furthermore, several different types of bacteria can both coexist and replicate in glycocalyx-enclosed microcolonies in the interstitial spaces of connective tissue associated with dead bone sequestra, causing mixed infections.

CLINICAL FINDINGS

Clinical signs of osteomyelitis vary with the type and duration of disease. Acute osteomyelitis, either hematogenous or post-traumatic in origin, has swelling and localized pain. The animal is usually febrile. Elevated leukocyte counts are common. Various signs of systemic illness include lethargy and inappetence.[6, 19, 23] Chronic post-traumatic osteomyelitis is a localized disease with rare systemic manifestations; the most common of these is a history of trauma or surgery with a subsequent draining tract and lameness.

DIAGNOSIS

History, physical examination, and radiography will localize the site of the lesion. Nonspecific laboratory findings may include variable leukocytosis and increased serum concentrations of calcium and phosphorus or high alkaline phosphatase (ALP) activity. Radiography will localize and determine the type of lesion. In an acute case, the only finding may be

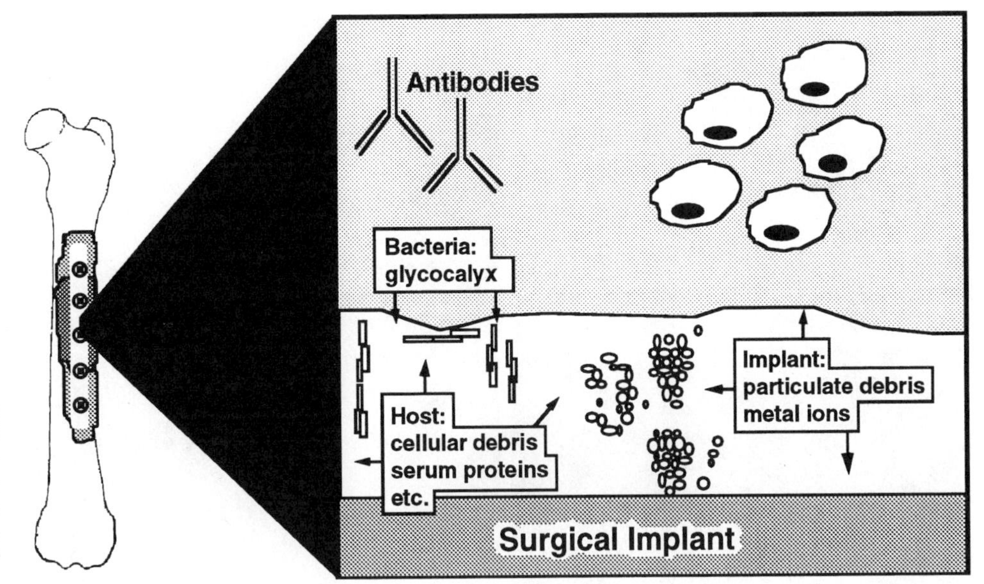

Figure 86–1. Schematic drawing showing osteomyelitis involving the femur and associated surgical implant. Bacteria produce glycocalyx, which, combined with host-derived and implant-derived materials, forms a biofilm. This biofilm protects bacteria from host defenses.

soft tissue swelling. As the infection progresses, radiographic changes include, but are not limited to, periosteal bone proliferation, bone resporption, and increased medullary density. In chronic cases, radiography can demonstrate the presence of loose or broken implants or nonviable bone (sequestra).

Technetium-99m-methylene diphosphonate (MDP), indium-111 leukocyte, and IgG scintigraphy are radionuclide imaging techniques that can provide additional diagnostic information if radiographic findings are equivocal.[26] However, these tests are used sparingly in veterinary medicine and require the specialized equipment of referral centers.

Cytologic evaluation of exudates is informative, whereas microbiologic culture of an infectious agent is definitive. Specimens from a sterile aspirate of the lesion through intact skin or from sequestra, local necrotic tissue, or implant at the time of debridement provide the most valuable material for culture. Organisms isolated from discharges of draining tracts may be contaminants. Proper collection and transport of both aerobic and anaerobic samples is also imperative (see Chapter 33). In cases of hematogenous osteomyelitis, blood should be cultured as well as the secondary site of infection.

Anaerobic infections should be suspected when affected tissue is characterized by a foul odor, sequestra, or presence of multiple bacterial species suggested by impression smears or histologic specimens (see Chapter 41).[35] Further suspicion of an anaerobic infection should be raised if no organism is cultured from material in which cytologic findings indicate infection. Multifocal sterile pyogranulomatous osteomyelitis has been reported in dogs[9] but probably is caused by immune dysregulation rather than infection.

THERAPY

The infective agent, local tissue environment, and blood supply should always be considered in any therapeutic strategy. Treatment is customized to each patient, but certain principles must be followed. Mere use of antimicrobial drugs will not eradicate the chronic infection associated with osteomyelitis. The local environment must be improved by debridement, drainage, fracture stabilization, dead space obliteration, and antimicrobial therapy. Regardless of the situation, every effort should be made to obtain a culture and susceptibility testing for both aerobic and anaerobic bacteria.

Hematogenous Osteomyelitis

Animals with hematogenous osteomyelitis are often septic. The infections usually involve the metaphyseal region of the bone and do not extend into the adjacent joint (Fig. 86–2*A*). However, synoviocentesis and radiography are strongly recommended to make this determination. If joints are affected, aggressive management should be undertaken as described later for monoarthropies. If no joint involvement can be demonstrated, any fluctuant, warm, or painful area around the affected bone can be aspirated for culture and susceptibility testing. If there is an obvious fluctuant area, attempts should be made to open and copiously lavage the region with a sterile isotonic solution and to perform debridement. Systemic IV antibiotics should be given for a minimum of 3 to 5 days before switching to the oral route. Oral administration should continue for a minimum of 21 days. Bactericidal agents that are active against β-lactamase–producing *Staphylococcus* should be used (Tables 86–2 and 86–3). Systemic treatment for sepsis should be addressed if necessary (see Chapters 38 and 87). Radiographs taken 2 to 3 weeks after treatment can help evaluate progression and response to therapy (Fig. 86–2*B*). Systemic manifestations and presence of joint involvement are indicators of poorer prognoses.[20]

Acute Post-Traumatic Osteomyelitis

Osteomyelitis developing within 2 to 5 days after an insult may be difficult to differentiate from a soft tissue wound infection. However, most wound complications are restricted to soft tissues. Regardless, treatment is very similar, and absolute differentiation is not always necessary. Treatment should be aggressive in an effort to prevent these infections from developing into chronic processes. Modalities include drainage and debridement, systemic antimicrobial agents,

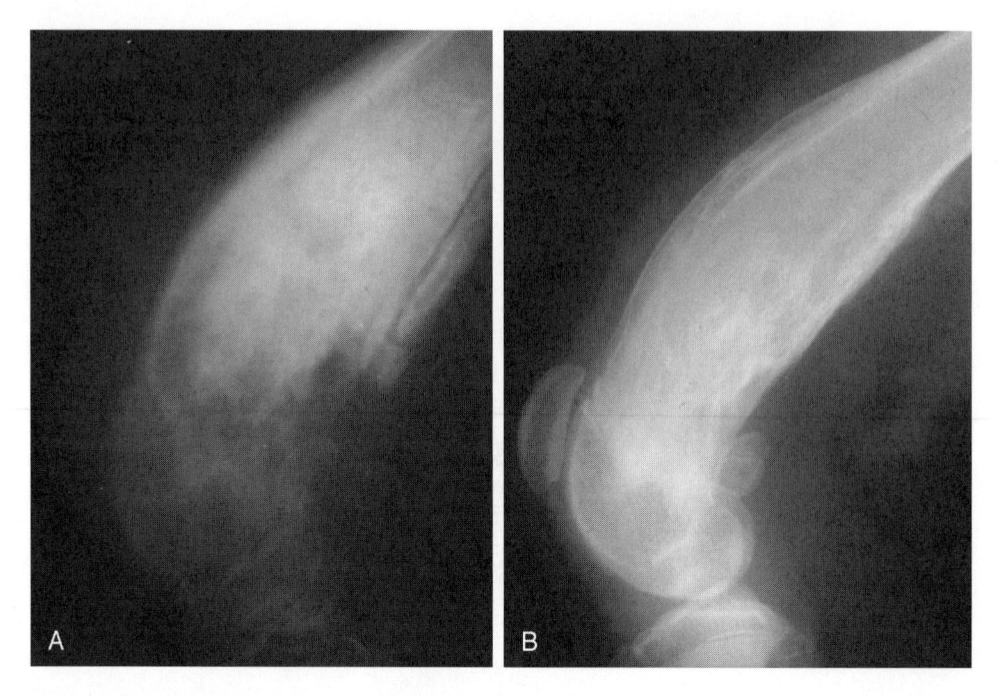

Figure 86–2. *A*, Pelvic limb radiograph of 4-month-old Doberman, with lameness and painful stifle swelling of 10 days' duration. Acute hematogenous osteomyelitis with metaphyseal lysis and extensive bony production within the distal diaphysis are evident. *B*, One month after surgical biopsy and culture of *Staphylococcus intermedius* and institution of systemic antibiotic treatment. There is remodeling of the femoral metaphysis with reduced sclerosis and periosteal proliferation.

rigid stabilization, direct bone culture, and delayed wound closure (Fig. 86–3*A*).[6, 19, 23]

Drainage and debridement of all necrotic tissues or bones, hematomas, and abscesses should be done first. Culture and biopsy samples are obtained at this time, followed by copious lavage of the area with lactated Ringer's solution or saline. Drainage by closed suction units or open wound management with daily flushing are options to be considered. Initial antimicrobial therapy is similar to that of hematogenous osteomyelitis; the most common bacterium is β-lactamase–producing *Staphylococcus* (see Tables 86–2 and 86–3). Drugs should be given parenterally (preferably IV) for the first 3 to 5 days followed by oral therapy for a minimum of 4 weeks; many cases require 8 weeks. Therapeutic agents may be adjusted as culture results become available. Patient monitoring must be intense and regular. In all cases, radiographs should be taken 2 to 3 weeks after intervention and then sequentially as needed (Fig. 86–3*B*).

Chronic Post-Traumatic Osteomyelitis

This is the most common type of osteomyelitis seen in veterinary practice. Because of devitalized tissues, therapy with antibiotics alone is usually not successful. Drugs cannot enter the tissue in which they are most needed. Without improving the ischemic, necrotic environment, success in bacterial eradication is minimal. Treatment is based on the same

Table 86–2. Recommended Therapy for Musculoskeletal Infections in Dogs and Cats

ORGANISM (Chapter Reference)	USUAL CONDITION	SYSTEMIC ANTIBIOTICS[a]
Staphylococcus intermedius (36)	D, A, O	Amoxicillin-clavulanate, cephradine,[b] oxacillin[c]
Brucella canis (40)	D	Tetracycline[d] and streptomycin[e]
Streptococcus sp. (β-hemolytic) (35)	D, A	Ampicillin, penicillin[f]
Proteus, Pseudomonas (37)	I, O	Quinolones, gentamicin, second- or third-generation cephalosporins
Erysipelothrix (35)	D, A	Penicillin[b, c]
Pasteurella multocida (53, 88)	I	Ampicillin, tetracycline
Anaerobes (41)	M, O, I	Amoxicillin-clavulanate, clindamycin, metronidazole, chloramphenicol
Mycoplasma (32)	A	Tetracycline,[d] quinolones
Borrelia (45)	A	Ampicillin, tetracycline
Toxoplasma (80)	M	Clindamycin, pyrimethamine and sulfonamides, azithromycin
Aspergillus (65)	D	Itraconazole, amphotericin B
Cryptococcus (61)	A	Itraconazole, ketoconazole, fluconazole, amphotericin B
Coccidioides (62), *Blastomyces* (59)	O	Itraconazole, ketoconazole, amphotericin B

[a]Drugs are listed in order of most desirable choice first.
[b]Substitute any first-generation cephalosporin.
[c]Substitute any β-lactam–resistant penicillin.
[d]Substitute minocycline or doxycycline.
[e]Substitute gentamicin or amikacin.
[f]Substitute amoxicillin, first-generation cephalosporin, or erythromycin.
D = diskospondylitis; A = arthritis; M = myositis; O = osteomyelitis; I = otitis media/interna.

Table 86–3. Drug Dosages for Treatment of Musculoskeletal Infections[a]

DRUG	SPECIES	DOSE[b]	ROUTE	INTERVAL (HOURS)
Amikacin	B	7.5 mg/kg	V, IM, SC	12
Ampicillin	B	22 mg/kg	IV, IM, SC, PO	6–8
Amoxicillin	B	22–30 mg/kg	IV, IM, SC, PO	6–8
Amoxicillin-clavulanate	B	22 mg/kg	PO	8
Cefazolin	B	22 mg/kg	IV, IM, SC	6–8
Cefotetan	B	30 mg/kg	IV, IM, SC	12
Cefoxitin	B	30 mg/kg	IV, IM, SC	8
Cephalexin	B	22–30 mg/kg	PO	8
Cephradine	B	22–30 mg/kg	PO	8
Chloramphenicol	D	25–50 mg/kg	IV, PO	8
	C	25–50 mg/kg	IV, PO	12
Ciprofloxacin	B	11 mg/kg	IV, PO	12
Clindamycin	B	11 mg/kg	IV, IM, PO	8–12
Cloxacillin	B	10–15 mg/kg	IV, IM, PO	6–8
Doxycycline	B	10 mg/kg	PO	12
Enrofloxacin	B	5–11 mg/kg	SC, PO	12
Gentamicin	B	3.3 mg/kg	IV, IM, SC	12
Minocycline	B	10 mg/kg	PO	12
Oxacillin	B	22–30 mg/kg	IV, IM, SC, PO	6–8
Penicillin G (aqueous)	B	20,000–40,000 IU	IV	6
Penicillin V	B	40 mg/kg	PO	6
Streptomycin	B	20 mg/kg	IM	12
Tetracycline	B	22 mg/kg	PO	8

[a]Duration of therapy is dependent on the tissue, site, and duration of infection; see text for guidelines.
[b]Dose per administration at specified intervals.
B = dog and cat; D = dog; C = cat.

fundamental objectives of debridement of necrotic tissue, bony sequestra, and all foreign material, including old implants. Attempted bacterial isolation, obliteration of dead space, establishment of drainage, and rigid stabilization of bone should be done. Bone will actually heal in the presence of infection if it can be stabilized.

Debridement and sequestra removal are essential to management. During and after the surgical procedure, copious lavage is performed. Fracture stability should be evaluated intraoperatively; implants must be removed if they are loose. Rigid fixation of fractures is imperative for healing and eradication of infection. Removal of all implants, if the fracture is healed, or of implants that are not adding to the stabilization eliminates sites for biofilm formation. Eradication of dead space and removal of unnecessary foreign material, including sutures, should be performed. Establishment of drainage can be accomplished by a number of different techniques. Closed suction units, saucerization, and treating an open wound without suturing the skin to the soft tissues are all viable methods. Placement of vascularized muscle flaps over the defect after infection has been controlled can also be considered.

Antimicrobial therapy must be based on culture and susceptibility results; however, there is often a lack of correlation of clinical response and in vitro susceptibility of some microorganisms. These failures can be attributed in part to the inability of antibiotics to achieve sufficient concentrations in affected tissue. With this limitation, the best chance to reach and maintain levels at consistent concentrations would be IV infusions over a treatment period of a minimum of 4 to 6 weeks. Unfortunately, in practice, financial constraints usually limit treatment to short parenteral regimens followed by orally administered antimicrobials. Antibiotics that can be used orally for long-term treatment that are effective against β-lactamase–producing *Staphylococcus* should be considered (see Tables 86–2 and 86–3). Placement of local infusion drug delivery systems is currently receiving a great deal of research interest. Use of implants impregnated with antibiotics is common in human medicine and less frequent in veterinary medicine. Carriers are usually either a form of bone cement or a biodegradable polymer.[7, 45]

Management of open wounds or suction systems dictates initial postoperative management. Once this early phase is complete, weekly checks and radiographs at 3-week intervals are advised. Antibiotics must be continued for 6 to 8 weeks regardless of any early positive response. Owners should be advised that the animal's chronic osteomyelitis can remain quiescent for weeks, months, or years with potential for relapse or reinfection.

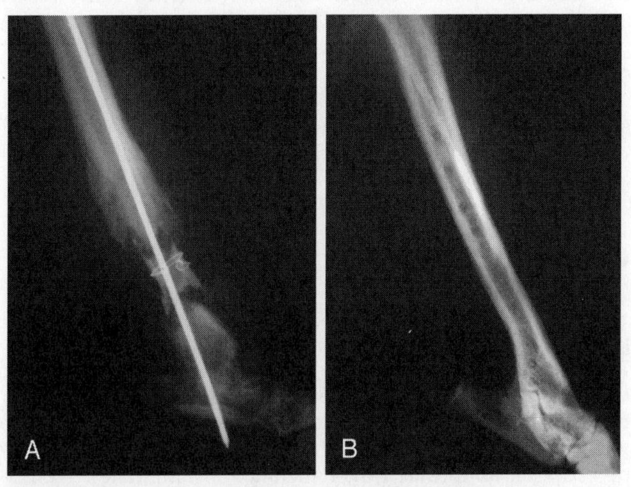

Figure 86–3. *A*, Radiograph of a 4-year-old dog with open segmental fracture of tibia, in which an IM pin was placed 3 months previously. Osteomyelitis with a nonunion and large sequestrum of bone are present in the mid tibia. *B*, Radiograph 2 years later after surgical removal of implant and bony sequestrum, obtaining tissue for culture and susceptibility, debridement, lavage, stabilization with a bone plate, cancellous bone graft, open wound management, and systemic antimicrobial therapy. (Courtesy of Dr. Dennis Aron, University of Georgia.)

Diskospondylitis

Diskospondylitis is defined as inflammation of an intervertebral disk and adjacent vertebral end plates and bodies. In comparison, infections located in the vertebral body usually caused by penetrating wounds or foreign bodies are termed *vertebral osteomyelitis* and are less frequent in dogs and cats. The most common cause of diskospondylitis is bacterial infection (see Table 86–1).[34] Any vertebral space can be affected; the thoracic and lumbar sites are the most commonly involved.

ETIOLOGY

Staphylococcus intermedius is the most common causative bacterium identified in the dog.[24, 25, 34] Other frequently documented bacterial pathogens include *Streptococcus, Brucella canis*, and *E. coli*.[24, 25, 34] The wide variety of other bacterial species underscores the need to attempt to obtain bacterial isolation and susceptibility testing in each case. Fungi are involved in some infections, and genera have included *Aspergillus, Fusarium*, and *Paecilomyces*.[8, 24, 34] In addition to hematogenous exposure, migrating foreign bodies have produced spinal infections with vertebral body osteomyelitis (see Actinomycosis, Chapter 49). Plant materials have been the most widely associated foreign bodies, and geographic regional differences influence the specific causative agent.[34] Epidural abscess and diskospondylitis can develop after epidural injections.[38] Spinal column and disk infection have also been sequelae of spinal surgery or disk fenestration.

PATHOGENESIS

Diskospondylitis is thought to arise from hematogenous spread of the organism into the disk space and subsequently into the adjacent vertebrae. The most commonly incriminated sources include urogenital tract and skin infections, dental disease, and valvular endocarditis. However, in many cases, no other site of infection is detected. Preferential hematogenous localization in the disk space probably occurs as a result of retrograde blood flow into vertebral sinuses or as a result of subchondral vascular loops in the vertebral epiphysis that slow blood flow.[24, 25, 34] Predisposing factors have included immunosuppression and previous trauma, including surgical intervention.[24, 25]

CLINICAL SIGNS

Clinical presentation can vary; however, in general, signs progress slowly. Although any dog or cat is susceptible to this disease, the most common signalment is that of a young to middle-aged male large-breed dog.[24, 25] Signs can vary from those of systemic infection (depression, anorexia, fever, weight loss) to musculoskeletal dysfunction (paraspinal hyperesthesia, abnormal gait, reluctance to ambulate). Neurologic signs are those of extradural compression, paresis and ataxia, or paralysis and are dependent on the vertebral site and severity of the lesion (Fig. 86–4). Paraspinal hyperesthesia is often noticed earliest, although some dogs are stoic and do not show overt signs of discomfort. Neurologic dysfunction can develop gradually with osteoproliferation or suddenly with intervertebral disk rupture from weakened ligaments. The reported most common sites of infection are L7-S1, caudal cervical area, and midthoracic spine.[24, 25] Monoparesis or monoparalysis can result from nerve root involvement in patients with infection, causing chronic asymmetric osteoproliferation.

DIAGNOSIS

A tentative diagnosis is made from the patient history and the physical and neurologic examinations. Definitive diagnosis is made with spinal radiographs. Changes include concentric lysis of adjacent vertebral end plates early, with later vertebral body osteolysis or proliferative sclerosis, vertebral body shortening, narrowed disk spaces, and ventral osseous bridging (Fig. 86–5). Extensive vertebral body infection may result in vertebral body collapse or subluxation.[5] Radiographic changes associated with diskospondylitis can take 2 to 4 weeks to develop after the initiation of the infection.[25] Thus, sequential radiographs may be needed to confirm the diagnosis in an animal with initial signs of hyperesthesia. Clinical signs and radiographic severity of lesions do not always correlate.

When hyperesthesia and neurologic dysfunction are absent, diskospondylitis may be overlooked. Spinal radiographs should be considered in animals with chronic, recurrent urinary tract infection or fever of unknown origin. Dogs with confirmed diskospondylitis should always be immediately screened serologically for *B. canis* (see Chapter 40). Should serologic test results be negative, disk space culture provides the most consistent recovery of the offending organism. However, culturing the disk is often impractical because of the inaccessibility of the lesion unless decompressive surgery is performed. If the lesion is caudal to the thoracolumbar junction and fluoroscopy is available, guided direct aspiration of the disk can be attempted.[17a] Blood and urine cultures should be performed, therefore, in an attempt to

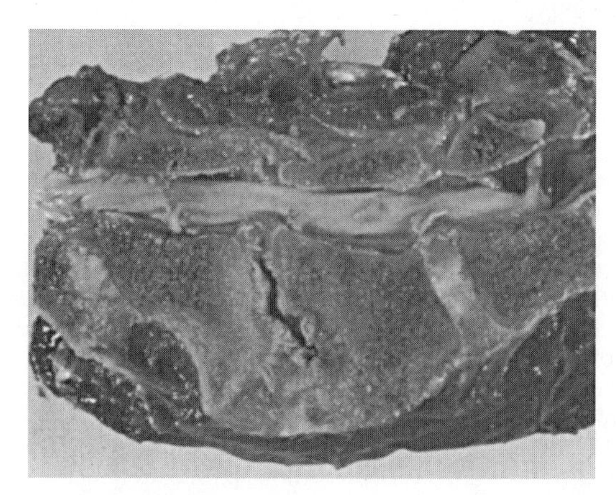

Figure 86–4. Lateral view of transected vertebral column from a 6-year-old female Great Dane with tetraparesis and depression of 6 weeks' duration. The C6-C7 interspace is at the center of the picture. The caudal aspect of the vertebral body of C6 and the cranial aspect of the vertebral body of C7 are irregular in appearance, suggesting vertebral lysis. Fibrous tissue and new bone present dorsal to the disk space compress the spinal cord ventrally. The intervertebral disk at C6-C7 is absent. There is considerable new bone ventral to the C6-C7 disk space and sclerosis of the caudal aspect of the vertebral body of C6 and the cranial aspect of the vertebral body of C7. A diagnosis of diskospondylitis was made. (From Kornegay JN: *Compend Cont Educ Pract Vet* 1:931, 1979. Used with permission.)

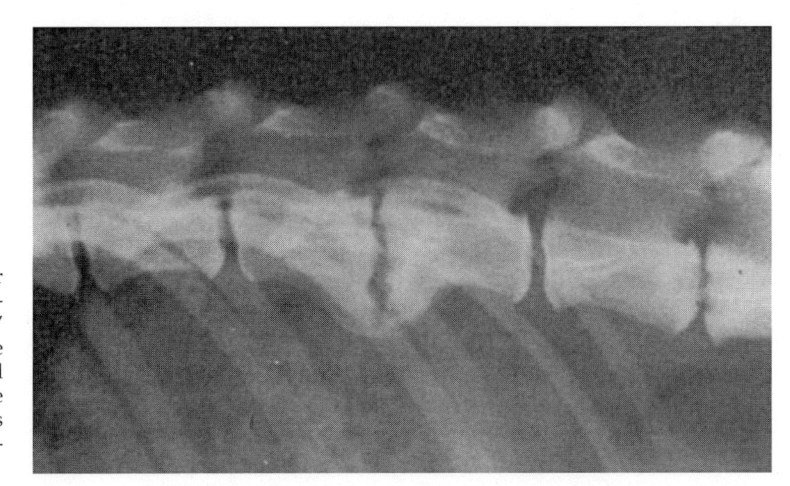

Figure 86–5. Lateral radiograph of the thoracolumbar spine from a 2-year-old female mixed-breed dog with spinal hyperesthesia and mild posterior ataxia of 2 weeks' duration. The T13-L1 interspace is at the center of the picture. There is lysis and associated sclerosis of the cranial end plate of L1 and the caudal end plate of T13. Note the new bone ventrally. Similar but less pronounced changes are evident at L2-L3. A diagnosis of multifocal diskospondylitis was made.

recover the organism before instituting therapy. Positive blood culture results range from 45% to 75% and should be considered in all cases. This approach is especially warranted in dogs with increased rectal temperatures or animals with signs of sepsis in hematologic parameters.[25] Organisms may be cultured from urine approximately 40% of the time.[25] Other sources of infection from which possible dissemination has occurred may be investigated. If infection is detected in urine and blood, the entire urinary tract and heart valves, respectively, may be evaluated by radiologic or ultrasonographic testing.

Other imaging techniques may aid in the diagnosis of early radiographically undetectable diskospondylitis. Computed tomography (CT), magnetic resonance imaging, and radionuclide scans, including MDP, gallium-67, and indium-111–labeled leukocytes, may become more routine in veterinary referral centers to augment the diagnosis of occult diskospondylitis.

THERAPY

Ideally, antimicrobial treatment should be based on culture results from blood, urine, or optimally affected bone. Initial empiric treatment is recommended while culture results are still pending. The initial assumption should be that the offending bacterium is a *Staphylococcus*-producing β-lactamase, rendering penicillin, amoxicillin, and ampicillin ineffective. Use of a bactericidal, β-lactamase–resistant drug that is primarily effective against gram-positive bacteria is preferred. Several drugs fit these criteria (see Table 86–2). First-generation cephalosporins have been clinically most effective in this regard. Table 86–3 lists dosages of recommended drugs.

The next decision is route of administration, which is dictated by clinical presentation and disease progression. Treatment in patients with minimal to no neurologic dysfunction should begin with the appropriate oral antimicrobial drug. Parenteral therapy should be the initial step in dogs with moderate neurologic dysfunction, including ataxia and paresis. In rare instances, initial therapy may include relieving extradural cord compression with surgical decompression. Analgesics may be needed in dogs with intense hyperesthesia early in the course of treatment. For instance, with acute and rapidly progressive severe neurologic dysfunction, regardless of length of onset, IV administration of antibiotics is needed for 5 to 7 days, followed by a course of oral administration. In more slowly progressive situations, a single loading dose of parenterally administered antibiotics may be followed by oral treatment. Length of oral treatment is a minimum of 6 to 8 weeks, regardless of favorable patient response in the early period. If *B. canis* titers come back positive, switching to a combined regimen of tetracyclines and aminoglycosides is advisable (see Chapter 40). *Brucella* test–positive dogs should always be neutered before treatment.

In all cases of bacterial diskospondylitis, improvement should begin within 3 to 5 days after initiation of therapy. If no response is noted and results of cultures of blood and urine are negative, the class of antimicrobial may be switched. In addition, attempts at surgical curettage of the lesion may be considered to obtain a direct bone culture.

The patient should be closely monitored over the first few days after institution of antimicrobial therapy and then be evaluated at 2-week intervals once improvement is noted. Follow-up radiography for monitoring patient progress is controversial. Radiographs have been recommended as frequently as every 2 weeks, but subtle changes are difficult to interpret. A more pragmatic evaluation routine is to obtain radiographs 1 month after initiation of treatment and once again after cessation of therapy.[6] Therapy is usually at least 2 to 4 months. Resolution of clinical signs occurs well before radiographic improvement. Resolving lesions are characterized by decreased osteolysis and osteoproliferation and new bone formation with intervertebral bridging. Radiographs are usually more of a benefit to document cases of aggressive, spreading infections that are not responsive to treatment.

In animals with complete paralysis, intensive, aggressive, parenteral antibiotic therapy must be instituted. If signs do not improve dramatically in 24 to 72 hours, changing of the antimicrobial agents or possible decompressing of the spinal cord and stabilizing of the vertebral column may be necessary. If vertebral fracture or dislocation is present, surgical intervention is mandatory and prognosis is guarded. If a single disk is affected, on the basis of neurologic and myelographic findings, and paralysis is severe, surgery might be recommended. However, if multiple lesions are causing compression, surgical intervention, including decompression, may not be feasible or advisable *unless* the goal of surgery is biopsy for microbiologic culture and susceptibility testing.[6] Cases of fungal diskospondylitis usually involve *Aspergillus terreus* infections in German shepherd dogs (see Chapter 65). The dogs usually have complicating signs of systemic infection and respond poorly to treatment.

Otitis Media/Interna

Clinical signs of otitis media/interna usually reflect neurologic rather than musculoskeletal disease.[25] However, it is discussed with musculoskeletal infection because the infection is a form of osteomyelitis in bone of the middle ear and the bony labyrinth of the inner ear. Therapeutic considerations are based on principles for treating osteomyelitis. In contrast, otitis externa is considered as an integumentary infection (see Chapter 85).

ANATOMY

Knowledge of the anatomic interrelations of the compartments of the ear is important in understanding the pathogenesis of otitis media/interna and its treatment (Fig. 86–6). Both middle and inner ears are housed in the petrous temporal bone. The middle ear is separated from the horizontal portion of the external ear canal by the tympanic membrane. Together with the incus and stapes, the malleus connects the tympanic membrane to the oval window of the inner ear. The auditory ossicles are situated in a small dorsal concavity of the middle ear, the epitympanic recess. The larger, air-filled tympanic bulla forms the remainder of the middle ear and contains the round foramen and the aural opening of the auditory tube. The osseous bulla is a major site of localization of infection and a concern for therapeutic intervention. The aural opening is covered by the secondary tympanic membrane and communicates with the cochlea of the inner ear. The cochlea contains the peripheral sense organs of hearing. In addition to the auditory cochlea, the inner ear consists of semicircular canals and the utricle and saccule of the vestibule. These structures are concerned with balance.[25]

ETIOLOGY AND PATHOGENESIS

Otitis media/interna in dogs and cats usually is caused by extension of otitis externa. Accordingly, *S. intermedius, Pseudomonas aeruginosa, Proteus,* and *Streptococcus* are the most common bacterial pathogens, and fungi such as *Malassezia* and *Candida* may occasionally be isolated (see Chapter 85). Less frequently, otitis media/interna results from ascension of bacteria from the oral cavity through the auditory tube. Conversely, infections originating in the middle ear may reach the oral cavity through this same route. Rarely, hematogenous spread of blood-borne bacteria or fungi to the middle and inner ears has been observed. Cats may have otitis externa as the nidus of otitis media/interna; however, cats also develop inflammatory polyps within the middle ear. These polyps are often associated with bacterial infections; yet the order of occurrence or the association between these findings is not understood.[16]

CLINICAL FINDINGS

Clinical signs of simple otitis media are similar to those of otitis externa. Aural hyperesthesia is manifested by head shaking or cocking, pawing of the involved ear, and discomfort on manipulation of the animal's pinna, auditory canal, or face. When the infection has followed otitis externa, the external ear canal is inflamed and usually contains debris. On otoscopic examination, the tympanic membrane may be absent or obscured by debris. When visible and intact, the membrane is usually discolored and often bulges outward. Occasionally, a fluid line is observed, indicating the presence of serum or exudate in the middle ear. Some animals subsequently may have evidence of facial nerve paralysis and Horner's syndrome because of the involvement of the facial nerve and ocular branch of the sympathetic trunk, respectively, as they pass through the middle ear.[25] Horner's syndrome can also be seen in cats with middle ear polyps.[16]

With chronicity, there is increased likelihood that the causative organism of otitis media will spread to the inner ear. In these cases, evidence of peripheral vestibular disease occurs. Clinical signs include head tilt toward the affected side; horizontal nystagmus with the fast component in a direction opposite the involved side; and asymmetric ataxia manifest variably by falling, rolling, and circling in the direction of the lesion. Most affected animals also have clinical evidence

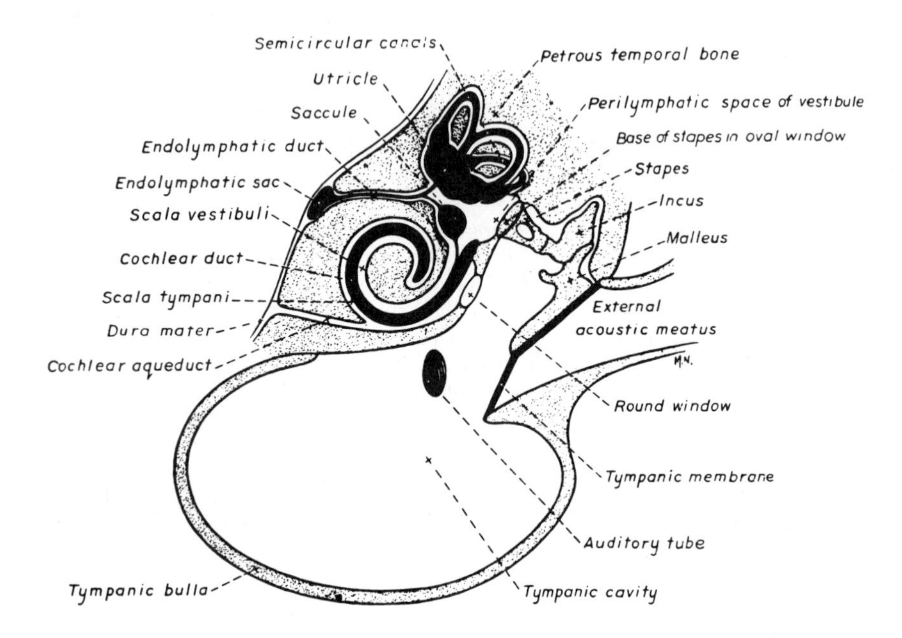

Figure 86–6. Diagram of the middle and inner ears of the dog. (From Getty R et al: *Am J Vet Res* 17:364–375, 1956. Used with permission.)

of otitis, both media and externa. When concomitant external ear disease is absent in either dogs or cats and only vestibular peripheral nerve dysfunction is noted, idiopathic peripheral vestibular disease or ascending infection from the oropharynx should be considered. If there is evidence of central vestibular disease (postural reaction involvement, vertical or variable direction nystagmus, involvement of cranial nerves other than facial, or mental depression), extension to the brain stem or subarachnoid space may have occurred or meningitis is the primary problem with involvement of the eighth cranial nerve.

Nystagmus and ataxia usually resolve despite the occasional irreversible destruction of the peripheral vestibular sense organs or nerves. Reasons why these signs resolve are not clear. However, affected animals probably compensate through accommodation of the vestibular system and reliance on other sensory modalities such as vision and conscious proprioception. Head tilt may remain, but this usually is a cosmetic rather than a functional handicap.[25] In the dark, and after anesthesia or various other stress factors, the head tilt or imbalance may be noticeably worse.

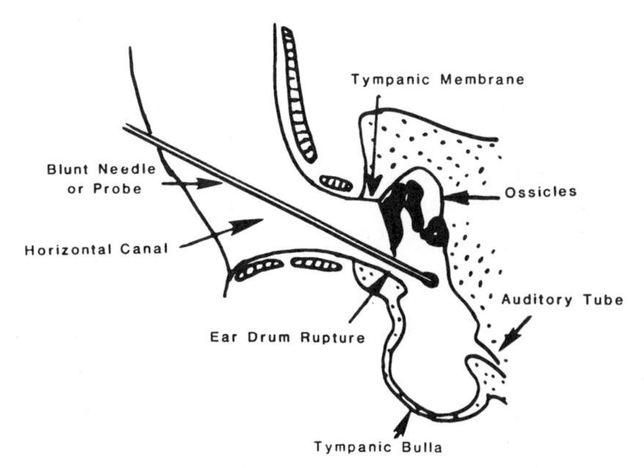

Figure 86–7. Diagram depicting proper placement of a needle for myringotomy and flushing of the tympanic bulla. (Modified from Lane G: *In Pract* 1:5–15, 1979. Used with permission.)

DIAGNOSIS

Animals with clinical evidence of otitis media/interna should be anesthetized so that an otoscopic examination can be completed and radiographs taken. If the tympanic membrane is obscured by debris, the external ear canal should be gently flushed with a sterile saline or lactated Ringer's solution. While dilute chlorhexidine or aqueous povidone-iodine solutions have been advocated, these should be used with caution because they can be detrimental to deeper tissues if the tympanic membrane is ruptured (see Otitis Externa, Chapter 85). The external canal is then suctioned and dried. This step aids in the visualization of the tympanic membrane. If observed changes suggest middle ear disease, both open-mouth and lateral radiographs of the tympanic bullae should be taken. Radiographically, fluid accumulation will be reflected by increased density within the affected bullae. Radiography is more insensitive in early disease when inflammation or some effusion can be present without notable changes. In advanced cases, there may be radiographic evidence of osteomyelitis of the bulla and, on rare instances, the adjacent temporomandibular joint. If available, CT offers a more definitive means of identifying these changes.

THERAPY

Choice of treatment for otitis media/interna is dependent on the stage of the disease. If concurrent chronic otitis externa is not present, systemic administration of a broad-spectrum antibiotic, such as a first-generation cephalosporin or chloramphenicol, is recommended for a minimum of 14 days. However, most dogs and cats with otitis media/interna usually also have chronic otitis externa and will benefit from myringotomy or ventral bulla osteotomy. Alternatively, in very chronic cases, total ear canal ablation with a concurrent bulla osteotomy may be necessary. If the tympanic membrane is intact, myringotomy should be accomplished using anesthesia at the time of otoscopic examination and radiography. Either a blunted 17-gauge needle or myringotomy knife is utilized for the procedure. The needle allows simultancous collection of fluid for culture and flushing. The needle is passed along the ventral horizontal ear canal so that it penetrates the ventral aspect of the pars tensa (Fig. 86–7). Performing the procedure in this manner helps to prevent iatrogenic damage to the auditory ossicles. After fluid has been withdrawn for bacterial culture and cytologic evaluation, the middle ear is repeatedly but gently flushed until the fluid recovered by suction is clear of debris and blood, and an antibiotic is then instilled. Selection of the antibiotic is based on prior culture results of the external ear. It should be changed if follow-up culture results of middle ear fluid indicate unresponsiveness. When culture and susceptibility results are unavailable, a broad-spectrum antibiotic should be chosen (see Tables 86–2 and 86–3). Aminoglycosides might be avoided because they potentially impair auditory or cochlear nerve function, if these have not already been lost (see Aminoglycosides, Chapter 34). Antibiotics should be applied topically for 10 to 14 days.

Animals with cytologic or cultural evidence of yeast infection should receive a topical antifungal agent for a similar period of time (see Otitis Externa, Chapter 85). Systemic antibiotics or antifungal agents are not usually indicated, unless the disease is recurrent or establishment of drainage through the external ear is impossible. Animals with nystagmus and vertigo from acute otitis interna also may benefit from antihistamines or benzodiazepines.

Many dogs and cats with otitis media respond to a single session of middle ear irrigation, together with daily cleaning and topical antibiotic application. This approach is particularly effective in animals with recent onset because the inner ear often is either unaffected or only minimally affected. Care should be taken during irrigation, because excessive trauma during cleaning can cause complete damage to middle and inner ear structures. Some animals with clinical evidence of otitis interna may respond rapidly after myringotomy, suggesting that the clinical signs are associated with either increased pressure within the bony labyrinth or reversible inflammation of the sensory end-organs. Animals that fail to respond or have a chronic repetitive history and radiographic evidence of osteomyelitis are candidates for bulla osteotomy. This procedure allows for removal of proliferative tissue and more complete drainage. Operative techniques for this procedure can be found elsewhere.[16] Ventral bulla osteotomy is the treatment of choice for cats with inflammatory polyps.

The greatest danger of otitis media/interna is extension of the infection to the meninges and CNS along the cranial nerves. This situation usually is avoided if proper treatment is initiated early. Collection and evaluation of CSF should be done when the animal is anesthetized for the myringotomy procedure if neurologic signs suggest intracranial involvement.

Joint Infections

Inflammatory joint disorders are defined as and characterized by inflammation in the synovial membrane and fluid. Systemic signs are variable and may include lethargy, fever, and leukocytosis. The causes of inflammatory joint diseases in dogs and cats are diverse and include both infectious and noninfectious disorders. This section focuses only on infectious arthropathies.

ETIOLOGY

Infectious inflammatory arthritis may be caused by bacteria, mycoplasmas, rickettsiae, spirochetes, fungi, and viral agents (see Table 86–1). Bacteria are the most common infective agents. Bacterial contamination occurs by either direct inoculation (surgery, penetrating wound, or extension from surrounding tissues) or hematogenous seeding of a distant infective nidus. With direct inoculation, *Staphylococcus* and *Streptococcus* are the most common agents.[4] Direct inoculation induces a monoarticular septic arthritis. If polyarthropathy is diagnosed, hematogenous spread of bacteria directly or immune-mediated disease secondary to a chronic distant infection should be considered. Hematogenously spread bacterial arthritis is uncommon in the dog and cat. It is usually limited to neonates or debilitated patients. Young puppies and kittens may develop suppurative bacterial polyarthritis as a result of congenital or neonatal exposure. *S. canis* has been most commonly incriminated (see Chapter 35). Immunodeficient Shar peis or Akitas may develop chronic polyarthritis (see Chapters 95 and 100). The most common distant sites of infection include skin, heart, lungs, prostate, anal sacs, umbilicus, and digestive tract.[3, 4] Polyarthropathies of an infectious nature, other than bacterial, are being recognized more and more with the overall improvement of diagnostic abilities. Diseases such as ehrlichiosis, Rocky Mountain spotted fever, and Lyme borreliosis have been associated with polyarthropathies.[11, 39, 43, 44] Mycoplasma-induced polyarthritis occurs in cats.[10] Fungal, viral, and protozoal (leishmaniasis) arthritis are rare and are usually signs of systemic disorders.[2] See the respective chapters for specifics on diagnosis and treatment of each infection.

PATHOGENESIS

Polyarthritis secondary to infectious diseases can result either from systemic spread of organisms to the joints, with subsequent inflammatory reactions, or from development of immune complexes that circulate systemically, eventually depositing in joint tissues with resultant immune complex–mediated injury. If the organisms involved in the primary disease cannot be recovered from the joints, this failure suggests an immune complex–mediated cause for the polyarthritis rather than a direct spread of microorganisms.

After direct bacterial invasion, an acute inflammatory response occurs within the joint. There is a complex set of interactions between host defenses and various bacterial components, including enzymes, exotoxins, and endotoxins. Synovial fluid levels increase, causing higher intra-articular pressure, ischemia, and release or activation of cartilage matrix–damaging enzymes. Cartilage damage occurs quickly and is irreversible. Glycosaminoglycan depletion occurs within the first 5 days followed by cartilage softening and fissuring. This sequence of events leads to the mechanical weakening of the subchondral bone as well as the cascade of changes within the synovial fluid, articular cartilage, and cartilage matrix.

Arthritis can develop in infectious diseases in the absence of detectable organisms in synovial tissues. Immune complex deposition in joints usually occurs in more chronic, persistent infections. Circulating antibody levels increase, resulting in formation of soluble antigen-antibody complexes that circulate from the site of infection and deposit in joints. Furthermore, after recovery from infections, when organisms had entered synovial tissues by local spread or hematogenous means, persistent inactivated antigens or bacterial fragments may perpetuate the inflammatory process. Antibacterial therapy may also produce cell wall–free bacteria (L forms) that are difficult to detect and that can persist, causing continued inflammation (see Chapter 32).

CLINICAL SIGNS

Monoarthropathies cause an acute limb lameness and have been most common in medium- and large-breed male dogs.[4] The affected joint is usually swollen, warm, and often painful. Systemic signs, including fever, anorexia, and lethargy, are uncommon or variable. Most signs follow some type of insult to the affected joint. In cases of **polyarthropathies**, secondary to hematogenous spread, there are often systemic signs along with joint abnormalities. Onset of illness may be the classic acute form or the more chronic, local, and low grade. Lameness may vary from mild to severe; however, swelling is usually present in the joints distal to the shoulder and hip.

DIAGNOSIS

In most cases, clinical signs allow a presumptive diagnosis; however, the definitive diagnosis is based on evaluation of synovial fluid obtained via arthrocentesis. The synovial fluid will have increased turbidity and a poor mucin clot and may have an abnormal color. Cytologic examination will reveal increased total WBC counts with a shift in the cell population to polymorphonuclear leukocytes. Bacteria may be visualized; however, in many septic joints no organisms are detected. Direct synovial fluid culture samples should be taken. These cultures do not always yield bacterial growth even when bacteria are seen microscopically. Thus, inoculation of blood culture media with the synovial fluid sample should also be done to improve the chances for bacterial growth. These blood culture samples should be allowed to incubate for 24 hours at 37°C before they are placed on culture media.[33] In cats, L-form and feline syncytium-forming arthritis is erosive, whereas mycoplasmal, caliciviral, feline infectious peritonitis, and borrelial arthritis are nonerosive.[10] Negative results from a joint with changes typical of infective arthritis may be caused by an anaerobe that is difficult to culture. For handling specimens for anaerobic culture, see Chapters 33 and 41. Culture of biopsied synovial tissue may be more sensitive than that of synovial fluid.

Hematologic and biochemical abnormalities may indicate systemic inflammatory or infectious diseases associated with arthritis. Inflammatory leukograms may be associated with systemic infections or may be seen secondary to the inflammation of an infected joint. Thrombocytopenia may be observed in animals with blood stream infections or rickettsial diseases. Biochemical features of bacteremia may include increased serum alkaline phosphatase activity, hypoalbuminemia, and hypoglycemia. Proteinuria can be associated with glomerular diseases that may result from the same diseases causing immune complex or embolic polyarthritis.

Radiographs can also be of some use; however, early signs are usually too nonspecific to allow a diagnosis. By the time substantive radiographic signs appear, there is severe loss of bone mineral, intra-articular cartilage erosion, and cartilage matrix breakdown. Early signs include joint effusion and associated periarticular soft tissue swelling. Later signs include joint surface pitting or irregularities and subchondral bony lysis. Nuclear scintigraphy can provide supportive data earlier than conventional radiography; however, it is impractical in most practice settings.

THERAPY

Goals of treatment are eradication of the causative agent and preservation of the articular cartilage. Regardless of the cause, infectious arthritis warrants aggressive early treatment. In animals with **monoarthropathy**, treatment should include the adequate drainage of suppurative material, debridement of the accessible necrotic tissue, and copious lavage of the joint. A further benefit in the immature patient is decompression of the joint to avoid further vascular embarrassment of the epiphysis. Initial antimicrobial therapy centers on parenteral bactericidal antibiotics.

Adequate drainage and debridement of the joint are best accomplished by arthrotomy. Needle aspirations are difficult and do not provide for adequate debridement, drainage, or extensive lavage. In acute infections, primary closure of the joint after copious lavage is usually adequate. In more advanced cases, partial closure or application of a drainage system may be considered. Both of these methods require intensive postsurgical management.

Choice for antimicrobial therapy should be based on culture and susceptibility results. Initially, before obtaining culture results or in cases with negative results, antimicrobial choices should be based on the empirical criteria (see Tables 86–2 and 86–3). The drug should be bactericidal, active against β-lactamase–producing *Staphylococcus*, parenterally administered, and broad spectrum. Initially, antibiotics should be given intravenously for 48 to 72 hours and then orally for a minimum of 21 days. In more advanced cases, the antibiotic should be administered for at least 6 to 8 weeks. Post-treatment joint aspiration for cytology and culture should be considered in all cases.

Passive flexion and extension of the affected joint are advisable as soon as the patient tolerates the procedure. Exercise should be restricted to walks on a leash during the antimicrobial treatment period. For an additional 6 to 10 weeks, exercise should be increased gradually, but the dog should always be on a leash. Alternatively, or in addition, swimming is an excellent mode of physical therapy and can be encouraged as soon as all skin incisions or wounds are healed.

The prognosis is primarily determined by the amount of destruction of the articular cartilage and is difficult to estimate. Clinical evaluation over the next 1 to 2 months with radiographs on the second visit may begin to define the amount and severity of changes that have occurred; however, degenerative changes to the point at which the patient is showing clinical signs may take months.

Distinguishing infectious **polyarthropathies** from immune-mediated causes is warranted because immunosuppression can lead to disastrous consequences if systemic infections are present. A further problem is that infectious processes may be responsible for inciting immune-mediated joint diseases through the deposition of immune complexes and/or persistence of foreign antigens in synovial tissues. Nevertheless, immunosuppression is often reserved as a final modality in cases in which infection cannot be definitively incriminated. Because of the high frequency of tetracycline-susceptible organisms that cause polyarthritis, such as *Borrelia, Ehrlichia, Mycoplasma*, and L-forms, these drugs are often instituted as first treatment. Caution should be taken in attributing a favorable clinical response to an infection because tetracyclines are known to reduce their inflammatory effects (see Tetracyclines, Chapter 34).

Treatment of polyarthropathies associated with hematogenous bacterial agents is far more difficult for complete resolution. In these cases, diagnosis of the cause of the septic event must be addressed simultaneously with management of joint infection. Multiple arthrotomies are not feasible in most cases, and needle aspiration may be the only viable option for removal of a portion of suppurative material. Antibiotic therapy is the mainstay of treatment and should be aggressive, as described previously. Follow-up evaluation, physical therapy, and prognosis are also similar to those described for single joint treatment.

Infectious Myositis

Inflammatory response in muscle can have infectious and noninfectious causes. Infectious inflammatory myositis can be divided into generalized or local disease. The majority of generalized infections are polymyopathies and are polysystemic. Muscular complications are part of the overall disease. In contrast, localized infectious myositis is usually a component of trauma-induced injury to the soft tissues of a confined region in which the regional musculature is involved. Noninfectious myopathies are usually classified as immune mediated; however, an underlying infectious agent may have provoked an antigenic response against the muscle. Classic examples of this syndrome in people are viral infections, which incite an immunologic attack against muscle. In either case, in this chapter discussion is limited to the management of muscle inflammation directly caused by infectious agents.

POLYMYOSITIS

Etiology

Infectious polymyopathies can be caused by bacteria, viruses, and protozoa (see Table 86–1). Examples of these include clostridial and spirochetal infections, hepatozoonosis, toxoplasmosis, and neosporosis.[1, 12, 13, 37]

Clinical Findings

Clinical signs vary depending on potential infective agents. The site of infection can also markedly influence the observed abnormalities. A puppy with myocarditis from parvovirus infection has signs that are far different from those in a cat with generalized toxoplasmosis or a dog with tetanus. Neosporosis of puppies may have less painful muscular involvement, which manifests clinically as paresis, paralysis, and rigid contracture of the affected area. Leptospirosis, hepatozoonosis, or toxoplasmosis may cause significant generalized muscle pain.[36] There may be associated neural tissue inflammation in some diseases, which amplifies clinical paresis. With acute inflammation, there is also swelling of the affected muscle regions. This is also seen in localized disease. Chronic disease is characterized by atrophy, fibrosis, and contracture.

Diagnosis

Polymyositis is determined on the basis of clinical signs, elevated serum muscle enzyme (creatine kinase [CK] and aspartate aminotransferase) activities, and electromyographic (EMG) changes. EMG findings can include continuous insertional discharges, high-frequency discharges, and normal nerve conduction velocities. Biopsy of the muscle can often provide valuable information. Histologic evidence of necrosis and inflammation confirms polymyositis but may not provide the specific cause. Biopsy samples can identify the source of the myositis, if infectious agents, such as *Hepatozoon* schizonts, *Toxoplasma* or *Neospora* tachyzoites, or clostridial organisms, are seen in the tissue.[1, 13, 30, 37] Serial serologic titers can provide valuable information in toxoplasmal and leptospiral infections. Additional information on most aforementioned organisms can be found in the chapters specifically dedicated to these infectious agents.

Therapy

Therapy should be directed toward the specific agent. For example, toxoplasmosis is treated with clindamycin. Initial treatment should be parenteral for the first week if the animal is severely affected. Only after clinical improvement is seen should oral administration be used. Antimicrobial treatment for myositis is usually continued for a minimum of 6 to 8 weeks. Supportive care is of equal importance in these cases because there is a protracted time frame of weeks for the resolution of signs. For further information on the treatment of specific infections consult Tables 86–2 and 86–3 and respective chapters. When infectious agents are not found and immune-mediated polymyositis is suspected, immunosuppressive therapy may be required.

LOCALIZED MYOSITIS

Localized infectious myopathies are not commonly diagnosed because they are usually part of extending soft tissue infections. These focal infections are the result of trauma, either blunt in nature or a penetrating wound such as a bite. Common bacterial agents include the normal skin flora (usually *S. intermedius*), oral flora, and occasionally *Clostridium perfringens*.[30, 40] Certainly other bacteria should be considered with penetrating wounds, and cultures are advised. Clinical signs include fever and local or regional pain. Swelling with crepitus may be noted in cases of gas formation. Fistulation with drainage of foul-smelling discharge will also be apparent with anaerobic infections. Leukocytosis, predominantly neutrophilia, and high CK activity are common. Drainage of any purulent material, surgical removal of the necrotic muscle, and lavage of the region are performed when possible with intrasurgical parenteral and subsequent antimicrobial therapy. Empiric therapy should be based on the type of wound and the most likely contaminant. In most instances, use of an agent that has gram-positive and anaerobic antibacterial activity is a good first choice. Penicillin and derivatives, metronidazole, and clindamycin are recommended for anaerobic infections.

References

1. Baneth G, Harmelin A, Presentey BZ. 1995. *Hepatozoon canis* infection in two dogs. *J Am Vet Med Assoc* 206:1891–1894.
2. Becker KM, Brown NO, Denardo G. 1994. Polyarthropathy in a cat seropositive for feline synctial-forming virus and feline immunodeficiency virus. *J Am Anim Hosp Assoc* 30:225–232.
3. Bennett D, Taylor DJ. 1987. Bacterial endocarditis and inflammatory joint disease in the dog. *J Small Anim Pract* 29:347–365.
4. Bennett D, Taylor DJ. 1988. Bacterial infective arthritis in the dog. *J Small Anim Pract* 29:207–230.
5. Braund KG. 1995. Comment on diskospondylitis. *Small Anim Digest* 1:110–111.
6. Budsberg SC. 1992. Musculoskeletal Diseases, pp 364–370. *In* Lorenz MD, Cornelius LM, Ferguson DC (eds), Small animal medical therapeutics. JB Lippincott, Philadelphia, PA.
7. Budsberg SC, Brown J. 1994. Distribution of clindamycin in cortical bone during direct local infusion of the canine tibia. *J Orthop Trauma* 8:383–389.
8. Butterworth SJ, Barr FJ, Pearson GR, et al. 1995. Multiple discospondylitis associated with *Aspergillus* species infection in a dog. *Vet Rec* 136:38–41.
9. Canfield PJ, Malik R, Davis PE, et al. 1994. Multifocal idiopathic pyogranulomatous bone disease in a dog. *J Small Anim Pract* 35:370–373.

9a. Carr AP. 1997. Infectious arthritis in dogs and cats. *Vet Med* 92:786–797.

10. Carro T. 1994. Polyarthritis in cats. *Compend Cont Educ Pract Vet* 16:57–67.
11. Carro T, Pedersen NC, Beaman BL, et al. 1989. Subcutaneous abscesses and arthritis caused by a probable bacterial L-form in cats. *J Am Vet Med Assoc* 194:1583–1588.
12. Craig TM. 1989. Parasitic myositis of dogs and cats. *Semin Vet Med Surg Small Anim* 4:161–167.
13. Dubey JP, Koestner A, Piper RC. 1990. Repeated transplacental transmission of *Neospora caninum* in dogs. *J Am Vet Med Assoc* 197:857–860.
14. Dunn JK, Dennis R, Houston JEF. 1992. Successful treatment of two cases of metaphyseal osteomyelitis in the dog. *J Small Anim Pract* 33:85–89.
15. Evans RP, Nelson CL, Harrison BH. 1993. The effect of wound environment on the incidence of acute osteomyelitis. *Clin Orthop* 286:289–297.
16. Faulkner JE, Budsberg SC, 1990. Results of ventral bulla osteotomy for treatment of middle ear polyps in cats. *J Am Anim Hosp Assoc* 26:496–499.
17. Feldman DG. 1994. Glucocorticoid-responsive idiopathic nonerosive polyarthritis in a cat. *J Am Anim Hosp Assoc* 30:42–44.

17a. Fischer A, Mahaffey MB, Oliver JE. 1997. Fluoroscopically guided percutaneous disk aspiration in 10 dogs with diskospondylitis. *J Vet Intern Med* 11:284–287.

18. Fitzgerald RH, Whalen JL, Petersen SA. 1992. Pathophysiology of osteomyelitis and pharmacokinetics of antimicrobial agents in normal and osteomyelitic bone, pp 387–390. *In* Esterhai JL, Gristina AG, Poss R (eds), Musculoskeletal infection. American Academy of Orthopedic Surgeons, Park Ridge, IL.
19. Fossum TW, Hulse DA. 1992. Osteomyelitis. *Semin Vet Med Surg* 7:85–87.
20. Gilson SD, Schwartz PD. 1989. Acute hematogenous osteomyelitis in a dog. *J Am Anim Hosp Assoc* 25:684–688.
21. Gristina AG, Naylor PT, Myrvik QN. 1992. Molecular mechanisms of musculoskeletal sepsis, pp 13–20. *In* Esterhai JL, Gristina AG, Poss R (eds), Musculoskeletal infection. American Academy of Orthopedic Surgeons, Park Ridge, IL.
22. Jaffe M, Kerwin SC, Fitch RB. 1997. Canine diskospondylitis. *Compend Cont Educ Pract Vet* 19:551–555.
23. Johnson KA. 1994. Osteomyelitis in dogs and cats. *J Am Vet Med Assoc* 204:1882–1883.
24. Kornegay JN. 1993. Discospondylitis, pp 1087–1094. *In* Slatter D (ed), Textbook of small animal surgery. WB Saunders, Philadelphia, PA.
25. Kornegay JN, Anson LW. 1990. Musculoskeletal infections, pp 84–96. *In* Greene CE (ed), Infectious diseases of the dog and cat. WB Saunders, Philadelphia, PA.
26. Lamb CR. 1987. Bone scintigraphy in small animals. *J Am Vet Med Assoc* 191:1616–1621.
27. Love DN. 1989. Antimicrobial susceptibility of staphylococci isolated from dogs. *Aust Vet Pract* 19:196–200.
28. Malik R, Dowden M, Davis PE, et al. 1995. Concurrent juvenile cellulitis and metaphyseal osteopathy: an atypical canine distemper virus syndrome. *Aust Vet Pract* 25:62–65.
29. Malik R, Latter M, Love W. 1990. Bacterial diskospondylitis in a cat. *J Small Anim Pract* 31:404–406.

30. Mane MC, Vives MA, Barrera R, et al. 1992. A putative clostridial myositis in a dog. *J Small Anim Pract* 33:345–348.
31. Mayberry-Carson KJ, Tober-Meyer B, Lambe DW, et al. 1986. An electron microscopic study of the effect of clindamycin therapy on bacterial adherence and glycocalyx formation in experimental *Staphylococcus aureus* osteomyelitis. *Microbios* 48:189–206.
32. Mee AP, Gordon MT, May C, et al. 1993. Canine virus transcripts detected in the bone cells of dogs with metaphyseal osteopathy. *Bone* 14:59–67.
33. Montgomery RD, Long IR, Milton JL, et al. 1989. Comparison of aerobic culturette, synovial membrane biopsy, and blood culture medium in detection of canine bacterial arthritis. *Vet Surg* 18:300–303.
34. Moore MP. 1992. Discospondylitis. *Vet Clin North Am Small Anim Pract* 22:1027–1034.
35. Muir R, Johnson KA. 1992. Anaerobic bacteria isolated from osteomyelitis in dogs and cats. *Vet Surg* 21:463–466.
36. Poncelet L, Fontaine M, Balligand M. 1991. Polymyositis associated with *Leptospira australis* infection in a dog. *Vet Rec* 129:40.
37. Poonacha KB, Donahue JM, Nightengale JR. 1989. Clostridial myositis in a dog. *J Am Vet Med Assoc* 194:69–70.
38. Remedios AM, Wagner R, Caulhett NA, et al. 1996. Epidural abscess and discospondylitis in a dog after administration of a lumbosacral epidural analgesic. *Can Vet J* 37:106–107.
39. Roush JK, Manley PA, Dueland RT. 1989. Rheumatoid arthritis subsequent to *Borrelia burgdorferi* infection in two dogs. *J Am Vet Med Assoc* 195:951–953.
40. Seddon ML, Barry SJ. 1992. Clostridial myositis in dogs. *Vet Rec* 131:84.
41. Smith KR, Kerlin RM, Mitchell G. 1994. Diskospondylitis attributable to gram-positive filamentous bacteria in a dog. *J Am Vet Med Assoc* 205:428–432.
42. Smith MM, Vasseur PB, Saunders HM. 1989. Bacterial growth associated with metallic implants in dogs. *J Am Vet Med Assoc* 195:765–767.
43. Stockhom SL, Schmidt DA, Curtis KS, et al. 1992. Evaluation of granulocytic ehrlichiosis in dogs of Missouri, including serologic status to *Ehrlichia canis, Ehrlichia equi* and *Borrelia burgdorferi*. *Am J Vet Res* 53:63–68.
44. Straubinger RK, Straubinger AF, Harter L, et al. 1997. *Borrelia burgdorferi* migrates into joint capsules and causes up regulation of interleukin-8 in synovial membranes of dogs experimentally infected with ticks. *Infect Immun* 65:1273–1285.
45. Wei G, Kotoura Y, Oka M, et al. 1991. A bioabsorbable delivery system for antibiotic treatment of osteomyelitis. *J Bone Joint Surg Br* 73:246–252.
46. White SD, Rosychuk RA, Stewart LJ, et al. 1989. Juvenile cellulitis in dogs: 15 cases (1979–1988). *J Am Vet Med Assoc* 195:1609–1611.
47. Wolf AM, Troy GC. 1989. Deep mycotic diseases, pp 341–372. *In* Ettinger SJ (ed), Textbook of veterinary internal medicine, ed 3. WB Saunders, Philadelphia, PA.

Chapter **87**

Cardiovascular Infections

Clay A. Calvert

Bacteremia and Endocarditis

Bacteremia indicates the presence of bacteria in the blood, and, although a presumptive diagnosis can be offered on the basis of clinical findings, it can be proved only by positive blood culture results. The term *septicemia* is often used interchangeably with bacteremia and implies "toxemia" and associated inflammation along with pulmonary, cardiovascular, hepatic, and intestinal dysfunction or involvement.

ETIOLOGY

Bacteria normally are excluded from the blood stream by effective host defenses. On occasion, they do circumvent these barriers, gain access to the blood, and cause a transient bacteremia, an event that is often unnoticed in clinically healthy individuals. Bacteremia, particularly in the presence of immunosuppression, can lead to disastrous and overwhelming infection. This is referred to as sepsis, which produces a constellation of clinical signs. Sepsis often leads to decreased organ perfusion characterized by tachycardia, GI damage, liver dysfunction, lactic acidosis, and oliguria. Hypotension is consistent with septic shock, and the latter is associated with high mortality.

Any heavily colonized mucous membrane surface or localized site of infection can serve as a source for direct bacterial extension into lymphatics or blood vessels. Many procedures in hospitals circumvent or alter host defense mechanisms. The use of IV and bladder catheters or respiratory, GI, and percutaneous endoscopic biopsies allow a direct means by which bacteria may gain access to body sites that are normally protected against such invasion. Prolonged surgical procedures, such as neurologic and orthopedic ones, may lead to infection. Commonly used medical treatments such as glucocorticoids, cytotoxic drugs, and radiation therapy exert a deleterious effect on host defense mechanisms. Thus, the modern hospital provides the optimal conditions for opportunistic bacterial infections.

Bacteremia often leads to sepsis, which may lead to septic shock. If attended to quickly and aggressively, septic shock may be reversible, but it may quickly become irreversible. Irreversible shock is often associated with endotoxemia caused by gram-negative organisms, but mortality can just as easily result from gram-positive sepsis.[12] Bacterial virulence and likelihood of septic shock depend on the presence of cell capsules isolating cell wall antigens from host inflammatory cells; microbial enzyme production facilitating rapid tissue penetration; and concentration of bacteria in the blood stream, which is related to size of the inoculum and duration of bacteremia.[26, 33]

Treatment outcome is related to whether or not irreversible changes have occurred. Often bacteremia in dogs and cats is diagnosed when it is fairly advanced. The release of mediators of septic shock, such as endotoxin, exotoxin, tumor necrosis factor (TNF), and some interleukins, is associated with hypotension, hepatic failure, and breakdown of the GI mucosa-blood barrier, all of which are associated with high mortality. Rapid and aggressive intervention not only with appropriate antibiotics but also with fluid therapy is required to increase the likelihood of survival. Prevention of bacteremia, identification of high-risk patients (e.g., chemotherapy patients, otherwise immunosuppressed or debilitated patients, patients undergoing invasive procedures), and early recognition of sepsis are critical to reducing overall mortality.

EPIDEMIOLOGY

Prevalence

Aerobic bacteremia in a veterinary hospital population was found to occur in approximately 1% of the internal medicine case load and 0.3% of the general hospital accessions when blood cultures were procured because of suspected sepsis. It is safe to assume that the incidence of bacteremia in dogs and cats is significantly underestimated, particularly in referral and emergency hospitals. Affected dogs can be any age. Although there are equal numbers of male and female dogs with bacteremia, there is approximately a 2:1 male-female ratio of dogs with bacterial endocarditis and diskospondylitis.

A predisposition of large male dogs to bacterial endocarditis has been observed. Although chronic or subacute bacterial prostatitis has been identified in some bacteremic male dogs, a causal relationship is difficult to prove. Nonetheless, the prostate gland should be suspected as a potential nidus of bacteremia in large middle-aged or older male dogs. Chronic seeding of the blood stream by sites of infection such as bone and the prostate gland probably predisposes them to bacterial endocarditis. Bacteriuria, commonly associated with bacteremia, diskospondylitis, and bacterial endocarditis, may indicate a possible source or a consequence of bacteremia.

Various factors influence the relative frequency of etiologic agents among different hospitals. Surgical and trauma practices may experience a higher incidence of gram-negative and anaerobic infections. The site of local infection and prior antibiotic therapy and whether the infection is nosocomial or community acquired determine the most likely offending microbes. The percentages of isolation of various organisms from dogs and cats with bacteremia and bacterial endocarditis are summarized in Table 87–1. Because the recognized prevalence of bacteremia in cats has not equaled that of dogs, most of the discussion that follows concerns the disease in dogs. Much of the information can be extrapolated for diagnosing and treating feline cardiovascular infections.

Staphylococcus

Coagulase-positive staphylococci are among the most common pathogens. Manifestations of their infection vary from trivial, as in some pyodermas, to overwhelming sepsis. Coagulase-positive *S. intermedius* (also see Etiology, Chapters 36 and 85) have been the most common bacteria isolated from blood cultures of dogs with intravascular infections, diskospondylitis, and bacterial endocarditis. Staphylococcal bacteremia is not, however, synonymous with endocarditis, especially when an obvious extravascular source for the bacteremia can be identified. Common sources for blood stream infection include abscesses and skin and wound infections. Staphylococci tend to spread from localized abscesses, wounds, and deep pyodermas into the blood stream by invading blood vessels and producing septic thrombi or by lymphatics and incompetent lymph nodes. Metastatic foci of infection are common and often involve the kidneys, bones, joints, and heart valves.

S. intermedius is normally present on canine hair and skin, and an association of cutaneous infections with staphylococcal bacteremia in dogs is to be expected. These staphylococci also may gain entry into the blood stream of dogs from foci such as acute osteomyelitis, diskospondylitis, septic arthritis, aspiration pneumonia, and genitourinary infection.

Coagulase-negative staphylococci, commonly called *S. epidermidis*, may be cultured from blood specimens but are often not fully identified in clinical microbiology laboratories.

Table 87–1. Frequency of Isolation of Bacteria From Positive Blood Culture[a]

BACTERIA	CANINE ENDOCARDITIS (n = 58)	CANINE BACTEREMIA (n = 73)	FELINE BACTEREMIA (n = 13)
Gram Positive			
Staphylococcus intermedius	6–33	11–36	0
Streptococcus spp.	12–26	18–21	0
Enterococcus	0	4	0
Gram Negative			
Escherichia coli	6–30	18–71	14
Klebsiella pneumoniae	0	6–28	14
Salmonella	0	11–13	29
Enterobacter cloacae	0	3–8	7
Pseudomonas aeruginosa	0	6–7	0
Proteus	0	14	0
Anaerobic			
Clostridium perfringens	0	20	0
Propionibacterium acnes	6	0	14
Bacteroides spp.	0	4	14
Fusobacterium spp.	0	0	0
Pasteurella	0	3	0
Moraxella	0	2	0
Erysipelothrix rhusiopathiae	19	0	0
Corynebacterium spp.	19	3	0
Multiple species	0	53	0

[a]Values are expressed as a percentage of organisms isolated.
0 = not reported.

The majority of these are either contaminants or of no clinical importance. However, significant coagulase-negative staphylococcal bacteremia can occur in immunocompromised patients with indwelling IV catheters or profound neutropenia.

Intact skin and mucous membranes provide defense against staphylococcal invasion. When these defenses are breached, blood invasion can arise from any site but most often from localized skin or soft tissue infections, surgical wounds, catheters, bones, and joints. Although coagulase-positive staphylococci produce toxins and enzymes, none has been proved to be of importance to the development of bacteremia. Strains isolated from the blood are no more virulent than other strains. Various conditions may predispose animals to *Staphylococcus* bacteremia. Debilitation resulting from malignancies, renal failure, diabetes mellitus, and liver disease are examples. Glucocorticoids, cytotoxic drugs, and other immunosuppressive agents also contribute to such infections.

Clinical Manifestations. Staphylococcal bacteremia can vary from a fulminating infection characterized by higher fever, trembling, and tachycardia to, perhaps more commonly, a subacute syndrome characterized by more subtle, nonspecific signs. Septic shock is less frequent than that with gram-negative septicemia.

Sequelae. Perhaps the most serious complication of staphylococcal bacteremia is valvular endocarditis. Although experimental *S. aureus* endocarditis requires damage to the heart valves, in veterinary and human medicine, endocarditis usually occurs in the absence of known prior valvular disease. Congenital subaortic stenosis is the most common comorbid heart disease associated with endocarditis. It is often difficult to differentiate bacteremia alone from endocarditis.

Septic embolization of the kidneys may occur with staphylococcal bacteremia and is consistently present with valvular endocarditis of the left side of the heart. Infarcts can be detected by excretory urograms and ultrasonograms. Proteinuria and pyuria are often present, and immune complex glomerulonephritis may be a further complication. Other sites of septic embolization or abscess formation are the spleen, brain, joints, and lungs, including pulmonary arterial thromboembolism.

Disseminated intravascular coagulation (DIC) is another sequela of staphylococcal bacteremia, but its incidence is probably less than that associated with gram-negative bacteremia. Thrombocytopenia; prolongation of the activated coagulation time, prothrombin time (PT), and activated partial thromboplastin time (APTT); decreased plasma fibrinogen; and the presence of fibrin degradation products (FDPs) are consistent with the diagnosis. *S. aureus* bacteremia in people occasionally triggers a septic shock syndrome ("toxic shock") virtually indistinguishable from gram-negative bacillary endotoxic shock.

Streptococcus

Systemic streptococcal infections are common in dogs and cats (see Chapter 35). Streptococcal pneumonia may be associated with a high incidence of subsequent bacteremia. As many as one fourth of bacterial endocarditis in dogs may be the result of β-hemolytic streptococci. In bacteremic dogs with a variety of underlying illnesses, approximately 5% of blood culture results may be positive for β-hemolytic *S. canis* and 5% positive for non-β-hemolytic *S. viridans* and enterococci. Most β-hemolytic streptococci enter the blood stream via the skin, whereas α-hemolytic streptococci usually enter via breaks in the mucous membranes. Non-β-hemolytic streptococci are normal skin commensals and occasionally may contaminate improperly collected blood culture specimens.

Group B streptococci can cause sepsis in both dogs and cats. In puppies, group B streptococci have been incriminated as a cause of bacteremia and death in fading puppies. *S. agalactiae* was associated with valvular endocarditis, septic endocarditis, and DIC in a dog.[25] In people, bacteremia caused by group D streptococci (enterococci), including *S. faecium* and *S. faecalis*, usually originates from the urinary tract but also can occur after manipulation of the lower bowel. Enterococcal endocarditis, which has been reported in dogs, is especially serious because, unlike most other streptococci, enterococci are often resistant to penicillins and cephalosporins.

Gram-Positive Aerobic Bacilli

Diphtheroids, a heterogenous group of bacteria including the genus *Corynebacterium*, are often interpreted as contaminants when isolated from blood culture because they normally inhabit skin and mucous membrane surfaces. *Corynebacterium* may account for approximately 5% of cases of bacteremia in dogs and has been associated with endocarditis. *Corynebacterium* spp. are common isolates from dogs with endocarditis of the aortic valve. *Erysipelothrix* is occasionally incriminated (see Chapter 35). *Bacillus* spp. are frequent blood culture contaminants. In the immunocompromised host, however, *B. cereus* and *B. subtilis* can cause serious septicemias. *Corynebacterium* and *Bacillus* should be isolated from multiple blood cultures before bacteremia is diagnosed.

Gram-Negative Bacilli

The term *gram-negative bacteremia* is typically applied to bacteremias associated with the Enterobacteriaceae and Pseudomonadaceae. Bacteremias resulting from other gram-negative agents, such as *Pasteurella*, *Brucella*, and *Salmonella*, although producing similar clinical manifestations, are usually considered discrete clinical entities. *Salmonella enteritidis* was the most common organism isolated from bacteremic cats in one study.[12] Gram-negative bacillary bacteremia usually represents a serious opportunistic infection that has developed subsequent to significant depression of host defenses, because these bacteria are rarely considered primary invaders. Gram-negative bacteremia is often associated with high mortality, and the number of such infections has increased along with the use of new antibiotics, the greater use of invasive medical devices, and the trend toward more immunosuppressive therapy for malignancies and inflammatory diseases.

Gram-negative bacilli are ideally suited for opportunistic infections. Ubiquitous in the environment, they are major components of the fecal flora, are normal skin inhabitants, and are present in all hospital environments. They tend to be relatively resistant to moisture, drying, and some disinfectants. Some may persist and multiply in water. These agents tend to develop antibiotic resistance to a greater degree than gram-positive bacteria. Although antibiotic exposure per se does not induce resistance, it does provide a selective reproductive advantage to bacteria that are resistant.

Of bacteria of the family Enterobacteriaceae, *Escherichia coli* is the most common blood stream isolate from animals. *E. coli* is abundant in the lower GI tract, which often serves as a reservoir for infection of other body sites. The urinary tract and large intestine are common sources for gram-negative bacteremias. The respiratory tract and infections of the skin and wounds can also serve as portals of entry to the blood stream for gram-negative microbes.

Oropharyngeal and fecal colonization with gram-negative bacilli may increase progressively in seriously ill hospitalized patients as their clinical status deteriorates. Gram-negative bacteria not only gain access to the blood from extravascular foci, but also may originate from IV catheters and urinary catheters and from septic thrombophlebitic conditions. In extravascular infections, bacteria often gain access to the blood via lymphatics or invasion of small blood vessels within a site of infection. Other sources for blood stream invasion include drainage tubes, contaminated IV fluids, and contaminated aerosolization devices; disrupted mucosal barriers (e.g., after dental procedures or endoscopic examinations) and decubitus ulcers. In contrast to staphylococcal bacteremia, gram-negative bacteremia in dogs and cats rarely is associated with septic thrombosis and metastatic abscess formation. Presumably, this finding can be explained by the rapidly progressive course of gram-negative bacteremia that is associated with endotoxemia (also see Chapter 38). Animals are cured or do not survive to develop embolic complications.

Although common in the environment and occasionally present on mucosal surfaces, *Pseudomonas* has rarely been isolated from deeper tissues of healthy patients. It has been more common in otitis externa, dermatitis, cystitis, and respiratory infections of dogs. Because *Pseudomonas* is an opportunist, its rapid colonization with subsequent development of bacteremia is much more likely to occur after disruption of host defenses, especially cutaneous barriers (surgery, IV catheters, and burns) and depletion of neutrophils, as occurs with cancer chemotherapy patients.[8] Extensive antibiotic use or contaminated IV fluids may also predispose patients to *Pseudomonas* bacteremia. Most cases of *Pseudomonas* bacteremia in dogs have been nosocomial.[8]

Clinical Manifestations. Although there may be considerable case-to-case variation in the severity of disease, the signs and symptoms of gram-negative bacteremia are virtually identical. In the classic case, fever, trembling, and sometimes vomiting are early signs. These may develop within hours after manipulation or biopsy of an area of focal infection or after manipulation, insertion, or removal of IV or urinary catheters. Often, however, the clinical manifestations of bacteremia are subtle. Fever is almost always present at the onset but may be minimal in patients receiving glucocorticoids or cytotoxic drugs and in uremic and debilitated patients. Tachypnea, tachycardia, hypotension, and oliguria are consistent with sepsis and septic shock. Thrombocytopenia of a mild to moderate degree is common. When a pre-existing local infection exists, the emergence of bacteremia may be obscured by the associated signs and preoccupation of attending clinicians with that infection.

Prevention is easier than treatment of gram-negative bacteremia. The use of IV and urinary catheters should be limited to instances in which they are absolutely necessary. They should be inserted under scrupulously sterile conditions and removed or changed within 2 to 3 days. Strict aseptic precautions in the management of wounds, use of tube drainage systems, prevention of decubitus, and limitation of prophylactic antibiotics are all important in preventing opportunistic infections for all patients, particularly those with reduced defense capabilities.

Anaerobic Bacteria

Anaerobic bacteria, particularly anaerobic gram-negative rods, are now considered serious bacteremic pathogens. Development of anaerobic blood stream infections may be encouraged by the presence of periodontal disease, deep abscesses, granulomas, peritonitis, osteomyelitis, septic arthritis, and septic pleural effusion (also see Chapter 41). *Clostridium perfringens* is the most common canine isolate. Both *Bacteroides* and *Fusobacterium* are more commonly isolated from cats. A mechanically correctable lesion (abscess, perforated bowel, necrotic tissue) is often the source of anaerobic bacteremia, although impaired host defenses are not a prerequisite for infection. In people, *Bacteroides* usually enters the blood stream via intra-abdominal sources, such as GI and genital inflammatory diseases. *Fusobacterium* bacteremia often originates from infections of the respiratory tract. Characteristics of anaerobic bacteremia include variable (sometimes absent) fever, thrombophlebitis, and icterus, particularly with *Bacteroides* bacteremia. Sequelae to anaerobic bacteremia include metastatic abscess formation and endocarditis. Clostridial bacteremia tends to have a relatively insidious clinical course without obvious signs of sepsis, although septic shock may occur occasionally.

Polymicrobial Bacteremia

Blood stream infection with multiple species of bacteria occur in up to 20% of dogs and 30% of cats with positive blood culture results. Anaerobic bacteria, especially *Bacteroides* and *Clostridium*, are often components of polymicrobial infection in people and dogs. Clinical implications of polymicrobial compared with monomicrobial bacteremia are not clearly established. Higher mortality rates have not been observed in dogs or cats with polymicrobial bacteremia compared with those with monomicrobial bacteremia. Factors that predispose patients to polymicrobial bacteremia include neutropenia, GI and urogenital tract obstruction and infection, bowel perforation and surgery, and prostatic surgery.

PATHOGENESIS

Bacteremia develops as a normal but transient phenomenon whenever bacteria-laden mucosal surfaces such as the nasopharynx and the GI and genital mucosae are traumatized. Clinically important bacteremia may occur when the blood stream is seeded with high numbers of bacteria via venous and lymphatic drainage from sites of infections. Fluid accumulation, high tissue pressure, surgical or physical manipulation of abscesses, areas of cellulitis, or other infected tissues all favor lymphatic and venous spread of bacteria to the systemic circulation. In most healthy individuals, bacteria are removed from the blood stream rapidly and effectively through phagocytosis by fixed tissue macrophages in the spleen and liver. Persistent bacteremia ensues when bacteria multiply at a rate that exceeds the mononuclear phagocyte system's ability to remove them. Serum from healthy patients is bactericidal largely because of the presence of a number of humoral defense factors, including specific antibacterial antibodies of the IgM and IgG classes as well as complement proteins, properdin, and fibronectin. Bacterial capsules and other virulence factors may delay clearance of blood-borne bacteria, whereas bacteria that activate complement via the alternate (antibody-independent) pathway are cleared rapidly. Glucocorticoids apparently do not affect clearance of bacteria from the blood stream but may allow greater multiplication in extravascular tissues, thereby facilitating increased blood stream entry.

Bacteremia associated with clinical findings such as fever; hepatic, intestinal, renal, pulmonary, and cardiovascular dysfunction; and evidence of inflammation is referred to as sepsis. Signs of severe sepsis include hypothermia, oliguria, respiratory failure, and lactic acidosis. Bacterial toxins are responsible for sepsis and can lead to septic shock, the hallmarks of which are decreased cardiac output and hypotension. Endotoxin produced by gram-negative bacteria has been the most studied. Endotoxin is composed of lipid, polysaccharide, and protein, and it is the lipid portion (lipid A) that is responsible for toxicity. Endotoxins interact with macrophages, neutrophils, and vascular endothelia by binding to cell receptors, causing release of mediators of sepsis, the magnitude of which is directly related to the endotoxin concentration.[3, 26]

Numerous mediators of sepsis and septic shock exist. Cytokines, released primarily from macrophages, include interleukins and TNF.[2, 11, 16, 26] Lipid mediators, arising principally from neutrophils, platelets, and vascular endothelia, include leukotrienes, prostaglandins, and platelet-activating factors.[3, 30, 36] Normally, these mediators interact with inflammatory cells, vascular endothelia, and platelets in a complex fashion that modulates immune function.[3] However, high concentrations of endotoxin stimulate high concentrations of mediators, which produce both specific actions and potentiating actions on other mediators. TNF has been associated with hypotension, respiratory dysfunction, anorexia, and cachexia. Interleukin-1 causes fever, neutropenia followed by neutrophilia, and pulmonary vascular sequestration of granulocytes.[2] Platelet-activating factor causes platelet activation and aggregation; neutrophil activation, aggregation, and chemotaxis; vasodilation and hypotension; vasoconstriction in the heart and lungs; increased vascular permeability; and GI ulceration. Thromboxane, a product of the prostaglandin cascade, is associated with vasoconstriction and platelet aggregation.[3, 28] Leukotrienes are chemotactic and increase vascular permeability.[30] Cytokines and lipid mediators invoke secondary mediators of sepsis such as vasopressin, angiotensin II, catecholamines, histamine, and serotonin.[16] Organ failure associated with septic shock is the result of hypoxia, free radical and lysozyme damage, thrombosis, and necrosis.[6, 16]

Sources of Infection and Risk Factors

The most common sources of bacteremia include infections of the GI and genitourinary tracts, skin and wounds, respiratory tract, abdomen, and biliary tract. IV catheter–associated infections also occur. The sources of infection are not always identified.

A variety of factors, summarized in Table 87–2, have been cited as predisposing patients to bacteremia. When considering mortality from bacteremia and sepsis, the single most important factor influencing outcome after infection is the severity of the patient's underlying disease. Death from bacteremia is much less likely to occur if the animal was previously healthy.

Neutropenic patients are very susceptible to sepsis. Cancer chemotherapy–neutropenia is particularly dangerous because the destruction of GI crypt epithelial cells is a concomitant problem. Enteric bacteria gain access to the blood via the damaged mucosal barrier, and the neutropenia renders phagocytosis of these bacteria ineffective. To complicate matters, fever may be absent or minimal as a clue to the presence of bacteremia, because neutrophils are a component of the inflammatory process. The febrile neutropenic patient is a medical emergency if sepsis is the suspected cause. Splenectomized patients are also predisposed to bacterial sepsis because the spleen was an important component of the host's defense mechanisms.

Table 87–2. Factors Predisposing to Bacteremia in Dogs and Cats

SPECIFIC INFECTIOUS DISEASES
Ehrlichiosis
Feline immunodeficiency virus infection
Feline leukemia virus infection
Canine parvoviral enteritis
Feline panleukopenia
SITES OF INFECTION
Abscesses
Burns
Colitis
Stomatitis
Pyoderma
Urogenital infections
Penetrating wounds
Abdominal surgery
Protracted surgery (i.e., spinal and orthopedic)
Perianal surgery
Musculoskeletal infections
IMMUNODEFICIENCIES
Diabetes mellitus
Glucocorticoids
Phagocyte defects
Hepatic failure
Renal failure
Solid tumors
Hematologic malignancies
Splenectomy
Old age
Shock
IATROGENIC MANIPULATIONS
Dental prophylaxis
Endoscopic procedures
IV catheterization
Antimicrobial therapy
Urogenital tract manipulations

Bacterial Endocarditis

It is assumed that prior heart valve damage is an important predisposing factor for development of valvular bacterial endocarditis. Experimentally, it is difficult to induce bacterial endocarditis of heart valves in dogs unless the valves have been physically or chemically damaged or unless highly virulent bacteria are used. The most common congenital heart defect associated with valvular bacterial endocarditis in dogs is subaortic stenosis. However, most dogs with confirmed valvular bacterial endocarditis have no history of valvular disease or congenital heart defect.

Stress or endothelial injury leading to collagen exposure on the valve surface has been shown to result in platelet aggregation. Subsequent bacteremia may result in colonization of the platelet-fibrin thrombus. The pathogenesis of subacute bacterial endocarditis may involve these platelet-fibrin thrombi. In addition, a high titer of agglutinating antibody against the infective bacteria may predispose a patient to bacterial endocarditis. Certain pathogenic bacteria, such as some staphylococci, streptococci, and *Pseudomonas,* may produce endocarditis in the absence of predisposing factors because of their ability to adhere to normal canine heart valves.

Time Course of Bacteremia

Relating the time course of bacteremia to the infecting organism is not always possible. Peracute bacteremia, which

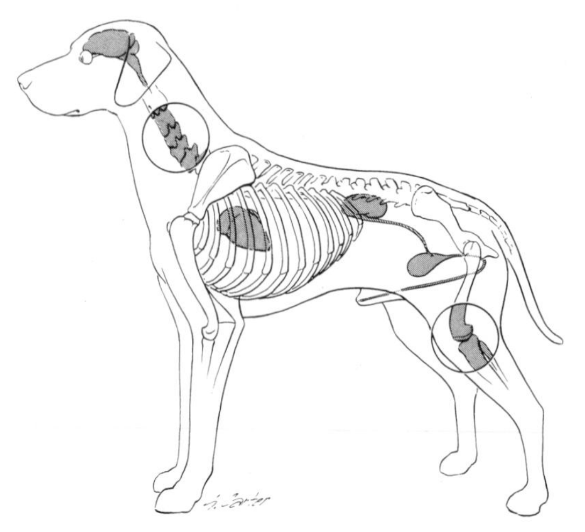

Figure 87–1. Sites of predilection (shaded areas) for bacterial embolization in bacteremia include the meninges, intervertebral disc spaces, heart valves, urinary tract, and joints.

Table 87–4. Frequency of Various Heart Valve Involvement in 44 Dogs With Necropsy-Proved Bacterial Endocarditis[a]

AFFECTED VALVES	DOGS AFFECTED (%)
Mitral	71
Aortic and others	34
Aortic only	23
Mitral and aortic	14
Pulmonic	2
Tricuspid	14

[a]Recent trends indicate a preponderance of aortic valve infections and less mitral valve involvement.

develops over several hours often in debilitated or immunosuppressed patients, may be the result of either gram-positive or gram-negative infection. Acute bacteremia develops over 12 to 24 hours and is usually the result of gram-negative or staphylococcal infection. Subacute bacteremia develops and persists for several weeks or longer and is often the result of gram-positive and sometimes anaerobic infections, although acute sepsis can also occur in the susceptible host. Chronic bacteremia lasting weeks to months may result from infections with microorganisms of low toxicity (e.g., *Brucella canis* and *S. intermedius*); sequestration of bacterial colonies on heart valves or in bone; abscess formation in the liver, spleen, kidneys, or muscles; or partial response to antibacterial therapy. The time course also is associated with the seriousness of clinical signs, how quickly the patient is presented to the attending clinician, how quickly the bacteremia is suspected, and the appropriateness of treatment.

Sequelae

Secondary embolic abscesses, splenomegaly, hematuria, and proteinuria are more often associated with bacterial endocarditis than with bacteremia alone (Fig. 87–1 and Table 87–3). Metastatic infection can result in life-threatening complications. Virtually all dogs with bacterial endocarditis of the left side of the heart experience multiple continuous embolizations and renal infarctions, which may lead to renal failure (Fig. 87–2). Septic embolization of the spleen occurs in most dogs with bacterial endocarditis, although clinically apparent complications are uncommon. Subacute and chronic bacteremia can result in sustained antigenic stimulation of the immune system and increased circulating immunoglobulin. Circulating immune complexes may be deposited in many tissues, leading to development of polyarthritis, myositis, vasculitis, and glomerulonephritis. In animals of any age, diskospondylitis may occur, whereas younger, growing animals may develop metaphyseal embolization with resultant hypertrophic osteodystrophy.[34]

Valvular damage and dysfunction, myocardial microembolization, and cardiac rhythm disturbances are the principal cardiac consequences of bacteremia and bacterial endocarditis. The mitral and aortic valves are most often affected (Table 87–4 and Fig. 87–3). Vegetations of the aortic or mitral valve lead to valvular regurgitation (insufficiency), which induces volume overload of the heart and left-sided congestive heart failure. Arrhythmias are the primary consequences of myocardial embolization. Major coronary artery occlusion and myocardial infarction are unusual in dogs with bacterial endocarditis.

Aortic valvular endocarditis may lead to a dissecting valve-ring abscess with infection of the septum or a major component of the atrioventricular (AV) conduction system. AV heart blocks have been found in dogs with endocarditis but are uncommon.

Table 87–3. Sequelae to Bacteremia

AUTOIMMUNE DISORDERS
Positive ANA, LE, Coombs' testing
IMMUNE COMPLEX DISEASES
Glomerulonephritis, polyvasculitis, polyarthritis
BACTERIAL EMBOLIZATION
Meningitis, polyarthritis, renal microembolization
DISKOSPONDYLITIS
Hyperesthesia, spinal cord compression
BACTERIAL ENDOCARDITIS
Valvular insufficiency, cardiac arrhythmias, congestive failure
ENDOTOXEMIA
Shock, hypotension, coagulopathy

ANA = antinuclear antibody; LE = lupus erythematosus.

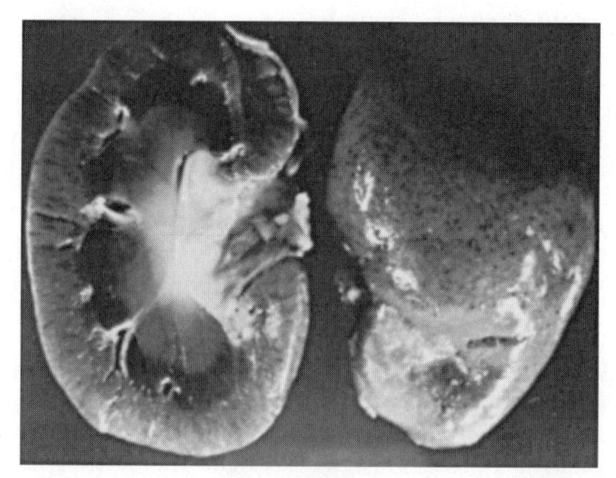

Figure 87–2. Kidney specimens of a dog with bacterial endocarditis demonstrating renal infarction resulting from embolization.

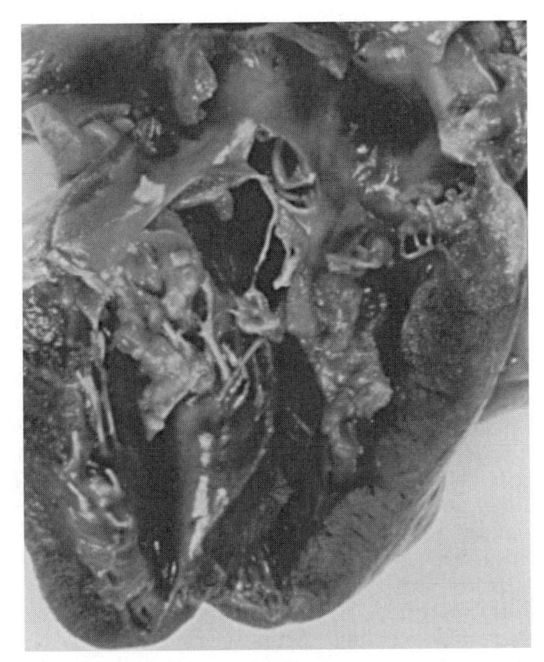

Figure 87–3. Severe proliferative lesions of the mitral valves from a dog with vegetative endocarditis.

CLINICAL FINDINGS

The clinical signs associated with bacteremia and bacterial endocarditis are similar (Table 87–5). The prevalence of lameness, heart murmurs, cardiac rhythm disturbances, embolic complications, and immune-mediated phenomena is greater with bacterial endocarditis. Gram-negative sepsis usually manifests peracute or acute clinical signs. Bacterial endocarditis tends, however, to be subacute or chronic and is manifest by low-grade or episodic fever, although body temperature is sometimes normal.

Fever, tachycardia, tachypnea, pale or "mud"-colored mucous membranes are the hallmarks of sepsis. Fever is most often associated with gram-positive or polymicrobial bacteremia and least often associated with anaerobic bacteremia.[12]

Reversible septic shock in patients with adequate intravascular volume is often associated with brick-red mucous membranes, tachycardia, high cardiac output, and normal or low blood pressure. Hypodynamic shock occurs in patients with decreased intravascular fluid volume, and affected individuals tend to be pale, cold, tachycardic, and hypotensive. The latter can be corrected with rapid, aggressive fluid therapy, unless the stage of irreversible shock (elevated blood lactate concentration, hepatic failure, oliguria, hypotension, cold extremities) has developed. Patients with irreversible shock cannot be stabilized by fluid therapy because of massive fluid leakage through permeable endothelium, vasodilation, and possible myocardial failure.[9] Cardiac output may be increased in such patients with rapid-acting, powerful inotropes such as dopamine and dobutamine.[19, 24]

Table 87–5. Clinical Signs in 122 Dogs With Either Bacteremia Alone or Bacterial Endocarditis

CLINICAL SIGNS	BACTEREMIA (n = 77)	BACTERIAL ENDOCARDITIS (n = 45)
Fever (> 39.4°C [102.9°F])	75	70
Lameness		
Total	19	34
Shifting	6	18
Vomiting	17	35
Heart murmur	6	74
Ventricular arrhythmia	5	27

Dogs with bacteremia usually display some combination of lethargy, anorexia, and GI disturbances, such as vomiting and diarrhea, at the time of initial bacteremia. After the initial clinical signs, dogs with gram-positive bacteremia or early bacterial endocarditis variably manifest fever, lameness, myalgia, lethargy, and anorexia. Dogs with subacute or chronic bacterial endocarditis may exhibit signs of left-sided congestive heart failure, especially if the aortic valve has been damaged. Heart failure usually develops from 2 to 6 months after the onset of clinical signs of bacteremia when the aortic valve is involved. Mitral insufficiency alone seldom results in heart failure within the first year after the diagnosis. Acute cardiogenic pulmonary edema occurring in breeds not normally affected by mitral valve endocardiosis, cardiomyopathy, or congenital subaortic stenosis is often the result of bacterial endocarditis. In such cases, there is usually no history of a pre-existing heart murmur, or the heart murmur may be absent at the time of presentation.

Organ failure in bacteremic septic patients can quickly lead to septic shock. In the dog, the GI tract, liver, kidneys, and lungs, in order, are most affected. Mucosal sloughing, characterized by vomiting and bloody diarrhea, often with mucosal remnants, is commonly seen with advanced sepsis. Hepatic failure is characterized by vomiting, anorexia, and icterus. Oliguria is usually the result of hypotension and shock. In the cat, respiratory failure can occur early in the course of sepsis.

Physical examination findings from patients with bacterial endocarditis vary with the stage of disease and associated sequelae. In some dogs, lameness or polyarthritis may be the dominant clinical sign. However, lameness is an inconsistent finding in dogs with bacterial endocarditis. In some, heart failure or renal failure may distract the clinician's attention from an infectious disease.

Although often absent early in the disease course, systolic heart murmurs have been detected in most dogs with bacterial endocarditis. The murmur usually is of recent onset or latent in these animals. The systolic murmur of rapidly changing character, described in association with endocarditis in people, is less common in dogs. The presence of a systolic murmur in which intensity increases over a short period of time and evidence of a diastolic murmur are ominous signs. A diastolic murmur is often due to aortic valve regurgitation and is suggestive of vegetative endocarditis.

The presence of lameness, joint pain, muscle pain, and stiffness may suggest either immune-mediated disease or septic embolization of various tissues in dogs with bacteremia alone or endocarditis. Infective and immune-mediated arthritis may coexist. Bilaterally symmetric joint involvement is more typical of the immune-based arthritis. Lumbar or abdominal pain on palpation may suggest renal or splenic inflammation secondary to septic embolization, infarction, or abscess formation or diskospondylitis. Diskospondylitis can also result in paresis or paralysis, depending on the location and degree of spinal cord compression (see Musculoskeletal Infections, Chapter 86). In younger animals, hypertrophic osteodystrophy causing malaise, fever, anorexia, swollen limbs, and reluctance to move has been observed.

Occasionally, erosion of an artery occurs after septic embolization, and hemorrhage results. Thrombophlebitis also may produce pain and edema of an extremity. Vasculitis has commonly been associated with bacteremia, and although petechiae and ecchymoses of the mucous membranes or retina are possible, such findings in spontaneous cases have been uncommon.

DIAGNOSIS

Clinical Laboratory Findings

The leukograms of dogs with bacteremia alone and with bacterial endocarditis are similar. A neutrophilic leukocytosis with an appropriate left shift and monocytosis are present in most dogs with gram-positive or anaerobic bacteremia and in virtually all dogs with chronic bacterial endocarditis at some point during the course of disease. However, in one study, 19% of dogs with bacterial endocarditis did not have leukocytosis at any time during the course of the clinical evaluation. Leukopenia and an inappropriate left shift have been more common with bacteremia alone, usually in association with peracute and acute gram-negative infections.

A normocytic normochromic anemia commonly has been seen with subacute or chronic bacteremia and usually has been nonregenerative. A regenerative anemia occasionally has been encountered with bacterial endocarditis and probably is the result of erythrocyte destruction from physical forces associated with vegetative lesions or blood flow turbulence. Coombs' test results occasionally have been positive. Thrombocytopenia usually develops.

With advanced sepsis, hemoconcentration occurs after fluid losses from the intravascular space. Hematocrits as high as 60% to 70% may develop in severe, acute sepsis. Serum total solids tend to decrease owing to the loss of protein from the intravascular compartment.

Serum chemistry abnormalities are commonly, but not exclusively, associated with bacteremia and bacterial endocarditis. The main findings in affected dogs have been hypoalbuminemia (<2.5 mg/dl), a twofold or greater elevation of alkaline phosphatase (ALP) activity, and hypoglycemia (<80 mg/dl). Hyperglycemia occurs during the early phase (hyperdynamic phase) of septic shock.

The liver is an important site of removal of bacteria from the blood. Increased serum ALP activity is associated with both gram-positive and gram-negative infections. Bacterial toxins are associated with impaired bile metabolism and cholestasis. Hyperbilirubinemia, bilirubinuria, and icterus can occur (reactive hepatopathy of sepsis, see Chapter 90).

Hypoalbuminemia has been a common manifestation of most types of bacteremia. Subacute and chronic bacteremia may result in transcapillary leakage as a result of immune-mediated or embolic vasculitis or bacterial toxins. Sepsis also has been associated with reduced hepatic synthesis of albumin, and as many as 50% of bacteremic dogs may have increased BSP retention, suggesting reduced hepatic function. Hypocalcemia is often observed and is usually attributed to hypoalbuminemia.

Hypoglycemia may occur, and in the absence of seizures, the clinician should consider the possibility of a bacteremic episode. The mechanism of hypoglycemia is uncertain at this time; however, it may partly result from the effects of bacteria or bacterial toxins on the intermediary metabolism of glucose. In contrast, hyperglycemia has been correlated with a higher postoperative mortality in dogs than in normoglycemia or hypoglycemic septicemic dogs and cats. This finding may be related to the fact that hyperglycemia has been seen in early severe septicemia, and hypoglycemia develops in more chronically affected cases.

Hypercoagulability leading to DIC is a common sequela of bacteremic sepsis. Evidence of DIC (low fibrinogen, prolonged PT and APTT, and increased FDPs) is consistent with advanced sepsis. Major organ failure as well as cardiovascular collapse may be imminent.[19, 20, 24]

Septic patients often have metabolic acidosis with respiratory compensation. The carbon dioxide tension can decrease severely to compensate for acidemia. Hypoxemia is uncommon in awake patients. Cats suffering from endotoxemia exhibit hypoxemia, hypercarbia, and metabolic acidosis.

Blood lactate levels are often increased in septic patients. Hemoconcentration and shock cause decreased oxygen delivery to the tissues, resulting in anaerobic metabolism. Cellular oxidative respiration is inhibited by an endotoxin or a mediator.[32] Furthermore, septic patients tend to be in a hypermetabolic state, requiring increased oxygen delivery to tissues.

Proteinuria, occult hematuria, and pyuria may occur in association with bacteremia or, more commonly, with bacterial endocarditis in which renal infarction, glomerulonephritis, and renal microabscess formation are common sequelae. Urinary tract infections may be either a cause or an effect of bacteremia, and urine cultures should be submitted when abnormalities are found on urinalysis.

Test results for immune-mediated diseases, such as antinuclear antibody titer, rheumatoid factor, and lupus erythematosus cell preparation, occasionally are positive in bacteremic patients, particularly those with bacterial endocarditis.

Bacteremia is only occasionally diagnosed by direct microscopic examination of leukocytes in blood smears. Direct Gram's stains of peripheral blood are usually unrewarding, because the number of microorganisms present is often much lower than the 10^5/ml necessary for detection. Wright's stains of buffy coat smears may increase the rate of detection. Acridine orange is more sensitive than Gram's stain, because organisms can be detected at 10^4/ml concentrations. Slides must be handled carefully to prevent inadvertent contamination, which may be revealed as extracellular bacteria.

A simple method of performing leukocyte smears involves placing one drop of freshly collected, nonclotted venous blood on a clean glass coverslip and incubating it in a moist Petri dish for 25 minutes at 37°C. The clot on the coverslip is gently washed off with normal (0.9%) saline, and the coverslip with attached leukocytes is immersed in fixative (methanol or glutaraldehyde) before Giemsa staining and microscopic examination.

Radiographic and Electrodiagnostic Testing

Thoracic radiographs are usually of little value in the diagnosis of bacteremia and bacterial endocarditis, because left-sided congestive heart failure (e.g., left atrial enlargement, pulmonary edema, distention of the lobar veins) is apparent only in late stages of bacterial endocarditis. Rarely have radiopaque densities identified as valvular vegetations been visualized.[23] Bacterial endocarditis of the tricuspid or pulmonic valve is uncommon, although it produces multiple embolization of the pulmonary arterial system that appears as focal areas of mixed interstitial and alveolar lung disease.

ECGs of dogs with bacterial endocarditis are frequently abnormal. Ventricular tachyarrhythmias, the most common arrhythmias, are in most cases not life threatening. AV blocks, supraventricular arrhythmias, evidence of chamber enlargement, and ST-segment changes are observed occasionally.

Cardiac ultrasonography is an important diagnostic test for identifying bacterial endocarditis and for monitoring cardiac function in surviving dogs. Lesions of the aortic valve are not difficult to detect. Ultrasonography has made possible the presumptive diagnosis of valvular endocarditis in the absence of positive blood culture results and diastolic heart murmurs.

Blood Culture

The definitive diagnosis of bacteremia requires compatible clinical signs and laboratory data and the isolation of the offending microbe from blood cultures. As primary or secondary sites of infection, urine, CSF, and joint fluid may also contain the organism. Preferably, the bacteria should be isolated from more than one blood sample. In addition, a source of infection should be sought and attempts made to isolate an organism from that site. Negative blood culture results in bacteremic patients can occur as a result of antimicrobial therapy, chronic low-grade infections such as diskospondylitis and endocarditis, uremia, right-sided endocarditis, or nonbacterial endocarditis.

In addition to that for bacteremia, the definitive antemortem diagnosis of bacterial endocarditis requires the presence of a cardiac murmur of recent onset. The presence of ECG abnormalities indicative of bacterial endocarditis are extremely useful.

When an etiologic diagnosis is established with positive blood culture results, more appropriate and effective antibiotic therapy can be used. Low blood culture yields are a frequent complaint but probably reflect the effects of poor patient selection, improper blood culturing techniques (e.g., timing, volume, number of specimens), and inadequate laboratory processing (e.g., failure to culture for anaerobes). By adhering to recommended guidelines for obtaining and processing blood culture specimens, the diagnostic yield from blood cultures is rewarding.

Although empiric multiple antibiotic therapy often has been instituted in critically ill patients before obtaining culture results, the effort and expense required for blood culture have been justifiable because improper treatment may increase mortality from bacteremia. Furthermore, prior administration of antimicrobials appears to slow but not prevent bacterial isolation.[12]

Indications. Blood culture is indicated in acutely ill patients with fever or hypothermia; with leukocytosis, especially with a marked left shift; with neutropenia; and with unexplained tachycardia, hypoglycemia, circulatory collapse, tachypnea or dyspnea, anuria or oliguria, icterus, thrombocytopenia, or DIC. Complementary cultures of urine and any other obvious sites of infection should be obtained. Blood cultures are also indicated in animals with unexplained fever, intermittent or shifting lameness, recent or changing cardiac murmur, or other signs of bacterial endocarditis.

Bacteremia in animals with endocarditis or other intravascular infections is usually continuous, although low level, and fewer blood cultures are necessary for a positive diagnosis. Intermittent bacteremia or fungemia usually reflects established infections extrinsic to the blood stream. Generally, it is suggested that a maximum of three blood cultures obtained over a 24-hour period is usually sufficient to diagnose endocarditis. Culturing blood during febrile episodes does not increase the frequency of positive results from patients with endocarditis. Prior antibiotic therapy rarely results in negative blood cultures and more often simply delays bacterial growth.

Timing of blood cultures becomes more critical when bacteremia originates from an extravascular source. Ideally, blood cultures should be drawn within the hour before the onset of fever, because there typically is a delay between the influx of bacteria into the blood stream and the onset of fever.[38] Because it is usually impossible to predict a fever spike, multiple blood cultures obtained over a 24-hour span are sufficient in most instances to detect intermittent bacteremia. When an infectious cause for fever of unknown origin is suspected, two blood cultures are recommended initially followed by two additional cultures over 24 to 36 hours. In the case of critically ill, acutely septic patients, three blood cultures should be obtained over a 30- to 60-minute period before instituting antimicrobial treatment.

At least 5 to 10 ml of blood should be collected for each culture, because the chances of obtaining a positive result are directly related to the volume of blood cultured. The concentration of organisms is relatively low (<5/ml) in the blood of most patients with bacteremia. A blood–culture broth ratio of 1:10 must be maintained to counteract the bactericidal activity of serum. Anticoagulant and antiphagocytic effects of broth additives are diminished if dilution of blood in media is less than 1:8.

Technique. Before venipuncture, thorough skin antisepsis as for surgery is the most effective means of avoiding culture contamination.[17] Small numbers of bacteria may persist inside hair follicles and sweat and sebaceous glands, which may be penetrated by the needle. If the vein must be palpated after skin disinfection, a sterile glove should be worn. To minimize the risk of contamination, blood samples should not be drawn through indwelling IV catheters unless it is a recently and appropriately placed jugular catheter. Arterial blood specimens offer no advantage over venous blood specimens except that they may be helpful for the detection of fungemia. Although collection of blood from separate veins is unnecessary, unless a catheter-related infection or phlebitis is suspected, finding the same organism at two different surgically prepared sites reduces the likelihood of the same contaminant, especially when sampling intervals are close. Blood for culture has also been taken through newly inserted IV catheters without increasing the risk of false contamination.[18]

Blood is inoculated immediately and directly into culture media, using a syringe and needle or a blood transfer set. A new needle should be utilized to introduce blood into the culture bottle after the culture bottle diaphragm has been disinfected with alcohol or iodine. Changing needles reduces the contamination rate by 2% to 5% but does increase the risk of stick injuries.[17, 21] Only commercial culture bottles packed under vacuum and fitted with rubber diaphragms should be used for routine blood cultures to minimize the risk of contamination. Air must not be allowed to enter into vacuum bottles during blood injection. The blood should be dispersed in the culture medium by gently inverting the bottle two or three times. Blood culture bottles should be inoculated and can be maintained at room temperature to avoid killing temperature-sensitive bacteria; however, incubation at 37°C is often used in the laboratory.

For suspected sepsis, the catheter should be removed aseptically with a sterile forceps after local antisepsis of the insertion site with a 70% alcohol-soaked swab. A blood sample can be taken at the same time for culture. After removal of the catheter, the distal segment should be cut off and placed in a sterile dry tube to be sent to the laboratory. Methods for quantitating catheter-associated bacteria should be done to differentiate contamination of the catheter from clinically significant infection.

Liquid Media. Commercial multipurpose nutrient broth media, such as tryptic soy broth, trypticase soy broth, Columbia broth, and brain-heart infusion broth (Difco Laboratories, Detroit, MI) are all suitable for *qualitative* recovery of both aerobic and anaerobic bacteria. Thioglycolate and thiol broth (Difco), intended for anaerobic blood culture only, should not be relied on for multipurpose cultures because aerobic (especially *Pseudomonas*) and facultative anaerobic bacteria are not reliably isolated. Most liquid media are bottled under vacuum with carbon dioxide added and usually are suitable to support the growth of clinically important anaerobes. The use of special anaerobic broth is rarely necessary.

Most commercial blood culture media contain 0.025% to 0.05% sodium polyanethol sulfonate (SPS), a polyanionic anticoagulant that also inhibits complement and lysozyme activity, interferes with phagocytosis, and inactivates therapeutic serum levels of aminoglycosides. Dilution of blood with liquid media is essential to neutralize serum and cellular antimicrobial properties. Even at 1:10 dilutions, serum may be bactericidal to coliforms, an effect that is counteracted by addition of SPS. SPS is inhibitory to mycoplasmas and should not be in media intended for their isolation. Dilution of blood in culture broth will usually lower therapeutic concentrations of antibiotics to noninhibitory levels. When high levels of β-lactam antibiotics are present in blood before culture, β-lactamase can be added to the culture media. Para-amino benzoic acid, available in some commercial blood culture media, competitively antagonizes the actions of sulfonamides and increases the blood culture yields from patients receiving sulfonamide drugs.

Bacterial growth can be suppressed in blood culture vials containing blood from patients' receiving antibiotics. Anionic and cationic resins have been incorporated into blood collection vials for antibiotic removal before broth culture. The effectiveness of removal is variable based on the resin and antibiotic.[10]

In the laboratory, culture bottles are examined daily for evidence of microbial growth: turbidity, hemolysis, gas production, or colony formation. In aerobic culturing, the broth should appear turbid within 24 hours of inoculation. In 95% of all instances wherein bacteria are isolated from blood culture media, such isolation occurs within 7 days. Longer incubation may be necessary for specimens from patients' receiving prior antibiotic therapy or from patients with endocarditis caused by fastidious organisms. In addition to visual inspection, routine (blind) subcultures onto solid culture media usually are performed for antimicrobial susceptibility testing between 7 and 14 hours after blood collection and again after 48 hours of incubation.

Lysis-Centrifugation. Although broth-based blood culture methods are sensitive, they provide no *quantitative* information as to the number of microorganisms. In contrast, inoculation of blood on solid agar allows for colony enumeration. Direct plating of freeze-thawed specimens of anticoagulated blood improves the sensitivity by freezing intracellular and phagocytized organisms. Only small volumes (1.0 ml) of blood can be directly plated. Lysis-centrifugation methods, with commercially prepared tubes (e.g., Wampole Isolator-tubes, Carter-Wallace Inc., Cranbury, NJ), allow for lysis of cellular elements followed by microbial concentration through centrifugation. These methods may also shorten the time to isolation of blood-borne organisms, but they are associated with an increased risk of bacterial contamination. Lysis methods also enhance the ability to recover intracellular organisms such as *Brucella*, *Mycobacterium*, *Histoplasma*, and *Bartonella*.

Interpretation of Results. It may be difficult to determine whether a positive culture result signifies actual bacteremia or simply contamination. Contamination is best distinguished from bacteremia by culturing multiple blood specimens. Multiple isolations of the same organism imply significance because of repeatability. Knowledge of the normal canine and feline bacterial skin flora is helpful in interpreting blood culture results. Coagulase-negative staphylococci, α-hemolytic streptococci, *Micrococcus*, and *Acinetobacter* are normal skin commensals on the dog. *S. intermedius* is normally present on canine hair, whereas *Micrococcus*, α-hemolytic streptococci, and *Acinetobacter* are normally present on feline skin. Recovery of diphtheroids, *Bacillus* sp., and coagulase-negative staphylococci usually signifies contamination unless they are isolated from multiple specimens. Nonhemolytic streptococci and α-hemolytic streptococci from single cultures are also of uncertain significance. Clostridia in the blood stream of dogs occasionally have been unassociated with clinical signs of sepsis, and the true significance of their presence is uncertain. The presence of bacteria of the family Enterobacteriaceae or Bacteroidaceae, *P. aeruginosa*, *S. intermedius*, β-hemolytic streptococci, or yeasts in the blood stream is nearly always clinically significant. In all cases, the significance of positive blood culture results should be interpreted in light of the patient's clinical status and the potential sources for bacteremia.

THERAPY

IV access lines are essential to the management of the bacteremic patient not only for fluid and antibiotic administration but also for blood sampling. A urinary catheter is helpful in patients at risk of septic shock in order to monitor urine output. Core and toe-web temperature readings should be monitored to assess peripheral blood flow and vasoconstriction.

Blood cultures and bacterial antibiotic susceptibility tests are essential for the proper treatment of bacteremia and bacterial endocarditis. It is important to choose a bactericidal antibiotic that has good tissue penetration and to use high (when permissible) IV doses for the first 4 to 10 days. Antimicrobial therapy may be continued orally for at least 3 weeks for treatment of bacteremia and for 6 to 8 weeks for bacterial endocarditis. Blood cultures need not be repeated after antibiotics have been discontinued if endocarditis was not suspected and recovery was complete.

Despite the primary concern with the infectious agent, concomitant disorders should not be overlooked. In fact, the severity of comorbid disease is as important in treatment outcome as the invading organism. The ability to treat or control concomitant disease effectively may exert a more favorable influence on outcome than the antibiotic regimen chosen. Sources of infection should be identified and managed. Urinary and IV catheters should be removed when sepsis is suspected, and potential sites of infection should be drained, debrided, and otherwise treated.

In critically ill patients, antibiotic therapy should be started before the return of blood culture results, although this approach has inherent shortcomings, such as selection for microbial resistance. Subsequent therapeutic adjustments may be made on the basis of culture results. Several antibiotics may have to be given in sequence for treatment of bacterial endocarditis. Bacteriostatic antibiotics, if administered at all, should conclude rather than initiate this sequence.

On the basis of predisposing infections or other factors, time course of infection, known patterns of associated bacteria, and their antimicrobial susceptibility patterns, the antibiotics most likely to be effective can be predicted (Table 87–6). This knowledge is important when blood culture results are negative and in critically ill patients before the return of blood culture results. Subsequently, appropriate adjustments in therapy may be necessary based on antibiotic susceptibility results.

In dogs and cats, staphylococci and streptococci are the most commonly encountered gram-positive pathogens,

Table 87–6. Choice of Antimicrobial Therapy for Bacteremia

ORGANISM	SITES	FIRST CHOICE	SECOND CHOICE(S)
Staphylococcus intermedius	Pyoderma	cep, brp	amg, vanc
Escherichia coli	Bowel compromise, peritonitis	amg, tms	3rd-gen cep, quin
β-hemolytic *Streptococcus*	Genital, navel, and skin infections	pen, amp	1st-gen cep, chlor, ery
Pseudomonas	Chronic wounds, leukopenia, burns, tracheostomy	amg,[a] quin	carb, ticar
Anaerobes	Abscesses, oral cavity lesions, bowel compromise, body cavity exudates	pen, met, clin	amp, chlor

[a]May combine aminoglycoside with ticarcillin or carbenicillin for maximum efficacy.
cep = cephalosporins; brp = β-lactamase–resistant penicillin; amg = aminoglycoside; vanc = vancomycin; tms = trimethoprim-sulfonamide; 3rd-gen cep = 3rd-generation cephalosporins; quin = quinolone; pen = penicillin; amp = ampicillin; 1st-gen cep = 1st-generation cephalosporins; chlor = chloramphenicol; ery = erythromycin; carb = carbenicillin; ticar = ticarcillin; met = metronidazole; clin = clindamycin.

whereas the Enterobacteriaceae, such as *E. coli, Klebsiella, Proteus,* and *Pseudomonas,* are the most common gram-negative offenders.

Antibiotics

For additional information on specific drugs discussed next, see Chapter 34 and the Drug Formulary, Appendix 8. The penicillin family of antibiotics include the narrow-spectrum penicillin G; intermediate spectrum ampicillin; and the extended-spectrum carbenicillin, ticarcillin, ticarcillin-clavulanate, and piperacillin. A common misconception is that ampicillin is a broad-spectrum antibiotic. Most coagulase-positive staphylococcal isolates are resistant to penicillin and ampicillin, and these are poor choices for serious and life-threatening infections, in which such organisms are isolated or suspected, without antibiogram evidence of susceptibility. Penicillin G should be restricted to streptococcal and possibly some anaerobic infections.

The extended-spectrum penicillins, carbenicillin, ticarcillin, ticarcillin-clavulanate, and piperacillin are useful agents but are usually provided after antibiogram results indicate their effect against a highly resistant microbe. These antibiotics have a spectrum that includes that of ampicillin plus activity against *Pseudomonas* and *Proteus*. Ticarcillin is more potent than carbenicillin, and piperacillin is active against many anaerobes. With the exception of ticarcillin-clavulanate, these penicillins lack resistance to β-lactamase produced by staphylococci.

The cephalosporins are very helpful in the treatment of potentially life-threatening infections because of their activity against *Staphylococcus* and *Streptococcus* as well as a greater spectrum of activity against gram-negative bacteria compared with ampicillin. These antibiotics include cephalothin, cefazolin, and cephapirin, but, like many antibiotics, are not effective against enterococci and *Pseudomonas* and are susceptible to the β-lactamase activity of *Bacteroides fragilis*. Second- and third-generation cephalosporins (cefoxitin and cefotaxime, respectively) are generally effective against gram-negative bacteria that are resistant to the first-generation family. However, cefoxitin is generally reserved for resistant anaerobes, and cefotaxime is generally reserved for bacterial infections involving the CNS and gram-negative infections wherein resistance to aminoglycoside and fluoroquinolone antibiotics has been demonstrated. They are also useful when the nephrotoxic aminoglycosides are contraindicated. The third-generation cephalosporins, with the exception of ceftazidime, are generally ineffective against *Pseudomonas*. Cost is often a factor limiting the administration of the third-generation family. Fluoroquinolones are often a good choice over the third-generation cephalosporins for gram-negative bacteremias not involving the CNS.

Ceftiofur is a near third-generation cephalosporin that has an antibacterial spectrum similar to that of cefotaxime but with a longer half-life[4, 37] and less expense. It should be given at least twice daily, however, for bacteremia (see Drug Formulary, Appendix 8). Ceftiofur is variably effective against *S. intermedius* and ineffective against *Pseudomonas* spp. or *Bordetella,* and its anaerobic spectrum is narrow. In vitro activity against *Fusobacterium* is generally good, but it is poor against *Bacteroides* spp. It is variably effective against S. *intermedius* and there are inadequate data concerning streptococcal species.

Aminoglycosides are highly effective against *Staphylococcus* and many gram-negative bacteria. They are not effective against anaerobes and *Streptococcus* and have limited activity in necrotic tissue and acid pH milieu. The useful drugs for bacteremia are gentamicin, amikacin, and tobramycin. Their primary limitation is nephrotoxicity; therefore, other agents are required for extended antibiotic therapy. The incidence of gentamicin-associated acute renal failure has increased markedly since three times daily administration has been used for systemic infections. Dehydration and sodium and potassium depletion predispose patients to nephrotoxicosis as does administration for longer than 5 to 7 days. Aminoglycosides demonstrate rapid bactericidal action for severe sepsis compared with that of the penicillins and cephalosporins. They also invoke post-antibacterial effects (i.e., bactericidal action after the serum concentration has decreased below the minimum inhibitory concentration).

The fluoroquinolones are very useful for the treatment of bacteremia, having bactericidal action at achievable concentrations. Like the aminoglycosides, they exhibit post-antibacterial effects. They are effective against *Pseudomonas* and Enterobacteriaceae but are generally ineffective against anaerobes and enterococci. Efficacy against streptococci is limited. Ciprofloxacin is approved for IV administration in humans, and enrofloxacin solution has been IV diluted and given slowly. A combination of enrofloxacin plus clindamycin may be as effective as and less toxic than ampicillin, gentamicin, and metronidazole for life-threatening sepsis due to unknown bacteria.

In general, first-generation cephalosporins and penicillins, especially β-lactamase–resistant types, are most effective in vitro for gram-positive bacteria, whereas aminoglycosides, first-generation cephalosporins, and fluoroquinolones are most effective against gram-negative agents. Thus, a combination of an aminoglycoside, such as gentamicin or amikacin, with ampicillin, ticarcillin, piperacillin, or first-generation cephalosporin is the logical choice for immediate treatment of life-threatening bacteremia in the absence of laboratory identification of an organism or its antibiotic susceptibility. The combination of first-generation cephalosporins and aminoglycosides, however, is not very effective against anaerobic bacteria. When an anaerobic infection is suspected, clindamycin, metronidazole, or cefoxitin is recommended. Despite in vitro susceptibility testing, trimethoprim-sulfonamide is a poor choice for anaerobic infections. Penicillin formerly was the preferred drug for anaerobic bacteremia. However, those infections caused by *Bacteroides* spp. are becoming increasingly resistant to both penicillins and first-generation cephalosporins.

A highly effective triple therapy for dogs with sepsis, particularly for intra-abdominal infections, is a β-lactam drug (ampicillin, ticarcillin, piperacillin, or first-generation cephalosporin) with an aminoglycoside and metronidazole. For cats, an antimicrobial spectrum encompassing gram-negative and anaerobic bacteria such as *Bacteroides* and *Propionibacterium acnes* is recommended. The combination of enrofloxacin and clindamycin is suggested when renal function is impaired.[12]

To ensure adequate serum antibiotic concentrations, the upper limit of the usual recommended dosage range of antimicrobial drugs is indicated (Table 87–7). Parenteral treatment is desirable for up to 14 to 21 days, especially for bacterial endocarditis, although this approach is not always practical. SC administration of ampicillin, cephalothin, or ceftiofur or SC or IM administration of gentamicin may be substituted for the IV route when necessary or after 4 to 10 days of IV treatment. Except in animals with endocarditis or other internal sources of infection, such as bone, lung, and prostate gland, most bacteremic episodes are usually short lived. Ideally, oral antibiotic therapy should be instituted only after 4 to 7 days of IV therapy and even then only after clinical and hematologic evidence of improvement.

Combination antibiotic therapy is often provided for gram-negative infections because they may be associated with rapid progression and high mortality. Although clinical evidence supports the use of carbenicillin or ticarcillin with aminoglycosides for *Pseudomonas* and *Proteus*, these drugs must be given separately because of known in vitro incompatibilities. Amikacin, unlike tobramycin and gentamicin, is not inactivated in vitro by penicillins. Administration of some antibiotics such as aminoglycosides, cephalosporins, metronidazole, and enrofloxacin is recommended by infusion in a compatible solution over 30 to 60 minutes.

Bactericidal rather than bacteriostatic antibiotics have been shown to result in higher concentrations of circulating endotoxin in animals with experimental gram-negative septicemia. However, clinical signs have not been more severe in animals treated with bactericidal antibiotics, and these animals have had more suppression of bacterial replication and seeding from extravascular sites.

Patients with bacteremia must be closely monitored (see also Endotoxemia, Chapter 38). Although clinical and hematologic evidence of improvement often occurs initially, relapse is common. Acquired antimicrobial resistance may develop rapidly. Clinical signs of resurging bacteremia include fever, which may be transient, deterioration of mucous membrane color, increasing capillary refill time, increasing rectal to toe-web temperature differential, decreasing blood pressure, and tachycardia. Detection of these signs of early deterioration indicates a need for intensification of therapy, including adjustments of antibiotic. It also should prompt a search for a persistent focus of infection (e.g., abscess, catheter) that may be treatable.

Septic Shock

Rapid restoration of organ perfusion and tissue oxygen delivery are essential for the management of the patient in septic shock (see also Endotoxemia, Chapter 38). Oxygen therapy can be administered by cage, mask, or intranasal catheter. Rapid fluid therapy (crystalloid fluid, colloid-crystalloid mixture, or hypertonic solution[1]) is required to raise the central venous pressure to 2 to 5 cm of water within 15 minutes. High volumes of fluids are required for the treatment of septic shock, and crystalloid fluid volumes can be decreased with colloids. Hetastarch 120 or dextran 70 is usually administered for this purpose. At high dosages, both can prolong clotting times by decreasing platelet function and fibrin clot strength. Colloids should be used with caution if

Table 87–7. Antimicrobial Dosages for Bacteremia With or Without Endocarditis in Dogs and Cats

DRUG	SPECIES	DOSE[a]	ROUTE	INTERVAL (HOURS)	DURATION (DAYS)[b]
Penicillin	B	$20–40 \times 10^3$ U/kg	IV	4–6	4–7
Imipenem	B	10 mg/kg	IV	8	4–7
Carbenicillin	B	40–50 mg/kg	IV	6–8	4–7
Piperacillin	B	30 mg/kg	IV	6	4–7
Ticarcillin	D	30–40 mg/kg	IV	6	4–7
Ampicillin	B	20–40 mg/kg	IV	6	4–7
Cephalothin	B	20–40 mg/kg	IV	8	4–7
Cefazolin	B	20–30 mg/kg	IV	8	4–7
Cefoxitin	B	20 mg/kg	IV	8	4–7
Cefapirin	B	10–30 mg/kg	IV	8	4–7
Cefotaxime	B	20–80 mg/kg	IV	8	4–7
Gentamicin[c]	B	2–4 mg/kg	IV	8	4–7
Amikacin[c]	B	7–10 mg/kg	IV	8	4–7
Tobramycin[c]	B	2–4 mg/kg	IV	8	4–7
Trimethoprim-sulfonamide	D	15 mg/kg	IV	8–12	4–7
Metronidazole	B	8–15 mg/kg	IV, PO	8	5–7
Chloramphenicol	D	15–25 mg/kg	IV	6–8	4–7
	C	10–15 mg/kg	IV	6–8	4–7
Ciprofloxacin[d]	B	10–15 mg/kg	PO	12	14
Norfloxacin[d]	B	22 mg/kg	PO	12	14
Enrofloxacin[d]	B	5–7 mg/kg	IV	12	4–7
		5–15 mg/kg	PO	12	14

[a]Dose per administration at specified interval.
[b]After the animal is stabilized, oral therapy should be continued when possible for periods of 3 to 6 weeks; see text.
[c]Renal function and urinalysis must be closely monitored for signs of nephrotoxicity at this dosage and frequency. Reduce dose to 1–2 mg/kg every 8 hours if renal compromise is anticipated.
[d]For dosages of other quinolones, see Chapter 34 and the Drug Formulary, Appendix 8.
B = dog and cat; D = dog; C = cat.

Table 87–8. Fluid Therapy In Septic Shock

FLUID	VOLUME	COMMENTS
Hypertonic saline	4 ml/kg	Once
Glucose-insulin potassium (K) (1 g glucose, 1 U insulin, 0.25 mEq K/kg in 250 ml of lactated Ringer's solution, or mixed in 0.45% NaCl to 5% glucose)	10% volume bolus, remainder infused over 4–5 hrs	May be repeated as needed
Colloids	Maximum: 20 ml/kg over 24 hrs, then 10 ml/kg/24 hrs	Slow infusion
Hetastarch 120		
Dextran 70		

the serum albumin concentration is less than 1 g/dl. Another treatment for cardiovascular support is the administration of hypertonic solutions. Glucose-insulin-potassium also improves cardiovascular function as well as hypoglycemia. Hypertonic saline and glucose-insulin-potassium are the two most often administered hypertonic solutions (Table 87–8). After the hypertonic solutions are provided, crystalloid administration is continued. Serum albumin, potassium, and RBC concentrations decrease after aggressive fluid therapy. Peripheral edema is a common sequela. Colloids are superior to crystalloids in maintaining hemodynamic function and reducing the volume of crystalloids required.

Rapid-acting, powerful inotropes, such as dopamine and dobutamine, are indicated only if fluid therapy fails to establish or maintain adequate tissue oxygen perfusion. Monitoring of heart rate and rhythm, core/toe-web temperature differential, central venous pressure, and urine output is required.

DIC is a risk of sepsis.[31] If the clotting time and platelet count are normal or nearly normal, prophylaxis is recommended. Synthetic colloids assist in this regard, but if crystalloids alone are administered, low-dose heparin (75–100 U/kg SC every 8 hours) is suggested in an attempt to inhibit coagulation and maintain blood flow in the microcirculation.[36] Acute and end-stage DIC is more difficult to treat, requiring more intense heparinization and coagulation factor replacement, respectively.

PROGNOSIS

Many factors influence the natural course of bacteremic disorders, including adequacy of therapy, severity of bacteremia, source of infection, delay before treatment, and concomitant disorders, plus the age and prior health status of the patient. The prognosis is better when abscesses, cellulitis, and skin and wound infections are the sources of bacteremia than when gram-negative bacteria and endotoxemia are present. Mortality of bacteremic dogs with hypoalbuminemia, high serum ALP, and hypoglycemia is significantly higher than that of dogs without or with only one of these abnormalities. Late relapse and death have occurred in some dogs, usually when bacteriostatic antibiotics were chosen for treatment. Premature termination of antibiotic therapy may also result in relapse and death in bacteremic dogs, particularly those associated with bacterial endocarditis, antimicrobial-restricted sites, abscesses, and cellulitis. Relapse after IV antibiotic therapy that was maintained for only 1 to 2 days followed by oral antibiotics is common. Oral antibiotic therapy alone is not recommended as initial treatment for patients with suspected bacteremia.

Aortic valvular insufficiency caused by endocarditis usually results in intractable left-sided congestive heart failure within 2 to 6 months. Bacterial endocarditis affecting only the mitral valve is associated with a better prognosis. Renal failure related to septic embolization-infarction is a latent complication or one that can be present at the time of diagnosis of chronic bacterial endocarditis.

The indiscriminate use of glucocorticoids (even with antibiotics) as prophylaxis is detrimental to bacteremic patients. A common reason that glucocorticoids are administered to bacteremic dogs is the similarity in clinical manifestations of bacteremic and immune-mediated diseases. The survival rate of dogs with bacterial endocarditis given glucocorticoids is lower than that of dogs not given glucocorticoids. Prophylactic antibiotic treatment usually is ineffective unless it is used when surgical or dental procedures (see Chapters 55 and 89) are done or when the type of bacteria and its susceptibility are known. Bacterial resistance to frequently administered antibiotics, such as ampicillin, is common. Thus, effective prophylactic antibiotic therapy usually requires combinations of antibiotics, often including an aminoglycoside. Even then, the tendency to select for resistant bacteria is increased.

Infectious Myocarditis

Myocarditis (inflammation of the myocytes, interstitium, and vasculature) may result from primary or secondary causes. Both active and chronic myocardial disease may be associated with infectious diseases of dogs (Table 87–9). Indicated respective chapters should be consulted for additional information. Myocarditis secondary to infectious agents may be subclinical if the inflammation is focal and limited. Severe or diffuse myocarditis results in fever, malaise, weakness, cardiac arrhythmia, and congestive heart failure. Congestive heart failure caused by necrotizing myocarditis can be a lethal complication of neonatal canine parvovirus infection but is currently a rare occurrence. Dogs in the southwestern United States infected with Chagas' disease develop granulomatous myocarditis that can cause heart failure and heart rhythm disturbance.

Neospora caninum and *Borrelia burgdorferi* can infect the myocardium, but the disease is usually mild and overshadowed by clinical signs associated with other organ or system involvement.

The diagnosis of myocarditis is usually made when ventricular tachyarrhythmias, with or without ST-segment changes, are detected in patients with evidence of systemic diseases. The interpretation of elevated levels of the myocardial fraction of serum muscle enzymes such as creatine kinase (CK), lactic dehydrogenase, and AST has not been evaluated in dogs. Specific serologic testing is available for some of the underlying diseases. Therapy is directed at the primary infectious agent, control of cardiac arrhythmia, and treatment of congestive heart failure.

TRANSMISSIBLE MYOCARDITIS-DIAPHRAGMITIS OF CATS

This disease is a sporadic disease, affecting mainly adult cats, that occurs most commonly in the summer months. It has been reported in California[29] and Florida.[15]

Although the disease can be experimentally transmitted between cats, the organism has not been identified.[29] A viral agent may be involved, and the disease resembles Coxsackie B virus infection of people and other animals.[22] Clinical signs in cats include transient fever occurring 9 to 30 days after inoculation and usually lasting for 1 to 3 days. Some cats have a second fever spike during this interval. Lethargy, rough hair coat, and anorexia correlate with the fever. Hematologic and biochemical abnormalities are absent except for high serum CK activity in some cats. Gross necropsy findings during the febrile period are pale foci surrounded by hemorrhage in the ventricular myocardium and diaphragm. Gross lesions were absent in recovered cats. Myonecrosis and cellular infiltration with predominantly neutrophils and sometimes macrophages have been found in heart and diaphragmatic muscle. In acutely infected cats, lymphoid tissues showed reactive changes and mild neutrophilic-histocytic infiltrates in the liver and renal interstitium. There is some evidence in people that viral myocarditis may result in development of chronic inflammatory heart disease and cardiomyopathy. Whether this infection in cats has any relationship to some cases of feline cardiomyopathy remains to be determined.

Table 87–9. Infectious Causes of Myocarditis

VIRUSES
Canine distemper virus (neonate) (Chapter 3)
Canine parvovirus (prenatal, neonate) (Chapter 8)
Canine herpesvirus (Chapter 5)
RICKETTSIAE
Rickettsia rickettsii (Chapter 29)
BACTERIA
Numerous genera
Borrelia burgdorferi (Chapter 45)
ALGAE
Prototheca spp. (Chapter 69)
FUNGI
Cryptococcus neoformans (Chapter 61)
Coccidioides immitis (Chapter 62)
Aspergillus terreus (Chapter 65)
Paecilomyces varioti (Chapter 68)
PROTOZOANS
Trypanosoma cruzi (Chapter 72)
Toxoplasma gondii (Chapter 80)
Hepatozoon canis (Chapter 74)
Neospora caninum (Chapter 80)
UNKNOWN
Transmissible myocarditis-diaphragmitis of cats[29]

Infectious Pericardial Effusion

ETIOLOGY

There are many causes of pericardial effusion in dogs and cats (Tables 87–10 and 87–11). Pericarditis (inflammation of the fibrous and serous layers of the pericardium) due to infectious agents is uncommon. Pericarditis may result from local (pleural or pulmonary) infections or from hematogenous spread of microorganisms.[13] *Actinomyces, Nocardia, Mycobacterium*, and anaerobic infections are most likely to spread from pleural infections or migrating foreign bodies (see Chapter 49). *Pasteurella multocida*, introduced by a bite wound, caused purulent pericarditis in a puppy.[14] Hematogenous infections of the pericardium can occur when infectious organisms embolize in the myocardial or pericardial vasculature. Bacteremias and viral infections, such as feline infectious peritonitis (see Chapter 11), can cause effusive pericarditis.

Table 87–10. Causes of Pericardial Effusion in 42 Dogs

CAUSE	DOGS WITH SIGNS (%)
Neoplasia	24 (57)
Idiopathic hemorrhagic	8 (19)
Cardiac	6 (14)
Traumatic	2 (5)
Uremic	1 (2)
Infectious	1 (2)

Data from Berg RJ, Wingfield W: *J Am Anim Hosp Assoc* 20:721–730, 1994.

Pericarditis may be effusive or constrictive, but in the dog and cat it is usually effusive. Effusions of infectious pericarditis are either modified transudates or exudates and are usually serosanguineous or bloody.

CLINICAL FINDINGS

The infectious nature of the underlying agent and the severity of pericardial effusion determine the findings of the patient's history. Weight loss, weakness, dyspnea, and mild

Table 87–11. Causes of Pericardial Effusion in 84 Cats

CAUSE	CATS WITH SIGNS (%)
Cardiac	20 (24)
Feline infectious peritonitis	16 (19)
Neoplasia	13 (15)
Infectious[a]	12 (14)
Renal failure	9 (11)
Coagulopathies	7 (8)
Miscellaneous	5 (6)
Iatrogenic	2 (2)

[a]Other than feline infectious peritonitis.

Data from Rush JE et al: *Proc Am Coll Vet Intern Med* 5:922, 1987; Harpster NK: *In* Holzworth J (ed), *Disease of the Cat: Medicine and Surgery*. WB Saunders, Philadelphia, 1987, p 820.

abdominal effusion are the earliest signs. Fever is an inconsistent finding, varying with the infectious agent and time course of the disease. As the severity of the pericardial effusion worsens, dyspnea, weakness, and abdominal effusion become pronounced.

The principal physical findings reflect external cardiac compression. As the effusion becomes more extensive, the intrapericardial pressure rises to or exceeds right atrial and left ventricular diastolic pressures. Intracardiac pressure increases, ventricular diastolic filling is impaired, and stroke volume is reduced. The central venous pressure is increased, and venous return to the right atrium is impaired, resulting in right-sided heart failure. Jugular pulses and distention of the jugular veins are often present. Subsequently, increased venous pressure can lead to pleural and abdominal effusions. The triad of increased central venous pressure, as with evident jugular pulses, weak peripheral arterial pulses, and muffled heart sounds, is strongly suggestive of pericardial effusion.

When the effusion is severe, the heart and lung sounds are not clearly audible. Mucous membrane color is often pale, and the peripheral pulses are weak because of decreased cardiac output. A reflex tachycardia is often present.

DIAGNOSIS

Thoracic radiographs will always be abnormal when pericardial effusion is severe enough to produce cardiovascular impairment. However, because the pericardial and cardiac silhouettes cannot be distinguished by simple radiographs, the size of the heart and the severity of effusion cannot be accurately determined. In some cases, pleural effusion may partially obscure the pericardial-cardiac silhouette.

Massive effusion is characterized by a greatly enlarged, round cardiac silhouette in which the borders are smooth without the normal protrusions produced by the chambers. The silhouette is flattened where it contacts the thoracic walls. The parenchymal lung fields are not affected unless the lungs are involved as the primary source of infection. The lobar arteries may appear small because of decreased right-ventricular output. Contrast radiography (positive or negative) may be performed after removal of the effusion in an attempt to identify mass lesions.

ECG changes may be present, particularly when the degree of effusion is severe. Low-voltage complexes, electrical alternans, and ST-segment changes may be present. Echocardiography is an accurate means of determining the presence and severity of effusion and cardiac function. Two-dimensional ultrasound examination is helpful in many cases in the detection of intrapericardial masses.

Pericardiocentesis is performed immediately if severe cardiovascular impairment has occurred secondary to severe effusions. Otherwise, pericardiocentesis is performed after radiographic, electrocardiographic, and echocardiographic examinations.

Cytologic analysis and microbial culture of the effusion should always be performed. Infectious pericardial effusion is either serosanguineous or (more often) bloody. The protein content is greater than 2.5 mg/dl and is often in excess of 3.5 mg/dl. Neutrophils and, to a lesser extent, erythrocytes are the predominant cell types. Macrophages and reactive mesothelial cells are usually present, especially when the effusion is chronic. Erythrophagia and hemosiderocytes may be observed. Degenerate neutrophils and infectious agents may be detected. When the latter are absent, hemorrhagic effusions caused by neoplasia, idiopathic benign (hemorrhagic) pericardial effusion, and infectious pericarditis cannot be distinguished by cytology. The presence of pyrexia, inflammatory leukogram, or other biochemical data associated with bacteremia or sepsis are variably and inconsistently associated with infectious pericarditis.

THERAPY

If the cause of a systemic infection is evident, aggressive antimicrobial therapy is indicated as soon as appropriate samples for culture are procured. In some cases, the infectious nature of the effusion is not appreciated until the results of cytology and culture are obtained.

Continuous drainage via an indwelling pericardial catheter or preferably surgical intervention, along with antimicrobial therapy, is recommended. Subtotal pericardectomy is suggested because surgically created pericardial fenestrations may adhere to the epicardium postoperatively, thus resealing the pericardium.

Constrictive pericarditis-epicarditis may occur and is recognized at surgery. Although pericardectomy can be performed, extensive fibrin deposition on the epicardium is difficult to remove. Stripping of the epicardium is tedious and associated with complications, such as tearing of the myocardium and heart rhythm disturbances.

Bacterial infection, although producing fibrinous pericarditis and epicarditis, can often be treated successfully once the pericardium is removed. In my experience, *Staphylococcus* and *Streptococcus* organisms are most often incriminated. Antimicrobial therapy should involve broad-spectrum, bactericidal drugs administered IV at high dosages when feasible and should always be guided by antimicrobial susceptibility results.

References

1. Armistead CW, Vincent JL, Preiser JC, et al. 1989. Hypertonic saline solution-hetastarch for fluid resuscitation in experimental septic shock. *Anesth Analg* 69:714–720.
2. Beutler B. 1989. Cachetin in tissue injury, shock, and related states. *Crit Care Clin* 5:353–367.
3. Braquet P, Hosford J, Braquet M, et al. PAF/cytokine auto-generated feedback networks in microvascular immune injury: consequences in shock, ischemia, and graft rejection. *Int Arch Allergy Appl Immunol* 88:88–100, 1989.
4. Brown SA, Arnold TS, Hamlow PJ, et al. 1995. Plasma and urine disposition and dose proportionality of ceftiofur and metabolites in dogs after subcutaneous administration of ceftiofur sodium. *J Vet Pharmacol Ther* 18:363–369.
5. Calvert CA, Dow SW. 1990. Cardiovascular infections, pp 97–113. *In* Greene CE (ed), Infectious diseases of the dog and cat. WB Saunders, Philadelphia, PA.
6. Cerra FB. 1990. The systemic septic response: concepts of pathogenesis. *J Trauma* 30:S169–S174.
7. Cockerill FR, Hughes JG, Vetter EA, et al. 1997. Analysis of 281,797 consecutive blood cultures performed over an eight-year period: trends in microorganisms isolated and the value of anaerobic culture of blood. *Clin Infect Dis* 24:403–418.
8. Court EA, Watson AD, Martin P. 1994. *Pseudomonas aeruginosa* bacteraemia in a dog. *Aust Vet J* 71:25–27.
9. Creasey AA, Stevens P, Kenny J, et al. 1991. Endotoxin and cytokine profile in plasma of baboon challenged with lethal and sublethal *Escherichia coli*. *Circ Shock* 33:84–91.
10. Crepin O, Roussel-Delvallez M, Martin GR, Courcol RJ. 1993. Effectiveness of resins in removing antibiotics from blood cultures. *J Clin Microbiol* 31:734–735.
11. Dinorello CA. 1991. Interleukin-1 and interleukin-1 antagonism. *Blood* 177:1627–1652.
12. Dow SW, Curtis CR, Jones RL, et al. 1989. Bacterial culture of blood from critically ill dogs and cats: 100 cases (1985–1987). *J Am Vet Med Assoc* 195:113–117.
13. Forrester SD, Fossum TW, Miller MW. 1992. Pneumothorax in a dog with a pulmonary abscess and suspected infective endocarditis. *J Am Vet Med Assoc* 200:351–354.
14. Fuentes VL, Long KJ, Darke PGG, et al. 1991. Purulent pericarditis in a puppy. *J Small Anim Pract* 32:585–588.

15. Hall GG. 1995. Personal communication. Schering Animal Health, Orlando, FL.
16. Hardie EM, Krus-Ellliot K. 1990. Endotoxic shock: Part I. A review of causes. *J Vet Intern Med* 4:258–266.
17. Isaacman DJ, Karasic RB. 1990. Lack of effect of changing needles on contamination of blood cultures. *Pediatr Infect Dis J* 9:274–278.
18. Isaacman DJ, Karasic RB. 1990. Utility of collecting blood cultures through newly inserted intravenous catheters. *Pediatr Infect Dis J* 9:815–818.
19. Jardin F, Brun-Ney D, Auvert B, et al. 1990. Sepsis-related cardiogenic shock. *Crit Care Med* 18:1055–1060.
20. LaRue MJ, Murtaugh RJ. 1978. Pulmonary thromboembolism in dogs: 47 cases. *J Am Vet Med Assoc* 1368–1372.
21. Leisure MK, Moore DM, Schwartzman JD, et al. 1990. Changing the needle when inoculating blood cultures. A no-benefit and high-risk procedure. *JAMA* 264:2111–2112.
22. Leslie K, Blay R, Haisch C, et al. 1989. Clinical and experimental aspects of viral myocarditis. *Clin Microbiol Rev* 2:191–203.
23. Malik R, Church DB, Allan GS. 1992. What is your diagnosis? Left-sided heart failure attributable to chronic vegetative endocarditis of the mitral and aortic valves. *J Am Vet Med Assoc* 200:1391–1393.
24. Martin C, Saux P, Eon B, et al. 1990. Septic shock: a goal-directed therapy using volume loading, dobutamine and/or norepinephrine. *Acta Anaesthesiol Scand* 34:413–417.
25. Messier S, Daminet S, Lemarchand T. 1995. *Streptococcus agalactiae* endocarditis with embolization in a dog. *Can Vet J* 36:703–704.
26. Natanson C. 1990. A canine model of septic shock. In Parillo JE (moderator), Septic shock in humans: advances in the understanding of pathogenesis, cardiovascular dysfunction, and therapy. *Ann Intern Med* 1113:227–282.
27. Nostrandt AC. 1990. Bacteremia and septicemia in small animal patients. *Probl Vet Med* 2:348–361.
28. Olson NC, Joyce B, Fleisher LN. 1990. Role of platelet-activating factor and eicosanoids during endotoxin-induced lung injury in pigs. *Am J Physiol* 258:H1674–H1686.
29. Pedersen NC, Griffey SM, Grahn R, et al. 1993. A transmissible myocarditis/diaphragmitis of cats manifested by transient fever and depression. *Feline Pract* 21:13–19.
30. Petrak RA, Balk RA, Bone RC. 1989. Prostaglandins, cyclooxygenase inhibitors, and thromboxane synthetase inhibitors in the pathogenesis of multiple systems organ failure. *Crit Care Clin* 5:303–314.
31. Rana MW, Ayala A, Dean RE, et al. 1990. Heparin administration before or after hemorrhagic shock protects microvascular patency. *Circ Shock* 13:59.
32. Seigel JH. 1990. Through a glass darkly: the lung as a window to monitor oxygen consumption, energy metabolism, and severity of critical illness. *Clin Chem* 35:1585–1593.
33. Sheagren JN. 1989. Mechanism-oriented therapy for multiple systems organ failure. *Crit Care Clin* 5:393–409.
34. Shultz KS, Payne JT, Aronson E. 1991. *Escherichia coli* bacteremia associated with hypertrophic osteodystrophy in a dog. *J Am Vet Med Assoc* 199:1170–1173.
35. Slattum MM, Maggio-Price L, DiGiacomo RF, et al. 1991. Infusion related sepsis in dogs undergoing acute cardiopulmonary surgery. *Lab Anim Sci* 41:146–150.
36. Sprague RS, Stephenson AH, Dahms TE, et al. 1989. Proposed role for leukotrienes in the pathophysiology of multiple systems organ failure. *Crit Care Clin* 5:315–329.
37. Technology Transfer Document. 1992. Use of ceftiofur sodium for canine urinary tract infections. The Upjohn Company, Kalamazoo, MI.
38. Yagupsky P, Nolte FS. 1990. Quantitative aspects of septicemia. *Clin Microbiol Rev* 3:269–279.

Chapter **88**

Respiratory Infections

Craig E. Greene

The respiratory system is divided into the upper and lower respiratory tracts and the pleural cavity. The upper respiratory tract consists of the nasal passages, nasopharynx, pharynx, larynx, and extrathoracic trachea. The lower respiratory tract consists of the intrathoracic trachea, bronchi, and alveoli. Specific diseases caused by viruses, fungi, protozoa, rickettsiae, *Mycoplasma*, and certain bacteria such as *Actinomyces* and *Nocardia* that primarily infect the respiratory system are covered in other chapters. This discussion focuses on bacterial infections of the respiratory system produced by invasion of normal microflora, by specific bacterial pathogens, or after impairment of normal host defense mechanisms. The normal microflora of the respiratory tract are discussed because these organisms frequently become involved in both upper and lower respiratory tract infections.

Normal Bacterial Flora

UPPER RESPIRATORY TRACT

Surveys of the bacterial microflora of the nasal cavities, tonsils, and pharynx of clinically healthy dogs and cats have found many types of aerobic and facultative anaerobic bacteria (Tables 88–1 and 88–2). Greater numbers of organisms are routinely cultured from the rostral than from the caudal nasal cavity. Because of marked individual variations, it is not possible to expect to find the same organisms as flora of the nasal cavity and pharynx in each animal, but the presence of a certain range of flora can be predicted.

LOWER RESPIRATORY TRACT

Bacteria are prevented from entering the lower respiratory tract by filtration of inspired air in the nasal turbinates, sneezing or coughing of inhaled particulate matter, and mucociliary clearance mechanisms. Despite these barriers, the normal tracheobronchial tree and lung are not continuously sterile. Airways down to the first bronchial division are contaminated with low numbers of organisms in clinically healthy animals. Studies using guarded culture swabs or tissue samples of the lower trachea of clinically healthy dogs

Table 88–1. Bacterial Isolates From Nasal Swabs of Clinically Healthy Animals [a]

DOGS	CATS
Gram-Positive Aerobic or acultative	**Gram-Positive Aerobic or Facultative**
Staphylococcus (coagulase negative)	*Streptococcus*
Streptococcus (α- and nonhemolytic)	*Staphylococcus*
Corynebacterium	*Corynebacterium*
Bacillus	*Micrococcus*
Staphylococcus (coagulase positive)	**Gram-Negative Aerobic or Facultative**
Streptococcus (β-hemolytic)	*Pasteurella multocida*
Gram-Negative Aerobic or Facultative	*Escherichia coli*
Neisseria	*Pseudomonas aeruginosa*
Escherichia coli	*Proteus*
Enterobacter	*Klebsiella*
Pasteurella multocida	*Enterobacter*
Moraxella	*Bordetella bronchiseptica*
Proteus	*Moraxella*
Pseudomonas aeruginosa	*Mycoplasma*
Alcaligenes	
Bordetella bronchiseptica	
Obligate Anaerobes	
Clostridium	

[a]Bacteria are listed in approximate order of frequency of isolation.

Table 88–2. Bacterial Isolates From Tonsillar and Pharyngeal Swabs of Clinically Healthy Dogs [a]

Streptococcus (α- and nonhemolytic)	*Proteus* spp.
Staphylococcus (coagulase negative)	*Pseudomonas* spp.
Neisseria spp.	*Corynebacterium* spp.
Escherichia coli and *Enterobacter* spp.	*Staphylococcus* (coagulase positive)
Pasteurella multocida	*Clostridium* spp.
Bacillus spp.	*Bacteroides* spp.
Streptococcus (β-hemolytic)	*Propionibacterium* spp.
Alcaligenes spp.	*Peptostreptococcus* spp.
Klebsiella pneumoniae	*Fusobacterium* spp.

[a]Bacteria are listed in approximate order of frequency of isolation.

Table 88–3. Bacterial Isolates From Tracheal Swabs and Lungs of Clinically Healthy Dogs

Staphylococcus (coagulase positive and negative)	*Enterobacter aerogenes*
Streptococcus (α- and nonhemolytic)	*Acinetobacter* spp.
Pasteurella multocida	*Moraxella* spp.
Klebsiella pneumoniae	*Corynebacterium* spp.

have found some bacteria in 40% to 50% of samples (Table 88–3). Oropharyngeal bacteria are frequently aspirated and may be present for an unknown interval in the normal tracheobronchial tree and lung. Aerobic bacteria were isolated from 37% of lung tissue samples, whereas only 10% of dogs examined had no growth from cultures of multiple samples of their lung tissues. Most of the bacteria cultured from the trachea and lungs are identical to those found in the pharynx of those same dogs. This bacterial population has the potential to cause or complicate clinical respiratory infection and clouds interpretation of airway and lung cultures. Finding large (>10^5 CFU/ml) concentrations of bacteria or cytologic evidence of inflammatory cells in tracheobronchial washings makes their presence of more concern to the clinician.

Upper Respiratory Tract Infections

BACTERIAL RHINITIS

Primary bacterial rhinitis is rare in the dog and cat. Bacterial rhinitis commonly is secondary to nasal trauma or inhalation of foreign material; reflux of liquids or food into the nose due to pharyngeal or esophageal dysfunction; viral, fungal, or parasitic infections; neoplasia; dental disease; oronasal fistula; and bacterial bronchopneumonia. Fungi such as *Aspergillus* and *Penicillium* may colonize airways diseased by bacteria or other processes (see Chapter 65) and *Cryptococcus* produces infection in this area in immunocompromised dogs and cats (see Chapter 61).

Clinical signs of bacterial rhinitis include sneezing, mucopurulent nasal discharge, ocular discharge secondary to nasolacrimal duct obstruction, and cough with gagging or retching. Epistaxis occurs infrequently with primary bacterial rhinitis, but may be associated with underlying disease such as fungal rhinitis or neoplasia. Pawing at the face or nose indicates severe nasal irritation, often caused by foreign bodies or food lodged in the nasal cavity. Ulceration of the external nares and accumulation of crusted exudate occur in severe or chronic cases.

Because primary bacterial rhinitis is uncommon, a thorough search for underlying problems should be performed. Diagnostic techniques include skull and nasal radiographs, endoscopic examination of the nasal passages, thorough oropharyngeal examination, cytologic examination of exudate, bacterial culture, and biopsy. These techniques are usually performed with the patient under general anesthesia. Computed tomography is available at referral centers as a noninvasive method for determining the source of chronic nasal discharge.[11]

The radiographic features of chronic rhinitis are increased density of the nasal cavity as a result of excessive secretion accumulation. The turbinates are rarely destroyed, and the vomer bone is intact unless the disease is advanced. The frontal sinuses usually do not have increased density. Oblique views of the skull should be taken to evaluate the upper dental arcade.

The potential of rhinoscopy to detect significant abnormalities depends on the instrument and the amount of exudate or hemorrhage obscuring the field of view. Rhinoscopy is invaluable in evaluating fungal rhinitis and foreign bodies but is less so in nasal neoplasia. Purulent exudate and friable, hyperemic mucosa with or without ulceration are seen in bacterial rhinitis.

Cytologic specimens of lesions or exudates will be consistent with septic, purulent exudates. Bacterial cultures are difficult to interpret because they often yield a mixed population similar to that of the normal nasal flora. Occasionally, a pure culture of a pathogen is helpful in choosing an appropriate antimicrobial on the basis of susceptibility testing. Biopsy of nasal turbinates and mucosae may be helpful in identifying nasal diseases associated with bacterial rhinitis.

Bacterial rhinitis will often resolve if the underlying problem, such as a foreign body, oronasal fistula, or dental disease, is corrected. In many patients, signs of rhinitis are temporary and may improve without treatment. Persistent or recurring signs require drug therapy for a limited period of time.

The external nares should be cleansed of exudate frequently. In the absence of specific culture results, administration of broad-spectrum antibacterials is indicated. Nebulization or vaporization helps mobilize secretions in the clogged nasal passages and soothes irritated mucous membranes. Sympathomimetic nasal decongestants such as phenylephrine and oxymetazoline in patients with copious serous or mucoid nasal discharges may be indicated. However, nasal decongestants are contraindicated in patients with thick tenacious, mucopurulent nasal discharges, because the exudates may become more viscous and difficult to expel. Glucocorticoid-responsive rhinitis associated with lymphoplasmacytic infiltrates of nasal mucosa, which may mimic bacterial rhinitis, has been described. The decision to institute glucocorticoid therapy is made after antibacterial therapy fails to improve clinical signs and no evidence of a primary infectious process is found during diagnostic evaluation.

CHRONIC SINUSITIS

Chronic bacterial sinusitis is uncommon in the dog, although mucous accumulation does occur when nasal diseases occlude normal drainage of the frontal sinus through the sinus ostium. Chronic sinusitis in cats occurs as a result of mucosal and bone damage secondary to feline viral respiratory infections (Chapter 16). Severe mucosal ulceration and turbinate destruction allow secondary bacterial infection of the nose and frontal sinuses. This syndrome is often called the "chronic snuffler" because the clinical signs in cats include chronic snorting and snuffling breathing, purulent nasal discharge, and sneezing. Many young cats with this syndrome are infected with feline leukemia virus (Chapter 13), which may influence their response to treatment.

Treatment of bacterial rhinitis is often frustrating because the underlying pathogenesis of the disease syndrome is poorly understood, and many patients fail to respond to all forms of symptomatic therapy. The nasal cavity can be vigorously flushed with saline with or without antiseptic solutions to remove the exudate and inhibit bacterial growth. Drug penetration into the normal canine sinus is poor for the few antibacterials that have been evaluated, and this is probably similar in cats. Drug penetration will obviously increase with inflammation, but actual levels are unknown. Broad-spectrum antibacterials are used for prolonged periods (2–4 months) after bacterial culture and susceptibility testing. Nasal decongestants may be helpful in individual cats, but they can exacerbate the problem by drying the exudate. Surgical turbinectomy and sinus trephination may be helpful in establishing drainage of these areas and removing inspissated pockets of exudate. Nasal flushing and systemic antibacterials can be used subsequent to surgical intervention. More aggressive surgical approaches have included sinus obliteration and reconstruction of apertures into the frontal sinuses.

TONSILLITIS AND PHARYNGITIS

Tonsillitis is usually bilateral but occasionally may occur as a unilateral disease when a foreign body is trapped in the tonsillar crypt. Primary tonsillitis usually occurs in young, small-breed dogs that exhibit clinical signs of malaise, gagging cough with retching, fever, and inappetence. Inspection will often reveal a bright-red tonsil with an associated pharyngitis. Punctate hemorrhages on the tonsil itself and purulent exudate in the tonsillar crypt may also be visible. The tonsil will be friable and will easily bleed on manipulation. Tonsillitis is not always associated with gross enlargement of the tonsil; in fact, the benign appearance of the tonsil in some cases may be in sharp contrast to the severity of clinical signs. Specific bacteria associated with primary tonsillitis have not been studied.

Tonsillitis most commonly occurs secondarily to a pre-existing disease process. Primary diseases commonly associated with a secondary tonsillitis include chronic vomiting or regurgitation, chronic gingivitis or periodontitis, tracheobronchitis, and nasopharyngeal irritation owing to rhinitis.

Inflamed swollen tonsils are not an absolute indication for treatment. Elimination of pre-existing problems usually results in resolution of the tonsillitis. If clinical signs are severe or persistent, then broad-spectrum antibacterial therapy for 10 to 14 days should be considered. Tonsillectomy is indicated when primary tonsillitis is a recurrent problem or hyperplastic tonsils protrude from the crypts, causing mechanical interference with breathing and swallowing.

Primary pharyngitis is uncommon but may occur concurrently with tonsillitis. Pharyngitis is usually a secondary problem as part of a widespread oral or systemic disease. Pharyngitis often accompanies viral or bacterial upper respiratory tract infections, pharyngeal foreign bodies, and retropharyngeal abscesses. Treatment is aimed at underlying diseases such as removal of foreign bodies or surgical drainage of abscesses. Broad-spectrum antibacterial therapy may be used for 7 to 14 days.

LARYNGITIS

Laryngitis usually occurs as part of a widespread viral or bacterial respiratory infection such as canine tracheobronchitis or feline rhinotracheitis. Other common causes of acute noninfectious laryngitis are trauma to the larynx during endotracheal intubation and prolonged barking or dyspnea. Treatment is aimed at the coexisting infectious problem.

Lower Respiratory Tract Infections

TRACHEOBRONCHITIS

Canine infectious tracheobronchitis is a highly contagious respiratory disease of dogs and is characterized by coughing. This syndrome is associated with a wide variety of viral, mycoplasmal, and bacterial agents. The diagnosis is usually made on the basis of history and physical examination alone. Chapter 6 discusses this syndrome in detail. Feline bordetellosis is discussed in Chapter 16. *Bordetella bronchiseptica* is the bacterial pathogen that can be a primary respiratory pathogen in dogs and cats without accompanying viral or *Mycoplasma* infection.[2, 38] Human infections with *B. bronchiseptica* have been reported, although the organism has a preference for infecting animals, whereas *B. pertussis* and *B. parapertussis* cause whooping cough in people (see Public Health Considerations, Chapter 6).[45, 68] When human infections with *B. bronchiseptica* occur, they are often acquired through animal contact and typically involve immunocompromised patients.

CHRONIC BRONCHIAL DISEASE

Chronic infectious or allergic inflammation of the lower airways can result in colonization with secondary bacteria. A variety of aerobic or facultatively anaerobic bacteria or mycoplasmas may be involved in chronic bronchitis, which can result in secondary bronchiectasis and emphysema. Whether the infection is primary or secondary is difficult to determine. Cats are especially prone to develop bronchial disease manifest by coughing, wheezing, dyspnea, and open mouth breathing. The role of infection in feline bronchial disease is uncertain. Although it may develop initially as an allergic or asthmatic problem, many cats chronically develop bronchiectasis and emphysema with secondary bacterial infections. Cultures of tracheal and bronchial exudates of clinically healthy cats often reveal a mixed pattern of low numbers of organisms ($<5 \times 10^3$ organisms/ml), which probably reflects airway contamination rather than infection when greater than 10^5 organisms/ml is expected (Table 88–4).[46] The role of *Mycoplasma* is intriguing because these organisms can be isolated in up to 25% of airway washings from cats with chronic bronchial disease but not in those from healthy cats.[49] *Mycoplasma* degrade neutral endopeptidase and prolong the effect of substance P, a potent bronchoconstrictor,[57] which may be involved in feline asthma. *Mycoplasma* may damage airway epithelium, resulting in chronic inflammation. Inflammation in airways results in bronchial infiltration, edema, and smooth muscle constriction and hypertrophy. Eosinophilic infiltration of varying degrees develops in later stages as a component of the chronic (not necessarily allergic) inflammatory response. For these reasons, treatment of unresponsive chronic feline bronchial disease with antimicrobials is unjustified with the exception of *Mycoplasma* infections.

BACTERIAL PNEUMONIA

Etiology

Many infectious agents cause pulmonary alveolar inflammation (Table 88–5). This section focuses on bacterial infections; information on other infections can be found in respective chapters. Bacteria enter the lower respiratory tract primarily by inhalation or aspiration of aerosols, oropharyngeal flora, foreign materials, or gastroesophageal contents or by hematogenous spread of extrapulmonary infections. Normal clearance mechanisms are effective unless the inoculum is greater than 10^7 organisms/ml or gastric acid is aspirated concurrently. Whether or not a respiratory infection will develop after bacterial colonization depends on the complex interplay of many factors, including size of the inoculum, virulence of the organism, and resistance of the host. Clinical conditions that predispose the animal to bacterial pneumonia include pre-existing viral, mycoplasmal, or fungal respiratory infections; regurgitation, dysphagia, and vomiting; reduced levels of consciousness (stupor, coma); severe metabolic disorders (diabetes mellitus, uremia, hyperadrenocorticism); thoracic trauma or surgery; immunosuppressive therapy (anticancer chemotherapeutic agents, glucocorticoids); and functional or anatomic disorders (tracheal hypoplasia, primary ciliary dyskinesia). IV catheter–associated bacteremia is probably the most common cause of hematogenous pneumonia, especially in patients with severe underlying disease.

For aspiration pneumonia, risks are increased by recumbency or sedation, nasogastric or endotracheal intubation, debilitation, and esophageal or neuromuscular paralysis. Other factors are mechanical ventilation, concurrent illness, old age, and abdominal or thoracic surgery.[30]

Bacterial pneumonia is more common in the dog than in the cat. *B. bronchiseptica* appears to be the principal primary

Table 88–4. Bacterial Isolation From Lower Respiratory Tract of Cats

HEALTHY[a, 27, 49]	CHRONIC BRONCHIAL DISEASE[b, 17, 39, 46]
Gram Positive	
Staphylococcus	*Staphylococcus*
Streptococcus	*Corynebacterium*
Micrococcus	*Streptococcus*
Gram Negative	
Escherichia coli	*Pasteurella multocida*
Pasteurella multocida	*Moraxella*
Pseudomonas aeruginosa	*Pseudomonas aeruginosa*
Klebsiella	*Bordetella bronchiseptica*
Enterobacter	*Mycoplasma*
Proteus	
Haemophilus felis	

[a]Collected by bronchoscopic alveolar lavage. Organisms isolated from the upper respiratory tract are found in lesser concentrations in the lower airways down to first bronchial division of healthy cats. Colony counts $< 2 \times 10^3$ CFU/ml. No anaerobic bacteria or *Mycoplasma* isolated in healthy cats.

[b]Collected by endotracheal tube bronchial lavage, transtracheal lavage.

Table 88–5. Infectious Agents Causing Pneumonia

AGENT	CHAPTER
Viruses	
Canine distemper virus	3
Canine parainfluenza virus	6
Canine adenovirus-2	4
Canine herpesvirus	5
Feline rhinotracheitis virus	16
Feline calicivirus	16
Rickettsia	
Rickettsia rickettsii	29
Ehrlichia canis	28
Bacteria[a]	
Bordetella	6, 16
Streptococcus	35
Escherichia coli	37
Klebsiella	37
Pasteurella	53
EF-4	88
Mycobacteria	50
Yersinia	47
Pseudomonas mallei	37
Mycoplasma	32
Fungi	
Blastomyces	59
Histoplasma	60
Cryptococcus	61
Coccidioides	62
Aspergillus	65
Penicillium	65
Protozoa	
Toxoplasma	80
Acanthamoeba	79

[a]See Table 88–6 for additional isolates.

bacterial pathogen of canine pneumonia. *Streptococcus zooepidemicus* may also be a primary pathogen (see Group C Streptococcal Infections, Chapter 35). Most isolates in dogs with pneumonia are thought to be opportunistic invaders, the most common of which are staphylococci, streptococci, *E. coli*, *P. multocida*, *Pseudomonas* spp., and *Klebsiella pneumoniae* (Table 88–6).[60] A single pathogen is isolated in the majority of cases, but mixed infections are common. Gram-negative isolates predominate in both single and mixed infections.

As in dogs, most organisms causing pneumonia in cats are resident microflora. Bacterial pathogens in feline pneumonia are poorly documented. Of aerobic organisms, *B. bronchiseptica* and *Pasteurella* spp. are reported most frequently, with *Proteus* and *Pseudomonas* less frequently reported. Isolates are generally similar to those listed for chronic bronchial disease (see Table 88–4).

Bordetella bronchiseptica. This upper respiratory tract inhabitant is the most common bacterial agent associated with tracheobronchitis in dogs and can cause pneumonia and bacteremia. *B. bronchiseptica* can be a significant cause of pneumonia and mortality in cats, especially in congregated cats and in kittens.[65, 67] For further information on lower respiratory tract disease caused by this organism in dogs and cats, see Chapters 6 and 16, respectively.

Streptococcus. As facultatively anaerobic gram-positive cocci, they are isolated from tracheal washings in 14% to 47% of dogs with pneumonia. Although less pathogenic α-hemolytic strains have been isolated, the predominant pathogens are β-hemolytic, with groups C and G being most important in dogs and cats (see also Chapter 35). Some virulence factors identified for hemolytic group A streptococci, which affect people, are capsular polysaccharides; surface protein A; and pneumolysin, a toxin that inhibits cilia, disrupts the alveolar capillary barrier, and interferes with neutrophil chemotaxis and lymphocyte function. Some of these are probably important in animal infections. In addition, nonvirulence products include neuraminidases that promote attachment, immunoglobulin proteases, adhesins, erythrogenic toxins, hyaluronidases, streptokinases, and streptolysins.[6]

Once streptococci reach the alveoli, development and progression of pneumonia depend on virulence factors of the offending agent. With the most virulent strains, vascular leakage and edema are mediated by pneumolysin and hyaluronidase. This fluid exudation facilitates spread of organisms throughout lung lobes. Less virulent strains damage some type 1 epithelial cells, whereas more virulent strains denude large areas of the epithelial surface from the basement membrane. More extensive epithelial loss results in type 2 pneumocyte proliferation and fibroplasia, leading to permanent pulmonary scarring.

Severe pneumonia with high mortality associated with group C streptococci has been reported in dogs, usually secondary to concurrent viral infection. Many persistent streptococcal pneumonias occur in dogs with concurrent immunodeficiencies. Streptococcal pneumonias may be associated with hematogenous spread of infection to meninges, joints, kidneys, heart valves, spleen, lymph nodes, and other organs.

Escherichia coli. These facultatively anaerobic bacilli are commensal flora of predominantly the lower GI tract and are isolated from 17% to 43% of transtracheal washes from dogs

Table 88–6. Bacteria Isolated in Tracheal Aspirates From Dogs With Bacterial Pneumonia[a]

BACTERIA	% RANGE
Gram Negative	
Escherichia coli	17–43
Klebsiella	3.9–23
Bordetella	3–23
Pseudomonas	4.9–33
Pasteurella	0–45
Enterobacter	0–5
Acinetobacter	0–7
Moraxella	2–26
Other gram-negative rods	4.4–12
Gram Positive	
Staphylococcus	5.4–27
Streptococcus	13.8–47
Nonhemolytic	0–13
α-hemolytic	3–30
β-hemolytic	0–16
Corynebacterium	0–5
Mycoplasma[b]	2.9–100
Anaerobes[c]	
Total	18.7
Bacteroides	23.7
Clostridium perfringens	5.3
Eubacterium	2.6
Fusobacterium	15.8
Peptostreptococcus	23.7
Prevotella	5.3
Porphyromonas	15.8
Propionibacterium	2.6

[a]Data taken from Creighton & Wilkins, 1974, 30 dogs; Harpster, 1981, 30 dogs; Thayer & Robinson, 1983, 42 dogs; Hirsh, 1991, 105 dogs; Jameson et al, 1995, 48 dogs; Angus et al, 1997, 203 dogs.

[b]From pharyngeal isolates *Mycoplasma* are isolated 85.7–100% of the time representing normal microflora. From transtracheal washings (34–69%) and from bronchiolar washings (7.1–26.9%). Jameson et al, 1995; Randolph et al, 1993.

[c]A range is not listed because data are from one study of 203 dogs (Angus et al, 1997).

with pneumonia. As gram-negative organisms, they contain endotoxin and can form antiphagocytic polysaccharide capsules and cell-injurious exotoxins. They also form fimbrial adhesins to bind to respiratory epithelial cells and siderophores, which allow them to compete for iron from the bound iron in host tissues and secretions.

E. coli usually enters the lower respiratory tract through aspiration from colonized nasal and oropharyngeal areas. In addition, bacteremic spread from the genitourinary or GI tracts is possible but less frequently documented in dogs. Pneumonia has also occurred in dogs secondary to viral infections, with long-term antibiotic or glucocorticoid therapy or with myelosuppressive or immunodeficiency diseases.[32] Persistent pneumonias have involved mixed infections with other organisms in dogs with immunodeficiencies. Complications of *E. coli* pneumonia are dissemination of infection to other organs such as the meninges, joints, uveal tracts, or glomeruli; DIC; and endotoxin-induced lung injury, resulting in acute respiratory distress.

Pasteurella. These facultatively anaerobic coccobacilli are isolated in up to 45% of transtracheal washings from dogs with pneumonia. *Pasteurella* are among the indigenous microflora of the nasopharynx and large airways of dogs and cats (see also Bite Infections, Chapter 53). Concurrent viral infections and other stresses to the host lead to proliferation and subsequent migration of *Pasteurella* to lower airways. Reduced defense mechanisms lead to impaired bacterial clearance from the lung with resultant pneumonia. *Pasteurella* form adhesin, promoting their epithelial attachment, and polysaccharide capsule, which interferes with phagocytosis. Exotoxin production has not been documented as a feature of *Pasteurella* infections in dogs and cats, as in other animals. However, gram-negative endotoxin decreases the quantity of and increases the surface tension of pulmonary surfactant, altering pulmonary mechanics and gas exchange. Bacterial proliferation results in an influx of inflammatory cells and cytokine mediators, resulting in fibrinopurulent exudation typical of *Pasteurella* pneumonia. Once they develop, such pneumonias may be slow to resolve, and abscesses or pleuritis may develop.

Eugonic Fermenter-4 (EF-4) Infection. Group EF-4 is a collection of unclassified bacterial strains designated by the Centers for Disease Control and Prevention, Atlanta, GA. These bacteria, ecologically and culturally similar to *Pasteurella* species, have been isolated as commensal and opportunistic flora from the oral cavity of dogs and cats (see Table 89–1) and from local infections in people as contaminating organisms of dog and cat bite wounds (see Chapter 53). The precise means by which EF-4 organisms produce respiratory, local, or systemic infections is unknown. Localized infections in dogs and cats have primarily involved cranial infections such as keratitis, retrobulbar abscess, otitis, sinusitis, and stomatitis. Infections probably arise as a result of contamination from the oropharyngeal area. When pneumonia develops, inhalation or hematogenous dissemination of the organism from an oral site is suspected. Concurrent immunosuppression may be important for the organism to colonize other regions of the body.

Both domestic and exotic cats and domestic dogs have been affected.[12, 56] Anorexia, hypersalivation, and dyspnea have been the main clinical signs of respiratory infection. Sudden death, with or without premonitory signs, has been noted in some cases. Abdominal distention from exudative peritonitis was noted in one pup. An epizootic outbreak of fatal pneumonia was identified in a closed research colony of cats.[66]

Diagnosis has been made primarily by culture of the abscess wounds at necropsy. The organism can be cultivated on blood agar, incubated aerobically or anaerobically, and classified by its biochemical reactions. In a few cases in cats, premortem leukopenia and nonregenerative anemia have been found. Multifocal nodular abscess formation is the typical pathologic finding in the lungs. The lesions are grossly indistinguishable from multifocal neoplasms or granulomas. Extrapulmonary lesions have included similar multifocal abscesses in the liver, peritoneal cavity, and lymph nodes. The abscesses are histologically characterized by neutrophilic and mononuclear infiltrates sometimes surrounding visible colonies of gram-negative bacteria.

Therapy for this type of infection is unknown but can be expected to be similar to that for yersiniosis (see Chapter 47 and Table 47–1).

Pathogenesis

Bacteria enter the distal airways and alveoli and are phagocytized by alveolar macrophages. In some cases, neutrophils participate. Virulence of organisms is important in their colonization and persistence in respiratory tissues. Adherence of organisms occurs through specific binding of ligands or adhesins to complementary receptors on mucosal surfaces. Bacterial pili are adhesive structures, whereas cell surface glycoproteins, glycolipids, and proteoglycans are the cell receptors.[9, 53] In addition to attachment of organisms to respiratory surfaces, failure of host defenses such as mucociliary clearance is a primary mechanism that contributes to infections of the upper respiratory tract and bronchi. The mucosal surface is covered by a thin mucous layer that is propelled toward the larynx at up to 1 cm/min by ciliated epithelial cells. Mucus reaching the larynx is usually swallowed or sometimes coughed up. Some pathogenic bacteria, such as *Pseudomonas aeruginosa*, *B. bronchiseptica*, *Mycoplasma pneumoniae*, coagulase-positive staphylococci, and β-hemolytic streptococci, interfere with ciliary movement or affect respiratory epithelial function.[28] Some organism by-products act on neutrophils, which produce ciliastatic hydrogen peroxide. Viruses such as canine distemper virus, canine parainfluenza virus type 2, and canine adenovirus-2 damage ciliated epithelial cells, resulting in decreased mucociliary clearance.

Mucociliary clearance requires functional cilia and appropriate levels and consistency of mucus, which is formed of glycoproteins, glycolipids, and other proteins. Two active ion transport mechanisms adjust the level of periciliary fluid to maximize the mucociliary clearance.[5] Bacterial infection makes mucus more voluminous, less compliant, and more difficult to propel the embedded bacteria, which remain stationary.[18, 58]

Bacterial pneumonia after aspiration of contaminated materials occurs frequently as a nosocomial event from intubation associated with surgery or after recovery from anesthesia. Disorders that predispose patients to aspiration are swallowing impairment, laryngeal paralysis, megaesophagus, hiatal hernia, and regurgitation or vomiting from any cause. Antacids are often given in disorders when vomiting is anticipated to reduce the threat of gastric acid inhalation. However, paradoxically, raised gastric pH increases gastric microbial replication, making aspiration pneumonia worse.[42] Conditions such as periodontal disease and intestinal stasis also increase the bacterial load in aspirated GI secretions.

Clinical Findings

History and clinical signs of canine bacterial pneumonia include cough (usually moist, productive), variable fever, dyspnea, serous or mucopurulent nasal discharge, anorexia, depression, weight loss, and dehydration. Auscultation usually reveals abnormal lung sounds, including increased intensity of bronchial breath sounds, crackles, and wheezes. Aspiration pneumonia should be suspected in any animal that develops these signs while hospitalized or after episodes of vomiting or regurgitation.

Diagnosis

The diagnosis of bacterial pneumonia is suspected on the basis of history and physical examination and is confirmed by hematologic findings, thoracic radiography, and microbiologic and cytologic examination of material from the tracheobronchial tree or lung. A neutrophilic leukocytosis with a left shift is frequently found on a CBC, but may be present in only 60% of animals. Arterial blood gas values correlate well with the degree of physiologic disruption in patients with bacterial pneumonia and are sensitive monitors of progress during treatment. Thoracic radiographs reveal an alveolar pattern characterized by increased pulmonary density in which margins are indistinct and in which air bronchograms may be seen. A patchy or lobar alveolar pattern will be present in a cranial ventral lung lobe distribution.

The definitive method of establishing a diagnosis of bacterial pneumonia is to obtain aspirates, washings, or brushings for microbiologic and cytologic examinations. Multiple procedures that bypass the oropharynx have been recommended to obtain these specimens. Blood cultures can also be helpful in identifying the etiologic agent causing bacterial pneumonia.

Transtracheal Aspiration. Because animals are unable to expectorate sputum, and because it bypasses the oropharyngeal area, the method of transtracheal washing and aspiration is safe, simple, and clinically valuable for obtaining tracheobronchial and pulmonary material for culture and cytologic examination. The technique is well tolerated by most dogs and cats and requires only minimal restraint of the unanesthetized patient.

Materials needed to perform transtracheal aspiration are listed in Table 88–7. Sedation is not required in most dogs, with the exception of the hyperexcitable miniature and toy breeds, for which narcotics are the drugs of choice. After the catheter is inserted into the airway, the effects of the sedative can be reversed, allowing the cough reflex to return, thereby increasing the probability of obtaining a diagnostic-based specimen from the lower airway. Ketamine, used to sedate cats, does not interfere with the cough reflex. The animal is allowed to sit or is placed in sternal recumbency with its neck extended. The area of the larynx is clipped and scrubbed as for surgery. The cricoid cartilage, identified by palpating the tracheal rings from the midcervical region toward the larynx, is the first prominent ventral ridge at the larynx. Cranial to the cricoid cartilage and between the thyroid cartilages is the cricothyroid ligament (Fig. 88–1). From 1/2 to 1 ml of 2% lidocaine is injected SC over the cricothyroid ligament. The needle and catheter are then directed caudoventrally through the skin and cricothyroid ligament into the larynx in a single motion. In larger dogs, the catheter can be inserted into the lower regions of the trachea between cartilage rings to facilitate recovery of flushing solutions. The catheter is passed into the trachea, and the needle is withdrawn from the larynx (Fig. 88–2). The needle guard is then applied to prevent the catheter from being cut by the needle. Paroxysms of coughing can be expected as the catheter is passed into the trachea.

A syringe generally containing up to 15 to 20 ml of sterile, nonbacteriostatic saline is attached to the catheter, and 2 to 4 ml of fluid is injected. As the animal coughs, suction is applied with the syringe. Resistance suggests that secretions are being collected in the catheter. If only air is aspirated, the syringe is disconnected, the air is expelled, and another 8 to 10 ml of fluid is injected and reaspirated. This procedure is repeated until respiratory secretions, which will appear as a cloudy fluid, are aspirated into the syringe. Up to 1 ml/kg of solution can be safely injected into the airway during a single flush without causing significant respiratory insuffi-

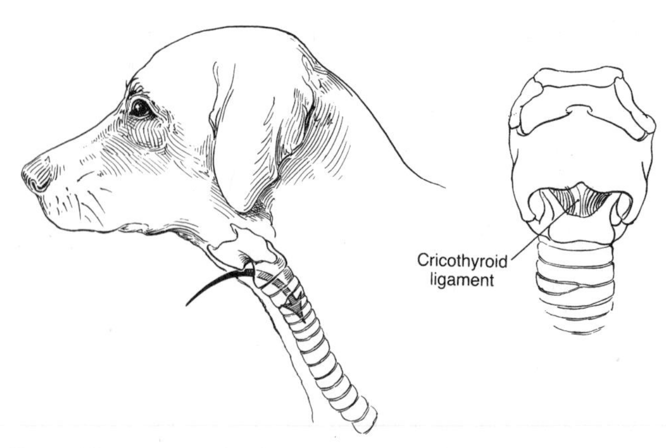

Figure 88–1. Transtracheal aspiration. The needle is inserted through the cricothyroid ligament. For larger dogs, the needle may be inserted at a lower point through the tracheal rings.

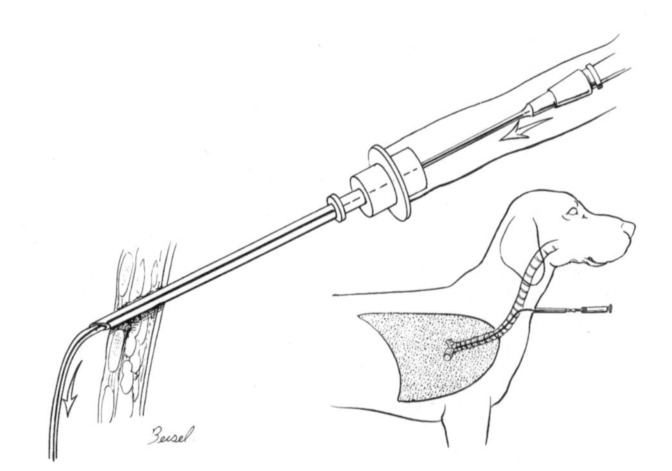

Figure 88–2. Transtracheal aspiration. After the needle is inserted into the tracheal lumen, the catheter is advanced through the needle. The needle is withdrawn from the trachea, and the needle guard is attached before flushing with sterile fluids. Note the ventral position of the needle bevel.

Table 88–7. Materials Required for Performing Transtracheal Aspiration

Materials
16-gauge × 12-inch through-the-needle IV catheter[a] or 18.5-gauge × 8-inch through-the-needle IV catheter[b] (for small dogs and cats)
Clippers
Surgical scrub
1 ml 2% lidocaine
20-ml syringe
Sterile water or saline (nonbacteriostatic)
Surgical gloves (optional when using a through-the-needle catheter)

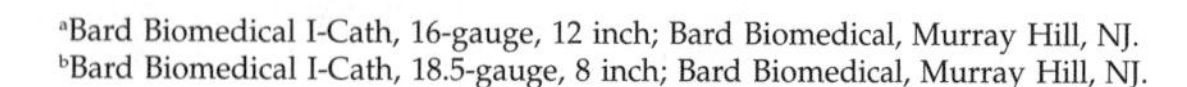

[a]Bard Biomedical I-Cath, 16-gauge, 12 inch; Bard Biomedical, Murray Hill, NJ.
[b]Bard Biomedical I-Cath, 18.5-gauge, 8 inch; Bard Biomedical, Murray Hill, NJ.

ciency. The largest amount of aspirate will be collected when the animal is coughing. When the specimen has been obtained, the syringe is detached and capped to prevent contamination. The catheter is removed, and a light bandage is applied to prevent SC hemorrhage or emphysema. The specimen is mixed in the syringe and divided into aliquots for cytologic and microbiologic examination (see later).

Although complications from transtracheal washing and aspiration are uncommon, the procedure is not without risk. As with the majority of invasive diagnostic procedures, risk is significantly decreased with experience. The procedure is considerably more difficult in cats and small dogs than in larger dogs. Transtracheal washing should not be attempted in the fractious or uncooperative patient without adequate chemical and manual restraint.

The most common complication associated with transtracheal washing is subcutaneous emphysema. This occurs when persistent coughing or dyspnea causes air to leak from the puncture site into the cervical subcutaneous tissues. Other complications include endotracheal hemorrhage, tracheal laceration, cardiac arrhythmia, and infection at the puncture site.

Endotracheal Wash. This technique involves general anesthesia and short-acting barbiturates. After endotracheal intubation with a sterilized endotracheal tube, a fine, flexible urinary catheter or feeding tube is passed down through the lumen to the level of the carina. Two or more 5- to 10-ml aliquots of sterile 0.9% saline solution are administered through the catheter, each followed immediately by aspiration attempts. There are several advantages: washings can be obtained without producing tracheal injury and minimal equipment is needed, and it is technically simpler to perform in small dogs and cats. Disadvantages are oropharyngeal contamination, as for bronchoscopy (see later), and airway visualization is not possible.

Bronchoalveolar Lavage (BAL). This technique is performed using general anesthesia with or without the aid of an endoscope.[24] Without endoscopy, the animal is positioned in lateral recumbency, and a single lumen endotracheal tube is placed just rostral to the carina. The cuff is inflated, and a syringe adaptor is connected to the end of the tube. Aliquots (5 ml/kg) of warmed sterile 0.9% saline are infused via syringe. Immediately after each aliquot, mild suction is applied to the syringe. The animal is tilted with its head caudal end elevated to assist in fluid recovery. The syringe is immediately disconnected after the fluid is taken, and 100% oxygen is given through the endotracheal tube for 5 minutes. The advantage of BAL is that it provides specimens of cells and proteinaceous materials from the deeper portions of the lungs.[23] An alternative procedure is to use a double-lumen endotracheal tube with which one side of the lung can be ventilated and the other lavaged. These tubes are not available in small sizes, are expensive, and are designed for either left or right lung lobes.

Bronchoscopy. Tracheobronchoscopy is valuable for obtaining brush catheter specimens for cytologic and microbiologic examination. The procedure requires that the patient be maintained under general anesthesia, which may be of concern in those with bacterial pneumonia. IV anesthetic agents and a speculum will allow a thorough tracheobronchial examination with a rigid bronchoscope passed through the mouth. Brush catheters and suction cannulas may be passed through the lumen of the rigid bronchoscope to obtain specimens.

The transoral approach with a flexible fiberoptic bronchoscope inserted through an endotracheal tube is preferred. The patient is anesthetized, using standard procedures, intubated, and maintained on inhalation anesthesia. An endotracheal tube T-adapter allows oxygen and anesthetic gas to flow to the patient, whereas the flexible endoscope passes through the endotracheal tube and into the trachea. This technique is successful in moderate- to large-sized dogs during lengthy procedures. Small dogs and cats are given an IV anesthetic, and a flexible or small-diameter rigid fiberoptic endoscope is passed directly into the trachea and wedged in a terminal bronchus. During wedge lavage in cats and small dogs, oxygen is infused alongside the bronchoscope through a 5-French diameter tube. Brush catheters are passed through the biopsy channel of the endoscope to obtain specimens. BAL lavage of individual lobes or segments can be performed by inserting small catheters through the channel into terminal airways and flushing saline in and aspirating fluids out.[35]

The advantages of tracheobronchoscopy are numerous when compared with other diagnostic techniques. Endoscopy allows the direct visualization of the tracheobronchial tree and the lesions associated with bacterial pneumonia, thereby allowing a better assessment of the patient's clinical status and prognosis. The cytologic preparations obtained by mucosal brushings or by BAL lavage through the endoscope are superior to those obtained by transtracheal washing and aspiration. When indicated, transbronchial biopsy specimens may also be taken.

Because of contamination from the oropharynx, bacterial cultures obtained with sterile, open-end, brush-in-catheter systems passed through the endoscope have been considered unreliable in the past. A commercially available catheter (Microbiology Specimen Brush, Microvasive Inc., Milford, MA) that enhances the ability to obtain reliable cultures of lower airway secretions through a bronchoscope has been developed. This system consists of a sterile brush contained within a telescoping double catheter occluded by a polyethylene glycol plug. This system is passed through the instrumentation channel of the bronchoscope. The brush is extended into the secretions to be cultured and then retracted into the inner catheter. The entire brush-in-telescope, double-catheter system is removed from the endoscope. The brush is advanced out of the catheter, where the wire is transected with sterile scissors. The brush is placed in trypticase soy broth. The only disadvantage is the expense of a catheter system that can be used only once.

Fine-Needle Lung Aspiration. Transthoracic fine-needle aspiration can be utilized to procure material for microbial culture and cytologic examination directly from the lung. Fine-needle aspiration is best performed after routine diagnostic procedures, such as transtracheal washing, have proved negative. The technique, contraindications, and complications are well documented elsewhere.

A study of diagnostic procedures in a canine model of streptococcal pneumonia found that transthoracic fine-needle lung aspiration had the highest sensitivity and specificity for bacterial recovery compared with transtracheal washing, flexible fiberoptic bronchoscopy, transbronchial lung biopsy, and blind catheter brushing. Sensitivity was enhanced when "dog-side" culturing was performed rather than sending the samples to the microbiology laboratory. Complications of percutaneous fine-needle aspiration are common and potentially serious. Pneumothorax is the primary complication; a 10% to 30% incidence rate was reported in one study.

Cytologic and Microbiologic Examination. Preparation of material for cytologic evaluation can be done by several methods. Visible strands of exudate may be teased onto a microscope slide, smeared, and stained. Small quantities of material can be centrifuged and smears made of the sediment. New methylene blue wet mounts and Wright-Giemsa's or Gram's stain of air-dried smears can be used for identification of cellular elements and bacteria. Bacterial infections are associated with degenerate neutrophils and intracellular bacteria; excess mucus, proteinaceous material, and alveolar macrophages may be present. Bacteria are only demonstrable in one third of washings from pneumonic animals, and their absence in cytologic specimens from transtracheal aspirations does not rule out bacterial pneumonia.

All collection methods of airway washings can be associated with pharyngeal contamination. This is one explanation for why many lower airway washings contain artifact, resident nasopharyngeal microflora. Pharyngeal contamination is detected by the presence in cytologic preparations of squamous epithelium or *Simonsiella (Caryophanon)*, a characteristic genus of oral bacteria, which appears as "stacked coins."

Because of the delay in bacterial culture, the organisms are classified as being rods or cocci or other recognizable bacterial or fungal elements. Anaerobes, *Actinomyces*, and *Nocardia* are often larger, pleomorphic, or filamentous. Acid-fast staining will help detect *Nocardia* or *Mycobacterium*. Specific yeast or filamentous fungi may be identified by additional staining (see Chapter 56). Mycoplasmas may be obtained if special media is used (see Chapter 32.)

Bacteriologic Culture. An aliquot of aspirated material can be cultured directly for aerobic and anaerobic bacteria. Gram-negative organisms are most commonly cultured, whereas gram-positive and anaerobic bacteria and *Mycoplasma* are less commonly isolated. Anaerobic culture is indicated only when aspiration pneumonia or pulmonary abscess formation is suspected, but still may not add information that alters treatment. Secretions that coat the distal end of the catheter can be cultured if the amount of aspirated material is minimal. Sensitivity of transtracheal washing and aspiration for recovery of bacteria is good, but because larger airways may contain low levels of microflora, specificity for infection rather than contamination cannot be determined. If clinical features suggest infection, and organisms can be visualized cytologically or grow readily in large numbers without enrichment, they are thought to be clinically significant.[22] False-negative results may be obtained if antimicrobial therapy has not been discontinued for at least 1 week before sampling.

Blood Cultures. These have been recommended in people with bacterial pneumonia to help isolate the infectious agent. Documented bacteremia is also thought to be a poor prognostic finding. No studies in animals that document the value of blood cultures in establishing a prognosis or isolating the bacterial agent in cases of pneumonia exist. Up to 50% of dogs with experimentally induced streptococcal pneumonia have been blood culture–positive within 48 hours of onset of clinical signs.[56]

PULMONARY ABSCESS

Pulmonary abscesses, necrotic areas of lung parenchyma containing purulent material usually produced by pyogenic infection, are uncommon in dogs and cats. Most arise from aspiration of oropharyngeal or gastric contents and are termed primary lung abscess. Secondary lung abscess results from a primary underlying process such as bronchial obstruction, septic or heartworm thromboembolism, airway parasite, foreign body, bullous emphysema, tuberculous cavity, or neoplasia. Obligate anaerobic bacteria are identified more frequently than aerobic, but mixed infections are common. *Mycoplasma* spp. have also been recovered in cats.

The clinical signs in pulmonary abscess formation depend on the cause but closely resemble those of chronic bacterial pneumonia. Clinical findings include weight loss, chronic fever, cough, and hemoptysis. Hematologic findings include leukocytosis with a left shift, anemia, and rarely hypoproteinemia. An abscess usually will appear on a thoracic radiograph as an ill-defined pulmonary nodule or mass with or without cavitation. Abscesses are often indistinguishable from granulomas, traumatic bullae, tumors, and pneumatocysts. Cytologic examination of brushings or aspirations is consistent with a septic or nonseptic purulent exudate.

THERAPY OF LOWER AIRWAY INFECTIONS

Unlike treatment of upper airway infections, that for lower tract infections must be aggressive. Systemically effective antimicrobials must be used. Drug penetration into consolidated lung tissues is more effective systemically than by topical means.

Antibiotics

Drug dosages for lower and other airway infections are summarized in Table 88–8. Specific information on each drug is available in the Drug Formulary, Appendix 8. Oral or parenteral antibacterials are the principal therapies for lower airway bacterial infections. It is unrealistic to expect any single antibacterial to be routinely effective against the wide variety of organisms causing bacterial pneumonia. The most important criterion for selection of an antibacterial is identification of the bacterial organism. Substantially more patients recover if antibacterial therapy is administered according to culture results and in vitro susceptibility testing than not.[60]

Penetration of antimicrobial drugs into airway secretions and pulmonary tissues is favored by high lipophilicity and low molecular weight. Drugs enter normal bronchial secretions at a fraction of their serum concentrations. Trimethoprim, clindamycin, fluoroquinolone, erythromycin, and doxycycline enter in highest proportions. Penicillins have the lowest penetration; cephalosporins and aminoglycosides have intermediate distribution. With inflammation, penetrance is increased, but antibiotic distribution through the airway may be impaired in exudates.

Initial choices of antibacterials can be based on the morphology of bacteria noted on airway or lung cytologic preparation. Cocci are usually staphylococci or streptococci. Rods are usually members of the family Enterobacteriaceae, which are most unpredictable with respect to antibacterial agents (Table 88–9). The aminopenicillanic derivatives have a broader spectrum than penicillin, including activity against gram-positive, many gram-negative, and some anaerobic bacteria. *E. coli*, *Proteus*, *Klebsiella*, and *Pasteurella* are usually susceptible. Resistance is often present in *Enterobacter*, *Serratia*, and *Pseudomonas*. Resistance can be overcome in some instances by use of a β-lactamase inhibitor such as clavulanate or sulbactam. Fluoroquinolones or aminoglycosides are recommended if resistant gram-negative infections are suspected. If cytologic information is not available, initial treatment with amoxicillin-clavulanate is recommended. Later therapy should be based on the susceptibility spectrum indicated by cultural results. With severe clinical signs, respiratory distress, or evidence of bacteremia, IV therapy is recommended until the patient stabilizes. Levels of antibacterials

Table 88–8. Recommended Dosages of Antibacterial Drugs for Respiratory Disease[a]

DRUG	SPECIES	DOSE	ROUTE	INTERVAL (HOUR)
Amikacin	B	5.0–7.5 mg/kg	IV, IM, SC	12
	B	15 mg/kg	IV, IM, SC	24
Amoxicillin	B	15–20 mg/kg	PO, IM, SC	8
Amoxicillin-clavulanate	B	15 mg/kg	PO	8
	B	20 mg/kg	PO	12
Ampicillin	B	22–30 mg/kg	PO, IV, SC	8
Ampicillin-sulbactam	D	20 mg/kg	IV, IM	6–8
Carbenicillin	D	10–30 mg/kg	IV, IM	6–8
Cefazolin (1st)	B	10–30 mg/kg	IV, IM, SC	6–8
Cefotaxime (3rd)	B	25–50 mg/kg	IV, IM	6–8
Cefotetan (2nd)	B	25–30 mg/kg	IV, SC	8
Cefoxitin (2nd)	B	10–20 mg/kg	IV, IM	6–8
Ceftiofur (3rd)	B	4.4 mg/kg	SC	12
Cephalexin (1st)	B	22–44 mg/kg	PO	8
Cephradine (1st)	B	22–44 mg/kg	IV, SC	8
Chloramphenicol	D	50 mg/kg	PO, IV, SC	8
	C	50 mg total	PO, IV, SC	12
Clindamycin	D	10 mg/kg	PO, SC	12
	C	10–15 mg/kg	PO, SC	12
Doxycycline[b]	B	5–10 mg/kg	PO	12
Enrofloxacin[c]	B	5–11 mg/kg	PO, SC, IV[d]	12
Gentamicin[e]	B	2 mg/kg	IV, IM, SC	8–12
	B	8 mg/kg	IM, IV	24
Imipenem-cilastatin	B	3–10 mg/kg	IV, IM	8
Kanamycin[e]	B	5–7.5 mg/kg	IV, IM, SC	8
Piperacillin	B	25–50 mg/kg	IV	8
Tetracycline	D	22 mg/kg	PO	8
Ticarcillin	B	40–75[d] mg/kg	IV	6–8
Ticarcillin-clavulanate	B	30–50[d] mg/kg	IV	6–8
Tobramycin[e]	B	2 mg/kg	IV, IM, SC	8
Trimethoprim-sulfonamide	B	15 mg/kg	PO, SC	12

[a]For more information on all drugs, see Drug Formulary, Appendix 8. Dose per administration at specified interval. Duration is for at least 1 week after clinical response is noted. Responses should be noted within 3–5 days, and therapy should continue for at least 14 days.
[b]Also can substitute minocycline.
[c]Also can substitute ciprofloxacin.
[d]Highest levels for treating *Pseudomonas*.
[e]Potentially nephrotoxic. Must monitor urine sediment and serum urea concentration.
B = both; D = dog; C = cat.

in airway secretions after oral or parenteral administration are much lower than serum levels. Systemic antibacterials, therefore, should be administered in high doses for long periods of time so that maximum concentrations are reached in lung tissues and airway secretions. For usually self-limiting **tracheobronchitis**, antibiotics are not usually indicated unless complicating *Bordetella* infection is suspected. Of antibiotics tried in tracheobronchitis, only trimethoprim-sulfonamide or ampicillin-amoxicillin had some benefit in reducing the duration of coughing.[62] Treatment for most lower respiratory tract infections is recommended for at least 1 week beyond resolution of clinical illness or at least a 2-week minimum. With **bronchiectasis** or **chronic bronchitis**, treatment is usually much longer.

Table 88–9. Antimicrobial Therapy for Lower Airway Bacterial Infections[a]

Gram-positive cocci:	Amp(amox)icillin, chloramphenicol, gentamicin, trimethoprim-sulfonamide, first-generation cephalosporins
Gram-negative rods:	Amikacin, chloramphenicol, gentamicin, trimethoprim-sulfonamide, fluoroquinolones, second- and third-generation cephalosporins, ampicillin-sulbactam, imipenem-cilastatin, piperacillin, ticarcillin, carbenicillin
Pasteurella:	Ampicillin, gentamicin, trimethoprim-sulfonamide, enrofloxacin
Bordetella:	Tetracycline, gentamicin, chloramphenicol, trimethoprim-sulfonamide, tylosin, kanamycin, fluoroquinolones, amoxicillin-clavulanate, azithromycin
Anaerobes:	Amp(amox)icillin-clavulanate, penicillin, second- or third-generation cephalosporins, clindamycin, metronidazole,[b] ticarcillin, carbenicillin
Mycoplasmas:	Doxycycline, chloramphenicol, gentamicin, fluoroquinolones, tylosin, clindamycin

[a]Consult Appendix 8 for appropriate dosages and further information on each drug.
[b]Despite in vitro efficacy, metronidazole does poorly in treatment of anaerobic pulmonary infections because of the high oxygen tension in these tissues.

Particularly severe or resistant gram-negative or anaerobic bacterial pneumonia must be treated parenterally with drugs such as the extended-spectrum penicillin, ticarcillin, combined with clavulanate. The combination is effective against gram-negative bacteria and anaerobes, as are imipenem-cilastatin or second- or third-generation cephalosporins. Aminoglycosides are effective against gram-negative organisms.

Pneumonia secondary to bacteremia is often due to gram-negative sepsis in immunocompromised people or animals. If clinical improvement occurs and blood culture results are negative after 4 days, parenteral therapy can be discontinued.

With **aspiration pneumonia**, use of antimicrobials should be delayed until the animal becomes ill because of the increased chance of developing bacterial resistance, which delays the clinical response. When antibiotics are given, combination therapy may be required because of the multiplicity of aerobic and anaerobic organisms that are involved. Prevention of aspiration pneumonia involves reducing the proliferation of gastric microflora and their entry into the airways. This is accomplished by keeping the patient's body positioned in sternal recumbency or by keeping the cranial part elevated (especially with paralysis, gastric intubation, or history of vomiting or regurgitation); minimizing gastric volume by frequent feedings or keeping feeding tubes in the small bowel rather than the stomach or esophagus; keeping gastric pH below 3.5 by use of sucralfate rather than antacid preparations, which promote gastric bacterial overgrowth; and using small-bore feeding tubes if feeding via the esophagus.[42] To prevent aspiration and infection during anesthesia, aspiration of oropharyngeal secretions, maintenance of endotracheal tube pressure, and avoidance of cross-contamination between patients by using sterilized equipment are recommended. For nebulization, disposable sterile tubing and fluid chambers should be utilized and nebulizers should be disinfected after each patient (see Chapter 94).

Pulmonary consolidation or **abscesses** are common with airway obstruction from severe infection, certain bacteria such as *Actinomyces* or *Nocardia*, or from foreign material. Lung abscesses are usually treated without drainage, but with long-term antibacterial therapy. Choice of antibacterials should be based on culture and susceptibility findings. Response to antimicrobial therapy is often temporary or incomplete, and relapse of fever and coughing occurs once treatment is discontinued, even after months of such treatment. Furthermore, evidence of a persistent pattern of alveolar consolidation may be apparent in thoracic radiographs. Bronchoscopy can be used to localize affected lobes and, if performed early, can be used to remove foreign material such as plant awns. With long-standing occlusion, scarring, and abscess formation, thoracotomy and lobectomy must be done to effect a resolution. Lobectomy is most effective in resolving pneumonias, and postoperative complications are least in pneumonias that are localized to individual lobes.[40]

Hydration

Maintenance of normal systemic hydration is an important therapeutic objective in patients with bacterial pneumonia. Dehydration hinders mucociliary clearance and secretion mobilization because normal respiratory secretions are more than 90% water.

Aerosol

The goal of aerosol therapy is to mobilize secretions by adding water to the mucociliary blanket. A nebulizer that produces particles between 0.5 to 3.0 μm ensures that water is deposited in the lower airways. Water vaporizers or humidifiers are inadequate for this reason. The animal is placed in an enclosed chamber, and a bland aerosol (normal saline) is nebulized into the chamber. The animal should be treated two or three times daily for 20 minutes per treatment. Because bronchoconstriction invariably develops, pretreatment with bronchodilators is recommended.

Nebulization with bland aerosols has subjectively resulted in more rapid resolution of cases of canine bronchopneumonia in conjunction with physiotherapy and systemic antimicrobials. For aerosol administration, 50 mg of gentamicin is diluted in 3 ml of saline and is added to the nebulizer chamber. Antimicrobial aerosolization decreases the bacterial counts in airways and the duration and severity of coughing in dogs with experimentally induced tracheobronchitis. Routine intratracheal or aerosol administration of antibacterials is not recommended unless pneumonia is caused by a difficult to treat organism (e.g., *Pseudomonas*). With severe alveolar consolidation in pneumonia, airway penetration of antimicrobials is inferior to systemic administration. Physiotherapy should always be performed immediately after aerosolization to enhance secretion clearance. Methods include mild forced exercise, increased cough frequency by chest wall coupage or tracheal manipulation, and postural drainage.

Supportive

Animals with severe tachypnea, dyspnea, or marked hypoxemia (arterial oxygen tension <60 mm Hg) require oxygen therapy. The early period of highest mortality with bacterial pneumonia corresponds to the period of greatest hypoxemia. The oxygen should be humidified to prevent drying of respiratory membranes. Oxygen can be administered by cage, mechanical ventilator, intratracheal cannula, or nasal catheter. Drugs such as antitussives and antihistamines that inhibit mucokinesis and exudate removal from the respiratory tract are contraindicated with bacterial pneumonia. Long-term therapy with systemic bronchodilators is recommended in animals with evidence of chronic bronchial inflammation, but caution should be taken in concurrent use of chloramphenicol or fluoroquinolones, which increase serum theophylline concentration. Terbutaline can be given at 0.01 mg/kg SC for emergency treatment of bronchospasm and acute respiratory distress. Cyproheptadine (2 mg PO given twice daily) has been administered in cats with bronchoconstriction that do not tolerate terbutaline.[47]

Pleural Infections

Purulent pleuritis, pyothorax, and thoracic empyema describe septic processes of the pleural cavity resulting in exudate accumulation.

ETIOLOGY

Despite the results from bacterial culture, pleural infections are almost always polymicrobic in nature. This factor is evident when comparing the cytologic findings and culture results. There is a high incidence of obligate anaerobic bacteria as sole pathogens or in combination with aerobic-facultative and anaerobic bacteria. Obligate anaerobic bacteria and gram-positive filamentous organisms such as *Nocardia* and *Actinomyces* are most commonly isolated from dogs with pyothorax (see Chapter 49). Feline pyothorax is associated with a high incidence of pure obligate anaerobic bacteria, including *Actinomyces* and *Bacteroides* and infection with *Pasteurella*.[61] Other bacterial, fungal, and yeast organisms isolated from pleural exudate of the dog and cat are summarized in Table 88–10. Sources of bacterial pleural infections are not identified in most cases, but include penetrating thoracic wounds; migrating foreign bodies; esophageal perforation; hematogenous spread; lung parasites; extension from cervical, lumbar, mediastinal, or pulmonary infections; and iatrogenic causes.

CLINICAL FINDINGS

Pyothorax occurs most commonly in young adult, male, nonpurebred cats and adult large-breed dogs. Clinical signs

Table 88–10. Specific Etiologic Agents Isolated From Pleural Infections in Dogs and Cats

MOST COMMON	LESS COMMON
Anaerobes	**Anaerobes**
Actinomyces	*Clostridium*
Bacteroides	**Aerobes**
Fusobacterium	*Escherichia coli*
Peptococcus	*Enterobacter*
Propionibacterium	*Proteus*
Aerobes	*Pseudomonas*
Corynebacterium	**Fungi**
Nocardia	*Aspergillus*
Pasteurella	*Blastomyces*
Staphylococcus	*Candida*
Streptococcus	*Cryptococcus*

result from restrictive respiratory disease, including increased respiratory rate, shallow respirations, dyspnea, and orthopnea. Other signs include exercise intolerance, lethargy, anorexia, and fever. Physical examination reveals muffled heart sounds, decreased breath sounds, and hyperresonant (dull) percussion sounds, especially over the ventral portions of the thorax. Chronic or severe infections result in a dehydrated, debilitated, or hypothermic patient.

DIAGNOSIS

A diagnosis of pyothorax is confirmed by hematology, thoracic radiography, and thoracocentesis with cytologic evaluation and culture of pleural fluid. Neutrophilic leukocytosis with or without a left shift is the most common hematologic finding. Leukogram results do not correlate with the severity of the underlying infection, however, and leukocyte counts within or lower than the reference range are found with some frequency. Radiographic signs of free pleural fluid include increased hazy density of the lung fields (ventral portions of lung fields on lateral view), which obscures the cardiac silhouette; retraction of the lobar borders from the chest wall; visibility of the interlobar fissures; and rounding or filling of the costophrenic angles.

Cytologic evaluation of pleural fluid is usually consistent with a septic or nonseptic exudate. Degenerate neutrophils and mixed populations of bacteria are often observed. Cytomorphology of the neutrophil is most helpful for determination of whether pleural fluid should be cultured and for interpretation of the results of culture. Aerobic and anaerobic cultures of pleural fluid should be made, if available, whenever neutrophil degeneration is observed, regardless of whether bacteria are seen cytologically.

THERAPY

Treatment of pyothorax should be prompt and aggressive. Initial goals include relief of respiratory embarrassment via thoracocentesis, appropriate fluid therapy, supportive care, and systemic antibacterials. Pleural drainage and lavage are essential as for any accumulation of pus. Disadvantages of delay in pleural lavage are incomplete resolution of signs and formation of loculated abscesses and fibroses, which will necessitate later thoracotomy. Pleural drainage and lavage are achieved by tube thoracostomy. Advantages of closed chest drainage and lavage include avoiding frequent needle thoracocentesis, facilitating pleural fluid sampling to monitor therapeutic response, and allowing direct instillation of isotonic lavage fluid into the pleural space. Disadvantages include maintaining drain placement and patency and risking pneumothorax and chest wall infection. Mortality appears to be higher in patients treated with multiple thoracocentesis and antibacterials than in those treated with tube thoracostomy alone. The average length of chest tube drainage is 3 to 7 days.

For tube placement, the patient is first given fluid therapy, and specimens for cytologic and microbiologic examination can be withdrawn for analysis by needle aspiration. After sedation with local anesthetic infusion or general anesthesia, a tube is placed in the intercostal space by tunneling under the skin a few interspaces and penetrating the pleura with the tube by hemostat or stylet. After fluid removal, radiographs should be taken to assess whether drainage is complete, especially on the contralateral side. If removal is incomplete, another tube may be required. The tubes are clamped and wrapped to prevent inadvertent air leakage into the pleural space. When available or practical, one-way continuous suction or intermittent suction every 2 hours may be applied. A less frequent and intensive approach involves twice-daily instillation of IV saline into the pleural space with mild coupage followed by immediate removal of whatever fluid can be obtained. Fluid is infused through the tip of an IV administration set wedged firmly into the lumen of the tube's orifice. The clamp is used to control infusion rate. Fluid volumes for infusion are usually 100 ml for small dogs and cats, 500 ml for intermediate sized dogs, and 1000 ml for large dogs. This method rinses the pleural surfaces and facilitates removal of accumulated pus and bacteria. Lavage is continued for up to 7 days or until the removed fluid looks clear of pus. Cytologic improvement is manifest by decreasing cell count, with loss of degenerative changes in neutrophils, and absence of bacteria.

Systemic antimicrobial therapy can be considered concurrently, but it is *ineffective* without lavage or drainage of the infected pleural cavity (see Table 88–8). No single antibacterial agent will inhibit the wide variety of facultative and obligate anaerobic bacteria associated with pyothorax. Penicillin or penicillin derivatives are often given because they are effective against obligate anaerobic, *Pasteurella*, and *Actinomyces* infections.

Systemic antibacterial therapy should be continued for at least 4 to 6 weeks. Regardless of the anaerobic or facultative anaerobic bacteria that are cultured, the regimen should always contain drugs effective against anaerobes. Lack of significant improvement in fluid consistency during lavage, formation of lung abscesses, or radiographic evidence of fluid encapsulation indicates surgical exploration or lobectomy. Foreign bodies are often involved in persistent pulmonary abscesses. Radiographic re-evaluation should be performed when the chest tube is removed and when systemic antibacterial therapy is completed.

References

1. Angus JC, Jang SS, Hirsh DC. 1997. Microbiological study of transtracheal aspirates from dogs with suspected lower respiratory tract disease: 264 cases (1989–1995). *J Am Vet Med Assoc* 218:55–58.
2. Bemis DA. 1992. *Bordetella* and *Mycoplasma* respiratory infections in dogs and cats. *Vet Clin North Am* 22:1173–1186.
3. Bonten MJ, Gaillard CA, de Leeuw PW, et al. 1997. The role of colonization of the upper intestinal tract in the pathogenesis of ventilator associated pneumonia. *Clin Infect Dis* 24:309–319.
4. Boothe DM. 1997. Principles of drug selection for respiratory infections in cats. *Suppl Compend Cont Educ Pract Vet* 19:5–15.
5. Boucher RC. 1994. Human airway ion transport. Part 1. *Am J Respir Crit Care Med* 150:271–281.

6. Boulnosis GJ. 1992. Pneumococcal proteins and the pathogenesis of disease caused by *Streptococcus pneumoniae*. *J Gen Microbiol* 138:249–259.
7. Brownlie SE. 1990. A retrospective study of diagnosis in 109 cases of canine lower respiratory disease. *J Small Anim Pract* 31:371–376.
8. Cape L. 1992. Feline idiopathic chronic rhinosinusitis. A retrospective study of 30 cases. *J Am Anim Hosp Assoc* 28:149–155.
9. Carnoy C, Scharfman A, Van Brussel E, et al. 1994. *Pseudomonas aeruginosa* outer membrane adhesions for human respiratory mucus glycoproteins. *Infect Immun* 62:1896–1900.
10. Ceyssens K, Devriese LA, Maenhout T. 1989. Necrotizing pneumonia in cats associated with infection by EF-4a bacteria. *J Vet Med* 36:314–316.
11. Codner EC, Lurus AG, Miller JB, et al. 1993. Comparison of computed tomography with radiography as a noninvasive diagnostic technique for choice nasal discharge in dogs. *J Am Vet Med Assoc* 202:1106–1110.
12. Corboz L, Ossent P, Gruber H. 1993. Isolation and characterization of Group EF-4 bacteria from various lesions in cat, dog and badger. *Zbl Bakt* 279:140–145.
13. Corcoran BM, Fuentes VL, Clarke CJ. 1992. Chronic tracheobronchial syndrome in eight dogs. *Vet Rec* 130:485–487.
14. Creighton SR, Wilkins RJ, 1974. Bacteriologic and cytologic evaluation of animals with lower respiratory tract disease using transtracheal aspiration biopsy. *J Am Anim Hosp Assoc* 10:227–232.
15. Creighton SR, Wilkins RJ. 1974. Transtracheal aspiration biopsy: technique and cytologic evaluation. *J Am Anim Hosp Assoc* 10:219–225.
16. Dambro NN, Grad R, Witten ML, et al. 1992. Bronchoalveolar lavage fluid cytology reflects airway inflammation in beagle puppies with acute bronchiolitis. *Pediatr Pulmonol* 12:213–220.
17. Dye JA, McKiernan B, Rozanski EA, et al. 1996. Bronchopulmonary disease in the cat. Historical, physical, radiographic, clinicopathologic, and pulmonary functional evaluation of 24 affected and 15 healthy cats. *J Vet Intern Med* 10:385–400.
18. Fung DCK, Somerville M, Richardson DS, et al. 1995. Mucus glycoconjugate complexes released from feline trachea by a bacterial toxin. *Am J Respir Cell Mol Biol* 12:296–306.
19. Gibson KL, Hedlund CS. 1992. Aspirated dental calculus in a dog. *J Am Vet Med Assoc* 200:514–516.
20. Harpster NK. 1981. The effectiveness of the cephalosporins in the treatment of bacterial pneumonias in the dog. *J Am Anim Hosp Assoc* 17:766–772.
21. Hawkins EC. 1995. Diseases of the lower respiratory system, pp 767–811. *In* Ettinger S (ed), Textbook of veterinary internal medicine. WB Saunders, Philadelphia, PA.
22. Hawkins EC. 1996. Antibiotic therapy for respiratory infections in clinical practice, pp 23–28. *In* Proceeding of the Comparative Respiratory Society Symposium, North American Veterinary Conference, Orlando, FL.
23. Hawkins EC, Davidson MG, Meuten DJ, et al. 1997. Cytologic identification of *Toxoplasma gondii* in bronchoalveolar lavage fluid of experimentally infected cats. *J Am Vet Med Assoc* 210:648–650.
24. Hawkins EC, DeNicola DB. 1989. Collection of bronchoalveolar lavage fluid in cats using an endotracheal tube. *Am J Vet Res* 50:855–859.
25. Hirsh DC. 1986. Bacteriology of the lower respiratory tract, pp 247–250. *In* Kirk RW (ed), Current veterinary therapy IX. WB Saunders, Philadelphia, PA.
26. Hoskins JD, Taboada J. 1994. Specific treatment of infectious causes of respiratory disease in dogs and cats. *Vet Med* 89:443–452.
27. Inzana TJ, Johnson JL, Shell L, et al. 1992. Isolation and characterization of a newly identified *Haemophilus* species from cats: *Haemophilus felis*. *J Clin Microbiol* 30:2108–2112.
28. Jackowski JT, Szepfalusi ZS, Wanner DA, et al. 1991. Effects of *P. aeruginosa*–derived bacterial products on tracheal ciliary function: role of radicals. *Am J Physiol* 260:L61–L67.
29. Jameson PH, King LA, Lappin MR, et al. 1995. Comparison of clinical signs, diagnostic findings, organisms isolated, and clinical outcome in dogs with bacterial pneumonia—93 cases (1986–1991). *J Am Vet Med Assoc* 206:206–209.
30. Johnson JA, Murtaugh RJ. 1997. Preventing and treating nosocomial infection: part 1. Urinary tract infections and pneumonia. *Compend Cont Educ Pract Vet* 19:581–603.
31. Kapatkin AS. 1990. Results of surgery and long term follow-up in 31 cats with nasopharyngeal polyps. *J Am Anim Hosp Assoc* 26:387–391.
32. King RR. 1996. Nonresolving pneumonias: causes and complications, pp 29–36. *In* Proceedings of the Comparative Respiratory Society Symposium, North American Veterinary Conference, Orlando, FL.
33. King RR. 1996. Pathogenesis of lower respiratory tract infections, pp 13–15. *In* Proceedings of the Comparative Respiratory Society Symposium, North American Veterinary Conference, Orlando, FL.
34. Kirchner BK, Port CD, Magoc TJ, et al. 1990. Spontaneous bronchopneumonia in laboratory dogs infected with untyped *Mycoplasma* sp. *Lab Anim Sci* 40:625–628.
35. Lecuyer M, Dube P-G, DiFruscia R, et al. 1995. Bronchoalveolar lavage in normal cats. *Can Vet J* 36:771–773.
36. Lotti U, Niebauer GW. 1992. Tracheobronchial foreign bodies of plant origin in 153 hunting dogs. *Compend Cont Educ Pract Vet* 14:900–904.
37. Malik R, Love DN, Hunt GB, et al. 1991. Pyothorax associated with a *Mycoplasma* species in a kitten. *J Small Anim Pract* 32:31–34.
38. McArdle HC, Dawson S, Coutts AJ, et al. 1994. Seroprevalence and isolation role of *Bordetella bronchiseptica* in cats in the UK. *Vet Rec* 135:506–507.
39. Moise NS, Wi D, Yeager AC, et al. 1989. Clinical, radiographic and bronchial cytologic features of cats with bronchial disease: 65 cases (1980–1986). *J Am Vet Med Assoc* 194:1467–1473.
40. Murphy ST, Ellison GW, McKiernan BC, et al. 1997. Pulmonary lobectomy in the management of pneumonia in dogs: 59 cases (1972–1994). *J Am Vet Med Assoc* 210:235–239.
41. Nagy B, Katona E, Erdei J, et al. 1991. Fibronectin in bronchoalveolar lavage fluid and plasma of dogs with acute inflammation of the lungs. *APMIS* 99:387–396.
42. Niederman MS, Craven DE. 1997. Editorial response: devising strategies for preventing nosocomial pneumonia—should we ignore the stomach? *Clin Infect Dis* 24:320–323.
43. Norsworthy GD. 1993. Surgical treatment of chronic nasal discharge in 17 cats. *Vet Med* 88:526–537.
44. Norsworthy GD. 1995. Treating chronic nasal discharge in cats. *Vet Med* 90:1048–1054.
45. Novotny P. 1990. Pathogenesis in *Bordetella* species. *J Infect Dis* 161:581–582.
46. Padrid P. 1996. Distinguishing chronic bronchitis from bacterial pneumonia, pp 47–48. *In* Proceedings of the Comparative Respiratory Society Symposium, North American Veterinary Conference, Orlando, FL.
47. Padrid P. 1996. New strategies for cats with exacerbations of asthma, pp 49–51. *In* Proceedings of the Comparative Respiratory Society Symposium, North American Veterinary Conference, Orlando, FL.
48. Padrid P, Amis TC. 1992. Chronic tracheobronchial disease in the dog. *Vet Clin North Am* 22:1203–1229.
49. Padrid PA, Feldman BF, Funk K, et al. 1991. Cytologic, microbiologic and biochemical analysis of bronchoalveolar lavage fluid obtained from 24 healthy cats. *Am J Vet Res* 52:1300–1307.
50. Padrid PA, Hornof WJ, Kurpenshoek CJ, et al. 1990. Canine chronic bronchitis. A pathophysiologic evaluation of 18 cases. *J Vet Intern Med* 4:172–180.
51. Padrid PA, Mitchell RW, Cozzi P, et al. 1994. Cyclosporine treatment in vivo inhibits the development of airway hyperresponsiveness and histologic alterations after chronic antigen challenges in cats. *Am Rev Respir Dis* 149:A771.
52. Perry AW, Schlingman DW. 1988. Pneumonia associated with eugonic fermenter-4 bacteria in two Chinese leopard cats. *Can Vet J* 29:921–922.
53. Prince A. 1992. Adhesions and receptors of *Pseudomonas aeruginosa* associated with infections of the respiratory tract. *Microb Pathog* 13:251–260.
54. Randolph JF, Moise NS, Scarlett JM, et al. 1993. Prevalence of mycoplasmal and ureaplasmal recovery from tracheobronchial lavages and prevalence of mycoplasmal recovery from pharyngeal swab specimens in dogs with or without pulmonary disease. *Am J Vet Res* 54:387–391.
55. Rodriguez CO, Moon ML, Leib MS. 1993. *Salmonella choleraesuis* pneumonia in a cat without signs of gastrointestinal disease. *J Am Vet Med Assoc* 202:953–955.
56. Roudebush P. 1990. Bacterial infections of the respiratory system, pp 114–124. *In* Greene CE (ed), Infectious diseases of the dog and cat. WB Saunders, Philadelphia, PA.
57. Solway J, Leff A. 1991. Sensory neuropeptides and airway function. *J Appl Physiol* 71:2077–2087.
58. Somerville M, Taylor GW, Watson D, et al. 1992. Release of mucus glycoconjugates by *Pseudomonas aeruginosa* rhanolipids into feline trachea in vivo and human bronchus in vitro. *Am J Respir Coll Mol Biol* 6:116–122.
59. Stone MS, Pook H. 1992. Lung infections and infestations. *Probl Vet Med* 4:279–290.
60. Thayer GW, Robinson SK. 1984. Bacterial bronchopneumonia in the dog: a review of 42 cases. *J Am Anim Hosp Assoc* 20:731–735.
61. Thompson JC, Gartrell BM, Butler S, et al. 1992. Successful treatment of feline pyothorax associated with an *Actinomyces* species and *Bacteroides melaninogenicus*. *N Z Vet J* 40:73–75.
62. Thrusfield MV, Aitken CGG, Muirhead RH. 1991. A field investigation of kennel cough: efficacy of different treatments. *J Small Anim Pract* 32:455–459.
63. Thrusfield MV, Aitken CGG, Muirhead RH. 1991. A field investigation of kennel cough: incubation period and clinical signs. *J Small Anim Pract* 32:215–220.
64. Turnquist SE, Ostlund E. 1997. Calicivirus outbreak in a Missouri feline colony. *J Vet Diagn Invest* 9:195–198.
65. Welsh RD. 1996. *Bordetella bronchiseptica* infections in cats. *J Am Anim Hosp Assoc* 32:153–158.
66. Weyant RS, Burris JA, Nichols DK, et al. 1994. Epizootic feline pneumonia associated with Centers for Disease Control group EF-4a bacteria. *Lab Anim Sci* 44:180–183.
67. Willoughby K, Dawson S, Jones RC, et al. 1991. Isolation of *Bordetella bronchiseptica* from kittens with pneumonia in a breeding cattery. *Vet Rec* 129:407–408.
68. Woolfrey BF, Moody JA. 1991. Human infections associated with *Bordetella bronchiseptica*. *Clin Microbiol Rev* 4:243–255.

Chapter **89**

Gastrointestinal and Intra-Abdominal Infections

Craig E. Greene

Oral Cavity

ORAL MICROFLORA

The resident microbial flora of the canine and feline oral cavity is composed of a wide variety of both aerobic and facultative and obligate anaerobic bacteria (Tables 89–1 and 89–2). In most studies, *Streptococcus* and *Actinomyces* are the most frequently reported bacteria that are not obligate anaerobes. The frequency with which individual species are isolated depends on culture methods, sampling sites, and breed and individual differences. From a clinical standpoint, bacterial culture of specimens from the oropharyngeal region is meaningless because of the diversity of commensal organisms and the lack of accurate quantitative methods. However, antimicrobial agents used in treating oral infections such as gingivitis and stomatitis should be chosen with the composition of the resident microflora in mind. Organisms found in soft-tissue (see Chapter 53), pleural (see Chapter 88), and peritoneal (see Intra-Abdominal Infections later) bite-inflicted wound infections reflect the composition of the oral microflora.

Table 89–1. Microflora Most Commonly Isolated From the Oral Cavities of Clinically Healthy Dogs

ORGANISM	SITES
Aerobic and Facultative Anaerobic	
Gram Negative	
Neisseria	B
Escherichia coli	B
Pasteurella	B
Pseudomonas	B
Proteus	T
Moraxella	N
Acinetobacter	N
Capnocytophaga	N
EF-4	N
Weeksella zoohelcum	N
Gram positive	
Actinomyces	N
Nonhemolytic streptococci	B
β-Hemolytic streptococci	B
Staphylococcus epidermidis	B
S. intermedius	B
Corynebacterium	N
Lactobacillus	B
Obligate Anaerobic	
Bacteroides	U
Fusobacterium	U
Propionibacterium	U
Peptostreptococcus	U
Bifidobacterium	U
Clostridium	U
Bacillus	U
Veillonella	U
Eikenella corrodens	N
Simonsiella	N
Others	
Candida	T
Mycoplasma	T

B = both tonsillar and nontonsillar; T = tonsillar; N = nontonsillar, supragingival scrapings; U = unspecified sites.

GINGIVITIS AND PERIODONTITIS

Inflammation and recession of perialveolar gum margins are common finding in dogs and cats.[24] They are initially caused by excessive accumulation of dental plaque resulting from deposition of by-products from breakdown of foodstuffs and saliva by normal resident microflora. Plaque is an organic matrix of salivary glycoproteins and polysaccharides adhering to the tooth surface that provides sites for oral bacteria to proliferate. Microflora involved with supragingival and subgingival plaque in healthy mucosal sites in dogs are resident streptococci and *Actinomyces*.[35, 36] At first, these gram-positive, nonmotile aerobic cocci and bacilli predominate. As periodontal inflammation progresses with associated calculus (tartar) formation, gram-negative motile, obligate anaerobic rods and spirochetes proliferate (Fig. 89–1).[69, 107] Early bacterial damage occurs in the gingival epithelial tissues with penetration of the interdental retes. Proliferating spirochetes may disrupt the intercellular junctions, creating a portal of entry for other bacteria.[69] Microflora from anaerobic plaque of dogs with periodontal disease are *Porphyromonas (Bacteroides) gingivalis*–like isolates and *Prevotella* and *Wolinella* species that are pigmented gram-negative rods, and *Actinobacillus actinomycetemcomitans*, *Clostridium*, and *Fusobacterium*. Reduced numbers of streptococci, enterococci, and staphylococci are found compared with normal flora (Table 89–3).[24, 35, 36, 85] In cats, differences in the microflora between clinically healthy animals and those with gingivitis have not been appreciated (see Table 89–2).[26] Salivary microflora, which differs from plaque microflora, remains relatively constant in the presence of periodontal disease.

Calculus is mineralized dental plaque that adheres to tooth surfaces, facilitating further plaque formation and periodontal inflammation. Complete removal of all supragingival and subgingival calculi is essential in control of periodontal disease. Gingival hypertrophy and alveolar abscess formation are sequelae of calculus formation. The type of microflora present, the diet, and the animal's chewing habits may be important in the formation of calculus.[100] Advancing age is a predisposing factor in dogs.[40] Leukopenia and bacteremia are sometimes observed as secondary effects.[59]

Table 89–2. Facultative and Obligate Anaerobic Flora of the Gingival Margin of Cats

ORGANISM	CLINICALLY HEALTHY % OF ALL ISOLATES (Love et al.[63])	CLINICALLY HEALTHY % OF ALL ISOLATES (Gruffydd-Jones[26])	GINGIVITIS % OF ALL ISOLATES (Gruffydd-Jones[26])
Aerobic and Facultative			
α-Hemolytic streptococci	NC	82[a]	NC
Enterococci	NC	50	NC
Corynebacterium	NR	75	NC
Bergeyella (Weeksella) zoohelcum	NR	75	NC
Pseudomonas	NC	69	NC
Moraxella	NC	62	NC
Flavobacterium	NR	46	NC
Nocardia	NC	50	NC
Actinomyces spp.	12[b]	42	NR
Pasteurella multocida	9.3	72	NR
Other bacteria	NC	< 10[c]	NC
Anaerobic			
Propionibacterium spp.	6	NR	NR
Bacteroides spp.	36.7[d]	7–57[e]	2–31
Fusobacterium spp.	19.3[f]	11	20
Clostridium spp.	8.7[g]	< 10[h]	3
Wolinella spp.	4.6[i]	NR	NR
Peptostreptococcus	3.3	< 10	14

[a]Includes *Micrococcus* spp., *Streptococcus sanguis, S. mutans, S. mitis.*
[b]*A. viscosus, A. hordeovulneris, A. denticolens.* In one other study,[75] *Lactobacillus fermentum* and *Veillonella parvula* were also isolated.
[c]Includes *S. epidermidis, Alcaligenes* spp., *Actinobacter* spp., *Achromobacter* spp., and group G β-hemolytic streptococci.
[d]*B. tectum, B. fragilis, B. heparinolyticus, B. salivosus, Porphyromonas gingivalis,* other *Bacteroides* pigmented group, including *Prevotella, B. gracilis.*
[e]Includes *B. asacchardyticus, B. melaningenicus, B. oralis, B. fragilis, B.* unspeciated.
[f]*F. alocis, F. nucleatum, F. russii, F.* unspeciated.
[g]*C. villosum, C. novyi.*
[h]*C. perfringens.*
[i]*W. recta, W.* nonmotile.
NR = not reported; NC = no attempted culture.

Hard diets, regular tooth brushing, and oral hygiene chews have been shown to reduce the incidence of calculus accumulation.[21, 22, 74] Treatment includes the extraction of severely affected teeth, debriding necrotic or proliferative gum margins, and scaling of calculi from the remaining involved dental surfaces. Systemic antimicrobials such as tetracycline, metronidazole, and tinidazole and topical chlorhexidine have been evaluated for treatment of periodontitis in experimentally affected dogs.[24] For drug dosages, see Table 89–4 and the Drug Formulary, Appendix 8. Tetracycline and metronidazole have been beneficial in reducing dental calculus or preventing its reformation when they have been given with or without mechanical cleansing. After 1 year of tetracycline therapy, dogs with periodontal disease had less alveolar bone resorption than untreated controls.[24] A topically applied polymer-containing doxycycline is available for treatment and control of periodontal disease in dogs (Heska, Fort Collins, CO). Metronidazole therapy has had similar beneficial effects.[24] Tinidazole had good efficacy against *P. gingivalis*–like bacteria, which are periodontal pathogens.[86] Flushing dental surfaces once daily with 0.1% to 0.2% chlorhexidine[24] or alternate-day brushing[24] may delay accumulation of calculi. Unfortunately, chlorhexidine may stain teeth light-blue, but a commercial product formulated especially for dental purposes (Nolvadent, Fort Dodge Labs, Fort Dodge, IA) does not stain. When monoperoxyphthalic acid was applied prior to chlorhexidine, reduced dental staining was noted.[10a] With twice daily application, nisin, an antimicrobial peptide, was as effective as chlorhexidine in preventing calculus in dogs.[43a] Numerous cleansers and brushes have been developed for daily brushing of dogs' teeth, and they warrant consideration when there is a tendency to form calculi.

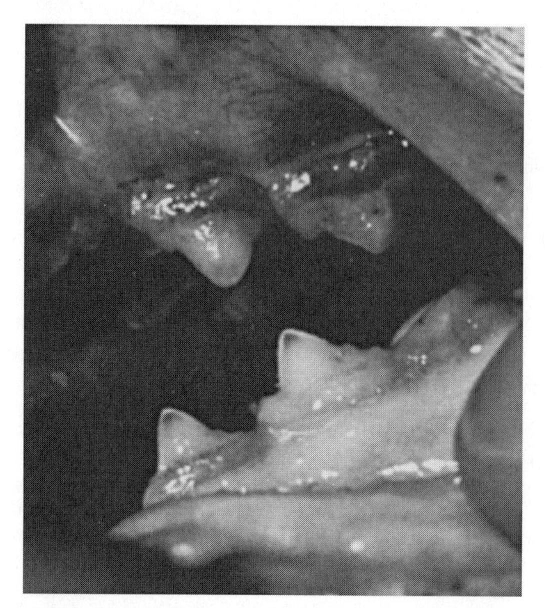

Figure 89–1. Accumulation of dental tartar and resulting perialveolar gingivitis in a cat.

Systemic complications of periodontal disease, including cerebral and myocardial infarction and early mortality, have been linked in people. Similar relationships to heart, liver, and kidney disease have been made in dogs.[14] Ophthalmic manifestations can occur from dental disease because of the close proximity of the caudal maxillary teeth and the orbit. See Table 89–5.[73]

GINGIVITIS IN KITTENS

A syndrome of gingival hypertrophy and associated plaque formation has been observed in Abyssinian and Persian kittens around the time of eruption of their adult teeth.[111] It may be caused by inborn immunodeficiency with secondary proliferation of gingival and plaque-forming bacteria.

Table 89–3. Percentage Distribution of Gingival Microflora From Dogs With Healthy and Diseased Gingival Tissues [a, 35, 36, 55, 101]

VARIABLE	HEALTHY DOGS	GINGIVITIS DOGS	PERIODONTITIS DOGS
Aerobic and Facultative	**36.5**	**27**	**3.8**
Streptococcus			
Esculin positive[b]	ND	5.8	3.2
Esculin negative[c]	ND	6.45	23.2
Actinomyces[d]	ND	41.9	13.0
Other aerobes and microaerophiles	17–30	ND	7–15
Anaerobic	**48**	**70**	**95**
Gram-positive cocci	3	7	5–12
NP *Bacteroides*[e] group	16	ND	19
P *Bacteroides*[f] group	6	15	20–34
Fusobacterium[g]	7	25	10–40
Gram-positive *bacilli*	5	10	6–25
Spirochetes	+	++	+++

[a]Supra and subgingival collection sites. Values are expressed as percentage of isolates.
[b]Esculin positive, streptococci (*S. faecalis*, group D streptococci, enterococci).
[c]Esculin negative, streptococci (*S. mitis*; includes facultative and anaerobic species).
[d]Includes both aerobic and facultative species.
[e]Nonpigmented *B. fragilis* group.
[f]Pigmented group containing *Porphyromonas*, including *P. asaccharolyticus*, *P. gingivalis*, *P. endontalis*, *P. canoris*, and *P. circumstantaris*; *Prevotella*, including *P. intermidia*, *P. loescheii*, *P. melaninogenica*, and *P. denticola*; *Bacteroides nodosus* (*Dichelebacter nodosaus*); *Wolinella* (*Campylobacter*) *curus* and *Wolinella* (*Campylobacter*) *rectus*.
[g]*Fusobacterium necrophorum* (ss *Funduliforme* and *Necrophorum*); *F. pseudonecrophorum*; *F. nucleatum* (ss *animalis*, *fusiforme*, *nucleatum*, *polymorphum* and *vincentii*).
ND = not determined; NP = nonpigmented; P = pigmented.

Treatment involves gingival tissue debridement, plaque removal, and frequent dental prophylaxis. Systemic antibacterial therapy may temporarily halt the progression, but it cannot be used indefinitely. Fortunately, most cats have a reduction in the severity of proliferation as they mature.

BACTEREMIA AND DENTAL DISEASE

Bacteremia associated with dental manipulations may be clinically nonsymptomatic, may cause acute septicemia, or subsequently may result in bacterial endocarditis or localized embolic tissue infections (see Chapter 87).[76] The severity of bacteremia frequently correlates with the degree of periodontitis present. In cats with periodontitis having dental scaling and extraction, 36% had positive blood culture results at the time of the dental procedures.[30] Bacteria most commonly isolated were *Propionibacterium acnes*, *Pasteurella multocida*, and *Staphylococcus epidermidis*. None of the cats became ill after the dental procedures. Positive blood culture results of resident microflora have also been found in up to 40% of

Table 89–4. Systemic Therapy for Oral Infections

DRUG	SPECIES	DOSE[a]	ROUTE	INTERVAL (HOURS)	DURATION (DAYS)
Gingivitis-Stomatitis					
Metronidazole[b]	D	10–15 mg/kg	PO	12	10–28
	C	8 mg/kg	PO	12	7–14
	C	5–10 mg/kg	PO	8	7–14
Tinidazole	D	15 mg/kg	PO	12	7–14
Tetracycline	D	20–40 mg/kg	PO	12–24	14–21
Clindamycin	B	5–10 mg/kg	PO	12	7–10
Amp(amox)icillin	B	20 mg/kg	PO	12	14–21
Amoxicillin-clavulanate	B	15–20 mg/kg	PO	12	14–21
Ketoconazole	B	5–10 mg/kg	PO	12	7–10
Prednis(ol)one	B	0.5–2 mg/kg	PO	12	7–14
Triamcinolone	C	4 mg total	PO	24–48	28
Methylprednisolone acetate	C	2 mg/kg	IM	7–30 days	3–12 months
Methylprednisolone acetate	C	0.5–1 mg/kg	IL[d]	Once	28
Triamcinolone acetonide	C	0.1–0.2 mg/kg	IL[d]	Once	28
Aurothioglucose	C	1 mg/kg	IM	7 days[e]	prn
Dental Prophylaxis					
Amp(amox)icillin	B	10–20 mg/kg	IV, SC	[f]	1
Amoxicillin-clavulanate	B	12.5 mg/kg	SC, PO	[f]	1
Chloramphenicol	B	15–25 mg/kg	IV	[f]	
Clindamycin	B	5 mg/kg	IV, SC, PO	[f]	1
Metronidazole	B	10–20 mg/kg	IV, PO	[f]	1
Enrofloxacin	B	5 mg/kg	SC, PO	[f]	1
Gentamicin	B	2 mg/kg	IV, SC	[f]	1
Cephapirin	B	20 mg/kg	IV	[f]	1

[a]Dose per administration at specified interval. For additional information, see Drug Formulary, Appendix 8.
[b]Metronidazole and spiramycin are available in combination (Stomorgyl) outside the United States for treatment of oral infections.
[c]Not available in The United States.
[d]Injection done under anesthesia as a last resort.
[e]Give every 7 days until improvement, then once every 14 to 35 days as needed.
[f]Only given once beginning just before or during anesthesia for dental procedures. In general, the desired spectrum is against anaerobic bacteria. For gram-negative facultative anaerobes in severe pyorrhea, combine whatever drug is chosen with the aminoglycoside (gentamicin) or fluoroquinolone (enrofloxacin).
D = dog; C = cat; B = dog and cat; IL = intralesional.

Table 89–5. Ophthalmic Manifestations of Dental Infections[a]

Orbital Cellulitis
Exophthalmos, reduced retropulsion
Protrusion of membrana nictitans
Pain on opening mouth
Chemosis
Conjunctival hyperemia
Fever, anorexia
Oral mucosal swellings
Periapical Abscess
Infraorbital swelling and drainage
Alveolar mucosal swelling
Conjunctival
Hyperemia, chemosis
Chronic mucopurulent conjunctivitis
Nasolacrimal
Chronic unilateral nasal discharge
Lacrimal fistula
Neuro-ophthalmologic Signs
Deficits cranial nerve II, III, IV, VI, lacrimal, ciliary nerve, optic neuritis, retinal degeneration, blindness, ophthalmoplegia, anisocoria, reduced tear production, Horner's syndrome
Uveitis, Endophthalmitis

[a]Information adapted from Ramsey et al.[73]

dogs with periodontal disease having dental scaling and tooth extraction, and none showed clinical evidence of bacteremia.[29] Dental procedures should not be performed at the same time as other surgical procedures, because surgical wounds have been infected by bacteria released when simultaneous dentistry is performed. Oral microflora may establish themselves in tissue injured or devitalized by routine surgical procedures, sutures, or foreign implants. Whenever dentistry is performed, prophylactic administration of antimicrobial drugs has been recommended (see Table 89–4). Routine use of antimicrobials for dental procedures should be mandatory in immunocompromised animals. Penicillin is the drug of choice for humans undergoing dental cleaning; however, IV administration of aqueous penicillin during ultrasonic dentistry in dogs did not alter the prevalence of bacteremia before or after dental manipulation.[24] In dogs and cats, pretreatment with clindamycin at 5.5 mg/kg for 5 days decreased plaque and reduced aerosolization of bacteria during ultrasonic teeth cleaning.[117] Ampicillin (amoxicillin) has been recommended empirically beginning 1 hour before dental procedures.[42] On the basis of in vitro susceptibility testing, chloramphenicol, cephalosporin, erythromycin, or gentamicin have also been recommended. With the exception of erythromycin, all can be given parenterally while the animal is anesthetized. Gentamicin should never be administered alone because it is relatively ineffective against anaerobic bacteria. For these reasons, ampicillin (amoxicillin), chloramphenicol, clindamycin, metronidazole, or cephalosporin with or without gentamicin or rarely fluoroquinolone is recommended for dental prophylaxis. Appendix 8 and Table 89–4 should be consulted for drug information and appropriate dosages. Therapy should begin no earlier than 4 hours before the dental procedure and preferably should be continued during it by IV infusion. The most critical period is throughout the procedure. Drug administration should be terminated no longer than 12 hours after the procedure because no further benefits are gained, and the risk for antibiotic-resistant bacteria causing infections are increased.

Public Health Considerations

Because of the large numbers of bacteria in the mouth and especially the gingival crevices, face masks and ocular shields should always be worn by people who clean an animal's teeth. In addition, biofilms that form on the inside surface of water lines of ultrasonic scalers may harbor *Legionella* sp., which might produce acute pneumonia in susceptible individuals.[113]

GINGIVOSTOMATITIS AND PHARYNGITIS

In people **necrotizing ulcerative gingivostomatitis (NUG)** or "trench mouth" is a syndrome with multiple causes, characterized by oral ulcerations and secondary infections. NUG may be a manifestation of systemic or immunosuppressive illness. Opportunistic overgrowth of oral microflora occurs in many diseases when immune defenses are impaired or oral ulcerations develop.[24] Similar to periodontitis, motile (predominantly anaerobic) bacteria, including spirochetes, often proliferate and may invade tissues in advance of necrotic lesions.[77] The causes of NUG in dogs and cats are equally diverse and include many acquired immunosuppressive conditions, such as diabetes mellitus, persistent neutropenia, feline leukemia virus (FeLV) and feline immunodeficiency virus (FIV) infections, and canine Cushing's disease. Exogenous glucocorticoid administration in dogs also increases their susceptibility to NUG.[69] It is common in Maltese terriers.[33] A virus antigenically related to feline calicivirus (FCV) was found to cause transient gingivitis and glossitis in a dog.[24] Calicivirus appears to be especially prevalent in affected cats. As in people, psychological and physical stresses may be involved in some animals. Bristles of plant awns can induce a similar syndrome when they become embedded in gingival tissues.[24] Fungal stomatitis can result from infection with *Candida*. Candidiasis can be associated with diffuse oral inflammation, especially on the tongue and at mucocutaneous junctions. See Chapter 66 for further information concerning its diagnosis and treatment.

Cats subclinically infected with FCV and feline rhinotracheitis virus may develop oral ulceration with or without respiratory signs after stress or immunosuppression, such as with concurrent FIV infection. Stress also appears to reduce the amount of fibronectin, a receptor protein, on epithelial cells for gram-positive organisms. Thus, overgrowth with gram-negative bacteria may develop. Hard, dry cat food also appears to have a role in exacerbating palatine ulceration in cats with acute FCV infection.[24] Proliferative stomatitis (see following discussion of faucitis) has been associated with persistent FCV infection sometimes as a result of concurrent FIV infection.[24, 105] The prevalence of FeLV infection in affected cats with stomatitis is lower than that of FIV. As a common but poorly understood syndrome with diverse causes, NUG often has uniform histopathologic features of lymphoplasmacytic infiltration.[105]

The pattern of oral ulceration may be helpful in determining its underlying cause (Table 89–6). Regardless of its cause, oral ulceration has a particular clinical syndrome characterized by reluctance to eat, hypersalivation, halitosis, and evidence of pain on opening the mouth. Hemorrhage may occur spontaneously or after oral manipulation. Although rare, systemic signs may include fever, lymphadenomegaly, and depression. Ulcers may be distributed throughout the oral cavity but are usually concentrated on the dental, labial, and gingival surfaces (Fig. 89–2). Ulcers may be covered by a pseudomembranous exudate. White pseudomembranous plaques can be found in cases of candidal stomatitis. In many neutropenic cats infected with FeLV, the ulcers characteristically have minimal exudation; some can progress rapidly with sloughing of large portions of the caudal oropharynx or larynx.

Table 89–6. Comparison of Ulcerative Lesions in Oral Cavities of Dogs and Cats

CAUSE	SPECIES	LESION LOCATION	THERAPY
Excessive licking (eosinophilic ulcer)	C	Upper incisor or carnassial area of lip, near philtrum, roof of mouth (hard palate)[a]	Intralesional or systemic glucocorticoids
Autoimmune diseases, bullous pemphigoid	D	Roof of mouth, lips, cheeks, often symmetric; other mucocutaneous regions, foot pads	Systemic glucocorticoids
Irritants, uremia	B	Tip of tongue	Systemic antibacterial; amputation
Viral (parvoviral, Chapters 8 and 10), rickettsial (RMSF, Chapter 29)	D	Multifocal lingual	Systemic antibacterials; antirickettsials
Maltese terrier stomatitis	D	Ulcerative lesions, lateral tongue and buccal mucosae	Systemic antibacterials
Dental tartar, periodontal disease	B	Periodontal regions (gingival margins); fusospirochetal proliferation	Systemic antibacterials; tartar removal; tooth extraction; chlorhexidine rinses, hard diets
Herpesvirus (Chapter 5)	C	Tongue, palate, multifocal	Systemic antibacterials
Calicivirus (Chapter 16)	C	Acute: tongue, palate, multifocal	Systemic antibacterials
		Chronic: fauces (glossopharyngeal reflection, upper last molar region; occasionally extends rostrally; occasionally roof of mouth (hard palate)[b]	Antibacterials; soft food diet; intralesional or systemic glucocorticoids; occasionally remove molars
Immunosuppression; hyperadrenocorticism, leukopenia, FeLV, FIV (Chapters 13 and 14) Abyssinian, Persians	B	Periodontal region, may spread to gums and cheeks[c]	Systemic antibacterials; low-dose oral interferon, oral lactoferrin

[a]Eosinophilic infiltration on biopsy.
[b]Lymphocytic-plasmacytic infiltration on biopsy and polyclonal hyperglobulinemia are usually present. FIV coinfection can exacerbate.
[c]Sometimes observed as an idiopathic syndrome in young cats. See text discussion of gingivitis in kittens. Retroviral infections are occasionally associated with a rapidly spreading gingival necrosis.
C = cat; D = dog; B = both dog and cat; RMSF = Rocky Mountain spotted fever; FeLV = feline leukemia virus; FIV = feline immunodeficiency virus.

Faucitis is characterized by vesicular, ulcerative, and later proliferative lesions in the mucosa, usually accompanied by lymphoplasmacytic or eosinophilic infiltrations in the tissue of the caudal pharynx at the glossopharyngeal arch (fauces).[24] Faucitis frequently appears among a number of cats within a household and tends to be recurrent after the initial treatment or is unresponsive to treatment. In chronic stages, proliferation of granulation tissue forms large masses in the caudal pharynx (Fig. 89–3). FCV has been isolated in a high percentage of cats with this syndrome compared with clinically healthy cats or those with oral ulcers at other locations. It is likely a hypersensitivity phenomenon to persistent FCV infection.

Diagnosis of animals with persistent stomatitis-pharyngi-

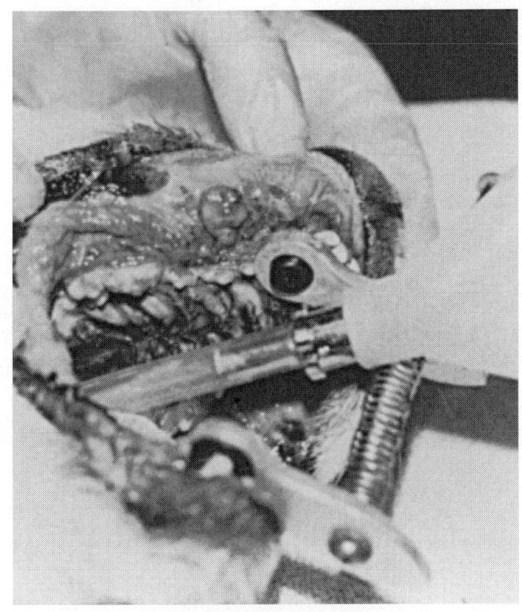

Figure 89–2. Diffuse necrotizing ulcerative gingivostomatitis in a dog. (Courtesy of Dr. D. W. Scott, New York State College of Veterinary Medicine, Cornell University, Ithaca, N.Y.)

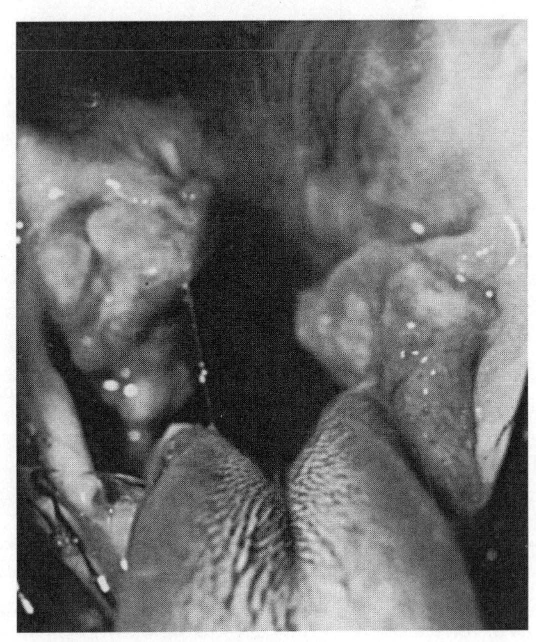

Figure 89–3. Chronic proliferative stomatitis in the oral cavity of a cat.

tis first involves examination for excessive accumulation of dental tartar. Systemic or underlying diseases will usually be apparent from the results of urinalysis and routine hematology, biochemistry, and FeLV and FIV testing. Neutropenia or neutrophil function defects are a common underlying cause of oral ulceration. Hyperproteinemia and polyclonal hyperglobulinemia is often present in cats affected with chronic stomatitis (faucitis) and lymphoplasmacytic infiltration. Monoclonal gammopathy may occur in some cats.[63a] Specimens for FCV isolation can be taken by rubbing sterile swabs on the gums, soft palate, and oropharynx (especially palatine tonsillar region) and by placing them directly into viral transport or culture media (see Chapter 1). Results of bacterial cultures and susceptibility testing are useless because most isolated organisms are merely commensals proliferating in already damaged tissues. Clinical features should be correlated with cytologic and histologic findings. Lymphoplasmacytic infiltration may be present in chronic inflammation from many different causes but has been most commonly associated with chronic faucitis in cats.

Underlying disease processes and other causes of NUG should be eliminated or treated when they are encountered. Plant awns or foreign material embedded in the gums can be scraped away with a scalpel when the gum margins are debrided. Symptomatic therapy of stomatitis includes changing the diet to soft or bland foods to encourage eating and to lessen the mechanical irritation of ulcers. With chronic, nonhealing ulcers, it is often beneficial to remove dental tartar and normal or diseased teeth in affected regions of the mouth.[8] Although dentistry may reduce pain and discomfort, it is not by itself sufficient in controlling faucitis in many cats.[105] In some cats, removal and biopsy with histologic examination of chronic proliferative lesions may be required. Some lesions that arise adjacent to or later involve the tonsillar crypt may originate as, or later develop into, squamous cell carcinomas.

Topical therapy such as swabbing and flushing of teeth, gums, and lesions throughout the oral cavity with 1% hydrogen peroxide has been recommended for gingivitis and stomatitis; however, excessive use of peroxide may cause vomiting. Astringents or disinfectants have also been advocated but can be irritating and distasteful. Cauterization with silver nitrate or dilute acid solutions also has been recommended but may interfere with healing and epithelization. Vitamins B and C administration has been recommended on an empiric basis without adequate documentation of efficacy.

Systemic therapies for stomatitis are summarized in Tables 89–4 and 89–6. Topical or systemic antimicrobial therapy appears to hasten the resolution of NUG significantly, perhaps by inhibiting the overgrowth of anaerobic and spirochetal bacteria that colonize and impair healing of ulcerated lesions in the oral cavity. Oral administration of lactoferrin, an iron-chelating agent, was effective in treating intractable stomatitis in cats with and without FIV infections (see Drug Formulary, Appendix 8).[89] Improvement was presumably due to its antibacterial effects. Candidal stomatitis is best treated by topical application of antifungal drugs, such as clotrimazole and nystatin (see also Table 57–3) or with systemic ketoconazole. Historically, tetracycline, chloramphenicol, ampicillin, and penicillin solutions have been applied topically for bacterial stomatitis, although the first two drugs may cause anorexia in cats. Systemic antibiotic therapy directed primarily against anaerobic bacteria appears to be more efficacious in treating stomatitis. Relapse may occur in some cases after termination of antimicrobial therapy, and a repeated course of therapy may be required.

Prednisone or other glucocorticoids (see Table 89–4) may be administered when antimicrobial therapy is being discontinued in an attempt to break the cycle of recurrent chronic stomatitis or faucitis in cats. Glucocorticoid therapy may be needed if an autoimmune disease such as pemphigus is suspected; however, the immunosuppression induced by glucocorticoids can itself cause or exacerbate some cases of NUG.

In cats with refractory faucitis, therapy with hypoallergenic diets, progesterones, or intralesional injections of repositol (water-insoluble) glucocorticoids using general anesthesia may be attempted as a last resort. Another systemic treatment with variable success has been parenteral administration of gold salts. Because faucitis is likely a hypersensitivity phenomenon to FCV, immunosuppression, rather than immunostimulation, gives the most benefit.

TONSILLITIS

Chronic tonsillar inflammation is most commonly recognized in dogs and is usually accompanied by pharyngeal irritation initiated by foreign bodies, chronic gingivitis or periodontitis, chronic coughing, persistent vomiting or gastroesophageal reflux of acid, and licking of infected sites, such as lesions caused by anal sacculitis. Dogs may have inappetence, hypersalivation, or sneezing and oculonasal discharge; they may scratch at their ears or repeatedly shake the head. Fever and malaise do not usually accompany tonsillitis unless it is secondary to underlying systemic infection or neoplasia.

Diagnosis is based on a thorough oral examination, which usually requires sedation. The pharyngeal mucosa is reddened, and tonsils are enlarged and frequently protrude from the crypts as the tongue is pulled rostrally. Culture is unnecessary, and antibacterial therapy with amoxicillin, tetracycline, or trimethoprim-sulfonamide is recommended. Low anti-inflammatory dosages of glucocorticoids have shown temporary benefit in reducing the severity of clinical signs in conjunction with antimicrobial therapy.[24] Surgical removal of the tonsils, followed by histologic examination, is usually the best course of action when antibacterial therapy has been ineffective or transiently curative. Chronic tonsillar enlargement, if not corrected by surgery, usually serves as a nidus for continual infection and sometimes chronic bronchitis (see also Tonsillitis and Pharyngitis, Chapter 88).

Esophagus and Stomach

The oral cavity and ingested material are the primary sources of microorganisms that colonize the lower portions of the GI tract (Fig. 89–4). The esophagus and stomach contain a transient population of organisms after saliva or food is swallowed. Once the stomach has been emptied of food, the low pH usually destroys most of the bacteria that remain. Those that persist during the fasting period are strains adapted to survival at low pH (Table 89–7). The oral cavity, esophagus, stomach, and proximal small intestine are colonized primarily by gram-positive aerobic and anaerobic bac-

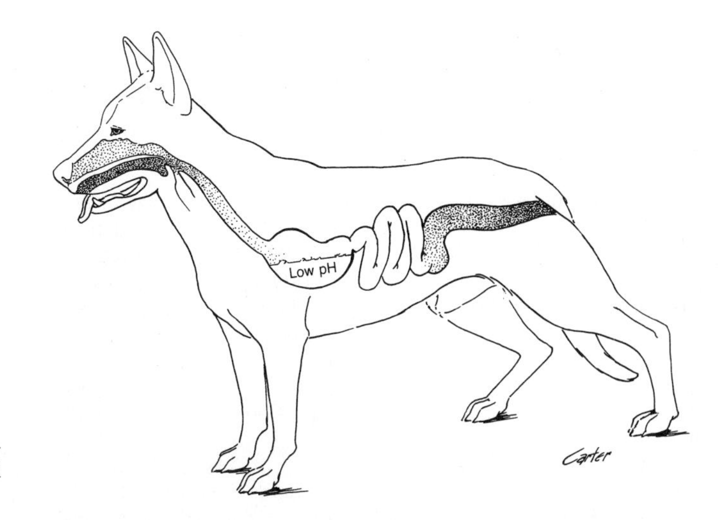

Figure 89–4. Concentration of microorganisms throughout the intestinal tract of a fasting dog. Numbers are highest in the oral cavity and colon and lowest in the midportion of the bowel.

teria, which are usually susceptible to penicillin or its derivatives. This susceptibility is the rationale for the clinical use of such drugs in treating ulcerations and perforations and for antimicrobial prophylaxis involving surgery of these portions of the GI tract.

Exudates from abscesses or cellulitis that develop after perforating lesions of the oral cavity or upper GI tract should be collected with sterile syringes that are capped or sealed immediately after collection. The latter method will increase the chances of detecting anaerobic bacteria, although cultures must be performed soon after specimen collection (see Chapters 33 and 41). A variety of organisms, including gram-positive rods and cocci, gram-negative rods and cocci, yeasts, and spirochetes, have been found in the stomach of most normal dogs.[24] Nontoxigenic *Clostridium perfringens* was found in the gastric contents of normal dogs and those with acute gastric dilation. The type and prevalence of organisms in clinically healthy dogs did not differ from those in dogs with acute gastric dilation. For a discussion of gastric helicobacteriosis, see Chapter 39.

Table 89–7. Major Microflora of the GI Tract of Dogs and Cats[a]

VARIABLE	ORAL CAVITY[c]	STOMACH[d]	SMALL BOWEL Proximal[d]	SMALL BOWEL Distal	CECUM/COLON	FECES
Total counts[b]						
Fasting	10^7	10^1–10^2	10^1–10^2	10^3–10^7	10^9–10^{10}	10^{10}–10^{11}
Postprandial	10^7	10^4–10^5	10^2–10^3	10^3–10^7	10^9–10^{10}	10^{10}–10^{11}
Aerobic organisms						
Gram positive[e]	+	$10^{0.4}$–10^1	$10^{0.4}$–10^2	$10^{1.4}$–10^3	10^4–10^9	10^4–10^9
Gram negative[f]	+	10^1–10^2	10^2	10^2–10^6	10^7–10^8	10^7–10^8
Anaerobic Organisms						
Gram positive[g]	+	$10^{0.3}$–10^2	$10^{0.1}$–10^3	10^2–10^6	10^7–10^8	10^7–10^{10}
Gram negative[h]	+	–	+	10^1	10^6–10^{10}	10^8–10^{10}
Other Organisms						
Spirochetes	+	+	+	+	+ + +	0
Mycoplasma	+	–	–	–	–	–
Yeasts	+	–	–	–	10^5	+

[a]Data derived from studies in people, dogs, and cats.
[b]Values expressed as organisms per milliliter or gram of intestinal contents.
[c]See Table 89–1 for information concerning frequency of isolation.
[d]All values listed are for fasting animals except when the postprandial state is indicated.
[e]*Streptococcus, Staphylococcus, Bacillus, Corynebacterium.*
[f]Enterobacteriaceae (primarily *Escherichia coli, Enterobacter, Klebsiella*), *Pseudomonas, Neisseria, Moraxella.*
[g]*Clostridium, Lactobacillus, Propionibacterium, Bifidobacterium.*
[h]*Bacteroides, Fusobacterium, Veillonella.*
+ = present but absolute quantity uncertain; + + + = present in large numbers; – = absent or data not available; 0 = normally absent.

Small Intestine

INTESTINAL MICROFLORA

Concentrations of bacteria in the proximal small bowel are relatively low because of the influence of gastric acid and bile, and they gradually increase toward the ileocecal region (see Table 89–7 and Fig. 89–4). Numbers of microorganisms in the distal small bowel or the large bowel are not affected by feeding but remain relatively constant after meals. Increased numbers of resident organisms may be found in the stomach and upper small intestine, or pathogenic organisms may proliferate when normal bowel defenses are impaired. Excessive use of antacids, obstruction or stasis of intestinal or bile flow, or decreased mucosal or IgA secretions can result in bacterial overgrowth of the small intestine.

The normal microflora of the small intestine plays an important role in preventing colonization by pathogenic bacteria by competing for available nutrients, maintaining oxygen levels, and producing antibacterial substances. In addition, the normal intestinal microflora assist the body in metabolizing bile acids and drugs and have a role in synthesizing volatile fatty acids and vitamins. Puppies and kittens lacking normal microflora at birth derive their microflora from exposure to their dam and littermates or from their environment by 2 to 3 weeks of life.[24] Organisms that initially colonize the intestinal tract (which may vary somewhat between individuals) permanently colonize the intestinal tract and remain relatively stable in composition throughout the life of the individual. High-meat diets ingested by most carnivores result in a predominance of streptococci and *C. perfringens* and a suppression of *Lactobacillus*. Lactose in the diet of nursing animals contributes to acidification of the colonic contents, with a resultant increase in *Enterobacter* and a decrease in *Escherichia coli* and *Bacteroides*.

Greater knowledge of the composition of the intestinal microflora has been gained because of improved techniques for culture of anaerobic bacteria. Anaerobes are known to make up a majority of the intestinal microflora, greatly outnumbering aerobes (see Table 89–7). The duodenum and upper jejunum primarily harbor gram-positive bacteria, including streptococci and lactobacilli. Anaerobes and gram-negative organisms predominate in the distal portions of the small bowel and colon. Numbers of microorganisms reach their maximum in the cecum, colon, and feces.

Quantifying organism numbers is important in determining whether bacterial overgrowth may be occurring (see Small Intestinal Bacterial Overgrowth, later). In contrast, clinically healthy cats have much higher concentrations of bacteria in the duodenal or proximal jejunal region, ranging from 2.2×10^5 to 1.6×10^8 CFU/ml of fluid, with anaerobes predominating.[52] Most common anaerobes in cats were *Bacteroides, Eubacterium*, and *Fusobacterium*, whereas *Pasteurella* was most common among aerobic flora. In another study on cats,[70b] in which similar numbers of bacteria were found, the most common anaerobes were *Clostridium, Fusobacterium*, and *Bacteroides*. The most common aerobes were gram-negative rods, streptococci, enterococci, and staphylococci. In studies on healthy dogs, results of quantifying proximal small intestinal bacteria have been variable, with some showing numbers of $<10^5$/ml[104] and others with populations comparable to those in cats.[9, 13, 91]

The composition and distribution of the normal fecal flora can be altered by disease, such as diarrhea.[24] Decreased transit time of intestinal contents and evacuation of fluid feces result in decreased numbers of lactobacilli with concomitant increased numbers of *Bacteroides* and members of the Enterobacteriaceae. Organisms such as *Enterobacter*, which normally reside in the small intestine, may appear in the feces of dogs with diarrhea. The concentration of many anaerobes is reduced in the feces during diarrhea because these organisms normally require intestinal stasis and low oxygen tension for growth.

Bacterial Translocation

The GI tract is a known reservoir of microorganisms, which under certain circumstances can spread by portal blood vessels or intestinal lymphatics to extraintestinal sites, including the mesenteric lymph nodes, liver, spleen, pancreas, and, by systemic circulation, other organs. Bacterial isolation from mesenteric lymph node tissue of 50 clinically healthy dogs having ovariohysterectomies yielded bacteria in lymph nodes of 26 dogs, including *Staphylococcus intermedius* (n = 3), nonhemolytic *Streptococcus* (n = 4), *Bacillus* spp. (n = 5), *Escherichia coli* (n = 6), *Salmonella* spp. (n = 3), *Pseudomonas* (n = 2), *Enterococcus* (n = 2), *Clostridium sodelli* (n = 1), *Micrococcus* spp. (n = 1), *Lactobacillus* spp. (n = 1) and *Propionibacterium acnes* (n = 1).[12a] Corresponding peripheral venous and portal venous blood cultures yielded a gram-positive coccus and a coagulase-negative *Staphylococcus* from the peripheral blood of one dog. Mesenteric lymph node culture needs to be evaluated further in ill dogs before conclusions can be drawn as to its clinical usefulness. Conditions associated with bacterial translocation migration are hemorrhagic shock, intestinal obstruction, intestinal resection, abdominal trauma, burns, abdominal radiation therapy, and obstructed biliary disease.[9a] For a further discussion of this problem, see Chapter 55.

PATHOPHYSIOLOGIC MECHANISMS OF INFECTIOUS DIARRHEA

Enteropathogenic organisms, unlike resident and nonpathogenic transient microflora, have acquired means of overcoming the host defense mechanisms and the inhibitory properties of the normal microflora. Adherence factors (e.g., somatic pili) that permit intestinal pathogens to establish infection also allow them to attach to, multiply on, and colonize the intestinal mucosa. Some pathogenic bacteria that cause diarrhea remain on the mucosal surface and produce potent enterotoxins that disrupt fluid flux across the intestinal mucosa. Others are able to penetrate intact epithelial cells, producing inflammatory damage in the underlying mucosa. Enteric viruses damage the intestine by replicating within and destroying selected populations of epithelial cells. Various mechanisms by which microorganisms produce intestinal injury are covered in the following sections.

Normal Function of Intestinal Villi

Intestinal epithelial cells are produced by germinal epithelium located in the intestinal crypts (Fig. 89–5). Younger, undifferentiated, and primarily secretory epithelial cells, produced by the germinal epithelium of the intestinal glands (crypts), migrate up the intestinal villus as the older, differentiated, absorptive cells at the tip eventually slough into the intestinal lumen. Most of the absorptive process is confined

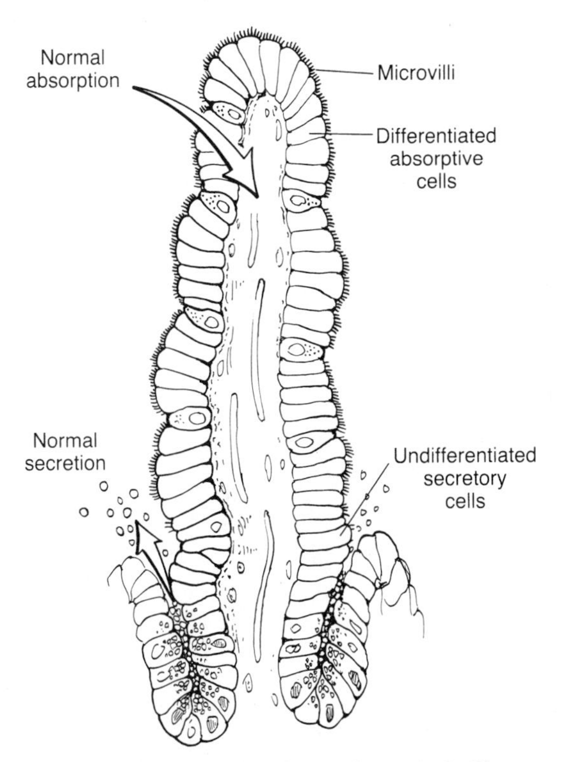

Figure 89–5. Structure of normal intestinal villus.

to the differentiated cells at the villous tip, which also produce locally active intestinal enzymes that aid in the digestive process. The preponderance of intestinal secretion is confined to specialized goblet cells and undifferentiated cells that line the sides and depths of the crypts.

Noninvasive Enterotoxigenic Organisms

After attachment to the intact epithelial surface, noninvasive organisms produce powerful heat-labile exotoxins that bind to surface receptors on the small intestinal epithelial cells. Toxin acts at the cellular level to stimulate adenyl cyclase and other unknown mechanisms to increase intracellular cyclic adenosine monophosphate (AMP) (Fig. 89–6*A*). The net effect of cyclic AMP is to increase secretion of chloride and to decrease absorption of sodium by intestinal epithelium, resulting in loss of large quantities of water and electrolytes in feces in the absence of morphologic injury to intestinal mucosa.

Many bacterial species that infect dogs and cats not only produce enterotoxin-induced diarrhea after initial colonization but also produce mucosal invasion (Table 89–8 and Chapters 37 and 39). Strains of some species, such as *E. coli*, can produce diarrhea by either mechanism. Several enterotoxin-producing strains of bacteria such as *Staphylococcus*, *C. perfringens*, and *E. coli*, which commonly cause food-borne diarrhea and acute gastroenteritis, are harbored in the colons of clinically normal dogs and cats.[24] Presumably, the bacteria and toxin cause clinical illness only after being ingested or during bacterial overgrowth or intestinal stasis, when they proliferate in the small intestine. Enterotoxigenic *E. coli* have been recovered from dogs with acute diarrhea, but their importance as a primary cause of illness has been uncertain (see Neonatal Colibacillosis below and Chapter 37). Similar isolation of enteropathogenic strains has been made from cats.[24] *Clostridium difficile*, a bacterium associated with diarrhea in people and animals (see Acute Colitis, later), produces both an enterotoxin and a cytotoxin, which induces diarrhea and frequently mucosal ulceration and hemorrhage.

Enteroadherent Organisms

Some organisms, notably adherent streptococci classified as enterococci, have been reported to be present on the intestinal epithelial surfaces of dogs and cats with diarrhea (see Table 89–8). See Enterococcal Infections, Chapter 35 and the respective chapters for other organisms. Microscopically, diffuse colonization of intestinal enterocytes with mild inflammatory changes has been observed.[11, 49] Bacterial attachment has not usually been seen in the upper small intestine.

Mucosal-Invading Organisms

After invasion of the mucosa, some bacteria produce hemorrhagic (dysenteric) stools (see Table 89–8). Two bacterial genera that classically produce dysentery are *Salmonella*, which usually has an affinity for the ileum, and *Shigella*, which has an affinity for the ileum and the colon. After they penetrate submucosal tissue, both produce a marked inflammatory response characterized by the influx of neutrophils. *Shigella* and many strains of *Salmonella* are phagocytized and killed, although some may persist, causing a chronic carrier state. Refer to Chapter 39 for more detailed information concerning these two genera.

Submucosal Invading Organisms

The same organisms that invade mucosally can penetrate deeper into submucosal tissues (see Table 89–8). Host defenses are usually impaired, and systemic spread may occur. Submucosal invasion is characterized by hemorrhagic diarrhea, increased fecal leukocytes, leukopenia, leukocytosis, or leukopenia with a left shift and positive blood culture results. Clinical evidence of bacteremia is manifest by fever, hemorrhagic diarrhea, and shock. Fungal or protozoal pathogens or opportunists may also invade the submucosal layers, producing chronic granulomatous enterocolitis.

Villous Atrophy

The well-differentiated apical absorptive cells of the intestinal villus are responsible for producing digestive enzymes that act locally at the intestinal brush border. Reoviruses, rotaviruses, and coronaviruses have a selective affinity for replication within and destruction of these cells, resulting in villous atrophy (Fig. 89–6*B*). Impaired absorption and digestion are characteristic of this type of diarrhea. A relative increase in intestinal secretion is usually associated with terminal villous atrophy because of continued replication of the undifferentiated germinal crypt epithelial cells, which have more secretory than absorptive functions.

Intestinal Crypt Degeneration

Because canine and feline parvoviruses require rapidly dividing cells for replication, they selectively damage mitotically active intestinal gland epithelium so that absorptive cells at the tips of the villi are not replaced, which leads to intestinal gland degeneration and eventual mucosal collapse

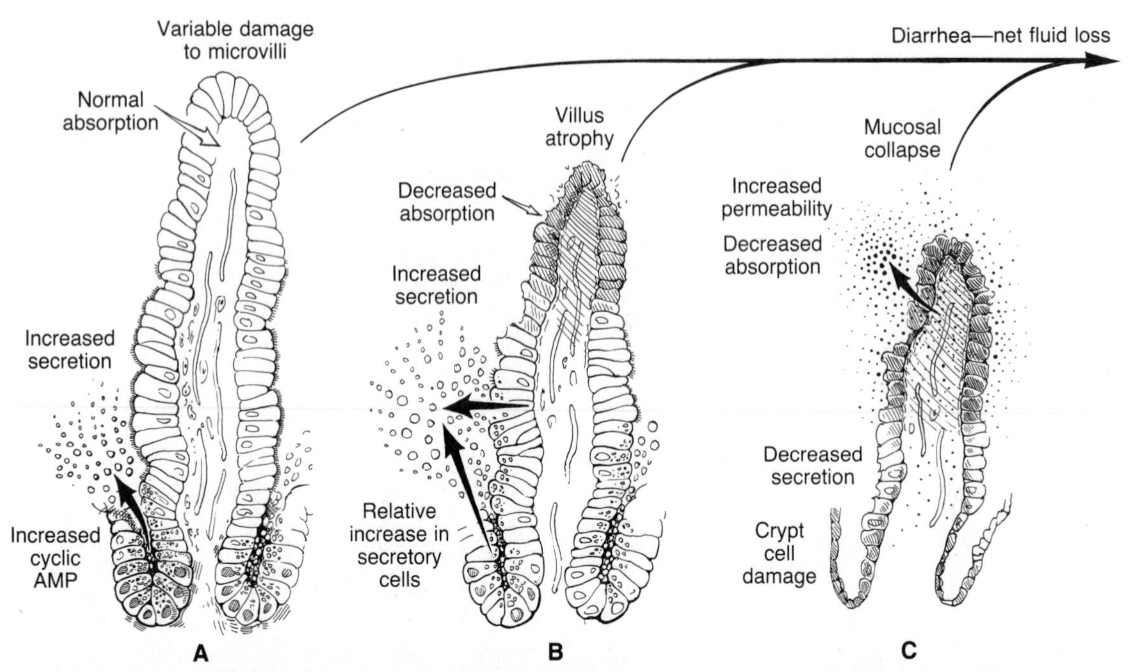

Figure 89–6. Pathogenesis of infectious diarrhea. *A*, Noninvasive enterotoxigenic bacteria (e.g., vibrios, staphylococci, and clostridia) primarily stimulate cyclic adenosine monophosphate (AMP). *B*, Villous atrophy results from selective infection of apical epithelial cells with certain viruses (e.g., coronaviruses and rotaviruses). *C*, Intestinal gland degeneration and mucosal collapse occur when viruses (e.g., paroviruses) damage the germinal intestinal gland epithelium.

(Fig. 89–6C). The primary defect is in absorption; however, secretory processes are also inactivated. Damage to the mucosal barrier in most cases also results in an influx of inflammatory cells and increase in vascular permeability, with the eventual exudation of serum proteins.

DIAGNOSIS OF ACUTE INFECTIOUS GASTROENTERITIS

Collection of fecal samples for culture of aerobic bacteria is easier when commercially prepared, sterile, cotton-tipped applicators are used. These are supplied with transport media or enrichment broth in which the swab is placed immediately following specimen collection (see Chapter 33). Additional care can be taken to clean the anus with 70% alcohol or dilute organic iodine solution before inserting the cotton-tipped applicator. When organisms such as *Salmonella, Shigella, Helicobacter,* or *Campylobacter* are suspected, the laboratory can be notified because selective media or special cultural conditions may improve yield (see Diagnosis, Chapter 39).

Cytologic examination of fecal mucus or exudate can be an effective way to determine the integrity of the bowel mucosa. Infectious processes that cause damage to mucosal surfaces result in the appearance of large numbers of neutrophils and macrophages in feces. Diarrhea caused by parvoviruses and invasive bacteria can be distinguished by the presence of these inflammatory cells and erythrocytes.

Like cultures of specimens from the oral cavity, cultures of feces or other intestinal contents yield ambiguous results. Disturbances in the composition of microflora will not be detected unless quantitative cultures are performed. Primary pathogens such as *Salmonella* and *Shigella* require selective media if they are to be isolated. Enterotoxigenic strains of bacteria require specific identification techniques that are not routinely available to most veterinarians.[72] Finding a potentially pathogenic organism is not the same as identifying the cause of diarrhea, because there is a high prevalence of subclinical carriers of *Salmonella, Campylobacter,* and other enteropathogenic bacteria in dog and cat populations (see Chapters 37 and 39). Cultures should always be performed when zoonotic exposure to these pathogens is suspected.

THERAPY FOR ACUTE INFECTIOUS GASTROENTERITIS

Antibacterial therapy is indicated in selected instances of intestinal disease when it is usually combined with supportive care such as dietary modification, fluid therapy, motility modification, and antiemetics. Antimicrobials should be used when episodes of diarrhea or vomiting are accompanied by signs of systemic illness, including fever, depression, and impending shock, and the presence of leukopenia or leukocytosis with a marked left shift. These findings indicate that there has been an absorption of microbes or, more likely, their toxins.[24] In some instances, routine use of antimicrobials may be harmful, altering the composition and number of intestinal microorganisms that normally serve to inhibit the growth of pathogenic varieties or the induction of resistant strains. The choice of drugs depends on a knowledge of the susceptibilities of both the usual pathogens and the normal intestinal flora. For further information on indicated drugs, see the discussion of therapy for intra-abdominal sepsis that appears later in this chapter. See the Drug Formulary, Appendix 8, for appropriate dosages and features of recommended antimicrobial drugs.

Antimotility agents have been routinely used in the treatment of infectious diarrhea. However, slowing intestinal transit may be counterproductive to the defense mechanism of diarrhea, which acts to eliminate harmful microorganisms and their toxins. Antimotility drugs have resulted in increased morbidity and persistence of infection in bacterial enteritis (see *Salmonella* Therapy, Chapter 39).

Table 89–8. Mechanism and Site of Action of Enteropathogenic Microorganisms[a]

MECHANISM AND ORGANISM	SITE
Enterotoxin Production	
Vibrio cholerae	SI
Staphylococcus (36)	Stomach and SI
Clostridium perfringens (39)	SI
Bacillus cereus (87)	SI in initial stages
Vibrio parahaemolyticus	SI
Escherichia coli (37)	Some strains in SI
Yersinia enterocolitica (39)	SI and colon
Klebsiella pneumoniae (88)	SI
Campylobacter jejuni (39)	SI
Salmonella typhimurium (39)	SI in initial stages
Entamoeba histolytica (78)	
Enteroaderence	
Enterococci (35)	SI and colon
E. coli (37)	SI
Giardia (78)	SI
Mucosal Invasion	
Salmonella (39)	Ileum in later stages
Shigella (39)	Colon
B. cereus (87)	SI in later stages
V. parahaemolyticus	SI in later stages
E. coli (37)	Some strains in colon
Campylobacter (39)	SI
Helicobacter (39)	Stomach, SI, colon[b]
Coccidia (81)	SI
Balantidium coli (78)	Colon
Entamoeba histolytica (78)	Colon
Submucosal Invasion	
Salmonella (39)	SI
Shigella (39)	SI and colon
E. coli (37)	SI
Mucor, Absidia, Rhizopus (68)	Stomach and SI
Candida (66)	Colon
Histoplasma (60)	Colon
Aspergillus (65)	Colon
Villous Atrophy	
Coronaviruses (8 and 11)	SI
Reoviruses (12)	SI
Rotaviruses (8 and 12)	SI
Crypt Degeneration	
Canine parvovirus (8)	Primarily SI
Feline panleukopenia virus (10)	Primarily SI

[a]Chapter references appear in parentheses.
[b]Site depends on species.
SI = small intestine.

Fluid therapy is probably one of the most important treatments of the symptoms of the diarrheic animal. Fluids should be given IV when severe shock and hypotension, semicoma, or persistent vomiting or ileus accompanies the diarrheal episode. Less affected animals with these complications should receive subcutaneous fluids. The majority of animals with acute nonhemorrhagic diarrhea without vomiting can be treated with specific oral fluid preparations.[68] Oral fluid therapy is based on the observation that glucose is actively absorbed by the normal small bowel and that sodium is carried with it in about an equimolar ratio. Hypertonic oral antidiarrheal fluid replacement solutions can be prepared that contain sodium and glucose in an equimolar ratio, in addition to bicarbonate and potassium in a composition similar to that of the fluid lost in diarrheic stool (Table 89–9). In most situations, amino acids commercially marketed for veterinary use such as glycine have been added to facilitate absorption. Solutions containing glucose or sodium, either alone or in an imbalanced ratio of lesser concentration, are *not* effective in reversing fluid and electrolyte flux across the intestinal mucosa. Similarly, polyionic, isotonic fluids such as lactated Ringer's solution, Pedialyte (Ross Laboratories, Columbus, OH), and Gatorade (Stokey–Van Camp, Indianapolis, IN) are helpful only for oral fluid maintenance or electrolyte supplementation and do little to stop ongoing or existing losses. Oral antidiarrheal solutions are effective only when the integrity of the intestinal mucosa is intact. This can be assessed in practice by looking for gross and microscopic evidence of blood and leukocytes in stools.

Promoted by the World Health Organization (WHO) for treating human cholera, "WHO juice" can be made by veterinarians or their clients (Table 89–10). The ingredients can be mixed and stored in a powered state and reconstituted when necessary. Unused portions can be stored in a refrigerator for several days or weeks. WHO juice is voluntarily accepted by most dogs and some cats, although some animals require gavage by syringe or stomach tube. The volume of WHO juice to be administered depends on the circumstances, but a range of 50 to 100 ml/kg/day is usually given, according to the fluid losses, until the diarrhea stops. Vomiting, which may occur when use of these hypertonic solutions begins, can usually be obviated by giving small amounts more frequently. Although they facilitate fluid absorption, large volumes of hypertonic fluids may cause a transient increase in stool water volume because of residual unabsorbed electrolytes in the feces. Hypertonic oral fluids can also cause serum hyperosmolality and hyperosmolar coma when adequate volumes of water or isotonic fluids are not provided orally. Parenteral isotonic fluid therapy may have to be given concurrently with hypertonic fluids in small or young animals.

Protectants and **adsorbents** such as kaolin and pectin are limited because they are relatively ineffective in absorbing toxins produced by enteropathogenic bacteria. Kaolin (hydrated aluminum silicate) is a potent coagulation activator and may be of some benefit in treating diarrhea associated with mucosal disruption and hemorrhage. Pectin is polymeric carbohydrate that is thought to act as an absorbent; however, large amounts may produce diarrhea.

Nonsteroidal anti-inflammatory drugs such as aspirin have been shown to be beneficial in the management of infectious diarrhea. Clinical studies in people and experimental studies in dogs and cats have shown that salicylates interfere with the mechanism of enterotoxin-induced intestinal hypersecretion, presumably by blocking production of cyclic AMP and prostaglandin synthesis. Subsalicylate preparations (Pepto Bismol, Norwich Eaton Pharmaceuticals, Norwich, NY) that are commonly provided in the treatment of diarrhea are thought to work in a similar manner. Further studies have shown that bismuth subsalicylate has antibacterial activity because of the binding and killing of exposed pathogenic bacteria. Administration at a dose of 0.25 ml/kg every 4 to 6 hours, early in the course of disease, may be helpful in treating diarrhea that results from the mechanism of increased secretion.

INFECTIOUS SMALL INTESTINAL DISORDERS

A number of defined syndromes attributed to alterations in intestinal microflora have been described and are discussed in the following sections. In many instances, the pathophysiologic mechanisms are not completely elucidated.

Neonatal colibacillosis caused by *E. coli* has been described in many species, including dogs and cats[24] (see also Chapter 37). Characteristically, puppies are affected within the first week of life and have a high mortality rate. They show acute depression, weakness, hypothermia, cyanosis,

Table 89–9. Chemical Composition of Various Orally Administered Fluids for Infectious Diarrhea

FLUID (MANUFACTURER)	Na (mEq/L)	K (mEq/L)	Cl^- (mEq/L)	HCO_3^- (mEq/L)	GLUCOSE (g/L)[a]	AMINO ACIDS (mmol/L)[b]	ENERGY (kJ/L)	OSMOLARITY (mOsm/L)
Body Fluids								
Normal plasma[c]	142	4.5	105	25	1.0	ND	ND	300
Cholera stool[c]	140	13	104	44	ND	ND	ND	ND
Replacement								
WHO juice[c]	90	20	80	30	20	0	336	330
Rehydrate solution (Ross)	75	20	65	30[d]	25	0	378	ND
Pedialyte RS (Ross)	75	20	ND	ND	25	0	ND	285
Gastrolyte Oral (USV)	90	20	80	30[d]	20	0	336	ND
Ion-Aid (Diamond)	89	28	ND	0	24	125	559	480
Entrolyte (Pfizer)[e]	105	26	51	80	23	63	399	490
Resorb (Pfizer)[e]	80	30	27	0[h]	22	0	370	315
HY-SORB (Sandofi)	120	10	70	40	56	0	941	ND
Biolyte (UpJohn)	184	31	104	111	68	0	1142	ND
Maintenance								
Pedialyte (Ross)	45	20	35	30[d]	25	0	378	250
Infalyte (Pennwalt)	50	20	40	30	20	0	269	260
Enterim-5 (Schering-Plough)	90	20	80	ND	31	0	521	ND
Supplementation								
Gatorade (Stokey–Van Camp)[f]	21	3	11	3[d]	20	0	336	330
Apple juice[g]	1.7	26	0	0	ND	0	ND	ND

[a]Multiply by 5.5 to get millimoles per liter glucose.
[b]Supplied primarily as glycine.
[c]Data from Pierce NF, Hirshorn N: *WHO Chronicle* 31:87–93 1977; Sack et al: *Bull WHO* 43:351–360, 1970.
[d]Anion supplied as citrate instead of bicarbonate.
[e]Data from Lewis and Phillips. 1980. *Norden News* 55:4–8.
[f]Stokey–Van Camp, Indianapolis, IN, personal communication, December 1982.
[g]Data from Dupont and Pickering: Infections of the gastrointestinal tract. Plenum Medical, New York, pp 247–267.
[h]Buffering capacity supplied as citrate.
ND = no data, do not use in cases of GI obstruction or moribund animals; Na = sodium; K = potassium; Cl^- = chloride; HCO_3^- = bicarbonate.

and CNS signs before death. Older puppies that survive for several weeks may have persistent diarrhea, abdominal discomfort, weight loss, and dehydration. Gross necropsy findings include hemorrhagic lesions on serosal surfaces of all body cavities and throughout the GI mucosa. Septicemia can be confirmed by bacterial culture from the blood or from many organs. Histologic examination reveals gram-negative bacilli in many tissues of septicemic newborns.

The cause of *E. coli* septicemia in newborn puppies may be associated with their immunologic incompetency rather than the virulence of a particular strain of organism. Enterotoxic, attaching, and effacing bacterial strains of *E. coli* exist. Furthermore, intestinal epithelial cells of newborn puppies are highly and nonselectively permeable to a variety of proteins (including bacteria) that are absorbed by pinocytosis. Exposure of newborns to *E. coli* before colostrum ingestion or their failure to obtain sufficient colostrum may further predispose these puppies to infection. *E. coli* is also able to cross the intestinal epithelial barrier 48 to 72 hours after birth, after which the cells also cease to absorb immunoglobulins. Puppies appear to be completely resistant to intestinal exposure to *E. coli* at 2 weeks of age. Enteropathogenic *E. coli* may cause disease in animals of any age.

Small intestinal bacterial overgrowth (SIBO) is a syndrome of bacterial proliferation in the upper intestinal lumen accompanied by chronic or recurrent small-bowel diarrhea. It has been most commonly observed in German shepherd dogs.[6, 24] Causes for SIBO in this and other breeds are impaired motility or obstruction of the GI tract, secretory IgA deficiency, and reduced gastric or pancreatic secretion. Dogs with SIBO have generally been between 5 months and 2 years of age. They are usually bright and alert but show variable weight loss, which becomes apparent with time, and they consistently have foul-smelling, watery feces lasting for months. Results of quantitation of bacteria in duodenal secretions from affected animals have revealed increased numbers of *E. coli* and enterococci, typically normal flora of this site, and proliferation of anaerobes such as clostridia, which are unusual inhabitants.[24]

Although disordered motility and hypochlorhydria are

Table 89–10. Composition of WHO Juice

DRY INGREDIENTS[a]	AMOUNT: Grams	AMOUNT: Teaspoons	SUBSTITUTES
Sodium chloride (table salt)	3.5	0.64	None
Sodium bicarbonate (baking soda)	2.5	0.55	None
Glucose powder (dextrose)	20.0	6.0	Sucrose (table sugar): 40.0 g (8 tsps) or equivalent amount of honey or corn syrup
Potassium chloride	1.5	0.31	Apple juice: 0.47 liter (1 U.S. pint)

[a] In 1 liter of water (1.05 U.S. quarts).
Data modified from World Health Organization: Treatment and Prevention of Dehydration in Diarrheal Diseases, Geneva, WHO, 1976; Gangarosa EJ: *Postgrad Med* 62:113–117, 1977; and Pierce NF, Hirschhorn N: *WHO Chron* 31:87–93, 1977.

possible causes of SIBO, a secretory IgA immune deficiency is considered most important (see Chapter 95).[6, 24, 109, 110] Histochemical analysis suggests that German shepherd dogs have defective synthesis or secretion of IgA despite the presence of IgA-committed plasma cells.[6] Duodenal bacterial overgrowth also occurs in German shepherd dogs with pancreatic exocrine insufficiency (PEI). Furthermore, similar clinical features of PEI and bacterial overgrowth make these syndromes difficult to differentiate. Bacterial overgrowth in the jejunum has developed in dogs after surgical reconstruction of the biliary tract.[115]

Anaerobic bacterial overgrowth in the proximal small intestine leads to increased breath hydrogen concentration in most dogs and variably increased serum folic acid concentration.[109] Increased serum folate results from increased synthesis of this compound by the large numbers of intestinal bacteria with greater amounts available for absorption. In addition, reduced serum B_{12}, found in up to 25% of these dogs, is thought to be caused by bacterial binding of the vitamin within the intestine, preventing its absorption. Steatorrhea is usually mild or absent unless concurrent PEI is present. Xylose absorption has been variably reduced in affected dogs, presumably as a result of bacterial utilization of xylose in the proximal small bowel, thereby decreasing the amount being absorbed. In some cases, abnormal xylose absorption may be corrected by prior administration of antibiotics. Differential sugar absorption testing has been used to confirm the presence of SIBO and to monitor the response to treatment.[81] Serum trypsin–like immunoreactivity and absorption of bound para-aminobenzoic acid have been within reference ranges unless concurrent PEI is present. Minimal histologic abnormalities have been found in affected dogs, and the activities of some brush border intestinal enzymes have been altered depending on whether anaerobic or aerobic bacteria predominate and whether PEI is present.[24] Chronic SIBO may result in protein-losing enteropathy, which can be controlled by antimicrobial therapy.

Although difficult to perform in routine practice, quantitative culture of duodenal or proximal jejunal fluid from dogs with overgrowth shows bacterial counts greater than 10^5 organisms/ml.[13, 15] Proliferating organisms in dogs often consist of small intestinal microflora such as *E. coli*, *Enterobacter*, *Enterococcus*, and *Lactobacillus*, but sometimes unusual species for that location, such as clostridia, predominate.

When possible, underlying causes of SIBO should be determined and eliminated. Response to antimicrobial therapy supports the diagnosis (see Table 89–11). Oxytetracycline and tylosin are recommended for dogs and metronidazole for cats.[112] Because of the development of overgrowth in some dogs with PEI, antimicrobial therapy may be required in those that do not respond to enzyme supplementation alone. In addition, a bland diet, such as cottage cheese or chicken and boiled rice or specialized diets (I/D, Hills Foods, Topeka, KS) have often been recommended during the treatment period to obtain more consistent responses. Increased-fiber diets actually reduced transit time and intestinal bacterial populations. Feeding IgA-deficient dogs with SIBO fructo-oligosaccharides reduced bacterial populations in their proximal small intestines.[109]

Inflammatory Bowel Diseases (IBD)

Chronic intestinal inflammation, characterized by bowel inflammation, have been attributed to pathogenic microorganisms (Table 89–12). In idiopathic forms, normal or opportunistic microflora may be involved in immunoderanged hosts or those with immunodeficiency diseases (see Chapter 95). There are also numerous helminthic and noninfectious causes for these inflammatory intestinal disorders. The following discussion focuses on microbiologic causes. For specific agents, see the respective chapters indicated in Table 89–12. For a more general review of these syndromes, see other sources.[27]

Lymphocytic-plasmacytic enteritis (LPE) is the most frequent inflammatory bowel condition reported in dogs and cats.[16, 24, 31, 45, 95, 108, 114] It is characterized by diffuse mucosal infiltration of lymphocytes, plasma cells, eosinophils, and neutrophils. Variants of inflammatory bowel disorders are eosinophilic and granulomatous infiltrations. LPE may or may not involve the stomach and colon. In cats, it has been observed in association with cholangiohepatitis and pancreatitis.[102] The cause of this syndrome is probably multifactorial, and the infiltration is probably a general response of the GI tract to chronic immune stimulation and immunoreactive or autoreactive intestinal injury. Chronic infection with enteropathogens such as *Helicobacter*, *Yersinia*, or *C. perfringens* may be involved in some cases. Similarly, small intestinal bacterial

Table 89–11. Antimicrobial Therapy for Bacterial Overgrowth, Lymphoplasmacytic Enteritis, and Enteropathogenic Bacteria[a]

DRUG	USE	SPECIES	DOSE (mg/kg)[b]	ROUTE	INTERVAL (HOURS)	DURATION (DAYS)
Tylosin	SIBO, LPE, EPB	B	10–15	PO	12	7–14
Tetracycline[e]	SIBO	D	20	PO	8	28
Metronidazole	SIBO, LPE	D	15	PO	12	7–14
		D	10	PO	8	7–14
		C	30	PO	24	7–14
Sulfasalazine[c]	LPE	D	12.5	PO	6	21–28
		D	10–25	PO	8	21–28
		C	5–10	PO	8	14–21
		C	25	PO	24	14–21
Prednisolone	LPE	B	0.5–1.5	PO	12	14–21
Azathiopine	LPE	D	2–2.5[d]	PO	24	14–21
		C	0.3	PO	48	14–21
Erythromycin	EPB	D	10	PO	8	7–14
Enrofloxacin	EPB	B	2.5–5.0	PO	12	7–14
Gentamicin	EPB	B	2.2	IV, IM, SC	12	7
Trimethoprim-sulfonamide	EPB	B	15	PO	12	7–14

[a]For additional information on each drug, see Drug Formulary, Appendix 8.
[b]Dose per administration at specified interval.
[c]Azulfidine.
[d]Dose also expressed as 40 mg/m², based on body surface area.
[e]Or oxytetracycline.
D = dog; C = cat; B = dog and cat; SIBO = small intestinal bacterial overgrowth; LPE = lymphoplasmacytic enteritis; EPB = enteropathogenic bacteria (see Chapter 39).

overgrowth of resident microflora may be involved. In cats, even protozoa such as *Toxoplasma gondii* have been implicated in some cases.[71] Evidence for resident microflora alone, in the pathogenesis of the inflammation, is unlikely.[95] Interactions between microorganisms in hosts having particular immunologic and genetic composition is the most logical cause. Chronic exposure of GI-associated lymphoid tissue to ingested or endogenous microfloral antigens or toxins may be responsible. Immunohistochemical studies suggest that IgG is the major antibody in the immune response in the lamina propria of affected dogs.[66a]

In contrast to bacterial overgrowth, no dog breed is predisposed to this syndrome, and affected animals are usually older than 2 years. The disease generally affects older purebred cats. Chronic or intermittent intractable diarrhea is noted in dogs. Stools may vary in consistency, but gross evidence of hemorrhage is usually lacking. With long-standing and severe disease, weight loss develops. In contrast, vomiting and weight loss are major signs in affected cats; vomiting is often unrelated to eating and may occur in sporadic episodes.[114] Diarrhea is less common and variable and can occur from small- or large-bowel origin. Some cats have colonic localization with signs of large-bowel diarrhea with hematochezia.[16] Appetite may be reduced, corresponding to the episodic nature of vomiting and diarrhea. Some dogs and cats with significant weight loss have voracious appetites similar to those in PEI. Thickening or discomfort may be found on palpation of the intestine. Hepatomegaly has been observed in some cats. Edema, hydrothorax, or ascites may be found in animals with severe hypoproteinemia.

Neutrophilia, sometimes with a left shift, or stress leukogram and hypoproteinemia are seen in dogs with moderate to severe disease. Cats may have high serum activities of alanine aminotransferase and serum alkaline phosphatase.[31] Clinical laboratory evaluation for malabsorption or maldigestion is generally within reference ranges. As a measure of bowel inflammation, high concentrations of IgG and nitrates can be detected in colonic lavage analytes.[27a] In addition, tests for absorption of inert sugars show altered values in dogs with IBD.[91a] Contrast radiographic findings are variable and of low yield. Intestinal biopsy by endoscopy or exploratory laparotomy is the *only* means of definitive diagnosis. Biopsies of mesenteric lymph nodes should be taken if they are enlarged.

Caution should be taken when interpreting biopsy reports of mild lymphocytic-plasmacytic infiltrations in the intestinal mucosae. Pathologists may vary in their interpretations of mild infiltrates, which may be found in intestinal biopsy specimens of clinically healthy animals. Therapy of lymphocytic-plasmacytic enteritis is very similar to that of chronic colitis, which is covered under that section later. Bacterial overgrowth may be involved, especially in long-standing cases, and should be addressed in some treatments. Other organisms or food ingredients may be associated with the pathogenesis, and hypoallergenic diets are recommended for initial treatment. Because immune-mediated and infectious causes may be involved, both antimicrobial (metronidazole, tylosin, sulfasalazine) and anti-inflammatory or immunosuppressive (glucocorticoid or azathioprine) therapies are recommended if dietary management fails or cannot be implemented (see Table 89–11). When the diagnosis is uncertain, antimicrobial therapy should be instituted first because of potential complications of immunosuppression of dogs with bacterial overgrowth.

Table 89–12. Microorganisms Causing Chronic Inflammatory Bowel Diseases in Dogs and Cats[a]

SUPPURATIVE	
Bacterial:	*Salmonella* (39), toxigenic *Escherichia coli* (37), *Yersinia* (39)
LYMPHOPLASMACYTIC	
Viral:	Immunosuppression induced by FIV (14) or FeLV (13)
Bacterial:	*Helicobacter* (39), *Campylobacter* (39), *Clostridium perfringens* (39) and resident microflora (overgrowth, SIBO)
Protozoal:	*Cryptosporidium* (82)
GRANULOMATOUS	
Viral:	Feline coronavirus (11)
Bacterial:	*Mycobacterium* (50)
Fungal:	*Histoplasma* (60), *Cryptococcus* (61), *Zygomycetes* (68), *Pythium* (68)
Algal:	*Prototheca* (69)
Protozoal:	*Leishmania* (73), *Toxoplasma* (80)

[a]Respective chapter for reference appears in parentheses.
FIV = feline immunodeficiency; FeLV = feline leukemia virus; SIBO = small intestinal bacterial overgrowth.

Hemorrhagic gastroenteritis (HGE), a syndrome characterized by the sudden onset of vomiting and production of profuse, mucoid, bloody diarrhea, was primarily described in small house dogs between 2 and 4 years of age.[24] The syndrome is also marked by hematologic findings that include relative polycythemia, with normal or low plasma protein concentration, and coagulation test results suggestive of disseminated intravascular coagulation (DIC) and, occasionally, acute oliguric renal failure.

The pathogenesis of the syndrome of acute HGE is unknown, but many clinical and laboratory findings are similar to those produced in dogs by experimental administration of bacterial endotoxin or enterotoxins with resultant DIC (see Chapters 37 and 38). Whether a cause or an effect, DIC may explain many of the clinical features that have been observed in dogs. Allergic, hereditary, autoimmune, and infectious causes for HGE have been proposed. The high prevalence of the syndrome in certain breeds, such as schnauzers and miniature poodles, has been explained by their hereditary predisposition to such causative factors. Dogs have been reported to develop hemolytic-uremic syndrome as well, which may be related to enterotoxigenic bacteria.[41] The influence on microbial flora of the highly digestible meat-based protein diets commonly fed to house dogs that are well cared for should be examined. Diagnosis of the syndrome of HGE is based on historical, clinical, and laboratory findings. Treatment is essentially similar to that for endotoxemia (see Chapter 38). Rehydration and diuresis with polyionic isotonic fluids are the most important components of treatment. Antimicrobial therapy for enteropathogens is recommended because of the damaged mucosal integrity (see Table 89–11). Some enteropathogenic bacteria, including members of *Clostridium*, *Escherichia*, and *Salmonella*, can also cause similar appearing, acute hemorrhagic diarrhea (see Chapters 37 and 39).[4, 97]

Large Intestine

MICROFLORA

The cecum and colon are the richest sources of intestinal microflora, and a single gram of feces contains up to 10^{11} organisms, approximately 100 times the human population of the world. Organisms that inhabit the lower bowel are primarily gram-negative aerobes and spore- and non-spore-forming anaerobes (see Table 89–7 and Table 89–13). Anaerobic bacteria, which usually comprise more than 90% of the colonic microflora, include clostridia, lactobacilli, *Bifidobacterium*, and *Bacteroides*. Aerobic or microaerophilic bacteria primarily consist of streptococci, members of the Enterobacteriaceae, and spirochetes.

ACUTE COLITIS

A number of acute inflammatory diseases of the colon have been described in dogs and cats. Colitis, whether acute or chronic, usually involves the microflora as a secondary phenomenon. As with stomatitis, many cases of acute colitis in dogs and cats can be associated with the stressful circumstances or immunosuppressive diseases. Acute colitis has been reported in cats experimentally infected with panleukopenia virus, although the colonic lesions were milder than those in the small intestine.[24] One case of mycotic colitis in a cat was assumed to be a sequela to panleukopenia virus infection.[24] Acute ulcerative colitis of undetermined cause has also been recognized in young cats.[24]

Antimicrobial Drug-Associated Pseudomembranous Colitis

This syndrome can be caused by species of *Clostridium* (especially *C. difficile*) and staphylococci in people. Suppression of normal flora by antimicrobial agents, immunosuppression, or nosocomial acquisition is a possible predisposition. Although this syndrome has been well documented in people and horses, especially those given macrolides, it is not well recognized in dogs and cats. Carriage of *C. difficile* with a proportion of toxigenic strains has been documented in cats housed in a veterinary teaching hospital.[64a] Those cats with toxigenic strains had at least one risk factor, and half of the cats had diarrhea. Treatment for this disease in people involves vancomycin or metronidazole.

Table 89–13. Colonic Bacterial and Fungal Microflora[a]

MICROFLORA AEROBIC AND FACULTATIVE	CONCENTRATION
Gram Negative	
Escherichia coli	10^7–10^8
Enterobacter (Aerobacter)	ND
Klebsiella	10^7–10^8
Proteus	ND
Pseudomonas	ND
Gram Positive	
Staphylococcus	$10^{4.7}$
Streptococcus	10^8–10^9
Lactobacillus	10^8–10^9
Ruminococcus	ND
Corynebacterium	$10^{8.7}$
Obligate Anaerobes	
Bacteroides	10^8–10^{10}
Bifidobacterium	$10^{6.6}$
Fusobacterium	ND
Veillonella	$10^{5.9}$
Eubacterium	ND
Bacillus	$10^{5.4}$
Clostridium	10^7–$10^{9.1}$
Spirochetes	ND
Yeasts	10^5

[a]Numbers are expressed as organisms per milliliter of contents.
ND = no data.
Data adapted from Strombeck DR: *In* Guilford WS et al (eds), Strombeck's small animal gastroenterology. WB Saunders, 1996. Used with permission.

Spirochetal Diarrhea

In the veterinary literature, there are numerous reports of spirochetes as a cause of diarrhea in dogs and cats.[23] These organisms are known to be a part of the normal microflora throughout the GI tract of dogs and cats, with the greatest numbers in the oral cavity (see NUG previously discussed), cecum, and colon. Because spirochetes are not demonstrable by H and E staining, they have been overlooked in biopsy specimens by pathologists. Some confusion has also occurred in histologic examination of spiral helicobacters such as in the gastric mucosa (see Gastric Helicobacters, Chapter 39). Scanning or transmission EM and special staining procedures can help to confirm the presence of spirochetes, which are usually attached to the intestinal epithelia at the base of crypts.

Because of intestinal adherence, spirochetes are not shed in formed feces of dogs and cats. During diarrheal episodes, they dislodge from the epithelia and appear in large numbers in feces. Spirochetes in stool cannot be incriminated as the cause of diarrhea, despite their close relationship with *Serpulina (Treponema) hyodysenteriae*, the cause of swine dysentery[19] and spirochetes from people with diarrhea.[56, 58] A specific pathogen-free beagle pup with a history of chronic diarrhea and concurrent giardiasis had suspected colonic spirochetosis.[18a, 19] Spirochetes were attached to the lamina propria in areas of superficial mucosal erosions, similar to those in swine and human intestinal spirochetosis.

CHRONIC COLITIS

Chronic colitis is a common syndrome recognized in dogs, characterized by intermittent diarrhea with hematochezia and tenesmus, weight loss, occasional vomiting, and abdominal pain. Fever is not a consistent finding with large-bowel inflammation. The colitis that occurs in boxers is granulomatous associated with infiltrates of periodic acid–Schiff–positive histocytes. It may be a secondary result of chronic ulceration and a reaction to intestinal microflora. Granulomatous inflammation of the bowel can also occur with feline infectious peritonitis, protothecosis, mycobacteriosis, zygomycosis, and pythiosis. Respective chapters should be consulted. Chronic ulcerative colitis does not appear to be associated with primary bacterial pathogens but probably results from stress, debilitation, or immunosuppression. That the lesions are invaded by intestinal microflora after mucosal disruption may explain the apparent beneficial effect of antibiotics and the occasional deleterious effect of glucocorticoids in treating this disease.

Older cats appear to be affected by a chronic ulcerative colitis similar to that of dogs.[24] Cats infected with FeLV or

Table 89–14. Therapy for Colitis

DRUG	SPECIES	DOSE[a] (mg/kg)	ROUTE	INTERVAL (HOURS)	DURATION (DAYS)
Antimicrobials					
Sulfasalazine (Azulfidine)	D	12.5	PO	6	21–28
	D	10–25	PO	8	21–28
	C	5–10	PO	8	14–21
	C	25	PO	24	14–21
Chloramphenicol	D	25	PO	8	14–21
	C	15–25	PO	12	7–14
Metronidazole	B[b]	10–20	PO	12	14–21
	B[b]	7.5–10	PO	8	14–21
	B[b]	30	PO	24	14–21
Tylosin	D	10–25	PO	8	14–21
Motility Modifiers					
Clidinium and chlordiazepoxide[c]	D	0.1	PO	6–12	prn
Diphenoxylate	D	0.5–1	PO	8–12	prn
Loperamide	D	0.1	PO	6	prn
Diazepam	B	5 mg total	PO	8–12	prn

[a]Dose per administration at specified interval. For additional information on each drug, see Drug Formulary, Appendix 8.
[b]Most cats get one quarter of a 250-mg tablet per day.
[c]Librax, Roche Products Inc, Marrati, PR.
D = dog; C = cat; B = dog and cat.

FIV can develop chronic ulcerative colitis, presumably as an immunosuppressive phenomenon. Lymphocytic-plasmacytic colitis, a chronic IBD, has been described in cats with chronic large-bowel diarrhea.[24]

Acute or chronic colitis should be suspected in any animal presented with large-bowel diarrhea. A stained fecal smear and rectal scraping and a parasite examination are helpful in eliminating parasitism, neoplasia, and algal and fungal disorders as causes of the diarrhea and, in many cases, they help to confirm a diagnosis. A presumptive diagnosis of colitis should be confirmed by proctoscopy and biopsy when possible.

The antibiotics that have been useful in treating canine and feline ulcerative colitis are primarily those that are effective against anaerobic bacteria (Table 89–14). The lesions usually do not resolve spontaneously. Dietary management is usually attempted first in dogs and cats. Food should be withheld for 24 to 48 hours, and the animal should then be started on a bland diet in multiple, small feedings. A nonallergenic diet low in fat, such as boiled rice, meat, and potatoes is satisfactory.[24] For dogs, prescription diets (I/D or D/D, Hills, Topeka, KS) are indicated. Drugs that have been most effective in dogs and cats include oral sulfasalazine, oral chloramphenicol, and oral metronidazole. In addition to its antibacterial effect, sulfasalazine inhibits intestinal hypersecretion by interfering with leukotriene and prostaglandin synthesis. After several weeks of therapy, the dosage should be reduced, and in animals requiring long-term therapy, the minimum effective dose should be determined. Cats with lymphocytic-plasmacytic colitis have responded to sulfasalazine with or without concurrent metronidazole and glucocorticoid therapy or to dietary management of lamb and rice or a prescription diet (c/d DIET, Hills, Topeka, KS).[24] Glucocorticoids should be provided at anti-inflammatory doses with caution and only if relapses have occurred after clinical improvement has been noted with antimicrobial therapy. When stress is suspected to be a problem or diarrhea is incessant, clidinium and chlordiazepoxide, diphenoxylate, loperamide, or diazepam may be added to the regimen. Because colonic motility is already depressed in colitis, there is no need for routine anticholinergic or opiate drugs, unless given for relief of acute straining. Antispasmodic drugs, such as diphenoxylate and loperamide, must be used with caution in invasive bacterial infections of the bowel because of the increased risk of sepsis or toxemia. In acute experimental colitis in dogs, drugs such as desferrioxamine, verapamil, and disulfiram, which are oxygen free radical scavengers, were effective in preventing mucosal ulceration.[54a]

Intra-Abdominal Infections

PANCREATITIS

Pancreatic infection by bacteria develops in less than 10% of humans with acute pancreatitis but in up to 40% of those with severe pancreatitis. Bacterial contamination may arise from hematogenous spread from the systemic circulation, duodenal reflux up the pancreatic duct, contamination from the biliary tree, or bacterial translocation from the lower bowel via the portal circulation. Common enteric organisms are usually involved, causing secondary infection of acutely inflamed or necrotic pancreatic tissue. People with severe acute pancreatitis that receive prophylactic antibiotics IV have a lower mortality rate than those that do not.[38] Dogs with intestinal colonization by genetically labeled *E. coli* had spread of organisms to the pancreas and mesenteric lymph nodes after experimentally induced pancreatitis.[54] Secondary ischemic damage to jejunal and ileal mucosa was noted in affected dogs and was probably responsible for portal venous bacteremia. In cats, experimental inoculation of pancreatic ducts with *E. coli* resulted in infection with concurrent pancreatitis, whereas bacteria were cleared in cats with healthy pancreatic tissue.[106] Antimicrobial therapy with cefotaxime (50–100 mg/kg IM every 8 hours) was started 12 hours after inoculation. Infection developed in 73% of animals receiving no antibiotic and in none of those cats receiving antibiotic.

In dogs with acute experimental pancreatitis, significant differences in bioactive levels were found between antibiotics in pancreatic tissue.[96] Ampicillin, gentamicin, and cefazolin reached therapeutic levels in blood, but not in normal or inflamed pancreatic tissue. Of other drugs tested, clindamycin, metronidazole, and chloramphenicol achieved penetrance in normal and inflamed pancreas. Consult Table 89–15 for suggested dosages.

PERITONITIS AND INTRA-ABDOMINAL ABSCESSES

Etiology and Clinical Findings

Peritonitis and intra-abdominal abscess formation are frequent complications of intestinal perforation caused by postsurgical wound dehiscence of the GI tract, foreign bodies, severe ulcerative enteritis, penetrating abdominal wounds, and rupture of abscesses of intra-abdominal organs.[24, 43, 95a] Infection of ascitic fluid may occur from hematogenous, lymphogenous, and transmural migration from the GI or genitourinary tract. Animals with peritonitis may become depressed, weak, and hypotensive after GI illness or abdominal wounds. Fever, abdominal distention, and abdominal pain are variable findings.

Diagnosis

Peritonitis should be suspected when a severe, inappropriate left shift in the leukogram is found. Radiography may be misleading in early or localized disease. Confirmation of intra-abdominal sepsis is best achieved through abdominal paracentesis.

Abdominal Paracentesis. The skin of the abdomen is clipped free of hair and prepared as for surgery from the umbilicus to the inguinal region. An 18-gauge, 1-inch needle fitted to a 20-ml syringe can be used to make the tap. Plastic IV catheters or metal teat cannulas are less likely than metal needles to penetrate intra-abdominal structures accidentally and they allow sampling at greater depths. The use of needles and IV catheters is frequently unrewarding because of occlusion, too small a volume of abdominal fluid being recovered, and localization of the inflammatory process. Multiple collection attempts in each of the four abdominal quadrants are recommended. Peritoneal lavage should be attempted if no material can be aspirated.[24] Peritoneal dialysis catheters or cutting fenestrated openings in flexible Teflon vascular catheters facilitates administration and withdrawal of fluid. Lavage is performed by inserting the large catheter through the caudal ventral abdominal wall in the direction of the pelvic canal. A negative aspiration is followed by rapid infusion of isotonic saline through an IV drip set at a volume of 20 ml/kg. After the animal has been gently rotated, the fluid can be removed by placing the still-connected fluid bottle on the floor to allow gravity drainage. A portion of the fluid that runs back into the bottle should be analyzed for protein concentration and examined cytologically. If an inflammatory exudate is detected, an aliquot should be submitted for culture. The presence of degenerative neutrophils with nucleated cell counts greater than 9000 cells/μl, intracellular bacteria, or organic debris indicates bacterial peritonitis. A portion of the fluid should be kept in a sealed syringe to preserve anaerobes during transport to the laboratory. Immediate inoculation of an aliquot of fluid into a blood culture bottle improves the isolation rate of aerobic bacteria, even compared with centrifugation-lysis methods.[90]

Table 89–15. Antimicrobial Therapy for Intra-Abdominal Infections

DRUG	SPECIES	DOSE[a] (mg/kg)	ROUTE[b]	INTERVAL (HOURS)	DURATION (DAYS)
Pancreatitis					
Cefotaxime	C	50–100	IV, IM, SC	8	3–5
	D	20–80	IV, IM, SC		
Clindamycin	B	5–11	IV, SC, PO	8–12	3–5
Metronidazole	B	7–15	IV, PO	8–12	3–5
Chloramphenicol	D	25–50	IV, IM, SC, PO	8	3–5
	C	50	IV, IM, SC, PO	12	
Intra-Abdominal Sepsis					
Combination					
Clindamycin	B	5–11	IV, SC, PO	8–12	5–7
or					
Metronidazole	B	10–15	IV, SC, PO	8–12	5–7
or					
Amoxicillin	B	20–25	IV, IM, SC, PO	8	5–7
combined with					
Gentamicin	B	4.4	IV, SC	12	5–7
	D	8–12	IV, SC	24	5–7
or					
Cefotaxime[c]	C	50–100	IV, SC	8	5–7
	D	20–80	IV, SC	8	5–7
or					
Enrofloxacin[d]	B	5–10	SC, PO, IV[e]	12	5–7
Single agent					
Ticarcillin-clavulanate	B[f]	30–50	IV	6–8	5–7
Piperacillin-tazobactam	B[f]	50	IV, IM	4–6	5–7
Ampicillin-sulbactam	B[f]	20	IV, IM	6–8	5–7
Imipenem-cilastatin	B[f]	3–5	IV	8	5–7

[a]Dose per administration at specified interval. For additional information on these drugs, see Drug Formulary, Appendix 8.
[b]Oral route recommended for pancreatitis and only in intra-abdominal sepsis when animals are not vomiting.
[c]Or other third-generation cephalosporin.
[d]Or other fluoroquinolone.
[e]Must be diluted 10-fold before IV administration, and then given very slowly over 10 minutes.
[f]Extrapolation of human dose with limited studies in dogs and cats.
C = cat; D = dog; B = both dog and cat.

Therapy

Antibiotic therapy is important in the management of intra-abdominal infections (see Table 89–15).[24] Mixed infections caused by indigenous flora are associated with GI leakage. With gastric leakage, lower concentration of bacteria result in lower prevalence of infection unless microbial overgrowth is present from decreased gastric acid output and gastric motility or from gastric ulcers or malignancies.[70] With biliary leakage, contamination rates are intermediate. With lower small intestinal and colonic leakage infection is certain. Organisms in all cases are a mixture of facultative anaerobic bacteria, usually Enterobacteriaceae, and obligate anaerobes.

A combination of antimicrobial therapy and surgical drainage is required for treating most cases of intra-abdominal infections. Therapy against facultative enteric gram-negative bacteria (e.g., *E. coli*) and anaerobes (e.g., *Bacteroides fragilis*) is essential when leakage occurs from the small intestine, cecum, or colon. Aerobes are important in producing bacteremia and early mortality in intra-abdominal infections, whereas the obligate anaerobes, which outnumber them, are instrumental in leading to abscess formation. Drugs such as aminoglycosides have been recommended because of their effect against gram-negative bacteria.[24, 50] In animals with experimentally induced intra-abdominal sepsis, the administration of aminoglycosides alone greatly reduces the mortality associated with gram-negative sepsis, although the prevalence of postoperative adhesions and abscess formation are unaffected. Under similar experimental circumstances, the use of drugs effective against anaerobic bacteria such as clindamycin resulted in death from gram-negative septicemia, even though the prevalence of intra-abdominal abscesses was reduced. This finding indicates that antimicrobial drugs or combinations used in treating intra-abdominal sepsis must be effective against both aerobic and anaerobic intestinal flora to decrease both mortality and abscess formation after peritonitis. Regimens in which a third-generation cephalosporin is substituted for the aminoglycoside or metronidazole is substituted for clindamycin give similarly favorable results. A summary of antimicrobial drug combinations recommended for experimental abdominal sepsis is presented in Table 89–15.

Antimicrobial Prophylaxis. To reduce postoperative complications, antimicrobial agents can be administered to animals without established infections when they undergo abdominal surgery in which spillage of ingesta is anticipated. Preoperative and intraoperative administration of cephalosporins or penicillin derivatives combined with aminoglycosides has been effective in reducing the complications of intestinal leakage and peritoneal contamination in people. Total sterilization of the bowel before surgery, however, is impossible in a conventional environment. Bowel sterilization has been achieved only experimentally in dogs that have been kept in a germ-free environment, fed sterilized food, and given combination therapy with large dosages of nonabsorbable antibiotics.[24] Even with these elaborate procedures, decontamination was incomplete, and the microflora was re-established within 1 week after termination of therapy. Administration of prophylactic antimicrobial therapy for GI surgery should begin 12 to 24 hours before the operation and terminate on the day of surgery if the bowel contents are not spilled. One week of therapy is indicated if contamination occurs during the surgical procedure.

Management of Surgical Contamination. Spillage of intestinal contents during experimental surgery in dogs has been best controlled by rinsing the peritoneal cavity with an irrigation solution of neomycin (500 mg), polymyxin (500,000 U), and bacitracin (50,000 U) mixed in 1 liter of saline.[24] Similar broad-spectrum antimicrobial activity can be achieved by rinsing the peritoneal cavity with organic iodine solutions diluted 1:10 to 1:20 with physiologic saline. Intra-abdominal instillation of povidone-iodine solutions can cause peritonitis and hepatotoxicity in dogs.[24] Dosages of 3.5 ml/kg of a 10% solution caused neutrophilic leukocytosis, increased hepatic enzyme activity, icterus, and death. Lower dosages (2 ml/kg) had fewer side effects. Although beneficial when given with antimicrobial therapy or drainage, saline alone to rinse the abdominal cavity has been less successful in preventing infection, despite its diluting effect on the spilled material. See Iodophors, Chapter 94 for further information on their use as lavage fluids.

Management of Established Peritonitis. Antimicrobial therapy is essential for animals with acute septic peritonitis. Broad-spectrum antimicrobial therapy is less important than lavage in the management of established peritonitis. This procedure involves the placement of intra-abdominal tubes and daily infusion and removal of isotonic saline solutions. Antimicrobial agents can be placed in the infusion fluid to reach higher concentrations than when they are given orally or parenterally. Only small amounts of many systemically administered antibiotics reach the peritoneal cavity, whereas most of the drug introduced into the abdominal cavity enters the systemic circulation.

Open peritoneal drainage has usually been successful for treatment of established generalized peritonitis in dogs and cats.[12, 24] The technique involves exploratory laparotomy, surgical correction of the cause, lavage of the abdominal cavity, and incomplete closure of the ventral midline incision with supportive wraps. The abdominal cavity is treated like one large abscess that can drain through the open incision. When the bandage is changed, additional lavage is performed. Complications are loss of fluids, proteins, and electrolytes. Absorbent abdominal pads are applied under a supportive wrap to draw fluid away from the incision. This method is reserved for advanced cases of septic peritonitis in which all the tissues cannot be debrided and sepsis is expected from residual intra-abdominal inflammation. Closure of the peritoneal cavity was usually done 3 to 4 days after surgery. Antimicrobial therapy was continued until the time of final closure.

Aminoglycosides, such as gentamicin IM, and cephalosporins orally or IM result in minimal peritoneal concentrations. Higher concentrations, should they be desired, might be added in restricted therapeutic doses to the peritoneal lavage fluid. When given orally, metronidazole, a relatively effective drug for anaerobic infections, reaches a higher concentration in peritoneal effusions than most other antimicrobial agents.[24]

References

1. Allaker RP, Langlois T, Hardie JM. 1994. Prevalence of *Eikenella corrodens* and *Actinobacillus actinomycetemcomitans* in the dental plague of dogs. *Vet Rec* 134:519–520.
2. Anderson JG. 1991. Approach to diagnosis of canine oral lesions. *Compend Cont Educ Pract Vet* 13:1215–1226.
3. Ashkenazi S, Cleary TG. 1991. Antibiotic treatment of bacterial gastroenteritis. *Pediatr Infect Dis J* 10:140–148.
4. Badcoe LM. 1992. Haemorrhagic enteritis in a dog associated with *Clostridium* sp. *N Z Vet J* 40:34.
5. Batt RM. 1996. Enteric bacteria: friend or foe? *J Small Anim Pract* 37:261–267.
6. Batt RM, Barnes A, Rutgers HC, et al. 1991. Relative IgA deficiency and small intestinal bacterial overgrowth in German shepherd dogs. *Res Vet Sci* 50:106–111.
7. Batt RM, Hall EJ, McLean L, et al. 1992. Small intestinal bacterial over-

growth and enhanced intestinal permeability in healthy Beagles. *Am J Vet Res* 53:1935–1940.
8. Bellows J. 1996. Tooth extraction for treatment of feline stomatitis. *Vet Forum* April: p 56.
9. Benno Y, Nakao H, Uchida K, et al. 1992. Impact of the advances in age on the gastrointestinal microflora of Beagle dogs. *J Vet Med Sci* 54:703–706.
9a. Bibbo C, Petschenik AJ, Reddell MT, et al. 1996. Bacterial translocation after mesenteric ligation in dogs. *J Invest Surg* 9:293–303.
10. Boosinger TR, Dillon AR. 1992. *Campylobacter jejuni* infections in dogs and the effect of erythromycin and tetracycline therapy on fecal shedding. *J Am Anim Hosp Assoc* 28:33–38.
10a. Charbonneau DL, Snider AG. 1997. Reduced chlorhexidine tooth stain coverage by sequential administration of monoperoxyphthalic acid in the beagle dog. *J Dent Res* 76:1596–1601.
11. Collins JE, Bergeland ME, Lindeman CJ, et al. 1988. *Enterococcus (Streptococcus) durans* adherence in the small intestine of a diarrheic pup. *Vet Pathol* 25:396–398.
12. Culvenor JA. 1997. Peritonitis following intestinal anastomosis and enteroplication in a kitten with intussusception. *Aust Vet J* 75:175–177.
12a. Dahlinger J, Marks SL, Hirsh DC. 1997. Prevalence and identity of translocating bacteria in healthy dogs. *J Vet Intern Med* 11:319–322.
13. Davenport DJ, Ludlow CL, Hunt J, et al. 1994. Effect of sampling method on quantitative duodenal cultures in dogs: endoscopy vs permucosal aspiration. *J Vet Intern Med* 8:152.
14. DeBowes LJ, Mosier D, Logan E, et al. 1996. Association of periodontal disease and histologic lesions in multiple organs from 45 dogs. *J Vet Dent* 13:57–60.
15. Delles EK, Willard MD, Simpson RB, et al. 1994. Comparison of species and numbers of bacteria in concurrently cultured samples of proximal small intestinal fluid and endoscopically obtained duodenal mucosa in dogs with intestinal bacterial overgrowth. *Am J Vet Res* 55:957–964.
16. Dennis JS, Kruger JM, Mullaney TP. 1993. Lymphocytic/plasmacytic colitis in cats: 14 cases (1985–1990). *J Am Vet Med Assoc* 202:313–318.
17. De Rycke J, Gonzalez EA, Blanco J, et al. 1990. Evidence for two types of cytotoxic necrotizing factor in human and animal clinical isolates of *Escherichia coli*. *J Clin Microbiol* 28:694–699.
18. Diehl K, Rosychuk RAW. 1993. Feline gingivitis-stomatitis. *Vet Clin North Am* 23:139–153.
18a. Duhamel GE, Hunsaker BD, Mathiesen MR, et al. 1996. Intestinal spirochetosis and giardiasis in a beagle pup with diarrhea. *Vet Pathol* 33:360–362.
19. Duhamel GE, Muniappa N, Mathlesen MR, et al. 1995. Certain canine weakly β-hemolytic intestinal spirochetes are phenotypically and genotypically related to spirochetes associated with human and porcine intestinal spirochetosis. *J Clin Microbiol* 33:2212–2215.
20. Farmer RG. 1990. Infectious causes of diarrhea in the differential diagnosis of inflammatory bowel disease. *Med Clin North Am* 74:29–38.
21. Gorel C, Rawlings JM. 1996. The role of a dental hygiene chew in maintaining periodontal health. *J Vet Dent* 13:31–34.
22. Gorel C, Rawlings JM. 1996. The role of tooth brushing and diet in the maintenance of periodontal health in dogs. *J Vet Dent* 13:139–143.
23. Greene CE. 1984. Gastrointestinal, intra-abdominal, and hepatobiliary infections, pp 247–268. *In* Greene CE (ed), Clinical microbiology and infectious diseases of the dog and cat. WB Saunders, Philadelphia, PA.
24. Greene CE. 1990. Gastrointestinal and intra-abdominal infections, pp 125–137. *In* Greene CE (ed), Infectious diseases of the dog and cat. WB Saunders, Philadelphia, PA.
25. Greenfield CL, Walshaw R. 1987. Open peritoneal drainage for treatment of contaminated peritoneal cavity and septic peritonitis in dogs and cats: 24 cases (1980–1986). *J Am Vet Med Assoc* 191:100–105.
26. Gruffydd-Jones TJ. 1991. Gingivitis and stomatitis, pp 397–402. *In* August JR (ed), Consultations in feline internal medicine. WB Saunders, Philadelphia, PA.
27. Guilford WG. 1996. Idiopathic inflammatory bowel diseases, pp 451–486. *In* Guilford WG et al (eds), Strombeck's small animal gastroenterology, ed 3. WB Saunders, Philadelphia, PA.
27a. Gunawardana SC, Jergens AE, Ahrens FA, et al. 1997. Colonic nitrite and immunoglobulin G concentrations in dogs with inflammatory bowel disease. *J Am Vet Med Assoc* 211:318–321.
28. Hall JA, Washabau RJ. 1997. Gastrointestinal prokinetic therapy: motilin-like drugs. *Compend Cont Educ Pract Vet* 19:281–288.
29. Harari J, Besser TE, Gustafson SB, et al. 1993. Bacterial isolates from blood cultures dogs undergoing dentistry. *Vet Surg* 22:27–30.
30. Harari J, Gustafson S, Meinkoth K. 1991. Dental bacteremia in cats. *Feline Pract* 19:27–29.
31. Hart JR, Shaker E, Patnaik AK, et al. 1994. Lymphocytic-plasmacytic enterocolitis in cats: 60 cases (1988–1990). *J Am Anim Hosp Assoc* 30:505–514.
32. Harvey CE. 1991. Antibiotic therapy in oral diseases. *Prac Vet Dent* 5:133–138.
33. Harvey CE, Carter D, Bennett G, et al. 1989. Ulcerative stomatitis in maltese dogs. *Proc Vet Dent* 44:7–8.
34. Hennet P. 1991. Utilization of spiramycin and metronidazole in periodontal diseases of the dog. *Rec Med Vet* 167:1029–1036.
35. Hennet PR, Harvey CE. 1991. Aerobes in periodontal disease in the dog: a review. *J Vet Dent* 8:9–11.
36. Hennet PR, Harvey CE. 1991. Anaerobes in periodontal disease in the dog. A review. *J Vet Dent* 8:18–21.
37. Hennet PR, Harvey CE. 1992. Natural development of periodontal disease in the dog: a review of clinical, anatomical, and histological features. *J Vet Dent* 9:13–19.
38. Ho HS, Frey CF. 1997. The role of antibiotic prophylaxis in severe acute pancreatitis. *Arch Surg* 132:487–493.
39. Hoffmann T, Gaengler P. 1996. Clinical and pathomorphological investigation of spontaneously occurring periodontal disease in dogs. *J Small Anim Pract* 37:471–479.
40. Hoffmann T, Gaengler P. 1996. Epidemiology of periodontal disease in Poodles. *J Small Anim Pract* 37:309–316.
41. Holloway S, Senior D, Roth L, et al. 1993. Hemolytic uremic syndrome in dogs. *J Vet Intern Med* 7:220–227.
42. Holstrom S, Belmont CA. 1994. Rational antibiotic therapy in veterinary dentistry. *Vet Forum* May: p 54.
43. Hosgood G, Salisbury SK. 1988. Generalized peritonitis in dogs: 50 cases (1975–1986). *J Am Vet Med Assoc* 193:1448–1450.
43a. Howell TH, Fiorellini JP, Blackburn P, et al. 1993. The effect of a mouthrinse based on nisin, a bacteriocin, on developing plaque and gingivitis in beagle dogs. *J Clin Periodontol* 20:335–339.
44. Isogai E, Isogai H, Miura H, et al. 1989. Oral flora of mongrel and Beagle dogs with periodontal disease. *Jpn J Vet Sci* 51:110–118.
45. Jacobs G, Collins-Kelly L, Lappin MR, et al. 1990. Lymphocytic-plasmacytic enteritis in 24 dogs. *J Vet Intern Med* 4:45–53.
46. Jensen L, Logan E, Finney O, et al. 1996. Reduction in accumulation of plaque, stain and calculus in dogs by dietary means. *J Vet Dent* 12:161–163.
47. Jergens AE. 1994. Rational use of antimicrobials for gastrointestinal disease in small animals. *J Am Anim Hosp Assoc* 30:123–131.
47a. Jergens AE, Moore FM, Kaiser MS, et al. 1996. Morphometric evaluation of immunoglobulin A-containing and immunoglobulin G-containing cells and T cells in duodenal mucosa from healthy dogs and from dogs with inflammatory bowel disease or nonspecific gastroenteritis. *Am J Vet Res* 57:697–704.
48. Jergens AE, Moore FM, March P, et al. 1992. Idiopathic inflammatory bowel disease associated with gastroduodenal ulceration-erosion: a report of nine cases in the dog and cat. *J Am Anim Hosp Assoc* 28:21–26.
49. Jergens AE, Moore FM, Prueter JC, et al. 1991. Adherent gram-positive cocci on the intestinal villi of two dogs with gastrointestinal disease. *J Am Vet Med Assoc* 198:1950–1952.
50. Johnson CC, Baldessarre J, Levison ME. 1997. Peritonitis: update on pathophysiology, clinical manifestations, and management. *Clin Infect Dis* 24:1035–1047.
51. Johnson KA, Powers PE, Withrow SE, et al. 1989. Splenomegaly in dogs: predictions of survival after splenectomy. *J Vet Intern Med* 3:160–166.
52. Johnston K, Lamport A, Batt RM. 1993. An unexpected bacterial flora in the proximal small intestine of normal cats. *Vet Rec* 132:362–363.
52a. Johnston KL, Lamport A, Batt RM. 1994. Effects of metronidazole on intestinal bacteria and disaccharidase activities in normal cats. *Gastroenterology* 106:A242.
53. Karjalainen J, Kanervo A, Vaisanen ML. 1993. *Porphyromonas*-like gram-negative rods in naturally occurring periodontitis in dogs. *FEMS Microbiol Immunol* 6:207–212.
54. Kazantsev GB, Hecht W, Rao R. 1994. Plasmid labeling confirms bacterial translocation in pancreatitis. *Am J Surg* 167:201–207.
54a. Koksoy FN, Kose H, Soybir GR, et al. 1997. The prophylactic effects of superoxide dismutase, catalase, desferrioxamine, verapamil and disulfiram in experimental colitis. *J R Coll Surg Edinb* 42:27–30.
55. Koopman MBH, Kasbohrer A, Beckman G, et al. 1993. Genetic similarity of intestinal spirochetes from humans and various animal species. *J Clin Microbiol* 31:711–716.
56. Lee JI, Hampson DJ. 1994. Genetic characterization of intestinal spirochetes and their association with disease. *J Med Microbiol* 40:365–371.
57. Lee JI, Hampson DJ. 1996. The prevalence of intestinal spirochaetes in dogs. *Aust Vet J* 74:466–467.
58. Lee JI, McLaren AJ, Lymbery AJ, et al. 1993. Human intestinal spirochetes are distinct from *Serpulina hyodysenteriae*. *J Clin Microbiol* 31:16–21.
59. Lonsdale T. 1995. Periodontal disease and leucopenia. *J Small Anim Pract* 36:542–546.
60. Loret J. 1990. Studies of the in vivo and in vitro efficacy of combined spiramycin-metronidazole on the periodontal flora of dogs after experimental periodontitis. Doctoral thesis in pharmacy, University Paul Sabatier, Toulouse, France.
61. Love DN, Bailey GD, Bastin D. 1992. Chromosomal DNA probes for the identification of asaccharolyticus anaerobic pigmented bacterial rods from the oral cavity of cats. *Vet Microbiol* 31:287–295.
62. Love DN, Johnson SL, Moore LVH. 1989. *Bacteroides* species from the oral cavity and oral-associated diseases of cats. *Vet Microbiol* 19:275–281.
63. Love DN, Vekselstein R, Collings S. 1990. The obligate and facultatively anaerobic bacterial flora of the normal feline gingival margin. *Vet Micorbiol* 22:267–275.
63a. Lyon KF. 1994. Feline lymphoplasmacytic stomatitis associated with

monoclonal gammopathy and Bence-Jones proteinuria. *J Vet Dent* 11:25–27.
64. Macintire DK, Smith-Carr S. 1997. Canine parvovirus: part II. Clinical signs, diagnosis and treatment. *Compend Cont Educ Pract Vet* 19:291–302.
64a. Madewell BR, Bea JK, Kraegel SA, et al. 1998. *Clostridium difficile* fecal carriage in cats. Abstract, Proceedings, 16th Ann Vet Med Forum, San Diego, CA, May 1998.
65. Manfra Marretta S. 1992. Chronic rhinitis and dental disease. *Vet Clin North Am Small Anim Pract* 22:1101–1117.
66. Mauterer JV, Abood SK, Buffington CA, et al. 1994. New technique and management guidelines for percutaneous nonendoscopic tube gastrostomy. *J Am Vet Med Assoc* 205:574–579.
66a. Mayoral I, Pena L, Rodriguez-Franco F, et al. 1996. Immunohistological study of IgA, IgG and IgM in endoscopic biopsies of dogs with plasmacytic-lymphocytic colitis. *Zbl Vet B* 43:613–620.
67. McConkey S, Briggs C, Solano M, et al. 1997. Liver torsion and associated bacterial peritonitis in a dog. *Can Vet J* 38:438–439.
68. Michell AR. 1994. Small animal fluid therapy: 1. Practice principles. *J Small Anim Pract* 35:559–565.
69. Mikx FHM, Maltha JC, Campen GJ, et al. 1990. Spirochetes in early lesions of necrotizing ulcerative gingivitis experimentally induced in Beagles. *Oral Microbiol Immunol* 5:86–89.
70. Nord CE. 1990. Incidence and significance of intraperitoneal aerobic and anaerobic bacteria. *Clin Ther* 12:9–20.
70a. Norris JM, Love DN. 1995. Serum responses of cats with periodontal/gingival disease to members of the genus *Porphyromonas*. *Clin Infect Dis* 20:S314–S316.
70b. Papasouliotis K, Sparkes AH, Werrett G, et al. 1998. Assessment of the bacterial flora of the proximal part of the small intestine in healthy cats, and the effect of sample collection method. *Am J Vet Res* 59:48–51.
71. Peters JL, Willard MD, Lees GL, et al. 1991. Toxoplasmosis in two cats with inflammatory bowel disease. *J Am Vet Med Assoc* 199:473–476.
72. Prada J, Baljer G, DeRycke J, et al. 1991. Characteristics of α-hemolytic strains of *Escherichia coli* isolated from dogs with gastroenteritis. *Vet Microbiol* 29:59–73.
73. Ramsey DT, Manfra Marreta S, Hamor RE, et al. 1996. Ophthalmic manifestations and complications of dental disease in dogs and cats. *J Am Anim Hosp Assoc* 32:215–224.
74. Rawlings JM, Gorrel C, Markwell PJ. 1997. Effect of two dietary regimens on gingivitis in the dog. *J Small Anim Pract* 38:147–151.
75. Rayan GM, Downard D, Cahill S, et al. 1991. A comparison of human and animal mouth flora. *J Okla State Med Assoc* 84:510–515.
76. Richardson EF, Brown NO. 1996. Hematological and biochemical changes and results of aerobic bacteriological culturing in dogs undergoing splenectomy. *J Am Anim Hosp Assoc* 32:199–210.
77. Riviere GR, Weisz KS, Simonson LG, et al. 1991. Pathogen-related spirochetes identified within gingival tissue from patients with acute necrotizing ulcerative gingivitis. *Infect Immun* 59:2653–2657.
78. Runkel NSF, Moody FG, Smith GS, et al. 1991. The role of the gut in the development of sepsis in acute pancreatitis. *J Surg Res* 51:18–23.
79. Rutgers HC, Batt RM, Elwood CM, et al. 1995. Small intestinal bacterial overgrowth in dogs with chronic intestinal disease. *J Am Vet Med Assoc* 2:187–193.
80. Rutgers HC, Batt RM, Hall EJ, et al. 1995. Intestinal permeability testing in dogs with diet-responsive intestinal disease. *J Small Anim Pract* 36:295–301.
81. Rutgers HC, Batt RM, Proud FJ. 1996. Intestinal permeability and function in dogs with small intestinal bacterial overgrowth. *J Small Anim Pract* 37:428–434.
82. Rutgers HC, Lamport A, Simpson RW, et al. 1993. Bacterial overgrowth in dogs with chronic intestinal disease. *J Vet Intern Med* 7:133.
83. Salman T, Buyruk MN, Gurler N, et al. 1992. The effect of surgical trauma on the bacterial translocation from the gut. *J Pediatr Surg* 27:802–804.
84. Sarkiala E. 1993. Treatment of periodontitis in dogs with tinidazole. *J Small Anim Pract* 34:90–94.
85. Sarkiala E, Asikainen S, Wolf J, et al. 1993. Clinical radiological and bacteriological findings in canine periodontitis. *J Small Anim Pract* 34:265–270.
86. Sarkiala E, Asikainen SEA, Kamervo A, et al. 1993. The efficacy of tinidazole in naturally occurring periodontitis in dogs: bacteriological and clinical results. *Vet Microbiol* 36:273–278.
87. Sarkiala E, Harvey C. 1993. Systemic antimicrobials in treatment of periodontitis in dogs. *Semin Vet Med Surg* 8:197–203.
88. Sarkiala E, Jarvinen A, Sippola T, et al. 1992. Penetration of tinidazole into the gingival crevicular fluid in dogs. *Res Vet Sci* 52:391–393.
88a. Sarkiala-Kessel E, Jarvinen A, Nokelainen M, et al. 1996. Concentrations of tinidazole in gingival crevicular fluid and plasma of dogs after multiple dose administration. *J Vet Pharmacol Ther* 19:171–175.
89. Sato R, Inanami O, Tamaka Y, et al. 1996. Oral administration of bovine lactoferrin for treatment of intractable stomatitis in FIV positive and FIV-negative cats. *Am J Vet Res* 57:1443–1446.
90. Siersema PD, deMarie S, van Zeijl JH, et al. 1992. Blood culture bottles are superior to lysis-centrifugation tubes for bacteriologic diagnosis of spontaneous bacterial peritonitis. *J Clin Microbiol* 30:667–669.
91. Simpson KW, Batt RM, Jones D, et al. 1990. Effects of exocrine pancreatic insufficiency and replacement therapy on the bacterial flora of the duodenum in dogs. *Am J Vet Res* 51:203–206.
91a. Sorensen SH, Proud FJ, Rutgers HC, et al. 1997. A blood test for intestinal permeability and function: a new tool for the diagnosis of chronic intestinal disease in dogs. *Clin Chim Acta* 264:103–115.
92. Spangler WL, Culbertson MR. 1992. Prevalence, type and importance of splenic diseases in dogs: 1480 cases (1985–1989). *J Am Vet Med Assoc* 200:829–834.
93. Spangler WL, Kass PH. 1997. Pathologic factors affecting post splenectomy survival in dogs. *J Vet Intern Med* 11:166–171.
94. Strombeck DR. 1996. Microflora of the gastrointestinal tract and its symbiotic relationship with the host, pp 14–19. *In* Guilford WS et al (eds), Strombeck's small animal gastroenterology. WB Saunders, Philadelphia, PA.
95. Thayer WR, Chitravis V. 1994. The case for an infectious etiology in inflammatory bowel disease. *Med Clin North Am* 78:1233–1247.
95a. Tilgner SL, Anstey SI. 1996. Nocardial peritonitis in a cat. *Aust Vet J* 74:430–432.
96. Trudel JL, Wittnich C, Brown RA. 1994. Antibiotics bioavailability in acute experimental pancreatitis. *J Am Coll Surg* 178:475–479.
97. Turk J, Fales W, Miller M, et al. 1992. Enteric *Clostridium perfringens* infection associated with parvovirus enteritis in dogs: 74 cases (1987–1990). *J Am Vet Med Assoc* 200:991–993.
98. Turk J, Miller M, Brown T, et al. 1990. Coliform septicemia and pulmonary disease associated with canine parvoviral enteritis: 88 cases (1987–1988). *J Am Vet Med Assoc* 196:771–773.
99. Waters L, Hopper CD, Gruffydd-Jones TJ, et al. 1993. Chronic gingivitis in a colony of cats infected with feline immunodeficiency virus and feline calicivirus. *Vet Rec* 132:340–342.
100. Watson ADJ. 1994. Diet and periodontal disease in dogs and cats. *Aust Vet J* 7:313–318.
101. Watts J. 1995. Microbiology of the mouth–a toothy issue, pp 8–11. *In* Proceedings of the Pharmacia and Upjohn Worldwide Companion Animal Veterinary Dental Forum, Augusta, MI.
102. Weiss DJ, Gagne JM, Armstrong PJ. 1996. Relationship between inflammatory hepatic disease and inflammatory bowel disease, pancreatitis and nephritis in cats. *J Am Vet Med Assoc* 209:1114–1116.
103. Westermarck E, Myllys V, Aho M. 1993. Effect of treatment on the jejunal and colonic bacterial flora of dogs with exocrine pancreatic insufficiency. *Pancreas* 8:559–562.
104. Westermarck E, Siltanen R, Maijala R. 1993. Small intestinal bacterial overgrowth in seven dogs with gastrointestinal signs. *Acta Vet Scand* 34:311–314.
105. White SD, Rosychuk RAW, Janik TA, et al. 1992. Plasma cell stomatitis-pharyngitis in cats: 40 cases (1973–1991). *J Am Vet Med Assoc* 200:1377–1380.
106. Widdison AL, Karanjia ND, Reber HA. 1994. Antimicrobial treatment of pancreatic infection in cats. *Br J Surg* 81:886–889.
107. Wiggs RB. 1995. Multifactorial and oral host factors, pp 4–7. *In* Proceedings of the Pharmacia and Upjohn Worldwide Companion Animal Veterinary Dental Forum. Augusta, MI.
108. Willard MD. 1992. Inflammatory bowel disease: perspective on therapy. *J Am Anim Hosp Assoc* 28:27–32.
109. Willard MD, Simpson B, Delles EK, et al. 1994. Effects of dietary supplementation of fructooligosaccharides on small intestinal bacterial populations of dogs with spontaneous small intestinal bacterial overgrowth. *Am J Vet Res* 55:654–659.
110. Willard MD, Simpson RB, Fossum TW, et al. 1994. Characterization of naturally developing small intestinal bacterial overgrowth in 16 German shepherd dogs. *J Am Vet Med Assoc* 204:1201–1206.
111. Williams C, Aller MS. 1991. Feline stomatology. *Vet Dent* 91:101–116.
112. Williams DA. 1996. Malabsorption, small intestinal bacterial overgrowth, and protein losing enteropathy, pp 367–380. *In* Guilford WG et al (eds), Stombeck's small animal gastroenterology. WB Saunders, Philadelphia, PA.
113. Williams JE. 1995. Microbial contamination of denta lines, pp 8–1. *In* Proceedings of the Pharmacia and Upjohn Worldwide Companion Animal Veterinary Dental Forum, Augusta, MI.
114. Wolf AM. 1992. Feline lymphocytic-plasmacytic enterocolitis. *Semin Vet Med Surg (Small Anim)* 7:128–133.
115. Yamamoto T, Harnaka Y, Suzoki T. 1991. Intestinal microflora and bile acids following biliary tract reconstruction. *Nippon Geka Gakkai Zasshi* 92:1288–1291.
116. Zenger E, Willard MD. 1989. Oral rehydration therapy in companion animals. *Comp Anim Pract* 19:6–10.
117. Zetner K, Thiemann G. 1993. The antimicrobial effectiveness of clindamycin in diseases of the oral cavity. *J Vet Dent* 10:6–9.

Chapter **90**

Hepatobiliary Infections

Sharon A. Center

NORMAL FLORA

Bacteriologic studies of portal vein blood of the mature dog have shown that alimentary flora commonly circulates to the liver.[12, 13] It is suspected, but has not been proven, that this also occurs in the cat. Enteric organisms delivered to the liver in the healthy animal are extracted by the hepatic Kupffer's cells and either killed or excreted in bile. Liver disorders associated with ischemic injury, impaired hepatic artery perfusion, reduced macrophage function, and cholestasis can be complicated by infections derived from this normal enteric flora.[7]

SUSCEPTIBILITY TO INFECTION

Given the dual blood supply and strategic location of the liver, its exposure to gut-derived particulate debris, toxins, microorganisms, and immunoreactive substances from the systemic circulation is considerable. The hepatic mononuclear phagocyte system (MPS), comprised largely of Kupffer's cells, provides a major component of the systemic phagocytic clearance capacity. This MPS is the largest source of fixed macrophages in the body and provides a first line of defense against bacterial organisms derived from enteric translocation and resultant portal venous bacteremia. The liver protects against systemic bacteremia by cleansing blood delivered via the hepatic artery. Integrity of hepatic MPS influences systemic resistance to shock associated with hemorrhage, endotoxemia, trauma, and bowel ischemia.[38] Failure of this MPS may result in hepatic infection with or without systemic complications. In dogs with experimentally induced multiple portosystemic shunts, intraoperative portal venous bacteremia was greater (75%) than in sham-operated controls (60%).[25a] Similar studies in dogs with naturally occurring shunts did not show this correlation.[45b] In addition to the unique susceptibility to infection imposed by the circulatory exposure to infectious agents, the large mass of hepatic sinusoidal endothelium provides a site for invasion by agents targeting endothelial surfaces.

Hepatobiliary production of bile and IgA is important for maintaining the health of the biliary and GI systems. A normal biliary-enterobacterial cycle permits rapid elimination of bacteria in bile. Local IgA production protects against invasion by infectious agents.[7, 43] Cholestasis compromises these protective mechanisms. In experimental studies of complete biliary obstruction in dogs, small intestinal bacterial overgrowth and bacterial translocation to mesenteric lymph nodes and liver were observed.[11a] Mechanical resolution of cholestasis, as with surgical alleviation of major bile duct occlusion, allows mobilization of bacteria from sites of hepatic sequestration, resulting in the sudden appearance of bacteria in bile. Failure to provide adequate antibiotic coverage during such corrective surgery increases the risk of postoperative infection.

Despite the susceptibility of the liver to infectious disease, increased liver enzyme activity and hepatic dysfunction seem to develop more often as secondary effects of systemic bacterial infection rather than hepatotropic infection.[37, 39] Pyrexia, anoxia, nutritional deficits, released toxins, and inflammatory mediators each contribute to the development of clinicopathologic abnormalities. "Innocent bystander" injury from pathologic conditions initiated elsewhere in the body can lead to inappropriate diagnostic emphasis on the hepatobiliary system. On occasion, a self-perpetuating form of chronic active hepatitis may develop as a complication of infection with bacterial or viral agents. Examples include chronic hepatitis in dogs after infection with leptospirosis or canine adenovirus-1.[3, 20]

Systemic Infections

SEPSIS AND ENDOTOXEMIA

Hepatic dysfunction and cholestatic liver injury have been documented in people as a result of systemic bacterial infection.[14] Intrahepatic cholestasis has also been associated with severe extrahepatic bacterial infection in dogs.[46] The response of the liver to systemic sepsis has been studied in dogs experimentally infused with endotoxin and/or live gram-negative bacteria.[17, 22, 24] Acute morphologic changes include dilation and congestion of sinusoids and hepatic veins, central and midzonal hepatocellular necroses, fatty vacuolations, acute diffuse influx of inflammatory cells (neutrophils and monocytes), and microabscess formation. Kupffer cell hyperplasia occasionally develops, and, with chronicity, canalicular stasis becomes apparent. Hepatocellular dysfunction results in a shift to anaerobic metabolism, impaired gluconeogenesis, and mobilization of lipid from adipose stores. In dogs, acute increases in serum concentrations of triglyceride and cholesterol are speculated to reflect energy dependency on fat metabolism.

Clinical Findings

Hepatomegaly, splenomegaly, fever, icterus, and lethargy are common clinical signs. The hemogram may depict a leukopenia, degenerative left shift, and nonregenerative anemia. Hyperglobulinemia, hyperfibrinogenemia, hypoalbuminemia, and hypoglycemia may develop rapidly, as may variable increases in the serum activity of alanine aminotransferase (ALT) and aspartate aminotransferase (AST). In the dog, serum alkaline phosphatase (ALP) activity consistently increases after several days and hyperbilirubinemia after 36 to 48 hours. Although certain bacterial organisms can directly induce jaundice without causing substantial hepatic injury, generally the development of jaundice portends a poor prognosis. Disseminated intravascular coagulation (DIC), acute renal failure, and myocardial dysfunction may develop in terminal cases.

Therapy

The cornerstone of treatment is the provision of adequate fluid therapy, including colloids, parenteral antibiotics effective against involved organisms, glucose supplementation, and identification and correction of associated conditions (see Endotoxemia, Chapter 38).

Hepatobiliary Infections

Bacterial infections restricted to the hepatobiliary system are uncommon. These may assume the form of multifocal microabscess formation, diffuse cholangitis-cholangiohepatitis, cholecystitis, and choledochitis, or they may be associated with discrete, unifocal suppuration and necrosis.

PYOGENIC ABSCESS

Unifocal pyogenic hepatic abscesses are rare.[16] These may develop as a result of trauma, extension of sepsis from adjacent viscera or the peritoneal cavity, hematogenous distribution, or ascending biliary tract infection. Patients with solitary abscesses may have no discernible underlying predisposing conditions, whereas those with multiple abscesses usually have some other disease of the abdominal cavity or bacteremia. Because of the dynamics of the portal circulation to the liver lobes, focal abscess formation is most common in the right lobes. Lethal hepatic abscesses have been reported in neonates with omphalogenic infections,[25] in which *Staphylococcus* has been the most common isolate (Fig. 90–1).

The pathogenesis of hepatic abscess formation is linked to portal bacteremia and extension from biliary tract infections.[4, 31] Impaired hepatic perfusion augments development of infection. Portal thromboembolism related to enteric and mesenteric disease processes or necrosis of tumor tissue are likely causes. Immunocompromised patients are at greatest risk. In humans, polymicrobial infections and anaerobic bacteria are isolated from approximately 50% of large solitary abscesses.[36] Organisms retrieved from liver and bile cultures from dogs and cats with suppurative hepatic inflammation and abscesses are shown in Table 90–1. Approximately 40% of these were confirmed polymicrobial.

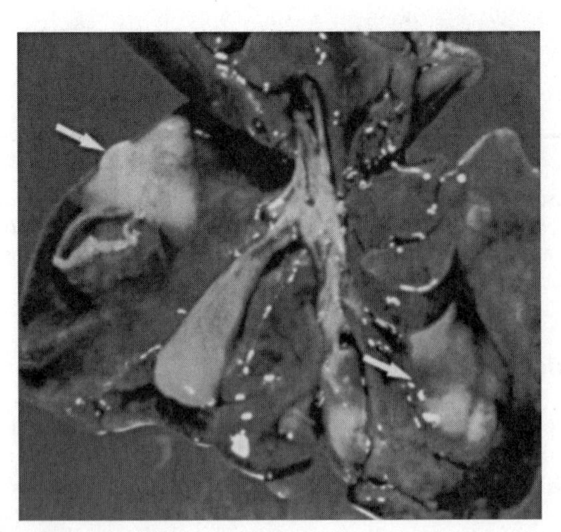

Figure 90–1. Gross appearance of hepatic abscesses *(arrows)* associated with a *Staphylococcus* omphalitis in a neonatal puppy. (Photomicrograph courtesy of the Department of Pathology, New York State College of Veterinary Medicine, Cornell University, Ithaca, NY.)

Multifocal microabscess formation has been described in conjunction with a variety of organisms associated with systemic infection, such as *Listeria, Salmonella, Brucella, Escherichia coli, Yersinia pseudotuberculosis, Bacillus piliformis, Actinobacillus lignieresii, Actinomyces, Nocardia,* and *Pasteurella* (Fig. 90–2).

Clinical Findings

When a hepatic abscess is the isolated focus of infection, clinical signs may remain vague and include fever, lethargy, anorexia, vomiting, diarrhea, and weight loss. Early diagnosis is difficult. Physical abnormalities may include hepatomegaly, abdominal tenderness, and abdominal effusion. Animals with systemic infections often demonstrate signs attributable to other organ systems, and the hepatobiliary system is secondarily and less overtly affected.

Diagnosis

Most patients demonstrate a neutrophilic leukocytosis intermittently associated with a left shift, toxic neutrophils,

Table 90–1. Bacteria Isolated From Suppurative Inflammation and Abscesses in Dogs and Cats[a]

Aerobic Cultures (Positive Cultures: n = 54)	Anaerobic Cultures (Positive Cultures: n = 26)
n = ≥ 3 each	*Propionibacterium acnes*
Escherichia coli	*Clostridium perfringens*
Staphylococcus intermedius	*Closridium*
S. aureus	*Bacteroides melaninogenicus*
S. epidermidis	*Corynebacterium* spp.
Streptococcus group D enterococci	*Actinomyces*
Streptococcus β-hemolytic	*Peptostreptococcus*
Enterococcus	*Fusobacterium*
Enterobacter aerogenes	Anaerobic streptococci
E. agglomerans	**Additional Microbes Reported Elsewhere**
Pseudomonas aeruginosa	*Bacillus piliformis*
n = 1 each	*Corynebacterium* spp.
Pseudomonas fluorescens	*Proteus* spp.
Klebsiella pneumoniae	*Francisella tularensis*
Bacillus spp.	*Listeria monocytogenes*
Acinetobacter calcoacetius	Eugenic fermenter-4 bacilli
Citrobacter freundii	
Moraxella phenylpyruvica	
Pasteurella multocida	
Bordetella bronchiseptica	
Nocardia	
Salmonella	
Campylobacter jejuni	

[a]In order from most to least common. Data acquired from case records, Companion Animal Hospital, College of Veterinary Medicine, Cornell University, Ithaca, NY 1985–1996.

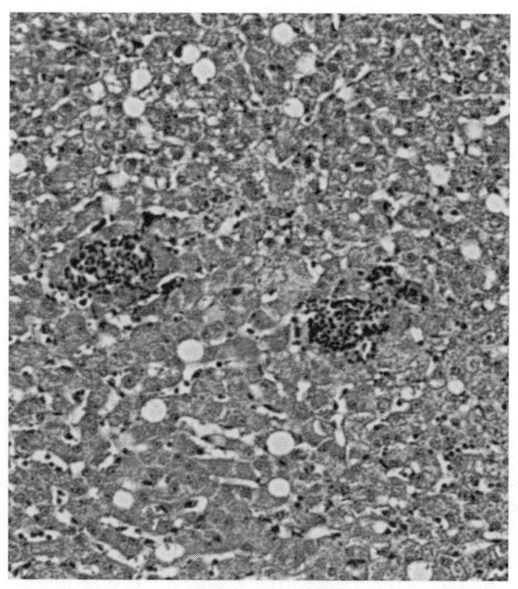

Figure 90–2. Hepatic microabscess formation in a mature dog associated with an *Escherichia coli* septicemia. (Photomicrograph courtesy of the Department of Pathology, New York State College of Veterinary Medicine.)

and monocytosis. Some become thrombocytopenic. Increased serum ALT, AST, and ALP activities and hyperglobulinemia are common. Hyperfibrinogenemia indicates the presence of an appropriate acute-phase response. Hyperbilirubinemia is inconsistent and usually mild. Septic animals may become hypoglycemic. Abscess formation with a gram-negative organism may produce the laboratory features of endotoxemia. Septic peritonitis develops on abscess rupture. Blood cultures are more likely to be positive in patients with multiple abscesses.

Ultrasonographic examination provides the best chance for early diagnosis of unifocal abscess formation. Ultrasonographic imaging can disclose focal lesions larger than 0.5 cm in diameter. Echogenic patterns vary: they may appear *hypoechoic*, consistent with liquefaction necrosis without marginal granulation; *heteroechoic*, reflecting a hyperechoic abscess rim surrounding an hypoechoic center; or *hyperechoic*, representing a caseated abscess.[26] Dystrophic mineralization and the presence of gas associated with an emphysematous nidus will appear hyperechoic. These changes may also be evident on abdominal radiographs. Miliary abscess formation cannot be distinguished from other multifocal hepatic parenchymal lesions using ultrasonography or radiography. Thoracic radiographs may reveal evidence of pneumonia possibly resulting from increased MPS activity in the lung.

Blood cultures may identify the causative organisms, especially if anaerobic organisms are grown. Urine culture may also be used to harvest the infectious organism.

Cytologic examination of abscess contents, including Gram's stain, anaerobic and aerobic cultures of affected as well as normal tissues, and routine histopathologic evaluations, are essential diagnostic evaluations. Anaerobic organisms may be difficult to culture and should be suspected if a polymicrobial population is seen on cytologic preparations of abscess contents, although none are cultured or only a few aerobic organisms are grown.

Therapy

Successful treatment of unifocal abscesses requires early diagnosis, aggressive surgical drainage and/or lobectomy, and long-term administration (minimum of 6–8 weeks) of an appropriate antibiotic. Response to antibiotic therapy is monitored with serial body temperatures and measurements of liver enzymes and repeated ultrasonographic evaluation of lesions. Because polymicrobial infections involving anaerobes are common, antibiotics effective against both aerobic and anaerobic organisms should be initially administered. Anaerobes have been shown to act synergistically with other pathogens in altering the course of infection and the prevalence of other pathogens. This modifies the abscess environment such that control of infection and eradication of bacterial organisms are impaired. Anaerobes can enhance the virulence of other bacteria in a polymicrobial infection by inhibiting phagocytosis with impaired opsonization and neutrophil chemotaxis and by locally interfering with the efficacy of antibacterial therapy.[35, 45, 45a] *Bacteroides fragilis* is one of the worst offenders, producing β-lactamases, which can overwhelm the function of β-lactamase inhibitors combined with some penicillins.

Initial therapy with a combination of a penicillin and an aminoglycoside is suggested. Metronidazole or clindamycin can be substituted for penicillin to provide activity against anaerobes. (Consult Therapy sections and Tables 90–2, 90–3, and 90–4.) Fluoroquinolones can be used in place of an aminoglycoside. First-generation cephalosporins, potentiated sulfonamides, and aminoglycosides are uniformly ineffective against anaerobes.

Treatment of hepatic microabscesses requires extensive supportive care and long-term effective antibiotic therapy against the involved pathogen and identification and management of the underlying cause. Disseminated sepsis should initiate a search for an underlying immunocompromised condition such as feline leukemia virus (FeLV) infection or neoplasia.

GRANULOMATOUS HEPATITIS

Granulomatous infiltration in the liver is an uncommon histologic diagnosis in dogs and cats. Causes in dogs include metazoal (e.g., schistosomiasis, dirofilariasis), fungal (e.g., histoplasmosis, paecilomycosis), and bacterial (e.g., tuberculosis, nocardiosis) infections and noninfectious disorders (lymphangiectasis, histiocytosis, lymphosarcoma).[11] In some idiopathic cases, reactions to infectious agents are suspected. Clinical signs are hepatomegaly, icterus, and ascites. Laboratory features are hyperbilirubinemia and high serum ALP activity and prolonged coagulation time (ACT). Hepatomegaly or reduced liver size may be seen on radiographs. Results of abdominal ultrasonography will show normal echogenicity of the liver and hyperechoic, irregularly hyperechoic, or hypoechoic hepatic parenchyma. Splenomegaly and abdominal lymphadenomegaly or peritoneal effusion may also be detected. The pathologic changes in the liver are variable degrees and character of granuloma formation depending on the underlying cause.[11] When causes can be detected, specific therapy is indicated. In idiopathic cases, clinical signs may respond to glucocorticoid therapy; however, the induced immunosuppression may increase susceptibility to an undetected microorganism.

FELINE HEPATOBILIARY INFECTIONS

Cholangitis-Cholangiohepatitis

The cholangitis-cholangiohepatitis syndrome is one of the most common hepatobiliary disorders in cats.[10, 19, 28] Inflam-

Table 90–2. Guidelines for Selection of Initial Antimicrobials for Anaerobic Hepatobiliary Infections Based on Gram's Stain Characteristics[1, 2, 42]

ANTIMICROBIAL	GRAM-NEGATIVE RODS NON-SPORE-FORMING: *Bacteroides*	GRAM-POSITIVE RODS SPORE-FORMING: *Clostridium*	GRAM-NEGATIVE RODS NON-SPORE FORMING: *Propionibacterium*	GRAM-NEGATIVE RODS NON-SPORE FORMING: *Actinomyces*	GRAM-POSITIVE COCCI: *Peptostreptococcus*
Penicillin G	−	− to + +	+ + +	+ + +	+ + +
Penicillin and β-lactamase inhibitor	− to +	+ + +	+ + +	+ + +	+ + +
Ticarcillin	+ + +	+ + +	+ + +	+ + +	+ + +
Cephalosporins					
Cephalothin (1st generation)	−	−	−	+ +	−
Cefoxitin (2nd generation)	+ +	− to + +	+ + +	−	+ + +
Metronidazole	+ + +	+ + +	−	+ + +	+ + to + + +
Clindamycin	+ + to + + +	+ + +	+ + +	+ + +	+ + +
Chloramphenicol	+ + +	+ + +	+ + +	−	+ + +
Tetracycline	−	− to + +	−	−	−
Doxycycline	−	− to + +	−	−	−
Fluoroquinolones	−	−	−	−	−
Aminoglycosides[a]	−	−	−	−	−
Trimethoprim-sulfonamide[b]	−	−	−	−	−
Vancomycin	−	+ + +	−	−	NA

[a]Aminoglycosides require transport enzyme systems to gain entrance to the interior of the bacteria; these are lacking in anaerobes.
[b]Sulfonamides are usually not effective despite in vitro sensitivity testing results. Tissue necrosis and suppuration commonly associated with anaerobic infections result in competitive inhibition of sulfonamide activity.
NA = not available; − = not effective; + = slight efficacy; + + = effective; + + + = very effective.

mation of intrahepatic bile ducts (cholangitis) is frequently associated with chronic interstitial pancreatitis because of the anatomic fusion of their common bile and pancreatic ducts. Cholangiohepatitis develops when cholangitis involves surrounding hepatic parenchyma. Inflammation of intrahepatic portions of the biliary tree develops in cats infected with a variety of infectious agents, including trematodes, *Toxoplasma* (see Chapter 80), an organism resembling *Hepatozoon canis* (see Chapter 74), gram-negative intestinal bacteria, and *Clostridium (Bacillus) piliformis* (see Chapter 39) (Fig. 90–3). Although infectious agents may initiate inflammation, it may become a chronic and self-perpetuating disorder because of immunologic processes. Feline hepatobiliary infections are separated into two forms: suppurative and nonsuppurative.

Suppurative Cholangitis

Suppurative cholangitis is less commonly diagnosed than nonsuppurative hepatitis.[9, 10, 19, 27] Most cats are middle aged or younger, and significantly more males than females are affected. Many cats have only a short duration of clinical

Table 90–3. Guidelines for Selection of Initial Antimicrobials for Aerobic Hepatobiliary Infections Based on Gram's Stain Characteristics[1, 2, 15, 42]

VARIABLE	GRAM-POSITIVE COCCI: *Staph.*	GRAM-POSITIVE COCCI: *Strep.*	GRAM-POSITIVE COCCI: *Enteroc.*	GRAM-NEGATIVE RODS: *E. coli*	GRAM-NEGATIVE RODS: *Past.*	GRAM-NEGATIVE RODS: *Enterob.*	GRAM-NEGATIVE RODS: *Pseud.*[e]	GRAM-NEGATIVE RODS: *Kleb.*
Penicillin G	−	+ + +	−	+ to + + +[c]	+ + +	−	−	−
Penicillin and β-lactamase inhibitor	+ to + + +	+ + +	− to + +[c]	− to + +[c]	+ + +	+ to + + +[c]	−	−
Extended spectrum Penicillin								
Ticarcillin and	−	+ + +	+ +[c]	− to + +[c]	+ + +	+ + +[c]	− to + + +[c]	− to + + +[c]
β-lactamase inhibitor	+ to + + + +	+ + +	+ +[c]	− to + +[c]	+ + +	+ + +[c]	− to + + +[c]	− to + + +[c]
Cephalosporins								
Cephalothin (1st generation)	− to +	+ + +	−	+ +	+ + +	−	−	+ + +
Cefoxitin (2nd generation)	− to +	+ + +	−	+ +	+ + +	− to + +	−	+ + +
Metronidazole	−	−	−	−	−	−	−	−
Clindamycin	− to + + +	+ +	−	−	−	−	−	−
Chloramphenicol	− to +	+ + +	−	+ + +	+ + +	− to + +	+ + to −	+ + + to −
Tetracycline	−	NA	−	−	+ + to −	−	− to + +	−
Doxycycline	−	− to + + +	−	−	+ + +	−	− to + +	−
Fluoroquinolones	+ to −	− to +	− to +	+ + +	+ + +	+ + +	+ +[d]	+ + +
Aminoglycosides[a]	+ to −	−	− to +	+ + +	+ + +	+ + +	NA	+ + +
Trimethoprim-sulfonamide[b]	+ to −	− to +	−	− to + + +	NA	+ + +	−	+ + +
Vancomycin	+ + +	+ + +	+ + +	−	−	−	−	−

[a]Aminoglycosides require transport enzyme systems to gain entrance to the interior of the bacteria; these are lacking in anaerobes.
[b]Sulfonamides are usually not effective despite in vitro susceptibility testing results. Tissue necrosis and suppuration commonly associated with anaerobic infections result in competitive inhibition of sulfonamide activity.
[c]Synergistic with aminoglycosides.
[d]Not *Pseudomonas fluorescens*.
[e]Pseudomonas: may require parenteral 3rd-generation cephalosporins, antipseudomonal penicillins: ticarcillin, carbenicillin, ticarcillin clavulanate, or lastly, a fluoroquinolone.
Staph. = *Staphylococcus*; *Strep.* = *Streptococcus*; *Enteroc.* = *Enterococcus*; *E. coli* = *Escherichia coli*; *Past.* = *Pasteurella*; *Enterob.* = *Enterobacter*; *Pseud.* = *Pseudomonas*; *Kleb.* = *Klebsiella*; NA = data not available; − = not effective, + = slight efficacy; + + = effective; + + + = very effective.

Table 90–4. Dosages of Drugs for Treatment of Hepatobiliary Infections and Modifications for Hepatic Insufficiency or Jaundice[a]

DRUG	STANDARD DOSE	LIVER-IMPAIRED DOSE (mg/kg)	ROUTE	INTERVAL (HOURS)	TOXICITY WITH ACCUMULATION[b]
Antimicrobials					
Penicillin G	20,000–40,000 U/kg	—	IV, IM, SC	4	Low
Amoxicillin-clavulanate	10–20 mg/kg	—	PO	12	Low
Ticarcillin	55–110 mg/kg	—	IV, IM, SC	8	Low
Cephalosporin					
1st generation	10–30 mg/kg	—	PO, IV, IM, SC	8	Low
2nd generation	10–20 mg/kg	—	IM, IV	8	
Metronidazole	15 mg/kg	7.5	PO	12	Neurotoxic
Clindamycin	10–16 mg/kg	5	SC	24	Anorexia, vomiting,
	5–10 mg/kg	5	PO	12	diarrhea
Chloramphenicol	25–50 mg/kg	12–25	PO, IV, IM, SC	8	Myelosuppression
	16–22 mg/kg	8–11	PO, IV, IM, SC	8	
Tetracycline	10–20 mg/kg	—	PO	8	Potential hepatotoxic
Doxycycline	2.5–5 mg/kg	—	PO	12	Low
Enrofloxacin	2.5 mg/kg	—[c]	PO, IM, SC	12	Drug interactions, seizures
Gentamicin	2.2–4.4 mg/kg	—	IV, IM, SC	12	Nephrotoxic, ototoxic
Amikacin	10 mg/kg	—	IV, IM, SC	8–12	Nephrotoxic, ototoxic
Trimethoprim-sulfonamide	30 mg/kg	15	PO, SC	12–24	Cholestasis, immune complex disease
Vancomycin	20 mg/kg	—	IV (slowly)	12	Nephrotoxic, painful IM
Supportive Therapy					
Vitamin K_1	1–1.5 mg/kg	—	SC	12[d]	Anaphylaxis, hemolysis
Vitamin C	100–500 mg total	—	PO, IV	24	Low
Vitamin E	10–15 U/kg		PO	24	Low
Dehydrocholic acid	15–20 mg/kg	—	PO	8–24[e]	Pruritus[f]
Ursodeoxycholic acid	2.5–7.5 mg/kg	—	PO	12	Pruritus[f]
Crystalloids	66 ml/kg	—	IV, SC	24	Edema, hypertension
Hetastarch					
Dogs	10–20 mg/kg	—	IV	24	Hypertension
Cats	10–15 mg/kg	—	IV	24	Hypertension

[a]For further information on antimicrobial drugs, see Drug Formulary, Appendix 8.
[b]For additional information on toxicity, see Drug Formulary, Appendix 8.
[c]Data on dose reduction not established.
[d]Use for 1–3 doses, then dose every 7–10 days. Too frequent administration or too high a dose will cause Heinz body hemolytic anemia in cats.
[e]Use 24-hr frequency for chronic therapy.
[f]Avoid use until complete biliary obstruction is relieved.

illness (<5 days). Less than 50% have hepatomegaly, and most are jaundiced, febrile, lethargic, and dehydrated. Abdominal pain is frequent. Vomiting or diarrhea is reported in 50%.

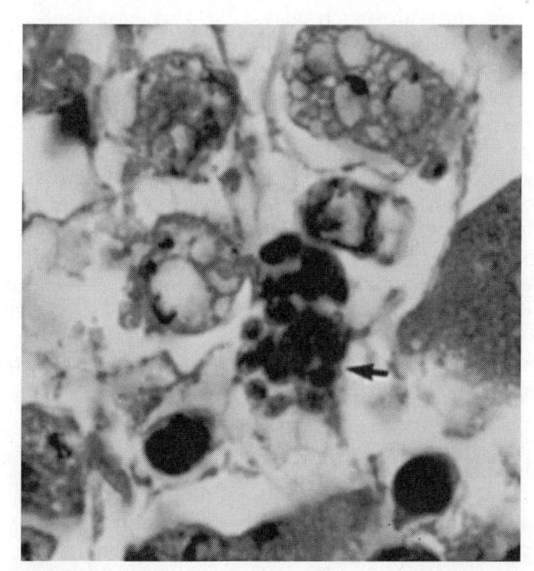

Figure 90–3. Photomicrograph of hepatic tissue demonstrating *Toxoplasma*-like organisms *(arrow)* in a cat with cholangiohepatitis (× 960). (Photomicrograph courtesy of the Department of Pathology, New York State College of Veterinary Medicine, Cornell University, Ithaca, NY.)

Most cats have underlying disorders of the biliary system associated with bile stasis, such as extrahepatic bile duct occlusion, cholelithiasis, periductal pancreatic and biliary duct fibrosis associated with ascending infection or pancreatitis, trematode infection, or congenital biliary tract malformation. Several cats have had histologically confirmed cholecystitis, and some have concurrent inflammatory bowel disease. Culture of tissue, bile, and choleliths have revealed bacterial infections with *E. coli*, *Enterobacter*, α-hemolytic *Streptococcus*, *Enterococcus*, *Klebsiella*, *Actinomyces*, *Clostridium*, and *Bacteroides*. Unfortunately, when an organism is isolated by bacterial culture, the question remains unanswered whether its presence is causal or is a result of an underlying disorder. Many affected cats have histories of intermittent vomiting and diarrhea, which could be associated with portal bacteremia or reflux of enteric flora into the bile or pancreatic ducts. Once enteric organisms gain access to bile, they may dehydroxylate certain bile acids, resulting in the formation of lithocholic acid, a hepatotoxin capable of producing cholestasis and hepatobiliary inflammation.

Suppurative cholangitis is characterized by a neutrophilic infiltration around and within intrahepatic bile ducts, hepatocellular cholestasis, and eventually periportal fibrosis. It is possible that suppurative cholangitis precedes the development of chronic nonsuppurative cholangitis. If this is true, biliary tract infection may initiate the cholangitis syndrome.

Nonsuppurative Cholangitis

Nonsuppurative cholangitis is more common in middle-aged to old cats and is associated with variable clinical signs and slow, insidious progression. There is no sex or breed predisposition. FeLV infection is rare. Most cats have been ill more than 3 weeks, many more than 2 months. Intermittent anorexia, vomiting and/or diarrhea, weight loss, cyclic fever, hepatomegaly, and jaundice develop in 70% of cats. Most are not profoundly lethargic. Chronic disease may lead to polyphagia seemingly associated with maldigestion induced by impaired bile flow. Common concurrent disorders include inflammatory bowel disease, chronic fibrosing pancreatitis, and cholecystitis. Frequently, there has been a history of extrahepatic bile duct obstruction. In some, cholangitis is the only disease process identified.

Retrospective study of affected cats in North America suggests that there are several different histologic categories included in the morphologic description of nonsuppurative cholangitis: *lymphoplasmacytic cholangitis, lymphocytic cholangitis, lymphoproliferative disease* (low-grade lymphosarcoma confined to the liver), and *sclerosing cholangitis*.[9, 10] Discussion of each subset of these disorders is beyond the scope of this chapter. Histologically, nonsuppurative cholangitis is characterized by bile duct hyperplasia, biliary fibrosis, lymphoid or lymphoplasmacytic aggregates in the portal triads, and, with chronicity, biliary cirrhosis. Sclerosing cholangitis is characterized by obliteration of small and medium-sized bile ducts. Only in rare cases has nonsuppurative cholangitis been associated with active infection. Because cholangitis is uncommon in nonsuppurative infiltrates, the term *lymphocytic portal hepatitis* may be a more appropriate pathologic description.[19]

Clinical Laboratory Findings

Suppurative cholangitis is more commonly associated with a moderate to severe neutrophilic leukocytosis accompanied by a left shift. Nonsuppurative cholangitis may be associated with a mild nonregenerative anemia, normal leukogram, neutrophilic leukocytosis, or lymphocytosis. Variable magnitudes of increased serum activities of ALT, AST, ALP, and γ-glutamyltransferase (γGT) develop, depending on the duration and degree of tissue inflammation and cholestasis. Hyperglobulinemia and prerenal azotemia are common. Overt hyperbilirubinemia is more consistent in cats with nonsuppurative cholangitis. In the anicteric cat, detection of bilirubinuria is a sensitive measure of impending hyperbilirubinemia. Measurement of serum bile acids can also be utilized to detect cholestasis before hyperbilirubinemia develops. Abnormal coagulation test results and bleeding tendency responsiveness to vitamin K_1 are observed when cholangitis is severe and chronic or is accompanied by major bile duct occlusion.

Therapy

Surgical exploration is necessary for definitive diagnosis of feline hepatobiliary disorders, because it allows visual and mechanical inspection of the biliary tree and tissue biopsy. If the common bile duct is occluded, a biliary diversion is necessary. Inspissated bile should be removed. Hydrocholeresis can be used to improve bile flow.

A therapeutic strategy is formulated after examination of liver and bile for sepsis. Aggressive antibiotic therapy should be implemented if infection is suspected. Samples of tissue and bile should be cultured for aerobic and anaerobic bacteria. Hepatic tissue should be submitted for routine histologic evaluation and reviewed for infectious agents. If flukes are considered a possibility, bile and feces should be examined for eggs.

Management of cholangitis-cholangiohepatitis requires long-term supportive care, including fluid therapy, forced nutritional supplementation with a balanced feline ration, supplemental water-soluble vitamins, antibiotics tailored to the involved organisms, ursodeoxycholic acid (Actigall, CIBA-Geigy, Summit, NJ) for its immunomodulatory-antifibrotic-choleretic effects, and, in some cases, anti-inflammatory doses of prednisolone.[9, 10] Suppurative cholangitis should be treated with antibiotics for at least 6 to 8 weeks. Periodic re-evaluation (every 2– 3 weeks) of hemogram, liver enzyme activities, and bilirubin concentration is advised. The response to treatment is based on the physical status of the patient, absence of fever, and resolution of leukocytosis, increased liver enzyme activities, and jaundice. Re-evaluation of hepatic biopsy is desirable but often cannot be justified. In some cases, repeated aspiration of hepatic parenchyma and bile, under ultrasonographic guidance, permits re-evaluation of the status of the infectious agent.

Cats with nonsuppurative cholangitis should be prophylactically treated with antibiotics for possible initiating bacterial infections. If peribiliary fibrosis is observed and culture results are negative, prednisolone is given at a dose of 2.0 to 4.0 mg/kg orally once per day. The initial dose of prednisolone is tapered after the first 1 to 4 weeks if the animal demonstrates improvement. Chronic administration of anti-inflammatory and chemotherapeutic drugs may be necessary to control this form of feline cholangitis.[9, 10]

CHOLECYSTITIS

Septic inflammation of the bile ducts and gallbladder occurs in dogs and cats.[18] The pathogenesis of acute cholecystitis is not clearly understood, although a variety of associated causes are implicated. Acute cholecystitis is experimentally produced by introduction of pepsin, activated proteolytic pancreatic enzymes, neutrophils, or bacteria into the bile duct.[21, 44] Spontaneous reflux of such initiating factors into the bile duct is probably more common in the cat. Biliary tract obstruction and septicemia are the most commonly implicated causes of biliary infection.[9] Cholelithiasis and choledocholithiasis have been associated with septic and nonseptic cholangitis, cholecystitis, and choledochocystitis (duct inflammation) in both dogs and cats.[30] In dogs, aged, small-breed females are most commonly affected with stone formation. Bile stasis, biliary inflammation, biliary infection, and changes in bile composition (increased cholesterol or bilirubin concentrations) are associated with stone formation. Insidious duct occlusion by choleliths or slow-growing biliary neoplasia augments development of septic inflammation, because cholestasis impairs normal biliary elimination of portal vein-derived bacteria. *E. coli* has been a common bacterial isolate from biliary tissue and bile from affected animals. Chronic cholecystitis has been associated with *Salmonella* (dogs) and *Pasteurella* (cats). Acute cholecystitis has been observed in dogs with *Campylobacter* (likely *Helicobacter*) infections (see Chapter 39).

Clinical Signs

Infection involving the bile ducts and gallbladder is associated with fever, anorexia, vomiting, abdominal tenderness, hepatomegaly, and jaundice. These signs can be persistent, intermittent, or episodic. If complete occlusion of the biliary tract is chronic (>2 weeks), pale acholic feces, absence of urinary urobilinogen, and bleeding tendencies resulting from vitamin K depletion may also be observed.

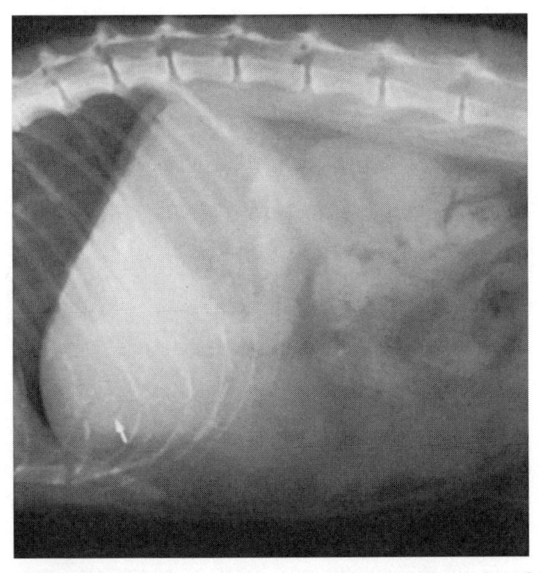

Figure 90–4. Radiodense microcholedocholithiasis *(arrow)* within the intrahepatic biliary tree in a mature cat that 2 years previously underwent cholecystotomy for cholelith removal. Chronic cholangitis, biliary infection, and sludged bile were contributing causes of cholelith development.

Diagnosis

Cholecystitis is frequently associated with clinicopathologic abnormalities typical of major bile duct occlusion. A nonregenerative anemia of chronic inflammation may also develop. A strongly regenerative anemia may develop in animals that have experienced substantial GI hemorrhage from pyloric or duodenal ulcers. Alimentary ulcerations are common in patients with compromised hepatic function and severe cholestasis, seemingly caused by impaired mucosal perfusion and repair. A marked leukocytosis with a left shift is common. Liver enzyme activities, especially ALP and γGT, are markedly increased (5–10-fold reference values). Severe cholestasis is common, with hyperbilirubinemia reaching as much as 20-fold reference values. Serum concentrations of total cholesterol may be increased 2- to 4-fold reference values. Increased prothrombin time, activated partial thromboplastin time, or ACT may develop owing to vitamin K_1 depletion or DIC. Septic bile peritonitis may prevail if the biliary system ruptures. Abdominocentesis yielding yellowish-orange fluid containing bile or bacteria indicates the need for immediate abdominal lavage and surgical intervention. Abdominal radiographs may show the presence of abdominal effusion, and, in exceptional cases, radiodense calcium containing choleliths may be observed (Fig. 90–4). In most instances, choleliths in dogs and cats are radiopaque and cannot be visualized on survey abdominal radiographs.

Ultrasonography can provide important diagnostic information because it can reveal evidence of biliary tract occlusion within the first 72 hours, thickening and distention of the biliary structures, obstruction-induced tortuousity of the common bile duct, and choleliths within the gallbladder.[41, 47] Choleliths located within the common or cystic ducts are less easily visualized. Care must be taken to avoid confusion caused by commonly visualized "bile sludge or sediment" in the gallbladder associated with anorexia. Ultrasonography can also detect the presence and permit the accurate sampling of small quantities of loculated pericholecystic effusion.

Therapy

Treatment of septic cholecystitis includes prolonged administration of antibiotics effective against the involved aerobic and anaerobic organisms. Laparotomy is usually undertaken to confirm the diagnosis, to define the underlying etiologic factors, and to perform a cholecystectomy and biliary diversion (e.g., provision of an alternate route of bile drainage; cholecystoenterostomy, and choledochoenterostomy). Cholecystectomy is advised if the gallbladder appears devitalized or neoplastic. Emergency laparotomy is essential if biliary rupture or septic bile peritonitis has developed. Management of bile peritonitis is discussed later. Hydrocholeresis may be used in conjunction with antibiotics to diminish bile stasis. See General Treatment Considerations for Hepatobiliary Infections.

EMPHYSEMATOUS CHOLECYSTITIS

Emphysematous cholecystitis is an uncommon condition that has been diagnosed in dogs with and without diabetes mellitus.[5, 23, 33, 34] Diagnosis in the cat is rare. The most common precipitating factor is believed to be cystic duct obstruction. Ischemia of the gallbladder wall as a result of tense distention promotes development of an anaerobic environment. Gas-producing organisms gaining access to the hepatic circulation or parenchyma can proliferate in the wall of the gallbladder and spread to the surrounding tissues. Left untreated, the gallbladder may rupture and the organisms may spill into the abdominal cavity. Pneumoperitoneum associated with septic peritonitis follows (Fig. 90–5).

Clinical Findings

Clinical signs associated with emphysematous cholecystitis include abdominal tenderness, fever, jaundice, anorexia, and vomiting. Neutrophilic leukocytosis; hyperbilirubinemia; increased serum ALP, γGT, ALT, and AST activities; and prerenal azotemia are common. When the gallbladder ruptures, the abdomen may become tympanic. Initially, radiographic features consist of gas infiltrates in the gallbladder wall.

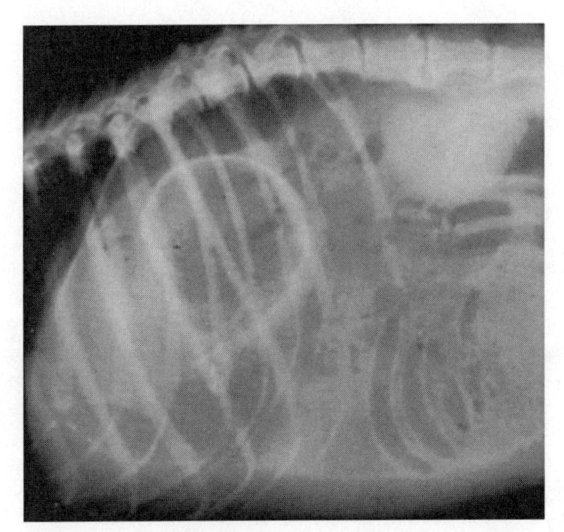

Figure 90–5. Radiograph of a mature dog demonstrating pneumoperitoneum associated with septic bile peritonitis. A clostridial organism was suspected on the basis of Gram's stain characteristics and was subsequently confirmed by anaerobic bacterial culture.

These spread to fill the gallbladder lumen completely and then progresses to involve the pericholecystic tissues. A sufficient volume of gas for radiographic detection will accumulate within 24 to 48 hours. The most common bacteria isolated from humans and dogs with emphysematous cholecystitis are *Clostridium* spp.

Therapy

Management of emphysematous cholecystitis involves cholecystectomy combined with prolonged administration of antibiotics effective against anaerobes, but even then the prognosis is poor. Only rarely have patients with emphysematous cholecystitis survived without surgical intervention. Medical and surgical treatment for septic peritonitis is usually also indicated.

BILE PERITONITIS

Bile peritonitis is a serious complication of biliary tree infection, inflammation, ischemia, or trauma. The toxicity of bile on tissues and hypovolemic shock associated with the pooling of fluid in the peritoneal cavity are responsible for the major clinical signs. Pleural effusion of a similar composition may also occur.[1a] Bacterial contamination of biliary ascites spontaneously develops and is the usual cause of death.[6, 9, 40] Bile-induced permeability changes in the intestinal wall promote the passage of enteric flora into the peritoneal effusion. Anaerobic organisms (*Clostridium* spp.) have been shown to spontaneously invade experimentally created biliary ascites in dogs.

Clinical Findings

Animals with bile peritonitis usually have histories of anorexia, vomiting, abdominal tenderness and distention, fever, and lethargy. Most patients are jaundiced. Emphysematous peritonitis may develop when gas-producing bacteria produce a tense tympanic abdomen (see Fig. 90–5).

Diagnosis

Usual hematologic abnormalities include a neutrophilic leukocytosis with a regenerative left shift, although in some cases a degenerative left shift develops. Biochemical abnormalities are characteristic of the underlying disease process. Increased serum activities of liver enzymes and moderate to severe hyperbilirubinemia are expected. Hypercholesterolemia may exist if complete bile duct occlusion preceded biliary tree rupture. Hypoalbuminemia may rapidly develop owing to sequestration of protein-rich fluid in the abdominal cavity. Prerenal azotemia is common because of the hypovolemic shock that frequently accompanies the syndrome. Prolonged hypovolemia may result in acute renal failure.

Abdominal radiography reveals a diffuse lack of visceral detail owing to the presence of peritoneal fluid. Free gas within the peritoneal cavity or migrating within the biliary tree usually indicates anaerobic bacterial infection. Cholangiography rarely delineates the site of biliary rupture because the competition between bilirubin and iodinated contrast prohibits adequate dye uptake and concentration in the biliary tree. Cholescintigraphy utilizing an iminodiacetic analog can provide a noninvasive method of documenting the site of bile leakage.[32]

Abdominocentesis reveals a yellowish-orange or golden-green effusion. Cytologic examination reveals neutrophils, macrophages, erythrocytes, and bilirubin crystals (Fig. 90–6). The presence of bacteria is detected using Wright-Giemsa's or new methylene blue stains. Gram's stain elucidates the morphology of organisms as well as the presence of spores. Aerobic and anaerobic cultures should be initiated regardless of organism visualization.

Therapy

Whenever bile peritonitis is suspected, surgical intervention is indicated. The presence of sepsis makes the situation urgent. Before general anesthesia and laparotomy, the patients must receive aggressive supportive care, including colloid administration to reinstate deficient oncotic pressure. Visual inspection usually reveals the site of biliary rupture and provides important information with which the surgeon can formulate an appropriate operative approach. If the gallbladder is severely inflamed or devitalized, a cholecystectomy is appropriate. If a portion of the common bile duct is damaged, a biliary diversion such as a cholecystoduodenostomy or cholecystojejunostomy may be appropriate. If the cystic duct is damaged, placement of a T-tube or choledochoenterostomy may be appropriate. The biliary tree should be examined for patency and bile fluidity. Identified choleliths should be removed. Biopsy specimens of the liver and involved portions of the biliary tree should be collected for histopathologic examination and for aerobic and anaerobic bacterial cultures.

If peritoneal sepsis is present, the abdominal cavity may generate a fetid odor at surgery. Lavage with sterile saline is

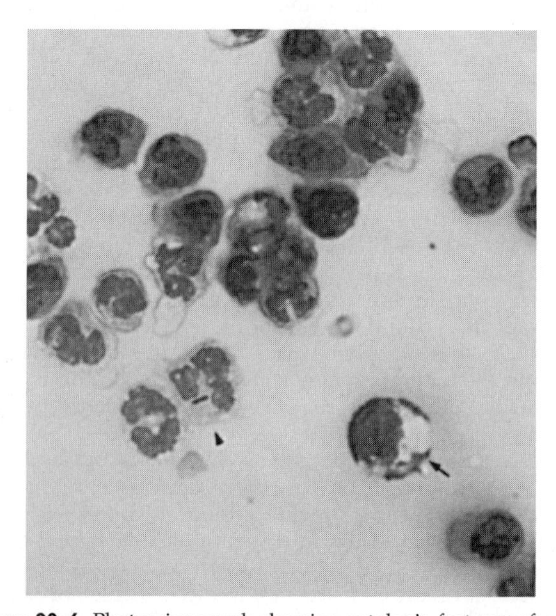

Figure 90–6. Photomicrograph showing cytologic features of an abdominal effusion observed in the same dog as shown in Figure 90–5 with septic bile peritonitis. Neutrophils, macrophages, erythrocytes, intracytoplasmic large Gram's stain–positive rod-form bacteria *(arrowhead)*, and golden bilirubin crystals *(observed in the cell with arrow)* were observed (Wright-Giemsa's stain, × 680). (Photomicrograph courtesy of the Department of Pathology, New York State College of Veterinary Medicine, Cornell University, Ithaca, NY.)

recommended before abdominal closure. Appropriate antibiotics should be continued for 4 to 6 weeks. Repeated administration of colloids to maintain plasma oncotic pressure may become necessary during recovery from peritonitis because of the prodigious loss of plasma proteins from continued abdominal drainage.

GENERAL TREATMENT CONSIDERATIONS

Supportive Care

Initial management of the animal with hepatobiliary infection involves provision of fluid therapy and a calorically and nutritionally adequate diet. Polyionic crystalloid fluids are given to correct dehydration, to cover contemporary losses, and to provide maintenance needs. Commercially available colloids (Hetastarch, Hespan, Dupont Pharma, Wilmington, DE), are given to reinstate colloid oncotic pressure when necessary. If present, hypoglycemia is treated with fluids supplemented to a 2.5% or 5.0% dextrose concentration, as necessary. If hypoalbuminemia, hepatic insufficiency, ascites, or a tendency for sodium retention exists, mixed solutions containing 2.5% dextrose with one-half strength mixed crystalloid (e.g., Ringer's, lactated Ringer's, and 0.45% sodium chloride solution) may be appropriate combined with colloid administration.

Anorexia is managed by forced oral alimentation, nasogastric or esophageal intubation, or placement of a gastrostomy or enterostomy tube. Total parenteral or enteral alimentation may be required if vomiting is persistent despite the administration of metoclopramide (0.2–0.4 mg/kg SC or IM TID or IV constant infusion drip of 0.01–0.02 mg/kg/hr). Caloric intake should achieve at least 70–90 Kcal/kg/day. The diet should not be restricted in protein content unless signs of hepatic encephalopathy are overt. It is imperative that animals with hepatobiliary infections or bile peritonitis maintain a positive nitrogen balance such that maintenance and tissue regeneration needs are satisfied. One finding is that forced tube feeding failed to improve malnutrition in complete obstructive jaundice in dogs and was associated with higher mortality than ad lib feeding.[11a] The use of benzodiazepines to stimulate the appetite will not ensure adequate caloric intake. Furthermore, in the circumstance of hepatic insufficiency and encephalopathy, these drugs are contraindicated. Water-soluble vitamins should be provided at a doubled conventional daily dose whether the patient is eating or not. Antioxidant activity of additional vitamins C and E may also be beneficial.

Vitamin K_1 should be administered by SC injection when prolonged coagulation times, hemorrhage, and icterus are noted (see Table 90–4). Increased PIVKA (proteins invoked by vitamin K antagonism or absence) seem to develop rapidly in patients with cholestatic liver disorders treated with long-term oral antimicrobials. Bleeding tendencies recognized before or during surgical procedures should be managed by administration of a fresh, compatible blood transfusion. The patient may also benefit from administration of synthetic vasopressin (desmopressin, DDAVP, Rhone Poulenc Rorer Pharm., Collegeville, PA; 1 μg/kg SC 30 minutes before expected result, one time therapy). Whole blood rather than plasma is usually better because the possibility of thrombocytopenia or acquired thrombopathia. DDAVP treatment of the blood donor may assist in arresting pathologic bleeding in the recipient. The mechanism of action of DDAVP in patients with hepatic insufficiency is ill defined, but is clearly more complex than simple elaboration of von Willebrand's factor from vascular endothelium.[29]

Antibiotics

Antibiotics for hepatobiliary infections should possess the relevant activity against enteric organisms commonly cultured from liver tissue and bile (see Tables 90–1 to 90–4).[1, 2, 15, 42, 45] Culture and susceptibility of involved organisms remain the best measures for correct antibiotic selection. In every case in which tissue biopsy and bile are collected for culture and histologic evaluation, cytologic evaluation should also be pursued. This permits rapid verification of infection with simple Wright-Giemsa's staining. Infectious organisms are difficult to visualize on routinely prepared histologic specimens and cultures can be erroneously negative. Morphologic characterization of bacteria on the basis of Gram's stain will help select the best initial course of antimicrobial therapy (see Tables 90–1 to 90–3).[1, 2, 10, 15, 42] Although selection of an antimicrobial having good penetration into the biliary tract is recommended (Table 90–5),[42] systemic activity of the antibiotic may be more important. Antibiotics administered during complete bile duct occlusion do not attain therapeutic concentrations in bile because of the cessation of bile flow. It is critical that therapeutic concentrations of an effective antimicrobial be achieved in tissues before manipulation occurs at surgery. In patients with extrahepatic cholestasis, it is essential that bile flow be reinstated by removal of obstructing calculi, inspissated bile, and other luminal obstructions or by creation of a biliary-enteric anastomosis.

In the absence of culture and susceptibility results or cytologic evaluation, selected antibiotics should be effective over the expected range of aerobic and anaerobic enteric organisms. A combination of drugs is usually provided. β-Lactamase–resistant penicillin, clindamycin, chloramphenicol, and

Table 90–5. Achieved Biliary Concentrations of Certain Antimicrobial Agent in the Absence of Major Bile Duct Occlusion[a]

ANTIMICROBIAL AGENT	RATIO OF ANTIBIOTIC BILE-SERUM
Aminoglycosides	
Amikacin	0.3
Gentamicin	0.3–0.6
Kanamycin	1
Streptomycin	0.4–3.0
Cephalosporins	
Cefazolin (1st gen)	0.7–3.0
Cephalothin (1st gen)	0.4–0.8
Cefoxitin (2nd gen)	2.8
Ceftriaxone (3rd gen)	10
Penicillins	
Ampicillin	1.0–2.0
Penicillin G	0.5
Oxacillin	0.2–0.4
Piperacillin	10–15
Mezlocillin	10
Nafcillin	40
Tetracyclines	
Tetracycline	5–10
Doxycycline	10–20
Miscellaneous	
Chloramphenicol	0.2
Clindamycin	2.5–3
Ciprofloxacin	2.0
Erythromycin	8–25
Metronidazole	1
Trimethoprim/sulfonamide	1–2/0.4–0.7
Vancomycin	0.5

[a]Data derived from experimental literature and from work in human beings.[1, 35]

Table 90–6. Influence of Hepatic Disease on Disposition of Selected Antibacterials in Humans With Severe Hepatic Disease–Insufficiency[1, 2]

ANTIBACTERIALS	PLASMA CLEARANCE	VOLUME OF DISTRIBUTION	T1/2
Amikacin	—	↑ 200%	No change
Ampicillin	No change	↑ 46–200%	↑ 30–45%
Carbenicillin	—	—	↑ 90%
Cefoperazone	↓ 0–40%	↑ 150%	↑ 200%
Cefotaxime	↓ 30–40%	—	Increased
Chloramphenicol	↓ 65–70%	↓ 20%	↑ 130–150%
Clindamycin	↓ 25–60%	↓ 40%	↑ 15–40%
Erythromycin	↓ 30%	↑ 50%	↑ 60–65%
Gentamicin	—	No change	↑ 85%
Metronidazole	No change	No change	↑ 40–150%
Mezlocillin	↓ 50%	—	↑ 170%
Norfloxacin	No change	—	No change
Pefloxacin	↓ 70%	↓ 20%	↑ 255%
Vancomycin	↓ 70%	No change	↑ 130%

T1/2 = half-life.

metronidazole are given IV as good first-choice antibiotics for anaerobic organisms. One of these is used in combination with either an aminoglycoside or enrofloxacin against aerobic organisms. Aminoglycosides should not be given until the patient's hydration status and prerenal azotemia are corrected. Aminoglycoside nephrotoxicity should be monitored by urine sediment examination for granular casts on an alternate-day schedule.

Antibiotics that require extensive hepatobiliary activation, biotransformation, or excretion or those that have been associated with adverse effects on the hepatobiliary system are considered poor first-choice selections for patients with compromised hepatic function. These drugs include hetacillin, tetracycline, doxycycline, lincomycin, erythromycin, sulfonamides, trimethoprim-sulfonamide, chloramphenicol, and metronidazole. Severe jaundice contraindicates the use of antibiotics that are excreted predominantly in bile, such as chloramphenicol, erythromycin, doxycycline, rifampin, clindamycin, and nafcillin. If metronidazole or chloramphenicol is administered to a jaundiced patient, the conventional dose is usually reduced by 50% to avoid toxic effects (Table 90–6).[1, 2] Tetracycline is avoided whenever possible because of its ability to produce hepatocellular lipid vacuolation in all species and hepatic encephalopathy in those with insufficient liver function. When circumstances warrant use of "contraindicated" drugs, Table 90–6 should be consulted.

Surgery

Laparotomy is indicated in most cases of hepatobiliary sepsis. Surgical intervention is imperative if hepatobiliary abscess, septic peritonitis, bile peritonitis, or major bile duct occlusion is suspected. Hepatic or bile aspirate or biopsy is the only definitive method of confirming an infectious process. Biopsy is required for definitive diagnosis. At surgery, the abdominal viscera should be inspected for a primary disease process. Mesenteric and hepatic lymph nodes should be visualized and biopsy specimens taken for histologic evaluation and culture, if a diagnosis remains uncertain. Liver specimens from one or more sites should be taken for biopsy. If entire lobes of liver seem to be involved in an abscess or appear to be necrotic, they should be resected. These areas should be manipulated minimally before resection. Venous outflow from the tissues should be ligated as early in resection as possible to avoid release of toxins from infected or devitalized tissues. The biliary tract should be evaluated for patency by gentle compression on the gallbladder, and bile fluidity should be assessed. The gallbladder and major bile ducts should be carefully palpated for choleliths, intraluminal or mural masses, and sludged bile. If abnormalities are detected, a cholecystotomy should be done, a biopsy of the gallbladder taken, and any abnormalities inspected and removed. Extrahepatic bile ducts may be surgically flushed with a soft rubber catheter and sterile saline solution to remove choleliths and sludged bile, taking care to avoid peritoneal contamination. Cholecystectomy is advised if the gallbladder wall appears devitalized or has suspected neoplastic involvement.

Samples of tissue and bile should be cultured anaerobically and aerobically. Bile for culture and cytology should be collected by fine-needle (22-gauge) aspiration into a syringe. The needle should enter the gallbladder at an oblique angle to reduce the chance of bile leakage after collection. If cholecystitis or cholangitis is suspected, biopsy and culture of a portion of the gallbladder wall and liver are frequently more reliable than culture of bile alone. Choleliths should also be submitted for culture.

Cytologic smears should be made from each tissue biopsy, lesion, and sample of bile, because bacteria are better visualized on cytologic preparation. Gram's staining assists in the selection of initial antibacterial therapy. Aerobic and anaerobic bacterial cultures should be requested on representative samples. Strict attention must be paid to the methods of handling and transporting specimens for anaerobic bacterial cultures (see Chapter 33). Cytologic evaluation serves as an important quality control indicator of transport and culture procedures. If organisms are identified on smears made at surgery and yet are not grown, transport or culture methods were probably inadequate. If trematode infection is possible, bile and feces should be examined cytologically for trematode eggs. Hepatic tissue should always be submitted for routine histologic evaluation, and the pathologist should be prompted to examine tissues for infectious agents with special stains.

Hydrocholeresis

After the patency of the biliary tract has been established at surgery, hydrocholeresis can improve bile flow in patients having considerable cholestasis, cholelithiasis, or inspissated bile. Resolution of bile stasis assists in the clearance of biliary infection and prohibits further stone formation. Ursodeoxycholic acid (Actigall, CIBA-Geigy, Summit, NJ) (see Table 90–4) is usually recommended as a long-term therapeutic agent in patients with persistent cholestatic liver injury. More substantial short-term hydrocholeresis, however, can be accomplished with dehydrocholic acid (Decholin, Bayer Corp, West Haven, CT; Cholan-HMB, CIBA-Geigy, Summit, NJ). This is a synthetic bile acid that increases the liquid or water component of ductular secretions.[9] It should be initially provided in conjunction with fluid therapy to ensure adequate patient hydration, which optimizes hydrocholeresis.

References

1. American Society of Hospital Pharmacists. 1996. APHIS formulary. American Hospital Formulary Service, Bethesda, MD.
1a. Barnhart MD, Rasmussen LM. 1996. Pleural effusion as a complication of extra hepatic biliary tract rupture in a dog. *J Am Anim Hosp Assoc* 32:409–412.
2. Bass NM, Williams RL. 1990. Hepatic function and pharmacokinetics, pp 235–254. *In* Zakim D, Boyer TD (eds), Hepatology: a textbook of liver disease. WB Saunders, Philadelphia, PA.

3. Bishop L, Strandberg JD, Adams RJ, et al. 1979. Chronic active hepatitis in dogs associated with leptospires. *Am J Vet Res* 40:839–844.
4. Branum GD, Tyson GS, Branum MA, et al. 1990. Hepatic abscess: changes in etiology, diagnosis, and management. *Ann Surg* 212:655–662.
5. Burk RL, Johnson GF. 1980. Emphysematous cholecystitis in the nondiabetic dog: three case histories. *Vet Radiol* 21:242–245.
6. Cain JL, Labat JA, Cohn I. 1967. Bile peritonitis in germ-free dogs. *Gastroenterology* 53:600–603.
7. Cardoso V, Pimenta A, da Fonseca JC, et al. 1982. The effect of cholestasis on hepatic clearance of bacteria. *World J Surg* 6:330–334.
8. Center SA. 1990. Hepatobiliary infections, pp 146–183. *In* Greene CE (ed), Infectious diseases of the dog and cat. WB Saunders, Philadelphia, PA.
9. Center SA. 1996. Diseases of the gallbladder and biliary tree, pp 860–888. *In* Guilford G, Center SA, Strombeck D, et al. (eds), Strombeck's small animal gastroenterology, ed 3. WB Saunders, Philadelphia, PA.
10. Center SA, Rowland PH. 1994. Cholangitis/cholangiohepatitis complex in the cat, pp 766–771. *In* Proceedings of the 12th ACVIM Forum, San Francisco, CA.
11. Chapman BL, Hendrick MJ, Washabau RJ. 1993. Granulomatous hepatitis in dogs. Nine cases (1987–1990). *J Am Vet Med Assoc* 203:680–684.
11a. Chuang JH, Chen WJ, Lo SK, et al. 1997. Adverse metabolic and microbiologic effects of tube feeding in experimental canine obstructive jaundice. *J Parenter Enteral Nutr* 21:36–40.
12. Cobb LM, McKay KA. 1962. A bacteriological study of the liver of the normal dog. *J Comp Pathol* 72:92–96.
13. Dineen P. 1978. The importance of the route of infection in experimental biliary tract obstruction. *Surg Gynecol Obstet* 119:1001–1008.
14. Dirix LY, Polson RJ, Richardson A, et al. 1989. Primary sepsis presenting as fulminant hepatic failure. *QJ Med* 73:1037–1043.
15. Dow SW, Jones RL. 1987. Anaerobic infections: part II. Diagnosis and treatment. *Compend Cont Educ Pract Vet* 9:827–839.
16. Farrar ET, Washabau RJ, Saunders HM. 1996. Hepatic abscesses in dogs: 14 cases (1982–1994). *J Am Vet Med Assoc* 208:243–247.
17. Filkins JP, Cornell RP. 1974. Depression of hepatic gluconeogenesis and the hypoglycemia of endotoxic shock. *Am J Physiol* 227:778.
18. Forrester SD, Rogers KS, Relford RL. 1992. Cholangiohepatitis in a dog. *J Am Vet Med Assoc* 200:1704–1706.
19. Gagne JM, Weiss DJ, Armstrong PJ. 1996. Histopathologic evaluation of feline inflammatory liver disease. *Vet Pathol* 33:521–526.
20. Gocke DJ, Morris TQ, Bradley SE. 1970. Chronic hepatitis in the dog. The role of immune factors. *J Am Vet Med Assoc* 156:1700–1705.
21. Gonciarz A, Trusz-Gluza M, Kusmierski S, et al. 1974. Leukocytic proteases in gallbladder pathology. Experimental acute cholecystitis in dogs. *Digestion* 10:65–72.
22. Griffiths J, Groves AC, Leung FY. 1973. Hypertriglyceridemia and hypoglycemia in gram-negative sepsis in the dog. *Surg Gynecol Obstet* 136:897.
23. Grooters AM, Sherding RG, Biller S, et al. 1994. Hepatic abscesses associated with diabetes mellitus in two dogs. *J Vet Intern Med* 8:203–206.
24. Groves AC, Woolf LI, O'Regan PJ, et al. 1974. Impaired gluconeogenesis in dogs with *E. coli* bacteremia. *Surgery* 76:533.
25. Hargis AM, Thomassen RW. 1980. Hepatic abscesses in Beagle puppies. *Lab Anim Sci* 30:689–693.
25a. Howe LM, Boothe DM, Boothe HW. 1997. Endotoxemia associated with experimentally induced multile portosystemic shunts in dogs. *Am J Vet Res* 58:83–88.
26. Ito K, Ito S, Naito A, et al. 1988. Ultrasonographic manifestations of liver abscesses: an experimental study. *Hiroshima J Med Sci* 37:63–69.
27. Jackson MW, Panciera DL, Hartmann F. 1994. Administration of vancomycin for treatment of ascending bacterial cholangiohepatitis in a cat. *J Am Vet Med Assoc* 204:602–605.
28. Kaufman AC. 1994. Infectious causes of feline hepatobiliary disease. *Vet Med* 89:869–873.
29. Kelly DA, Summerfield JA. 1987. Hemostasis in liver disease. *Semin Liver Dis* 7:182–191.
30. Kirpensteijn J, Fingland RB, Ulrich T, et al. 1993. Cholelithiasis in dogs: 29 cases. *J Am Vet Med Assoc* 202:1137–1142.
31. Klatchko BA, Schwartz SI. 1989. Diagnostic and therapeutic approaches to pyogenic abscess of the liver. *Surg Gynecol Obstet* 168:332–336.
32. Krishnamurthy S, Krishnamurthy GT. 1989. Technetium-99m-iminodiacetic acid organic anions: review of biokinetics and clinical application in hepatology. *Hepatology* 9:139–153.
33. Lord PF, Carb A, Halliwell WH, et al. 1982. Emphysematous hepatic abscess associated with trauma, necrotic nodular hyperplasia and adenoma in a dog: a case history report. *Vet Radiol* 23:46–49.
34. Lord PF, Wilkins RJ. 1972. Emphysema of the gallbladder in a diabetic dog. *J Am Vet Radio Soc* 13:49–52.
35. Lykkegaard NM, Asnaes S, Justesen T. 1976. Susceptibility of the liver and biliary tract to anaerobic infection in extrahepatic biliary tract obstruction: III. Possible synergistic effect between anaerobic and aerobic bacteria. *Scand J Gastroenterol* 11:263–272.
36. McDonald MI, Corey GR, Gallis HA, et al. 1984. Single and multiple pyogenic liver abscesses. Natural history, diagnosis and treatment with percutaneous drainage. *Medicine* 63:291–302.
37. Miller DJ, Keeton GR, Webber BL, et al. 1976. Jaundice in severe bacterial infection. *Gastroenterology* 71:94–97.
38. Niehaus GD, Schumacker PR, Saba TM. 1980. Reticuloendothelial clearance of blood-borne particulates. *Ann Surg* 191:479–487.
39. Nolan JP. 1978. Bacteria and the liver. *N Engl J Med* 299:1069–1070.
40. Nora PF, Bransfield JJ, Laufman H. 1969. Hyperbaria in experimental bile peritonitis. *Arch Surg* 98:235–238.
41. Nyland TG, Gillett NA. 1982. Sonographic evaluation of experimental bile duct ligation in the dog. *Vet Radiol* 13:252–260.
42. Sanford JP, Gilbert DN, Gerberding JL, et al. 1995. The Sanford guide to antimicrobial therapy. Antimicrobial Therapy, Dallas, TX.
43. Scott AJ, Khan GA. 1967. Origin of bacteria in bile duct bile. *Lancet* 2:790–792.
44. Stephenson S, Nagel C. 1963. Acute cholecystitis. An experimental study. *Ann Surg* 157:687–694.
45. Styrt B, Gorbach SL. 1989. Recent developments in the understanding of the pathogenesis and treatment of anaerobic infections: part I. *N Engl J Med* 321: 240–246.
45a. Styrt B, Gorbach SL. 1989. Recent developments in the understanding of the pathogenesis and treatment of anaerobic infections: part II. *N Engl J Med* 321:298–302.
45b. Swalec-Tobias KM, Besser TE. 1997. Evaluation of leukocytosis, bacteremia, and portal vein partial oxygen tension in clinically normal dogs and dogs with portosystemic shunts. *J Am Vet Med Assoc* 211:715–718.
46. Taboada J, Meyer DJ. 1989. Cholestasis associated with extrahepatic biliary bacterial infection in five dogs. *J Vet Intern Med* 3:216–221.
47. Zeman RK, Raylor KJW, Rosenfield AT, et al. 1981. Acute experimental biliary obstruction in the dog: sonographic findings and clinical implications. *Am J Radiol* 136:965–967.

Chapter 91

Genitourinary Infections

Jeanne A. Barsanti

Bacterial infections of the urogenital system are among the most frequently encountered infections in small animal practice. Urinary tract and genital infections can occur separately or concomitantly. Infections range in severity from nonsymptomatic to life threatening. *Escherichia coli* is the most common agent associated with these infections. Infections with other types of organisms, especially fungi, are found but are much rarer than those with bacteria.

NORMAL FLORA

The vagina, vestibule, prepuce, and distal urethra have a normal microflora. The clinical importance of this microflora is twofold: first, it must be considered when the results of cultures of urine, semen, and preputial and vaginal discharges are interpreted; second, the normal microflora is thought to be an important factor in host defense against pathogenic organisms.

Bacteria are not normally found in the upper urinary tract, bladder, proximal urethra, or prostate gland. Bacteria are not normally found in the uterus, except during proestrus and estrus.[23, 105]

Dogs

In healthy male dogs, commensal organisms cultured from the distal urethra and prepuce include both gram-positive and gram-negative organisms (Tables 91–1 and 91–2).[8] Mycoplasmas are found in the distal urethra and the prepuce and have also been isolated from the canine prostate (see Chapter 32). When sampling the prepuce, usually more than one organism is recovered; however, only a single organism is obtained in about 20% of preputial and semen samples.[17] The prostatic fraction of a cleanly collected ejaculate from healthy, fertile stud dogs will usually be sterile (70% of samples).[17]

The normal flora of the vagina of the bitch includes the same types of bacteria (Table 91–3).[8, 16] Although the same types of organisms are found throughout the vagina, the nearer they are to the cervix, the lower the number of organisms.[8] Two or more bacterial species are usually recovered from vaginal cultures; however, 18% of vaginal cultures from healthy bitches contain only one organism, and repeated cultures from most dogs will yield a pure culture on at least one occasion.[16] Mycoplasmas can also be isolated from the vagina of healthy bitches.[8, 16] Changes in the microflora occur with stages of the estrous cycle, but the change is mainly in the frequency of organism isolation rather than the type of organism.[16] Few changes are associated with neutering.[8] *Staphylococcus* has been isolated more frequently from prepuberal and postpartum bitches than from postestrual bitches.[8, 16] The same organisms are found in the uterus during proestrus and estrus as are found in the vagina, with the exception that mycoplasmas were not found in the uterus.[105]

Treatment with either ampicillin or trimethoprim-sulfamethoxazole altered the normal microflora of the vagina in healthy bitches.[95] The normal microflora was suppressed in only two of five ampicillin-treated dogs. In three ampicillin-treated dogs and in all dogs treated with trimethoprim-sulfamethoxazole, bacteria sensitive to the antimicrobial tended to be eradicated, whereas resistant bacteria remained or appeared. Thus, the use of these antimicrobial agents to "sterilize" the vagina before mating is irrational and ineffective. Commensal bacteria are sometimes transferred between dog and bitch during mating.[16, 17] This transfer does not affect the fertility of either the male or the female.

Table 91–1. Bacteria Isolated From the Distal Urethra of Clinically Healthy Male Dogs[8]

Staphylococcus intermedius	*Klebsiella* spp.
Staphylococcus epidermidis	*Streptococcus canis*
Corynebacterium spp.	*Streptococcus viridans*
Escherichia coli	*Mycoplasma* spp.
Flavobacterium spp.	*Ureaplasma* spp.
Haemophilus spp.	

Table 91–2. Bacteria Isolated From the Prepuce of Clinically Healthy Male Dogs[8, 17]

Staphylococcus intermedius	*Proteus* spp.
Staphylococcus epidermidis	*Pasturella* spp.
Corynebacterium spp.	Bacillus spp.
Escherichia coli	*Streptococcus* spp.
Flavobacterium spp.	*Streptococcus equisimilis*
Haemophilus spp.	*Streptococcus canis*
Klebsiella spp.	*Streptococcus viridans*
Moraxella spp.	*Streptococcus faecalis* (*Enterococcus* spp.)
Acinetobacter spp.	*Pseudomonas* spp.
Mycoplasma spp.	
Ureaplasma spp.	

Table 91–3. Bacteria Isolated From the Vagina of Clinically Healthy Bitches[8, 16, 95]

Staphylococcus intermedius	*Moraxella* spp.
Staphylococcus epidermidis	*Micrococcus* spp.
Streptococcus viridans	*Neisseria* spp.
Streptococcus canis	*Bacteroides* spp.
Streptococcus faecalis (*Enterococcus* spp.)	*Bacillus* spp.
Streptococcus zooepidemicus	*Enterobacter* spp.
Streptococcus spp.	*Klebsiella* spp.
Escherichia coli	*Flavobacterium* spp.
Pasteurella spp.	*Citrobacter* spp.
Proteus spp.	*Mycoplasma* spp.
Haemophilus spp.	*Ureaplasma* spp.
Acinetobacter spp.	*Corynebacterium* spp.
	Pseudomonas spp.

Cats

Bacteria isolated from voided or catheterized urine samples from female and male cats without bacteria in bladder urine were, in decreasing order of frequency, *E. coli*, *Staphylococcus*, *Streptococcus*, *Corynebacterium*, *Pasteurella*, and *Flavobacterium*.[8]

Similar organisms were isolated from the vagina of healthy female cats; *E. coli*, *Staphylococcus* spp., and *Streptococcus* were the most common.[23] Relative numbers of vaginal organisms were greater in young cats (<1 year), in cats in estrus, and in pregnant cats.[23] Bacteria were also found in 2 of 29 uterine cultures, both from cats in estrus.[23]

Urinary Tract Infections

ETIOLOGY

Urinary tract infection (UTI) refers to microbial colonization of the urine or of any urinary tract organ, except the distal urethra, which has a normal bacterial flora. Infection of the urinary tract may affect more than one organ or may be localized to the upper tract (kidney and adjacent ureter; bacterial pyelonephritis) or to the lower tract (bladder and adjacent urethra; bacterial cystitis; bacterial urethrocystitis). Infections of the lower urinary tract in intact male dogs are considered to concomitantly affect the prostate gland (bacterial prostatitis). Infection of one part of the urinary tract increases the likelihood that the rest of the tract will become infected.[71, 72] It has been estimated that 14% of all dogs develop a UTI during their lifetime.[8] Infection rate in 237 dogs submitted for necropsy was 6% in males and 27% in females, most of which were reproductively intact. Infection rates were highest in those younger than 2 years and in those older than 6 years.[8]

Each infection is usually caused by a single bacterial species, except in complicated infections secondary to anatomic or functional abnormalities of the urinary tract. The most common gram-negative organisms are *E. coli*, *Proteus*, *Klebsiella*, *Pseudomonas*, and *Enterobacter*. Gram-positive organisms (*Staphylococcus*, *Streptococcus*, *Enterococcus*) account for approximately 25% of naturally occurring UTIs.[8] Infection with *Staphylococcus* or *Proteus* is often associated with struvite calculi because of alkalinization of the urine by the organisms' metabolism of urea. Although mycoplasmas have been reported as causes of UTI in dogs, their significance remains obscure because most of the reported cases were complicated by multiple disease processes (see Chapter 32).[8]

Bacterial UTIs are much less common in cats than in dogs. Numerous studies have shown that young adult cats having signs of lower urinary tract problems (dysuria with hematuria) rarely have bacterial UTIs.[8, 57] Bacterial UTIs may develop secondary to urinary catheterization or to urinary tract surgery, such as perineal urethrostomy, in cats with urethral obstruction.[7, 27, 38] When bacterial infection occurs in cats, the organisms most frequently involved are the same as those in dogs, except *Pasteurella* organisms are more commonly reported in cats.[8] Viruses and mycoplasmas have been considered as potential causes of lower urinary tract signs in cats. Investigators have been unable to find evidence of viral infections in clinical cases and experimental viral infections have not induced clinical signs in cats.[54–56] *Mycoplasma felis* and *M. gateae* could not survive in osmotic conditions present in normal feline urine, although a *Ureaplasma* sp. could.[19] However, ureaplasmas were not isolated from any cats with signs of lower urinary tract diseases.[57]

Fungal UTI is uncommon, but may be found secondary to abnormalities in host defenses (see Chapter 66). Antibiotics in animals with urinary obstruction, urinary tract foreign bodies (including catheters), hyperadrenocorticism, and diabetes mellitus have been factors in the development of fungal UTI in cats and dogs.[18, 34, 36, 112]

PATHOGENESIS

UTIs are usually caused by bacterial organisms that are constituents of the microflora of the intestinal or lower urogenital tracts. Dogs with UTI associated with *E. coli* or *Proteus mirabilis* were likely to carry the same organism in their intestinal tracts and prepuce or vagina.[35, 63] The usual method of infection of the bladder is by organisms ascending the urethra.[8] Pyelonephritis is believed to be most commonly caused by ascending infection from bladder urine. The renal cortex is much more resistant to infection than the renal medulla, decreasing the likelihood of hematogenous infection.[65]

Development of UTI indicates an alteration in the host and bacterial flora inter-relationship.[76] To accomplish infection, bacteria must attach to and colonize the mucosa of the urethral orifice and transport themselves up the urethra, adhering to the uroepithelium. Both bacterial virulence properties and host defense mechanisms are important in determining whether infection occurs as well as what part of the urinary tract is affected (Table 91–4).

Bacteria adhere poorly to normal bladder epithelium owing to the presence of a glycosaminoglycan coating.[76] This coating, which can be replaced within 24 hours if injured, is extremely hydrophilic, so that a layer of water forms at the surface. This aqueous layer provides a barrier between the transitional epithelium and the urine, explaining in part why bladder epithelium can tolerate constant exposure to a substance as irritating as urine. Infection is more likely to occur if this surface coating is damaged as by uroliths, neoplastic transformations, or exposures to chemical irritants such as cytoxan.

Important host factors in resistance to infection are normal, frequent emptying of the urinary bladder and normal urinary tract anatomy. Any condition that impairs normal micturition or obstructs urine flow will predispose the animal to infection. Treatment of UTI with antibiotics in animals with abnormal micturition can predispose them to highly antibiotic-resistant infections, especially in a hospital environment, because susceptible organisms are killed and resistant organisms are selected.[30] Lower urinary tract obstruction with secondary vesicoureteral reflux of infected urine is a contribut-

Table 91–4. Major Host Defenses Against Urinary Tract Infection[78]

Normal micturition	Antimicrobial properties of urine
Normal anatomy	Hyperosmolality-concentration
Intact mucosal defense	Tamm-Horsfall mucoprotein
Surface glycosaminoglycans	Systemic immunocompetence
Cell exfoliation	
Normal microflora	
Local antibody production	
Epithelial cell antimicrobial properties	

From Osborne CA, Finco DR (eds): Canine and Feline Nephrology and Urology. Williams & Wilkins, 1995, with permission.

ing factor to the development of pyelonephritis.[89] Approximately 17% of dogs with ectopic ureters were found to have pyelonephritis.[40]

Virulence properties of organisms infecting the urinary tract, particularly *E. coli*, are also important in the development of UTI. These properties include resistance to the bactericidal properties of serum, ability to produce hemolysin, and ability to attach to urinary tract epithelium.[76] Fimbriae on *E. coli* and *P. mirabilis* are important in adherence to canine uroepithelial cells.[14, 35, 92] *E. coli* isolated with canine UTI cluster within certain serotypes.[92] Differences in virulence properties have been found among strains of *E. coli*, causing pyelonephritis, acute cystitis, or nonsymptomatic bacteriuria in people.[8] In comparison with human urinary isolates, canine *E. coli* was more likely to be antibiotic resistant and to have a higher R-plasmid transmissibility rate.[8]

One iatrogenic cause for UTI is urinary tract catheterization. Even a single catheterization can result in UTI in female dogs.[76] Risk of infection is greater if the catheter is left in place (indwelling).[8, 62, 76] Bacteria can readily ascend either around or through the catheter. Closed, sterile systems can prevent bacterial access within the catheter lumen, which is the most rapid route of entry, but no method to date has been effective to prevent access up the extraluminal side of the catheter.[73, 87, 88] Consequences of bacteriuria arising from indwelling catheterizations include pyelonephritis, bacteremia, prostatitis, and epididymitis (see also Nosocomial Urinary Tract Infections, Chapter 94). Because of the risk of iatrogenic infection, an indwelling urinary catheter should be placed only when needed: after relief of urethral obstruction, when rapid reobstruction would compromise survival; in the preoperative and postoperative management of lower urinary tract trauma; in neurologic bladder dysfunction; and in monitoring urine output in possible oliguric renal failure.

CLINICAL FINDINGS

Nonsymptomatic Bacteriuria

UTIs in dogs and cats are often nonsymptomatic.[61] Because of the lack of historical and physical signs, such infections are difficult to localize to the upper or lower urinary tract. In one study, 6 of 12 clinically nonsymptomatic female dogs with UTI had infection localized to one or both kidneys whereas 6 had bladder infections.[8] Despite the absence of clinical signs, 3 of the dogs with renal infection and 3 of the dogs with bladder infection had mild to moderate inflammation in the infected organ. Animals with few historical signs have had severe tissue injury, such as renal or prostatic abscess formation. Duration of nonsymptomatic infection or other host factors may be important in determining the degree of tissue injury. This situation emphasizes the importance of routine analysis of cystocentesis-collected urine in health screening.

Pyelonephritis

In acute bacterial pyelonephritis, dogs may be systemically ill with fever, depression, anorexia, renal pain, and leukocytosis. GI signs, particularly vomiting, may be seen. In humans, GI signs have been attributed to a secondary paralytic ileus.[98] All signs are inconsistent and, in experimentally induced disease, transient (<5 days).[8, 71, 72]

Chronic pyelonephritis may be nonsymptomatic or associated with polyuria and secondary polydipsia. Polyuria can occur before the onset of renal lesions and can resolve with eradication of infection. With chronic, bilateral pyelonephritis, signs of renal failure may eventually occur, especially if infection is associated with other structural abnormalities such as urolithiasis. Diseases reported to occur secondarily to pyelonephritis include diskospondylitis[104] and distal renal tubular acidosis.[103]

Cystitis and Urethritis

The bladder and proximal urethra are so closely associated that inflammation in one is thought to affect the other. Infection of the distal urethra unassociated with infection in the rest of the lower urinary tract is uncommon unless an anatomic abnormality exists.

Urethrocystitis is characterized by dysuria (straining) and pollakiuria (frequent voiding of urine). The urine is often cloudy and hemorrhagic and may have a foul odor. Gross hematuria at the end of urination suggests that the blood is from the bladder. Gross hematuria at the beginning of urination or a urethral discharge may be associated with urethral or prostatic disease. Prostatic disease is a more common cause of a urethral discharge independent of urination than is urethral disease in dogs. Signs of systemic illness, such as fever and leukocytosis, are not associated with bacterial urethrocystitis. The bladder may be painful on abdominal palpation, and with chronic infection the wall becomes thickened.

DIAGNOSIS

Examination of bladder urine is the method by which UTI is confirmed. Samples of urine for urinalysis and culture should be collected before initiation of antimicrobial therapy.

Table 91–5. Terms Used to Categorize Urinary Tract Infection

BY LOCATION

Pyelonephritis: kidney
Cystitis: bladder
Urethritis: urethra
Prostatitis: prostate

BY RESPONSE TO THERAPY

Persistent: Bacteriuria with the same organism continues during therapy with appropriate antimicrobial agent.
Relapsing: Infection with the same microorganism recurs within several weeks of cessation of antimicrobial therapy.
Reinfection: Infection with initial microorganism responds to therapy, but infection by a different organism occurs weeks to months after cessation of that therapy.
Superinfection: Infection with new organisms develops during therapy for the initial infecting organism; usually associated with an indwelling catheter, severe anatomic abnormalities, or surgical diversion techniques.

BY COMPLEXITY

Simple-uncomplicated: No underlying structural or functional abnormality is suspected or found.
Complicated: Infection associated with structural or functional abnormalities within the urinary tract or with impaired immunocompetence:
- Urinary obstruction
- Incomplete bladder emptying
- Congenital abnormalities (urachal diverticula, ectopic ureters)
- Surgical diversion procedures
- Urolithiasis
- Indwelling urinary catheters
- Neoplasia
- Cytotoxic drugs (cyclophosphamide)
- Hyperadrenocorticism or glucocorticoid therapy
- Diabetes mellitus
- Renal failure

Table 91–6. Guidelines to Diagnostic Tests and Therapy Indicated in Urinary Tract Infection

CLINICAL CLASSIFICATION	DIAGNOSTIC TESTS	THERAPY
Simple, cystitis or nonsymptomatic, initial episode	Urinalysis, urine culture	Antimicrobial agent for 10 days in cats and female or neutered male dogs; 21 days for intact male dogs
Relapsing or persistent	Urinalysis, urine culture, radiography, ultrasonography, prostatic fluid examination in intact males	Antimicrobial agent for 6 weeks; treatment of any underlying disease process
Reinfection	Urinalysis, urine culture	As for simple; consider prophylactic therapy if frequent reinfections
Suspect pyelonephritis	Urinalysis, urine culture, CBC, BUN, serum creatinine, radiography, excretory urography, nephrosonography	Antimicrobial agent for 4 weeks; longer if chronic
Suspect prostatitis	Urinalysis, urine culture, CBC, radiography, prostatic ultrasonography, prostatic fluid examination	Antimicrobial agent for 4 weeks; longer if chronic

CBC = complete blood cell count; BUN = blood (serum) urea nitrogen.

If antimicrobial therapy was initiated only on the basis of clinical signs and the diagnosis of UTI is in doubt, it should be discontinued for 3 to 5 days before urine culture to minimize inhibition of bacterial growth.[75]

The presence of bacteria in urine collected from the bladder confirms UTI, but does not localize the infection. The bacteria could be originating from the kidneys, bladder, and/or prostate gland. Diagnostic tests in addition to history and physical examination, which help localize infection to an anatomic site in the urinary tract, include radiography, ultrasonography, and prostatic fluid evaluation. Tests such as antibody coating of bacteria in urine and bladder washout techniques are unreliable.[75]

Because of the difficulty in localizing a UTI to an anatomic site in the urinary tract, UTIs are also subdivided on the basis of response to initial antimicrobial therapy (Table 91–5). The extensiveness of the diagnostic evaluation required on each case varies with response to initial antimicrobial therapy as well as severity of illness (Table 91–6).

Urine Collection

Because the distal urethra, vagina, and prepuce have a normal bacterial flora, the method of urine collection is important for accurate assessment of the results of urinalysis and urine culture. Whenever a urine sample is collected, the method of collection should be recorded.

Cystocentesis. Cystocentesis is the preferred method of urine collection for culture, because lower genitourinary tract contamination is avoided. Any bacteria present in such samples are indicative of infection unless inadvertent bowel penetration or skin contamination occurs. Because of the possibility of inadvertent contamination, diagnosis is more certain if urine is cultured quantitatively, with evaluation of the number of organisms found, as well as qualitatively, to identify the infecting species. For a laboratory to do a quantitative culture, a small volume of urine must be submitted. Sterile swabs dipped in urine are not suitable.

Before cystocentesis is performed, a small area of skin around the site of needle insertion should be clipped free of hair and cleansed. The bladder should be palpated and immobilized against the pelvis with one hand. A 21-gauge or smaller needle is inserted into the bladder at an oblique angle, and urine is withdrawn into a syringe. The palpating hand releases pressure on the bladder, and negative pressure on the syringe is discontinued. The needle is withdrawn.

Cystocentesis is performed with the animal in the position in which it seems most comfortable (standing, lying down, or suspended by the front or rear limbs) (Figs. 91–1 to 91–3). The only serious potential complication is leakage of urine from the puncture hole in the bladder. This is rare, unless the bladder is distended secondary to inability to voluntarily void urine. In animals with distended bladders that are unable to urinate, their bladders should be emptied as soon as possible after cystocentesis. Cystocentesis can result in a mild degree of hematuria being detected on urinalysis.

Catheterization. If the bladder is not palpable or if cystocentesis fails, urine should be collected for culture in male dogs by catheterization. Catheterization techniques should always be performed as aseptically and gently as possible. The prepuce should be retracted and the penis cleansed and dried. A sterile, disposable catheter should be used. The catheter should be passed employing only sterile instruments

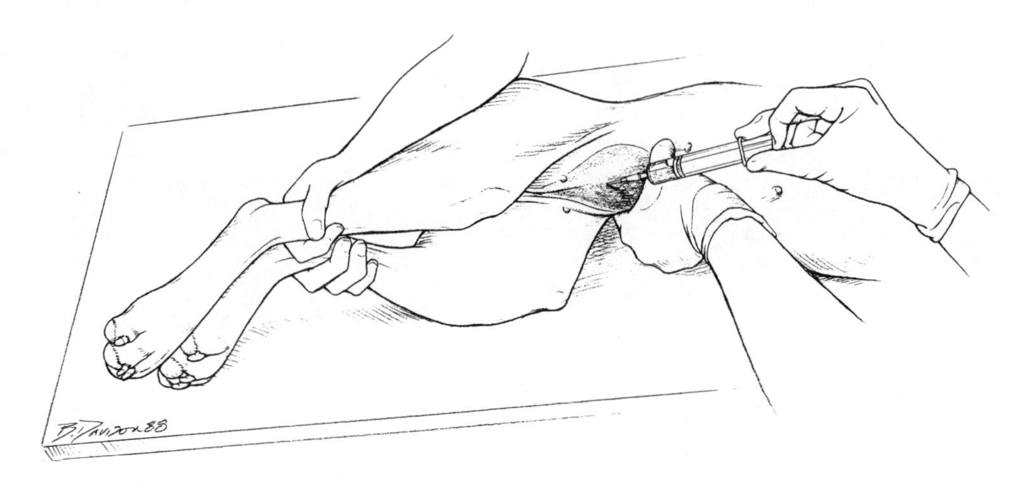

Figure 91–1. Cystocentesis with the animal in lateral recumbency. The palpating hand is positioned so that the bladder is pushed back toward the pelvis to immobilize it. (From Stone EA, Barsanti JA: Urologic Surgery of the Dog and Cat. Lea & Febiger, 1992, with permission.)

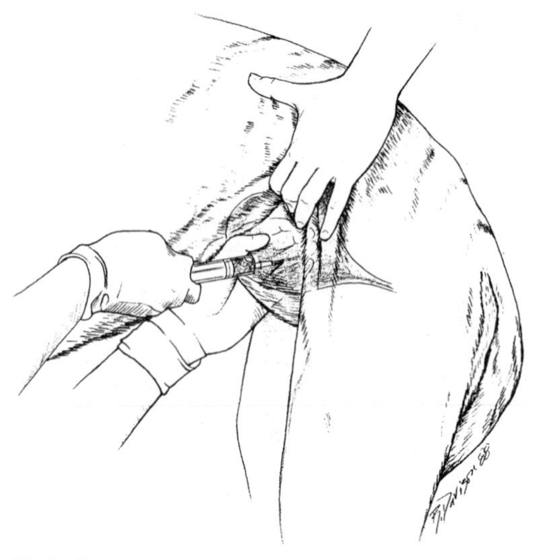

Figure 91–2. Cystocentesis with the animal standing. The palpating hand holds the bladder back against the pelvic brim. (From Stone EA, Barsanti JA: Urologic Surgery of the Dog and Cat. Lea & Febiger, 1992, with permission.)

or gloves. Catheterization done in this way results in introducing bacteria into urine only in low (<10^3/ml) numbers.[8]

In contrast, catheterization of female dogs, even during as aseptic a technique as possible, introduces bacteria approximately 50% of the time. Occasionally, there are large (10^5/ml) numbers of organisms.[8] Experimentally, introduction of large numbers of bacteria into the bladders of normal female dogs by catheterization does not usually result in persistent UTI unless a complicating factor, such as a bladder foreign body, is present.[8] However, because of the difficulty in distinguishing infection from contamination and because of the small risk of inducing UTI, catheterization is not an adequate substitute for cystocentesis in female dogs. Diuretics such as furosemide (1 mg/kg, SC) to distend the bladder for cystocentesis are preferable to evaluate UTI, although the effect on specific gravity must be noted.

In normal cats, catheterized samples have fewer than 10^3 bacteria/ml in both males and females.[8] However, unsedated cats may be difficult to catheterize atraumatically. As in female dogs, diuretics may be needed to distend the bladder so that cystocentesis can be accomplished.

Samples may be obtained through an indwelling urinary catheter for quantitative culture. In this situation even low numbers of bacteria suggest infection, because the numbers increase if the catheter is left in place.[8]

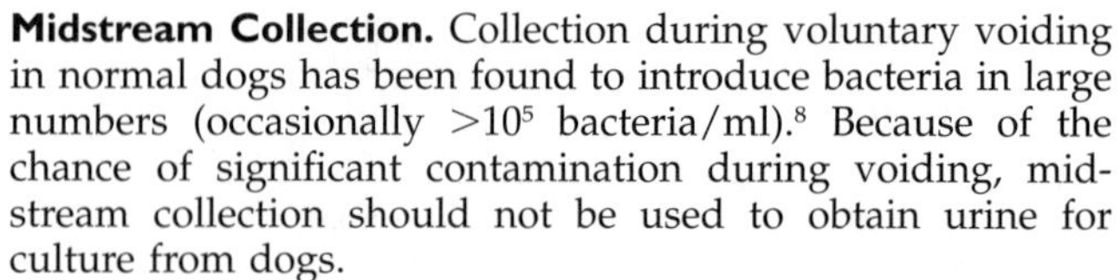

Midstream Collection. Collection during voluntary voiding in normal dogs has been found to introduce bacteria in large numbers (occasionally >10^5 bacteria/ml).[8] Because of the chance of significant contamination during voiding, midstream collection should not be used to obtain urine for culture from dogs.

Midstream-collected urine occasionally must be utilized for culture in severely dysuric cats. The bladder may not fill sufficiently for successful cystocentesis, even after administration of diuretics. In these cases, urine should be expressed as cleanly as possible into a sterile container. The urine should be cultured quantitatively. A urinalysis should also be performed so that the sediment findings can be correlated with the culture results.

Handling of Urine Samples

Once urine is collected for culture, it must be handled properly to prevent changes in bacterial numbers. Specimens should be refrigerated and cultured within 6 hours.[8] However, tubes with preservatives have been shown to maintain types and numbers of bacteria in urine for up to 72 hours with refrigeration.[8] Before culture, urine should not be incubated, kept at room temperature, or frozen.

If a veterinary practice cannot deliver urine samples to a laboratory in a timely manner, the practice can use calibrated loops to inoculate blood agar plates.[75] The plates are incubated at 37°C for 24 hours. If bacteria grow, either the plates or swab cultures from the plates can be sent to a commercial laboratory for species identification and antimicrobial susceptibility tests.

Interpretation of Urinalysis

To evaluate a dog or cat for infection, a complete urinalysis, *including sediment examination*, must be performed. Findings on a urine dipstick that may occur with infection are positive occult blood and protein, but these indicate only hemorrhage, which has many causes. Infection can also occur without hemorrhage and can be associated with a normal dipstick evaluation. Dipstick leukocyte assays and dipstick assays for bacteria are inaccurate in companion animals.[8]

Findings on a urine sediment examination that suggest UTI are pyuria, hematuria, and bacteriuria. Of these, the most specific is bacteriuria. False-positive bacteriuria on cystocentesis samples can only arise as a consequence of contamination or misinterpretation of brownian movement or amorphous debris. False-negative results are possible because

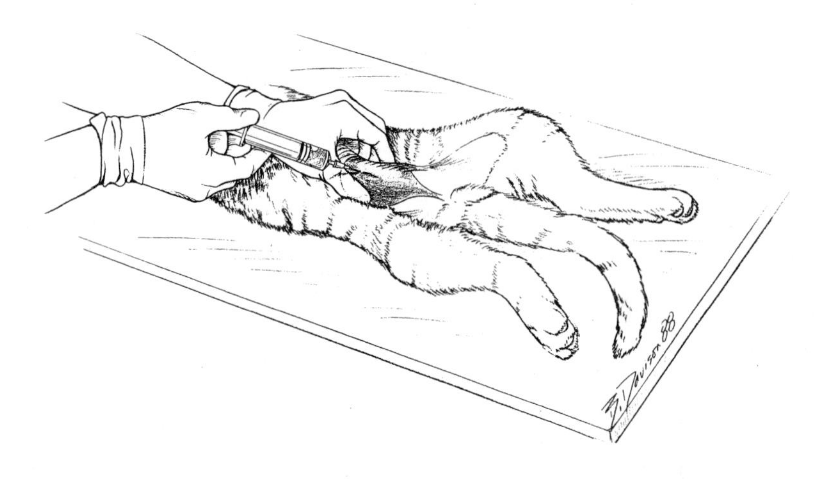

Figure 91–3. Cystocentesis with the animal in dorsal recumbency. The palpating hand is positioned to hold the bladder back against the pelvic brim. (From Stone EA, Barsanti JA: Urologic Surgery of the Dog and Cat. Lea & Febiger, 1992, with permission.)

Table 91–7. Criteria for Determining Infection in Urine Specimens Based Upon Method of Collection

METHOD	CONTAMINATION (bacteria/ml)	INFECTION
Midstream voided		
Culture	$< 10^5$	Cannot distinguish in dogs $> 10^5$ in cat[a]
Catheterization		
Culture[b]	$< 10^3$ in male dogs	$> 10^5$ in male dogs $> 10^3$ in cats
Cystocentesis		
Culture	< 1000 Multiple bacteria[c]	$> 10^3$

[a]Small numbers of clinically healthy cats had 10^5 bacterial/ml by this collection method.
[b]10^3 to 10^5 may indicate either contamination or infection.
[c]In the absence of cytologic correlation, may be inadvertent bowel contamination.

large numbers of organisms must be present in order to be consistently visualized. Correlation of Gram's-stained smears of canine urine with culture results was good, whereas that of unstained smears was poor.[8]

Pyuria is defined as greater than 3 WBCs/high power field (40× objective; hpf) on cystocentesis samples and greater than 8 WBCs/hpf on catheterized or voided urine samples.[75] Pyuria is often, but not always, present in association with bacteriuria. Pyuria without bacteriuria indicates inflammation, and a culture of urine is indicated to determine whether infection is the cause of the inflammation. Bacteria are more difficult to detect than WBCs. Infection with minimal tissue invasion may not induce pyuria, and the magnitude of the WBC response seems to vary markedly, even in the same animal.[61] Hypercortisolemia inhibits pyuria. In dogs treated with glucocorticoids or dogs with hyperadrenocorticism, urine culture is essential to evaluate for infection.

Interpretation of Urine Culture Results

Dogs and Cats. The definitive test for UTI in dogs and cats is isolation of bacteria from a properly collected cystocentesis sample (Table 91–7). Most UTIs (80%) involve a single bacterial species, present in high numbers (>100,000/ml).[61] Urine culture that results in isolation of multiple types of bacteria or low (<1000/ml) numbers must be assessed carefully. Artifactual contamination of urine with intestinal contents leads to the presence of multiple bacterial species. Contamination from the skin or in the laboratory leads to low numbers of organisms. Isolation of multiple types of bacteria may occur in UTIs, which are secondary to indwelling catheters or marked anatomic abnormalities.

Dogs. In male dogs, more than 10^5 bacteria/ml in a catheterized sample indicates infection (see Table 91–7). Fewer than 10^3 bacteria/ml suggests contamination. Intermediate (10^3–10^5/ml) numbers may indicate either contamination or infection. Other case information such as history, physical examination, urinalysis results, and degree of potential contamination during catheterization can help guide a decision as to whether infection exists when culture results are inconclusive. Midstream or expressed urine samples and catheterization of female dogs should not be used for culture because of the likelihood of contamination.

Cats. In samples of urine obtained by catheterization, bacterial counts greater than 10^3/ml are considered indicative of infection in both male and female cats (see Table 91–7).[8] If midstream samples must be utilized in a dysuric cat, greater than 10^5 bacteria/ml is suggestive of infection if contamination during collection was minimal. Even counts greater than 10^5 bacteria/ml would not confirm infection, because counts this high were found in a small number of urine specimens from cats with negative culture results by cystocentesis.[8] Urinalysis results should be correlated with culture results in making a final determination as to whether the bacteria are due to infection or contamination.

Bacterial Pyelonephritis

Bacterial pyelonephritis may be suspected on the basis of history and physical examination as reviewed previously or on the basis of the UTI being persistent or relapsing (see Table 91–5). The diagnosis of bacterial pyelonephritis is supported by laboratory tests, radiography, excretory urography, and nephrosonography. The diagnosis can be confirmed only by pyelocentesis or renal biopsy. Because treatment can be based on a presumptive diagnosis, definitive diagnosis is usually sought only if the case is difficult or unusual or if anesthesia or surgery is to be performed for another reason, such as to remove nephroliths.

Laboratory Findings. A CBC may show a neutrophilic leukocytosis with or without a left shift in acute or complicated chronic pyelonephritis, especially with renal abscess formation or ureteral or renal pelvic obstruction (see Table 91–5). An inflammatory leukogram may also indicate bacteremia secondary to acute pyelonephritis or complicated, chronic pyelonephritis. A normal CBC does not eliminate the possibility of pyelonephritis.

Abnormalities in renal function (abnormal creatinine clearance, inadequate urine concentrating ability in spite of demand, azotemia) in association with UTI suggest that the UTI may be of renal origin. However, further tests are indicated because the UTI may be a lower tract infection in an animal with decreased concentrating ability due to renal disease that is noninfectious in origin. The presence of hypoalbuminemia, greater than normal concentrations of liver enzymes, and hypoglycemia suggest secondary bacteremia.

On urinalysis, hematuria, pyuria, and bacteriuria are often noted but are not specific for pyelonephritis. Consistently low urine specific gravity readings should increase the suspicion of pyelonephritis. Concentrated urine (>1.035) does not rule out pyelonephritis because the infection may be unilateral. The degree of concentrating defect depends on how diffusely and severely the renal medulla is affected. The presence of leukocyte casts suggests renal infection; however, such casts are rarely seen.[76]

Survey Abdominal Radiography. An abnormality in renal size or contour may be seen with pyelonephritis. Normal renal size is determined by comparison with the second vertebral body (L2): canine kidneys are 2.5–3.5 × L2 and feline kidneys are 2.4–3.0 × L2.[32] Most textbooks state that acute pyelonephritis is associated with renomegaly; however, this has not been reported in experimentally induced infections in dogs. Renomegaly may be noted with renal abscess formation. With chronic pyelonephritis without abscess formation, renal size decreases and renal contour may become irregular.[8] These changes are nonspecific for pyelonephritis. Survey abdominal radiographs help to detect radiopaque nephroliths. The concurrent findings of UTI and nephroliths are suggestive of pyelonephritis.

Excretory Urography. Signs suggestive of pyelonephritis are decreased opacity of the vascular nephrogram, decreased

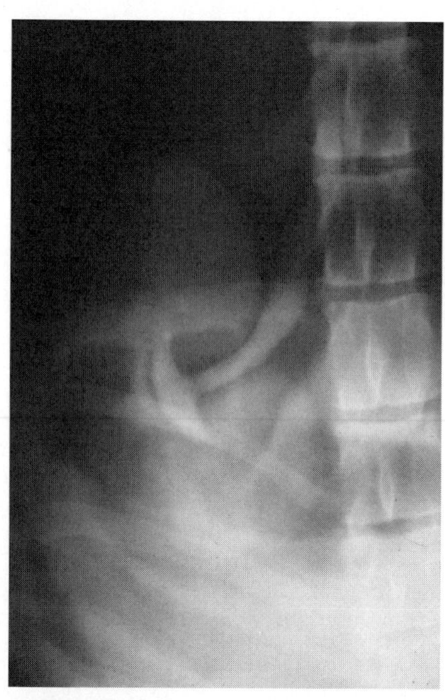

Figure 91–4. Excretory urogram showing dilation of the renal pelvis with lack of opacification (blunting) of the pelvic recesses and dilation of the proximal ureter. These signs are consistent with pyelonephritis.

opacity and blunting of the pelvic recesses, and renal pelvic and ureteral dilatation (Fig. 91–4).[8] The size of infected kidneys progressively decreases over weeks in experimental infections.[8] Absence of these findings does not rule out renal infections, especially in acute cases (<10 days duration).[8, 72]

Nephrosonography. The major sonographic findings in pyelonephritis are pelvic dilatation and proximal ureteral dilatation and a hyperechoic line within the renal pelvis or proximal ureter.[72] Other common findings are a generalized hyperechoic renal cortex, focal hyperechoic areas within the medulla, focal hyperechoic or hypoechoic areas in the renal cortex, and poor corticomedullary differentiation.[72] These abnormalities were found within 2 days of inducing infection.[71] Some of these findings, such as a hyperechoic renal cortex, are nonspecific and common with most types of renal disease as well as occasionally being normal. Others such as renal pelvic dilatation can be seen with other conditions such as hydronephrosis. The combination of such findings, however, in a case with UTI and appropriate clinical signs or relapsing infections are highly suggestive of pyelonephritis. As with excretory urography, a normal nephrosonogram does not rule out pyelonephritis.[72]

There are many advantages to ultrasonography to examine the kidneys: there is no ionizing radiation, no contrast agent is required, it is unaffected by renal dysfunction, and it is safe in animals with azotemia. However, performance and evaluation of ultrasound examination are very operator dependent, and the accuracy of the outcome is directly related to the skill of the examiner. The animal's body size and lack of cooperation may also limit the value of ultrasonography. It does not reliably detect small renal or ureteral calculi or determine the cause of hydronephrosis.[67] The renal pelvis is difficult to consistently visualize.[32]

Pyelocentesis. Percutaneous nephropyelocentesis allows collection of urine for culture directly from the renal pelvis.[8, 89] The renal pelvis is visualized by means of excretory urography and fluoroscopy and dilated by application of an abdominal compression band. A 20-gauge disposable arterial needle is then directed through the skin of the lateral flank into the dilated renal pelvis. A positive culture result confirms renal pelvic infection.

Renal Biopsy. Renal biopsy is rarely performed to confirm a diagnosis of pyelonephritis, because the lesions are often focal and medullary; thus, they may be missed on renal biopsy samples, which are only a small, cortical part of the kidney. If surgery is performed for another purpose, such as nephrolith removal, culture of urine from the renal pelvis and culture and histologic examination of renal tissue samples should be performed to confirm a diagnosis of bacterial pyelonephritis.

Bacterial Cystitis-Urethritis

The diagnosis of acute bacterial cystitis is usually based on history and clinical signs and on confirming UTI by results of urinalysis and urine culture. In cases of relapsing or persistent UTI, a complicated infection should be suspected (see Table 91–5). In these cases, survey radiography, contrast cystourethrography, and bladder ultrasonography may be indicated to detect uroliths and structural abnormalities. On cystography, mucosal irregularity and thickened bladder wall indicate cystitis (Fig. 91–5). These are better seen on double-contrast cystography than on positive-contrast studies.[64] Mild to moderate cystitis may be missed if the bladder is completely distended during cystography.[64] Long-standing chronic cystitis may result in the development of polyps (polypoid cystitis), which require biopsy for differentiation from neoplasia.

Biopsy of the bladder wall should be performed in difficult cases.[41] Biopsy specimens should be cultured for bacteria as well as processed for histologic evaluation. Gram's stain may be helpful in examining bladder tissue for bacteria.[41]

Emphysematous cystitis is particularly severe. It is usually diagnosed radiographically by finding air bubbles within a thickened bladder wall as well as within the bladder lumen, although it may be suspected by the sound of air being voided during urination or by the palpation of crepitus within the bladder on physical examination. Although diabetes mellitus may predispose an animal to emphysematous

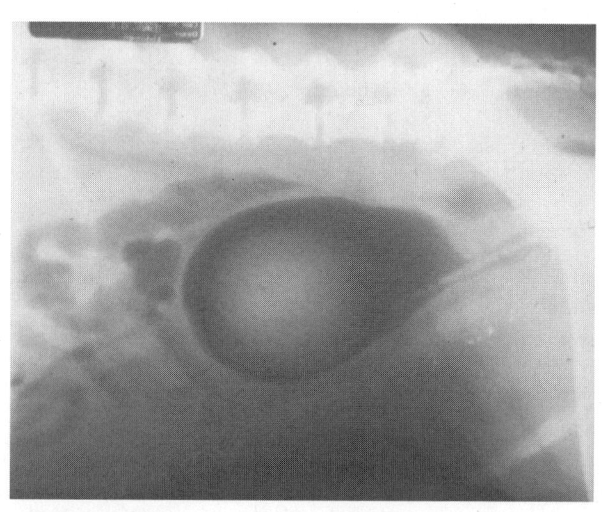

Figure 91–5. Double-contrast cystogram showing a thickened bladder wall.

Table 91–8. Mean Urine Concentrations of Antimicrobial Agents Used in Management of Canine Urinary Tract Infection[a, 61]

DRUG	DOSAGE (mg/kg)[b]	ROUTE	INTERVAL (HOURS)	MEAN URINE CONCENTRATION (μg/ml)
Ampicillin	22	PO	8	309
Amoxicillin	11	PO	8	201.5
Chloramphenicol	33	PO	8	124
Nitrofurantoin	4.4	PO	8	100
Trimethoprim-sulfonamide	13	PO	12	26/79[c]
Gentamicin	2	SC	8	107
Amikacin	5	SC	8	342
Cephalexin	8	PO	8	225
Enrofloxacin	2.5	PO	12	40
Tetracycline	18	PO	8	138

[a]Values were determined in hydrated dogs with normal renal function. To determine the efficacy of a drug, multiply the minimum inhibitory concentration of the bacteria isolated by 4. If the total is less than the mean urine concentration for that drug, the drug has a 90–95% chance to be efficacious.
[b]Dose per administration at specified interval. For duration, see Table 91–6. For further information on these drugs, see Drug Formulary, Appendix 8.
[c]Mean concentration of trimethoprim in urine is 26 and mean concentration of sulfonamide is 79.
Most of the data determined by and supplied courtesy of Dr. Gerald Ling, University of California, Davis, CA. Permission to reproduce these data granted by Dr. Ling.

cystitis, it also occurs in nondiabetics. Because of bacterial fermentation, the absence of glucosuria does not exclude a diagnosis of diabetes mellitus, which should be determined by measurement of the blood glucose.[84] In nondiabetics, urine proteins are suspected to be the substrate for gas formation.[84] Cases in nondiabetics are usually complicated,[27] and the usual infecting organism is *E. coli*.[27, 84, 110]

THERAPY

Urine Concentration of Antimicrobial Agents

The major difference between therapy for UTIs and for infections in other organ systems is that most antimicrobials are present in urine in high concentrations as a result of renal excretion (Table 91–8).[8] Because most antimicrobial disks contain serum concentrations, routine antimicrobial susceptibility results should be considered only as rough guidelines for treatment of UTIs. If the infecting organism is reported to be susceptible to a certain antimicrobial agent, that agent will probably be effective if it is excreted in active form by the kidney and if renal function is normal. Furthermore, an antimicrobial to which the organism is reported to be resistant may also give good results in vivo because of significantly higher urine than serum concentrations in animals which can concentrate the urine.

Another method of choosing an effective therapeutic agent for UTIs is to determine the minimum inhibitory concentration (MIC) of antimicrobials for the infective agent (see also Chapter 34). The MIC is defined as the least amount of an antimicrobial agent that causes complete inhibition of growth of the infecting bacteria under standardized conditions. This is most accurately measured by microdilution analysis with varying antimicrobial concentrations, but can be estimated from the diameter of the zone of inhibition of Kirby-Bauer plates.[2] Rather than absolute susceptibility or resistance, the concentration of antimicrobial that will inhibit the growth of the organism is reported. The MIC is then compared with the concentration reached by that antimicrobial in urine. If the mean urine concentration (see Table 91–8) exceeds the MIC by at least four times, the antimicrobial agent should be effective. In renal parenchymal and prostatic infections, special considerations apply to antimicrobial penetration, which is discussed under Bacterial Pyelonephritis and Prostatitis, respectively.

Antibiotic Choice

Determination of organism type and its in vitro antimicrobial susceptibility is the optimal way to proceed with therapy in UTI. One usually begins therapy pending culture results. By examining urine pH and whether the organisms in the urine are rods or cocci on urine sediment examination, one can make an educated guess as to the type of organism present and a reasonable first choice of antimicrobial agent (Table 91–9). With recurrent UTI, one should compare the findings on the current urinalysis with those on prior urinalyses and urine cultures to determine the most likely causative organism and its susceptibility, pending results.

On the basis of MIC determinations for common urinary tract pathogens, usually effective antimicrobials have been determined (Table 91–10). Ciprofloxacin may have greater antimicrobial activity than enrofloxacin against *Pseudomonas*.[29] UTIs caused by *Staphylococcus* seem to be increasingly antibiotic resistant, especially to ampicillin and penicillin.[74]

Nitrofurantoin has efficacy against gram-positive and gram-negative organisms, but administration is confined to females and neutered males because it does not penetrate the

Table 91–9. Guide to the Type of Organism Most Likely to be Causing an Initial Urinary Tract Infection[a] *and to Initial Antibiotic Choice*[b]

URINE pH	BACTERIAL CHARACTERISTICS	LIKELY ORGANISM	INITIAL ANTIBACTERIAL CHOICE
Acidic	Rods	*Escherichia coli*	Trimethoprim, enrofloxacin
	Cocci	*Enterococcus-Streptococcus*	Ampicillin[c]
Alkaline	Rods	*Proteus mirabilis*	Ampicillin
	Cocci	*Staphylococcus*	Cephalexin

[a]Based on urine pH and bacterial characteristics on urine sediment examination.
[b]This may need to be modified once the causative organism and its antibiotic susceptibility are determined by urine culture.
[c]Enterococci may often show antibacterial resistance.

Table 91–10. Guidelines to Antimicrobial Choice in Genitourinary Infections Based on Identification of the Causative Bacteria[a, 8, 29, 74, 77, 91]

ORGANISM	ANTIMICROBIALS RECOMMENDED
Escherichia coli	Trimethoprim-sulfonamide, amoxicillin–clavulanate, enrofloxacin, chloramphenicol
Staphylococcus	Amoxicillin–clavulanate, first-generation cephalosporin, chloramphenicol
Streptococcus-Enterococcus	Ampicillin, amoxicillin
Proteus	Ampicillin, amoxicillin
Pseudomonas[b]	Tetracycline, ciprofloxacin, enrofloxacin
Klebsiella[b]	First-generation cephalosporin, trimethoprim-sulfonamide, amoxicillin–clavulanate
Enterobacter	Trimethoprim-sulfonamide

[a] Highly antibiotic-resistant urinary tract infections can be a problem with any of these organisms, especially in animals that have received antimicrobial therapy. For this reason, this table is provided for general guidelines only. Identification of the organism and its susceptibility is important in each clinical case for appropriate antimicrobial selection. In highly resistant gram-negative infections, quinolones, third-generation cephalosporins, and extended-spectrum penicillins may be needed.

[b] *Pseudomonas* and *Klebsiella* infections are the most difficult to predict susceptibility. Although these organisms are usually susceptible to aminoglycosides, aminoglycosides are not usually used because of nephrotoxicity. Repeated urine evaluation during and after therapy is essential to determine treatment efficacy in infections with these organisms.

prostate gland. Nitrofurantoin should be given only as the macrocrystalline formulation to decrease adverse GI effects and to maximize efficacy.

Ceftiofur sodium has been approved for dogs with lower urinary tract infections.[21] Its efficacy is for gram-negative aerobic organisms except *Pseudomonas* and *Enterobacter.* It does not penetrate the prostate gland and thus would not be a good choice in intact males. Twice the recommended dose may be needed for some *E. coli* infections.[78] Ceftiofur is metabolized to desfuroylceftiofur, which is less potent than ceftiofur against staphylococci and *Proteus*.[29] Susceptibility tests with ceftiofur may overestimate efficacy against these organisms because of the differences in activity of the parent compound and its major metabolite.[29]

Although selection of an antimicrobial agent by organism identification and susceptibility test usually correlates with success of therapy in vivo, the correlation is not 100%. Various factors such as GI absorption, location of infection, renal function, polyuric state, and urine characteristics will influence antimicrobial urine concentrations. The only way to be certain that the chosen drug is effective is to re-examine the urine during and after therapy. Urine should be recultured, or the sediment should be examined cytologically after a few days of therapy. If the antibiotic eliminates bacteria from the urine within a few days, the drug's efficacy against that bacterial species is confirmed. However, a longer course of therapy is necessary to eliminate the organism from infected bladder, renal, or prostatic tissues.

Whenever any antimicrobial is dispensed, adverse reactions are possible. One client survey found the highest rate of adverse reactions in dogs to be with erythromycin (52%, most commonly vomiting); the lowest with amoxicillin (7.5%).[58] Even though there are reports of serious toxicity with trimethoprim-sulfadiazine, this drug had a relatively low percentage of adverse reactions (18%, most commonly anorexia, lethargy, and polyuria-polydipsia) despite being the most commonly prescribed drug in the survey.[58] An approximately 15% incidence of keratoconjunctivitis sicca (KCS) was found with trimethoprim-sulfadiazine; dogs weighing less than 12 kg were at greater risk.[10] Enrofloxacin should not be given to immature dogs, to dogs prone to seizures, or to uremic animals without dosage modification.[1, 77, 91] For additional specific information on antibacterials, see Chapter 34 and Drug Formulary, Appendix 8.

Therapy in Different Types of UTI

Optimal duration of therapy in different types of UTI in dogs and cats has not been determined by clinical studies. The duration of therapy will vary with anatomic location of the infection. It also varies as to whether the infection is complicated or not and whether it is an initial infection, a relapsing one, or a persistent one (see Tables 91–5 and 91–6). It is best to classify a UTI by as many of these characteristics as possible to determine the optimal therapeutic course. For example, an uncomplicated initial cystitis requires much less intensive diagnostic and therapeutic efforts than a complicated, relapsing pyelonephritis.

Nonsymptomatic Bacteriuria. A diagnostic effort should be made to determine whether an underlying cause of immunosuppression exists, such as glucocorticoid therapy or hyperadrenocorticism. Nonsymptomatic infections should be treated based on urine culture results (see Table 91–6). A urine culture should be repeated approximately 1 week after concluding therapy. If the infection remains, a diagnostic effort should be made to localize the tissue source (kidney, bladder, prostate) and any underlying disease (urolithiasis, neoplasia, congenital defect). Treatment should be reinstituted and urine cultured during therapy. If the chosen drug is effective during therapy, duration should be extended to at least 6 weeks. Lack of resolution of infection should prompt further diagnostic efforts to determine why the organism persists despite appropriate therapy.

Acute Pyelonephritis. Antibiotic therapy should be started on the basis of urinalysis and pending culture results (see Tables 91–6 and 91–9). Although aminoglycosides also have excellent renal tissue penetrance, nephrotoxicity makes their administration difficult. Other drugs that can diffuse into renal tissue are preferred (Table 91–11).[8] Nitrofurantoin should not be given in acute pyelonephritis because it is ineffective for bacteremia, which may accompany acute pyelonephritis.[25]

If the animal is systemically ill, initial therapy should consist of parenteral antibiotics as well as IV fluid support. Parenteral therapy should be continued until response is indicated by normalization of body temperature and appetite.

If the organism is reported to be resistant to the initially chosen antimicrobial but the animal is better, a urinalysis should be checked again before changing therapy to determine whether the drug is efficacious in vivo. If the drug is not efficacious, therapy should be changed. If the drug is efficacious, initial therapy should be continued for at least 4 weeks, with follow-up cultures made during and 1 to 2 weeks after the conclusion of treatment. Urine cultures should be performed monthly for several months to detect recurrence (Table 91–12).

Table 91–11. Guidelines to Antimicrobial Choice in Genitourinary Infections Based on the Site of Infection

SITE	ANTIMICROBIAL AGENT
Kidney	Trimethoprim, chloramphenicol, quinolones, nitrofurantoin
Prostate	Trimethoprim, chloramphenicol, quinolones, erythromycin, clindamycin
Uterus	Enrofloxacin, chloramphenicol, trimethoprim
Mammary gland	Ampicillin, amoxicillin-clavulanate, cephalosporin (first generation)

Table 91–12. Time of Therapy at Which Urine Cultures Should be Repeated to Ensure Efficacy of Urinary Infection Therapy

NONCOMPLICATED	COMPLICATED
1 week after conclusion	1 week after conclusion
	1 month
	2 months
	3 months
	6 months
	9 months
	12 months
	18 months
	24 months

Chronic Pyelonephritis. Antibiotics with the ability to penetrate renal tissue are preferred if the causative organism is susceptible to one of them (see Table 91–11). Sulfonamides do not reach effective intrarenal concentrations, so that only the trimethoprim component of trimethoprim-sulfonamide is effective in renal infections.[11] Nitrofurantoin can be used for chronic renal infections, but not in animals with renal dysfunction.[25] Efficacy of the chosen antimicrobial agent should be checked by urinalysis and urine culture after the first 2 weeks of therapy. If the urine is not sterile at this point, therapy should be changed. If the urine is sterile, the antimicrobial agent should be continued for a total of at least 6 weeks. Urine cultures should be repeated on a periodic basis after finishing therapy (see Table 91–12).

If conservative therapy is unsuccessful and if the infection appears to be unilateral (usually determined by abnormalities on excretory urography), one can consider nephrectomy. Unilateral nephrectomy has been reported to be effective in humans,[12] although it is not done very often.[11] Surgery may not be as effective in dogs. A 1996 study indicated that UTI continued to be a problem in all five dogs that underwent nephrectomy in an attempt to eliminate unilateral pyelonephritis.[37]

Nephrectomy may be necessary if renal abscess formation is present. The remaining kidney must be able to maintain renal function. Crude indicators of adequate renal function are normal serum urea nitrogen, normal serum creatinine, concentrated urine, normal radiographic and ultrasonographic appearance, normal excretion of dye on excretory urography, and normal appearance at surgery. One needs to recognize that all these tests are insensitive, and normal findings do not confirm normal function.[37] Renal scintigraphy is recommended to more thoroughly assess individual kidney function before surgery.[37] Even with all these tests, 9 of 21 dogs undergoing nephrectomy became azotemic, albeit mildly so, after nephrectomy.[37] At surgery, urine should be collected from the renal pelvis or ureter of the remaining kidney and cultured for bacteria to direct future therapy and to provide a more accurate prognosis to the owner.

Acute Cystitis, Initial Episode. Acute, uncomplicated bacterial cystitis in female dogs, neutered male dogs, and cats should be treated for 7 to 10 days (see Tables 91–6 and 91–9). Because clinical signs often improve within 48 hours, the client must be instructed to give all medication as directed. One week after therapy is concluded, a urine sample should be collected for culture to ensure efficacy. Such follow-up is important to prompt an early search for an underlying predisposing cause for treatment failure, such as uroliths, pyelonephritis, abnormal bladder or urethral function, renal failure, urinary tract neoplasia, or hyperadrenocorticism. Whenever one part of the urinary tract is infected, the entire tract is at risk; pyelonephritis may be present along with cystitis.

In intact male dogs, prostatitis often occurs in conjunction with cystitis, necessitating longer therapy (see Table 91–6). Re-examinations should include evaluation of prostatic fluid as well as urine. Drugs with prostatic penetrance are preferred (see Table 91–11). However, one study indicated no difference in clinical response between ampicillin (little prostatic penetrance) and trimethoprim-sulfonamide (good prostatic penetrance) in UTIs in intact male dogs.[8]

Reinfections. In some dogs, acute cystitis recurs frequently. The causative organism must be determined by urine culture to differentiate reinfection from relapse (see Table 91–5). Reinfection suggests a problem with host defenses (see Table 91–4). A careful history should be taken and complete physical examination performed to determine whether micturition and urinary tract anatomy are normal. Hyperadrenocorticism and glucocorticoid therapy are predisposing causes of reinfections. Some bitches have recurrent cystitis with no other discernible abnormalities.

Each episode of reinfection is treated individually. If infections recur frequently (> three to four episodes per year), low-dose, prophylactic therapy can be provided (see Prophylactic Therapy).

Chronic Cystitis. Chronic bacterial cystitis requires protracted treatment. Urine should be recultured or checked by sediment examination approximately 7 days after therapy is begun. If the urine is sterile, that antimicrobial agent should be continued for 4 to 6 weeks. If it is not sterile, another antimicrobial should be chosen. Culturing should be repeated after approximately 7 days of treatment until an effective agent is found. Urine should be recultured after the conclusion of therapy (see Table 91–12).

Relapsing or Persistent UTIs. Relapse or persistence of UTI, despite therapy that should have been effective, should prompt a diagnostic investigation to determine the site of tissue infection and any underlying disease process that is causing the infection to be complicated (see Tables 91–5 and 91–6). Any underlying factors discovered should be treated.

Antimicrobial therapy should be continued at least 6 weeks (see Table 91–6). Urine cultures should be evaluated during and after therapy (see Table 91–12). If antimicrobial therapy eliminates bacteriuria during therapy but bacteriuria recurs with discontinuation of therapy, a longer course of therapy (4–6 months) should be considered. When providing antimicrobials for this duration, consideration must be given to side effects. Prolonged use of drugs with significant potential side effects, such as chloramphenicol, should be avoided. The risk of KCS and other toxicities with trimethoprim-sulfonamide should be conveyed to the owner (see Drug Formulary, Appendix 8).

Suppressive Therapy. If the patient experiences relapses each time antimicrobial therapy is stopped, suppressive therapy can prevent extension of the infection and control symptoms.[89] Once the urine is sterile from full-dose therapy, suppressive therapy is begun. A single dose per day of an antimicrobial is administered, preferably when the animal will be confined (usually evening) so that urination is prevented for several hours. Drugs to consider for suppressive therapy are trimethoprim, nitrofurantoin, cephalexin, and enrofloxacin. Risks include antimicrobial toxicity and induction of bacterial resistance. Urine should be cultured monthly during suppressive therapy to ensure that the drug remains effective.

UTI Associated With Catheterization. Treatment of UTIs

developing during indwelling urinary catheterization should be delayed until the catheter is removed, unless systemic signs of infection develop. When the urinary catheter is removed and the animal is again urinating normally, urine should be cultured and appropriate antimicrobial therapy should be started if infection is found. Treatment should continue at least 10 days, with reculture of urine approximately 1 week after therapy is discontinued.

Catheter-induced infections may involve more than one bacterial species with different antimicrobial susceptibility patterns. In these cases, one species is treated first. Urine is re-evaluated after treatment, and if infection persists with another species, that infection is treated. Except for combinations such as trimethoprim-sulfonamide, simultaneous administration of two or more antimicrobial agents is avoided in UTI.

Fungal UTI

Fungal UTIs are fortunately rare because they are difficult to treat. The first and most important step is to eliminate or control any underlying factors: for example, remove indwelling urinary catheters, correct any anatomic abnormalities, control diabetes mellitus, and stop unnecessary antibacterial therapies. Antifungal therapy can be provided in conjunction, although reports of such an approach are scarce in the veterinary literature. 5-Fluorocytosine was used in one cat with candidal urethrocystitis in addition to correction of a urethral stricture (see Chapter 66).[34] In humans, nonsymptomatic infections are usually treated with removal of predisposing factors without antifungal therapy, whereas symptomatic ones are treated with antifungal therapy even though an optimal therapy is not known.[109] Bladder irrigation with amphotericin B was most effective and ketoconazole the least effective in one review.[109] Fluconazole, which is largely excreted in urine in the active form, has been successful in clinical cases of candidal UTI in men.[97]

PROPHYLACTIC THERAPY

Prophylactic therapy is defined as the administration of antimicrobial drugs to prevent establishment of infection in uninfected sites.[107] In relation to the urinary tract, such therapy is provided to prevent bacterial reinfections in animals that have a history of frequent reinfection (>2–3 times a year), to prevent sepsis during surgery in animals with UTI, and to prevent bacterial UTI as a result of urinary tract manipulation and catheterization. Prophylaxis is effective only if the antimicrobial drug is present at the time of bacterial inoculation.[107] Prophylaxis with drugs cannot replace aseptic technique in importance in preventing infections related to medical procedures.

Reinfections

Infections should be treated until urine is sterile before prophylactic therapy is begun. Drug choice is based on the susceptibility of the latest isolate.[61] The chosen drug is given once just before a 6- to 12-hour period when urine will be retained in the bladder, such as at night in house dogs. The dose is one half to one third of the usual total daily dose. Therapy is continued for 6 months. Urine should be cultured every 4 weeks to be sure UTI is prevented. If the urine remains sterile for 6 months, prophylactic therapy can be discontinued and the animal monitored for reinfection (see Table 91–12). If reinfections do occur, each is eliminated with full-dose therapy and prophylactic therapy is reinstituted. Potential adverse effects of prophylactic therapy include induction of antimicrobial resistance and drug toxicity. All urine samples for culture should be collected by cystocentesis in animals on prophylactic therapy, because they may be more susceptible to induction of infection when catheterization is performed.[61]

Cranberry juice may be effective in prevention of reinfections in older women.[3] I have used cranberry juice with some apparent success in one female dog. However, experimentally in dogs, a cranberry extract did not inhibit bacterial adherence to canine uroepithelial cells, the proposed method by which cranberry juice prevents infection.[96]

Perioperative Therapy

If surgery is to be performed on an animal with a urogenital infection, antibiotics should be administered before and during surgery to reduce the possibility of sepsis. If the animal's condition permits, determination of the causative organism and its susceptibility before surgery is recommended.

Urinary Tract Manipulation

To prevent introduction of UTI in animals without infection, short-term administration of a broad-spectrum antimicrobial may be helpful during urinary tract procedures such as cystoscopy, urethroscopy, contrast urethrocystography, electrodiagnostic procedures, urohydropulsion, and prostatic massage.[13] Its use for 24 to 72 hours beginning a few hours before the procedure should be sufficient. Drugs to consider include amoxicillin-clavulanate, trimethoprim-sulfonamide, macrocrystalline nitrofurantoin, a first-generation cephalosporin, or enrofloxacin.

Indwelling Urethral or Cystic (Cystostomy Tube) Catheterization

Antibiotics should not be given prophylactically to prevent UTI developing during indwelling catheterization unless the duration of catheterization is to be short (<3 days). Although antibiotics may delay onset of bacteriuria, they will not prevent infection if the catheter remains in place. This approach will predispose the animal to infection with multi-drug-resistant organisms.[9, 62, 102] Bacteria initiate the growth of biofilms on the catheter surface, which protects the bacteria from antibiotics.[94] Even in short-term catheterization, urinalysis, urine culture, and treatment after catheter removal may be preferable to prophylactic antibiotics.

Two principles are most important in preventing UTI in the catheterized animal: maintenance of a closed catheter system and minimization of the duration of catheterization.[62, 102] In humans of both sexes, intermittent catheterization is less conducive to infection than indwelling catheters.[94] This may also be true for male dogs, but is less likely to be true in female dogs in which the urethral orifice is intravestibular. In humans on intermittent catheterization, UTI has been reduced by bladder irrigation with a solution of neomycin and polymyxin (Neosporin G.U. Irrigant, Burroughs Wellcome, Research Triangle Park, NC) or by oral methenamine hippurate or nitrofurantoin.[5, 25, 94]

Whether any local therapy into the bladder is beneficial during indwelling catheterization is controversial. In general, the short contact time plus the necessity of disconnecting the closed catheter system to infuse the antimicrobial substance abrogates any beneficial effect. No benefit was found with intravesicular dimethyl sulfoxide with indwelling urinary catheters in cats.[9] Silver-impregnated urinary catheters did not seem beneficial in reducing catheter-associated UTIs in humans.[87]

Glucocorticoids, even at anti-inflammatory doses, should be avoided in animals with indwelling urinary catheters. In cats with indwelling urinary catheters, oral prednisolone at 5 mg/day predisposed the cats to bacterial pyelonephritis with no benefit in reducing catheter-associated inflammation.[9]

Male Genital Infections

Organisms associated with genital infections in male dogs are the same as those associated with UTIs.[53] Anaerobes are occasionally associated with abscess formation. Fungal infections, especially with disseminated infections, are rarely reported.[52, 108] A parainfluenza virus was isolated from the prostatic fluid of a dog; however, the dog was nonsymptomatic (see Chapter 7).[100] Genital infections in male cats are uncommon, with the exceptions of those occurring in scrotal injury during fighting and in feline infectious peritonitis.

PROSTATITIS

Etiology and Pathogenesis

Prostatitis is an inflammatory disease of the prostate gland, most commonly associated with bacterial infection. The infection may be acute or chronic. The chronic infections are more common.[53] Abscesses develop when the infection is severe and encapsulation of purulent material occurs. Prostatic infections are mainly a problem in intact male dogs. If infection is present before neutering, that infection may persist.

Of the male dog's genital organs, the prostate gland is in closest proximity to indigenous microflora of the distal urethra. Migration of bacteria up the urethra to the prostate is inhibited by urine flow during micturition, urethral pressure, characteristics of the urethral mucosa, normal secretion of the prostatic fluid, and the antibacterial nature of the normal prostatic fluid. The prostate gland can also produce IgA as a local response to bacterial infection. The higher prevalence of UTI in castrated male dogs than in intact ones may reflect the importance of prostatic defense mechanisms.[8]

The pathogenesis of prostatic infections is incompletely understood. Most infections are assumed to be secondary to migration of bacteria up the urethra, although spread via blood, urine, semen, and rectal flora (via direct extension or lymphatics) is also postulated. The close anatomic relationship between the bladder, proximal urethra, and prostate gland is reflected in the high frequency with which all three are simultaneously infected. Prostatic fluid normally refluxes into the bladder, and urine can enter prostatic ducts during micturition. Whether prostatic infection usually precedes, follows, or develops simultaneously with bladder infection cannot be determined. Any condition that increases bacterial numbers in the prostatic urethra predisposes the animal to infection. Examples include urethral urolithiasis, neoplasia, trauma, stricture, or lower UTI. Diseases that interfere with normal prostatic fluid formation and excretion also predispose the animal to infection. An example is squamous metaplasia of the prostate secondary to hyperestrogenism.[68, 79]

Acute bacterial prostatitis and abscess formation may result in septicemia, which is responsible for the severity of clinical signs in some cases. Chronic prostatitis may be a sequela to acute infection or may develop insidiously. Abscess formation is thought to result from chronic infection and from prostatic cyst infection. Abscesses may rupture, leading to peritonitis.

Clinical Findings

Signs associated with acute bacterial prostatitis include fever, depression, anorexia, urethral discharge, and pain on prostatic palpation. Vomiting is possible because of localized peritonitis. Less common signs are constipation from avoidance of defecation because of pain and a stiff, stilted rear-limb gait. The size, symmetry, and contour of the prostate gland are normal, unless enlarged as a result of hyperplasia.

Chronic bacterial prostatitis is usually not associated with signs of systemic illness, although some dogs may be more lethargic than normal.[53] A purulent or hemorrhagic urethral discharge may be present. In some dogs, the only indication of chronic bacterial prostatitis is recurrent UTI or mild hematuria. Chronic prostatitis should be considered in stud dogs with signs of infertility. The prostate gland is not painful on palpation and infection alone does not affect prostatic size, although there may be some variation in consistency associated with increased fibrous tissue.

The most common signs of prostatic abscess formation are depression and lethargy, associated with caudal abdominal pain.[69] The prostate is often enlarged and asymmetric, causing tenesmus and constipation. A constant or an intermittent urethral discharge, which is hemorrhagic and/or purulent, may be present. Affected dogs are often febrile. Dysuria can occur as a result of interference with normal urethral function. Chronic partial urethral obstruction resulting from abscess formation can lead to a distended bladder, eventual detrusor dysfunction, and overflow urinary incontinence. About 10% of dogs have signs of septic shock (tachycardia, pale mucous membranes, delayed capillary refill, and weak pulse).[69] Icterus due to hepatic compromise may be present (see Chapters 38 and 90). Rupture of a prostatic abscess can cause localized or diffused peritonitis with signs of abdominal pain and vomiting. If the abscess is secondary to squamous hyperplasia due to hyperestrogenism, other signs of hyperestrogenism such as pendulous prepuce, truncal alopecia, hyperpigmentation, and gynecomastia may be seen.

Diagnosis

The main diagnostic techniques employed to determine whether bacterial prostatitis is present are history and prostatic palpation, CBC, urinalysis and urine culture, prostatic fluid evaluation, ultrasonography, and prostatic aspiration and biopsy. Associated clinical signs and physical examination findings in conjunction with CBC and urinalysis and urine culture results are often sufficient to establish a tentative diagnosis of acute prostatitis. Further tests are necessary in cases of chronic prostatitis to localize the site of infection to the prostate gland, because clinical signs are minimal. Prostatic ultrasonography or aspiration during surgery is often necessary to confirm the presence of an abscess.

Laboratory Findings. An inflammatory leukogram with or without a left shift is often associated with acute bacterial prostatitis and with prostatic abscess formation. The CBC is usually normal in dogs with chronic prostatitis without abscess formation.[8] Urinalysis and urine culture indicate UTI in most, but not all, cases.

Blood chemistry is usually normal with acute and chronic prostatitis, but may be abnormal with abscess formation and bacteremia secondary to acute infection. Serum bilirubin concentration and liver enzyme activities (especially alkaline phosphatase [ALP]) may be increased. Even in the absence of icterus, liver function tests such as BSP (Bromsulphalein) retention or bile acids may be abnormal. Hypoglycemia was found in 40% of cases with abscess formation.[69]

Prostatic Fluid Evaluation. Prostatic fluid is usually not evaluated in dogs with acute prostatitis or abscess formation because affected dogs are often in too much pain to ejaculate and because of the difficulty in interpreting prostatic massage samples when UTI is present. However, an *ejaculate* is usually essential for diagnosis of chronic prostatic infection. The prostatic fluid is the last and largest fraction of the ejaculate, following the sperm-rich fraction. In collecting the ejaculate, the dog is allowed to urinate and is then returned to his run or to a quiet environment. Any preputial discharge is removed from the sheath by gentle, minimal cleansing with moistened gauze sponges. The area is gently dried. The ejaculate is collected with a sterile funnel and tube; a large, sterile plastic syringe case; or a sterile urine cup. If a dog's semen cannot be collected after manual manipulation, he can be teased by an estrous bitch or an anestrous bitch to whose vulva *p*-methyl hydroxybenzoate (Eastman Kodak, Rochester, NY) has been applied. Part of the ejaculate is used for cytologic study and part for quantitative culture. Quantitative culture is essential because of the normal flora of the distal urethra.

Both ejaculate cytology and culture results must be considered in determining whether infection is present. Normal dogs occasionally have leukocytes and positive culture results. Bacteria number fewer than 10^5/ml and are usually gram positive. In dogs with bacterial prostatitis, the prostatic fluid is usually purulent and septic and may be hemorrhagic. Quantitative culture of urine and prostatic fluid should yield significant numbers of the same organism. Dogs with experimental chronic bacterial prostatitis had greater than 1000 organisms/ml, but establishing a definitive number to distinguish infection from urethral or preputial contamination is difficult. High numbers of gram-negative organisms with large numbers of leukocytes indicate infection. Large numbers of gram-positive organisms with large numbers of leukocytes also indicate infection if preputial contamination did not occur. Lower numbers of gram-negative or gram-positive organisms must be correlated with clinical signs and ejaculate cytologic findings to determine their significance. If results of culture and cytology are questionable, a second sample should be evaluated. The finding of macrophages in prostatic fluid correlated with prostatic infection in experimentally induced prostatitis.

Evaluation of prostatic fluid collected by ejaculation is preferred for detection of chronic prostatitis over the fluid collected after prostatic massage. The results of prostatic massage in dogs with UTI are difficult to interpret because of the large number of bacteria already in the urinary tract. To effectively use prostatic massage to diagnose bacterial prostatitis, UTI must be controlled first with prior antimicrobial therapy. Prostatic massage in normal dogs yields only a few erythrocytes and transitional epithelial cells.

With **prostatic massage**, the dog is allowed to empty the bladder by normal voiding. A urinary catheter is then passed to the bladder with aseptic technique. Residual urine volume should be measured as the bladder is emptied. The bladder is flushed several times with sterile saline to ensure that all urine is removed. The last flush of 5 to 10 ml is saved as the premassage sample. The catheter is then retracted distal to the prostate, as determined by rectal palpation, and the prostate is massaged rectally or abdominally for 1 to 2 minutes. After massage, sterile physiologic saline is injected slowly while the urethral orifice is occluded around the catheter to prevent reflux of the fluid. The catheter is slowly advanced to the bladder with repeated aspiration in the prostatic urethra. The bulk of the fluid will be aspirated from the bladder. Both the premassage and postmassage samples are examined by cytology and quantitative culture. It is important to compare the postmassage sample with the premassage sample to ensure that any abnormality arose in the prostatic fluid and did not pre-exist in the bladder or urethra.

Radiography. The only radiographic sign of acute prostatitis is an indistinct cranial prostatic border. This is not noted in all cases. Contrast radiography is not often performed in acute prostatitis, because the diagnosis can usually be made without it.

A change associated with some cases of chronic prostatitis is granular, parenchymal mineralization, but the prostate is often radiographically normal with chronic infection, and prostatic mineralization occurs more commonly with prostatic neoplasia.[32] Infection without abscess formation does not cause marked prostatomegaly. With abscess formation, the prostate is usually enlarged and irregular.[8] There may be poor contrast in the caudal abdomen. The iliac lymph nodes may be enlarged. Gas within the prostate gland on radiography indicates emphysematous prostatitis owing to infection with gas-forming bacteria, most commonly *E. coli*.[51]

Radiography is important to detect bone lesions due to metastasis from prostatic neoplasia and to detect diskospondylitis due to bacteremia from associated UTI.[32] With chronic prostatitis, greater than normal urethroprostatic reflux may be noted on retrograde urethrography, but this is not specific and occurs with most other prostatic diseases. With abscess formation, periurethral asymmetry and narrowing of the prostatic urethra may be observed in addition to urethroprostatic reflux.[51] Urethroprostatic reflux is not present in all cases. The prostatic urethral lumen may appear undulant, but is not distorted or destroyed.[8] A prominent colliculus seminalis is sometimes seen with squamous metaplasia of the prostate gland. The colliculus seminalis appears like a protuberance into the urethra; it is differentiated from a neoplasm by its smooth, round borders.

Ultrasonography. Ultrasonography provides more information about prostatic internal structure than radiography. Ultrasonography of the canine prostate gland has been most often performed transabdominally. A transrectal approach allows a higher resolution transducer to be placed closer to the prostate gland, resulting in a better image.[79] Ultrasonography is less sensitive in imaging the prostatic urethra; thus, in dogs that are dysuric, urethrocystography should be performed in addition to ultrasonography.[32]

Either a uniform prostatic echo pattern or a pattern of focal, multifocal, or diffuse hyperechogenicity is associated with prostatic inflammation, whereas a neoplasm tends to produce a complex combination of hyperechoic and hypoechoic areas with some unaffected parenchyma.[32] With abscess formation, the prostate gland is usually hyperechoic with parenchymal hypoechoic cavities, irregular outlines, and asymmetric shapes. The cavitary areas exhibit distal enhancement, suggestive of being fluid filled, but these cannot be distinguished from noninfected prostatic cysts, cavitary neoplasias, or hematomas.[32]

Needle Aspiration or Biopsy. Diagnosis of prostatic disease can also be approached by needle aspiration or biopsy by the perirectal or transabdominal route, depending on the location of the prostate. Transrectal fine-needle aspiration with a Franzen needle guide (Precision Dynamics, Burbank, CA) and a 22-gauge needle has also been described.[79] Ultrasonography, if available, can guide the process. If the prostate contains fluid-filled spaces, these should be aspirated before a needle biopsy. If the prostate is solid, both aspiration and biopsy can be performed. If ultrasonography is not available, fine-needle aspiration should always be performed before needle biopsy because of the possibility of an occult abscess.

Before aspiration and biopsy, hair at the site should be clipped and the site prepared aseptically. If done under ultrasound guidance, the transducer should be covered with a sterile sleeve and sterile acoustic gel used. Clean, but not aseptic, technique for prostatic aspiration resulted in conversion of a prostatic cyst to a prostatic abscess in one dog.[6]

Needle aspiration is performed with a 21-gauge, 1- to 2½-inch needle, depending on animal and prostatic size. In the perirectal approach, the needle should have a stylet (such as a spinal needle) and is guided by rectal palpation. The procedure can be performed in most dogs with mild tranquilization. Perirectal aspiration is best avoided in dogs with suspected abscesses, because bacteria may be seeded along the needle track. After aspiration of abscesses, some dogs have developed signs of localized peritonitis that required parenteral antibiotic therapy to resolve. Cytology should be performed on all aspirates. If pus is aspirated, aerobic and anaerobic bacterial cultures are indicated.

Prostatic biopsy can be performed perirectally or transabdominally or via a caudal abdominal surgical exposure. Nonsurgical biopsy procedures require tranquilization and local anesthesia. A biopsy needle such as the Tru-Cut (Travenol Laboratories, Deerfield, IL) is used. An automatic spring-loaded biopsy device (Biopty gun, Radiplast AB, Uppsala, Sweden), with a 14- to 18-gauge needle makes the procedure less difficult. Closed biopsy can be directed by palpation or by ultrasonography. The only complication reported from blind prostatic biopsy is mild hematuria, although significant hemorrhage is possible in any blind biopsy procedure. The dog should always be monitored closely for several hours after biopsy. Biopsy samples can be cultured for bacteria as well as examined histologically.

Ultrasound-guided aspiration and/or biopsy of the prostate resulted in an accurate diagnosis in 14 of 17 cases (82%) in one survey.[6] In the remaining cases, neoplasia was confirmed or suspected, but aspiration revealed hemorrhage or abscess formation. One difficulty with diagnosis by closed aspiration or biopsy is that the prostate may be affected by more than one disease process. This possibility necessitates that all the data about a clinical case be evaluated together. A diagnosis must be reconsidered if response to therapy is not as predicted. Open biopsy samples should be collected if surgery is performed.

Therapy

Acute Bacterial Prostatitis. In acute bacterial prostatitis, an antibiotic should be administered for 28 days (see Table 91–6). The choice of antibiotic can be based on urine culture results, because the organism in the urine probably originated from the prostate. Because the blood–prostatic fluid barrier is damaged in acute inflammation, a wide choice of antibiotics, similar to that for UTI, may be considered for initial treatment (see Tables 91–9 and 91–10). If the presenting signs are severe, the antimicrobial is initially given IV. Supportive therapy should be given as necessary for systemic illness. Once the dog's condition is stable, an oral antimicrobial with prostatic penetrance is preferred for the remainder of therapy (see Table 91–11). Because acute infections may become chronic, re-examination should be performed 7 days after antibiotic therapy is finished. This examination should include physical examination, urinalysis, urine culture, and prostatic fluid cytology and culture.

Chronic Bacterial Prostatitis. Cases of chronic bacterial prostatitis are very difficult to treat effectively because of a blood–prostatic fluid barrier. This barrier is related to the pH difference between the blood and prostatic interstitium and the prostatic fluid, the characteristics of the prostatic acinar epithelium, and the plasma protein-binding characteristics of antibiotics.

The pH of the blood and the prostatic interstitium is 7.4, whereas the pH of normal and infected prostatic fluid in dogs is less than 7.4.[8] When prostatic fluid is acidic, basic antibiotics (pK_a >7) such as erythromycin, clindamycin, and trimethoprim will cross the barrier more readily than other antibiotics (see Table 91–11; Fig. 91–6).[8] In men, infected prostatic fluid is alkaline; thus, drug efficacy in men cannot be directly extrapolated to dogs. Fluoroquinolones are more active in alkaline environments (pH >7.4) for gram-negative bacteria and thus may be more effective in chronic prostatitis in men than in dogs.[20]

Lipid solubility is also an important factor in determining drug movement across the prostatic epithelium. Chloramphenicol, macrolide antibiotics, trimethoprim, and enrofloxacin are examples of lipid-soluble drugs that can cross the barrier effectively.[20, 28] Drugs with low lipid solubility, such as penicillin, ampicillin, cephalosporin, and aminoglycoside, cannot cross into the prostatic acini.

Protein binding in plasma also determines the amount of drug that enters prostatic fluid. The more protein bound the

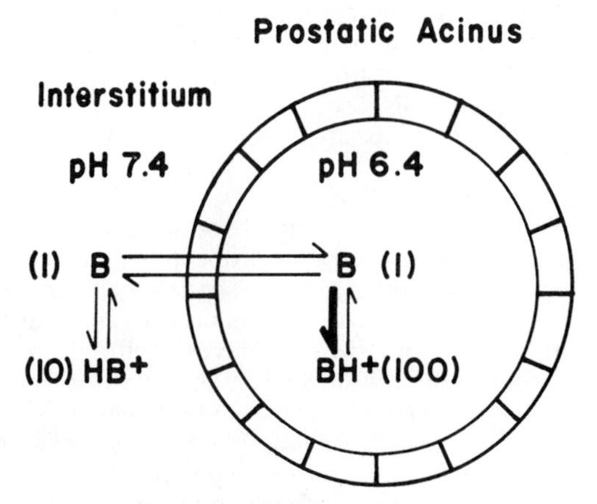

Figure 91–6. The diffusion into the prostate of an antibiotic that is a weak base (ionization constant pK_a of 8.4) is shown at equilibrium. With more acid pH within the prostate, the drug becomes more ionized and hence cannot leave the prostatic fluid. The prostatic fluid/plasma ratio is 101:11 (B = basic drug [pK_a > 7]; BH, HB = ionized drug). (From Barsanti JA, Finco DR: *Vet Clin North Am* 9:679–699, 1979, with permission.)

drug is, the less that is available to cross the prostatic epithelium. This factor is probably less important than lipid solubility or ionization, because biologic systems rarely reach equilibrium. Examples of drugs with significant protein binding are clindamycin and chloramphenicol.

In general, diffusion of tetracyclines into canine prostatic fluid is minimal. Although clinical studies in men with prostatitis demonstrated efficacy of minocycline and doxycycline, these lipid-soluble drugs did not penetrate well into canine prostatic fluid.

Current recommendations for the treatment of chronic bacterial prostatitis are based on whether a gram-positive or gram-negative organism is the infective agent. If the causative organism is gram positive, erythromycin, clindamycin, chloramphenicol, or trimethoprim can be given, depending on the organism's susceptibility. If the causative organism is gram negative, chloramphenicol, enrofloxacin, or trimethoprim is best. Although trimethoprim is often combined with a sulfonamide drug, they do not diffuse into the prostate gland.[4]

Antibiotic therapy should be continued for at least 6 weeks (see Table 91–6). If UTI is present, urine should be re-evaluated by culture during therapy to be sure that the administered drug has eliminated the UTI. After discontinuing antibiotics, urine should be recultured (see Table 91–12) to ensure that the infection has been eliminated, not merely suppressed. If initial therapy fails, a 3-month course of therapy should be instituted, bearing in mind potential adverse effects of the drug chosen. For such long-term therapy, trimethoprim and enrofloxacin are the best current choices. Trimethoprim is the most cost effective. However, trimethoprim-sulfonamide can result in KCS or mild anemia because of folate deficiency. Folic acid should be supplemented when administering trimethoprim-sulfonamide at full dosage for longer than 6 weeks. Because of the propensity for adverse effects, either trimethoprim only should be used (3–4 mg/kg BID PO) or the dose of trimethoprim-sulfonamide should be 15 mg/kg BID. There is no evidence that higher doses are needed. The prognosis for cure, based on experience in human medicine, is only fair. The long-term cure rate in humans is less than 70%.[4] If prostatic infection cannot be eliminated, suppressive therapy must be used continuously to prevent recurrent UTI (see discussion of therapy of persistent UTI).

Castration is recommended as adjunctive therapy to control infection. Limited studies indicate that castration in dogs is beneficial in resolution of prostatic infection.[24] Estrogens used as chemical castration are not recommended as therapy for prostatitis because estrogens can induce squamous metaplasia and thus predispose the dog to infection.[8] Estrogen therapy can also be associated with significant bone marrow toxicity.

Prostatic Abscesses. Prostatic abscesses require surgical drainage or prostatectomy. Complications are common. Drainage procedures often result in septic shock immediately after surgery and in ascending infection with antibiotic-resistant bacteria. Marsupialization leaves a chronic draining stoma in some dogs. Postoperative survival for at least 1 year with drainage procedures was approximately 50%.[8, 69] A common long-term complication of prostatectomy is urinary incontinence, especially in dogs with preoperative abnormalities in micturition. Removal of the prostate with an ultrasonic surgical aspirator has fewer complications, but the equipment is expensive.[85]

If prostatic enlargement has resulted in partial urethral obstruction, bladder and urethral function should be carefully assessed. Prolonged bladder distension may have resulted in bladder atony. An indwelling urinary catheter may be necessary to allow the detrusor muscle to recover. If the bladder wall has been chronically distended and infected, it may be irreversibly damaged.

Castration is recommended as adjunctive therapy. Castration without abscess drainage leads to reduction of prostatic tissue but continuation of the abscess pockets.

The dog should be treated with antibiotics as described previously for chronic prostatitis. The antibiotic choice should be modified based on the results of culture and susceptibility and the presence or absence of bacteremia. IV antimicrobials should be provided when the dog is systemically ill and during surgery. If possible, surgery should be delayed until after culture results are obtained. The prostate gland should be re-examined by palpation and ultrasonography at monthly intervals until abscess resolution is confirmed.

Polyuria and polydipsia, similar to those expected with nephrogenic diabetes insipidus, have been noted in a few dogs after surgical treatment for prostatic abscesses.[8] These problems resolved within 1 month after surgery. Evidence of hepatopathy also resolved postoperatively.

If the owners decline surgery, the dog can be managed with long-term suppressive antibiotic therapy after the UTI is controlled with at least 6 weeks of standard, full-dose therapy (see discussion of treatment of persistent UTI). The owners must realize that the abscess will persist and will potentially result in life-threatening infection.

EPIDIDYMITIS AND ORCHITIS

Etiology

Bacterial infection is the most common cause of epididymo-orchitis.[8] As in UTI, *E. coli* is a common causative organism. *Brucella canis* infection should always be a consideration in dogs. Infection may be caused by a secondary finding of trauma, by breeding to an infected female, by hematogenous spread of a systemic infection, or by spread from a UTI or prostatic infection. The cause may not be able to be determined.

Clinical Findings

Any age or breed of dog may be affected, although dogs younger than 2 years were most common in one small series of cases.[82] Both the testicle and the epididymis are usually involved. Infection may be unilateral or bilateral. Clinical signs in acute infections include pain (which may manifest as rear limb lameness), heat, and swelling, which is doughy to firm in consistency. The dog will often lick the edematous scrotum, which may cause development of dermatitis. Systemic signs, such as fever, are variable. With chronic infection, fibrosis will produce increased firmness and contracture. Localized areas of abscess formation may feel soft.

Diagnosis

Orchitis or epididymitis is usually strongly suspected on the basis of physical examination. Diagnostic tests should include CBC, urinalysis, urine culture, and brucellosis testing. The CBC may show leukocytosis if the inflammation is active. Urinalysis and urine culture determine whether there is an associated UTI. If there is a UTI, the organism is assumed to be the cause of the epididymitis-orchitis. In dogs with brucellosis, urine may contain the organism, although usually only in low numbers (<1000/ml).[22] Although semen is more productive for *Brucella* culture, handling it has greater public health risk (see Chapter 40).

If there is no UTI and the dog will ejaculate, cytologic examination and quantitative culture of semen should be performed. With semen, the cytologic finding of bacteria and neutrophils and the culture of more than 10^5 gram-negative organisms per milliliter suggest infection. Because of the urethral microflora, quantitative cultures are mandatory for assessment of results.

If the urine is not infected and semen cannot be collected, aspiration of the testicle or epididymis with a 21- to 23-gauge needle and a 12-ml syringe can be performed for cytology and culture. Ultrasonography can guide aspiration to abnormal areas of the epididymis or testicle.

Ultrasonography can also be used to determine whether a palpable abnormality in the scrotal contents is testicular or epididymal or both or whether it is outside the testicles-epididymides. A cause of swelling can be defined as being due to fluid or a solid mass.[31, 51] It may be possible to differentiate an inflammatory disease from testicular torsion, traumatic rupture, or neoplasia.[82] Ultrasonographic findings associated with acute orchitis-epididymitis include a diffuse, patchy, hypoechoic pattern, testicular and/or epididymal enlargement, and occasionally extratesticular fluid.[82]

Therapy

Bilateral orchidectomy is the treatment of choice for orchitis and epididymitis. If the dog is a valuable sire and the condition is unilateral, the testicle on the affected side should be removed to save the other from thermal degeneration.[31] If unilateral orchidectomy is performed, the owner should be advised that a subclinical infection of the apparently normal testicle and epididymis or a concurrent prostatic infection could cause future problems for the dog.

Antibiotics should be given whether or not surgery is performed. Isolation of the causative organism and antimicrobial susceptibility testing should guide therapy. Therapy should be continued at least 2 weeks. While culture results are pending, an antibiotic such as enrofloxacin, chloramphenicol, or trimethoprim-sulfonamide should be started. Adjunctive soaks in cool water may help to reduce testicular degeneration from the hyperthermia of inflammation.

BALANOPOSTHITIS

Balanoposthitis is usually caused by bacteria normally present in the prepuce (see Table 91–2). Herpesvirus infections and blastomycosis also have caused balanoposthitis.

Mild balanoposthitis is so common that it is considered normal in male dogs. It is characterized by a purulent exudate within or dripping from the prepuce with variable degrees of inflammation of the preputial mucosa. There are no signs of systemic illness. Dogs usually are nonsymptomatic, but some will lick the prepuce.

There is no specific diagnostic test for balanoposthitis except cytologic examination of preputial exudate. Bacteria and large numbers of degenerate and nondegenerate neutrophils are seen. A culture of pus can be performed, but results are impossible to interpret because of the abundant normal flora. Culture is not required for successful management of most cases.

Balanoposthitis is not a serious medical problem but may be an annoyance to the owner. Cleansing antiseptic douches or local antibacterials may be of benefit. Neutering affected animals may help reduce the amount of secretion produced.

Female Genital Infections

VAGINITIS

Etiology

Inflammation of the vagina can be due to bacterial or viral infections, immaturity, or irritation from urine, foreign material, neoplasia, or anatomic abnormalities. Bacterial infection can develop secondarily to these causes of irritation. Vaginitis is more common in bitches than in queens. So-called juvenile or puppy vaginitis is common in otherwise normal, healthy prepubertal bitches and resolves spontaneously with physical maturity in most. Vaginitis in the young dog (<1 year) is more likely a problem with immaturity than with bacterial infection.[44] Bacterial organisms recovered from bitches with vaginitis are the same organisms found in the normal flora, although the numbers of bacteria may be higher in mature dogs with vaginitis.[44, 99] Isolation of a single bacterial species occurs in about 25% of bitches with vaginitis; *E. coli*, *Streptococcus*, and *Staphylococcus* are the most common.[15]

Viral infections of the canine or feline vagina are uncommon. Herpesviruses (canine herpesvirus, feline rhinotracheitis virus) cause vesicular lesions and erythema when inoculated intravaginally.[43] Although genital tract infection readily occurs after experimental inoculation, genital herpesvirus infection is an uncommon clinical entity.[83] Vaginal lymphoid follicular hyperplasia, which could result from any inflammatory process, may be mistaken for vesicle formation. Confirmation of genital herpesvirus infection should include viral isolation and histologic examination of the vesicular lesions (see Chapter 5).

Clinical Findings

The most common historical and physical finding associated with vaginitis is the presence of a vulvar discharge in an otherwise healthy animal. The discharge is mucus, mucopurulent, or purulent, varying in color from cloudy white to yellow to green.[44] Blood is rare.[44] The discharge may attract male dogs and may cause the affected dog to lick the vulvar area. The perineal hair may be discolored by saliva and exudate. Pollakiuria occurs in about 10% of affected bitches.[44] Signs of systemic illness are not expected.

Diagnosis

The diagnosis of vaginitis is strongly suggested by the history and physical abnormalities and by the vaginal cytology. This approach is sufficient for dogs younger than 1 year without urinary tract signs. In older dogs, especially those with chronic vaginitis, vaginoscopy, as well as urinalysis and urine culture, should be performed. The most important diagnostic considerations are whether the vulvar discharge is abnormal and whether the inflammatory process is confined to the vagina.

CBCs are normal in dogs with vaginitis.[44] UTI was found in approximately 20% of mature bitches with vaginitis.[44] UTI was not found in puppies with vaginitis, but urine from only a few puppies was examined.[44] At least a urinalysis and optimally a urine culture are indicated in mature dogs with vaginitis and in puppies with signs of pollakiuria.

To avoid contamination from the skin and the vestibule, samples for bacterial culture from the cranial vagina should be obtained with a guarded swab or through a sterile speculum. The results of vaginal cultures must be interpreted cautiously, because the most common pathogens of the vagina and uterus are *E. coli*, *Streptococcus*, and *Staphylococcus*, which are also commensal organisms (see Table 91–3). Bacterial cultures will *not* confirm the diagnosis of vaginitis, because some bacterial growth *is* expected. Heavy growth of a single organism is more convincing of the possibility that the organism is causing the clinical signs.

Cytologic evidence of inflammation (neutrophils; possibly lymphocytes and macrophages in chronic cases) with or without bacteria is expected from animals with vaginitis.[83] Vaginal cytology must be interpreted with regard to the stage of the estrous cycle. WBCs are often numerous during the first few days of diestrus. This normal phenomenon can be distinguished from inflammation because the number of WBCs declines markedly in 24 to 48 hours of diestrus, whereas it persists with vaginitis. A mucoid vulvar discharge is normal during the early postpartum period in the bitch and queen. A hemorrhagic vulvar discharge is normal during proestrus and estrus in the bitch.

Vaginoscopy helps determine the source of the discharge and the nature and extent of vaginal lesions. Sedation or general anesthesia may be necessary for a thorough examination. With vaginitis, the vaginal mucosa is hyperemic. There is exudate in the vaginal lumen. Ulcers or lymphoid follicles may be seen. The inciting cause of the vaginitis may be identified (Table 91–13). Vaginal cultures are easily obtained during vaginoscopy. Vaginal biopsy samples are taken when discrete lesions are seen.

Therapy

Treatment of puppy vaginitis is either none or conservative (perivulvar cleaning only), because the condition subsides with or without therapy in at least 90% of cases.[44] Some recommend that the affected animal be allowed to experience an estrous cycle to increase the chance of spontaneous recovery[99]; however, the majority of young bitches recover before experiencing an estrous cycle.[44, 46] Estrogen in the maturing bitch induces antibacterial activity in the vaginal mucosa, which facilitates recovery. The current recommendation is that young bitches with clinically significant vaginitis not undergo ovariohysterectomy (OHE) until they have experienced estrus or until the vaginitis has resolved.[46, 83]

Most mature bitches with vaginitis have a predisposing abnormality (see Table 91–13).[44, 46] Recovery from vaginitis requires correction of the underlying disorder.

In mature bitches with no underlying abnormality, vaginitis, even if chronic, resolves spontaneously in 75% of cases, although full recovery may take months.[46] The remaining 25% of cases are frustrating for owners and veterinarians because no current therapy is consistently effective.[44] In intact bitches, OHE does not improve clinical signs of vaginitis.[44]

The relative efficacy of various treatments for vaginitis has yet to be investigated in small animals. Antiseptic douches, instillation of antibiotic suppositories, ointments, or solutions, and systemic antibiotic therapy have been tried.[43] Solutions that alter pH, such as vinegar (0.25%) or most commercial douches, may discourage the overgrowth of vaginal bacteria. Douching should not be performed during proestrus or estrus.[46] Many owners are unable to douche their pets effectively.

Systemic antibiotics may diminish clinical signs in mature bitches with chronic vaginitis. The antimicrobial should be chosen on the basis of urine and cranial vaginal cultures. Antibiotics usually provided are ampicillin, trimethoprim-sulfonamide, amoxicillin-clavulanate, cephalosporin, and chloramphenicol.[46] Although ampicillin did not concentrate in the vaginal secretions of bitches, it did eradicate susceptible bacteria within 24 hours in healthy bitches.[95] Trimethoprim, which was shown to concentrate in vaginal secretions, did not eradicate all in vitro susceptible organisms in healthy bitches.[95] During therapy with either ampicillin or trimethoprim-sulfonamide, organisms were still present in the vaginal secretions of 8 of 10 bitches and additional organisms emerged.[95]

If vaginitis is concurrent with pregnancy, the possible teratogenic or abortifacient effects of therapy must be considered. If vaginitis occurs in proestrus or estrus and the bitch is scheduled for breeding, the possibility of transmission of infection to the stud and the effects of therapy on sperm survival should be considered.

Table 91–13. Underlying Causes of Vaginitis

Atresia	Clitoral hypertrophy
Strictures	Foreign objects
Septa	Urinary incontinence
Neoplasia, granuloma	Urinary tract infection

METRITIS

Etiology and Pathogenesis

Metritis is acute ascending bacterial infection of the uterus.[43] Metritis may follow abortion, dystocia, obstetric manipulation, retention of fetal or placental parts, or normal parturition. Rarely, metritis may occur after natural or artificial insemination.

Many organisms cross the canine placenta and infect fetuses but do not infect the uterus per se. They may, however, be transiently recovered from uterine or vaginal cultures of parturient or periparturient bitches. These organisms include canine herpesvirus, adenovirus, distemper virus, *Brucella canis*, and *Toxoplasma gondii*.[43] Experimental, intrauterine inoculation of *Mycoplasma canis* can cause uterine disease in bitches,[43] but the role of mycoplasmal infection in spontaneous disease is uncertain (see Chapter 32). In cats, FeLV, panleukopenia virus, and herpesviruses can be transmitted to the fetuses of viremic queens.

Clinical Findings

Animals with metritis are febrile and have a fetid, septic, purulent vaginal discharge. Dehydration, sepsis, and endotoxemia can occur. Neonates of affected dams are usually neglected and crying from hunger.

Diagnosis

A presumptive diagnosis is based on the history and physical findings. Cytology and bacterial culture and susceptibility should be performed on the discharge. Cytology shows a hemorrhagic, septic, purulent exudate. Cytologic evidence of endometrial cells or uteroverdin indicates uterine involvement, but these are not consistently present. Abdominal radiography and/or uterine ultrasonography should be performed to locate fetal remnants and to assess the integrity of the uterus. Ultrasonographic diagnosis of metritis is not very accurate because the changes are subtle. The uterus may be slightly enlarged and echogenicity may be abnormal.[111]

Therapy

IV fluids should be administered if needed to maintain normal hydration. A systemic, broad-spectrum antimicrobial should be given, pending the uterine culture results. An antimicrobial that is usually effective against *E. coli* should be chosen (see Tables 91–10 and 91–11). Antibiotic therapy is reassessed when the culture results are returned. Therapy should continue for 7 to 10 days if the uterus is removed and 2 to 4 weeks if it is not. Neonates are usually hand reared until the mother is sufficiently recovered to care for them.

A decision must be made as to whether therapy of the infected uterus will be surgical or medical on the basis of the severity of the illness and the owner's desire to maintain reproductive capability. OHE should be performed if the uterus has ruptured. OHE or hysterotomy with lavage is necessary if placental or fetal tissues are in the uterus.

Medical management involves stimulation of evacuation of uterine contents. If the animal is within 24 hours of parturition, oxytocin can be administered at 5 to 20 units once or twice.[47] Natural prostaglandin $F_{2\alpha}$ ($PGF_2\alpha$ Lutalyse, Upjohn Company, Kalamazoo, MI) can be given any time post partum at a dose of 0.1 mg/kg SC once a day for 2 to 3 days.[47] Adverse effects include vomiting, panting, restlessness, vocalization, and change in pupil size. Neither oxytocin nor $PGF_2\alpha$ affects lactation or neonatal health.[47]

Intrauterine infusion of antiseptic or antibiotic solutions is of questionable value. The canine cervix is extremely difficult to cannulate; therefore, most infusions via the vagina are probably intravaginal rather than intrauterine. Intrauterine infusion of nitrofurazone may actually decrease subsequent fertility in some species.[43] Surgical placement of drains within the uterus and subsequent flushing is usually not successful.[43]

PYOMETRA

Etiology and Pathogenesis

Pyometra is a bacterial infection of the uterus secondary to uterine pathology induced by progesterone over successive heat cycles or by exogenous therapy.[43] Pyometra occurs more frequently in dogs than cats. Affected dogs tend to be middle-aged or older, but administration of estradiol cypionate or megestrol acetate can induce pyometra in young dogs.[93, 106] Age of affected cats has varied from young adults, 3 to 6 years of age,[26, 60, 106] to older than 5 years,[81] to an average age of 7 years.[50] In queens, no correlation was found among development of pyometra and age at first breeding, age at first queening, or number of litters produced.[81] Pyometra involving the uterus masculinus of hermaphrodites can occur in dog and cats.[43]

Because progesterone initiates the sequence of events leading to pyometra, it occurs during the luteal phase of the cycle in dogs (diestrus) or after the administration of progestins.[101] Progesterone causes cystic endometrial hyperplasia, fluid accumulation within the endometrial glands and uterine lumen, and decreased myometrial activity. The uterine disease and decreased contractility favor secondary ascending bacterial infection. *E. coli* also binds to the endometrium more effectively during the luteal phase of the estrous cycle. Although bacteria do not initiate pyometra, secondary infection causes most of the morbidity and mortality.

E. coli isolates from dogs that suffer from pyometra and/or urinary infections have been biochemically compared with corresponding fecal isolates.[101a] Strains from infected uteri and urinary tracts were biochemically similar, confirming the hypothesis of fecal contamination of the genitourinary tract.

A correlation between the presence of a corpora lutea and pyometra is also found in cats. Because cats are induced ovulators, pyometra occurs after nonfertile matings, drug-induced ovulation, and treatment with progestins. Some cats have been found to be in the luteal phase of the ovarian cycle, even though they were isolated from male cats and received no therapy, suggesting that the luteal phase must be able to be induced by other factors as well.[60] Progesterones are not the only factors involved in cats, because some affected cats are in the follicular phase of the ovarian cycle.[60, 81]

Clinical Findings

Affected dogs and cats are usually presented 2 months after estrus or breeding or have been given estrogens or progestogens. Owners may note vulvar discharge, lethargy, vomiting, and polyuria-polydipsia in dogs.[93, 106] Vaginal discharge (mucopurulent to hemorrhagic) and abdominal distention were the most common signs in cats.[26, 81] Nonspecific signs of illness such as anorexia, weight loss, unkempt appearance, lethargy, and vomiting are seen in some cats.[49] Polyuria and polydipsia are seen less commonly in cats than in dogs.[49]

Uterine enlargement is found on physical examination. Fever is uncommon.[50, 93, 106] Open pyometra (the cervix is open and draining) is more common than closed pyometra.[66, 93, 106] Approximately one third of affected cats are dehydrated.[49] Septicemia or endotoxemia may develop at any time, in which case animals may have tachycardia, tachypnea, poor peripheral perfusion, and subnormal body temperature. Animals with closed-cervix pyometra are at greater risk for development of septicemia and endotoxemia.[43]

Diagnosis

The diagnosis is established by the history, stage of the estrous cycle, physical examination, and laboratory and radiographic abnormalities.[43] A CBC, biochemical profile, and urinalysis are essential to detect the metabolic abnormalities associated with septicemia or toxemia and to evaluate renal function. Urine collection by any means should be done carefully, because of the risks of perforating the enlarged uterus during cystocentesis or introducing the organisms from the reproductive tract into the bladder during catheterization.

Results of vaginal cytology show degenerate neutrophils and bacteria.[26, 43] Endometrial cells may also be found.[43]

Leukocytosis with a left shift is often present in the CBC,[26, 81, 106] but approximately 25% of dogs had normal WBC and differential counts in one survey.[93] Leukopenia with a degenerative left shift and neutrophil toxicity may be found in animals with septicemia. Anemia, hyperglobulinemia and hyperfibrinogenemia, and azotemia may be detected.[26, 43] Abnormalities are most severe in animals with closed-cervix pyometra. Most dogs with pyometra have a concentration of serum ALP above normal.[93, 106] This finding may reflect reactive hepatopathy, secondary to bacteremia or toxemia, as in dogs with prostatic abscess formation (see Chapters 38 and 87).

Concurrent UTI has been detected in up to 69% of affected bitches.[93] The organism in the urine is usually the same as that in the uterus.[90] Isosthenuria and proteinuria are found in 30% of bitches with pyometra. Isosthenuria is thought to be a result of endotoxin-induced unresponsiveness to antidiuretic hormone and to renal tubular injury. Mild tubulointerstitial nephritis is the most consistent pathologic finding.[43] Most affected bitches, with or without azotemia, have reduced glomerular filtration rates that are not correlated with structural alteration in glomeruli.[43] Proteinuria may be the result of tubular injury; however, proteinuria may also be due to glomerular lesions characteristic of immune complex deposition, which are found in some bitches with pyometra.

The most important diagnostic consideration is the differentiating of pyometra from pregnancy with associated vaginitis. Abdominal radiography will confirm the presence of uterine enlargement, but the nature of the uterine contents cannot be determined from radiographs until calcified fetal structures are present at approximately 40 to 45 days of gestation. Ultrasonography is useful in differentiating fetal structures, solid masses, and luminal fluids. A large, fluid-filled uterus (anechoic or hypoechoic) with no fetuses is characteristic of pyometra.[26, 86] Fetal structures may be identified by ultrasonogram as early as 10 days after breeding and are readily identifiable by 28 days.[66] Because pyometra occurs more than 28 days after estrus, ultrasonography is helpful in differentiating pregnancy from pyometra.

Therapy

Treatment should be prompt and aggressive because rapid deterioration can occur in animals with pyometra. Therapy consists of administration of IV fluids and an appropriate antibiotic and evacuation of uterine contents. Fluid therapy should be continued throughout surgical or medical management to ensure adequate tissue perfusion.

Antimicrobial therapy should be chosen on the basis of culture and susceptibility testing of the uterine exudate. Samples should be obtained directly from the uterine lumen at the time of OHE. If surgery is not performed, specimens should be obtained from the cranial vagina. Pending the return of culture results, an antibiotic effective against *E. coli* should be administered (see Table 91–10). In one survey, *E. coli* isolated from bitches with pyometra was most commonly susceptible to enrofloxacin, trimethoprim-sulfonamide, chloramphenicol, and aminoglycosides.[33] *E. coli* tended to be resistant to ampicillin, cephalothin, and tetracycline. In another report, *E. coli* was isolated from 77% of uteri with susceptibility to amoxicillin-clavulanate, cephalexin, enrofloxacin, and gentamicin.[110a] Enrofloxacin and other fluoroquinolones may reach higher uterine fluid concentrations than serum concentrations.[20]

Evacuation of uterine contents can be accomplished surgically (OHE) or medically with prostaglandin therapy. If the animal is in critical condition, if there is evidence of uterine rupture or peritonitis, or if the pyometra is closed (no vaginal discharge), OHE is recommended. The prognosis for recovery from pyometra is good after surgery. Intraoperative and immediate postoperative death occurs in 5% to 8% of cases.[49, 106] If the uterus ruptures, the mortality increases to 50%.[106] Severely azotemic dogs (BUN >150 mg/dl) also have poor prognoses. Postoperative complications in dogs with pyometra include intracranial thromboembolism, septicemia, and osteomyelitis secondary to septicemia.[106]

OHE may be unacceptable to owners who wish to preserve the animal's reproductive ability. In these cases, prostaglandin therapy may be given. The beneficial effects of prostaglandins (PGs) are due to evacuation of uterine contents rather than to changes in the endometrium or ovarian function. Naturally occurring $PGF_{2\alpha}$ is given at a dose of 0.1 mg/kg SC per day for 3 to 5 days until the uterus is empty and the vaginal discharge is resolving.[26, 43] Synthetic $PGF_{2\alpha}$ should not be used because it is much more potent, and a safe dose is not established for dogs and cats.[26] A prolonged vaginal discharge should prompt re-evaluation of the patient and the choice of antibiotics. The most common side effects of prostaglandin therapy are restlessness, pacing, hypersalivation, vocalization, panting, vomiting, diarrhea, abdominal discomfort, tachycardia, mydriasis, and fever; these signs usually resolve within 1 hour of therapy.[26, 43] Adverse reactions tend to diminish in severity and duration with repeated administration.[26] When prostaglandin therapy is used, the animal should be bred on the next estrus.[66]

$PGF_{2\alpha}$ is usually successful in treating open-cervix pyometra in both dogs and cats (93–100% for resolution of clinical signs; 55–87% for subsequent pregnancy).[26, 50] However, recurrence of pyometra can be expected.[50] $PGF_{2\alpha}$ is less successful in dogs with closed-cervix pyometra (only about 25–34%).[50, 66] There are no reports of successful medical management of closed-cervix pyometra in the queen.

MASTITIS

Etiology

The usual cause is bacterial infection; *E. coli*, *Staphylococcus*, and *Streptococcus* are most common.[45] A damp, humid environment is a predisposing factor.[59]

Clinical Findings

Mastitis is most common in postpartum dogs. It is uncommon in queens and in pseudopregnant, lactating bitches.[42] Mastitis may develop anytime during lactation and up until approximately 1 week past weaning.[59] Heavily lactating bitches are more likely to develop postweaning mastitis, especially if food intake is not restricted during the early weaning period.[59]

The classic clinical signs are mammary gland heat, pain, redness, and swelling, which may be edematous or firm. Milk expressed from infected glands is discolored, hemorrhagic, or purulent. One or multiple glands may be affected. The animal may be systemically ill with fever, anorexia, dehydration, and neglect of offspring. Mastitis is usually acute; abscesses or gangrenous changes may occur secondarily.

Diagnosis

Diagnosis is usually based on physical findings plus examination of milk. A hemogram may show a neutrophilic leukocytosis. Reactive thrombocytopenia, possibly secondary to DIC, was found in one case of gangrenous staphylococcal mastitis.[39] Cytology of milk confirms septic, purulent inflammation. Bacterial culture and susceptibility of milk are recommended to determine the causative organism and the most efficacious antimicrobial therapy.

Therapy

Therapy includes systemic, broad-spectrum antibiotics, warm packs and frequent milking of affected glands, and fluid therapy if dehydration is present. When choosing an antibiotic, one must consider the susceptibility of the organism, its ability to reach the milk, and the effects on nursing neonates. Initial drugs of choice pending culture results are ampicillin, amoxicillin-clavulanate, or first-generation cephalosporin.[45] Antibiotic therapy should be continued for several days after mastitis resolves. Most animals require therapy for at least 1 week.[45]

Occasionally, a severely abscessed gland may require surgical drainage. This should be done carefully because hemorrhage is a potential complication.[59] Abscessed or ruptured glands should be debrided of devitalized tissue and allowed to drain, with at least twice-daily flushing of an antibacterial solution.

Whether offspring need to be removed from the dam if she is ill is not known. If the mother is not systemically ill, offspring do not need to be removed.[59] Affected animals often have decreased milk production, so that supplemental feeding of offspring is required.

References

1. Altreuther P. 1992. Safety and tolerance of enrofloxacin in dogs and cats, pp 15–20. *In* Proceedings of the First International Baytril Symposium, Bonn, Germany.
2. Aucoin DP. 1990. Rational approaches to the treatment of first time, relapsing, and recurrent urinary tract infections. *Probl Vet Med* 2:290–297.
3. Avorn J, Monane M, Gurwitz JH, et al. 1994. Reduction of bacteriuria and pyuria after ingestion of cranberry juice. *JAMA* 271:751–754.
4. Baert L, van Poppel H, Vandeursen H. 1991. Review of modern trends in the treatment or chronic bacterial prostatitis. *Infection* 19:S157–S159.
5. Bakke A, Vollset SE. 1993. Risk factors for bacteriuria and clinical urinary tract infection in patients treated with clean intermittent catheterization. *J Urol* 149:527–531.
6. Barr F. 1995. Percutaneous biopsy of abdominal organs under ultrasound guidance. *J Small Anim Pract* 36:105–113.
7. Barsanti JA, Finco DR, Brown SA. 1994. Diseases of the lower urinary tract, pp 1769–1823. *In* Sherding RG (ed), The cat: diseases and clinical management. Churchill Livingstone, New York, NY.
8. Barsanti JA, Johnson CA. 1990. Genitourinary infections, pp 157–183. *In* Greene CE (ed), Infectious diseases of the dog and cat. WB Saunders, Philadelphia, PA.
9. Barsanti JA, Shotts EB, Crowell WA, et al. 1992. Effect of therapy on susceptibility to urinary tract infection in male cats with indwelling urethral catheters. *J Vet Intern Med* 6:64–70.
10. Berger SL, Scagliotti RH, Lund EA. 1995. A quantitative study of the effects of tribrissen on canine tear production. *J Am Anim Hosp Assoc* 31:236–241.
11. Bergeron MG. 1995. Treatment of pyelonephritis in adults. *Med Clin North Am* 79:619–649.
12. Bergman B, Norrgard O. 1990. Nephrectomy in unilateral chronic pyelonephritis: a long-term follow-up study. *Int Urol Nephrol* 22:209–214.
13. Bhatia NN, Karram MM, Bergman A, et al. 1992. Antibiotic prophylaxis following lower urinary tract instrumentation. *Urology* 39:583–585.
14. Bijlsma IG, van Dijk L, Kusters G, et al. 1995. Nucleotide sequences of two fimbrial major subunit genes, pmpA and uca A, from canine-uropathogenic *Proteus mirabilis* strains. *Microbiology* 141:1349–1357.
15. Bjurstrom L. 1993. Aerobic bacteria occurring in the vagina of bitches with reproductive disorders. *Acta Vet Scand* 34:29–34.
16. Bjurstrom L, Linde-Forsberg C. 1992. Long-term study of aerobic bacteria of the genital tract in breeding bitches. *Am J Vet Res* 53:665–669.
17. Bjurstrom L, Linde-Forsberg C. 1992. Long-term study of aerobic bacteria of the genital tract in stud dogs. *Am J Vet Res* 53:670–673.
18. Brain PH. 1993. Urinary tract candidiasis in a diabetic dog. *Aust Vet Pract* 23:88–91.
19. Brown MB, Stoll M, Maxwell J, Senior D. 1991. Survival of feline mycoplasmas in urine. *J Clin Microbiol* 29:1078–1080.
20. Brown SA. 1996. Fluoroquinolones in animal health. *J Vet Pharmacol Ther* 19:1–14.
21. Brown SA, Arnold TS, Hamlow PJ, et al. 1995. Plasma and urine disposition and dose proportionality of ceftiofur and metabolites in dogs after subcutaneous administration of ceftiofur sodium. *J Vet Pharmacol Ther* 18:363–369.
22. Carmichael LE, Joubert JC. 1988. Transmission of *Brucella canis* by contact exposure. *Cornell Vet* 78:63–73.
23. Clemetson LL, Ward ACS. 1990. Bacterial flora of the vagina and uterus of healthy cats. *J Am Vet Med Assoc* 196:902–906.
24. Cowan LA, Barsanti JA, Crowell WA, et al. 1991. Effects of castration on chronic bacterial prostatitis in dogs. *J Am Vet Med Assoc* 199:346–350.
25. Cunha BA. 1988. Nitrofurantoin—current concepts. *Urology* 32:67–71.
26. Davidson AP, Feldman EC, Nelson RW. 1992. Treatment of pyometra in cats, using prostaglandin F2a: 21 cases (1982–1990). *J Am Vet Med Assoc* 200:825–828.
27. Davies NL, Williams JH. 1993. Emphysematous cystitis in a non-diabetic cat. *J S Afr Vet Assoc* 64:162–164.
28. Dorfman M, Barsanti JA, Budsberg SC. 1995. Enrofloxacin concentrations in dogs with normal prostate and dogs with chronic bacterial prostatitis. *Am J Vet Res* 56:386–390.
29. Dowling PM. 1996. Antimicrobial therapy of urinary tract infections. *Can Vet J* 37:438–441.
30. Elad D, Aizenberg I, Shamir M, et al. 1992. Isolation of *Corynebacterium* Group D2 from two dogs with urinary tract infections. *J Clin Microbiol* 30:1167–1169.
31. Ellington J, Meyers-Wallen V, Suess R, et al. 1993. Unilateral bacterial epididymitis in the dog. *J Am Anim Hosp Assoc* 29:315–319.
32. Feeney DA, Johnston GR, Walter PA. 1991. Ultrasonography of the kidney and prostate gland. *Probl Vet Med* 3:619–646.
33. Franklin A, af Rantzien MH, Morner AP. 1996. Antibiotic sensitivity of bacterial isolates from urinary tract infections and metritis in dogs. *Suppl Compend Contin Educ Pract Vet* 18:96.
34. Fulton RB, Walker RD. 1992. *Candida albicans* urocystitis in a cat. *J Am Vet Med Assoc* 200:524–526.
35. Gaastra W, van Oosterom RA, Pieters EW, et al. 1996. Isolation and characterisation of dog uropathogenic *Proteus mirabilis* strains. *Vet Microbiol* 48:57–71.
36. Gerding PA, Morton LD, Dye JA. 1994. Ocular and disseminated candidiasis in an immunosuppressed cat. *J Am Vet Med Assoc* 204:1635–1638.
37. Gookin JL, Stone EA, Spaulding KA, et al. 1996. Unilateral nephrectomy in dogs with renal disease: 30 cases (1985–1994). *J Am Vet Med Assoc* 208:2020–2026.
38. Griffin DW, Gregory CR. 1992. Prevalence of bacterial urinary tract infection after perineal urethrostomy in cats. *J Am Vet Med Assoc* 200:681–684.
39. Hasegawa T, Fujii M, Fukada T, et al. 1993. Platelet abnormalities in a dog suffering from gangrenous mastitis by *Staphylococcus aureus* infection. *J Vet Med Sci* 55:169–171.
40. Holt PE, Hotston-Moore A. 1995. Canine ureteral ectopia: an analysis of 175 cases and comparison of surgical treatments. *Vet Rec* 136:345–349.
41. Itkin RJ, Krawiec DR, Cloran JA. 1994. Ulcerative urocystitis in a dog associated with a *Nocardia*-like organism. *J Am Anim Hosp Assoc* 30:296–299.
42. Johnson CA. 1986. Non-neoplastic disorders of the mammary gland. *Vet Clin North Am Small Anim Pract* 16:539–542.
43. Johnson CA. 1990. Female genital infections, pp 177–181. *In* Greene CE (ed), Infectious diseases of the dog and cat. WB Saunders, Philadelphia, PA.
44. Johnson CA. 1991. Diagnosis and treatment of chronic vaginitis in the bitch. *Vet Clin North Am Small Anim Pract* 21:523–531.
45. Johnson CA. 1992. Disorders of the mammary gland, pp 665–668. *In* Nelson RW, Couto CG (eds), Essentials of small animal internal medicine. CV Mosby, St. Louis, MO.
46. Johnson CA. 1992. Disorders of the vagina and uterus, pp 654–664. *In* Nelson RW, Couto CG (eds), Essentials of small animal internal medicine. CV Mosby, St. Louis, MO.
47. Johnson CA. 1992. False pregnancy, disorders of pregnancy, parturition, and the postpartum period, pp 669–683. *In* Nelson RW, Couto CG (eds), Essentials of small animal internal medicine. CV Mosby, St. Louis, MO.
48. Johnson CA. 1992. Medical management of feline pyometra, pp 969–971. *In* Kirk RW, Bonagura JD (eds), Current veterinary therapy XI. WB Saunders, Philadelphia, PA.
49. Johnson CA. 1994. Female reproduction and disorders of the female reproductive tract, pp 1855–1876. *In* Sherding RG (ed), The cat: diseases and clinical management, Churchill Livingstone, New York, NY.
50. Johnson CA. 1995. Cystic endometrial hyperplasia, pyometra, and infertility, pp 1636–1642. *In* Ettinger SJ, Feldman EC (eds), Textbook of veterinary internal medicine, ed 4. WB Saunders, Philadelphia, PA.
51. Johnston GR, Feeney DA, Rivers B, et al. 1991. Diagnostic imaging of the male canine reproductive organs. *Vet Clin North Am Small Anim Pract* 21:553–589.
52. Kadota K, Uchida K, Nagatomo T, et al. 1995. Granulomatous epididymitis related to *Rhodotorula glutinis* infection in a dog. *Vet Pathol* 32:716–718.

53. Krawiec DR, Helfin D. 1992. Study of prostatic disease in dogs: 177 cases (1981–1986). *J Am Vet Med Assoc* 200:1119–1122.
54. Kruger JM, Osborne CA. 1990. The role of viruses in feline lower urinary tract disease. *J Vet Intern Med* 4:71–78.
55. Kruger JM, Osborne CA, Goyal SM, et al. 1990. Clinicopathologic analysis of herpesvirus-induced urinary tract infection in specific-pathogen-free cats given methylprednisolone. *Am J Vet Res* 51:878–885.
56. Kruger JM, Osborne CA, Goyal SM, et al. 1990. Clinopathologic and pathologic findings of herpesvirus-induced urinary tract infection in conventionally reared cats. *Am J Vet Res* 51:1649–1655.
57. Kruger JM, Osborne CA, Goyal SM, et al. 1991. Clinical evaluation of cats with lower urinary tract disease. *J Am Vet Med Assoc* 199:211–216.
58. Kunkle GA, Sundlof S, Keisling K. 1995. Adverse side effects of oral antibacterial therapy in dogs and cats: an epidemiologic study of pet owners' observations. *J Am Anim Hosp Assoc* 31:46–55.
58a. Kyles AE, Douglass JP, Rottman JB, 1996. Pyelonephritis following inadvertent excision of the ureter during ovariohysterectomy in a bitch. *Vet Rec* 139:471–472.
59. Lawler DF. 1991. Canine and feline periparturient problems, pp 20–51. *In* Cain J, Lawler DF (eds), Small animal reproduction and pediatrics. Ralston Purina, St. Louis, MO.
60. Lawler DF, Evans RH, Reimers TJ, et al. 1991. Histopathologic features, environmental factors, and serum estrogen, progesterone, and prolactin values associated with ovarian phase and inflammatory uterine disease in cats. *Am J Vet Res* 52:1747–1753.
61. Ling GV. 1995. Urinary tract infections, pp 116–128. *In* Lower urinary tract diseases of dogs and cats. Mosby–Year Book, St. Louis, MO.
62. Lippert AC, Fulton RB, Parr AM. 1988. Nosocomial infection surveillance in a small animal intensive care unit. *J Am Anim Hosp Assoc* 24:627–636.
63. Low DA, Braaten BA, Ling GV, et al. 1988. Isolation and comparison of *Escherichia coli* strains from canine and human patients with urinary tract infections. *Infect Immun* 56:2601–2609.
64. Mahaffey MB, Barsanti JA, Crowell WA, et al. 1989. Cystography: effect of technique on diagnosis of cystitis in dogs. *Vet Radiol* 30:261–267.
65. Measley RE, Levison ME. 1991. Host defense mechanisms in the pathogenesis of urinary tract infection. *Med Clin North Am* 75:275–286.
66. Memon MA, Mickelsen WD, Johnson CA, et al. 1993. Diagnosis and treatment of closed-cervix pyometra in a bitch. *J Am Vet Med Assoc* 203:509–512.
67. Merenich WM, Popky GL. 1991. Radiology of renal infection. *Med Clin North Am* 75:425–469.
68. Metzger FL, Hattel AL, White DG. 1993. Hematuria, hyperestrogenemia, and hyperprogesteronemia due to a Sertoli-cell tumor in a bilaterally cryptorchid dog. *Canine Pract* 18:32–35.
69. Mullen HS, Matthiesen DT, Scavelli TD. 1990. Results of surgery and postoperative complications in 92 dogs treated for prostatic abscessation by a multiple Penrose drain technique. *J Am Anim Hosp Assoc* 26:369–379.
70. Nemzek JA, Homco LD, Wheaton LG, et al. 1992. Cystic ovaries and hyperestrogenism in a canine female pseudohermaphrodite. *J Am Anim Hosp Assoc* 28:402–406.
71. Neuwirth L, Kuperus JH, Calderwood-Mays M, et al. 1995. Comparative study of indium-111 leukocytes and nephrosonography for detection of experimental pyelonephritis in dogs. *Vet Radiol Ultrasound* 36:253–258.
72. Neuwirth L, Mahaffey M, Crowell W, et al. 1993. Comparison of excretory urography and ultrasonography for detection of experimentally induced pyelonephritis in dogs. *Am J Vet Res* 54:660–669.
73. Nickel JC, Downey J, Costerton JW. 1992. Movement of *Pseudomonas aeruginosa* along catheter surfaces. *Urology* 39:93–98.
74. Oluoch AO, Weisiger R, Siegel AM, et al. 1996. Trends of bacterial infections in dogs: characterization of *Staphylococcus intermedius* isolates (1990–1992). *Canine Pract* 21:12–19.
75. Osborne CA. 1995. Three steps to effective management of bacterial urinary tract infections: diagnosis, diagnosis, diagnosis. *Comp Cont Educ Vet Med* 17:1233–1249.
76. Osborne CA, Lees GE. 1995. Bacterial infections of the canine and feline urinary tract, pp 759–797. *In* Osborne CA, Finco DR (eds), Canine and feline nephrology and urology. Williams & Wilkins, Baltimore, MD.
77. Osborne CA, Lulich JP. 1992. Control of chronic relapsing feline bacterial pyelonephritis with the aid of enrofloxacin, pp 27–32. *In* Proceedings of the First International Baytril Symposium, Bonn, Germany.
78. Papich MG. 1996. Comments on ceftiofur sodium. *Adv Small Anim Med Surg* 9:1–2.
79. Peter AT, Steiner JM, Adams LG. 1995. Diagnosis and medical management of prostate disease in the dog. *Semin Vet Med Surg* 10:35–42.
80. Polzin DJ. 1994. Management of recurrent urinary tract infections. *Compend Cont Educ Pract Vet* 16:1565–1571.
80a. Polzin DJ. 1997. Management of recurrent bacterial urinary tract infections. *Suppl Compend Cont Educ Pract Vet* 19:47–52.
81. Potter K, Hancock DH, Gallina AM. 1991. Clinical and pathologic features of endometrial hyperplasia, pyometra, and endometritis in cats: 79 cases (1980–1985). *J Am Vet Med Assoc* 198:1427–1431.
82. Pugh CR, Konde LJ. 1991. Sonographic evaluation of canine testicular and scrotal abnormalities: a review of 26 case histories. *Vet Radiol* 32:243–250.
83. Purswell BJ. 1995. Vaginal disorders, pp 1642–1648. *In* Ettinger SJ, Feldman EC (eds), Textbook of veterinary internal medicine. WB Saunders, Philadelphia, PA.
84. Quint HJ, Drach GW, Rappaport WD, et al. 1992. Emphysematous cystitis: a review of the spectrum of disease. *J Urol* 147:134–137.
85. Rawlings CA, Crowell WA, Barsanti JA, et al. 1994. Intracapsular subtotal prostatectomy in normal dogs: use of an ultrasonic surgical aspirator. *Vet Surg* 23:182–189.
86. Renton JP, Boyd JS, Harvey MJA. 1993. Observations on the treatment and diagnosis of open pyometra in the bitch (*Canis familiaris*). *J Reprod Fert Suppl* 47:465–469.
87. Riley DK, Classen DC, Stevens LE, et al. 1995. A large randomized clinical trial of a silver-impregnated urinary catheter: lack of efficacy and staphylococcal superinfection. *Am J Med* 98:349–356.
87a. Ritt MG, Fossum TW. 1997. Successful treatment of uterine torsion and fetal retention in a postparturient Great Pyrenees bitch with septic peritonitis and post-thrombotic complications. *J Am Anim Hosp Assoc* 33:537–539.
88. Roberts JA, Kaack MB, Fussell EN. 1993. Adherence to urethral catheters by bacteria causing nosocomial infections. *Urology* 41:338–342.
89. Schaer M, Ackerman N, Ellison G, et al. 1992. Bilateral pyonephrosis, hydroureter, renal failure, and urethral obstruction in a cat. *Feline Pract* 20:19–23.
90. Schwarz K. 1991. Zur beteiligung von *E. coli* an erkrankungen des urogenitaltraktes des hundes. *Kleintierpraxis* 36:179–184.
91. Senior DF. 1996. The use of enrofloxacin in the management of urinary tract infections in dogs and cats. *Suppl Compend Cont Educ Pract Vet* 18:89–95.
92. Senior DF, deMan P, Svanborg C. 1992. Serotype, hemolysin production, and adherence characteristics of strains of *Escherichia coli* causing urinary tract infections in dogs. *Am J Vet Res* 53:494–498.
93. Sevelius E, Tidholm A, Thoren-Tolling K. 1990. Pyometra in the dog. *J Am Anim Hosp Assoc* 26:33–38.
94. Stamm WE, Hooton TM. 1993. Management of urinary tract infections in adults. *N Engl J Med* 329:1328–1334.
95. Strom B, Linde-Forsberg C. 1993. Effects of ampicillin and trimethoprim-sulfamethoxazole on the vaginal bacterial flora of bitches. *Am J Vet Res* 54:891–896.
96. Suksawat J, Cox HU, O'Reilly KL, et al. 1996. Inhibition of bacterial adherence to canine uroepithelial cells using cranberry juice extract (abstract). *J Vet Intern Med* 10:167.
97. Tacker JR. 1992. Successful use of fluconazole for treatment of urinary tract fungal infections. *J Urol* 148:1917–1918.
98. Tenner SM, Yadven MW, Kimmel PL. 1992. Acute pyelonephritis. *Postgrad Med* 91:261–268.
99. Van Duijkeren E. 1992. Significance of the vaginal bacterial flora in the bitch: a review. *Vet Rec* 131:367–369.
100. Vieler E, Herbst W, Baumgartner W, et al. 1994. Isolation of a parainfluenzavirus type 2 from the prostatic fluid of a dog. *Vet Rec* 135:384–385.
101. Von Berky AG, Townsend WL. 1993. The relationship between the prevalence of uterine lesions and the use of medroxyprogesterone acetate for canine population control. *Aust Vet J* 70:249–250.
101a. Wadas B, Kuhn I, Lagerstedt AS, et al. 1996. Biochemical phenotypes of *Escherichia coli* in dogs: comparison of isolates isolated from bitches suffering from pyometra and urinary tract infection with isolates from faeces of healthy dogs. *Vet Microbiol* 52:293–300.
102. Warren JW. 1991. The catheter and urinary tract infection. *Med Clin North Am* 75:481–493.
103. Watson ADJ, Culvenor JA, Middleton DJ, et al. 1986. Distal renal tubular acidosis in a cat with pyelonephritis. *Vet Rec* 119:65–68.
104. Watson E, Roberts RE. 1993. Discospondylitis in a cat. *Vet Radiol Ultrasound* 34:397–398.
105. Watts JR, Wright PJ, Whithear KC. 1996. Uterine, cervical, and vaginal microflora of the normal bitch throughout the reproductive cycle. *J Small Anim Pract* 37:54–60.
105a. Wendt K, Stellmacher H. 1996. Infectious burdens of reproduction of female dogs. *Tierarztl Prax* 24:79–84.
106. Wheaton LG, Johnson AL, Parker AJ, et al. 1989. Results and complications of surgical treatment of pyometra: a review of 80 cases. *J Am Anim Hosp Assoc* 25:563–568.
107. Wilke JR. 1990. Use of antimicrobial drugs to prevent infections in veterinary patients. *Probl Vet Med* 2:298–311.
108. Wilson SM, Odeon A. 1992. Disseminated *Aspergillus terreus* infection in a dog. *J Am Anim Hosp Assoc* 28:447–450.
109. Wong-Beringer A, Jocobs RA, Guglielmo J. 1992. Treatment of funguria. *JAMA* 267:2780–2785.
110. Wuggenig K, Koppel E. 1992. Emphysematous cystitis in a Cocker Spaniel bitch. *Wien Tierarztl Wochenschr* 79:38–40.
110a. Yates DG. 1996. The antimicrobial sensitivity of bacteria isolated from 30 cases of pyometra in the bitch. *Irish Vet J* 49:709–710.
111. Yeager AE, Concannon PW. 1995. Ultrasonography of the reproductive tract of the female dog and cat, pp 1040–1052. *In* Bonagura JD (ed), Kirk's current veterinary therapy XII. WB Saunders, Philadelphia, PA.
112. Zanotti S, Kaplan P, Garlick D, et al. 1989. Endocarditis associated with a urinary bladder foreign body in a dog. *J Am Anim Hosp Assoc* 25:557–561.

Chapter 92

Central Nervous System Infections

William R. Fenner

ETIOLOGY

CNS inflammation may be caused by infections, immune disorders, or idiopathic mechanisms. Such inflammation is described as encephalitis, myelitis, and meningitis on the basis of whether the process affects brain, spinal cord, and meninges, respectively. Rapid and accurate diagnosis is desired in patients with CNS inflammations, because they may be either controlled or cured by using appropriate therapy.

In comparison with infections involving other organ systems, CNS infections are uncommon in animals. The frequency of various causes of meningoencephalitis in dogs was reported, in decreasing order, as viral (e.g., canine distemper virus [CDV] and parainfluenza virus encephalitis; see Chapters 3 and 7), presumed immune meningitis (steroid-responsive meningitis-arteritis, juvenile polyarteritis-meningitis; see Chapter 84), protozoal (neosporosis, toxoplasmosis; see Chapter 80), idiopathic (granulomatous meningoencephalitis, Pug encephalitis; see Chapter 84), bacterial (this chapter), and rickettsial (see Chapters 28 and 29).[43] The low prevalence of CNS infections results from its protection by barriers rather than a scarcity of infectious agents. To infect the CNS, organisms must either elude the host's barrier system (e.g., CDV via lymphocytes) or the barrier system must be disrupted (e.g., CNS ischemia with vasculitis)[10, 23, 26] More infections result from an organism's ability to bypass CNS defense mechanisms than result from an organism's unique neurotropism.

Bacterial meningitis is an inflammatory response to bacterial invasion of meninges and CSF. Such infections can rapidly disseminate and, on the basis of the virulence of the pathogen, lead to serious illness and death.[23] Bacterial meningitis, which can be localized or diffuse, occurs when pathogenic organisms overcome (or elude) host defense mechanisms and reach the subarachnoid CSF. Meningitis typically causes diffuse or multifocal lesions in dogs and cats, although the clinical signs may not reflect the disease's diffuse nature.[43] Brain abscesses, which result from a focal pyogenic infection, appear to result from contiguous spread of infections, such as progression of otitis interna, more than from hematogenous spread of organisms. Brain abscesses are uncommon in the dog and cat.[10, 25] This finding may in part be due to the inability of the CNS to form scar tissue, which in other tissue restricts the spread of pyogenic infections. Because epidural abscess develops outside the parenchyma of the CNS, true abscess formation can occur. Spinal epidural abscesses are more common than cranial epidural abscesses because of the greater available space in the spinal canal.

Although bacterial and rickettsial meningoencephalitis are relatively infrequent (e.g., bacterial infections account for about 7% of meningoencephalitis patients),[43] they are the most likely to be cured by antimicrobial therapy. This chapter focuses on bacterial infections. Other infectious causes of CNS inflammation are covered in other chapters. Bacteria commonly associated with meningoencephalitis in dogs and cats include *Staphylococcus intermedius, S. epidermidis, S. albus, Pasteurella multocida, Actinomyces, Nocardia,* and various anaerobes, including *Bacteroides, Fusobacterium, Peptostreptococcus,* and *Eubacterium.*[8] *Flavobacterium breve* has been isolated from one dog.[12a] In patients in which multiple organisms are identified, it is probable that one or more organisms will be anaerobic.[8]

Prospective data from large case series of appropriately diagnosed and treated dogs or cats with meningitis or meningoencephalitis are lacking in the veterinary literature. Most relatively large published case series are retrospective and pathology based; the patient's antemortem evaluation is thereby frequently incomplete. Owing to this lack of case series, it cannot be stated with certainty whether bacterial meningoencephalitis is actually less frequent in veterinary patients than in human patients or just not as well recognized. Clinicians must also depend on either limited veterinary clinical trials or careful extrapolation from the human literature when establishing therapeutic protocols. Knowledge learned in treatment of animal infections has been beneficial in the development of current human therapeutic protocols.

PATHOGENESIS

Location of an infection in the CNS is determined by the interplay among several factors, including the etiologic agent, its route of entry into the CNS, whether the infection remains focal or becomes generalized, and the character of the host's immune response.[10] The most common route of infection is hematogenous, with direct invasion, contiguous effect, and parameningeal spread and entry along nerve roots also serving as routes of infection (Table 92–1).

Several barriers limit a microorganism's entry into the CNS. The principal barrier to hematogenous entry is the blood-brain barrier (BBB), which provides an anatomic and physiologic barrier between the systemic circulation and the CNS parenchyma. The anatomic BBB is created by the CNS capillaries, which have tight junctions between endothelial cells, lack basement membrane fenestrations, and are enveloped by astroglial foot processes (Fig. 92–1).[10] Hematogenous infections must penetrate this barrier to enter the sub-

Table 92–1. Source and Localization of Nonneurotrophic Infections of the CNS

POINT OF ENTRY	USUAL LOCATION OR TYPE OF INFECTION
Hematogenous	Diffuse subarachnoid infection Focal parenchymal abscess or granuloma
Spinal cord	Diffuse subarachnoid infection
Paranasal sinuses	Frontal lobes Focal epidural abscess Diffuse epidural empyema
Petrous temporal bone (otitis media)	Temporal lobe (cerebrum) Cerebellum Brain stem (cerebellopontomedullary junction)
Cranial nerves	Basilar meninges Most frequently cranial nerves VII and VIII

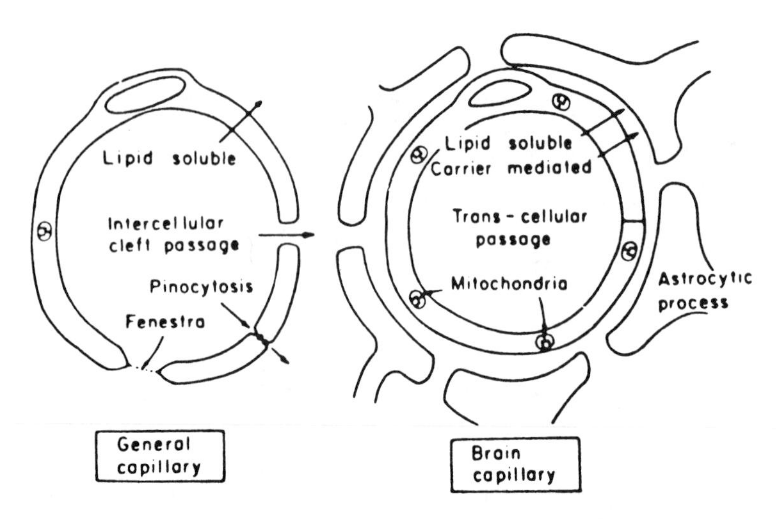

Figure 92–1. Comparison of features of systemic capillaries and the capillary endothelial cells of the brain. (From Oldendorf WH: *In* Bito LL, Dauson H, Fenstermacher JD: Experimental Eye Research. Supplement, Vol 25; The Ocular and Cerebrospinal Fluids. Academic Press, 1977, pp 177–190. Reprinted with permission).

arachnoid space. In viral infections, this activity occurs when infected lymphocytes are transported across the BBB. In general, the site and mechanism for bacterial invasion across the BBB remain poorly understood. Certain bacteria may have the capacity to adhere to the BBB because of their pili or cell wall components. Others may be transported across the BBB inside phagocytic cells, a process similar to that used by many viruses.[45, 47] The BBB is also important when determining a drug's capacity to enter the CNS and is discussed further under Therapy.

Barriers to direct or contiguous (parameningeal) infections include the meninges, spinal column, and skull. Direct invasion by microorganisms is usually preceded by some injury that provides access across these protective membranes. Contiguous spread is a fairly common cause of bacterial infections of the spinal column (i.e., diskospondylitis), but the infection rarely invades the CNS itself. Contiguous brain infections, such as migration from an inner ear infection, are also seen. In dogs and cats, bacterial migration along a nerve appears to be a relatively rare method of entry into the CNS. *Listeria monocytogenes* is an organism that may use this route. Refer to gram-positive bacterial infections, Chapter 35.

Whereas hematogenous spread predisposes the patient to meningitis, contiguous transaxonal infections are more likely to cause pyogenic encephalitis (brain abscesses). Contiguous spread typically arises from otitis media, chronic sinusitis, or epidural abscesses.[43, 48] When hematogenous spread does cause pyogenic encephalitis, it is usually in the presence of some event (e.g., vasculitis) that has caused an area of focal brain necrosis where the infection becomes established. Once an infection is established in the CNS, host defense mechanisms are essentially absent, allowing for rapid progression of the infection. Opsonic activity, even in infected CSF, is quite low; therefore, mechanisms to promote bacterial phagocytosis are highly inefficient.[23]

In short, a successful CNS pathogen must pass the host's mucosal epithelium, invade and survive in the intravascular space, cross the BBB, and finally survive and reproduce in the CNS and CSF.[26] Systemic infections, which may ultimately lead to CNS bacterial infections, arise from splenic abscesses, pleuritis, lung abscesses, vegetative endocarditis, bite wounds, urinary tract infections, pneumonia, infected cranial sinuses, and middle ear infections.[2, 9, 19, 23, 39, 43] Circumstances that facilitate a systemic infection in establishing a CNS infection include a sustained bacteremia, bacterial adhesion to BBB components and/or transport within phagocytes that have the capacity to cross the BBB, injury to the BBB or meningeal barrier system (e.g., head trauma), immune deficiency states, vasculitis, parameningeal localization of infections, and virtual absence of host humoral defense mechanisms inside the CNS.[23, 43]

Meningeal inflammation is largely responsible for the clinical signs seen in meningitis, more than the direct effects of organisms. Bacterial cell wall components in CSF stimulate local production and release of cytokines in CSF, including interleukin-1, tumor necrosis factor (TNF), and macrophage inflammatory proteins 1α, 1β, and 2.[21, 23, 36] These factors attract WBCs and promote meningeal and ependymal inflammation. CSF pleocytosis, which occurs with bacterial infections, is largely neutrophilic in acute stages. Pleocytosis may lead to further chemotactic attraction of leukocytes, creating a positive feedback cycle with worsening disease. Changes caused by meningeal inflammation include increased BBB permeability, vasculitis of penetrating vessels, CNS edema, and secondary inflammation of tissues adjacent to meninges. Vasculitis may lead to local tissue infarction, a phenomenon seen in steroid-responsive meningitis-arteritis of young dogs (see Chapter 84).[14, 38, 44] Ependymal inflammation may lead to obstructed CSF flow with secondary hydrocephalus, a phenomenon well demonstrated in feline infectious peritonitis (FIP), virus meningoencephalitis of cats (see Chapter 11), and parainfluenza virus meningoencephalitis of dogs (see Chapter 7). Once sufficient numbers of bacteria proliferate in the subarachnoid space, they may pass through the pores of the arachnoid villi, enter the venous sinuses, and enter the systemic circulation. Bacteremia may be either the cause or result of meningitis.

Organism effects are determined by whether the bacteria produce toxins (e.g., *Clostridium*) or vasculitis (e.g., *Haemophilus*) or is neurotropic. Bacterial toxins may produce more CNS injury than the primary inflammation surrounding the organism, resulting in severe clinical dysfunction even with low-grade infection. Vasculitis produced by organisms may result in CNS infarctions with peracute worsening of clinical signs. Certain bacteria, especially gram-negative rods, produce more damage to the meninges than do gram-positive organisms. Organisms such as *Corynebacterium* spp., *Nocardia*, and *Serratia marcescens* are of low virulence and usually only produce infection in immunocompromised hosts. If an organism is neurotropic (e.g., CDV, FIV), it will cause direct destruction of neural elements.

Because few bacteria are neurotropic, most produce secondary neural damage. Secondary effects of CNS infection may be profound. Compression of healthy tissue by the accumulation of pyogenic exudates may produce mass lesions. Inflammation results in fibrin deposition, vein thrombosis, and arteritis. Degenerating leukocytes release toxins producing further vasospasm, local ischemia, and tissue edema. In some cases of encephalitis, there is a high risk for brain herniation.[10] With meningitis, there is marked resistance to CSF outflow through the arachnoid granulations, resulting in elevations of CSF pressure. The potential for herniation is high with increased CSF pressure and may be reduced with glucocorticoids.

Several mechanisms may alert the peripheral immune system to the presence of foreign antigens in the CNS. CSF may eventually drain via lymphatic pathways to the retropharyngeal lymph nodes. Choroid plexus epithelial cells may take up foreign antigens on their apical surfaces exposed to the CSF. They then process antigen to circulating T cells that enter the extracellular space through fenestrated vascular endothelial cells in capillaries. Once significant populations of lymphocytes reach the CSF, astrocytes and potentially microglia may act as antigen-presenting cells.

During meningitis, tight junctions of the BBB open, which facilitates antibody entry into CSF, as does elevated plasma antibody levels. Some immunoglobulins found in CSF are the result of extravasation across an open BBB. Infection with some organisms (CDV, *Toxoplasma*, *Borrelia*) results in local production of immunoglobulins by blood-derived plasma cells that migrate into CNS. Most phagocytic cells present in CNS inflammation also originate from blood. The peak inflammatory response occurs about 72 hours after the infection begins and is neutrophilic with bacterial infections. After a CNS infection becomes established, repair of the BBB may isolate the CNS from systemic immune responses, delaying or preventing infection control.

CLINICAL FINDINGS

Systemic Signs

Many patients with CNS infections have nonspecific clinical signs of systemic illness in addition to signs of CNS involvement.[43] Some patients also have concomitant (often primary) infections in other organ systems with respective clinical signs. For meningitis, fever may result from the inflammatory process, or hyperthermia may be present because of muscle tremors, seizures, or exertional activity. Some animals with meningitis have ophthalmic inflammation, including retinitis, choroiditis, uveitis, and vasculitis of retinal vessels. Abnormalities of heart rate and rhythm or vomiting may occur either as a result of elevated intracranial pressures or of direct brain stem involvement. In advanced disease, with severe brain edema or mass effect, brain herniation with acute respiratory insufficiency may be seen. Sepsis may be noted in some of these patients, with associated shock, hypotension, and/or disseminated intravascular coagulation (DIC).[25] If the patient has endocarditis as the source of the CNS infection, the patient might be expected to have a heart murmur.[9]

CNS Signs

Classically, meningitic or meningoencephalitic patients are described as having diffuse or multifocal signs; however, many such patients will have focal abnormalities on examination.[43] The presence of multifocal or diffuse signs should be a cardinal indicator of inflammation. The presence of focal signs does not exclude inflammation from consideration.

Classic signs of meningitis include paraspinal discomfort, paraspinal muscle rigidity, and decreased vertebral mobility, combined with a stiff, short-strided gait.[39] Hyperesthesia on muscle palpation or traction on limbs is frequent. Vomiting, photophobia, nuchal rigidity, and depressed mental status are often associated with meningeal inflammation. Additional signs of neurologic dysfunction vary according to the CNS area involved. Forebrain diseases are principally characterized by behavioral or personality changes and seizures. Other cerebral abnormalities include circling, menace deficit, upper motor neuron facial muscle weakness, reduced facial pain sensation, and abnormal postural reaction. Brain stem involvement is manifest by depressed consciousness, head tilt, loss of balance, ataxia, limb weakness, and multiple cranial nerve deficits, especially pathologic nystagmus. Cerebellar disorders are usually characterized by ataxia, tremor, and pathologic nystagmus. Spinal cord involvement results in limb ataxia and weakness.

DIAGNOSIS

Any dog or cat with progressive, multifocal CNS dysfunction, with or without meningeal irritation, should be evaluated for meningoencephalitis. If a patient has meningitis without parenchymal CNS signs, steroid-responsive meningitis-arteritis and bacterial or eosinophilic meningitis should be considered. With parenchymal CNS involvement, viral, fungal, protozoal, and idiopathic causes of meningoencephalitis become statistically more probable than bacterial causes. Bacterial encephalitis, as opposed to bacterial meningitis, is more likely to cause signs of a space-occupying mass than typical signs of meningitis.[8, 48] Hematologic and biochemical changes, when seen, are nonspecific (e.g., leukocytosis with or without a left shift) and simply reflect the presence of an inflammatory process. Because of the BBB, the absence of leukocytosis does not eliminate meningitis from consideration.

CSF Evaluation

The crucial diagnostic test for meningitis remains early CSF evaluation with both cytologic examination and protein evaluation, which includes electrophoresis. Testing both serum and CSF either for antigens (e.g., cryptococcal antigen) or antibodies against infectious agents plays an increasing role in the diagnosis of meningoencephalitis, but is of less value in establishing a cause in bacterial meningitis. Examination for organism-specific antigens or antibodies is also valuable in certain diseases (e.g., canine distemper).

CSF evaluation remains crucial in meningoencephalitis patients because of the expanded role of glucocorticoids in treating meningitis. Diseases in which glucocorticoid use probably remains absolutely or relatively contraindicated include fungal and protozoal infections. Glucocorticoid treatment is controversial but sometimes beneficial with viral meningoencephalitis (e.g., FIP and canine distemper). Short-term glucocorticoid therapy may be beneficial when combined with an antimicrobial drug (e.g., bacterial meningitis). Glucocorticoids are the treatment of choice for some immune-mediated conditions (e.g., eosinophilic meningitis, steroid-responsive meningitis-arteritis, and granulomatous meningoencephalitis). Currently, CSF analysis is the best tool for distinguishing between inflammatory causes and choosing the most appropriate therapy.

CSF analysis can help confirm the presence of an inflammatory process, determine the nature of the inflammation, often determine a specific cause, and, in some cases, monitor therapeutic effectiveness. False-negative CSF results occur for several reasons. First, bulk flow of CSF tends to be from cranial to caudal. CSF collected from the cerebellomedullary cistern may be normal in a patient with a focal spinal cord infection. Second, inflammation must involve the ventricular system or subarachnoid space for cells to be shed into CSF. Deeply seated inflammations may disrupt the BBB, allowing protein leakage without cell migration into the CSF. In such patients, even though cell numbers may be normal, cytologic examination may reveal abnormal cell distribution.[7] Bacterial infections are more likely to involve the ventricular and subarachnoid spaces and produce marked neutrophilic pleocytosis, and the chance of a missed diagnosis is lessened. With chronic bacterial meningitis or with antibacterial treatment, fewer cells that are of more mononuclear types are found in CSF. Predominantly nonsuppurative cytologic findings, therefore, should not eliminate bacterial infection from consideration.

CSF may be collected at the cerebellomedullary cistern or the lumbar space. The lumbar space is more difficult to enter, yields smaller volumes, and has a higher rate of blood contamination; therefore, the cerebellomedullary cistern is the preferred collection site. However, analysis of CSF collected at the cerebellomedullary cistern may not always demonstrate abnormalities in lower spinal cord inflammatory diseases.

Technique

The equipment needed for both the collection and the analysis includes a small-gauge (20 or 22), 1.5- to 2.5-inch spinal needle; a container for the fluid; and, if pressure will be measured, a three-way stopcock and manometer. In cats, because pressures are rarely measured, a scalp infusion (butterfly) catheter may be used instead of a spinal needle. These catheters allow better control over the needle and allow the clinician to identify blood contamination in the tubing before it contaminates the entire sample.

All patients should be anesthetized and intubated during the collection process. Complications of CSF collection include anesthetic accidents, damage to the CNS with the needle, and brain herniation after anesthesia and/or CSF removal. Any animal that has a deterioration of consciousness before CSF collection or papilledema on fundic examination is at increased risk for herniation. If during the CSF collection the fluid pressure appears elevated, collection should be stopped, and the patient should be allowed to recover from anesthesia. Hyperventilation with oxygen before fluid removal may help decrease intracranial pressure.[10]

For collection from the cerebellomedullary cistern, hair on the cranial portion of the dorsal neck and back of the skull is clipped from between the pinnae caudally to the second or third cervical vertebra. The animal is placed in lateral recumbency, and the clipped area is prepared for a sterile procedure. If necessary, padding is used to straighten the cervical spine. The head is held at 90 degrees to the long axis of the body (Fig. 92–2).[10] Overflexion of the neck may obstruct the patient's airway as well as occlude the jugular veins. Jugular venous occlusion artifactually elevates intracranial pressure. Landmarks for penetration are the wings of the atlas (C1) and the occipital protuberance. An imaginary T is drawn, using the line between the cranial aspect of the two wings of the atlas for one bar and the midline of the neck as determined by the occipital protuberance for the other. The point at which the two lines cross is the site where the needle is inserted (see Fig. 92–2). The skin is pinched up, and the needle is inserted through it to prevent sudden, inadvertent needle advancement. The needle bevel is pointed cranially toward the occipital protuberance. The needle is advanced through the muscle layers on a line approximately perpendicular to the spine's long axis. When the needle advances through the subarachnoid space, a sudden loss of resistance is felt. Muscle twitching is rarely noted when the dura is penetrated at this site. As soon as the change in resistance is felt, the stylet is removed and CSF should flow.

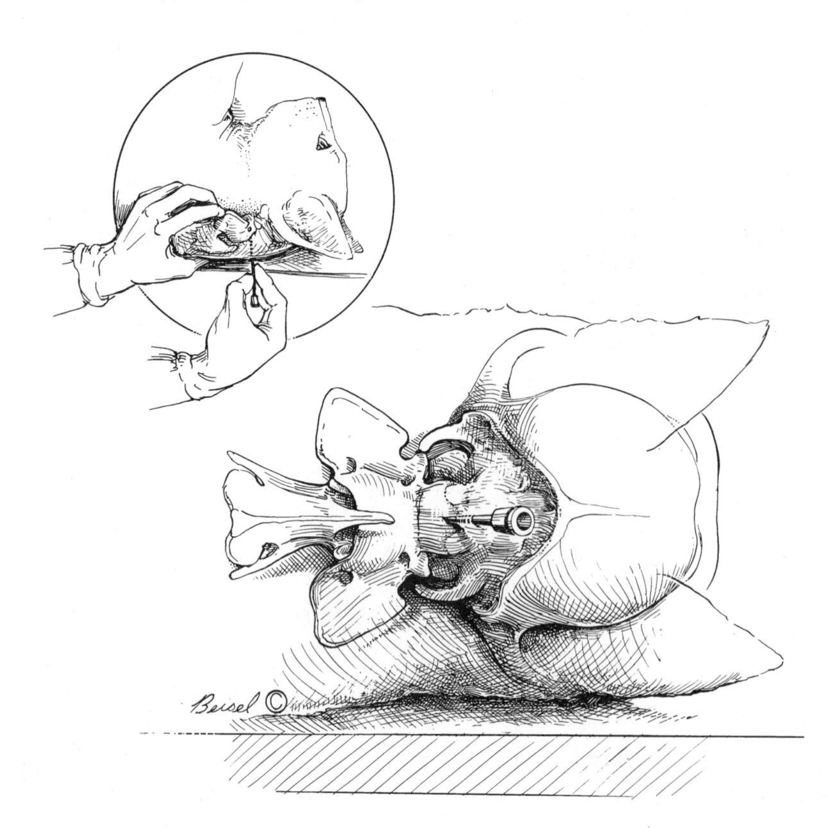

Figure 92–2. One landmark for CSF collection is the intersection of a line drawn transversely between the wings of the atlas on the cranial aspect and a midline drawn through the occipital protuberance. (From Greene CE, Oliver JE: *In* Ettinger SJ (ed): Textbook of Veterinary Internal Medicine: Diseases of the Dog and Cat, ed 2. WB Saunders, 1983, pp 419–460. Reprinted with permission).

CSF will flow immediately if a butterfly catheter is utilized, and the cap on the line is loosened. To prevent accidental needle advancement, the needle should be held with thumb and forefinger each time the stylet is removed. If CSF does not appear after a few seconds, the stylet is replaced and the needle advanced further. If the location feels correct and still no CSF flows, the jugular veins are occluded to increase CSF pressures. If there is still no flow, it is possible that the animal has suffered brain herniation and CSF flow is blocked.

If the needle hits bone, the needle tip is advanced cranially or caudally a few millimeters. If that does not work, the needle is removed, and the entire collection process is started over. The average distance between skin and subarachnoid space varies with patient size. Distances are 0.5 inch for cats or for dogs smaller than 4.5 kg; 0.75 inch for dogs 4.5 to 9.1 kg; 1 inch for dogs 9.1 to 22.7 kg; 1.5 inches for dogs 22.7 to 50.9 kg; and 2 inches for dogs larger than 50.9 kg.[10] When fluid begins to flow, it is best to collect it by allowing it to drip into a container or syringe. CSF should always be collected in plastic containers because WBCs adhere to glass.

The *lumbar subarachnoid space* is the ideal site to collect CSF when there are spinal cord diseases or when it is impossible to collect it from the cerebellomedullary cistern. Collection sites will be the L7 to S1 interspaces in the cat and the L5 to L7 interspaces in the dog. Before anesthesia, the area is clipped on the back between the last rib and the tuber coxae for a distance of 2 to 3 inches on each side of the midline. After anesthesia is induced, the animal is placed in lateral recumbency and the spine flexed. The forelimbs are drawn back between the pelvic limbs or vice versa. The spine should be parallel to the table, with padding if needed to ensure a straight line. A 20- or 22-gauge needle is adequate, but for this procedure it generally should be 2.5 to 3 inches long. The vertebra's dorsal spinal process is chosen for a landmark. The needle bevel faces cranially and should also be inserted just cranially to the dorsal spinous process of the caudal vertebra along a line perpendicular to the spine's long axis. The needle is advanced until bony resistance is felt and then moved cranially or caudally a few millimeters to find the interspace. When the needle passes through the interarcuate ligament, a sudden loss of resistance is felt. As the needle penetrates the dura, the pelvic limbs may suddenly twitch. The needle stylet is removed and the orifice observed for CSF to appear. Because lumbar pressures are often quite low and the needle is longer (2.5 inches), the wait is longer than the 4 to 5 seconds needed during cerebellomedullary collection. If no CSF appears, the stylet is replaced and the needle advanced through the spinal cord until it contacts the bony floor of the spinal canal. The needle is withdrawn slightly; the stylet is removed; and the opening is observed for CSF flow. Spinal cord penetration is not ideal because it may produce cord injury and artifactual hemorrhage in the CSF sample. If pressures are adequate, CSF should always be collected by allowing it to drip into a plastic container. If the pressure is low, the needle too long, or the gauge of the needle too small, CSF flow may not be sufficient for spontaneous collection. In those cases, a syringe is used to aspirate CSF. The syringe increases the potential for blood contamination. Although CSF pressures can be measured with a manometer,[10] they are not as helpful as cytology and protein assessment in the evaluation of CNS infections.

Complications

Blood contamination, the most common problem with accurate CSF evaluation, is generally the result of penetration of meningeal vessels. If the fluid contains a trace of blood at the beginning of the collection process, the stylet is replaced and the needle left in place. After waiting 30 to 60 seconds, the stylet is removed to see whether the fluid has cleared. If there are still small traces of blood, CSF is collected in at least two portions, with the samples in separate containers. Often contamination will diminish during collection, leaving a second sample that is adequate for interpretation.

The most serious reported complication of CSF collection is brain herniation. In the presence of elevated intracranial pressure, the pressure shift created by CSF removal may precipitate a shift in intracranial contents (brain herniation). This sudden movement of intracranial contents may result in the patient's death; it may also be nonsymptomatic.[41] Brain herniation in dogs and cats has occurred in association with CSF collection and anesthesia.[10] In reports of anaerobic bacterial infections, three of four patients had CNS herniations, although it appeared that the herniations occurred before CSF collection rather than as a result of collection.[8] Progressive sensory and motor paralysis, pupillary size changes, sudden onset of pathologic nystagmus, and reflex abnormalities signal that brain herniation is occurring. The actual relationship between herniation and CSF collection is not as conclusive as once believed, so fear of herniation should not prevent CSF collection in a patient with suspected meningoencephalitis.[41]

Analysis

All CSF analyses should include a gross visual examination, cytologic analysis, biochemical analysis, and, when indicated by cytology, cultural or serologic evaluation. Typically, cerebellomedullary cisternal fluid has slightly more cells and lower protein concentrations than fluid from the lumbar space.[10]

Normal CSF is clear and colorless on gross examination. An increase in the number of WBCs and/or protein generally causes CSF to become turbid and assume an off-white to grayish color. Turbidity usually indicates cell count elevations above 500/μl. Centrifuge or sediment of CSF should take place before color is evaluated because blood contamination produces a pink discoloration. Persistence of the pink color indicates free hemoglobin and suggests previous subarachnoid hemorrhage rather than contamination during fluid collection. Yellow-orange (xanthochromic) fluid generally indicates hemorrhage, typically 1 or more days before CSF collection, or marked elevation of CSF protein (>100 mg/dl). Xanthochromia may occasionally be observed in patients with protracted icterus. In patients with pigment-producing bacteria such as *Pseudomonas*, the CSF may acquire a greenish tint.

The cytologic evaluation should include a total cell count on an unconcentrated CSF and slide preparation from a concentrated CSF sample for evaluation of cell types and differential numbers. It is essential to perform differential cytologic examinations on all CSF samples, even those with normal total cell counts.[7] Total cell count should be performed as soon as possible after collection, because CSF cells begin to degenerate rapidly after collection.[10] Refrigeration slows WBC lysis, if analysis cannot be done immediately. An aliquot of freshly collected CSF can also be mixed with 10% volume of bovine serum albumin or cell-free serum to help preserve cell number and morphology for longer periods. For the most accurate differential cell evaluation, cell-concentrating techniques are employed. In cytocentrifugation, the CSF is spun at 1500 *g* for 10 minutes in a conventional centrifuge[10] or 100 *g* for 10 minutes in a cytocentrifuge (Cytospin, Shandon Southern Instruments, Sewickley, PA).[7] Supernatant is removed, and the cells are resuspended by adding a drop of normal serum or 20% albumin. The protein provides better cell adherence to the slide and prevents cell-drying artifact. Staining is generally done with Wright or Giemsa stains.

In sedimentation, equal volumes of CSF and normal serum are combined in a hollow cylinder placed on the slide, and time is allowed for the cells to undergo sedimentation. The liquid is pipetted, the cylinder is removed, and the slide is stained. In a variation of this technique, filter paper is used to remove fluid. Sedimentation techniques require larger CSF volumes, although they preserve CSF cell architecture better than centrifugation techniques. For general practitioners, the sedimentation technique is simple and reliable.

Membrane filtration is another, less commonly used technique. It allows good cell architecture preservation but requires different staining techniques. Experience is needed for the reading of membrane filtration cytology for reliable results.

Normally, there are fewer than 5 WBCs/μl in the CSF regardless of collection site. Typically, with CNS inflammation, WBC numbers in CSF increase. The cell type and number reflect the type of inflammation, thus providing etiologic information, especially in acute, untreated CNS infections. Because not all infections cause ventriculitis or meningitis, normal cell counts do not exclude infectious processes. Artifactual increases in WBC counts can result from blood contamination. For each 500 RBCs/μl present as a result of blood contamination, WBC numbers in CSF increase by approximately 1 WBC/μl and protein by 1 mg/dl.[10] A more accurate correction factor can be determined by taking a sample of the patient's blood at the time of CSF collection and determining hematologic values. Plasma WBC-RBC ratio is multiplied by RBC concentration in CSF to obtain the expected number of WBCs from contamination. The expected contamination WBC count is used to determine the significance of the measured WBC count in CSF. The adjusted WBC count (observed minus expected contamination), or the observed-expected WBC ratio in CSF can be measured. Overall, the observed-expected WBC ratio is more accurate than the adjusted count in determining true WBC elevation. The observed-expected count appears more accurate in recognizing bacterial meningitis than viral or aseptic meningitis in humans, probably because there are higher WBC counts in bacterial meningitis. A ratio of 10 or greater is considered predictive of culture-positive bacterial infections.[24] Correcting for contamination may allow valid conclusions to be drawn in cases with mild contamination,[13a] but marked contamination makes most CSF uninterpretable.

Suppurative meningitis is diagnosed on the basis of an increased number of neutrophils in CSF (Table 92–2). In the early stages of bacterial infection, the predominant CSF cytology will be a neutrophilic pleocytosis. Similarly, neutrophilic pleocytosis may be observed in patients with steroid-responsive meningitis-arteritis and in patients with meningiomas. Features that may distinguish these diseases are patient age,

Table 92–2. Representative CSF Changes Seen in Various CNS Inflammatory Diseases of Dogs and Cats[a]

DISEASE (CHAPTER)	WBC[b] COUNT	WBC TYPE[c]	TOTAL PROTEIN CONCENTRATION (mg/dl)[d]	ALBUMIN PROPORTION	GLOBULIN PROPORTION	CSF ANTIBODIES DETECTED	ORGANISMS SEEN
Bacterial meningitis (92)	+ + (+ + +)	PMN (mixed)	+ + (+ + +)	+ +	+ +	Varies	Yes (Varies)
Steroid-responsive meningitis/arteritis (84)	+ + + (+ +)	Mixed (mono)	+ + + (+ +)	+ +	+ (+ +)	No (IgA)	No
Tumor (e.g., meningioma)-associated pleocytosis[e]	+ (+ +)	PMNs (mixed)	+ (+ +)	+ (+ +)	WNL	No	No
Granulomatous meningoencephalitis (84)	+ + (+ + +)	Mixed—PMN, mono	+ + (+ + +)	+ +	+ +	No	No
Feline infectious peritonitis (11)	+ + + (+ +)	Mixed—PMNs, some mono	+ + +	+ +	+ +	Yes (?)	No
Fungal meningoencephalitis (58–69)	+ +	Mixed—PMN, eos, mono	+ +	+ +	+ (+ +)	Varies	Varies
Protozoal meningoencephalitis (72–84)	+	Mixed—PMN, eos, mono	+ (+ +)	+	+ (+ +)	Variable	Rarely
Ehrlichiosis (28)	+ (+ +)	Mono	+	+	+	?	Varies
Rocky Mountain spotted fever (29)	+	Mixed (neutrophils)	+ (WNL)	+	+	?	No
Eosinophilic meningitis	+ (+ +)	Eos	+	+	+	No	No
Canine distemper (3)							
Inflammatory	+	Both mono	+	WNL	+	Yes	No
Noninflammatory	WNL (+)	(lymphocytes)	WNL	WNL	WNL (+)	No (varies)	No
Other viral encephalitis (7 and 26)	+	Mono	+ (+ +)	WNL	+	?	No
Necrotizing encephalitis, Yorkshire terriers (84)	+	Mono	+	+	+	No	No

[a]Symbols in parentheses indicate less frequent variations; for example, + (+ +) indicates that typically the test results are mildly elevated but in some patients are moderately elevated.
[b]WNL = <4/μl; + = 5–80/μl; + + = 81–500/μl; + + + = > 500/μl.
[c]Mono = lymphocytes, plasma cells, monocytes, and macrophages; mixed = mononuclear cells, neutrophils and eosinophils; PMN = neutrophils predominate; Eos = eosinophils predominate.
[d]WNL is < 25 mg/dl; + is mild elevation, 25–100 mg/dl; + + = moderate elevation, 100–300 mg/dl; + + + = marked elevation is > 300 mg/dl.
[e]For neoplasia, typically protein increase is greater than that of leukocytes (albuminocytologic dissociation); for lymphoma in subarachnoid space, greater number of cells are present of mononuclear variety.
WNL = within normal limits; + = mild elevation; + + = moderate elevation; + + + = marked elevation; ? = uncertain (see below for specifics on WBC count, WBC type and protein concentration).
Data from various sources, including Fenner,[10] Tipold,[43] Rand et al,[30] Chrisman.[6]

presence of organisms, character of neutrophils, levels of CSF protein as compared with cells, and history of illness. High levels of TNF-α in CSF has been an indicator of bacterial meningitis in people.[11a]

Steroid-responsive meningitis-arteritis (see Chapter 84) is typical when animals are younger than 2 years, when no organisms are seen in CSF, when the neutrophils are nontoxic, and when the disease has a waxing and waning course. The animals are often in more pain than those with bacterial meningitis as well. In this condition, there are typically disease-free intervals during which CSF is normal. These are punctuated by acute clinical exacerbations, often with a marked CSF pleocytosis and higher protein and IgA concentrations (see Table 92–2).

Bacterial meningoencephalitis is most likely to occur in dogs between 1 and 7 years of age. In some patients with bacterial meningitis, the organisms may be seen to be phagocytized within WBCs, the neutrophils are more likely to be toxic, and the clinical course is progressive. The dogs are generally in less pain and are less febrile than those with steroid-responsive meningitis. Free, nonphagocytized organisms in the CSF may be the result of contamination in the stain in slide preparation, so that the presence of nonphagocytized bacteria on stained slides should be interpreted cautiously. Many cases of antibiotic-responsive meningitis have no organisms visualized or cultured from CSF but are presumed to be caused by bacterial infection. Some of these cases are mistakenly identified as steroid-responsive meningitis because treatment is with glucocorticoids alone or in combination with antibiotics. Signs of bacterial meningitis can subside for indefinite periods with glucocorticoids. Antibiotics should therefore be tried alone first.

Patients with neutrophilic pleocytosis secondary to meningiomas have focal CNS signs, typically are older than 8 years, and have a progressive course. The neutrophils are usually mature and not toxic in appearance. Generally, the patients are neither febrile nor in pain. Neutrophilic pleocytosis is also rarely observed with meningeal carcinomatosis or meningeal sarcomatosis. Malignant cells may be observed, especially if multiple CSF collections are performed.[46]

In a mixed inflammatory process, CSF is composed of multiple cell types, including macrophages, lymphocytes, neutrophils, and sometimes plasma cells (see Table 92–2). In those patients with a mixed CSF cytology, nonbacterial diseases become more likely. These common causes of meningoencephalitis include viral, fungal, protozoal, and rickettsial infections and several noninfectious conditions.[10, 25, 39, 42, 43] Nonsuppurative inflammation is typified by increased numbers of mononuclear cells, especially lymphocytes, in the CSF. Nonsuppurative CSF is most typical of viral encephalitis. Rarely, patients with bacterial meningitis will have a primary, nonsuppurative CSF cytology. As any meningitis or meningoencephalitis becomes chronic, the CSF cytology will shift from a suppurative (neutrophilic) to either a mixed or a nonsuppurative cytologic pattern.[46] Additionally, with bacterial meningitis, as the disease becomes chronic, the total cell count in CSF decreases.[23] Thus, accurate knowledge of the duration of signs is crucial in evaluating CSF cytology. Because CSF cytology normally changes during the progression of meningoencephalitis, serial CSF collections are the most reliable diagnostic and prognostic methods.[10] The need for anesthesia, however, makes this difficult in dogs and cats. Table 92–2 reviews the expected CSF changes in the more common causes of meningoencephalitis in dogs and cats.[10, 25, 39, 42, 43]

If organisms are seen, the cytologic preparation should be stained with Gram's stain to aid in further identification. Negative Gram's stain results may be due to the effects of previous therapy or to low organism numbers in CSF.[23] False-positive identification of organisms may result from bacterial contamination of the staining reagent. With cytologically evident inflammation, the CSF sample should be inoculated into culture media. In veterinary medicine, negative culture results are common, even with known bacterial meningoencephalitis. Negative culture results may occur because of too few organisms in CSF, improper sample storage or transport, improper choice of culture technique, or inadequate culture media nutrients to support growth. Substances present in CSF may also actively inhibit organism growth.[10] Anaerobic cultures should be performed if there is radiographic evidence of a mass lesion or evidence of multiple organisms in CSF. Culturing CSF without evidence of inflammation is of little value.

Although CSF contains essentially the same biochemical constituents as plasma, they are present in different concentrations in the two fluids. Generally, CSF constituent levels are lower than corresponding serum levels. The two constituents most commonly measured are protein and glucose. In dogs and cats, protein from a cerebellomedullary cisternal tap is generally less than 25 mg/dl, whereas that from a lumbar puncture may be as high as 45 mg/dl.[10] CSF protein is usually increased in patients with meningoencephalitis, although the values remain much lower than the 5 to 8 g/dl of protein normally seen in plasma. Because storage of CSF does not significantly affect protein content, CSF may be sent to an outside laboratory for protein evaluation.

In encephalitis and meningitis, CSF protein elevations may result from increased BBB permeability, intrathecal immunoglobulin production, or a combination of both.[10, 40] Because many noninflammatory conditions also elevate CSF protein levels, quantitative and qualitative analysis utilizing electrophoresis or immunoelectrophoresis is desirable.[10] Unfortunately, routine screening tests (Pandy and Nonne-Appelt) do not identify specific CSF protein constituents. The relative CSF protein proportions provide some answers to questions about the causes of the protein changes (see Table 92–2). When globulins are the primary protein present, an inflammatory disease or CNS lymphoreticular neoplasm is likely, even with inconclusive cytology. Mixed CSF protein elevations support inflammation as a partial, but not the sole, cause of the protein elevation and further suggest that the meninges are involved in the inflammation. When albumin is the principal protein, a noninflammatory BBB injury is likely.[10, 40]

Normally, CSF glucose levels are about 60% to 80% of serum levels. In humans, the ratio between blood glucose and CSF glucose is routinely lower in bacterial meningoencephalitis. A similar relationship between bacterial meningoencephalitis and CSF–serum glucose ratios has not been established in dogs and cats.

Immunologic Testing

Detection of the presence of specific antibodies or antigens may be helpful in the diagnosis of viral, fungal, and rickettsial diseases but is less helpful in bacterial encephalitis. In most circumstances, the presence of antibodies is an indication of local immunoglobulin production, which suggests that the organism to which the antibodies are directed is the cause of the encephalitis. Yet, false-positive antibody levels can be caused by leakage of plasma proteins into the CSF as a result of fever or collection techniques. Antibodies may also be the result of previous infections. Increased albumin on CSF electrophoresis would support a false-positive diagnosis. The accuracy of CSF serology can be increased by evaluating parallel CSF and corresponding serum titers. Organism-specific antibody indexes or CSF-IgG indexes have been used for detection of specific infections[1] (see Diagnosis, Chapters 3, 45, 80, and 84).

Where available, countercurrent immunoelectrophoresis, coagglutination, or latex agglutination (LA) tests may help to identify bacteria by detection of bacterial antigens.[18] Patients with the highest quantity of CSF antigen carry guarded prognoses. These tests must be performed before therapy. There is no correlation between antigen quantity and prognosis once drug therapy has been initiated. CSF titers are probably more reliable in nonbacterial than bacterial causes of meningitis. CSF titers may also be more reliable indicators of active CNS involvement than serum titers, especially with protozoal, spirochetal, and rickettsial diseases.[46] Although measurement of bacterial antigen has been uncertain, cryptococcal antigens can be detected in CSF by the LA procedure (see Diagnosis, Chapter 61). CDV viral antigen has been detected in CSF cells utilizing immunofluorescent methods (see Chapter 3). Polymerase chain reaction has also been employed in detection of microorganisms in CSF.[28]

Other Diagnostics

Because bacterial meningoencephalitis normally originates from other body sites, the patient should be carefully examined for other sites of infection. This evaluation should include hemograms, urinalysis, and radiographs of structures adjacent to the suspected site of CNS infection. Culturing other body fluids, especially blood and urine, in addition to CSF may help identify the organism. Overall, such culture results are negative in more than half the cases with pathologically confirmed bacterial meningitis. In dogs with heart murmurs, echocardiography is indicated to screen for vegetative endocarditis.[9] Electroencephalopathy has been used to predict those animals likely to manifest seizures.[22a]

Magnetic resonance imaging (MRI) or computed tomography (CT) are the best tools available for identifying a space-occupying mass in meningoencephalitic patients. MRI and CT may also reveal complications such as secondary hydrocephalus. Evidence suggests a role for contrast-enhanced MRI in demonstrating meningeal inflammation.[22, 33] The changes seen may not be specific for bacterial meningitis, rather than simply reflecting meningeal inflammation from any cause.

THERAPY

Treating CNS infections requires controlling specific causative agents and providing supportive care for life-threatening complications such as brain edema. In some cases, presumptive therapy, on the basis of Gram's stain or intuition, may be instituted before cultures. If the organism can be isolated, subsequent treatment should be based on the culture and susceptibility results. In all cases, those drugs with better CNS penetration should be provided. Drugs that are active in infected fluid should also be used.

Antimicrobial Therapy

Ideal treatment involves the single least toxic, most effective, bactericidal drug. The chosen drug achieves therapeutic CNS levels during the acute, inflammatory phase and maintains them in the infection's healing phase.[3, 10] Bactericidal antimicrobials are essential for adequate therapy in bacterial meningoencephalitis because of the host's inefficient CNS immune defense mechanisms.[3, 27] As an example, CSF of rabbits with pneumococcal meningitis becomes sterile during the first 5 days of treatment with ampicillin or bactericidal chloramphenicol doses. If, however, chloramphenicol was given in bacteriostatic doses, the therapy consistently failed.[10]

A drug's ability to reach and maintain therapeutic blood levels is of special consideration in treating CNS diseases because the BBB limits the entry of many therapeutic agents into CSF. As a result, there are often significant discrepancies between serum and CSF drug concentrations. Although BBB permeability to drugs increases during acute inflammation, as it resolves, the barrier to drug entry is restored. Unless the chosen drug can maintain adequate levels in the presence of a normal barrier, the risk of incomplete therapy exists. Ideal drugs have low albumin binding, a low degree of ionization at physiologic pH, and a high lipid solubility (Table 92–3).

Higher CSF antibiotic concentrations may be required for maximum effect than those expected from the minimum inhibitory concentration (MIC) determined in vitro. This occurrence may be due to lowered CSF pH in meningitis, which reduces certain antimicrobials activity (e.g., aminoglycosides). The greater CSF protein levels in meningitis may increase a drug's protein binding (e.g., cephalosporins), lowering the clinically active free drug fraction. Another factor that may explain the need for higher drug doses is slower bacterial growth in CSF than in broth, when susceptibility testing is performed.

If possible, a drug available in a parenteral formulation is recommended because initial IV therapy may allow more rapid therapeutic CNS and CSF drug concentrations to be achieved. The drugs recommended for specific bacterial infections are presented in Table 92–4.[10] The recommended dose and routes of antimicrobials administered for treating

Table 92–3. Antimicrobial Drugs Penetrating Blood-Brain Barrier and Blood CSF Barriers

DRUG ACTION	GOOD PENETRATION	INTERMEDIATE PENETRATION	POOR PENETRATION
Microbiocidal drugs	Trimethoprim Metronidazole	Penicillin Ampicillin Methicillin Oxacillin Carbenicillin Ceftriaxone Ceftazidime Ceftizoxime Moxalactam Fluoroquinolones	1st-generation cephalosporins Aminoglycosides Clindamycin
Microbiostatic drugs	Chloramphenicol Sulfonamides	Tetracyclines Flucytosine	Amphotericin B Erythromycin Ketoconazole Itraconazole

Table 92–4. Recommended Antimicrobials for Specific Agents or Settings [10]

ORGANISM	FIRST CHOICES	SECOND CHOICES
Staphylococcus	Nafcillin	Vancomycin, vancomycin + rifampin, ampicillin, trimethoprim-sulfonamide
Streptococcus	Penicillin, ampicillin	Ceftriaxone, vancomycin
Actinomyces	Ampicillin	Minocycline
Gram-negative bacteria	Cefotaxime + ampicillin	Gentamicin + ampicillin, gentamicin + ceftriaxone
Pseudomonas	Ceftazidime + aminoglycoside[a]	Piperacillin + aminoglycoside,[a] carbenicillin + gentamicin[a]
Pasteurella	Ampicillin	Trimethoprim
Brucella	Minocycline	Gentamicin[a]
Salmonella	Ceftriaxone	Ampicillin, chloramphenicol
Enterococcus	Ampicillin	Minocycline
Bacteroides	Metronidazole	Chloramphenicol, piperacillin

[a]Fluoroquinolone can be substituted.

CNS infections are listed in Table 92–5.[3] Therapy should initially be started with ampicillin and/or a third-generation cephalosporin.[3, 23] After Gram's stain or culture results, therapy may be modified as appropriate.

Penicillins. These drugs reach therapeutic CSF concentrations in the presence of meningeal inflammation but penetrate noninflamed meninges poorly. Without meningeal inflammation, CSF penicillin concentrations are only 1% to 2% serum levels as contrasted with 10% to 18% in the presence of inflammation.[10] Meningeal inflammation is not as important a factor in order for ampicillin to reach high CSF concentrations.[10] High activity along with their low toxicity maintains their value in treating CNS bacterial infections.[3, 23, 49] Ampicillin and penicillin, therefore, remain first-choice drugs for treatment of meningitis in dogs and cats.[10] Gram-positive infections such as streptococcal infections are generally treated with penicillin. Because of reduced efficacy once the meningeal inflammation subsides, treatment may be switched to better-penetrating drugs such as trimethoprim-sulfonamide once clinical signs improve. Anaerobic and gram-negative infections may be treated with other members of the β-lactam family (see also Penicillins, Chapter 34). Newer drugs include aztreonam and imipenem.

Vancomycin. This drug is effective against methicillin-resistant staphylococci and streptococci.[3, 23] Vancomycin is poorly absorbed and has relatively poor penetration of noninflamed meninges, so that it is more likely to reach therapeutic CSF concentrations in the presence of meningeal inflammation. It is given primarily as an alternative therapy after other drugs have failed.

Chloramphenicol. Chloramphenicol reaches high CSF concentration (45–99% of serum concentrations) regardless of meningeal inflammation.[10] This drug also appears to concentrate in the CNS, reaching levels that exceed those in serum; however, large doses are required for bactericidal effects in the CNS.[10] There is a high relapse rate with this drug, suggesting it is not bactericidal at dosages used in dogs and cats. This drug is provided for treating gram-negative infections but is not a first-line drug. There appears to be no therapeutic difference between IV and oral chloramphenicol administration, although the oral form has a higher bioavailability.

Cephalosporins. The earliest generations of cephalosporins did not cross the BBB well, even in meningitic patients. Newer (third-generation) cephalosporins (e.g., moxalactam, ceftriaxone, and cefotaxime) cross both the normal and inflamed meninges.[3, 23] In addition to these, ceftizoxime and ceftazidime have been shown to be effective in the treatment of bacterial meningitis in people. This group of drugs is now considered first-line in the treatment of meningitis if the animal is severely affected and the client can afford the cost.

Trimethoprim-Sulfonamide. This drug combination is effective against several organisms causing human meningitis, such as *Pneumococcus*, *Meningococcus*, *Listeria*, *Haemophilus*, some *Staphylococcus*, and many gram-negative organisms.

Table 92–5. Antimicrobial Drug Dosages for CNS Bacterial and Fungal Infections of Dogs and Cats[a]

DRUG	DOSE[b]	ROUTE	INTERVAL (HOURS)
Penicillin (aqueous)	10–22 × 10^3 U/kg	IV	4–6
Ampicillin	5–22 mg/kg	IV	6
Carbenicillin	10–30 mg/kg	IV, IM	4–6
Oxacillin (or cloxacillin)	8.8–20 mg/kg	IV, PO	4–8
Trimethoprim-sulfonamide[c]	15–20 mg/kg	IV, PO	8–12
Gentamicin[c]	2 mg/kg	IV, IM	8
Chloramphenicol	10–15 mg/kg	PO	4–6
Cefalexin	20 (10–30) mg/kg	PO	8
Cephapirin	20–30 mg/kg	IV, IM	8
Amphotericin B[c]	0.15–0.50 mg/kg	IV	48
Flucytosine	50 mg/kg	PO	8
Rifampin	10–20 mg/kg	PO	8–12
Metronidazole	10–15 mg/kg	PO	8
Cefotaxime	6–40 mg/kg	IM, IV	4–6
Enrofloxacin[d]	5–10 mg/kg	PO	12

[a]See discussion of drug administration for recommended duration of therapy and precautions. See respective chapters for dosages in treating viral, protozoal, and some fungal infections.
[b]Dose per administration at specified interval. For further information on those drugs, see Drug Formulary, Appendix 8.
[c]Potential for renal toxicity is greatest in cats and young or dehydrated dogs. Closely monitor renal functions and use lowest dosage under these circumstances.
[d]Other fluoroquinolones such as orbifloxacin or marbofloxacin can be substituted.

These drugs penetrate both the normal and inflamed meninges at therapeutic levels. This drug combination has not been widely given for treating CNS infections in veterinary practice, although it probably should be more regularly. It is recommended that animals that respond to ampicillin be switched to this drug for extended therapy.

Metronidazole. Metronidazole crosses both normal and inflamed meninges in therapeutic concentrations. This drug is primarily indicated for the treatment of anaerobic CNS infections. The drug obtains bactericidal CSF concentrations.

Aminoglycosides. Aminoglycosides do not readily cross the normal or inflamed BBB. For aminoglycosides to be consistently bactericidal in CSF, they must be present at levels 10 to 20 times the MIC as determined in vitro. In people, aminoglycosides are effective in neonates but not in older patients. The situation in canine and feline meningitis is uncertain. There are some synergistic combinations of antimicrobials with aminoglycosides for treating bacterial infections (see Table 92–4). The inability of aminoglycosides to cross the BBB and their diminished effectiveness at low pH may limit the expected synergistic effect. High CSF concentrations are reported with intrathecal administration of aminoglycosides, but this route is not routinely recommended.

Fluoroquinolones. These drugs are primarily active against gram-negative bacteria and penetrate CNS tissues and CSF with reasonable concentrations. They can be considered as safer alternatives to aminoglycoside therapy.

Clindamycin. Clindamycin does not appear as useful for CNS anaerobic infections as for anaerobic infections in other locations, because it does not cross the intact BBB.[3, 23] In spite of this problem, it has been used for treating CNS protozoal infections with mixed results.[13, 15, 20]

Glucocorticoid Therapy

Many complications of meningitis arise from the inflammatory process, not the infection itself or the organism's direct effects. Massive bacterial lysis, releasing high concentrations of inflammatory bacterial fragments, follows antimicrobial administration to patients with bacterial meningitis.[32] These bacterial cell wall components may severely exacerbate the meningeal inflammation, worsening the patient's condition. As a result, adjunct anti-inflammatory drug therapy, especially with glucocorticoids, has become increasingly advocated. Administering dexamethasone at 0.15 mg/kg at 15 to 20 minutes before initiating antimicrobial therapy and then continuing the dexamethasone at the same dose four times daily for a maximum of 4 days has been associated with lower intracranial pressures, lower CSF cytokine concentrations, less CNS inflammation (as measured by normalization of CSF glucose levels), and fewer neurologic sequelae when dexamethasone-treated patients are compared with patients not receiving dexamethasone.[3, 16, 23, 34, 35] These studies looked primarily at human patients with *Haemophilus* infections, but preliminary reports in other bacterial infections suggest similar benefits.

The beneficial effects of glucocorticoids were not observed if steroid use was delayed for 12 or more hours after the first antimicrobial dose.[16] Empiric treatment before diagnostics remains contraindicated. Glucocorticoids may affect CSF values, obscuring the diagnosis. More importantly, although many patients may benefit from their use, patients with viral, fungal, protozoal, and rickettsial meningoencephalitis may be adversely affected. As such, the drugs should be given to patients only when the benefits outweigh the risks.

Drug Administration

After choosing an appropriate drug, the major variable determining drug efficacy is the peak CSF concentration. In humans, if the peak concentration is more than 10 times the minimum bactericidal concentration, a cure will occur in greater than 90% of cases. For this reason, IV administration is desirable for at least 3 to 5 days and then PO administration can be used. Administration frequency is less important than achieving periodic high CSF drug concentrations. Treatment should be continued for a minimum of 10 to 14 days after the patient becomes nonsymptomatic. If CSF can be collected before ending therapy, glucose normalization and lowering of both the WBC count and the protein concentration are expected. Patients receiving appropriate therapy, based on organism identification, that show improvement of CNS signs but remain febrile should be screened for other causes of the fever before changing drugs. In these patients, the persistent fever may be due to vasculitis from an indwelling catheter, a new (e.g., catheter-related) infection, or an adverse reaction to the antibiotics.

Supportive Therapy

Direct supportive therapy is directed toward treating or preventing brain edema. Fluid restriction has been advocated unless the patient is hypovolemic or has systemic illness. Fluid restriction may lead to higher mortality and more serious sequelae.[37] The risk of brain edema appears lower than the sequela of fluid restriction, and therefore appropriate, maintenance fluid therapy should always be used.[5] Data are not available regarding the effects of fluids at greater than maintenance levels.

If the animal is being anesthetized for CSF collection, controlled hyperventilation to lower carbon dioxide tension levels may alleviate or prevent brain swelling.[10] If brain herniation develops, osmotic diuretics such as mannitol (1.25 g/kg) may be given.

Hyperthermia from tremors or seizures should be treated with cool water baths, ice packs, or topical applications of alcohol. Patients that develop seizures should be treated with anticonvulsants. Recumbent animals should be kept on a waterbed, if available. Frequent turning to prevent formation of decubital ulcers and passive pulmonary congestion is essential. The bladder may need to be expressed, and, if necessary, suppositories should be given to prevent constipation. Management of systemic infections is covered in Endotoxemia, Chapter 38, and Cardiovascular Infections, Chapter 87.

If enhanced imaging confirms the presence of an epidural or a subdural mass lesion, surgical drainage may be considered. Otherwise, therapy should be strictly medical.

PROGNOSIS

Prognosis in CNS infections is determined by several factors. The most important are the ability to identify the causative agent and to select an effective antimicrobial that will enter the CNS. The speed with which specific therapy is instituted plays a large role in determining the prognosis. In children, those with lowest initial CSF cell counts, longest duration of signs before therapy, hypothermia at presentation, and/or history of seizures had the poorest prognosis.[17]

Conversely, high pretreatment CSF WBC counts have been associated with a favorable prognosis. Continued post-treatment CSF pleocytosis suggests a worsening prognosis.[10]

In summary, the antemortem diagnosis of bacterial meningitis rests on a combination of the following: 1) finding a neutrophilic pleocytosis in CSF, preferably with phagocytized organisms present; 2) having positive culture results of CSF or other bodily fluids; 3) experiencing clinical recovery when treated with appropriate antimicrobials; 4) finding an extraneural site for the infection; and 5) experiencing a rapidly deteriorating course before antimicrobial therapy.

At necropsy, the diagnosis rests on the presence of suppurative inflammation of the meninges with bacteria confirmed in the tissues. Regardless of cause, many CNS inflammatory diseases are expensive to treat. Relapses may occur when treatment is discontinued. Even when the infection is successfully treated, the potential for residual neurologic deficits may discourage clients. Overall, a success rate of about 13% is reported for dogs and cats.[43]

References

1. Andiman WA. 1991. Organism-specific antibody indices, the cerebrospinal fluid-immunoglobulin index and other tools: a clinician's guide to the etiologic diagnosis of central nervous system infection. *Pediatr Infect Dis J* 10:490–495.
2. Bachur R, Caputo G. 1995. Bacteremia and meningitis among infants with urinary tract infections. *Pediatr Emerg Care* 11:280–284.
3. Bell W, McGuinness G. 1993. Antibacterial and antifungal therapy for CNS infections, pp 305–353. *In* Tyler KL, Martin JB (eds), Infections of the CNS. Contemporary neurology series, vol 41. FA Davis, Philadelphia, PA.
4. Brass DA. 1994. Pathophysiology and neuroimmunology of bacterial meningitis. *Comp Cont Educ Pract Vet* 16:45–54.
5. Brown L, Feigin R. 1995. Bacterial meningitis: fluid balance and therapy. *Pediatr Ann* 23:93–98.
6. Chrisman CL. 1992. Cerebrospinal fluid analysis. *Vet Clin North Am* 22:781–811.
7. Christopher MM, Perman V, Hardy RM. 1988. Reassessment of cytologic values in canine cerebrospinal fluid by use of cytocentrifugation. *J Am Vet Med Assoc* 192:1726–1729.
8. Dow SW, LeCouteur RA, Henik RA, et al. 1988. Central nervous system infection associated with anaerobic bacteria in two dogs and two cats. *J Vet Intern Med* 2:171–176.
9. Elwood C, Cobb M, Stepien R. 1993. Clinical and echocardiographic findings in 10 dogs with vegetative bacterial endocarditis. *J Small Anim Pract* 34:420–427.
10. Fenner WR. 1990. Bacterial Infections of the central nervous system, pp 184–196. *In* Greene CE (ed), Infectious diseases of the dog and cat. WB Saunders, Philadelphia, PA.
11. Gaillard J, Abadie V, Cheron G, et al. 1994. Concentrations of ceftriaxone in cerebrospinal fluid of children with meningitis receiving dexamethasone therapy. *Antimicrob Agent Chemother* 38:1209–1210.

11a. Glimaker M, Kragsbjerg P, Forsgren M, et al. 1993. Tumor necrosis factor-α (TNFα) in cerebrospinal fluid from patients with meningitis of different etiologies: high levels of TNFα indicate bacterial meningitis. *J Infect Dis* 167:882–889.

12. Gray LD, Fedorko DP. 1992. Laboratory diagnosis of bacterial meningitis. *Clin Microbiol Rev* 5:130–145.

12a. Habujak JJ, Schubert TA. 1997. *Flavobacterium breve* meningitis in a dog. *J Am Anim Hosp Assoc* 33:509–512.

13. Hay WH, Shell LG, Lindsay DS, Dubey JP. 1990. Diagnosis and treatment of *Neospora caninum* infection in a dog. *J Am Vet Med Assoc* 197:87–89.

13a. Hurtt AE, Smith MO. 1997. Effects of iatrogenic blood contamination on results of cerebrospinal fluid analysis in clinically normal dogs and dogs with neurologic disease. *J Am Vet Med Assoc* 211:866–867.

14. Irving G, Chrisman CL. 1990. Long-term outcome of five cases of corticosteroid-responsive meningomyelitis. *J Am Anim Hosp Assoc* 26:324–328.
15. Jacobson LS, Jardine JE. 1993. *Neospora caninum* infection in three Labrador littermates. *J S Afr Vet Assoc* 64:47–51.
16. Jafari H, McCracken GJ. 1994. Dexamethasone therapy in bacterial meningitis. *Pediatr Ann* 23:82–88.
17. Kaaresen P, Flaegstad T. 1995. Prognostic factors in childhood bacterial meningitis. *Acta Paediatr* 84:873–878.
18. Kiska DL, Jones MC, Mangum ME, et al. 1995. Quality assurance study of bacterial antigen testing of cerebrospinal fluid. *J Clin Microbiol* 33:1141–1144.
19. Kornegay JN. 1991. Multiple neurologic deficits. Inflammatory diseases. *Probl Vet Med* 3:426–439.
20. Lappin MR, Greene CE, Winston S. et al. 1989. Clinical feline toxoplasmosis. Serologic diagnosis and therapeutic management of 15 cases. *J Vet Intern Med* 3:139–143.
21. Lauritsen A, Oberg B. 1995. Adjunctive corticosteroid therapy in bacterial meningitis. *Scand J Infect Dis* 27:431–434.
22. Lowrie CT, Kumar K, Moore JB, et al. 1989. A preliminary study of magnetic resonance imaging (MRI) in experimental canine meningitis. *Comp Anim Pract* 19:3–6.

22a. Mariscoli M, Jaggy A. 1997. Clinical and electroencephalographic findings of inflammatory and infectious diseases of the central nervous system in dogs: a retrospective study. *Zentralbl Vet Med B* 44:1–18.

23. Martin JB, Tyler KL, Scheld WM. 1993. Bacterial meningitis, pp 176–187. *In* Tyler KL, Martin JB (ed), Infections of the CNS. contemporary neurology series, vol 4. FA Davis, Philadelphia, PA.
24. Mayefski J, Roghmann K. 1987. Determination of leukocytosis in traumatic spinal tap specimens. *Am J Med* 82:1175–1181.
25. Meric JM. 1988. Canine meningitis: a changing emphasis. *J Vet Intern Med* 2:26–35.
26. Quagliarello V, Scheld WM. 1992. Bacterial meningitis: pathogenesis, pathophysiology, and progress. *N Engl J Med* 327:864–872.
27. Quagliaerollo VJ, Scheld WM. 1997. Drug therapy: treatment of bacterial meningitis. *N Engl J Med* 336:708–716.
28. Radstrom P, Backman A, Qian N, et al. 1994. Detection of bacterial DNA in cerebrospinal fluid by an assay for simultaneous detection of *Neisseria meningitidis, Haemophilus influenzae* and streptococci using a seminested PCR strategy. *J Clin Microbiol* 32:2738–2744.
29. Rand JS, Parent J, Jacobs R, et al. 1990. Reference intervals for feline cerebrospinal fluid: cell counts and cytologic features. *Am J Vet Res* 51:1044–1047.
30. Rand JS, Parent J, Percy D, et al. 1994. Clinical, cerebrospinal fluid, and histological data from twenty-seven cats with primary inflammatory disease of the central nervous system. *Can Vet J* 35:103–110.
31. Rockowitz J, Tunkel A. 1995. Bacterial meningitis. Practical guidelines for management. *Drugs* 50:838–853.
32. Roos K. 1993. New treatment strategies for bacterial meningitis. *Clin Neuropharmacol* 16:373–386.
33. Runge V, Wells J, Williams N, et al. 1995. Detectability of early brain meningitis with magnetic resonance imaging. *Invest Radiol* 30:484–495.
34. Schaad U, Kaplan S, McCracken GJ. 1995. Steroid therapy for bacterial meningitis. *Clin Infect Dis* 20:685–690.
35. Schaad U, Lips U, Gnehm H, et al. 1993. Dexamethasone therapy for bacterial meningitis in children. Swiss Meningitis Study Group. *Lancet* 342:457–461.
36. Seebach J, Bartholdi D, Frei K, et al. 1995. Experimental *Listeria* meningoencephalitis, macrophage inflammatory protein-1 alpha and -2 are produced intrathecally and mediate chemotactic activity in cerebrospinal fluid of infected mice. *J Immunol* 155:4367–4375.
37. Singhi S, Singhi P, Srinivas B, et al. 1995. Fluid restriction does not improve the outcome of acute meningitis. *Pediatr Infect Dis J* 14:495–503.
38. Snyder P, Kazcos E, Scott-Moncrieff J, et al. 1995. Pathologic features of naturally occurring juvenile polyarteritis in Beagle dogs. *Vet Pathol* 32:337–345.
39. Sorjonen D. 1992. Myelitis and meningitis. *In* Moore M (ed), Diseases of the spine. WB Saunders, Philadelphia, PA: Vet Clin North Am: Small Anim Pract 22:951–964.
40. Sorjonen DC. 1987. Total protein, albumin quota, and electrophoretic patterns in cerebrospinal fluid of dogs with central nervous system disorders. *Am J Vet Res* 48:310–315.
41. Speciale J. 1996. Brain herniation, pp 673–675. *In* Proceedings of the 14th ACVIM Forum, San Antonio, TX.
42. Stalis I, Chadwick B, Dayrell-Hart B, et al. 1995. Necrotizing meningoencephalitis of Maltese Dogs. *Vet Pathol* 32:230–235.
43. Tipold A. 1995. Diagnosis of inflammatory and infectious diseases of the central nervous system in dogs: a retrospective study. *J Vet Intern Med* 9:304–314.
44. Tipold A, Jaffy A. 1994. Steroid responsive meningitis arteritis in dogs: long-term study of 32 cases. *J Small Anim Pract* 35:311–316.
45. Townsend GC, Scheld WM. 1995. Microbe-endothelium interactions in blood-brain barrier permeability during bacterial meningitis. *ASM News* 61:294–298.
46. Tucker T, Ellner J, 1993. Chronic meningitis, pp 188–215. *In* Tyler KL, Martin JB (eds), Infections of the CNS. Contemporary neurology series, vol 41. FA Davis, Philadelphia, PA.
47. Tunkel AR, Scheld WM. 1993. Pathogenesis and pathophysiology of bacterial meningitis. *Clin Microbiol Rev* 6:118–136.
48. Tyler K, Martin J, Scheld W. 1993. Focal suppurative infections of the central nervous system, pp 157–175. *In* Tyler KL, Martin JB (eds), Infections of the CNS. Contemporary neurology series, vol 41. FA Davis, Philadelphia, PA.
49. Whitby M, Finch R. 1986. Bacterial meningitis. Rational selection and use of antibacterial drugs. *Drugs* 31:266–278.

Chapter **93**

Ocular Infections

Charles L. Martin and Jean Stiles

Extraocular Infections

NORMAL FLORA

Despite the fact that all dogs probably have indigenous conjunctival bacteria in their conjunctival cul-de-sac, positive isolation rates between 46% and 91% of clinically healthy dogs have been reported (Table 93–1).[19, 33] Variables in the type of isolate and the frequency may be due to geography, culturing technique, breed, and season.

In contrast to the dog, the cat has a relatively lower isolation rate of cultivable bacteria from their conjunctival flora.[17] Bacteria or mycoplasmas have been isolated from 34% of the conjunctival samples and from 25% of the samples from the lid margins.[33] In one study of 50 cats, no organisms were isolated from 42% of the cats, bacteria were isolated from the conjunctiva of 34% of the cats or 47% of the eyes, and 26% of the cats or 14% of the eyes had fungal isolates from the conjunctiva (Table 93–2). No anaerobes were isolated.[18]

OCULAR SURFACE

Most surface bacterial infections are not strictly primary; other debilitating conditions often potentiate the pathogenicity of organisms that are indigenous to the ocular surface. Other local nidi of infection, such as in the lacrimal sac and meibomian glands or adjacent structures to the eye (ears, lip folds), should be sought and corrected to overcome persistent or recurring infection. Control of the normal ocular flora is maintained by rinsing of the ocular surface with tears and blinking, which pushes the tears into the nasolacrimal system. Tears also contain IgA and other antibacterial substances such as lactoferrin. Competitive interaction between the indigenous flora helps to keep the organisms in lower numbers, whereas disrupting this balance may cause an overgrowth of one species. Debilitating conditions to the ocular surface such as reduced tear secretions, UV radiation, systemic states with immune suppression such as diabetes mellitus and Cushing's syndrome, and trauma creating breaks in the epithelial barrier may allow indigenous bacteria to adhere and/or overgrow to produce disease. To become established, bacteria must adhere, replicate, and then invade the tissue. Adherence is the first step, and the same bacteria may have a differential ability to adhere to varying epithelial surfaces, thus explaining why certain organisms are relatively specific for different tissues. In most cases, adherence does not occur with healthy cells but only with injured cells, thus the frequent association with prior trauma. The factors involved with adhesion are incompletely understood, but require both a bacterial component such as fimbriae or pilus and host cellular receptors. Cellular injury may expose these cellular receptors, or the bacteria may adhere to fibronectin bound to the damaged cell. Once adhered, the bacteria are engulfed by the cell and then invade the stroma, where inflammation is stimulated. Tissue damage with infection is a combination of toxins liberated by the organism and enzymes such as collagenase, elastase, and cathepsins liberated by the neutrophilic response.[51] Bacteria, such as *Pseudomonas aeruginosa*, that have a variety of proteolytic enzymes typically produce rapidly progressive corneal ulcers.

Table 93–1. Frequency of Isolation of Bacteria From the Conjunctival Sacs of Clinically Healthy Dogs[19, 33]

ORGANISM	ISOLATION (%)[a]
Staphylococcus (total)	57–70
Coagulase positive	24–45
Coagulase negative	46–55
Streptococcus (total)	6–43
Nonhemolytic	12–51
α-Hemolytic	4–34
β-Hemolytic	2–7
Corynebacterium (total)	30–75
Undifferentiated	11
C. pseudodiphtheriticum	9
C. xerosis	13
Neisseria (total)	26
Undifferentiated	4
N. catarrhalis	9
N. pharyngis	4
N. sicca	3
N. caviae	3
N. lactamica	3
N. flavescens	3
Pseudomonas	14
Moraxella	7
Bacillus	6–18

[a]Percentages are based on the numbers of animals from which organisms were isolated.

Dogs

Bacterial. Conjunctivitis and, to a lesser extent, keratitis are common syndromes in the dog, and the isolated agents are usually similar to the indigenous flora. Isolates, in decreasing order of prevalence, have included coagulase-positive *Staphylococcus aureus (intermedius)*, α- or β-hemolytic streptococci, *S. epidermidis*, *Escherichia coli*, and *Proteus mirabilis*.[33] Infectious keratitis or conjunctivitis should be considered in any animal with a strong leukotactic response. This is recognized as a dense, creamy white infiltrate at a nidus or around the periphery of an ulcer. In addition, infected corneal ulcers typically stimulate a strong corneal neovascular response, have some purulent ocular discharge, and carry a history and potential for rapid progression.

Fungal. Keratomycosis in small animals is a rare syndrome and usually has a predisposing cause such as long-term glucocorticoid therapy, diabetes mellitus, long-term topical

Table 93–2. Bacterial Isolates From Clinically Healthy Cats[a, 17, 18]

LOCATION	ORGANISM	%
Conjunctiva	*Staphylococcus* spp.	27
	Corynebacterium spp.	1.3–5
	Bacillus spp.	3–5
	Streptococcus spp.	2–2.5
	Mycoplasma	0–5
	Fungal isolates	13
Lids	*Staphylococcus* spp.	23–28
	Streptococcus spp.	0–2
	Bacillus spp.	2–5
	Corynebacterium spp.	1.6

[a]Percentages are based on the numbers of animals from which organisms were isolated.

antibacterial therapy, lack of tears, or exposure keratitis. Both filamentous fungi and yeasts may produce ocular disease. Filamentous organisms have included *Aspergillus, Scedosporium, Acremonium, Fusarium, Cephalosporium, Alternaria, Pseudallescheria,* and *Curvularia*.[32] *Candida* are the most commonly isolated yeasts. Keratomycosis is typically chronic, and the yeast may produce plaque formation on the surface of the cornea. The dematiaceous fungi may produce a brown pigmentation of the lesion.[38] A corneal ulcer or plaque with associated fluffy white or yellow to brown pigmented appearance should be suspected. Deep corneal scrapings should be obtained for cytologic and cultural examination. Topical treatment usually involves ocular miconazole or nystatin solutions with concurrent antibacterials such as aminoglycosides (see Therapy).

Cats

Conjunctivitis. This is probably the most common feline clinical ophthalmic disorder. Determining the underlying cause of conjunctivitis in cats can be extremely difficult. In a study of 91 cats with chronic conjunctivitis, only 37% of cats had positive diagnostic test results that helped pinpoint a cause for the conjunctivitis.[43] Following is a discussion of the most common infectious agents known to cause conjunctivitis in the cat.

Feline herpesvirus-1 (FHV-1) is a frequent cause of ocular disease in cats. Young cats with respiratory tract disease generally have conjunctivitis with marked conjunctival hyperemia, chemosis, and serous to purulent ocular discharge (Fig. 93–1). The condition is usually self-limiting and resolves over 1 to 2 weeks, although in severe cases symblepharon may occur. In addition to general supportive care, the eyes

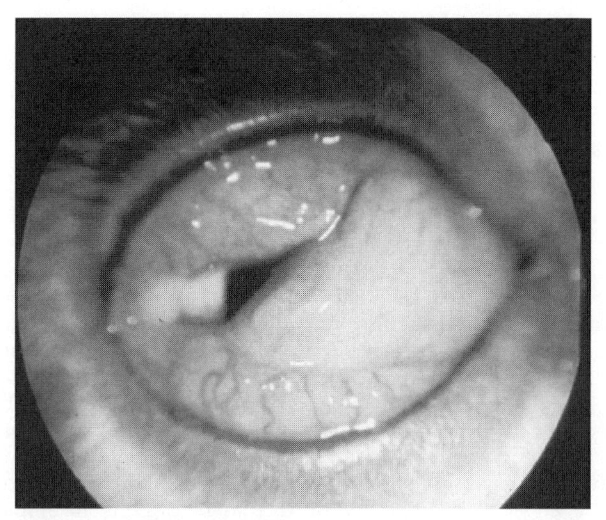

Figure 93–1. Acute conjunctivitis secondary to feline herpesvirus. Note chemosis and conjunctival hyperemia. A lack of tear production was also present that resolved with resolution of the chemosis.

should be cleansed frequently and a broad-spectrum topical antibiotic applied to minimize secondary bacterial infection as the conjunctival surface sloughs. Cats become latent carriers of FHV-1 once infected and may have recurrences of ocular disease, including conjunctivitis and corneal ulcers. Many cats will have transient episodes of conjunctivitis, with conjunctival hyperemia, serous or purulent ocular discharge, and blepharospasm. Most cases are self-limiting and do not require treatment. If a topical antibiotic is used, tetracycline is the most appropriate choice for its efficacy against *Chlamydia psittaci* and *Mycoplasma felis*, which are common feline conjunctival pathogens that may contribute to conjunctivitis along with FHV-1.

Cats may develop chronic conjunctivitis secondary to FHV-1. Keratoconjunctivitis sicca (KCS) has also been associated with FHV-1 in cats.[52] Laboratory diagnostic tests, such as virus isolation from the conjunctiva and conjunctival scrapings for fluorescent antibody, to prove FHV-1 as a cause of conjunctivitis in cats are frequently negative, making the diagnosis uncertain.[43] Treatment with an ophthalmic antiviral medication, such as idoxuridine or trifluridine, can be used in cats with chronic conjunctivitis, although results are variable (Table 93–3). Many cats are irritated by topical antiviral agents. Treatment for KCS in cats with FHV-1 conjunctivitis can include topical 0.2% cyclosporine ointment in addition

Table 93–3. Topical Ophthalmic Antiviral Medications

DRUG	AVAILABLE PREPARATION	BRAND NAME (MANUFACTURER)	DOSING INTERVAL (HOURS)	DURATION OF TREATMENT	COMMENT
Trifluridine	1% solution (refrigerate)	Viroptic (Burroughs Wellcome)	4	1 week beyond clinical resolution	Most efficacious against FHV-1 in vitro[42]
Idoxuridine	0.1% solution	Herplex (Allergen)	4	1 week beyond clinical resolution	Second most efficacious against FHV-1 in vitro
Vidarabine	3% ointment	Vira-A (Parke-Davis)	4	1 week beyond clinical resolution	Third most efficacious against FHV-1 in vitro
Acyclovir[a]	3% ointment	Zovirax (Burroughs-Wellcome)	4–6	1 week beyond clinical resolution	Least efficacious against FHV-1 in vitro
IFN-α-2	3×10^6 IU/vial[b] (Reconstitute in artificial tears)	Roferon-A (Roche)	4–6	1 week beyond clinical resolution	Efficacy unknown

[a]Available in the United Kingdom.
[b]Based on human literature; final concentrations in artificial tears have ranged from $1–30 \times 10^6$ IU/ml.
IFN = interferon; FHV = feline herpesvirus.

to antiviral therapy. Recombinant interferon has also been administered to cats with chronic FHV-1–related ocular disease, although no studies document effectiveness. Both oral administration (see Chapter 100) and topical administration of interferon have been utilized (see Table 93–3).[36, 55, 56]

Treatment with oral lysine has been of some benefit in humans in accelerating recovery from herpes simplex infection and in suppressing recurrence.[20] In vitro studies with FHV-1 have shown that L-lysine does suppress viral replication but only in conjunction with low arginine levels.[8] Anecdotal reports indicate that 200 mg of lysine given once or twice daily may benefit cats with chronic or recurring ocular herpesvirus disease. Gastric upset has also been noted with administration of lysine.

C. psittaci is a common cause of conjunctivitis in cats. The typical clinical picture is one of unilateral conjunctivitis with involvement of the second eye a few days later. The clinical presentation is indistinguishable from conjunctivitis caused by FHV-1, and the two organisms may be present simultaneously. Diagnosis is based on seeing the typical elementary body in the cytoplasm of conjunctival epithelial cells (Fig. 93–2) or obtaining a positive fluorescent antibody test result on a conjunctival scraping. Elementary bodies are often few in number and diminish with chronicity, making them easy to miss. In an experimental study of chlamydial conjunctivitis, infection with feline immunodeficiency virus (FIV) prolonged the duration of clinical signs and led to chronic conjunctivitis.[44] Conjunctivitis caused by *Chlamydia* should be treated with tetracycline applied to both eyes four times daily for 1 to 2 weeks after clinical resolution. This organism has the potential to be transmitted to humans, so that washing of hands after treating an affected cat is advised. Oral tetracycline or doxycycline may be necessary to treat refractory infections and may be advisable to clear the GI tract of infection.[44]

M. felis has been variably implicated as a cause of conjunctivitis in cats. Some studies have recovered *Mycoplasma* as normal flora from feline conjunctiva,[33] whereas others have not. Similarly, experimental infections of healthy, young cats have produced conjunctivitis in some studies[21] and not in others. *Mycoplasma* may require a stressor, such as another conjunctival pathogen or injury, to cause disease. *Mycoplasma* are sensitive to many topical antibiotics, including tetracycline.

Keratitis. Keratitis in cats has been most frequently associated with invasion of the corneal epithelium by FHV-1. The most common corneal abnormality is punctate or linear epithelial erosions (Fig. 93–3), which may enlarge to form larger ulcers.[52] Conjunctivitis often accompanies the corneal ulcers.

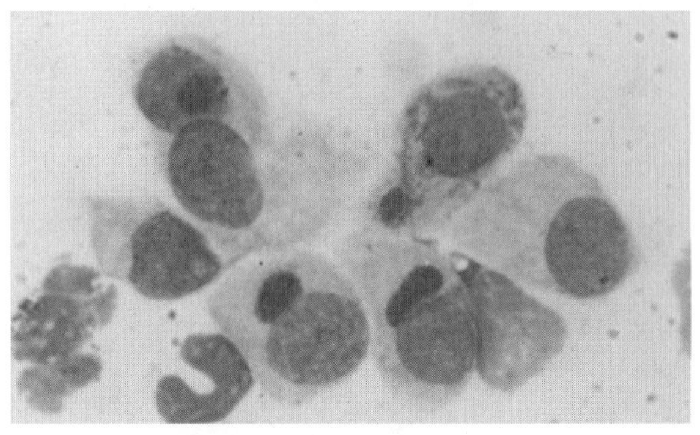

Figure 93–2. Intracytoplasmic chlamydial inclusions in conjunctival epithelial cells of a cat with conjunctivitis. Giemsa stain, × 330.

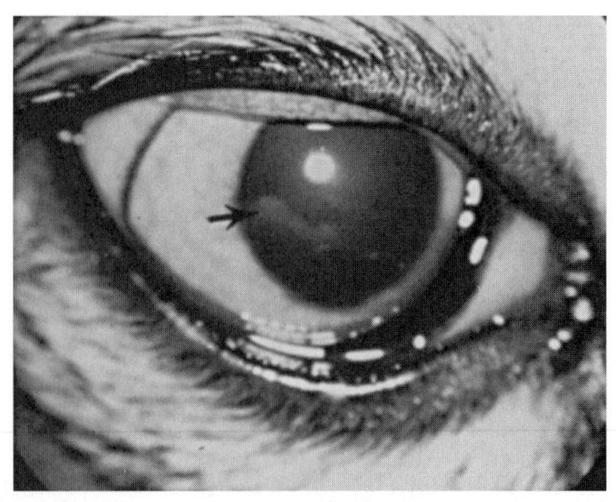

Figure 93–3. Linear epithelial ulcer (*arrow*) in a young adult cat without obvious respiratory disease. Note the chemosis from the dorsal conjunctiva.

Mechanical debridement of the epithelium to remove virus and treatment with a topical antiviral agent have been the most successful therapies, although many of these ulcers will heal without antiviral agents. Antiviral agents, such as idoxuridine or trifluridine, are virostatic and should be given six times daily until the ulcer heals and for approximately 1 week afterward (see Table 93–3). Many cats are irritated by topical antiviral agents.

Stromal keratitis is one of the most serious manifestations of FHV-1 corneal infection and is thought to primarily be a result of an immune reaction to the virus. Experimentally, subconjunctival dexamethasone caused cats infected with FHV-1 to develop stromal keratitis.[40] Stromal keratitis may develop with or without a corneal ulcer. Vascularization and cellular infiltrate of the deeper layers of the cornea, often accompanied by chronic discomfort, are typical at presentation. Antiviral agents alone usually do not improve the keratitis. A topical anti-inflammatory agent, such as glucocorticoids or cyclosporine, may help the inflammatory response but risks exacerbating the viral infection. It should be used only in conjunction with an antiviral agent. Glucocorticoids may predispose cats to the development of corneal sequestration. Topical interferon has been used in people with herpetic keratitis and may be of benefit in cats (see Table 93–3).[36, 55, 56] Lysine for ocular herpetic disease is discussed under feline conjunctivitis.

Corneal sequestration is a common disorder in cats, particularly Persians and Himalayans, and may follow chronic corneal ulcers or keratitis caused by FHV-1 (Fig. 93–4). It has been noted to occur after topical glucocorticoid treatment in FHV-1 experimentally infected cats.[41] We have also noted this in naturally infected cats. The condition is characterized by an area of corneal degeneration with a brown to black discoloration. The lesions vary from pinpoint sequestra to those that occupy more than half the cornea; vascularization may be intense or absent; and ocular pain ranges from none to marked. Like stromal keratitis, sequestrum can be one of the most serious and potentially blinding sequela of FHV-1. Most ophthalmologists recommend keratectomy followed by a graft (corneal or conjunctival) as the therapy for sequestra.

Florida spots, or "Florida keratopathy," is a corneal condition in cats in the southeastern part of the United States. The lesions are characterized by focal gray-white opacities in the anterior stroma (Fig. 93–5). The lesions are presumed to be caused by a *Mycobacterium* species, although definitive proof is lacking. Treatment has not been successful and is usually

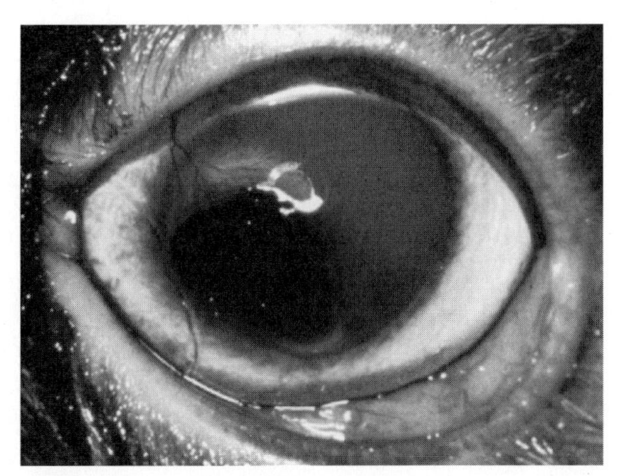

Figure 93–4. Corneal sequestrum in a cat. Note also the corneal blood vessels.

not attempted because the condition remains nonsymptomatic.

DIAGNOSIS

The decision to perform cultures from the ocular surface should be made early in the examination before various eyedrops have been administered and manipulations performed. The use of a moist or calcium alginate swab improves the recovery rate.[33] Because the volume of material collected is usually small and subject to drying, swabs should be inoculated quickly onto appropriate media or placed in transport media.

Cytologic examination of conjunctival and corneal scrapings is an important and rapid diagnostic aid. A topical anesthetic is applied, and the appropriate surface is scraped with a small, flat spatula. Excessive ocular discharges should be removed before scraping. Only a small amount of material is collected, and it is tapped directly onto the slides and air dried. Multiple slides should be prepared, because some slides may not have adequate numbers of cells. The slides are stained with a modified Giemsa method for cytologic evaluation and a Gram's stain to evaluate the type of bacteria that might be present. Slides can also be made for examination by indirect FA for distemper virus, herpesvirus, and *Chlamydia.*

An alternate technique is to roll a small nylon bristle brush applicator (Microbrush, IDE Interstate, Amityville, NY) over the appropriate surface and then roll it onto a slide (Fig. 93–6). The nylon bristles repel the negatively charged cells when rolled onto the slide. Preparations made with this method have fewer cells that are spread out and not found in clumps or multilayers.[60, 62] This method is less traumatic and easier to perform on the cat and small dogs with tight lid-globe conformations.

Small snip biopsy specimens of the conjunctiva are readily obtained under topical anesthesia and plaquelike lesions can often be removed from the cornea without general anesthesia. These small pieces of tissue should be spread out on a piece of paper before placing in fixative.

THERAPY

Specific anti-infective therapy is initially selected on the basis of cytology and later on the results of culture and susceptibility testing. If the condition is severe or has corneal involvement that is progressive, both the frequency and concentration of antibiotic therapy are usually increased. Therapy for prophylaxis or mild problems includes the application of commercial ophthalmic preparations three to four times a day. Further problems may require hospitalization to monitor and ensure frequent therapy. Hourly therapy is not unusual for progressive bacterial ulcers. The antibiotic concentration of commercial ophthalmic preparations is often augmented by systemic preparations of the antibiotic to three or four times the concentration of the ophthalmic preparations. If resistant gram-positive bacteria are involved, few appropriate commercial ophthalmic preparations are available, and it is necessary to formulate drops from systemic preparations (Table 93–4).

In the rare instance of fungal infection in small animals, the only specific therapy that is commercially available is 5% natamycin suspension (Natacyn, Alcon Lab, Forth Worth, TX) but, because of expense and lack of widespread availability, it is usually not administered. Antifungal preparations used systemically or topically are often given as ophthalmic preparations. Agents such as 1% miconazole IV solution or topical cream, 1% clotrimazole dermatologic cream, 1% silver sulfadiazine cream, amphotericin B (0.15–1%), and povidone-io-

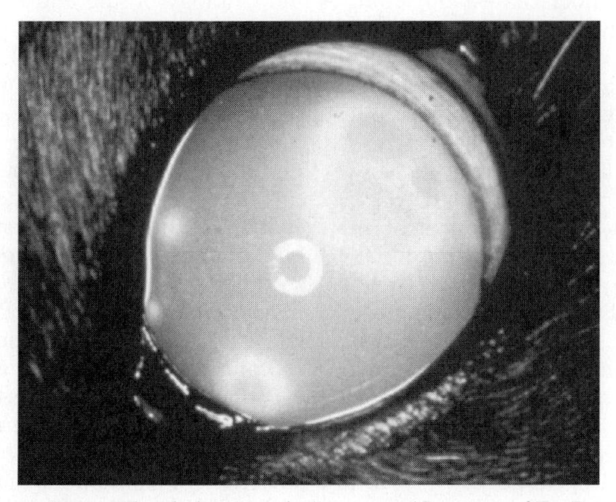

Figure 93–5. "Florida keratopathy" in a cat. (Courtesy of Dr. Patricia Smith, Freemont, CA.)

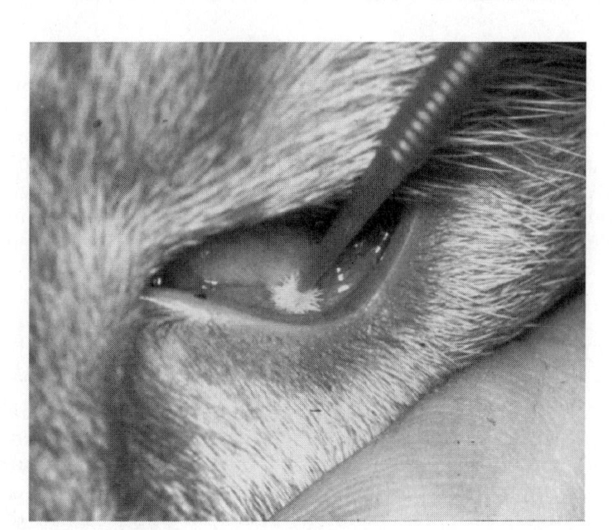

Figure 93–6. Nylon bristle brush used to obtain conjunctival cytology specimen. (Courtesy of Dr. Michelle Willis, Ohio State University, Columbus, OH.)

Table 93–4. Concentrations and Dosages of Locally Used Ocular Antibacterial Agents[a]

AGENT	TOPICAL	SUBCONJUNCTIVAL	INTRAVITREAL
Ampicillin	—	50–250 mg	500 μg
Bacitracin	10,000 U/ml	10,000 U	—
Carbenicillin	4 mg/ml	100 mg	250 μg–2 mg
Cefazolin	50 mg/ml	100 mg	2.25 mg
Cephalothin	50 mg/ml	50–100 mg	2 mg
Chloramphenicol	5 mg/ml	1–2 mg	2 mg
Clindamycin	—	15–40 mg	1 mg
Colistin	5–10 mg/ml	15–37.5 mg	—
Erythromycin	50 mg/ml	100 mg	500 μg
Gentamicin	8–15 mg/ml	10–20 mg	100–400 μg
Lincomycin	—	150 mg	1.5 mg
Methicillin	—	20–100 mg	2 mg
Neomycin	5–8 mg/ml	250–500 mg	—
Penicillin G	100,000 U/ml	0.5–1 million U	—
Polymyxin B	16,250 U/ml	10 mg	—
Streptomycin	—	50–100 mg	—
Sulfacetamide	100–300 mg/ml	—	—
Tobramycin	3 mg/ml	—	0.2–0.4 mg
Vancomycin	50 mg/ml	25 mg	1 mg

[a]For dosage recommendations for systemic administration, see Drug Formulary, Appendix 8.
Adapted from Copyright © *Physician's Desk Reference for Ophthalmology,* 1989 Edition. Published by Medical Economics Co, Inc, Oradell, NJ 07649. With permission.

dine solutions have been successful in treating fungal keratitis in humans and animals.[39] Because susceptibility testing for fungi is not widely available and is time consuming, the clinician is usually not aware of the best antifungal preparation for the specific case. If the condition is not ulcerative, removal of the epithelium by lamellar keratectomy or penetrating keratoplasty enhances drug absorption, because most antifungals do not penetrate an intact cornea.[45] Therapy by killing the organisms may transiently enhance the inflammatory reaction.

ANCILLARY

Ocular pain should be treated with topical 1% atropine two to three times daily. Ocular discharge should be cleansed frequently to remove neutrophils and their proteolytic enzymes. In ulcerative states, topical autogenous serum may be provided every 1 to 2 hours to try to inhibit further enzymatic digestion of the corneal collagen and proteoglycan. This is kept in a refrigerator and replenished frequently (every other day) to avoid bacterial contamination. If tear production is inadequate, topical 0.2% cyclosporine (Optimmune 0.2% ointment, Schering-Plough Animal Health Corp, Kenilworth, NJ) and artifical tears should be administered to supplement and stimulate lacrimation. Physical protection may be provided by application of a collagen insert or a soft contact lens. Both of these will also act as a reservoir for the slow release of topical drugs. Closing the lids should be avoided because this inhibits drainage of discharge and increases the temperature of the environment, thus promoting bacterial and/or fungal growth. Deep ulcerations will require surgical splinting of the ulcer with conjunctival flaps or corneal transplantation.

Intraocular Infections

Intraocular bacterial infections may be exogenous or endogenous in origin. Endogenous infections are discussed along with systemic ocular infections and uveitis. The source of an exogenous infection from a penetrating ocular injury may be obvious from the history and appearance of the eye or occult, such as a self-sealing cat claw injury through the conjunctiva and sclera. Exogenously induced infections are usually unilateral, whereas endogenous infections are often bilateral.

LOCAL INJURY

All recent perforating ocular injuries should be considered septic and treated intensively with bactericidal broad-spectrum antibiotics until susceptibility data are obtained. A surprising number of perforating missiles (BBs, pellets) and cat claw injuries do not result in infection, but, because the intraocular consequences of infection are so devastating, it is preferable to err on the side of overtreatment.

Most active intraocular inflammations associated with perforating injuries should have centesis performed. Anterior chamber centesis for cultures and cytology is safe and easy and may yield specific information to guide future therapy. Aqueous centesis is not as reliable as vitreous centesis in demonstrating bacterial growth in endophthalmitis; consequently, negative culture results from an aqueous sample are not definitive evidence of sterile inflammation.[33] Sepsis is indicated on oculocentesis by the finding of degenerate neutrophils and bacteria. Nondegenerate neutrophils may indicate a sterile purulent inflammation such as phakoclastic uveitis (phacoanaphylaxis, lens-induced inflammation) caused by lenticular capsular laceration.

Exogenous intraocular infections associated with intraocular surgery such as cataract surgery are a dreaded complication. On the basis of reviews of complications of relatively small series of cases, infectious endophthalmitis appears to be an infrequent occurrence despite the ability to culture bacteria from the aqueous from 24% of canine eyes at the end of surgery.[11, 48, 58] Despite bacterial contamination, there were no reported cases of endophthalmitis. As might be anticipated, the small incision and closed system of phacoemulsification had an aqueous contamination rate of 9% versus 37% with an "open sky" or large incision approach. The latter figures are comparable to humans in whom bacterial contamination was present in 24% of aqueous samples and was not influenced by preoperative antibiotics.[6] Another potential compounding factor in cataract surgery is that bacteria adhere to the surface of the methyl methacrylate intraocular lenses. Simply exposing the lens in the "sterile" surgical field for several minutes produced a contamination rate of 65%.[13] How much additional risk for endophthalmitis is produced by the implantation of intraocular lenses is unknown, but the presence of low grade pathogens may contribute to the smoldering chronic inflammation observed in some postoperative eyes. In an attempt to minimize this surface contamination, topical antibiotics are routinely given preoperatively by most surgeons, although numerous studies have emphasized the difficulty in sterilizing the conjunctival cul-de-sac. Preoperative norfloxacin did not affect the rate of aqueous contamination during surgery.[6] Dilute povidone-iodine (1:10–1:100) has been reported to be highly effective in temporarily sterilizing the ocular surface in dogs and decreasing the number of bacterial colonies for 24 hours when given postoperatively.[1, 50] Despite this finding, the previously cited studies in humans and dogs of postoperative aqueous contamination used preoperative povidone-iodine scrubs and irrigation.

SYSTEMIC DISEASE

In addition to local ocular infections, the eye frequently is affected by systemic infectious agents. It is not unusual for a systemic disease to remain occult and have the presenting complaint as an ocular lesion. It is important to recognize the systemic involvement to give an accurate prognosis and adequate therapy. Conversely, dogs with systemic disease should have ocular examinations, which may provide rapid diagnostic clues and prognostic information for function. Most infectious agents access the eye via the uveal or vascular tunic. Typically, infectious agents become established in the uvea, producing a posterior uveitis or chorioretinitis, an anterior uveitis, or, if overwhelming, an endophthalmitis (all of the inner tunics as well as the vitreous). See Table 93–5 for a list of known infectious causes for canine uveitis.

Dogs

Distemper. Catarrhal signs of distemper (see Chapter 3) are usually associated with a bilateral conjunctivitis that prog-

Table 93–5. Possible Ocular Tissue Involvement With Systemic Infectious Diseases

INFECTIOUS AGENT	CONJUNCTIVA[a]	LACRIMAL SYSTEM[b]	CORNEA[c]	ANTERIOR CHAMBER[d]	ANTERIOR UVEA[e]	LENS[f]	VITREOUS[g]	RETINA/ CHOROID[h]	OPTIC NERVE[i]
Viruses									
Canine distemper virus	C	M	—	—	—	—	—	M	N
Infectious canine hepatitis virus	—	—	I, E	G	U	—	—	—	—
Canine herpesvirus									
Neonate	—	—	K	—	U	C	—	C, R	N
Adult	C	—	—	—	—	—	—	—	—
Feline herpesvirus	C, S	E	U, N, S	—	U (rare)	—	—	—	N (rare)
Feline panleukopenia virus	—	—	—	—	—	—	—	D, A	H
Feline leukemia virus	—	—	I	T, G, H, F	U, P	C	—	I, H, V, X	—
Feline infectious peritonitis virus	—	—	—	G, F	U	C	—	X, C	N
Rabies virus	E	—	—	—	A	—	—	C	—
Rickettsiae									
Chlamydia psittaci	C	—	—	—	—	—	—	—	—
Ehrlichia canis	H	—	—	H	U	—	B	E, P, X	—
Rickettsia rickettsii	C, H	—	I	—	U	—	—	H, L	—
Haemobartonella felis & *canis*	—	—	—	—	—	—	—	P, H	—
Bacteria									
Leptospira	C, H, I	—	—	—	U	—	—	—	—
Brucella canis	—	—	I	—	U	C	H	C	—
Clostridium tetani	E	—	—	—	—	—	—	—	—
Mycobacterium bovis	—	—	I	—	U	—	—	C, X	—
Bacterial septicemia	—	—	I	S	—	—	—	C, H	—
Systemic Fungi	—	—	—	S	U	C	H	C, X	N
Algae (*Prototheca*)	—	—	—	—	—	—	—	C, X	N
Protozoa									
Toxoplasma gondii	—	—	—	—	U	—	H	C	N
Leishmania donovani	C	—	K	S	U	—	H	—	—

[a]C = conjunctivitis; S = symblepharon; E = prolapsed third eyelid; H = hemorrhage; I = icterus.
[b]M = mucopurulent secretions; E = epiphora.
[c]I = interstitial keratitis; E = edema; K = keratitis; U = ulcerative keratitis; N = nonulcerative keratitis; S = symblepharon.
[d]G = glaucoma; T = tumor mass; H = hyphema; F = fibrin; S = secondary glaucoma.
[e]U = uveitis; P = paradoxical pupil size; A = anisocoria.
[f]C = cataract.
[g]B = hemorrhage; H = hyalitis.
[h]M = multifocal chorioretinitis; C = chorioretinitis; R = retinal dysplasia; D = dysplasia; A = atrophy; I = multifocal infiltrates; H = hemorrhages; V = pale vessels; X = detachment; E = vascular engorgement; P = perivascular infiltrates; L = vasculitis.
[i]N = neuritis; H = hypoplasia.

resses from serous to mucopurulent in nature. The palpebral conjunctiva is primarily involved, and lacrimal adenitis or dehydration may result in a marked reduction in tear production (sicca), which in turn results in more profound signs of blepharospasm and corneal ulceration. Sicca usually resolves if the animal recovers from systemic infection. Occasionally, conjunctival or lacrimal involvement occurs with such mild systemic signs that distemper is not suspected.

Distemper often produces a multifocal, nongranulomatous chorioretinitis that does not usually cause blindness. The incidence of chorioretinitis is unknown but probably varies, as do the neurologic signs, with strain of virus and immunocompetency of the host. Dogs with neurologic forms of distemper had an overall prevalence of chorioretinal lesions of 41%, but specifically 83% of the dogs with chronic leukoencephalopathy syndromes had chorioretinal lesions.[59] Occasionally, chorioretinitis is diffuse and blinding and may mimic the genetic syndrome of progressive retinal atrophy. Acute focal lesions in the tapetum have hazy or ill-defined borders with mild to moderate disruption of the mosaic texture and color changes. Acute lesions in the nontapetum have hazy borders and are white in color (Fig. 93–7).[33] Chorioretinal scars resulting from distemper have sharply demarcated borders, are hyperreflective in the tapetum, and are depigmented in the nontapetum. Histologically, retinal changes are characterized by degeneration of the retina with perivascular cuffing in some instances. Lesions may be focal or diffuse degeneration of ganglion cells, proliferation of retinal pigment epithelium, atrophy of photoreceptors, disorganization of retinal layers, focal gliosis, and distemper inclusion bodies in glial cells.

The most dramatic clinical ocular problem associated with distemper is optic neuritis.[33] This syndrome is characterized by an acute onset of bilateral blindness and mydriasis. If inflammation extends rostrally to the optic papilla, ophthalmoscopic signs of peripapillary hemorrhages and edema, retinal vascular congestion, and elevation of the papilla are observed (Fig. 93–8).[33] If the neuritis remains retrobulbar, the diagnosis is made by exclusion (i.e., blind eyes with dilated pupils and normal retinal function as tested by electroretinography). The optic neuritis syndrome may be isolated, prodromal, or concurrent with other neurologic distemper signs. Distemper-associated blindness also may occur with inflammation of the occipital cortex or optic radiations, but pupillary reflexes are usually normal under such circumstances.

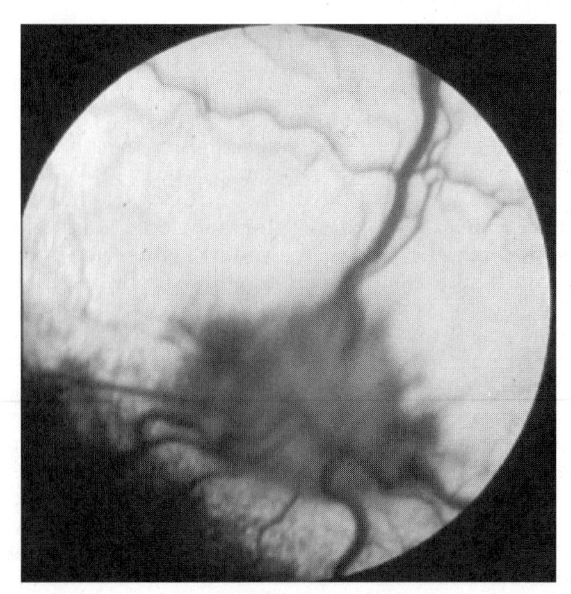

Figure 93–8. Acute optic neuritis–papillitis recognized by elevated disc, peripapillary hemorrhages, and loss of vision. Distemper is one cause for this syndrome.

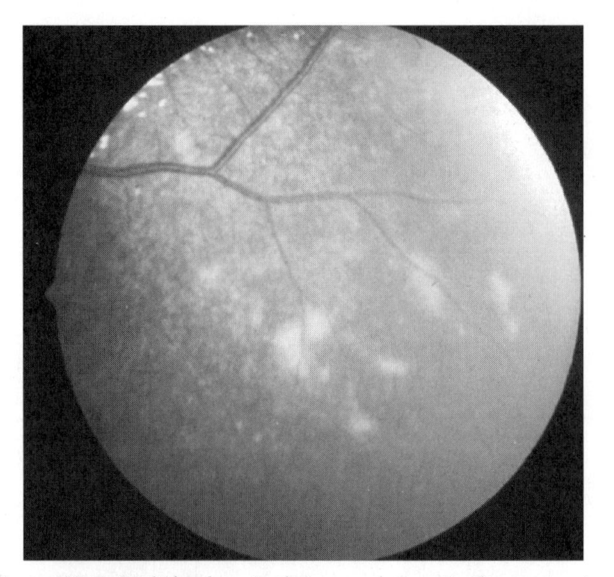

Figure 93–7. Multifocal acute distemper lesions in the nontapetum of a dog. Active lesions are recognized by hazy borders.

Ocular signs are suggestive but not definitive for distemper. Acute lesions of chorioretinitis usually correlate well with concurrent systemic disease, but chorioretinal scars do not. Finding distemper inclusions or positive immunofluorescence on conjunctival scraping may be of diagnostic help early in the course of systemic disease (5–21 days after inoculation), but a negative finding is inconclusive. Distemper should be considered in any acute optic neuropathy or acute onset of KCS.

Because no specific antiviral therapy is available, treatment is mainly symptomatic. Acute optic neuritis syndromes are treated with systemic anti-inflammatory dosages of glucocorticoids if other distemper signs are absent.

Infectious Canine Hepatitis. Canine adenovirus-1 (CAV-1) infection has been estimated to produce ocular lesions in approximately 20% of dogs recovering from natural infections, whereas a 0.4% or less prevalence has been noted in CAV-1–vaccinated dogs (see Chapter 4). The universal use of CAV-2 for immunization has made the postvaccinal reaction of corneal edema and uveitis a syndrome that is rarely observed today. The lesion, considered to be an immune complex Arthus reaction, occurs 10 to 21 days after vaccination and requires about an equal time to resolve. The condition is bilateral in 12% to 28% of the cases. The Afghan hound has been reported to have an increased prevalence,[33] and other sight hounds and Siberian huskies may share a similar high frequency of ocular reactions to CAV-l.

The most visible ocular lesion is stromal corneal edema resulting from inflammatory cell damage to the corneal endothelium (Fig. 93–9). Occasionally, a dog will have blepharospasm, miosis, hypotony, and anterior chamber flare 1 to 2 days before the corneal edema is manifest. Corneal edema may be focal or generalized and is usually transient. In some instances, the edema is permanent or may require several months to clear. A marked hypotony combined with altered corneal rigidity may result in a keratoconus. Glaucoma, the most significant sequela, usually results in blindness, because

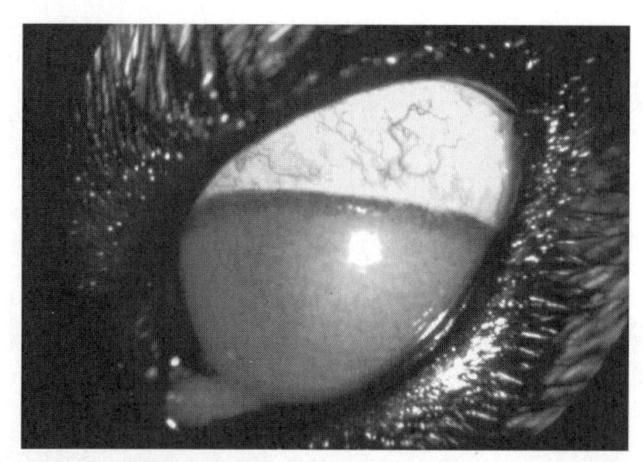

Figure 93–9. Diffuse corneal edema induced by vaccination with adenovirus-1 live vaccine. Note the early corneal neovascularization, mucoid discharge, and conjunctival hyperemia.

it is masked in the early stages by the pre-existing corneal edema and conjunctival hyperemia. The syndrome is usually diagnosed by the typical ocular lesions combined with the history of recent vaccination or illness in a puppy or young (<2 years of age) dog. Other causes of corneal edema, such as a congenital pupillary membrane syndrome, glaucoma, or corneal ulceration, should be ruled out. Therapy is similar to that for other forms of nonseptic anterior uveitis, specifically, topical glucocorticoids and atropine.

Herpesvirus Infection. Canine herpesvirus (CHV) infection (see Chapter 5) in the adult has produced only a transient conjunctivitis and vaginitis of 4 to 5 days duration. Occasional dendritic ulceration patterns are seen in the dog, but their cause has not been determined. Neonatal CHV infection produces a bilateral panuveitis with keratitis, synechiae, cataracts, retinal necrosis and disorganization, retinal atrophy and dysplasia, and optic neuritis and atrophy.[33]

Ehrlichiosis and Rocky Mountain Spotted Fever (RMSF). Either *Ehrlichia canis* or *E. platys* may produce ocular lesions (see Chapter 28). Ocular findings in canine ehrlichiosis may result from thrombocytopenia-induced hemorrhages or inflammatory reactions. Hemorrhages vary from petechiae to massive orbital or ocular hemorrhages with ehrlichiosis. Experimentally, transient, large perivascular retinal infiltrates have been observed during the first 2 months of infection, but they have not been described in clinical cases.[33] Typical ocular signs are bilateral anterior uveitis, often with ocular hemorrhages, secondary glaucoma, rhegmatogenous and exudative retinal detachments, chorioretinitis, and papilledema

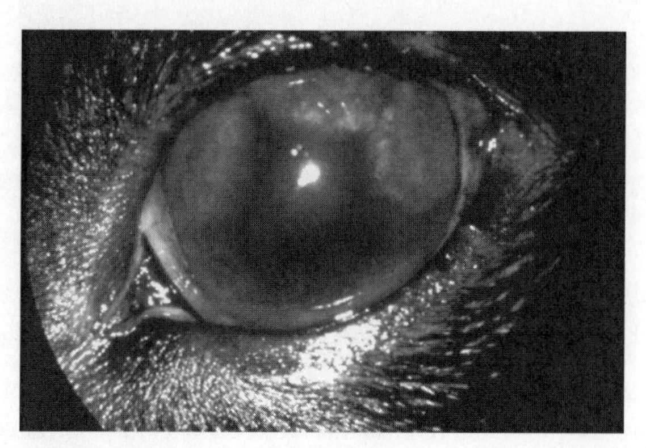

Figure 93–10. *Ehrlichia canis*–induced anterior uveitis with hyphema. Iris bombé is present, and the condition was bilateral.

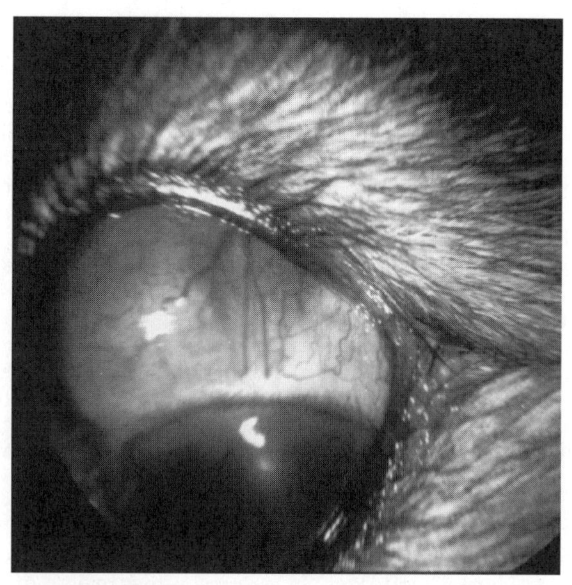

Figure 93–11. Acute scleral perforations with subconjunctival uveal prolapse associated with *Ehrlichia canis*. The initial presenting problem was anterior uveitis. The condition was bilateral.

(Fig. 93–10).[33] An unusual infrequently observed ocular lesion has been bilateral subconjunctival melting scleral lesions (scleral malacia perforans) that result in perforation and uveal tract prolapse (Fig. 93–11).

Rickettsia rickettsii produces ocular lesions that are similar to, albeit much milder than, *E. canis*. Signs of conjunctivitis; chemosis; petechiae of the conjunctiva, iris, and retina; retinal vasculitis; and anterior uveitis are common, occurring in 9 of 11 dogs in one series (Fig. 93–12).[9]

Diagnosis and antimicrobial therapy of these diseases are discussed in Chapters 28 and 29. The inflammatory lesion of the anterior ocular segment should be treated with topical or subconjunctival glucocorticoids in addition to systemic antibiotics. The ocular lesions of RMSF usually resolve quickly with therapy, but the sequelae of glaucoma, retinal

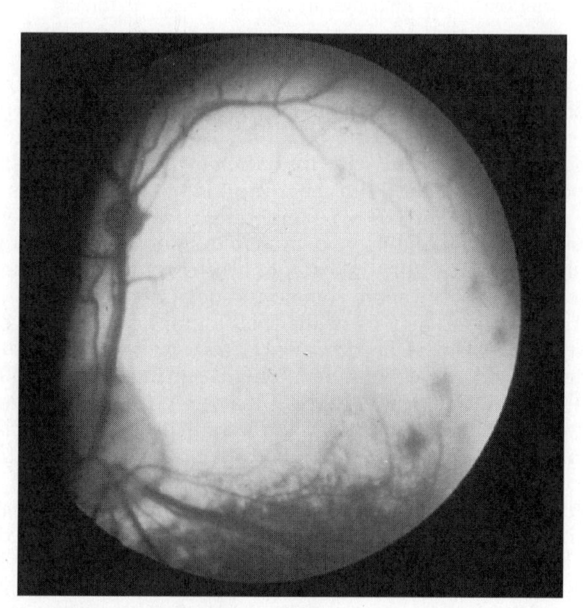

Figure 93–12. Multifocal intraretinal hemorrhages in a dog with Rocky Mountain spotted fever.

detachment, and severe ocular hemorrhage with ehrlichiosis may be blinding.

Brucellosis. *Brucella canis* has been a documented cause of unilateral or bilateral anterior uveitis and endophthalmitis, often accompanied by hemorrhage. This syndrome is often severe and blinding (see also Chapter 40).[33] Testing for *B. canis* should be performed in sexually intact or neutered dogs with unexplained uveitis or ocular hemorrhage.

With the exception of *B. canis* infection, the diagnosis of intraocular bacterial infection is usually based on cultures of centesis samples from the eye or on the association with systemic signs. Blood cultures from a septicemic animal may help identify a bacterial agent that has seeded the eye. Therapy consists of systemic and often intraocular antibiotics, because the inflammatory reaction is rapidly devastating to ocular structures. Refer to respective chapters to determine the proper therapy.

Borreliosis. Lyme disease or borreliosis produced by the spirochete *Borrelia burgdorferi* may cause ocular lesions in humans, horses, and dogs. In a retrospective review of 132 seropositive dogs, 5 had the primary complaint of ocular lesions. Ocular lesions were undoubtedly under-represented owing to the study design. Ocular lesions reported were conjunctivitis, anterior uveitis, corneal edema, retinal petechia, chorioretinitis, and retinal detachment.[7] Although ocular involvement in horses has been confirmed by isolation of the organism, such documentation is lacking in dogs. New developments in testing may confirm that ophthalmic disease occurs in infected dogs. Because of the limitations of current tests that measure antibody response, the diagnosis of borreliosis is based on compatible signs, ruling out other causes, endemic area, and response to antibiotic therapy.[31]

Other Bacterial Infections. Septicemias caused by a variety of bacteria may localize in the eyes. Examples are embolization from local infections such as bacterial endocarditis, urinary tract infection, pyometra, and dental infection. The simultaneous procedures of teeth scaling and intraocular surgery should be avoided to minimize the risk of a transient bacteremia localizing in injured ocular tissue. Contagious bacterial infections such as leptospirosis, tuberculosis, and salmonellosis may also manifest with ocular lesions.

Mycoses. The systemic mycoses in North America are frequently associated with a granulomatous anterior and/or posterior uveitis in the dog. The ocular signs are often the presenting complaint with occult systemic signs. The ocular syndromes associated with the different mycotic organisms are clinically similar. With the exception of cryptococcosis in the cat, systemic mycoses are important to rule out if bilateral uveitis-endophthalmitis and systemic signs are simultaneously observed. With the exception of cryptococcosis, these diseases have been more common in dogs than cats.

In indigenous regions of the Mississippi and Ohio Rivers and the central Atlantic states, *Blastomyces dermatitidis*–induced ocular infections commonly occur in more than 40% of the cases. Ocular involvement may vary from a relatively occult focal granulomatous chorioretinitis to a panophthalmitis syndrome (Fig. 93–13).[33] Secondary glaucoma is a frequent complication (see also Chapter 59).

As evidenced by published reports, ocular involvement with histoplasmosis is relatively rare in dogs.[33] In the cat, the ocular syndrome of histoplasmosis occurs in association with a systemic wasting or neurologic disease and will mimic feline infectious peritonitis (FIP) and feline leukemia virus (FeLV) infection. In the cat, the predominant lesion is a granulomatous choroiditis with minimal anterior segment inflammation (see also Chapter 60).[33]

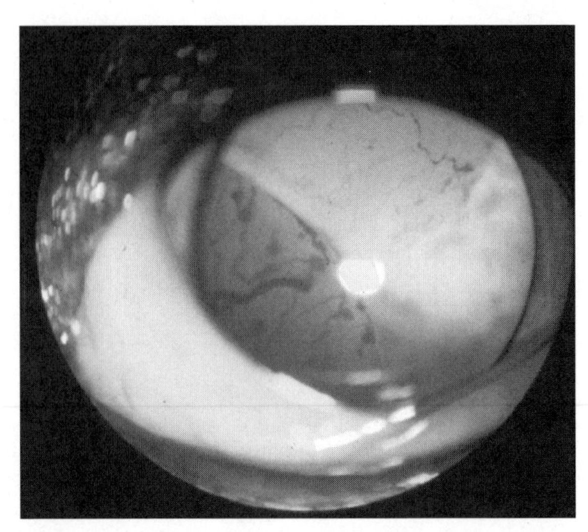

Figure 93–13. Complete exudative retinal detachment with retinal hemorrhages caused by blastomycosis. The condition was bilateral.

Coccidioides immitis is endemic in the southwestern United States. It produces a characteristic granulomatous posterior uveitis that frequently extends to the anterior segment. Organisms are found predominantly in the retina and choroid. The lesions are usually unilateral (80%), and ocular signs may be present without systemic signs (40%) (see also Chapter 62).[33]

Ocular infection with *Cryptococcus neoformans* has occurred in the dog and cat via direct extension from nasal or CNS involvement. However, hematogenous spread appears to be the most important route. Posterior uveitis is the predominant lesion, and the organisms are readily demonstrable (Fig. 93–14). Anterior uveal inflammation is less frequent, and when present, the organisms may not be demonstrable at this site, resulting in speculation that the anterior lesions may be a sterile immune-mediated inflammation.[33] Orbital and optic nerve granulomatous inflammation may also occur (see also Chapter 61).

Bilateral granulomatous chorioretinitis or endophthalmitis

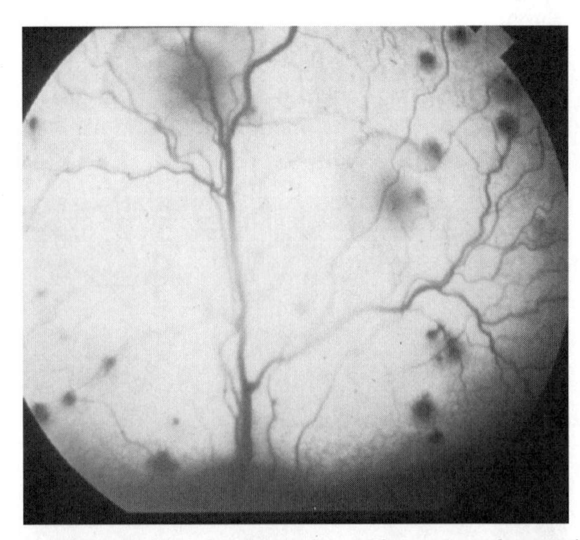

Figure 93–14. Multifocal subretinal granulomas in a dog resulting from cryptocococcis. The larger lesions are producing small bullous detachments.

should suggest the possibility of systemic mycoses. Associated systemic signs of fever and respiratory, skeletal, dermatologic, or CNS involvement are often present. The specific diagnosis is often made by finding the organism in tissue aspirates. If the systemic disease is occult, vitreal centesis may be the method of diagnosis.

Specific therapy for ocular involvement with the systemic mycoses is either systemic amphotericin B (AMB) and/or an imidazole antibiotic as discussed in Chapter 57. Subconjunctival injections of 125 μg or intraocular injection of 1 to 5 μg of AMB may augment systemic therapy but are of questionable value. Most ocular conditions that are considered severe enough for local ocular therapy have such extensive structural alterations that blindness results no matter how intensively they are treated. In many instances, the ocular inflammatory reaction continues to worsen with systemic therapy presumably owing to reaction to the killed organisms. Enucleation of blind eyes has also been proposed as a means of eliminating a nidus of infection that may cause relapses. Although it is justifiable to remove a blind, painful eye for humane reasons, the logic of recommending enucleation for infectious reasons is questionable when probably numerous other nidi remain that are not recognized.

Protothecosis. *Prototheca* are ubiquitous algae in soil and water that are occasionally pathogenic to animals (see Chapter 69). More than 50% of affected animals may have ocular involvement.[33] Most ocular syndromes are associated with systemic signs, but in some instances the systemic signs are occult. Lesions include a granulomatous posterior uveitis (Fig. 93–15) or panuveitis that is usually bilateral and blinding. Lesions are often dramatic, but will have to be differentiated from the more common causes of granulomatous uveitis. Definitive diagnosis is usually made by finding the organism on ocular aspirates, exudates, excretions, or biopsy samples. No efficacious therapy has been reported.

Toxoplasmosis. Ocular disease associated with *Toxoplasma gondii* is more commonly observed in cats than in dogs and is usually not associated with overt manifestation of the disease. In experimental and natural infections with *T. gondii* in the dog, the ocular lesions, in order of decreasing frequency, were a mononuclear anterior uveitis (35/60), retinitis (27/60), choroiditis (18/60), extraocular myositis (12/60), scleritis (3/60), and optic neuritis (3/60).[33] We have also noted episcleritis in the dog and cat as the presenting and only clinical sign with elevated and raising *Toxoplasma* titers. Although systemic disease production with *T. gondii* is relatively rare, when it occurs in the dog it is usually associated with other diseases such as distemper or other systemic debilitating states. *T. gondii* appears to be a very significant cause of ocular lesions in systemically healthy dogs and cats on the basis of the correlation of lesions with positive serology findings. The pathogenesis of the ocular inflammation is unknown, because histopathology of uveitis of the eyes rarely demonstrates the organism.

Because of the ubiquitous presence of *T. gondii*, it should be considered in the differential diagnosis of endogenous anterior uveitis and chorioretinitis whether or not systemic signs are present. A diagnosis of toxoplasmosis is usually based on serologic testing, preferably with species-specific anti-immunoglobulins (see Chapter 80).

Toxoplasmosis may be a self-limiting disease that does not require therapy, but if systemic signs or active intraocular inflammation is present, systemic therapy is usually advised. Oral clindamycin at 12.5 mg/kg given every 12 hours for 21 to 30 days and topical glucocorticoids and atropine are recommended for surface and anterior uveal inflammation and clindamycin and oral glucocorticoids for posterior uveal inflammation. In cats with uveitis, the combination therapy of clindamycin and glucocorticoids was more successful in suppressing ocular inflammation than glucocorticoids alone.[27]

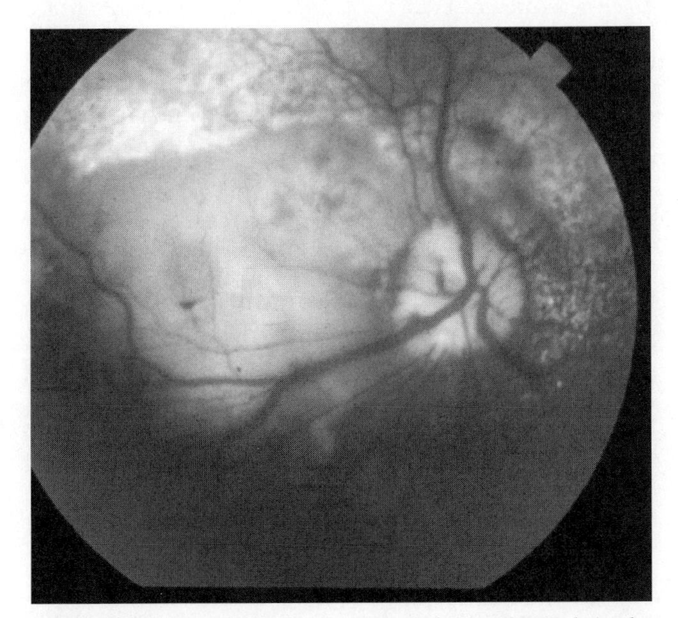

Figure 93–15. Large bullous detachment from subretinal exudate associated with protothecosis. The organism was isolated from the urine sediment.

Neosporosis. *Neospora caninum* is a protozoan parasite that is morphologically similar to *T. gondii*. Currently, the only identified mode of transmission is the transplacental route; consequently, reports in the dog have often involved neonate infections. Although puppies die or are euthanized because of neurologic signs, ocular lesions are present in most cases. The ocular lesions are mainly a retinitis with extension into the choroid (retinochoroiditis). A mild anterior uveitis was also reported.[14] Further reports are necessary to determine the importance and extent of this syndrome in the dog (see also Chapter 80).

Leishmaniasis. The dog is a reservoir host for *Leishmania donovani* in endemic areas of the Mediterranean region, Africa, and Asia, and may produce ocular lesions of blepharitis, scleritis, keratitis, anterior uveitis, and secondary glaucoma. Whereas the anterior vitreous may have an inflammatory reaction, the posterior choroid and retina are usually spared. Uveitis may be exacerbated with therapy. The inflammation is mononuclear, and the organism can be found in the histiocytes. The majority of cases reported in North America have been in dogs imported from endemic areas, but reports involving a closed research colony of English foxhounds in Ohio and Oklahoma indicate that, once introduced, it can be transmitted in the United States.[57] Therapy with IV pentavalent antimonial compounds every 48 hours for 20 to 30 treatments produces remission of clinical signs, but the relapse rate is high (75%) (see Chapter 73).[25]

Cats

Anterior uveitis is a common disorder in the cat and may be related to a variety of underlying mechanisms. Uveitis, unilateral or bilateral, may be the only presenting clinical

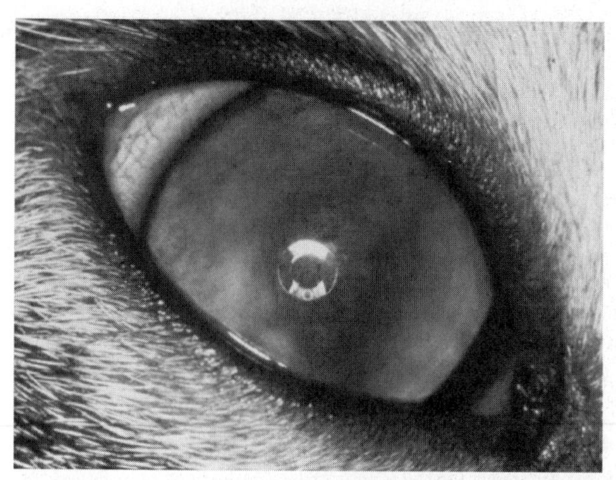

Figure 93–16. Anterior uveitis in a cat with blood-tinged fibrin in the anterior chamber. Note the obscurity of the pupil and iris surface detail.

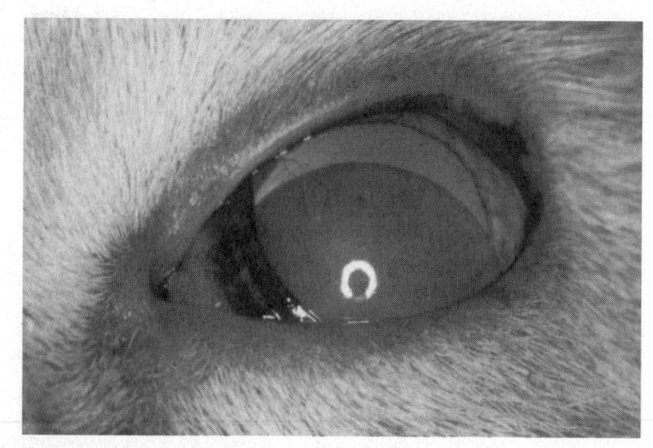

Figure 93–18. Cataract and anterior lens luxation in a cat with toxoplasmosis and uveitis.

sign, even if systemic infection with an organism is present. Signs of uveitis may include aqueous flare, keratic precipitate, miosis, posterior synechia, iridal hyperemia or neovascularization, and ocular pain (Figs. 93–16 and 93–17). Many cats do not exhibit ocular pain, which may allow the uveitis to advance without detection, leading to glaucoma in many instances. Lens luxation is also a potential sequela to uveitis in the cat (Fig. 93–18) and has been associated with toxoplasmosis and FIV infection, which are discussed next (see also Chapters 14 and 80).[46, 47] The cause of many cases of feline uveitis remains unknown despite extensive testing. In a study of 53 cats with anterior uveitis that were tested for infectious disease known to cause uveitis in cats, 37 (70%) had no underlying cause established.[10] Another study of 124 cats with uveitis found positive serologic results in 83% of samples tested for infectious agents.[28] Following is a discussion of infectious agents that are known to cause uveitis in cats.

Toxoplasmosis. *T. gondii* has been implicated over the past few years as a major contributor to uveitis in the cat.[4, 14, 27–29] The diagnosis of toxoplasmosis-related uveitis is generally based on a positive serum *T. gondii* antibody titer, although sensitive tests designed to identify the organism in biologic samples have been developed.[25a, 54] Laboratory tests that measure both *T. gondii*–specific IgM and IgG are most helpful, because the IgM class of antibody has been shown to rise and fall over approximately 3 to 4 months after infection, whereas the IgG class of antibody may rise more slowly and remain elevated in cats for years after exposure to *T. gondii*.[26] Additionally, cats coinfected with FIV and *T. gondii* may develop a positive IgM antibody titer, whereas the IgG antibody titer remains negative.[28] Cats with toxoplasmosis-induced uveitis should be treated with oral clindamycin hydrochloride, 12.5 mg/kg every 12 hours for 21 to 30 days, in addition to a topical glucocorticoid, such as 1% prednisolone acetate every 6 hours, and atropine (as needed to maintain mydriasis).[27] Long-term use of topical prednisolone acetate may be needed to control the uveitis.

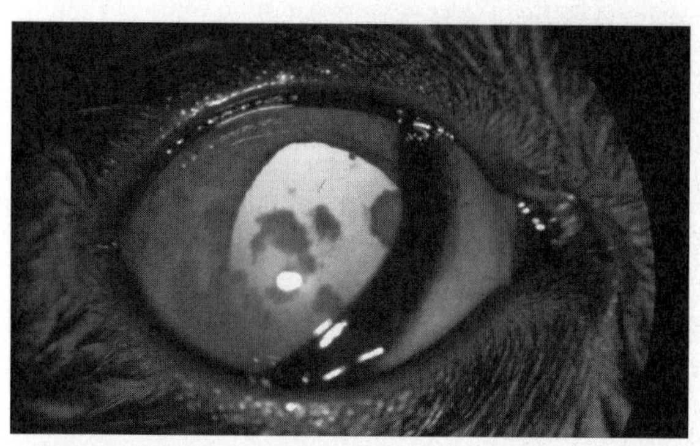

Figure 93–17. Anterior uveitis with large keratic precipitates in a cat with feline infectious peritonitis.

FIV. Infection with FIV has also been associated with uveitis. In an experimental study, 3 of 20 cats developed anterior uveitis and conjunctivitis after infection with FIV.[3] In a study of 9 cats with naturally occurring FIV infection, all had ocular disease; anterior uveitis was the most frequent clinical diagnosis.[16] Pars planitis was seen in 4 of these 9 cats and was evidenced by anterior vitreal and pars planitis inflammatory cell infiltrates. In a study of 54 clinically ill cats that were seropositive for antibody to FIV, 19 cats (35%) had ocular disease. Anterior uveitis and chorioretinitis were the most common findings. Serologic evidence of coinfection with *T. gondii* was present in 28 (57%) of 49 FIV-positive cats tested for toxoplasmosis. Of the 19 cats with ocular disease, 14 (74%) were coinfected with *T. gondii*.[47] Approximately 43% of cats coinfected with both FIV and *T. gondii* had positive *T. gondii*–specific IgM serum antibody titers without a positive *T. gondii*–specific IgG titer, emphasizing the need for a laboratory test that includes both antibody classes.

Cats with uveitis should always be tested for both toxoplasmosis and FIV infections simultaneously. Treatment of uveitis in cats with both FIV and toxoplasmosis should be as that for toxoplasmosis. Cats with uveitis associated only with FIV should be treated with topical prednisolone acetate. Some cats may also benefit from oral prednisolone. Long-term topical prednisolone acetate may be needed to control the uveitis. In our experience, response of pars planitis to oral and topical prednisolone has been poor.

FIP. The most common ocular manifestation of infection with FIP is bilateral granulomatous anterior uveitis, often accompanied by chorioretinitis (see also Chapter 11). There are frequently large keratic precipitates and a fibrinous exudate into the anterior chamber (see Fig. 93–17). The nature of the disease is a vasculitis, and it is common to see a pyogranulomatous exudate sheathing the retinal vessels (Fig. 93–19). Retinal hemorrhages and detachments may also occur.

Ocular disease is more common with the noneffusive or

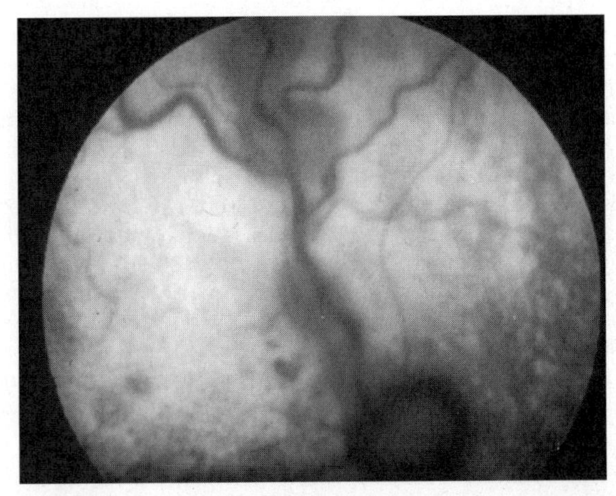

Figure 93–19. Chorioretinitis and retinal perivascular sheathing in a cat with feline infectious peritonitis.

dry form of FIP and may be the initial presenting sign. Diagnosis of FIP-associated ocular disease is difficult because of the nonspecific nature of available coronavirus serum antibody tests. Rising serum antibody titers in the presence of characteristic ocular lesions is suggestive.

Because there is no effective treatment at this time for FIP, treatment of ocular disease is symptomatic and includes topical, subconjunctival, or systemic glucocorticoid and topical atropine. Temporary amelioration of ocular disease may occur, but it will usually rebound in a short period of time.

FeLV. The predominant ocular manifestation of FeLV is lymphosarcoma.[2] The uveal tract is a common site for metastasis of neoplastic lymphocytes via hematogenous spread. Cats with ocular lymphosarcomas may present initially with signs of mild uveitis, including miosis, aqueous flare, and keratic precipitates. As the disease progresses, the iris becomes greatly thickened and distorted with the infiltration of tumor cells. Glaucoma is a common sequela as tumor cells infiltrate the iridocorneal angle. Aqueous centesis may be helpful in making the diagnosis, because neoplastic lymphocytes exfoliate into the aqueous humor. In addition to intraocular involvement, we have frequently seen concurrent invasion of the orbit by lymphosarcoma. Aggressive treatment of cats with ocular lymphosarcoma with topical glucocorticoids, such as 1% prednisolone acetate, as well as systemic therapy with glucocorticoids or other chemotherapeutic protocols, can result in temporary improvement.

Spastic pupil syndrome has been seen in some FeLV-positive cats. It is characterized by anisocoria, which may be changing in nature, with no other ocular abnormalities present. The syndrome is thought to occur because of viral invasion of the ciliary ganglion and short ciliary nerves.

Mycoses. Systemic fungal infections are less common in the cat than the dog. Ocular lesions may accompany systemic mycoses and may be the presenting signs. *Cryptococcus neoformans* is the most commonly reported feline mycotic infection and enters the body through the respiratory tract (see also Chapter 60). Chorioretinitis, with granulomatous inflammation and retinal detachment, is the most common manifestation; anterior uveitis is less frequent. Optic neuritis may also occur, particularly if the CNS is involved. A case of adnexal cryptococcus in a cat, without intraocular or systemic lesions, has been described.[35]

Granulomatous chorioretinitis has also been infrequently described in cats with *Blastomyces dermatitidis*, *Histoplasma capsulatum*, and *Coccidioides immitis*. In the cat, ocular histoplasmosis occurs in association with a systemic wasting or neurologic disease that may mimic the more common diseases of FIP and FeLV infection. In the cat, the predominant lesion is a granulomatous choroiditis with minimal anterior segment inflammation.[33] Itraconazole has been administered successfully to treat cats with histoplasmosis.[22a]

Diagnosis of ocular mycotic infections is best made by cytologic examination of aspirated samples from open skin lesions, the respiratory system, the lymph nodes, or the eye itself. Vitreous centesis is often the most rewarding sample for obtaining fungal elements for identification, although the risk of damaging the eye is greater (see discussion of canine ocular mycotic infections) than with aqueous centesis. Serum antigen titers are helpful for identifying cats affected by cryptococcosis and for monitoring response to therapy.[37]

The treatment of systemic mycotic infections is described in Chapter 57. If anterior uveitis is present, it should also be treated with a topical glucocorticoid, such as 1% prednisolone acetate, and atropine. Treatment of chorioretinitis must be delivered parenterally and may include the judicious use of oral glucocorticoids to damp the severe inflammatory response that accompanies ocular fungal infection along with appropriate antifungal therapy. Treatment of cryptococcosis in cats with itraconazole has the benefit of a high efficacy and a lower rate of adverse side effects than does ketoconazole or AMB.[37]

DIAGNOSIS

Aqueous Centesis

This procedure is performed using heavy sedation or general anesthesia. A 25- to 30-gauge needle on a tuberculin syringe is utilized with the "seal" broken so that movement of the plunger does not require a jerky effort. The site of centesis is usually in the dorsal or lateral limbus because it is the most accessible. Forceps applied to the conjunctiva close to the limbus fixates the globe and applies counterpressure to the needle. The needle enters the cornea just rostral to the limbus and parallel to the plane of the iris. The operator must be careful to avoid the iris, lens, and corneal endothelium (Fig. 93–20). The procedure may be more hazardous

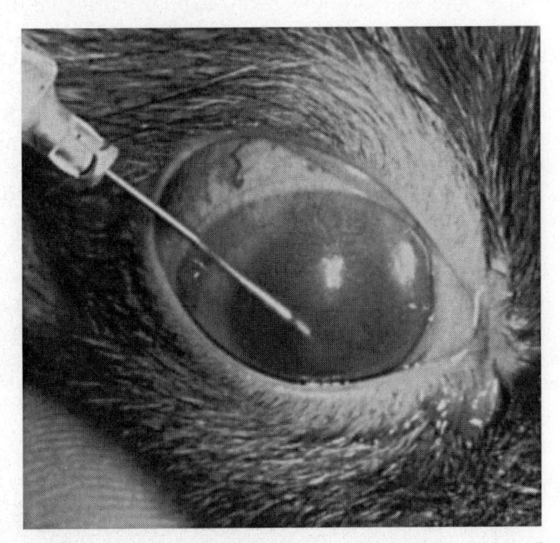

Figure 93–20. Aqueous centesis being performed on a cat with feline leukemia–associated anterior uveitis.

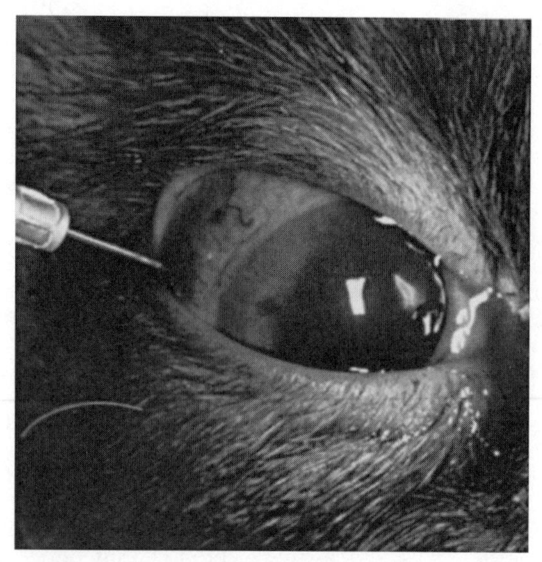

Figure 93–21. Vitreous centesis being performed on a cat. The needle enters 6 mm posterior to the limbus and is directed to the center of the globe.

in the diseased cornea because the needle point is obscured, and the increased corneal thickness results in a longer, beveled tract before the needle enters the anterior chamber. Unless the anterior chamber is collapsed, the volume that can be removed in the dog is about 0.3 ml, and in the cat about 0.5 ml. A culture swab is saturated with a portion of the aspirated aqueous, and the remaining aliquot is prepared for cytology by centrifugation or fine filtration (Milipore, Bedford, MA). An antibiotic is frequently injected after aspiration of the aqueous (see Table 93–4). If fibrin clots and adhesions of less than 4 days' duration are present, 25 μg of tissue plasminogen activator (tPA) may be injected to dissolve clots and break adhesions.[34]

Vitreous Centesis

Centesis of the vitreous cavity has more potential complications than aqueous centesis and is usually reserved for eyes that have lost considerable visual function. Vitreous hemorrhage and retinal hole formation are the two most likely complications. A 25-gauge needle with a 3-ml syringe for added suction is utilized. The site of entry is 6 mm caudal to the limbus in the dorsolateral quadrant. Forceps are employed to apply counterpressure, and the needle point is aimed at the center of the globe (Fig. 93–21). The needle should be short (0.5 inch) so that it is not inadvertently passed completely across the vitreous to tear the opposite retina. If fluid cannot be obtained, minor positioning changes of the needle point are attempted. If unsuccessful, the procedure is repeated with a 22-gauge needle. The syringe is removed while the needle is kept in place, and the aspirated fluid is placed on a culture swab. The remainder is concentrated by centrifugation for cytology. A bactericidal antibiotic is injected at the appropriate dose if a bacterial endophthalmitis is suspected (see Table 93–4).

THERAPY

The therapeutic routes available for treating ocular infections are topical, subconjunctival, intraocular, retrobulbar, and systemic. The routes selected will depend on the location, severity of the infection, and the drug being given. The eye has three rather formidable barriers to drug penetration: the intact cornea for topical penetration and the blood-aqueous and blood-retinal barriers for systemic drug penetration. In general, drugs with a differential solubility in water and lipids and small molecular size are better able to penetrate these barriers. Inflammation or ulceration will negate these barriers to a variable degree and allow better penetration. Table 93–6 summarizes the ability of a variety of antibacterials to penetrate into the normal eye.[33] The vitreous is a large, rather inert structure; this results in low drug levels by any route of drug administration except direct intravitreal injection, in which the vitreous acts as a depot for the relatively slow release of the drug.

Topical

Depending on the drug and whether the cornea is intact, topical therapy may provide adequate drug levels only on the surface or as deep as the iris and ciliary body. Epithelial defects of 25% to 50% increase drug penetration into the corneal stroma and aqueous by nine times, but larger defects do not produce an additional increase.[23] Other variables influencing drug concentrations via topical administration are the frequency of application, drug contact time, and drug concentration. In general, ointments have a longer contact time than solutions, but some drugs (dexamethasone) bind to the ointments, resulting in decreased drug availability. To a point, a higher drug concentration will increase the absorption. However, concentrated drugs may increase reflex lacrimation and become diluted by osmotically drawing fluid from the tissues.

When drops are provided, about 20 μl of a preparation is adequate. Multiple or rapidly repeated instillations of the same or different preparations simply increase the rate of loss via the nasolacrimal duct or mutually dilute each preparation, thereby reducing the availability of each drug. An interval of 2 to 5 minutes should be observed between instillation of multiple drugs to allow reflex tearing to subside and to avoid diluting the previous drop.

Treatment of routine surface infections of the conjunctiva or prophylactic antibacterial therapy of corneal ulcers should

Table 93–6. Intraocular Penetration of Antibacterial Agents in the Noninflamed Eye

	PENETRATION BY ROUTE		
AGENT	Systemic	Topical	Subconjunctival
Penicillin	Poor	Poor	Good
Ampicillin	Poor	Poor	Good
Methicillin	Good (multiple dose)	—	Good
Erythromycin	Poor	Good	Good
Cephalosporins	Poor	Poor	Good
Colistin	Poor	Poor	Good
Gentamicin	Poor	Poor	Good
Tobramycin	Poor	Poor	Good
Lincomycin	Good	—	—
Neomycin	—	Poor	—
Chloramphenicol	Fair	Good	Good
Tetracycline	Poor	Good	—
Bacitracin	—	Poor	Poor
Polymyxin B	—	Poor	—
Trimethoprim-sulfadiazine	Good	Good	Good
Sulfonamides (in general)	Good	Good	Good
Ciprofloxacin	Good	Fair	Good
Ofloxacin	—	Good	Good

include topical broad-spectrum antibiotics, such as neomycin-polymyxin-bacitracin, that are not applied systemically. This rationale is based on minimizing bacterial resistance to antibiotics that are beneficial in systemic therapy and avoiding sensitization of a patient by a topical antibiotic that might have potential in systemic therapy. In practice, routine bacterial conjunctivitis is not initially cultured due to the cost and the ambiguous results.

Subconjunctival

Subconjunctival administration is used primarily for anterior segment disease and can achieve therapeutic intraocular levels of water-soluble antibiotics that normally do not penetrate into the eye. The major limitations of subconjunctival injections are drug irritation and ocular manipulation. The means by which a subconjunctivally injected drug reaches the interior of the eye are controversial, but both direct diffusion through the sclera, which has no epithelial barrier, and vascular uptake and leakage through the needle hole with topical absorption have been demonstrated. Except for long-acting drugs, most others must be readministered at 12- to 24-hour intervals to maintain therapeutic levels. Whereas significant posterior segment levels of drugs can be achieved when injecting near the equator of the globe, the subconjunctival route is *not* adequate for bacterial infections of the vitreous or optic nerve. Table 93–4 gives the subconjunctival dosages for various antibiotics.[33]

Intraocular

Intracameral or intraocular injection of antibiotics is a heroic and extremely effective means of achieving high levels of antibiotics. To preserve vision, the decision to use the intracameral route must be made early to avoid rapidly devastating inflammation to delicate intraocular structures. Because culture and susceptibility testing results are not available, a broad-spectrum bactericidal antibiotic is usually administered. The intraocular injection in itself has an inherent risk, but, in addition, the drug concentration is critical owing to toxicity to the retina, lens, and corneal endothelium. Historically, gentamicin (350–500 μg), cephaloridine (250 μg), and cephalothin (2 mg), either alone or in combination, have been the drugs recommended for intraocular administration.[33] Intravitreal injection of cephalothin and gentamicin produce therapeutic levels for 32 and 96 hours, respectively. However, the combination of gentamicin and cephalosporins in the vitreous may be of questionable value because aminoglycosides are inactivated when incubated in vitro with β-lactam antibiotics. With the emergence of gentamicin-resistant organisms, other aminoglycosides have been advocated. Amikacin is inactivated by β-lactam antibiotics to a lesser degree than gentamicin and tobramycin. The aminoglycoside with greatest retinal toxicity is gentamicin followed by, in decreasing order, netilmicin, tobramycin, amikacin, and kanamycin. The relative lack of resistant organisms combined with decreased toxicity has resulted in amikacin (400 μg) being advocated over gentamicin for intraocular injection.[33] However, amikacin has a 20% to 50% higher incidence of falsely resistant organisms than gentamicin and tobramycin when tested with Kirby-Bauer disks.[33] Systemic and topical antibiotics are often administered concurrently with intraocular antibiotics, although it is doubtful that they add to the therapeutic effectiveness. Intraocular injections of dexamethasone in conjunction with antibiotics have been recommended to minimize the inflammation and ocular tissue disruption, although this practice is controversial.

Adjunctive

In addition to specific antimicrobial therapy, standard nursing care involves cleansing of the ocular surface and lids with warm, moist swabs or using hot packing, if lid and orbital swelling is evident, to remove accumulated discharges. Antiprostaglandin preparations such as flunixin, phenylbutazone, and aspirin provide analgesia and lessen the inflammatory reaction. Topical atropine minimizes ocular pain due to ciliary muscle spasms and pupil adhesions and is usually standard therapy with intraocular inflammation. Injection of 25 μg tPA into the anterior chamber is an effective and dramatic means of breaking down adhesions and dissolving fibrin clots if given within 3 to 4 days of formation. Once the clot is organized, the efficacy is lost and, if hemorrhage is present, rebleeding may occur after injection. Injections may be repeated if necessary. Injection of tPA into the vitreous is not as safe due to retinal toxicity.

References

1. Apt L, Isenberg SJ, Yoshimore R, et al. 1995. The effect of povidone-iodine solution applied at the conclusion of ophthalmic surgery. *Am J Ophthalmol* 119:701–705.
2. Brightman AH, Ogilvie GK, Tompkins M. 1991. Ocular disease in FeLV-positive cats: 11 cases (1981–1986). *J Am Vet Med Assoc* 6:1049–1051.
3. Callanan JJ, Thompson H, Toth SR, et al. 1992. Clinical and pathological findings in feline immunodeficiency virus experimental infection. *Vet Immunol Immunopathol* 35:3–13.
4. Chavkin MJ, Lappin MR, Powell CC, et al. 1994. Seroepidemiologic and clinical observations of 93 cases of uveitis in cats. *Vet Comp Ophthalmol* 2:29–36.
5. Chavkin MJ, Lappin MR, Powell CC, et al. 1994. *Toxoplasma gondii*-specific antibodies in the aqueous humor of cats with toxoplasmosis. *Am J Vet Res* 55:1244–1249.
6. Chitkara DK, Manners T, Chapman F, et al. 1994. Lack of effect of preoperative norfloxacin on bacterial contamination of anterior chamber aspirates after cataract surgery. *Br J Ophthalmol* 78:772–774.
7. Cohen ND, Carter CN, Thomas MA, et al. 1990. Clinical and epizootiologic characteristics of dogs seropositive for *Borrelia burgdorferi* in Texas: 110 cases (1988). *J Am Vet Med Assoc* 197:893–898.
8. Collins BK, Nasisse MP, Moore CP. 1995. In vitro efficacy of L-lysine against feline herpesvirus type-1. *Trans Am Coll Vet Ophthalmol* 26:141.
9. Davidson MG, Breitschwerdt DB, Nasisse MP, et al. 1989. Ocular manifestations of Rocky Mountain spotted fever in dogs. *J Am Vet Med Assoc* 194:777–781.
10. Davidson MG, Nasisse MP, English RV, et al. 1991. Feline anterior uveitis: a study of 53 cases. *J Am Anim Hosp Assoc* 27:77–83.
11. Davidson MG, Nasisse MP, Jamieson VE, et al. 1993. Phacoemulsification and intraocular lens implantation: a study of surgical results in 182 dogs. *Prog Vet Comp Ophthalmol* 1:233–238.
12. Donnenfeld ED, Schrier A, Perry HD, et al. 1994. Penetration of topically applied ciprofloxacin, norfloxacin, and ofloxacin into the aqueous humor. *Ophthalmology* 101:902–905.
13. Doyle A, Beigi B, Early A, et al. 1995. Adherence of bacteria to intraocular lenses: a prospective study. *Br J Ophthalmol* 79:347–349.
14. Dubey JP, Carpenter JL. 1993. Histologically confirmed clinical toxoplasmosis in cats: 100 cases (1952–1990). *J Am Vet Med Assoc* 203:1556–1566.
15. Dubey JP, Koestner A, Piper RC. 1990. Repeated transplacental transmission of *Neospora caninum* in dogs. *J Am Vet Med Assoc* 197:857–860.
16. English RV, Davidson MG, Nasisse MP, et al. 1990. Intraocular disease associated with feline immunodeficiency virus infection in cats. *J Am Vet Med Assoc* 196:1116–1119.
17. Espinola MB, Lilenbaum W. 1996. Prevalence of bacteria in the conjunctival sac and on the eyelid margin of clinically normal cats. *J Small Anim Pract* 37:364–366.
18. Gerding PA, Cormany K, Weisiger R, et al. 1993. Survey and topographic distribution of bacterial and fungal microorganisms in eyes of clinically normal cats. *Feline Pract* 21:20–23.
19. Gerding PA, Cormany K, Weisiger R, et al. 1993. Survey and topographic distribution of bacterial and fungal microorganisms in eyes of clinically normal dogs. *Canine Pract* 18:34–38.

20. Griffith RS, Norins AL, Kagan C. 1978. A multicentered study of lysine therapy in herpes simplex infection. *Dermatologica* 156:257–267.
21. Haesebrouck F, Devriese LA, van-Rijssen B, et al. 1991. Incidence and significance of isolation of *Mycoplasma felis* from conjunctival swabs of cats. *Vet Microbiol* 26:95–101.
22. Mauger TF, Craig EL (eds). 1994. Havener's ocular pharmacology, ed. 6. CV Mosby, St Louis, MO.
22a. Hodges RD, Legendre AM, Adams LG, et al. 1994. Itraconazole for the treatment of histoplasmosis in cats. *J Vet Intern Med* 8:409–413.
23. Johnson D. 1995. The relationship of corneal epithelial defect size to drug penetration. *Arch Ophthalmol* 113:641–644.
24. Jones SMP, Bedford PCG. 1989. Ocular antimicrobial therapy in small animal practice. *J Small Anim Pract* 30:550–578.
25. Kontos VJ, Koutinas AF. 1993. Old world canine leishmaniasis. *Compend Cont Educ Pract Vet* 15:949–959.
25a. Lappin MR, Burney DP, Dow SW, et al. 1996. Polymerase chain reaction for detection of *Toxoplasma gondii* in aqueous humor of cats. *Am J Vet Res* 57:1589–1593.
25b. Lappin MR, Dow SW, Reif JS, et al. 1997. Elevated interleukin 6 activity in aqueous humor of cats with ureitis. *Vet. Immunol Immuno pathol* 58:17–26.
26. Lappin MR, Greene CE, Prestwood AK, et al. 1989. Diagnosis of recent *Toxoplasma gondii* infection in cats by use of an enzyme-linked immunosorbent assay for immunoglobulin M. *Am J Vet Res* 50:1580–1585.
27. Lappin MR, Greene CE, Winston S, et al. 1989. Clinical feline toxoplasmosis. Serologic diagnosis and therapeutic management of 15 cases. *J Vet Intern Med* 3:139–143.
28. Lappin MR, Marks A, Greene CE, et al. 1992. Serologic prevalence of selected infectious diseases in cats with uveitis. *J Am Vet Med Assoc* 201:1005–1009.
29. Lappin MR, Roberts SM, Davidson MG, et al. 1992. Enzyme-linked immunosorbent assays for the detection of *Toxoplasma gondii*-specific antibodies and antigens in the aqueous humor of cats. *J Am Vet Med Assoc* 201:1010–1016.
30. Lesk MR, Amman H, Marcil G, et al. 1993. The penetration of oral ciprofloxacin into the aqueous humor, vitreous, and subretinal fluid of humans. *Am J Ophthalmol* 115:623–628.
31. Levy SA, Dombach DM, Barthold SW, et al. 1993. Canine Lyme borreliosis. *Compend Cont Educ Pract Vet* 15:833–846.
32. Marlar AB, Miller PE, Canton DD, et al. 1994. Canine keratomycosis: a report of eight cases and literature review. *J Am Anim Hosp Assoc* 30:331–340.
33. Martin C. 1990. Ocular infections, pp 197–212. *In* Greene CE (ed), Infectious diseases of the dog and cat. WB Saunders, Philadelphia, PA.
34. Martin C, Kaswan R, Gratzek A, et al. 1993. Ocular use of tissue plasminogen activator in companion animals. *Prog Vet Comp Ophthalmol* 3:29–36.
35. Martin C, Stiles J, Willis M. 1996. Ocular adnexal cryptococcus in a cat. *Vet Comp Ophthalmol* 6:225–229.
36. McLeish W, Pflugfelder SC, Crouse C, et al. 1990. Interferon treatment of herpetic keratitis in a patient with acquired immunodeficiency syndrome. *Am J Ophthalmol* 109:93–94.
37. Medleau L, Greene CE, Rakich PM. 1990. Evaluation of ketoconazole and itraconazole for treatment of disseminated cryptococcosis in cats. *Am J Vet Res* 51:1454–1458.
38. Miller DM, Blue JL, Winston SM. 1983. Keratomycosis caused by *Cladosporium* sp in a cat. *J Am Vet Med Assoc* 182:1121–1122.
39. Mohan M, Gupta SK, Vajpayee RB, et al. 1988. Management of keratomycosis with 1% silver sulfadiazine: a prospective controlled clinical trial of 110 cases, pp 495–498. *In* Cavanagh HD (ed), The cornea: transactions of the world congress on the cornea III. Raven Press, New York, NY.
40. Nasisse MP, English RV, Tompkins MB, et al. 1995. Immunologic, histologic, and virologic features of herpesvirus-induced stromal keratitis in cats. *Am J Vet Res* 56:51–55.
41. Nasisse MP, Guy JS, Davidson MG, et al. 1989. Experimental ocular herpesvirus infection in the cat. Sites of virus replication, clinical features and effects of corticosteroid administration. *Invest Ophthalmol Vis Sci* 30:1758–1768.
42. Nasisse MP, Guy JS, Davidson MG, et al. 1989. In vitro susceptibility of feline herpesvirus-1 to vidarabine, idoxuridine, trifluridine, acyclovir or bromovinyldeoxyuridine. *Am J Vet Res* 50:158–160.
43. Nasisse MP, Guy JS, Stevens JB, et al. 1993. Clinical and laboratory findings in chronic conjunctivitis in cats: 91 cases (1983–1991). *J Am Vet Med Assoc* 203:834–837.
44. O'Dair HA, Hopper CD, Gruffydd-Jones TJ, et al. 1994. Clinical aspects of *Chlamydia psittaci* infection in cats infected with feline immunodeficiency virus. *Vet Rec* 134:365–368.
45. O'Day DM, Ray WA, Head WS, et al. 1984. Influence of the corneal epithelium on the efficacy of topical antifungal agents. *Invest Ophthalmol Vis Sci* 25:855–859.
46. Olivero DK, Riis RC, Dutton AG, et al. 1991. Feline lens displacement: A retrospective analysis of 345 cases. *Vet Comp Ophthalmol* 4:239–244.
47. O'Neil SA, Lappin MR, Reif JS, et al. 1991. Clinical and epidemiological aspects of feline immunodeficiency virus and *Toxoplasma gondii* coinfections in cats. *J Am Anim Hosp Assoc* 27:211–222.
48. Peiffer R. 1991. Posterior chamber intraocular lens implantation in the dog: results of 65 implants in 61 patients. *J Am Anim Hosp Assoc* 27:453–462.
49. Peiffer RL, Wilcock BP. 1991. Histopathologic study of uveitis in cats: 139 cases (1978–1988). *J Am Vet Med Assoc* 198:135–138.
50. Roberts SM, Severin GA, Lavach JD. 1986. Antibacterial activity of dilute povidone-iodine solutions used for ocular surface disinfection in dogs. *Am J Vet Res* 47:1207–1210.
51. Snyder R, Hyndiuk R. 1995. Mechanisms of bacterial invasion of the cornea, pp 1–7. *In* Tasman W, Jaeger E (eds), Duane's foundations of clinical ophthalmology. Lippincott-Raven, Philadelphia, PA.
52. Stiles J. 1995. Treatment of cats with ocular disease attributable to herpesvirus infection: 17 cases (1983–1993). *J Am Vet Med Assoc* 207:599–603.
53. Stiles J, McDermott M, Bigsby D, et al. 1997. Use of nested polymerase chain reaction to identify feline herpesviruses in ocular tissue from clinically normal cats and cats with corneal sequestra or conjunctivitis. *Am J Vet Res* 58:338–342.
54. Stiles J, Prade RA, Greene CE. 1996. Detection of *Toxoplasma gondii* in feline and canine biological samples by use of the polymerase chain reaction. *Am J Vet Res* 57:264–267.
55. Sundmacher R, Cantell K, Neumann-Haefelin D. 1978. Combination therapy of dendritic keratitis with trifluorothymidine and interferon. *Lancet* 2:687.
56. Sundmacher R, Mattes A, Neumann-Haefelin D, et al. 1987. The potency of interferon-alpha 2 and interferon-gamma in a combination therapy of dendritic keratitis. A controlled clinical study. *Curr Eye Res* 6:273–276.
57. Swenson CL, Silverman J, Stromberg PC, et al. 1988. Visceral leishmaniasis in an English foxhound form an Ohio research colony. *J Am Vet Med Assoc* 193:1089–1092.
58. Taylor M, Kern TJ, Riis RC, et al. 1995. Intraocular bacterial contamination during cataract surgery in dogs. *J Am Vet Med Assoc* 206:1716–1720.
59. Thomas W, Sorjonen D, Steiss J. 1993. A retrospective evaluation of 38 cases of canine distemper encephalomyelitis. *J Am Anim Hosp Assoc* 29:129–133.
60. Tsubota K, Kajiwara K, Ugajin S, et al. 1990. Conjunctival brush cytology. *Acta Cytol* 34:233–235.
61. Wiedbrauk DL, Werner JC, Drevon AM, et al. 1995. Inhibition of PCR by aqueous and vitreous fluids. *J Clin Microbiol* 33:2643–2646.
62. Willis M, Bounous D, Hirsh S, et al. 1997. Conjunctival brush cytology: evaluation of a new cytological collection technique in dogs and cats with a comparison to conjunctival scraping. *Vet Comp Ophthalmol* 7:74–81.

Chapter 94

Environmental Factors in Infectious Disease

Craig E. Greene

MEANS OF TRANSMISSION

The **reservoir** of an infectious disease is the natural habitat of its causative agent. Organisms such as *Clostridium* and *Salmonella* can survive and multiply in inanimate reservoirs such as soil and water. Animate reservoirs, known as **carriers**, can be clinically or subclinically infected with and shed microorganisms that cause disease. Reservoirs and carriers are distinguished from the **source** of infection, which can be any vertebrate, invertebrate, inanimate object, or substance that enables the infectious agent to come into immediate contact with a susceptible individual. In many cases, the source is the reservoir.

The **transmissibility** or **communicability** of an infection refers to its ability to spread from infected to susceptible hosts. "Contagion" and "transmissibility" have been used interchangeably; however, the former implies spread after intimate contact. Transmission can occur between members of the same population (horizontal) or succeeding generations through the genetic material (vertical). Spread of infection to offspring by the placenta, from genital contact at birth, or in the milk is actually horizontal transmission. Not all infectious diseases are transmissible (e.g., systemic mycotic infections originate from soil rather than spreading between individuals).

Direct contact transmission is probably the most frequent and important means of spread of infection. This transmission involves direct physical contact or close approximation between the reservoir host and the susceptible individual. Venereal transmission of *Brucella canis* between dogs or bite transfer of feline immunodeficiency virus between cats are examples of direct physical contact transmission. Aerosol droplets from respiratory, fecal, or genitourinary secretions of dogs and cats generally do not travel farther than 4 or 5 feet; therefore, droplet spread can be considered a form of direct transmission. The spread of infection under such circumstances usually can be limited, as long as fomite transmission is prevented, by ensuring adequate distance between affected and susceptible animals.

Vehicle, or indirect, transmission involves the transfer of infectious organisms from the reservoir to a susceptible host by animate or inanimate intermediates known as **vehicles** or **fomites**. Indirect transmission is dependent on the ability of the infectious agent to temporarily survive adverse environmental influences. The most common animate fomites involved in indirect transmission in veterinary practice are human hands. Inanimate fomites can include anything by which an agent indirectly passes from infected to susceptible individuals, such as food dishes, cages, and surgical instruments. Canine and feline parvoviruses are often spread in this manner owing to the short shedding period in infected animals and the relatively long period of environmental persistence of these viruses.

Common-source transmission involves the simultaneous exposure of a number of individuals within a population to a vehicle contaminated by an infectious agent. The vehicles of common-source infections usually are blood products, drugs, food, and water. Food-source outbreaks of *Salmonella* gastroenteritis have been observed in small animal practice.

Air-borne spread of infection depends on the ability of resistant microorganisms to travel for relatively long distances or to survive in the environment for extended periods until they encounter susceptible hosts. Freshly aerosolized particles containing microbes rarely remain air-borne for more than 1 m unless they are smaller than 5 μm in diameter. **Droplet nuclei**, which are desiccated aerosolized particles containing resistant microbes, may also be carried alone or on dust particles by air currents for extended periods and distances. Resistant respiratory pathogens such as *Mycobacterium tuberculosis* and *Histoplasma capsulatum* are commonly spread by this means.

Vector-borne disease may be considered a specialized form of vehicular or indirect contact spread in which invertebrate animals transmit infectious agents. Vectors are generally arthropods that transmit infection from the infected host or its excreta to a susceptible individual, to its food and water, or to another source of immediate contact. Vectors such as flies may transfer organisms externally, or **mechanically**, on their feet or internally within their intestinal tracts. The ability of organisms to survive in the vector without further propagation has been demonstrated with *Shigella* and *Salmonella* infections. **Propagative transmission** means that the infectious agent multiplies in or on the vector before transfer. Transmission of the plague bacillus, *Yersinia pestis*, by fleas occurs in this manner. **Transovarial** transmission results when the vector transfers the organism to its progeny, as in the case of ticks transmitting *Rickettsia rickettsii*, the agent of Rocky Mountain spotted fever. **Transtadial transmission,** the transfer of infection only between molting stages in the life cycle of the vector, occurs in canine ehrlichiosis. True biologic (**developmental** or **cyclopropagative**) transmission by arthropod vectors involves an obligate developmental stage in the life cycle of the vector. Some of the protozoal pathogens of the dog and cat (e.g., *Hepatozoon*, *Trypanosoma*, *Leishmania*) have a developmental life cycle in the vector.

A pathogenic organism must evolve a mechanism that enables it to spread from one infected animal via the reservoir or carrier to other animals to perpetuate the cycle of infection. Generalized spread of the infection to many body tissues results in contamination of many body secretions. Acute localized respiratory and GI infections usually result in heavily contaminated secretions or excretions, such as aerosols produced during coughing and sneezing or diarrhea and vomitus, respectively. Genitourinary infections are transmitted in urine, uterine or vaginal discharges, and semen. Occasionally, infectious organisms may be shed from open, draining wounds.

Clinical illness is not always encountered in animals that are shedding. Many subclinical carriers exist; they are usually in the chronic or convalescent stage of disease. Latent carriers may shed organisms intermittently in association with reactivation of infection. Infection potential, however, generally varies inversely with the length of time over which a disease is communicable. Acute, severe illnesses usually are associated with highly contagious secretions because transmission occurs over a short time.

ENVIRONMENTAL CONTROL OF MICROBES

The health of both humans and domestic animals depends on the ability to control microorganisms that cause or have the potential to cause disease. Destruction of the organisms occurs when the microenvironment is changed adversely by physical or chemical means. Several levels of microbial disinfection are recognized. Good decontamination always requires initial cleaning to remove organic residues and debris. With prior cleaning, most of the organisms are removed and disinfectants are more effective.

Sterilization is the process by which microorganisms are completely destroyed by chemical or physical means. All life forms, including heat-resistant spores, are killed. Sterility is an absolute condition. There is no partial sterilization process.

Disinfection is the destruction of most pathogenic microorganisms, especially the vegetative forms, but not necessarily bacterial spores. Although disinfection may be brought about by physical as well as chemical agents, a disinfectant is usually a chemical used on inanimate objects. **Antisepsis**, a special category of disinfection, is the inhibition or destruction of pathogenic microbes on the skin and mucous membranes. It is assumed that all pathogenic vegetative microbes are destroyed; however, resident flora may persist. It is important that the antiseptic not be toxic to animal tissues. To reduce tissue toxicity, chemicals must be either diluted or applied for a shorter period than would be necessary to produce sterility.

Sanitation is the reduction of the number of bacterial contaminants to a safe level. A sanitizer is not concentrated enough, nor is it in contact with the organisms long enough, to effect disinfection.

In practice, in the absence of bacterial spores, sterilization and disinfection produce identical results. However, when spores are present, only the harshest of measures can ensure sterility. Unless the item to be treated can withstand sterilization procedures via autoclave or ethylene oxide (EO), either physical or chemical disinfection must be relied on to reduce the number of microorganisms to a safe level.

Protozoal cysts, coccidial oocysts, mycobacteria, and bacterial spores are highly resistant to disinfection and sanitation. Prions, the proteinaceous agents that cause transmissible degenerative encephalopathies (see Chapter 84), are the most resistant infectious agents known. Some loss of infectivity of prions accurs at 100°C; however, 130°C for 30 to 60 minutes is required for their inactivation. Prions are not affected by sterilizing levels of radiation, formalin, nonpolar organic solvents, burial for years, or passage through 0.1μ filters. Their infectivity is destroyed by 1M sodium hydroxide at 55°C or sodium hypochlorite (household bleach) diluted 1:1.

Physical Agents

Heat. Use of either **moist** or **dry heat** is one of the oldest physical controls of microorganisms. Of the two, moist heat, especially under pressure, is more efficient, requiring shorter exposure at a lower temperature than is needed for disinfection by dry heat. When utilized correctly, steam under pressure is the most efficient means of achieving sterility. The recommended temperature-pressure-exposure time to produce sterilization with an autoclave is 121°C at 15 psi for 15 minutes or 126°C at 20 psi for 10 minutes. Steam heat is also most effective for the elimination of resistant protozoal cysts, such as *Toxoplasma* and coccidia. Hot-air ovens are the most common dry heat sterilizers, but to be effective, they must provide a consistent heat source. Dry heat sterilization can be assumed if objects are maintained at 160 ± 10°C for a minimum of 1 hour but preferably 2 hours. Microwave oven sterilization times of dry materials are similar to those of dry ovens once the sterilization temperature is reached. The only advantage of the microwave is the shorter time it takes to achieve these temperatures. Dry heat is recommended for sterilizing cutting instruments and glassware or items that might be damaged by moisture, such as glass syringes and reusable needles.

Radiation. Ionizing or high-energy radiation can be produced by radioactive elements, which are sources of γ-rays, or by a cathode-ray tube that produces X-rays. γ-Rays and X-ray radiations induce ionization of the vital cell components, especially nuclear DNA. Owing to the cost and dangers of handling this equipment, this type of microbial control has found practical application chiefly in the industrial field. Pharmaceuticals, plastic disposables, and suture materials generally are sterilized by the manufacturer by means of ionizing radiation. Foodstuffs can be sterilized or disinfected of pathogenic microbes by use of ionizing radiation. This process is safe and efficient but has met with resistance by the public. There is an unfounded misconception concerning residual radioactivity in treated foods. Nonionizing, or low-energy, radiation, in the form of UV light, has found practical application in the destruction of air-borne organisms. Because low-energy rays do not penetrate well, they are used primarily as surface-active agents. The bactericidal range of UV light is 240 to 280 nm. UV lamps usually produce radiation in the range of 254 nm and work at maximum efficiency at temperatures of 27° to 40°C. They depend on air convection currents to circulate air-borne organisms. Germicidal lamps must be positioned above eye level to prevent retinal burns. For best efficiency, the lamps can also be placed in air conditioning or heating ducts. (See Air-Borne Contaminants, under Prevention of Nosocomial Infections.)

Chemical Agents

Biocides (germicides) denote chemical agents having antiseptic, disinfectant, or preservative properties. In addition to the environmental control of infection, many of these agents are used to preserve food, pharmaceuticals, and medical supplies. Typically, biocides lack selective toxicity to microorganisms. The antimicrobial properties of various chemical disinfectants are summarized in Table 94–1. Table 94–2 describes the uses of the compounds to disinfect hospital equipment.

Alcohols. Ethyl and isopropyl alcohol are rapidly bactericidal against vegetative bacteria but have little effect against spores. Alcohols can be virucidal, provided there is adequate exposure time. Ethyl alcohol is more effective against the nonenveloped viruses than isopropyl alcohol, whereas the reverse is true for the enveloped viruses. Ethyl alcohol is effective against *Proteus* and *Pseudomonas*, whereas isopropyl has a broader antibacterial spectrum. Alcohol is effective only as long as it remains in contact with the item to be disin-

Table 94–1. Antimicrobial Properties of Common Classes of Chemical Disinfectants

CLASS OF DISINFECTANT	BACTERIA				FUNGI	VIRUSES	
	Gram Positives	Gram Negatives	Acid Fast	Spores		Enveloped	Nonenveloped
Alcohols							
Ethyl	+	+	+	−	−	+	+
Isopropyl	+	+	+	−	−	+	−
Halogens							
Chlorine (hypochlorite)	+	+	+	+	+	+	+
Iodine	+	+	+	±	+	+	±
Aldehydes							
Formaldehyde	+	+	+	+	+	+	+
Glutaraldehyde	+	+	+	+	+	+	+
Phenolics	+	+	+	−	+	+	±
Surface-Active Compounds							
QUATs (cationic)	+	±	−	−	+	±	−
Amphoterics (anionic)	+	±	+	−	+	±	−
Biguanides	+	+	−	−	−	?	?
Ethylene Oxide	+	+	+	+	+	+	+

+ = effective; ± = somewhat effective; − = not effective; ? = effectiveness not known; QUATs = quaternary ammonium compounds.

Table 94–2. Treatment Time Required for Chemical Disinfection of Hospital Equipment

EQUIPMENT	TYPE OF DISINFECTION[a]	DISINFECTANT[b]	EXPOSURE TIME[c]
Objects with smooth hard surfaces	H	17	3–12
	H	8–10	15–18
	H	11	5
	I	1–3, 6, 8–10, 12	30
	L	1, 4, 7, 13, 14–16	10
	L	8–10	5
Rubber tubing (completely filled) and catheters	H	17	3–12
	I	6, 10, 12	30
	L	7, 13, 14–16	10
Polyethylene tubing (completely filled) and catheters	H	17	3–12
	H	8–10	15–18
	I	1, 2, 6, 10, 12	30
	L	1, 7, 13–16	10
Thermometers (wiped thoroughly clean)	H	8–10	10–12
	I	2, 5, 10	30
	L	6	10
Lensed instruments	H	9–11	10–12
	I	9, 10	30
	L	7, 13–16	10
Hinged instruments (free of organic material)	H	9, 10	10–12
	I	2, 8–10	20
	I	6, 12	30
	L	8–10	10
	L	1, 7, 13–16	20
Inhalation, anesthetic, and endoscopic equipment	H	9, 11	10
	H	17	3–12
	I	2, 10	20
	L	1, 14–16	20
	L	10, 11	5
Housekeeping (floors, furnishings, and walls)	I	3, 6, 12	20
	L	4, 7, 13–16	10

[a]H = high-level disinfection (free of all microorganisms; equivalent to sterilization); I = intermediate-level disinfection (free of all vegetative bacteria and fungi, tubercle bacilli, and most viruses); L = low-level disinfection (free of vegetative bacteria and fungi and most enveloped viruses).

[b]1 = 70–90% ethyl or isopropyl alcohol; 2 = 70–90% ethyl alcohol; 3 = hypochlorite (1000 ppm); 4 = hypochlorite (100 ppm); 5 = 0.2% iodine + alcohol; 6 = iodophors (500 ppm); 7 = iodophors (100 ppm); 8 = 20% formalin + alcohol; 9 = 20% formalin aqueous; 10 = 2% activated glutaraldehyde aqueous; 11 = 0.13% activated glutaraldehyde + phenate complex; 12 = 2% phenolic aqueous; 13 = 1% phenolic aqueous; 14 = quaternary ammonium compounds; 15 = amphoterics; 16 = chlorhexidine; 17 = ethylene oxide.

[c]For H time in hours; for I and L time in minutes.

fected. Because it evaporates readily, repeated applications may be needed to ensure adequate effect. Alcohol is applied primarily on viable tissues as an antiseptic agent but only on intact skin. Alcohols inactivate hexachlorophene, but are utilized as a diluent for iodine to enhance its disinfection properties. Alcohol has often been used as a rinse for povidone-iodine or chlorhexidine in skin decontamination. Because water is essential for the antimicrobial action, absolute (100%) alcohol has no disinfecting qualities. Concentrations found to be most bactericidal are between 50% and 95% by volume. The two most widely employed concentrations are 70% and 85%. The alcohols are inactivated by organic soil, and they are ineffective if diluted to less than 50%. Alcohols are not effective for cold sterilization of instruments, and they dissolve lens-mounting cements, blanch asphalt tiles, and harden plastics on long-term exposure.

Halogens. These compounds are ineffective or unstable in the presence of organic material, soap, or hard water. They are active against a wide variety of viruses and resistant bacteria, such as *Proteus* and *Pseudomonas*.

Household bleach ,a 5.25% sodium hypochlorite solution diluted to a maximum of 1:30 (vol/vol), is a common form of chlorine for disinfection. The germicidal activity of chlorine compounds is most active at alkaline pH of the solution. Increasing the temperature of the solution decreases the exposure time needed. Other than aldehydes, this is one of the few chemicals that will inactivate parvoviruses. Solutions of bleach are deactivated by light. They should be kept in opaque containers and diluted fresh daily.

Iodine is only slightly soluble in water; therefore, disinfectant solutions are made by dissolving it in alcohol or combining it with organic compounds. Iodine is sporicidal, fungicidal, protozoacidal, and somewhat virucidal, depending on exposure time and concentration of free iodine. Destruction of bacterial spores requires moist contact for more than 15 minutes. Unlike chlorine, iodine exerts its effect over a wide range of pH.

Iodophors are iodine solutions complexed with surfactants or polymers, which help to increase the contact of the iodine with the surface to be disinfected while limiting the concentration of free iodine. The advantages of iodophors over iodine are that they are nonstaining and produce minimal tissue damage. Organic matter may reduce their activity, especially with dilute solutions, but the effect is less marked than with hypochlorites. Rinsing with alcohol will reduce their residual antibacterial activity. Povidone-iodine is a complex of polyvinylpyrrolidone and iodine (Betadine solution, Purdue Frederick, Norwalk, CT). Such iodine compounds have been used for presurgical preparation, topical wound therapy, and joint or body cavity lavage. Solutions of 10% (undiluted) to 1% (1:9) povidone-iodine have been applied for skin and wound disinfection. Dilutions (1:4 to 1:100) of 10% stock solution result in increased bactericidal activity owing to increased concentrations of free iodine, more so than in the undiluted stock solution. A 1:50 dilution of povidone-iodine is recommended as an ocular surface disinfectant in presurgical situations.[15, 16] A 7.5% scrub containing an anionic detergent damages tissues and should be used only on intact skin. Bacterial concentrations are reduced on canine skin for up to 1 hour after scrub application.[15] Polyhydroxydine is a potent iodine-containing wound and skin antiseptic (Xenodine, Squibb Animal Health Division, Princeton, NJ). It has been effective in treating canine wounds when used undiluted (100%) or as a 1:9 dilution (10%). As long as the iodophor solution maintains its color, it is effective.

Systemic absorption of iodine may result in transient reduction in serum thyroxine or bicarbonate concentrations. Contact dermatitis that persists for several hours may occur in dogs.[15–17, 19] The skin irritation may lead to inactivation of the iodine through weeping proteins and increased postsurgical infection. Iodophors are also damaging to deeper tissue fibroblasts and must be diluted to 0.001% to be applied as wound or body cavity rinses.[11] Concentrations of 0.5% to 1% have been effective but may be too strong for lavage of contaminated peritoneal cavities. Peritoneal lavage with 10% povidone-iodine can be fatal to dogs if 8 ml/kg is infused with intact peritoneum or 2 ml/kg with peritonitis. Concentrations of greater than 0.1% should not be used in joint irrigation.

Aldehydes. These have been employed as gaseous sterilants as well as chemical disinfectants. The exposure time needed for **formaldehyde** to effect sterilization is long because the gas does not penetrate well and has been replaced by more efficient gases. A 100% formalin solution is approximately 40% formaldehyde in water. A 20% formalin solution (8% formaldehyde) is a high-level disinfectant (sporicidal), and its biocidal activity can be increased by addition of 70% alcohol, but the solution is irritating to tissues and mucous membranes.

Glutaraldehyde is chemically related to formaldehyde but is more reactive, even in the presence of organic materials, soaps, and hard water. A 2% aqueous alkaline solution is equivalent to 20% formalin in alcohol in biocidal activity. The alkaline solution is much more biocidal but less stable. Stability is maintained for about 2 weeks at pH 7.5 to 8.5. At the dilution at which it is used, glutaraldehyde is slightly irritating to the skin and mucous membranes and very irritating to the eyes. Both glutaraldehyde and formalin are high-level disinfectants for cold sterilization of instruments that are unable to withstand steam or EO gas, including lensed instruments, such as endoscopes, and plastic tubing and catheters. After disinfection, items should be rinsed thoroughly with sterile distilled water. A glutaraldehyde-phenate complex (Sporicidin, Sporicidin International, Washington, DC) has been shown to be as effective at 1:16 dilution as undiluted glutaraldehyde and as stable and less irritating.

Phenolics. These are good housekeeping disinfectants because they remain stable when heated and, after prolonged drying, will redissolve on contact with water. They remain active in the presence of organic soil, soap, and hard water and usually are the disinfectant of choice in treating fecal contamination, such as with *Salmonella*. They must be thoroughly rinsed from areas contacted by cats because of greater toxicity in this species, and they are irritating to the skin and mucous membranes.

Hexachlorophene, a phenolic derivative commonly formulated with hand soap, is utilized as a degerming agent for the skin and mucous membranes because it causes little tissue irritation. Used only once, hexachlorophene is no more effective than soap in eliminating microorganisms. It takes longer than chlorhexidine or povidone-iodine to be effective. Its activity is reduced by organic material, and it is inactivated by alcohol. Hexachlorophene is also neurotoxic when absorbed from the skin, and it should be avoided over extensive areas and in neonates and animals with severely abraded skin.

Hydrogen Peroxide. This common irrigant has been advocated for flushing directly into contaminated or infected wounds. Owing to its lack of antibacterial activity and potential cytotoxicity, it is recommended as an initial flush in wounds for its effervescent action and increased oxygenation, which retard anaerobic bacteria. It works best as a disinfectant for nebulizer and anesthetic equipment.

Surface-Active Agents. These are chemicals that alter the surface tension of the organism and are classified as cationic or anionic. The **quaternary ammonium compounds** (QUATs) are cationic detergents that have been utilized for disinfection and antiseptic purposes, although their activity as disinfectants may have been overrated. They are inactivated by organic material, soap, and hard water. They should not be used in preparation of skin for surgery because they are inactivated by detergents in surgical scrubs. QUATs are algicidal, fungicidal, bactericidal, and virucidal (against some enveloped viruses) at medium concentrations. Virucidal activity of newer QUATS such as dodecyl dimethyl ammonium chloride or *N*-alkyl dimethyl benzyl ammonium chloride is incomplete against viruses (even herpesviruses) in contrast to the claims of manufacturers.[9] When properly used, QUATs are effective bactericides against both gram-positive and gram-negative bacteria; however, they display greater activity against gram-positive organisms. They have an unusual ability to kill *Giardia* cysts at refrigerator and room temperatures (see Prevention, Chapter 78). They are ineffective against tubercle bacilli, *Proteus*, *Pseudomonas*, bacterial spores, and nonenveloped viruses even at high concentrations. When the temperature is increased from 20° to 37°C, the concentration of the solution can be reduced by half. Benzalkonium chloride is the most common compound of this group.

As an environmental or skin disinfectant, concentrations of 0.001% to 1% benzalkonium chloride are generally used. Benzalkonium chloride has also been employed in medicine as an antiseptic and in flushing infected wounds at very low (≤.007%) concentrations. QUATs are thought to form a film over the skin, with the inactive part of the compound directed toward the skin, possibly trapping bacteria but not killing them. The germicidal part is directed toward the environment, preventing further contamination. Degerming the skin with a more effective antiseptic before applying a QUAT may overcome the problem. Care must be taken not to allow undiluted QUATs to contact exposed tissues. Chemical burns occurred after applying undiluted (10–17%) benzalkonium chloride on skin surfaces or 0.1% to 0.5% on conjunctivae or mucosae of dogs and cats. Cats also developed oral and esophageal ulcerations after licking treated skin areas, and oral ingestion should be avoided. Concentrations as low as 0.002% to 0.007% must be used on wounds, but other agents such as chlorhexidine or povidone-iodine are preferred.

Anionic surfactants or **amphoterics**, organic acids that have the detergency of anionic compounds, are effective against both gram-negative and gram-positive bacteria, and are reported to be fungicidal but not sporicidal. Unlike QUATs, they are effective against *Proteus* and *Pseudomonas*. Amphoterics are effective in one application and are not inactivated by serum or hard water, although soaps and detergents affect them adversely. Like QUATs, they leave a film on the skin that will block the transfer of organisms from unwashed to washed hands. Amphoterics are nontoxic to tissues and noncorrosive to moist surfaces, and they have a deodorizing ability. They can greatly reduce the total number of bacteria on hospital floors.

Biguanides. Chlorhexidine, the most common disinfectant of this class, has gained popularity for surgical skin preparation and as a wound antiseptic because of its low tissue toxicity.[15, 16] It is effective against *Proteus*, *Escherichia coli*, staphylococci, and *Pseudomonas*. In the skin it binds to stratum corneum, giving up to 2 days residual activity after a single application. It has been shown to be an effective and a nonirritating antiseptic for irrigation of canine wounds. Concentrations of chlorhexidine of 0.5% in water, saline, lactated Ringer's solution, or alcohol have been shown to reduce bacterial contamination in canine wounds or as a surgical antiseptic, but they retard granulation tissue formation and epithelization. Lower concentrations of chlorhexidine (0.05–0.1%) were less antiseptic but could be used as a lavage for tissues or joints and did not inhibit wound repair. Chlorhexidine has not been effective in the treatment of dermatophytosis (see Chapter 58). Because of irritation, even low concentrations should never be placed in the eye or in the ear canal with a damaged tympanum, although use with a damaged tympanum has been shown to be safe in dogs.[11] These compounds retain some activity in the presence of organic material and hard water but are inactivated by soaps. They are more effective at an alkaline pH.

EO. When properly applied, this gas is the most effective chemical sterilant. Like other chemical disinfectants, EO is subject to limitations imposed by temperature, moisture content, concentration, and exposure time. It has been recommended that routine sterilization be performed at 30° to 55°C. If the temperature is not properly maintained, the gas may condense, or if the exposure time is too short, sterility failures can occur. Most EO sterilizers in hospitals are designed to produce 50% to 60% relative humidity; it must not fall below 30%, or sterility failure will occur.

EO sterilization is not recommended for some plastics and pharmaceuticals or for animal feeds and beddings. The gas reacts with or is absorbed by these items. Solutions in sealed glass containers cannot be sterilized because the gas cannot penetrate glass. Instruments and other items should be clean, dry, and as free of contamination as possible before EO sterilization. Items are placed in semipermeable plastic wraps. After the sterilization process, articles must be aerated to allow the residual gas to dissipate, because the absorbed gas is irritating to skin and mucous membranes. Recommended routine aeration procedures are as follows: at room temperature, 48 to 168 hours, depending on the items sterilized and their use; with forced-air cabinets, 8 to 12 hours, depending on the cabinet temperature.

NOSOCOMIAL INFECTIONS

Nosocomial (hospital-acquired) infections can arise endogenously from the spread of indigenous microflora or exogenously from contact with organisms on external sources. Exogenous sources of infection commonly include other animals and fomites such as human hands, rodents, arthropods, food dishes, catheters, and hospital cages. Transmission can occur by air-borne, contact, or vehicle routes. Many nosocomial infections result from opportunistic spread of the normal microflora rather than newly acquired agents. The prevalence rate of nosocomial infections in humans and probably veterinary hospitals is 5% to 10% of hospitalized patients.

Not all infections that develop in the hospital environment are nosocomial in origin. Infections that are present or incubating at the time of admission are excluded. Moreover, nosocomial infections may not become clinically evident until after the patient has been discharged from the hospital. Hospitalized animals are more prone to infection because of increased exposure to pathogens, concurrent immunosuppressive illness, and the increased stress imposed by technologic advances in medical practice (Table 94–3). Excessive antimicrobial therapy may increase the risk of colonization with antimicrobial-resistant pathogens. Nosocomial patho-

Table 94–3. Classification of Infectious Diseases Based on Zoonotic and Nosocomial Potential

CLASS 1[a]	CLASS 3[d]
Systemic herpesvirus infection (puppies)	Drug-resistant bacterial infections (*Klebsiella, Pseudomonas*)[c]
Canine distemper (neurologic form)	Canine brucellosis[c]
Histoplasmosis	Leptospirosis[c]
Cryptococcosis	Giardiasis[c]
Coccidioidomycosis	Cryptosporidiosis[c]
Protothecosis	Toxoplasmosis (feline enteroepithelial)[c]
CLASS 2[b]	Campylobacteriosis[c]
Drug-susceptible bacterial infections	Dermatophytosis[c]
Feline leukemia and other viral neoplasias	Sporotrichosis[c]
Feline immunodeficiency virus infection	**CLASS 4[e]**
Canine viral papillomatosis	Canine parvoviral diarrhea
Feline infectious peritonitis	Other enteric infections
Haemobartonellosis	Feline panleukopenia
Canine ehrlichiosis	Infectious canine hepatitis
Babesiosis	Canine distemper (multisystemic form)
Pneumocystosis	Canine viral respiratory diseases
American trypanosomiasis	Feline viral respiratory diseases
Leishmaniasis	Feline chlamydiosis[c]
Rocky Mountain spotted fever[c]	Rabies
Lyme disease (canine borreliosis)	Salmonellosis[c]
Atypical mycobacterial infections	Shigellosis[c]
Blastomycosis	*Mycobacterium tuberculosis* infections[c]
	Plague

[a]Acquired from the environment or limited shedding or susceptibility period.
[b]Close contact or vector transmission required of environmentally nonresistant organisms.
[c]Zoonotic potential with direct transmission to people.
[d]Transmission by infected body secretions with organism of moderate environmental resistance and zoonotic potential.
[e]Serious zoonotic pathogens or high level of transmission.

gens are either naturally resistant to antimicrobial drugs or develop resistance during hospital therapy.

Development of Antibacterial Resistance

Microorganisms have evolved means of overcoming the effects of antimicrobial drugs. Most resistance mechanisms are under genetic control. Spontaneous chromosomal mutations are relatively rare in bacterial populations; extrachromosomal transfer of genetic material or plasmids is more important. Plasmid transfer occurs most frequently during bacterial conjugation, although alterations in bacterial nucleic acid may also occur through bacteriophages (via transduction), acquisition from naked nucleic acid (via transformation), or exchange between bacterial and host DNA (via translocation). Plasmid transfer also commonly occurs between bacteria of different genera.

Genetic acquisition of bacterial resistance to antimicrobials may manifest in a variety of ways, including changes in permeability to the drug, in receptors for the drug, or in metabolic pathways. Plasmid resistance is frequently associated with cross-resistance among a number of structurally related antimicrobials.

The prevalence of antibiotic resistance commonly increases in proportion to the frequency of use. Resistance very often develops with streptococci, staphylococci, *E. coli, Salmonella, Proteus,* and *Klebsiella.* Suppression of normal enteric flora and proliferation of antimicrobial-resistant strains occur with partially absorbed antimicrobials or those that are excreted in the bowel in active form, such as tetracycline, chloramphenicol, ampicillin, metronidazole, furazolidone, amoxicillin, and cloxacillin. Antibiotic resistance in fecal coliform bacteria has been documented in domestic pets in association with the increased use of antibacterial drugs in such animals. Heightened antibacterial resistance among pets in rural environments was correlated with the increased use of antibiotics in livestock feeds. These findings should caution veterinarians against indiscriminate administration of antimicrobials; moreover, similar resistance patterns have been identified in human contacts of both types of animals.

Antimicrobial resistance in human medicine has been shown to be more of a problem in hospitalized patients, in whom antibiotic usage is widespread, than among patients in general.[21] Similar findings probably exist in veterinary practices. The development of new antibacterial drugs has just barely kept ahead of evolving resistance patterns. Widespread or indiscriminate usage of gentamicin, trimethoprim-sulfonamide, and fluoroquinolone by veterinarians may threaten the efficacy of these antibiotics in the near future. The availability of a large number of antibacterial drugs should not give the veterinarian a sense of security, because many drugs have become obsolete as a result of evolving bacterial resistance.

Development of bacterial resistance can be prevented by certain adjustments during antimicrobial therapy. Measures include restricted prophylactic drug therapy, fully effective doses at adequate intervals, narrow-spectrum antibacterials specific for the isolated organisms, isolation of animals receiving long-term antibacterial therapy, selection of antibacterials against which the isolated organisms are not prone to develop resistance, changing of antibacterials after an effective treatment period, restriction of indiscriminate use of antibacterial drugs, and topical or local rather than systemic therapy whenever possible.

Conditions Associated With Nosocomial Infections

In human and probably veterinary hospitals, the most common nosocomial infections are urinary tract infections, followed by pneumonias, surgical site infections, and bacteremias.[2] For surgical and wound related infections, see Chapter 55.

Urinary Catheterization. This procedure is probably the most common cause of nosocomial infection in veterinary practice. Fluid washout from urine flow is a primary defense mechanism of the urinary tract. Catheters upset this barrier by permitting entry of organisms at the urethral meatus and catheter junction. The distal urethra and prepuce or vagina are normally inhabited by commensal organisms. When catheters are left in place, these bacteria can migrate in retrograde fashion and infect the rest of the urinary tract, which is normally sterile. Transient bacteremia also may occur after manipulation of urinary catheters in infected patients. To prevent infection, the external genitalia must be thoroughly cleansed, after which catheterization must be performed under strict aseptic conditions. A short-term, repeated, nontraumatic catheter is preferable to placement of a long-term indwelling catheter. Prophylactic topical or systemic antimicrobial therapy does not reduce the prevalence of infection unless the catheter is left in place for fewer than 4 days (see Indwelling Catheters, Chapter 91). Antimicrobial therapy should not begin until the catheter is removed. At this time the urine can be cultured, the sediment examined, and the animal started on therapy, which should be modified when the culture results are received. Antimicrobial therapy instituted while the catheter is in place merely selects for resistant infections. Periodic instillation of a disinfectant such as hydrogen peroxide into closed urinary drainage systems has not been effective in preventing catheter-associated bacteriuria in people.

IV Catheterization. IV infusions are both essential and life saving in veterinary practice. Since the development of flexible plastics, IV catheters are maintained in the patient for longer periods; however, the possibility that the infusion system can become contaminated is greater. The improper use of indwelling catheters has resulted in a high prevalence of nosocomial bacteremias. IV catheter–related infections are more common than realized in veterinary practice. Infusion bottles, bags, or administration sets can become contaminated from hairline cracks produced during manufacturing. Organisms may enter infusion systems when the administration set is inserted into the bottle, allowing the influx of room air when the vacuum is released or when medicaments are added. Organisms can also be introduced at the connection of the infusion set with the hub of the IV catheter.

Bacteria can also enter the IV infusion system at the site of penetration of the catheter tip by migrating between the catheter and skin surfaces. The prevalence of local infection is greatly increased when IV cutdown sites are used and catheters are in place for longer than 24 to 48 hours. Organisms producing localized infection at the catheter site can be infused systemically during the administration of fluid or during flushing of clogged catheters. Bacteria can also migrate in retrograde fashion, even against gravity flow, from the contaminated catheter to the infusion bottle.

Organisms such as coagulase-negative staphylococci have been shown to adhere to plastic catheters with subsequent replication and production of catheter-associated infections.[4] Some investigators believe that the slime-producing strains of bacteria are more effective in catheter colonization. Inserted catheters develop a biofilm (glycocalyx) containing large numbers of organisms. This layer may offer a physical barrier to host defenses or antibiotics in eliminating the bacteria.

Organisms of the family Enterobacteriaceae, such as *Klebsiella, Enterobacter, Serratia,* as well as *Citrobacter,* proliferate readily at room temperature in 5% dextrose and can reach concentrations of 10^5 and 10^6 organisms/ml without producing obvious clouding of the solution. Many other common contaminants, such as *Staphylococcus, Pseudomonas, E. coli,* and *Proteus,* do not survive or proliferate in 5% dextrose, although *Candida* can grow very slowly. *Serratia marcescens* has been incriminated as the most common cause of IV catheter infection in small animal practice. Benzalkonium chloride solutions should not be used for skin preparation, because these antiseptic solutions can support the growth of *S. marcescens* and other microorganisms. In one instance, this organism was isolated from alcohol-soaked cotton balls used for skin decontamination.[6] *Pseudomonas* can grow in distilled water, normal saline, and even iodophors.[4] *Candida* grow well in protein hydrolysates, whereas *Candida* and *Malassezia* proliferate in lipid emulsions.

Lactated Ringer's solution, normal saline, other isotonic fluids, and hypertonic saline solution have been less commonly incriminated as the causes of nosocomial bacteremia than have dextrose solutions; however, they can support the growth of a variety of organisms. Parenteral hyperalimentation fluids and other hypertonic solutions readily support the growth of *Candida.* Blood products, even when stored at refrigerated temperatures, can become contaminated and support the growth of cold-growing microorganisms such as *Pseudomonas* and some coliforms, such as *S. marcescens. S. marcescens* was responsible for contamination of feline blood units.[6] Bacterial growth in the blood units caused slight brown discoloration of the blood.

Clinical signs of catheter-associated infection include localized swelling and warmth at the insertion site and venous cording. The systemic spread of infection is characterized by fever, hypotension, tachycardia, and GI and CNS signs. Overwhelming infections associated with endotoxemia are more likely to occur when gram-negative organisms are involved and in immunosuppressed patients. Clinical signs in such cases are shock, collapse, coma, and death. In cats receiving blood contaminated with *S. marcescens,* vomiting, collapse, diarrhea, icterus, panting, fever, and death were variable findings.

Diagnosis of IV infusion–associated infection is frequently made when the clinical signs improve suddenly after termination of fluid therapy. However, because bacteremia may seed many organs, clinical signs can persist after the infusion is discontinued. Culture or Gram's staining of catheter tips has been recommended and is a more rapid and practical means of determining presence of infection. After removal, the IV or intracutaneous segment of the catheter is rolled across an agar plate, and the resultant colonies that grow are counted. A count greater than 15 colony-forming units is often associated with bacteremia.[4] However, this finding alone may not always confirm the presence of bacteremia. When blood cultures are performed, organisms found should correspond to those found at the catheter site. It is also possible for pseudobacteremia to occur when the infected catheter site locally seeds the venous effluent being sampled. At least two to three blood samples should be taken from different sites at intervals of at least 10 minutes once the catheter has been removed. Once catheter-related infection is suspected and the catheter tip or blood cultures are taken, the offending catheter should be removed. The animal should be started on antimicrobial therapy. Most infections can be eliminated with a 10- to 14-day course of antibacterials if the appropriate drug is selected.

IV catheter–associated infections can be prevented with adequate precautions. Adequate skin preparation and antisepsis at the collection sites are essential. Hands should be washed before catheter placement. A large area of fur at the catheter site should be removed by carefully clipping to avoid microabrasions of the skin. Gentle mechanical cleansing of the skin with an iodophor or with soap and water for 2 to 5 minutes should be followed by alternate disinfection using 70% alcohol and 1% to 2% tincture of iodine or iodophor solutions or, preferably, 2% chlorhexidine-gluconate.[13] Iodine-containing antiseptics are effective against most bacteria and fungi, with the exception of spores. Tincture of iodine preparations, superior to iodophors for the final application, are frequently too irritating for repeated application.

To restrict movement, catheters should be firmly stabilized with adhesive tape. A small amount of a broad-spectrum antimicrobial ointment, such as one containing organic iodine or neomycin-bacitracin-polymyxin, should be applied at the point of catheter penetration through the skin, and the site should be covered with a sterile occlusive dressing. If only tape is to be used, it must be sterile. The date and time of catheter insertion should be recorded. No catheter should be left in place longer than 72 hours. If the catheter must remain in place for longer periods, the IV site should be inspected and dressed with a new sterile dressing at 48- to 72-hour intervals. Disconnecting the IV catheters for sampling or administering medicines should be minimized. Concurrent administration of antibiotics does little to prevent IV catheter–associated infection, but causes the development of an antimicrobial–resistant infection.

When long-term IV catheterization is required, special

catheters such as the Broviac or Hickman type should be considered.[1a, 4] These have been designed to reduce migration of bacteria toward the implanted portion by a built-in cuff and subcutaneous tunneling of the proximal portion. These catheters are made of more flexible and nonreactive silicone, which is less irritative and thrombogenic, reducing the chance for a nidus of infection. Unfortunately, these catheters do not overcome the less common hematogenous seeding of bacteria on the catheter tips, which may occur from distant sites of infection.

When a small volume or slow infusion rate is required, multiple small infusion bottles are preferred to one large bottle. The rationale is that should the system become contaminated, the time for microorganism multiplication is minimized. Infusion bottles should be checked for turbidity and vacuum, and infusion bags should be squeezed before use to detect leaks. Infusion filters 0.22 μm in diameter are available to restrict the flow of microorganisms through the fluid catheter into the patient; however, they will not prevent passage of endotoxins and pyrogenic factors. Drugs should be added to infusion fluid containers in uncontaminated surroundings after proper disinfection of the site of addition to the infusion fluid.

Respiratory Infections. The upper respiratory tract passages have anatomic defense mechanisms that prevent most inhaled particles from reaching the lower airways. However, invasive procedures such as tracheostomy, fiberoptic endoscopy, transtracheal catheterization, nebulization, and endotracheal intubation bypass these defense mechanisms and expose the respiratory tract to increased numbers of organisms, especially gram-negative organisms. The occurrence of nosocomial pneumonias was *much* higher in endotracheally intubated human patients receiving histamine H_2-receptor antagonist. Retrograde contamination of the oropharynx with gram-negative bacteria from the stomach was thought to be responsible.

Decreased respiratory clearance function has also been associated with an increased risk of nosocomial respiratory infections. Decreased clearance activity can occur with CNS depression, neuromuscular paralysis, chronic obstructive lung disease, and impairment of pulmonary alveolar macrophage function. Inhalation anesthesia, nebulization, humidification, and ventilatory support increase the risk of nosocomial infection resulting from cross-contamination. Appropriate disinfection protocols for the equipment in these procedures are discussed later (see Prevention of Nosocomial Infections).

GI Infections. Enteric pathogens, such as parvoviruses, coronaviruses, *Salmonella*, and *Giardia*, may spread among dogs or cats in a veterinary hospital or animal-holding facility. Outbreaks are usually the result of poor sanitation, inadequate disinfection, and crowding of animals. Wards, treatment areas, waiting rooms, cages, exercise runs, thermometers, and feeding utensils are all sources of infection. All outbreaks of gastroenteritis among recently hospitalized patients should be investigated as to the cause and possible source of infection. Fecal examinations and cultures for protozoa and parvovirus should be performed when economically feasible.

Prevention of GI infections requires intense cleaning and disinfection procedures. All feces within the hospital should be removed as soon as possible, and the contaminated surface should be thoroughly disinfected with a diluted (1:32) chlorine bleach solution. Smooth, impervious floor and cage surfaces will facilitate disinfection and cleaning. Crowding of animals in waiting rooms and in hospital wards should be avoided. Use of gloves and hand washing should be enforced. Hospitalized animals should not be moved from cage to cage, but each should be assigned to one cage. Those having episodes of acute vomiting or diarrhea either before or after being admitted to the hospital should be isolated.

Decubital Ulcers. These are the most common nosocomial skin infections to develop in incapacitated animals maintained in immobile or recumbent positions on unpadded surfaces. Abrasion and continuous pressure over bony surfaces cause devitalization of skin and secondary bacterial invasion. Immunosuppressed animals may develop septicemia as a result of decubital sores. *Pseudomonas* commonly contaminates these wounds. Identification of the invading microorganism and antibacterial therapy usually are of little benefit unless the primary cause is eliminated. Prevention is easier than cure; it involves frequent turning of recumbent patients and the placement of padding in their cages.

Prevention of Nosocomial Infections

Most nosocomial pathogens, whether acquired endogenously or exogenously, do not produce disease by themselves. The risk of nosocomial infections is greatest for immunocompromised or surgery patients and for newborns. Prevention of these infections can be achieved only by strict monitoring of the known predisposing causes. Attempts should be made to reduce the contact of high-risk patients with potential pathogens by segregating them from the general hospital population or minimizing their hospital stay. Additional measures include placing indwelling catheters only when necessary, minimizing surgical procedures, and practicing routine disinfection. Chemical disinfection procedures in veterinary hospitals are reviewed in the following section and are summarized in Table 94–2.

Antimicrobial Prophylaxis. Prophylactic antimicrobial drugs are controversial. The unnecessary use of antibiotics has caused justifiable concern because of the increased prevalence of resistant microorganisms. Antibiotics alter the patient's microflora and allow infection by resistant bacteria. It has long been thought that microflora were responsible for bacterial superinfections after prophylactic administration of antimicrobial drugs; however, invasion by exogenous, resistant organisms is more likely. Prolonged antibiotic administration may not lessen an animal's susceptibility to infection but may merely alter the microbial flora that cause the problem.

Certain justifications exist for instituting treatment with antimicrobial drugs before documenting that an infectious process exists. Immunosuppressed hosts that have been exposed to disease may require antimicrobial therapy; however, most clinicians would argue that close monitoring of the patient should be followed by IV administration of antimicrobials only if fever or other signs of infection appear. High-risk conditions associated with immunosuppression and with secondary infection include diabetes mellitus, persistent neutropenia, Cushing's disease, immunosuppressive or cancer chemotherapy, and chronic bronchopulmonary disease. Traumatic or contaminated wounds and burns may require topical or systemic chemotherapy. For information on antimicrobial prophylaxis in wounds, burns, and surgical procedures, see Chapter 55.

Isolation Precautions. Restricting animal movement and contact within a veterinary hospital is important in controlling spread of nosocomial infections. As a general rule, animals entering the hospital should be currently vaccinated (see Chapter 100) or should be vaccinated if their status is uncertain. Any animal infested with ectoparasites should be dipped on admission if its condition permits. Immunosuppressed patients should not be housed in the hospital or, if admitted, should be moved to a separate area. If an infection is identified in an animal, four categories are proposed for which isolation precautions are indicated (see Table 94–3).

Class 1 infections have very little chance of spread between individuals, and the zoonotic potential is low. Systemic mycotic and algal infections are primarily contracted by environmental exposure. Systemic herpesvirus infection is a threat only to young neonates, and dogs showing only neurologic signs with canine distemper are unlikely to spread disease. No additional precautions are needed, and routine cage cleaning, hand washing, and disinfection of hospital equipment are all that is necessary.

Class 2 infections are of greater risk of transmission than class 1. Close contact is required between animals with papillomatosis or feline leukemia virus infection or feline infectious peritonitis. Many of these infections can be spread by contact with infected body fluids. Most other infections in this group are vector transmitted, so that proper arthropod control will minimize the risk of spread from infected individuals. Most of the organisms cannot survive outside the host and are susceptible to routine disinfectants.

Class 3 infections are spread by close or direct contact with infected individuals or their excreta, but the risk of transmission via body fluids and excreta can be minimized by sanitary measures. These animals can be admitted to the general hospital population, but they should remain in their cages so as to restrict the contact of their urine and feces with other animals. Their cages should be identified as to the particular illness. Hand washing and cage cleaning must be critically practiced between animals, and feces or diarrhea, urine, and vomitus should be removed immediately. Dilute (1:30) bleach for viruses and phenolic compounds for bacteria should be used for disinfection. *Toxoplasma* and *Cryptosporidium* oocysts are inactivated by 10% ammonia solutions or by boiling water or steam cleaning. *Giardia* cysts are most susceptible to some dilute (1:100 or greater) QUAT disinfectants.

Animals with *Class 4* infections should be strictly isolated in a separate ward and should not be admitted to the general animal population. Infections in this category have a high degree of zoonotic risk with potentially serious complications or they are rapidly spread between susceptible animals. Animals with upper respiratory tract infections are preferably not admitted to the hospital and should be treated as outpatients. These highly contagious diseases are spread by air or contact. The animal's body exudates or secretions are highly infectious or the organisms are too resistant to enable control of spread. Persons handling these animals should wear protective outer garments, shoe covers, and rubber gloves. Contaminated wastes from these areas should be double-bagged in plastic and disposed of separately. Cages should be thoroughly disinfected once the animal is discharged. If the patient had *Salmonella*, the treated cage surface should have negative culture results before being used again.

Hands. These are the most common reservoirs or fomites for microorganisms associated with nosocomial infection, and hand washing is probably the *single most important* and immediate way of reducing its hospital-acquired infections. Hands should be washed routinely with water and mild, noncaustic soap or detergent after handling or examining patients and especially after contact with blood, secretions, and excretions. The mechanical effect of soap and water cleansing is most important in reducing the numbers of transient bacteria on the skin surface. Frequent use of antiseptics should be avoided because they can burn or dry the skin. Pre-existing dermatitis will result in the persistent carriage of large numbers of microorganisms, which negates the effect of hand washing. Bar soaps, allowed to dry between uses, appear to have a lower prevalence of contamination than liquid soaps. Liquid soap canisters can become contaminated and must routinely be emptied, cleaned, and disinfected before being refilled.

Iodine-containing soaps are superior as scrubbing agents before surgery; however, they may produce dermatitis in sensitive individuals. A comparison of the available hand-washing soaps and antiseptics appears in Table 94–4. Hand-washing sinks and bathing tubs in all areas of a veterinary hospital can be disinfected with chlorine bleach to reduce contamination with organisms such as *Pseudomonas*. Rubber gloves may be used as an adjunctive means of reducing spread of infection when hand washing must be done so frequently as to prove impractical or irritating to the skin.

Air-Borne Contaminants. These can be reduced by having impervious floor coverings and using wet mops or filtered vacuums throughout the hospital. Air conditioning systems should be electronically filtered if possible and should be designed to reduce turbulent airflow. The best ventilation systems have air inlets near the ceiling and air outlets near the floor, allowing air to travel downward toward the heavily contaminated floor region. Air exchange rates of 6 to 10 times per hour have been shown to efficiently reduce the number of air-borne microorganisms in animal-holding facilities while producing minimal air turbulence. Electronic purification and reduction in air-borne bacteria can be achieved with installation of ozone-producing devices that are mounted in a given room or in the supply air plenum (Aqua-Mist Inc, Winston-Salem, NC). A UV radiation decontamination device that is effective in inactivating environmentally resistant organisms, such as *Pseudomonas aeruginosa* and *Mycobacterium*

Table 94–4. Comparison of Commonly Used Topical Soaps and Antiseptics

AGENT	ADVANTAGES	DISADVANTAGES
Hand soap	Noncaustic, inexpensive	Liquids and moist bars support bacterial growth
Hexachlorophene (phenolic)	Good for *Staphylococcus*	Must use daily, CNS toxicity with absorption, minimal effect on gram-negative bacteria and fungi
Benzalkonium chloride (QUAT)	Inexpensive	Ineffective, harbors opportunistic bacteria (e.g., *Serratia*)
Alcohol	Relatively inexpensive, need 70% aqueous, ethanol superior	Volatile, flammable, drying, bacterial resistance common
Iodine (halogen)	Good for viruses, fungi, and vegetative and sporulated bacteria; most effective as tincture; sustained germicidal action	Irritating, hypersensitivity, stains skin, drying
Iodophors (halogen)	Water soluble, low irritation, less staining	Reduced potency compared with iodine, drying

Table 94–5. Susceptibility of Bacteria to Heat Disinfection

PROCEDURE	ORGANISMS KILLED	TEMPERATURE °C	TEMPERATURE °F	TIME	COMMENTS
Dishwashing					
Automatic wash	Most vegetative	60	140	20 sec	Add detergent
Sterilization	All vegetative, most spores	82	180	10 sec	Add detergent
Manual wash	Some vegetative	43–49	110–120	10–20 sec	Add detergent
	All but spores	76.5	170	30 sec	Add disinfectant
Cage Cleaning	Gram-negative rods, gram-positive cocci	49	120	2–4 min	Steam or hot water
	Gram-negative rods	48–60	120–140	Instantaneous	Steam or hot water
	Gram-positive cocci	71	160	2–4 min	Steam or hot water
	All but *Bacillus* spores	82	180	Instantaneous	Steam or hot water
	Bacillus spores	82	180	> 1 min	Steam or hot water
Anesthetic Tube Cleaning					
Mild disinfection	Most vegetative	55	132	3 min	Hot water
Pasteurization	All but spores	80	176	15 min	Hot water
Clothes Washing (Automatic)	All spores	>71	>160	25 min	Add detergent, add bleach to increase cidal activity

tuberculosis, in air ducts is commercially available (Sterilite, AB-medica, Milan, Italy).[1]

Surgical Equipment. This should be appropriately sterilized with steam autoclaves or EO rather than cold disinfection, and it should be stored in dust-free enclosed cabinets. Cold disinfection should be avoided when possible because it may be associated with the increased risk of infections from soil saprophytes such as *Clostridium tetani.* All surfaces in operating rooms that do not contact the patient should be routinely disinfected with phenolic compounds. Floors can be washed with disinfectants and wet mopped or polished. Wet mops or vacuums with filtered exhaust elements can pick up excess disinfectant and loosening debris. Built-up disinfectant films can be removed with a solution of 0.12 L (one-half cup) of vinegar in 3.8 L (1 gallon) of water. Dry mops and brooms should never be used to clean hospital floors because they disseminate microorganisms in dust. Personnel should wear face masks to minimize aerosol contamination in surgery areas. Hand washing and gloving for surgery are superior to hand washing alone in minimizing the spread of skin microflora to the patient. Antisepsis of the skin at the incision site is similar to that in preparing IV catheter sites, but there is a final application of tincture of iodine or iodophor solution just before the animal is draped.

Anesthesia and Nebulizer Equipment. This should be washed with water and detergents. This equipment may be heat sensitive, and it may need to be sterilized with EO gas or soaked in 2% glutaraldehyde for 30 minutes followed by aeration or sterile water rinse, respectively. All equipment should be completely dry before it is used. Solid rubber face masks that can withstand heat disinfection may be flash autoclaved at 56°C for 3 minutes.

Rubber anesthesia circuits can be disinfected by immersion in 80°C water for 15 minutes. Soda lime canisters should be completely emptied and disinfected by similar means when needed.

Nebulizers and humidifiers can be disinfected by flushing hydrogen peroxide (20% by volume in water) through the system. Acetic acid at a concentration of at least 2% has been utilized, but it is somewhat ineffective against the more resistant gram-negative bacteria. Chlorhexidine (0.02%) is better for this purpose, especially at a temperature of 50°C. Temperature-controlled nebulizers that can be maintained at 45°C have the lowest prevalence of contamination. Periodic disinfection of nebulizer chambers with chlorine bleach or sterilization with EO gas is also recommended.

Endoscopic Equipment. This should be cleaned with soap and water as soon as possible after each use to remove gross soil, rinsed thoroughly with clean water, then rinsed with a disinfectant solution. Iodophors and bleach are corrosive to metal parts. Flexible endoscopes should be effectively disinfected or sterilized between uses whenever possible, particularly if they are employed to examine normally sterile areas such as the respiratory and genitourinary tracts. Flexible endoscopes can be sterilized by soaking in alkaline glutaraldehyde for 10 minutes and then rinsed with sterile water. Sterilization can be achieved with EO gas, but many endoscopes cannot withstand the 63°C aeration temperature that is commonly utilized and require more prolonged aeration at lower temperatures. Unlike rigid metal endoscopes, most flexible endoscopes cannot tolerate sterilization by steam autoclaving.

Cages. Animal-holding facilities must receive adequate disinfection. Mere cleansing of cages with liquid disinfectants between uses is insufficient. Steam cleaning on a monthly basis is the most effective means of ward and cage sanitation. Transient washing at 82°C is considered optimal for cage disinfection except against spores of *Bacillus,* which can be killed if the washing is prolonged for a minute or more. Lower temperatures may be effective in destroying vegetative bacteria (Table 94–5).

Clothes and Dishes. Disinfection of these articles requires higher temperatures that can be achieved with automatic clothes washers, and dishwashers are preferred to manual rinsing (see Table 94–5). At high temperatures, most organisms will be killed; bacterial spores are the exception. Low-temperature (22°C) washing using laundry chemicals and bleach followed by drying is as effective as high-temperature (71°C) washing to eliminate pathogenic bacteria.

References

1. Allegra L, Blasi F, Tarsia P, et al. 1997. A novel device for the prevention of airborne infections. *J Clin Microbiol* 35:1918—1919.
1a. Blaiset MA, Couto CG, Evans KL. 1995. Complications of indwelling Silastic central venous access catheters in dogs and cats. *J Am Anim Hosp Assoc* 31:379–384.

2. Emori TG, Gaynes RP. 1993. An overview of nosocomial infections, including the role of the microbiology laboratory. *Clin Microbiol Rev* 6:428–442.
3. Freeman MJ, Kirby BM, Panciera DL, et al. 1994. Hypotensive shock syndrome associated with acute *Babesia canis* infection in a dog. *J Am Vet Med Assoc* 204:94–96.
4. Goldmann DA, Pier GB. 1993. Pathogenesis of infections related to intravascular catheterization. *Clin Microbiol Rev* 6:176–192.
5. Greene CE. 1990. Environmental factors in infectious diseases, pp 3–20. *In* Greene CE (ed), Infectious diseases of the dog and cat. WB Saunders, Philadelphia, PA.
6. Hohenhaus AE, Drusin LM, Garvey MS. 1997. *Serratia marcescens* contamination of feline whole blood in a hospital blood bank. *J Am Vet Med Assoc* 210:794–798.
7. Johnson JA, Murtaugh RJ. 1997. Preventing and treating nosocomial infection: part I. Urinary tract infections and pneumonia. *Compend Cont Educ Pract Vet* 19:581–603.
8. Johnson JA, Murtaugh RJ. 1997. Preventing and treating nosocomial infections: part II. Wound, blood, and gastrointestinal infections. *Compend Cont Educ Pract Vet* 19:693–703.
9. Kennedy MA, Mellon VS, Caldwell G, et al. 1995. Virucidal efficacy of the newer quaternary ammonium compounds. *J Am Anim Hosp Assoc* 31:254–258.
10. Kruth SA, Prescott JF, Welch MK, et al. 1989. Nosocomial diarrhea associated with enterotoxigenic *Clostridium perfringens* infection in dogs. *J Am Vet Med Assoc* 195:331–333.
11. Lemarie RJ, Hosgood G. 1995. Antiseptics and disinfectants in small animal practice. *Compend Cont Educ Pract Vet* 17:1339–1352.
12. Lozier S, Pope E, Berg J. 1992. Effects of four preparations of 0.05% chlorhexidine diacetate on wound healing in dogs. *Vet Surg* 21:107–112.
13. Maki D, Ringer M, Alvarado CJ. 1991. Prospective randomized trial of povidone-iodine, alcohol, and chlorhexidine for prevention of infection associated with central venous and arterial catheters. *Lancet* 338:339–343.
14. Mathews KA, Brooks MJ, Valliant AE. 1996. A prospective study of intravenous catheter contamination. *J Vet Emerg Crit Care* 6:33–43.
15. Osuna DJ, De Young DJ, Walker RL. 1990. Comparison of three skin preparation techniques in the dog: part 1. Experimental trial. *Vet Surg* 19:14–19.
16. Osuna DJ, De Young DJ, Walker RL. 1990. Comparison of three skin preparation techniques in the dog: part 2. Clinical trial in 100 dogs. *Vet Surg* 19:20–23.
17. Osuna DJ, De Young DJ, Walker RL. 1992. Comparison of an antimicrobial adhesive drape and povidone-iodine preoperative skin preparation in dogs. *Vet Surg* 21:458–462.
18. Phillips MA, Vasseur PB, Gregory CR. 1991. Chlorhexidine diacetate versus povidone-iodine for preoperative preparation of the skin: a prospective randomized comparison in dogs and cats. *J Am Anim Hosp Assoc* 27:105–108.
19. Rochat MC, Mann FA, Berg JN. 1993. Evaluation of a one-step surgical preparation technique in dogs. *J Am Vet Med Assoc* 203:392–395.
20. Russell AD. 1990. Bacterial spores and chemical sporicidal agents. *Clin Microbiol Rev* 3:99–119.
21. Shah PM, Schafer V, Knothe H. 1993. Medical and veterinary use of antimicrobial agents: implications for public health. A clinician's view on antimicrobial resistance. *Vet Microbiol* 35:269–274.
22. Swaim SF, Riddell KP, Geiger DL, et al. 1991. Evaluation of surgical scrub and antiseptic solutions for surgical preparation of canine paws. *J Am Vet Med Assoc* 198:1941–1945.
23. Wise LA, Jones RL, Reif JS. 1990. Nosocomial canine urinary tract infections in a veterinary teaching hospital (1983–1988). *J Am Anim Hosp Assoc* 26:148–152.
24. Zimmerman FA. 1990. Comparison of three skin preparation techniques in the dog (letter). *Vet Surg* 19:405.

Chapter 95

Immunodeficiencies and Infectious Diseases

Urs Giger and Craig E. Greene

Immunodeficiencies are a large heterogenous group of hereditary and acquired disorders of host immunity that can be associated with an increased risk of infection.[14, 33, 39, 44] They can arise through disturbances in antigen-specific defense mechanisms mediated by lymphocytes and/or the nonspecific defense system, which includes phagocytes, plasma proteins, and physical barriers. Although the exact pathogenesis of many canine and feline immunodeficiencies remains unknown, the molecular defects for some forms have been elucidated. Because many effective preventive and therapeutic measures are now available to control infectious diseases in individuals with intact host defense mechanisms, animals with persistent, antimicrobial-unresponsive infections likely suffer from an immunodeficiency disorder. A few hereditary immunodeficiency disorders are prevalent within certain breeds of dogs and cats, whereas others have been described once and may currently exist only in research animal colonies.

Some major clinical features suggest that a patient has an impaired immune system (Table 95–1). Specific organisms and medical conditions often implicated in immunocompromised hosts are listed in Table 95–2. A definitive diagnosis often requires specific immune testing in addition to routine laboratory tests, and therapeutic interventions are limited. Immunodeficiencies can be divided into primary or secondary forms depending on whether they are inherited or acquired.

PRIMARY OR HEREDITARY IMMUNODEFICIENCIES

Many genetically determined immune defects have been described in the dog, whereas only a few are known in cats.

Table 95–1. Major Clinical Signs of Immunodeficiency Disorders

1. Recurrent and/or chronic protracted course of infection
2. Infection with common nonpathogenic (opportunistic) or unusual infectious agents
3. Severe and often atypical infectious disease manifestations
4. Delayed, incomplete, or lack of response to antimicrobial therapy
5. Adverse reactions to modified live virus vaccines

Table 95–2. Organisms and Medical Problems Commonly Implicated in Immunocompromised Hosts

OPPORTUNISTIC ORGANISMS

Viruses: feline herpesvirus, feline infectious peritonitis virus, feline calicivirus, canine papillomavirus, canine herpesvirus
Rickettsia: *Haemobartonella*
Bacteria: *Citrobacter* sp., *Escherichia coli, Enterobacter, Klebsiella pneumoniae, Mycobacterium* spp., *Nocardia asteroides, Proteus, Pseudomonas aeruginosa, Serratia marcescens, Staphylococcus intermedius*
Fungi: *Aspergillus* sp., *Candida* sp., *Cryptococcus, Histoplasma, Mucor*
Protozoa: *Pneumocystis carinii, Toxoplasma gondii, Cryptosporidium*
Metazoa: *Demodex canis, Otodectes notoedres*

MEDICAL PROBLEMS

Recurrent skin infections
Recurrent mucosal infections
Neonatal sepsis and mortality
Reactive amyloidosis
Vasculitis, arteritis, polyarthritis
Recurrent bacteremia
Granulomatous infections
Chronic hypersensitivity reactions
Autoimmune diseases
Persistent intracellular rickettsial or bacterial infections
Disproportional leukocytosis
Persistent lymphopenia

They occur rarely and are summarized in Table 95–3; some are discussed next in more detail under Specific Primary or Inherited Immunodeficiencies. They can be broadly classified into defects of the specific or nonspecific immune system as well as combinations thereof.[31] The nonspecific immune system, also known as innate or natural immunity, should be functional at birth and available on short notice to protect the host from invasion by all sorts of organisms. It includes physicochemical barriers, phagocytes, complement and other plasma proteins, and natural killer cells. Congenital barrier defects particularly involve the skin and mucous membrane surfaces and are associated with infections of particular organs. The Ehlers-Danlos syndrome, causing fragile, hyperextendable skin in many dogs and cats as well as the myxedematous skin and immunodeficiencies of Shar peis, predisposes the animals to pyoderma, whereas ciliary dyskinesia in dogs increases the susceptibility to rhinosinusitis and pneumonia. Disorders of the phagocytic system involve defects of neutrophils and monocytes as well as the complement system and can lead to pyogenic and granulomatous infections. The granulomatous reaction can occur when neutrophils malfunction and mononuclear cells are recruited. A wide variety of pyogenic bacteria (e.g., staphylococci, *Escherichia coli, Klebsiella, Enterobacter*) are usually involved, most of which are normal microflora or pathogens of relatively low virulence. Recurrent infections of the skin, respiratory tract, and oral cavity are common, and recurrent bacteremia and overwhelming sepsis are also seen. Multisystemic amyloidosis, vasculitis, or immune complex disease are complications that can occur as a result of chronic persistent infection. Cyclic hematopoiesis and leukocyte adhesion deficiency (LAD) are examples of quantitative and qualitative phagocytic defects, respectively.

The specific immune system can be divided into humoral and cell-mediated immune systems and includes B and T lymphocytes, immunoglobulins, and cytokines.[31] Deficiencies of B lymphocytes or humoral immunity affect the production of immunoglobulins and lead to increased susceptibility to pyogenic bacterial infections. Deficiencies of T lymphocytes or cell-mediated immunity (CMI) are associated with viral and fungal infections, but intracellular bacterial infections may also occur. Animals with cellular immunodeficiencies may have smaller thymic and tonsillar tissues as well as intestinal and peripheral lymph nodes and decreased numbers of circulating lymphocytes.

The degree of immunodeficiency varies greatly between defects. Infections may be systemic or restricted to a particular organ system like the skin or respiratory tract. Some immunodeficiencies lead to overwhelming infections and death within the first few days to weeks of life, whereas others, such as morphologic leukocyte changes, are not consistently associated with any noticeable predisposition to infection. Chédiak-Higashi syndrome in smoke-colored Persian cats, characterized by abnormally large eosinophilic granules in polymorphonuclear leukocytes, causes no immunodeficiency but a bleeding tendency resulting from a platelet storage pool disease. Similarly, Birman cats with acidophilic granulation of neutrophils and dogs and cats with various lysosomal storage diseases (e.g., mucopolysaccharidosis, gangliosidosis, mannosidosis) have granulation or vacuolation of leukocytes without being immunocompromised. Pelger-Huët anomaly characterized by hyposegmentation of granulocytes causes no immunodeficiency despite the fact that these dogs' and cats' leukograms reveal the most severe left shift with a normal leukocyte count. In foxhounds, in vitro chemotactic response of these neutrophils was diminished,[6, 57, 58] whereas in basenjis no functional abnormalities have been found.

Although there is an increased susceptibility to opportunistic infections, the type of infection varies depending on the type of defect within the immune system. A few immunodeficiency disorders predispose animals to a restricted group of unusual infectious agents. Male dachshunds appear predisposed to *Pneumocystis* pneumonia, and German shepherd dogs may be prone to systemic aspergillosis or rickettsioses. Dobermans and rottweilers are more likely to develop parvoviral disease. Basset hounds have an increased susceptibility to systemic avian mycobacteriosis, toxoplasmosis, and neosporosis. A genetic predisposition to demodicosis has been proposed in various canine breeds and families. The mechanisms predisposing them to specific infections remain unknown in many breeds.

The previously mentioned key signs of infection (see Table 95–1) occur in animals with primary immunodeficiency generally early in life. Non-colostrum-deprived neonates to juvenile animals develop recurrent and overwhelming infections that lead to severe debilitation and death before 1 year of age. Several animals, but typically not all in a litter, may be affected, whereas the parents are usually healthy. A genetic predisposition to infection is rarely noted after 1 year of age (e.g., avian tuberculosis in basset hounds). Furthermore, animals with primary immunodeficiencies may have other special clinical manifestations. Hypersensitivity reactions may occur and reflect an overall dysregulation of the immune system caused by a lack of one or more components or a chronic antigen stimulation due to inadequate clearance of infections. Chronic systemic infections may also hamper the growth rate. Characteristic coat color dilutions and increased tendency for surface bleeding are seen in collies with cyclic hematopoiesis, Persian cats with Chédiak-Higashi syndrome, and Weimaraners with an incompletely defined immunodeficiency.

The mode of inheritance of primary immunodeficiencies has not yet been determined in all cases. Autosomal recessive transmission, with affected males and females born to healthy parents, is usual, but there are a few exceptions. Pelger-Huët anomaly is inherited as an autosomal dominant trait. Severe combined immunodeficiency due to different mutations in the common γ-chain interleukin-2 (IL-2) receptor in basset hounds and Cardigan Welsh corgis is X-chromo-

Table 95–3. Primary or Hereditary Immunodeficiencies of Dogs and Cats[a]

DISEASE (SYNONYMS)	INHERITANCE	BREEDS	DEFECT	CHARACTERIZATION (CHAPTER REFERENCE)
Dog				
Ciliary dyskinesia (immotile cilia syndrome)[16, 29, 35]	AR	Many breeds[b]	Functional/morphologic cilia abnormalities	Rhinosinusitis, bronchopneumonia with bronchiectasis, situs inversus
Respiratory infections[59]	U	Irish wolfhound	Unknown, IgA defect?	Rhinitis, pneumonia
Bactericidal neutrophil defect[7]	U	Doberman	Unknown	Upper respiratory tract infections, reduced bactericidal activity, ciliary dyskinesia not excluded
Cyclic hematopoiesis (cyclic neutropenia)[54, 61]	AR	Gray collie	Hematopoietic growth factors	Severe neutropenia every 12–14 days, reactive amyloidosis
Leukocyte adhesion deficiency (canine granulocytopathy)[9b, 60, 71, 91, 92]	AR	Irish setter	CD11/18 deficiency, β-chain (CD18) deficiency	Severe leukocytosis, limited pus formation, lack of neutrophil adhesion
Complement component 3 (C3 deficiency)[4, 97, 98]	AR	Brittany spaniel	C3 deficiency	Pyogenic infections, lack of C-mediated phagocytosis in colony of dogs with neuromuscular disease
Selective cobalamin malabsorption[36, 37, 69]	AR	Giant Schnauzer Border collie	Ileal cobalamin receptor defect	Weight loss, inappetence, leukopenia with hypersegmentation, megaloblastic bone marrow Methylmalonic aciduria
Increased susceptibility to avian mycobacteriosis[15, 21, 45, 88]	U	Basset hound	RAMP deficiency?	Systemic avian tuberculosis (Chapter 50), toxoplasmosis and neosporosis (Chapter 80)
Increased susceptibility to Pneumocystis pneumonia[5, 13, 30]	XR	Dachshund	Unknown	Pneumocystis pneumonia, male dogs (Chapter 83)
Pelger-Huët anomaly[6, 57]	AD	Australian shepherd, foxhound, others	Unknown	No immunodeficiency, hyposegmented granulocytes
Susceptibility to fungal and rickettsial infections, pyoderma[10, 18, 65, 77, 99]	U	German shepherd	Macrophage?, T cell?	Severe ehrlichiosis (Chapter 28), RMSF (Chapter 29), disseminated aspergillosis (Chapter 65), deep pyoderma
Severe combined immunodeficiency[22, 33, 34, 47, 51, 82–85]	XR	Basset hound Cardigan Welsh corgi	Common gamma chain of IL-2 and other cytokines	Severe bacterial/viral infections, no IgG and IgA, deficient lymphocyte blastogenesis
Selective IgA deficiency[32, 42, 67, 96]	U	Beagle, Shar pei, German shepherd	IgA deficiency	Respiratory and GI infections
Thymic abnormalities and dwarfism[78, 79]	U	Weimaraner	Unknown	Reduced growth (thymosin responsive)
Recurrent infections[15, 21, 45, 88]	U	Weimaraner	Reduced IgG	Pyoderma, severe abscess formation, bleeding tendency (HOD Chapter 100)
Combined immunodeficiency[74]	U	Shar pei	T cell, B cell, low IL-6 and IL-2	Skin, respiratory, and GI infections
Amyloidosis[26, 53, 60, 64, 75, 76]	U	Shar pei	Elevated IL-6	Arthritis, amyloidosis, renal failure, hepatic rupture, hypoproteinemia
Lethal acrodermatitis[52]	AR	Bull terrier	Zinc metabolism defect	Zinc deficiency, hyperkeratosis
Increased susceptibility to parvoviral infection	U	Rottweiler Doberman	Unknown	Parvovirus infection (Chapter 8)
Vaccine-exacerbated immune disturbance[27]	U	Akita	Unknown	Variable meningitis, polyarthritis, amyloidosis (Chapter 100)
Cat				
Hypotrichosis, congenital and thymic aplasia[9]	AR	Birman	Unknown	Nude kittens, neonatal death, no thymus
Thymic and lymphoid atrophy[44a]	U	Ragdoll	Unknown	Neonatal death or fatal infections at weaning, lack lymph nodes and thymus
Leukocyte granulation[48]	U	Birman	Unknown	No immunodeficiency, acidophilic granules
Pelger-Huët anomaly[58]	AD	Domestic shorthair	Unknown	No immunodeficiency, hyposegmented granulocytes
Chédiak-Higashi syndrome[12, 55]	AR	Persian	Unknown	No immunodeficiency, large granules in phagocytes, bleeding tendency
Reactive AA amyloidosis[24, 25, 46]	U	Abyssinian, Siamese, Oriental short hair	Unknown	Reactive AA amyloidosis, renal or hepatic failure

[a]For additional references, see Greene[44] (pp 55–63). In addition to the listed syndromes, bone marrow dyscrasias have been described in miniature and toy poodles and transient hypogammaglobulinemia in Samoyeds, but less is known of these disorders.
[b]e.g., Springer spaniel, Old English sheepdog, English setter, West Highland white terriers, pointers.
AR = autosomal recessive; U = unknown; RAMP = resistance against mycobacterial protein; XR = X-linked recessive; AD = autosomal dominant; RMSF = Rocky Mountain spotted fever; IL = interleukin; HOD = hypertrophic osteodystrophy; ? = suspected.

somal recessively inherited (i.e., only males are affected and the dams and half of the female littermates are carriers). Thus, the breed, gender, age of onset, and type of infections, and other special characteristics may well suggest a particular immunodeficiency.

SECONDARY OR ACQUIRED IMMUNODEFICIENCIES

All components of the immune system of animals with secondary immunodeficiencies are initially intact and functional, but become transiently or permanently impaired during or after an underlying disease condition or exposure to certain agents. Thus, secondary immunodeficiencies occur much more commonly than primary forms. They are associated with organ impairment, whereby infectious agents are allowed to enter the body. This infection may further compromise the function of the particular organ or lead to systemic infectious diseases. A variety of barrier disturbances lead to surface infections, such as upper respiratory tract, urogenital, and GI infections, and dermatitis. Furthermore, certain infections, particularly viral diseases, directly impair the immune system, predisposing animals to secondary bacterial infections.

Puppies and kittens are particularly vulnerable to infections because of incompletely developed immune competency. Colostrum intake during the first day of life transfers maternal immunoglobulins and provides maternal protection during the first few weeks of life in small animals. Although colostrum deprivation has been shown in large animals to result in major neonatal losses, neonatal kittens and puppies kept in good catteries or kennels appear to be not predisposed to infections. However, a transient hypoglobulinemia after the decline of maternal antibodies in the plasma and before the immunocompetency of 2- to 4-month-old animals may increase the susceptibility to various infections.[81] Similarly, aged animals may again become immunocompromised. A variety of drugs and chemicals as well as nutritional deficiencies may drastically impair the production and function of leukocytes. Known secondary immunodeficiencies in companion animals are listed in Table 95–4, and some are covered in detail at the end of this chapter.

DIAGNOSTIC STUDIES

Although an immunodeficiency may be suspected on the basis of clinical evidence, specific laboratory tests are generally required to reach a definitive diagnosis.[38] A minimum data base including CBC, serum chemistry screen, and urinalysis is always indicated and may suggest a specific disorder. The differential WBC count is the most important test result. Leukopenia in the presence of an active bacterial infection is by far the most feared condition. Neutropenia may be transient, as with cyclic hematopoiesis every 12 to 14 days, or persistent, as with cobalamin deficiency and with overwhelming infections (sepsis). Lymphopenia may be observed in dogs with T-cell or severe combined immunodeficiency. Although leukocytosis is expected during periods of infection, defects in leukocyte adhesion and egress from blood circulation at sites of infection may be associated with disproportionately high leukocytosis for the degree of infection as with hereditary LAD and glucocorticoid usage. Dachshunds with *Pneumocystis* pneumonia also have very marked leukocytosis. The WBC count may be in the normal range despite active infections as well as during periods of treatment and remission. Careful review of a blood smear may reveal leukocyte abnormalities such as granulation and vacuolation resulting from lysosomal storage diseases or Chédiak-Higashi syndrome,[55] acidophilic granulation of leukocytes in Birmans,[48] phagocytized microorganisms, or toxic leukocyte changes suggesting overwhelming infections.

Serum globulin concentrations are generally increased during chronic infections. Low to normal globulin levels in infected animals may suggest major external losses or diminished production from a humoral (B-cell) immune defect. Indeed, specific immunoglobulin deficiencies have been recognized in dogs. Serum protein electrophoresis may identify a γ-globulin deficiency, but immunoelectrophoresis is required to detect the class and degree of immunoglobulin deficiency. Maternal immunoglobulins influence the values during the first few weeks of life. IgM can be synthesized very early in life, whereas the development of IgA may be delayed for months. Thus, it is important to compare values with data from age-matched controls. Titers against specific antigens can be measured, followed by evaluation of the antibody response to vaccination against particular agents. Biopsy specimens of lymph nodes may reveal disorganization with loss of germinal centers and normal paracortical lymphocytes. Decreases in plasma cell populations may be evident.

With T-cell or combined immunodeficiencies, there will be defective CMI responses. There may be decreased delayed-type hypersensitivity to skin testing with viral vaccines, tuberculin, or dinitrochlorobenzene (DNCB)[68] and prolonged allograft rejection times. Reduced in vitro lymphocyte stimu-

Table 95–4. Secondary or Acquired Immunodeficiencies

Immature Animals	**Barrier Damage**	**Chemical and Drug-Induced Suppression**[28]
Colostrum deprivation	Burns	Myelosuppression
Neonatal hypothermia	Invasive or indwelling catheters	Cytotoxic agents
Transient hypoglobulinemia (between 2–6 months)	Endoscopic devices	Chloramphenicol
Aged Animals	Splenectomy	Griseofulvin
Weakened immune system in very young and old[43, 80, 81]	Centesis	Estrogens (dogs and ferrets)
Organ Disorders	**Whole Body Irradiation**	Immunosuppression
Hyperadrenocorticism	**Immunosuppressive Viral Agents**	Glucocorticoids[23]
Diabetes mellitus	FeLV[49, 56, 62]	Cytotoxic agents
UTI	FIV[1, 8, 17, 49, 63, 72, 73, 89, 100]	Anesthetics
Skin diseases	Feline and canine parvovirus	**Antibiotic and Antacid Usage for GI Diseases**
Pulmonary diseases	CDV	**Nutritional Disorders**
GI diseases	Canine retrovirus?[3, 66, 70, 86, 87]	Vitamin A deficiency
Malnutrition	**Other Infections**	Vitamin E deficiency
Systemic lupus erythematosus	Demodicosis[2]	Protein-caloric restriction
Chronic hemolytic anemias	Ehrlichiosis	Zinc deficiency
Dysproteinemias	Protracted bacterial infections	Hematopoietic neoplasia
Cancer		

URI = urinary tract infection; FeLV = feline leukemia; FIV = feline immunodeficiency; CDV = canine distemper virus.

lation results may also be due to a primary lymphocyte defect or secondary to the infection found.

The identification of the agents infecting an animal is important for diagnostic as well as therapeutic considerations. Appropriate cultures of tissues, body fluids, and excretions for microorganisms and antigen and serologic blood tests are covered in the chapters on specific infectious agents. Antibody titers may also be used to assess a response to vaccines and humoral immunity. For instance, Rottweilers appear to respond late to parvovirus vaccines and have an increased susceptibility to the infection.

Gross and microscopic histopathology and cytology may discover certain microorganisms, but are also most helpful in characterizing the architecture, morphology, maturation, and function of the immune system such as leukocytes, bone marrow, lymph nodes, thymus, and spleen as well as other barrier systems. In ciliary dyskinesia, morphologic abnormalities of cilia may be identified by EM, but functional studies by imaging techniques or on respiratory epithelial biopsy specimens are also indicated.

To characterize the immunodeficiencies further, special leukocyte studies are often required. Surface marker studies by fluorescent-assisted cell sorters or flow cytometers can differentiate between T and B cells or determine T- and B-cell ratio and the presence or absence of leukocyte adhesion proteins (CD11/18) or IL-2 receptors. Lymphocyte function studies include lymphocyte stimulation and plaque-forming assays for in vitro immunoglobulin production. Phagocyte function studies assess leukocyte adhesion, migration, chemotaxis, phagocytosis, "respiratory burst," and bactericidal activity. All functional assays should be performed on fresh blood cells and compared simultaneously to an age- (and breed-) matched control. Furthermore, in vitro lymphocyte functions are generally impaired and phagocyte functions are enhanced during periods of active infection. It is advisable, whenever possible, to control the infection before studying leukocyte function.

TREATMENT AND PREVENTION

Successful control of infection in immunodeficient animals depends on the underlying disease as well as the type and severity of the immune defect. In immunocompromised patients, early and aggressive antimicrobial therapy is indicated even for mild infections with usually nonpathogenic agents. Because of the immunodeficient host's potential inability to kill bacteria, bactericidal antibiotics are recommended until bacterial infections are controlled. If the underlying disorder causing a secondary immunodeficiency can be corrected, the infection is often easily controlled. The underlying disorder should be treated and triggering agents such as drugs removed immediately.

Currently, no practical treatments for primary immunodeficiencies exist. Immunocompromised animals with infection generally have a guarded to poor prognosis. Despite aggressive antimicrobial therapy, their infections are difficult to control, leading to overwhelming infections, protracted courses, and recurrences. Some leukocyte defects cause death before 1 year of age, whereas others may not lead to a markedly increased predisposition to infection. In experimental studies, bone marrow transplantation has corrected several leukocyte defects.

Fresh whole blood may be transfused repeatedly to animals with overwhelming infections and neutropenia or neutrophil dysfunction, but the effect is very transient. Plasma transfusions or immunoglobulin injections may support humoral immunodeficiencies. However, these products should not be used in animals with IgA deficiency because they may experience anaphylactic reactions. There is currently no commercial canine γ-globulin available, and the human γ-globulin preparations are exorbitantly expensive and may cause allergic reactions upon repeated use. There are no data to support their use in immunodeficient infected small animals, although they have been given to treat autoimmune anemias. Nonspecific immunostimulators have not been documented to be beneficial in animals with cell-mediated immunodeficiencies. However, immunocompromised animals with active infections should not be vaccinated. Furthermore, modified live virus (MLV) vaccines should be avoided in animals with inherited or acquired T-cell defects, because they may develop clinical disease from the vaccine virus.

The potential zoonotic risks involved must be considered in keeping an immunodeficient animal with infections that may be contagious to humans, particularly immunosuppressed humans (see Chapter 99).

SPECIFIC PRIMARY OR INHERITED IMMUNODEFICIENCIES

Dogs

Primary Ciliary Dyskinesia. This is also known as immotile cilia syndrome. Primary ciliary dyskinesia is caused by a variety of functional and ultrastructural ciliary abnormalities, including lack of outer or inner dynein arms, abnormal microtubular pattern, random ciliary orientation, and electron-dense cores in the basal body. Owing to impaired mucociliary clearance, affected animals suffer from recurrent bacterial rhinitis, sinusitis, and bronchopneumonia with bronchiectasis. Poorly motile or immotile live sperms lead to male infertility, and although evidence is lacking, dysfunction of ependymal cilia may cause hydrocephalus. Otitis media may also occur. The lack of coordinated cilia motility during embryogenesis is responsible for the 50% prevalence of concurrent situs inversus. The clinical triad of rhinosinusitis, bronchiectasis, and situs inversus is known as Kartagener's syndrome.[29]

Primary ciliary dyskinesia is inherited by an autosomal recessive trait. It represents a heterogenous group of defects that have been described in more than a dozen breeds. Clinical signs typically begin at an early age, and recurrent respiratory infections lead to death or euthanasia before 1 year of age. However, a few dogs have remained nonsymptomatic for months to years.[35] A diagnosis is reached by documenting an absence of ciliary clearance of a technetium Tc 99m–labeled microaggregated albumin placed through a catheter into the nasal cavity or the tracheal bifurcation, and tissue biopsy of ciliated mucosae with ultrastructural analysis.[16]

Irish Wolfhound Rhinitis and Pneumonia. Chronic recurrent respiratory infections have been observed in Irish wolfhounds.[59] As puppies, the disease begins with a serous rhinitis that later becomes catarrhal to hemorrhagic with turbinate ulceration and destruction. Pneumonia and generalized lymphadenomegaly are apparent in later stages. Although the disease is responsive to antimicrobial treatment, it may progress in intervening periods. Although a familial relationship exists, the exact mode of inheritance and the underlying defect are uncertain.

Neutrophil Bactericidal Defect Associated With Respiratory Infection. Neutrophil dysfunction was described in a family of Doberman pinschers from which a young animal had chronic recurrent respiratory tract infections.[7] Oxygen radical formation and bactericidal activity of neutrophils were reduced despite normal phagocytosis of bacteria. The specific defect has not yet been identified, and primary ciliary dyskinesia has not been completely ruled out. The cilia morphology appeared normal, but no functional studies have been performed. Affected Doberman pinschers develop clinical signs of upper respiratory tract infections at a few weeks of age. They respond to antibiotics, but the prognosis is guarded.

Cyclic Hematopoiesis. This is characterized by a periodic production and maturation defect of hematopoietic cells in the bone marrow. In affected dogs all blood cell counts cycle precisely at a 12- to 14-day interval, whereas in human patients the cycle is 21 days. Because of the short half-life of granulocytes, severe neutropenia (<1000/µl) is seen every 12 to 14 days and lasts for 3 to 4 days, explaining the synonym "cyclic neutropenia syndrome." Serial blood counts are used to reach a definitive diagnosis. During periods of severe neutropenia, dogs are highly susceptible to bacterial infections. Clinical features start at 6 to 8 weeks of age with regularly recurring bacterial infections. The chronic exposure leads to systemic amyloidosis, and death may be due to organ failure (kidney and others) and sepsis before 1 year of age. Furthermore, gingival bleeding may occur from an associated platelet storage pool disease. Affected collies have a silver gray or light-beige to tan color, and secondary hormonal cycling has also been observed.[54, 61]

Cyclic hematopoiesis was the first reported canine immunodeficiency observed and has only been clearly described in collies that are hypopigmented, hence the term "gray collie syndrome." It is inherited as an autosomal recessive trait, but no clinical case has been reported since the 1970s. The basic reason for the cycling remains unknown.[61] Experimentally, bone marrow transplantation completely corrects this syndrome, including the coat color dilution. Furthermore, administration of lithium carbonate, at extremely high and otherwise toxic doses, is known to induce a leukocytosis and ameliorates the cyclic neutropenia in affected animals. Similarly, injections of granulocyte colony-stimulating factors, alone or in combination with steel factor, abolish the cycling, suggesting a signaling defect in the proliferation and maturation of hematopoietic cells.

Leukocyte Adhesion Deficiency (LAD). This has previously been described as canine granulocytopathy syndrome in Irish setters.[71] Today, it is known to be caused by an absence of a family of three leukocyte integrins.[40, 91, 92] These surface proteins are heterodimers (CD11a-c/CD18) with a specific α-chain (CD11a-c) and a common β-chain (CD18). In LAD, the β-subunit is missing (CD18 deficiency), resulting in a lack of surface expression and function of all three leukocyte integrins. The CD11b/18 is the most critical integrin because this is the CR3 receptor and binds C3bi and ICAM-1 of activated endothelium, thereby mediating tight adhesion leukocytes. Because of this deficiency, granulocytes are unable to marginate, migrate randomly or by chemotaxis, and kill microorganisms, resulting in an impaired inflammatory response despite marked leukocytosis. Furthermore, the in vitro lymphocyte stimulation response is reduced.

Affected dogs have a severely increased susceptibility to bacterial and fungal infections. Signs of pyogenic infections develop during the first weeks to months of life, are often recurring, and are poorly responsive to antibiotics. Omphalophlebitis and gingivitis are often the first infections and might be followed by pyoderma, pododermatitis, thrombophlebitis, pneumonia, pyometra, osteomyelitis (especially craniomandibular and metaphyseal), and fatal sepsis. Pups are often stunted or in poor body condition. The sites of infections exhibit only minimal inflammation and pus formation despite a most severe persistent leukocytosis of 25,000 to 500,000/µl. Regional lymphadenomegaly and poor wound healing are commonly noted. Long-term therapy with bactericidal antibiotics is required to keep affected animals alive.

LAD has been reported in Irish setters from the United States and Sweden and is inherited by an autosomal recessive mode. This defect also has been documented in red Holstein cattle and in humans. The diagnosis is made by demonstrating a lack of neutrophil adherence to glass, plastic, or wool and confirmed by a deficiency of leukocyte glycoproteins CD11/CD18 by flow cytometry analysis.

Complement C3 Deficiency. In a colony of Brittany spaniels with spinal muscular atrophy, a C3 deficiency was found.[4, 97, 98] This is a key factor of the complement system required in opsonizing bacteria. Affected dogs have defective chemotaxis and bacterial phagocytosis owing to a complete deficiency of C3 (0.1%) and less than 1% plasma complement activity. The immunodeficiency is generally mild, but serious infections may occur, including pneumonia, sepsis, pyometra, and septic arthritis. Affected dogs may develop renal failure with amyloidosis. This is an autosomal recessively inherited disorder, and a diagnosis can be reached by documenting a lack of serum complement activity.

Selective Cobalamin Malabsorption. Chronic neutropenia and megaloblastic anemia have been described in giant Schnauzers and border collie pups.[37, 69] Affected animals fail to thrive and present with lethargy, inappetence, and cachexia, but are only rarely predisposed to infection with fever, lameness, or diarrhea. Blood smears show neutropenia with hypersegmented neutrophils. Affected animals have low serum cobalamin concentrations and methylmalonic aciduria. A cobalamin ileal receptor defect was documented in affected giant Schnauzers.[37] Treatment with parenteral administration of cobalamin once monthly is highly effective.

Miscellaneous Defects in Dogs. Increased susceptibility to avian mycobacteriosis has been recognized in Basset hounds and miniature Schnauzers (see Chapter 50). The underlying defect is unknown, but it may represent a defect in resistance against mycobacterial protein (RAMP). Dachshunds have a predisposition to develop pneumocystosis (Chapter 83). Although Pelger-Huët anomaly has been observed in dogs, it has not been associated with clinical illness.

German Shepherd Infections. These dogs are more severely infected with *E. canis* (Chapter 28), *R. rickettsii* (Chapter 29), and *Aspergillus* (Chapter 65). Some German shepherd dogs also are predisposed to pyoderma.[10, 18] These predispositions may involve separate as yet undefined defects. Affected dogs have pruritus with a deep pyoderma over the lumbosacral region, which may spread to other regions.[77] Coagulase-positive *Staphylococcus intermedius* is most commonly cultured. Proposed mechanisms for this susceptibility include hypothyroidism, cell-mediated immunodeficiency associated with serum inhibitors or defective helper T cells, and bacterial hypersensitivity reactions to staphylococci.[10, 18, 19, 99] Although the inciting causes may be multivariate, the condition responds favorably to long-term administration of systemic antibacterials.

X-Linked Severe Combined Immunodeficiency (XSCID). This severe combined immunodeficiency is characterized by a failure in humoral immunity and CMI.[31, 34] Defects in the γ^c chain lead to deficiency of several cytokine receptors (IL-

2, IL-4, IL-7, IL-9, and IL-15). The shared usage of a γ^c chain explains the profound immunologic abnormalities. The ability of lymphocytes to bind and proliferate to IL-2 is severely impaired, and the development of thymocytes is drastically reduced with an increased proportion of CD4-/CD8-thymocytes.[84, 85] Serum IgG and IgA concentrations are low, but IgM values are normal.[51] Because of X-chromosomal recessive mode of inheritance, male dogs are affected, whereas females (dam and some littermates of those affected) are carriers. The gene defect for this disease in dogs and people has been located on the proximal short arm of the X chromosome (Xq13). Bassets with XSCID have a four–base pair deletion that produces a frame shift and subsequent premature stop codon in exon 1.[47] Affected Cardigan Welsh corgis have an insertion of cytosine, resulting in a premature stop codon.[70a, 83]

After the decline of maternal immunity, affected male dogs will develop bacterial skin, GI, and respiratory infections. Puppies will fail to thrive and grow and die within a few months. The most characteristic clinical features are a lack of lymph nodes and thymus. A diagnosis is reached by histopathology, immunologic testing, or polymerase chain reaction–based test to identify the specific mutation in Bassets and corgis.

Bone marrow transplantation from unaffected littermates was effective in re-establishing normal T- and B-cell function in affected dogs.[32a]

Selective (IgA) Deficiency. Various forms of selective IgA deficiency have been described in several breeds, including beagles,[31, 42] Shar peis,[67] and German shepherd dogs,[96] but the mode of inheritance remains unknown. Serum IgA concentrations may be completely absent or markedly reduced and only very slowly developing over the first year of life. Thus, serum IgA concentrations need to be compared with those of age-matched controls. The serum IgG and IgM concentrations are normal. Affected juvenile dogs are predisposed to mucocutaneous infections such as chronic recurrent respiratory infections (involving parainfluenza and *Bordetella bronchiseptica*), gastroenteritis, pyoderma, and otitis. IgA-deficient dogs may have a positive rheumatoid factor and/or anti-IgA antibodies and may develop allergies and autoimmune diseases.

Immunodeficiencies in Weimaraners. Two distinct syndromes of immunodeficiency have been observed in this breed. In the first, which has been reported only once, growth hormone deficiency has been associated with wasting and thymic hypoplasia.[78, 79]

The second involves recurrent bacterial infections, which often become systemic.[15, 21, 45, 88] Clinical signs of recurrent disease start at a few months to several years of age, characterized by intermittent fever, lymphadenomegaly, pyogranulomatous disease, large abscesses in muscle, stomatitis, osteomyelitis, surface bleeding, and coat color dilution. Inconsistencies exist in the immunologic studies performed on these dogs. Neutrophilia, which is often marked with a left shift, has been observed. Decreased neutrophil phagocytosis of opsonized bacteria and chemiluminescence, and slightly low serum IgG and IgM concentrations have been reported in some dogs with increased amounts of circulating immune complexes (CICs).[15] In other reports, reduced serum IgG, IgA, and IgM have been observed with no increase in CICs. The lack of CICs in most reports suggests that primary decreased production rather than secondary immunoglobulin consumption is responsible for the defect. No specific diagnostic tests are currently available. Despite antibiotic and supportive therapy (draining of abscesses), the prognosis remains guarded. Some Weimaraners also appear to have an increased tendency to develop hypertrophic osteodystrophy, which has been associated as a postvaccination reaction (see Chapter 100). Whether this predisposition is involved with the same syndrome is uncertain.

Immunodeficiencies in Shar Peis. Two distinct syndromes have been characterized in the Shar pei dog, one involving combined antibody and cell-mediated immune defects and the other involving renal amyloidosis and swollen joints.

The **combined immunodeficiency syndrome** may have been confused with the selective IgA deficiency described in this breed (see Selective (IgA) Deficiency, above). Dogs 7 months to 7 years of age suffer recurrent infections involving respiratory, skin, and GI systems.[74] Chronic bronchitis, gastroduodenal or colonic ulceration, diarrhea and vomiting, adult-onset pyoderma, demodicosis, and bacterial and fungal otitis are observed. In addition, the dogs have a predilection to develop GI neoplasia, lymphoma, and other malignancies. Single to multiple immunoglobulin class deficiency is observed in dogs, with IgM deficiency and decreased IL-2 synthesis predominating. Dogs with GI signs or malignancy usually had reduced IgM. Decreased lymphocyte stimulation test results were found in most of the dogs, suggesting a combined T- and B-cell defect.[74] In addition, peripheral blood mononuclear cells had reduced IL-6 synthesis.

Recurrent fever of unknown origin and **swelling of the tibiotarsal joints** constitute another immune-based syndrome in this breed: "Shar pei fever" or "Shar pei hock."[26, 64, 76] The lameness can be monoarticular or can involve multiple joints, usually affecting the tibiotarsal joints and sometimes the carpus. Predominant mononuclear cell and cellulitis, with or without synovial inflammation, can occur. Clinical signs reflecting renal failure, as a result of amyloid deposition in the kidney, and the nephrotic syndrome (proteinuria, hypercholesterolemia, and hypoproteinemia) eventually develop. Although a majority of the dogs have amyloid deposition in the renal medulla, glomerular involvement from amyloid or membranous glomerulitis occurs in only 60% to 80% of affected dogs.[26] Polydipsia, polyuria, weight loss, dehydration, ascites, and peripheral edema may occur. Thromboembolism may occur as a sudden complication in some dogs with the nephrotic syndrome. Radiographic changes are soft tissue swelling, with periarticular bone erosion and bone production. Recurrent fever, joint pain, and swelling often resolve within 24 hours.[64] Postpartum metritis has developed in intact female dogs and may be another inflammatory feature of this illness.[26] Hyperglobulinemia and increased levels of IL-6 are found in affected dogs.[75] This syndrome is similar to familial Mediterranean fever, a human hereditary disorder characterized by polyserositis and reactive amyloidosis. Treatment with colchicine early in the course of disease may reduce amyloid deposition in people and has been proposed for affected dogs.

Lethal Acrodermatitis. This is also known as "zincers" among Bull terrier breeders. This syndrome is characterized by hyper- and parakeratosis and thymus and lymph node hypoplasia, leading to increased susceptibility to infection and failure to thrive.[52] Growth retardation, hard and cracked footpads, pyoderma around body orifices, and aggressive to unresponsive behavior are hallmark features at a few weeks of age. The disease resembles zinc deficiency but is unresponsive to zinc therapy. Thus, affected dogs die or are euthanized before 6 months of age.

Susceptibility to Parvovirus Infection. A number of purebred dogs have an increased prevalence rate of parvovirus infection. These include Dobermans, Rottweilers, American pitbulls, and Dalmatians, among others (see Chapter 8). The reason for this apparent susceptibility is unknown.

Akita Polyarthritis. This syndrome has been observed in related Akita dogs and is exacerbated by MLV vaccines (see Chapter 100).

Cats

Hypotrichosis Congenita with Thymic Aplasia in Cats. This defect is characterized by the birth of nude athymic kittens with severe immunodeficiency similar to the well-known laboratory nude mice. This lethal syndrome has been recognized in the Birman breed and is inherited by an autosomal recessive trait.[9] I (CEG) have observed a syndrome in Ragdoll kittens characterized by fatal infections in the neonatal to weaning period. Use of MLV panleukopenia vaccine may have accelerated the mortality. Some kittens died of that disease at an earlier age. By weaning, others developed a number of systemic fatal infections. Thymic, splenic, and lymphoid hypoplasia were observed in these affected kittens.

Other Defects in Cats. Neutrophil abnormalities have been observed in Birman cats with leukocyte granulation, Persian cats with Chédiak-Higashi syndrome, and domestic shorthaired cats with Pelger-Huët anomaly. Clinical immunodeficiencies have not been recognized with these defects. Other purebred cats have had more problems with viral respiratory (Chapter 16) and coronavirus (Chapter 11) infections, but specific defects have not been elucidated.

Reactive Amyloidosis in Abyssinian Cats. Cats in this breed have a predisposition to develop reactive amyloidosis in many organs but clinical signs are referable to renal dysfunction. A genetic basis is suspected, but the mode of inheritance is uncertain. This syndrome is similar to amyloidosis in Shar pei dogs and familial Mediterranean fever in people. Splenic inflammatory diseases, often related to secondary infections from immunodeficiency, are responsible for the amyloid deposition in reactive amyloidosis. However, in some affected cats, concurrent inflammatory disease is not detected.[25] Generalized amyloidosis has also been observed in Siamese and oriental cats but clinical features and amyloid protein composition differ.[93] Reactive amyloidosis has also been detected in Siberian tigers *(Panthera tigris altaica)*[79a] and cheetahs *(Acinonyx jobatus)*.[69a] It may be related to genetic homogenicity with increased susceptibility to infectious disease.

SPECIFIC SECONDARY OR ACQUIRED IMMUNODEFICIENCIES

Acquired or secondary immunodeficiencies can develop at any time as a result of interference in host defense mechanisms. Immune defects secondary to many infectious diseases, metabolic disturbances, intoxications, and drug therapies[11a, 64a] have been reported (see Table 95–3), and some are described in more detail next.

Infectious Diseases

Canine Distemper. Disseminated viral infections that involve replication in and damage to lymphoid tissue, such as canine distemper, are associated with depression of CMI. Persistent immunodeficiency caused by canine distemper virus (CDV) usually occurs when infection develops prenatally or within the first weeks of neonatal life, when full immunocompetence has not been established.[44] Affected dogs frequently are stunted and may develop chronic infections with protozoans such as *Giardia* and rickettsiae such as *Haemobartonella*. They can also be expected to be more susceptible to viral and fungal pathogens, and they frequently have pronounced lymphopenia and hypogammaglobulinemia.[44] Persistent suppression of CMI in neonatal puppies can be detected by decreased lymphocyte stimulation test results and decreased synthesis of T cell–dependent antibodies (IgG and IgA). IgM is also reduced if thymic hypoplasia results from early in utero infection. Transient depression of CMI has been reported in older neonates that are infected with virulent CDV. Some of this suppression has been shown to be caused by lymphocyte immunoregulatory factors in serum. Depression of immunoresponsiveness after vaccination is minimal if it occurs at all. See Chapter 3 for additional information.

Canine Parvovirus Infection. This virus has an affinity for replicating in rapidly dividing cells and produces severe lymphopenia and immunosuppression in neonates (see Chapter 8). An increased risk of secondary infections, including greater susceptibility to canine distemper vaccine–induced encephalitis, has been reported in 3-week-old pups (see Chapter 100). Lymphocyte stimulation assay results were depressed in adult mongrel dogs shedding canine parvovirus in the feces.[44]

Canine Ehrlichiosis. Depression of in vitro lymphocyte stimulation and skin hypersensitivity with DNCB have been reported in canine ehrlichiosis several months after initial infection, when hyperglobulinemia develops. The depression does not appear to alter the course of infection at this time, although certain breeds (e.g., German shepherds) have more severe illness and greater depression of CMI before and after infection than other breeds. No increased susceptibility to infection has been documented in dogs with acute ehrlichiosis as yet; however, they are susceptible to pyogenic infections during the chronic neutropenic phase of the disease (see also Chapter 28).

Canine Demodicosis. Dogs with generalized demodicosis have decreased in vitro lymphocyte stimulation, T-lymphocyte deficiency, and random neutrophil movement.[2, 74] Serum proteins with apparent immunoregulatory roles are responsible for the findings. No increased susceptibility to infection has been documented in vivo, although many dogs do develop severe secondary pyoderma. Secondary bacterial infection rather than the mite *Demodex canis* has been thought to be responsible for the suppressed immune response, because neutrophilic chemotactic movement has been decreased in bacterial (staphylococcal) pyoderma in dogs. In some cases, with antimicrobial therapy, these abnormal test results return to normal and are accompanied by clinical improvement. Histologically, mural folliculitis is a consistent lesion of active demodecosis. Histochemical studies indicate a preponderance of $CD3^+$ and $CD8^+$, infiltrating lymphocytes, and a low $CD4^+$: $CD8^+$ ratio in follicular lesions and peripheral blood.[9a] These cytotoxic lymphocytes may induce the inflammatory lesions or represent a deleterious response in dogs that develop this disease.

Feline Panleukopenia. Feline panleukopenia virus has a predilection for rapidly dividing cells and produces permanent cell-mediated immunosuppression and thymic atrophy in kittens infected in utero. Lymphoid depletion, mild depression of in vitro lymphocyte function, and neutropenia are characteristic in neonatally infected cats, which may have a transiently increased susceptibility to infection. Overwhelming sepsis from gram-negative enteric microflora, which accompanies feline panleukopenia, may be related to the immunosuppression caused by the virus (see also Chapter 10).

Feline Leukemia Virus (FeLV) Infection. Immunodeficiency in FeLV infection often occurs before malignant transformation of T lymphocytes. A reduction in $CD4^+$ and $CD8^+$ lymphocyte subset ratios has been shown to occur in FeLV-infected cats, similar to that of feline immunodeficiency virus (FIV)–infected cats.[49] FeLV-infected cats have impaired T cell–mediated immunity as characterized by reduced in vitro lymphocyte stimulation, prolonged retention of cutaneous allografts, and impaired response to delayed hypersensitivity skin testing. Secondary hyperglobulinemia and complement depletion have also been found. Immune complex formation may also interfere with lymphocyte function, because immune complex removal has improved the clinical condition of infected cats. Infected cats that do not develop neoplasia have a high mortality rate and increased susceptibility to concurrent infection with other organisms, such as commensal bacteria, pathogenic fungi, *Haemobartonella*, and feline infectious peritonitis (FIP) virus. Certain forms of FeLV infection also result in severe neutropenia, which increases the risk of secondary bacterial infection. Persistent neutropenia may also develop in some cats latently infected with FeLV. A panleukopenia-like syndrome can develop in cats that are coinfected with FeLV and FIV (see also Chapter 13).[62]

FIV Infection. Cats naturally affected with this syndrome develop fever, variable neutropenia, and chronic infections of the skin and mucosal surfaces (see Chapter 14). Experimentally inoculated cats develop generalized peripheral lymphadenomegaly and transient neutropenia followed by a disease-free period. In natural circumstances, opportunistic infectious agents, normally controlled by CMI, are also involved in producing disease. Calicivirus, FIP, *Toxoplasma*, and systemic fungi are notable examples.[17, 73] Compared with uninfected cats, FIV-infected cats have a higher frequency of isolation of *Cryptococcus neoformans* and *Candida albicans* from oropharyngeal mucosa and *Microsporum canis* from skin.[63] Defective natural killer cell cytotoxic activity has been detected.[100] Incidental and opportunistic infections may accelerate the progression of infected cats to develop acquired immunodeficiency.[72] Cats with FIV must be vaccinated with killed vaccines (see Chapter 100).

Retroviruses Isolated From Diseased Dogs. Anorexia, depression, and multiple lymphadenomegaly have been described in a Rottweiler. A cell line from this dog contained an identifiable C-type retrovirus.[3] Retroviral elements have been isolated from cells derived from canine lymphosarcoma and endogenous sequences from normal canine cells.[86, 87] A novel canine lentivirus has been isolated from buffy coat of a leukemic dog.[70] Whether canine retroviruses cause clinical illness in dogs remains to be determined.

Overwhelming Bacteremia. Severe endotoxemia or sepsis has been shown to impair CMI of dogs and to decrease neutrophil bactericidal function (also see Chapter 38).

Metabolic Disturbances

Many biochemical processes that occur in noninfectious disease states interfere with normal immune mechanisms. Failure of neonates to ingest colostrum and dysproteinemia are both associated with impaired humoral antibody function. Decreased complement concentration has been noted with endotoxemia, immune-mediated hemolysis, and malnutrition. Age has a marked influence on CMI. Newborn puppies and kittens experience a hypothermic state during the first week of life that suppresses T-cell function. A decline in CMI, which is also seen in older dogs and cats, may explain their increased susceptibility to infectious and neoplastic disorders. Lymphocyte stimulation by various mitogens is depressed in older dogs, and male dogs were more profoundly affected. A decline in B-cell percentages was also noted.[43] Proper nutrition is also an important determinant of immunoresponsiveness. Protein and caloric restriction has resulted in premature thymic atrophy and decreased cell-mediated, humoral, and phagocytic responses in animals. In contrast, overfed, obese dogs have had an increased susceptibility to infection and severe clinical illness.

Vitamin E and selenium deficiencies in dogs have been associated with decreased in vitro lymphocyte responsiveness, decreased serologic response to vaccination, and increased susceptibility to infection with opportunistic pathogens. The deficit can be accentuated by excessive intake of polyunsaturated fats (strong oxidants that counteract the effects of vitamin E). Vitamin E deficiency causes the animal to produce a suppressor serum factor capable of decreasing lymphocyte responsiveness to antigenic stimulation. Increased incidence of distemper infection has been noted in a kennel of dogs that developed "brown fat" disease as a result of a vitamin E–deficient ration.

Vitamin A deficiency can cause immunosuppression with opportunistic infections similar to that of vitamin E deficiency. In areas of the world where vitamin A deficiency exists, human measles virus infection produces a high mortality. A similar phenomenon might be expected to occur in dogs with canine distemper. Zinc deficiency during prenatal and neonatal periods can result in impaired CMI responses and thymic atrophy. Immunosuppression caused by dietary deficiencies can be relieved by adequate supplementation.

Depressed phagocyte function has also been reported in humans with diabetes mellitus, systemic lupus erythematosus, and renal failure. Similarly, poorly regulated or untreated diabetic dogs had reduced neutrophil adherence compared with controlled diabetic and nondiabetic dogs. Any cause of permanent neutropenia, such as bone marrow aplasia, will significantly impair phagocyte function. Intestinal lymphangiectasia is associated with depressed CMI because of lymphocyte loss.

References

1. Barr MC, Zou L, Holzschu DL, et al. 1995. Isolation of a highly cytopathic lentivirus from a nondomestic cat. *J Virol* 69:7371–7374.
2. Barriga OO, Al-khalidi NW, Martin S, et al. 1992. Evidence of immunosuppression by *Demodex canis*. *Vet Immunol Immunopathol* 32:37–46.
3. Bleakley JS, Gilmore WH, Kelly DF, et al. 1996. Retroviral infection in a canine cell line, p 192. *In* Proceedings of the British Small Animal Veterinary Association meeting, Birmingham, UK.
4. Blum JR, Cork LC, Morris JM, et al. 1985. The clinical manifestations of a genetically-determined deficiency in the third component of complement in the dog. *Clin Immunol Immunopathol* 24:304–317.
5. Botha WS, van Rensburg IBJ. 1979. Pneumocystosis: a chronic respiratory distress syndrome in the dog. *J S Afr Vet Assoc* 50:173–179.
6. Bowles CA, Alsaker RD, Wolfle TL. 1979. Studies of the Pelger-Huet anomaly in Foxhounds. *Am J Pathol* 96:237–246.
7. Breitschwerdt EB, Brown TT, DeBuyssher EV, et al. 1987. Rhinitis, pneumonia, and defective neutrophil function in the Doberman pinscher. *Am J Vet Res* 48:1054–1062.
8. Buonavoglia C, Marsilio F, Tempesta M, et al. 1993. Use of a feline panleukopenia modified live virus vaccine in cats in the primary-stage of

feline immunodeficiency virus infection. *Zentralbl Veterinarmed B* 40:343–346.
9. Casal M, Straumann U, Sigg C, et al. 1994. Congenital hypotrichosis with thymic aplasia in nine birman kittens. *J Am Anim Hosp Assoc* 30:600–602.
9a. Caswell JL, Yager JA, Parker WM, et al. 1997. A prospective study of the immunophenotype and temporal changes in the histologic lesions of canine distemper. *Vet Pathol* 34:279–287.
9b. Cauvin A, Connolly D. 1997. Immunodeficiency syndrome in Irish setters. *Vet Rec* 141:556.
10. Chabanne L, Marchal T, Denerolle P, et al. 1995. Lymphocyte subset abnormalities in German shepherd dog pyoderma (GSP). *Vet Immunol Immunopathol* 49:189–198.
11. Cheeseman MT, Kelly DF, Horsfall KL. 1995. Multisystemic inflammatory disease in a Borzoi dog. *J Small Anim Pract* 36:22–24.
11a. Cohn LA. 1997. Glucocorticosteroids as immunosuppressive agents. *Semin Vet Med Surg* 12:150–156.
12. Colgan SP, Blancquaert A-M B, Thrall MA, et al. 1992. Defective in vitro motility of polymorphonuclear leukocytes of homozygote and heterozygote Chediak-Higashi cats. *Vet Immunol Immunopathol* 31:205–227.
13. Copeland JW. 1974. Canine pneumonia caused by *Pneumocystis carinii*. *Aust Vet J* 50:515–518.
14. Couto CG, Giger U. 1989. Congenital and acquired neutrophil function abnormalities in the dog, pp 521–525. *In* Kirk RW (ed), Current veterinary therapy X. WB Saunders, Philadelphia, PA.
15. Couto CG, Krakowka S, Johnson G, et al. 1989. In vitro immunologic features of Weimaraner dogs with neutrophil abnormalities and recurrent infections. *Vet Immunol Immunopathol* 23:103–112.
16. Daniel GB, Edwards DF, Harvey RC, Kabalka GW. 1995. Communicating hydrocephalus in dogs with congenital ciliary dysfunction. *Dev Neurosci* 17:230–235.
17. Davidson MG, Rottman JB, English RV, et al. 1993. Feline immunodeficiency virus predisposes cats to acute generalized toxoplasmosis. *Am J Pathol* 143:1486–1497.
18. Day MJ. 1994. An immunopathological study of deep pyoderma in the dog. *Res Vet Sci* 56:18–23.
19. Day MJ, Mazza G. 1995. Tissue immunoglobulin G subclasses observed in immune-mediated dermatopathy, deep pyoderma and hypersensitivity dermatitis in dogs. *Res Vet Sci* 58:82–89.
20. Day MJ, Penhale WJ. 1992. Immune-mediated disease in the old English sheepdog. *Res Vet Sci* 53:87–92.
21. Day MJ, Power C, Oleshko J, et al. 1997. Low serum immunoglobulin concentrations in related Weimaraner dogs. *J Small Anim Pract* 38:311–315.
22. Deschenes SM, Puck JM, Dutra AS, et al. 1994. Comparative mapping of canine and human proximal xq and genetic analysis of canine X-linked severe combined immunodeficiency. *Genomics* 23:62–68.
23. Dhabhar FS, Miller AH, McEwen BS, et al. 1995. Effects of stress on immune cell distribution: dynamics and hormonal mechanisms. *J Immunol* 154:5511–5527.
24. DiBartola SP, Benson MD, Dwulet FE, et al. 1985. Isolation and characterization of amyloid protein AA in the Abyssinian cat. *Lab Invest* 52:485–489.
25. DiBartola SP, Tarr MJ, Benson MD. 1986. Tissue distribution of amyloid deposits in Abyssinian cats with familial amyloidosis. *J Comp Pathol* 96:387–398.
26. DiBartola SP, Tarr MJ, Webb DM, Giger U. 1990. Familial renal amyloidosis in Chinese Shar Pei dogs. *J Vet Med Assoc* 197:483–487.
27. Dougherty SA, Center SA, Shaw EE, et al. 1991. Juvenile-onset polyarthritis syndrome in Akita. *J Am Vet Med Assoc* 198:849–856.
28. Dowling PM. 1995. Immunosuppressive drug therapy. *Can Vet J* 36: 781–783.
29. Edwards DF, Patton CS, Kennedy JR. 1992. Primary ciliary dyskinesia in the dog. *Probl Vet Med* 4:291–319.
30. Farrow BRH, Watson ADJ, Hartley WJ. 1972. Pneumocystis pneumonia in the dog. *J Comp Pathol* 82:447–453.
31. Felsburg PJ. 1994. Overview of the immune system and immunodeficiency disease. *Vet Clin North Am* 24:629–653.
32. Felsburg PJ, Glickman LT, Jezyk PF. 1985. Selective IgA deficiency in the dog. *Clin Immunol Immunopathol* 36:297–305.
32a. Felsburg PJ, Somberg RL, Hartnett BJ, et al. 1997. Full immunologic reconstitution following nonconditioned bone marrow transplantation for canine X-linked severe combined immunodeficiency. *Blood* 90:3214–3221.
33. Felsburg PJ, Somberg RL, Krakowka GS. 1994. Acute monocytic leukemia in a dog with X-linked severe combined immunodeficiency. *Clin Diagn Lab Immunol* 1:379–384.
34. Felsburg PJ, Somberg RL, Perryman LE. 1992. Domestic animal models of severe combined immunodeficiency: X-linked severe combined immunodeficiency in the dog and severe combined immunodeficiency in the horse. *Immunodeficiency Rev* 3:277–303.
35. Foodman MS, Giger U, Stebbins K, Knight D. 1989. Kartagener's syndrome in an old miniature Poodle. *J Small Anim Pract* 30:96–100.
36. Fyfe JC, Giger U, Hall CA, et al. 1990. Inherited selective intestinal cobalamin malabsorption and cobalamin deficiency in dogs. *Pediatr Res* 29:24–31.
37. Fyfe JC, Jezyk PF, Giger U, et al. 1989. Inherited selective malabsorption of vitamin B12 in giant Schnauzers. *J Am Anim Hosp Assoc* 25:533–539.
38. Gershwin LJ. 1992. Immunologic assessment of the small animal patient, pp 441–448. *In* Kirk RW (ed), Current veterinary therapy XI. WB Saunders, Philadelphia, PA.
39. Giger U. 1994. Primäre Immundefekte beim Kleintier. *Kleintierpraxis* 39:433–438.
40. Giger U, Boxer LA, Simpson PJ, et al. 1987. Deficiency of leukocyte surface glycoproteins Mo1, LFA-1 and Leu M5 in a dog with recurrent bacterial infections: an animal model. *Blood* 69:1622–1630.
41. Giger U, Felsburg PJ. 1997. Immunodeficiency disorders, pp 779–785. *In* Morgan R (ed), Handbook of small animal medicine. Churchill Livingstone, New York, NY.
42. Glickman LT, Shofer FS, Payton AJ, et al. 1988. Survey of serum IgA, IgG and IgM concentrations in a large Beagle population in which IgA deficiency had been identified. *Am J Vet Res* 49:1240–1245.
43. Greeley EH, Kealy RD, Ballam JM, et al. 1996. The influence of age on the canine immune system. *Vet Immunol Immunopathol* 55:1–10.
44. Greene CE. 1990. Immunodeficiency and infectious disease, pp 55–63. *In* Greene CE (ed), Infectious diseases of the dog and cat. WB Saunders, Philadelphia, PA.
44a. Greene CE. 1997. Unpublished observations. University of Georgia, Athens, GA.
45. Hansen P, Clercx C, Henroeaux M, et al. 1995. Neutrophil phagocyte dysfunction in a Weimaraner with recurrent infections. *J Small Anim Pract* 36:128–131.
46. Harats N, DiBartola SP, Benson MD, et al. 1991. Abyssinian cat model of AA amyloidosis: SAA gene analysis, pp 32–35. *In* Natvig JB (ed), Amyloid and amyloidosis. Kluwer, Dordrecht, the Netherlands.
47. Henthorn PS, Somberg RL, Fimiani VM, et al. 1994. IL-2R gamma gene microdeletion demonstrates that canine X-linked severe combined immunodeficiency is a homologue of the human disease. *Genomics* 23:69–74.
48. Hirsch VM, Cunningham TA. 1984. Hereditary anomaly of neutrophils granulation in Birman cats. *Am J Vet Res* 45:2170–2174.
49. Hoffmann-Fezer G, Mortelbauer W, Mysliwietz J, et al. 1996. Comparison of T-cell subpopulations in cats naturally infected with feline leukaemia virus or feline immunodeficiency virus. *Res Vet Sci* 61:222–226.
50. Houston DM, Clark EG, Matwichuk CL, et al. 1993. A case of cutaneous sterile pyogranuloma/granuloma syndrome in a Golden retriever. *Can Vet J* 34:121–122.
51. Jezyk PF, Felsburg PJ, Haskins ME, Patterson DF. 1989. X-linked severe combined immunodeficiency in the dog. *Clin Immunol Immunopathol* 52:173–189.
52. Jezyk PF, Haskins ME, MacKay-Smith WE, Patterson DF. 1986. Lethal acrodermatitis in Bull terriers. *J Am Vet Med Assoc* 188:833–839.
53. Johnson KH, Sletten K, Hayden DW, et al. 1995. AA amyloidosis in Chinese Shar pei dogs: immunohistochemical and amino acid sequence analyses. *Int J Exp Clin Invest* 2:92–99.
54. Jones JB, Lange RD. 1983. Cyclic hematopoiesis: animal models. *Exp Hematol* 11:573–580.
55. Kramer JW, Davis WC, Prieur DJ. 1977. The Chediak-Higashi syndrome in cats. *Lab Invest* 36:554–562.
56. Lafrado LJ, Dezzutti CS, Lewis MG, et al. 1989. Immunodeficiency in latent feline leukemia virus infections. *Vet Immunol Immunopathol* 21:39–46.
57. Latimer KS, Prasse KW. 1982. Neutrophilic movement of a Basenji with Pelger-Huet anomaly. *Am J Vet Res* 43:525–527.
58. Latimer KS, Rakich PM, Thompson DF. 1985. Pelger-Huet anomaly in cats. *Vet Pathol* 22:370–374.
59. Leisewitz AL, Spencer JA, Jacobson LS, et al. 1997. Suspected primary immunodeficiency syndrome in three related Irish wolfhounds. *J Small Anim Pract* 38:209–212.
59a. Loeven KO. 1994. Hepatic presentations of familial amyloidosis in two Chinese Shar-pei dogs. *J Am Vet Med Assoc* 204:1212–1216.
60. Loeven KO. 1994. Spontaneous hepatic rupture secondary to amyloidosis in a Chinese Shar-pei. *J Am Anim Hosp Assoc* 30:577–579.
61. Lothrop C. 1997. Unpublished results. Auburn University, Auburn, AL.
62. Lutz H, Castelli I, Ehrensperger F, et al. 1995. Panleukopenia-like syndrome of FeLV caused by co-infection with FeLV and feline panleukopenia virus. *Vet Immunol Immunopathol* 46:21–33.
63. Mancianti F, Giannelli C, Bendinelli M, et al. 1992. Mycological findings in feline immunodeficiency virus-infected cats. *J Med Vet Mycol* 30:257–259.
64. May C, Hammill J, Bennett D. 1992. Chinese Shar pei fever syndrome: a preliminary report. *Vet Rec* 131:586–587.
64a. Miller E. 1997. Immunosuppression—an overview. *Semin Vet Med Surg* 12:144–149.
65. Miller WH. 1991. Deep pyoderma in two German shepherd dogs associated with a cell mediated immunodeficiency. *J Am Anim Hosp Assoc* 27:513–517.
66. Modiano JF, Getzy DM, Akol KG, et al. 1995. Retrovirus-like activity in an immunosuppressed dog: pathological and immunological findings. *J Comp Pathol* 112:165–183.
67. Moroff SD, Hurvitz AI, Peterson ME, et al. 1986. IgA deficiency in Sharpei dogs. *Vet Immunol Immunopathol* 13:181–188.
68. Otto CM, Brown CA, Lindl PA, et al. 1993. Delayed hypersensitivity testing as a clinical measure of cell-mediated immunity in the cat. *Vet Immunol Immunopathol* 38:91–102.
69. Outerbridge CA, Myers SL, Giger U. 1996. Hereditary cobalamin defi-

ciency in Border Collie dogs, p 751. *In* Proceedings of the American College of Veterinary Internal Medicine, San Antonio, TX.
69a. Papendick RE, Munson L, O'Brien TD, et al. 1997. Systemic AA-amyloidosis in captive cheetahs *(Acinonyx jubatus)*. *Vet Pathol* 34:549–556.
70. Perk K, Safran N, Dahlberg JE. 1992. Propagation and characterization of novel canine lentivirus isolated from a dog. *Leukemia* 6(Suppl 3):155S–157S.
70a. Pullen RP, Somberg RC, Felsburg PJ, et al. 1997. X-linked severe combined immunodeficiency in a family of Cardigan Welsh corgis. *J Am Anim Hosp Assoc* 33:494–499.
71. Renshaw HW, Davis WC. 1979. Canine granulopathy syndrome: an inherited disorder of leukocyte function. *Am J Pathol* 95:731–744.
72. Reubel GH, Dean GA, George JW, et al. 1994. Effects of incidental infections and immune activation on disease progression in experimentally feline immunodeficiency virus-infected cats. *J Acquir Immune Defic Syndr* 7:1003–1015.
73. Reubel GH, George JW, Higgins J, et al. 1994. Effect of chronic feline immunodeficiency virus infection on experimental feline calicivirus-induced disease. *Vet Microbiol* 39:335–351.
74. Rivas AL, Tintle L, Argentieri D, et al. 1995. A primary immunodeficiency syndrome in Shar-pei dogs. *Clin Immunol Immunopathol* 74:243–251.
75. Rivas AL, Tintle L, Kimball E, et al. 1992. A canine febrile disorder associated with elevated interleukin-6 (IL-6). *Clin Immunol Immunopathol* 64:36–45.
76. Rivas AL, Tintle L, Meyers-Wallen V, et al. 1993. Inheritance of renal amyloidosis in Chinese Shar-pei dogs. *J Hered* 84:438–442.
77. Rosser EJ. 1997. German shepherd dog pyoderma: a prospective study of 12 dogs. *J Am Anim Hosp Assoc* 33:355–363.
78. Roth JA, Kaeberle ML, Grier RL, et al. 1984. Improvement in clinical condition and thymus morphologic features associated with growth hormone treatment of immunodeficient dwarf dogs. *Am J Vet Res* 45:1151–1155.
79. Roth JA, Lamox LG, Altszuler, et al. 1980. Thymic abnormalities and growth hormone deficiency in dogs. *Am J Vet Res* 41:1256–1262.
79a. Schulze C, Brugmann M, Boer M, et al. 1998. Generalized AA-amyloidosis in Siberian tigers *(Panthera tigris altaica)* with predominant renal medullary amyloid retention. *Vet Pathol* 35:70–74.
80. Sellon RK, Levy JK, Jordan HL, et al. 1996. Changes in lymphocyte subsets with age in perinatal cats: late gestation through eight weeks. *Vet Immunol Immunopathol* 53:105–113.
81. Shofer FS, Glickman L, Payton AJ, et al. 1990. Influence of parental serum immunoglobulins on morbidity and mortality of Beagles and their offspring. *Am J Vet Res* 51:239–243.
82. Snyder PW, Kazacos EA, Felsburg PJ. 1993. Histologic characterization of the thymus in canine X-linked severe combined immunodeficiency. *Clin Immunol Immunopathol* 67:55–67.
83. Somberg RL, Pullen RP, Casal ML, et al. 1995. A single nucleotide insertion in the canine interleukin-2 receptor gamma chain results in X-linked severe combined immunodeficiency disease. *Vet Immunol Immunopathol* 47:203–213.
84. Somberg RL, Robinson JP, Felsburg PJ. 1994. T lymphocyte development and function in dogs with X-linked severe combined immunodeficiency. *J Immunol* 153:4006–4015.
85. Somberg RL, Tipold A, Hartnett BJ, et al. 1996. Postnatal development of T cells in dogs with X-linked severe combined immunodeficiency. *J Immunol* 156:1431–1435.
86. Squires RA, Gorman NT, Onions DE. 1989. Endogenous retroviral elements in the canine genome (abstract 60), p 127. *In* Proceedings of the 7th Annual Meeting of the American College of Veterinary Internal Medicine, San Diego, CA.
87. Squires RA, Gorman NT, Padua RA. 1989. Defective endogenous retroviral elements in a canine lymphosarcoma cell line (abstract 9), p 127. *In* Proceedings of the 7th Annual Meeting of the American College of Veterinary Internal Medicine, San Diego, CA.
88. Studdert VP, Phillips WA, Studdert MJ, et al. 1984. Recurrent and persistent infections in related Weimeraner dogs. *Aust Vet J* 61:261–263.
89. Torten M, Franchini M, Barlough JE, et al. 1991. Progressive immune dysfunction in cats experimentally infected with feline immunodeficiency virus. *J Virol* 65:2225–2230.
90. Trautwein G, Hewicker-Trautwein M. 1994. Immunopathogenesis of viral diseases in cats and dogs. *Tierarztl Prax* 22:63–72.
91. Trowald-Wigh G, Hakansson L, Johannisson A, et al. 1992. Leucocyte adhesion protein deficiency in Irish setter dogs. *Vet Immunol Immunopathol* 32:261–280.
92. Trowald-Wigh G, Johannisson A, Hakansson L. 1993. Canine neutrophil adhesion proteins and Fc-receptors in healthy dogs and dogs with adhesion protein deficiency, as studied by flow cytometry. *Vet Immunol Immunopathol* 38:297–310.
93. Van der Linde-Sipman JS, Niewold TA, Tooten PCJ, et al. 1997. Generalized AA-amyloidosis in Siamese and oriental cats. *Vet Immunol Immunopathol* 56:1–10.
94. Weiss RC. 1992. Immunologic responses in healthy random-source cats fed N, N-dimethylglycine-supplemented diets. *Am J Vet Res* 53:829–833.
95. Weiss RC, Cox NR. 1989. Evaluation of immunity to feline infectious peritonitis in cats with cutaneous viral-induced delayed hypersensitivity. *Vet Immunol Immunopathol* 21:293–301.
96. Whitbread TJ, Batt RM, Garthwaite G. 1984. Relative deficiency of serum IgA in the German shepherd dog: a breed abnormality. *Res Vet Sci* 37:350–352.
97. Winkelstein JA, Cork LC, Griffin DE. 1981. Genetically determined deficiency of the third component of complement in the dog. *Science* 212:1169–1170.
98. Winkelstein JA, Johnson JP, Swift AJ, et al. 1982. Genetically determined deficiency of the third component of complement in the dog: in vitro studies of the complement system and complement-mediated serum activities. *J Immunol* 129:2598–2602.
99. Wisselink MA, Bernadina WE, Willense A, et al. 1988. Immunologic aspects of German Shepherd dog pyoderma (GSP). *Vet Immunol Immunopathol* 19:67–77.
100. Zaccaro L, Falcone ML, Silva S, et al. 1995. Defective natural killer cell cytotoxic activity in feline immunodeficiency virus-infected cats. *AIDS Res Hum Retroviruses* 11:747–752.

Chapter **96**

Fever

John K. Dunn and Craig E. Greene

Fever is a common presenting sign of many infectious, metabolic, immune-mediated, and neoplastic disease processes. In general practice, most fevers are due to transient viral or bacterial infections, which resolve spontaneously or respond to appropriate therapy. In referral centers, however, a much higher percentage of cases presenting with unresolved febrile episodes are associated with immune-mediated disorders or neoplasia (see Fever of Unknown Origin later).

PATHOPHYSIOLOGY

Normal body temperature is determined by the set-point of the thermoregulatory center located in the preoptic region of the rostral hypothalamus. The thermoregulatory center consists of two subcenters; a rostral (parasympathetic) heat loss center and a caudal (sympathetic) heat production center.

The sensory arm of the thermoregulatory reflex consists of peripheral neural thermoreceptors located in the skin; internal receptors are also present in the abdomen and CNS (hypothalamus and spinal cord).

A delicate equilibrium exists between the body's heat production and heat loss mechanisms. Physiologic and behavior effector mechanisms ensure that the core body temperature of dogs and cats fluctuates less than 2°C over a 24-hour period. Body heat is lost to the environment through alter-

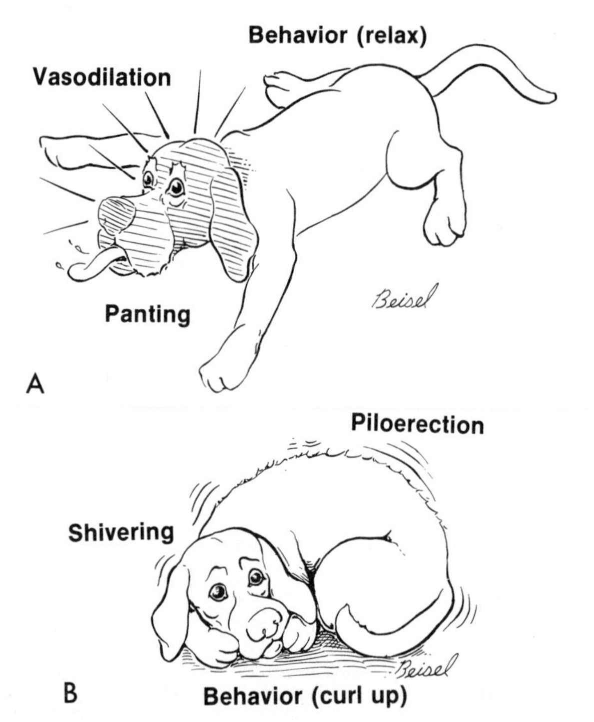

Figure 96–1. Behavioral mechanisms of decreasing body temperature (*A*) and increasing body temperature (*B*).

ations in conduction, convection, and radiation. Excess heat is dissipated through the skin (primarily cutaneous vasodilation because dogs and cats do not sweat) and via the respiratory tract (panting) (Fig. 96–1*A*). Behavioral means of lowering body temperature include seeking shelter and remaining inactive. Heat can be gained from the environment by heat transfer and metabolically through increased muscle activity (shivering) and catabolism of body fat. Body heat may be further conserved by cutaneous vasoconstriction, piloerection, and postural alterations (curling up) (Fig. 96–1*B*).

Fever occurs when the hypothalamic set-point is raised. Endogenous heat production increases, but the balance between heat gain and heat loss is nevertheless maintained (compare Figs. 96–2*A* and 96–2*B*). Numerous infectious and noninfectious agents (exogenous pyrogens) elicit a febrile response by inducing the synthesis and release of a number of low-molecular-weight peptide mediators known as endogenous pyrogens. The list of exogenous pyrogens is extensive. It includes gram-negative and gram-positive bacteria, bacterial endotoxins (lipopolysaccharides), viruses, fungi, parasites, bile acids, toxins, certain tumors, and drugs. Endogenous pyrogens are produced by circulating monocytes and fixed mononuclear phagocytes (e.g., Kupffer's cells, splenic and alveolar macrophages), activated lymphocytes, and polymorphonuclear cells.

Several immunologic mediators released by endotoxin-activated macrophages can be classified as endogenous pyrogens. These include interleukin (IL)-1, tumor necrosis factor (TNF), interferon, and platelet-activating factor (PAF). Numerous chemical mediators—for example, prostaglandins (PGs), cyclic AMP, 5-hydroxytryptamine, and norepinephrine—may also contribute to fever. The mechanism by which endogenous pyrogens increase the hypothalamic set-point is uncertain. TNF is known to elicit the production and release of other cytokines and PGE_2 precursors, which are themselves capable of inducing a febrile response. Although IL-1 and TNF are structurally distinct, IL-1 has many of the same biologic properties as TNF; both IL-1 and TNF are involved in the generation of the acute-phase response and may be directly responsible for the anorexia and depression usually associated with fever. Some tumor cells release endogenous pyrogen without prior stimulation by an exogenous agent. The pathogenesis of fever is summarized in Figure 96–3.

Hyperthermia

True fever should be differentiated from hyperthermia in which the hypothalamic set-point is not altered (see Fig. 96–2C). Under normal circumstances, the effects of exercise or excitement on body temperature are usually insignificant, and increases of more than 1.0°C to 1.5°C [4.5°F] are unusual. Dehydration may raise body temperature, but any increase is usually mild and corrected by rehydration. Body temperature may increase transiently and then decrease below normal after a meal. More severe and possibly life-threatening increases in body temperature may occur if dissipation of the excess heat is inadequate. Causes of hyperthermia are listed in Table 96–1.

Hyperthermia, unlike fever, requires prompt and aggressive emergency treatment in the form of total body cooling to prevent irreversible damage to vital organs. A variety of methods can be used, including hosing with cold water, ice bath, cold water enema, cold water gastric lavage, and alcohol bath, and the use of fans to increase ventilation.

Adverse and Beneficial Effects

Fever is usually associated with nonspecific signs of depression, anorexia, and generalized stiffness. Heart rate increases and mild tachypnea may become evident. Experimentally, pyrogens initially cause increased thirst and water diuresis in dogs. Thereafter, with sustained fever, the thirst center becomes more refractory to osmotic stimuli, and the affected animal stops drinking and becomes severely dehydrated. Extremely high body temperatures (e.g., those associated with heat stroke) may lead to disseminated intravascular coagulation and irreversible damage to the CNS. Because it is not under thermoregulatory control, hyperthermia, and not true fever, is usually associated with these higher (>41°C [106°F]) body temperatures.

Firm evidence supports the view that fever represents a protective adaptation to the effects of infection. Animals with experimentally induced sepsis have a higher mortality rate if they do not develop a febrile response.[9] Many endogenous

Table 96–1. Causes of Hyperthermia

Impaired Heat Loss
Exposure to high ambient temperatures in a closed, poorly ventilated environment (heat stroke)
Strenuous exercise especially if concurrent respiratory embarrassment (e.g., if animal is brachycephalic or has laryngeal paralysis)
Hypermetabolic Disorders
Malignant hyperthermia
Hyperthyroidism
Pheochromocytoma
Increased Muscle Activity
Tetanus
Seizure activity
Miscellaneous Causes
Hypothalamic tumor
Certain drugs (phenothiazines, cholinergics)

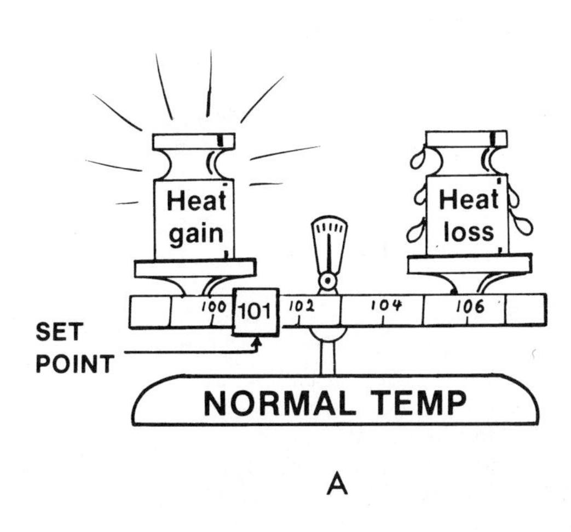

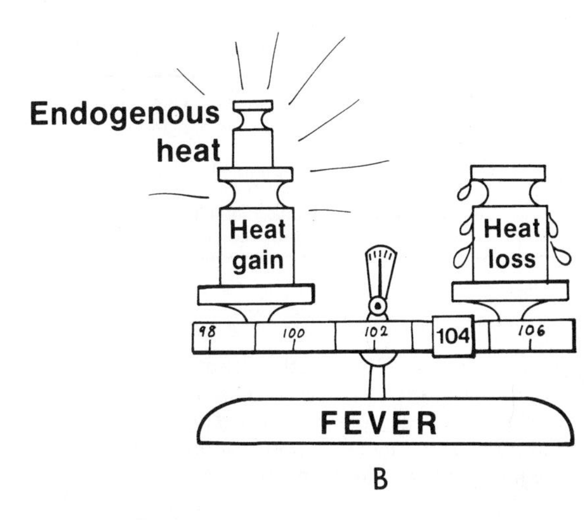

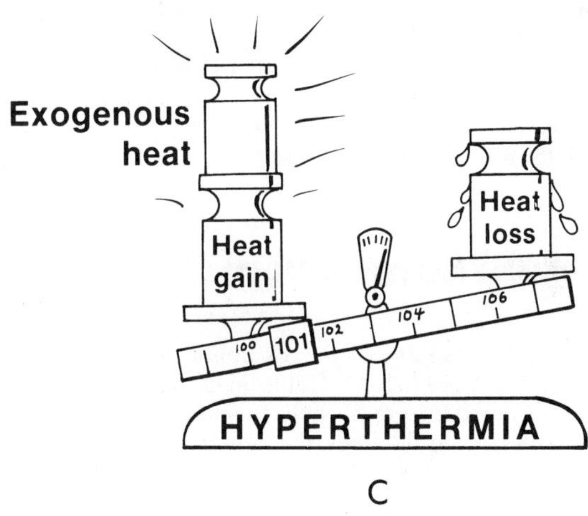

Figure 96–2. *A,* Temperature regulation in the normal animal showing a thermal set-point of 38.3°C (101°F) with balanced heat gain and heat loss mechanisms. *B,* Mechanism of fever involves a rise in set-point to 40°C (104°F), which increases endogenous heat production and conservation while maintaining a balance between heat gain and heat loss. *C,* Mechanism of hyperthermia, in contrast to that of fever, involves an increase in heat load on a normal set-point. Increased heat gain can be from exogenous (environmental) or endogenous (muscle activity) sources.

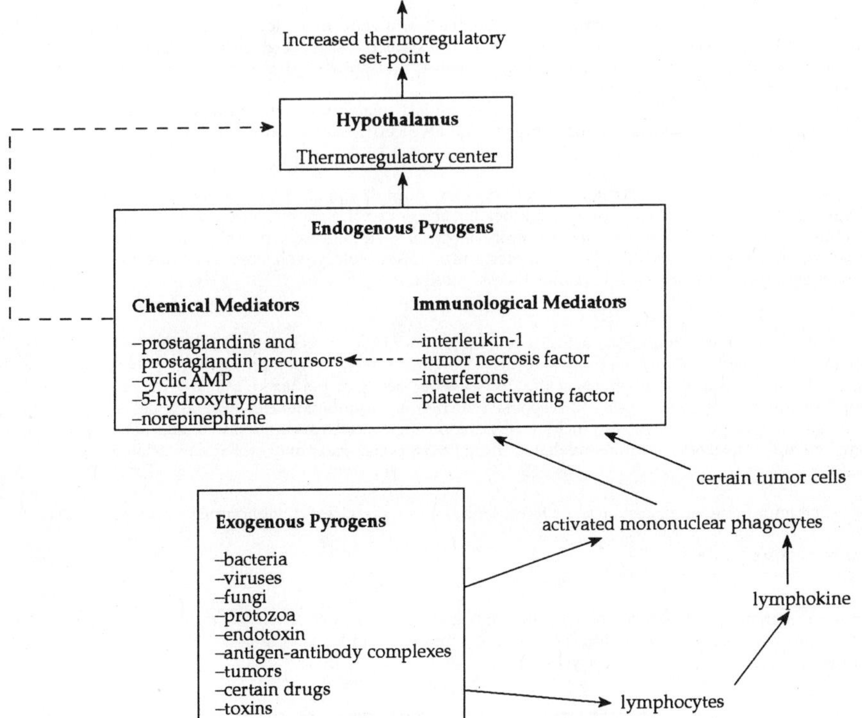

Figure 96–3. Pathogenesis of fever. (AMP = adenosine monophosphate.)

Table 96–2. Criteria Used to Define Fever of Unknown Origin[a]

1. Prolonged fever of more than 3 weeks duration associated with vague nonspecific signs of illness such as lethargy, weight loss, and anorexia
2. Temperature more than 1.5°F (0.8°C) above normal on several occasions
3. Diagnosis uncertain after 1 week of hospitalization involving repeated physical examinations and routine laboratory tests

[a]Established for humans.

pyrogens increase granulocyte function and mobility. Both IL-1 and TNF, for example, activate T cells and enhance T-cell responses during antigen presentation. The sequestration of iron by mononuclear phagocytes and resultant decrease in plasma iron concentration are features of the acute-phase response. This decrease in available iron is thought to play an important role by inhibiting microbial growth. It appears, therefore, that the beneficial effects of fever outweigh the adverse effects and a strong argument exists for allowing moderate fevers to run their course. When specific antimicrobial therapy is available, monitoring rectal temperature can be used to determine treatment efficacy.

FEVER OF UNKNOWN ORIGIN

The criteria in human medicine to define fevers of unknown origin (FUOs) are listed in Table 96–2. Although these criteria may not be strictly applicable to small animal medicine, they are helpful guidelines that eliminate short-lived fevers associated with infections, postoperative fevers, and other nonpyrogenic causes of hyperthermia such as heat stroke. Undiagnosed fever can be classified as intermittent or sustained. Bacterial infections, particularly those that result in bacteremia, are more often associated with intermittent temperature "spikes" with interspersed periods of normal temperature.

Etiology

FUO presents a considerable diagnostic challenge. Many unexplained fevers are due to early atypical manifestations of what are often relatively common diseases. Most diagnoses are made because new clinical or clinicopathologic abnormalities develop. Many cases, therefore, require repeated physical examinations and ancillary testing.

The list of differential diagnoses for FUO, in the absence of localizing signs of disease, is extensive. The major causes of FUO can be categorized into four groups (Table 96–3): systemic and localized infections, immune-mediated disorders, neoplasia, and miscellaneous disorders. Immunodeficiency syndromes are discussed in Chapter 95 (Table 95–3).

A retrospective survey of dogs with FUO was performed at the Cambridge Veterinary School.[6a] The distribution of these cases was as follows: 16% infections, 26% immune-mediated disorders (mostly polyarthropathies), 23% primary bone marrow disorders (including myeloproliferative disorders, lymphoproliferative disorders, and myelodysplastic syndromes), 10% solid neoplasms, 8% miscellaneous, and 17% undiagnosed cases (i.e., considered to be true FUO). The most common causes of FUO in the dog and cat are discussed next.

Table 96–3. Conditions Associated With Fevers of Unknown Origin

ANIMAL	CONDITION
Systemic Infections	
Dogs	Bacterial endocarditis, bacteremias from an inapparent focus (e.g., secondary to persistent neutropenia or a congenital/acquired immunodeficiency syndrome); Lyme borreliosis (acute); leptospirosis; brucellosis infection; mycobacterial infections; rickettsial disease (e.g., ehrlichiosis, RMSF, haemobartonellosis); protozoal infections (e.g., babesiosis, leishmaniasis, disseminated toxoplasmosis, neosporosis); disseminated mycotic infections (e.g., histoplasmosis, blastomycosis, cryptococcosis, coccidioidomycosis, aspergillosis)
Cats	FIV infection; FeLV infection; feline infectious anemia *(Haemobartonella felis);* feline infectious peritonitis; bacteremias from an inapparent focus (see opposite); systemic mycoses (e.g., histoplasmosis, cryptococcosis); mycobacterial infections (often atypical); atypical calicivirus infection
Localized Infections	
Dogs	Bacterial endocarditis; urogenital infections (e.g., pyelonephritis, chronic prostatitis/prostatic abscess, stump pyometra); pyothorax and lung infections (e.g., inhaled pulmonary foreign bodies/pulmonary abscess, bronchopneumonia); occult hepatic abscess or cholangitis; localized peritonitis; diskospondylitis; juvenile metaphyseal osteomyelitis; retrobulbar or tooth root abscess; oropharyngeal stick injuries, septic thrombi
Cats	Pyothorax and lung infections (e.g., pulmonary abscess, bronchopneumonia), upper respiratory infections; occult hepatic abscess or cholangiohepatitis; urogenital infections (e.g., pyelonephritis); localized peritonitis; osteomyelitis; cat bite abscess/cellulitis
Immune-Mediated Diseases	
Dogs	Systemic lupus erythematosus. Immune-mediated polyarthropathies: rheumatoid arthritis (erosive); nonerosive, nonseptic polyarthritis Idiopathic; polyarthritis-meningitis complex (Weimaraner, Newfoundland, German shorthaired pointer, boxer, beagle); polyarthritis-polymyositis complex (spaniel breeds); polyarthritis of Akitas; polyarthritis and amyloidosis of the Chinese Shar pei (Shar pei hock); polyarteritis nodosa Autoimmune hemolytic anemia and immune-mediated thrombocytopenia; steroid-responsive meningitis; immunodeficiency syndromes
Cats	Systemic lupus erythematosus (rare in cats); chronic progressive polyarthropathy, includes the ankylosing (periosteal proliferative) and luxating (erosive) forms; autoimmune hemolytic anemia (rare; may be FeLV associated); immune-mediated thrombocytopenia (rare; may be FeLV associated)
Neoplasia	
Dogs	Solid neoplasms (especially those that are necrotic, elicit an inflammatory response, or have widespread metastases); lymphoproliferative or myeloproliferative disease
Cats	FeLV-related lymphoproliferative and myeloproliferative disorders
Miscellaneous Disorders	
Dogs	Metaphyseal osteopathy, panosteitis; inflammatory-granulomatous bowel disease; liver disease (e.g., hepatic necrosis, cirrhosis, portosystemic shunts); pulmonary emboli; nodular panniculitis; drug reactions (tetracyclines, penicillin, sulfonamides, amphotericin B, quinidine)
Cats	Pansteatitis (cats on fish-rich diets); hypervitaminosis A; drug reactions (e.g., tetracycline, levamisole)
Immunodeficiencies (see Chapter 95 and Tables 95–3 and 95–4)	

RMSF = Rocky Mountain spotted fever; FIV = feline immunodeficiency virus; FeLV = feline leukemia virus.

Bacterial Infections

Bacterial Endocarditis. Although a common cause of FUO in the dog, it appears to be rare in the cat (see also Chapter 87). Vegetative lesions form on the valve cusps (the mitral valve or less frequently the aortic valve) or mural endocardium and thromboembolic spread of infection throughout the body and bacteremia (see later) are common sequelae. Immune complexes may be deposited in the joints and glomeruli. Affected animals are usually depressed and anorexic. Immune-mediated polyarthritis may manifest as a vague shifting lameness or generalized stiffness. A cardiac murmur may be present, although this may develop later in the course of the disease.

Bacteremias From an Inapparent Focus. Bacteremia may occur in association with primary or secondary immunodeficiency syndromes, lymphoproliferative or myeloproliferative disorders, aplastic anemias (e.g., chronic ehrlichiosis and hyperestrogenism), or other causes of bone marrow suppression resulting in persistent neutropenia. For example, the myelodysplastic effects of feline leukemia virus (FeLV) predispose infected cats to recurrent bacterial infections. The presence of intermittent fever in association with a neutrophilic leukocytosis (with or without a left shift), monocytosis, hypoalbuminemia, hypoglycemia, and increased alkaline phosphatase (ALP) activity (or various combinations of these clinicopathologic abnormalities) is suggestive of bacteremia (see Chapter 87).[2, 3]

Localized Urogenital or Respiratory Infections. In dogs, FUO may be associated with localized urogenital infections (e.g., stump pyometra, prostatic abscess, and pyelonephritis). Early cases of pyothorax, pulmonary abscess, or inhaled pulmonary (bronchial) foreign bodies may occur without obvious respiratory signs.

Diskospondylitis. Bacterial infection of one or more intervertebral spaces results in stiffness and a focal area of pain over the affected discs. Some animals with diskospondylitis may have neurologic deficits. Large-breed dogs appear to be more susceptible, and the lumbosacral disc space is most commonly involved. *Staphylococcus aureus*, coliforms, and *Brucella canis* are the organisms most frequently isolated from the lesions (see Chapter 86).

***Borrelia burgdorferi* Infection (Lyme Borreliosis).** Infection with the tick-borne spirochete *Borrelia burgdorferi* may be associated with fever, especially in young dogs. Polyarthritis resulting in lameness is a common manifestation of this disease (see Chapter 45).

Viral Infections

Most of the common viral diseases of the dog and cat induce fever during the peracute or acute phases of infection. Most of these infections are associated with other clinical signs that help to establish a diagnosis. Some cases of feline infectious peritonitis (FIP), particularly the "dry" (noneffusive) form, have few clinical signs other than fever, anorexia, and depression.

The classic signs of *feline calicivirus* infection are oral ulceration, conjunctivitis, and rhinitis. In some cases, these signs may be absent and the animal may show fever and lameness, making diagnosis difficult. Some kittens may develop similar signs 5 to 7 days after they are vaccinated with modified live calicivirus for the first time (see Chapters 16 and 100). These signs are usually transient, however, lasting no more than a few days.

The immunosuppressive effects of FeLV or feline immunodeficiency virus (FIV) predispose the affected animal to recurrent infections (chronic gingivitis, recurrent abscess formation, viral respiratory infection, feline infectious anemia, and FIP), all of which may be associated with fever. The direct myelodysplastic effects of FeLV on the bone marrow may result in persistent or, less frequently, cyclic neutropenia, which also predisposes the animal to recurrent infections.

Fungal Infections

Systemic mycotic infections such as blastomycosis, histoplasmosis, cryptococcosis, and coccidioidomycosis follow a prolonged course, and fever is often associated with marked weight loss. Many body systems, including the skin, joints, bones, and eyes, may be affected. Dogs with nasal aspergillosis, especially with extensive turbinate destruction and severe concurrent bacterial infection, may have intermittent pyrexia.

Protozoal Infections

Fever is an uncommon feature of *Toxoplasma gondii* infection in dogs and cats. Clinical signs are variable and may be quite vague and nonspecific. The organism may infect the CNS, eyes (chorioretinitis), and muscle (see Chapter 80).

A similar protozoal infection caused by *Neospora caninum* has been described in the dog. Although clinical signs may be similar, affected animals often have an acute onset of hind limb paresis or paralysis (see Chapter 80).

Visceral leishmaniasis in the dog is a chronic, debilitating disease characterized by weight loss, enlargement of the liver and spleen, and polyarthritis. Cutaneous involvement may be associated with generalized enlargement of peripheral lymph nodes. The causative organism, *Leishmania donovani*, is transmitted by sand flies. The disease may remain latent for as long as 5 years (see Chapter 73).

Babesia canis is a tick-borne protozoan parasite of dogs. The organism infects red blood cells, resulting in intravascular hemolysis, icterus, and hemoglobinuria (see Chapter 77).

Rickettsial Infections

The rickettsial organism *Ehrlichia canis* is transmitted by the brown dog tick, *Rhipicephalus sanguineus*. The chronic phase of the disease is characterized by severe bone marrow suppression and pancytopenia. Affected dogs have a tendency to bleed and are susceptible to recurrent sepsis (Chapter 28).

Haemobartonellosis occurs in dogs and cats. In the cat, *Haemobartonella felis* infection is also referred to as feline infectious anemia. Fever is a common feature of the acute parasitemic phase of the disease. *H. canis* infection occurs most frequently in splenectomized dogs or as a result of prolonged immunosuppression (see Chapter 30).

The infectious agent that is responsible for Rocky Mountain spotted fever (RMSF; tick fever), *Rickettsia rickettsii*, is transmitted from rodents by a number of ticks. Clinical signs include fever, lethargy, anorexia, oculonasal discharge, lymphadenomegaly, splenomegaly, and thrombocytopenia (see Chapter 29).

Immune-Mediated Disease

Immune-Mediated Polyarthritis. Fever is a common clinical sign of a spectrum of canine immune-mediated polyarthropathies, including rheumatoid arthritis and idiopathic (nonerosive nonseptic) polyarthritis. Antigen-antibody complexes deposited in the synovial membrane activate complement, leading to the release of a number of potent inflammatory mediators. Endogenous pyrogen is released by activated macrophages and neutrophils attracted to the sites of immune complex deposition. Polyarthritis may occur as a manifestation of systemic lupus erythematosus and several other immune-mediated syndromes (e.g., polyarthritis-polymyositis syndrome, polyarthritis-meningitis syndrome, and polyarteritis nodosa) (see Table 96–3). Erosive and nonerosive (periosteal proliferative) forms of polyarthritis occur in the cat; both forms may be associated with feline syncytium virus infection (see Chapter 17). Clinical signs include periarticular swelling and pain on manipulation of the joints.

Immune-Mediated Hemolytic Anemia and Thrombocytopenia. Fever may be associated with the release of RBC pyrogens into circulation and activation of splenic and hepatic macrophages. The immune-mediated destruction of platelets may also induce a febrile response.

Immunodeficiency Syndromes. Immunodeficiency may be either primary (hereditary) or secondary (acquired) (see Chapter 95). Primary immunodeficiency should be suspected if a young animal has a history of recurrent bacterial infections, especially if the infections involve organisms of relatively low virulence, and/or if the infections become refractory to conventional antimicrobial therapy. The infections most frequently involve the skin and urinary and GI tracts, and affected animals often have a marked neutrophilia with or without a left shift. Similar infections in littermates or previous litters or evidence of a concurrent immune-mediated disorder may further increase the index of suspicion.

A number of primary immunodeficiency syndromes have been recognized in the dog; many of these occur in certain breeds (see Table 95–3). They may affect nonspecific immunity (e.g., neutrophil function and mucosal barrier function) or specific components of the immune system (humoral immunity, cellular immunity, complement function).

Acquired immunodeficiency may occur secondary to infection (e.g., generalized demodicosis, certain fungal infections, and protracted bacterial infections), drugs (cyclophosphamide, doxorubicin [Adriamycin], glucocorticoids, estrogens), toxins, nutritional factors, stress, endocrine abnormalities (e.g., hyperadrenocorticism and diabetes mellitus), or other systemic diseases.

Neoplasia

The interaction of tumor-related antigens with sensitized lymphocytes results in the release of soluble lymphokines, which stimulate the production of endogenous pyrogen by macrophages and granulocytes. Solid tumors may be associated with a febrile response, particularly if they become necrotic, elicit an inflammatory response, or have widespread metastases (e.g., metastatic carcinomas). Tumors involving the lungs, stomach, liver, gallbladder, kidneys, and bone are more frequently associated with fever and are often hard to localize. Fever is also a common sign of myeloproliferative or lymphoproliferative disorders. Affected animals may have defective humoral and/or cellular immune function. The proliferation of neoplastic cells in the bone marrow may lead to persistent neutropenia and predisposition to recurrent infections. Some tumor cells release endogenous pyrogen without prior stimulation by exogenous pyrogen.

Table 96–4. Fever of Unknown Origin: Important Points in the History and Clinical Examination

History
Age, sex, breed
Vaccination status
Previous illness or recent operations
Recent trauma or evidence of pain
Drug administration
Previous response to antibiotics
Duration and periodicity of clinical signs
Localized or shifting leg lameness
Geographic location, travel history
Exposure to infectious agents
Lifestyle (free roaming or house cat)
Exposure to ticks
Diet (pansteatitis in cats on all fish diets)
Clinical Examination
Lymphadenomegaly
Enlargement of liver, spleen, or kidneys
Petechial, ecchymotic hemorrhages (skin, mucosae, retinae)
Cardiac murmurs (systolic or diastolic)
Localized pain (neck, back, or abdomen)
Ulcerative, vesicular skin lesions or oral ulcers
Joint pain, periarticular soft tissue swelling, or joint effusion
Evidence of penetration injury in oropharyngeal region (e.g., stick injuries)
Rectal examination (prostatomegaly)
Ophthalmoscopy (chorioretinitis, retinal detachment or hemorrhage, anterior uveitis)

Miscellaneous Diseases

A number of painful orthopedic conditions, including metaphyseal osteopathy and panosteitis, may be associated with fever. In cats hypervitaminosis A may be associated with fever, lameness, or generalized stiffness. Liver disease (e.g., acute hepatocellular necrosis and less frequently portosystemic shunts) may result in intermittent endotoxemia and fever.

CLINICAL FINDINGS

Because the list of differential diagnoses for FUO is extensive, normal history and clinical findings can be extremely informative and may help to rule out many of the possible causes. The important aspects of the history and clinical examination are summarized in Table 96–4.

The type of fever should be established early in the course of the investigation by recording the animal's temperature two to three times daily over at least a 72-hour period. Initial signs are usually vague and nonspecific, and localizing signs of disease, at least initially, are often absent. The intensity of some clinical signs (e.g., shifting lameness associated with the immune-mediated polyarthropathies) may spontaneously wax and wane. An attempt should be made to rule out infectious causes of fever first.

To identify any septic, inflammatory, or neoplastic focus that may be present, a series of preliminary screening tests should be performed. The indiscriminate use of antibiotics, glucocorticoids, and nonsteroidal anti-inflammatory drugs not only may mask clinical signs but may significantly interfere with the results of many laboratory tests. Although therapeutic trials should generally be undertaken only if the cause of the fever cannot be established, knowledge of a previous response to antibiotics alone is helpful and should prompt more extensive investigation for a septic focus.

DIAGNOSIS

Initial diagnostic investigations should include full hematologic examination, including platelet count; complete serum biochemical screen, including urea, creatinine, glucose, bile salt, sodium, potassium, chloride, calcium, and phosphate concentrations and alanine aminotransferase, ALP, aspartate aminotransferase, and creatine kinase activities; total plasma protein and fibrinogen concentrations; routine urinalysis, including microscopic examination of sediment; urine culture and susceptibility; lateral thoracic and abdominal radiographs, including long bones and joint surveys if there has been a history of a shifting leg type of lameness; FeLV and FIV status in cats; and fecal examination for parasitic ova and occult blood. Feces should be submitted for bacteriologic culture if there has been a history of diarrhea.

The requirement for additional diagnostic procedures should be based on the results of preliminary screening tests and/or the presence of new clinical signs. The major indications for each procedure are summarized in Table 96–5.

Blood cultures are indicated in most unresolved FUO cases. More specific indications include the presence of a systolic or diastolic heart murmur, history of shifting leg lameness or back, bone or joint pain (especially if these signs are accompanied by neutrophilia, with or without a left shift), or neutropenia.

Peracute bacteremia associated with endotoxemia is nearly always caused by gram-negative organisms, particularly *Escherichia coli* and *Salmonella* spp. In comparison, subacute or chronic bacteremia is more often the result of a gram-positive or anaerobic infection and is usually associated with a persistent focus of infection (e.g., vegetative endocarditis and diskospondylitis).[2]

Conditions most frequently associated with bacteremia are malignant neoplasms and infections of the skeletal, cardiovascular, and urogenital systems.[10] The most frequently isolated bacteria are Enterobacteriaceae and coagulase-positive staphylococci (particularly *S. aureus*) and β-hemolytic streptococci.[2, 10] Enterobacteriaceae, if present in the blood, are often isolated elsewhere in the body.[10] Concurrent urinary tract infections involving the same organisms cultured from the blood may occur in some bacteremic dogs; however, it has not been established whether this is cause or effect.[2] For additional information on blood culture techniques and interpretation, see Chapter 87.

Bone marrow aspiration is indicated to rule out myeloproliferative and lymphoproliferative disease when fever is associated with an unexplained cytopenia or leukocytosis. **Multiple synovial fluid aspirates** are indicated in animals with a history of intermittent or shifting leg lameness, back or joint pain, or periarticular soft tissue swelling, especially if these findings are accompanied by neutrophilia and hyperfibrinogenemia.

Electrocardiography (ECG) should be performed in any animal showing signs of congestive heart failure or having cardiac arrhythmia or pulse deficit. Valvular vegetations occasionally result in thromboembolic myocarditis and premature ventricular contractions. Echocardiography is the most

Table 96–5. FUO: Indications for Diagnostic Procedures

PROCEDURE	INDICATIONS BASED ON PROBLEMS IDENTIFIED FROM HISTORY, CLINICAL EXAM, INITIAL LABORATORY-RADIOGRAPHIC PROCEDURES
Diagnostic Procedures	
Blood culture	Systolic or diastolic cardiac murmur; neutropenia or neutrophilia (± left shift); shifting leg lameness; back, bone, or joint pain
Bone marrow aspiration	Anemia, thrombocytopenia, and/or neutropenia; leukocytosis/suspect leukemia (e.g., unexplained neutrophilia, lymphocytosis, or large numbers of atypical WBC in peripheral blood)
Multiple joint aspirates	History of shifting leg lameness with back or joint pain and periarticular swelling; neutrophilia ± hyperfibrinogenemia
Electrocardiography	Congestive heart failure, especially if dysrhythmia (e.g., myocarditis)
Echocardiography	Cardiac murmur ± dysrhythmia suggestive of bacterial endocarditis
Immunodiagnostic Screening Tests	
Rheumatoid factor	As for joint aspirates and blood culture
Antinuclear antibodies	As for joint aspirates and blood culture; ulcerative or vesicular cutaneous or oral lesions; persistent proteinuria
Direct antiglobulin (Coombs') test	Hemolytic anemia; thrombocytopenia (especially if positive for antiplatelet antibodies)
Antiplatelet antibodies	Thrombocytopenia; Coombs' positive anemia
Serum protein electrophoresis ± immunoelectrophoresis	Abnormal total serum/plasma proteins; hypergammaglobulinemia; immunodeficiency syndrome suspected
Serology (toxoplasmosis, neosporosis, borreliosis, FIP, ehrlichiosis, RMSF, leishmaniasis, brucellosis, aspergillosis, and other systemic mycoses)	Fundic lesions (e.g., chorioretinitis, retinal detachment [toxoplasmosis, FIP, systemic mycoses]; anterior uveitis [FIP, toxoplasmosis, systemic mycoses]; diskospondylitis *[Brucella canis]*; polyarthropathy [Lyme borreliosis, RMSF, leishmaniasis]; increased total serum/plasma proteins, especially if increased globulin fraction [FIP, ehrlichiosis, leishmaniasis])
Specialized Radiographic Techniques	
Double-contrast cystography (with abdominal ultrasound examination)	Prostatomegaly
Barium meal	Persistent melena
Neutrophil function tests	Unable to establish cause of FUO; indicated especially if an immunodeficiency syndrome is known to exist in the breed
Radiolabeled leukocyte scan	Unable to establish cause of FUO
Exploratory laparotomy	Abdominal mass; enlarged spleen or liver; unexplained abdominal pain
Tissue biopsy	Abnormal renal or hepatic function tests; ulcerative or vesicular cutaneous or oral lesions (additional immunofluorescent studies may be indicated)
Therapeutic trial	Diagnosis cannot be established after extensive investigation

FUO = fever of unknown origin; FIP = feline infectious peritonitis; RMSF = Rocky Mountain spotted fever.

useful diagnostic aid for confirming or ruling out the presence of vegetative lesions on the heart valves or mural endocardium.

Indications for the most common immunodiagnostic screening tests to detect anti-red cell antibodies, antiplatelet antibodies, antinuclear antibodies, and rheumatoid factors are given in Table 96–5. None of these tests can be regarded as completely reliable because both false-negative and false-positive results occasionally occur. For example, a number of chronic inflammatory, infectious, and neoplastic diseases may be associated with low antinuclear antibody titers. It is important to interpret positive titer results in association with clinical signs and results of other laboratory tests. The diagnostic significance of a positive titer result depends not only on the type of test but the methodology employed to perform it.

Serum protein electrophoresis/immunoelectrophoresis should be performed when the total plasma protein concentration is abnormal (usually increased) or when a chronic inflammatory or infectious process is suspected. Polyclonal increases in the globulin fractions are most commonly associated with persistent intracellular viral, rickettsial, and protozoal infections (e.g., feline infectious peritonitis (FIP), ehrlichiosis, and leishmaniasis), chronic bacterial infections, and immune-mediated disorders. A monoclonal γ-globulin peak is more consistent with plasma cell myeloma, although similar peaks are occasionally seen with ehrlichiosis, functional B-cell lymphomas, and some chronic inflammatory conditions in cats.

Decreased serum concentrations of γ-globulin usually occur with a concomitant decline in the concentrations of other protein fractions and are associated with numerous debilitating disorders, including lymphoma and other malignant neoplasms. Low serum concentrations of specific immunoglobulin subclasses may occur with various primary immunodeficiency syndromes. For example, a syndrome characterized by chronic rhinitis and pneumonia occurs in association with low serum IgA levels in Irish wolfhounds. Chronic recurrent bacterial infections have been reported in Weimaraners with low serum levels of IgA and IgG (see Chapter 95).

Serologic tests for antibody measurements are currently available for toxoplasmosis, FIP, FIV, borreliosis, brucellosis, ehrlichiosis, RMSF, leishmaniasis, aspergillosis, and other systemic mycotic diseases. The first of paired serum samples should be collected early in the evaluation of a patient with FUO and stored at −20°C. Single positive-titer results are diagnostic for FIV, brucellosis, ehrlichiosis, and leishmaniasis. A fourfold increase in the titer of a sample taken 2 to 3 weeks later is usually significant for toxoplasmosis, borreliosis, and RMSF and indicates recent exposure to the infectious agent. For FIP and mycotic diseases, antibody titers are compatible with exposure to the agent but must be performed along with other clinical parameters to establish infection.

Neutrophil function tests require sophisticated equipment and must be performed on fresh cells within 2 hours of collection. For these reasons, its use is restricted to referral institutions or research laboratories. Confirmation of neutrophil dysfunction requires in vitro assessment of chemotaxis, adhesion, and bactericidal properties. The nitroblue tetrazolium dye reduction test assays the respiratory burst of neutrophils after phagocytosis. Fluorescent activated cell scanning has been used to investigate surface expression of leukocyte adhesion molecules (heterodimers CD18 and CD11) on neutrophils from some related dogs, with repeated bouts of pyrexia.[6] Pyrexic episodes in two of these dogs were related to a transient decrease in neutrophil adhesion molecule expression. Dogs that had no history of pyrexia had a normal distribution of these adhesion molecules. **Complement activity** can be measured with a 50% hemolytic complement (CH50) assay, and specific components of the complement cascade (e.g., C3) can be assayed by radial immunodiffusion. The cell-mediated arm of the immune system can be evaluated in vitro by measuring **lymphocyte stimulation** by uptake of tritiated thymidine in response to various mitogens.

Radiolabeled leukocyte scans are used in human medicine to localize inflammatory and infectious diseases; examples include inflammatory bowel disease, acute and chronic osteomyelitis, and intra-abdominal and soft tissue sepsis. Radionucleotide scans for investigation of FUO in humans is also well established; however, the disease process must be associated with a purulent inflammatory response. Preliminary studies in the dog have suggested that, although technetium Tc99m–labeled leukocyte studies may detect areas of hidden infection, other nuclear medicine techniques such as gallium scintigraphy may be more appropriate screening tests for detecting chronic inflammation. Unlike technetium Tc99m, gallium[67] enters inflamed tissues nonspecifically through "leaky" capillaries, and its localization is less related to leukocyte activity.[5]

THERAPY

The beneficial effects of "true fever" often outweigh the adverse effects. The main objective in the management of the febrile animal is to identify and treat the primary disease. Mild to moderate fevers (increases in body temperature less than 41°C) are rarely fatal, and antipyretic therapy should be considered only if the cause of pyrexia cannot be established or the associated clinical signs such as anorexia and weight loss become particularly severe. The indiscriminant administration of steroidal or nonsteroidal anti-inflammatory agents

Table 96–6. Doses of Antipyretic Agents Used in Dogs and Cats

DRUG	SPECIES	DOSE (mg/kg)[a]	ROUTE	INTERVAL (HOURS)	DURATION (DAYS)
Acetylsalicylic acid	D	10–25	PO	8–24	
(aspirin)	C	10	PO	48–72	
Acetaminophen[b]	D	10–20	PO	12–24	
Dipyrone	B	25	IV, IM, SC	8	
Flunixin meglumine	D	0.5–1.0	IV, IM, PO	24	Maximum 3 days

[a]Dose per administration at specified interval. For further information on these drugs, see Drug Formulary, Appendix 8.
[b]Contraindicated in cats.
D = dog; C = cat; B = dog and cat.

masks clinical signs, making accurate clinical monitoring and assessment of response to more specific forms of therapy difficult.

Most antipyretic drugs used in veterinary medicine, including salicylates, acetaminophen, dipyrone, and flunixin meglumine, are inhibitors of prostaglandin synthesis that act centrally to lower the thermoregulatory set-point (see Table 96–6 for doses). Acetylsalicylic acid (aspirin) has the lowest expense and toxicity of common nonsteroidal analgesic antipyretic agents. Toxic effects of salicylates include vomiting, gastric ulceration, acid-base imbalance, and CNS disturbance. Cats are especially susceptible to salicylate toxicity because of slow hepatic clearance. The antipyretic activity of acetaminophen in dogs is equal to that of aspirin. The drug is hepatotoxic at high doses and is contraindicated in severe liver disease. It can also induce Heinz body formation and methemoglobinemia, particularly in cats. Cats may show signs of toxicity after the administration of as little as half of a 325-mg tablet; therefore, acetaminophen is contraindicated in this species. Dipyrone has potent antipyretic activity in dogs and cats. It is recommended for short-term therapy (i.e., 4–5 days) because prolonged administration of this drug may cause bone marrow suppression. Flunixin meglumine, one of the newer prostaglandin synthetase inhibitors currently licensed for use in small animals, has more potent antipyretic properties than aspirin, but its use has been associated with similar GI side effects.

References

1. Calvert CA. 1982. Valvular bacterial endocarditis in the dog. *J Am Vet Med Assoc* 180:1080–1084.
2. Calvert CA, Greene CE. 1986. Bacteraemia in dogs: diagnosis, treatment and prognosis. *Compend Cont Educ Pract Vet* 8:179–186.
3. Calvert CA, Greene CE, Hardie EM. 1985. Cardiovascular infections in dogs: epizootiology, clinical manifestations and prognosis. *J Am Vet Med Assoc* 187:612–616.
4. Dow SW, Jones RL. 1989. Bacteraemia: pathogenesis and diagnosis. *Compend Cont Educ Pract Vet* 11:423–443.
5. Dunn KJ. 1996. Personal communication. University of Cambridge.
6. Dunn KJ, Bujdoso R, Herrtage ME. 1995. Decrease in cell-surface expression of CD11 and CD18 by neutrophils isolated from dogs with pyrexia, p 62. *In* Proceedings of the 5th Annual Congress of the European Society of Veterinary Internal Medicine, Cambridge, England.
6a. Dunn KJ, Dunn JK. 1998. Diagnostic investigations in one hundred and one dogs with pyrexia of unknown origin. *J Small Anim Pract.* In press.
7. Elwood CM, Cobb, MA, Stepien RL. 1993. Clinical and echocardiographic findings in 10 dogs with vegetative bacterial endocarditis. *J Small Anim Pract* 34:420–427.
8. Greene CE. 1990. Fever, pp 64–71. *In* Greene CE (ed), Infectious diseases of the dog and cat. WB Saunders, Philadelphia, PA.
9. Hardie EM, Rawlings CA, Calvert CA. 1986. Severe sepsis in selected small animal patients. *J Am Anim Hosp Assoc* 22:33–41.
10. Hirsch DC, Jang SS, Biberstein EC. 1984. Blood culture of the canine patient. *J Am Vet Med Assoc* 184:175–178.
11. Hirschmann JV. 1997. Fever of unknown origin in adults. *Clin Infect Dis* 24:291–302.
12. MacKowiak PA, Bartlett JG, Borden EC, et al. 1997. Concepts of fever: recent advances and lingering dogma. *Clin Infect Dis* 25:119–138.
13. Pinals RS. 1994. Polyarthritis and fever. *N Engl J Med* 330:769–774.

Chapter 97

Prevention and Management of Infection in Catteries

Dennis F. Lawler

Cattery populations can be described as being stable or transient. They can be defined by intended purpose. Relatively stable populations include catteries that conduct breeding for professional, enthusiast, research, or commercial markets, some research catteries, and multicat households. Transient populations usually are associated with veterinary hospitals, grooming and boarding establishments, retail outlets, shelters, suppliers, some research facilities, and feral environments. Neighborhood populations, relocated feral populations, and shelters that do not euthanize have some characteristics of both stable and transient populations.

ALL CATTERY ENVIRONMENTS

General Characteristics

Characteristics shared by congregated feline populations include species, proximity, goal or purpose for existing, means of confinement (except feral populations), system for sanitation and management, some level of health care for most, and environmental influences. Some degree of exposure to infectious agents is inevitable, given the ubiquitous nature of viruses such as rhinotracheitis (FRV-1) and calicivirus (FCV) and the environmental persistence of others such as feline panleukopenia virus (FPV). Even specific pathogen–free facilities have to be repopulated occasionally, because ubiquitous disease agents can be inadvertently introduced and disseminated after small lapses in maintenance of environmental barriers and sterility.

Transmission and Management of Diseases

Infectious diseases may be transmitted directly by immediate or close contact between reservoir and susceptible host. Indirect transmission includes inanimate vehicle (fomite), air or droplet, or various mechanical or biologic vectors. Variable but unique environmental factors also affect transmission by influencing interactions among source, organism, and host (see Chapter 94).[11, 35, 39] Season, crowding, ventilation, and sanitation are among the most important environmental factors. Recognizing these interactions is an important part of developing effective preventive medicine strategies.

Depending on logistic and economic factors, efforts at disease management may be directed toward prevention (i.e., a disease does not occur) or acceptable suppression (i.e., a disease occurs with control). Feline leukemia virus (FeLV) is an example of the former, and the latter is represented by upper respiratory tract disease. Host factors that influence expression of infections as clinical disease in individuals and populations include age, inbreeding, health and resistance of hosts, and nutritional status. Organism factors include virulence and dose of the infecting strain, route of inoculation, and environmental influences and stressors.[11, 35, 39] Consulting clinicians need to understand these interactions in individual catteries and must consider the potential role of each component, because the ways in which these factors are expressed are not universal. However, the key factor is interrupting the transmission of microorganisms, and the essential element is knowing the biology or life cycles of identified target infectious agents.

Environmental Management

The primary goal of environmental management is to maintain surroundings that harbor the lowest possible number of infectious organisms and that reduce stress as much as possible. The sanitary state of the cattery influences infectious diseases directly by providing or by preventing access to concentrations of microorganisms and indirectly by modulating stress. Disinfection alone is not a substitute for good overall management. The nonspecific effectiveness of chemical disinfection depends more on type of environment and manner of use.[19, 23, 26]

Rapid changes in environment, temperature, and humidity can facilitate development of infectious diarrhea and respiratory disease, especially in crowded environments or when young kittens are present. Increased stress and easier transmission of infectious organisms are the most likely explanations. Cages, pens, feeding equipment, and litter pans should be cleaned and disinfected daily and between occupants. Cats should not be replaced in wet cages or pens because of the risk of physical injury and direct exposure to disinfectant. Animal handling ordinarily should be done on an age-priority basis, such as youngest first, progressing through the older groups.[23]

Nutritional fads and extremes should be avoided. Nutritional supplementation increases overhead costs and seldom is necessary or particularly effective if a good-quality commercial product is fed. Anecdotal reports of effectiveness of unusual diets or supplements should be regarded suspiciously until results of controlled studies can be produced. Nutritionally complete and balanced commercial products should be chosen for applicable life stages, and manufacturers' claims should be supported by controlled feeding studies and not simply by analytic results based on National Research Council guidelines.

STABLE ENVIRONMENTS

General

Stable environments such as breeding catteries offer greater opportunity for point-of-entry control of some, but not all, infectious diseases. New residents in larger catteries should be isolated for about 4 weeks for observation, vaccination, parasite control, and selected surveillance laboratory procedures. See Appendix 5 and chapters concerning specific microorganisms for preferred diagnostic and screening procedures. Isolation should be outside of usual traffic patterns in large catteries, and isolated cats should be cared for after other residents or by other personnel.[23] When this guideline is not possible, hand washing and clothing change may reduce risk for introducing some infectious agents. In smaller catteries where time, space, and funding do not permit isolation, careful evaluation of the infectious disease status of the source cattery should precede entry to the destination cattery. Vaccination, parasite control, and physical examination should be completed 2 to 4 weeks before entry.

Programs for population health maintenance need to be individualized, because the biologic and environmental factors that interact to influence occurrence of infectious diseases can result in varying patterns of morbidity and mortality. Identifying and targeting offending organisms do not differ procedurally from individual clinical presentations, but population-based problems occur in magnitude commensurate with population size and density. Management programs should not be designed or modified on the basis of results of empiric diagnosis or therapy. Most populations harbor several infectious agents, and these often act and interact in cyclic fashion. All target agents must be recognized if effective long-term management is to be achieved.

Mortality

Veterinarians sometimes are reluctant to recommend postmortem examination, and clients may be reluctant to agree. However, in breeding and research catteries, causes of mortality must be identified. Most kitten mortalities occur as stillbirths or during days 0 to 3 of the neonatal period. Variations in expected patterns should prompt investigation. Neonates react in limited scope to dissimilar insults, whether infectious, physiologic, environmental, or genetic (anatomic or metabolic) in origin.[21] When infectious causes are suspected, laboratories should be advised of tentative diagnoses before necropsy, if possible. Correct procedures must be followed for taking diagnostic samples and for proper sample preservation, shipping, and processing.[23] Refer to Chapters 1, 33, 56, 70 and Appendix 5 for specific submission and handling requirements.

Increased morbidity and mortality in specific age groups within populations should increase suspicion for genetic or infectious causes.[21, 23, 28] However, clinical findings should be considered in light of overall cattery health and management, because transmission of infectious agents has an environmental component. Patterns of morbidity and mortality, established over time, can be used along with specific diagnoses to develop preventive strategies.[23, 21]

Inbreeding

Inbreeding frequently is practiced to concentrate traits that are perceived to be superior. However, excessive emphasis on aesthetic desirability or on any single trait can be hazardous. Excessive inbreeding can be associated with compromised immunity, increased susceptibility to infection, and reduced reproductive efficiency.[1, 2, 12] Increased cattery incidence of FeLV, feline immunodeficiency virus (FIV), feline infectious peritonitis (FIP), and dermatophytosis often results.

Age

Advanced age is a theoretical risk factor for infections because of naturally declining immune function.[10] However, practical experience in well-managed catteries has shown that occurrence of, and death from, infectious diseases does not increase with advancing age. Maintaining older cats in stable populations seems to pose no significant infectious risk to individuals or catteries. The highest risk for infections occurs after weaning, consequent to the relationship between decline of passive antibody and exposure to infectious organisms by animal or environmental contact.[13]

Research Catteries

Research catteries that maintain long-term residents without a reproductive purpose should be managed according to the nonreproductive components of a breeding cattery. The control programs may be somewhat less intense than those necessitated by a kitten population, but consulting clinicians should remember that size and density of adult populations and environmental sanitation also influence stress and ease of transmission of infectious agents.

In research catteries, careful attention should be given to the nature of the research and the potential for undiagnosed infections to influence and compromise experimental data. Cats in research catteries often originate from transient populations. Recognition of new diseases in destination catteries should prompt evaluation of source catteries as well. If a source cattery is to continue to act as a supplier, eradication or acceptable control must be achieved at both catteries.

Households

Extensive evaluations are less the custom for entry of new pets into multipet households. Vaccination and parasite control should be current before entry, and physical examination should be conducted for external parasites and dermatophytes. Sanitation should be strict with respect to fecal wastes, but the home environment usually limits use of disinfectants. If pet cats are raised and maintained indoors with a restricted population density, many traumatic, toxic, and infectious exposures may be avoided.

Specific Infectious Diseases

Respiratory Disease. It is difficult to exclude cats from breeding catteries on the basis of history of respiratory disease, because of (1) the ubiquitous nature of FRV-1 and FCV, (2) the fact that carrier cats are common, and (3) the fact that completely effective vaccines do not exist.[4, 8, 9, 18] However, several practical guidelines for control can be provided. FRV-1 and FCV are transmitted primarily by direct contact or close proximity (i.e., by sneezing). Indirect transmission may occur in some situations.[18] FRV-1 survives no longer than 24 to 48 hours outside the host. FCV also is labile in the environment but can survive up to 10 days.[35] However, a high proportion of cattery residents usually are infected and may shed FRV-1 intermittently or shed FCV continuously.[18] A cattery environment may be continually contaminated, therefore, and transmission becomes facilitated by crowded conditions and stress. Recurrent symptoms in breeding catteries may indicate overcrowding or inattention to preventing environmental contamination. Many activities associated with kitten production impose significant stress, especially travel for breeding or shows, lactation, weaning, and periodic regrouping for housing purposes. All of these activities facilitate virus shedding, reshedding by carrier cats, and transmission.[18]

Respiratory disease in breeding catteries usually can be controlled by identifying and managing important contributing factors and means of transmission.[18, 35] In breeding catteries, vaccination with inactivated products is recommended, with boosters given to breeding queens before mating (see also Chapters 16 and 100). Traditional vaccination schedules usually are effective for small catteries with infrequent litter production. For larger catteries, vaccination schedules may need to be individualized and supplemented with more strict sanitation policies. Colostrum intake should be ensured for neonatal kittens. If early weaning and isolation are to be practiced as part of control measures, body weight and condition of kittens must be evaluated individually. Kittens weaned at less than 550 g body weight are much more likely to develop wasting syndromes and to die from the same infections that early weaning is designed to prevent.[20]

Queens that develop clinical signs during gestation or lactation, and those that repeatedly produce litters that develop significant respiratory disease, should be removed from production. If suspected carrier queens are to remain in production, early vaccination of kittens, and possibly early weaning and isolation, should be considered.

On the basis of available evidence, IN vaccination should be implemented before weaning in catteries that experience significant disease in preweaning or weanling kittens. Local immunity provides rapid (48–96 hours) protection, can prevent serious morbidity and mortality, but is short lived.[18, 35] IN vaccination may be associated with mild clinical signs of ocular and nasal discharge and some sneezing.[13, 18] These signs may occur in kittens that are vaccinated shortly before leaving the facility, but advantages clearly outweigh disadvantages in terms of morbidity and mortality. More serious clinical signs may represent concurrent natural infection, secondary bacterial or viral infection, or effects of stress associated with weaning or transport.[18] Prevention of crowding will minimize many problems associated with respiratory disease.

Feline Coronaviruses. Feline coronaviruses (FCoVs) are transmitted mainly by fecal-oral means.[15, 16, 33, 34] Close contact seems to be important for transmission, because coronaviruses are not environmentally resistant. Drying and disinfection readily inactivate coronaviruses, but fomite transmission over short times and distances, in close confinement housing, may be possible.[1] Currently, control is based principally on avoiding exposure.[41] However, serologic studies have shown that congregated cats have high exposure rates ranging from 40% to 85%. Because of the ambiguity of antibodies to FCoV, serotesting alone is not a viable exclusionary policy in multicat environments.[1, 2] For further information on control of feline coronavirus infection in catteries, see Chapter 11.

In brief, seropositivity does indicate exposure to FCoV in the environment. Seronegative cats should not be sent to seropositive catteries for breeding, or bred with seropositive cats, if seronegative catteries are to be protected.[41] Admission to seronegative catteries should be based on seronegative status of the source cattery and negative individual serology results before entry and 4 to 6 weeks later.[1, 2] Whether to admit seronegative cats from seropositive catteries, with or without history of FIP, is a risk-benefit decision that must be approached thoughtfully.

Breeding stock that produce offspring that develop clinical FIP should be removed from production.[1, 2] Common food sources should be avoided, and highly communal litter pans should be kept clean.[30] Breeding catteries that experience increased incidence of FIP should be evaluated for excessive inbreeding and for concurrent retrovirus infection.

FPV. Parvoviruses such as FPV resist environmental extremes; therefore, environmental contamination and fomites are important modes of transmission.[14] FPV also is shed from all body secretions of infected cats, facilitating transmission by direct or close contact.[14] Control in stable environments is achieved by vaccination. Standard vaccination protocols generally are adequate, and inactivated virus products are recommended for breeding catteries. Cats with clinical signs should not be maintained in breeding or research catteries, but control based on serologic evaluation is impractical, unnecessary, and undesirable. Reports of FPV causing neonatal mortality in catteries having well-vaccinated queens have increased, suggesting that vaccine breaks may occur with some current practices (see Chapter 10).

FeLV and FIV Infections. Retroviruses are associated with an array of direct and indirect clinical manifestations and have very complex biologic characteristics.[3, 37, 38] However, a significant factor in population management is that they are quite labile outside the host. Horizontal transmission via bite wounds seems to be most important for FIV; secondary roles are played by prolonged close contact, social behaviors, and fomites.[32] Congenital transmission has been documented experimentally but is not a major factor under natural circumstances. Horizontal transmission from queens to kittens, perhaps through milk, may occur occasionally, but germ cell transmission has not been documented.[3, 40, 43] FeLV also is horizontally transmitted postnatally, primarily through saliva and respiratory secretions.[3] Fighting and oronasal contact in prolonged close confinement housing seem to be the most important modes of transmission.[3]

Control in breeding and research catteries is based on exclusion (or strict observation of research protocols if the viruses are the subject of research). FeLV- or FIV-positive cats should not be kept in breeding catteries, and no seropositive cat should be used in a breeding program. Test and removal programs should be implemented for positive breeding catteries. For further information, see Chapters 13 and 14.

Bacterial Infections. These should occur relatively infrequently in well-managed catteries. Frequent diagnosis of the same type of bacterial infection in a cattery should prompt evaluation for management errors or additional undiagnosed diseases and attention to the possibility of inbreeding in production catteries. For example, in kittens, lower respiratory tract disease often is caused by *Bordetella bronchiseptica*. Low incidence may occur in many catteries. However, increased incidence may result from crowding, wasting syndromes associated with poor kitten growth during lactation, or poor management of reproduction and breeding stock selection.[20]

Pyothorax is not unusual in middle-aged to older cats that are maintained in catteries, even if management generally is good. Pyothorax may be caused by a variety of bacteria, including *Actinomyces*, *Bacteroides*, *Clostridium*, *Fusobacterium*, *Klebsiella*, *Nocardia*, *Pasteurella*, and *Pseudomonas*.[7] Currently, associated epidemiologic factors are not understood well. For a discussion of group G streptococcal infections in catteries, see Chapter 35.

Bacterial infections of the reproductive system include mastitis, metritis, endometritis, and pyometra. Mastitis and metritis tend to occur during warm, damp conditions but should occur infrequently. Endometritis and pyometra are consequences of extended diestrus.[24] Upward of 35% of intact queens housed in catteries may ovulate without mating.[25, 36] Cattery operators should be counseled that, although pyometra is not necessarily a consequence of poor breeding or management, intact queens not intended for breeding should be spayed.

Dermatophytosis. *Microsporum canis* causes more than 95% of feline dermatophytosis cases.[29] Transmission is favored by crowding, mixed age grouping, high population turnover, free roaming within an environment, common exercise areas, nonsymptomatic carriers, poor sanitation practices and inattention to ventilation systems, circulating fans that disseminate infected hairs, poor screening of source catteries and new residents, inattention to preventive health planning, and resistance of *M. canis* spores.[29, 31] Persistence within populations is by acute, active infections (which usually are recognizable), nonsymptomatic carriers, and environmental contamination. Nonsymptomatic carrier states may persist for weeks to years.[27, 42]

Control in catteries should emphasize prevention as the least expensive and most practical measure. Cats should not be purchased or otherwise imported from known positive catteries. New arrivals or returning cats may be isolated and examined by Wood's light and brush culture.[6] In the case of known exposure or positive examination or culture, antifungal shampoos and total body dips may be added, along with prophylactic oral therapy.[6]

In positive catteries, all cats should receive Wood's light examination and brush culture.[29] Environmental contamination is almost certain and must be addressed. Nonsymptomatic carriers also must be identified, so that infected and uninfected cats can be segregated completely.[29] The cattery should be closed to further breeding, show activity, or other traffic (entry and exit) until affected cats and the environment have been treated successfully (see Chapter 58).

TRANSIENT ENVIRONMENTS

Management of infectious diseases in transient environments is much more difficult. Maintenance is short term, and sources usually are random. Residents often are stressed by illness or anxiety. In all transient facilities, sanitation should be extremely strict. Practices used can be similar to those for dogs (see Chapter 98).

Veterinary Hospitals

The major problems in reducing the prevalence of infectious diseases are proximity, illness, and stress, all of which facilitate transmission of infectious microorganisms. Potentially contagious patients should be isolated, with rapid removal of their wastes and careful attention to possible routes of fomite transmission. Disinfectants should be chosen for broad spectrum of activity and should be used in outdoor and indoor areas (see Chapter 94). All cats should be examined carefully for signs of infectious diseases, and elective entries should be admitted only after vaccinations are current. Cats with highly contagious illnesses that require hospitalization should be isolated from others. Veterinary associations should pursue education about vaccination programs with clients and community.

Boarding Catteries

Populations vary constantly, population density may be high, residence usually is brief, and stress from separation anxiety is very significant. Direct, aerosol, and fomite modes of transmission are facilitated by these conditions. Individual caging minimizes direct contact, and strict sanitation should help minimize fomite transmission. Transmission of organisms such as FeLV, FIV, and FCoV should be minimal, but respiratory diseases and external parasitism often remain significant problems. *Giardia* also may be transmitted among cats housed individually if sanitation is not strict. Younger cats appear to be at greater risk for acquiring new *Giardia* infection.[17] Most boarded cats are owned pets; therefore, requirements for current vaccinations before entry can be enforced.[18] Proper ventilation, age segregation, prevention of crowding, daily disinfection, and washing hands frequently (especially after handling residents suspected of having active infection) are practical preventive steps.

Kittens should be boarded only in emergencies and should be kept isolated from older residents. The cattery staff, especially supervisors, should be taught to conduct examinations for external parasites on all entries and should recognize clinical signs that suggest dermatophytosis. All staff members should understand how the major infectious agents are transmitted and maintained in the environment. Grooming and feeding equipment should be kept meticulously clean and disinfected after each use. Animal wastes should be disposed of promptly.

Shelters

Most shelters house random-source populations with high turnover and high incidence of infectious diseases. Point-of-entry control essentially is impossible, and crowding occurs frequently, unavoidable circumstances that greatly increase risk for repeated introduction and transmission of infectious diseases.

All clinically healthy entering cats should be vaccinated and wormed. IN vaccines for respiratory diseases should be given. Unhealthy entries should be segregated for triage. Those that have severe clinical signs of infection, and especially those with high potential for transmission and low potential for survival, should be euthanized unless they can be isolated very effectively for treatment.[5] Animal control officers should be trained to recognize general clinical signs that suggest infection, so that accidental introduction of infectious agents is minimized. In large shelters, daily veterinary attention is essential. In smaller shelters, disease control policies should be understood by all supervisors, and veterinary consultation should be available at all times.

Retail Outlets

Residents usually are young kittens that are shipped from distant sources shortly after weaning. Residence is short term, and stress associated with weaning, shipping, separation anxiety, and anorexia is significant. Some level of direct or indirect contact with other species frequently occurs.

Point-of-entry control is possible, but must be based on accurate individual diagnosis and records that clearly establish source and means of transportation. Control is established by working with suppliers and their veterinarians to implement improved programs. Bilateral changes may be needed, such as better means of transportation, adjusted allowable population density at the destination cattery, revised management procedures at the source *and* the destination outlets, and use of different suppliers, if necessary. Each work shift should have at least one employee trained to recognize clinical signs of viral, bacterial, parasitic, and dermatophyte infections. Species segregation should be as strict as practical.

Research Catteries

Research catteries that maintain short-term residents usually depend on suppliers. Attending veterinarians must understand the health programs utilized by suppliers and must recognize the potential for undetected infections to influence research protocols. In general, other principles that apply to long-term research facilities and other short-term populations also apply to transient research populations.

Suppliers

Suppliers usually work with random-source adult cats, using various conditioning programs. Effective isolation may be precluded by small facility size and brief residence. Operators should be taught to recognize general indicators of infectious diseases, such as upper respiratory tract and GI signs, poor appetite, and depression. They should be able to screen cats for intestinal and external parasitism and for signs of dermatophytosis. All conditioned cats should be vaccinated and wormed. Preferably, they should be tested for FeLV and FIV.

References

1. Barlough JE, Stoddart CA. 1990. Feline coronaviral infections, pp 300–312. *In* Greene CE (ed), Infectious diseases of the dog and cat, ed 1. WB Saunders, Philadelphia, PA.
2. Barlough JE, Stoddart CA. 1991. Feline coronaviruses: interpretation of laboratory findings and serologic tests, pp 557–561. *In* August JR (ed), Consultations in feline internal medicine, ed 1. WB Saunders, Philadelphia, PA.
3. Cotter SM. 1990. Feline viral neoplasia, pp 316–345. *In* Greene CE (ed), Infectious diseases of the dog and cat, ed 1. WB Saunders, Philadelphia, PA.
4. Crandall RA. 1973. Feline viral rhinotracheitis (FVR). *Adv Vet Sci Comp Med* 17:201–224.
5. Edwards MA. 1989. The practice of veterinary medicine in humane society facilities, pp 85–90. *In* Kirk RW, Bonagura JD (eds), Current veterinary therapy X. WB Saunders, Philadelphia, PA.
6. Fortney WD. 1994. Control of dermatophytes in catteries, pp 627–635. *In* August JR (ed), Consultations in feline internal medicine, ed 2. WB Saunders, Philadelphia, PA.
7. Fossum TW, Relford RL. 1994. Pleural effusion: physical, biochemical, and cytologic characteristics, pp 287–296. *In* August JR (ed), Consultations in feline internal medicine, ed 2. WB Saunders, Philadelphia, PA.
8. Gaskell RM. 1985. Viral induced upper respiratory tract disease, pp 257–270. *In* Chandler EA, Gaskell CJ, Hilbery ADR (eds), Feline medicine and therapeutics, ed 1. Oxford, England, Blackwell Scientific.
9. Gaskell RM, Wardley RC. 1978. Feline viral respiratory disease: a review with particular reference to epizootiology and control. *J Small Anim Pract* 19:1–16.
10. Greeley EH, Kealy RD, Ballam JM, et al. 1993. The influence of age on the canine immune system (abstract). Presented at the Midwest Autumn Immunology Conference, Chicago, IL.
11. Greene CE. 1990. Environmental factors in infectious disease, pp 3–20. *In* Greene CE (ed), Infectious diseases of the dog and cat, ed 1. WB Saunders, Philadelphia, PA.
12. Greene CE. 1990. Immunodeficiency and infectious disease, pp 55–63. *In* Greene CE (ed), Infectious diseases of the dog and cat, ed 1. WB Saunders, Philadelphia, PA.
13. Greene CE. 1990. Immunoprophylaxis and immunotherapy, pp 21–54. *In* Greene CE (ed), Infectious diseases of the dog and cat, ed 1. WB Saunders, Philadelphia, PA.
14. Greene CE, Scott FW. 1990. Feline panleukopenia, pp 291–299. *In* Greene CE (ed), Infectious diseases of the dog and cat, ed 1. WB Saunders, Philadelphia, PA.
15. Hayashi T, Watabe Y, Nakayama H, et al. 1982. Enteritis due to feline infectious peritonitis virus. *Jpn J Vet Sci* 44:97–106.
16. Hayashi T, Watabe Y, Takenouchi T, et al. 1983. Role of circulating antibod-

ies in feline infectious peritonitis after oral infection. *Jpn J Vet Sci* 45:487–494.
17. Kirkpatrick CE. 1985. Giardiasis in a cattery. *J Am Vet Med Assoc* 187:161–162.
18. Knowles JO, Gaskell RM. 1991. Control of upper respiratory diseases in multiple cat households and catteries, pp 563–569. *In* August JR (ed), Consultations in feline internal medicine, ed 1. WB Saunders, Philadelphia, PA.
19. Lawler DF. 1989. Disinfection of animal environments, pp 90–95. *In* Kirk RW, Bonagura JD (eds), Current veterinary therapy X. WB Saunders, Philadelphia, PA.
20. Lawler DF. 1991. Wasting syndromes of young cats, pp 52–68. *In* Cain J, Lawler DF (eds), Small animal reproduction and pediatrics. Ralston Purina, St. Louis. MO.
21. Lawler DF. 1995. The role of perinatal care in development. *Semin Vet Med Surg* 10:59–67.
22. Lawler DF. 1996. Unpublished observations. Ralston Purina Company, St Louis, MO.
23. Lawler DF, Bebiak DM. 1986. Nutrition and management of reproduction in the cat. *Vet Clin North Am* 16:495–519.
24. Lawler DF, Evans RH, Reimers TJ, et al. 1991. Histopathologic features, environmental factors, and serum estrogen, progesterone, and prolactin values associated with ovarian phase and inflammatory uterine disease in cats. *Am J Vet Res* 52:1747–1753.
25. Lawler DF, Johnston SD, Hegstad RL, et al. 1993. Ovulation without cervical stimulation in domestic cats. *J Reprod Fertil Suppl* 47:57–61.
26. Lemarie RJ, Hosgood G. 1995. Antiseptics and disinfectants in small animal practice. *Compend Cont Educ Vet Pract* 17:1339–1351.
27. Merchant SR. 1990. Zoonotic diseases with cutaneous manifestations. *Compend Cont Educ Vet Pract* 12:515–522.
28. Meyers-Wallen VN. 1994. Selecting breeding stock and screening for genetic diseases in catteries, pp 607–619. *In* August JR (ed), Consultations in feline internal medicine, ed 2. WB Saunders, Philadelphia, PA.
29. Moriello KA. 1990. Management of dermatophyte infections in catteries and multiple cat households. *Vet Clin North Am* 20:1457–1474.
30. Pedersen NC. 1987. Coronavirus disease (coronavirus enteritis, feline infectious peritonitis), pp 193–214. *In* Holzworth J (ed), Diseases of the cat. WB Saunders, Philadelphia, PA.
31. Pedersen NC. 1991. Feline husbandry: diseases and management in the multiple-cat environment, pp 254–261. American Veterinary, Goleta, CA.
32. Pedersen NC, Barlough JE. 1991. Clinical overview of feline immunodeficiency virus. *J Am Vet Med Assoc* 199:1298–1305.
33. Pedersen NC, Boyle JF, Floyd K, et al. 1981. An enteric coronavirus infection of cats and its relationship to feline infectious peritonitis. *Am J Vet Res* 42:368–377.
34. Pedersen NC, Floyd K. 1985. Experimental studies with three new strains of feline infectious peritonitis virus: FIPV-UCD2, FIPV-UCD3, and FIPV-UCD4. *Compend Cont Educ Pract Vet* 7:1001–1011.
35. Povey RC. 1990. Feline respiratory diseases, pp 346–357. *In* Greene CE (ed), Infectious diseases of the dog and cat, ed 1. WB Saunders, Philadelphia, PA.
36. Romagnoli S, Vannozzi I, Ferdeghini M, et al. 1996. Spontaneous ovulation in domestic queens kept in a laboratory environment (abstract). Presented at the International Congress on Animal Reproduction, Sydney, Australia.
37. Shelton GH. 1991. Clinical manifestations of feline immunodeficiency virus infection. *Feline Pract* 19:14–20.
38. Sparger EE. 1991. Feline immunodeficiency virus, pp 543–550. *In* August JR (ed), Consultations in feline internal medicine, ed 1. WB Saunders, Philadelphia, PA.
39. Stoddart CA, Barlough JE. 1991. Feline coronaviruses: spectrum of virus strains and clinical manifestations of infection, pp 551–556. *In* August JR (ed), Consultations in feline internal medicine, ed 1. WB Saunders, Philadelphia, PA.
40. Wasmoen T, Armiger-Luhman S, Egan C, et al. 1991. Transmission of feline immunodeficiency virus from infected queens to kittens, p 6. *In* Proceedings of the First International Conference of Feline Immunodeficiency Virus Researchers, Davis, CA.
41. Weiss KC. 1994. Feline infectious peritonitis virus: Advances in therapy and control, pp 3–12. *In* August JR (ed), Consultations in feline internal medicine, ed 2. WB Saunders, Philadelphia, PA.
42. Wright AI. 1989. Ringworm in dogs and cats. *J Small Anim Pract* 30:242–249.
43. Yamamoto JK, Sparger EE, Ho EW, et al. 1988. Pathogenesis of experimentally induced feline immunodeficiency virus infection in cats. *Am J Vet Res* 49:1246–1262.

Chapter **98**

Prevention and Management of Infection in Kennels

Dennis F. Lawler

Dog kennel populations can be described as being stable or transient and can be defined by their purpose. Relatively stable adult canine populations are found in kennels that support purebred interests (breeding or sporting), in those that provide puppies for commercial pet channels, in research kennels that maintain long-term residents, and in multipet households. Transient populations usually are associated with veterinary hospitals, grooming and boarding facilities, shelters, retail outlets, suppliers that acquire and condition dogs for resale, and research kennels that do not maintain long-term residents. Shelters that do not euthanize have characteristics of both stable and transient kennels.

ALL KENNEL POPULATIONS

General Characteristics

Regardless of their intended purpose, all kennel populations share general features, including close proximity of residents, some means of confinement, a system for sanitation and husbandry, a level of health care, and environmental effects. Yet each possesses unique features that influence occurrence of infectious diseases. For example, in most geographic areas, nearly all dogs housed in kennels are exposed to the same environmentally stable agents, such as canine parvovirus (CPV). However, kennels that produce many litters of puppies are likely to experience greater incidence of clinical CPV infection because of environmental contamination and sequential passage to susceptible younger litters. Clinical diseases caused by more labile agents are influenced by interactions between environmental stressors and the natural biology of the agents. Seasonal tracheobronchitis in crowded boarding kennels is an example of the latter. In *all* environments, planned preventive management is far more efficient and cost effective than purely therapeutic or reactive management.

Transmission

Transmission of infectious agents can be direct, by immediate or close contact between reservoir hosts and susceptible subjects. Microorganisms also spread by inanimate vehicle (fomite), by air or droplet, or by various mechanical or biologic vectors.[4] Host factors that influence expression of infection as clinical disease include age, inbreeding coefficient, nutritional status, and health. Organism factors include virulence and dose of the infecting strain and route of inoculation. Variable but unique environmental factors (season, crowding, ventilation, sanitation) influence the interaction among source, organism, and host and often strongly influence the outcome.[12, 13] Recognizing the nature of this interaction in individual kennels is an extremely important part of developing effective preventive management strategies.

Disease Management

Depending on logistic and economic circumstances, the goal may be to prevent one or more diseases (i.e., disease does not occur) or to maintain acceptable suppression (i.e., disease occurs with control of morbidity and mortality). The key factor is interrupting transmission of microorganisms, and the essential element is knowing the biology or life cycles of target infectious agents. Associated management procedures include vaccination and parasite control, ongoing surveillance, disinfection, and genetic supervision of breeding kennels. Long-term successful management is possible only if major target organisms have been identified.

The sanitary state of the kennel influences occurrence of infectious disease directly by providing or preventing access to concentrations of microorganisms and indirectly by modulating stress. Disinfection alone is not a substitute for good overall management. Often, kennel operators simply wish to know which disinfectant should be purchased. (See Chapter 94.) However, the nonspecific effectiveness of chemical disinfection depends substantially on the intended environment and manner of use.[1, 7, 11] The primary goal of environmental management is to maintain surroundings that harbor the lowest possible number of infectious agents and that reduce stress as much as possible.

Disinfection and effective parasite control are essentially impossible in kennels with dirt flooring, especially in warm, humid climates or during wet seasons. Increased environmental microorganism load can compromise reproductive or work performance, and additional parasite burden can be devastating for puppies. Facilities that use grass surfaces ultimately face the same problems unless these areas can be rotated regularly; the household is the lone possible exception.[1, 7]

Gravel runs provide drainage and are not prohibitively expensive, and sanitation can be managed reasonably well for small numbers of dogs if preventive health care is adequate. For larger facilities, gravel maintenance and disease control require more effort. Digging by dogs is followed by accumulation of standing water, providing a reservoir for some infectious agents such as enteropathogenic bacteria. Chemical disinfection is more difficult because of the large surface area provided by several inches of gravel and because large amounts of organic material accumulate readily, reducing the effectiveness of many disinfectants. Weed control and wasted feed removal must be aggressive to control external parasites and rodents. Regular worming schedules should be implemented and monitored frequently with fecal examinations. Scrupulous daily removal of feces is imperative. Complete replacement of gravel materials at intervals may solve these problems but adds greatly to investments of time, money, and labor.[1, 7]

Concrete pens are more expensive to construct, but sanitation and disease control can be managed more effectively. A surface that is slightly roughened (to minimize injuries) and gradually sloped for drainage can be disinfected regularly and kept clean daily without difficulty. Cracks and other damage need to be repaired as they occur. Environmental management programs designed to maximize effectiveness of disinfecting agents in individual kennels still must be based on knowledge of primary target disease agents, but broadly applicable general principles of sanitation greatly facilitate this process (Table 98–1).[1, 7]

Pens of any design should be dry and sheltered from prevailing winds during inclement weather, and puppies should not be allowed to become wet or chilled. Rapid changes in temperature and humidity can facilitate development of infectious diarrhea and respiratory disease, especially when the environment is crowded or when young dogs are present. Increased stress and easier transmission of infectious organisms are the most likely explanations for disease outbreaks. Cages should be cleaned and disinfected daily and between occupants. Periodic steam cleaning is helpful when available.[4] Animals should not be placed in wet cages or pens because of the risk of injury or direct

Table 98–1. General Principles of Environmental Management in Kennels

1. Regular cleaning and disinfecting schedule should be established.
2. Surfaces should be cleared of wastes and other organic material before disinfectants are applied. Organic materials compromise the effectiveness of many disinfectants.
3. Disinfectants and other cleaning products such as soaps should be combined only by, or on direction of, the manufacturer. Inappropriate combinations can cause loss of effectiveness. Manufacturer's directions for product use should be followed exactly. Dogs should be removed from pens that are being disinfected and reintroduced when pens are dry.
4. Many products are more effective in hot water and less effective in hard water or when combined inappropriately with other agents. Municipal water supplies usually are safe for drinking, but wells, ponds, and other nonstandard water sources should be monitored for bacterial and protozoal (i.e., *Giardia*) contamination as well as for mineral content.
5. Bedding should be clean and dry. Access by insects, rodents, and birds should be prevented. Bedding should be changed as often as needed to maintain sanitation. Some litters of puppies may require multiple changes daily.
6. Feed should be stored in containers that prohibit access by insects, birds, and rodents (i.e., metal cans with tight-fitting lids). Great caution must be used with home-formulated feeds, especially in large kennels, from nutritional and disease perspectives.
7. Fecal waste should be disposed of daily, and waste containers should be disinfected frequently. Fecal wastes should not be disposed of within animal areas.
8. Equipment such as heating and cooling systems and vacuums should be cleaned and serviced regularly by qualified persons to avoid creating habitats for microorganisms.
9. Stored equipment, debris, weeds, and other items not critical to kennel function should not be allowed to accumulate.

exposure to disinfectant. Animal handling ordinarily should be done on an age-priority basis, such as youngest first, progressing through older groups.

Nutrition

Nutritional fads and extremes should be avoided. Nutritional supplementation adds considerably to overhead costs and seldom is necessary or particularly effective. In studies of vitamin-mineral supplementation or excessive protein supplementation of growing puppies, no beneficial effects on immunologic measures were found.[10] Anecdotal reports of effects of unusual diets or supplements should be regarded suspiciously until results of controlled studies can be produced. Good-quality, nutritionally complete and balanced commercial products should be chosen for applicable life stages, and manufacturers' claims should be supported by feeding studies and not simply by analytic results based on National Research Council guidelines.

STABLE KENNEL ENVIRONMENTS

Breeding Kennels

Isolation. Stable facilities usually have low adult population turnover and, therefore, offer opportunity for point-of-entry control of infectious diseases. Entering dogs in larger breeding kennels should be isolated for about 4 weeks for observation, worming, vaccination, and selected surveillance laboratory procedures. (See Appendix 5 and respective chapters for testing for specific microorganisms and preferred diagnostic and screening procedures.) Brucellosis testing always should be done before departure from the source kennel, and repeated one or more times at 30-day intervals in the destination kennel (see Chapter 40). Isolation should occur outside of usual traffic patterns. Isolated dogs should be cared for after other residents or by different personnel. When this is not possible, hand washing, clothing change, and separate footwear may be indicated if there is high risk of introducing new infectious agents.[1]

In smaller kennels where time, space, and funding do not permit isolation, careful evaluation of the infectious disease status of the source kennel should precede entry to the destination kennel. Vaccinations, parasite checks, and other surveillance procedures should be completed 2 to 4 weeks before entry, and veterinary examination also should be completed before entry.

Inbreeding. Inbreeding frequently is practiced to concentrate traits that are perceived to be superior. However, excessive emphasis on aesthetic desirability (such as coat color or conformation) or on any individual trait can be hazardous. Excessive inbreeding can be associated with immunocompromise and increased susceptibility to infection (see Chapter 95),[5] which may explain in part why certain breeds seem to have disproportionate susceptibility to diseases such as CPV. Declining reproductive efficiency also may be observed consequent to excessive inbreeding, resulting in smaller litters and greater neonatal mortality.[9]

Age. Advanced age represents a theoretical risk factor for infections because of naturally declining immune function.[3] However, practical experience in kennels that are managed well has shown that occurrence of, and death from, infectious diseases does not increase with advancing age. Maintaining older dogs in stable populations seems to pose no significant infectious risk to individuals or to the kennel.

Poorly managed breeding kennels may experience increased neonatal mortality, usually from bacterial infections. However, the highest risk for infection in most kennels occurs after weaning, as a consequence of the relationship of maternal antibody decline and exposure to infectious organisms by animal or environmental contact.[6] Deficient vaccination and parasite control, environmental mismanagement, and poor breeding selection policies become evident, but recognizing these contributing factors is more difficult in kennels that retain few puppies past the immediate postweaning period. Information about problems that occur at destination kennels may be necessary when planning corrective strategies in some source kennels, but multiple-source or poorly managed destination kennels can present interpretive dilemmas. In the latter instances, evaluation of multiple facilities may be necessary.

Health Maintenance. Vaccination and parasite control need to be individualized by kennel, because the biologic and environmental factors that interact to influence occurrence of infectious diseases can result in varying patterns of morbidity and mortality.

Identifying and targeting offending infectious microorganisms do not differ procedurally from individual clinical presentations, but population-based problems almost always occur in magnitude commensurate with population size and density. Investments into determining the type and extent of specific infectious disease prevalence are worthwhile. Clinical signs and response to empiric therapy alone should not be used as criteria for designing or modifying management programs. Most kennel populations harbor several infectious agents that induce clinical disease variably and often in cyclic fashion. Transmission can be interrupted effectively when all offending agents are identified and when their season and environment-based influences are understood.

Mortality. Veterinarians sometimes are reluctant to recommend postmortem examination, and clients may be reluctant to agree. However, in breeding kennels, causes of mortality must be identified. Most puppy mortalities occur as stillbirths (30%) or during the 0- to 3-day neonatal period (50%).[8] Variations in this expected pattern should prompt investigation. Neonates react in limited scope to dissimilar insults, whether infectious, physiologic, environmental, or genetic (anatomic or metabolic) in origin. When infectious causes are suspected, consulting laboratories should be advised of tentative diagnoses before necropsy, if possible. Appropriate procedures must be followed for taking correct diagnostic samples. Successful diagnosis also depends on proper sample preservation, shipping, and processing.[1] See Chapters 1, 33, 56, 70, and Appendix 5 for pertinent information.

Increased morbidity and mortality in specific age groups within populations should increase suspicion for genetic or infectious causes. However, clinical findings should be considered in light of overall kennel health and management status, because transmission of infectious agents has an environmental component. Patterns of morbidity and mortality, established over time, can be used along with specific diagnoses to develop preventive strategies.

Research and Sporting Kennels

In research and sporting kennels that maintain long-term residents with minimal reproductive activity, isolation on entry, parasite control, vaccination, and surveillance should be practiced aggressively, as for breeding kennels. The intensity of the control program usually is less than in kennels with high puppy populations, although the size and density of the adult population do influence stress and ease of transmission of infectious agents.

In research kennels, valid interpretation of experimental data depends on having a complete data base. Careful attention should be given to the type of work in progress and the potential for undiagnosed infections to compromise experimental data. For example, nutritional or GI research should be accompanied by aggressive monitoring for enteric viral, bacterial, and parasitic agents. Cardiovascular research necessitates continuing evaluation for bacterial diseases, especially those that have systemic potential. The quality and outcome of studies involving immunity, such as vaccine research, depend on documenting that only the experimental agent is introduced (i.e., potentially interfering infectious agents are surveyed and not found), on knowing the status of control subjects with respect to the experimental agent, and on knowing the immunocompetence of dogs in control and test groups.

Specific pathogen-free dogs can be purchased for research kennels; however, in many circumstances, these dogs originate from more transient types of kennels. When new diseases are recognized in destination kennels, investigation of the status of source kennels can facilitate early diagnosis, which in turn supports rapid implementation of control measures to minimize further transmission. At times, alternate-source kennels may need to be sought, but accurate records are essential to support exclusion of problem sources on factual grounds only.

Households

Extensive evaluations are less the custom for entry of new pets into multipet households. Vaccination and parasite control should be current before entry, and physical examination should be conducted for external parasites. Sanitation should be strict with respect to fecal wastes, but the home environment usually limits use of disinfectant chemicals. When two or more dogs in the same household have similar clinical signs, it is important to remember that proximity often means common exposure to infectious agents. However, individual characteristics, such as behavior, age, or immune status, also may influence clinical expression. Illness in one dog in a multidog household does not rule out group exposure.

TRANSIENT ENVIRONMENTS

Management of infectious diseases in transient environments is much more difficult. Maintenance is short term, and sources usually are random. Residents often are stressed by illness or anxiety. In all transient facilities, sanitation should be extremely strict.

Veterinary Hospitals

Disinfectants are very important because of the high frequency of presentation of animals with infectious diseases and the risk of transmitting to other hospitalized patients or establishing nosocomial infections.[4] Disinfectants should be chosen for broad-spectrum activity unless specific agents are being targeted (see Chapter 94).[1, 7, 11] Hospital personnel should be taught to clean and disinfect table surfaces and equipment between patients, to wash hands or rubber gloves after each hospitalized or boarded patient is handled, and to recognize clinical signs of major internal and external infections. The outdoor area of the hospital should be cleaned regularly to prevent exposure of patients by environmental contamination.

Patients with potentially contagious diseases should be isolated as well as possible, with rapid removal of wastes from animal areas. Careful attention to fomite transmission of environmentally stable *and* unstable agents is needed, because transmission distances usually are very short. Special care should be taken to protect individuals that might be immunodeficient.[5]

Thorough vaccination programs should be pursued with all clients individually and through community education by local veterinary associations. Current vaccinations should be required for elective surgery and boarding patients, updated before admission. Every entry, whether inpatient or outpatient, should be checked carefully for external parasites and for signs of dermatophytosis.

Grooming and Boarding Kennels

Population turnover is high and constant; residence usually is very brief. Separation anxiety, close proximity or crowding, and poor ventilation often facilitate transmission of infectious agents by direct, aerosol, and fomite routes. Some opportunity for control is afforded by the fact that dogs and cats in these kennel populations nearly always are owned pets. Appropriate vaccinations can be required before entry. Veterinarians should play active roles in helping to establish policies for vaccination requirements.

Grooming and other equipment that is utilized in common among dogs should be kept meticulously clean and disinfected after each use. Operators of grooming and boarding facilities should be trained to recognize external parasites such as fleas, ticks, and lice and to note clinical signs suggesting sarcoptic mange and dermatophytosis. In addition, all personnel involved should understand how these diseases, as well as major viral and bacterial diseases, are transmitted.

Shelters

Most shelters house random-source populations with high turnover and high incidence of infectious diseases. Point-of-entry control essentially is impossible and crowding occurs frequently, unavoidable circumstances that greatly increase risk for repeated introduction and transmission of infectious diseases.

All clinically healthy dogs should be vaccinated and wormed. IN vaccines for respiratory diseases should be provided. Unhealthy animals should be segregated for triage. Those that have severe clinical signs of infection, and especially those with high potential for transmission and low potential for survival, should be euthanized unless they can be isolated very effectively for treatment.[2] Animal control officers should be trained to recognize general clinical signs that suggest infection, so that accidental introduction of infectious agents is minimized. In large shelters, daily veterinary attention is essential. In smaller shelters, disease control policies should be understood by all supervisors, and veterinary consultation should be available at all times.

Retail Outlets

Residents usually are young puppies that are shipped from distant sources shortly after weaning. Residence is short term, and stress associated with weaning, shipping, anxiety, and anorexia is significant. Some level of direct or indirect contact with other species frequently occurs.

Point-of-entry control is possible, but must be based on accurate individual diagnosis (either in-house or after sale) and records that clearly establish source and means of transportation. Control is established by working with suppliers and their veterinarians to implement improved breeding programs. Preshipping management changes also may be needed, as well as improved means of transportation, adjusted allowable population density at the destination kennel, revised management procedures at the source *and* the destination outlet, and use of different suppliers, if necessary. Each work shift should have at least one employee trained to recognize clinical signs of viral, bacterial, parasitic, and dermatophyte infections. Species segregation should be strict.

Research Kennels

Research kennels that maintain short-term residents must understand the conditioning or health programs used by suppliers and must have aggressive and thorough in-house veterinary service. If residence duration is sufficiently short, time for development of clinical signs of infectious diseases may be insufficient. Negative effects on research protocols and their results may therefore be unrecognized. In general, the principles that apply to influence of infectious diseases on research projects in long-term facilities also apply to transient research populations.

Suppliers

Suppliers usually work with adult dogs from random sources and have varying conditioning programs. At minimum, these should include vaccination, parasite control, and behavioral evaluation. Facilities usually are too small and residence terms too short to permit effective isolation of all new entries. Operators should be trained, therefore, to recognize general signs of internal and external infectious diseases. The ability to conduct routine screening of feces for intestinal parasites also is helpful.

References

1. Bebiak DM, Lawler DF, Reutzel LF. 1987. Nutrition and management of the dog. *Vet Clin North Am* 17:505–533.
2. Edwards MA. 1989. The practice of veterinary medicine in humane society facilities, pp 85–90. *In* Kirk RW, Bonagura JD (eds), Current veterinary therapy X. WB Saunders, Philadelphia, PA.
3. Greeley EH, Kealy RD, Ballam JM, et al. 1993. The influence of age on the canine immune system (abstract). Presented at the Midwest Autumn Immunology Conference, Chicago.
4. Greene CE. 1990. Environmental factors in infectious disease, pp 3–20. *In* Greene CE (ed), Infectious diseases of the dog and cat. WB Saunders, Philadelphia, PA.
5. Greene CE. 1990. Immunodeficiency and infectious disease, pp 55–63. *In* Greene CE (ed), Infectious diseases of the dog and cat. WB Saunders, Philadelphia, PA.
6. Greene CE. 1990. Immunoprophylaxis and immunotherapy, pp 21–54. *In* Greene CE (ed), Infectious diseases of the dog and cat. WB Saunders, Philadelphia, PA.
7. Lawler DF. 1989. Disinfection of animal environments, pp 90–95. *In* Kirk RW, Bonagura JD (eds), Current veterinary therapy X. WB Saunders, Philadelphia, PA.
8. Lawler DF. 1990. The role of perinatal care in development. *Semin Vet Med Surg* 10:59–67.
9. Lawler DF. 1996. Unpublished observations. Ralston Purina Company, St Louis, MO.
10. Lawler DF, Goff BSL, Roth JA, et al. 1995. Immune function in growing dogs fed increased or decreased dietary protein, or excess vitamins and minerals, pp 223-235. *In* Proceedings of the Society of Theriogenology, San Antonio, TX.
11. Lemarie RJ, Hosgood G. 1995. Antiseptics and disinfectants in small animal practice. *Compend Cont Educ Vet Pract* 17:1339–1351.
12. Povey RC. 1990. Feline respiratory diseases, pp 346–357. *In* Greene CE (ed), Infectious diseases of the dog and cat. WB Saunders, Philadelphia, PA.
13. Stoddart CA, Barlough JE. 1991. Feline coronaviruses: spectrum of virus strains and clinical manifestations of infection, pp 551–556. *In* August JR (ed), Consultations in feline internal medicine, ed 1. WB Saunders, Philadelphia, PA.

Chapter 99

Immunocompromised People and Pets

Craig E. Greene

IMMUNODEFICIENCIES

Immunodeficiency occurs in people owing to a variety of physiologic and pathologic reasons (Table 99–1). Age is one determinant; fetuses, neonates, and young children have underdeveloped immune systems. Similarly, elderly persons, especially those in nursing homes or hospitals, have apparent increased risks of developing infections. Concurrent conditions such as other illnesses, pregnancy, burns, or indwelling tubes, catheters, or implants increase the risk of the host by breaching natural barriers to infectious agents. Immunodeficiency is also a result of cancer chemotherapy and leukopenic disorders and may be the result of congenital or hereditary defects in the immune system. The most rapidly advancing cause of immunodeficiency in people is AIDS, resulting from infection with HIV.

An estimated 1 million people in the United States are HIV positive and up to 50% own companion animals,[11, 25] as is

Table 99–1. Conditions Associated With Immunocompromised People

Age: fetus, neonate (infant), preschooler, elderly
Health conditions: hospitalization, concurrent illnesses, diabetes mellitus, chronic renal failure, pregnancy, burns, leukopenia, congenital immunodeficiencies, hepatic cirrhosis, malnutrition
Therapeutic agents: cancer chemotherapy, autoimmune disease therapy
Instrumentation: catheters, indwelling tubes, synthetic implants, splenectomy
HIV infection: AIDS complex

typical for the population at large.[32] The estimated prevalence of companion animals in all U.S. households is 60%, with the following representation: dogs, 38.2%; cats, 30.5%; birds, 5.7%; and horses, 2.8%. The psychological benefits that these companion animals provide are great, and the risk for acquiring infections from animals is low. Nevertheless, certain precautions that are taken in handling and caring for pets will further reduce any inherent risks. The information presented herein will stress documented AIDS-related zoonoses, although people with immunodeficiencies from any cause should apply similar guidelines in handling their pets. Furthermore, because zoonoses can develop in immunocompetent people, many of the principles and practices can be applied by anyone with pets.

ZOONOTIC RISK

Zoonoses are defined as infectious diseases shared by people and animals; however, not all zoonoses that occur in the immunocompromised are transmitted directly from animals to humans (Table 99–2). Those zoonoses that can be contracted from companion animals pose a potential risk for immunocompromised people exposed to pets. Inhalation and ingestion are the common means by which many zoonotic infections may be transmitted. Transmission can occur by bites or scratches or by arthropod vectors. Many zoonotic agents are maintained in nature in soil, water, and vegetation.

Table 99–2. Means of Transmission of Zoonotic Infections of Immunosuppressed People

DIRECT ZOONOSES FROM PETS[a]

Bite, saliva: rabies, pasteurellosis, capnocytophagiosis, helicobacteriosis
Scratch, contact: dermatophytosis, bartonellosis
Inhaled, aerosols: plague (cat), tularemia, bordetellosis
Feces: toxoplasmosis, cryptosporidiosis, campylobacteriosis, helicobacteriosis, salmonellosis, giardiasis, ancylostomiasis, toxocariasis
Urine: brucellosis (dog), leptospirosis (dog)
Transport of insect vector: bartonellosis, tularemia, plague, RMSF, dipylidiasis
Other animal hosts: *Rhodococcus equi* infection (horse), *Mycobacterium marinum* infection (fish), psittacosis (birds), salmonellosis (reptiles and amphibians)

ENVIRONMENTALLY ACQUIRED ZOONOSES

Saprophytic: pneumocystosis, microsporidiosis, *Mycobacterium avium*-complex infection, cryptococcosis, coccidioidomycosis, histoplasmosis, blastomycosis, aspergillosis
Vector acquired: ehrlichiosis, borreliosis, babesiosis, plague, RMSF, tularemia, bartonellosis

NONZOONOTIC INFECTIONS

Unique to people: cytomegalovirus disease, herpes simplex virus disease, varicella-zoster virus infection, human papillomavirus infection, hepatitis B infection, influenza virus infection
Indigenous microflora: candidiasis, *Streptococcus pneumoniae* infection, other bacteria associated with sepsis

[a]Predominantly dog and cat, except where otherwise indicated.
RMSF = Rocky Mountain spotted fever.

In these zoonoses, people and animals acquire infections simultaneously and independently of each other.

The importance of zoonotic diseases has become more apparent owing to the AIDS epidemic in the human population. In fact, the appearance of unusual zoonotic infections in people was one way that AIDS was first recognized. The increasing incidence of zoonotic infections in immunosuppressed people makes it imperative that veterinarians keep current on their knowledge of these diseases. Most physicians are not as well trained in zoonoses compared with veterinarians, and their advice, when given, is often to give up pets altogether.[1, 16] Veterinarians may be in a better position to advise immunocompromised persons about the relative risk of pets and provide them with accurate information on precautionary measures. There was a significant difference in the type of opportunistic infections that developed in people with AIDS, depending on whether or not they owned a pet.[11] Although veterinarians are among the best educated concerning animal infections, few have taken an active role in educating their immunodeficient clients.[1, 26] AIDS patients most frequently consult physicians, nurses, and community health personnel, who give conflicting advice, whereas only few consult their veterinarians.[1, 11, 15] Many AIDS patients have misconceptions about zoonoses and have received misleading or no information concerning the transmission risks.[11] Surveys have shown that more than 60% to 90% of HIV-infected people have been advised by human health professionals to give up their pets, whereas only 5% have followed this advice.[6, 26] The latest guidelines from the U.S. Public Health Service and the Infectious Disease Society of America indicate that immunocompromised people should not give up their pets but rather take simple precautions.[3, 3a, 19a]

At first glance, the risk of acquiring animal infections may appear to dominate the medical literature and media reports, but a relatively small fraction of infections in people can actually be attributed to pet contact. People with immunosuppression are at increased risk for acquiring all types of infections, including zoonoses. People are more likely to acquire infections from other people than from animals. Furthermore, some of the highly publicized zoonoses in AIDS patients such as toxoplasmosis are due to reactivation of previously acquired infection and are not related to current pet exposure.

PET BENEFITS

Pets offer important physiologic and psychological benefits for people, especially the infirm. Important bonds of friendship exist between people and their pets. Although illness and disability often alienate homebound AIDS victims from their family, friends, and acquaintances, pets provide continued companionship and overcome the deleterious effects of loneliness.[9] Pets also provide pleasure, protection, and a sense of worth.[9] It may be more detrimental to the well-being of isolated immunocompromised people to lose their pet companions than to risk the potential of acquiring a zoonotic infection.

SUPPORT GROUPS

Immunodeficient people may develop emotional and physical limitations that prevent them from adequately caring for their pets. Extended unanticipated hospitalization and physical or financial limitations are often present. In addition, needs for preventive and disease-related veterinary care and feeding are expected. Veterinarians can advise their clients

Table 99–3. Resources for Pet Owners Infected with HIV

Local Groups by State

Pets Are Wonderful Support (PAWS), 539 Castro St, San Francisco, **CA** 94114, (415) 241-1460
Dan Griffith, DVM, Sunset Pet Clinic, 3926 Sunset Blvd, Los Angeles, **CA** 90029
Marin Humane Society: SHARE Program, 171 Bell Marin Keys Blvd, Novato, **CA** 94949, (415) 883-4621
Pets Are Loving Support (PALS), P.O. Box 1539, Guerneville, **CA** 95446, (707) 887-2729
PAWS/LA, 7327 Santa Monica, Blvd, West Hollywood, **CA** 90046-6615, (213) 876-7297
PAWS, Orange County, 14 Misty Creek Ln, Laguna Hills, **CA** 92653, (714) 583-0078
PAWS, San Diego, P.O. Box 178, 1278 University Ave, San Diego, **CA** 92103, (619) 234-7297
PAWS, Denver, P.O. Box 13616, Denver, **CO** 80201, (303) 861-7297
Projects for Pets Helping People Inc., 311 Benham Ct, Newark, **DE** 19711
Pets, Washington D.C., 2001 O St, NW, Washington, **DC** 20009, (202) 234-7387
PAWS, Tampa, 1917 E. Clinton St, Tampa, **FL** 33610, (813) 237-8089
PALS Inc., 1438 Peachtree St, Suite 176, Atlanta, **GA** 30309, (404) 876-7257
Hawaiian Humane Society: PALS Project, 2700 Waialea Ave, Honolulu, **HI** 96826, (808) 955-5122
Maui PAWS, P.O. Box 111, Kula, **HI** 96790, (808) 876-0000
PAWS, Chicago, 47 W. Division, Suite 117, Chicago, **IL** 60610, (312) 465-3741
PAWS, Indiana, 3951 N. Meridian St. Suite 101, Indianapolis, **IN** 46208
Companion Animal Support & Assistance Network (CASAN), c/o AIDS Service Center, 810 Barrett Ave, Rm 263, Louisville, **KY** 40204, (502) 574-5490
PAWS, Maine, P.O. Box 5305, Portland, **ME** 04101, (207) 874-0091
Pet Owners With AIDS/ARC Resource Services (POWARS), Baltimore, 38 Parkin St, Baltimore, **MD** 21202
PAWS, St. Louis, 1425 Hampton Ave, St. Louis, **MO** 63139, (314) 781-7976
Pet PALS of Southern New Jersey, c/o ACSNJ, 607 S. White Horse Pike, Audubon, **NJ** 08106, (609) 310-0334
POWARS, New York, 1674 Broadway, Suite 7A, New York, **NY** 10019, (212) 246-6307
Philly PAWS, P.O. Box 30262, Philadelphia, **PA** 19103, (215) 985-0206
Pittsburgh PAWS, 210 Scarborough Dr, Cheswick, **PA** 15024
Pet Pals, P.O. Box 190869, Dallas, **TX** 75219, (214) 521-5124
The Pet Patrol, P.O. Box 980255, Houston, **TX** 77098, (713) 522-1954
Humane Society/SPCA: Pet Project, 13212 S.E. Eastgate Way, Bellevue, **WA** 98005, (206) 649-7566
The Pet Project, 20454 S.E. 264th St, Kent, **WA** 98042
Pet Support Network, c/o Broadway Veterinary Hospital, 1824 12th Ave, Seattle, **WA** 98122, (206) 270-1015

General Resources

California VMA, 5321 Madison Ave, Sacramento, **CA** 95841, (916) 344-4988
Center for Animals in Society, University of California, Davis, **CA** 95616, (916) 752-3602
The Latham Foundation, 1826 Clement Ave, Alameda, **CA** 94501, (510) 521-0920
AAHA, P.O. Box 150899, Denver, **CO** (303) 986-2800
AVMA, 1931 N. Meacham Rd, Suite 100, Schaumberg, **IL** 60173, (800) 248-2862
Delta Society, 321 Burnett Ave, S, 3rd Fl, Renton, **WA** 98055, (205) 226-7357

Recommended Brochures for Affected Clients

PAWS, *Questions you may have about toxoplasmosis and your cat.* PAWS of San Francisco, **CA** 94114.
PAWS, *Safe Pet Guidelines. Toxoplasmosis and Your Cat, Cat Scratch Disease, Zoonoses and your Bird.* PAWS, San Francisco, **CA** 94114.
American Animal Hospital Association, *Pet Owner Guidelines for People with Immunocompromised Conditions.* For members of AAHA (800) 252-2242, ask for Member Service Center.

regarding the relative risks and care necessary to contain zoonoses and direct them to support groups to help them with home pet care. Veterinarians can also assist by channeling donations of money and by offering their time and professional expertise to these local groups. Veterinarians can demonstrate their willingness to participate in a zoonoses prevention program in a discrete fashion by having signs or brochures in their waiting room. They must recognize that the increased cost of surveillance and treatment to prevent zoonoses will add an increased financial obligation to the client. In addition to home pet care, support groups can provide speakers, slide shows, newsletters, and brochures concerning pet care, zoonoses, and personal hygiene. They can provide assistance in screening of suitable pets, financing pet health care, and educating pet assistants for routine care and emergencies. Numerous organizations are available to help with these needs. Pets Are Wonderful (PAWS), originating in San Francisco, and Pet Owners With AIDS/ARC Resource Services (POWARS), based in New York City, are nonprofit volunteer organizations dedicated to providing information and "at-home" support for immunocompromised people who want to keep their pets. PAWS publishes a brochure from their San Francisco office entitled "Safe Pet Guidelines," which gives immunocompromised owners background information on keeping their pets and themselves healthy. A list of a national network of support organizations and brochures is provided in Table 99–3.[19, 22]

DISEASES

More than 250 organisms are known to cause zoonotic infections and approximately 30 to 40 involve companion animals. Of these, a selected few have been reported with greater frequency in people with immunodeficiency and AIDS (see Table 99–2).[2] The appearance of a few of these infections (cryptosporidiosis, *Mycobacterium avium*–complex infection, cryptococcosis, salmonellosis) has been used to define the onset of AIDS in HIV-infected people. Some of the AIDS-related zoonoses are acquired directly from companion animals, and others are probably acquired from environmental exposure rather than from pets. The zoonoses described next are restricted to those that have been associated with exposure of immunodeficient people to companion animals.

Toxoplasmosis is the most publicized zoonotic disease acquired from pets due in part to the emphasis physicians receive in their training in animal diseases. Approximately 30% of childbearing women in the United States have antibodies to *T. gondii* and are protected against congenital transmission. If one of the remaining 70% of women should become pregnant and infected during pregnancy, there is a 20% to 50% probability that the fetus will be infected. The most severe complications in the fetus occur between the second and sixth months of gestation.

Toxoplasmosis occurs in 10% of AIDS patients and is thought to be responsible for at least 30% of CNS complications in this immunodeficient population.[15] Most cases of CNS toxoplasmosis are due to reactivation of quiescent infections rather than recent exposure. *Toxoplasma* antibody seroconversion is unusual in HIV-infected adults and appears unrelated to cat exposure.[29] Although it can be acquired by ingestion of oocysts shed by infected cats, infection in people living in industrialized countries usually occurs by ingestion of undercooked meats, especially goat, mutton, or pork. Actually, the overall risk of becoming infected from cats in the household is comparatively low except for young children, who contract infection from soil exposure in rural environments.[29] Isolated outbreaks of disease have also been reported after handling or inhaling soil or dust contaminated by cat feces. Cats usually only shed oocysts for 2 weeks after their first exposure to the organism and generally do not shed them again. Oocysts must sporulate to be infectious, a process that takes from 1 to 5 days. Because the feces neither remain on the fur nor do oocysts appear to sporulate on the fur, handling of cats is an unlikely source of infection (see Chapter 80).

Immunosuppressed persons should wear gloves and wash their hands after contact with soil or raw meat. The cat litter box should be changed daily, preferably by an immunocompetent, nonpregnant person. Hands should be thoroughly washed after changing the litter box. The person's cats should be kept inside and fed only commercial diets or well-cooked table food. Patients need not be advised to part with their cats or have them separately tested for toxoplasmosis.

Cryptosporidiosis is an intestinal infection caused by a ubiquitous, relatively non-host-specific coccidian parasite of vertebrates that can be acquired from young domestic herbivores (calves, lambs, kids, and piglets) or less commonly from pets (see Chapter 82). Kittens, especially those with diarrhea or with concurrent immunosuppressive infections with feline leukemia virus (FeLV) or feline immunodeficiency virus (FIV), or puppies are more likely to have clinical illness manifest by diarrhea and shedding of organisms. Healthy mature animals are often unaffected. Human-to-human transmission occurs without animal reservoirs, and outbreaks have been noted in day care centers and family groups. The usual source of outbreaks from environmental exposure is raw sewage or contaminated water sources. Water run-off from land with grazing animals, animal-holding facilities, or sewage treatment facilities can contaminate surface water supplies. Chlorination of water does not kill these parasites, and filtration systems for municipal water must be of high caliber to eliminate these organisms. Water can also be boiled for 1 minute. *Cryptosporidium* oocysts can be found in 90% of untreated municipal water supplies and in 30% of treated systems. As a result, most people contact this organism independent of exposure to their pets, and approximately 15% of AIDS patients develop this complication.[7]

Newborn and young pets are of some risk in transmitting this infection; stray or any pets with diarrhea should not be adopted. Puppies or kittens younger than 6 months should have their stools examined by a veterinarian for *Cryptosporidium* oocysts. In addition, immunosuppressed people should avoid exposure to calves and lambs and should not drink untreated water directly from lakes or rivers.

Immunocompetent people show signs of abdominal pain and a self-limiting diarrhea of 5 to 10 days duration. Immunodeficient individuals have a severe, watery, debilitating, chronic diarrhea that is refractory to therapy. Oocysts in feces are small (2–4 μ) and are difficult to demonstrate without concentration procedures and special staining.

Giardiasis is caused by a ubiquitous protozoal enteropathogen found in animals and people, although it is not well established whether interspecies transmission is common. As with cryptosporidiosis, outbreaks are usually water borne or involve young children in day care centers. Signs of infection in immunocompetent people are a watery, foul-smelling diarrhea with flatus, and abdominal distention or nonsymptomatic shedding can occur. Immunocompromised hosts have a greater risk of infection and may develop chronic diarrhea with malabsorption. The diagnosis in people may be difficult to make because the chance of finding the parasite on up to three stool examinations is no greater than 50%.[23] For this reason, treatment is often empiric (see Chapter 78).

Salmonellosis develops in approximately 5% of AIDS patients. Food-borne episodes from contaminated meat account for many exposures, but a few pet-related exposures have involved turtles. Severe recurrent diarrhea and bacteremia are common in AIDS patients. Reptiles and amphibians should be avoided as pets. For further information on the epidemiology and prevention of infection in dogs and cats, see Chapter 39.

Campylobacteriosis is caused by a microaerophilic group of gram-negative, curved motile rods that are commensal flora of animals. Although *Campylobacter jejuni* has been the incriminated organism, studies have shown that a wide variety of related, potentially zoonotic *Helicobacter* species exist in domestic and wild animals (see Chapter 39). *C. jejuni* is frequently isolated from dogs or cats recently acquired from pet stores, kennels, animal shelters, or pounds. Pups and kittens with diarrhea have been most commonly associated with household infections. Uncooked meat, especially poultry, is probably a more important source of infection for people. Fecal-oral, food-borne, and water-borne modes of transmission are the principal avenues for infection. Contaminated water supply, possibly due to migrating waterfowl or herbivores, may be a source of infection for outdoor pets. Children younger than 5 years with a newly acquired puppy have the highest prevalence of infection.[21] Signs of infection in people are intense abdominal discomfort, bloody diarrhea, fever, tenesmus, and fecal leukocytosis. Immunosuppressed individuals with AIDS develop recurrent diarrhea, dehydration, and bacteremia.

Bartonellosis is caused by a group of small gram-negative bacteria that infect people and animals. *Bartonella henselae* causes a variety of illnesses, including cat-scratch disease or regional lymphadenitis, neuroretinitis, Parinaud's oculoglandular syndrome, and aseptic meningitis (see Chapter 54). Immunodeficient people can also develop bacteremia, aseptic meningitis, peliosis hepatis, and bacillary angiomatosis. *B. henselae* can be isolated from clinically healthy cats, and exposure to cats is associated with many of these diseases in people. Other *Bartonella* species have been isolated from people and animals, but a zoonotic association with cats has not been made with other than for *B. henselae* and *B. clarridgeiae*.

There is an association of fleas with transmission of infection between cats. Eliminating and controlling fleas are essential for reducing the spread of infection among cats. Because the means of transmitting infection from cats to people is uncertain but possibly involves flea excreta, cat bites or scratches should not be rubbed with uncleaned hands and should be washed immediately.

Rhodococcus equi infections (see Chapter 35) have been reported in AIDS patients with exposure to horses or farm animals or environmental exposure to this soil saprophyte. The organism is found in greatest numbers in soil contaminated by herbivore manure. Clinical signs are usually related to a pneumonia with pulmonary abscess.

Listeriosis, caused by a saprophytic gram-positive bacillus, occurs most commonly in pregnant women, the old or very young, those taking immunosuppressive drugs, or those with AIDS. The organism can be isolated in the environment from soil, and humans may contract it from contaminated meat or vegetable sources (see Chapter 35).

In regard to **mycobacteriosis**, although people and pets become infected with *M. avium* complex (MAC) organisms, their infections are related to common environmental exposure rather than spread between animals or human hosts (see Chapter 50). Treatment of MAC infection is possible. Nevertheless, in households with immunocompromised persons, the decision to remove the infected pet is understandable. *M. marinum* infection is acquired by immunosuppressed people who clean fish aquariums or those who are exposed to other aquatic environments.

Dermatophytosis from pet animals is caused by two zoophilic fungi: *Microsporum canis* and *Trichophyton mentagrophytes*. Cats and dogs, respectively, are inapparent carriers of these fungi. People develop classic lesions with circular alopecia, scaling, crusting, and ulceration. Topical therapy of lesions in people is often rewarding, but topical and systemic therapy of pets and environmental decontamination are often needed to prevent recurrence (see Chapter 58).

Psittacosis is an endemic infection of birds worldwide caused by *Chlamydia psittaci*. It may be transmitted by direct contact with birds or indirectly by their feces or feathers. Infected birds may remain carriers. Animal care workers have a high risk of becoming exposed. Affected people develop pneumonia with a variety of systemic manifestations, including arthralgia and myalgia. The risk of infection has been greatly reduced through the introduction of tetracycline in poultry feeds; however, this practice has the undesirable consequence of producing antimicrobial-resistant strains and does not reduce the prevalence of infection in pet birds. Dogs and cats may become infected with the strains from birds as do people (see Chapter 31). The risk of this infection does not appear any greater for immunocompromised people as compared with those who are clinically healthy.

Bordetellosis caused by *Bordetella bronchiseptica* has been reported in immunocompromised people.[34] This is a commensal and pathogen of animals, and people have been infected from close animal contact (see Chapter 88). Exposure of such people or their pets to kennels, catteries, or shows is not advised. If necessary, vaccination may be considered. Swine are another major source of infection that should be avoided.

Bite infections with *Pasteurella* and *Capnocytophaga* (DF-2) are a risk to immunosuppressed people. These two bacteria are the most documented species involved in bite wounds (see Chapter 53). Splenectomy or other immunosuppressive diseases are associated with an increased risk of fatal sepsis from these bacteria. Signs are acute severe cellulitis and bacteremia, which may develop within 24 to 48 hours of the bite. Cats and dogs should not be allowed to lick open cuts or wounds.

Cryptococcosis has been identified as a respiratory illness in people with AIDS. Immunocompetent people are subclinically infected. As with the other systemic mycoses, these organisms are acquired from contact with contaminated soil. Pigeon and other bird droppings enrich the soil and transport organisms into new areas. Areas with large congregations of birds should be avoided. Although cats and sometimes dogs develop cutaneous infections, aerosols are not sufficient from these lesions to infect people in the immediate environment (see Chapter 61). See respective chapters for other systemic mycoses that are similarly contracted from the environment rather than from pets.

Microsporidiosis has been reported with increasing frequency as a cause of chronic watery diarrhea in AIDS patients. These protozoan parasites are a heterogenous group in the phylum Microspora (see Chapter 75). Although various microsporidia infect animals, none of the infections in humans (primarily *Enterocytozoon bieneusi*) have been traced to household pets or any animal reservoir. A wide variety of environmental exposures exist, and a number of species of farm animals, monkeys, rodents, rabbits, and fish have been shown to become infected. The premise that pets are involved has not been well substantiated. Owing to the ubiquitous nature of microsporidians, no specific precautions, other than attention to hand and food washing, can be justified.

A number of other zoonoses have not been documented with any greater frequency in immunosuppressed individuals compared with the general population. The references at the end of this chapter and the Public Health Considerations section of other chapters in this book should be consulted for a more extensive review of all companion animal–associated zoonoses.

RECOMMENDATIONS

According to guidelines established by medical experts,[3] human health care providers should advise HIV-infected persons of the potential risk posed by pet ownership. However, those giving advice should be sensitive to the possible psychological benefits of pet ownership and should not routinely advise HIV-infected persons to part with their pets. Handling pets offers no greater danger of acquiring infection for an immunosuppressed person than would contacting other people or the environment. Simple hygienic measures by immunosuppressed owners will greatly reduce the risk of exposure to zoonoses (Table 99–4). Factors that make animals poten-

Table 99–4. Guidelines for People With Immunodeficiencies to Reduce Public Health Risk of their Dogs and Cats

Pets can have zoonoses, which are infections that also occur in people. Having an immunodeficiency means that you are more susceptible to develop infections. In some instances, zoonoses can spread to people from pets; and in other zoonoses, people contract these infections from the same sources, which include contaminated food, soil, water, or other people. There is no evidence that pets can become infected with or transfer HIV between people. People need not be advised to part with their pets if they follow simple precautions.

SELECTION

Choose a pet whose energy level matches yours. Choosing a young (<6 months old) puppy or kitten has greater risk because of their increased susceptibility to infections. Similarly stray, exotic, wild, ill, or debilitated animals are more likely to carry zoonotic infections. Sources of pets that have poor hygiene, unsanitary facilities, and crowded conditions should be avoided. Your veterinarian can help advise you in pet selection, screen it for infectious agents, and begin a vaccination and parasite control program. In contemplating a new pet, do not acquire any that have diarrhea. Should you or your pet develop illness, friends and local support groups can help with caring for your pet.[a]

FEEDING

Feed your pet commercial rations or pelleted feeds. If used, all meat should be cooked until no longer pink (>150°F). If dairy products are given, they should always be pasteurized. Restrict your pet's access to carrion or hunting. Allow your pet to drink tap water but not from the toilet. Control fleas, flies, and cockroaches in your pet's environment.

PERSONAL HYGIENE

Your pet's mouth contains organisms that might infect you should they enter your body through open wounds or by biting or scratching. You should avoid activities that might induce such behavior or exposure to their saliva, such as licking your face or wounds. Wear gloves or have others give them oral medications or brush their teeth. As a general rule, wash your hands after handling your pet. Bite or scratch sites should be washed promptly. You should wear gloves and a face mask when cleaning up the litter box or diarrhea from your pet or have others assist you. You should minimize your contact with your pet's excreta (urine, feces, and vaginal or seminal discharges). Litter boxes should be emptied daily; liners make this job easier and minimize exposure. The litter box should be kept out of food preparation or eating areas.

PARASITE CONTROL

Your veterinarian can assist you in controlling external parasites such as fleas or ticks, which potentially can transmit zoonotic infections to people. Gloves should be worn when removing ticks from your pet. Testing for and treating intestinal parasites are also warranted because they can cause diarrhea or, in some cases, infect people.

DISEASE TESTING

Cats do not need to be serologically or microscopically tested for toxoplasmosis. The stool of dogs and cats can be checked for *Cryptosporidium* oocysts (see Chapter 82). Feces can also be cultured for *Salmonella* and *Campylobacter* (see Chapter 39). Cats can be tested for and treated for *Bartonella*, although the need for this is controversial (see Chapter 54).

[a]Your veterinarian can provide you with names of assistance programs that can provide some of the following services: In-home pet care; changing litter boxes; walking dogs; home flea control; care or medication of pet if hospitalized or ill; pet bathing; foster care and adoption; delivery of pet food.

Recommendations compiled from various sources including references 1, 3, 3a, 16 and 17.

Table 99–5. Veterinary Guidelines for Handling Dogs and Cats for Directly Transmitted Zoonoses Most Commonly Affecting Immunocompromised People

DISEASE, PET	DIAGNOSIS	TREATMENT	PRECAUTIONS
Toxoplasmosis C (Chapter 80)	NR: fecal exam—rarely found; serology—cannot predict oocyst shedding; seropositive generally protected because of previous exposure	NR: clindamycin—reduces oocyst shedding; bathing—feces not often on fur	R: litter box hygiene—daily cleaning by immunocompetent assistant; prevent cat from hunting or eating raw meat
Giardiasis: C, D (Chapter 78)	R: test pups, kittens, diarrheic pets; zinc sulfate method	R: metronidazole, albendazole, fenbendazole	R: litter box hygiene; handle feces with gloves
Cryptosporidiosis: C, D (Chapter 82)	R: acid-fast or FA staining of feces	R: paromomycin; untreated may shed 2 weeks	R: litter box hygiene; handle feces with gloves
Campylobacteriosis, helicobacteriosis: C, D (Chapter 39)	R: fecal culture NR: culture stomach contents or biopsy, histopathology with silver stains	R: I—erythromycin, chloramphenicol R: G—metronidazole, ampicillin, bismuth subsalicylate	R: prevent ingestion of raw meat
Salmonellosis: C, D (Chapter 39)	R: fecal culture, selective media	NR: fluoroquinolones	R: prevent hunting, carrion, or raw meat ingestion. If positive, temporarily remove from household
Bartonellosis: C (Chapter 54)	R: blood culture NR: serologic testing	R: fluoroquinolones, doxycycline, rifampin	R: strict flea control, screen or avoid kittens, avoid bites or scratches, wash immediately if they occur
Bordetellosis: C, D (Chapters 6, 16, and 88)	NR: endotracheal wash and culture	R: tetracyclines	R: avoid exposure to boarding kennel dog shows, congregated dogs, vaccination if exposure likely

R = recommended; NR = not recommended; C = cat; D = dog; I = intestinal *Campylobacter*; G = gastric *Helicobacter*.

tially greater risks are some of the unique organisms they can harbor and the lack of sanitary behavior often practiced by pets. Owners can often institute routines in their own behavior that will make it unlikely that they will contract a disease from their companion animals. Veterinarians can institute certain screening procedures to identify potential zoonoses and initiate treatment or prevention protocols where indicated (Table 99–5).

Screening

In general, precautions should be taken if an immunosuppressed person decides to acquire a pet for companionship or if a pet is being used to provide companionship for people in hospitals or nursing homes. In a survey of U.S. and Canadian animal-assisted therapy programs, 94% used dogs or cats.[30] Two thirds visited elderly in nursing homes, one fourth were taken to schools, and another one fourth were taken to hospitals. Although unfounded, the major zoonotic concerns were rabies, ringworm, and external parasites.[30] Less than half of these groups consulted veterinary professionals, and only 10% had written guidelines for zoonoses transmission.

With dogs and cats, infectious diseases, including zoonoses, are more frequently a problem in puppies or kittens. Exotic or wild animals are not as tractable and may inflict injuries or harbor unusual parasites or infections. Furthermore, those animals coming from high population densities, as exist in humane shelters, pet-breeding facilities, pounds, or crowded pet stores, or stray animals may have a greater chance of harboring pathogens. Acquiring a new adult pet from a single pet household may be the best consideration. Any newly acquired pet should be thoroughly examined by a veterinarian before being introduced. It should be clinically healthy and have no evidence of illness (especially diarrhea) or immunosuppression. Any animal with diarrhea should be examined by a veterinarian for *Cryptosporidium*, *Salmonella*, or *Campylobacter* (see Table 99–5 and respective chapters).

Handling

Immunosuppressed people should wash their hands frequently during the course of the day and consistently after handling their pets or excretions. This is especially important before eating, smoking, performing dental hygiene, and putting in corrective lenses. The pet's environment should also be kept clean and free of dirt, uneaten foods, and excrement.

Health Care

Newly acquired cats should have their vaccinations and routine anthelminthic therapy for roundworms and hookworms. Serologic testing for FeLV and FIV is recommended. Although FeLV and FIV pose no chance of infecting people, cats affected with these immunosuppressive viruses are more likely to develop other infectious diseases. Measuring IgG toxoplasmosis titers might help determine prior exposure in cats but is not definitive. Younger kittens are more likely to be seronegative and are at risk of shedding oocysts after their first exposure to *T. gondii*. IgG seropositivity indicates prior exposure and minimal risk, because cats rarely re-shed oocysts after initially being infected (see Chapter 80). Prophylaxis for dirofilariasis should be given to pets in endemic areas. Yearly physical examinations, current vaccinations, and fecal parasite examinations are indicated to prevent the possibility of the pet contracting highly infectious illnesses. Illness in any pet should be an important reason to seek veterinary care without delay.

Grooming

The animal's hair coat and skin should be kept in good condition by weekly baths and brushing and trimming of matted fur. Nails of dogs and cats should be trimmed frequently to reduce the chance of scratch injuries. If cats scratch when handled, declawing should be considered. Fleas should be managed with regular bathing and dipping with insecticides and intensive environmental treatment in the area that the animals frequent. This includes indoor floors and carpets, especially where they sleep, their sheltered roaming areas, and other animals in contact. Environment treatment using flea bombs or spraying should include larvicidal growth inhibitors as well as adulticide compounds. Flea collars, powders, sprays, or topical application of concentrated residual insecticides are adjunctive measures but should be used while observing for toxicity. Newer oral or topical products that interfere with flea development and reproduction are warranted. More effective control of fleas in the environment may require a professional exterminator.

To control ticks, routine daily checking of pets or checking immediately after leaving tick-infested areas is indicated. Prior application of DEET-containing compounds or newer long-term topical inhibitors is indicated. Any attached ticks should be removed with rubber gloves, tweezers, or facial tissues, and protected hands should be washed after removal. Ticks should not be removed or crushed with bare, exposed hands. For further information on tick removal and prevention, see Chapters 29 and 45. Flies, cockroaches, and vermin may also transport infectious organisms. Pets should be restricted from areas where rodents burrow, and measures should be taken to eliminate areas near the home where vermin may nest.

Excrement

Immunosuppressed individuals should try to avoid direct contact with pets excretions and wear gloves when handling fecal material. When possible, diarrhea should be handled by others. Diarrheic stools are particularly challenging to remove without becoming exposed to pathogens they may contain. Feline litter boxes should be kept out of eating areas and should be cleaned by an immunocompetent, nonpregnant adult. Litter box dust can be avoided by supplying bag liners and dust-free litters and by moistening litter before sealing bags. Although the litter box should be emptied outdoors or in well-ventilated areas to avoid inhalation, the litter should not be disposed in the outdoors. Because a minimum of 24 hours is required for *Toxoplasma* oocyst maturation for infectivity, the litter box should be cleaned at least every 24 to 48 hours when possible. The litter box can be disinfected of coccidian oocysts once monthly by filling it for 10 minutes with boiling water from the stove or dilute (10%) ammonia solutions.

Dogs should be discouraged from coprophagia, and cat litter boxes should be isolated from other nonfeline pets. Within communities, animals should be restricted from defecating in playgrounds, parks, and walkways, or provisions should be made for owners to remove their pets' excrement from public places.

Improved health education of children should be provided. Children should be educated not to practice geophagia or pica and to wash their hands after playing in soil. For those with aquatic or cold-blooded pets, rubber gloves should be used for cleaning aquariums or terrariums. Diarrheic pets should not be exposed to the general household and should not contact young children of immunosuppressed members in a household. Animals suffering from diarrhea should be bathed as needed to decontaminate their hair coat. Pet owners should be instructed to wear rubber gloves during cleaning of diarrheic or other stools and to use sodium hypochlorite (bleach) at a dilution of 1 ounce per quart of water for disinfection. Similar precautions can be recommended for other body fluids, including blood, urine, and saliva. Hands should be washed after the gloves are removed.

Oral Hygiene

Immunocompromised owners should be advised not to let pets lick them on the mouth and to practice good preventive dental hygiene for themselves and their pets. Pets should not be kissed on the mouth. Routine dental prophylaxis with scaling or brushing is recommended for pets exposed to immunocompromised people. Veterinarians or other household members or assistants should assume these responsibilities. Saliva should be washed from hands or open wounds. Rubber gloves should be worn when oral medication is given to pets, or someone else should assume these responsibilities.

Bite wounds are probably the most frequent health risk faced by immunocompromised individuals. Pets that are aggressive in behavior or play should not be kept under these circumstances. People who are inadvertently bitten should immediately wash the wound with soap and water and rinse with dilute organic iodine solutions or quaternary ammonium compounds as an alternative. A physician should promptly examine any injuries. Pets should not be allowed to lick human wounds. Children should be taught not to startle feeding or sleeping animals. A physician should be immediately notified of any bites or scratches from pets that do occur. Prophylactic antimicrobial therapy may be considered by physicians who know the patient's immunocompromised status.

Nutrition

The diet of pets is extremely important in limiting fecal-oral pathogens. Only commercial diets that have been cooked or pelleted should be fed. Raw or unprocessed meat or offal or unpasteurized dairy products should not be provided. Pets should be prevented from coprophagy, scavenging, hunting, and feeding on carrion or garbage. They may have to be leashed or confined or have outdoor supervision. Bells can be placed on cat's collars to reduce their success at hunting. Water from the tap should always be available to pets. Commercial bottled water is advisable if the tap water has been shown to be unhealthy from inadvertent contamination with bacteria or protozoa. Access to outside surface water or toilet bowl water should be restricted.

References

1. Angulo FJ, Glaser CA, Juranek DD, et al. 1994. Caring for pets of immunocompromised persons. *J Am Vet Med Assoc* 205:1711–1718.
2. Anonymous. 1990. Aids patients can acquire some infections from animals. *J Am Vet Med Assoc* 197:1268–1269.
3. Anonymous. 1995. Centers for Disease Control and Prevention. USPHS/ISDA guidelines for the prevention of opportunistic infection in persons infected with HIV: a summary. *MMWR Morb Mortal Wkly Rep* 44:1–34.

3a. Anonymous. 1997. USPHS/IDSA guidelines for the prevention of opportunistic infections in persons infected with human immunodeficiency virus: disease specific recommendations. *Clin Infect Dis* 25:S313–S335.

4. Anonymous. 1995. Informing clients about zoonotic disease transmission: a legal and public health issue. *Vet Forum* 12:37–38.
5. Baxter DN, Leck I. 1984. Deleterious effects of dogs on human health 2. Canine zoonoses. *Commun Med* 6:185–197.
6. Bixler T. 1992. Two new human-animal bond studies begin to break ground. *DVM Magazine* March:18–21.
7. Buckley RM, Braffman MN, Stern JJ. 1990. Opportunistic infections in the acquired immunodeficiency syndrome. *Semin Oncol* 17:335–349.
8. Burton BJ. 1989. Pets and PWAS: claims of health risks exaggerated. *AIDS Patient Care* 2:34–37.
9. Carmack BJ. 1991. The role of companion animals for persons with AIDS/HIV. *Holist Nurs Pract* 5:24–31.
10. Clavin T. 1995. Your pet can be hazardous to your health. *Readers Digest* 39:33–41.
11. Conti L, Lieb S, Liberti T, et al. 1995. Pet ownership among persons with AIDS in three Florida counties. *Am J Public Health* 85:1559–1561.
12. Current WL, Reese NC, Ernst JV, et al. 1993. Human cryptosporidiosis in immunocompetent and immunodeficient persons: studies of an outbreak and experimental transmission. *N Engl J Med* 308:1252–1257.
13. Delafuente J, Albo C, Rodriguez A, et al. 1994. *Bordetella bronchiseptica* pneumonia in a patient with AIDS. *Thorax* 49:719–720.
14. Deutz A, Fuchs K, Hinterdorfer F, et al. 1996. Serological examination on

zoonoses in veterinarians. Basic data and prevalence of antibodies against bacterial zoonoses. *Wien Tierarztl Monatasschr* 83:283–288.
15. Gill DM, Stone DM. 1992. The veterinarian's role in the AIDS crisis. *J Am Vet Med Assoc* 201:1683–1684.
16. Glaser CA, Angulo FJ, Rooney JA. 1994. Animal associated opportunistic infections among persons infected with the human immunodeficiency virus. *Clin Infect Dis* 18:14–24.
17. Goldstein EJC. 1991. Household pets and human infections. *Infect Dis Clin North Am* 5:117–130.
18. Greene CE (ed). 1990. Infectious diseases of the dog and cat. WB Saunders, Philadelphia, PA.
19. Griffith D. 1996. Group helps Los Angeles residents with HIV/AIDS keep and care for their pets. *Top Vet Med* 7:35–36.
19a. Kaplan JE, Masur H, Holmes KK (eds). 1997. Prevention of opportunistic infections in persons infected with human immunodeficiency virus. *Clin Infect Dis* 25(Suppl):S299–S335.
20. McCrindle CME, Hay IT, Odendaal JSJ, et al. 1996. An investigation of the relative morbidity of zoonoses in paediatric patients admitted to Ga-Rankuwa hospital. *J S Afr Vet Assoc* 67:151–154.
20a. Meslin FX. 1997. Global aspects of emerging and potential zoonoses: a WHO perspective. *Emerg Infect Dis* 3:223–228.
20b. Noah DL, Kramer CM, Verbsky MP, et al. 1997. Survey of veterinary professionals and other veterinary conference attendees for antibodies to *Bartonella henselae* and *B. quintana*. *J Am Vet Med Assoc* 210:342–344.
20c. Nowotny N, Deutz A, Fuchs K, et al. 1997. Prevalence of swine influenza and other viral, bacterial, and parasitic zoonoses in veterinarians. *J Infect Dis* 176:1414–1415.
21. Salfield NJ, Pugh EJ. 1987. *Campylobacter enteritis* in young children living in households with puppies. *BMJ* 294:21–22.
22. Scheck J, Lewis LA, Lane TJ. 1996. A model program for assisting pet owners infected with human immunodeficiency virus. *J Am Vet Med Assoc* 208:483–484.
23. Scully RE, Mark EJ, McNeely BU. 1985. Case records of the Massachusetts General Hospital, case 39-1985. *N Engl J Med* 313:805–815.
24. Sorvillo FJ, Lieb LE, Waterman SH. 1991. Incidence of campylobacteriosis among patients with AIDS in Los Angeles county. *J Acquir Immune Defic Syndr* 4:598–602.
25. Spencer L. 1992. Pets prove therapeutic for people with AIDS. *J Am Vet Med Assoc* 201:1665–1668.
26. Spencer L. 1992. Study explores health risks and human/animal bond. *J Am Vet Med Assoc* 201:1683–1684.
27. Stefanelli P, Mastrantonio P, Hausman SZ, et al. 1997. Molecular characterization of two *Bordetella bronchiseptica* strains isolated from children with cough. *J Clin Microbiol* 12:1550–1555.
28. Stryler-Gordon R, Beall N, Anderson RK. 1985. Facts and fiction: health risks associated with pets in nursing homes. *J Delta Soc* 2:74–75.
28a. Tan JS. 1997. Human zoonotic infections transmitted by dogs and cats. *Arch Intern Med* 158:1933–1943.
29. Wallace MR, Rossetti RJ, Olson PE. 1993. Cats and toxoplasmosis risk in HIV-infected adults. *JAMA* 269:76–77.
30. Waltner-Toews D. 1993. Zoonotic disease concerns in animal-assisted therapy and animal visitation programs. *Can Vet J* 34:549–551.
31. Wilson JF, Lacroix C, Allen C. 1996. Zoonotic parasitic diseases: a legal and medical update. *Vet Forum* 13:40–46.
32. Wise JK, Yang JJ. 1992. Veterinary service market for companion animals 1992: part 1. Companion animal ownership and demographics. *J Am Vet Med Assoc* 201:990–992.
33. Wong MT, Dolan MJ, Lattuada CP, et al. 1995. Neuroretinitis, aseptic meningitis, and lymphadenitis associated with *Bartonella* (*Rochalimaea*) *henselae* infection in immunocompetent patients and patients infected with human immunodeficiency virus type 1. *Clin Infect Dis* 21:352–360.
34. Woodard DR, Cone LA, Fostvedt K. 1995. *Bordetella bronchiseptica* infection in patients with AIDS. *Clin Infect Dis* 20:193–194.

Chapter 100

Immunoprophylaxis and Immunotherapy

Craig E. Greene

Immunoprophylaxis

Immunoprophylaxis involves enhancement of a specific immune response in an animal in an attempt to protect it against infectious disease. This response can be actively induced through vaccines containing microorganisms, their components, or their metabolic by-products. Immunity can also be passively transferred by the administration of humoral or cellular factors obtained from a previously sensitized donor. Immunoprophylaxis also implies pre-exposure immunopotentiation, and it should be differentiated from immunotherapy, which is the attempt to increase nonspecifically the immune response in an already infected animal. Immunoprophylaxis is more commonly used and is successful in the prevention of viral and bacterial diseases because of the relatively few antigens responsible for immunologic control of such infectious agents. Fungal, protozoal, and metazoan pathogens and neoplasms, all containing more complex antigenic determinants, are often controlled immunologically with nonspecific immunotherapy. Nevertheless, vaccines are being developed for some of these infections of dogs and cats, and a fungal vaccine exists for dermatophytosis.

PASSIVE IMMUNIZATION

Artificial (passive) transfer of specific antibodies or other immunoreactive substances from one individual to another has been classically used to treat a variety of infectious diseases in humans and animals. Passive immunization itself has been decreasing in use. Currently, it is found in small animal veterinary practices only in a few special instances (Table 100–1).

Passive administration of serum or immunoglobulin has a beneficial role in protecting colostrum-deprived neonates (<2 days old) against certain diseases such as parvoviral infections. Active immunization must be avoided because of the

Table 100–1. Comparison of Passive and Active Immunoprophylaxis

VARIABLE	PASSIVE	ACTIVE
Advantages	Immediate protection Works for agents that are poor immunogens	Stronger protection Longer protection Anamnestic response
Disadvantages	Allergic reactions Immune reactions Delays ability to vaccinate Short-lived protection Transfer of disease more likely	Delayed response
Indications	Exposed susceptible neonates Colostrum-deprived neonates Exposed immunosuppressed animals	Unexposed susceptible neonates Routine immunization Booster vaccinations

risk of inducing disease with modified live vaccines and because of the weaker response to noninfectious vaccines at this age. Antisera given to older kittens (<8 weeks) that become inadvertently exposed to feline panleukopenia virus (FPV) provide protection much sooner than that produced after vaccination. Passive immunization may also temporarily benefit severely immunosuppressed dogs and cats receiving cancer chemotherapy that may become exposed to infectious agents during a course of hospitalization.

Immune sera may be of prophylactic or therapeutic benefit in treating litters of puppies that are clinically affected with neonatal herpesvirus infections (see Treatment, Chapter 5). Serum, in such cases, should be prepared from recovered bitches that have previously had affected litters. Hyperimmune serum has been beneficial in treating parvovirus-infected dogs within 4 days PI (first days of clinical illness).[53] A commercial, multivalent, homologous hyperimmune immunoglobulin preparation (Stagloban P, Hoechst Veterinär Gmb, Munich) is available in Germany for this purpose. Endotoxemia and tumor necrosis factor increases in serum have been observed in dogs with naturally occurring parvoviral enteritis.[114] Heterologous antiserum produced in horses for *Salmonella typhimurium* endotoxin is commercially available (Septiserum, Immvac, Columbia, MO), and it has shown benefit in treating endotoxemia in dogs associated with experimental parvoviral infection (see Chapters 8 and 38 and Drug Formulary, Appendix 8).[34] Passive immunization with heterologous (equine or human) antitoxin is used in the initial treatment of dogs and cats with tetanus (see Chapter 43). Monoclonal antibodies have been provided as specific passive immunotherapy for infectious agents, but because they are usually produced in rodents, tolerance is low to systemically administered foreign immunoglobulins.

The efficacy of passive immunization depends on many factors, including the antibody titer to the specific agent involved and volume administered, the relative importance of serum antibody in controlling the particular infection involved, and the timing of administration of antibody compared with exposure. Owing to the large amounts of foreign protein that are administered, allergic reactions are more likely with passive immunization. Transfer of infectious agents is more likely with administration of serum when noncommercially prepared products are used. Unfortunately, the administration of immunoglobulins also delays the ability to stimulate active immunity in the host by vaccination. Large amounts of exogenously administered antibody may negate endogenous antibody production by tying up exogenous antigens or by direct feedback mechanisms that are not clearly understood. The duration of protection received from passively administered antisera is short lived. The amount received is finite and, like all exogenous proteins, undergoes accelerated elimination from the body, especially if it originates from a different species.

Although not readily available commercially, canine and feline immune sera can be prepared in veterinary practices by sterilely harvesting serum or plasma. Immune serum (or plasma) is derived from healthy individuals or from groups of animals that have recovered from the disease in question, whereas hyperimmune serum comes from animals that have been repeatedly vaccinated against specified infectious agents. Veterinarians who prepare their own serum must carefully screen donors for insidious blood-borne infectious diseases such as bartonellosis, feline leukemia virus (FeLV) or feline immunodeficiency virus (FIV) infections, and canine brucellosis or ehrlichiosis.

Oral administration of sera, either alone or in the milk substitute, is probably the most effective means of treating colostrum-deprived neonates in their first hours of life. Immunoglobulins, rapidly absorbed by neonates for up to 72 hours, also provide some local protection from intestinal pathogens. This local protection afforded by orally administered sera is only temporary because unstable serum antibodies are destroyed by proteolytic enzymes once the neonate develops improved digestive function. IgA in the milk offers continued protection against mucosal pathogens in the nursing animal. Other routes for the serum administration in

Table 100–2. Comparison of Maternal Immunity for Selected Canine and Feline Infectious Diseases[a]

DISEASE	SERUM TITER OF NEONATE: % of Dam's Titer, Presuckle	SERUM TITER OF NEONATE: % of Dam's Titer, Postsuckle	SERUM TITER OF NEONATE: % of Neonate's Titer (Obtained in Utero, Colostrum)	HALF-LIFE MATERNAL ANTIBODY (DAYS)
Canine distemper	3	77	4/96	8.4
Infectious canine hepatitis	NR	92	NR/NR	8.6
Feline panleukopenia	<1	97	1/99	9.6
Canine parvoviral infection	5.7	60	10/90	9.7

[a]For references, see Greene CE.[53]
NR = not reported.

Table 100–3. Effect of Maternal Immunity on Vaccination for Selected Canine Infectious Diseases[a]

DISEASE	MINIMUM TITER PREVENTING REPLICATION (METHOD DETERMINED)[b]		MINIMUM AGE (WEEKS)		
	Virulent Virus	Vaccine Virus	To Begin Vaccinating Colostrum Deprived	To Begin Vaccinating Colostrum Recipients	To Stop Vaccinating Colostrum Recipients
Canine distemper	20–30 (SN)	30 (SN)	2–3	6	12–14
Infectious canine hepatitis	NR	5 (SN)	2–3	6	12
Canine parvoviral infection	80 (HI)	<10 (HI)	5	6–9	10–20[c]

[a]For references, see Greene CE.[53]
[b]Absolute titers will vary among laboratories.
[c]Twelve to 16 weeks with high-titer lower passage (potentiated) parvoviral vaccines unless titers are exceptionally high.
SN = serum neutralization (viral neutralization); NR = not reported; HI = hemagglutination inhibition.

neonates are IM, SC, intramedullary, and intraperitoneal. The dose of 2 to 4 ml/kg varies, depending on the titer of the preparation. Immune sera is not usually administered IV to small puppies or kittens because of the tendency to produce immunologic or coagulatory reactions in the recipient and because of the difficulty in cannulating a vein. If given IV, plasma anticoagulated with citrate is more desirable than serum.

MATERNAL IMMUNITY AND VACCINATION

Newborn pups and kittens have the inherent capacity to respond immunologically to numerous antigens at birth, but this response is slower and inferior compared with that of older animals. Under normal circumstances, protection against infection during these early weeks of life is afforded by passive transfer of immunoglobulins and small amounts of cellular material from the dam. The amount (2–18% of total) of antibody transferred in utero from an immune dam protects colostrum-deprived puppies or kittens but makes them refractory to immunization for several weeks. Subsequently, that immunoglobulin absorbed in colostrum gives the neonate a titer that may almost equal that of the dam in some instances (Tables 100–2 and 100–3). The decline of maternal antibody in neonates is similar to that for passively administered immunoglobulins. Each disease has a characteristic half-life for elimination (Table 100–4).[70] Antibody class is also important with respect to titer loss. Serum maternally derived IgA, IgM, and IgG in neonates are usually lost in the order given.

The absolute titer of maternal immunoglobulin in the serum of a neonate depends on the quantity of immunoglobulin received during nursing and the absolute titer of the dam. The amount is also inversely proportional to the size of the litter. Titers may be increased by vaccination of the dam just before conception or during pregnancy, although caution should be exercised with attenuated products. Titer values are so variable among individual animals that quantitative predictions cannot be made short of direct measurement of serum immunoglobulins of the dam or puppy. A commercially available ELISA test kit is available for canine parvoviral vaccination (Immunocomb, Biogal, Kibbutz Gal'ed Israel; see Appendix 6).[166] Such measurements (nomogram determinations) are usually impractical. Veterinarians therefore use multiple vaccines, given at 2- to 4-week intervals, in an attempt to break through maternal immunity before exposure to virulent organisms (Figs. 100–1 and 100–2). Frequently given vaccines may also accelerate the depletion of the maternal antibody present in the neonate's circulation. Attempts to overcome the interfering effects of maternal antibody on vaccination have included antigenically related vaccines, such as measles for canine distemper virus (CDV); alternate routes, such as intranasal administration for canine or feline respiratory viruses or *Bordetella;* and different vaccine strains or types that are able to overcome maternal immunity at a younger age as with higher titer, lower passage canine parvoviral vaccine.

Table 100–4. Half-Life of Maternally Derived Immunoglobulins in Neonatal Dogs and Cats

DISEASE	HALF-LIFE (DAYS)	USUAL DURATION OF PROTECTION AGAINST DISEASE (WEEKS)[a]
Canine distemper	8.4	9–12
Canine parvovirus	9.7	10–14
Infectious canine hepatitis	8.4	9–12
Feline panleukopenia	9.5	8–14
Feline leukemia	15.0	6–8
Feline rhinotracheitis	18.5	6–8
Feline calicivirus infection	15.0	10–14
Feline coronavirus infection	7.0	4–6

[a]The duration of maternal antibody protection against disease usually corresponds to the interval over which vaccines are ineffective. In some diseases, such as canine parvovirus infection, 3 to 5 weeks additional time may be needed for maternal antibody interference with vaccination to disappear. For references, see Greene CE.[53]

ACTIVE IMMUNIZATION

Vaccination, the production of an active immune response, involves stimulating the host with antigenic extracts or whole cultures of microorganisms. Clinical vaccination in small animals has been limited to diseases caused by viruses, bacteria, and dermatophytes. Vaccines for some protozoal infections have been developed on an experimental or limited clinical basis.

Types of Vaccines

Classic vaccines have generally been derived from whole organisms and are either live attenuated or noninfectious inactivated. The advantages and disadvantages of these conventional whole agent products are summarized in Table 100–5. To increase potency and remove nonessential, potentially allergenic proteins, newer vaccines are being developed. Live agents are being modified by genetic deletion or recombination or use of naked nucleic acids. Newer noninfectious vaccines are utilizing subunit fractions of purified agents or synthetic peptides produced by genetic recombination or anti-idiotypes. Table 100–6 compares these newer vaccines.

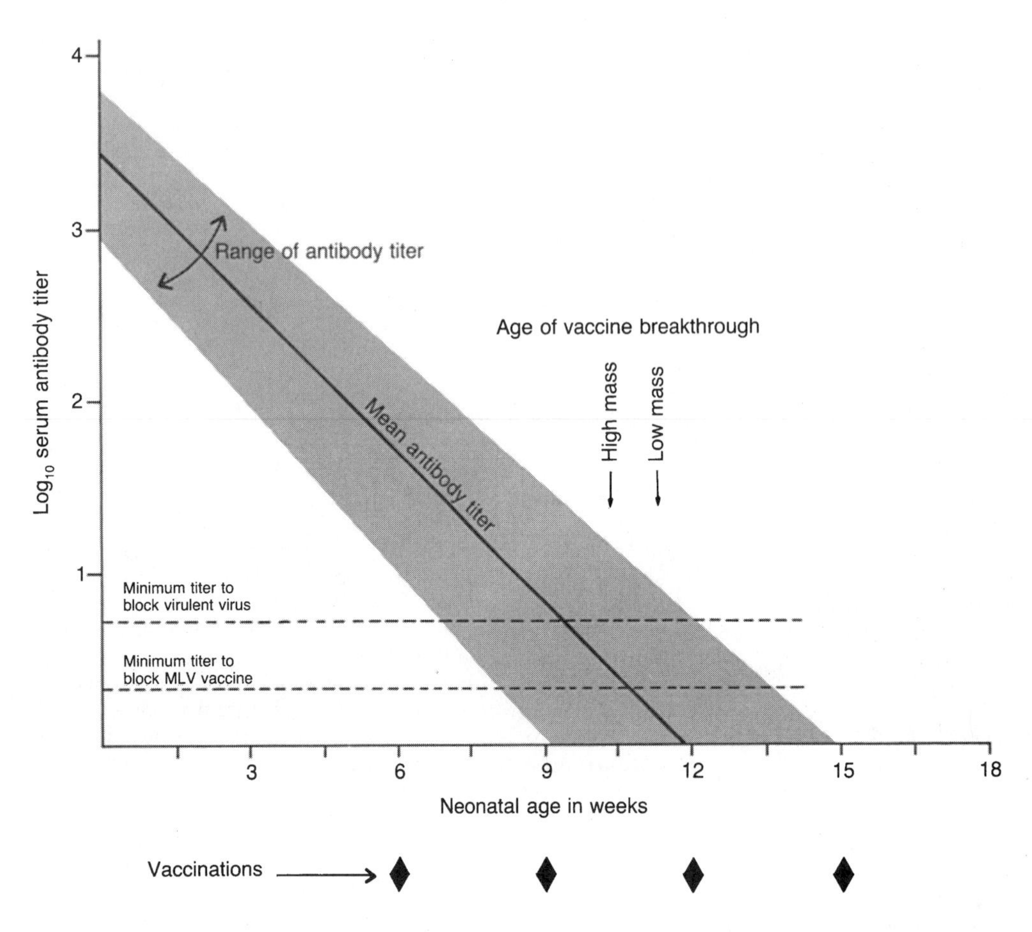

Figure 100–1. Elimination of maternal antibody in the neonate in relation to vaccination. At a critical period, the antibody titer may block a modified live virus (MLV) vaccine but fail to protect against infection with virulent virus. Higher antigen mass or less-attenuated vaccines break through this maternal antibody barrier sooner than lower antigen mass or more attenuated products.

Live

Live whole agents in vaccines must be modified (attenuated) so that they retain immunogenicity and ability to replicate in the intended host but do not produce illness. Attenuated vaccines produce cell-mediated and long-lived humoral immune responses compared with noninfectious (inactivated or purified antigen) vaccines. T-cell stimulation is superior with attenuated products. Because they replicate in the host, initial antigenic content is of low importance; however, any factor that neutralizes or inactivates the vaccine will make it ineffective. Attenuation of agents is usually achieved by adapting them to unusual hosts, by subjecting them to prolonged storage, or by serial passage in tissue culture. Vaccines also have been developed by inoculating only partially attenuated strains of organisms at sites other than those of their tissue tropism. Use of an alternate vaccination site has been used to produce parenteral vaccines against respiratory pathogens. The agents undergo limited replication at the alternative sites, but, unfortunately, they may produce a more systemic than local antibody response.

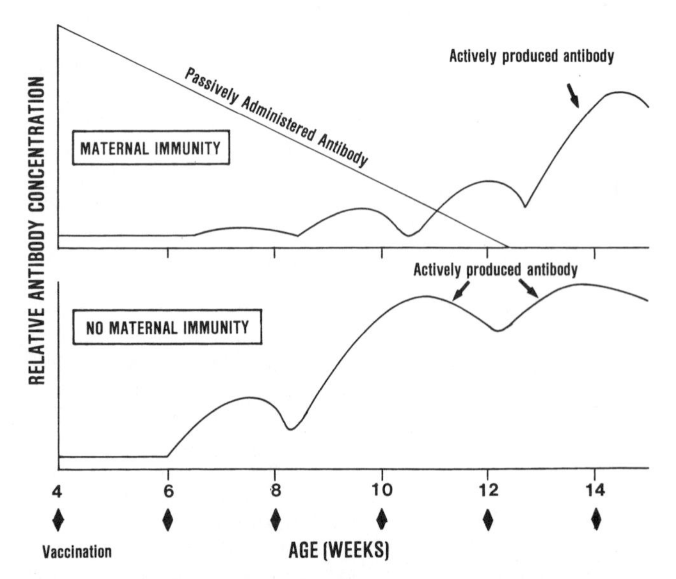

Figure 100–2. Comparison of response to sequential (2-week interval) vaccination in neonates with *(top)* and without *(bottom)* maternal antibody protection. The presence of maternal antibody delays the neonate's ability to produce successful active immunization.

Quality control is an essential factor in biologics production to ensure that cell lines used in attenuating vaccine agents do not contain latent pathogens, especially because veterinary vaccine production usually involves primary and secondary cell cultures (see Adventitious Agents later). Primary cell cultures are those derived from tissues harvested directly from an animal. Secondary cultures originate from further cultivation of primary cell lines. Established (continuous) cell lines that are employed for routine diagnostic virology are usually too anaplastic for vaccine production. Unlike human vaccines, those for animals are usually produced in cell lines of the species for which the vaccine is intended, which increases the risk of contamination with potentially pathogenic, latent, or passenger viruses.

Live vaccines are usually lyophilized, which increases their stability and storage life span. Temperature is another important factor determining storage life span, and vaccines should always be stored refrigerated at 4°C. Commercially prepared live vaccines usually contain excess antigen, because some deterioration is expected.

Genetic deleted recombinant involves removing genetic

Table 100–5. Comparison of Two Main Types of Conventional Whole Agent Vaccines

ADVANTAGES	DISADVANTAGES	INDICATIONS	DISEASES WHERE USED
Modified Live (Attenuated) Vaccine			
Rapid protection Prolonged protection Lower antigen mass needed Can administer by natural route Stimulate secretory antibody Better able to stimulate cell-mediated immunity Can administer locally (intranasal, oral) Better stimulator of interferon Overcome maternal antibody interference Single administration can protect	Risk of adventitious agents Can produce vaccine-induced illness in immunosuppressed hosts Susceptible to inactivation Require more rigorous testing for potency and reversion to virulence Require replication in host Might revert to virulence No preservatives for storage	Outbreaks For production of mucosal immunity Routine vaccination Reduced allergenicity	Canine: Parvoviral enteritis Hepatitis Bordetellosis (intranasal) Parainfluenza Distemper Feline: Panleukopenia Calicivirus Rhinotracheitis Infectious peritonitis (intranasal)
Noninfectious Whole Agent (Inactivated) Vaccine			
No reversion to virulence Increased activity with added adjuvants Stability in storage Safe in immunosuppressed	Primarily stimulates humoral immunity Minimum of two doses needed for maximum protection Increased risk of allergic complications Shorter duration of immunity than modified live vaccines Higher antigen mass needed Restricted to parenteral use Adjuvants frequently required More hypersensitivity reactions (local and systemic)	Pregnant animals Debilitated or immunosuppressed animals Colostrum-deprived neonates (passive immunization preferred)	Canine: Lyme borreliosis Coronaviral enteritis Parvoviral enteritis Hepatitis Bordetellosis (parenteral) Leptospirosis Feline: Panleukopenia Calicivirus Rhinotracheitis Leukemia Canine and feline: Rabies

Table 100–6. Comparison of Newer Types of Vaccines

TYPE	PRODUCTION METHOD	ADVANTAGES/DISADVANTAGES	EXAMPLES
Attenuated (Modified Live)			
Genetic deletion	Selected genome removed to reduce virulence	A: Controlled attenuation D: Only certain organisms can be modified this way; costly to produce	Experimental FHV-1[81]
Recombinant vector	Genomic portion encoding for immunogen of pathogenic organism inserted into an avirulent "vector" organism	A: Stimulate immunity without disease-producing potential; may coexpress immunomodulators or multiple agents simultaneously D: May produce persistent immunopathologic response; may spread environmentally; may produce genetic instability of vector or host; costly to produce; vector can be cytolytic	Oral and parenteral rabies; experimental FIP, panleukopenia, feline leukemia, canine distemper, canine parvovirus infection[33, 126, 153, 155]; Recombitek CDV (Merial) Recombitek-R/F rabies (Merial)
Nucleic acids (DNA, RNA)	Naked genes encoding for antigen inserted into a plasmid carrier	A: Triggers cell-mediated immunity; yields protein antigens in natural form; easy to manufacture D: Potential antinucleic responses; introduces foreign genes into host	Experimental canine distemper
Noninfectious			
Purified subunit	Organism propagated in vitro with purification of selected components; otherwise chemical synthesis of specific immunogenic proteins	A: Purified proteins; less allergenic; no postvaccinal illness D: Works primarily for humoral immune protection; costly to produce	Bordetellosis (cell wall); Leukocell 2-FeLV; leptospirosis (envelope) Duramune; experimental CPV-V_2 protein[84]
Recombinant protein	Desired gene cloned into organism that produces it in vitro, followed by harvesting and purification	A: Highly purified immunogen; higher potency possible D: Primarily stimulates humoral immune protection	Leucogen (Vibrac) Recombitek Lyme (Merial)
Anti-idiotypes	Immunoglobulins produced against antigen-combining sites on immunoglobulin directed against the infectious agent	A: Highly specific immune response; stimulates cell-mediated immunity D: Foreign proteins potentially reactive	None

FHV-1 = feline herpesvirus-1; FIP = feline infectious peritonitis; CDV = canine distemper virus; FeLV = feline leukemia virus; CPV = canine parvovirus.

code for virulence factors while maintaining reproductive function and is the basis for these vaccines. A gene-deleted feline herpesvirus-1 vaccine has been developed experimentally.[81] This method allows for selective attenuation of a variety of infectious agents when existing modified live agent vaccines are effective.

Live agent recombinant vector vaccines use expression vectors, which are organisms in which genetic code has been inserted to produce key immunogenic proteins on a sustained basis after inoculation of the host. Vector systems can also be genetically altered to elicit killer T-cell or cytotoxic T-lymphocyte activity. Multiple genes may be inserted, including those for cytokines such as interleukin (IL)-2, which may enhance the immune response to the simultaneously generated immunogenic proteins.

Expression vectors have included poxvirus, simian virus 40, bovine papillomavirus, adenovirus, and herpesvirus.[8, 174] Bacterial vectors such as *S. typhimurium* and *Mycobacterium bovis* bacille Calmette-Guérin (BCG) can also be utilized. All vectors must be attenuated for the host. Poxviruses such as vaccinia work well because of their large genome and wide host range. One potential problem with recombinant vector vaccines is that the host may mount an immune response to the vector. A recombinant vaccinia virus expressing FeLV gp70 envelope protein was not successful in producing antiviral antibodies in cats.[53] Instead, inoculated cats developed neutralizing antibody against the vaccinia virus. Experimental recombinant vaccinia virus products have been capable of inducing immune responses in dogs to human influenza virus, rabies virus, herpesvirus, and hepatitis virus.[53]

Commercially available oral rabies vaccines with poxviruses as vectors have been employed to protect wildlife. Canary pox has been as an effective vector in vaccines for canine distemper, rabies, and feline leukemia.[153, 155, 156] A canine canary pox–vectored distemper vaccine is commercially available.[115] Pups vaccinated with canary pox–rabies vaccine could be protected at a young age despite the negating influence of maternal antibodies.[155] Parenteral canary pox–FeLV recombinant vaccine, expressing the envelope and gag genes, was protective against oronasal challenge with virulent FeLV.[155] A recombinant baculovirus was utilized to express the VP2 capsid component of canine parvovirus (CPV), and the respective vaccine produced titers in dogs that were higher than those in commercially available inactivated vaccine.[33, 34, 129]

Nucleic acids (RNA and DNA), when inoculated as naked or plasmid-containing molecules containing complete coding, can stimulate production of immunogenic proteins by the host without being permanently incorporated into the host cell genome. Nucleic acid vaccines are stable, resisting extremes in temperature, making their storage and preservation more practical and less expensive. They can be utilized to develop broader antigenic subtypes and induce both humoral and cell-mediated responses. Direct IM inoculation of DNA from pathogenic organisms is a promising method for vaccination against some diseases. Apparently, the injected DNA stimulates long-lasting cytotoxic T cells and variable antibody responses against the immunogens.

Noninfectious

Noninfectious whole agent (inactivated or killed) vaccines are produced in a similar fashion to live vaccines. Because noninfectious vaccines fail to replicate in the host, the antigenic mass present is a critical determinant in the efficacy of a particular product. Inactivated whole-agent products contain agents subjected to various forms of denaturation without destroying their immunogenicity. Heat and light treatments have been relatively ineffective because, in many cases, they destroy immunogenicity without complete inactivation. Chemical inactivation with formalin produces slight modification in antigenic composition of the product, reduction in immunogenicity, and severe irritation to the animal at the site of injection. Ethylenediamine and β-propiolactone are inactivating agents that overcome many of these disadvantages. Having greater antigenic mass and added adjuvants, inactivated vaccines have more of a tendency to produce local and systemic allergic reactions.

In general, noninfectious vaccines must be given at least twice to produce an anamnestic response that equals one attenuated vaccination (Fig. 100–3). Full protection may not develop until 2 to 3 weeks after the last immunization. Despite this shortcoming, immunity that is stimulated by noninfectious products is commonly sufficient for clinical protection and routine use. After vaccination with noninfectious vaccines, many partially protected animals probably become infected when exposed to virulent agents. They develop a mild or subclinical infection that further boosts their immunity to the disease.

Purified subunit vaccines are composed of purified immunogenic components of infectious agents in an attempt to increase the specificity and quantity of the immunogen while reducing its allergenicity. The components are recognized by the host immune system as foreign and elicit an antibody-based immune response. Examples of subunit vaccines are Pfizer Leukocell 2 vaccine for FeLV, which is produced by harvesting cell-free supernatants from cell culture; parenteral lipopolysaccharide (LPS)-extracted cell wall *Bordetella* vaccine; and Fort Dodge Duramune, containing a purified outer membrane protein, leptospiral vaccine.

Recombinant protein vaccines, developed using DNA technology, also allow for in vitro production of large quantities of immunogenic proteins by introducing coding into bacteria, yeasts, and continuous cell lines. These differ from recombinant vectors in that the preformed antigen is produced in large amounts ex vivo and then administered to the animal as a purified component. The FeLV vaccine (Genetivac, Schering-Plough; Leukogen, Virbac) consists of synthetic glycoprotein for FeLV (gp70) subgroup A expressed in *Esche-*

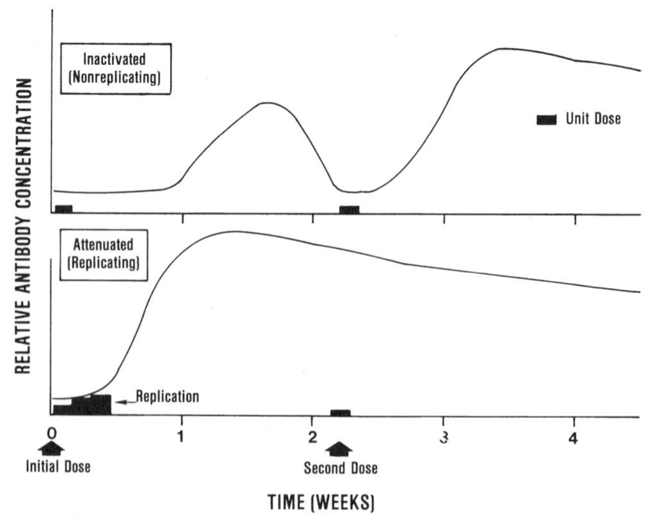

Figure 100–3. Comparison of antibody response after inoculation with noninfectious *(top)* and live attenuated *(bottom)* virus vaccines. One dose of the live attenuated virus vaccine continues to drive the immune response. Two doses of noninfectious vaccine are required to produce a similar effect. Modified from Mims CA: The pathogenesis of infectious disease. Academic Press, 1977, p 225. Used with permission.

richia coli.[102] Recombinant OspA protein vaccine is also available for vaccination of dogs for Lyme borreliosis (RM Recombitek Lyme, Merial, Iselin, NJ). Synthetic antigens can be produced by identifying the antigenic or genetic determinants using monoclonal antibodies. Once the nucleotide and amino acid sequences have been determined, the protein can be synthesized. Unfortunately, many antigenically active peptides by themselves are weak antigens requiring adjuvants. Recombinant subunit protein vaccines have a similar duration of immunity as inactivated whole-agent vaccines, which is shorter than live attenuated products. A synthetic peptide VP2 has been effective in protecting dogs against canine parvovirus-2 infection.[84]

Adjuvants have been added to noninfectious biologics in an attempt to increase their duration and amount of immunostimulation to a level comparable with that of MLVs. Adjuvants are of two types: vehicles and immunomodulating compounds. ***Vehicles*** can be composed of metallic salts, oils, liposomes, emulsions, and immunostimulating complexes (ISCOMs). For a further discussion of liposomes and ISCOMs, see later discussion under Immunotherapy. Vehicles maintain antigen at a specific site and intensify the body's reaction to the antigen. Purified subunit or recombinant products are poorly immunogenic without inclusion of an adjuvant. Emulsified water in oil (Freund's incomplete adjuvant) and mineral gels or metallic salt adjuvants such as aluminum hydroxide, aluminum phosphate, and alum have been used.

Aluminum-based adjuvants are frequently associated with granulomatous reactions at vaccination sites. These reactions have been linked with sarcoma development in cats (see Postvaccinal Complications). The amount of aluminum can vary from 350 ppm for some FeLV vaccines to 800 ppm for some rabies products.[96] Highest levels are contained in rabies vaccines having a 3-year duration of immunity. One-year vaccines have approximately half as much adjuvant, and some 3-year vaccines are sold under separate label as 1-year products. To reduce the amount of adjuvant load, 3-year intervals of vaccination are recommended where legally approved.

Immunomodulators include substances such as muramyl dipeptides, copolymers, and saponins, which stimulate local secretion of cytokines. They may enhance cell-mediated immunity (CMI), provide for slowed antigen degradation and release, and stimulate the function of the mononuclear phagocyte system to produce IL-1. This cytokine stimulates T cells to release IL-2, which in turn potentiates cellular defense mechanisms. Some cytokines have been given directly in an attempt to boost the immune response (see discussion of cytokines, under Immunotherapy).

Saponins are plant-derived extracts that are glycosides with hydrophobic moieties. Quil A (Spikoside, Isotec AB, Sweden) has been given alone and in combination with aluminum hydroxide in a variety of veterinary vaccines. Quil A stimulates both humoral immunity and CMI by enhancing recognition of both soluble and membrane-bound antigens. Quil A is also a component of ISCOMs.

Adjuvants have also been evaluated in stimulating protective immunity at mucosal surfaces.[94] Adjuvants such as cholera toxin β-subunits, muramyl dipeptides, saponins, and phorbol esters have been utilized. Combinations of antigens with these substances produce specific secretory IgA responses.

One disadvantage of adjuvants is that they may evoke local tissue reactions, granulomas, or abscess formations at the site of injection. Systemic manifestations of polyarthritis, uveitis, and autoimmune reaction have been documented in vaccinated people. Another concern is the potential development of vaccine-induced sarcoma (see Postvaccinal Complications).

Anti-idiotypic antibodies are immunoglobulins produced against antigen-combining sites on specific immunoglobulins directed against the infectious agent. The anti-idiotypic antibody actually resembles the antigen itself and stimulates T cells in a manner similar to that of a vaccine. Although veterinary vaccines of this type are only in experimental stages, anti-idiotypic vaccines have the advantages of being produced by genetic manipulation and are safe because they lack the risk of the infectious agents in attenuated vaccines.

Alternative Routes

Secretory IgA, produced by mucosa-associated lymphoid tissue, is effective in local protection against mucosal infection or penetration by infectious agents. Vaccination for respiratory infections in dogs and cats and feline coronaviral (FCoV) disease in cats makes use of this locally protective immune response. Intranasal vaccines are commercially available. Alternate delivery methods are also being considered to reduce side effects of parenteral inoculation, stimulate mucosal immunity, and increase effectiveness.

Microencapsulation involves placing antigens into hydrogels or microspheres to protect orally administered antigens from GI degradation. This approach sustains the antigenic stimulation and allows them to be exposed to the intestinal lymphoid tissues. Biodegradable microspheres are inert synthetic polymers (often poly DL-lactide-Co-glycolide) used to coat antigen and are similar to those used in absorbable suture material. The type and size of the coating determine the duration of the antigenic stimulus. The primary and secondary waves of antigen release can be modified with coatings to simulate repeated vaccination after single-dose administration. Microspheres also have a potential usefulness in oral vaccines where they protect against antigen degradation by gastric acid, allowing the antigens to reach intestinal lymphoid tissues in Peyer's patches. Intraperitoneal administration of adjuvanted vaccines may also have a regional effect on stimulating local intestinal lymphoid tissues.

Vaccine Efficacy

Immunity after vaccination takes several days to develop, but it may last for years. After first-time or primary exposure to an antigen, the initial protection is usually provided by interferon and later by an immunoglobulin response. The primary response is slower in onset than a secondary or an anamnestic response and initially is predominantly composed of IgM (Fig. 100–4). A secondary response that follows re-exposure to the antigen is characterized primarily by IgG.

Fortunately, veterinary vaccines, unlike their human counterparts, can be more extensively tested in the species for which they will be used, and appropriate challenge tests can be performed. The efficacy of a vaccine is determined by subsequently exposing vaccinated and unvaccinated animals to the same challenge dose and measuring the incidence and severity of clinical disease that follows. Both humoral and CMI responses are important in protection from infection. Vaccines have an important role in stimulating both mechanisms. Unfortunately, humoral immune responses have often been measured after vaccination and thus equated with protection of an animal from infection. Some animals may actually be protected even in the absence of a serologic response. The significance of an absolute antibody titer is meaningful only when standardized serologic procedures are used and when this absolute titer is related to titers of protected animals following challenge infections. The correlation between

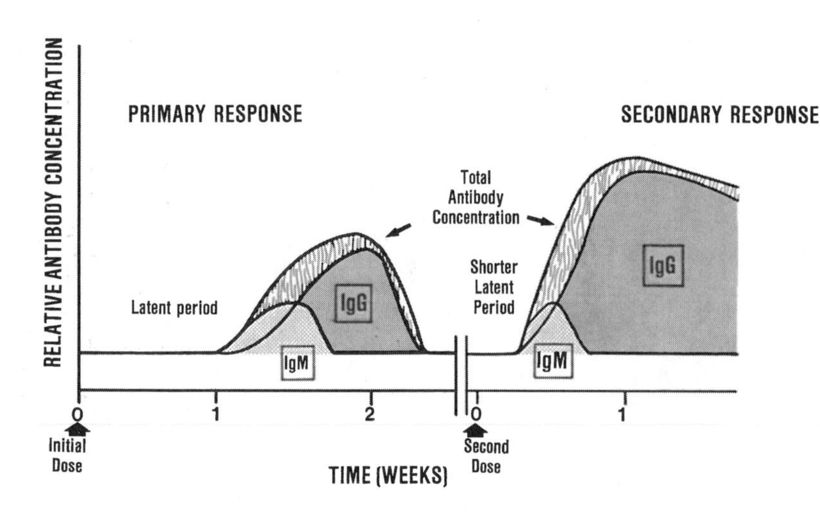

Figure 100–4. Primary and secondary humoral immune responses. Modified from Bellanti JA (ed): Immunology II. WB Saunders, 1978, p 155. Used with permission.

antibody titers and protection from disease is good for self-limiting systemic infections such as CDV and CPV infections and FPV (Table 100–7). Absolute titers may vary among laboratories and methodologies, making interlaboratory comparisons difficult.[54, 146, 160] In contrast, protection against many respiratory and GI mucosal surface infections is based on secretory rather than serum immune responses. Protection against persistent intracellular infections is more dependent on effective CMI. Challenge of the animal with a virulent agent is therefore a more reliable measure of vaccine efficacy. Cellular memory of past exposure to an antigen may persist long after serum antibody titers decline.

The development of tissue culture of viruses has greatly improved both the quality and the means of manufacturing veterinary vaccines. Commercial production, licensing, and marketing of biologics is rigidly controlled by the U.S. Department of Agriculture (USDA), the Ministry of Agriculture in the United Kingdom, the Bureau of Animal Health in Australia, the Department of Agriculture in Canada, and similar bureaus in other countries. Current testing guidelines include duration of immunity, potency, and safety studies. Vaccines are evaluated for safety as demonstrated by tests for sterility, toxicity, and adventitious agents. Efficacy of products marketed in the United States is subsequently confirmed by challenge studies.

Serologic responses are monitored in some instances for extended periods but, unfortunately, do not represent an absolute measure of protection in all types of infectious diseases. Subsequently, vaccines are subjected to field testing by a limited number of practicing veterinarians before they are released for general usage. Many products had been initially marketed without complete knowledge of duration of immunity or adverse side effects. Manufacturers are receptive to reports of complications encountered by practicing veterinarians, and in turn keep the veterinary profession informed of continuing efficacy studies and potential complications. (For a listing of available vaccines and manufacturers in the United States, see Appendix 3.)

Duration of immunity is important in determining the timing for booster vaccinations. Annual revaccination has been traditional. With the exception of rabies vaccines, the duration of immunity of many previously marketed vaccines is not available, because most challenge infections were performed 2 to 3 weeks after the last vaccination in a series. Manufacturers had been under no legal obligation to demonstrate longer duration of immunity. USDA guidelines now require actual duration of immunity challenge studies for vaccines containing "novel" antigens for which no other products are available. Animals are held in isolation for the labeled period and are subsequently challenged or tested for serum antibody titers. Findings of longer term studies must be comparable to challenge studies obtained a few weeks after vaccination.

The efficacy of a vaccine to withstand challenge infection is expressed in terms of **preventable fraction,** which accounts for the proportion of vaccinated animals that do not develop a disease after challenge compared with those that do develop a disease that are not vaccinated. The formula is calculated as follows:

$$\frac{\text{Prevalence (\%) of disease in nonvaccinates} - \text{Prevalence (\%) in vaccinates}}{\text{Prevalence (\%) in nonvaccinates}}$$

Directions given by the manufacturers for handling of vaccines should always be followed accurately because of the labile and occasionally harmful nature of biologic products and the liability risk to the veterinarian. If lyophilized products are used, vaccines should always be mixed with the diluents provided. Serial numbers of vaccines and sites of vaccination should be entered in medical records to assist in tracing vaccine breaks or vaccine-induced illnesses. Some veterinarians split doses of vaccine for smaller animals to reduce proportionally the amount of extraneous proteins that might cause allergic reactions (see discussion of type I immunologic complications, postvaccinal reactions). Although reducing antigen by 50% of the original amount is probably

Table 100–7. Classification of Canine and Feline Infectious Diseases by Protective Immune Response

TYPE OF INFECTION	EXAMPLES	PROTECTIVE MOIETY
Systemic spread, self-limiting	Canine and feline parvoviral infections; infectious canine hepatitis; canine distemper	Serum antibody
Mucosal	Canine and feline coronaviral infections; canine parainfluenza; feline rhinotracheitis and caliciviral infections	Secretory IgA
Persistent intracellular	Canine ehrlichiosis and brucellosis; feline leukemia and immunodeficiency virus infections	Cell-mediated immunity (antibody nonprotective)

inconsequential, this practice voids implicit warranties of the manufacturer and shifts the liability to the veterinarian should a break in protection occur. The only recognized reduction in vaccine dose that has been recommended is in the intranasal-intraocular vaccination of neonatal kittens for upper respiratory tract disease. Here a few drops are administered in the nostrils and eyes of each kitten rather than giving an entire dose.

Commercial production of combined vaccines has made vaccine protocols less expensive and more convenient for both the veterinary profession and pet owners, increasing the likelihood that animals will be properly vaccinated. Interference testing, required for licensing, helps assure the veterinarian that antigens in multivalent products will produce immunity equal to individual antigens administered separately without risk of complications. Separate vaccine products may result in exposure to more extraneous proteins and allergenic components than the same antigens in combination. When individual vaccines were combined and given SC at one site, the antibody responses were inferior compared with the responses when antigens were given at separate sites.[28] For this reason, only licensed combination products (which have been screened for compatibility) should be administered, and multiple vaccines given at the same time should be given at *separate* sites. Different products should *never* be mixed to produce combination vaccines. As a general guideline, veterinarians should administer as few antigens as they believe necessary by profiling patients and giving those antigens as multivalent products when possible. The only disadvantage is that more than one multivalent combination vaccine may be needed in inventory.

Vaccination Failures

The many causes of vaccination failure in dogs and cats are summarized in Table 100–8. A few of the more pertinent features are discussed in this section. Veterinarians should realize the difference between vaccination and immunization. Not all vaccines will effectively immunize those patients to which they are given because of inherent host factors, difficulties with the vaccine, or errors made in the process of administration. Vaccination in the presence of **maternal antibody** is the most common cause of vaccine interference in young animals and has been discussed previously.

Cytotoxic agents or **glucocorticoids** may be associated with a decreased response to vaccination, depending on the dosage and duration of treatment. When glucocorticoids are given long-term, alternate-day therapy is less likely to cause immunosuppression. Although glucocorticoids are less likely to interfere with booster vaccinations, they are not recommended when the primary immune response to a particular antigen is being elicited. Moderate dosages of prednisolone were administered to previously unvaccinated 13-week-old puppies for a 3-week period before vaccination for CDV.[53] Dosages of 1 or 10 mg/kg were given every 12 hours for the first week, once daily for the second week, followed by alternate-day therapy for the last week. The dogs were challenged with virulent virus 3 days after vaccination. Although in vitro lymphocyte stimulation testing showed a depressed response compared with that in control dogs, all vaccinated puppies receiving glucocorticoid therapy were immune to challenge.

Antibody responses to measles and CDV vaccination have also been studied in dogs more severely immunosuppressed with concurrent methotrexate and antithymocyte sera.[53] Dogs immunosuppressed before CDV vaccination developed vaccine-induced systemic illness and encephalitis and died. Dogs immunosuppressed after CDV vaccination and later challenged with virulent CDV resisted challenge, but they had no increase in neutralizing antibody titer.

Dexamethasone, at a daily dosage of 0.25 mg/kg (equivalent to 1.25 mg/kg prednisolone), was given to dogs before and after their first vaccination with rabies vaccine.[53] There was no decrease in the serum antibody titer of treated compared with untreated animals.

Changes in **body temperature** may influence the immune response. Elevated rectal temperature, artificially induced by high environmental temperature and humidity, has been shown to inhibit the serologic response of 8- to 12-week-old puppies to canine distemper vaccination. Puppies with elevated rectal temperatures (≥39.8°C [103.6°F]) that were kept under these conditions developed clinical illness after subsequent challenge with virulent CDV, whereas those with lower rectal temperatures were protected.[53] The serologic response after vaccination for infectious canine hepatitis (ICH) was not affected by these conditions. Hypothermia is also known to decrease the measured in vitro CMI response of dogs, and probably cats, to vaccination.[53]

There are a few reports of the effects of **anesthesia** and surgery on concurrent vaccination. General anesthesia or surgery causes a suppression of the response in lymphocyte stimulation testing, but the clinical significance of such results is probably minimal and the serologic response is unaffected.[53] Vaccination before and after surgery had no effect on the humoral or CMI vaccine response to CDV or CPV-2 in dogs and did not predispose them to vaccine-induced illness.[108]

Inactivation of **modified live vaccine** is less commonly a cause of vaccine failure because of the current manufacture and lyophilization of vaccines, refrigerated storage, and utilization of heat-sterilized disposable syringes rather than chemically disinfected syringes. Vaccines must be handled according to label directions. Vaccines should always be

Table 100–8. Causes of Vaccination Failure

HOST FACTORS	VACCINE FACTORS	HUMAN ERROR
Immunodeficiencies	Rendered noninfectious during handling	Improper mixing of products
Maternal antibody interference	Improper storage	Exposed at time of vaccination
Age: very young or very old	Vaccines do not protect 100% of population (biologic variation)	Concurrent use of antimicrobials or immunosuppressive drugs
Pregnancy	Disinfectant used on needles and syringes	Simultaneous use of antisera
Stress, concurrent illness	Wrong strain	Too frequent administration (<2-week interval)
Pyrexia, hypothermia	Excessive attenuation	Disinfection of skin?
Incubating disease at time of vaccination	Overwhelming exposure	Wrong route of administration
Drugs: cytotoxic, glucocorticoids		Delay between vaccines in initial series
Anesthesia?		Omit booster vaccination
Hormonal fluctuations		
General debilitation, malnutrition		

? = uncertain.

stored at the manufacturer's recommended temperature away from UV light. They should be reconstituted only with the supplied diluent and should be administered soon after reconstitution. Most vaccines have adequate particle numbers to overcome possible reductions in antigen mass or organism numbers that occur during handling and storage.

Vaccination does not equal immunization. Even with all factors taken into consideration, no vaccine produces immunity in 100% of the population to which it is administered. Compared with the degree of severity of illness in unvaccinated animals, some licensed vaccines may reduce severity of clinical disease or the number of ill animals after challenge infection rather than provide complete protection. Even with vaccines that are highly protective, biologic variation is responsible for vaccine breaks in a low percentage of vaccinates. Protection of 70% of the population may be effective in reducing the prevalence of diseases when communicability is low, such as has occurred with rabies; however, it is unacceptable in preventing rapidly transmitted diseases such as canine parvoviral enteritis. Depending on the disease, the acceptable efficacy of protection allowed for most vaccines is between 65% and 95%, meaning a certain percentage of animals will be unprotected in any vaccinated population. Unfortunately, from an individual animal standpoint, one vaccine break constitutes a failure.

Veterinarians are often blamed for animals developing disease after apparently adequate vaccinations. It is possible that the animal was incubating the disease before vaccination. Puppies and kittens from animal shelters are often exposed to high levels of pathogens before vaccination. Other factors, however, are under direct control of the veterinarian. Many of these vaccine breaks may be caused by inattention to precautions that should have been taken during the vaccination procedure. Dogs and cats may contact pathogenic agents, such as parvoviruses, for the first time when they enter the veterinary hospital for vaccination. This may occur in the hospital waiting room or ward area because of improper traffic flow or inadequate disinfection or isolation procedures for already infected animals. Vaccination of animals with existing mild illness or immunodeficiencies may not be contraindicated. In such situations, inactivated or other noninfectious products are recommended. For further information, see later discussion of Postvaccinal Complications, vaccine-induced illnesses, and Chapter 95 concerning immunodeficiency disorders.

Vaccine **interference** can occur whenever attenuated antigens are administered at too frequent an interval. It is better to administer several attenuated vaccines simultaneously than to give them 1 to 4 days apart because of the blocking effect that the first vaccine may have on the second. This interference may be related, in part, to the production of interferon by infected cells. Whenever possible, modified live vaccines should not be administered in the presence of other infectious diseases for this reason. Postponement of vaccinations for at least 2 to 3 weeks after illness or before sequential vaccinations with the same or a different product has been shown to be sufficient to overcome this interference. Animals with pre-existing fever, debilitation, or multisystemic illness should not be vaccinated because immunization may fail and vaccine-induced illness or further immunosuppression is possible. Some have suggested that immunosuppression occurs with use of vaccine strains of CPV-2 because they induce lymphopenia, lymphocyte depletion, and suppressed lymphocyte stimulation responses to mitogen, but these responses are likely just a reflection of the expected response to a live agent.

Delayed completion of a primary vaccination series is another potential for vaccination failures. Many times this is beyond veterinary control because of poor client compliance or client relocation. Under such circumstances, delays of longer than 2 to 3 months between initial vaccination should be corrected by at least two vaccines, given 2 to 3 weeks apart, even if animals are beyond the age of maternal antibody interference. Should the brand or formulation (recombinant vs. inactivated vs. attenuated) of vaccine be significantly different or should the vaccination status be unknown or uncertain, a similar protocol of two vaccinations can be followed. Multivalent combination products are recommended in these older animals receiving their primary vaccination series with respect to complications, and simplicity will, one hopes, ensure client compliance for the return visit. Some veterinarians prefer to administer rabies vaccine on the second visit to ensure further compliance.

In some circumstances, the **route** of vaccination is also critical in maximizing the immune response because MLV rabies vaccines, feline respiratory vaccines, and measles vaccines are more effective when given IM rather than SC. For MLV rabies vaccines (which have been discontinued in most countries), this discrepancy may be explained by the fact that vaccine virus replicates better in innervated muscle as opposed to less innervated subcutaneous tissue. For other products, the difference may be related to greater blood supply or better tissue environment. Unfortunately, IM, versus SC, vaccination is more painful and is associated with a higher risk of postvaccinal type I immunologic reactions (see Postvaccinal Complications later).

VACCINATION RECOMMENDATIONS FOR SPECIFIC DISEASES

The diseases to be discussed are those for which vaccines are commercially available to small animal practitioners. Specific chapters on each disease should be consulted for additional information. Overall recommendations for canine and feline initial immunization protocols are summarized in Appendices 1 and 2, respectively. Appendix 3 lists veterinary biologics available in many countries.

Canine Vaccination Recommendations

See also Appendices 1 and 3.

Canine Distemper. (Also see Prevention, Chapter 3.) In the past, only MLV vaccines have been effective in protecting dogs against CDV. Distemper vaccination is presently performed in combination with other antigens at 3- to 4-week intervals, beginning at 5 to 8 weeks of age. Most currently used vaccines are able to break through maternal immunity by the time the animal is 12 weeks old. Colostrum-deprived puppies should be vaccinated with distemper vaccine beginning at 2 to 3 weeks of age with less virulent products.

Measles vaccination, alone and in combination with that for distemper, has been recommended in the first vaccination given to puppies between 6 and 9 weeks of age. It creates a heterotypic immune response in the presence of a high concentration of maternally derived distemper antibody, at a time when vaccination with MLV distemper vaccine would fail. Six-week-old pups may respond to measles antigen, whereas only 50% may respond to CDV antigen. Measles virus does not typically produce as strong a humoral response to virulent CDV as does homologous vaccine virus. Distemper antigen has been combined with measles by some vaccine manufacturers with the assumption that it would produce a superior homotypic response in those puppies whose maternal immunity is weak. Measles vaccines should never be given to bitches older than 12 weeks. It is usually not recommended after 9 weeks of age. Maternal antibodies to measles antigen, present in bitches' colostrum if they are bred and have a litter after the first heat, will interfere with the effectiveness of measles vaccine subsequently given to the pups. Furthermore, by 12 weeks of age, maternal immunity will have waned sufficiently that distemper vaccine alone should be effective.

Immunity to distemper in a previously unvaccinated, unexposed dog lasts for 10 months when only one CDV vaccine is given or when a distemper-measles vaccine is followed by one distemper vaccine. To ensure protection until a yearly booster is given, at least two vaccinations with CDV antigen should follow in the puppy vaccination series whenever measles or combined distemper-measles antigens are given as the first vaccine. At least two vaccinations with CDV vaccine should also be given, 3 to 4 weeks apart, whenever dogs older than 12 weeks are presented for their first vaccination. Vaccination of dogs with MLV CDV vaccine IV may be effective in preventing disease when it is given within 3 to 4 days after initial exposure to virulent distemper virus (see Prevention, Chapter 3). Dogs should be given one MLV vaccination booster whenever such exposure occurs, regardless of their vaccination history. In general, boosters could be given alternate years or every third year when exposure is low. With less protective vaccine strains, immunity may wane with time in dogs that do not receive periodic boosters.[80a]

Distemper is a disease that can develop from virulent virus infection after stress, concurrent illness, or immunosuppression of currently vaccinated dogs. Attenuated distemper vaccines give the strongest immunity and long-term protection; unfortunately, these vaccines have the greatest risk of producing disease of any canine biologic. Distemper vaccine–induced illness, also termed inclusion body polioencephalitis, usually occurs 7 to 15 days after vaccination and develops in immunosuppressed dogs or with particular lots or strains of vaccine (see Chapter 3 and Postvaccinal Complications later). The illness may be caused by a nonproductive CDV infection of neurons by vaccine virus.[110] As a result, it usually affects gray matter in the diencephalon, mesencephalon, and medulla oblongata, although cortical and spinal cord involvement has been observed.[24] Systemic signs are uncommon. Unlike conventional CDV infections, the CNS progression may subside, and dogs may survive with clinical improvement or residual neurologic deficits.[24] The Snyder Hill and Rockborn strains produce the strongest immunity but have the greatest risk of producing postvaccinal disease. Care must be taken, therefore, not to vaccinate dogs against distemper, especially neonates younger than 3 months that have a known or suspected parvoviral infection or other immunodeficiency (see Prevention, Chapters 3 and 8).

A recombinant canary pox–vectored distemper vaccine expressing H and F antigens (see Chapter 3) is available (Recombitek CDV, Merial, Iselin, NJ) that is safe for immunocompromised pups and wild carnivores.[115, 147] Because the duration of long-term immunity is uncertain with noninfectious vaccines, yearly boosters might be recommended with this product. For a summary of strains of CDV in canine vaccines, see Table 100–9. Measles vaccine might be administered in lieu of distemper vaccine under such circumstances because it is less likely to produce vaccine-induced encephalitis. There has been some concern that poor immunity in some dogs after vaccination may be caused by genetic diversity of the field isolates and the vaccine strains. Although differences were found in the naturally occurring strains,[10] cross-protection studies have not been evaluated.

Infectious Canine Hepatitis. (Also see Chapter 4.) Vaccination for ICH is usually performed in combination with that for distemper and other diseases, beginning at 6 to 9 weeks of age. Modified live adenovirus vaccines are generally used in the United States because of their ability to produce a superior immune response. Vaccination for ICH has brought about a marked reduction in the prevalence of this disease that was once widespread. Outbreaks or isolated cases still occur when vaccination of puppies is delayed or incomplete. The shedding of modified viruses and viral stability outside the host have been responsible for inadvertent immunization of many dogs. Vaccines for ICH contain either homologous canine adenovirus (CAV)-1 or a closely related respiratory isolate, CAV-2. CAV-1 is shed in the urine and CAV-2 in upper respiratory tract secretions; however, the amount that is shed varies between individual products. Another side effect of MLV CAV-1 vaccine is its ability to produce anterior uveitis (blue eye) in a small percentage of dogs. The prevalence of this complication can be increased if the vaccine is inadvertently given IV. CAV-2 vaccines do not frequently cause this potential complication. Intranasal CAV-2 vaccines can protect puppies, despite maternal antibody interference, by stimulating local immune responses.

Adjuvanted inactivated CAV-1 and CAV-2 vaccines have been provided more commonly in the United Kingdom. Although inactivated vaccines produce a lesser serologic response, they are not shed by the host and do not produce uveitis. A booster dose must be given annually, whereas in many cases the MLV products produce more lasting immunity. Inadvertent exposure to virulent virus may provide longer duration of protection to dogs given noninfectious vaccines.

Canine Infectious Tracheobronchitis. (Also see Prevention, Chapter 6.) Infectious tracheobronchitis, or kennel cough, is incited by a number of respiratory pathogens with variable degrees of virulence and immunogenicity. They can infect dogs alone and in combination. MLV CDV and CAV-2 viruses, both of which can cause respiratory tract infections, are included in routine parenteral vaccines, and CAV-2 is

Table 100–9. Distemper Viral Strains in Commercially Available Vaccines[a]

STRAIN	BRAND	MANUFACTURER	IMMUNITY	RISK OF POSTVACCINAL DISEASE
Rockborn MLV	Duramune	Fort Dodge	+ + +	+ +
	Commander	BioCor		
Snyder Hill MLV	Vanguard	Pfizer	+ + +	+ +
Onderstepoort MLV	Progard	Intervet	+ +	+
	Galaxy	Schering-Plough		
Recombinant vector	Recombitek CDV	Merial	+ +	–

[a]Refer to Appendix 3 for additional information on these vaccines and manufacturers.
+ + + = more protective; + + = protective or possible; + = low likelihood; – = does not occur; MLV = modified live virus.

available in some intranasal vaccines. Modified live parainfluenza virus and *Bordetella bronchiseptica* bacterin may be added in parenteral combinations; however, herpesvirus- and reovirus-containing products are not available. The duration of immunity produced by respiratory vaccines against most primary respiratory pathogens, such as parainfluenza virus and *Bordetella,* has not been well established. Serum antibody titers that last for relatively long periods after parenteral vaccination with these antigens have little role in providing protection against infections of the respiratory or other mucosal surfaces. Secretory antibody and other local immune mechanisms are more important. Vaccination with parenteral products can begin at 6 weeks of age and is safe for pregnant animals. It is recommended that animals receive at least two doses 2 to 4 weeks apart.

Parenteral canine respiratory vaccines usually do not produce protection until 2 to 3 weeks after the second vaccination. Originally, parenterally administered *Bordetella* bacterins contained LPS, which produced fever, swelling, pain, or abscess formation at the site of injection. Newer parenteral products have modified whole cell or purified cell wall components that obviate these side effects. Some reduction in efficacy and duration of immunity has been associated with the purification process. Despite this disadvantage, they are more convenient to administer parenterally, combined with distemper and parvoviral antigens. Parenteral products can be used for initial vaccination in the puppy series and subsequently in booster vaccinations. Intranasal vaccine may be used prior to anticipated exposure to infection.

Intranasal vaccines, including both modified live parainfluenza virus and *B. bronchiseptica,* have been developed in an attempt to increase the local immune response to vaccination (see Table 6–2 and Appendix 3). Intranasal *Bordetella* vaccine has been shown to protect against clinical illness and to reduce the shedding of organisms after challenge exposure.[53] Most animals were protected against infection by 4 to 14 days after vaccination. Intranasal parainfluenza and *Bordetella* vaccines may protect beginning 72 hours after their administration, so that they can help to prevent illness in an outbreak in a kennel or in pets before hospitalization or boarding. The clinical illness resulting from intranasally administered canine respiratory vaccine is generally mild or unnoticeable compared with that of topically applied feline respiratory vaccines.

Vaccines against canine tracheobronchitis are recommended when an increased risk of respiratory infection is known or suspected. When anticipated, naive dogs initially should be vaccinated with at least two parenteral or one intranasal vaccine at least 10 to 14 days before possible exposure at dog shows, kennels, or veterinary hospitals. With intranasal vaccines, the animal could be vaccinated immediately before exposure as a less desirable but practical alternative. Puppies as young as 2 to 3 weeks can be given intranasal vaccine, because it is not as affected by maternal antibody as parenteral products. Some of the products are also recommended as being safe for pregnant bitches. Annual or more frequent boosters are recommended in animals that are exposed to a high prevalence of tracheobronchitis. Up to 10 months of protection has been demonstrated for some products. Parenteral parainfluenza virus and *Bordetella* vaccines have minimal side effects. Because they are marketed in combination with distemper vaccines, additional intranasal administration for dogs with minimal exposure is not required.

Canine Parvoviral Enteritis. (Also see Prevention, Chapter 8.) Vaccination for canine parvoviral enteritis is an essential part of the vaccination program in dogs. Parvovirus is as contagious as CDV, but it is much more stable in the environment. This means that more than 90% to 95% of dogs in the population may have to be successfully immunized to break the chain or spread of infection. Produced from canine origin CPV-2 isolates, they are available as either inactivated or MLV vaccines (Table 100–10).

In CPV infection as with other diseases, MLV vaccines offer a longer duration of immunity. Although antibody titers may wane earlier with inactivated products, under field conditions, dogs may be partially protected and, when subsequently exposed to virulent virus, may become subclinically infected, which boosts their immunity. Equal protection can be provided by one MLV CPV-2 injection. MLV products also offer relatively better protection against shedding of virulent virus after challenge than do inactivated vaccines. For this reason, older dogs that will be housed with younger suscepti-

Table 100–10. Comparison of Vaccines Available for Canine Parvovirus Infection

VARIABLE	INACTIVATED VIRUS	MODIFIED LIVE VIRUS	
		Conventional	Potentiated
Recommended for use in pregnancy	Yes	No	No
Shedding of vaccine virus	No	Yes	Yes, consistent
Protects contacts of vaccinates	No	Variable	Frequently
Positive test results for fecal vaccine virus	No	3–5 days	5–7 days
Prevents shedding of virulent virus	No	Yes	Yes
Relative magnitude of humoral response	Low	High	High
Relative particle mass of vaccine	High	Low	High
Breakthrough of maternal antibody			
Start vaccinating (weeks)	9	6–9	5–8
Generally protected (weeks)	18–20	16–18	12
Stop vaccination series (weeks)	18–20	16–18	12–16
Stop vaccination in problem breeds[a] (weeks)	16–22	16–22	16
Single dose protects naive dog[b]	No	Yes	Yes
Selected examples of products	Adenomune, Parvocine (BioCor) Durvet Performer (Agri Labs) Vanguard (Pfizer) RXV Vac (RXV)	Parvocine (BioCor) Vanguard (Pfizer) Puppy Protector (Agri Labs) Solo-Jec (Anchor) CPV/LP (Vaccicel)	Commander (BioCor) Progard, Nobivac (Intervet) Vanguard puppy (Pfizer) Canine Parvo XL (Merial) Galaxy (Schering-Plough) Duramune (Fort Dodge)[c]

[a]Rottweiler, Doberman pinscher, American Staffordshire terrier, German shepherd.
[b]Assuming no interference from maternal antibody.
[c]Originally formulated product protects similar to potentiated products.

ble animals should be vaccinated with MLV vaccines. In case of an outbreak, MLV vaccines should always be used. MLV CPV-2 products themselves are consistently shed in the feces of vaccinated dogs, albeit at a lower level than that after natural infection. The amount of fecal shedding, which decreases with attenuation, is of no clinical significance, although accidental exposure of other dogs to vaccine virus with seroconversion may occur. MLV strains shed in the feces can cause weak positive reactions on the fecal parvovirus ELISA tests.

Vaccination for parvovirus might seem indicated earlier than 6 to 8 weeks of age when the prevalence of the disease is high or when puppies are colostrum-deprived. However, only inactivated products are generally recommended in puppies younger than 5 weeks because of potential damage to rapidly dividing cells, such as those in the myocardium. MLV products are also not recommended in immunosuppressed or pregnant dogs. If previously unvaccinated young or immunosuppressed animals are presented, inactivated vaccine or immune sera (see Passive Immunization) should be considered. Experimentally, an intranasal MLV CPV-2 vaccine was given to successfully vaccinate pups with maternal antibody, at a level that is associated with vaccine blockade of parenteral products.[13] However, parenteral vaccination still provides the highest degree of protection against CPV-2 infection. Parenteral products (Progard, Intervet, Millsboro, DE; or Nobivac, Boxmeer, The Netherlands) have been recommended in puppies 4 weeks of age if the parvovirus monovalent product is used. Ideally, bitches should be vaccinated with MLV CPV-2 products at least 2 weeks before breeding. If already pregnant with an uncertain level of antibody, the bitch can be given two doses of inactivated CPV-2 vaccine 3 to 4 weeks apart in the last trimester.

Lack of vaccinations and incomplete vaccination series are important factors in the development of CPV enteritis. Vaccine breaks that occur with a seemingly "good" vaccine schedule in young dogs (<2 years) are probably accounted for by maternal antibody blockade. However, increased virulence of the newer parvoviral isolates may be responsible for more severe illness that has been observed in dogs becoming infected.

Maternal antibody may fall below protective levels, requiring earlier vaccination, in areas of high environmental contamination. Attenuated vaccine strains do not break through maternal immunity as effectively as virulent parvovirus. In the past, manufacturers claimed that their **"conventional"** CPV-2 vaccines would break through maternal immunity as early as 6 weeks of age with one dose. Although it has been difficult to compare parvoviral titers among laboratories, prevaccination titers were low in the litters reported to be protected at such young ages by vaccines. Manufacturers have been able to overcome the susceptibility period when vaccines are ineffective by using more immunogenic strains, raising the virus titer per dose of vaccine, and lowering the serial passage, thus creating **"potentiated"** CPV-2 vaccines (see Table 100–10).[17, 85–87] Regardless of high efficacy of these potentiated products at 12 weeks in laboratory puppies, for puppies in household environments, recommendations are to give a complete series of vaccinations, with doses given every 3 to 4 weeks until pups are 16 weeks old.[103] In contrast, pups born to bitches with high antibody titers or certain breeds of pups may not respond to conventional CPV-2 vaccines until up to 20 weeks of age. The manufacturers are switching to the more effective potentiated products for all of their vaccines. Puppies can then be given their vaccination in the series between 12 and 16 weeks of age. Although these potentiated products are new to the United States and other countries, they have been available in Europe for many years.

Certain breeds appear to be more susceptible to CPV-2 infection; current recommendations dictate that these dogs be vaccinated up to 16 weeks of age. Breeds including Doberman pinschers, American Staffordshire terriers, Rottweilers, and German shepherd dogs are at greater risk for developing infection than are mixed-breed dogs.[68] Certain Rottweilers do not develop a significant titer to CPV vaccines but nevertheless may be protected, and up to 98% experience seroconversion with potentiated vaccines by 12 weeks of age.[67] Rather than being only poorly immunoresponsive to vaccine, Dobermans and Rottweilers may develop severe signs if they do become infected.

Because of the large amount of virus excreted by infected dogs, vaccination alone is inadequate in breaking the parvovirus infection cycle. Pups may be isolated at 4 to 6 weeks from outside exposure. They should be kept away from parks, boarding facilities, other litters, and shows until the vaccination series is complete. Suspected parvovirus-infected dogs that may contaminate waiting rooms and hospital wards should be prevented from coming into contact with susceptible puppies in that environment.

Although combined vaccination with MLV CDV and CPV-2 vaccines has been rumored to cause immunosuppression, more controlled experimental studies have refuted these claims.[53, 120, 121, 152] Despite the safety of combined products, recommendations have been made by some breeders not to use them together for the first vaccinations of puppies younger than 9 to 10 weeks. These same recommendations state that CPV-2 vaccine be administered alone for the first immunization (6 weeks of age), to be followed by subsequent distemper vaccination 3 weeks later (9 weeks of age) or vice versa. Unfortunately, during this 3-week interval, puppies with reduced maternal immune protection will be highly susceptible to infection with either virulent distemper or parvovirus, depending on which is omitted. Another recommendation by breeders has been to give the vaccines alternatively on a weekly basis, although spacing MLV inoculations too closely may cause vaccine interference. In summary, alternating between distemper and parvoviral vaccines in young puppies on a weekly or greater interval is *not* recommended. Measles vaccine alone, or Onderstepoort distemper strain, or recombinant distemper vaccines are recommended as alternatives in the first vaccination of very young puppies (<9 weeks of age) when concurrent virulent parvoviral outbreaks or debilitation is present. This approach will reduce the chance of potential CDV vaccine–induced encephalitis (see Canine Distemper earlier).

Cases of CPV-2 infection in older dogs are uncommon. Older dogs may not require annual boosters for parvovirus; however, polyvalent products are usually given because of convenience. If a dog recovers from CPV-2 infection, it is best to wait 4 weeks before vaccinating it so that the immune response is recovered. Immunity to parvovirus after natural infection is probably lifelong. Because it is never certain that parvoviral infection was responsible, vaccination is always recommended.

A shifting of antigenic determinants and genetic composition of CPV-2 began taking place about 1981 (CPV-2a) and again in 1985 (CPV-2b). Despite marketing claims, cross-protection still exists between the old strains in the vaccine and the new field isolates. Molecular virology has shown that the most common viral type isolated now is 2b. In all instances, there is cross-protection among CPV-2, 2a, and 2b. Similarly, immunodiagnostic tests based on monoclonal antibodies to original isolates are still sensitive in detecting newer strains of virus. Of significance is that CPV-2b can infect and cause clinical illness in cats (see Feline Panleukopenia later and Chapter 10).

CPV-1. The so called "minute virus of canines" can cause illness in very young puppies (see Chapter 8). CPV-1 outbreaks have been associated with neonatal and in utero mortality and may be responsible for diarrhea and reported vaccine breaks in very young puppies. Because the CPV-1 disease looks grossly and histologically like CPV-2 infection, cultural diagnosis is essential to distinguish them. Puppies younger than 6 weeks dying of parvoviral disease should be presumed to have CPV-1 infection because of the general presence of high levels of CPV-2 maternal antibodies in this age group. Because of lack of serologic cross-reactivity, there is currently no vaccine that protects against CPV-1, and immunologic tests for CPV-2 do not detect this virus.

Coronaviral Infection. (Also see Prevention of Coronaviral Infections, Chapter 8.) Canine coronavirus (CCV) generally produces less morbidity and minimal mortality compared with CPV-2; nevertheless, combined infections with CPV-2 and CCV can be more severe than with either infection alone. There may be some justification in vaccinating dogs against CCV as a means of protecting them against severe CPV-2 infections. Vaccination against CCV is recommended when clients desire all possible means of protection against viral diarrhea or in endemic areas. Currently, several products are nationally licensed for protection against CCV infection. Most are canine-origin inactivated virus (A.M. Biotechniques, Fort Dodge, Pfizer, and BioCor), one is a feline-origin inactivated virus (Schering-Plough), and the other is a canine-origin MLV vaccine (Merial) (see Appendix 3).

Inactivated CCV vaccines require at least two doses for adequate protection in the naive animal, and protection may not be complete for 2 to 3 weeks after the last injection. Previously unvaccinated animals may not respond in time during an outbreak. Inactivated vaccines appear to be safe and not to cause interference when given simultaneously with other biologics. The CCV vaccine has been combined with distemper, adenovirus, parainfluenza virus, and parvovirus multivalent products. Combination of *Leptospira* bacterins or potentiated CPV-2 products and inactivated CCV antigen in the same vaccine has caused some difficulties. Increased allergic reactions have been found when CCV adjuvants are present. Manufacturers have had to purify the leptospiral products to remove foreign proteins. There does not appear to be a problem with administering *Leptospira* bacterin at another site at the same time. To avoid potential interactions or if allergic reactions are noted, combined inactivated CCV vaccine and *Leptospira* bacterins can be avoided in puppies between 6 and 9 weeks of age. These products can be administered alone or in combination for the subsequent vaccines in the puppy series. Similarly, if allergic reactions are noted in young puppies given potentiated CPV-2 products, CCV should be delayed. Within time, manufacturers will incorporate the CCV antigen into all of the newer, higher potency parvoviral vaccines. CCV vaccine on a routine basis depends on the cost to the client for this additional protection and the inconvenience to the practitioner of maintaining inventories of separate preparations. Otherwise, routine use of these inactivated CCV vaccines can help reduce the severity of infection, and adverse reactions appear few.

The first MLV vaccine against CCV infection that was approved and released for dogs in the United States was withdrawn soon after its release because of a suspected coronavirus-induced vasculitis similar to feline infectious peritonitis (FIP).[53] Unlike the previously marketed MLV CCV vaccine, the MLV vaccine strain manufactured by Merial produces no neurologic or systemic disease or lesions or fecal shedding.[117]

Manufacturers of CCV vaccines recommend that two vaccines be given 2 to 3 weeks apart, beginning at 6 weeks of age. However, because of the potential maternal antibody interference, puppies completing their vaccination schedule when younger than 12 weeks should be given an additional dose between 12 and 16 weeks. As with many vaccines, immunity studies of only 2 to 3 weeks duration after the second dose are available, but clinical protection may be longer. Protection is not complete in that only a reduction of viral proliferation occurs. Serum and intestinal antibody concentrations, although potentially less conclusive measures of protection, have been evaluated for longer periods. Inactivated vaccines for CCV do not totally prevent infection of exposed dogs but reduce the degree of viral replication throughout the intestinal tract. In contrast, MLV CCV vaccine protects most challenged dogs against clinical signs, intestinal lesions, viral replications, and fecal shedding, with a preventable fraction of 88%.[116] Secretory IgA has been increased in challenged vaccinated animals compared with unvaccinated controls. Because secretory antibody titers are generally short lived—or if a parenteral inactivated product is being used—booster vaccines are recommended yearly or sooner if the need for confirmed protection arises.

Leptospirosis. (Also see Prevention, Chapter 44.) *Leptospira* vaccines for dogs contain inactivated bacterins of *L. canicola* and *L. icterohaemorrhagiae.* Vaccination with these products is not recommended in animals younger than 9 weeks because of the allergenic nature of the vaccines and the suppression of antibody responses to other antigens in puppies vaccinated at 6 weeks for leptospirosis. Anaphylaxis may be noted within 1 hour after the second or third vaccination in puppies given the initial series (see later discussion of type 1 immunologic complications). A prior allergic reaction to a combination booster in any dog is probably enhanced by *Leptospira* bacterin, which should be eliminated or administered cautiously in subsequent vaccinations. Similarly, its use should be avoided in miniature dachshunds, which have a high rate of allergic reactions. Combination of *Leptospira* vaccine with noninfectious adjuvanted vaccines, such as those for CCV disease, increases the risk of anaphylaxis. *Leptospira* bacterin is marketed in a liquid form and is usually used to reconstitute the lyophilized components in combination vaccines. Sterile diluent provided by the manufacturer may be substituted for the *Leptospira* fraction when there is a reason to omit it.

Unfortunately, *Leptospira* bacterins do not produce as high a level or as long a duration of immunity as other agents in canine vaccines. Certain *Leptospira* products would have to be administered two or three times over 2- to 3-week intervals to produce an immunity that might last 6 months. Such protocols of vaccination are impractical under most circumstances, because this vaccination is usually performed in conjunction with routine distemper and hepatitis vaccination. A few manufacturers have products that are claimed to provide protection from challenge for up to 12 to 14 months. Unfortunately, none of the present *Leptospira* vaccines protect against the carrier state, which may develop after exposure to virulent organisms; they only decrease the development of clinical illness. None of the vaccines protect against serovars other than *L. canicola* and *L. icterohaemorrhagiae* that are now known to cause most cases of canine leptospirosis. Some manufacturers are considering adding new serovars to their vaccines. Newer subunit vaccines containing the immunogenic envelope of *Leptospira* are being evaluated to overcome the disadvantages of currently available products. An envelope vaccine is currently found in Duramune from Fort Dodge (see Appendix 3). Leptospiral vaccines have been considered optional by veterinarians in many areas because of the perceived rarity of the disease, short duration of immunity, and risk of postvaccinal hypersensitivity.

Lyme Borreliosis. (See also Prevention, Chapter 45.) Two commercial inactivated whole cell bacterins (Galaxy Lyme, Schering-Plough; LymeVax, Fort Dodge) and one recombinant subunit outer surface protein A vaccine (RM Recombitek, Merial) are available for protection against Lyme borreliosis. Studies by the various manufacturers have shown protection when dogs were challenged at times ranging from 156 to 366 days after the second vaccination. Vaccines protect dogs from spirochetemia and clinical limping episodes after challenge with virulent organisms compared with unvaccinated control dogs. Although the numbers of dogs have been small, these vaccines appear to offer advantages for high-risk dogs (predisposed to tick exposure) in high-prevalence regions. It cannot be recommended for routine vaccination unless dogs are in or travel to endemic regions and spend considerable time outdoors. The vaccine interferes with accurate interpretation of serologic titers for months to years unless immunoblotting is used (see Chapter 45). Concern has been expressed regarding immune-mediated complications such as hypersensitivity reactions or accentuating polyarthritis from Lyme vaccine.[94a] These claims have not been well substantiated and might be less of a concern with recombinant OspA product. Another concern is that the vaccines contain a limited number of strains that may not cross-protect against the known varieties of *Borrelia* species and serovars.

Despite the controversy that exists, Lyme vaccines appear to be effective in challenge studies. Vaccination induces production of bactericidal antibodies against the organism that appear to develop late or not at all in the natural infection. These antibodies interfere with the organism in the attached tick's midgut before it can infect the host (see Chapter 45). Because *B. burgdorferi* is virtually impossible to eradicate from tissues once infection is established,[149] profiled pups determined to be at risk should be vaccinated on two of the later visits in their initial vaccination series. Lyme vaccines are recommended for use beginning at 9 to 12 weeks of age, depending on the product, and primary vaccination consists of two inoculations 3 weeks apart (see Appendix 1). Vaccination of dogs at potential risk should *not* be postponed until booster age.

Babesiosis. A commercial vaccine against *Babesia canis* infection (Pirodog, Merial, Lyon, France) is available in Europe (see Appendix 3 and Chapter 77). An experimental vaccine, using soluble parasite antigens (SPAg) from cell cultures, was effective in eliciting antibody production to SPAg while reducing the degree of anemia that developed in infected dogs as compared with corresponding control dogs.

Rabies Vaccination Recommendations

(Also see Prevention, Chapter 22.) Rabies vaccines have been extremely effective in reducing the prevalence of this disease in dogs. As a result, the incidence of human disease has decreased substantially, whereas the relative incidence of feline rabies has increased. The first vaccines for rabies, derived from nervous tissue of infected animals, evoked severe autoimmune reactions in the CNS. Subsequently, more purified, extraneurally produced MLV vaccines were cultivated in avian embryo and tissue culture media. Unfortunately, certain MLV vaccines produced postvaccinal rabies in dogs and cats (see discussion of postvaccinal encephalomyelitis). Because of this problem, the trend was to switch to the inactivated rabies vaccines. There are no more MLV vaccines currently USDA approved for dogs and cats in the United States. A similar situation exists worldwide (see Appendix 3). The *Compendium of Animal Rabies Vaccines* published by the National Association of State Public Health Veterinarians should be consulted (see Appendix 4).

Inactivated virus vaccines can provide a duration and level of protection comparable with MLV products.[7] To give similar immunity, inactivated rabies vaccines must contain high viral content and adjuvants such as aluminum hydroxide. Combination products containing rabies antigen have been licensed for cats. These modifications may be associated with a greater degree of allergic and neoplastic reactions, especially in cats (see Postvaccinal Complications later).

All MLV rabies vaccines must be given IM at one site in the thigh. MLV requires fixation to nerve endings to be effective and these are more plentiful in muscle compared with subcutaneous tissue. In general, inactivated rabies virus vaccines given IM often give stronger immune responses than those given SC, but the former is associated with more systemic allergic reactions. An avipoxvirus-vectored recombinant rabies vaccine (Recombitek F/R, Merial, Iselin, NJ) will be marketed that should produce few, if any, allergic or neoplastic reactions. Consult the *Compendium* (Appendix 4) for the approval recommendations for the route of administration and duration of protection afforded by particular products.

Both dogs and cats should receive their first rabies vaccine no earlier than 3 months of age. This is frequently given on the last visit of the neonatal vaccination series (Appendices 1 and 2). Subsequent boosters are administered 1 or 3 years later, depending on the age of the animal, the vaccine, and the local public health laws. Animals that receive their first vaccine before 1 year of age should be revaccinated 1 year later for their first booster. Although inactivated vaccines generally require at least two vaccinations in a series to offer full protection, a decision to complete this series at the first booster was made to facilitate pet owner compliance. Thereafter, triennial vaccination is sufficient when the appropriate product is used. Because of the confusion it might cause in diagnosis and management, rabies vaccination is not recommended for wild animals that are kept as pets; however, when needed, only noninfectious or recombinant vector products should be considered.

Feline Vaccination Recommendations

(See also Appendices 2 and 3.)

Feline Panleukopenia. (Also see Prevention, Chapter 10.) Both inactivated virus and MLV vaccines are effective in preventing this disease. In the absence of maternal antibody interference, at least two doses of inactivated vaccine are required in kittens to equal the protection afforded by one dose of MLV vaccine. At least two MLV or three inactivated vaccine doses should be given at 3- to 4-week intervals when kittens are presented for the initial series at 8 to 9 weeks of age. The second MLV vaccine ensures that an anamnestic response will occur if the first vaccine was blocked by maternal antibody, which is usually passed by 12 weeks of age.

Although FPV infection has been considered as a disease of unvaccinated shelter kittens, it has been documented in fading kittens from well-vaccinated pedigree breeding catteries.[1] Virus was detected in the feces by CPV-2 and FPV ELISA tests. Further studies indicated that the virus was FPV and not CPV, and that vaccine breaks were occurring because of exposure of kittens to large amounts of virus in a contaminated environment.

Both parenteral and intranasal vaccines are available. The

intranasal vaccine (Heska, Fort Collins, CO) is combined with the feline respiratory virus components. As with canine parvoviral infection, parenteral vaccination may offer stronger protection than intranasal vaccine because serum rather than secretory antibody titers are more important in defense against systemic viremia. However, intranasal vaccine offers less risk of allergic or neoplastic complications.

Genetic modification of the CPV-2 virus to the CPV-2b strain has been associated with an adaptation of CPV-2b strain to infect cats and produce disease identical to feline panleukopenia (see Chapters 8 and 10 and prior discussion of canine parvoviral infection). Although not documented, potential complications of virus alterations are changes in feline vaccine efficacy or in diagnostic test accuracy.

Both MLV and inactivated virus vaccines are effective when administered as yearly boosters, although one MLV vaccine probably provides longer protection. Antibody titers after vaccination persist for at least 3 to 4 years (see Overvaccination later). After the initial series in kittens and boosters 1 year later, vaccination can be every 3 years to minimize the number of boosters. MLV vaccines would be recommended over inactivated virus products if vaccine breaks are observed. Because of the risk of producing vaccine-induced illness, inactivated virus vaccines are preferred if immunization is warranted in pregnant queens, in severely immunosuppressed (e.g., FIV-infected) or diseased cats, and in kittens younger than 4 weeks. Newborn kittens are immunologically responsive to feline panleukopenia virus by 7 days of age; however, MLV vaccine must be avoided before 4 weeks of age because of its potential for producing cerebellar damage. Colostrum-deprived kittens can receive vaccinations between 2 and 4 weeks of age, but inactivated virus vaccines should be used at this time. Routine parenteral or intranasal vaccination of 4- to 6-week-old kittens is recommended in endemic catteries or shelters to reduce the prevalence of disease. Homologous immune serum can also be administered to provide immediate protection to exposed unvaccinated kittens (see Passive Immunization earlier); however, subsequent vaccination should be delayed for at least 2 weeks.

Feline Respiratory Disease. (Also see Prevention, Chapter 16.) Feline calicivirus (FCV) and herpesvirus (FHV-1 rhinotracheitis virus [FRV]) vaccines are available as MLV and inactivated parenteral and as MLV intranasal products. Intranasal products provide more rapid and superior protection, longer lasting immunity, and better breakthrough of maternal immunity. Parenteral vaccination for respiratory infections produces a slower response to protection, usually requiring at least two vaccines a minimum of 3 to 4 weeks apart. In contrast, intranasal vaccines may provide protection within 48 hours in a susceptible cat, but they may typically produce a high incidence of mild contagious respiratory illness after vaccination.

Despite the improved efficacy, veterinarians dislike the intranasal and conjunctival route of vaccination because of the high prevalence of postvaccinal disease they produce. Intranasal vaccine should therefore not be chosen if the disease is already of low prevalence. Although intranasal vaccine has been recommended for cats that suffer from chronic persistent respiratory infection, there are no studies to document its effectiveness in resolving persistent infections. Parenteral products are less attenuated than intranasal vaccines. When giving parenteral vaccine, care should be taken to prevent accidental oronasal exposure of cats to aerosols or spilled vaccine. Postvaccinal respiratory disease may be more severe with parenteral compared with intranasal products. A recommended method of administering intranasal vaccine to adult cats is to have an assistant raise the muzzle at 45 degrees. One hand of the administrator covers the eyes and the other delivers the vaccine.[10a]

Protection afforded against the development of respiratory diseases is usually incomplete and temporary whether parenteral or intranasal vaccination is administered. Vaccination does not prevent infection or all manifestations of disease. Cats that contract respiratory viruses after vaccination may have milder clinical illness than they would have had without vaccination. Outbreaks have occurred, even in households or catteries where all animals have been vaccinated.[161] Attenuated vaccine strains may colonize the vaccinated cat's respiratory tract in a persistent carrier state.

When respiratory disease is endemic in closely congregated cats, it is likely that kittens will be exposed and become ill early in life before successful immunization can be achieved. Colostric immunity to feline respiratory viruses is thought to last for approximately 6 to 14 weeks, depending on the virus (see Table 100–4). Early vaccination may protect kittens in congregated environments in which respiratory disease is endemic and affects the youngest animals. Intranasal vaccines can break through maternal immunity earlier because of the reduced importance of serum antibodies to protection against infection or inactivation of vaccine virus on the respiratory mucosa. Early vaccination, before weaning, between 4 and 6 weeks of age with intranasal or parenteral vaccines, may be beneficial in controlling endemic respiratory disease in problem catteries. When outbreaks occur at an earlier age, small doses of intranasal vaccine to 2- to 4-week-old kittens have been recommended.

Parenteral feline respiratory vaccines given during gestation were more beneficial than before conception in protecting against outbreaks of respiratory disease in kittens.[69] Although MLV and inactivated virus vaccines were administered in this study, the latter type is recommended. Kittens born to queens vaccinated during gestation had reduced morbidity and mortality from respiratory infections without any adverse effects on reproductive performance. When it is impossible to vaccinate queens during pregnancy, the interval between vaccination of the queen and conception should be as short as possible.

A recombinant strain of FHV-1 with virulence genes deleted was developed experimentally.[81] Recombinant vaccine produced mild clinical signs when given oronasally compared with a commercially available FHV-1 vaccine, which produced typical clinical respiratory illness. When given SC, the recombinant vaccine was less effective than the commercial product in reducing signs of clinical illness after virulent challenge. Oronasal recombinant vaccine also reduced virus shedding after virulent challenge.

Parenteral inactivated respiratory virus vaccines are safe for debilitated cats, in kittens younger than 4 weeks that have been deprived of colostrum, and in pregnant queens, although protection is generally weaker than that provided by MLV products. With these exceptions, MLV vaccines should always be used to protect cats in case of an outbreak. Intranasal vaccine may be preferred. Because they contain adjuvants, inactivated virus vaccines have a greater risk of producing allergic or neoplastic complications so that the frequency of their utilization as boosters should be reduced (see Postvaccinal Complications later). Because chronic ulcerative gingivostomatitis appears to be a hypersensitivity reaction to persistent caliciviral carriage, repeated booster vaccination against respiratory viruses is not recommended in affected cats.

Chlamydial vaccines are available as MLV products for parenteral administration. Routine vaccination is not essential because of the relatively lower prevalence of infection and milder clinical illness produced by *Chlamydia* compared with the viruses. Vaccines offer some degree of protection against clinical illness caused by *C. psittaci,* but immunity is not complete; exposed vaccinated cats develop milder clinical illness than unvaccinated cats. Maternal antibody interference does not appear to be important with this vaccine, and no teratogenic effects are known. Kittens can be vaccinated as early as 3 weeks of age when neonatal conjunctivitis is a problem (see Chapter 16). Certain parenteral chlamydial vaccines have been shown to produce protective immunity for 6 months to 1 year. Attenuated chlamydial vaccines have produced postvaccinal fever and malaise, and some have had to be further attenuated. With combination products, vaccination for chlamydiosis, although it is probably not essential, can be accomplished without much additional expense or inconvenience to cat owners. The overall low prevalence of chlamydial respiratory disease, or the potential for postvaccinal reactions, makes these products less essential or desirable on a routine basis. Nevertheless, inclusion of these products provides the potential for more complete protection. Should the disease be endemic, yearly boosters are recommended. A higher prevalence of feline chlamydiosis has been observed in the United Kingdom, justifying routine vaccination. Routine vaccination against all of the feline respiratory diseases is often necessary in cats that are stressed or congregated in catteries, research facilities, and multiple cat households.

Feline Leukemia. (See also Prevention, Chapter 13.) Of the licensed FeLV vaccines, most contain noninfectious whole virus and one is a genetically engineered subunit type. Varying types and quantities of adjuvant are present in each (Table 100–11). The FeLV vaccines currently available are not 100% effective. Challenge studies of the vaccines, completed by their respective manufacturers using specific pathogen-

Table 100–11. Comparison of Commercially Licensed FeLV Vaccines[a]

VARIABLE	LEUCAT/VACSYN	FEL-O-VAX	FEVAXYN	LEUCOGEN/ GENETIVAC[b]	LEUKOCELL-2
Manufacturer	Merial/Synbiotics	Fort Dodge	Schering-Plough (Solvay) Solvay-Duphar	Virbac, Intervet	Pfizer[c] (Norden, SmithKline)
Composition					
Viral subgroups	A, B, C	A	A, B	A	A, B, C
Adjuvant	None	Yes Dual proprietary	Yes Aqueous proprietary	Yes ALOH and Quil A/QS21	Yes ALOH and Quil A
Formulation	Whole virus	All viral antigens	Whole virus	Gp70(p45) env. Ag purified recombinant	Viral subunits from culture supernatant
Propagation	Feline FL-74 cell line	Genetically cloned feline cell line	Tissue culture cell line	Genetically produced in *E. coli* plasmid	FeLV transformed lymphocytes
FOCMA Ab claims	Yes	No	No	No	Yes
Licensing Studies					
Vaccine route	SC	SC	SC, IM	SC	SC
Vaccine strain/ challenge strain	UCD-1[d]/Rickard	61E-A/Rickard	?/Rickard	Jarrett/Jarrett	UCD-1[d]/Rickard
Challenge route	ON, IM	IP	ON	IP	IN
Prechallenge immunosuppression	Yes	Yes	Yes	No	Yes
Latency examined[e]	No	No	Yes	No	Yes
Vaccinates infected	9% (4/44)	9% (8/90)	9% (8/88)	15% (3/20)	28% (7/25)
Controls infected	85% (17/20)	93% (54/58)	82% (18/22)	70% (14/20)	60% (6/10)
Preventable fraction (calculated efficacy)	85–9/85 = 89%	93–9/93 = 90%	82–9/82 = 89%	70–15/70 = 79%	60–28/60 = 53%
Other Studies					
Literature and advertisements[e, f] vaccinated protected	91	91	91	85	>70
Independent studies preventable fraction[e,f]	14–93	85–100	90–100	52–93	5–100
References	71, 90, 119, 141	64, 65, 90, 141	62, 118	22, 71, 92	55, 71, 90, 122, 141, 159
Exposure route	ON, N	ON, IP	ON	IP	N
Latency examined in some studies	Yes	Yes	Yes	?	Yes
Administration					
First, age (wks)	9–10	≥10	≥9	≥8	≥9
Interval to second (wks)	2–3	3–4	3–4	2–3	3–4
Recommended booster	Annual	Annual	Annual	Annual	Annual

[a]Although the vaccines are listed here for comparative purposes, the conditions of testing for licensing and experimental studies have varied between products, making absolute comparisons difficult. For additional information on available vaccines and manufacturers, see Appendix 3.

[b]*Leucogen*® (Virbac Ltd) in countries outside the United States.

[c]Parentheses indicate previously designated manufacturer.

[d]UCD-1 is Kawakami-Theilen strain.

[e]Examining for latency is a more critical assessment of whether a cat is infected. Unfortunately, the time for examining for latency viremia after challenge varies among the studies, making exact comparison of percentages difficult.

[f]Preventable fraction has not been calculated for all of these studies, making exact comparison of percentages difficult.

ALOH = aluminum hydroxide; ON = oronasal; IN = intranasal; IP = intraperitoneal; N = natural exposure; ? = uncertain or not reported; FeLV = feline leukemia virus; FOCMA = antibody to feline oncornavirus cell membrane antigen.

free cats, represent ideal laboratory conditions that may not be met in the field. Many studies involve immunosuppression, which reduces the number of cats needed to demonstrate efficacy by increasing the proportion of viremic cats, but this approach may differ from protection of cats under natural circumstances. Unfortunately, challenge conditions have been variable, and no independent study exists to compare all FeLV vaccines on an equal basis.[145] Manufacturers' licensing studies (see Table 100–11) may represent the best case scenario for measured protection. Laboratory challenge models generally show higher degrees of protection than occur with natural exposure challenge models, and they may explain some of the discrepancies in various vaccine studies conducted between manufacturers and independent researchers. Natural exposure studies involve placing vaccinated and unvaccinated, nonimmunosuppressed control cats directly in an environment with FeLV-positive cats. Despite the challenge method, some degree of protection is induced in vaccinated cats compared with unvaccinated controls. None of the vaccines produces sufficient mucosal protection against transient viremia in challenge exposed cats.

Vaccination for FeLV has some controversial aspects. Questions have arisen about the efficacy, administration, and safety of FeLV vaccines. Some practitioners have resorted to vaccination without testing of clinically healthy cats. This practice may result from the extra amount of time for client education and cost of prevaccination screening for infection. With FeLV antigen testing, a positive result is definitive for infection. Cats that have FeLV-positive test results should *not* be vaccinated because there is *no* benefit in vaccinating already viremic cats. For general guidelines concerning FeLV and FIV testing, see Table 100–12.

FeLV vaccination should be recommended for *all* kittens in their initial vaccine series. Vaccine recommendations are to begin at 8 to 10 weeks of age with a second dose 2 to 4 weeks later (see Table 100–11). Manufacturers recommend annual boosters. Because of potential allergic and neoplastic complications, veterinarians are decreasing the routine administration of these products and their booster frequency. FeLV boosters are optional for older cats, depending on their environmental risk of exposure.

In efficacy studies for FeLV vaccines, challenge has involved glucocorticoid-induced immunosuppression before oronasal exposure to virulent virus so that a high proportion of unvaccinated controls become infected. Results of challenge studies are better indicators of protection than serum antibody titers; however, as with most vaccines, challenge has been done only 2 weeks after the second immunization. Antibody titers to gp70 and feline oncornavirus cell membrane antigen (FOCMA) have been measured as potential alternatives to challenge studies at various intervals. These antibodies seem to be important in protection against viremia (gp70) and tumor development (FOCMA). However, not all antibodies to gp70 measured by ELISA or indirect FA are virus neutralizing. Only virus neutralizing antibodies have been directly correlated with protection against FeLV infection. Although increases in neutralizing and gp70 antibodies after vaccination have been variable, increases in FOCMA antibodies have been more consistent. Still, the relationship of FOCMA antibodies to protection against neoplasia is not absolute. Furthermore, although helpful as a research tool, the measurement of serum antibodies to gp70 or FOCMA is impractical and unnecessary in clinical practice.

PROTECTION AGAINST LATENCY. Cats can harbor FeLV in their cell genome without complete viral expression (see Pathogenesis of FeLV, Chapter 13). Latency appears to be a phase in the course of elimination of infection in viremic cats. Most cats that are only transiently viremic gradually eliminate this latent virus within a 6- to 30-month period. Not all vaccines have been tested for protection against viral latency.[118]

Table 100–12. Recommendations for Testing for FeLV and FIV[a]

FeLV Viremia

1. **When:**
   a. FeLV status of *all* cats of *all* ages desirable
   b. Positive cats should not be vaccinated
   c. Allows disease prevention and elimination
2. **Timing:**
   a. When cat is first acquired and before introduced
   b. If cat has never tested before and is first presented
   c. Maternal antibody in young kittens does not interfere[b]
   d. Before *any* FeLV vaccination
3. **Repeating:**
   a. Positive or equivocal results; if serology results are positive or equivocal
   b. To confirm positive blood, saliva, or tear test results
   c. After two ELISA-positive tests, perform indirect FA
   d. Discordant results: repeat ELISA and indirect FA
   e. Annual retest of high-risk cats, which includes those going outdoors; in open households; in closed households with test-positive cats

FIV Antibody

1. **When:**
   a. Test all cats older than 6 months
2. **Timing:**
   a. When cat is first acquired and before introduction
   b. When newly adopted
   c. Any previously untested cats
   d. After known exposure (2–3 mos for seroconversion)
   e. With unexplained fevers or recurrent infections
3. **Repeating:**
   a. ELISA is screen; indirect FA or immunoblot is more discriminating for positive results
   b. Passively acquired maternal antibody may cause false-positive results in kittens; retest after 6 mos of age
   c. Periodic retesting of at-risk cats recommended for fighting, strays, unexplained wounds, routinely outdoors, mating to unknown male, known positive cat in household

[a]For further information, consult American Association of Feline Practitioners/Academy of Feline Medicine, *Recommendations for Feline Retrovirus Testing* (6808 Academy Parkway East NE, Suite B-1, Albuquerque, NM 87109).[42a]

[b]Less than 10 to 12 weeks old, false-negative results from maternal antibody suppression of viremia might occur, although this is controversial.

FeLV = feline leukemia virus; FIV = feline immunodeficiency virus.

VACCINE SAFETY. Adverse reactions to FeLV vaccines have primarily been of an allergic or a neoplastic nature. They do not cause immunosuppression in uninfected cats or any change in the course of illness of already viremic cats, nor do they appear to activate latent infections. They are noninfectious vaccines and will *not* produce FeLV infection or cause cats to have positive test results. No data exist on the prevalence of allergic reactions, but IM is more likely than SC administration to produce anaphylaxis because of the more rapid absorption of antigen. The amount and composition of adjuvants vary among the products (see Table 100–11 and prior discussion of Adjuvants). Precautions should be taken to limit the number of antigens given simultaneously to cats if such allergic reactions are noted. Limited safety studies have involved these vaccines in exotic cats.

PREVACCINATION TESTING. Only clinically healthy and FeLV-negative cats should be vaccinated. Low-risk groups for infection include cats from single-cat households, FeLV-negative catteries, and isolated environments (see Table 100–12). Whether these individuals should be tested is usually based on the practitioner's decision or advice given to the client and the client's reaction to the cost involved. Testing itself may cost as much or more than the vaccine. Although there is some expense and inconvenience to prevaccination testing of all cats, it is not always comparable to the cost to the client of the complete vaccination series. In this regard, it could be recommended that all cats of all ages be tested for FeLV viremia before vaccination. The ELISA test results can usually be utilized as the criteria for response to vaccine. Vaccines do not seem to benefit ELISA-tested viremic cats; their use under such circumstances would be wasteful and misleading. However, latently infected cats that have negative test results with ELISA may still be able to benefit from vaccination. The FA test for initial vaccination screening may miss some ELISA-positive immune carrier cats that may not benefit from vaccine and may later develop persistent viremia or disease.

Cats can become infected at a very early age or in utero, and the background of their dam is often unknown. Testing of young kittens should be first done at 8 weeks of age or younger, when they are presented for their first vaccinations, although hidden infections may reactivate once maternal antibody has waned at 10 to 12 weeks of age. There is an additional expense to retest kittens at subsequent visits once the vaccination protocol has already been started. If testing is not performed before vaccination, clients become concerned if their already vaccinated cat has a positive test result. Some cats can be latently infected at the time of vaccination but remain undetected by FeLV testing until a later date; however, these cats may benefit from vaccination. The decisions of whether or not and when to vaccinate cats with the currently available products rest with the practitioner. Existing vaccines may boost a cat's immune response against a very harmful viral infection; however, clients should be advised of potential protection breaks that can occur.

If cats are first presented at 8 to 10 weeks of age or older, a prevaccination blood sample can be obtained and the animal can be given the first dose. This saves the client an additional visit. If the test result is negative, the vaccination series can be continued. If the result is positive, the series must be discontinued and a second ELISA test should be performed 4 to 8 weeks later. If the second test result is negative, the cat may be presumed to have recovered from natural infection, and the need for vaccination is optional. If the second result is positive, a FA test should be done. This result will determine whether the bone marrow is infected, because most FA-positive cats have a poor prognosis and remain persistently viremic (see Chapter 13).

NUMBER OF VACCINE DOSES. As with other noninfectious products, antigen mass and repetitive vaccination offer the best assurance of protective response. Cats receiving only one dose of the initial series and not revaccinated within a 3-month period should have the vaccination series started over, although no data are available. Although studies on duration of immunity are not available, subsequent annual revaccination with a single dose is recommended when need for ongoing protection is justified.

VACCINATION OF HIGH-RISK CATS. Multicat households, catteries, and research facilities allow for close contact and, therefore, greater risk that FeLV infection will be spread. Because efficacy of vaccines is never 100% under natural circumstances, clients should be advised not to place FeLV-vaccinated cats in the same environment with viremic cats. Similarly, in established FeLV-free populations, vaccination should not be a substitute for routine FeLV testing and elimination or quarantine of viremic cats. Because of the short period of residence compared with the time and expense to induce protective immunity, vaccination of all cats entering humane shelters may not be justifiable. Testing and removal of all incoming viremic cats may be of more benefit. Studies that have claimed a reduction in FeLV in infected populations in which vaccination is instituted have been misleading. The initial prevalence of infection cannot be accurately compared with subsequent incidence data because vaccination has been coupled with removal of infected cats.

FIP. (See also Chapter 11.) An intranasal product is available for vaccination (Primucell FIP, Pfizer, Exton, PA). The vaccine consists of a temperature-sensitive restricted replicating mutant that produces local secretory antibody and systemic CMI responses to FCoV. The intranasal vaccine produces local protection against viral invasion, a prerequisite to the development of FIP. Previous use of parenteral vaccines caused sensitization of the humoral immune response and acceleration and precipitation of illness in vaccinates compared with controls (antibody-dependent enhancement). The intranasal vaccine causes only a self-limiting infection; because it does not enter the body, it does not cause persistently high antibody titers, which might confuse a diagnosis of active disease. There was initial concern from laboratory studies that high aerosol or intranasal viral challenge doses allowed virulent virus to gain entry into the body despite intranasal vaccination.[138, 140] When such high challenged doses were administered, animals developed antibody-dependent enhancement of disease. In contrast with lower oral challenge doses, which probably correlate with natural exposure rates, the vaccine is protective. In three controlled challenge studies, preventable fractions ranged from 67% to 82%.[52] The perceived low prevalence of disease, prolonged incubation period, and required intranasal administration make the routine use of a vaccine for FIP questionable. However, the vaccine has been shown to be beneficial in controlled studies in which naive animals are vaccinated before entering contaminated catteries.[46a, 123a] Vaccinated animals had a lower subsequent incidence of FIP than unvaccinated animals. Cats having low or no antibody titer at the time of vaccination may benefit while those already infected that have a high FCoV antibody titer or infection may develop FIP despite vaccination.[46a] Vaccination is recommended in cats from environments in which FIP has been diagnosed. In one survey,[9a] owners of less than five breeding cats were more willing to vaccinate their cats as compared with larger professional cat breeders. In addition to vaccination, other husbandry and control measures may be equally if not more important in reducing the prevalence of FIP-related illnesses in such catteries.

Feline Bordetellosis. Similar to canine kennel cough, feline respiratory disease can be caused or complicated by bordetellosis. *B. bronchiseptica* infection is usually associated with pneumonia and systemic manifestations. Outbreaks have been reported in closely congregated catteries. Intranasal live attenuated vaccines, similar to those for dogs, are available for cats in the United States. A purified subunit vaccine is available in some European countries (see Chapter 16 and Appendix 3).

Feline Dermatophytosis. A killed cell wall *Microsporum canis* vaccine (Fel-O-Vax MC-K, Fort Dodge Labs, Fort Dodge, IA) has been licensed as an adjunct to treatment and prevention of *M. canis* infection in cats. When administered to affected cats, clinical lesions and evidence of infection as detected by Wood's lamp fluorescence are reduced. In controlled experimental and clinical trials, vaccination reduces the size and amount of inflammation and the duration of lesions compared with those in unvaccinated cats. The vaccine should not be given to pregnant or immunosuppressed cats. Vaccination by itself will be ineffective in controlling the disease in catteries unless additional adjunctive measures are employed (see Chapter 58). The vaccine may induce a local cutaneous inflammatory reaction characterized by swelling and alopecia in some cats. Organisms and adjuvant may be observed in a biopsy specimen of the lesion. This vaccine is recommended for adult cats as a series of three SC doses with intervals of

12 to 16 and 26 to 30 days between respective doses. It should primarily be given to affected or contact cats when infection has been confirmed. Duration of immunity has not been established.

Feline Bartonellosis. Cats are known reservoirs for *Bartonella* species that cause cat-scratch disease and related illness in people. Experimentally, *B. henselae* vaccines have been protective in some studies (see Chapter 54). Because young kittens are more likely reservoirs for infection, a vaccine for this disease should be included in the primary vaccination series. At least two doses of a noninfectious vaccine product would have to be given at 2- to 3-week intervals.

Feline Giardiasis. An experimental vaccine containing inactivated, adjuvanted *Giardia lamblia* tachyzoites was given to kittens in two doses at a 3-week interval.[112a] Vaccinated animals had greater body weight gain, less diarrhea, and reduced prevalence and quantity of cyst shedding as compared with control unvaccinated kittens.

Feline Toxoplasmosis. An MLV *Toxoplasma gondii* vaccine is being developed as an aid in the prevention of oocyst shedding by cats.[19] It consists of tissue culture–propagated bradyzoites that have been purified. The vaccine is given orally with two doses at 3- to 4-week intervals. The vaccine prevents oocyst shedding after challenge. It appears to be a phenotypically stable mutant, which does not itself produce oocysts (see Chapter 80).

FIV. Experimental vaccines have been developed for FIV infection. Noninfectious whole cell vaccines and purified viral vaccines have shown efficacy. Limited testing against heterologous strains has been performed.[46b] The duration of immune protection has been short lived and difficult to boost.[102a] The existence of multiple virus subtypes and their genetic recombination is one of the significant obstacles to development of an effective vaccine.[159a] As with vaccines for HIV infections, the diverse nature and shifting of antigenic determinants may limit the potential effectiveness of prevention through immunization (see Chapter 14).

OVERVACCINATION

A concern has been raised about too-frequent vaccination of dogs and cats. With current vaccines, a minimum three-injection series of kittens and puppies, ending at 12 and 16 weeks, respectively, can be recommended. One year later, a booster can be given, but subsequent boosters can be given triennially. In a survey of veterinarians and their clients in the United States, more than 96% of the veterinarians recommended annual vaccination for distemper, hepatitis, and parainfluenza and parvovirus infections.[111] Clients of these same veterinarians recognized that their dogs were receiving rabies (86%), distemper (84%), and parvovirus (84%). Fewer realized that antigens for hepatitis (58%), parainfluenza infection (55%), and leptospires (53%) were included. Veterinary opinion, not public pressure, is responsible for the antigenic content and frequency of vaccines given to pets.

A number of concerns exist with regard to routine annual vaccination booster recommendations for dogs and cats.[5, 111] In general, the trend has been to combine all vaccine antigens within a single product. This approach provides convenience for administration but may result in some loss of efficacy from potential interference or increase the amount of adjuvants and foreign proteins that may cause allergic or neoplastic complications. Some vaccines may have short-term ($\leq$1 year) protection, such as those for canine parainfluenza virus, *Bordetella,* and *Leptospira.* With MLV vaccines, others have long-term, possibly lifelong immunity, such as for CPV-2, CDV, and canine adenoviruses. Noninfectious FCV, FHV, and FPV vaccines produce evidence of humoral antibody protection for up to 6 years.[139] Vaccines for FeLV and FIP have an uncertain degree and duration of immunity. Attenuated live FPV vaccines produce long-term and possibly lifelong immunity.

Annual vaccines have been given without question in the past, but now, with the increased incidence of side effects, this policy is being questioned. Overvaccination has been compared with minimal vaccination protocols in greyhound puppies, and no detriment to the immune response was detected by extending vaccination intervals in the latter protocol.[105] On the side of the argument for annual vaccination, pets may be more stressed and exposed to unsanitary conditions in their natural environment than in the research laboratories where challenge studies are performed. Dogs and cats may smell and lick excreta of other animals. Furthermore, it may be impractical, expensive, and inaccurate to serotest pets each year to determine whether boosters are needed rather than to administer them (see Vaccine Efficacy earlier). Annual or periodic vaccination allows for regular clinical examinations for detection and prevention of incipient illnesses. Older dogs and cats have a noticeable decline in their immunity after 10 years of age. A compromise would be to extend booster immunizations every 3 years in adult animals for recommended vaccines in dogs such as distemper, parvovirus, and infectious hepatitis and rabies and in cats for panleukopenia, respiratory viruses, and rabies. Optional vaccines are for feline leukemia, *Chlamydia* infection, FIP, and ringworm in cats and for Lyme borreliosis, coronavirus, and upper respiratory tract infections in dogs. Recommended guidelines for vaccination boosters for dogs and cats with various backgrounds are summarized in Tables 100–13 and 100–14, respectively.

VACCINATION OF EXOTIC CARNIVORES

Many nondomestic carnivores are vaccinated for diseases of dogs and cats with commercially available canine and feline vaccines. Only noninfectious rabies vaccines should be administered. Recombinant vectored vaccines are orally available for wildlife, but the licensing of a parenteral product for exotic pets is uncertain. Susceptibility to canine and feline infections and recommendations for vaccinating wild or exotic carnivores are summarized in Table 100–15. Because of the risk of vaccine-induced infection, there is a concern for vaccinating nondomestic carnivores with MLV CDV vaccine; however, noninfectious whole viral products have been ineffective. Chicken embryo–derived CDV vaccines appear to be safer in this regard for species such as the ferret. Recombinant vectored CDV vaccine has been safe and effective in ferrets.[147]

VACCINATION REQUIREMENTS FOR TRANSPORT OF ANIMALS

Interstate shipment of animals that are affected with or have recently been exposed to infectious diseases is prohibited within the United States. Each state has established guidelines that normally include a physical examination and current rabies vaccination. General information is available in the current regulations of the USDA, Animal Health and Plant Inspection Service; Department of Agriculture in Can-

Table 100–13. Recommended Booster Vaccination for Dogs Based on Their Lifestyles and Habits[a]

CANINE CLASSIFICATION	HABITS	FREQUENCY, BOOSTER TYPE
Outdoor enthusiast	Most of the time outdoors running unrestrained; unsupervised roaming and supervised or unsupervised hunting or fieldwork	Annual: D, H, Pv, L, PI, Bd, R,[b] CCV,[c] Lyme[c] Triennial: R[b]
Outdoor socialite	Some of time outdoors; may contact other strange dogs on a periodic basis	Annual: D, H, Pv, L, PI, Bd,[c] R[b] Optional: CCV,[c] Lyme[c] Triennial: R[b]
Indoor socialite	Multidog household, mostly indoors or confined but frequent contact with other known dogs through feeding, elimination, boarding, showing	Annual: D, H, Pv, L, PI, Bd, CCV[c], R[b] Triennial: R[b] None: Lyme
Indoor elitist	One- or two-dog household. Indoors mostly, but comes into contact with unknown dogs by occasional escape	Triennial: D, H, Pv, R[b] Optional: L, PI, Bd, CCV[c] None: Lyme
Indoor pampered pooch	Strictly indoor, never comes into contact with other dogs; sits in the lap for hours at a time; rarely touches bare earth, a real couch potato.	Triennial: D, H, Pv, R[b] None: L, PI, Bd, CCV, Lyme

[a]An annual booster is given the first year after the primary immunization series of all puppies. Use these guidelines for subsequent boosters. These guidelines could vary based on the animal's source, breed, age, reproductive status, geographic location, boarding and travel, recreational or work use, disease prevalence or past diseases, and particular vaccine efficacy or complications. As an alternative to triennial vaccination, antigens can be separated with some being given each year.

[b]Recommendations will be superseded by local public health laws. Rabies booster can be annual or triennial based on vaccine labeling.

[c]Use of this vaccine also depends on prevalence in a given region.

D = distemper; H = hepatitis (adenovirus-2); Pv = parvovirus infection; L = leptospirosis; PI = parainfluenza; Bd = bordetellosis (canine infections tracheobronchitis); R = rabies; CCV = coronavirus infection.

ada; Bureau of Animal Health in Australia; Ministry of Agriculture in the United Kingdom; and similar bureaus in other countries.

In the European Economic Community (EEC), animals may move between member countries provided they show no signs of disease; are identified by tattoo or microchip; are vaccinated using a World Health Organization–approved vaccine certified by an official veterinarian; and are accompanied by an individual passport clearly identifying the animal.[6]

Amendments have been added to protect the importation of animals into rabies-free areas of the United Kingdom and Ireland. Animals originating outside the EEC need an import license and a minimum of 6 months postimport quarantine in approved premises. From EEC member nations, animals must originate from a registered holding and must have been born and kept in captivity there since birth, with no contact with wildlife. The animals must be identified with a microchip and be vaccinated against rabies at least 6 months before shipping and at an age of at least 12 weeks. After vaccination, an internationally agreed serologic test must demonstrate a protective titer of at least 0.5 IU/ml. If the test is carried out after the first vaccination, it must be between the 1st and 3rd months after vaccination. Further changes in this law are being considered.[4]

POSTVACCINAL COMPLICATIONS

Many immune-mediated and nonimmune complications are severe enough to restrict or eliminate the routine periodic use of particular vaccines. Repeated annual revaccination of

Table 100–14. Recommended Booster Vaccination for Cats Based on Their Lifestyles and Habits[a]

FELINE CLASSIFICATION	HABITS	FREQUENCY, BOOSTER TYPE
Outdoor enthusiast	Most of the time outdoors; frequent contact with strange cats; multicat open household, with new stray or feral cats being admitted	Annual: FHV, C, P, Chlam,[a] R,[b] FeLV,[c] FIP[d] Triennial: R[b]
Outdoor socialite	Some of time outdoors; may contact other strange cats; fewer than 3 other cats in household	Annual: FHV, C, P, R,[b] FeLV Optional: Chlam,[c, d] FIP[c, d]
Indoor socialite	Multicat household, mostly indoors or confined but frequent contact with other known disease-free cats when feeding, eliminating, boarding, showing	Triennial: FHV, C, P, R[b] Optional: Chlam,[d] FeLV,[c, d] FIP[c, d]
Indoor elitist	One- or two-cat household; indoors mostly, but comes into contact with unknown cats by occasional escape	Triennial: FHV, C, P, R[b] Optional: Chlam,[d] R,[b] FeLV,[c, d] FIP[c, d]
Indoor window watcher	Strictly indoor, never comes into contact with other cats; sits in the window for hours at a time	Triennial: FHV, C, P, R[b] None: Chlam, R,[b] FeLV, FIP

[a]Annual booster is given the first year after the primary immunization of all kittens. Use these guidelines for subsequent boosters. These guidelines could vary based on the animal's source, breed, age, reproductive status, geographic location, boarding or hunting and travel, disease prevalence or past diseases, and particular vaccine efficacy or complications. FeLV-infected and FIV-infected cats should only receive noninfectious vaccines. As an alternative to triennial vaccination, antigens can be separated with some being given each year.

[b]Recommendations will be superseded by local public health laws. Rabies booster is given annually or triennially based on vaccine labeling.

[c]Disease prevalence and/or serotesting will determine need for routine use.

[d]Annual vaccination recommended for this optional product.

FHV = feline herpesvirus (feline rhinotracheitis virus [FRV]); C = calicivirus infection; P = panleukopenia; Chlam = chlamydiosis; R = rabies; FeLV = feline leukemia virus infection; FIP = feline infectious peritonitis.

Table 100–15. Vaccination of Families of Terrestrial Carnivores and Their Susceptibility to Infectious Diseases of the Dog and Cat[a]

DISEASE	SUSCEPTIBILITY/WHETHER TO VACCINATE						
	Canidae[b]	Felidae[c]	Procyonidae[d]	Ursidae[e]	Mustelidae[f]	Viverridae[g]	Hyenidae[h]
Canine distemper[i]	+/+	−/−	+/+	+/−	+/−	?/±	+/+
Feline panleukopenia[i]	−/−	+/+	+/+	?/−	+/+	?/±	−/−
Infectious canine hepatitis[i]	+/+	−/−	−/−	+/−	−/−	−/−	?/±
Feline respiratory disease	−/−	+/+	−/−	−/−	−/−	−/−	−/−
Parainfluenza	+/+	+/−	?/?	?/?	?/?	?/?	?/?
Rabies	+/+	+/+	+/+	+/+	+/+	+/+	+/+
Leptospirosis	+/+	+/−	+/±	+/−	+/±	+/±	+/±

[a]For reference sources, see Greene.[53]
[b]Coyote, dingo, domestic dog, jackal, raccoon dog, wolf, red fox, gray fox. Only modified live virus (MLV) chicken tissue culture vaccines or noninfectious or vectored recombinant distemper vaccines should be used on the gray fox.
[c]Cheetah, lion, jaguar, margay, ocelot.
[d]Bassariscus, coati, kinkajou, raccoon, lesser panda. Only noninfectious or vector recombinant distemper vaccines should be used on the lesser panda.
[e]Bears.
[f]Ferret, fisher, grison, marten, mink, otter, sable, skunk, wolverine, badger. Only MLV chicken tissue culture or vectored recombinant vaccines should be used on ferrets.
[g]Binturong, fossa linsang, mongoose, civet.
[h]Hyena.
[i]Noninfectious vaccines are preferred when available.
+ = yes, − = no, ± = optional, ? = uncertain.

veterinary patients cannot always be justified with respect to all the components included in currently available combination products. Veterinarians should be aware of potential complications caused by each vaccine component so that particular antigens can be deleted from subsequent boosters if problems arise. They should consider educating clients, either verbally or in writing, of potential vaccine complications to facilitate early recognition and treatment. For reporting such reactions in the United States, one should contact the USDA's Veterinary Biologic Division Consumer Hotline: (515) 232-5789; in Canada, the Veterinary Biologics and Biotechnology, Agriculture: (613) 952-8000. For a summary of the immunologic and nonimmunologic complications described next, consult Table 100–16. For a summary of preventive measures to avoid vaccine-induced complications, see Table 100–17. For a list of manufacturers to report specific vaccine or drug reactions, see Appendix 3.

Immunologic Complications

Immunologic reactions that can develop after vaccination are those related to either hypersensitivity or autoimmunity.

Table 100–16. Postvaccinal Complications Associated With Canine and Feline Biologics

TYPE OF PROBLEM	MECHANISM OF PRODUCTION	RESPONSIBLE VACCINES
Immunologic		
Type I	Immediate hypersensitivity; allergy, anaphylaxis	*Leptospira* bacterin; inactivated adjuvanted rabies, FeLV and respiratory vaccines
Type II	Cytotoxicity (hypersensitivity or autoimmunity)	
	Hemolytic anemia	MLV parvoviral vaccine
	Thrombocytopenia	MLV distemper vaccine
Type III	Immune complex (hypersensitivity)	
	Uveitis	MLV CAV-1 vaccine
	Generalized serum sickness	Passive immunization
Type IV	Cell-mediated (hypersensitivity or autoimmunity)	
	Granuloma	BCG immunotherapy
	Encephalitis	Nervous tissue–derived rabies vaccine
	Polyradiculoneuritis	Inactivated neonatal mouse brain rabies vaccine
Nonimmunologic		
Local reaction at injection site, cutaneous granulomas or sarcomas (especially cats)	Adjuvants, preservatives, inactivators	Bacterins such as for *Bordetella* and *Leptospira*; inactivated adjuvanted viral vaccines such as for rabies and FeLV
Systemic fever and malaise	Local lymphoid replication of MLV products	Any MLV vaccine
Neurologic complications	Viral	MLV rabies and distemper vaccines
Abortion, infertility, congenital malformation	In utero or early neonatal infection	Any MLV vaccine during pregnancy Parvoviral vaccines during neonatal period
Clinical disease in vaccinates	Incomplete attenuation or local administration of attenuated vaccines	IN vaccines Feline calicivirus, herpesvirus (IN or parenteral product); canine parainfluenza virus (mild) or canine *Bordetella* vaccine (mild)
	Feline limping	MLV caliciviral vaccine
	Polyarthritis in Akitas	Combined MLV or inactivated adjuvanted vaccines
	HOD and juvenile cellulitis	MLV distemper vaccine
Postvaccinal shedding	Virus localization	Canine parvovirus—GI, CAV-1 vaccine—renal, CAV-2 vaccine—respiratory
Postvaccinal encephalitis	Immunosuppressed animal or relatively unattenuated virus enters the nervous system where immune defenses are poor	Canine distemper vaccine, measles vaccine, MLV, rabies vaccine

CAV-1 = canine adenovirus-1 (hepatitis); BCG = bacille Calmette-Guérin; CAV-2 = canine adenovirus-2 (respiratory); MLV = modified live virus; HOD = hypertrophic osteodystrophy; FeLV = feline leukemia virus; IN = intranasal.

Table 100–17. Contraindications to Routine Vaccination of Dogs and Cats

DISEASES OR CONDITION	VACCINES TO AVOID	RECOMMENDED ALTERATIONS
Genetic immunodeficiencies (see Chapter 95): Weimaraners and Akitas	MLV vaccines, especially Rockborn or Snyder Hill CDV	Inactivated or other noninfectious products Onderstepoort or preferably recombinant CDV
Acquired immunodeficiencies (see Chapter 95): FIV, FeLV, cancer, chemotherapy, cytotoxic or myelosuppressive drugs[a]	Modified live vaccines	Inactivated or other noninfectious products
Immune-mediated diseases: uveitis, glomerulitis, polyarthritis, polyradiculoneuritis	Annual vaccination	Triennial rabies and minimize other antigens
Immune-mediated diseases: hemolytic anemia or thrombocytopenia	MLV parvoviral or combination vaccines	Triennial vaccination
Type I hypersensitivity vaccine reaction: Dachshunds	Inactivated, adjuvanted vaccines, IM administration	Modified live vaccines (see text for additional precautions)
Mild or one-system disease, fever	Modified live vaccines	Control disease or use noninfectious vaccines
Pregnancy or lactation	Modified live vaccines	Inactivated or other noninfectious products
Vaccine-induced sarcoma	Inactivated, adjuvanted vaccines	Nonadjuvanted inactivated or noninfectious products, modified live vaccines, triennial vaccination
Chronic feline ulcerative gingivostomatitis and faucitis (see Chapter 84)	Inactivated adjuvanted calicivirus vaccine	Reduce vaccine booster frequency, or use modified live vaccines when necessary

[a]Methotrexate, azathioprine, cyclophosphamide in dogs or cats; or extended use of chloramphenicol, sulfonamides, trimethoprim, dapsone, griseofulvin, or sulfadiazine in cats.
CDV = canine distemper virus; MLV = modified live virus.

They can be classified as types I, II, III, or IV (see Table 100–16).

Type I. Type I reactions involve an interaction with cytophilic IgE and antigen with resultant degranulation of circulating basophils and tissue mast cells releasing large amounts of heparin, chemotactants, prostaglandins, histamines, and biogenic amines into the systemic circulation. Anaphylaxis may occur after the use of any vaccine, although it is most commonly associated with the use of adjuvanted or multivalent products containing large amounts of foreign protein, such as inactivated rabies vaccine, canine coronavirus vaccine, FeLV vaccine, and *Leptospira* bacterin. Foreign proteins, such as fetal bovine serum, utilized in cell culture have also contributed to this problem. With the advent of inactivated and adjuvanted viral vaccines for rabies, feline respiratory disease, FPV, and FeLV infection, an increasing prevalence of type I hypersensitivity reactions has been noted, especially in cats. Miniature Dachshunds also have a disproportionally high reaction rate.

In the dog, signs are facial edema, pruritus, hypotensive shock, weakness, dyspnea, and diarrhea. Within minutes to hours (<24) of vaccination, cats have anaphylaxis, vomiting, and diarrhea. The diarrhea is usually watery but may become hemorrhagic if the diarrhea is severe or persistent. Respiratory distress, manifest by dyspnea and cyanosis, is the most severe reaction. A majority of cats will respond favorably to 0.2 ml IV of 10-fold diluted epinephrine (1:10,000) and systemic glucocorticoids, but those with severe progressive respiratory symptoms or hemoptysis usually die. Even with recovery, diarrhea may persist in some cats for several days thereafter.

Cats show facial pruritus, salivation, dyspnea, collapse, and respiratory distress from acute pulmonary edema. Local or systemic reactions may occur in young puppies within 1 to 24 hours after their second or third vaccination and may result in acute facial edema, vomiting, diarrhea, dyspnea, collapse, or death. Puppies that survive such episodes should not be revaccinated with known allergenic components such as inactivated leptospiral or coronaviral antigens in combined vaccines through the remainder of their initial vaccination series. If they are revaccinated with leptospiral antigen, it should be done only after they are at least 16 weeks of age and then with cautious monitoring immediately after the injection.

If anaphylaxis is a problem with some animals, it is advised to (1) modify the vaccination schedule to reduce the number of antigens given simultaneously; (2) switch to MLV instead of inactivated adjuvanted products; and (3) use SC or intranasal (when available) rather than IM inoculations, which decrease the rate of uptake of the product into the systemic circulation. Aspiration is essential before injecting any parenteral vaccine to determine whether a blood vessel has inadvertently been penetrated. Animals should be vaccinated early during the office visit to allow observation. Clients should also be advised to keep their pets inside for at least 1 hour after arriving home following vaccination. Antihistamines should always be given to those reactors before subsequent vaccinations, and these products can be administered separately to allow identification of the problematic component. Measurement of antibody titers to some infectious agents could determine whether and when revaccination is necessary (see Vaccine Efficacy previously). Pretesting animals by intradermal inoculation of 0.1 ml of the suspected vaccine may also determine immediate hypersensitivity to offending products. The site should be observed for at least 1 hour, and saline and histamine controls should be used for comparison.

Inbred atopic dogs have been shown to develop enhanced antipollen IgE responses when vaccinated with CDV, hepatitis, and leptospirosis vaccines just before, but not after, exposure to pollen extracts.[53] Because of this immunopotentiation, it is recommended that atopic dogs receive their booster vaccinations during nonallergic seasons or disease-free intervals.

Type II. Type II hypersensitivity or autoimmunity resulting in cellular injury has been suspected or reported after MLV vaccination in dogs. This reaction involves binding of antibody with or without complement with subsequent damage to host cells. Autoimmune hemolytic anemia (AIHA) and autoimmune nonregenerative anemias (autoimmunity to erythrocyte precursors) have been suspected to occur after MLV canine parvoviral vaccines in dogs. Affinity of the virus for erythrocytes may be explained by the hemagglutinating properties of the virus and the high antigen mass in some of these vaccines. This phenomenon might also occur after natural infections. One fourth of dogs studied with AIHA had been vaccinated with polyvalent products within 1 month of onset.[40] The dogs with this association had lower platelet counts, increased trend toward intravascular hemolysis and spontaneous microagglutination, and higher mortality than the other affected animals. The vaccine components may have induced autoantibody production or activated the immune system to destroy erythrocytes with pre-existing surface autoantibodies.

Transient thrombocytopenia also was reported after MLV combination vaccines in dogs.[53] Thrombocytopenia, which developed in most vaccinated dogs, was mild (>100,000 and <200,000 platelets/μl) and subclinical. Despite transient thrombocytopenia, no change in platelet function was detected. Whether this form of thrombocytopenia is caused by autoimmune or infectious mechanisms is uncertain. Only those animals with concurrent congenital or acquired bleeding tendencies may be expected to show hemorrhagic tendencies. Veterinarians may want to delay elective surgery on animals with known bleeding tendencies for a 1-week period after vaccination. Severe immune-mediated thrombocytopenia can also occur within 1 to 2 weeks after vaccination of some dogs. These animals have overt petechiae and hemorrhagic tendencies, with platelet counts less than 50,000/μl. Glucocorticoid therapy is usually required for several weeks thereafter to increase the platelet count, and subsequent boosters may have to be avoided or minimized to prevent a recurrence of the problem.

Type III. This hypersensitivity reaction, associated with immune complex formation and deposition, is responsible for the anterior uveitis that occurs in some dogs receiving the MLV CAV-1 vaccine. This local type III, or Arthus, reaction, results from virus-antibody complex formation within the eye (see Pathogenesis, Chapter 4). The process resolves spontaneously unless secondary complications such as glaucoma develop.

Generalized serum sickness is the result of widespread immune complex deposition throughout the walls of the microvasculature of certain structures, such as the renal glomeruli, joints, and uveal tracts. Usually this complication is seen only after the administration of large amounts of hyperimmune serum or globulin. Because passive immunization is used infrequently in dogs and cats, the prevalence of serum sickness is minimal. It has developed in a dog as a complication of *Propionibacterium acnes* immunotherapy.[53] Glomerulonephritis and amyloidosis can result from chronic or repeated antigenic exposure. One example would be vaccine-associated polyarthritis in Akitas (see Postvaccinal Complications later). This is one reason why humans are not given booster doses annually, as is the practice in veterinary medicine. Both amyloidosis and glomerulonephritis have been experimentally produced in animals after desensitization therapy protocols utilizing repeated injections of large quantities of foreign antigen. Although there is concern, neither disease has been attributed to repeated administration of biologics in immunocomponent dogs or cats. For a further discussion of vaccine-induced complications in immunodeficient dogs and cats, see Chapter 95 and Postvaccinal Complications.

Type IV. Cell-mediated, or type IV, hypersensitivity reactions can occur after BCG is used as an immunostimulatory compound (see Immunotherapy later). Large, exuding granulomas may develop at the site of injection. Postvaccinal encephalitis was an allergic reaction that occurred after nervous tissue–derived rabies vaccinations.

POLYRADICULONEURITIS. Known as coonhound paralysis in dogs and Guillain-Barré syndrome in humans, this immune-mediated inflammation of nerve roots has been a complication of a variety of vaccines given to dogs and cats.[53, 133] Coonhound paralysis is a disease caused by a filterable agent to which dogs become exposed after direct contact with raccoons. Although various vaccines can be incriminated, the highest frequency of this complication has been with some lots of suckling mouse brain–derived inactivated rabies vaccines.[53] The CNS of the newborn mouse, normally devoid of myelin, is well adapted to the production of large quantities of rabies virus needed to produce inactivated vaccine. A few older mice were apparently inadvertently used in production of the vaccine, or peripheral or cranial nerve myelin was accidentally included, and this resulted in transient acute lower motor neuron (LMN) paralysis 1 to 2 weeks after vaccination in a proportion of dogs.

This syndrome is similar whether it is caused by a vaccine or raccoon exposure. Rapid and progressive LMN weakness develops usually beginning in the pelvic limbs and progresses forward. Pain sensation remains intact, and animals are hypersensitive to muscle palpation. Cranial motor nerve abnormalities such as facial paralysis may be observed. Animals may have occasional swallowing and breathing difficulties or autonomic dysfunction.

The diagnosis of acute polyradiculoneuritis can be presumed on the basis of marked diffuse muscle atrophy, preserved pain and presence of hyperesthesia. When available, electromyographic changes show fibrillation potentials characteristic of LMN denervation, and nerve conduction velocities are variably reduced, depending on the degree and location of myelin loss. Clinical improvement with demyelination alone begins within 2 weeks of onset of paralysis, and recovery to normal results in 1 to 2 more weeks. With axonal injury, recovery may be delayed for several months or be incomplete. Subsequent exposure to the inciting cause may cause more severe and prolonged paralysis. Although glucocorticoid therapy has minimal effect on the course of this disease, I have found that one dose of cyclophosphamide (50 mg/m^2) given early in the course of illness may alleviate the severity of recurrent illness.

Local Reactions

Many complications have been associated with either local irritation or production of disease by canine and feline biologics. Local reactions after vaccination include pain, erythema, swelling, irritation, and abscess formation. These typically occur within 30 minutes to 1 week after inoculation. Pain can be caused by many components in the vaccine such as stabilizers, high or low pH, high osmolality, or preservatives. Swelling is most frequently noted with the noninfectious products containing adjuvants or with the bacterial vaccines containing large amounts of foreign protein derived from the culture media. Parenteral *Bordetella*- and *Leptospira*-adjuvanted bacterins and adjuvanted inactivated viral vaccines for rabies, FeLV, and feline respiratory diseases have most commonly been incriminated. Local reactions that persist or enlarge 2 to 3 months after vaccination should be evaluated by needle aspiration or biopsy.

Contamination

Local and systemic inflammatory reactions have occurred from the inadvertent inclusion or growth of pyrogens in vaccines. Multidose vials contribute to this problem. *Pseu-*

domonas and fungi can grow even during refrigerated storage. Endotoxin included in early inactivated whole cell, parenteral *Bordetella bronchiseptica* vaccines caused systemic manifestations in dogs, such as depression, shivering, tremors, and vomiting[11] and produced local reactions and abscesses. Newer purified cell wall products have alleviated this complication.

Adventitious Agents

Most viruses are grown in cell culture that must contain serum, and this is usually obtained from fetal calves. Vaccination of pregnant animals with MLV vaccines is not generally advised but may be done under some circumstances. Bluetongue virus grew undetected in one commercial release of canine vaccine and caused fatal illness in pregnant bitches vaccinated in the last trimester of gestation.[3, 170] Signs were abortion 7 to 9 days after vaccination and death within 48 to 72 hours with cardiac failure and respiratory distress. Necropsy findings were sanguineous pleural effusion, serous pericardial effusion, pulmonary congestion, splenomegaly, and enlarged mesenteric lymph nodes. Histologic features were multifocal vasculitis in parenchymal organs, interstitial pneumonia, multifocal myocardial edema, and myofiber degeneration.[46] No illness was found in any nonpregnant dogs, and no lesions were present in the aborted pups.[12] The virus was isolated from maternal organs and from a repository of the incriminated lot of vaccine.

Mycoplasmal DNA has been detected by polymerase chain reaction in a number of commercial veterinary vaccines.[79] Despite the presence of contaminating genetic maternal, viable *Mycoplasma* were not isolated.

Focal Cutaneous Granulomatous Reactions

Adjuvants of noninfectious vaccines potentiate the immune response by creating a depot effect, which sequesters antigen and stimulates a sustained inflammatory reaction. As a result, firm dermal or subcutaneous nodules may form at sites of vaccines given to dogs or cats.[58] These typically regress after 2 to 6 weeks. Such reactions have been more commonly reported after inactivated rabies vaccination of dogs and cats.[58] They produce visible hyperpigmented alopecic macules in the overlying dermis of breeds without undercoat such as the poodle and bichon frisé. A nonadjuvanted recombinant rabies-vectored vaccine would likely avoid this complication.

Histologically, the lesions were characterized by a local nonsuppurative vasculitis with rabies virus–specific fluorescence in the wall of the blood vessels. Central necrosis of tissue is surrounded by a granulomatous reaction with influx of macrophages and variable numbers of lymphocytes, plasma cells, and eosinophils. Lymphocytes are numerous, in many cases forming follicles. Globular gray-brown material within the necrotic zone and in macrophage cytoplasm represents residual vaccine adjuvant. Macrophages may transport this material to distant sites, perpetuating and disseminating the reaction. Dogs or cats suffering from such reactions may be more likely to develop anaphylaxis on subsequent boosters, should vaccine be inadvertently absorbed systemically at a rapid rate.

Vaccination Site Sarcomas

Persistent postvaccinal inflammatory reactions may be precursors of sarcoma development at vaccine sites.[38, 57–61, 76] Sarcomas have been reported with increasing frequency after the use of noninfectious adjuvanted vaccines in cats and with much lower frequency in dogs.[58] A similar problem of low-frequency occurrence has been reported in vaccinated people.[107, 150] Rabies and FeLV vaccines have been most commonly incriminated in cats, although combination inactivated adjuvanted products of other types have been associated with this reaction.[16, 93] The component thought to be associated with postvaccinal inflammation is the adjuvant.[95–97, 137] The inflammatory reactions to deposited aluminum and other proprietary adjuvants may predispose cats to a connective tissue reaction with proliferation of fibroblasts and myofibroblasts and eventually neoplastic transformations. In addition to fibrosarcomas, cats have developed osteosarcomas, liposarcomas, rhabdomyosarcomas, chondrosarcomas, and malignant histocytomas, among other neoplasms, at vaccination sites.

Postvaccinal inflammatory reactions have been evident in most cats receiving rabies vaccines.[98] Reactions were less frequent or consistent after FeLV vaccination, especially with nonaluminum adjuvanted and nonadjuvanted products. The epidemiologic link to inflammation, aluminum salts, and frequency of tumorigenesis is not clear. Sarcoma occurrence is not restricted to vaccines containing aluminum salts used as adjuvants. Other sources of trauma in cats can also lead to sarcoma development.[37] This finding may be related to the cat's unique response to chronic inflammation. Feline oncornaviruses do not appear to be involved in a cat's susceptibility.[41]

The estimated time course from vaccination to tumor development ranges from 3 months to 3.5 years. The estimated prevalence of occurrence based on biopsy submissions was 1:10,000 in vaccinated cats, although it may be as high as 1:1000 in vaccinated cats.[45, 76, 93, 97] In an epidemiologic survey of practicing veterinarians, the estimated prevalence was 2.1 cases per 10,000 cat visits or 3.6 cases per 10,000 cats.[26] Multiple vaccines at the same site and repeated yearly boosters may increase the risk. Unnecessary vaccines or boosters are not advised.

Three main avenues exist for reducing the prevalence of sarcomas that involve the veterinarian, the owner, and the vaccine manufacturer (Table 100–18). The site of sarcoma development has been most commonly in the interscapular area, presumably because this is a preferential location for veterinarians to inoculate cats. The interscapular area should be avoided because neoplasms in that location are hard to remove and drainage of inflammatory reactions is poor, resulting in sequestered adjuvants. Sarcomas can develop at IM and SC sites; the former is more difficult to detect and remove surgically. For this reason, recommendations have been made to give them at specified sites for future tracking of reactions and at extremities where they can be observed and removed. ***R***abies vaccine should be given SC in the ***R***ight rear leg as distal as possible on the extremity; ***L***eukemia is given on the ***L***eft leg at a corresponding site. Other products are given on the trunk just on either side of midline. Despite the potential complication of sarcoma development, the public health benefits of continuing rabies vaccination outweighs any complications. Restricting FeLV vaccination presents another alternative, because some studies have found an associated risk with these products. Manufacturers must work to provide less reactive feline vaccines.

Recommendations can also be made to monitor vaccination sites, because early detection and removal of sarcomas offer the best chance for a cure (Table 100–19). After inoculation, vaccine sites should be monitored by the owner for a 12-week period. Most masses that develop within 3 weeks of vaccination are granulomas that resolve in 1 to 2 months,

Table 100–18. Practices That May Reduce the Occurrence of Postvaccinal Sarcomas in Dogs and Cats

VETERINARIANS

1. Profile the pet and administer annual booster vaccines only for those agents for which animals are at risk for exposure.
2. Administer different vaccines at widely spaced apart sites, and use a consistent location for subsequent boosters. Use SC sites over extremities for easier detection or amputation.
3. Serotest, when applicable (see text), to determine whether vaccines are needed.
4. *R*abies *r*ight *l*imb, *l*eukemia *l*eft limb, and FHV-C-P on the lateral trunk on either side.
5. Map and record these sites, vaccine brand, and serial numbers.
6. Use MLV recombinant vector products, nonadjuvanted noninfectious, or intranasal when available and as effective.
7. Advise owners of risk and need for monitoring vaccine sites.
8. Massage vaccine sites immediately after inoculation to help disperse adjuvant (uncertain benefit).
9. Use single-dose rabies vaccines, always mix well, and preferably let vaccine warm up before using.
10. If multidose containers are used, mix them well before using to evenly disperse adjuvants.
11. Reduce use of combined multivalent products that compound the amount of adjuvants per dose.
12. Reduce the frequency and number of unnecessary vaccinations.
13. Booster doses should be administered at different sites over time.
14. Reduce the frequency of booster vaccines in adult animals.
15. Consider offering preventative health measures rather than vaccination for yearly visits.

OWNERS

1. Monitor vaccine sites for increased swelling.
2. Reduce animal co-mingling and sanitation to limit exposure and need for repeated boosters.
3. Return for annual physical examination regardless of need for vaccination.

MANUFACTURERS

1. Establish duration of immunity for products for proper booster frequency.
2. Develop vaccines for nonparenteral routes.
3. Reduce, alter, or eliminate sarcoma-inducing adjuvants.

FHV-C-P = feline herpesvirus (feline rhinotracheitis virus [FRV])-calicivirus-panleukopenia; MLV = modified live virus.

although some persist and enlarge, eventually to become sarcomas. Should they enlarge during a 3-month period or longer, wide local excision should be done. Removal of the early reactive granulomatous mass may reduce the overall immune response to the vaccine but will also reduce the chance of sarcoma development. After a 3-month period, progressive enlargement is probably related to a growing sarcoma. If this is suspected, a needle or an incisional wedge biopsy should be done if the patient will be referred. Alternatively, only extremely wide and deep mass removal should be considered. Excisional biopsy alone after this period is rarely curative because the neoplasm is locally invasive and recurs with more aggressive growth at the surgical site. Acemannan (see later discussion) with local irradiation before or after radical surgery has been advised and may need to be performed at a large referral center.[78] Sarcomas are usually locally invasive, but, uncommonly, distant metastasis has been reported.[44, 128, 130]

Table 100–19. Postvaccinal Sarcoma Recommendations

Site Monitoring

Local swelling < 3 months: observe
Enlarge > 3 months: wide excision
Usually invade locally, but rarely metastasize
Very enlarged: true cut or incisional biopsy and referral to determine whether granuloma or fibrosarcoma
Even aggressive surgery often incomplete, unless *very* early

Neoplasia Confirmed

Types usually fibrosarcomas, soft tissue osteosarcomas, chondrosarcomas, malignant fibrous histiocytomas, rhabdomyosarcoma
FeLV, FIV retesting
Aggressive surgery—wide excision; often reoccur
Acemannan
Radiation therapy
Doxorubicin (Adriamycin), 1 mg/kg every 3 weeks for five to six treatments
Vincristine

FeLV = feline leukemia virus; FIV = feline immunodeficiency virus.

Systemic Illness

Systemic illness characterized by fever and malaise may also occur from self-limiting infection with modified live vaccine within local lymphoid tissues without systemic spread. This illness commonly does not last longer than 1 to 2 days after vaccination, and it often explains the transient anorexia and depression noted in recently vaccinated animals. Rarely are anti-inflammatories, antipyretics, or other supportive therapies indicated. MLV FPV vaccine resulted in severe clinical disease characterized by fever, diarrhea, and leukopenia in kittens infected 60 days before with FIV.[14] Attenuated *Chlamydia* products can cause systemic illness in a low number of cats within 1 to 3 weeks after vaccination. Clinical signs include lethargy, weakness, anorexia, and stiffness. Short-term therapy with glucocorticoids or analgesics offers benefit.

Inadvertent parenteral inoculation of *B. bronchiseptica* and canine parainfluenza vaccine intended for intranasal use has caused localized pain and swelling, pyrexia, vomiting, mature leukocytosis, hypercholesterolemia, hypoalbuminemia, increased alkaline phosphatase and alanine aminotransferase activities, and hyperchloremia in an affected dog.[159b] Diffuse hepatocellular necrosis was found with liver biopsy. Management of this local and systemic reaction and acute hepatic necrosis involves symptomatic therapy with application of warm compresses daily to the injection site, systemic anti-inflammatory drugs as needed, and antibacterial drugs such as gentamicin, tetracycline, or trimethoprim-sulfonamide.

Neurologic Complications

Neurologic disease has been the most commonly documented postvaccinal reaction described in dogs and cats. This finding may be related to the overt nature of neurologic illness and to the decreased immunocompetence of the CNS against MLV agents. Rabies encephalomyelitis has been reported after vaccination with MLV vaccines, and, as a result, most licensed rabies vaccines for dogs and cats throughout the world are noninfectious. MLV rabies vaccines should never be used in exotic carnivores because of the uncertainty that exists with respect to their susceptibility to vaccine-induced disease.

Vaccine-induced rabies in dogs and cats after MLV vaccination begins with paralysis in the inoculated limb within 7 to 21 days and progresses bilaterally, in an ascending fashion.[53] Affected cats have had progressive LMN paralysis with unusual extensor rigidity of the limbs. Pain sensation and reflex function were decreased in an ascending fashion. Progression to forelimb and intracranial involvement was more common in affected cats, whereas dogs usually recovered completely within 17 days to 2.5 months. Injection in the cervical musculature, closer to the brain, has been associated with a much greater prevalence of neurologic complications. A peculiar feature of the paralysis in some cats is a sign of hyperextended limbs rather than flaccid paralysis. Animals with vaccine-induced rabies do not represent a health hazard because the virus is attenuated and is not shed in the saliva. Because of the difficulty in distinguishing the vaccine virus from virulent virus, expert virologists and public health officials should be contacted for recommendations concerning disposition of an affected animal (see Chapter 22 and Appendix 4).

Encephalomyelitis has been reported after CDV vaccination in dogs, especially in very young pups or immunosuppressed dogs (see Canine Distemper earlier and Prevention, Chapter 3). Postvaccinal distemper has been reported after immunosuppression of dogs with cytotoxic chemotherapy (see Vaccination Failures and Canine Distemper earlier) and in association with virulent parvoviral infection (see Canine Parvoviral Enteritis earlier). Atrophy of the Purkinje's cells in three of six pups given MLV measles vaccine at 6 weeks of age was reported.[53] Cerebellar signs were noted beginning 5 days after vaccination. MLV FPV vaccines and CPV vaccines should not be administered to animals younger than 4 to 5 weeks. Cerebellar degeneration and myocarditis may develop in kittens and puppies, respectively, from virulent parvovirus or MLV vaccine infection. Cases of cerebellar hypoplasia are rare from vaccination, because most veterinarians are aware of the problem. Parenteral vaccination with one of the first licensed attenuated canine coronaviral vaccines was associated with disseminated vasculitis and meningitis similar to FIP in affected dogs.[53] This was apparently a strain-related complication that does not occur with the current licensed product.

Prenatal and Neonatal Infections

If MLV vaccines are given during pregnancy, vaccine infections can result in fetal malformation or death or infertility and abortion in the dam. Neonatal infection can also occur after the use of MLV canine or feline parvoviral vaccines in puppies or kittens younger than 4 to 5 weeks. Although some vaccines may be safe, the general recommendation is never to give MLV vaccines to pregnant females.

Respiratory Disease

Clinical illness can develop as an expected postvaccinal event when intranasal vaccines are utilized for FCV, FHV-1 or canine parainfluenza virus, and *Bordetella bronchiseptica* infections. The mild clinical syndrome is usually self-limiting, but the organisms may produce a carrier state or spread to other susceptible animals. The secretory immune responses with intranasal vaccines are superior to those of parenteral vaccines. However, the clinical disease that these vaccines can produce has restricted their use by veterinarians. Parenteral MLV respiratory vaccines inadvertently or accidentally released into the environment or on the hair coat or aerosolized during administration can cause similar or more severe postvaccinal reactions. An outbreak may occur when large numbers of susceptible individuals are exposed. In some purebred catteries where inbred immunodeficiencies exist, the use of MLV respiratory vaccines may have to be avoided owing to the potential of vaccine-induced respiratory disease. Feline chronic ulcerative gingivostomatitis and faucitis (see Chapter 89) are likely caused by hypersensitivity to persistent calicivirus infection. Routine annual boosters, especially of adjuvanted noninfectious products, is not recommended in affected cats. In some cases, I have observed activation of oral ulceration after vaccine boosters of carrier cats.

Febrile Limping Syndrome of Cats

This problem is noted in kittens after the use of products containing attenuated calicivirus. The illness usually occurs in kittens younger than 6 months and within 21 days of first vaccination.[29, 30] Animals are lame, anorectic, and febrile 7 days after immunization. Pyrexia is commonly present, and some cats show concurrent signs of respiratory disease and/or oral ulceration. Kittens show a shifting leg lameness and hyperesthesia that cannot be localized to a particular joint. The lameness responds rapidly to low doses of analgesics. The clinical signs resolve with symptomatic therapy of fluids, antibiotics, and analgesics, and complete recovery is noted in 3 to 4 days. The kittens may have been incubating field virus at the time of vaccination, which triggers a hyperimmune response and resultant immune-mediated polyarthritis, or the vaccine virus may spread to the joints from viremia with a subsequent inflammatory response. Similar lameness occurs in lower frequency in unvaccinated cats that become naturally infected with FCV.

Vaccine-Associated Disease of Young Akitas

Related Akita dogs have developed immune-mediated polyarthritis 3 to 29 days after receiving MLV vaccines and less frequently or rapidly after noninfectious vaccines[36, 171] (see also Chapter 95). By 16 weeks of age, the dogs usually developed signs consisting of cyclic fever, joint pain, neutrophilic leukocytosis, and nonregenerative anemia. Elevated hepatic enzymes, creatine kinase, and azotemia have been observed. Joint fluid analysis reveals nonseptic, purulent polyarthritis. Treatment with glucocorticoids helps alleviate the clinical signs, but relapses are frequent and higher doses cause iatrogenic hyperadrenalism. The dogs usually have to be euthanized by 2 years of age because of progressive systemic disease, amyloidosis, and renal failure as a result of glomerular amyloidosis. The disease may be an immune-mediated disorder induced by an immunodeficiency with increased susceptibility to vaccine organisms or coincidental exposure to other environmental or commensal microflora.

Vaccine-Associated Hypertrophic Osteodystrophy (HOD) and Juvenile Cellulitis

After combination vaccines including MLV CDV, young Weimaraners (and less frequently, other large-breed dogs) 2 to 5 months of age develop fever, limb swelling, radiographic changes typical of HOD, and variable systemic manifestations such as coughing from pneumonia, lymphadenomegaly, diarrhea, pyoderma, and oral ulceration.[35] Typical cases of juvenile cellulitis have been associated with this syndrome.[100] In my experience, dogs with juvenile cellulitis may have radiographic evidence of HOD, even if the dermal lesions are the predominant manifestation. The concurrent occurrence of these two syndromes suggests that they may be related to infection with attenuated distemper vaccine virus in an immunocompromised host or infection with virulent distemper virus in dogs incompletely protected by vaccination. Distemper virus has been associated with metaphyseal osteodystrophy (see Chapter 3), and primary immunodeficiencies have been established in Weimaraners (see Chapter 95), which is also the most commonly affected breed developing postvaccinal HOD. Leukocytosis is the main laboratory abnormality. Signs usually begin 1 to 27 days after vaccination with a mean of 10.5 days. Treatment with anti-inflammatory dosages of glucocorticoids (0.5–1.0 mg/kg/day prednisolone) over 1 to 3 weeks at a gradually reduced level is adequate to cause a resolution of signs. In my experience, this syndrome has occurred most commonly with vaccination with the Rockborn or Snyder Hill strains of vaccines. Subsequent immunization of affected dogs or any vaccinations of Weimaraners, with the Onderstepoort strain or recombinant vectored distemper vaccine is recommended (see Table 100–9).

Shedding of Vaccine Agent

Shedding of vaccine virus, which occurs with the MLV intranasal products, can also occur after administration of parenteral vaccines such as MLV canine-origin parvoviral vaccine (feces), CAV-1 vaccine (urine), and CAV-2 vaccine (respiratory secretions). This shedding may serve to vaccinate other susceptible animals that come in contact with infected secretions. Reversion to virulence has not been demonstrated with any virus that is shed as a result of vaccination with commercially available veterinary vaccines, although the potential exists.

Influence on Drug Disposition

A potential influence of vaccines or viral infections on drug disposition exists in that they induce interferon synthesis, which in turn inhibits hepatic enzyme systems. This effect could prolong the effects of drugs eliminated by oxidative metabolism, such as aminophylline, barbiturate, lidocaine, propranolol, chloramphenicol, tylosin, griseofulvin, and trimethoprim.

False-Positive Test Results

Bovine serum or other proteins in cell culture can cause reactions that give false-positive ELISA results. This has been found in serotests for antibody in the diagnosis of toxoplasmosis, FIP, and FIV after routine herpesvirus, calicivirus, and panleukopenia virus vaccines.

Immunosuppression

Polyvalent vaccines can cause lymphopenia and suppress the response of lymphocytes to mitogens when testing is performed within the first week after vaccination. Individual antigen components do not cause this problem, and in dogs, distemper, adenovirus-1, and parvoviral antigens have been incriminated.[120] This problem is more of a laboratory dysfunction than of any practical significance; to be effective, many MLV products produce transient infection, which can lead to immunologic activation and temporary immune refractoriness.

Immunotherapy

In general, immunotherapy includes any form of treatment that alters the immune system. This discussion is limited to discussion of nonspecific means of stimulation of the immune system in an attempt to restore immunocompetence and control or treat infectious diseases (Table 100–20). Nonspecific immunotherapy has been employed to treat infections caused by facultative intracellular bacteria, viruses, fungal agents, or metazoan parasites for which vaccination or specific forms of chemotherapy are unavailable.

MICROORGANISMS

Microorganisms and their extracts have been used classically as nonspecific immunostimulators. Freund's complete adjuvant is a water-in-oil emulsion containing inactivated whole mycobacteria. The antigen is contained in the aqueous phase, and the mycobacteria are in the oil phase. Injection of this mixture induces CMI and humoral antibody formation. It produces a severe reaction of local inflammation and large granuloma formation. The adjuvant which is the active ingredient in Freund's is *N*-acetylmuramyl-L-alanyl-D-isoglutamine (muramyl dipeptide). Purified, it can produce a response without side effects. BCG is a nonpathogenic strain of *Mycobacterium bovis* that has been utilized in treating neoplasia in dogs and cats and in cats infected with FeLV. Ribigen-B and Ribigen-E (Ribi Immunochem Research, Hamilton, MA) are mycobacterial cell wall fractions that are given as adjuvants. Facultative intracellular organisms such as mycobacteria that are immunostimulators have a marked affinity for localizing in and stimulating mononuclear-phagocyte clearance mechanisms.

An emulsion of cell wall from a nonpathogenic species of mycobacteria (Regressin-V, Vetrepharm Inc, Athens, GA; Nomagen, Fort Dodge Labs, Fort Dodge, IA), which has been modified to decrease toxicity and antigenicity while retaining antineoplastic activity, has been licensed as a cell-mediated immune stimulant for treating equine sarcoids. It has been recommended for immunotherapy for other neoplasms, such as canine mammary tumors, lymphomas, or sarcomas, although studies demonstrating its efficacy for this purpose are not available at this time (Table 100–21). Various other bacteria, including *Propionibacterium acnes (Corynebacterium parvum)* and certain species of *Staphylococcus* and *Salmonella,* have also been proposed as immunostimulants. Immuno Regulin (ImmunoVet Inc, Tampa, FL) is a preparation of *P. acnes* that acts as a nonspecific immunostimulant. Clinical studies have involved the treatment of cats with FeLV infection, FHV infection, and canine staphylococcal pyoderma (see Drug Formulary, Appendix 8).

Modified inactivated, **rubeola virus immunomodulator** (Eudaemonic Corp, Omaha, NE) has been licensed as an immunomodulator to decrease the inflammatory reaction generated by activated T lymphocytes. It has not been adequately evaluated in controlled studies but has received conditional licensing for treatment of navicular disease in horses and ossifying spondylitis in dogs.[164]

Staphylococcus aureus phage lysate is a sterile preparation containing cell wall components of this bacteria. It has been licensed for the treatment of staphylococcal or polymicrobial pyoderma in dogs. It is thought to act through the stimulation of cytokine production. Local or systemic allergic reactions are potential side effects.

Staphylococcal protein A (SPA) is a polypeptide of *S.*

Table 100–20. Nonspecific Immunotherapy

EXAMPLE OR SOURCE	MODE OF ACTION	TYPE OF IMMUNE RESPONSE	DISEASE SPECIFIC	SPECIES SPECIFIC
Microorganisms				
Bacteria				
BCG, Freund's complete adjuvant (muramyl dipeptide) *Salmonella, Bordetella pertussis, Propionibacterium acnes*	Cell wall components: enhances phagocytosis and intracellular killing, increases macrophage chemotaxis and T-cell response	Cell mediated Humoral: primarily IgG	No	No
Viruses				
Newcastle disease virus, avian poxvirus	Interferon inducers	Interferon	No	Variable
Chemicals				
Macromolecules				
RNA, poly-IC, poly-AU	Interferon inducer, can enhance cellular and antibody response	Interferon Cell mediated	No	Variable
Interferons	Antiviral, immunostimulatory	Interferon	No	No
Small chemicals				
Organic: vitamin A, fatty acid, lipids, LPS, Freund's incomplete adjuvant, glycosides (Quil A)	Delays antigen absorption, alters antigen presentation	Humoral	No	No
Inorganic: beryllium, alum, silica	Prolongs release of antigen	Humoral: primarily IgE	No	No
Pharmacologic agents: Levamisole	Similar to thymic hormone: stimulates macrophage phagocytosis, immune killing, and chemotaxis Enhances T-cell cytotoxicity, lymphokine production, and nucleic acid synthesis	Cell mediated	No	No

BCG = bacille Calmette-Guérin; poly IC = polyriboinosinic-polyribocytidylic acid; poly AU = polyadenylic-polyuridylic acid; LPS = lipopolysaccharides.

aureus Cowan 1, which has the ability to bind to the Fc (non-antigen-binding) region of certain IgG subclasses. It may combine with immune complexes and stimulate complement activation, or it may induce T-cell activation, interferon (IFN)-γ production, and generation of cytotoxic responses. SPA has been given in the treatment of cats with FeLV infection. It has been given parenterally, causing increased serum interferon concentration and cytotoxic antibody to gp70. Antitumor, but no antiviral, effects were noted in other studies.[53] Extracorporeal immunoabsorption with SPA of plasma from FeLV-infected cats caused transient clearance of viremia and improved clinical signs associated with increased concentrations of interferon, complement, and cytotoxic antibody to gp70. The prognosis in neoplastic conditions is still poor. In clinically ill cats infected with FeLV, SPA treatment (10 μg/kg IP) given biweekly for up to 10 weeks was more effective than IFN-α (30 U, alone or in combination with the same SPA regimen) given orally once daily on alternate weekly intervals for 10 weeks.[102b, 102c] For further information on administering SPA, see Drug Formulary, Appendix 8.

IFNs

Interferons, a group of secretory glycoproteins produced by infected cells, inhibit subsequent replication of microorganisms in adjacent cells and stimulate lymphocytes for antitumor and antiviral responses via enhanced macrophage activity and lymphocyte-mediated cytotoxicity. There are three major classes of interferons: α, β, and γ. IFN-α and IFN-β are primarily responsible for antiviral effects, whereas IFN-γ is responsible for immunomodulation (see Antiviral Therapy, Chapter 2 and Drug Formulary, Appendix 8). Despite the broad range of effects against infections caused by many microorganisms, parenteral administration of preformed interferon substances is accompanied by complications. At first, it was thought to be relatively host specific, functioning only in the species in which it was produced; however, some interferons can protect a number of hosts. The major limitation to the clinical use of parenteral interferon has been the difficulty of production and purification of the large amounts that are required. The other disadvantage is that antibodies can develop to parenterally administered heterologous interferons. Recombinant feline IFN-α has been shown to be active in vitro,[124] and pharmacokinetics studies have been performed.[162] After IV administration, it is primarily distributed in the liver and kidneys; metabolism occurs with urinary excretion and minimal residual accumulation.

Many claims have been made on the efficacy of immunostimulants in cats with FeLV infection. Oral IFN-α has been shown in controlled studies to benefit cats with non-neoplas-

Table 100–21. Immunomodulators Licensed for Use in Dogs or Cats

PRODUCT	MANUFACTURER	ACTIVE PRINCIPLE	LICENSED INDICATIONS
Acemannan Immunostimulant	Carrington Labs	Complex carbohydrate from *Aloe vera*	Adjunctive therapy for canine and feline fibrosarcomas
ImmunoRegulin	Immunovet (Vetoquinol)	Killed *Propionibacterium acnes*	Adjunctive therapy with antibacterials for canine pyoderma
Regressin-V	Vetrepharm	Mycobacterial cell wall fraction	Treatment of canine mammary tumors
Nomagen[a]	Fort Dodge	Mycobacterial cell wall fraction	Treatment of equine sarcoid or bovine ocular carcinoma
Staphage Lysate	Delmont Labs	*Staphylococcus aureus* components with bacteriophage	Treatment of canine pyoderma
Rubeola virus[b]	Eudaemonic Corp	Inactivated rubeola virus	Treatment of ossifying spondylitis in dogs

[a]Same as Regressin-V, which is no longer available.
[b]Conditional license.

tic complications of FeLV infection. It has also been recommended for the treatment of cats with chronic herpetic corneal ulcers.[112] (See also Chapter 93, Table 93–3.) In conventional therapy, interferons are usually given IM and IV, whereas intranasal and oral administration of these drugs are not widely accepted. However, human IFN-α has been given orally in low doses (1.0–30 U/day) and has been beneficial in ameliorating the clinical course of FeLV-positive cats when given simultaneously with experimental inoculation of virus.[27, 169] Treated cats had improved survival rates, lowered weight loss, and increased appetite compared with untreated cats, although there was no effect on viremia.

Low-dose oral IFN-α may work across species lines, perhaps by stimulating oral lymphatic tissue. Interferon administration in small animal practice has primarily been provided in clinically ill FeLV-positive cats.[53] Although cats remained viremic, they showed signs of clinical improvement.[53] This finding contrasts with the 10^6-U doses per administration for IV administration in people, which in animals are associated with development of allergic reactions and refractoriness. High dose (2×10^4 to 2×10^6 U/kg) interferon has been used to treat cats with effusive FIP. Presumably, its beneficial effects are because of its immunosuppressive tendencies at these dosages.[105a, 168a] Because of the high expense, other immunosuppressive agents may be more practical. Low (30 U) doses of oral interferon, given daily on 7-day cycles, has shown some benefit in treating cats with the dry form of FIP.[168a]

IFN-α has pleiotropic adjuvant effects on host cell defenses. It is helpful in children in the treatment of chronic granulomatous disease by reducing life-threatening infections.[50] It has also been useful clinically to stimulate host cell–mediated immune defenses in treatment of persistent intracellular infections such as toxoplasmosis, leishmaniasis, systemic mycoses, and mycobacteriosis. For further information on interferons, see Antiviral Chemotherapy in Chapter 2; Therapy of FeLV Infection in Chapter 13, and Interferons in Drug Formulary, Appendix 8.

IFN Inducers

Several macromolecular compounds and certain viruses are known to produce antiviral and other antimicrobial activity in the host (see Table 100–20). These compounds induce interferon synthesis. Most of the substances known to induce the production of interferon have a structure similar to double-stranded RNA. Many viruses induce the formation of interferon naturally, but new synthetic nucleic acid polymers have been produced that also induce its synthesis. Interferon production occurred in healthy female dogs with mammary tumors that were given BCG cell wall emulsion. Synthetic interferon inducers have the advantage of continuing effectiveness after successive administrations. However, because the production of interferon is transient—lasting only for about 1 week—interferon inducers must be given repeatedly to be clinically helpful. Polyriboinosinic-polyribocytidylic acid (poly-IC) has been one of the most common chemical interferon inducers for dogs and cats. Toxic side effects of poly-IC in dogs and cats are lymphopenia, lymphoid necrosis, CNS depression, hemorrhagic gastroenteritis, and incoagulability. Poly-IC was reported to be effective in protecting dogs from ICH infection, although increased concentration of interferon could not be measured, and poly-IC was helpful in preventing herpesvirus infections in newborn puppies.[53] The concentration of interferon generally peaks 8 hours after administration of the inducer and declines gradually by 24 hours. Inhibition of interferon production is pronounced if inducers are readministered at a frequency greater than every 2 weeks. Because the duration of effect of interferon is less than 2 weeks, continuous protection cannot be maintained.

Other Cytokines

IL-2 is a lymphokine produced by activated helper T cells and is responsible for stimulating specific cell–mediated cytotoxicity. It has been synthesized in large quantities through recombinant DNA technology; however, it may cause toxicity. Its potential applications include treatment of neoplastic and viral diseases. IL-2 in low doses has been shown to increase the immune response to concurrent vaccination when it was given to immunodeficient people.[106] **IL-8,** a cytokine produced by monocytes and a variety of other tissue cells, has a role in activation of neutrophils and has been given to dogs to potentiate neutrophil chemotaxis.[176]

Granulocyte colony-stimulating factor (G-CSF) has been reported to be effective in reversing leukopenia; in profoundly leukopenic (<3000) dogs with parvoviral enteritis, improvement was noted within 24 hours.[48] G-CSF levels increased dramatically in parvovirus-infected dogs as neutropenia ensued.[125] Use of G-CSF in treating this disease is questionable. It has been beneficial in treatment of gray collies with cyclic hematopoiesis (see Chapter 95). The human recombinant product (rhG-CSF) is available as Neupogen (Amgen Inc, Thousand Oaks, CA) (see Drug Formulary, Appendix 8). The dosage is 5 μg/kg/day SC for 3 to 5 days and costs approximately $150 (U.S.). As with parenteral recombinant human interferon, therapy for 3 to 4 weeks is associated with resistance because of neutralizing antibodies. In people and experimental animals, G-CSF has shown preliminary benefit in adjunct therapy of bacterial pneumonia, sepsis, and some fungal infections. A commercial freeze-dried, heat-killed *Enterococcus faecalis* preparation (Nichi-Nichi Pharm, Tokyo, Japan) given orally at 100 mg/kg/day has been as effective as G-CSF in restoring cyclophosphamide-induced leukopenia in dogs.[75]

PHARMACOLOGIC AGENTS

Levamisole is a broad-spectrum anthelmintic that nonspecifically stimulates CMI in a variety of species. It potentiates mononuclear cells in the phagocytosis, chemotaxis, and intracellular destruction of bacteria. Toxicity of levamisole is relatively high; hypersalivation, vomiting, diarrhea, and CNS signs have been observed. Morphologic lesions, characterized by a perivascular, nonsuppurative, or granulomatous meningoencephalitis, were described in the CNS of treated dogs.[53] Potential facilitation of the cell-mediated immune system may produce the lesions in the CNS by causing the body to react against latent agents (e.g., distemper virus). Inosine (Isoprinosine) and muramyl dipeptide have also been provided as immunostimulants. The H_2-receptor antagonist cimetidine has been shown to be effective in potentiating CMI in people with common immunodeficiencies. It appears to block receptors on suppressor T cells.

LIPOSOMES

Liposomes are synthetic microscopic structures composed of multiple concentric lipid bilayers surrounding an equal number of aqueous layers. The lipid layers are relatively impermeable to aqueous substances trapped within. Immunologic mediators, antigenic substances, and drugs have been placed within the aqueous compartment of liposomes to facilitate delivery of these substances to selected tissues in the body. Liposomes themselves are relatively nonantigenic, nontoxic, and biodegradable because they are prepared from lipids normally found in cell membranes. As with microspheres, alterations in their physical properties can be used to modify antigen release. Liposomes may have potential to act as carriers of immunogens for purposes of vaccination. Immunogenicity can be increased by the addition of adjuvants within the liposomal membrane. Liposomal antigens, which normally stimulate only humoral immunity, can stimulate CMI if bacterial wall substances such as lipid A or muramyl dipeptide are added in the membrane. Liposomes also have been employed for selective in vivo delivery of drugs to cells of the mononuclear phagocyte system, which preferentially removes these compounds from the circulation. Intracellular parasites, such as systemic fungi, mycobacteria, *Babesia canis, Ehrlichia canis, Trypanosoma cruzi,* and *Leishmania donovani,* that reside in these cells may be more susceptible to chemotherapeutic agents delivered in liposomes (see also Lipid-Based Amphotericin B in Chapter 57 and Drug Formulary, Appendix 8).

IMMUNOSTIMULATORY COMPLEXES

Immunostimulatory complexes (ISOCOMs) are substances utilized to facilitate the immunologic recognition of membrane proteins of envelope viruses in subunit vaccines. The matrix of the ISOCOM has often been the glycoside Quil A (Spikoside, Isotec AB, Sweden), which in micelle form has accessible hydrophobic regions into which antigens are inserted. A hydrophobic region of the membrane glycoprotein can be attached to those sites on the ISOCOM matrix. ISOCOM preparations from enveloped viruses are highly immunogenic and have been used to prepare feline leukemia virus vaccines.

ACEMANNAN

This long-chained mannan is immunostimulatory by enhancing macrophage release of cytokines, which stimulate cell-mediated immune responses, including cytotoxicity. It can be used as an adjuvant in vaccines or by itself to enhance regression of tumors. Acemannan is utilized in the management of postvaccinal fibrosarcomas in cats. Acemannan has been used to treat spontaneous neoplasms in dogs and cats by intraperitoneal or intralesional routes.[56] Intralesional injections may cause marked tumor necrosis and liquefaction. In combination with radiation therapy and surgery, it is used in the treatment of postvaccinal fibrosarcomas.[78] Clinical studies suggest benefit to clinically ill FeLV-infected cats,[142] but corresponding prospective control cats were not evaluated. Acemannan may accelerate wound healing.[151] For further information on acemannan, see Drug Formulary, Appendix 8.

NOSODES

Nosodes are homeopathic preparations of tissues from animals with the disease for which they are intended to prevent. They have also been recommended to be given immediately after exposure to an infectious agent. These alternative medical therapeutic preparations have been claimed to protect animals as specific immunomodulators against a variety of infectious diseases. Their preparation consists of serial dilution with intervening agitation (succussion, potentiation, vortexing) of tissues, discharges or excretions from animals with corresponding diseases. They are administered orally. Clinical trials involving nosodes to prevent infectious disease[31, 131] have not been well controlled. In a controlled parvovirus challenge of puppies, nosodes were not protective.[135]

References

1. Addie DD, Jarrett O, Simpson J, et al. 1996. Feline parvovirus in pedigree kittens. *Vet Rec* 138:119.
2. Addie DD, Toth S, Thompson H, et al. 1998. Detection of feline parvovirus in pedigree kitten mortality. *Vet Rec* In press.
3. Akita GY, Ianconescu M, MacLachlan NJ, et al. 1994. Bluetongue disease in dogs associated with contaminated vaccine. *Vet Rec* 134:283–284.
4. Anonymous. 1993. Update on cat vaccines. BVA Congress. *Vet Rec* 133:409–411.
5. Anonymous. 1997. Is annual revaccination of pets appropriate? *Austr Vet J* 75:400–401.
6. Anonymous. 1997. Rabies and quarantine: report of the BVA working group. *Vet Rec* 141:79–81.
7. Baer GM. 1997. Evaluation of an animal rabies vaccine by use of two types of potency tests. *Am J Vet Res* 58:837–840.
8. Baer GM, Brooks RC, Foggin CM. 1989. Oral vaccination of dogs fed canine adenovirus in baits. *Am J Vet Res* 50:836–837.
9. Becker AM, Janik TA, Smith EK, et al. 1989. *Propionibacterium acnes* immunotherapy in chronic recurrent canine pyoderma. *J Vet Intern Med* 3:26–30.

9a. Bolcskei A, Bilkei G, Biro O, et al. 1995. Efficacy of the vaccine Primucell FIP and its acceptance by owners—OK as is. *Tierarztl Umschau* 50:851–853.

10. Bolt G, Jensen TD, Gottschalck E, et al. 1997. Wild-type distemper viruses differ from vaccine strains. *J Gen Virol* 78:367–372.

10a. Brent GS. 1997. Administering intranasal vaccines. *Vet Forum*, October, p 42.

11. Brooks R. 1991. Adverse reactions to canine and feline vaccines. *Aust Vet J* 68:342–344.
12. Brown CC, Rhyan JC, Grubman MJ, et al. 1996. Distribution of bluetongue virus in tissues of experimentally infected pregnant dogs as determined by in situ hybridization. *Vet Pathol* 33:337–340.
13. Buonavoglia C, Cavalli A, Gravino E, et al. 1994. Intranasal vaccination of pups with maternally derived antibodies with a modified live canine parvovirus. *J Vet Med B* 41:3–8.
14. Buonavoglia C, Marsilio F, Tempesta M, et al. 1993. Use of a feline panleukopenia modified live virus vaccine in cats in the primary stage of feline immunodeficiency virus infection. *Zentralbl Veterinarmed B* 40:343–346.
15. Buonavoglia C, Tollis M, Buonavoglia D, et al. 1992. Response of pups with maternal derived antibody to modified-live canine parvovirus vaccine. *Comp Immunol Microbiol Infect Dis* 15:281–283.
16. Burton G, Mason KV. 1997. Do postvaccinal sarcomas occur in Australian cats? *Aust Vet J* 75:102–106.
17. Carlson J, Mackowiak M. 1997. A new vaccine for canine parvovirus type-2: laboratory and field studies. (research report). Rhone Merieux, Athens, GA.
18. Chengalvala MV, Bhat BM, Bhat R, et al. 1994. Immunogenicity of high expression adenovirus-hepatitis B virus recombinant vaccine in dogs. *J Gen Virol* 75:125–131.
19. Choromanski L, Brown K, Bryant S, et al. 1995. Modified live *Toxoplasma gondii* (mutant strain) vaccine for cats, pp 137–172. *In* Proceeding of the American Association of Feline Practice and Academy of Feline Medicine, Washington, DC.
20. Church R. 1989. Lameness in kittens after vaccination. *Vet Rec* 125:609.
21. Clark KA, Wilson PJ. 1996. Postexposure rabies prophylaxis and preexposure rabies vaccination failure in domestic animals. *J Am Vet Med Assoc* 208:1827–1830.
22. Clark NC, Kushner NN, Barrett CB, et al. 1991. Efficacy and safety field trials of a recombinant DNA vaccine against feline leukemia virus infection. *J Am Vet Med Assoc* 199:1433–1443.
23. Clough NEC, Roth JA. 1995. Methods for assessing cell-mediated immunity in infectious disease resistance and in the development of vaccines. *J Am Vet Med Assoc* 206:1208–1216.
24. Coates JR, Carmichael KP, Roberts AW, et al. 1998. Vaccine-associated canine distemper viral encephalomyelitis in 14 dogs. *J Vet Intern Med.* Manuscript submitted for publication.
25. Cox WI. 1988. Examining the immunological hemopoietic properties of an immunostimulant. *Vet Med* 83:424–428.
26. Coyne MJ, Postorino-Reeves NC, Rosen DK. 1997. Estimated prevalence of injection site sarcomas in cats during 1992. *J Am Vet Med Assoc* 210:249–251.
27. Cummins JM, Tompkins MB, Olsen RC. 1988. Oral use of human alpha interferon in cats. *J Biol Respir Mod* 7:513–523.
28. Davies DH, Pidford S. 1991. Vaccination of dogs with multi-component vaccines. *Aust Vet J* 68:183–184.

29. Dawson S, Gaskell RM. 1993. Problems with respiratory virus vaccination in cats. *Compend Cont Educ Pract Vet* 15:1347–1369.
30. Dawson S, McArdle F, Bennett D, et al. 1993. Investigation of vaccine reactions and breakdowns after feline calicivirus vaccination. *Vet Rec* 132:346–350.
31. Day CEI. 1987. Isopathic prevention of kennel cough. Is vaccination justified? Faringdon, Oxon, England.
32. DeBoer DJ, Moriello KA, Thomas CB, et al. 1990. Evaluation of a commercial staphylococcal bacterin for management of idiopathic recurrent superficial pyoderma in dogs. *Am J Vet Res* 51:636–639.
33. De Turiso JAL, Cortes TE, Martinez C, et al. 1992. Recombinant vaccine for canine parvovirus in dogs. *J Virol* 66:2748–2753.
34. Dimmitt R. 1991. Clinical experience with cross-protective anti-endotoxin antiserum in dogs with parvoviral enteritis. *Canine Pract* 16:23–26.
35. Dodds WJ. 1995. Vaccine-associated disease in young Weimaraners, p 85. *In* Proceedings of the Annual Conference of the American Holistic Veterinary Medical Association, Snowmass, CO.
36. Dougherty SA, Center SA, Shaw EE, et al. 1991. Juvenile onset polyarthritis in Akitas. *J Am Vet Med Assoc* 198:849–855.
37. Dubielzig RR, Everitt J, Shadduck JA, et al. 1990. Clinical and morphologic features of post-traumatic ocular sarcomas in cats. *Vet Pathol* 27:62–65.
38. Dubielzig RR, Hawkins KL, Miller PE. 1993. Myofibroplastic sarcoma originating at the site of rabies vaccination in a cat. *J Vet Diagn Invest* 5:637–638.
39. Dubovi EJ. 1996. When serological testing is not enough: diagnosing disease in vaccinated animals. *Semin Vet Med Surg* 11:183–186.
40. Duval D, Giger U. 1996. Vaccine-associated immune-mediated hemolytic anemia in the dog. *J Vet Intern Med* 10:290–295.
41. Ellis JA, Jackson ML, Bartsch RC, et al. 1996. Use of immunohistochemistry and polymerase chain reaction for detection of oncoronaviruses in formalin-fixed, paraffin-embedded fibrosarcomas from cats. *J Am Vet Med Assoc* 209:767–771.
42. Elmslie RE, Dow SW, Ogilvie GK. 1991. Interleukins: biological properties of therapeutic potential. *J Vet Intern Med* 5:283–293.
42a. Elston T, Rodano I, Flemming D, et al. 1998. Report of the American Association of Feline Practitioners and Academy of Feline Medicine Advisory Panel on feline vaccines. *J Am Vet Med Assoc* 212:227–241.
43. England GCW, Allen WE. 1991. The lack of effect of parvovirus vaccination on the seminal characteristics of dogs. *Vet Rec* 128:611–612.
44. Esplin DG, Campbell R. 1995. Widespread metastasis of a fibrosarcoma associated with a vaccination site in a cat. *Feline Pract* 23:13–16.
45. Esplin DG, McGill LD, Meininger AC, et al. 1993. Postvaccination sarcomas in cats. *J Am Vet Med Assoc* 202:1245–1247.
46. Evermann JF, McKeirnan AJ, Wilbur LA, et al. 1994. Canine fatalities associated with use of a modified live vaccine administered during late stages of pregnancy. *J Vet Diagn Invest* 6:353–357.
46a. Fehr D, Holznagel E, Bolla S, et al. 1997. Placebo-controlled evaluation of a modified live virus vaccine against feline infectious peritonitis: safety and efficacy under field conditions. *Vaccine* 15:1101–1109.
46b. Flynn JN, Cannon CA, Neil JC, et al. 1997. Vaccination with a feline immunodeficiency virus multiepitopic peptide induces cell-mediated and humoral immune responses in cats, but does not confer protection. *J Virol* 71:7586–7592.
47. Fogleman RW, Chapdelaine JM, Carpenter RH, et al. 1992. Toxicologic evaluation of injectable acemannan in the mouse, rat and dog. *Vet Human Toxicol* 34:201–205.
47a. Fox J. 1997. Renewed signs immunomodulators help to overcome infections. *ASM News* 63:656–657.
48. Fox LM, Bruederle JB. 1996. Nearly foolproof parvovirus treatments. *Vet Forum* 13(April):36–38.
49. Fulton R, Gasper PW, Ogilvie GK, et al. 1991. Effect of recombinant human granulocyte colony-stimulating factor on hematopoiesis in normal cats. *Exp Hematol* 19:759–767.
50. Gallin JI, Farber JM, Holland SM, et al. 1995. Interferon-γ in the management of infectious diseases. *Ann Intern Med* 123:216–224.
51. Gaskell RM. 1989. Vaccination of the young kitten. *J Small Anim Pract* 30:618–624.
52. Gerber JD, Ingersoll JD, Gast AM, et al. 1990. Protection against feline infectious peritonitis by intranasal inoculation of a temperature-sensitive FIPV vaccine. *Vaccine* 8:536–542.
53. Greene CE. 1990. Immunoprophylaxis and immunotherapy, pp 21–63. *In* Greene CE (ed), Infectious diseases of the dog and cat. WB Saunders, Philadelphia, PA.
54. Greene RT, Hirsch DA, Rottman PL. 1991. Interlaboratory comparison of titers of antibody to *Borrelia burgdorferi* and evaluation of a commercial assay using canine sera. *J Clin Microbiol* 29:16–20.
55. Haffer KN, Koertje WD, Deer JT, et al. 1990. Evaluation of immunosuppressive effect and efficacy of an improved-potency feline leukemia virus vaccine. *Vaccine* 8:12–16.
56. Harris C, Pierce K, King G, et al. 1991. Efficacy of acemannan in treatment of canine and feline spontaneous neoplasms. *Mol Biother* 3:207–213.
57. Hendrick MJ, Brooks JJ. 1994. Postvaccinal sarcomas in the cat: histology and immunochemistry. *Vet Pathol* 34:126–129.
58. Hendrick MJ, Dunagan CA. 1991. Focal necrotizing granulomatous panniculitis associated with subcutaneous injection of rabies vaccine in cats and dogs: 10 cases (1988–1989). *J Am Vet Med Assoc* 198:304–305.
59. Hendrick MJ, Goldschmidt MH. 1991. Do injection site reactions induce fibrosarcoma in cats (letter)? *J Am Vet Med Assoc* 199:968.
60. Hendrick MJ, Goldschmidt MH, Shofer FS, et al. 1992. Postvaccinal sarcomas in the cat: epidemiology and electron probe microanalytical identification of aluminum. *Cancer Res* 52:5391–5394.
61. Hendrick MJ, Shofer FS, Goldschmidt MH, et al. 1994. Comparison of fibrosarcomas that developed at vaccination sites and at nonvaccination sites in cats: 239 cases (1991–1992). *J Am Vet Med Assoc* 205:1425–1429.
62. Hines DL, Cutting JA, Dietrich D, et al. 1991. Evaluation of efficacy and safety of an inactivated virus vaccine against feline leukemia virus infection. *J Am Vet Med Assoc* 199:1428–1430.
63. Hird DW, Ruble RP, Reagor SG, et al. 1992. Morbidity and mortality in pups from pet stores and private sources: 968 cases (1987–1988). *J Am Vet Med Assoc* 201:471–474.
64. Hoover EA, Mullins JI, Chu HJ, et al. 1995. Development and testing of an inactivated feline leukemia virus vaccine. *Semin Vet Med Surg* 10:238–243.
65. Hoover EA, Mullins JI, Chu HJ, et al. 1996. Efficacy of an inactivated feline leukemia virus vaccine. *AIDS Res Hum Retroviruses* 12:379–383.
66. Horber D, Mayr B. 1991. Paramunisierung FeLV-positiver katzen mit PIND-AVI. *Tierärztl Prax* 19:311–314.
67. Hoskins JD. 1997. Performance of a new generation canine parvovirus vaccine in Rottweiler puppies. *Canine Pract* 22:29–31.
68. Houston DM, Ribble CS, Head LL. 1996. Risk factors associated with parvovirus enteritis in dogs: 283 cases (1982–1991). *J Am Vet Med Assoc* 208:542–546.
69. Iglauer F, Gartner K, Morstedt R. 1989. Maternal protection against feline respiratory disease by means of booster vaccines during pregnancy. A retrospective clinical study. *Kleinterpraxis* 34:235–242.
70. Iida H, Fukuda S, Kawashima N, et al. 1990. Effect of maternally derived antibody levels on antibody responses to canine parvovirus, canine distemper virus and infectious canine hepatitis virus after vaccinations in Beagle puppies. *Exp Anim* 39:9–19.
71. Jarrett O, Ganiere JP. 1996. Comparative studies of the efficacy of a recombinant feline leukaemia virus vaccine. *Vet Rec* 138:7–11.
72. Johnston WB, Walden MB. 1996. Results of a national survey of rabies control procedures. *J Am Vet Med Assoc* 208:1667–1672.
73. Kahler S. 1993. Collective effort needed to unlock factors related to feline injection site sarcomas. *J Am Vet Med Assoc* 202:1551–1554.
74. Kahlon JB, Kemp MC, Yawei N, et al. 1991. In vitro evaluation of the synergistic antiviral effects of acemannan in combination with azidothymidine and acyclovir. *Mol Biother* 3:214–223.
75. Kanasugi H, Hasegawa T, Yamamoto T, et al. 1996. Optimal dose of enterococcal preparation (FK-23) supplemented personally for stimulation of leukocyte reconstriction in dogs treated with cyclophosphamide. *J Vet Med Sci* 58:563–565.
76. Kass PH, Barnes WG, Spangler WL, et al. 1993. Epidemiologic evidence of a causal relation between vaccination and fibrosarcoma tumorigenesis in cats. *J Am Vet Med Assoc* 203:396–405.
76a. Keil DJ, Fenwick B. 1998. Role of *Bordetella bronchiseptica* in infectious tracheobronchitis in dogs. *J Am Vet Med Assoc* 212:200–207.
77. Kent EM. 1993. Use of an immunostimulant as an aid in treatment and management of fibrosarcoma in three cats. *Feline Pract* 21:13–17.
78. King GK, Yates KM, Greenlee PG, et al. 1995. The effect of acemannan immunostimulant in combination with surgery and radiation therapy on spontaneous canine and feline fibrosarcomas. *J Am Anim Hosp Assoc* 31:439–447.
79. Kojima A, Takahashi T, Kijima M, et al. 1996. Detection of mycoplasma DNA in veterinary live virus vaccines by the polymerase chain reaction. *Jpn J Vet Med Sci* 58:1045–1048.
80. Kolbl S, Tschabrun S, Schuller W. 1995. Examination of the humoral immune response in puppies after first immunization with different combination vaccines: 1. Distemper virus component. *Kleintier Praxis* 40:851–865.
80a. Kommonen E, Sihovonen L, Pekkanen K, et al. 1997. Outbreak of canine distemper in vaccinated dogs in Finland. *Vet Rec* 141:380–383.
81. Kruger JM, Sussman MD, Maes RK. 1996. Safety and efficacy of a recombinant feline rhinotracheitis vaccine. *Virology* 220:299–308.
82. Lafrado L. 1990. Biological effects of staphylococcal protein A immunotherapy in cats with induced FeLV infection. *Am J Vet Res* 51:482–486.
83. Lafrado LJ. 1994. Evaluation of a feline leukemia virus vaccine in a controlled natural transmission study. *J Am Vet Med Assoc* 204:914–917.
84. Langeveld JPM, Casal JI, Osterhaus ADME, et al. 1994. First peptide vaccine providing protection against viral infection in the target animal: studies of canine parvovirus in dogs. *J Virol* 68:4506–4513.
85. Larson LJ, Schultz RD. 1996. Closing the window of susceptibility. *Top Vet Med* 7:22–26.
86. Larson LJ, Schultz RD. 1996. High-titer canine parvovirus vaccine: serologic response and challenge of immunity study. *Vet Med* 88:210–218.
87. Larson LJ, Schultz RD. 1997. Comparison of selected canine vaccines for their ability to induce protective immunity against canine parvovirus infection. *Am J Vet Res* 58:360–363.
88. Larson RL, Bradley JS. 1996. Immunologic principles and immunization strategy. *Compend Cont Educ Pract Vet* 18:963–971.

89. Lau RCH, Halliday AJ, Davies H. 1992. Evaluation of the immunogenicity of attenuated feline calicivirus vaccines by ELISA. *Vet Microbiol* 31:139–146.
90. Legendre AM, Hawks DM, Sebring R, et al. 1991. Comparison of the efficacy of three commercial feline leukemia virus vaccines in a natural challenge exposure. *J Am Vet Med Assoc* 199:1456–1462.
91. Legendre AM, Mitchener K, Potgieter L. 1990. Efficacy of a feline leukemia virus vaccine in a natural exposure challenge. *J Vet Intern Med* 4:92–98.
92. Lehmann R, Franchini M, Aubert A, et al. 1991. Vaccination of cats experimentally infected with feline immunodeficiency virus, using a recombinant feline leukemia virus vaccine. *J Am Vet Med Assoc* 199:1446–1452.
93. Lester S, Clemett T, Burt A. 1996. Vaccine site-associated sarcomas in cats: clinical experience and a laboratory review (1982–1993). *J Am Anim Hosp Assoc* 32:91–95.
94. Liao C, McVey DS. 1995. Immunity at mucosal surfaces. *Veterinary Scope* 3:1–2.
94a. Littman MP. 1997. Why I don't use Lyme disease vaccines. *Compend Cont Educ Pract Vet* 19:1269–1275.
95. Macy DW. 1995. The potential role and mechanisms of FeLV vaccine-induced neoplasms. *Semin Vet Med Surg* 10:234–237.
96. Macy DW. 1997. Vaccine adjuvants. *Semin Vet Med Surg* 12:206–211.
97. Macy DW, Bergman PJ. 1995. Vaccine-associated sarcomas in cats. *Feline Pract* 23:24–27.
98. Macy DW, Bergman PJ, Powers B. 1994. Postvaccination reactions associated with three rabies and three leukemia virus vaccines in cats. *Proc Annu Meet Vet Cancer Soc* 14:90–91.
99. Macy DW, Hendrick MJ. 1996. The potential role of inflammation in the development of postvaccinal sarcomas in cats. *Vet Clin North Am Small Anim Pract* 26:103–109.
100. Malik R, Dowden M, Davis PE, et al. 1995. Concurrent juvenile cellulitis and metaphyseal osteopathy: an atypical canine distemper virus syndrome. *Aust Vet Pract* 25:62–65.
101. Malik R, Kendall K, Cridland J, et al. 1997. Prevalences of feline leukemia virus and feline immunodeficiency virus infections in cats in Sydney. *Aust Vet J* 75:323–327.
101a. Mansfield PD. 1996. Vaccination of dogs and cats in veterinary teaching hospitals in North America. *J Am Vet Med Assoc* 208:1242–1247.
102. Marciani DJ, Kensil CR, Beltz GA, et al. 1991. Genetically-engineered subunit vaccine against feline leukemia virus: protective immune response in cats. *Vaccine* 9:89–96.
102a. Matteucci D, Pistello M, Mazzetti P, et al. 1997. Studies of AIDS vaccination using an ex vivo feline immunodeficiency virus model: protection by a fixed-cell vaccine against cell free and cell-associated challenge differs in duration and is not easily boosted. *J Virol* 71:8368–8376.
102b. McCaw DL. 1991. Advances in therapy for retroviral infections, pp 21–25. *In* August J. (ed), Consultations in feline internal medicine, ed 2. WB Saunders, Philadelphia, PA.
102c. McCaw DL, Boon GD. 1998. Immunomodulation therapy for FeLV: a comparison of two agents. Abstract. *Proc Am Coll Vet Intern Med*, San Diego, CA.
103. McCaw DL, Tate D, Dubovi EJ, et al. 1997. Early protection of puppies against canine parvovirus: a comparison of two vaccines. *J Am Anim Hosp Assoc* 33:244–250.
104. McGill LD. 1993. Vaccine associated sarcomas. Facing a real dilemma. *Vet Forum* June:26–28.
105. McMillen GL, Briggs DJ, McVey DS, et al. 1995. Vaccination of racing Greyhounds: effects on humoral and cellular immunity. *Vet Immunol Immunopathol* 49:101–113.
105a. McReynolds C, Macy D. 1997. Feline infectious peritonitis. Part II. Treatment and prevention. *Compend Cont Educ Pract Vet* 19:1111–1117.
106. Meuer SC, Dumann H, Buschenfelde KM, et al. 1989. Low dose interleukin-2 induces systemic immune responses against HBs Ag in immunodeficient non-responders to hepatitis B vaccination. *Lancet* 1:15–17.
107. Miliauskas JR, Mukherjee T. 1993. Postimmunization (vaccination) injection-site reactions. *Am J Surg Pathol* 17:516–524.
108. Miyamoto T, Taura Y, Une S, et al. 1995. Immunological responses after vaccination pre- and post-surgery in dogs. *J Vet Med Sci* 57:29–32.
109. Nakima S, Tamaka M, Tamaka T. 1990. Effects of halothane or pentobarbital anesthesia on blastogenesis of peripheral blood lymphocytes in dogs. *Jpn J Vet Anesth Surg* 21:71–77.
110. Nesseler A, Baumgärtner W, Gaedke K, et al. 1997. Abundant expression of viral nucleoprotein in mRNA and restricted translation of the corresponding viral protein in inclusion body polioencephalitis of canine distemper. *J Comp Pathol* 116:291–301.
111. New JC, Reinemeyer CR, Burr JHH. 1997. Results of a survey to assess knowledge and expectations of veterinarians and their clients regarding heartworm preventatives and vaccinations in dogs. *J Am Vet Med Assoc* 211:434–437.
112. Northsworthy GD. 1996. Interferon-alpha as an immunostimulant. *Vet Forum* October:27.
112a. Obradovich JE, Ogilvie GK, Stadler-Morris S, et al. 1993. Effect of recombinant canine granulocyte colony-stimulating factor on peripheral blood neutrophil counts in normal cats. *J Vet Intern Med* 7:65–67.
112b. Olson ME, Morck DW, Ceri H. 1996. The efficacy of a *Giardia lamblia* vaccine in kittens. *Can J Vet Res* 60:249–256.
113. Olson P, Hedhammar A, Klingeborn B. 1996. Canine parvovirus infection, canine distemper and infectious canine hepatitis: inclination to vaccinate and antibody response in the Swedish dog population. *Acta Vet Scand* 37:433–444.
114. Otto CM, Drobatz KJ, Soter C. 1997. Endotoxemia and tumor necrosis factor activity in dogs with naturally occurring parvoviral enteritis. *J Vet Intern Med* 11:65–70.
115. Pardo MC, Bauman JE, Mackowiak M. 1997. Protection of dogs against canine distemper by vaccination with a canary pox virus recombinant expressing virus fusion and hemagglutinin glycoproteins. *Am J Vet Res* 58:833–836.
116. Pardo MC, Mackowiak M. 1997. Efficacy of a new canine origin, modified live virus vaccine against canine coronavirus (research report). Rhone Merieux, Athens, GA.
117. Pardo MC, Mackowiak M. 1997. Safety of a new modified live virus vaccine against canine coronavirus (research report). Rhone Merieux, Athens, GA.
118. Pedersen NC. 1993. Immunogenicity and efficacy of a commercial feline leukemia virus vaccine. *J Vet Internal Med* 7:34–39.
119. Pedersen NC, Johnson L. 1991. Comparative efficacy of three commercial feline leukemia virus vaccines against methylprednisolone acetate. Augmented oronasal challenge exposure with virulent virus. *J Am Vet Med Assoc* 199:1453–1455.
120. Phillips TR, Jensen JL, Rubino MJ, et al. 1989. Effects of vaccine on the canine immune system. *Can J Vet Res* 53:154–160.
121. Phillips TR, Schultz RD. 1987. Failure of vaccine or virulent strains of canine parvovirus to induce immunosuppressive effects on the immune system of the dog. *Viral Immunol* 1:135–143.
122. Pollock RVH, Haffer KN. 1991. Review of the first feline leukemia virus vaccine. *J Am Vet Med Assoc* 199:1406–1409.
123. Pollock RVH, Scarlett JM. 1990. Randomized blind trial of a commercial FeLV vaccine. *J Am Vet Med Assoc* 196:611–615.
123a. Postorino Reeves NC. 1995. Vaccination against naturally occurring FIP in a single large cat shelter. *Feline Pract* 23:81–82.
124. Priosoeryanto B, Tateyama S, Yamaguchi R, et al. 1995. Antiproliferation and colony-forming inhibition activities of recombinant feline interferon (rFeIFN) on various cells in vitro. *Can J Vet Res* 59:67–69.
125. Rewerts JM, Cohn LA, McGaw D, et al. 1997. G-CSF levels in parvovirus infected puppies (abstract 118), p 680. *In* Proceedings of the American College of Veterinary Internal Medicine, Orlando, FL.
126. Richards JR. 1996. Advances in feline health research: impact of recent developments in vaccinology on feline levelfare. *J Am Vet Med Assoc* 208:505–512.
127. Rosenthal RC, Dworkis AS. 1990. Incidence of and some factors affecting adverse reactions to subcutaneous leukocell. *J Am Anim Hosp Assoc* 26:283–287.
128. Rudmann DG, VanAlstine WG, Doddy F, et al. 1996. Pulmonary and mediastinal metastases of a vaccination site sarcoma in a cat. *Vet Pathol* 33:466–469.
129. Saliki JT, Mizak B, Flore HP, et al. 1992. Canine parvovirus empty capsids produced by expression in a baculovirus vector: use in analysis of viral properties and immunization of dogs. *J Gen Virol* 73:369–374.
130. Sandler I, Teeger M, Best S. 1997. Metastatic vaccine associated fibrosarcoma in a 10-year-old cat. *Can Vet J* 38:374.
131. Saxton J. 1991. The use of canine distemper nosode in disease control. *Int J Vet Homeopathy* 5:8–12.
132. Scarlett JM, Pollock RVH. 1991. Year two of follow-up evaluation of a randomized blind field trial of a commercial feline leukemia virus vaccine. *J Am Vet Med Assoc* 199:1431–1432.
132a. Schetters TP, Scholtes NC, Kleuskens JA. 1996. Not peripheral parasitemia but the level of soluble parasite antigen in plasma correlates with vaccine efficacy against *Babesia canis*. *Parasite Immunol* 18:1–6.
133. Schrauwen E, van Ham L. 1995. Postvaccinal acute polyradiculoneuritis in a young dog. *Prog Vet Neurol* 6:68–70.
134. Schultz RD. 1995. Emerging issues: vaccination strategies for canine viral enteritis, pp 19–24. *In* Proceedings of the Symposium of Infectious Gastroenteritis, North American Veterinary Conference, Orlando, FL.
135. Schultz RD. 1997. Personal communication. University of Wisconsin, Madison, Madison, WI.
136. Schultz RD, Larson LJ. 1996. The new generation parvovirus vaccines. A comparison study. *Compend Cont Educ Pract Vet* 18:640–641.
137. Schultze AE, Frank LA, Hahn KA. 1997. Repeated physical and cytologic characterization of subcutaneous postvaccinal reactions in cats. *Am J Vet Res* 58:719–724.
138. Scott FW, Corapi WV, Olsen CW. 1992. Evaluation of the safety and efficacy of primucell-FIP vaccine. *Feline Health Topics* 7:6–8.
139. Scott FW, Geissinger C. 1997. Duration of immunity in cats vaccinated with an inactivated feline panleukopenia, herpesvirus, and calicivirus vaccine. *Feline Pract* 25:12–19.
140. Scott FW, Olsen CW, Corapi WV. 1995. Antibody-dependent enhancement of feline infectious peritonitis virus-infection. *Feline Pract* 23:77–80.
141. Sebring RW, Chu HJ, Chavez LG, et al. 1991. Feline leukemia virus vaccine development. *J Am Vet Med Assoc* 199:1413–1419.

142. Sheets MA, Unger BA, Giggleman GF, et al. 1991. Studies of the effect of acemannan on retrovirus infections: clinical stabilization of feline leukemia virus-infected cats. *Mol Biother* 3:41–45.
143. Smith CA. 1995. Are we vaccinating too much? *J Am Vet Med Assoc* 207:421–425.
144. Spaan W, Vennema H, de Groot R, et al. 1989. Early death after challenge with feline infectious peritonitis virus of kittens immunized with a recombinant vaccines virus expressing the FIPV spike protein, pp 491–495. *In* Vaccines 89, Cold Spring Harbor Laboratory, Cold Spring Harbor, NY.
145. Sparkes AH. 1997. Feline leukaemia virus: a review of immunity and vaccination. *J Small Anim Pract* 38:187–194.
146. Sparkes AH, Gruffydd-Jones TJ, Harbour DA. 1994. An appraisal of the value of laboratory tests in the diagnosis of feline infectious peritonitis. *J Am Anim Hosp Assoc* 30:345–350.
147. Stephensen CB, Welter J, Thacker SR, et al. 1997. Canine distemper virus (CDV) infection of ferrets as a model for testing morbillivirus vaccine strategies: NYVAC- and ALVAC-based CDV recombinants protect against symptomatic infection. *J Virol* 71:1506–1513.
148. Stockner PK. 1991. ML vaccine causes immune mediated symptoms in Great Danes. *DVM News Magazine* June:92–94.
149. Straubinger RK, Sumers BA, Yung-Fu C, et al. 1997. Persistence of *Borrelia burgdorferi* in experimentally infected dogs after antibiotic treatment. *J Clin Microbiol* 35:111–116.
150. Stringfellow HF, Howat AJ. 1994. Postimmunization (vaccination) injection site reactions. *Am J Surg Pathol* 18:1179–1180.
150a. Suliova J, Benisek Z, Svrcek S, et al. 1997. The effectiveness of inactivated purified and concentrated experimental rabies vaccine for veterinary use: immunogenic activity. *Vet Med (Praha)* 42:51–56.
151. Swaim SF, Riddell KP, McGuire JA. 1993. The effects of acemannan on wound healing models in the dog (abstract 63). *In* European Tissue Repair and Wound Healing Society, Amsterdam, The Netherlands.
152. Swango L, Barta R, Fortney B, et al. 1995. Choosing a canine vaccine regimen: part 1. *Canine Pract* 20:10–14.
153. Tartaglia J, Jarrett O, Neil JC, et al. 1993. Protection of cats against feline leukemia virus by vaccination with a canarypox virus recombinant, ALVAC-FL. *J Virol* 67:2370–2375.
154. Taylor J, Pincus S, Tartaglia J, et al. 1991. Vaccinia virus recombinants expressing either the measles virus fusion or hemagglutinin glycoprotein protect dogs against canine distemper virus challenge. *J Virol* 65:4263–4274.
155. Taylor J, Tartaglia J, Riviere M, et al. 1994. Applications of canarypox (ALVAC) vectors in human and veterinary vaccination. *Dev Biol Stand* 82:131–135.
156. Taylor J, Weinberg R, Tartaglia J, et al. 1992. Nonreplicating viral vectors as potential vaccines: recombinant canarypox virus expressing measles virus infection (F) and hemagglutinin (HA) glycoproteins. *Virology* 187:321–328.
157. Tizard I. 1990. Risks associated with the use of live vaccines. *J Am Vet Med Assoc* 196:1851–1858.
158. Tizard I. 1991. Use of immunomodulators as an aid to clinical management of feline leukemia virus-infected cats. *J Am Vet Med Assoc* 199:1482–1487.
159. Tizard I, Bass EP. 1991. Evaluation of a killed whole virion feline leukemia virus vaccine. *J Am Vet Med Assoc* 199:1410–1413.
159a. Torres B, Elyar JS, Okada S, et al. 1997. Fundamentals of FIV infection: is a vaccine possible? *Feline Pract* 25:6–12.
159b. Toshach K. Jackson M, Dubielzig RR. 1997. Hepatocellular necrosis associated with the subcutaneous injection of an intranasal *Bordetella bronchiseptica*-canine parainfluenza vaccine. *J Am Anim Hosp Assoc* 33:126–128.
160. Troy GC, Becker MJ, Greene RT. 1996. Proficiency testing of selected antigen and antibody tests for use in dogs and cats. *J Am Vet Med Assoc* 209:914–917.
161. Turnquist SE, Ostlund E. 1997. Calicivirus outbreak with high mortality in a Missouri feline colony. *J Vet Diagn Invest* 9:195–198.
162. Ueda Y, Sakurai T, Kasama K, et al. 1993. Pharmacokinetic properties of a recombinant feline interferon and its stimulatory effects on 2′,5′-oligoadenylate synthetase activity in the cat. *J Vet Med Sci* 55:1–6.
163. Van Kampen KR. 1997. Immunotherapy and cytokines. *Semin Vet Med Surg* 12:186–192.
164. Vasko KA, McMichael J, Smith B, et al. 1988. Use of an immunomodulating agent in the treatment of myofascial pain. *Vet Rev* 8:5.
165. Vennema H, de Groot RJ, Harbour DA, et al. 1990. Early death after feline infectious peritonitis virus challenge due to recombinant vaccinia virus immunization. *J Virol* 64:1407–1409.
166. Waner T, Naveh A, Wudovsky I, et al. 1996. Assessment of maternal antibody decay and response to canine parvovirus vaccination using a clinic-based enzyme-linked immunosorbent assay. *J Vet Diagn Invest* 8:427–432.
167. Wasmoen T, Chu HJ, Chavez L, et al. 1992. Demonstration of one-year duration of immunity for an inactivated feline *Chlamydia psittaci* vaccine. *Feline Pract* 20:13–16.
168. Weigland CM, Brewer WG. 1996. Vaccination site sarcomas in cats. *Compend Cont Educ Pract Vet* 18:869–878.
168a. Weiss RC. 1991. Feline infectious peritonitis: advances in therapy and control, pp 3–12. *In* Wolf AM, August JD (eds), Consultations in Feline Internal Medicine, ed 2. WB Saunders, Philadelphia, PA.
169. Weiss RC, Cummins JM, Richards AB. 1991. Low-dose orally administered alpha interferon treatment for feline leukemia virus infection. *J Am Vet Med Assoc* 199:1477–1481.
170. Wilbur LA, Evermann JF, Levings RL, et al. 1994. Abortion and death in pregnant bitches associated with a canine vaccine contaminated with bluetongue. *J Am Vet Med Assoc* 204:1762–1765.
170a. Woolhouse ME, Haydon DT, Bundy DA. 1997. The design of veterinary vaccination programs. *Vet J* 153:41–47.
171. Wynn SG, Dodds WJ. 1995. Vaccine-associated disease in a family of young Akita dogs, pp 81–84. *In* Proceedings of the Annual Conference of the American Holistics Veterinary Medicine Association, Snowmass, CO.
172. Yates KM, Rosenberg LJ, Harris CK, et al. 1992. Pilot study of the effect of acemannan in cats infected with feline immunodeficiency virus. *Vet Immunol Immunopathol* 35:177–189.
173. Yilma T. 1994. Genetically engineered vaccines for animal viral diseases. *J Am Vet Med Assoc* 204:1606–1615.
174. Yokoyama N, Maeda N, Mikami T. 1997. Recombinant viral vector vaccines for the veterinary use. *J Vet Med Sci* 59:311–322.
175. Zeidner N. 1990. Alpha interferon 2b in combination with zidovudine for treatment of presymptomatic feline leukemia virus-induced immunodeficiency syndrome. *Antimicrob Agents Chemother* 34:1749–1756.
176. Zwahlen RD, Spreng D, Wyder-Walther M. 1994. In vitro and in vivo activity of human interleukin-8 in dogs. *Vet Pathol* 31:61–66.

Appendices

Appendix I

Canine Immunization Recommendations

Craig E. Greene

AGE TO VACCINATE (weeks)	INITIAL AGE AT PRESENTATION (weeks): 6	7	8	9	10	11	>12
6	M/DM[a] or DA (Pi, Pv)[b]						
7	↓	M/DM[a] or DA[a] (Pi, Pv)[b]					
8	↓	↓	M/DM[a] or DA (Pi, Pv)[b]				
9	D, A, Pi, Pv (L, CoV)	↓	↓	D, A, Pi, Pv (L, CoV)			
10	↓	D, A, Pi, Pv (L, CoV)	↓	↓	D, A, Pi, Pv (L, CoV)		
11	↓	↓	D, A, Pi, Pv (L, CoV)	↓	↓	D, A, Pi, Pv (L, CoV)	
12	D, A, Pi, Pv (L, Bb[c], CoV, Ly[d])[e]	↓	↓	D, A, Pi, Pv (L, Bb[c], CoV, Ly[d])[e]	↓	↓	D, A, Pi, Pv (L, Bb[c], CoV[i], Ly[d])[e, f]
13	↓	↓	↓	↓	↓	↓	↓
14	↓	D, A, Pi, Pv (L, Bb[c], CoV[i], Ly[d])[e]	D, A, Pi, Pv (L, Bb[c], CoV[i], Ly[d])[e]	↓	D, A, Pi, Pv (L, Bb[c], CoV[i], Ly[d])[e]	D, A, Pi, Pv (L, Bb[c], Cov[i], Ly[d])[e]	↓
15	D, A, Pi, Pv[g], Ra[h] (L, Bb, CoV[i], Ly)	↓	↓	D, A, Pi, Pv[g], Ra[h] (L, Bb, CoV[i], Ly)	↓	↓	↓
16		Pv[g], Ra[h] (D, L, Pi, Bb, Ly)	↓		D, A, Pi, Pv[g], Ra[h] (L, Pi, Bb, CoV[i], Ly)	↓	↓
17			Pv[g], Ra[h] (D, L, Pi, Bb, Ly)			Pv[g], Ra[h] (D, L, Pi, Bb, Ly)	↓

Suggested optional antigens are in parentheses. Colostric immunity assumed; see Colostrum-Deprived Neonates footnote for that circumstance. For accompanying test, see Vaccination Recommendations for Specific Diseases, Chapter 100, and section on prevention in respective disease chapters. M = measles; D = distemper; A = adenovirus type 1 (hepatitis) or 2 (respiratory); Pi = parainfluenza; Pv = parvovirus; L = leptospirosis; CoV = coronavirus; Bb = bordetellosis; Ly = Lyme borreliosis; Ra = rabies; MLV = modified live virus; IN = intranasal; I = inactivated.

[a]M can be given up to 12 weeks of age, but preferably it should be reserved for pups about 6 weeks of age and should be used only for the first vaccination.

[b]Pv is essential for the initial vaccination series. There is no evidence that combining D and Pv as vaccine antigens is immunosuppressive, although it can be omitted in this age group if there is concern.

[c]If MLV-IN Bb is used, it can provide protection after one vaccination.

[d]Pups that are likely to be outdoors in endemic areas should be vaccinated for Ly during their initial vaccination series rather than waiting to adult age.

[e]L, CoV, and Ly vaccinations are often delayed until later in the series (>9–12 weeks) to reduce chance of severe allergic reactions. These are less life-threatening in older animals and less likely with fewer repetitive administrations.

[f]In pups of 12 weeks of age or older at first presentation, a second vaccination 2 to 3 weeks later with same antigens and also Ra antigen is recommended.

[g]Potentiated MLV-Pv products provide protection in most pups by 12 weeks. However, additional optional Pv vaccination may be given 2 to 3 weeks later when experience dictates that vaccine breaks will occur as a result of maternal antibody interference. Vaccination can stop between 12 to 16 weeks of age with these products. For conventional MLV- or I-Pv products, puppies may show this blockade up to 18 weeks of age (see Canine Vaccination Recommendations for Parvoviral Infection, Chapter 100).

[h]Ra can be given any time on or after 12 weeks. Veterinarians often delay rabies vaccination to ensure compliance.

[i]For CoV vaccination, at least two vaccinations are recommended, given 2 to 3 weeks apart. Pups completing this series before 12 weeks of age should be given an additional dose between 12 to 16 weeks of age.

Boosters

Manufacturers recommend the following:

D, A, Pi, Pv (L, Bb, CoV) yearly. Ra every 1 or 3 years, depending on product used, dog's age, and local public health laws (see Compendium of Animal Rabies Control, Appendix 4).

For profiling of a dog's lifestyle and booster modifications, see Table 100–13.

Pregnant Females

MLV vaccines are not recommended. The only effective I-products available for dogs are A, L, Pv, Ra, CoV, Ly, and Bb.

Colostrum-Deprived Neonates

Start D and A at 2 to 3 weeks of age and repeat every 3 weeks until the animal is 12 weeks old. Add L (Pi optional) between 9 to 12 weeks of age and Ra on the last visit. Use I-Pv until dog is older than 5 weeks and a live product thereafter along with the other antigens. Vaccination for Pv of certain breeds or in high-prevalence areas should continue until at least 12 or 16 weeks of age for potentiated or conventional products, respectively.

Outbreak

Distemper: vaccinate within 4 days of initial exposure.

Respiratory disease: booster with Pi or Bb (IN preferred).

Leptospirosis: two doses 2 to 3 weeks apart every 3 to 6 months.

Parvoviral enteritis: use potentiated MLV in exposed dogs.

Appendix 2

Feline Immunization Recommendations

Craig E. Greene

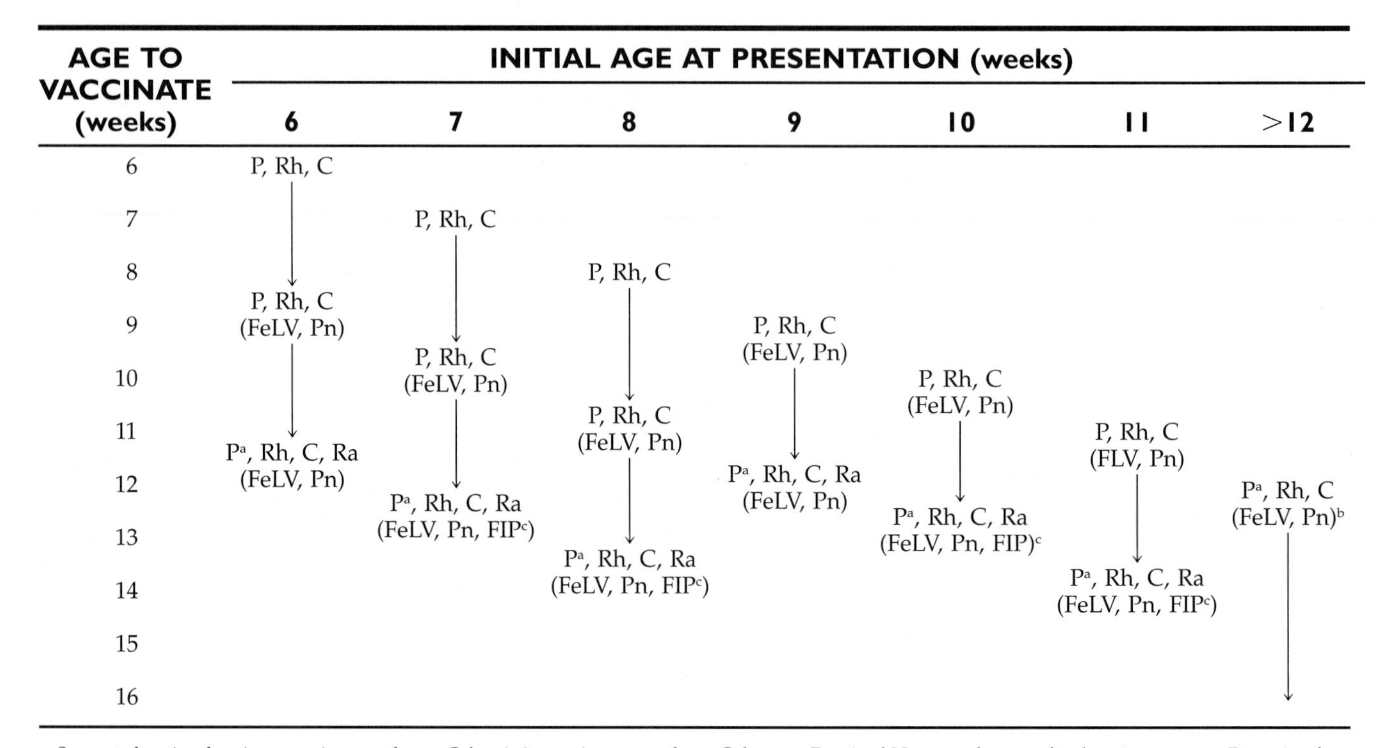

AGE TO VACCINATE (weeks)	INITIAL AGE AT PRESENTATION (weeks) 6	7	8	9	10	11	>12
6	P, Rh, C						
7	↓	P, Rh, C					
8	↓	↓	P, Rh, C				
9	P, Rh, C (FeLV, Pn)	↓	↓	P, Rh, C (FeLV, Pn)			
10	↓	P, Rh, C (FeLV, Pn)	↓	↓	P, Rh, C (FeLV, Pn)		
11	↓	↓	P, Rh, C (FeLV, Pn)	↓	↓	P, Rh, C (FLV, Pn)	
12	P[a], Rh, C, Ra (FeLV, Pn)	↓	↓	P[a], Rh, C, Ra (FeLV, Pn)	↓	↓	P[a], Rh, C (FeLV, Pn)[b]
13		P[a], Rh, C, Ra (FeLV, Pn, FIP[c])	↓		P[a], Rh, C, Ra (FeLV, Pn, FIP)[c]	↓	↓
14			P[a], Rh, C, Ra (FeLV, Pn, FIP[c])			P[a], Rh, C, Ra (FeLV, Pn, FIP[c])	↓
15							↓
16							↓

Suggested optional antigens are in parentheses. Colostric immunity assumed; see Colostrum-Deprived Neonates footnote for that circumstance. Pretesting for FeLV is recommended before considering vaccination. For accompanying text, see Vaccination Recommendations for Specific Diseases, Chapter 100, and section on prevention in respective disease chapters. P = panleukopenia; Rh = rhinotracheitis; C = calicivirus; FeLV = feline leukemia virus; Pn = pneumonitis *(Chlamydia)*; FIP = feline infectious peritonitis; Ra = rabies; MLV = modified live virus; IN = intranasal; I = inactivated; SC = subcutaneous; IM = intramuscular.

[a] If I product is used, then be sure to repeat this P antigen on or after 12 weeks of age.

[b] In kittens that are presented for their first vaccination at 12 weeks of age or older, give a second vaccination 2 to 3 weeks later with same antigens and also give Ra antigen. Only one P is essential if MLV is used; only one Rh and C if IN is used at this age.

[c] FIP IN vaccine is labeled for use beginning at 16 weeks of age with at least two inoculations given at a 2- to 3-week interval. Unfortunately, most kittens in endemic catteries seroconvert at 5 to 6 weeks of age. Extralabel use suggests starting earlier (6–9 weeks of age) vaccination in these circumstances. See FIP vaccination in Chapters 11 and 100.

Boosters

P, Rh, and C are recommended yearly; however, duration-of-immunity studies suggest intervals of at least 3 years are sufficient (see Chapter 100). Ra is either 1 or 3 years depending on local public health laws (see also Compendium of Animal Rabies Control, Appendix 4); Pn, FeLV, and FIP are optional, depending on incidence of disease in area. For profiling of a cat's lifestyle and booster modifications, see Table 100–14.

Pregnant Females

Two I-P, Rh, and C should be given 3 weeks apart with I-Ra on last visit. MLV vaccines are not recommended. Use of respiratory vaccines in pregnant queens has shown reduction in the prevalence of upper respiratory tract infection in kittens (see Chapter 100).

Colostrum-Deprived Neonates

Presented <4 weeks old: two I-P, Rh, C 3 weeks apart; then complete series as just listed.
Presented 4–6 weeks old: MLV-P, C immediately and 3 weeks later; then complete series as just listed.
Presented >6 weeks old: follow series as just listed.

Outbreak

Panleukopenia
- No colostral immunity or previous vaccination:
  - <6 weeks old; 2–4 ml/kg feline serum SC or IM; then 2 weeks later start series just listed.
  - >6 weeks old: MLV-P immediately.
- Vaccinated 1 year previously: MLV-P immediately.
- Outbreaks have been noted in catteries despite complete vaccination series (see Chapter 10).

Respiratory disease
- MLV-IN-Rh, C; MLV-Pn (optional). Use at an age earlier than disease occurrence (see Chapter 16).

Appendix 3

Canine and Feline Biologics Manufacturers and Products Available Worldwide

Craig E. Greene and Gerryll Gae Hall

U.S. Manufacturers/ Distributors	Address	Customer Service Phone	Technical Service Phone
Agri Laboratories Ltd.	20927 State Route K, P.O. Box 3103, St. Joseph, MO 64503	816-233-9533	800-542-8916
Anchor, Bio-Ceutic	Boehringer Ingelheim Animal Health, Inc., 2621 North Belt Hwy, St. Joseph, MO 64506	816-233-1385	800-325-9167
BioCor	Box 390, Shawnee Mission, KS 66201	800-633-3796	800-422-9874 800-255-6517
Delmont Laboratories, Inc.	715 Harvard Avenue, P.O. Box 269, Swarthmore, PA 19081	800-562-5541	800-562-5541
Durvet, Inc.	P.O. Box 279, 100 S. E. Magellan Dr, Blue Springs, MO 64014	800-821-5570	800-821-5570
Fort Dodge Animal Health	9401 Indian Creek Pkwy, P.O. Box 25945, Overland Park, KS 66225-5945	800-685-5656	800-477-1365
Heska Corp.	1825 Sharp Point Dr, Fort Collins, CO 80525	800-464-3752	888-437-5287
Hoechst-Roussel Vet	Box 4915, Warren, NJ 07059	800-247-4838	800-247-4838
Immvac, Inc.	6080 Bass La, Columbia, MO 65201	573-443-5363	573-443-5363
Intervet, Inc.	405 State St, P.O. Box 318, Millsboro, DE 19966	800-441-8272	800-992-8051
Merial Ltd.	2100 Ronson Rd, Iselin, NJ 08830	888-637-4251	888-637-4251
	Biological Division, 115 Transtech Dr, Athens, GA 30601	706-548-9292	706-548-9292
Pfizer Animal Health Inc.	Whiteland Business Park, 812 Springdale Dr, Exton, PA 19341	800-733-5500	800-366-5288
RX Veterinary Products	6301 Deramus, Kansas City, MO 64120	800-338-3362	800-338-3362
Schering-Plough Animal Health	1095 Morris Ave, Union, NJ 07083	800-521-5767	800-224-5318
Synbiotics Corp.	11011 Via Frontera, San Diego, CA 92127	800-379-6246	800-228-4305 800-796-2468
VacciCel, Inc.	P.O. Box 847, 101 Greenbriar St, Belton, TX 76513	254-939-7778	254-939-7778
Virbac, Inc.	P.O. Box 162059, Fort Worth, TX 76161	800-338-3659	800-338-3659

Selected International Manufacturers	Address	Voice Phone	Fax
Hoechst-Roussel Vet	Rheingaustrasse 190, D 65203 Wiesbaden, Germany	49-611-96205	49-611-9627896
Intervet International	P.O. Box 31, 5830AA Boxmeer, Netherlands	31-485-587600	31-485-577333
	Regional Offices in Belgium, Denmark, Finland, France, Germany, Greece, Hungary, Ireland, Italy, Netherlands, Norway, Poland, Portugal, Russia, Spain, Switzerland, Turkey, UK, Australia, Brazil, Canada, Colombia, Hong Kong, Indonesia, Japan, Malaysia, Mexico, Philippines, South Africa, Thailand		
Merial Ltd.	27 Knightsbridge, London SW1X7QT, UK	44-7171591-7400	44-7171591-7401
	Biologicals Division, 115 Transtech Dr, Athens, GA, USA	706-548-9292	706-543-1667
	Regional Offices: Europe—Belgium, Denmark, France, Germany, Italy, Netherlands, Portugal, Spain, UK; North America—Canada, Mexico, USA; South America—Argentina, Brazil, Colombia, Puerto Rico, Uruguay		
	International offices: Australia, Hong Kong, Japan, Singapore, Taiwan, Thailand		

Selected International Manufacturers	Address	Voice Phone	Fax
Virbac	Global Headquarters: 13ème Rue LID F-06511 Carros Cedex, France	33-49-208-7100	33-49-208-7165
Fort Dodge	Global Headquarters: 9401 Indian Creek Pkwy, Overland Park, KS, USA Regional Offices: Australia, Asia, Canada, Japan, and the Netherlands For Latin America, Africa, Eastern Europe, Singapore, Soviet Republics, and Middle East, use fax	913-664-7000	913-664-7062
Pfizer	Global headquarters: 235 E. 42nd St, New York, NY Regional offices: Argentina, Costa Rica for Central America, UK, Spain, New Zealand, Japan, South Africa, Belgium, Netherlands, Brazil, Mexico, Denmark, Germany, France, Venezuela, Chile, Sweden, Norway, Korea, Portugal, Italy, Colombia	212-573-2323	212-573-7851
Schering-Plough	Global headquarters, 1095 Morris Ave, P.O. Box 3182, Union, NJ, USA International offices: Argentina, Brazil, Colombia, Paraguay, Venezuela, Mexico, France, Germany, United Kingdom, Ireland, Spain, Singapore, Malaysia, Thailand, Norway, Australia, Philippines, Taiwan, Japan, New Zealand, Denmark, Greece, Portugal	908-298-4000	908-629-3365

Antigens	Route	Country	Manufacturers (Proprietary Names)
Canine and Feline			
Rabies (see also Compendium of Animal Rabies Control, Appendix 4)			
I	IM only	USA, Canada	Agri Labs (Champion Protector); Fort Dodge (Trimune, Annumune)
I	SC, IM	USA, Canada	Fort Dodge (Rabvac); Intervet (PRORAB); Merial (Imrab); Pfizer (Endurall, Defensor); Schering-Plough (Rabdomun)
I	SC, IM	Other countries	Fort Dodge (Latin America—Rai-Vac; Latin America, Asia—Rabvac, Trimune; Europe—Dohyrab, Unirab); Intervet (Europe, Asia, South Africa, New Zealand, Canada, Latin America—Nobivac); Merial (France—Rabisin, many countries—Imrab); Pfizer (Europe—Enduracell; Latin America, Asia—Endurall, Defensor); Schering-Plough (Rabdomun); Virbac (France—Rabigen)
VR	SC	USA, Canada	Merial (Recombitek F/R) (feline only)[a]
Rabies combined products-feline			
I	IM only	USA, Canada	Fort Dodge (Fel-O-Vax PCT-R)
I	SC, IM		Fort Dodge (Fel-O-Guard-R + FeLV-R); Merial (Feline + Imrab); Schering-Plough (Eclipse + FeLV/R)
I	SC, IM	Other countries	Merial (QUADRICAT); Virbac (Feligen RCP/R)
Rabies combined products-Canine			
	SC	Other countries	Virbac (Canigen DHPP/LR)
Canine			
Distemper (see also Table 100–9)			
L	SC, IM	USA, Canada	Agri Labs (Performer, Champion Protector, Puppy Protector); Anchor, Aspen (Solo-Jec); BioCor (Paramune, Commander, Adenomune); Durvet (Canine); Fort Dodge (Duramune, Puppyshot, Puppyshot Booster); Intervet (PROGARD); Pfizer (Vanguard); RXVet (RXV Vac); Schering-Plough (Galaxy)
L	SC, IM	Other countries	BioCor (Latin America, Eastern Europe, Middle East—Paramune, Adenomune); Fort Dodge (Europe, Latin America, Asia, Australia, New Zealand—Duramune; Europe—Kavak, Canlan; Europe, Japan—Dohyvac; Latin America, Asia—Galaxy; Australia, New Zealand—Protech; Latin America—Puppyshot, Puppyshot Booster); Intervet (many countries—Nobivac); Merial (Brazil—Eurican;

Antigens	Route	Country	Manufacturers (Proprietary Names)
			Europe—Caniffa, Hexadog; South America—Tetradog, Hexadog, Pentadog); Pfizer (Europe, Latin America, Australia, New Zealand, South Africa, Asia—Vanguard; Europe—Enduracell; Japan—Rescamune); Schering-Plough (many countries—Quantum, Epivax, Tissuvax); Virbac (France—Canigen)
VR	SC only	USA	Merial (Recombitek)
VR	SC only	Other countries	Merial (Latin America, Asia, New Zealand—Recombitek)
Measles			
L	IM only	USA, Canada	Pfizer (Vanguard) combined distemper antigen
L	IM only	Other countries	Pfizer (Latin America, South Africa, New Zealand, Asia—Vanguard)
Adenovirus-1			
L	SC, IM	USA	Agri Labs (Champion Protector, Performer, Puppy Protector); Anchor, Aspen (Solo-Jec); BioCor (Paramune, Adenomune); Durvet (Canine); RXVet (RXV Vac)
L	SC, IM	Other countries	BioCor (Latin America, Eastern Europe, Middle East—Paramune, Adenomune); Schering-Plough (many countries—Tissuvax)
Adenovirus-2			
L	SC, IM	USA	See L and VR under Distemper, previously
L	IN	USA	Fort Dodge (Bronchi-Shield III)
Adenovirus-2			
I	SC, IM	USA	Agri Labs (Performer); BioCor (Adenomune, Commander); Durvet (Canine); RXVet (RXV Vac)
I	SC, IM	Other countries	BioCor (many countries—Adenomune)
Parainfluenza (see also Table 6–2)			
L	SC, IM	USA	See L and VR under Distemper, previously
L	IN	USA	Bio-Ceutic (Naramune-2); Fort Dodge (Bronchi-Shield III); Intervet (PROGARD-KC); Schering-Plough (Intra-Trac II)
L	IN	Other countries	Schering-Plough (many countries—Intrac)
Leptospira			
I	SC, IM	USA	See L and VR under Distemper, previously
I	SC, IM	Other countries	See L and VR under Distemper, previously
Parvovirus-2 conventional[b] (see also Table 100–10)			
L	SC, IM	USA, Canada	Agri Labs (Puppy Protector, Champion Protector); Anchor, Aspen (Solo-Jec); BioCor (Parvocine, Adenomune)[c]; Pfizer (Vanguard, FirstDose CPV); VacciCel (CPV/LP)
L	SC, IM	Other countries	See L under Distemper for combination; BioCor (Latin America, Eastern Europe, Middle East—Adenomune); Fort Dodge (Latin America, Asia—Parvoid; Europe, Japan—Dohyvac); Merial (many countries—Parvodog, Canimid-P, Caniffa, EuricanPF); Pfizer (Europe—Enduracell; Japan—Rescamune; Latin America, Asia—Vanguard); Schering-Plough (many countries—Quanpar, Tissuvax, Quantum, Epivax); Virbac (Europe, Mexico—Parvigen; Central America—Canigen)
Parvovirus-2 potentiated[b] (see also Table 100–10)			
L	SC, IM	USA, Canada	BioCor (Commander); Fort Dodge (Duramune KF-11); Intervet (PROGARD); Merial (Parvo XL, Recombitek); Pfizer (Vanguard puppy, Vanguard Plus); Schering-Plough (Galaxy)
L	SC, IM	Other countries	Fort Dodge (Europe—Kavak; Europe, Latin America, Asia, Australia, New Zealand—Duramune; Latin America, Asia—Galaxy; Australia, New Zealand—Protech; Latin America—Puppyshot); Intervet (many countries—Nobivac); Merial (Latin America—Parvo XL, Primodog; Europe—Primodog, Eurican, Canimid-P forte); Pfizer (Europe—Vanguard; Brazil, Venezuela—Vanguard HTLP; Latin America, Asia, South Africa, New Zealand—Vanguard Puppy, Vanguard Plus)
Parvovirus-2			
I	SC, IM	USA	Agri Labs (Performer); BioCor (Adenomune, Parvocine); Durvet (canine parvovirus vaccine); Pfizer (Vanguard); RXVet (RXV Vac)

Antigens	Route	Country	Manufacturers (Proprietary Names)
I	SC, IM	Other countries	BioCor (Latin America, Eastern Europe, Middle East—Adenomune); Fort Dodge (Europe—Canlan); Pfizer (Mexico, Brazil, Argentina, Chile—Vanguard)
***Bordetella* canine** (see also Parainfluenza earlier and Table 6–2)			
I	SC only	USA, Canada	Agri Labs (Performer-Borde-Vac); BioCor (Bronchicine)
I	SC, IM	USA, Canada	Pfizer (Coughguard B, Vanguard 5/B)
I	SC, IM	Other countries	Merial (France—Pneumo dog); Pfizer (Korea—Coughguard B, Vanguard 5/B)
L	IN	USA, Canada	Bio-Ceutic (Naramune-2); Fort Dodge (Bronchi-Shield III); Intervet (PROGARD-KC); Pfizer (Nasaguard B); Schering-Plough (Intra-Trac II)
L	IN	Other countries	Schering-Plough (many countries—Intrac)
Borrelia burgdorferi			
I	SC, IM	USA, Canada	Fort Dodge (LymeVax, Puppyshot Plus LymeVax)
I	SC, IM	Other countries	Merial (Merilym)
I	IM only	USA	Schering-Plough (Galaxy Lyme)
SR	SC only	USA	Merial (Recombitek Lyme)
Coronavirus			
I	SC, IM	USA, Canada	Fort Dodge (Duramune CVK); Intervet (PROGARD, UnAMaX); Pfizer (FirstDose CV, Vanguard); Schering-Plough (Galaxy Cv)—feline origin; VacciCel (COR-1)
I	SC, IM	Other countries	Fort Dodge (Europe, Latin America, Asia—Duramune; Europe—Kavak, Canlan, Dohyvac; Latin America, Asia—Galaxy; Latin America—Puppyshot); Intervet (many countries—Nobivac); Pfizer (Latin America, Asia—FirstDose, Vanguard); Schering-Plough (Brazil—Tissuvax)
L	SC	USA, Canada	Merial (Canine Corona—MLV, Recombitek)
L	SC	Other countries	Merial (Latin America—Canine Corona—MLV, Recombitek)
Multivalent antisera			
Ab	IV, SC	Germany	Hoechst (Stagloban)
Antiendotoxin *(Salmonella)*			
Ab	IV, SC	USA	Immvac (SEPTI-Serum)
		Other countries	Immvac (Latin America, Taiwan, Japan, Korea—SEPTI-Serum)
Babesia			
I	SC, IM	Other countries	Merial (France, Italy, Switzerland, Belgium, Spain—Pirodog)
Staphylococcus aureus			
I	SC	USA	Delmont (Staphage Lysate SPL)
Feline			
Panleukopenia			
L	SC only	USA, Canada	Agri Labs (Performer, Champion Protector); BioCor (Rhinopan); Duravet (Feline); Synbiotics (PANACINE)
L	SC, IM	USA, Canada	Agri Labs (Champion Protector); Fort Dodge (Fel-O-Guard); Intervet (PROTEX); Merial Feline 3, Feline 4); Pfizer (Felocell); Schering-Plough (Eclipse)
L	SC, IM	Other countries	BioCor (Eastern Europe, Latin America—Rhinopan); Fort Dodge (Australia, New Zealand—Feline 3; Europe—Dohycat, Katavac; Latin America, Asia—Eclipse); Intervet (many countries—Nobivac Tricat); Pfizer (Europe, Latin America, Asia, South Africa, New Zealand—Felocell); Schering-Plough (Europe—Quantum, Fiovax); Virbac (France—Feligen)
L	IN/IO[d]	USA	Heska (Heska Trivalent Intranasal/Intraocular Vaccine)
I	SC only	USA	BioCor (Respomune); Duravet (Feline); RXVet (RXV Vac)
I	SC, IM	USA	Fort Dodge (Fel-O-Vax); Schering-Plough (FVRCP)
I	SC, IM	Other countries	Fort Dodge (Europe, Latin America, Asia, Australia, New Zealand—Fel-O-Vax; Europe—Pentofel, Fortvax; Dohycat; Australia, New Zealand—FPI; Asia, Latin America—Eclipse); Merial (Europe—Leocorffelin; France—Conifeline, QUADRICHI; South America—Feliniffa; many countries—QUADRICAT)
Rhinotracheitis			
L	SC only	USA	See L and I (SC only) under Panleukopenia previously
L	SC, IM	USA	See L under Panleukopenia previously
		Other countries	Fort Dodge (Australia, New Zealand—FR-FC, FPI) See L Panleukopenia previously

Antigens	Route	Country	Manufacturers (Proprietary Names)
L	IN/IO[d]	USA	Heska (Heska Trivalent, Bivalent Intranasal/Intraocular Vaccine); Pfizer (Felomune CVR)
I	SC, IM	USA	See I Panleukopenia previously
I	SC, IM	Other countries	See I Panleukopenia previously
Calicivirus			
L and I			See Rhinotracheitis previously
Chlamydia			
L	SC only	USA, Canada	Agri Labs (Performer); BioCor (Rhinopan); Durvet (Feline); Synbiotics (PANACINE)
L	SC, IM	USA, Canada	Fort Dodge (Fel-O-Guard); Merial (Feline 4); Pfizer (Felocell); Schering-Plough (Eclipse)
L	SC, IM	Other countries	BioCor (Eastern Europe, Latin America—Rhinopan); Fort Dodge (Europe—Dohycat, Katavac; Latin America, Asia—Eclipse)
I	SC, IM	USA, Canada	Fort Dodge (Fel-O-Vax)
I	SC, IM	Other countries	Fort Dodge (Europe, Latin America, Asia, Australia, New Zealand—Fel-O-Vax; Europe—Pentofel, Fortvax); Merial (Europe—EURIFEL)
***Bordetella* feline**			
L	IN	USA	Intervet (PROTEX Bb)[a]
PS	SC only	Other countries	Intervet (Netherlands, Spain—Nobivac Bb Cat)
Leukemia virus (includes combination products; see also Table 100–11 for individual products)			
I	SC only	USA, Canada	Agri Labs (Champion Protector Feline LK); Merial (Leucat); Synbiotics (PANACINE, VacSYN/FeLV)
I	SC, IM	USA, Canada	Fort Dodge (Fel-O-Vax LVK, Fel-O-Guard); Merial (Feline + Leucat); Pfizer (Leukocell 2); Schering-Plough (Fevaxyn, Eclipse)
I	SC, IM	Other countries	Fort Dodge (Europe, Latin America, Japan—Fevaxyn FeLV; Europe, Latin America, Asia, New Zealand—Fel-O-Vax; Europe—Pentofel; Dohycat, Katavac, Fortvax; Latin America—Eclipse); Intervet (UK—Nobivac FeLV); Merial (many countries—Leucat); Pfizer (Europe, Latin America, Asia, South Africa, New Zealand—Leukocell 2); Schering-Plough (many countries—Quantum Cat FeLV)
SR	SC	Other countries	Virbac (Europe—Leucogen)
Infectious peritonitis virus			
L	IN	USA, Canada	Pfizer (Primucell FIP)
		Other countries	Pfizer (Europe—Primucell FIP)
Microsporum canis			
I	SC	USA	Fort Dodge (Fel-O-Vax MC-K)

Monovalent and polyvalent products and brand names are listed together based on the antigen under consideration.
L = live, attenuated; I = inactivated; PS = purified subunit; SR = noninfectious subunit recombinant; VR = live vector recombinant; A = annual; T = triennial; Ab = antibody-containing sera.
[a]Licensing imminent USDA.
[b]Potentiated canine parvovirus vaccines generally have a higher infectious dose titer and lower culture passage than conventional vaccines, making them more protective than conventional products in breaking through maternally acquired immunity.
[c]Feline panleukopenia virus strain.
[d]Sometimes recommended intraocularly, with certain brands, and in young kittens.

Appendix 4

Compendium of Animal Rabies Control, 1998* National Association of State Public Health Veterinarians, Inc.

The purpose of this Compendium is to provide rabies information to veterinarians, public health officials, and others concerned with rabies control. These recommendations serve as the basis for animal rabies control programs throughout the United States and facilitate standardization of procedures among jurisdictions, thereby contributing to an effective national rabies control program. This document is reviewed annually and revised as necessary. Immunization procedure recommendations are contained in Part I; all animal rabies vaccines licensed by the United States Department of Agriculture (USDA) and marketed in the United States are listed in Part II; Part III details the principles of rabies control.

PART I: RECOMMENDATIONS FOR PARENTERAL IMMUNIZATION PROCEDURES

A. VACCINE ADMINISTRATION: All animal rabies vaccines should be restricted to use by, or under the direct supervision of, a veterinarian.
B. VACCINE SELECTION: In comprehensive rabies control programs, only vaccines with a 3-year duration of immunity should be used. This constitutes the most effective method of increasing the proportion of immunized dogs and cats in any population. (See Part II.)
C. ROUTE OF INOCULATION: All vaccines must be administered in accordance with the specifications of the product label or package insert. If administered intramuscularly, it must be at one site in the thigh.
D. WILDLIFE AND HYBRID VACCINATION: The efficacy of parenteral rabies vaccination of wildlife and hybrids (the offspring of wild animals crossbred to domestic dogs and cats) has not been established, and no such vaccine is licensed for these animals. Zoos or research institutions may establish vaccination programs which attempt to protect valuable animals, but these should not replace appropriate public health activities that protect humans.
E. ACCIDENTAL HUMAN EXPOSURE TO VACCINE: Accidental inoculation may occur during administration of animal rabies vaccine. Such exposure to inactivated vaccines constitutes no rabies hazard.
F. IDENTIFICATION OF VACCINATED ANIMALS: All agencies and veterinarians should adopt the standard tag system. This practice will aid the administration of local, state, national, and international control procedures. Animal license tags should be distinguishable in shape and color from rabies tags. Anodized aluminum rabies tags should be no less than 0.064 inches in thickness.

1. RABIES TAGS

YEAR	COLOR	SHAPE
1998	Orange	Oval
1999	Green	Bell
2000	Red	Heart
2001	Blue	Rosette

2. RABIES CERTIFICATE: All agencies and veterinarians should use the NASPHV form #51, "Rabies Vaccination Certificate," which can be obtained from vaccine manufacturers. Computer-generated forms containing the same information are acceptable.

THE NASPHV COMMITTEE
Suzanne R. Jenkins, VMD, MPH, Chair
Michael Auslander, DVM, MSPH
Robert H. Johnson, DVM
Mira J. Leslie, DVM
Grayson B. Miller, Jr., MD
F. T. Satalowich, DVM, MSPH
Faye E. Sorhage, VMD, MPH

***Address all correspondence to:**
Suzanne R. Jenkins, VMD, MPH
Virginia Department of Health
Office of Epidemiology
P.O. Box 2448, Room 113
Richmond, VA 23218

CONSULTANTS TO THE COMMITTEE
Deborah J. Briggs, PhD
James E. Childs, ScD; Centers for Disease Control and Prevention (CDC)
David W. Dreesen, DVM, MPVM
William L. Ingalls, DVM, MS; AVMA Council on Public Health and Regulatory Veterinary Medicine
Jim McCord, DVM; Animal Health Institute
Robert B. Miller, DVM, MPH; Animal and Plant Health Inspection Service, USDA
Charles E. Rupprecht, VMD, PhD; CDC
Charles V. Trimarchi, MS

ENDORSED BY:
American Veterinary Medical Association (AVMA)
Council of State and Territorial Epidemiologists (CSTE)

PART II: RABIES VACCINES LICENSED IN U.S. AND NASPHV RECOMMENDATIONS, 1998

Product Name	Produced by	Marketed by	For Use in	Dosage	Age at Primary Vaccination[1]	Booster Recommended	Route of Inoculation
A) Monovalent (inactivated)							
TRIMUNE	Fort Dodge Animal Health	Fort Dodge Animal Health	Dogs	1 ml	3 months & 1 year later	Triennially	IM[2]
	License No. 112		Cats	1 ml	3 months & 1 year later	Triennially	IM
ANNUMUNE	Fort Dodge Animal Health	Fort Dodge Animal Health	Dogs	1 ml	3 months	Annually	IM
	License No. 112		Cats	1 ml	3 months	Annually	IM
DURA-RAB 1	ImmunoMed	ImmunoMed, Vedco, Inc.	Dogs	1 ml	3 months	Annually	IM
	License No. 421		Cats	1 ml	3 months	Annually	IM
DURA-RAB 3	ImmunoMed	ImmunoMed, Vedco, Inc.	Dogs	1 ml	3 months & 1 year later	Triennially	IM
	License No. 421		Cats	1 ml	3 months & 1 year later	Triennially	IM
RABCINE-3	ImmunoMed	Pfizer, Inc.	Dogs	1 ml	3 months & 1 year later	Triennially	IM
	License No. 421		Cats	1 ml	3 months & 1 year later	Triennially	IM
CHAMPION PROTECTOR RABIES 3	ImmunoMed	AgriLaboratories	Dogs	1 ml	3 months & 1 year later	Triennially	IM
	License No. 421		Cats	1 ml	3 months & 1 year later	Triennially	IM
ENDURALL-P	Pfizer, Inc.	Pfizer, Inc.	Dogs	1 ml	3 months	Annually	IM or SC[3]
	License No. 189		Cats	1 ml	3 months	Annually	SC
RABGUARD-TC	Pfizer, Inc.	Pfizer, Inc.	Dogs	1 ml	3 months & 1 year later	Triennially	IM
	License No. 189		Cats	1 ml	3 months & 1 year later	Triennially	IM
			Sheep	1 ml	3 months	Annually	IM
			Cattle	1 ml	3 months	Annually	IM
			Horses	1 ml	3 months	Annually	IM
DEFENSOR	Pfizer, Inc.	Pfizer, Inc.	Dogs	1 ml	3 months & 1 year later	Triennially	IM or SC
	License No. 189		Cats	1 ml	3 months & 1 year later	Triennially	SC
			Sheep	2 ml	3 months	Annually	IM
			Cattle	2 ml	3 months	Annually	IM
RABDOMUN	Pfizer, Inc.	Schering-Plough	Dogs	1 ml	3 months & 1 year later	Triennially	IM or SC
	License No. 189		Cats	1 ml	3 months & 1 year later	Triennially	SC
			Sheep	2 ml	3 months	Annually	IM
			Cattle	2 ml	3 months	Annually	IM
RABDOMUN 1	Pfizer, Inc.	Schering-Plough	Dogs	1 ml	3 months	Annually	IM or SC
	License No. 189		Cats	1 ml	3 months	Annually	SC
SENTRYRAB 1	Pfizer, Inc.	Synbiotics Corp.	Dogs	1 ml	3 months	Annually	IM
	License No. 189		Cats	1 ml	3 months	Annually	IM
RABVAC 1	Fort Dodge Animal Health	Fort Dodge Animal Health	Dogs	1 ml	3 months	Annually	IM or SC
	License No. 112		Cats	1 ml	3 months	Annually	IM or SC
RABVAC 3	Fort Dodge Animal Health	Fort Dodge Animal Health	Dogs	1 ml	3 months & 1 year later	Triennially	IM or SC
	License No. 112		Cats	1 ml	3 months & 1 year later	Triennially	IM or SC
			Horses	2 ml	3 months	Annually	IM
PRORAB-1	Intervet, Inc.	Intervet, Inc.	Dogs	1 ml	3 months	Annually	IM or SC
	License No. 286		Cats	1 ml	3 months	Annually	IM or SC
			Sheep	2 ml	3 months	Annually	IM

Table continued on following page

PART II: RABIES VACCINES LICENSED IN U.S. AND NASPHV RECOMMENDATIONS, 1998 *Continued*

Product Name	Produced by	Marketed by	For Use in	Dosage	Age at Primary Vaccination[1]	Booster Recommended	Route of Inoculation
PRORAB-3F	Intervet, Inc. License No. 286	Intervet, Inc.	Cats	1 ml	3 months & 1 year later	Triennially	IM or SC
RM IMRAB 3	Rhone Merieux, Inc. License No. 298	Merial, Inc.	Dogs	1 ml	3 months & 1 year later	Triennially	IM or SC
			Cats	1 ml	3 months & 1 year later	Triennially	IM or SC
			Sheep	2 ml	3 months & 1 year later	Triennially	IM or SC
			Cattle	2 ml	3 months	Annually	IM or SC
			Horses	2 ml	3 months	Annually	IM or SC
			Ferrets	1 ml	3 months	Annually	SC
RM IMRAB 1 BOVINE PLUS	Rhone Merieux, Inc. License No. 298	Merial, Inc.	Cattle	2 ml	3 months	Annually	IM or SC
			Horses	2 ml	3 months	Annually	IM or SC
			Sheep	2 ml	3 months & 1 year later	Triennially	IM or SC
RM IMRAB 1	Rhone Merieux Inc. License No. 298	Merial, Inc.	Dogs	1 ml	3 months	Annually	IM or SC
			Cats	1 ml	3 months	Annually	IM or SC
B) Combination (inactivated rabies)							
ECLIPSE 3 + FeLV/R	Fort Dodge Animal Health License No. 112	Schering-Plough	Cats	1 ml	3 months	Annually	IM or SC[3]
ECLIPSE 4 + FeLV/R	Fort Dodge Animal Health License No. 112	Schering-Plough	Cats	1 ml	3 months	Annually	IM or SC
Fel-O-GUARD 3 + FeLV/R	Fort Dodge Animal Health License No. 112	Fort Dodge Animal Health	Cats	1 ml	3 months	Annually	IM or SC
Fel-O-GUARD 4 + FeLV/R	Fort Dodge Animal Health License No. 112	Fort Dodge Animal Health	Cats	1 ml	3 months	Annually	IM or SC
FEL-O-VAX PCT-R	Fort Dodge Animal Health License No. 112	Fort Dodge Animal Health	Cats	1 ml	3 months & 1 year later	Triennially	IM
RM FELINE 4 + IMRAB	Rhone Merieux, Inc. License No. 298	Merial, Inc.	Cats	1 ml	3 months & 1 year later	Triennially	SC
RM FELINE 3 + IMRAB	Rhone Meriux, Inc. License No. 298	Merial, Inc.	Cats	1 ml	3 months & 1 year later	Triennially	SC
RM EQUINE POTOMAVAC + IMRAB	Rhone Meriux, Inc. License No. 298	Merial, Inc.	Horses	1 ml	3 months	Annually	IM
MYSTIQUE II	Bayer Corp. License No. 52	Bayer Corp.	Horses	1 ml	3 months	Annually	IM
C) Oral (rabies glycoprotein, live vaccinia vector)—restricted to use in state and federal rabies control programs							
Raboral	Rhone Meriux, Inc. License No. 298	Merial, Inc.	Raccoons	N/A	N/A	To be determined	PO[4]

[1]Three months of age (or older) and revaccinated one year later.
[2]Intramuscularly.
[3]Subcutaneously.
[4]Per os.

PART III: RABIES CONTROL

A. PRINCIPLES OF RABIES CONTROL

1. HUMAN RABIES PREVENTION: Rabies in humans can be prevented either by eliminating exposures to rabid animals or by providing exposed persons with prompt local treatment of wounds combined with appropriate passive and active immunization. The rationale for recommending preexposure and postexposure rabies prophylaxis and details of their administration can be found in the current recommendations of the Immunization Practices Advisory Committee (ACIP) of the Public Health Service (PHS). These recommendations, along with information concerning the current local and regional status of animal rabies and the availability of human rabies biologics, are available from state health departments.
2. DOMESTIC ANIMALS: Local governments should initiate and maintain effective programs to ensure vaccination of all dogs, cats, and ferrets and to remove strays and unwanted animals. Such procedures in the United States have reduced laboratory-confirmed rabies cases in dogs from 6,949 in 1947 to 111 in 1996. Since more rabies cases are reported annually involving cats than dogs, vaccination of cats should be required. The recommended vaccination procedures and the licensed animal vaccines are specified in Parts I and II of the Compendium.
3. RABIES IN WILDLIFE: The control of rabies among wildlife reservoirs is difficult. Vaccination of free-ranging wildlife or selective population reduction may be useful in some situations, but the success of such procedures depends on the circumstances surrounding each rabies outbreak. (See C. Control Methods in Wildlife.)

B. CONTROL METHODS IN DOMESTIC AND CONFINED ANIMALS

1. PREEXPOSURE VACCINATION AND MANAGEMENT
   Parenteral animal rabies vaccines should be administered only by, or under the direct supervision of, a veterinarian. This is the only way to ensure that a responsible person can be held accountable to assure the public that the animal has been properly vaccinated. Within 1 month after primary vaccination, a peak rabies antibody titer is reached and the animal can be considered immunized. An animal is currently vaccinated and is considered immunized if it was vaccinated at least 30 days previously, and all vaccinations have been administered in accordance with this Compendium. Regardless of the age at initial vaccination, a second vaccination should be given one year later. (See Parts I and II for recommended vaccines and procedures.)
   (a) DOGS, CATS, AND FERRETS
   All dogs, cats, and ferrets should be vaccinated against rabies at 3 months of age and revaccinated in accordance with Part II of this Compendium. If a previously vaccinated animal is overdue for a booster, it should be revaccinated with a single dose of vaccine and placed on an annual or triennial schedule depending on the type of vaccine used.
   (b) LIVESTOCK
   It is neither economically feasible nor justified from a public health standpoint to vaccinate all livestock against rabies. However, consideration should be given to vaccination of livestock which are particularly valuable and/or may have frequent contact with humans.
   (c) OTHER ANIMALS
   (1) WILD
   No parenteral rabies vaccine is licensed for use in wild animals. Because of the risk of rabies in wild animals (especially raccoons, skunks, coyotes, foxes, and bats), the AVMA, the NASPHV, and the CSTE strongly recommend the enactment of state laws prohibiting the importation, distribution, relocation, or keeping of wild animals or hybrids as pets.
   (2) MAINTAINED IN EXHIBITS AND IN ZOOLOGICAL PARKS
   Captive animals not completely excluded from all contact with rabies vectors can become infected. Moreover, wild animals may be incubating rabies when initially captured; therefore, wild-caught animals susceptible to rabies should be quarantined for a minimum of 180 days before exhibition. Employees who work with animals at such facilities should receive preexposure rabies immunization. The use of pre- or postexposure rabies immunizations of employees who work with animals at such facilities may reduce the need for euthanasia of captive animals.
2. STRAY ANIMALS
   Stray dogs, cats, or ferrets should be removed from the community. Local health departments and animal control officials can enforce the removal of strays more effectively if owned animals are confined or kept on leash. Strays should be impounded for at least 3 days to give owners sufficient time to reclaim animals and to determine if human exposure has occurred.
3. QUARANTINE
   (a) INTERNATIONAL
   CDC regulates the importation of dogs and cats into the United States, but present PHS regulations (42 CFR No. 71.51) governing the importation of such animals are insufficient to prevent the introduction of rabid animals into the country. All dogs and cats imported from countries with endemic rabies should be currently vaccinated against rabies as recommended in this Compendium. The appropriate public health official of the state of destination should be notified within 72 hours of any unvaccinated dog or cat imported into his or her jurisdiction. The conditional admission of such animals into the United States is subject to state and local laws governing rabies. Failure to comply with these requirements should be promptly reported to the Division of Quarantine, CDC, 404-639-8107.
   (b) INTERSTATE
   Prior to interstate movement, dogs, cats, and ferrets should be currently vaccinated against rabies in accordance with the Compendium's recommendations (see B.1. Preexposure Vaccination and Management). Animals in transit should be accompanied by a currently valid NASPHV Form #51, Rabies Vaccination Certificate.

4. ADJUNCT PROCEDURES
   Methods or procedures which enhance rabies control include:
   (a) LICENSURE. Registration or licensure of all dogs, cats, and ferrets may be used to aid in rabies control. A fee is frequently charged for such licensure and revenues collected are used to maintain rabies or animal control programs. Vaccination is an essential prerequisite to licensure.
   (b) CANVASSING OF AREA. House-to-house canvassing by animal control personnel facilitates enforcement of vaccination and licensure requirements.
   (c) CITATIONS. Citations are legal summonses issued to owners for violations, including the failure to vaccinate or license their animals. The authority for officers to issue citations should be an integral part of each animal control program.
   (d) ANIMAL CONTROL. All communities should incorporate stray animal control, leash laws, and training of personnel in their programs.
5. POSTEXPOSURE MANAGEMENT
   ANY ANIMAL BITTEN OR SCRATCHED BY A WILD, CARNIVOROUS MAMMAL OR A BAT THAT IS NOT AVAILABLE FOR TESTING SHOULD BE REGARDED AS HAVING BEEN EXPOSED TO RABIES.
   (a) DOGS, CATS, AND FERRETS
   Unvaccinated dogs, cats, and ferrets exposed to a rabid animal should be euthanized immediately. If the owner is unwilling to have this done, the animal should be placed in strict isolation for 6 months and vaccinated 1 month before being released. Animals with expired vaccinations need to be evaluated on a case by case basis. Dogs, cats, and ferrets that are currently vaccinated should be revaccinated immediately, kept under the owner's control, and observed for 45 days.
   (b) LIVESTOCK
   All species of livestock are susceptible to rabies; cattle and horses are among the most frequently infected. Livestock exposed to a rabid animal and currently vaccinated with a vaccine approved by USDA for that species should be revaccinated immediately and observed for 45 days. Unvaccinated livestock should be slaughtered immediately. If the owner is unwilling to have this done, the animal should be kept under very close observation for 6 months.
   The following are recommendations for owners of unvaccinated livestock exposed to rabid animals:
   (1) If the animal is slaughtered within 7 days of being bitten, its tissues may be eaten without risk of infection, provided liberal portions of the exposed area are discarded. Federal meat inspectors must reject for slaughter any animal known to have been exposed to rabies within 8 months.
   (2) Neither tissues nor milk from a rabid animal should be used for human or animal consumption. However, since pasteurization temperatures will inactivate rabies virus, drinking pasteurized milk or eating cooked meat does not constitute a rabies exposure.
   (3) It is rare to have more than one rabid animal in a herd, or herbivore to herbivore transmission; therefore, it may not be necessary to restrict the rest of the herd if a single animal has been exposed to or infected by rabies.
   (c) OTHER ANIMALS
   Other animals bitten by a rabid animal should be euthanized immediately. Animals maintained in USDA-licensed research facilities or accredited zoological parks should be evaluated on a case by case basis.
6. MANAGEMENT OF ANIMALS THAT BITE HUMANS
   A healthy dog, cat, or ferret that bites a person should be confined and observed for 10 days; it is recommended that rabies vaccine not be administered during the observation period. Such animals should be evaluated by a veterinarian at the first sign of illness during confinement. Any illness in the animal should be reported immediately to the local health department. If signs suggestive of rabies develop, the animal should be euthanized, its head removed, and the head shipped under refrigeration (not frozen) for examination of the brain by a qualified laboratory designated by the local or state health department. Any stray or unwanted dog, cat, or ferret that bites a person may be euthanized immediately and the head submitted as described above for rabies examination. Other biting animals which might have exposed a person to rabies should be reported immediately to the local health department. Prior vaccination of an animal may not preclude the necessity for euthanasia and testing if the period of virus shedding is unknown for that species. Management of animals other than dogs, cats, and ferrets depends on the species, the circumstances of the bite, the epidemiology of rabies in the area, and the biting animal's history, current health status, and potential for exposure to rabies.

C. CONTROL METHODS IN WILDLIFE
The public should be warned not to handle wildlife. Wild mammals and hybrids that bite or otherwise expose people, pets or livestock should be considered for euthanasia and rabies examination. A person bitten by any wild mammal should immediately report the incident to a physician who can evaluate the need for antirabies treatment. (See current rabies prophylaxis recommendations of the ACIP.)
1. TERRESTRIAL MAMMALS
   The use of licensed oral vaccines for the mass immunization of free-ranging wildlife should be considered in selected situations, with the approval of the state agency responsible for animal rabies control. Continuous and persistent government-funded programs for trapping or poisoning wildlife are not cost effective in reducing wildlife rabies reservoirs on a statewide basis. However, limited control in high-contact areas (picnic grounds, camps, suburban areas) may be indicated for the removal of selected high-risk species of wildlife. The state wildlife agency and state health department should be consulted for coordination of any proposed vaccination or population reduction programs.
2. BATS
   (a) Indigenous rabid bats have been reported from every state except Hawaii, and have caused rabies in at least 28 humans in the United States. It is neither feasible nor desirable, however, to control rabies in bats by programs to reduce bat populations.
   (b) Bats should be excluded from houses and adjacent structures to prevent direct association with humans. Such structures should then be made bat-proof by sealing entrances used by bats.

Appendix 5

Laboratory Testing for Infectious Diseases of Dogs and Cats

Deborah C. Silverstein and Craig E. Greene

PART A: LABORATORIES PERFORMING COMMERCIAL ASSAYS FOR INFECTIOUS DISEASES

State/ Country	Laboratory	Address	City	Zip Code	Telephone
AL	1. Alabama State Veterinary Diagnostic Lab	P.O. Box 2209	Auburn	36831-2209	334-844-4987
AL	2. Auburn University	College of Veterinary Medicine, Department of Pathobiology, 166 Greene Hall	Auburn University	36849-5519	334-844-4539
AZ	3. Protatek Reference Laboratory	574 East Alamo St, Suite #90	Chandler	85225	602-545-8499
AZ	3A. Antech Diagnostics	13633 N. Cave Creek Rd.	Phoenix	85022	800-592-0503
AZ	4. Glen Zonger, Dawn Bueschel	Department of Veterinary Science, University of Arizona, 1117 E. Lowell St	Tucson	85721	520-621-2745
CA	5. University of California-Davis	Veterinary Medical Teaching Hospital, Clinical Pathology	Davis	95616	530-752-1393
CA	6. CA Veterinary Diagnostic Lab System	School of Veterinary Medicine, University of California-Davis, Box 1770	Davis	95617	530-752-8709
CA	6A. Antech Diagnostics	17672-A Cowan Ave, Suite 200	Irvine	92614	714-752-5612 800-542-1151 800-592-0503
CA	7. Engene Biotechnologies Incorporated, USA	16236 San Dieguito Rd, Suite 4-21, P.O. Box 9430	Rancho Santa Fe	92067-9430	619-759-9424
CA	7A. CVD[a]	2825 KOVR Dr	West Sacramento	95606	800-444-4210
CO	8. Veterinary Diagnostic Laboratory	Colorado State University	Fort Collins	80523	970-491-1281
CO	9. Plague Branch VBDD	Centers for Disease Control and Prevention, P.O. Box 2087	Fort Collins	80522	970-221-6465
CO	9A. Veterinary Services, Inc.[a] Corporate Office	2150 West 6th Ave, Suite H	Broomfield	80020	800-874-1983
CT	10. University of Connecticut	Department of Pathobiology, Box U-89, 61 N. Eagleville Rd	Storrs	06268	203-486-3736
FL	11. Animal Disease Laboratory	Florida Department of Agriculture, P.O. Box 460	Kissimmee	32742	407-846-5200
GA	12. Diagnostic Assistance Laboratory	College of Veterinary Medicine, The University of Georgia	Athens	30602	706-542-5568
GA	13. Tifton Veterinary Diagnostic Laboratory	P.O. Box 1389, Brighton Rd	Tifton	31793	912-386-3340
GA	14. Infectious Disease Laboratory	Department of Medical Microbiology, College of Veterinary Medicine, The University of Georgia	Athens	30602	706-542-5812
GA	15. Centers for Disease Control and Prevention	Mycology Unit or Bacteriology Unit, U.S. Department of Health & Human Services	Atlanta	30333	404-639-3311
IL	16. Department of Veterinary Pathobiology	2001 South Lincoln Ave, College of Veterinary Medicine, University of Illinois	Urbana	61801	217-333-1620
IL	17. Animal Disease Laboratory	Illinois Department of Agriculture, Shattic Road	Centralia	62801	618-532-6701

State/ Country		Laboratory	Address	City	Zip Code	Telephone
IL	18.	Animal Disease Laboratory	Illinois Department of Agriculture, 1455 Windish Dr, P.O. Box 2100X	Galesburg	61402-2100	309-344-2451
IL	18A.	Illinois Veterinary Laboratory[a]	650 Grand Ave	Elmhurst	60126	800-433-6928
IN	19.	Purdue University	1175 ADDL	West Lafayette	47907-1175	317-494-7440
IN	19A.	Antech Diagnostics	2351 South State Rd Z	Valparaiso	46383	219-464-1336 800-521-5849
IA	20.	Veterinary Diagnostic Laboratory	College of Veterinary Medicine, Iowa State University	Ames	50010	515-294-1950
KS	21.	Veterinary Diagnostic Laboratory	College of Veterinary Medicine, Veterinary Medical Center	Manhattan	66506	913-532-5650
KY	22.	Veterinary Diagnostic and Research Center	Murray State University, P.O. Box 2000, North Dr	Hopkinsville	42240	502-886-3959
KY	23.	Livestock Disease Diagnostic Center	University of Kentucky, 1429 Newtown Pike	Lexington	40511	606-253-0571
LA	24.	Louisiana Veterinary Medical Diagnostic Laboratory	School of Veterinary Medicine, Louisiana State University, P.O. Box 16570-A	Baton Rouge	70803	504-346-3193
ME	25.	IDEXX Laboratories[a]	One IDEXX Dr	Westbrook	04092	800-262-5801 1-888-Rx-IDEXX
MD	26.	Maryland Medical Laboratory, Inc.	1901 Sulfur Spring Rd	Baltimore	21227	410-247-9100
MD	27.	AnMed/Biosafe, Inc	7642 Standish Pl	Rockville	20855	301-762-0366
MA	28.	Division of Diagnostic Laboratories	Tufts University, 200 Westboro Rd	North Grafton	01536	508-839-7900
MI	29.	Animal Health Diagnostic Lab	Michigan State University, P.O. Box 30076	Lansing	48909-7576	517-353-0635
MN	30.	University of Minnesota	Veterinary Diagnostic Medicine, 1943 Carter Ave	St. Paul	55101	612-625-0256
MS	31.	Mississippi Board of Animal Health and Veterinary Diagnostic Laboratory	2531 North West St, P.O. Box 4389	Jackson	39216	601-354-6092
MO	32.	Dillavon, Tran, & Kline	National Reference Lab, Inc., 2200 S. Business 63	Kirksville	63501	816-665-1418
MO	33.	Veterinary Medical Diagnostic Lab	University of Missouri-Columbia	Columbia	65211	573-882-6811
MT	34.	State of Montana Animal Health Division	Box 997	Bozeman	59771	406-994-4885
NE	35.	Lincoln Diagnostic Laboratories	University of Nebraska	Lincoln	68583	402-472-1434
NJ	35A.	Cardiopet Incorporated[a] Cardiopet Veterinary Associates, P.A.	48 Notch Rd	Little Falls	07424	800-726-1212
NM	36.	New Mexico Department of Agriculture	Veterinary Diagnostic Services, 700 Camino de Salud, NE	Albuquerque	87106	800-432-9110 505-841-2576
NM	37.	New Mexico Department of Health	Scientific Lab Division, P.O. Box 4700	Albuquerque	87196	505-841-2535
NY	38.	Diagnostic Laboratory	New York State College of Veterinary Medicine, Box 5786, Cornell University	Ithaca	14852	607-253-3900
NY	38A.	Dr. Steve Barr (prior arrangement needed)	New York State College of Veterinary Medicine, Cornell University	Ithaca	14852	607-253-3043
NY	39.	Antech Diagnostics	10 Executive Blvd	Farmingdale	11735	516-753-4100 800-872-1001
NC	40.	North Carolina State University	School of Veterinary Medicine, 4700 Hillsborough St	Raleigh	27606	919-829-4347

State/ Country	Laboratory	Address	City	Zip Code	Telephone
NC	41. Roche Biovet	Division of Roche Biomedical Labs, P.O. Box 2230	Burlington	27215	800-334-5161 (Natl) 800-672-3646 (NC)
NC	42. Rollins Animal Disease Diagnostic Laboratory	NC Department of Agriculture, P.O. Box 12223, Cameron Village Station	Raleigh	27605	919-733-3986
NC	43. Lab Corp	Bioveterinary Testing Services, P.O. Box 2230	Burlington	27216	800-331-2843
ND	44. North Dakota State University of Agriculture & Applied Science	Veterinary Science	Fargo	58105	701-231-7522
OH	45. Ohio State University	College of Veterinary Medicine, 1925 Coffee Rd, Room 305	Columbus	43210-1089	614-292-5661
OH	46. Ohio Department of Agriculture	Division of Animal Health, 8995 E. Main St	Reynoldsburg	43068	614-866-6361
OK	46A. Veterinary Services of Oklahoma[a]	7601 Northwest 72nd, Suite 340	Oklahoma City	73132	405-721-3818
OK	47. Oklahoma Animal Disease Diagnostic Laboratory	Oklahoma State University	Stillwater	74078	405-744-6623
OK	47A. Cerodex Laboratory, Inc.	Route 1, Box 32T	Washington	73093	405-288-2383 800-654-3639
OR	47B. Antech Diagnostics	12616 Southeast Stark St	Portland	97233	800-485-8753
PA	48. Laboratory of Pathology	School of Veterinary Medicine, University of Pennsylvania	Philadelphia	19104	215-898-8859
PA	49. Immunology Service Center	VHUP, Room 2016, 3850 Spruce St	Philadelphia	19104-6010	215-898-6882
PA	50. PA Animal Diagnostic Lab System (PADLS)	Animal Health & Diagnostic Com., 2301 N. Camaron St	Harrisburg	17110-9408	717-787-2103
SD	51. Animal Disease Diagnostic Laboratory	South Dakota State University, P.O. Box 2175	Brookings	57007	605-688-5172
TN	52. C.E. Kord Animal Disease Laboratory	P.O. Box 40627, Melrose Station	Nashville	37204	615-360-0125
TN	53. Quest Diagnostic, Inc	210 12th Ave South	Nashville	37202-5110	615-255-5786
	54. Texas Veterinary Medical Diagnostic Laboratory	Drawer 3040	College Station	77841-3040	409-845-3414 888-646-5623
TX	55. Veterinary Medical Diagnostic Laboratory	Texas A&M University, P.O. Box 3200	Amarillo	79106	806-353-7478
TX	55A. VETLAB, Inc.[a]	5314 Broadway Ave	Forth Worth	76117	800-366-4184
VA	56. State of Virginia	Department of Agriculture and Consumer Services, Division of Animal Health, Bureau of Laboratory Services, 1 North 14th St, Room 162	Richmond	23219	804-786-9202
WA	56A. Dermatodiagnostics c/o HCS	85 SE 8th Ave, P.O. Box 1109	Oak Harbor	98277	425-775-6903
WA	57. Washington Animal Disease Diagnostic Laboratory	College of Veterinary Medicine, Washington State University, P.O. Box 2037, College Station	Pullman	99165-2037	509-335-9696
WA	58. VMRD, Inc.	NW 115 State St	Pullman	99163	509-334-5815
WI	59. Wisconsin Department of Agriculture, Trade, and Consumer Protection	Animal Health Division (Central Lab), 6101 Mineral Point Rd	Madison	53705-4494	608-266-2465
WI	60. Wisconsin Department of Agriculture, Trade, and Consumer Protection	Animal Health Division (Regional Lab), 1418 East LaSalle Ave	Barron	54812	715-537-3151

State/ Country		Laboratory	Address	City	Zip Code	Telephone
WY	61.	Wyoming State Veterinary Laboratory	1174 Snowy Range Rd	Laramie	82070	307-742-6638
Canada	62.	Guelph, Ontario, Ministry of Agriculture & Food	Veterinary Laboratory Services, Guelph Laboratories, Box 3612	Guelph, Ontario		519-823-8800
Canada	62A.	Dr. John Papp	Department of Pathobiology, University of Guelph	Guelph, Ontario		519-823-8800 Ext. 4758
England	63.	Liverpool University	Department of Clinical Pathology, P.O. Box 147	Liverpool		151-709-6022
England	63A.	The Liverpool School of Tropical Medicine		Liverpool		151-708-9393 Ext. 2220
England	64.	Diagnostic Laboratory	London School of Hygiene	London		44-171-636-8636
France	64A.	Rickettsial Unit, Center of Scientific Research	27 Boulevard Jean Moulin 13385	Cedex 05, Marseille		33-91-385517
Scotland	65.	Glasgow University	Department of Veterinary Pathology, University of Glasgow Veterinary School	Bearsden, Glasgow		041-330-5773

[a]These are divisions of IDDEXX Laboratories.

PART B: LABORATORY TESTS AND INTERPRETATION

Infectious Disease	Sample (Amount or Handling)	Detecting: Method Used (Laboratory, Reagents, or Test Kit)	Interpretation
Diagnosis of Viral, Rickettsial, Chlamydial, and Mycoplasmal Infections (see Chapter 1)			
Canine Distemper (see Chapter 3)			
Antemortem	Blood or buffy coat smear, conjunctival scraping, CSF, transtracheal wash (cytologic smears are air dried and refrigerated, alcohol- or acetone-fixed)	Ag: FA (many) Ag: ELISA (research)	Positive result confirms infection with proper technique; false-negative results possible in chronic (CNS) infections; false-positive results caused by lab technique.
	Serum: paired samples taken 10–14 days apart (2–3 ml, refrigerated)	Ab: VN (many) Ab: FA (many) Ab: ELISA (research, K6A)	Paired samples: rising (4-fold) IgG or high IgM titer confirms active infection; >100 single VN titer indicates relative immune protection against disease.
	CSF (1–3 ml), refrigerated	Ab: VN (38, 57) Ab: FA (research) Ab: ELISA (K6A)	Positive titer confirms CNS infection if serum contamination is excluded or if CSF titer is high relative to serum titer and titer to another infectious agent; some inconsistencies have been noted.
Postmortem	Lung, bladder, cerebellum, or conjunctival smear (refrigerated)	Ag: FA (many) Virus: VI (many, 38)	Positive result confirms infection.
	Lung, bladder, brain, liver, stomach (formalin-fixed)	Lesion: histol (many) Viral genome: PCR (research, 5) Ag: IHC (38)	Inclusion body detection with compatible histologic changes indicates infection; some false-positive and false-negative results.

Infectious Disease	Sample (Amount or Handling)	Detecting: Method Used (Laboratory, Reagents, or Test Kit)	Interpretation
Infectious Canine Hepatitis (see Chapter 4)			
Antemortem	Oropharyngeal swabs, urine, feces (refrigerated)	Virus: VI (many) Ab: HA-I (8)	Positive result confirms infection.
	Serum: paired samples taken 10–14 days apart (2–3 ml, refrigerated)	Ab: VN (many) Ab: FA (13, 19, 43, 52, 53)	Paired samples: rising (4-fold) titer confirms active infection.
Postmortem	Liver—fresh impression smear (refrigerated or alcohol-fixed)	Inclusions: cytol (many)	Presence of intranuclear inclusions supportive of diagnosis.
	Spleen, liver, brain (refrigerated)	Ag: FA (many)	Positive result confirms infection.
	Liver, gallbladder, kidney, lung, stomach, brain (formalin-fixed)	Lesions: histol (many)	Compatible histologic changes indicate infection.
Canine Herpesvirus Infection (see Chapter 5)			
Antemortem	Nasal swab, vaginal swab (refrigerated)	Virus: VI Ag: FA (many)	Positive result confirms infection.
	Serum: paired samples taken 10–14 days apart (2–3 ml, refrigerated)	Ab: VN (2, 38, 54, 57) Ab: FA (19, 44, 52)	Paired samples: rising (4-fold) titer confirms active infection; single-titer interpretation only determines prior exposure.
Postmortem	Neonates: lung, liver, kidney, CNS (refrigerated)	Virus: VI (many)	Positive result confirms infection.
	Brain, lymph node, liver, adrenal, kidney, spleen, lung (refrigerated)	Ag: FA (12, 38, 44, 52)	Positive result confirms infection.
	Tissue (formalin-fixed)	Ag: IHC (38)	Positive result confirms infection.
Canine Parainfluenza Infection (see Chapters 6 and 7)			
	Transtracheal washing, oropharyngeal swab, CSF (refrigerated)	Virus: VI (many)	Positive result confirms infection.
	Serum or CSF (2–3 ml, refrigerated)	Ab: VN (38, 57) Ab: FA (19, 43, 53)	Paired serum samples: rising (4-fold) titer confirms active infection; CSF positive titer confirms infection.
Canine Parvovirus Infection (see Chapter 8)			
Antemortem	Serum: paired samples taken 10–14 days apart (2–3 ml, refrigerated)	Ab: HA-I (many) Ab: VN (many) Ab: FA (many) Ab: ELISA (many, K1, K1A—quantitative)	Positive titers (level varies with lab) indicate protection; paired samples: rising (4-fold) titer confirms active infection; IgG titer usually increased by the time clinical signs are observed. As a single specimen, high serum IgM titer or fecal Ag examination is more diagnostic of active infection.
	Feces or rectal mucosa (refrigerated)	Ag: HA (many) Virus: EM (many) Ag: FA (many) Ag: ELISA (many, K1, K1B, K1C) Viral genome: PCR (research)	Positive result confirms infection; clinical disease associated with shedding of large quantities of virus; some shedders are subclinical carriers; false-negative result after 5–7 days of clinical illness.
Postmortem	Small intestine, heart (neonatal) (refrigerated)	Ag: FA (many) Virus: VI (many)	Positive result confirms infection.
	Intestine (formalin-fixed)	Lesions: histol (38)	Positive result confirms infection.
Canine Calicivirus Infection (see Chapter 8)			
	Oropharyngeal swab, fecal swab, trachea, lung, kidney, intestine (refrigerated)	Virus: VI (many)	Positive result confirms infection.

Infectious Disease	Sample (Amount or Handling)	Detecting: Method Used (Laboratory, Reagents, or Test Kit)	Interpretation
Canine Coronavirus Infection (see Chapter 8)			
Antemortem	Serum: paired samples taken 10–14 days apart (2–3 ml, refrigerated)	Ab: FA (many) Ab: VN (38)	Single high IgG titer indicates exposure only; serum titer does not reflect degree of protection against infection. Paired samples: rising (4-fold) IgG titer confirms infection.
	Feces (refrigerated)	Virus: VI (5, 12) Virus: EM (8, 12, 19, 33, 38, 52, 54, 59) Viral genome: PCR (research labs)	Positive result showing high particle numbers confirms infection; some shedders are subclinical carriers.
Postmortem	Intestine (refrigerated)	Ag: FA (many, 31, 33) Virus: VI (38)	Positive result confirms infection.
	Intestine (formalin-fixed)	Lesions: histol (38)	Compatible histologic changes indicate infection.
Canine and Feline Rotavirus Infection (see also Chapters 8 and 12)			
Antemortem	Feces (fresh, refrigerated)	Virus: VI (19) Virus: EM (19, 43, 52, 54, 59) Ag: ELISA (57, K3, K4, K5) Ag: LA (many, K2, K6)	Positive result confirms infection; some shedders may be subclinical carriers.
Postmortem	Tissue (intestine, refrigerated) (glutaraldehyde fixation)	Ag: FA (36) Virus: EM (52)	Positive result confirms infection.
Canine Papillomatosis (see Chapter 9)			
	Oral tissue (formalin fixed) (glutaraldehyde fixed)	Lesion: histol (many) Virus: EM (many)	Positive result suggests infection. Positive indicates viral-induced tumor.
Feline Panleukopenia (see Chapter 10)			
Antemortem	Serum: paired samples taken 10–14 days apart (2–3 ml, refrigerated)	Ab: FA, VN (many, 13, 19, 47, 52, 57) Ab: HA-I (8, 38)	Paired samples: rising (4-fold) IgG titer confirms active infection.
	Feces (fresh, refrigerated)	Virus: VI (8, 57) Ag: ELISA (many, K1, K1C) Virus: EM (8, 54, 57, 59) Viral genome: PCR (research labs)	Positive results confirms infection; some shedders (usually lower levels) are subclinical carriers.
Postmortem	Intestine, mesenteric lymph nodes, lung, pharyngeal swab (fresh or refrigerated)	Ag: FA (many) Virus: VI (many)	Positive result confirms infection.
	Intestine, feces, mesenteric lymph node (glutaraldehyde fixation)	Virus: EM (12)	Positive result confirms infection.
Feline Infectious Peritonitis (see Chapter 11)			
Antemortem	Serum, fluid effusion (1–2 ml, refrigerated)	Ab: FA (many) Ab: VM (many) Ab: ELISA (many, K7, K7A) Ab: PE (many) Ab: kinELISA (38)	Positive serum titer suggests exposure to FCoV; interpretation must be based on level of titer with knowledge of exposure of population of cats in environment. Titers vary among labs.
Postmortem	Liver, small intestine, kidney (refrigerated)	Ag: FA (many)	Positive result confirms infection.
	Kidney, liver, small intestine (formalin fixed)	Lesions: histol (many)	Compatible histologic changes indicate infection. Can do IHC to detect intralesional virus.
	Effusion fluid, lymphoid tissue, tissue sample (fresh refrigerated, fixed, or embedded)	Ag: IHC (38) Viral genome: PCR (5, 6a, 7, 39, K7B)	Positive result confirms lesions associated with this virus.

Infectious Disease	Sample (Amount or Handling)	Detecting: Method Used (Laboratory, Reagents, or Test Kit)	Interpretation
Feline Leukemia Virus Infection (see Chapter 13 and Table 13–3)			
Antemortem	Blood film or buffy coat or bone marrow smear (air-dried)	Ag: FA (many)	Positive result confirms infection; more specific for bone marrow infections than ELISA.
	Serum or anticoagulated whole blood (1–2 ml) Saliva (fresh or refrigerated)	Ag: ELISA (many, K8, K10, K11, K12, K13, K14, K15, K16) Ag: K15	Positive result confirms infection; more sensitive than FA; with saliva, some viremic cats are not positive.
	Serum (2–3 ml, refrigerated)	Ab: Not available commercially; only research laboratories	Positive result confirms current antitumor protection; may change with time.
Postmortem or antemortem	Blood (heparinized) or tissue, marrow (refrigerated, fresh)	Ag: FA (many)	Positive result confirms infection.
	Lymphoid tissue or bone marrow, anticoagulated blood (refrigerated)	Viral genome: PCR (7, 39)	Positive result confirms infection.
Feline Immunodeficiency Virus Infection (see Chapter 14)			
	Serum, anticoagulated whole, blood (1–2 ml, refrigerated)	Ab: ELISA (many, K9, K10, K12, K16a) Ab: kinELISA (38) Ab: (IgG) IFA (2, 5, 25, 52) Ab: immunoblot (5, 25, 38, 39, 53)	Positive result confirms exposure and probable infection with virus; few animals may test seropositive but be subclinical carriers.
	Lymphoid tissue, anticoagulated whole blood, bone marrow (refrigerated)	Virus: PCR (7)	Positive result confirms infection.
Feline Syncytium-Forming Virus Infections (see Chapter 17)			
	Serum (2 ml, refrigerated or frozen)	Ab: FA: not available commercially, research laboratories	Positive result indicates exposure.
Feline Papillomavirus Infections (see Chapter 21)			
Antemortem	Skin biopsies (formalin fixed)	Lesions: histol (many)	A histologic diagnosis suggestive.
	Skin biopsies (fixed or embedded)	FA or IHC (56a)	Positive staining indicates lesions from papillomavirus infection.
Rhinotracheitis Virus Infection (see Chapter 16)			
Antemortem	Serum: paired samples taken 10–14 days apart (2–3 ml, refrigerated)	Ab: FA (2, 19, 43, 52, 53) Ab: VN (many)	Paired samples: rising (4-fold) titer confirms active infection.
	Nasal swab (refrigerated)	Virus: VI (many)	Positive result indicates infection.
	Conjunctival smear (unfixed)	Ag: FA (5)	Positive result indicates infection.
Postmortem	Lung, liver, kidney (frozen or refrigerated)	Ag: FA (many) Virus: VI (many)	Positive result confirms infection.
	Lung, trachea, conjunctival smears, feces (glutaraldehyde fixed)	Virus: EM (12) Viral genome: PCR (research)	Positive result confirms infection.
Feline Calicivirus Infection (see Chapter 16)			
Antemortem	Serum: paired samples taken 10–14 days apart (2–3 ml, refrigerated)	Ab: FA (2, 52, 53) Ab: VN (many)	Paired samples: rising (4-fold) titer confirms active infection.
	Oropharyngeal swabs, intestinal and fecal swabs (refrigerated)	Virus: VI (many) Ag: FA (57)	Positive result confirms infection.
	Feces (refrigerated)	Ag: ELISA (8) Virus: EM (8)	Positive result confirms infection.
Postmortem	Trachea, lung, kidney, intestine (refrigerated)	Virus: VI (many) Viral genome: PCR (research)	Positive result confirms infection.

Infectious Disease	Sample (Amount or Handling)	Detecting: Method Used (Laboratory, Reagents, or Test Kit)	Interpretation
Feline Cowpox Infection (see Chapter 19)			
Antemortem	Scabs (dry, sterile vial) or lesions fluid (refrigerated)	Virus: EM (many, 65) Virus: VI (65)	Positive result confirms infection with poxvirus.
	Serum (2–3 ml refrigerated)	Ab: VN (63)	Positive titer confirms exposure but not necessarily active infection.
Rabies (see Chapter 22)			
Antemortem	Vibrissae biopsy (refrigerated, in dry sterile vial)	Research only; not considered as accurate as examination of CNS tissue	Positive result confirms infection.
	CSF (2–3 ml, refrigerated)	Ab: VN (many)	High titer means CNS is infected (vaccine or virulent virus); takes 1–2 weeks to develop a titer and must compare with serum value.
Postmortem	Brain (refrigerated)	Ag: FA (many) Ag: IHC (38)	Positive result confirms infection; more sensitive than Negri body detection.
	Brain (formalin fixed)	Lesion: histol (many) Ag: IHC (38)	Negri bodies not present in all cases; false-positive and false-negative results can occur; IHC makes testing more specific and sensitive.
Pseudorabies (see Chapter 23)			
Antemortem	Serum: paired samples taken 10–14 days apart (2–3 ml, refrigerated)	Ab: VN (many) Ab: LA (38)	Positive result indicates exposure; paired samples; rising (4-fold) titer confirms active infection.
Postmortem	Brain, tonsils, lung, cervical lymph nodes, salivary glands, spleen (refrigerated)	Ag: FA (many) Virus: VI (many)	Positive result confirms infection.
	Brain (formalin-fixed)	Lesions: histol (many)	Compatible histologic changes indicate infection.
Ehrlichiosis (see Chapter 28; see Table 28–3 for specific cross-reactivity)			
Antemortem	Blood films, bone marrow smears (refrigerated or alcohol-fixed)	Cells: cytol (many)	Positive result confirms infection; many false-negative results because of low numbers of organisms.
	Serum (2–3 ml, refrigerated)	Ab: PE (many)	Nonspecific hyperglobulinemia seen with other disorders.
	Serum: single sample (2–3 ml, refrigerated)	*Rickettsia:* RI (5, 45) Ab: FA (*Ehrlichia canis:* 1, 2, 5, 14, 16, 24, 29, 39, 40, 43, K20A, K21) (*E. platys:* 1, 2, 3, 5, 24, 54) (*E. risticii:* 3, 24, 29, 5, 8, 13, 25, 33, 38, 40, 45) (*E. equi:* 3, 5, 13, 38, 45, 54)	Positive titer confirms active infection unless animal was recently treated with appropriate drugs; must be infected for at least 30 days to have positive titer.
	Blood, EDTA anticoagulated 2–3 ml (sterile, refrigerated)	Rickettsial genome: PCR (*Ehrlichia canis:* 5, 7, 14, 38, 45) (*E. platys:* 5, 14) (*E. risticii:* 5, 14, 45) (*E. equi:* 5, 14, 38)	Positive result indicates active infection with specific *Rickettsia*.
Feline Ehrlichiosis (see Chapter 28)			
	Serum (2 ml, nonhemolyzed, refrigerated)	Ab: FA (*E. canis:* 3, 5, 8, 19a, 29, 40, 45) (*E. risticii:* 3, 5, 8, 19a, 40, 45)	Positive titer indicates exposure and, with antibiotic-responsive signs, probable infection.
	Blood, EDTA anticoagulated, 2 ml, refrigerated	PCR (5, 7, 14, 38, 45)	Positive result confirms infection.

Infectious Disease	Sample (Amount or Handling)	Detecting: Method Used (Laboratory, Reagents, or Test Kit)	Interpretation
Rocky Mountain Spotted Fever (see Chapter 29)			
Antemortem or postmortem	Skin biopsy or other tissue (formalin fixed)	Ag: FA (research)	Positive result confirms infection; many false-negative results; no need for species specificity.
	Serum: paired samples taken 10–14 days apart (1–2 ml, refrigerated)	Ab: FA-IgG (14, 25, 39, 40, 43, 53, 64A, K21, K23, K24)	Paired samples: rising (4-fold) IgG titer confirms active infection; species-specific testing required.
	Serum: single sample (1–2 ml, refrigerated)	Ab: FA-IgM (14, 40)	Single positive IgM titer indicates active infection; a second titer may be needed to clarify some low titers.
		Ab: LA (many)	Single positive latex titer indicates active infection since measures IgM.
	Anticoagulated whole blood, tissue	PCR: (7) Rickettsial genome (research)	Positive result confirms active infection.
Q Fever (see Chapter 29)			
Antemortem or postmortem	Serum (2–3 ml, refrigerated)	Ab: FA (36, 54) Ab: ELISA (26, 66) Ab: CF (59)	Acute: high phase II antibodies. Convalescent: intermediate to high phase I and II antibodies. Chronic: high phase I lipopolysaccharide antibodies.
Haemobartonellosis (see Chapter 30)			
	Blood films (unstained and unfixed)	Organism: cytol (many)	Positive result confirms infection; stained artifacts must be viewed cautiously.
		Ag: FA (43)	Positive result confirms infection without risk of false-positive results because of stain artifact.
	Blood, EDTA anticoagulated (refrigerated)	Organism genome: PCR (17, 16, 45, K22)	Positive result confirms active infection.
Chlamydial Infection (see Chapter 31)			
	Serum (2–3 ml, refrigerated)	Ab: CF (38, 47, 54, 59) Ab: LA (47) Ab: FA (5, 24, 47, 54) Ab: ELISA (K19A)	Paired samples: rising (4-fold) titer confirms active infection; single positive titer indicates exposure.
	Nasal and ocular swabs, lung (refrigerated)	*Chlamydia:* cult (2, 24, 29, 30, 38, 47, 54, 59) Ag: ELISA (K17, K18, K19)	Positive result confirms infection; large numbers of organisms more indicative of active infection.
	Conjunctival smear (refrigerated) or air-dried tissue smear (sterile container)	Ag: FA (52, K20) Ag: FA (38)	Positive result confirms infection; large numbers of organisms more indicative of active infection.
	Tissue (formalin fixed)	Ag: IHC (38)	Positive result confirms infection.
	Blood or tissue sample, fresh refrigerated or formalin fixed	Chlamydial genome: PCR (54)	Positive result confirms infection.
Mycoplasmal Infection (see Chapter 32)			
	Nasal swab, trachea (refrigerated)	*Mycoplasma:* cult (many)	Positive result confirms infection; many infections are subclinical since part of resident microflora.

Infectious Disease	Sample (Amount or Handling)	Detecting: Method Used (Laboratory, Reagents, or Test Kit)	Interpretation
Diagnosis of Bacterial Infections (see Chapter 33)			
Leptospirosis (see Chapter 44)			
Antemortem	Serum: paired samples taken 2–3 weeks apart (2–3 ml, refrigerated)	Ab: MA (many)	Paired samples: rising (4-fold) titer confirms active infection; single positive titer ≥400 confirms past exposure in nonvaccinate; lower or equivalent titers associated with vaccination; titer ≥800 by itself, or changing 4-fold titers over 2–3 weeks, suggests recent or active infection.
	Urine (1–2 ml, refrigerated)	Spirochetes: (many)	Positive result suggests infection; nonpathogenic spirochetes and artifacts make unreliable.
	Urine, blood (2–3 ml, refrigerated)	Spirochetes: cult (many)	Positive result confirms infection.
Postmortem	Urine, blood, kidney (in transport media)	Ag: FA (many) Spirochetes: cult (many)	Positive result confirms infection.
		Spirochetes: DF (many)	Positive result suggests infection; nonpathogenic spirochetes and artifacts make unreliable.
	Tissue: kidney, fetal fluid, placenta, or urine (refrigerated)	Spirochetal genome: GP (22)	Positive result confirms infection.
	Tissue (kidney), urine (refrigerated)	Spirochetal genome: PCR (54)	Positive result confirms infection.
	Tissue (formalin fixed)	Ag: IHC (38)	Positive result confirms infection.
Canine Lyme Borreliosis (Chapter 45)			
	Serum: paired samples taken 10–14 days apart (2–3 ml, refrigerated)	Ab: FA (many) Ab: ELISA-IgG (many, K21, K25A, K25, K26)	Paired samples: rising (4-fold) IgG titer confirms active infection with *Borrelia* spp.
		Ab: immunoblot IgG (14, 29, 38, 39, K26A)	Helps distinguish other spirochetal infections and vaccine responses from tissue exposure or infection.
		Ab: ELISA-IgM (8, 14, 39, 40) Ab: kinELISA (38) Ab: immunoblot IgM (14)	Single high IgM titer confirms recent or active infection with *Borrelia* spp., although IgM from other spirochetal infections such as *Leptospira* may cause some cross-reactivity.
	Blood, anticoagulated, tissue, joint fluid (2–3 ml, refrigerated)	PCR (7)	Positive result confirms infection.
	Tissue (formalin fixed)	IHC (38)	Positive result confirms infection.
Feline Lyme Borreliosis (see Chapter 45)			
Antemortem	Serum taken 10–14 days apart (0.5 ml, refrigerated)	Ab: FA (38, 39, 40, 43, 47)	Paired samples: rising (4-fold) IgG titer suggests active infection with *Borrelia* spp.
	Serum (0.5 ml refrigerated)	Ab: immunoblot (39)	Positive result helps distinguish true seroreactivity to *B. burgdorferi* from that with other spirochetes.
	Blood, anticoagulated, or body fluid (0.5 ml, refrigerated) or tissue (formalin-fixed, embedded)	Spirochetal genome: PCR (7, 38)	Positive result confirms infection.
		Ag: IHC (38)	Positive result confirms infection.
Botulism (see Chapter 42)			
	Feces, blood, serum, intestinal contents (5 ml, refrigerated)	MI (1, 47, 54)	Test performed with and without specific antisera for confirmation of toxin type involved.

Infectious Disease	Sample (Amount or Handling)	Detecting: Method Used (Laboratory, Reagents, or Test Kit)	Interpretation
Anaerobic Infections (see Chapter 41)			
	Lesion exudate (refrigerated in airtight or anaerobic transport system)	Bacteria: cult (many)	Positive result confirms infection but usually are contaminants of wounds from penetrating tissue injuries.
Gram-Negative Bacterial Infections (see Chapter 37)			
(Escherichia coli Infections)			
Antemortem	Feces: fresh fecal material (refrigerated)	Verotoxin (Shiga-like toxins): for enterohemorrhagic strains (many) LT toxin: enterotoxigenic strains (research)	Positive result with specific antisera neutralization of toxin confirms pathogenic strain.
	Feces, foods, tissues	Bacteria (O157:A7): cult, PCR (38)	Positive result confirms pathogenic strain.
	Fecal smears (refrigerated)	Pili Ag: FA	Positive result with fluorescence.
Postmortem or biopsy	Intestinal sections—fresh (refrigerated) and formalin fixed	Lesions: histol for attaching and effacing strain (many)	Bacterial attachment with associated pathologic changes characteristic for a presumptive diagnosis.
Enteric Bacterial Infections (see Chapter 39)			
Salmonellosis			
	Feces or fecal swab (3 g fresh or refrigerated)	Bacteria: cult (many)	Positive result confirms active infection; may be subclinical carrier.
	Blood (1–2 ml, sterilely collected in blood culture broth media), internal tissues collected aseptically	Bacteria: cult (many)	Positive result confirms clinically significant bacteremic or systemic infection.
Postmortem	Intestinal lymph nodes, spleen, many internal organs other than intestine (refrigerated)	Bacteria: cult (many)	Positive result confirms active systemic infection.
	Intestine, colon, lymph node, lung, spleen (formalin fixed)	Lesions: histol (many)	Compatible histologic changes indicate infection.
		Bacterial genome: PCR (38, 54)	Positive result confirms infection.
Campylobacteriosis/Helicobacteriosis			
	Gastric biopsy material in sterile screw cap w/saline or feces (2–3 g, fresh, in sterile airtight container; add thioglycolate medium)	Bacteria: cult (many) Ab: ELISA (K28, K29, K30)	Positive result confirms infection; may be subclinical carrier.
	Intestine, colon, lymph node, lung, spleen (formalin fixed)	Lesions: histol (many)	Compatible histologic changes indicate infection.
***Clostridium perfringens* Infection**			
	Feces or loops of intestine (2–3 ml, refrigerated)	Toxin: RPLA toxin A assay (5, 38) Toxin: MI (38)	Positive result confirms organism is producing toxins associated with clinical illnesses.
	Isolated organism (culture material)	Bacterial genome: PCR (4, 38)	Positive result confirms species of organisms.
Mycobacteriosis (see Chapter 50)			
	Tissue specimen or exudate (fresh or frozen)	Bacteria: cult (many)	Positive result confirms infection.
	Tissue (formalin fixed)	Lesions: histol (many)	Finding acid-fast bacteria must be combined with bacterial culture for determining organism involved.

Infectious Disease	Sample (Amount or Handling)	Detecting: Method Used (Laboratory, Reagents, or Test Kit)	Interpretation
Brucellosis (see Chapter 40)			
Antemortem	Serum: single sample (2–3 ml, refrigerated until sent)	Ab: SAT (many, K27)	Positive result confirms infection, but many false-positive results; do 2ME modification and TAT next to determine titer or AGID for increased specificity.
		Ab: TAT (many)	Titer of >50 suspicious; >100 positive; >200 usually bacteremic; some false-negative and false-positive results; do AGID or culture (if positive) for confirmation.
		Ab: FA (12, 47, 54, 57)	Has been used for screening to substitute for agglutination testing (see previously). Positive result may be confirmed by AGID and culture.
		Ab: AGID (11, 38)	May detect rare seronegatives, more specific test; use to check SAT and TAT positives.
Antemortem or postmortem	Anticoagulated blood (5–10 ml heparinized, refrigerated)	Bacteria: cult (38, 59)	Positive result confirms bacteremia; negative is uncertain.
	Tissue, fetus, testicles, placenta, semen, genital swabs (refrigerated)	Bacteria: cult (54, 59)	Positive result confirms infection; negative is uncertain.
Nocardiosis (see Chapter 49)			
Antemortem or postmortem	Peritoneal, pleural, and pericardial fluid	Bacteria: cult (many)	Positive result confirms infection.
Plague (see Chapter 47)			
Antemortem or postmortem	Serum (2–3 ml, refrigerated)	Ab: passive HA (9) Ab: HA-I (37)	Positive result confirms exposure; rising (4-fold) titer confirms active infection.
	Blood, sputum, fluid, or tissue smears, exudates (2–3 ml, refrigerated) (shipped with biohazard precautions)	Ag: FA (9, 37)	Positive result confirms infection.
	Exudates (swabs) tissue, blood (refrigerated, biohazard precautions)	Bacterial: cult (9, 37)	Positive result confirms infection.
Tularemia (see Chapter 48)			
	Serum: paired specimens taken 2–3 weeks apart (2–3 ml, refrigerated)	Ab: SAT (37) Ab: MA (37)	Positive result confirms exposure; rising (4-fold) titer confirms active infection.
	Swab or exudate (on ice) or tissue	Bacteria: cult (37)	Positive result confirms infection.
Bartonellosis (see Chapter 54)			
Feline *(Bartonella henselae)*			
Antemortem	Blood, EDTA, anticoagulated (aseptically collected)	Bacteria: cult: (14, 40, many) Bacterial genome: PCR (7, K31)	Positive result confirms infection.
	Serum, free of hemolysis (refrigerated)	Ab: FA (14, 40, 54)	Positive result indicates present or past exposure, useful for epidemiologic monitoring. Some bacteremic animals can be seronegative.

Infectious Disease	Sample (Amount or Handling)	Detecting: Method Used (Laboratory, Reagents, or Test Kit)	Interpretation
Canine *(B. vinsonii* subsp. *berkhoferii)*			
	Blood or serum (refrigerated)	Ab: FA (40)	Positive result indicates exposure.
	Blood (EDTA anticoagulated, aseptically collected) or material from culture plate	Bacteria: cult (many, as for *B. henselae)* PCR (7)	Positive result indicates infection.
Diagnosis of Fungal Infections **(see Chapter 56)**			
Fungal Identification and Susceptibility Testing			
	Tissue, exudate, or body fluid (refrigerated)	Fungus: cult (many)	Confirms infection.
	Organism from animal is isolated on fungal medium	Susceptibility: antifungal susceptibility testing (32, 38)	Determines susceptibility to drugs, which may not always correlate with in vivo efficacy.
	Serum, body fluids, or tissues (refrigerated)	Drug: antifungal drug concentrations (32)	Determines achieved concentrations of antifungal drug.
Dermatophytosis (see Chapter 58)			
Antemortem	Lesion (scabs or plucked hairs in sterile dry tubes)	Fungus: cult (many, K31)	Positive result confirms infection; some cats may be subclinical carriers.
Blastomycosis or Histoplasmosis (see Chapters 59, 60)			
Antemortem or postmortem	Serum: single sample (2–3 ml, refrigerated)	Ab: CF (many, K38) Ab: AGID (many; 12, 33, K37, K42) Ab: LA (histo only, K39)	Positive result confirms exposure but not necessarily active infection.
	Tissues or fluid aspirates (1–2 ml in sterile container)	Fungus: cult (12, 19) Fungus: cytol (many; can be done in practice)	Positive result confirms infection.
	Tissue biopsy (formalin fixed)	Lesions: histol (many)	Positive result confirms infection.
Cryptococcosis (see Chapter 61)			
	Serum or CSF: single sample (1–2 ml in sterile container, refrigerated)	Ag: ELISA (K32) Ag: LA (5, 8, 12, 14, 24, 29, 33, 38, 39, 47, 47a, 43, 52, 53, 54, K33, K34, K35)	Positive result confirms active infection. Level can be used to monitor treatment.
	Tissue or fluid aspirate (in sterile container, refrigerated)	Fungus: cult (many, 8, 12, 19)	Positive result confirms infection.
	Tissue or fluid aspirate on smear	Fungus: cytol (many; can be done in practice)	Positive result confirms infection.
	Tissue (in sterile container, refrigerated)	Ag: FA (15)	Positive result confirms infection.
Coccidioidomycosis (see Chapter 62)			
	Serum: single or paired samples (2–3 ml, refrigerated)	Ab: ELISA (K36) Ab: AGID (many, 3a, K37, K40) Ab: CF (2, 3a, 5, 47a, 54, K38)	See Table 62–1 for interpretation.
		Ab: LA (47a, K4, K39)	Positive result indicates current or recent infection.
	Tissue or fluid aspirate (1–2 ml, refrigerated)	Fungus: cult (8, 11)	Positive result confirms infection.
	Tissue (refrigerated)	Fungus: cytol (many; can be done in practice)	Positive result confirms infection.
Sporotrichosis (see Chapter 63)			
	Exudate from lymphatics (1–2 ml, refrigerated)	Fungus: cytol (many; can be done in practice)	Positive result confirms infection.
	Tissue (refrigerated)	Ag: FA (15) Fungus: cult (19, 29, 59, 60)	Positive result confirms infection.

Infectious Disease	Sample (Amount or Handling)	Detecting: Method Used (Laboratory, Reagents, or Test Kit)	Interpretation
	Serum (2–3 ml, refrigerated)	Ab: LA (47, 47a, K39)	Positive result confirms exposure but not necessarily active infection.
Aspergillosis (see Chapter 65)			
	Serum: single sample (2–3 ml, refrigerated)	Ab: ELISA (48) Ab: AGID (many, 47a, K37, K42) Ab: CF (many, K38)	Positive result confirms exposure but not necessarily active infection.
		Ag: ELISA (49)	Positive result confirms infection or colonization of skin or mucosal surface.
	Tissue or exudate (refrigerated)	Fungus: cult (many)	Positive result confirms infection; can be a contaminant. Histopathologic lesions in association with fungus help with confirmation.
Candidiasis (see Chapter 66)			
	Blood or tissue (refrigerated)	Fungus: cult (many)	Positive result of deeper tissues or body fluids confirms disseminated infection in association with microscopic lesions.
	Serum or CSF (refrigerated)	Ab: AGID (38, K40a, K36a)	Positive result indicates exposure to colonization of skin or mucosal surfaces or systemic infection. Need compatible microscopic lesion and culture findings for confirmation.
Protothecosis (see Chapter 69)			
	Tissue (refrigerated)	Ag: FA (15) Cult: (29, 59, 60)	Positive result confirms infection.
Diagnosis of Protozoal Infections (see Chapter 70)			
Trypanosomiasis (see Chapter 72)			
	Serum: single sample (2–3 ml, refrigerated)	Ab: ELISA (38a)	Positive result confirms recent or previous infection.
	Blood film (thick and thin)	Protozoa: cytol (many)	Positive result confirms infection.
	Tissue (formalin fixed or embedded)	IHC (38)	Positive result confirms infection.
Leishmaniasis (see Chapter 73)			
	Serum or dried blood spots (on filter paper)	Ab: FA (64)	Positive result confirms infection in animal with compatible signs; infection usually persists.
	Lymph node aspirate (fixed in methanol, stained with Giemsa)	Protozoa: cytol (many, 63A)	Amastigote in smear confirms infection.
	Serum (refrigerated)	Ab: ELISA (63A)	Positive titer seen with moderate or heavy infections.
		Ab: DA (K48a)	Positive result confirms infection in animal with compatible signs. Highly sensitive and specific.
Hepatozoonosis (see Chapter 74)			
	Blood film (air dried smears)	Protozoa: cytol (54)	Positive result confirms infection.
	Tissues, muscle biopsy (refrigerated) or formalin fixed	Protozoa: histol (many)	Positive result confirms infection.

Infectious Disease	Sample (Amount or Handling)	Detecting: Method Used (Laboratory, Reagents, or Test Kit)	Interpretation
Encephalitozoonosis (see Chapter 75)			
	Serum: single sample (2–3 ml, refrigerated)	Ab: ELISA (research only) Ab: IFA (54)	Positive result confirms previous exposure but not necessarily active infection.
Cytauxzoonosis (see Chapter 76)			
	Blood films, bone marrow (air-dried smears)	Protozoa: cytol (many, 33, 47)	Positive result confirms infection; may be uncommon in peripheral blood films.
Babesiosis (see Chapter 77)			
	Blood film (air-dried smears)	Protozoa: cytol (many)	Positive result confirms infection; may be uncommon in peripheral blood films.
	Serum: single sample (2–3 ml, refrigerated)	Ab: FA (5, 16, 24, 39, 40, 43, 53, 54)	Positive titer >40 indicates active or very recent infection. Some variation in titers exists among laboratories.
Enteric Protozoal Infections (see Chapter 78)			
	Feces (refrigerated)	Protozoa: float, sed (many) Protozoa: fecal smears, wet mounts	Positive result indicates infection; some animals may be subclinical carriers.
Giardiasis			
	Feces (refrigerated)	Ag: ELISA (K44, K47, K52, K55) Ag: FA (K48)	Positive result confirms infection.
Enterotest			
	Nylon string in capsule	Protozoa: adsorbed on string (K42b)	Allows obtaining duodenal specimen. Subsequent microscopic or immunologic detection methods used.
Entamoeba histolytica **Infection** (see Chapter 78)			
	Feces (refrigerated 2–3 ml)	Ag: ELISA (42a) Protozoal genome: PCR (5, 27)	Positive result confirms infection when fecal exam has detected a suspicious organism.
Toxoplasmosis (see Chapter 80)			
	Serum: paired samples taken 10–14 days apart (2–3 ml, refrigerated)	Ab: HA-I (many, K53) Ab: IFA-IgG (many 2, 29, 53, 54) Ab: CF (certain) Ab: ELISA-IgG (many, 8, 14, 39, K50A) Ab: LA (5, 12, 13, 16, 24, 25, 39, 44, 47, 59, K50) Ab: kinELISA (38)	Paired samples: rising (4-fold) IgG titer confirms active infection; single positive titer is nonspecific.
		Ab: ELISA-IgM (8, 14, 29) Ab: FA-IgM (24)	A single high IgM titer indicates active or recent infection; evaluation of IgG and IgM simultaneously is not informative.
	Feces (cat only, refrigerated)	Oocysts: float (many)	Oocyst identification is positive, although inoculation into intermediate host is often needed to confirm exact species.
	Tissue biopsy (lung, brain, lymphoid, liver, kidney (formalin fixed)	Histol (many) IHC (38, 57)	Positive for infection; if detected, clinical significance must be determined.

Infectious Disease	Sample (Amount or Handling)	Detecting: Method Used (Laboratory, Reagents, or Test Kit)	Interpretation
Neosporosis (see Chapter 80)			
	Serum: paired samples taken 10–14 days apart (2–3 ml, refrigerated)	Ab: IFA (2, 38, 52) Ab: ELISA (29, 59, 54, 57)	Paired samples: rising (4-fold) IgG titer confirms active infection; single positive titer indicates previous exposure.
	Tissue biopsy (brain, kidney, liver, muscle, skin) (formalin fixed or refrigerated)	Ag: FA (52, 58)	Positive result confirms infection.
	Tissue (formalin fixed)	IHC (38)	Positive confirms infection.
Coccidiosis (see Chapter 81)			
	Feces (refrigerated)	Oocysts: float (many)	Oocyst identification is positive.
Cryptosporidiosis (see Chapter 82)			
	Feces (refrigerated)	Oocysts: float (many)	Oocyst identification is positive.
	Feces (2–3 g; in 10% formalin)	Ag: FA (5, 30, 39, 54, K48) Ag: ELISA (38, K43, K45, K46, K51, K54)	Positive result confirms infection.
Pneumocystosis (see Chapter 83)			
	Sputum, lung aspirates (refrigerated)	Protozoa: cytol (many)	Positive result suggests infection; difficult-to-find and numerous artifacts make visualization difficult.
		Ag: FA (many, K49) Protozoal genome: PCR (27)	Positive result confirms infection.
Immunodeficiency Testing			
	Serum 3–5 ml (refrigerated)	IgG: radial diffusion (5, 24, 38, 49) IgM: radial diffusion (5, 24, 38, 49) IgA: radial diffusion (5, 24, 38, 49)	Low immunoglobulin concentration reflects humoral immunodeficiency.

2ME = 2-mercaptoethanol; Ab = antibody; Ag = antigen; AGID = agar-gel immunodiffusion; BI = bacterial isolation; CF = complement fixation; cult = culture of organism; cytol = cytology; DA = direct agglutination; DF = darkfield microscopy; EDTA = ethylenediaminetetra-acetic acid; FI = fungal isolation; GP = genetic probe; HA = hemagglutination; HA-I = hemagglutination-inhibition; histol = histology; IHC = immunohistochemistry; kinELISA = kinetic ELISA; LA = latex agglutination; MA = microscopic agglutination; MI = mouse inoculation; PCR = polymerase chain reaction; PE = protein electrophoresis; RI = rickettsial isolation; RPLA = reverse passive latex agglutination; RSAT = rapid slide agglutination test; SAT = slide agglutination test; TAT = tube agglutination test; VI = viral isolation; sed = fecal sedimentation.

Appendix 6

Manufacturers of Diagnostic Test Kits and Their Products

Deborah C. Silverstein and Craig E. Greene

PART A: MANUFACTURERS OF COMMERCIALLY AVAILABLE TEST KITS

Manufacturers	City	State/ Country	Zip Code	Telephone
Abbott Laboratories, Diagnostic Division	Abbott Park	IL	60064	800-323-9100
Addison Biologic Laboratory Inc. (Remel)	Fayette	MO	65248	816-248-2215
Alexon Biomedical	Sunnyville	CA	94089	800-366-0096
Bayer	West Haven	CT	06516	800-248-2637
HDC Corporation	San Jose	CA	95131	408-954-1909
IDEXX Corp	Portland	ME	04101	800-548-6733
Immunetics, Inc.	Cambridge	MA	02142	800-227-4765 617-492-5416
ImmunoMycologics, Inc (IMMY)	Norman	OK	73070	800-654-3639
Integrated Diagnostics (INDX)	Baltimore	MD	21227	301-247-2570 800-TEC-INDX
Meridian Diagnostics, Inc	Cincinnati	OH	45244	800-543-1980 513-271-3700
Life Sign	Somerset	NJ	08875-0218	732-246-3366
Seradyn	Indianapolis	IN	46225	800-428-4007 317-266-2000 317-266-2908
Synbiotics Corp	San Diego	CA	92127	800-228-4305
Tanabe	San Diego	CA	92111	619-571-8410
Trend Scientific, Inc	Ramsey	MN	55303	612-323-7800
Wampole Laboratories	Cranbury	NJ	08512	609-655-6000
Biogal-Galed Labs, Kibbutz Galed 19240	M.P. Megiddo	Israel		Telephone: 972-4-9898605 Fax: 972 49898690
European Vet Lab	Woerden	Netherlands		Telephone: 31 348 412 549 Fax: 31 348 414 626
SVM	Bilthoven	Netherlands		Telephone: 31 302 748 010 Fax: 31 302 250 610
ANGEN Biomedical	Brisbane	Australia		Telephone: 61-73370-6300 Fax: 61-73370-6370

PART B: TEST KITS COMMERCIALLY AVAILABLE FOR INFECTIOUS DISEASES

Kit No.[a]	Name of Test and Organism	Species	Specimen Tested	Type of Test	Manufacturer
Canine Enteric Viral Infections					
K1	CITE Parvovirus	D, C	Feces	Ag: ELISA	IDEXX
K1A	Immunocomb Canine Parvovirus	D	Serum	Ab: ELISA (quantitative)	Biogal Galed
K1B	Assure Parvovirus	D, C	Feces	Ag: ELISA	Synbiotics
K1C	CPV One Step Parvovirus	D, C	Feces	Ag: ELISA	European Vet
K2	Test Pack-Rotavirus	D, C	Feces	Ag: ELISA	Abbott
K3	MERITEC-Rotavirus	D, C	Feces	Ag: LA	Meridian
K4	Immunocard Rotavirus	D, C	Feces	Ag: ELISA	Meridian
K5	ProSpecT Rotavirus	D, C	Feces	Ag: ELISA	Alexon
K6	Rotatest Rotavirus	D, C	Feces	Ag: LA	Wampole

Kit No.[a]	Name of Test and Organism	Species	Specimen Tested	Type of Test	Manufacturer
Canine Distemper Virus					
K6A	Immunocomb Canine Distemper	D	Serum	Ab: ELISA (quantitative)	Biogal Galed
Feline Infectious Peritonitis					
K7	Snap FIP	C	Serum	Ab: ELISA	IDEXX
K7A	Immunocomb FIP	C	Serum	Ab: ELISA	Biogal Galed
K7B	FIPV PCR Assay	C	Fluid, blood	Genome: PCR	Synbiotics
Feline Retroviral Infections					
K8	CITE FeLV	C	Serum	Ag: ELISA	IDEXX
K9	CITE FIV	C	Serum	Ab: ELISA	IDEXX
K10	CITE FeLV/FIV	C	Serum	Ag–Ab: ELISA	IDEXX
K11	PetCheck FeLV	C	Serum	Ag: ELISA	IDEXX
K12	Snap FeLV/FIV	C	Blood, serum	Ag–Ab: ELISA	IDEXX
K13	ICT Gold FeLV	C	Serum	Ag: ELISA	Synbiotics
K14	UniTec FeLV	C	Blood, serum	Ag: ELISA	Synbiotics
K15	ViraCheck FeLV	C	Blood, serum	Ag: ELISA	Synbiotics
K16	Assure FeLV	C	Saliva, blood	Ag: ELISA	Synbiotics
K16A	Viracheck FIV	C	Serum	Ab: ELISA	Synbiotics (NA in USA)
K16B	Witness FIV, Witness FeLV	C	Serum	Ab: LA	AGEN Biomedical
K16C	Witness FeLV	C	Blood, serum	Ag: ELISA	Synbiotics
Rickettsial, Chlamydial, and Mycoplasmal Infections					
K17	Test Pack *Chlamydia*	D, C	Secretions	Ag: ELISA	Abbott
K18	Clearview *Chlamydia*	D, C	Secretions	Ag: ELISA	Wampole
K19	Premier *Chlamydia*	D, C	Secretions	Ag: ELISA	Meridian
K19A	Immunocomb *Chlamydia* (combined with *Toxoplasma*)	C	Serum	Ab: ELISA	Biogal Galed
K20	Meriflour *Chlamydia*	D, C	Secretions	Ag: FA	Meridian
K20A	Immunocomb *Ehrlichia canis*	D	Serum	Ab: ELISA	Biogal Galed
K21	Dip-S-Test *Rickettsia rickettsii, Ehrlichia canis, Borrelia burgdorferi*	D	Serum	Ab: ELISA (all on one stick)	Integrated Diagnostics
K22	PCR, *Haemobartonella felis*	C	Blood	Genome: PCR	Synbiotics
K23	Dip-S-Test *Rickettsia rickettsii*	D	Serum	Ab: ELISA	Integrated Diagnostics
K24	Latex *Rickettsia rickettsii*	D	Serum	Ab: LA	Integrated Diagnostics
Bacterial Infections					
K25	Canine *Borrelia burgdorferi* Antibody Test Kit	D	Serum	Ab: ELISA	Addison
K25A	Dip-S-Test *Borrelia burgdorferi*	D	Serum	Ab: ELISA	Integrated Diagnostics
K26	Lyme Check	D	Serum	Ab: ELISA	Synbiotics
K26A	Quali Code Canine Lyme Disease	D	Serum	Ab: immunoblot	Immunetics, Inc
K27	D-TEC-CB *(Brucella canis)*	D	Serum	Ab: RSAT	Synbiotics
K28	HM-CAP *(Helicobacter pylori)*	H[b]	Serum	Ab: ELISA	Alexon
K29	Premier *(H. pylori)*	H[b]	Serum	Ab: ELISA	Meridian
K30	Immunocard *(H. pylori)*	H[b]	Serum	Ab: ELISA	Meridian
K31	PCR *(Bartonella hensalae)*	C	Body fluids, tissue	Genome: PCR	Synbiotics
Fungal Infections					
K31	Fungassay	D, C	Hair	Culture	Synbiotics
K32	Premier Cryptococcal Antigen	D, C	Body fluids	Ag: ELISA	Meridian

Kit No.[a]	Name of Test and Organism	Species	Specimen Tested	Type of Test	Manufacturer
K33	"Calas"-Cryptococcal Latex	D, C	Body fluids	Ag: LA	Meridian
K34	Crypto-LA	D, C	Body fluids	Ag: LA	Wampole
K35	Latex-*Cryptococcus*	D, C	Body fluids	Ag: LA	IMMY
K36	Premier *Coccidioides*	H[b]	Serum	Ab: ELISA	Meridian
K36A	Candida ID Systems	D, C	Serum	Ab: AGID	Meridian
K37	*Histoplasma, Blastomyces, Coccidioides, Aspergillus*	D, C	Serum	Ab: AGID	Meridian
K38	*Histoplasma, Blastomyces, Coccidioides, Aspergillus*	H[b]	Serum	Ab: CF	Meridian
K39	*Coccidioides, Histoplasma, Sporothrix*	D, C	Serum	Ab: La	IMMY
K40	*Coccidioides*	D, C	Serum	Ab: AGID	IMMY
K40A	*Candida*	D, C	Serum	Ab: AGID	IMMY
K41	*Coccidioides*	D, C	Serum	Ab: LA	IMMY
K42	*Aspergillus, Blastomyces, Histoplasma, Paracoccidioides*	D, C	Serum	Ab: AGID	IMMY
Protozoal Infections					
K42A	ProSpecT *Entamoeba histolytica*	D, C	Feces	Ag: ELISA	Alexon
K42B	Enterotest	D, C	Duodenal fluid	Nylon string in capsule	HDC, Inc
K43	ProSpect/*Cryptosporidium*	D, C	Feces	Ag: ELISA	Alexon
K44	ProSpecT/*Giardia*	D, C	Feces	Ag: ELISA	Alexon
K45	ProSpecT/*Giardia* and *Cryptosporidium*	D, C	Feces	Ag: ELISA	Alexon
K46	Premier *Cryptosporidium*	D, C	Feces	Ag: ELISA	Meridian
K47	Premier *Giardia*	D, C	Feces	Ag: ELISA	Meridian
K48	Meriflour *Giardia*/Crypto	D, C	Feces	Ag: FA	Meridian
K49	Meriflour Pneumocystis	D, C	Feces	Ag: FA	Meridian
K50	Toxotest-MT	C	Serum	Ab: LA	Tanabe
K50A	Immunocomb *Toxoplasma* with *Chlamydia*	C	Serum	Ab: ELISA	Biogal Galed
K51	*Cryptosporidium* Test	D, C	Feces	Ag: ELISA	Trend
K52	*Giardia lamblia*	D, C	Feces	Ag: ELISA	Trend
K53	TPM-Toxotest	C		Ab: HA-I	Wampole
K54	Crypto. "Color Vue *Cryptosporidium*"	D, C	Feces	Ag: ELISA	Seradyn
K55	*Giardia* "Color Vue *Giardia* II"	D, C	Feces	Ag: ELISA	Seradyn
K55A	Dog-Dat *Leishmania*	D	Serum	Ab: DA	SVM
Bacteriuria Detection Kits[c]					
K56	Isocult	D, C	Urine	Bacteria: culture	Renel
K57	Bactercult	D, C	Urine	Bacteria: screening	Wampole
K58	Uricult	D, C	Urine	Bacteria: culture	Life Sign
K59	Microstix-3	D, C	Urine	Nitrite level, total bacteria count	Bayer
K60	Filtracheck-UTI	D, C	Urine	Bacteriuria, pyuria, yeast	Meridian

[a]These kit numbers are cited in Appendix 5 Part B where indicated for use in respective diseases.
[b]These tests have been manufactured for human antibody testing, reagents would require specific antibody conjugates for animal testing. Appropriate research data regarding their accuracy and significance is not available.
[c]The accuracy of such kits for detecting bacteriuria in dogs and cats has not been substantiated.
Ab = antibody; Ag = antigen; AGID = agar-gel immunodiffusion; C = cat; CF = complement fixation; D = dog; DA = direct agglutination; FeLV = feline leukemia virus; FIP = feline infectious peritonitis; FIV = feline immunodeficiency virus; H = human; HA-I = hemagglutination inhibition; LA = latex agglutination; RSAT = rapid slide agglutination test.

Appendix 7

Infectious Disease Rule-Outs for Medical Problems*

Craig E. Greene and Janet P. Calpin

INTEGUMENTAL PROBLEMS

Ulcerative, Fistulous, or Nodular Lesions

Canine viral papilloma (9)
Feline lymphosarcoma (13)
Feline sarcoma virus infection (13)
Felaine immunodeficiency virus infection (14)
Feline cowpox virus infection (19)
L-form infections (32)
Streptococcal infections (35)
Staphylococcal infections (36)
Canine brucellosis (40)
Glanders (46)
Melioidosis (46)
Plague (47)
Tularemia (48)
Actinomycosis (49)
Nocardiosis (49)
Feline leprosy (50)
Mycobacterial infections (50)
Opportunistic mycobacterial infections (50)
Dematophilosis (51)
Feline abscesses (52)
Bite infections (53)
Blastomycosis (59)
Histoplasmosis (60)
Cryptococcosis (61)
Coccidioidomycosis (62)
Sporotrichosis (63)
Aspergillosis, disseminated (65)
Candidiasis, disseminated (66)
Trichosporonosis (67)
Eumycotic mycetoma (68)
Hyalohyphomycosis (68)
Mucormycosis (68)
Phaeohyphomycosis (68)
Pseudallescheriosis (68)
Pythiosis (68)
Zygomycosis (68)
Protothecosis (69)
Leishmaniasis (73)
Caryosporiosis, cutaneous coccidiosis (81)
Sarcocystosis (81)

Pruritus

Rabies (22)
Pseudorabies (23)

Pustular or Vesicular Lesions

Canine distemper (3)
Canine herpesvirus infection, neonatal and adult (5)
Feline immunodeficiency virus infection (14)
Feline herpesvirus infection (16)
Streptococcal infections (35)
Staphylococcal infections (36)
Chrysomonas infection (46)
Dermatophytosis (58)
Bacterial skin infections (85)

Extremity Edema

Infectious canine hepatitis (4)
Canine ehrlichiosis (28)
Ehrlichiosis, granulocytic (28)
Rocky Mountain spotted fever (29)
Anthrax (35)
Aspergillosis, disseminated (65)
Zygomycosis, entomophthoromycosis (68)
Babesiosis (77)
Bacterial endocarditis (87)

MUSCULOSKELETAL PROBLEMS

Muscle Inflammation

Anaerobic bacterial infections (41, 86)
Dermatophilosis, feline (51)
Feline abscesses (52)
Trypanosomiasis (72)
Hepatozoonosis (74)
Toxoplasmosis (80)
Neosporosis (80)

Joint Inflammation

Infectious or Immune-Mediated

Feline calicivirus infection (16)
Feline syncytial virus infection (17)
Canine ehrlichiosis (28)
Feline ehrlichiosis (28)
Rocky Mountain spotted fever (29)
L-form infections (32)
Mycoplasmal infections (32)
Streptococcal infections (35)
Endotoxemia (38)
Canine Lyme borreliosis (45)
Actinomycosis (49)
Feline abscesses (52)
Coccidioidomycosis (62)
Aspergillosis, disseminated (65)
Leishmaniasis (73)
Bacterial skin infection (85)

Diskospondylitis

Streptococcal infections (35)
Staphylococcal infections (36)
Canine brucellosis (40)
Aspergillosis, disseminated (65)
Hyalohyphomycosis (68)
Other bacteremia or fungemias (86)

Bone Inflammation

Osteomyelitis, Periostitis

Staphylococcal infections (36)
Gram-negative infections (37)
Anaerobic bacterial infections (41)
Actinomycosis (49)
Nocardiosis (49)
Mycobacterial infections (50)
Feline abscesses (52)
Blastomycosis (59)
Histoplasmosis (60)
Coccidioidomycosis (62)
Aspergillosis, disseminated (65)
Candidiasis, disseminated (66)
Phaeohyphomycosis (68)
Leishmaniasis (73)
Hepatozoonosis (74)

CARDIOVASCULAR PROBLEMS

Heart Muscle

Cardiomyopathy, Myocarditis

Canine distemper, neonatal (3)
Canine parvovirus infection, neonatal or prenatal (8)
Pseudorabies (23)
Rocky Mountain spotted fever (29)
Streptococcal infection, neonatal (35)
Canine Lyme borreliosis (45)
Coccidioidomycosis (62)
Trypanosomiasis (72)
Hepatozoonosis (74)
Neosporosis (80)
Toxoplasmosis (80)
Bacterial endocarditis (87)

Endocarditis

Enterococcal infection (35)
Erysipelothrix infections (35)
Gram-positive bacterial infections (35)
Gram-negative infections (37)
Bartonellosis (54)

RESPIRATORY PROBLEMS

Upper Respiratory

Rhinitis, Sinusitis, Tracheobronchitis

Canine distemper (3)
Canine adenovirus-2 infection (4)
Canine herpesvirus infection (5)
Canine tracheobronchitis (6)
Bordetella infection (6)
Canine parainfluenza (6)
Feline immunodeficiency virus infection (14)
Feline calicivirus infection (16)
Feline rhinotracheitis (16)
Salmon poisoning disease (27)
Canine ehrlichiosis (28)
Rocky Mountain spotted fever (29)
Chlamydial infection (31)
Mycoplasmal infection (32)
Staphylococcal infection (36)
Cryptococcosis (61)
Rhinosporidiosis (64)
Aspergillosis, nasal (65)
Trichosporonosis (67)
Zygomycosis, entomophthoromycosis (68)
Bacterial respiratory infections (88)

Lower Respiratory
Radiographic/Pulmonary Pattern

Alveolar-Interstitial

Canine distemper (3)
Infectious canine hepatitis (4)
Canine infectious tracheobronchitis, complicated (6)
Mycoplasmal infections (6, 16, 32)
Feline reovirus infection (12)
Feline bordetellosis (16)
Feline calicivirus infection (16)
Streptococcal pneumonia (36, 88)
Endotoxemia (38)
Plague (47)
Nocardiosis (49)
Mycobacterial infections (50)
Acanthamebiasis (79)
Toxoplasmosis (80)
Pneumocystosis (83)
Bacterial pneumonia (88)
EF-4 infection (88)

Interstitial

Canine adenovirus-2 infection (4)
Canine herpesvirus infection (5)
Canine parainfluenza (6)
Feline calicivirus infection (16)
Canine ehrlichiosis (28)
Rocky Mountain spotted fever (29)
Leishmaniasis (73)

Interstitial-Nodular

Glanders (46)
Melioidosis (46)
Mycobacterial infections (50)
Blastomycosis (59)
Histoplasmosis (60)
Cryptococcosis (61)
Coccidioidomycosis (62)
Acanthamebiasis (79)

PLEURAL EFFUSION

Feline infectious peritonitis (11)
Feline viral neoplasia (13)
Anaerobic bacterial infections (41)
Actinomycosis (49)
Nocardiosis (49)
Feline abscesses (52)
Blastomycosis (59)
Toxoplasmosis (80)
Bacterial pyothorax (88)

GASTROINTESTINAL PROBLEMS

Oral Ulcerative or Vesicular Lesions

Canine herpesvirus infection (5)
Canine parvovirus infection (8)
Canine viral papillomatosis (9)
Feline panleukopenia (10)
Feline leukemia virus infection (13)
Feline immunodeficiency virus infection (14)
Feline calicivirus infection (16)
Feline rhinotracheitis (16)
Rocky Mountain spotted fever (29)
Leptospirosis (44)
Tularemia (48)
Candidiasis (66)
Chronic ulcerative stomatitis (89)

Dental Enamel Hypoplasia

Canine distemper (3)
Feline panleukopenia (10)

Icterus, Hepatomegaly, Hepatic Failure

Canine acidophil cell hepatitis (4)
Infectious canine hepatitis (4)
Canine herpesvirus infection, neonatal (5)
Feline infectious peritonitis (11)
Feline viral neoplasia (13)
Feline herpesvirus infection, neonatal (16)
Haemobartonellosis (30)
Rhodococcus equi infection (35)
Streptococcal infections, neonatal (35)
Salmonellosis (39)
Tyzzer's disease (39)
Leptospirosis (44)
Florida borreliosis (45)
Tularemia (49)
Mycobacterial infections (50)
Histoplasmosis (60)
Trypanosomiasis (72)
Encephalitozoonosis (75)
Cytauxzoonosis (76)
Babesiosis (77)
Neosporosis (80)
Toxoplasmosis (80)
Coccidiosis, intrahepatic biliary (81)
Cholangitis/Cholangiohepatitis (90)
Hepatic abscesses (90)

Vomiting

Canine distemper (3)
Canine acidophil cell hepatitis (4)
Infectious canine hepatitis (4)
Canine herpesvirus infection, neonatal (5)
Canine coronavirus infection (8)
Canine parvovirus infection (8)
Feline panleukopenia (10)
Feline infectious peritonitis (11)
Feline enteric viral infections (12)
Feline lymphosarcoma (13)
Elokomin fluke fever (27)
Salmon poisoning disease (27)
Rocky Mountain spotted fever (29)
Listeriosis (35)
Endotoxemia (38)
Campylobacteriosis (39)
Helicobacteriosis, gastric (39)
Salmonellosis (39)
Shigellosis (39)
Tyzzer's disease (39)
Leptospirosis (44)
Mycobacterial infections (50)
Aspergillosis, disseminated (65)
Mucormycosis (68)
Pythiosis (68)
Zygomycosis, entomophthoromycosis (68)
Toxoplasmosis (80)
Coccidiosis (81)
Intra-abdominal infections (89)
Cholangitis/Cholangiohepatitis (90)

Diarrhea

Canine distemper (3)
Infectious canine hepatitis (4)
Paramyxoviral infection (7)
Canine viral enteritis (8)
Feline panleukopenia (10)
Astroviral infection (12)
Feline enteric viral infections (12)
Rotaviral infection (12)
Feline lymphosarcoma (13)
Feline immunodeficiency virus infection (14)
Enterococcal infections (35)
Listeriosis (35)
Endotoxemia (38)
Campylobacteriosis (39)
Salmonellosis (39)
Clostridium perfringens infection (39)
Helicobacteriosis (39)
Shigellosis (39)
Tyzzer's disease (39)
Yersiniosis, intestinal (39)
Leptospirosis (44)
Protothecosis (69)
Trypanosomiasis (72)
Leishmaniasis (73)
Hepatozoonosis (74)
Amebiasis (78)
Balantidiasis (78)
Giardiasis (78)
Trichomoniasis (78)
Toxoplasmosis (80)
Coccidiosis (81)
Cryptosporidiosis (82)

Diarrhea *(Continued)*

Enterovirus infections (24)
Elokomin fluke fever (27)
Salmon poisoning disease (27)
Mycobacterial infections (50)
Histoplasmosis (60)
Pythiosis (68)
Bacterial overgrowth (89)
Enteric infections (89)

Acute Abdominal Pain

Canine acidophil cell hepatitis (4)
Infectious canine hepatitis, acute (4)
Canine herpesvirus infection, neonatal (5)
Feline panleukopenia (10)
Feline infectious peritonitis (11)
Rocky Mountain spotted fever (29)
Salmonellosis (39)
Tyzzer's disease (39)
Yersiniosis (39)
Leptospirosis (44)
Intra-abdominal infections (89)

Abdominal Effusion

Canine acidophil cell hepatitis (4)
Infectious canine hepatitis (4)
Feline infectious peritonitis (11)
Feline lymphosarcoma (13)
Streptococcal infections, neonatal (35)
Anaerobic bacterial infections (41)
Actinomycosis (49)
Nocardiosis (49)
Histoplasmosis (60)
Trypanosomiasis (72)
Toxoplasmosis (80)
Intra-abdominal infections (89)

Abdominal Mass

Feline infectious peritonitis (11)
Feline viral neoplasia (13)
Actinomycosis (49)
Nocardiosis (49)
Mycobacterial infections (50)
Histoplasmosis (60)
Coccidioidomycosis (62)
Eumycotic mycetoma (68)
Mucormycosis (68)
Pythiosis (68)
Zygomycosis (68)
Toxoplasmosis (80)
Intra-abdominal infections (89)
Hepatic abscesses (90)

URINARY PROBLEMS

Renal Failure

Feline lymphosarcoma (13)
Canine ehrlichiosis (28)
Rocky Mountain spotted fever (29)
Endotoxemia (38)
Leptospirosis (44)
Canine Lyme borreliosis (45)
Coccidioidomycosis (62)
Leishmaniasis (73)
Encephalitozoonosis (75)
Babesiosis (77)
Pyelonephritis (91)

GENITAL PROBLEMS

Scrotal Enlargement or Drainage

Feline infectious peritonitis (11)
Canine ehrlichiosis (28)
Rocky Mountain spotted fever (29)
Canine brucellosis (40)
Blastomycosis (59)
Rhodotorulosis (66)
Orchitis, epididymitis (91)

Reproductive Failure, Infertility, Abortion, Birth of Ill (Fading) Neonates

Canine distemper (3)
Canine herpesvirus infection (5)
Canine parvovirus-1 infection (8)
Feline panleukopenia (10)
Feline infectious peritonitis (11)
Feline leukemia virus infection (13)
Feline herpesvirus infection (16)
Q fever (29)
Listeriosis (35)
Streptococcal infection, neonatal (35)
Salmonellosis (39)
Canine brucellosis (40)
Neosporosis (80)
Toxoplasmosis (80)
Pyometra, endometritis (91)

HEMOLYMPHATIC PROBLEMS

Lymphadenomegaly

Canine distemper (3)
Infectious canine hepatitis, acute (4)
Canine viral papillomatosis (9)
Feline panleukopenia (10)
Feline infectious peritonitis, mesenteric (11)
Feline leukemia virus infection (13)
Streptococcal infections (35)
Salmonellosis (39)
Canine brucellosis (40)
Canine Lyme borreliosis (45)
Glanders (46)
Melioidosis (46)
Plague (47)
Sporotrichosis (63)
Aspergillosis, disseminated (65)
Candidiasis (66)
Trichosporonosis (67)
Mucormycosis (68)
Phaeohyphomycosis (68)
Pythiosis (68)

Lymphadenomegaly *(Continued)*

Feline immunodeficiency virus infection (14)
Feline syncytium-forming virus infections (17)
Mumps virus infection (25)
Salmon poisoning disease (27)
Canine ehrlichiosis (28)
Feline ehrlichiosis (28)
Q fever (29)
Rocky Mountain spotted fever (29)
L-form infections (32)
Rhodococcus equi infections (35)
Tularemia (48)
Actinomycosis (49)
Nocardiosis (49)
Mycobacterial infections (50)
Dermatophilosis, feline (51)
Feline abscesses (52)
Bite wound infections (53)
Bartonellosis (54)
Blastomycosis (59)
Histoplasmosis (60)
Cryptococcosis (61)
Coccidioidomycosis (62)
Zygomycosis (68)
Protothecosis (69)
Trypanosomiasis (72)
Leishmaniasis (73)
Hepatozoonosis (74)
Encephalitozoonosis (75)
Cytauxzoonosis (76)
Babesiosis (77)
Toxoplasmosis (80)
Bacteremia, any type (87)

Splenomegaly

Feline leukemia virus infection (13)
Feline immunodeficiency virus infection (14)
Canine ehrlichiosis (28)
Feline ehrlichiosis (28)
Q fever (29)
Rocky Mountain spotted fever (29)
Haemobartonellosis (30)
Endotoxemia (38)
Florida borreliosis (45)
Plague (47)
Tularemia (48)
Mycobacterial infections (50)
Histoplasmosis (60)
Trypanosomiasis (72)
Leishmaniasis (73)
Cytauxzoonosis (76)
Babesiosis (77)
Bacteremia, any type (87)

Immunodeficiency

See Table 95–3

Anemia

Regenerative
Feline leukemia virus infection (13)
Feline immunodeficiency virus infection (14)
Haemobartonellosis (30)
Hepatozoonosis (74)
Cytauxzoonosis (76)
Babesiosis (77)

Nonregenerative
Many chronic infections
Feline infectious peritonitis (11)
Feline leukemia virus infection (13)
Feline immunodeficiency virus infection (14)
Canine ehrlichiosis (28)
Feline ehrlichiosis (28)
Histoplasmosis (60)
Leishmaniasis (73)
Toxoplasmosis (80)

Circulating Cellular Inclusions

Canine distemper, lymphocytes, polychromatophilic erythrocytes (3)
Feline infectious peritonitis, neutrophils (11)
Elokomin fluke fever (27)
Canine ehrlichiosis, neutrophils, lymphocytes, or platelets (28)
Feline ehrlichiosis (28)
Haemobartonellosis, erythrocytes (30)
Histoplasmosis, monocytes or neutrophils (60)
Trypanosomiasis, monocytes (72)
Leishmaniasis, monocytes (73)
Hepatozoonosis, neutrophils and monocytes (74)
Cytauxzoonosis, erythrocytes (76)
Babesiosis, erythrocytes (77)
Toxoplasmosis, leukocytes (80)
Bacteremia (87)

Persistent Lymphopenia

Canine distemper, acute (3)
Canine parvovirus infection (8)
Feline leukemia virus infection (13)
Feline immunodeficiency virus infection (14)
Canine ehrlichiosis (28)
Bacteremia (87)

Leukocytosis

Canine herpesvirus infection, neonatal (5)
Feline infectious peritonitis (11)
Feline viral neoplasia (13)
Feline leukemia virus infection (13)
Salmon poisoning disease (27)
Q fever (29)
Rocky Mountain spotted fever (29)
Endotoxemia (38)
Campylobacteriosis (39)
Salmonellosis (39)
Canine brucellosis (40)
Anaerobic bacterial infections (41)
Leptospirosis (44)
Plague (47)
Actinomycosis (49)
Histoplasmosis (60)
Aspergillosis (65)
Candidiasis, disseminated (66)
Coccidioidomycosis (68)
Leishmaniasis (73)
Hepatozoonosis (74)
Encephalitozoonosis (75)
Acanthamebiasis (79)

Leukocytosis *(Continued)*

L-form infections (32)
Rhodococcus equi infection (35)
Streptococcal infections, neonatal (35)
Staphylococcal infections (36)
Nocardiosis (49)
Feline abscesses (52)
Blastomycosis (59)
Toxoplasmosis (80)
Pneumocystosis (83)
Bacteremia (87)

Neutropenia

Canine parvovirus infection (8)
Feline panleukopenia (10)
Feline leukemia virus infection (13)
Feline immunodeficiency virus infection (14)
Salmon poisoning disease (27)
Canine ehrlichiosis (28)
Endotoxemia (38)
Salmonellosis, acute (39)
Bacteremia (87)

Thrombocytopenia (Petechial Hemorrhages)

Primary
Feline leukemia virus infection (13)
Elokomin fluke fever (27)
Canine ehrlichiosis, chronic (28)
Feline ehrlichiosis (28)

Associated with DIC–Increased Consumption
Infectious canine hepatitis (4)
Canine herpesvirus infection, neonatal (5)
Canine parvovirus infection (8)
Feline panleukopenia (10)
Feline infectious peritonitis (11)
Feline leukemia virus infection (13)
Canine ehrlichiosis, acute or chronic (28)
Ehrlichia platys infection (28)
Rocky Mountain spotted fever (29)
Endotoxemia (38)
Salmonellosis (39)
Leptospirosis (44)
Plague (47)
Histoplasmosis (60)
Candidiasis (66)
Leishmaniasis (73)
Cytauxzoonosis (76)
Babesiosis (77)
Bacteremia (87)

MISCELLANEOUS LABORATORY PROBLEMS

Increased Liver Enzymes

Canine acidophil cell hepatitis (4)
Infectious canine hepatitis (4)
Canine herpesvirus infection, neonatal (5)
Feline panleukopenia (10)
Feline infectious peritonitis (11)
Feline lymphosarcoma (13)
Feline myeloproliferative disease (13)
Canine ehrlichiosis (28)
Rocky Mountain spotted fever (29)
Endotoxemia (38)
Helicobacteriosis, hepatic (39)
Tyzzer's disease (39)
Leptospirosis (44)
Histoplasmosis (60)
Aspergillosis, disseminated (65)
Candidiasis, disseminated (66)
Trypanosomiasis (72)
Hepatozoonosis (74)
Cytauxzoonosis (76)
Babesiosis (77)
Neosporosis (80)
Toxoplasmosis (80)
Cholangiohepatitis (90)
Hepatic abscesses (90)

Positive Coombs' Testing

Feline leukemia virus infection (13)
Canine ehrlichiosis (28)
Haemobartonellosis (30)
Canine brucellosis (40)
Leishmaniasis (73)
Babesiosis (77)

Azotemia

Canine herpesvirus infection, neonatal (5)
Feline leukemia virus infection (13)
Feline immunodeficiency virus infection (15)
Canine ehrlichiosis, chronic (28)
Rocky Mountain spotted fever (29)
Endotoxemia (38)
Leptospirosis (44)
Canine Lyme borreliosis (45)
Coccidioidomycosis (62)
Leishmaniasis (73)
Encephalitozoonosis (75)
Babesiosis (77)
Pyelonephritis (91)

Icterus

Infectious canine hepatitis (4)
Feline infectious peritonitis (11)
Feline leukemia virus infection (13)
Endotoxemia (38)
Hepatic helicobacteriosis/campylobacteriosis (39)
Tyzzer's disease (39)
Leptospirosis (44)
Histoplasmosis (60)
Zygomycosis, mucormycosis (68)
Cytauxzoonosis (76)
Babesiosis (77)
Toxoplasmosis (80)
Sarcocystosis (81)
Cholangiohepatitis (90)

Proteinuria

Infectious canine hepatitis (4)
Feline infectious peritonitis (11)
Feline leukemia virus infection (13)
Canine ehrlichiosis (28)
Rocky Mountain spotted fever (29)
Leptospirosis (44)
Canine Lyme borreliosis (45)
Coccidioidomycosis (62)
Leishmaniasis (73)
Toxoplasmosis (80)
Bacteremia (87)
Urinary tract infections (91)

Hyperfibrinogenemia

Feline infectious peritonitis (11)
L-form infections (32)
Leptospirosis (44)
Bacterial endocarditis (87)

Hypoalbuminemia

Canine parvovirus infection (8)
Feline infectious peritonitis (11)
Feline viral neoplasia (13)
Salmon poisoning disease (27)
Canine ehrlichiosis (28)
Rocky Mountain spotted fever (29)
Endotoxemia (38)
Salmonellosis (39)
Canine brucellosis (40)
Blastomycosis (59)
Histoplasmosis (60)
Coccidioidomycosis (62)
Leishmaniasis (73)
Bacteremia (87)

Hypoglobulinemia

Canine, distemper, neonatal or prenatal (3)
Hereditary immunodeficiency diseases (95)

Hyperglobulinemia

Feline infectious peritonitis (11)
Feline viral neoplasia (13)
Feline immunodeficiency virus infection (14)
Canine ehrlichiosis (28)
Feline ehrlichiosis (28)
L-form infections (32)
Canine brucellosis (40)
Actinomycosis (49)
Blastomycosis (59)
Histoplasmosis (60)
Cryptococcosis (61)
Coccidioidomycosis (62)
Leishmaniasis (73)
Encephalitozoonosis (75)
Bacteremia (87)
Chronic ulcerative stomatitis (89)
Cholangiohepatitis (90)

Hypoglycemia

Salmonellosis (39)
Actinomycosis (49)
Hepatozoonosis (74)
Bacteremia (87)

CNS PROBLEMS

Primary Meningitis, Secondary Encephalitis

Feline infectious peritonitis (11)
Canine ehrlichiosis (28)
Rocky Mountain spotted fever (29)
Listeriosis (35)
Canine brucellosis (40)
Anaerobic bacterial infections (41)
Actinomycosis (49)
Feline abscesses (52)
Blastomycosis (59)
Histoplasmosis (60)
Cryptococcosis (61)
Coccidioidomycosis (62)
Hyalohyphomycosis (68)
Mucormycosis (68)
Phaeohyphomycosis (68)
Zygomycosis (68)
Protothecosis (69)
Trypanosomiasis (72)
Encephalitozoonosis (75)
Babesiosis (77)
Acanthamebiasis (79)
Granulomatous meningoencephalitis (84)
Hydrocephalus with periventricular encephalitis (84)
Pug and Maltese encephalitis (84)
Steroid-responsive meningitis-arteritis (84)
Yorkshire terrier encephalitis (84)
Bacterial meningitis (92)
Brain abscesses (92)

Primary Encephalitis, Secondary Meningitis

Canine distemper (3)
Infectious canine hepatitis (4)
Canine herpesvirus infection, neonatal and prenatal (5)
Canine paramyxovirus encephalitis (7)
Feline panleukopenia, neonatal and prenatal (10)
Feline paramyxovirus infection (18)
Rabies (22)
Pseudorabies (23)
Arbovirus infections (26)
Louping ill (26)
Babesiosis (77)
Neosporosis (80)
Toxoplasmosis (80)
Sarcocystosis (81)
Feline poliomyelitis (84)
Feline spongiform encephalopathy (84)

CSF Results

(see also Table 92–2)

CSF Protein Increase and Mononuclear Cells
Canine distemper (3)
Paramyxoviral encephalitis (7, 18, 29)
Rabies (22)
Pseudorabies (23)
Arboviral infections (26)
Canine ehrlichiosis (28)
Granulomatous meningoencephalitis (84)
Feline polioencephalomyelitis (84)
Pug encephalitis (84)
Hydrocephalus with periventricular encephalitis (84)

CSF Protein Increase and Neutrophils
Feline infectious peritonitis (11)
Rocky Mountain spotted fever (29)
Canine brucellosis (40)
Leptospirosis (44)
Listeriosis (56)
Phaeohyphomycosis (68)
Steroid-responsive meningitis-arteritis (85)

CSF Protein Increase and Mixed (Mononuclear and Neutrophil) Cells
Blastomycosis (59)
Cryptococcosis (61)
Protothecosis (69)
Encephalitozoonosis (75)
Neosporosis (80)
Toxoplasmosis (80)
Granulomatous meningoencephalitis (84)
Yorkshire terrier encephalitis (84)

Epidural or Extradural Compression of Spinal Cord, Diskospondylitis

Feline lymphosarcoma (13)
Staphylococcal infections (36)
Canine brucellosis (40)
Actinomycosis (49)
Feline abscesses (52)
Aspergillosis (65)
Hyalohyphomycosis (68)
Paecilomycosis (68)

Hydrocephalus

Canine paramyxovirus encephalitis (7)
Feline infectious peritonitis (11)
Periventricular encephalitis (84)

OCULAR PROBLEMS

See Table 93–5

[a]For discussion, refer to chapters designated in parentheses.
DIC = disseminated intravascular coagulation.

Appendix 8

Antimicrobial Drug Formulary

Craig E. Greene and A. D. J. Watson

PROFESSIONAL FLEXIBLE LABELING

This practice of customized dosing of veterinary drugs has been adopted by the Food and Drug Administration in the United States. The concept of individualized dosing of an animal based on the animal and disease being treated is new to veterinary drugs where fixed-dosage regimens have been customary. Dosages given on antimicrobial labels in the past have often been based on licensing data obtained by using the antimicrobial on the most susceptible infection for the organ system under consideration. Thus, dosage information was the lowest level and ineffective for managing infections involving resistant organisms or other body systems. Future veterinary labels will provide the veterinarian with pharmacokinetic and pharmacodynamic information concerning each drug, and its microbiologic susceptibility data. Dosage ranges and specific dosage indications will also be provided.

The information in this formulary is intended to support the concept of flexible labeling. Information is provided on each drug to enable veterinarians to adjust dosages on the bases of clinical and toxicologic data. Recommendations for dosing with each drug are variable depending on the type and location of infection. The reader is referred to other dosage tables in their respective disease chapters for specific dosage regimens. An attempt has been made to include the majority of drugs available internationally to treat animal infections. Many of these drugs are approved for human use, but limited studies have been performed in dogs and cats. References to newer information are cited on the basis of information in the respective chapters on antiviral drugs (Chapter 2); antibacterial drugs (Chapter 34); antifungal drugs (Chapter 57), and antiprotozoal drugs (Chapter 71). References appear with the chapter number followed by a colon and the specific citation number.

Additional references used in completion of this work are as follows:

Compendium of Veterinary Products: Port Huron, MI, North American Compendium Inc, 1995.

Facts and Comparisons Staff: *Facts and Comparison: Loose-Leaf Drug Information Series.* St. Louis, MO, Facts and Comparisons Staff, 1997

Physicians' Desk Reference: Montvale, NJ, Medical Economics Co., 1997.

Plumb DC: *Veterinary Drug Handbook,* ed 2. Ames, IA, Iowa State University Press, 1995.

Reynolds JEF (ed): *Martindale, The Extra Pharmacopoeia.* London, Royal Pharmaceutical Society, 1996.

Micromedex Drug Information on Line 1997: www.micromedex. com.

MANUFACTURERS/ DISTRIBUTORS	ADDRESS	CITY	STATE/ COUNTRY	POSTAL CODE	TELEPHONE
3M Pharmaceutical	3M Center, Building 275-3E-09	St. Paul	MN	55133	612-736-4390
Abbott Laboratories	1 Abbott	Abbott Park	IL	60064-3500	800-255-5162
Allen & Hanburys Ltd.	Stockley Park West	Uxbridge, Middlesex	UK	UB11 1BT	081-990-9888
Allergan Herbert	2525 DuPont Dr	Irvine	CA	92715-9534	800-433-8871
Amgen	1840 Dehavilland Dr.	Thousand Oaks	CA	91320-1789	800-282-6436
Anthony Products Co.	5600 Peck Rd	Arcadia	CA	91006	818-357-8711
Apothecon	P.O. Box 4500	Princeton	NJ	08543-4500	609-897-2111
Astra USA, Inc.	50 Otis St	Westborough	MA	01581	800-225-4803
Bayer B.V.	Energieweg 1	3641 RT Mijdrecht	NL		02979-80666
Bayer Corporation Biological and Pharmaceuticals	400 Morgan Lane	West Haven	CT	06516	203-937-2000
Bayer Animal Health	P.O. Box 390	Shawnee	KS	66201	800-255-6517
Bayer Vet Ltd.	Eastern Way	Bury St. Edmunds, Suffolk	UK	IP32 7AH	01284-763200
Berlex Laboratories, Inc.	300 Fairfield Rd	Wayne	NJ	07470-2095	201-694-4100
Biocraft Laboratories, Inc.	18-01 River Rd	Fair Lawn	NJ	074100	800-631-0165
Boots Pharmaceuticals, Inc.	See Knoll Laboratories				
Bristol Laboratories	See Bristol-Myers Squibb				
Bristol-Myers Squibb	P.O. Box 4000	Princeton	NJ	08543-4000	609-252-4000
Burroughs Wellcome Co.	3030 Cornwallis Rd	Research Triangle Park	NC	27709	919-248-3000
The Butler Company	5000 Bradenton Ave	Dublin	OH	43017-0753	614-761-9095
Carrington Laboratories, Inc.	2001 Walnut Hill La	Irving	TX	75038	214-518-1300
Ciba Agriculture	Whittlesford	Cambridge	UK	CB2 4QT	0223-833621
Ciba-Geigy Pharmaceuticals	556 Morris Ave	Summit	NJ	07901	908-277-5000
Delmont Laboratories, Inc.	175 Harvard Ave, P.O. Box 269	Swarthmore	PA	19081	610-543-2747
Dista Products Co.	Lilly Corp. Center	Indianapolis	IN	46285	317-276-4000
DuPont Pharma	P.O. Box 800723	Wilmington	DE	19880	800-474-2762
Fleming & Co.	1600 Fenpark Dr	Fenton	MO	63026-2918	314-343-8200
Elanco Animal Health USA	A Div. of Eli Lilly & Co., Lilly Corporate Center	Indianapolis	IN	46285	317-276-3000
Elanco Animal Health	Dextra Court, Chapel Hill	Basingstoke Hants	UK	RG21 0EU	025653131
Elanco Animal Health	Divisie van Eli Lilly B.V., 4872 XL Etten-Leur	City Kantoren/Raadstede 15	NL	03402-79722	
Elkins-Sinn, Inc.	P.O. Box 8299	Philadelphia	PA	19101	215-688-4400
Fermenta Animal Health Co.	10150 N. Executive Hills Blvd	Kansas City	MO	64153	816-891-5500

MANUFACTURERS/ DISTRIBUTORS	ADDRESS	CITY	STATE/ COUNTRY	POSTAL CODE	TELEPHONE
Forest Pharmaceutical, Inc.	13622 Lakefront Dr	St. Louis	MO	63045	314-344-8870
Fort Dodge Laboratories	800-5th St, NW, P.O. Box 518	Fort Dodge	IA	50501	515-955-4600
Fujisawa USA, Inc.	3 Parkway North Center	Deerfield	IL	60015-2548	708-317-0600
Geigy Pharmaceuticals	556 Morris Ave	Summit	NJ	07901	908-277-5000
Genentech, Inc.	460 Point San Bruno Blvd	S. San Francisco	CA	94080	415-225-1000
Glaxo Wellcome, Inc.	Five Moore Dr	Research Triangle Park	NC	27709	918-248-2100
Glenwood, Inc.	83 Summit St	Tenafly	NJ	07670	201-569-0050
Hoechst Marion-Roussel Agri-Vet Co.	Animal Health Products, Route 202-206, Box 2500	Somerville	NJ	08876-1258	800-247-4838
Hoechst Marion-Roussel, Inc.	Route 202-206, P.O.Box 6800	Bridgewater	NJ	08807-0800	908-231-4000 800-981-2491
ICN Pharmaceuticals, Inc.	3300 Hyland Ave	Costa Mesa	CA	92626	714-545-0100
Immunovet (Vetoquinol)	5910-G Breckenridge Pkwy	Tampa	FL	33610-4253	800-627-9447
Imvac Inc.	RR 1, 6080 Bass Lane	Columbia	MO	65210	314-443-5363
Intervet Nederland B.V.	Kleine Broekstraat 1	5831 AP Boxmeer	NL		08855-87654
Intervet UK Ltd.	Science Park, Milton Rd	Cambridge	UK	CB4 4FP	01223-420221
Intervet USA	406 State Street	Millsboro	DE	19966	800-441-8272
Jacobus Pharmaceutical Co.	37 Cleveland Lane	Princeton	NJ	08540	609-921-7447
Janssen Pharmaceutical, Inc.	1125 Trenton-Harbourton Rd, P.O. Box 200	Titusville	NJ	08560-0200	609-730-2000
Knoll Laboratories	3000 Continental Dr North	Mt. Olive	NJ	07828-1234	201-426-5589
Lannett, Inc.	900 State Rd	Philadelphia	PA	19136	215-333-9000
Lederle Laboratories	North Middletown Rd	Pearl River	NY	10965-1299	914-732-5000
Lemmon Co.	650 Cathill Rd	Sellersville	PA	18960	215-256-8400
Lextron, Inc.	630 "O" St, P.O. Box 790	Greeley	CO	80632	303-353-2600
Eli Lilly and Co.	Lilly Corp. Center	Indianapolis	IN	46285	317-276-2000
Liposome Co.	One Research Way	Princeton	NJ	08540	609-452-7060
Lyphomed	See Fujisawa USA, Inc.				
Mallinckrodt Medical, Inc.	675 McDonnell Blvd., P.O. Box 5840	St. Louis	MO	63134	314-895-2000
Mallinckrodt Veterinary, Inc.	(see Schering-Plough, Inc.)				
Marion Merrell Dow, Inc.	P.O. Box 9627	Kansas City	MO	64134	800-362-7466
Mead Johnson Pharm.	See Bristol-Myers Squibb				
Merck AgVet Division	Merck & Co., P.O. Box 2000	Rahway	NJ	07065-0912	908-855-3800
Merck & Co.	P.O. Box 4	West Point	PA	19486	215-652-5000
Merial	115 Transtech Dr	Athens	GA	30601	706-548-9292
Miles, Inc.	See Bayer Corp				
Mycofarm Nederland B.V.	Ambachtstraat 2	3732 CN De Bilt	NL		030-212800
Mycofarm UK Ltd.	Science Park, Milton Rd	Cambridge	UK	CB4 4FP	0223-423971
Nexstar Pharmaceuticals, Inc.	650 Cliffside Dr	San Dimus	CA	91773	800-403-3945
North American Region, Animal Health Group	Pfizer Inc., Whiteland Business Park, 812 Springdale Dr	Exton	PA	19341	610-363-3100
Ortho Pharmaceutical Corp.	Route 202, P.O. Box 600	Raritan	NJ	08869	908-218-6000
Osborn					
Parke-Davis	201 Tabor Rd	Morris Plains	NJ	07950	800-223-0432
Parke-Davis Veterinary	Usk Rd	Pontypool, Gwent	UK	NP4 0YH	0495-762468
Pfizer Animal Health Ltd.	Ramsgate Road	Sandwich, Kent	UK	CT13 9NJ	0304-616091
Pfizer B.V.	Animal Health Division, Roer 266	2908 MC Capelle a/d IJs-sel	NL		010-4064200
Pharmacia Biotech	800 Centennial Ave P.O. Box 1327	Piscataway	NJ	08855-1327	800-526-3593
Pharmacia and Upjohn	700 Portage Rd	Kalamazoo	MI	49001	616-833-2690
Phoenix Pharm., Inc.	4621 Easton Road, P.O. Box 6457	St. Joseph	MO	64506-0457	816-364-5777
Procter & Gamble Pharm.	P.O. Box 191	Norwich	NY	13815-0191	607-335-2111
Prolabs Ltd., c/o Agri Laboratories, Ltd.	20927 State Route K, P.O. Box 3103	St. Joseph	MO	64503	816-233-9533
Purdue Frederick Co.	100 Connecticut Ave	Norwalk	CT	06856	203-853-0123
Rachelle Laboratories, Inc.	P.O. Box 187	Culver	IN	46511	219-842-3305
Reid Rowell	See Solvay				
Rhône-Merieux B.V.	Bovenkerkerweg 6-8	1185 XE Amstelveen	NL		020-5473933
Rhône-Merieux Ltd.	Pinnacles West, Spire Greene Centre	Harlow, Essex	UK	CM19 5TS	0279-439444
Rhône-Poulenc Rorer Pharmaceuticals, Inc.	P.O. Box 1200	Collegeville	PA	19426	610-454-8000
Roberts Pharmaceuticals	500 Acrola Rd, 4 Industrial Way West	Eatontown	NJ	07724	908-389-1182
Roche Laboratories	340 Kingsland St	Nutley	NJ	07110-1199	800-526-6367
Roche Animal Health	45 Waterview Blvd	Parsippany	NJ	07054-1290	800-526-0189
Roerig	235 E. 42nd St	New York	NY	10017	800-438-1985
Ross Laboratories, Inc.	P.O. Box 16532	Columbus	OH	43229	614-624-3333
Roussel-Uclaf					
RXV	6301 Deramus	Kansas City	MO	64120-1358	816-483-9220
Sandoz Pharmaceuticals	59 Route 10	E. Hanover	NJ	07936	201-503-7500
Sandoz Pharmaceuticals	Frimley Business Park, Frimley	Camberley, Surrey	UK	GU16 5SG	0276-692508
Sanofi Animal Health	7101 College Blvd	Overland Park	KS	66210	913-451-3434

MANUFACTURERS/ DISTRIBUTORS	ADDRESS	CITY	STATE/ COUNTRY	POSTAL CODE	TELEPHONE
Sanofi Animal Health Ltd.	P.O. Box 209 Rhodes Way	Watford, Herts	UK	WD2 4QE	0923-235022
Sanofi Sante B.V.	Govert van Wijnkade 48	3144 EG Maassluis	NL		01899-31399
Sanofi Winthrop Pharmaceuticals	90 Park Ave	New York	NY	10016	800-446-6267
Schering-Plough Animal Health	1095 Morris Ave	Union	NJ	07033	908-629-3346
Schiapparelli Searle	See SCS Pharmaceuticals				
SCS Pharmaceuticals	P.O. Box 5110	Chicago	IL	60680	800-323-1603
Searle	5200 Old Orchard Rd	Skokie	IL	60077	708-982-7000
Sequus Pharmaceuticals, Inc.	960 Hamilton Court	Menlo Park	CA	94025	650-323-9011
SmithKline Beecham Pharm.	P.O. Box 7929	Philadelphia	PA	19103	215-751-4000
Solvay Pharmaceuticals	901 Sawyer Rd	Marietta	GA	30062-2224	404-578-9000
Solvay Duphar Animal Health Benelux B.V.	Van Houten Industriepark 24	1381 MZ Weesp	NL		02940-65907
Solvay-Duphar Veterinary Ltd.	Solvay House, Flanders Road, Hedge End	Southampton, Hants	UK	SO3 4QH	01489-781711
E.R. Squibb & Sons, Inc.	See Bristol-Myers Squibb				
Stuart Pharmaceuticals	See Zeneca Pharmaceuticals				
Syntex Animal Health	4800 Westown Pkwy, Ste. 200	W. Des Moines	IA	50266-6711	515-224-2400
Teva Pharm.	1510 Delp Dr	Kulpsville	PA	19443	888-838-2872
UpJohn Co. Animal Health	7000 Portage Rd	Kalamazoo	MI	49001	616-323-4000
Upjohn Limited	Fleming Way	Crawley, West Sussex	UK	RH10 2LZ	0293-531133
Upjohn Nederland	Rubensstraat 167	6717 VE Ede	NL		08380-36802
Upsher-Smith Labs, Inc.	14905 23rd Ave, North	Minneapolis	MN	55447	612-473-4412
US Bioscience	100 Front St, Suite 400	W. Conshohocken	PA	19428	800-447-3969
Vedco, Inc.	Route 6, Box 35A	St. Joseph	MO	64504	816-238-8840
Vet Tek, Inc.	P.O. Box 279, 24010 Highway 40 Eastbound	Blue Springs	MO	64015	816-229-9101
Veterinary Pharm. Co.	Div. of Nylos Trading Co. Inc., Rte. 202 Professional Center, P.O. Box 2	Pomona	NY	10970	914-354-7077
Vetico Farma B.V.	Bovenheigraaf 101	8095 PB Wezep	NL		05253-3335
Vetoquinol B.V.	Postbus 3191	5203 DD's Hertogenbosch	NL		01834-1782
Vetoquinol USA	5910-G Breckenridge Pkwy	Tampa	FL	33610-4253	800-627-9447
Vetrepharm Res Inc.	119 Rowe Rd	Athens	GA	30601	800-265-5464
Vetrepharm of Canada VPC	383 Soverign Rd	London, Ontario	Canada	N6M IA3	519-453-3384
Willows-Francis Vet. Ltd.	3 Charlwood Court, County Oak Way	Crawley, West Sussex	UK	RH11 7XA	0293-61441
Winthrop Pharmaceuticals	See Sanofi Winthrop Pharmaceuticals				
Wyeth-Ayerst Laboratories	P.O. Box 8299	Philadelphia	PA	19101	610-688-4400
Zeneca Pharmaceuticals	1800 Concord Pike	Wilmington	DE	19897	302-886-3000

ACEMANNAN

CLASS. Complex carbohydrate (polymannose) extracted from *Aloe vera.*

ACTION. Immunostimulant and antiviral. Stimulates mononuclear phagocytes and T cells; interferes with viral glycosylation.

MORE INFORMATION. See Antivirals, Chapter 2, and Immunotherapy, Chapter 100; References: 2:4, 2:12, 2:19, 100:47, 100:56, 100:74, 100:77, 100:78, 100:102a, 100:142, 100:151, 100:172.

PHARMACOKINETICS. Uncertain.

SPECTRUM. Interferon inducer; has antitumor activity. Inhibits growth of HIV, Newcastle disease virus, and influenza virus in vivo.

INDICATIONS. Treatment of clinically affected, symptomatic FeLV-positive or FIV-positive cats (100:172). Intralesional injection into vaccine-induced fibrosarcomas. Prospective controlled studies on efficacy not available. Has been used in combination with surgery and radiation therapy for fibrosarcomas in dogs and cats (2:12).

APPROVED USES. Veterinary-adjunctive treatment for fibrosarcoma, nonspecific immunostimulant.

CONTRAINDICATIONS. Previous hypersensitivity reaction to the drug.

ADVERSE REACTIONS. IV causes tachypnea, tachycardia, salivation, weakness, collapse, pale mucosae. Avoid by using slow IV drip infusion rather than bolus infusion. Very high (80 mg/kg) IP doses in dogs cause transient abdominal discomfort, vomiting, and diarrhea (2:4). Histologic findings of mononuclear phagocyte infiltrates in liver, spleen, and peritoneal surfaces (atypical microgranulomatous peritonitis) when treated IP. When treated IV, mononuclear phagocytes accumulate in lungs (2:4). Increased WBC counts during treatments. Intralesional injections may cause discomfort and bleeding from injection sites. Sedation or anesthesia is recommended. Tumors will become enlarged and painful before regression, if any, is noted.

INTERACTIONS. Unknown.

Availability	Type	Sizes	Preparations (Company)
Veterinary	Lyophilized powder for injection	10-mg vial	*Acemannan Immunostimulant, Carrisyn* (Carrington)

HANDLING. Reconstitute to 1 mg/ml with 10 mL of 0.9% NaCl (supplied). Higher concentrations are insoluble and become gelatinous. Discard unused solution within 4 hr of reconstitution.

ADMINISTRATION. Intralesional and/or IP weekly injection given concurrently. Continue injections until necrosis and/or edema evident in mass (usually 4th–7th week). Then use surgery to remove mass by wide excision. May also consider radiotherapy using cobalt 60 teletherapy, immediately after surgery (2:12).

DOSAGE

Indications (Dogs & Cats)	Dose	Route	Interval	Duration
Immunostimulant	2 mg/kg	IP, SC	Weekly	6 wk
Fibrosarcoma				
Preoperative	1 mg/kg	IP	Weekly	4 wk (Weeks 1–4)
	2 mg	Intralesional	Weekly	4 wk (Weeks 1–4)
Surgical removal, week 5	1 mg	IP	Weekly	2 wk (Weeks 5, 6)
Postoperative	1 mg/kg	IP	Monthly	6 mo–1 yr (thereafter)

DISPENSING INFORMATION. IP: animal may have abdominal tenderness, observe for allergic reactions. Intralesional: may cause bleeding or necrosis of lesion with some exudation for days afterward.

ACYCLOVIR

CLASS. Nucleoside (guanosine) analog.

ACTION. Antiviral; interferes with DNA replication in herpesviruses types 1, 2, and some others. Accumulates and activates only in herpesvirus-infected cells. Affects only replicating virus. Best therapeutic index (efficacy/toxicity) of available antiviral drugs.

MORE INFORMATION. See elsewhere GANCICLOVIR (*Cytovene,* Syntex); Famciclovir (*Famvir,* SmithKline Beecham); Valacyclovir (*Valtrex,* Glaxo Wellcome). See Antivirals, Chapter 2; Table 2–1; for topical use, Chapter 93 and Table 93–3; references: 2:11, 2:21, 2:31.

PHARMACOKINETICS. IV gives good bioavailability; with PO use, bioavailability is 15%–30% of levels of those after the same parenteral dosage. Penetrates into most body tissues, including CNS. CSF concentrations are 50% of plasma. Minimal metabolism. 85% excreted unchanged in urine.

SPECTRUM. Herpesvirus infections. Some resistance has developed with extensive use.

INDICATIONS. In humans, for systemic, CNS, respiratory, or genital herpesvirus infections. Suppresses respiratory tract infections and mucosal eruptions. Does not prevent subclinical viral shedding. Should not be used in mild or self-limiting disease.

CONTRAINDICATIONS. Reduce dosage in renal failure. Use with caution in pregnant animals because it crosses placenta. High doses are fetotoxic.

ADVERSE REACTIONS. Nephrotoxic if given rapidly IV, transient renal tubular obstruction by crystals. CNS signs after IV infusion. Oral use may cause vomiting and diarrhea.

INTERACTIONS. If coadministered with zidovudine, may cause mental drowsiness and depression.

Availability	Type	Sizes	Preparations (Company)
Human	Topical (ophthalmic ointment)	5% polyethylene glycol ointment	*Zovirax* (Burroughs Wellcome)
	Oral	200-mg capsule; 400- and 800-mg tablets; 200-mg/5 ml suspension	*Zovirax*
	IV solution	500-mg vial	*Zovirax*

INTERNATIONAL PREPARATIONS. *Acicloftal, Aciyiran, Acyvir, Avyclor, Cusiviral, Cycloviran, Geavir, Herpotern, Maynar, Neviran, Vipral, Virmen, Zovir, Zyclir.*

HANDLING. For IV, dissolve powder in 10–20 ml of sterile preservative-free water. Add to calculated volume of IV solution to be given over 1 hr. Discard unused solution after 12 hr. Do not add to biologic or colloidial fluids.

ADMINISTRATION. IV use preferred to treat systemic infections. Must infuse slowly to avoid crystal precipitation in renal tubules. Rates lower than 5 mg/kg/hr have low toxicity. Give any dose over at least 1-hr time period. For cats, has been diluted to a concentration of 1 mg/ml with 0.9% NaCl and given SC (2:10).

DOSAGE

Indications	Dose	Route	Interval (hr)	Duration (days)
Human	500 mg/m^2	IV	8	7–10
Cats	10 mg/kg	SC	8	prn

DISPENSING INFORMATION. Animal may become depressed or drowsy or have vomiting and diarrhea. Notify veterinarian if persists.

ALBENDAZOLE

CLASS. Benzimidazole carbamate.

ACTION. Antinematodal, antiprotozoal by inhibiting parasite intestinal cell microtubular function.

MORE INFORMATION. See FENBENDAZOLE, MEBENDAZOLE (elsewhere). See Antiprotozoals, Chapter 71, and Giardiasis, Chapter 78; Table 78–2; references: 71:3, 71:33, 71:33a.

PHARMACOKINETICS. Poorly absorbed (<1%) from GI tract and passes through. Any absorbed drug is rapidly metabolized into sulfoxide and sulfone derivatives with antihelminthic activity. Metabolites are predominantly excreted in urine.

SPECTRUM. Various nematodes and cestodes. **Protozoa:** *Encephalitozoon; Pneumocystis; Giardia.* **Fungus:** *Cryptococcus* (in vitro). **More effective:** 50 times more active than metronidazole and 10–40 times more active than quinacrine against *Giardia.*

INDICATIONS. Microsporidiosis (encephalitozoonosis), pneumocystosis. Closely related fenbendazole (50 mg/kg PO once every 24 hr for 3 days) is also effective against giardiasis in dogs (71:3).

CONTRAINDICATIONS. Hepatic dysfunction, cholestasis, pregnancy, or lactation. Do not need to alter dosage in renal failure.

ADVERSE REACTIONS. Vomiting, diarrhea, liver enzyme activity increases, cholestatic hepatitis. Weight loss, myelotoxicity, and blood dyscrasias at 30–60 mg/kg daily for 26 weeks. Pancytopenia has been reported at therapeutic dosages (25 mg/kg) for 4 and 10 days in a cat and a dog, respectively (71:33a). Leukopenias may be associated with sepsis. They can be reversed with supportive antibiotic and fluid therapy. Embryotoxic and teratogenic in lab animals. Low systemic toxicity with short-term usage because poorly absorbed.

INTERACTIONS. Cimetidine increases its biliary excretion; dexamethasone increases its steady-state concentrations; albendazole potentially increases theophylline concentrations.

Availability	Type	Sizes	Preparations (Company)
Human	Oral tablets	200 mg, 400 mg	*Alben* (SmithKline Beecham)
Veterinary	Oral liquid suspension (cattle)	113.6 mg/ml	*Valbazen* (Pfizer Animal Health)

INTERNATIONAL PREPARATIONS. *Albenza, Eskazole, Zeben, Zentel.*

HANDLING. Store at controlled room temperature; shake well before using.

ADMINISTRATION. Give with fatty meals to increase (although variable) absorption. Poor absorption is a benefit in treating intestinal-restricted diseases such as giardiasis. For giardiasis, at least four doses must be given to be effective. For encephalitozoonosis in people, has been given concurrently with trimethoprim or pyrimethamine and sulfonamides. For longer (> 30 days) therapy, should have blood count checked every 3–4 weeks to detect myelotoxicity.

DOSAGE

Indications	Dose	Route	Interval (hr)	Duration (days)
Humans				
Encephalitozoonosis	200–400 mg/person	PO	8–12	14–28
Dogs				
Leishmaniasis	10 mg/kg	PO	24	30
Leishmaniasis	5 mg/kg	PO	6	60
Giardiasis	25 mg/kg	PO	12	2
Cats				
Giardiasis	25 mg/kg	PO	12	5

ADDITIONAL DOSAGES. Enteric protozoal infections, Table 78–2.

DISPENSING INFORMATION. Contact veterinarian if vomiting, diarrhea, abdominal tenderness, yellow mucous membranes, and skin are observed.

ALLOPURINOL

CLASS. Purine analog. Xanthine oxidase inhibitor.

ACTION. Interferes with purine and subsequent RNA synthesis.

MORE INFORMATION. References: 71:5, 71:9, 71:13, 71:17, 71:19, 71:21, 71:22, 73:58.

PHARMACOKINETICS. Absorbed from GI tract after PO administration, converted to oxypurinol in liver. Distributed in tissues and extracellular fluid spaces but less in CSF. Renal excretion of metabolite predominates, with some in feces.

SPECTRUM. **Protozoa:** *Leishmania, Trypanosoma cruzi.* **Others:** Treatment of gout or urate urolithiasis.

INDICATIONS. Inexpensive, less toxic, PO therapy for leishmaniasis. Also considered for American trypanosomiasis, because nifurtimox is more toxic.

APPROVED USES. For hyperuricemia and gout in people.

CONTRAINDICATIONS. Reduce dosing, increase interval of administration, or avoid in cases involving renal failure or hepatic dysfunction. Safety in breeding or pregnant animals not established.

ADVERSE REACTIONS. Vomiting, diarrhea, dermatologic eruption (pruritus and rash), myelosuppression, xanthine urolith formation (71:18a).

INTERACTIONS. May continue adjunctive therapy with meglumine antimonate or sodium stibogluconate in leishmaniasis. Increases myelotoxicity of cyclophosphamide. Urinary acidifiers increase risk of xanthine urolith formation. Increases toxicity of anticoagulant rodenticides and serum aminophylline concentrations. Dermatologic reactions are enhanced with coadministration of cytotoxic drugs and ampicillin.

Availability	Type	Sizes	Preparations (Company)
Human	Oral tablets	100 mg, 300 mg	*Zyloprim* (Glaxo Wellcome), generic (various)

INTERNATIONAL PREPARATIONS. *Alloprin, Allopur, Allopurin, Alloremed, Allural, Aloral, Aluline, Apurin, Caplenal, Capurate, Dabroson, Foligan, Jenapurinol, Lysuron, Novopurol, Purinol, Zyloric.*

HANDLING. Store at room temperature (59–77°F) in airtight container protected from light. A 120-ml suspension of 20 mg/ml may be prepared by taking 24 100-mg tablets *(Zyloprim)* crushed and adding glycerin or distilled water to levigate, methylcellulose 40 ml, and a sufficient quantity of a 2:1 simple syrup to bring the volume to 120 ml. The mixture should be refrigerated and labeled "shake well"; is stable for 8 weeks in the dark.

ADMINISTRATION. Check blood cell counts and serum hepatic enzymes, urea, and creatinine every 2 weeks. Use in combination with meglumine antimonate for the first 30 days to improve efficacy.

DOSAGE

Indications (Dogs)	Dose (mg/kg)	Route	Interval (hr)	Duration (days)
Leishmaniasis	10	PO	24	30*
	15	PO	12	240

*May treat for an extended period as needed to control infection.

ADDITIONAL DOSAGES. Antimicrobial therapy for canine leishmaniasis, Table 73–4.

DISPENSING INFORMATION. Give 1–2 hr after feeding.

AMANTADINE

CLASS. Adamantanamine.

ACTION. Antiviral against RNA viruses. Blocks viral penetration into host cells.

MORE INFORMATION. See Rimantidine and Chapter 2, Antivirals; Table 2–1.

PHARMACOKINETICS. Well absorbed from GI tract when given PO, not metabolized, excreted unchanged in urine, also in milk.

SPECTRUM. At achievable concentrations, only affects influenza A viruses. Resistance can develop.

INDICATIONS. Early (within 48 hr of onset of signs) or prophylactic use in influenza. Reduces severity of pulmonary lesions and clinical illness. Also augments dopaminergic activity, used to treat human parkinsonism.

CONTRAINDICATIONS. Reduce dose in renal failure; avoid in pregnancy, lactation, seizure-prone animals, gastric ulceration.

ADVERSE REACTIONS. Allergic reactions, ataxia, CNS manifestations with overdosage.

INTERACTIONS. Synergistic with anticholinergics.

Availability	Type	Sizes	Preparations (Company)
Human	Oral capsules	100 mg	*Symadine* (Solvay); *Symmetrel* (DuPont Pharma); generic (various)
	Syrup, raspberry flavor	50 mg/5 ml	*Symmetrel*

HANDLING. Store in airtight container.

ADMINISTRATION. Treat as early in illness as possible.

DOSAGE

Indications (Dogs and Cats)	Dose (mg/kg)	Route	Interval (hr)	Duration (days)
Dosage and toxicity uncertain*	4.4–8.8*	PO	24	5–7
	2.2–4.4*	PO	12	5–7

*Do not exceed 150 mg total/day. Extrapolated from human pediatric dose.

DISPENSING INFORMATION. Can be taken with or without food. Store capsules at room temperature, away from moisture and direct sunlight. Store syrup at room temperature.

AMICARBALIDE ISETHIONATE

CLASS. Aromatic diamidine.

ACTION. Antiprotozoal; interferes with nucleic acid metabolism.

MORE INFORMATION. See IMIDOCARB, DIMINAZENE, PHENAMIDINE, PENTAMIDINE; Chapter 71.

PHARMACOKINETICS. Similar to imidocarb.

SPECTRUM. *Babesia, Ehrlichia.*

INDICATIONS. Babesiosis, ehrlichiosis. Licensed to treat bovine anaplasmosis but has been used in dogs. Not available in U.S.

CONTRAINDICATIONS, ADVERSE REACTIONS, INTERACTIONS. See IMIDOCARB.

Availability	Type	Sizes	Preparation (Company)
Veterinary	Parenteral solution	Unknown	*Diampron* (Rhône-Poulenc Rorer)

HANDLING. See IMIDOCARB.

ADMINISTRATION. May repeat injection after 1 week because of relapses that may occur.

DOSAGE

Indications (Dogs)	Dose (mg/kg)	Route	Interval (hr)	Duration (days)
Babesiosis	20	IM	24	1

ADDITIONAL DOSAGES: Ehrlichiosis, Table 28–4.

DISPENSING INFORMATION: Watch for signs of weakness and neurologic dysfunction, and report them immediately to your veterinarian. See also IMIDOCARB and DIMINAZENE.

AMIKACIN

CLASS. Aminoglycoside.

ACTION. Antibacterial.

MORE INFORMATION. See GENTAMICIN, and Aminoglycosides, Chapter 34; Tables 34–5 and 34–6.

PHARMACOKINETICS. Not well absorbed PO; must give parenterally for systemic use. Distribution restricted to extracellular fluid because of low lipid solubility. Enhanced with inflammation. Reaches therapeutic concentrations in peritoneal, pleural, and synovial fluids, bile, and respiratory secretions. Concentrates in kidney tissues and excreted unchanged in urine. See also GENTAMICIN.

SPECTRUM. Gram positive: *Staphylococcus.* **Gram negative:** *Acinetobacter, Citrobacter, Enterobacter, Escherichia, Klebsiella, Proteus, Serratia, Salmonella, Yersinia.* **Others:** *Nocardia, Mycobacterium tuberculosis.* **More effective:** *Pseudomonas*: more effective than gentamicin. **Ineffective:** Obligate anaerobes.

INDICATIONS. For infections caused by gentamicin-resistant, gram-negative bacilli. Often shows broader antibacterial spectrum than gentamicin.

APPROVED USES. For *Mycobacterium avium-intracellulare*-complex infections in combination with other effective agents.

CONTRAINDICATIONS. Renal failure.

ADVERSE REACTIONS. Nephrotoxic in dogs and cats; the latter are more sensitive. See also GENTAMICIN; thought to be less nephrotoxic than gentamicin. Ototoxic, causing deafness, especially in cats.

INTERACTIONS. See GENTAMICIN.

Availability	Type	Sizes	Preparations (Company)
Human	Parenteral solution	250 mg/ml	*Amikin* (Apothecon), generic (various)
	Pediatric injectable solution	50 mg/ml	
Veterinary	Parenteral solution	50 mg/ml, 250 mg/ml	*Amiglyde-V (Fort Dodge)*

INTERNATIONAL PREPARATIONS. *Amicasil, Amikan, Amikine, Amiklin, Amukin, Biklin, Chemacin, Kanbine, Lukadin, Pierami.*

HANDLING. Compatible in 5% dextrose, 0.9% sodium chloride, and lactated Ringer's solutions. Stable for 24 hr. Should not premix or add to any other drug solutions. Solutions may change from colorless to pale yellow but no loss in potency occurs.

ADMINISTRATION. For IV give over a 30-min period in solutions. Maximum treatment duration usually 7–10 days. Important to monitor renal, vestibular, and auditory function. The greater the interval between doses, the less is its nephrotoxicity.

DOSAGE

Indications	Dose (mg/kg)	Route	Interval (hr)	Duration (days)
Dogs				
Urinary infections	2.3	IM, SC	12	7–10
Soft tissue infections	7.5	IV, IM, SC	12	7–10
	5	IV, IM, SC	8	7
Orthopedic infections	10	IV, IM, SC	8	7
Bacteremia, sepsis	7	IV	8	7
Cats				
Soft tissue infections	15–10	IV, IM, SC	24	7–10
Soft tissue infections	5–10	IM, SC	12	7
Bacteremia	10–12	IV, IM, SC	8–12	7

ADDITIONAL DOSAGES. None.

DISPENSING INFORMATION. Must be given SC; therefore, not advised for home administration. Monitoring for renal toxicity is also needed.

AMOXICILLIN

CLASS. Aminopenicillin.

ACTION. Bactericidal; inhibits bacterial cell wall synthesis.

MORE INFORMATION. See AMPICILLIN; Chapter 34, Aminopenicillins; Table 34–1.

PHARMACOKINETICS. See also AMPICILLIN. Better absorbed from GI tract than ampicillin and less affected by feeding. Rapidly absorbed after IM or SC. Injection site on body does not markedly affect this uptake from SC tissues. Longer serum half-life than ampicillin permits BID dosing. Mainly distributed in extracellular fluid compartment. Enters most tissues and body fluids except brain and CSF. With PO administration, liquid forms slightly better absorbed than tablets (bioavailability of suspension 77%; drops 68%; tablets 64%) (34:84). Most drug excreted unchanged in urine.

SPECTRUM. Same as ampicillin. **Gram positive:** *Streptococcus*, non–β-lactamase *Staphylococcus*. **Gram negative:** *Escherichia, Proteus, Pasteurella*. See also AMPICILLIN. **Anaerobes:** some efficacy but less than penicillin G. **Other:** borreliosis, leptospirosis. **Ineffective:** β-lactamase–producing bacteria.

INDICATIONS. Infections of nasopharynx, middle ear, urinary tracts, skin and soft tissue, upper and lower respiratory tracts, prophylaxis during dentistry, genitourinary infections.

CONTRAINDICATIONS. Previous hypersensitivity to penicillins.

ADVERSE REACTIONS. Dogs: diarrhea and vomiting; facial swelling, dermal rash; less diarrhea than with ampicillin; proximal renal tubular dysfunction (glucosuria, proteinuria, aminoaciduria, isosthenuria, hyposthenuria, with electrolyte loss and metabolic acidosis in one dog (34:6). **Cats:** vomiting, diarrhea, depression, anorexia, facial swelling, ocular irritation, polydipsia and polyuria, salivation, personality change (34:85).

INTERACTIONS. False-positive glucosuria result with Clinitest (Ames Laboratories, Elkhart, IN). See also AMPICILLIN.

Availability	Type	Sizes	Preparations (Company)
Human	Oral tablets	125 mg	*Amoxil* (SmithKline Beecham), generic (various)
	Oral capsules	250 mg, 500 mg	*Polymox* (Apothecon), *Wymoxl* (Wyeth-Ayerst)
	Powder for oral suspension (trihydrate)	125 mg/5 ml, 250 mg/5 ml, 500 mg/5 ml	*Amoxil, Polymox, Wymox*
Veterinary	Oral tablets	50 mg, 100 mg, 150 mg, 200 mg, 400 mg	*Amoxi-Tabs* (Pfizer Animal Health)
		50 mg, 100 mg, 200 mg, 400 mg	*Robamox-V,* Tablets (Fort Dodge)
	Powder for oral suspension	50 mg/ml	*Amoxi-Tabs* *Robamox-V, Qualamox* (Merial)
	Powder for parenteral suspension	3 gm (dilutes to 100 mg/ml or 250 mg/ml)	*Amoxi-Inject* (Pfizer Animal Health)
	Oral paste	20 mg/ml	*Vetrimoxin* (Sanofi)

INTERNATIONAL PREPARATIONS. *Amoxilan, Amoxina, Cilamox, Flemoxin, Helvamox, Polymox, Supramox, Trimox, Wymox.*

HANDLING. Store all tablets, capsules, and powders in airtight containers away from moisture at room temperature. Reconstituted oral suspension is stable for 2 weeks at refrigerated or room temperatures. Once reconstituted, parenteral suspension is stable for 3 mo at room temperature, 12 mo refrigerated.

ADMINISTRATION. Mix well before administering; food can reduce absorption. Continue treatment for 48 hr after all signs of infection are gone.

DOSAGE

Indications	Dose	Route	Interval (hr)	Duration (days)
Dogs				
Urinary infections	10–20 mg/kg	PO	12	5–7
	10 mg/kg	IM, SC	24	5
Systemic, bacteremia	22–50 mg/kg	PO	8	7
Orthopedic infections	22–30 mg/kg	IV, IM, SC, PO	6–8	7–10
Cats				
Urinary and soft tissue infections	50 mg/cat	PO	24	5–7
	11–22 mg/kg	PO	24	5–7
Sepsis	10–20 mg/kg	IV, SC, PO	12	prn

ADDITIONAL DOSAGES. Canine distemper, Table 3–5; feline panleukopenia, Table 10–1; streptococcal infections, Table 35–4; enteric bacteria, Table 39–1; anaerobic infections, Table 41–10; leptospirosis, Table 44–4; Lyme borreliosis, Table 45–3; actinomycosis, Table 49–1; dermatophilosis, Table 51–1; feline abscesses, Table 52–2; musculoskeletal infections, Table 86–3; respiratory infections, Table 88–8; oral infections, Table 89–4; intra-abdominal infections, Table 89–15; urinary infections, Table 91–8.

DISPENSING INFORMATION. Shake solution well before using. Give to fasted animal and no feeding for 2 hr before or after dosing. Keep refrigerated. Discard unused drug after 2 weeks.

AMOXICILLIN-CLAVULANATE

CLASS. Aminopenicillin and β-lactamase inhibitor in 4:1 ratio.

ACTION. Bactericidal; inhibits bacterial cell wall synthesis and bacterial β-lactamase.

MORE INFORMATION. See Chapter 34, Aminopenicillins; Tables 34–1 and 34–2.

PHARMACOKINETICS. Stable in the presence of gastric acid; absorption not influenced by food. Clavulanate does not affect the pharmacokinetics of amoxicillin. The only orally bioavailable-lactamase inhibitor and penicillin group combination. Widely distributed to most tissues *except* the CNS and CSF, where amoxicillin penetrates only with inflammation. Penetration of clavulanate into CNS is uncertain. High urinary levels of unchanged drug.

SPECTRUM. Gram positive: *Staphylococcus*, some *Streptococcus, Erysipelothrix, Corynebacterium*. **Gram negative:** *Escherichia, Klebsiella, Proteus, Enterobacter, Pasteurella, Bordetella.* **Anaerobes:** *Clostridium, Peptococcus, Peptostreptococcus*, others. **More effective:** Clavulanate has minimal antibacterial activity itself but extends the spectrum of amoxicillin to include β-lactamase producers, improving activity against *Escherichia, Salmonella, Klebsiella, Proteus, Staphylococcus*, and *Bacteroides* and other anaerobes. **Ineffective:** *Pseudomonas, Enterobacter.*

INDICATIONS. Otitis media, sinusitis, respiratory infections, urinary tract infections, anal sacculitis, gingivitis, pyoderma, soft tissue infections, osteomyelitis, bite wounds, *Proteus* urinary infections.

CONTRAINDICATIONS. Some dosage reduction in severe renal failure. Avoid with previous allergic reaction to β-lactam.

ADVERSE REACTIONS. Vomiting and diarrhea, depression, anorexia, dermal rash. Polyuria, polydipsia, lameness, personality change (34:85).

INTERACTIONS. False-positive glucosuria using Clinitest (Ames Laboratories). *See also* AMOXICILLIN.

Availability	Type	Sizes	Preparations (Company)
Human	Tablets	125 mg, 250 mg, 500 mg	*Augmentin; Clamoxyl; Synulox* (SmithKline Beecham)
	Oral suspension	125 mg/5 mL, 250 mg/5 ml	*Augmentin; Clamoxyl; Syrulox*
Veterinary	Tablets	62.5 mg, 125 mg, 250 mg, 375 mg total	*Clavamox* (Pfizer Animal Health)
	Oral solution	62.5 mg/ml	*Clavamox*

INTERNATIONAL PREPARATIONS. *Bimoxi, Ciblor, Clavepen, Clavucid, Clavulin, Duplamox.*

HANDLING. Oral suspension: powder should be stored in airtight container away from moisture at room temperature. Add water and shake to mix. Once reconstituted, must refrigerate; activity lasts 10 days. **Tablets:** supplied in sealed strips, maintain in moisture-proof foil wrapping for stability. Store at room temperature away from moisture.

ADMINISTRATION. Usual duration of treatment is extended for 21 days for deep pyoderma in dogs and 10–14 days in cats with resistant infections for a maximum of 30 days. Treat for at least 48 hr after signs have resolved.

DOSAGE

Indications	Dose	Route	Interval (hr)	Duration (days)
Dogs				
Urinary	12.5 mg/kg	PO	12	5–7
Skin, soft tissue infections	12.5 mg/kg	PO	12	5–7*
Deep pyoderma	12.5 mg/kg	PO	12	14–120
Systemic, bacteremia	22 mg/kg	PO	8–12	7
Cats				
Urinary tract	62.5 mg/cat	PO	12	10–30
Skin, soft tissue infections	62.5 mg/cat	PO	12	5–7
	10–20 mg/kg	PO	12	5–7
Sepsis, pneumonia	10–20 mg/kg	PO	8	7–10

*May have to treat 21 days with resistant infections for a maximum of 30 days.

ADDITIONAL DOSAGE. Tracheobronchitis, Table 6–1; gram-negative infections, Table 37–2; *Clostridium perfringens* diarrhea, Table 39–4; anaerobic infections, Table 41–10; nocardiosis, Table 49–5; canine pyoderma, Table 85–3; respiratory disease, Table 88–8; oral infections, Table 89–4; hepatobiliary infections, Table 90–4.

DISPENSING INFORMATION. Can be given with or without food; however, advisable to avoid use within 2 hr of mealtime. See AMOXICILLIN.

AMPHOTERICIN B

CLASS. Polyene antifungal.

ACTION. Amphotericin B (AMB) binds to sterols in fungal cell membrane, allows leakage of contents.

MORE INFORMATION. Chapter 57. See Table 57–2 for comparative features of the four formulations. All four preparations have different properties and dosage regimens. References: 57:1, 57:11, 57:12, 57:17, 57:19–21, 57:25, 57:28, 57:31, 57:39, 57:42, 57:43, 57:49, 57:53, 57:55, 71:16a, 71:39a, 73:30a, 73:40a.

PHARMACOKINETICS. Conventional drug is insoluble in water so prepared as a colloidal dispersion with the bile salt deoxycholate (ABD; *Fungizone*). Available in lipid-complex formulations, which include cholesteryl sulfate (ABCD; *Amphocil); encapsulated unilamellar liposomes (L-AMB; AmBisome) or lipid complexed (ABLC; Abelcet)*. ABD is not absorbed from GI tract after PO administration; given parenterally, usually IV. Initial rise in blood concentration in 24 hr is followed by prolonged elimination period over 2–3 weeks. Strongly bound to cell membranes. Use of AMB in lipid-complex formulations may be less nephrotoxic because of selective uptake by the mononuclear phagocyte system.
ABD. Poor oral absorption. Painful IM, so usually given IV. Widely distributed and penetrates many tissues and inflammatory exudates but is highly protein bound. Poor penetration into bones, brain and CSF (even with inflammation), aqueous and vitreous humor, amniotic fluid, muscle, respiratory secretions, pancreas, and salivary gland, and uninflamed body cavities (pleura, peritoneum, joints, pericardium). Accumulates in liver, kidneys, and lungs. Metabolism is uncertain; small amount of biliary excretion; slow urinary excretion (up to 2 mo) occurs with a small portion (<10%) as active drug. In dogs, up to 20% dose is excreted in bile over time. Does not accumulate to greater extent in renal failure, but is nephrotoxic (57:11, 57:53).
ABCD. Stable in plasma, not dissociating to free AMB; leads to mononuclear phagocyte uptake and lower renal concentrations and toxicity. In animal studies, compared with ABD, ABCD had lower plasma levels, higher liver concentrations, greater volume of distribution, and longer half-life. Highest drug concentration achieved in organs of the mononuclear phagocyte system (liver, spleen) and in lung, with lower concentrations in kidney, stomach, and small intestine. Lower concentrations in bone marrow and heart muscle, and little in brain and CSF (57:11, 57:53). With this preparation, concentrations are lower in kidneys, lungs, heart, brain, GI tract, and CSF than with deoxycholate. Most of the drug is concentrated in the liver with this formulation. Lower renal concentrations correlate with less nephrotoxicity of the liposomal-encapsulated derivative. Higher hepatic, splenic, and bone marrow concentrations resulting from increased mononuclear phagocyte concentrations were not associated with increased toxicity.
L-AMB. Highest serum levels are achieved with this formulation, presumably because of its small particle size and lower uptake by the mononuclear phagocyte system (MPS). Greatest concentrations in liver and spleen compared with ABD with similar levels in lung and kidney.
ABLC. Because of large molecular size and rapid uptake by the MPS, serum concentrations are lower than with ABD. Greatest concentration in dogs has been found in liver, spleen, and lung. Kidney concentrations are slightly lower than with ABD.

SPECTRUM. Fungi: *Histoplasma, Cryptococcus, Coccidioides, Paracoccidioides, Blastomyces, Candida, Sporothrix, Mucor, Aspergillus, Rhizopus, Absidia, Basidiobolus, Entomophthora.* **Others:** *Leishmania* (71:16a). **Ineffective:** dermatophytes.

INDICATIONS. Cryptococcosis, coccidioidomycosis, histoplasmosis, mucormycosis, sporotrichosis, aspergillosis, candidiasis, leishmaniasis. Primary drug for severe overwhelming systemic mycoses. Most effective antifungal for severe life-threatening infections of disseminated aspergillosis. Lipid formulations can be given at higher doses to enhance efficacy at a significantly greater cost. They are indicated over ABD when it has been ineffective or has caused nephrotoxicity if pre-existing renal impairment is evident.

CONTRAINDICATIONS. Renal failure, hepatic failure. Lipid formulations are associated with less nephrotoxicity.

ADVERSE REACTIONS. During infusion, can develop fever, vomiting, myalgia, phlebitis, occasional anaphylaxis. Lipid formulations have a greater tendency to cause these reactions, which can be reduced by slowing the infusion rate. Reduced nephrotoxicity may relate to lipid binding of drug in plasma and its direct uptake into the MPS. Nephrotoxicity is the dose-limiting factor; may have to interrupt therapy, reduce dosage, or use alternative drugs. Gradually increase dose if drug reinstated. The use of AMB deoxycholate is complicated by acute infusion-related toxicity and constitutional and chronic renal toxicities. These limit the dose and duration of AMB in clinical practice. Lipid formulations may be associated with infusion-related reactions. The theoretical advantage of the three lipid formulations is their ability to concentrate in the MPS and to be transported to the sites of infection. Larger doses of lipid formulations drug can be given with lower toxicity. AMB preparations are not advised in pregnancy, although there is no known toxicity. Can cause hypokalemia, which may affect cardiac, skeletal muscle, or renal function. Weight loss with long-term treatment. Nonregenerative normochromic normocytic anemia occurs with long-term therapy, presumably caused by nephrotoxicity or interference with erythropoietin. Increases renal vascular resistance without changing blood pressure, thereby reducing renal blood flow. To combat toxicity, renal dopamine DA1 receptors may be stimulated. Dopamine infusion has been used to reduce toxicity but has a nonselective effect. Fenoldopam (SmithKline Beecham), a specific DA1 agonist for receptors in renal tubules, might be more selective (57:39).

INTERACTIONS. AMB increases nephrotoxicity of cyclosporine, aminoglycosides, vancomycin, inhalation anesthetics, and cisplatin. Synergistic effects occur with combined use of rifampin against *Histoplasma, Aspergillus, Candida,* and tetracycline or fluorocytosine against *Candida* and *Cryptococcus.* AMB may alter the fungal cell membrane, allowing these other drugs to disrupt fungal metabolism. Combination therapy with azole antifungals may induce fungal resistance to AMB, although it is often recommended in rapidly advancing systemic mycoses.

Availability		Type	Sizes	Preparations (Company)
Human	**ABD**	Powder for injection (deoxycholate)	50 mg/vial	*Fungizone* (E.R. Squibb)
	ABCD	Powder for injection (colloidal dispersion)	50 mg/vial and 100 mg/vial	*Amphocil, Amphotec* (Sequus)
	L-AMB	Powder for injection (liposomal)	50 mg/vial	*AmBisome* (Fujisawa; Nexstar)
	ABLC	Solution for injection (lipid complex)	100 mg/20 ml vial (5 mg/ml)	*Abelcet* (Liposome Co.)

INTERNATIONAL PREPARATIONS. *Ampho-Moronal, Funganiline, Fungilin, Fungizona.*

HANDLING. ABD: Dilute powder with 10 ml sterile water (electrolyte or preservative free), shake until clear to give 5 mg/ml solution. Dilute further 1:50 with 5% dextrose to give final concentration of 10 mg/100 ml. Incompatible with many other fluids, but can use dilute heparin for flush. Precipitates will form if preservatives or saline are used. Stored powder is refrigerated in the dark in unopened vials. If accidentally left unrefrigerated; powder is stable for 2–4 weeks. Prepared 5-mg/ml solutions are stable for 24 hr in the dark at room temperature and for 1 week when refrigerated. When further diluted in 5% dextrose, solution is stable in PVC IV bags for 24 hr. Exposure to light during daily infusions (< 8 hr duration) does not affect potency enough to warrant concern. **ABCD:** As dry powder, stable at room temperature for at least 2 years. After reconstitution, vials can be stored refrigerated for 24 hr and should not be frozen. With further dilution to approximately 1 mg/ml in 5% dextrose, the stability is 24 hr refrigerated. **L-AMB:** Dry powder is stored under refrigeration. It is diluted with sterile water without preservatives to a 4-mg/ml solution. Shaking is necessary until the drug is completely dispersed. Reconstituted drug is stable up to 24 hr refrigerated, if not frozen. For further dilution to 1–2 mg/ml or lower concentrations, the drug is flushed through a 5-μm filter (provided) into 5% dextrose. Infusion into the patient should be within 6 hr of dilution. An in-line membrane filter may be used if the mean pore diameter is > 1 μm. **ABLC:** Shake vial to suspend yellow sediment, withdraw drug via 18-gauge needle into 20-ml syringes and infuse through the supplied 5-μm filter needle into 5% dextrose for infusion to a concentration of 1–2 mg/ml. Refrigerate suspension until used. Stable in 5% dextrose solution for 48 hr refrigerated and 6 hr at room temperature. Aseptic technique must be practiced because no bacteriostatic preservatives are included. Do not dilute with saline solutions or other drugs. Infusion catheters carrying such fluids can be flushed with 5% dextrose first. In-line filters should not be used. It should not be frozen.

ADMINISTRATION. ABD: Animals should be well hydrated before treatment, and pre-existing dehydration must be corrected by fluid therapy. Manufacturer of deoxycholate preparation recommends dose be given over 2–6 hr. When large-volume infusion is used, an IV catheter is placed and the dose (10 mg/100 ml) is given in 300–500 ml of 5% dextrose, depending on size of animal. Administration over this interval may reduce the likelihood or renal damage. However, clinical experience in dogs and cats has shown that more concentrated solutions, with the dose placed in a volume of 10 ml to 60 ml 5% dextrose, can be placed in a syringe and infused through a butterfly or indwelling catheter over a 5- to 10-min period. Ten milliliters of 5% dextrose flush should be infused immediately before and after administration of the drug. Although bolus infusions may have a higher risk of toxicity, this can be overcome by administering an equal or greater volume of lactated Ringer's or 0.9% NaCl (equal to that otherwise given with routine dilution of AMB) by IV or SC administration without the risks associated with extravasated drug. Supplemental fluid diuresis is highly recommended with each dose. For cats, indwelling catheters are preferable because of the difficulties of repeated venipuncture. Often test dose (1 mg) slowly IV to check for immediate systemic reactions. Coadministration of nonsteroidal anti-inflammatories, antihistamines, antiemetics, and/or small doses of IV glucocorticoids or heparin may reduce systemic reaction. Prevent thrombophlebitis by flushing catheters, using larger veins, rotating sites, adding heparin to the solution. The only way to reach the CNS is by intrathecal use of deoxycholate preparation, which can be irritating.

Renal toxic effects are monitored at least once if not twice weekly by checking serum urea concentrations and by examination of the urine for specific gravity, protein, casts, and hematuria. Serum creatinine and electrolytes (including magnesium, which may decrease) determinations are optional but may be required if screening tests or health becomes altered. Urine changes detect toxicity earlier than blood biochemical alterations. Therapy should be temporarily discontinued if anorexia or vomiting occurs or if serum urea increases to > 30 mg/dl. Therapy with AMB or alternative drug is reinstituted after signs and laboratory findings of nephrotoxicity disappear. Maintenance therapy with weekly or monthly injections of AMB or daily oral imidazoles has been used to avoid relapses that develop once therapy is discontinued.

Hypokalemia, a problem in people receiving AMB, has been documented in dogs and cats. Any potassium supplements should be given PO, SC, or by alternative IV route, because these solutions will precipitate the colloid.

Fever, nausea, and vomiting that occur during or immediately after treatment may be less severe if a physiologic dose of hydrocortisone sodium succinate (0.5 mg/kg, IV), diphenhydramine (0.5 mg/kg, IV or PO), or aspirin (10 mg/kg, PO) is given before administration of AMB. Anti-inflammatory or immunosuppressive doses of glucocorticoids should be avoided because they may lead to fungal dissemination. Muscular fasciculations and rigors that develop in people during IV infusions have been controlled with dantrolene sodium (10–50 mg, IV) or meperidine.

Attempts to avoid nephrotoxicity with ABD have been made using mannitol (0.5–1 g/kg, IV), sodium bicarbonate (1–2 mmol/kg, IV), and dopamine (3–10 μg/kg/min, IV), but controlled studies have not been done. Beneficial effects have been obtained when sodium-containing fluids or furosemide (5 mg/kg route) or aminophylline was given to dogs just before administration of AMB. SC administration is less nephrotoxic (see later).

Heparin has been added to ABD to control phlebitis that develops after repeated infusions, but there is no conclusive evidence that its use decreases the reaction. In-line micropore filters used to remove particulate matter and bacteria from IV solutions are less than 0.45 μm and will also remove the drug. Filters of greater than 1 μm can be used but will not remove bacteria.

Alternative Routes. Usual IV therapy requires repeated venous access, often necessitating catheter placement, especially in cats. ABD may be used topically, intra-articularly, or intrathecally or may be flushed in the bladder or renal pelvis if the infection site is accessible by these means. This will help achieve maximal concentrations with lower risk of systemic toxicity. **Intra-articularly**, 5 to 15 mg can be used to infuse one joint. For **bladder infusions**, AMB is mixed to a concentration of 30 to 50 mg in 50–100 ml sterile water and is infused once daily for 5–15 days. The bladder is distended, and the animal is permitted to void spontaneously. Alternatively, a constant-drip infusion of 50 mg/L has been used. For **intrathecal** use, 0.2–0.5 mg is diluted in 5 ml of 10% dextrose or CSF freshly removed from the animal under anesthesia. It is injected in the lumbar or cisternal space, and the head is lowered for a few minutes if signs of intracranial involvement are apparent. Unfortunately, this procedure must be repeated two to three times each week. For **aerosol** use, 50 mg divided into three doses has been used long term (3 weeks–2.5 years) in people for prophylaxis or treatment of pulmonary fungal infections. **Ocular injection:** Although intraocular mycotic infections are difficult to cure, enophthalmitis in people has been effectively treated by injecting simultaneously intravitreally 5 μg, peribulbar space 125 μg, and episclerally 5 mg. **Subcutaneous:** Route used in dogs and cats with cryptococcosis and potentially for other systemic mycoses. A daily dose of 0.5 to 0.8 mg/kg is added to 400 ml (cats) and 500 ml (dogs) of 0.45% saline/2.5% dextrose (57:31). This total fluid volume is given SC two or three times weekly to a cumulative level of 8–26 mg/kg, which is higher than IV regimen. Concentrations of > 20 mg/L are irritating, cause SC abscesses, and should be avoided. The method is suited for outpatient treatment and does not require IV catheter maintenance. Blood levels are lower but more sustained, reducing toxicity and allowing for increased efficacy. **Combined with fat emulsion:** This has been done in an attempt to decrease nephrotoxicity. AMB deoxycholate is stable in combination with fat emulsions. A concentration of 0.5 to 2 mg/ml is stable in a 20% fat emulsion for 4 days at 25°C in fluorescent lighting and 7 days at 4–8°C in the dark.

ABCD: Given by IV infusion at a rate of 1 mg/kg/hr. A test dose (10 ml) should be infused first to check for adverse reactions. The rate of infusion can be increased if it is tolerated.

L-AMB: Given by IV infusion over 60 to 120 min or longer with 5% dextrose as a diluent. Solution is diluted to 1–2 mg/ml.

ABLC: Given by IV infusion at 2.5 mg/kg/hr. With infusion times longer than 2 hr, the mixture should be shaken periodically to disperse any sediment.

DOSAGE. ABD: A wide range of systemic dosages has been described in the veterinary literature. The range has been a total (cumulative) dose of 4–12 mg/kg given as alternate day or Mon-Wed-Fri treatments. Dogs usually receive accumulative doses of 8–12 mg/kg and cats 4–6 mg/kg. Lower dosages are used if adjunctive therapy with oral flucytosine or an imidazole is used. Higher doses are given SC (see prior discussion). For IV use, the drug is given on these days at 0.15–0.5 mg/kg/day, which is continued until the final calculated total dosage is reached (usually 6 weeks) or when toxicity (elevated serum urea concentration) occurs. Daily doses are lower (0.15–0.25 mg/kg) for cats and higher (0.25–0.5 mg/kg) for dogs. The 0.5-mg/kg dose has a high risk of nephrotoxicity. Initial doses of 0.1 mg/kg for cats and 0.25 mg/kg for dogs are often given the first day and gradually increased to 0.25 mg/kg and 0.5 mg/kg, respectively. Doses up to 1 mg/kg/day given two to three times weekly have been used in particularly resistant infections in dogs that tolerate the drug well. Treatment often lasts for 2–3 mo or longer, and early discontinuance can lead to a relapse. Treatment may require 11 mo in aspergillosis and 9 mo in sporotrichosis. A recommended dose for long-term treatment of sporotrichosis is 0.2–0.5 mg/kg IV given every 48 hr (57:54). Higher dosages can be used with SC route; see previously under administration. **Lipid formulations—ABCD, L-AMB, ABLC:** higher dosages are tolerated and used as outlined in the table that follows. Rates of infusion and total doses are individualized to each animal to ensure maximum efficacy while reducing the potential for systemic toxicity or adverse reactions.

Indications	Initial Test Dose* (mg/kg)	Usual Dose (mg/kg)	Route	Interval (hr)	Duration
ABD (Fungizone)					
Dogs (mycoses)	0.25	0.25–0.5	IV	48†	6 weeks
Cats (mycoses)	0.1	0.1–0.25	IV	48†	6 weeks
Dogs and cats (mycoses)	—	0.5–0.8	SC	48†	3–10 weeks
Dogs (leishmaniasis)	—	0.5–0.8	IV	48†	See ‡

Table continued on following page

Indications	Initial Test Dose* (mg/kg)	Usual Dose (mg/kg)	Route	Interval (hr)	Duration
L-AMB (AmBisome)					
Dogs (leishmaniasis)	0.5	3.0–3.3	IV	72–96	See §
Dogs (mycoses)	0.5	1–2.5	IV	48†	4 weeks ‖
ABCD (Amphocil)					
Dogs (mycoses)	0.5	1–2.5	IV	48†	4 weeks ‖
ABLC (Abelcet)					
Dogs (mycoses)	0.5	1–2.5	IV	48†	4 weeks ‖

*Only use this dose first to test for potential adverse reactions or azotemia; animals developing azotemia usually tolerate subsequent administration at the usual dosage.
†Every 48 hours, or Monday (M), Wednesday (W), and Friday (F) on a weekly basis until the cumulative dosage is reached.
‡Every 48 hours, or MWF, until a cumulative dose of 8 to 16 mg/kg is reached (71:16a).
§Every 72–96 hours, until a cumulative dose of 15 mg/kg is reached (73:40a). May be possible to give the same cumulative dose with a lower level every 48 hours.
‖Every 48 hours, or MWF, or until a cumulative dose of 12 mg/kg is reached (59:16) by using 1 mg/kg dose for susceptible yeast or systemic (dimorphic) fungal infections. For more resistant filamentous fungal infections, such as pythiosis, use a 2–2.5 mg dose until a cumulative dose of 24–30 mg/kg is reached.

ADDITIONAL DOSAGES. Blastomycosis, Table 59–1; histoplasmosis, Table 60–1; cryptococcosis, Table 61–4; coccidioidomycosis, Table 62–3; disseminated aspergillosis, Table 65–4; candidiasis and trichosporonosis, Table 66–1; protothecosis, Table 69–1.

AMPICILLIN

CLASS. Aminopenicillin.

ACTION. Bactericidal; inhibits bacterial cell wall synthesis.

MORE INFORMATION. See AMOXICILLIN; Aminopenicillins, Chapter 34; Table 34–1.

PHARMACOKINETICS. Orally up to 50% absorbed, but decreased by ingesta. Oral trihydrate form is less efficiently absorbed than anhydrate. In cats, oral suspension has lower bioavailability (18%) than capsules (42%). IM and SC sodium salt better absorbed than trihydrate. Absorption of anhydrate form is comparable between SC and IM sites. Better absorbed from SC tissues in the dorsal neck region than over the thoracic wall (34:161). Penetrates body fluids and parenchymal organs (liver, lung). Only enters acutely inflamed meninges, CNS, eye, and prostate. One of few β-lactams that is metabolized and excreted by liver: biliary concentration is 40 times that in blood. About 50% excreted unchanged in urine.

SPECTRUM. Gram positive: Non–β-lactamase *Staphylococcus, Streptococcus.* **Gram negative:** *Escherichia, Proteus, Pasteurella.* No advantage using this drug in conjunction with trimethoprim-sulfonamide because it adds very little to spectrum. Has better gram negative, but less anaerobic spectrum, than to natural and β-lactamase–resistant penicillins. See also AMOXICILLIN. **Anaerobes:** Not as effective as penicillin. **Ineffective:** Rickettsiae, mycoplasmas, mycobacteria, and fungi. Not effective against β-Lactamase–producing organisms.

INDICATIONS. Gram-negative infections caused by *Proteus* and *Escherichia.* Appropriate first choice for bacterial meningitis in dogs and cats. Dental prophylaxis, septicemia, urinary, respiratory, and soft tissue infections; prophylaxis with GI surgery when combined with gentamicin.

CONTRAINDICATIONS. Avoid in resistant infections caused by *Klebsiella, Pseudomonas, Enterobacter.* β-Lactamase is main cause of resistance. Safe in pregnancy. In hepatic cirrhosis, clearance is increased, and dose may have to be increased. Increase dose interval to 12 hr or reduce dose in severe renal failure.

ADVERSE REACTIONS. Causes seizures with rapid IV administration; upsets normal intestinal microflora causing diarrhea.

INTERACTIONS. Reduces bioavailability of atenolol. Potential antagonism of activity when coadministered with chloramphenicol, tetracyclines, or erythromycin. See AMOXICILLIN.

Availability	Type	Sizes	Preparations (Company)
Human	Powder for injection (IV, IM)	125 mg, 250 mg, 500 mg, 1 g, 2 g, 10 g	*Omnipen-N* (Wyeth-Ayerst), *Polycillin-N* (Bristol)
	Oral capsules	250 mg, 500 mg	*Amcill* (Parke-Davis), *Principen* (Bristol-Myers Squibb),
	Powder for oral suspension	125 mg/5 ml, 250 mg/5 ml, 500 mg/5 ml	*Polycillin, Totacillin* (SmithKline Beecham)
Veterinary	Oral capsules (trihydrate) (dogs, cats)	125 mg, 250 mg, 500 mg	*Princillin* (Solvay)
	Oral suspension (trihydrate) (dogs, cats)	125 mg/5 ml	*Intracillin* (Intervet), *Princillin*
	Powder for parenteral (SC, IM) suspension (trihydrate) (dogs, cats, cattle)	10-g, 25-g vials	*Polyflex* (Fort Dodge)
	Powder for parenteral (IV, SC) injection (sodium salt) (horses)	1-g, 3-g vials	*Amp-Equine* (Pfizer Animal Health)

INTERNATIONAL PREPARATIONS. *Binotal, Jenampin, Novapen, Penbritin, Principen, Rimacillin, Spectracil, Vidopen.*

HANDLING. Reconstituted parenteral ampicillin sodium (30 mg/ml) in sodium chloride (0.9%) or lactated Ringer's is stable for 8 hr at room temperature and for 48 hr when refrigerated. More dilute concentrations (< 20 mg/ml, in 5% dextrose) are stable 2–4 hr at room temperature and 8 hr if refrigerated. Whenever possible, use freshly prepared solutions of ampicillin sodium. Parenteral trihydrate suspension is stable for 3 mo at room temperature or 12 mo if refrigerated. Oral suspensions are stable for 1 week at room temperature or 2 weeks when refrigerated and should be discarded thereafter. Capsules and nonreconstituted powders are stored at room temperature. Ampicillin sodium solutions are incompatible with macrolides, aminoglycosides, tetracyclines, phenothiazines, and various other drugs; therefore, mixing with other compounds is not advised.

ADMINISTRATION. Give PO on empty stomach. For IV, administer slowly over 10–15 min or as slower IV drip. IM or IV forms are used for severe infections that require highest dosages or when oral medication is contraindicated.

DOSAGE

Indications	Dose (mg/kg)	Route	Interval (hr)	Duration (days)
Dogs				
Urinary infections	12.5	PO	12	3–7
	6.6	SC, IM	12	3–7
Soft tissue infections	10–20	PO, IM, SC	8	7
Pneumonia, systemic	22	PO, IV, SC	8	7–14
Meningitis, orthopedics	22	IV, IM, SC, PO	6–8	prn
Bacteremia, sepsis	20–40	IV, IM, SC	6–8	prn
Neonatal sepsis	50	IV, intraosseous	4–6	prn
Cats				
Urinary infections	20	PO	8–12	7–14
Soft tissue infections	20–40	PO	8–12	14
Systemic infections	7–11	IV, IM, SC	8–12	prn

ADDITIONAL DOSAGES. Canine distemper, Table 3–5; canine viral enteritis, Table 8–1; feline panleukopenia, Table 10–1, feline infectious peritonitis, Table 11–3; streptococcal infection, Table 35–4; salmonellosis, Table 39–1; *Clostridium perfringens* diarrhea, leptospirosis, Table 44–4; Lyme borreliosis, Table 45–3; actinomycosis, Table 49–1; nocardiosis, Table 49–2; feline abscesses, Table 52–2; bartonellosis, Table 54–3; musculoskeletal infections, Table 86–3; bacteremia, Table 87–7; respiratory infections, Table 88–8; oral infections, Table 89–4; urinary infections, Table 91–8; CNS infections, Table 92–5.

DISPENSING INFORMATION. Give drugs to fasted (preferably > 5 hr) dogs or at least 1 hr before or 2 hr after feeding (34:82). Dry food interferes less with absorption than moist food.

AMPICILLIN-SULBACTAM

CLASS. Aminopenicillin and β-lactamase inhibitor in a 2:1 ratio.

ACTION. Bactericidal; inhibitor of bacterial cell wall synthesis and β-lactamase inhibitor.

MORE INFORMATION. Chapter 34; Table 34–2; reference: 34:90.

PHARMACOKINETICS. Therapeutic levels attained within 15 min of IV or IM dose. Good tissue levels and penetrates peritoneal and interstitial fluids. Up to 85% excreted in urine within 8 hr (39:90). Both drugs eliminated at similar rate in dogs. Sulbactam has no intrinsic antibacterial activity but extends spectrum of ampicillin.

SPECTRUM. **Gram positive:** *Staphylococcus, Streptococcus, Bacillus anthracis, Listeria monocytogenes.* **Gram negative:** *Escherichia, Klebsiella, Proteus, Salmonella, Enterobacter, Pasteurella, Acinetobacter.* **Anaerobes:** *Clostridium, Peptococcus, Peptostreptococcus, Bacteroides, Fusobacterium.* **Ineffective:** *Pseudomonas.*

INDICATIONS. Skin and soft tissue, intra-abdominal, orthopedic, and genitourinary infections caused by susceptible bacteria. Can substitute wherever amoxicillin-clavulanate is indicated and a parenteral formulation is desired.

CONTRAINDICATIONS. Reduce dose in renal failure. Animals with known penicillin hypersensitivity.

ADVERSE REACTIONS. Local pain with IM; thrombophlebitis or systemic allergic reactions with IV; diarrhea; vomiting; seizures with rapid IV infusions; increased hepatic transaminases. See also AMPICILLIN.

INTERACTIONS. Coadministration of ampicillin and sulbactam to dogs has no effect on the pharmacokinetics of either drug (34:90). Do not mix with aminoglycosides during administration.

Availability	Type	Sizes	Preparation (Company)
Human	Powder for injection (sodium)	1.5 g (total); 3.0 g (total)	*UnaSyn* (Pfizer)

HANDLING. Dilute in sterile water, 0.9% NaCl, 5% dextrose or lactated Ringer's. Stability of drug is shortest for dextrose (2 hr at room temperature and 4 hr when refrigerated) and 8 or 48 hr, respectively, for both NaCl or sterile water. Maximum storage time for lactated Ringer's is 24 hr refrigerated. Do not mix with aminoglycosides. For IM, can be reconstituted with 2% lidocaine (without epinephrine).

ADMINISTRATION. IV or IM. For IV dose, give slowly over 10–15 min or give with 50–100-ml infusion fluid over 15–30 min. For IM, give deep.

DOSAGE

Indications	Dose	Route	Interval (hr)	Duration (days)
Adult human	1.5–3 g/person	IV	6	prn
Dog and cat	50 mg/kg	IV	6–8	prn

AMPROLIUM

CLASS. Thiamine analogue.

ACTION. Antiprotozoal; inhibits parasite's thiamine utilization (first-generation schizont).

MORE INFORMATION. Chapter 81; Table 81–2; reference: 71:18.

PHARMACOKINETICS. Unavailable.

SPECTRUM. Coccidia.

INDICATIONS. Coccidiosis; especially convenient for treating litters of animals.

APPROVED USES. Veterinary: coccidiosis in lambs, calves, and poultry.

CONTRAINDICATIONS. Limit duration of therapy for 2 weeks.

ADVERSE REACTIONS. Anorexia, diarrhea, depression. Unpalatable as undiluted liquid or paste. Anorexia may develop in puppies that eat more than 300 mg of amprolium on a daily basis. Prolonged high dosages can cause neurologic signs of thiamine deficiency, characterized by cervical ventroflexion, anisocoria, seizures. Should these develop, stop treatment and administer thiamine 1–10 mg/day IM or IV immediately.

INTERACTIONS. Excess dietary thiamine can interfere with drug effectiveness.

Availability	Type	Sizes	Preparations (Company)
Veterinary	Oral crumbles	1.25%	*Corid* (Merck AgVet; Merial)
	Oral solution	9.6%	*Corid*
	Soluble powder	20%	*Corid*

HANDLING. Store all products at room temperature.

ADMINISTRATION. Can add soluble powder in food or water. Use only food or water additives, not both! If given in drinking water, offer this as the sole source of liquids to drink. For animals refusing food or water additive, place in gelatin capsules containing 20% powder. Can treat pups 6 weeks of age and older.

DOSAGE

Indications	Dose	Route	Interval (hr)	Duration (days)
Dogs				
Coccidiosis (in capsules) treatment				
Small pups (<10 kg adult weight)	100 mg total dose, 20% powder	PO, gelatin capsules	24	7–12
Large pups (≥ 10 kg adult weight)	200 mg total dose, 20% powder	PO, gelatin capsules		7–12
Coccidiosis (in food): pups or bitches	250–300 mg total dose, 20% powder, on food	PO, on food	24	7–12
Coccidiosis (in water): pups or bitches	30 ml of 9.6% solution, 3.8 L (1 gallon) of water; no other drinking water provided	PO, in water	24	7–10
Cats				
Coccidiosis (on food)	300–400 mg/kg	PO	24	5
	110–220 mg/kg	PO	24	7–12
Coccidiosis (in water)	1.5 teaspoon/gallon H_2O	PO	24	10
Coccidiosis (in combination)				
Amprolium	150 mg/kg	PO	24	14
and				
sulfadimethoxine	25 mg/kg	PO	24	14

Additional dosages: coccidiosis, Table 81–2.

DISPENSING INFORMATION. Report signs of diarrhea or neurologic problems immediately to your veterinarian.

ATOVAQUONE

CLASS. Hydroxynaphthoquinone.

ACTION. Antiprotozoal; blocks cytochromes, resulting in inhibited nucleic acid and adenosine triphosphate synthesis.

MORE INFORMATION. See Antiprotozoal Chemotherapy, Chapter 71; Table 71–1; Chapter 77; Table 77–3; Chapter 83; Table 83–2; reference: 71:15.

PHARMACOKINETICS. Highly lipid soluble. Low absorption from GI tract. Bioavailability is increased three times with food and especially fatty meals. Little or no metabolism. Very low CSF penetration. Enterohepatic cycling with prolonged fecal elimination. Minimal urinary excretion.

SPECTRUM. *Pneumocystis:* slightly lower efficacy than trimethoprim-sulfonamide (TMS). May add azithromycin for some *Babesia* infections. Effective against *Toxoplasma* bradyzoites experimentally. Not very effective against *Cryptosporidium.*

INDICATIONS. Pneumocystosis when resistance or toxicity to TMS has occurred. TMS is often used first because of lower toxicity.

APPROVED USES. Human: *Pneumocystis* pneumonia, malaria.

CONTRAINDICATIONS. Avoid in pregnancy, lactation. If cannot be taken with food owing to GI upsets, then use another drug.

ADVERSE REACTIONS. Nausea, vomiting, diarrhea, dermal hypersensitivity, fetotoxic, hypoglycemia, anemia, neutropenia.

INTERACTIONS. Competes for plasma protein binding with many drugs, but others such as diphenylhydantoin are not affected. Rifampin decreases activity. Rifampin and metoclopramide reduce its plasma concentrations.

Availability	Type	Sizes	Preparations (Company)
Human	Oral tablets	250 mg (discontinued in U.S.)	*Mepron* (Glaxo Wellcome)
	Oral solution	150 mg/ml	*Mepron*

INTERNATIONAL PREPARATIONS. *Wellvone.*

HANDLING. Store in airtight containers at controlled room temperature.

ADMINISTRATION. Absorption improved when given with meals (especially fatty). In people, > 23 g of fat per meal is recommended.

DOSAGE†

Indications (Dogs)	Dose	Route	Interval (hr)	Duration (days)
Pneumocystosis	13.3 mg/kg*	PO	8	21

*Extrapolated from human dose.
†Maximum dose per administration is 750 mg.

ADDITIONAL DOSAGES. Babesiosis, Table 77–3; pneumocytosis, Table 83–2.

DISPENSING INFORMATION. Administer tablet with fat such as butter, tuna oil, ice cream, or meat fat.

AZITHROMYCIN

CLASS. Macrolide.

ACTION. Bacteriostatic; inhibits bacterial RNA-dependent protein synthesis by binding to 50s subunit.

MORE INFORMATION. CLARITHROMYCIN; references: 34:69, 34:145.

PHARMACOKINETICS. Better absorption and tissue penetration than erythromycin; more stable in gastric acid than erythromycin. Food decreases bioavailability; 97% absorbed in dog (34:145); 58% absorbed PO in cats (34:69). Reaches higher concentrations in tissues, phagocytes, and macrophages than in blood, with slow release and antibacterial activity up to 4 days after single dose. Successive doses increase tissue saturation. Transported by neutrophils to sites of inflammation. Concentrations up to 150 times blood levels in sputum, lung, liver, tonsils, nasal sinuses, stomach, kidney, female genital tract, prostate. Levels in brain and eye are lower than in other tissues but exceed those in blood. Biliary excretion of unchanged drug is major route of elimination and metabolites are inactive. Only 6% urinary excretion.

SPECTRUM. **Gram positive:** Some *Streptococcus*, variable *Staphylococcus*. **Gram negative:** *Salmonella, Bordetella, Helico bacter.* **Anaerobes:** *Propionibacterium, Clostridium*, and *Bacteroides.* **Others:** *Mycoplasma, Chlamydia, Borrelia, Toxoplasma, Cryptosporidium, Babesia, Mycobacterium avium-intracellulare* complex but less active than clarithromycin. **More Effective:** Most active macrolide against *Toxoplasma*, in vitro activity against *Cryptosporidium* and *Pneumocystis*. **Ineffective:** Less active than erythromycin against *Staphylococcus* and *Streptococcus* but more active against gram negative and some anaerobes.

INDICATIONS. Cryptosporidiosis, toxoplasmosis (with pyrimethamine), Lyme borreliosis; *M. leprae* and *M. avium-intracellulare* infections. Lower respiratory tract infections, enteropathogenic bacterial infections. Substitute for erythromycin with less GI irritation, lower dosing, but higher cost.

CONTRAINDICATIONS. Some reduction in dosage with hepatic and/or biliary dysfunction. Less of a concern with renal failure. Avoid with previous macrolide hypersensitivity.

ADVERSE REACTIONS. GI irritation (vomiting, diarrhea, abdominal pain), hepatomegaly, cholestatic hepatitis, increased liver enzymes.

INTERACTIONS. Some reduction in serum concentration with oral antacids. See ERYTHROMYCIN.

Availability	Type	Sizes	Preparations (Company)
Human	Capsules (dihydrate)	250 mg	*Zithromax (Pfizer)*
	Oral suspension	100 mg/5 ml, 200 mg/5 ml	*Zithromax*

INTERNATIONAL PREPARATIONS. *Azithrocin, Azitromax, Ribotrex, Trozocina.*

HANDLING. Store capsules at controlled room temperature (<30°C). Reconstituted solution should be stored between 5°C and 30°C.

ADMINISTRATION. Do not mix with food or give oral antacids concurrently.

DOSAGE

Indications	Dose (mg/kg)	Route	Interval (hr)	Duration (days)
Dogs	5–10	PO	12	5–7
Cats	7–15	PO	12	5–7

ADDITIONAL DOSAGES. Lyme borreliosis, Table 45–3; babesiosis, Table 77–3; cryptosporidiosis, Table 82–1.

DISPENSING INFORMATION. Administer without food; give 1 hr before or 2 hr after a meal.

AZTREONAM

CLASS. Monobactam.

ACTION. Bactericidal; interferes with cell wall synthesis, especially gram-negative bacteria resistant to β-lactamases.

MORE INFORMATION. See Chapter 34; Table 34–1.

PHARMACOKINETICS. Poor GI absorption and must be given parenterally (IV or IM). Enters most body fluids, including CSF. Penetrates and effective in abscesses. Primarily renally excreted as unchanged drug. Widely distributed in body tissues, including gallbladder, liver, lungs, kidneys, heart, intestine, prostate. Reaches saliva, bronchial secretions, bile, pericardial, pleural, peritoneal, synovial fluids. Reaches CNS at therapeutic concentration. Eliminated by kidney with 60%–70% as active drug. Hepatic dysfunction does not alter excretion.

SPECTRUM. Gram positive: poor. **Gram negative:** *Pseudomonas, Escherichia, Enterobacter, Klebsiella, Proteus, Serratia, Citrobacter.* Wide activity against *only* gram-negative organisms. Synergistic with aminoglycosides in vitro against most strains of Enterobacteriaceae and other gram-negative aerobic and facultative bacilli. Little or no activity on gram-positive or anaerobic bacteria and intestinal microflora. **Anaerobes:** poor. **More effective:** gram negative. **Ineffective:** most other bacteria.

INDICATIONS. Serious gram-negative infections of the urinary and lower respiratory tracts, meningitis, septicemia, skin, soft tissue, intra-abdominal, genital infections. Could be considered as an alternative to aminoglycosides to avoid nephrotoxicity or to fluoroquinolones in young animals. Often as a single agent for resistant gram-negative pathogens such as *Escherichia, Klebsiella, Serratia, Pseudomonas.* Examples are nosocomial pneumonia and aspiration pneumonia (the latter use, in combination with clindamycin). With mixed infections, it should be used in combination with drugs against anaerobic and gram-positive bacteria. Can also combine with erythromycin, metronidazole, penicillins, vancomycin as a substitute for aminoglycosides.

CONTRAINDICATIONS. Must reduce dosages in renal dysfunction. No significant interactions with gentamicin, nafcillin, cephradine, clindamycin, metronidazole. Concurrent therapy needed if gram-positive aerobe or an anaerobe is suspected. Certain antibiotics (e.g., cefoxitin or imipenem) may induce β-lactamases in some gram-negative organisms making concurrent therapy with β-lactams such as aztreonam ineffective.

ADVERSE REACTIONS. Dermal hypersensitivity reactions, local phlebitis with IV, and swelling at injection site with IM. Nausea, vomiting, diarrhea, dermatologic eruptions, pancytopenia, seizures. Transient increase in hepatic transaminases; icterus from hepatotoxicity.

INTERACTIONS. Add to ampicillin for urinary tract infection caused by *Escherichia*. Use with clindamycin and metronidazole for intra-abdominal abscesses. Combination therapy with metronidazole for anaerobes and combine with vancomycin for gram positives.

Availability	Type	Sizes	Preparation (Company)
Human	Powder for injection	500 mg; 1 g or 2 g/vial	*Azactam* (Bristol-Myers Squibb)

INTERNATIONAL PREPARATIONS. *Primbactam.*

HANDLING. IV solutions of 2% (wt/vol) or less can be prepared with 0.9% NaCl or 5% dextrose. Can also add clindamycin phosphate, gentamicin, tobramycin sulfate, or cefazolin sodium. Stable for 48 hr at room temperature or 7 days when refrigerated. May be stored frozen at −20°C for 3 mo. Once thawed, should be used within 24 to 72 hr. Should not be refrozen. Incompatible in solution with amphotericin B, nafcillin, cephradine, metronidazole.

ADMINISTRATION. For IM use, give deep in large muscle. It is well tolerated and need not be mixed with local anesthetics. IV use recommended for animals with bacteremia, abscesses, severe overwhelming infections. Give IV infusion slowly over 20–60 min.

DOSAGE

Indications	Dose	Route	Interval (hr)	Duration (days)
Human*	1–2 g total	IV, IM	8–12	prn

*For dogs and cats, an established dose is not available; the pediatric human dose has not been established, but the drug has a wide margin of safety.

BAQUILOPRIM-SULFONAMIDE

CLASS. Sulfonamide and diaminopyridine in 1:5 ratio.

ACTION. Bactericidal, antibacterial, also antiprotozoal; folic acid synthesis inhibitors affecting two steps.

MORE INFORMATION. See TRIMETHOPRIM-SULFONAMIDE, ORMETOPRIM-SULFONAMIDE and Chapter 34.

PHARMACOKINETICS. Similar to trimethoprim-sulfonamide but longer half-life in dogs (15 hr baquiloprim; 13.2 hr sulfadimethoxine). Rapid and complete absorption; maintains antibacterial inhibitory effectiveness in plasma for up to 48 hr after a single dose. Both drugs are metabolized by the liver and are excreted in bile. Dogs do not acetylate sulfonamides, which reduces their nephrotoxicity. Unchanged drug is also excreted in the urine.

SPECTRUM. See ORMETOPRIM-SULFONAMIDE, TRIMETHOPRIM-SULFONAMIDE. **Aerobes:** Synergistic against *Staphylococcus intermedius, Streptococcus canis, E. coli,* and *Proteus mirabilis.* **Anaerobes:** in vitro, but not in vivo; therefore, not recommended for anaerobic infections. **Others:** *Coccidia.* **Ineffective:** anaerobic infections.

INDICATIONS. For coccidiosis, canine pyoderma and urinary tract infections.

CONTRAINDICATIONS. Not for use in dogs with sulfonamide hypersensitivity, hepatic dysfunction, blood dyscrasias, or pregnancy. Not for use in cats.

ADVERSE REACTIONS. Similar to TRIMETHOPRIM-SULFONAMIDE.

INTERACTIONS. See TRIMETHOPRIM-SULFONAMIDE.

Availability	Type	Sizes	Preparations (Company)
Human	Oral tablets*	600 mg (100 mg baquiloprim and 500 mg sulphamethoxine or sulphadimidine)	*Dazokan* (Merial)
		60 mg (10 mg baquiloprim and 50 mg sulphamethoxine or sulphadimidine)	*Zaquilan C* (Schering-Plough Animal Health)

*Not available in the USA.

HANDLING. Store in airtight, light-proof containers at room temperature.

ADMINISTRATION. Can be given with food. Supply plenty of water at all times.

DOSAGE

Indications (Dogs)	Dose (mg/kg)	Route	Interval (hr)	Duration (days)
Coccidiosis	30	PO	48	4
Urinary infections	30	PO	48	10
Pyoderma	30	PO	48	21*

*Give drug every 24 hr for the first 2 days.

DISPENSING INFORMATION. This drug can be given with food. Make sure the animal has unlimited access to drinking water while on this medication.

CARBENICILLIN

CLASS. Carboxypenicillin.

ACTION. Bactericidal; inhibits bacterial cell wall synthesis.

MORE INFORMATION. See Penicillins, Chapter 34; Table 34–1.

PHARMACOKINETICS. Carbenicillin is destroyed by gastric acid, resulting in poor GI absorption. Indanyl carbenicillin is more stable, being partially (30%–50%) absorbed. When given parenterally, enters many tissues and body fluids in therapeutic concentration but only in the CSF with meningeal inflammation. Primarily (80%) renal excretion of unchanged drug. Low biliary excretion. Difficult to achieve sufficient blood concentration when given PO so reserved for treatment of urinary tract infection. Carindacillin, the indanyl ester, is better absorbed from the GI tract and is hydrolyzed to the active drug after absorption. Its use is limited to treatment of urinary tract infections caused by *Pseudomonas* and other susceptible gram-negative organisms.

SPECTRUM. Gram positive: *Staphylococcus.* **Gram negative:** *Escherichia, Proteus, Salmonella, Enterobacter, Citrobacter, Pseudomonas, Serratia.* **Anaerobes:** *Clostridium, Peptococcus, Peptostreptococcus, Bacteroides, Fusobacterium.*

INDICATIONS. Parenteral formulation for treating systemic infections. Acute and chronic upper and lower urinary tract infection, including prostatitis and cystitis. Oral use should be restricted in treating urinary infections caused by gram-negative bacteria or *Pseudomonas* strains resistant to other drugs, but high dosages are needed for effective therapy. Ticarcillin or piperacillin are sometimes preferred over this drug.

CONTRAINDICATIONS. Dosage reduction in renal failure.

ADVERSE REACTIONS. Gastrointestinal side effects. Occasional hypersensitivity reactions, reversible neutropenia, occasional eosinophilia, hypokalemia. Neurotoxicity at high doses, with impaired renal excretion. In people, platelet malfunction can result in prolonged bleeding times.

INTERACTIONS. Inactivates aminoglycosides in vitro. Can be given with aminoglycosides by alternative route to enhance activity against *Pseudomonas.*

Availability	Type	Sizes	Preparations (Company)
Human	Film-coated oral tablets (indanyl sodium)	500 mg total containing 382 mg carbenicillin	*Geocillin* (Roerig)
	Parenteral powder (sodium)*	1-g, 2-g, 5-g, 10-g vials	*Geopen* (Roerig), *Pyopen* (SmithKline Beecham)

*No longer available in USA

INTERNATIONAL PREPARATIONS. *Carbapen, Carindapen.*

HANDLING. Oral tablets should be stored in dry, airtight containers at room temperature and are stable indefinitely. A suspension can be prepared by crushing six, 382-mg tablets and adding sufficient water to bring the volume to 60 ml. Shaken and refrigerated, the 38.2 mg/ml solution is stable for 3 days. Because of the bitter taste, the solution or crushed tablets can be added to a syrup before administration. The powder for parenteral injection is stored at room temperature and once reconstituted is stable for 24 hr at room temperature, 72 hr if refrigerated and 1 mo if frozen. With IV solution, up to 15% of solution activity is reduced in 4 hr at 25°F and NaCl but up to 8 hr in dextrose solutions. IV solution is incompatible with amphotericin B, chloramphenicol, gentamicin, kanamycin, carbenicillin, oxytetracycline.

ADMINISTRATION. Parenteral solution can be given IM and can be reconstituted with lidocaine (0.5% without epinephrine) or IV as a slow infusion. Minimum dilution is 1 g/7 ml given over a minimum of 15 min.

DOSAGE

Indications (Dogs and Cats)	Dose (mg/kg)	Route	Interval (hr)	Duration (days)
Urinary	22–33	PO	8	7–10
Systemic infections	22–33	IV	6–8	prn

ADDITIONAL DOSAGES. Gram-negative bacteria, Table 37–2; bacteremia and endocarditis, Table 87–7; respiratory disease, Table 88–8.

CEFACLOR

CLASS. Second-generation cephalosporin.

ACTION. Bactericidal; inhibits bacterial cell wall synthesis.

MORE INFORMATION. See Cephalosporins, Chapter 34; Table 34–4.

PHARMACOKINETICS. Well absorbed after oral administration to fasting animals, but absorption is delayed with feeding. The majority of drug is excreted in the urine unchanged.

SPECTRUM. Gram positive: *Staphylococcus, Streptococcus.* **Gram negative:** *Escherichia, Salmonella, Klebsiella, Proteus mirabilis.* **Anaerobes:** gram negatives, including *Bacteroides.* **Ineffective:** *Pseudomonas, Acinetobacter, Enterococcus, Serratia,* other *Proteus.*

INDICATIONS. Otitis media, sinusitis caused by β-lactamase–resistant organisms, lower respiratory tract infections, pyoderma, urinary infections. More active than first-generation drugs against gram-negative bacteria.

CONTRAINDICATIONS. Known cephalosporin or penicillin hypersensitivity. Reduce dosages in renal failure.

ADVERSE REACTIONS. Systemic allergy, previous hypersensitivity, vomiting, diarrhea, increased liver enzymes, mild eosinophilia.

INTERACTIONS. Potentiates anticoagulant rodenticides.

Availability	Type	Sizes	Preparations (Company)
Human	Oral capsules	250 mg, 500 mg	*Ceclor* (Eli Lilly), generic (various)
	Powder for oral suspension	125 or 325 mg/5 ml	*Ceclor;* generic

INTERNATIONAL PREPARATIONS. *Alfatil, Cefabiocin, Cef-Diolan, Distaclor, Kefolor, Pancef.*

HANDLING. Refrigerate suspension after reconstituting; stable for 2 weeks. No definitive data exist for freezing and thawing of oral suspension, but it is thought to be unstable after a similar time period after thawing. Store capsules at controlled room temperature (15–30°C).

ADMINISTRATION. Administer to fasting animal because food in stomach interferes with absorption. Maximum daily dose is 1 g. Twice-daily dosing has not been as effective as three-times daily dosing in human clinical studies.

DOSAGE

Indications (Dogs and Cats)	Dose (mg/kg)	Route	Interval (hr)	Duration (days)
Skin, soft tissue infections	7	PO	8	21–30
Systemic, lower respiratory tract infections	10–13	PO	8	14

DISPENSING INFORMATION. Store liquid in refrigerator and shake well before using. Discard unused portions after 2 weeks. Give at least 1 hr before or 2 hr after meals.

CEFADROXIL

CLASS. First-generation cephalosporin (longer acting derivative of cephalexin).

ACTION. Bactericidal; inhibits bacterial cell wall synthesis.

MORE INFORMATION. See Cephalosporins, Chapter 34; Tables 34–3 and 34–4.

PHARMACOKINETICS. Rapidly absorbed after oral administration even in presence of food. Stable in the presence of gastric acid. More than 90% excreted unchanged in the urine within 24 hr. Slower absorption and longer excretion period than cephalexin or cephradine, allowing for 12-hr dosing and higher serum levels.

SPECTRUM. Gram positive: β-hemolytic *Streptococcus, Staphylococcus,* and others. **Gram negative:** *Escherichia, Proteus mirabilis, Klebsiella, Pasteurella.* **Anaerobes:** poor activity. **Ineffective:** most *Enterococcus, Enterobacter,* other *Proteus, Acinetobacter.*

INDICATIONS. Urinary tract infections caused by susceptible gram-negative bacteria. Skin (pyoderma), respiratory, orthopedic, or systemic infections caused by *Staphylococcus* or *Streptococcus.* Good absorption and decreased frequency of administration are advantages over other first-generation cephalosporins.

CONTRAINDICATIONS. Known cephalosporin or penicillin hypersensitivity; reduce dose in renal failure.

ADVERSE REACTIONS. Vomiting, diarrhea, depression, anorexia, polydipsia, polyuria, salivation (34:85). Hypersensitivity reactions. No teratogenic or infertility problems have been seen in laboratory animals receiving high doses.

INTERACTIONS. False-positive Coombs' test results in people. False-positive urine glucose with copper reduction (Clinitest) methods.

Availability	Type	Sizes	Preparations (Company)
Human	Oral suspension (monohydrate)	125 mg, 250 mg, 500 mg/5 ml	*Duricef* (Mead-Johnson), *Ultracef* (Bristol), generics (various)
	Capsules (monohydrate)	50 mg, 100 mg, 200 mg, 500 mg	*Duricef, Utracef,* generics
	Tablets	1 g	*Duricef,* generics
Veterinary	Oral tablets	50 mg, 100 mg, 200 mg, 1 g	*Cefa-tabs* (Fort Dodge, Willows Francis Vet), *Cefa-cure* (Mycofarm)
	Oral liquid	50 mg/ml in 15-ml and 50-ml dropper bottles	*Cefa-drops* (Fort Dodge)

INTERNATIONAL PREPARATIONS. *Bidocef, Cefadril, Ceoxil, Cephos, Crenodyn, Duracef, Kefroxil, Moxacef, Oracéfal, Sedral.*

HANDLING. Shake suspension before use; keep container tightly closed in refrigerator; discard unused portion after 14 days. Store tablets in airtight, moisture-proof containers at room temperature.

ADMINISTRATION. Food does not reduce or delay absorption. Liquid has orange-pineapple flavor.

DOSAGE

Indications (Dogs and Cats)	Dose (mg/kg)	Route	Interval (hr)	Duration (days)
Urinary tract infections				
Cat	22	PO	24	≤21
Dog	11–22	PO	12	7–30
Skin, pyoderma	22–35	PO	12	3–30
Systemic, orthopedic infections	22	PO	8–12	30

ADDITIONAL DOSAGES. Canine pyoderma, Table 85–3.

DISPENSING INFORMATION. Can be given without regard to meals. Giving with food may help reduce gastrointestinal side effects.

CEFAZOLIN

CLASS. First-generation cephalosporin.

ACTION. Bactericidal; inhibits bacterial cell wall synthesis.

MORE INFORMATION. See Cephalosporins, Chapter 34; Table 34–4; references: 34:95, 34:132.

PHARMACOKINETICS. Not absorbed from GI tract. Given parenterally, it enters many tissues and body fluids. Primarily excreted by kidneys unchanged in urine. Some is excreted in bile to achieve therapeutic concentrations. Longer half-life and ability to reach higher tissue concentrations gives advantage for surgical prophylaxis over cephalothin and cephapirin in which aerobic infections are anticipated. Good levels achieved in bone, especially with inflammation. Does not penetrate CSF, even with inflamed meninges.

SPECTRUM. **Gram positive:** *Staphylococcus*, β-hemolytic *Streptococcus*. **Gram negative:** some *Enterobacter, Escherichia, Klebsiella, Proteus mirabilis*. **Anaerobes:** poor activity. **Ineffective:** *Proteus vulgaris, Enterobacter cloacae, Serratia, Pseudomonas*.

INDICATIONS. Surgical prophylaxis, for prolonged orthopedic procedures, for reducing postoperative infections of surgical wounds and intra-abdominal or biliary surgery. Greatest activity against *Escherichia* and *Klebsiella* compared with others in its class. Respiratory, genitourinary, biliary tract, bone, and joint infections, sepsis.

CONTRAINDICATIONS. Previous penicillin or cephalosporin hypersensitivity. Reduce dose in renal failure.

ADVERSE REACTIONS. Few; hypersensitivity to cephalosporins, diarrhea, neutropenia, leukopenia, eosinophilia, thrombocytopenia, increased liver enzymes, phlebitis with IV, pain on IM injection.

INTERACTIONS. False-positive urine glucose measurements with nonenzymatic methods.

Availability	Type	Sizes	Preparations (Company)
Human	Powder for injection	500 mg, 1 g, 5 g, 10 g, 20 g	*Ancef* (SmithKline Beecham), *Kefzol* (Eli Lilly)

HANDLING. Reconstitute in sterile water for IV; can also use 0.9% NaCl for IM; however, not advised because crystals may form in NaCl solution. Stable for 24 hr at room temperature and 96 hr when refrigerated; up to 12 weeks if frozen. Can be mixed with 5% dextrose, lactated Ringer's, 0.9% NaCl for infusion. Avoid admixture with many other drugs, including aminoglycosides, tetracyclines, macrolides, barbiturates. Powder has been mixed in acrylic bone cement for prophylaxis with surgical implants.

ADMINISTRATION. Inject IM in large muscle mass. Inject IV slowly into vein or through IV tubing access over 3–5 min. For surgical prophylaxis, give IV dose once immediately before surgical incision and repeat SC 6 hr later (34:132).

DOSAGE

Indications	Dose (mg/kg)	Route	Interval (hr)	Duration (days)
Dogs				
Surgical prophylaxis	8	IV	1	*
	20–22	IV	2	*
Systemic infections	5–25	IM, IV	6–8	prn
Orthopedic infections	22	IV, IM, SC	6–8	≤7
Sepsis, bacteremic	15–25	IV, IM, SC	4–8	≤7
Cats				
Systemic infections	33	IM, IV	8–12	prn

*Just before and during surgery.

ADDITIONAL DOSAGES. Parvoviral enteritis, Table 8–1; endotoxemia, Table 38–1; musculoskeletal infections, Table 86–3; bacteremia and endocarditis, Table 87–7; respiratory infections, Table 88–8; topical intraocular use, Table 93–4.

CEFEPIME

CLASS. Fourth-generation cephalosporin.

ACTION. Bactericidal; has enhanced ability to penetrate outer cell membrane of gram-negative bacteria. Has better gram-positive coverage than third-generation cephalosporins.

MORE INFORMATION. See Cephalosphorins, Chapter 34; Table 34–4.

PHARMACOKINETICS. Higher blood levels after IV than IM use. Penetrates blood-CSF barrier. Renal excretion with minimal metabolism.

SPECTRUM. **Gram positive:** many, including *Staphylococcus.* **Gram negative:** many Enterobacteriaceae. **Anaerobes:** variable activity. **Others:** *M. avium-intracellulare* complex. **Most effective:** resistant gram-negative bacteria. Similar to third-generation drugs; however, good antipseudomonal activity similar to ceftazidine. Good β-lactamase stability and good gram-positive activity. Has activity against some Enterobacteriaceae that are resistant to cefotaxime and ceftazidine. **Ineffective:** not active against methicillin-resistant strains of *Staphylococcus, Enterobacter, Clostridium, Bacteroides.*

INDICATIONS. Severe infections of lower respiratory, urinary, and female reproductive tracts; skin and soft tissue infections; pneumonia; meningitis.

APPROVED USES. Gram-negative pneumonia.

CONTRAINDICATIONS. Reduced dosage in renal failure. Previous hypersensitivity to cephalosporins.

ADVERSE REACTIONS. Eosinophilia, leukopenia, phlebitis, increased serum hepatic enzyme activities, gastrointestinal signs.

INTERACTIONS. In vitro synergy with quinolones, aminoglycosides, β-lactamase inhibitors. Antagonistic activity with imipenem or polymyxin B. Combine with metronidazole or clindamycin in intra-abdominal infections. Should closely monitor renal function in animals receiving cefepime with aminoglycosides.

Availability	Type	Sizes	Preparation (Company)
Human	Powder for injection (as hydrochloride)	500 mg, 1 g, 2 g	*Maxipime* (Bristol-Myers Squibb)

INTERNATIONAL PREPARATIONS. *Axépim.*

HANDLING. Reconstitute powder with 0.9% NaCl, 5% dextrose, 0.5%–1% lidocaine, or bacteriostatic water.

ADMINISTRATION. IV; give slowly over 30 min. Can add to 0.9% NaCl, 5% dextrose, and lactated Ringer's.

DOSAGE

Indications	Dose	Route	Interval (hr)	Duration (days)
Dogs and Cats*	50 mg/kg	IV, IM	8	prn

*Extrapolated human dose.

DISPENSING INFORMATION. Diarrhea may develop during use of this drug.

CEFIXIME

CLASS. Third-generation cephalosporin.

ACTION. Bactericidal; inhibits bacterial cell wall synthesis. Very stable to β-lactamase.

MORE INFORMATION. See CEFPODOXIME; references: 34:8, 34:87.

PHARMACOKINETICS. First third-generation *oral* cephalosporin—rapid oral absorption in absence of food; bioavailability is 40%–55%; suspension achieves higher blood concentrations than tablet; high serum protein binding; lower concentrations in tissues (uterus, ovaries) and fat; tissue concentration may increase with repeated dosing; very high levels in urinary tract. Eliminated in urine by glomerular filtration but reabsorbed by tubules to prolong activity (34:8).

SPECTRUM. **Gram positive:** *Streptococcus, Rhodococcus.* **Gram negative:** *Escherichia, Proteus, Klebsiella.* **Anaerobes:** minimal activity (unlike other third-generation drugs). **Ineffective:** *Pseudomonas, Enterococcus, Staphylococcus, Actinomyces, Bordetella, Listeria, Enterobacter, Clostridium, Bacteroides.*

INDICATIONS. Urinary and upper respiratory tract infections caused by susceptible organisms. One of few orally administered third-generation cephalosporins.

CONTRAINDICATIONS. Reduce dosage in renal failure.

ADVERSE REACTIONS. GI disturbances, abdominal pain, vomiting, dermal hypersensitivity (fever, urticaria, pruritus).

INTERACTIONS. False-positive results with nonenzymatic test results for urine glucose. False-positive urine ketone test results using nitroprusside.

Availability	Type	Sizes	Preparations (Company)
Human	Oral tablets (film coated as trihydrate)	200 mg, 400 mg	*Supran* (Teva Pharm), *Suprax* (Lederle)
	Oral suspension (strawberry flavor)	100 mg/5 ml	*Suprax*

INTERNATIONAL PREPARATIONS. *Aerocef, Cefspan, Cephoral, Denvar, Fixim, Necopen, Oroken, Tricef, Unixime.*

HANDLING. Store capsules in airtight containers at room temperature.

ADMINISTRATION. Possibly give once daily in urinary infections as a result of long half-life.

DOSAGE

Indications (Dogs)	Dose (mg/kg)	Route	Interval (hr)	Duration (days)
Urinary infections	5.0	PO	12–24	7–14*
Respiratory, systemic infections	12.5	PO	12	7–14*

*Duration may vary according to chronicity of infection.

DISPENSING INFORMATION. Give on an empty stomach.

CEFMETAZOLE SODIUM

CLASS. Cephamycin derivative.

ACTION. Bactericidal effect on cell wall synthesis; highly β-lactamase resistant.

MORE INFORMATION. See Cephalosporins, Chapter 34.

PHARMACOKINETICS. High binding to serum proteins after IV infusion. Approximately 85% excreted unchanged in the urine over 12 hr.

SPECTRUM. **Gram positive:** *Staphylococcus, Streptococcus.* **Gram negative:** *Escherichia, Klebsiella, Proteus.* **Anaerobes:** *Bacteroides, Fusobacterium, Clostridium.* **Ineffective:** *Enterococcus, Pseudomonas, Enterobacter.*

INDICATIONS. Recurrent or complicated urinary infections caused by *Escherichia;* serious intra-abdominal, lower respiratory, and cutaneous infections. Prophylaxis for intra-abdominal and pelvic surgery.

APPROVED USES. Human.

CONTRAINDICATIONS. Excretion is delayed, and dosage must be reduced in renal failure.

ADVERSE REACTIONS. Local: thrombophlebitis. Systemic: diarrhea, vomiting, occasional agranulocytosis, pancytopenia.

INTERACTIONS. May accentuate effects of anticoagulant rodenticides.

Availability	Type	Sizes	Preparation (Company)
Human	Sterile powder for reconstitution	1-g, 2-g vials	*Zefazone* (Pharmacia & Upjohn)

INTERNATIONAL PREPARATIONS. *Cefmetazon, Cemetol, Decacef, Metacaf, Metazol.*

HANDLING. Reconstitute with sterile water for injection or 0.9% NaCl to give 100–250 mg/ml. When reconstituted, maintains potency for 24 hr at room temperature, for 7 days when refrigerated, and for 6 weeks frozen (at or below −20°C). Thawed drug is stable for 24 hr but should not be refrozen. Can be further diluted to 1.0–20 mg/ml in 0.9% NaCl, 5% dextrose, or lactated Ringer's and stored for similar periods.

ADMINISTRATION. In people, given IV over 10–60 min as an infusion, or for presurgical prophylaxis as a bolus infusion of a maximum of 1–2 g over 3–5 min. As with most β-lactams, should not mix with aminoglycoside solutions. For surgical prophylaxis, give dose 30–90 min before surgery and repeat if procedure lasts longer than 4 hr.

DOSAGE

Indications	Dose (mg/kg)	Route	Interval (hr)	Duration (days)
Dogs				
Surgical prophylaxis	20	IV	*	*
Urinary infections	20	IV	12	7–14
Soft tissue infections	20	IV	8	7–14
Bacteremia	20	IV	6	prn

*Infused just before and during surgery; see Administration.

CEFOPERAZONE SODIUM

CLASS. Third-generation cephalosporin.

ACTION. Bactericidal; inhibits bacterial cell wall synthesis.

MORE INFORMATION. See Cephalosporins, Chapter 34; Table 34–4.

PHARMACOKINETICS. Longer half-life than others in its class permitting 12-hr dose interval. Not absorbed from the GI tract. After parenteral injection, distributed widely in tissues and body fluids. Erratic penetration of the CNS and CSF, better if meningitis present. Primarily (70%) excreted in bile; remainder unchanged in urine.

SPECTRUM. **Gram positive:** *Staphylococcus* spp, *Streptococcus,* but less active against these than other cephalosporins. **Gram negative:** *Escherichia, Klebsiella, Enterobacter, Proteus, Serratia, Pseudomonas.* Second most active cephalosporin against *Pseudomonas.* **Anaerobes:** *Peptococcus, Peptostreptococcus, Clostridium, Bacteroides.*

INDICATIONS. Severe infections, resistant to other drugs, in the lower respiratory tract, peritoneal cavity, skin, genital and urinary tracts, and septicemia. *Pseudomonas* infections.

CONTRAINDICATIONS. Avoid or reduce dosage with hepatic failure or biliary obstruction. Normal dosage in renal failure.

ADVERSE REACTIONS. Local or systemic hypersensitivity; vitamin K deficiency and hemorrhage or neutropenia with prolonged administration; transient diarrhea; azotemia or serum hepatic enzyme increases.

INTERACTIONS. Do not mix directly with an aminoglycoside, and if both are given through the same IV set, use this drug first and flush in between.

Availability	Type	Sizes	Preparation (Company)
Human	Sterile crystalline powder for injection or premixed iso-osmotic solution	1-g, 2-g vials	*Cefobid* (Pfizer, Roerig)

INTERNATIONAL PREPARATIONS. *Bioperazone, Cefazone, Céfobis, Cefogram, Cefoneg, Dardum, Ipazone, Mediper, Perocef, Zoncef.*

HANDLING. Protect sterile powder from light before reconstitution. Reconstitute with 5% dextrose or lactated Ringer's. Can dilute with epinephrine-free lidocaine for IM use. Stable for 24 hr at room temperature, 5 days if refrigerated, or 3–5 weeks when frozen. IM or IV solution is stable for 48 hr at room temperature and 5 days in refrigeration (5°C) and 3 weeks if frozen (−20°C). Do not refreeze once thawed.

ADMINISTRATION. Intermittent infusions should be given over 15–30 min. Continuous infusions should be given at a concentration of 2–25 mg/ml.

DOSAGE

Indications (Dogs)	Dose (mg/kg)	Route	Interval (hr)	Duration (days)
Soft tissue infections	22*	IV, IM	12	7–14
Bacteremia, sepsis	22*	IV, IM	6–8	prn

*Human dose extrapolation.

CEFOTAXIME SODIUM

CLASS. Third-generation cephalosporin.

ACTION. Bactericidal; inhibits bacterial cell wall synthesis.

MORE INFORMATION. See Chapter 34, Cephalosporins; Table 34–4.

PHARMACOKINETICS. Not absorbed from GI tract. Well absorbed after IM administration. When given parenterally, attains therapeutic concentration in many tissues, including prostate, bone, and both pleural and peritoneal fluids. Enters the aqueous humor and CSF. Metabolized by hepatic esterases to a biologically active form, desacetylcefotaxime, which prolongs the drug's clinical effect. Attains therapeutic levels in meninges with or without inflammation. Primarily renal excretion.

SPECTRUM. Gram positive: *Streptococcus* and *Staphylococcus* (with and without β-lactamase). More active than other third-generation drugs. **Gram negative:** most Enterobacteriaceae: *Acinetobacter, Citrobacter, Escherichia, Klebsiella, Proteus, Serratia,* some *Pseudomonas.* Synergistic with aminoglycosides. **Anaerobes:** variable activity against *Bacteroides, Clostridium, Fusobacterium, Peptococcus, Peptostreptococcus.* **Others:** *Borrelia.* **More effective:** most active third-generation drug against *Staphylococcus, Leptospira.* **Ineffective:** *Listeria.*

INDICATIONS. Initial empiric therapy in bacterial sepsis. Also good for problematic or recurrent lower respiratory tract, genitourinary, soft tissue, skin, and intra-abdominal infections, bone and joint and CNS infections, and surgical prophylaxis. Inconsistent against *Pseudomonas.*

CONTRAINDICATIONS. Reduce dose in renal failure.

ADVERSE REACTIONS. Local irritation, systemic hypersensitivity, GI signs. Altered bowel flora with diarrhea. Occasional granulocytopenia, increased nephrotoxicity when combined with aminoglycosides or other cephalosporins. Cardiac arrhythmias if infused too rapidly IV.

INTERACTIONS. Possibly synergistic with aminoglycosides but should not be mixed together for simultaneous administration.

Availability	Type	Sizes	Preparations (Company)
Human	Powder for injection	1 g, 2 g	*Claforan* (Hoechst-Roussel)
	Frozen, premixed in 5% dextrose in plastic containers	1 g, 2 g	*Claforan*

INTERNATIONAL PREPARATIONS. *Cefacron, Zariviz.*

HANDLING. Store powder at room temperature, reconstitute with sterile water. Stable for 24 hr at room temperature, 10 days when refrigerated, and 13 weeks if frozen. When mixed with IV fluids, only stable for 5 days if refrigerated. Unstable in alkaline solutions. Stable in 0.9 NaCl, 5% dextrose, lactated Ringer's. Powder and solutions darken with storage without affecting activity.

ADMINISTRATION. IV or IM, dosing interval shortens with increasing severity of infection. Never mix directly with aminoglycosides; can combine as separate infusions. Solution of 1 g Claforan in 14 ml of sterile water is isotonic. For IM give deep into large muscle and aspirate before injection. Use multiple sites with dose greater than 1 g. For IV infusion, 1 or 2 g may be reconstituted in 50 or 100 ml of 0.9% saline or 5% dextrose and be given over 30 min. IV preferred for septicemia, peritonitis, meningitis, or immunocompromised animals. Administer IV, 1 or 2 g in 10 ml sterile water over 3–5 min but not concurrently with other solutions. For surgical prophylaxis, give dose 30–90 min before operative incision. Maximum dose: 1 g medium-size dogs, 2 g for large dogs.

DOSAGE

Indications	Dose (mg/kg)	Route	Interval (hr)	Duration (days)
Dogs				
Soft tissue infections	22	IV, IM, SC	8	≤7
	50	IV, IM	12	≤7
Orthopedic infections	20–40	IV, IM, SC	6–8	≤7
Severe bacteremia	20–80	IV	6	prn
	10–50	IV	4–6	prn
Cats				
Severe bacteremia	20–80	IV, IM	6	prn

ADDITIONAL DOSAGES. Gram-negative infections, Table 37–2; Lyme borreliosis, Table 45–3; nocardiosis, Table 49–2; bacteremia and endocarditis, Table 87–7; respiratory infections, Table 88–8; intra-abdominal infections, Table 89–15; CNS infections, Table 92–5.

CEFOTETAN DISODIUM

CLASS. Cephamycin like CEFOXITIN, with similar properties to second-generation cephalosporin.

ACTION. Bactericidal; inhibits bacterial cell wall synthesis inhibitor.

MORE INFORMATION. See CEFOXITIN; Chapter 34; Table 34–4; reference: 34:122.

SPECTRUM. See CEFOXITIN.

INDICATIONS. Cost-effective replacement for cefoxitin. See CEFOXITIN.

CONTRAINDICATIONS. See CEFOXITIN; prior penicillin or cephalosporin hypersensitivity. Reduce dose in renal failure.

ADVERSE REACTIONS. Vomiting after IV bolus infusion. Cutaneous eruptions, angioedema. Coagulation disturbances with vitamin K antagonism. Neutropenia, anemia, eosinophilia.

INTERACTIONS. Potentiate aminoglycoside nephrotoxicity. Unpredictable synergism with penicillins.

Availability	Type	Sizes	Preparation (Company)
Human	Powder for injection	1 g, 2 g	*Cefotan* (Stuart Pharmaceuticals)

INTERNATIONAL PREPARATIONS. *Apacef, Apatef, Ceftenon, Cepan, Darvilen, Yamatetan.*

HANDLING. Reconstitute with sterile water; for IM use can add lidocaine. For IV infusion, can add to 5% dextrose or 0.9% NaCl. Stable for 24 hr at room temperature, 96 hr if refrigerated, and at least 1 week if frozen. In dextrose 10% or Ringer's, with cefotetan 0.5 to 30 mg/ml, can freeze at −20°C for 30 weeks and thaw in microwave oven before use. Do not mix in solutions containing aminoglycosides.

ADMINISTRATION. IV route preferred for bacteremia or severe infections. Bolus administration via IV catheter over 3–5 min. Flush catheter with heparinized saline (10 U/ml) after injection. Do not coadminister with other drugs. For surgical prophylaxis, begin infusion of 1 g 30 to 60 min before surgery.

DOSAGE

Indications (Dogs)	Dose (mg/kg)	Route	Interval (hr)	Duration (days)
Soft tissue infections	30	SC	12	≤7
Bacteremia, sepsis	30	IV, SC	8	prn

ADDITIONAL DOSAGES. Musculoskeletal infections, Table 86–3; respiratory infections, Table 88–8.

CEFOXITIN

CLASS. Cephamycin, like CEFOTETAN, with similar properties to second-generation cephalosporins.

ACTION. Bactericidal; bacterial cell wall synthesis inhibitor.

MORE INFORMATION. See CEFOTETAN; Chapter 34, cephalosporins, Table 34–4; surgical infections, Table 55–4; reference: 34:122.

PHARMACOKINETICS. Not absorbed from the GI tract. Must use parenteral administration. Reaches therapeutic concentrations in many tissues, including kidney and lung. Little penetration of CSF, even with inflamed meninges. Primarily excreted unchanged in the urine.

SPECTRUM. Gram positive: *Staphylococcus,* hemolytic *Streptococcus.* **Gram negative:** *Escherichia, Klebsiella, Proteus.* **Anaerobes:** *Bacteroides, Clostridium, Peptococcus, Peptostreptococcus.* **Ineffective:** *Salmonella, Pseudomonas, Enterococcus.* Has a similar spectrum to cefotetan.

INDICATIONS. Gram-negative sepsis, gingivitis, pyothorax, polymicrobial infections with renal impairment, surgical prophylaxis, intra-abdominal bowel rupture, osteomyelitis. Especially effective for surgical prophylaxis when anaerobic infections (e.g., *Bacteroides fragilis*) are expected (colon surgery).

CONTRAINDICATIONS. Reduce dosage in renal failure.

ADVERSE REACTIONS. Local tissue irritation when given IM or SC. Vomiting after IV bolus injection, cutaneous eruptions, angioedema. Can cause hemolytic anemia, thrombocytopenia, granulocytopenia, increased hepatic enzymes, azotemia.

INTERACTIONS. Increased nephrotoxicity has been observed when combined therapy with aminoglycosides has been used.

Availability	Type	Sizes	Preparation (Company)
Human	Powder for injection	1-g, 2-g vials	*Mefoxin* (Merck)

INTERNATIONAL PREPARATIONS. *Betacef, Cefaxicina, Cefociclin, Mefoxitin, Stovaren, Tifox.*

HANDLING. Store powder at room temperature. IV, reconstitute with 9.7 ml bacteriostatic water to 100 mg/ml solution; stable for 24 hr at room temperature, 1 week if refrigerated, 30 weeks when frozen. Times vary with other diluents. Powder and solutions darken with storage, but this does not affect potency. SC and IM, can dilute in 0.5% lidocaine (without epinephrine) to minimize irritation after injection.

ADMINISTRATION. Bolus administration via IV catheter over 3–5 min. Flush catheter with heparinized saline (10 U/ml) after injection.

DOSAGE

Indications	Dose (mg/kg)	Route	Interval (hr)	Duration (days)
Dogs				
Soft tissue infections	30	SC	8	prn*
	30	IV	5	prn*
Bacteremia	15–30	IV, IM, SC	6–8	prn*
Orthopedic infections	22	IV, IM	6–8	prn*
Cats				
Systemic infection	25–30	IV, IM	8	prn*

*Use to control initial infection, then switch to orally administered drugs for longer therapy.

ADDITIONAL DOSAGES. Anaerobic infections, Table 41–10; musculoskeletal infections, Table 86–3; bacteremia and endocarditis, Table 87–7; respiratory infections, Table 88–8.

CEFPODOXIME PROXETIL

CLASS. Third-generation cephalosporin.

ACTION. Bactericidal; inhibits bacterial cell wall synthesis.

MORE INFORMATION. See CEFIXIME; Chapter 34, cephalosporins; Table 34–4.

PHARMACOKINETICS. One of few oral drugs of its class. The oral form is given as the proxetil ester, which is hydrolyzed by the intestinal epithelium to active drug at the time of absorption. Excreted primarily unchanged in urine.

SPECTRUM. Gram positive: *Streptococcus, Staphylococcus.* **Gram negative:** *Escherichia, Klebsiella, Proteus.*

INDICATIONS. Upper respiratory and urinary tract infections, pyoderma, otitis media not responding to other drugs.

CONTRAINDICATIONS. Reduce dose in renal failure; no adjustment needed with hepatic dysfunction.

ADVERSE REACTIONS. Diarrhea, vomiting, eosinophilia, allergic reactions.

INTERACTIONS. Drugs that increase gastric pH interfere with absorption.

Availability	Type	Sizes	Preparations (Company)
Human	Oral tablets	100 mg, 200 mg	*Vantin* (Pharmacia & Upjohn)
	Granules for oral suspension; lemon cream flavored	500 mg/5 ml, 100 mg/5 ml	*Vantin*

INTERNATIONAL PREPARATIONS. *Banan, Biocef, Céfodox, Orelox, Ortreton, Podomexef.*

HANDLING. Store tablets in closed vials at controlled room temperature. Mix granules in distilled water, store in refrigerator for up to 2 weeks.

ADMINISTRATION. Food increases absorption.

DOSAGE

Indications (Dogs and Cats)	Dose (mg/kg)	Route	Interval (hr)	Duration (days)
Skin, soft tissue infections	10*	PO	24	8–10
	5*	PO	12	8–10

*Dose extrapolated from humans.

DISPENSING INFORMATION. Give drug with meals.

CEFTAZIDIME

CLASS. Third-generation cephalosporin.

ACTION. Bactericidal; inhibits bacterial cell wall synthesis.

MORE INFORMATION. See Chapter 34, cephalosporins, Table 34–4; CNS infections, Table 92–3.

PHARMACOKINETICS. Not absorbed PO; given parenterally. Highest levels in myocardium, bone, skeletal muscle. Good penetration into CSF and synovial, peritoneal, aqueous, lymphatic, and blister fluids. Primarily (80%–90%) excreted renally as unchanged drug.

SPECTRUM. Variable activity against gram-positive bacteria and anaerobes. See CEFTRIAXONE. **More effective:** most active cephalosporin against *Pseudomonas.*

INDICATIONS. Primarily for *Pseudomonas* sepsis; also gram-negative sepsis, meningitis, osteomyelitis, peritonitis, pneumonia. Used in immunosuppressed states (neutropenia) with fever of unknown origin and suspected bacteremia. May use with aminoglycosides or clindamycin for severe infections or when antimicrobial resistance is anticipated.

CONTRAINDICATIONS. Renal failure must reduce dosage. No adjustments for hepatic dysfunction.

ADVERSE REACTIONS. See CEFTRIAXONE.

INTERACTIONS. May increase risk of nephrotoxicity with coadministered aminoglycosides.

Availability	Type	Sizes	Preparations (Company)
Human	Powder for injection	500 mg, 1-g, 2-g vials	*Fortaz* (Glaxo Wellcome), *Tazicef* (SmithKline Beecham), *Tazidime* (Lilly)

INTERNATIONAL PREPARATIONS. *Ceftim, Ceptaz, Fortam, Fortum, Glazidim, Kefadim, Kefamin, Kefazim, Kefzim, Panzid, Potendal, Spectrum, Starcef.*

HANDLING. Reconstitute with sterile water, stable for 24 hr at room temperature and 7–10 days if refrigerated. Stable in 0.9% NaCl, Ringer's, or 5% dextrose. Less stable in bicarbonate. Not recommended to mix with aminoglycosides or metronidazole.

ADMINISTRATION. IV inject over 3–5 min. Administer separately from aminoglycosides. Can mix with 1% lidocaine (without epinephrine) for IM use.

DOSAGE

Indications	Dose (mg/kg)	Route	Interval (hr)	Duration (days)
Dogs				
Orthopedic infections	25	IV, IM	8–12	prn*
Soft tissue infections	30–50	IV, IM	8–12	prn*
Sepsis, bacteremia	15–30	IV, IM	6–8	prn*
Cats				
Systemic infections	25–30	IV, IM, intraosseous	8–12	prn*

*Use for initial control of infection, then switch to an orally administered drug with similar spectrum of activity.

ADDITIONAL DOSAGES. Gram-negative bacteria, Table 37–2.

CEFTIOFUR

CLASS. Third-generation cephalosporin.

ACTION. Bactericidal; inhibits bacterial cell wall synthesis.

MORE INFORMATION. See Chapter 34, Cephalosporins, Table 34–4; reference: 34:16.

PHARMACOKINETICS. Rapid blood levels after SC dose, approximately 50% of urinary excretion is metabolites (primarily desfuroylceftiofur) and 50% active drug. Half-life in dog is 6–7 hr.

SPECTRUM. Gram positive: some *Streptococcus, Staphylococcus.* **Gram negative:** *Escherichia, Proteus, Klebsiella, Salmonella, Pasteurella.* **Anaerobes:** some but inconsistent; in vitro effective against *Fusobacterium* but poor for *Bacteroides.* **Ineffective:** *Pseudomonas, Enterococcus, Bordetella.*

INDICATIONS. Urinary tract infections.

CONTRAINDICATIONS. Recommendations uncertain with previous hypersensitivity reaction, breeding, or pregnancy.

ADVERSE REACTIONS. Dose and duration related myelosuppression with anemia, leukopenia, and thrombocytopenia, especially at dosages of 6.6 mg/kg once daily.

INTERACTIONS. May expect synergistic antibacterial activity, but nephrotoxic potential is increased when used in combination with aminoglycosides.

Availability	Type	Sizes	Preparations (Company)
Veterinary			
Dogs, cattle	Sterile powder for injection	1-g and 4-g vials of 20 and 80 ml, respectively	*Naxcel* (Pharmacia & Upjohn)
Swine	Oil suspension as HCl	5 g	*Excenel* (Pharmacia & Upjohn)

HANDLING. Unreconstituted powder: stable if refrigerated for extended periods, avoid light. Reconstitute with sterile water for injection. Reconstituted solution: refrigerate for 7 days or room temperature for 12 hr; can be aliquoted in syringes and frozen (−20°C) for 8 weeks but thaw at room temperature (never warmer). Never use a single multidose vial more than 20 times.

ADMINISTRATION. Preferably, administer at least twice daily for other than urinary tract infections. At a single 2.2-mg/kg dose, plasma concentrations meet or exceed minimal inhibitory concentrations (MICs) for some organisms such as *Klebsiella, Proteus,* various *Streptococcus, Pseudomonas,* and *Escherichia* at 18 to 24 hr. With twice-daily dosing, MICs for *S. intermedius* might be adequate but insufficient for some *Streptococcus, Pseudomonas, Bordetella,* and *Klebsiella.* Higher than recommended dosages to affect these organisms may be myelotoxic.

DOSAGE

Indications (Dogs and Cats)	Dose (mg/kg)	Route	Interval (hr)	Duration (days)
Urinary infections	2.2	SC	24	5–14
Systemic, soft tissue infections	2.2	SC	12	5–14
	4.4	SC	24	5–14
Sepsis, bacteremia	4.4	SC	12	2–5

ADDITIONAL DOSAGES. Respiratory disease, Table 88–8.

DISPENSING INFORMATION. Return for recheck CBC count weekly.

CEFTIZOXIME

CLASS. Third-generation cephalosporin.

ACTION. Bactericidal; inhibits bacterial cell wall synthesis.

MORE INFORMATION. See Chapter 34, cephalosporins; CNS infections, Table 92–3.

PHARMACOKINETICS. Not absorbed by PO route. Penetrates many tissues and has therapeutic concentrations in virtually all body fluids. Penetrates meninges with and without inflammation. Not metabolized and primarily renal excretion of unchanged drug.

SPECTRUM. Similar to CEFOTAXIME. **Gram positive:** *Streptococcus, Staphylococcus* (methicillin susceptible). **Gram negative:** *Escherichia, Klebsiella, Proteus, Enterobacter;* low activity against *Pseudomonas.* **Anaerobes:** *Bacteroides.* **More effective:** most active cephalosporin against *Bacteroides.* **Ineffective:** *Enterococcus,* some *Pseudomonas.*

INDICATIONS. Primarily lower respiratory tract infections; urinary, intra-abdominal, skin, bone and joint infections; septicemia, meningitis.

CONTRAINDICATIONS. Allergies to this class. Reduce dose in renal failure.

ADVERSE REACTIONS. Hypersensitivities, local and systemic. Transient elevation in serum hepatic enzymes, anemia, leukopenia, thrombocytopenia.

INTERACTIONS. Although not reported, increased nephrotoxicity is expected with concurrent therapy with cephalosporins and aminoglycosides.

Availability	Type	Sizes	Preparations (Company)
Human	Powder or frozen solution for injection	1 g, 2 g	*Cefizox* (Fujisawa)

INTERNATIONAL PREPARATIONS. *Ceftix, Epocelin, Eposerin.*

HANDLING. Thaw plastic container at room temperature and squeeze bag to check for leaks. No additives should be introduced. After thawing, stable for 24 hr at room temperature or 10 days if refrigerated.

ADMINISTRATION. IM in a large muscle, 2-g doses should be divided at different sites. IV bolus infusion over 3–5 min or infusion in 50–100 ml of 0.9% NaCl, 5% or 10% dextrose, lactated Ringer's, or Ringer's. Stable for 24 hr at room temperature or 96 hr if refrigerated.

DOSAGE

Indications (Dogs)	Dose (mg/kg)	Route	Interval (hr)	Duration (days)
Urinary infections	50*	IV, IM	12	prn
Respiratory, systemic infections	25–50*	IV, IM	8	prn

*Extrapolated human dosage.

CEFTRIAXONE

CLASS. Third-generation cephalosporin.

ACTION. Bactericidal; inhibits bacterial cell wall synthesis.

MORE INFORMATION. See Chapter 34, cephalosporins, Table 34–4; CNS infections, Table 92–3.

PHARMACOKINETICS. Inactivated in stomach and must be given parenterally. Very soluble and can be given IV or IM. Highly protein bound. Achieves high levels in the CSF. Dual elimination, with 40% excreted in bile, 60% in urine. Longest half-life of third-generation drugs, making once-daily dosing possible.

SPECTRUM. **Gram positive:** some *Staphylococcus* (some β-lactamase–producing but not methicillin-resistant strains), some *Streptococcus*. **Gram negative:** *Enterobacter, Escherichia, Klebsiella, Proteus, Serratia, Citrobacter, Providencia, Shigella, Acinetobacter*, some *Salmonella* and *Pseudomonas*. **Anaerobes:** variable against *Bacteroides* and *Clostridium*. **Others:** *Borrelia*. **More effective:** *Borrelia*. **Ineffective:** *Enterococcus*.

INDICATIONS. Lower respiratory tract, skin and soft tissue, urinary tract, bone, joint, intra-abdominal, genital infections. It has been used to treat meningitis caused by susceptible strains (often gram negatives); gram-negative sepsis. Treatment of severe multisystemic gram-negative bacterial infections when toxicity of aminoglycosides or resistance to quinolones is of concern. Best option for treating systemic manifestations (meningitis, arthritis) of Lyme borreliosis. Used for surgical prophylaxis as a preoperative and interoperative infusion for abdominal contamination by bowel, genital, or biliary sources.

CONTRAINDICATIONS. Avoid with icterus. Reduce doses in renal failure. Previous cephalosporin or penicillin hypersensitivity.

ADVERSE REACTIONS. Diarrhea. Local pain on injection, systemic hypersensitivity, blood dyscrasias, diarrhea, rise in serum liver enzyme activity. Biliary crystal deposition and sludging, vitamin K antagonism, mild or transient azotemia, and hypercreatininemia.

INTERACTIONS. Incompatible with many other antimicrobials in solution.

Availability	Type	Sizes	Preparations (Company)
Human	Powder for injection in vials or infusion bottles	250 mg, 500 mg, 1g, 2g	*Rocephin* (Roche)

INTERNATIONAL PREPARATIONS. *Hosbocin, Rocephalin, Rocefalin, Rocefin, Rocephine.*

HANDLING. Store powder for injection away from light at controlled room temperature. Diluents can include sterile water, 0.9% NaCl, 5% dextrose. Solutions are stable for 1–3 days at room temperature, 3–10 days if refrigerated; concentrations at or below 100 mg/ml have the longest stability. Lower concentration (10–40 mg/ml) can be stored frozen (−20°C) for 36 weeks.

ADMINISTRATION. Avoid infusion or mixing with any other drugs. IV or IM administration for up to 14 days as necessary. For IM, may be diluted with lidocaine 1% without epinephrine. Available as IM convenience kit containing proper diluent. Use 0.9-ml diluent/250-mg drug. For IV, use 10–40 mg/ml and give by infusion over 30 min.

DOSAGE

Indications	Dose (mg/kg)	Route	Interval (hr)	Duration (days)
Dogs				
Meningitis, borreliosis	15–50*	IM, IV	12	4–14
Preoperative, intraoperative	25*	IM, IV	24	1
Skin, genitourinary infections	25	IM	24	7–14
Cats				
Systemic infections	25–50	IV, IM, intraosseous	12	prn

*Maximum dose per administration is 1 g for humans.

ADDITIONAL DOSAGES. Lyme borreliosis, Table 45–3.

CEFUROXIME AXETIL OR SODIUM

CLASS. Second-generation cephalosporin.

ACTION. Bactericidal; inhibits bacterial cell wall synthesis.

MORE INFORMATION. See Chapter 34, cephalosporins; Table 34–4.

PHARMACOKINETICS. Oral axetil ester: a prodrug that is hydrolyzed releasing cefuroxime by esterases in intestinal mucosa and blood. Better absorption with food. Parenteral sodium salt: only drug among the first- and second-generation classes to enter the CSF in absence of meningitis and good therapeutic levels with meningeal inflammation. Longer half-life than cefaclor allows twice-daily dosing. Excreted unchanged in urine.

SPECTRUM. Gram positive: *Staphylococcus* and *Streptococcus*. **Gram negative:** *Escherichia, Klebsiella, Enterobacter*. **Ineffective**: high-resistance β-lactamase–producing organisms. Ineffective against *Enterococcus* and methicillin-resistant *Staphylococcus*.

INDICATIONS. Oral, for penicillin-resistant gram-positive infections of skin and upper respiratory tract. Parenteral, also used to treat lower respiratory tract, CNS, and orthopedic infections.

CONTRAINDICATIONS. Reduce dose in renal failure. Previous hypersensitivity to penicillin or cephalosporin.

ADVERSE REACTIONS. Very bitter taste if tablet is bitten or ground up for administration. Adding to dairy products (milk or chocolate milk) may improve absorption and palatability. Some GI upsets may occur with oral axetil preparation. Neutropenia, leukopenia, and eosinophilia have been observed with parenteral sodium drug.

INTERACTIONS. Increased risk of nephrotoxicity when combined with aminoglycoside.

Availability	Type	Sizes	Preparations (Company)
Human	Oral tablets (as axetil)	125 mg, 250 mg, 500 mg	*Ceftin* (Glaxo Wellcome)
	Oral suspension (as axetil)	125 mg/5 ml	*Ceftin*
	Powder for injection (as sodium salt)	750 mg, 1.5 g, 7.5 g	*Kefurox* (Eli Lilly), *Zinacef* (Glaxo Wellcome)

INTERNATIONAL PREPARATIONS. *Biociclin, Biofurex, Bioxima, Cefamar, Cefoprim, Cefumax, Cefur, Cefurex, Cefurin, Cepazine, Ceurocef, Colifossim, Curoxim, Deltacef, Duxima, Elobact, Kefox, Nivador, Selan, Zinnat, Zoref.*

HANDLING. Powder and solutions should be stored protected from light; they darken with storage, but potency is unaffected. When reconstituted, stock solutions of parenteral drug are stable for 24 hr at room temperature and for 48 hr when refrigerated. Dilutions of stock for administration, can be added to 0.9% NaCl or 5% or 10% dextrose. These solutions (1–30 mg/ml) are stable for 7 days when refrigerated; when frozen (−20°C), the solution is stable for 6 mo and should be thawed slowly but not with a microwave, which destroys 85% of activity. Should not add to aminoglycoside-containing solutions, although these can be given separately.

ADMINISTRATION. Oral; advantage over cefaclor is that food enhances absorption and bioavailability. Tablets should be administered whole because of bitter taste, if dose needs are less, use oral suspension. Parenteral; IV is preferred route for systemic infections. IM; can give in large muscle mass; should aspirate first to avoid inadvertent IV inoculation.

DOSAGE

Indications (Dogs)	Dose (mg/kg)	Route	Interval (hr)	Duration (days)
Soft tissue infections	10*	PO	12	10
Systemic infections	15*	IV	8	prn
Meningitis	30*	IV	8	prn

*Extrapolated human dosage.

DISPENSING INFORMATION. Give tablets whole; do not break or crush if put on food. Give with meals.

CEPHALEXIN

CLASS. First-generation cephalosporin.

ACTION. Bactericidal; inhibits bacterial cell wall synthesis.

MORE INFORMATION. See Chapter 34, cephalosporins; Table 34–4; references: 34:76, 34:77.

PHARMACOKINETICS. Well absorbed orally (75% bioavailable). Distributed to most tissues, with highest concentrations in kidney, lung, trachea, and skin of dogs. Also penetrates muscle and bone in therapeutic concentrations. Excreted unchanged in urine and bile. Does not penetrate CNS or CSF.

SPECTRUM. Gram positive: *Staphylococcus, Streptococcus.* **Gram negative:** *Escherichia, Klebsiella, Proteus mirabilis.* **Ineffective:** *Pseudomonas, Aerobacter,* some *Proteus, Bacteroides, Enterococcus.*

INDICATIONS. Skin infections, chronic canine staphylococcal pyoderma; urinary tract infections, pneumonia, localized soft tissue infections, upper respiratory tract infections.

CONTRAINDICATIONS. Previous hypersensitivity to cephalosporins or penicillins. Some reduction in frequency of administration to every 12 to 24 hr in animals with renal failure.

ADVERSE REACTIONS. Dogs: vomiting, diarrhea, excitement or depression, anorexia, salivation (34:85). Cats: vomiting, diarrhea, pyrexia, salivation, occasional hypersensitivity reactions, cholestatic jaundice.

INTERACTIONS. Positive Coomb's tests have been seen in people treated with cephalosporins. False-positive urine glucose results with nonenzymatic test methods.

Availability	Type	Sizes	Preparations (Company)
Human	Powder for oral suspension	125 mg/5 ml, 250 mg/5 ml, 500 mg/5 ml	*Keflex* (Dista), generic (many)
	Capsules, tablets	250 mg, 500 mg, 1 g	*Keflex*
Veterinary	Oral tablets	50 mg, 250 mg	*Ceporex* (Mallinckrodt)
	Oral drops	100 mg/ml	*Ceporex*
	Injectable solution	18 mg/ml	*Ceporex*

INTERNATIONAL PREPARATIONS. *Abiocef, Biocef, Bioporina, Bioscefal, Cefact, Cefadina, Cefadine, Cefadros, Cefalorex, Cefanex, Ceferran, Cepexin, Cephalobene, Cepo, Ceporexin, Ceporexine, Cerexin, Cilicef, Coliceflor; Defaxina, Domucef, Efemida, Fexin, Ibilex, Janocilin, Keflet, Keforal, Keftab, Lafarin, Latoral, Lenocef, Lorexina, Novo-Lexin, Nu-Cephalex, Oracef, Ospexin, Talinsul, Ultralexin, Zartan, Zetacef.*

HANDLING. Oral suspension: refrigerate once reconstituted and discard after 14 days. Capsules: store away from moisture in airtight containers at room temperature.

ADMINISTRATION. Injectable for IM use: localized tissue reaction may occur, massage injection site. Food delays absorption and elimination to a minor degree.

DOSAGE

Indications	Dose (mg/kg)	Route	Interval (hr)	Duration (days)
Dogs				
Pyoderma	22–35	PO	12	14–28*
	22	PO	8	14–28*
Respiratory infections	20–40	PO	8	7–14*
Systemic infections	25–60	PO	8	14–28*
Orthopedic infections	22–30	PO	6–8	28*
Cats				
Soft tissue infections	30–50	PO	12	14–28*
Systemic infections	35	PO	6–8	14–28*

*Guideline: treat for 5–7 days beyond resolution of clinical disease or preferably negative culture.

ADDITIONAL INFORMATION. Streptococcal infections, Table 35–2; anaerobic infections, Table 41–10; canine pyoderma, Table 85–3; musculoskeletal infections, Table 86–3; respiratory disease, Table 88–8; urinary infections, Table 91–8.

DISPENSING INFORMATION. Food may be given with medication to prevent vomiting. Oral suspension should be shaken well before using.

CEPHAPIRIN

CLASS. First-generation cephalosporin.

ACTION. Bactericidal; inhibits bacterial cell wall synthesis.

MORE INFORMATION. See Chapter 34, Cephalosporins, Table 34–4.

PHARMACOKINETICS. Not absorbed from the GI tract after PO administration. Widely distributed into some body fluids (synovial, pleural, peritoneal) but poorly into aqueous humor and CSF. Penetrates many tissues, including bone but not prostate.

SPECTRUM. **Gram positive:** *Staphylococcus*, hemolytic *Streptococcus*. **Gram negative:** *Escherichia*, *Klebsiella*, *Proteus*.

INDICATIONS. Perioperative surgical prophylaxis, septicemia, pneumonia, osteomyelitis.

CONTRAINDICATIONS. Reduce dose in renal failure.

ADVERSE REACTIONS. Pain on injection, phlebitis.

INTERACTIONS. Use cautiously with nephrotoxic drugs such as aminoglycosides.

Availability	Type	Sizes	Preparations (Company)
Human	Powder for injection	500 mg, 1 g, 2 g, 4 g	*Cefadyl* (Bristol), generics (many)

HANDLING. Powder stored at room temperature is stable for 2 yr. Reconstitute with sterile water. Stable at room temperature for 24 hr or 10 days if refrigerated and 14 days if frozen. Compatible with 0.9% NaCl, dextrose, Ringer's, lactated Ringer's.

ADMINISTRATION. Infuse IV slowly over 3–5 min or give with IV fluids.

DOSAGE

Indications (Dogs and Cats)	Dose (mg/kg)	Route	Interval (hr)	Duration (days)
Soft tissue infections	10–20	IV, IM, SC	6–8	prn
Bacteremia, endotoxemia	11–30	IV	4–8	prn

ADDITIONAL DOSAGES. Canine distemper, Table 3–5; feline panleukopenia, Table 10–1; bacteremia or endocarditis, Table 87–7; oral infections, Table 89–4; CNS infections, Table 92–5.

CEPHAZOLIN

CLASS. First-generation cephalosporin.

ACTION. Bactericidal; inhibits bacterial cell wall synthesis.

MORE INFORMATION. See CEPHAPIRIN; Chapter 34, cephalosporins.

PHARMACOKINETICS. Poorly absorbed from GI tract. After IM or IV injection, enters many tissues and body fluids, including bone and peritoneal, pleural, and synovial fluids. Does not enter CSF appreciably. Predominantly excreted unchanged in urine.

SPECTRUM. See CEPHALEXIN, PENICILLIN G, or CEPHAPIRIN.

INDICATIONS. Surgical prophylaxis, biliary tract, and intra-abdominal infections and bacteremia.

CONTRAINDICATIONS. See CEPHALEXIN.

ADVERSE REACTIONS. IM injections are painful and IV can cause thrombophlebitis. See also CEPHALEXIN.

INTERACTIONS. See CEPHRADINE.

Availability	Type	Size	Preparations (Company)
Human	Powder for injection (as sodium)	1 g	*Ancef* (Smith Kline Beecham), *Kefzol* (Eli Lilly)

INTERNATIONAL PREPARATIONS. *Acef, Areuzolin, Baktozil, Biazolina, Brizolina, Caricef, Cefabiozim, Cefacidal, Cefadrex, Cefamezin, Cefazil, Cilicef, Elzogram, Fazoplex, Firmacef, Gramaxin, Izacef, Kefol, Recef, Sicef, Tasep, Totacef, Zolicef, Zolin, Zolival.*

HANDLING. Should reconstitute in sterile water. Store in light-proof containers. Incompatible with aminoglycosides and basic solutions in which hydrolysis occurs, and at pH < 4.5, the drug precipitates. Crystal formation occurs if reconstituted with 0.9% NaCl and should be avoided.

ADMINISTRATION. Give by deep IM injection or slow (3–5 min) IV infusion.

DOSAGE

Indications	Dose (mg/kg)	Route	Interval (hr)	Duration (days)
Soft tissue infections	22	IM, IV	8	prn
Surgical infections	22	IV	*	1

*Just before or during surgical procedure.

CEPHRADINE

CLASS. First-generation cephalosporin.

ACTION. Bactericidal; inhibits bacterial cell wall synthesis.

MORE INFORMATION. See Chapter 34, cephalosporins; Table 34–4.

PHARMACOKINETICS. See CEPHALEXIN. Better absorbed orally (90% bioavailable).

SPECTRUM. Gram positive: *Staphylococcus*, hemolytic *Streptococcus*. **Gram negative:** *Escherichia, Klebsiella, Proteus.*

INDICATIONS. Oral treatment of respiratory, skin, and urinary tract infections; parenteral treatment for septicemia, osteomyelitis, and perioperative prophylaxis.

CONTRAINDICATIONS. See CEPHALEXIN.

ADVERSE REACTIONS. Dogs: vomiting, diarrhea, anorexia, polydipsia, polyuria.

INTERACTIONS. False-positive results on urine protein tests using sulfosalicylic acid. Monitor renal function if used in combination with aminoglycosides.

Availability	Type	Sizes	Preparations (Company)
Human	Oral capsules	250 mg, 500 mg	*Velosef* (Apothecon), generics (many)
	Powder for oral suspension (fruit flavored)	125 mg/5 ml, 250 mg/5 ml	*Anspor* (SmithKline Beecham)
	Powder for injection	250 mg, 500 mg, 1 g, 2 g	*Velosef*

INTERNATIONAL PREPARATIONS. *Cefamid, Cefrasol, Cefril, Cefral, Celex, Cesporan, Ecosporina, Kelsef, Lisacef, Sefril, Septasef.*

HANDLING. Store powders and capsules below 86°F, and keep bottle closed tight away from light. Oral suspension stable 7 days at room temperature, 14 days if refrigerated. Compatible with most IV solutions except Ringer's or lactated Ringer's or calcium-containing solutions. Do not mix with other antibiotics given concurrently. Reconstituted solutions of less than 50 mg/ml are stable for 10 hr at room temperature and 48 hr if refrigerated. Solutions for injection can be stored frozen for 6 weeks.

ADMINISTRATION. Can be given orally without regard to meals. Food delays absorption but does not affect its extent.

DOSAGE

Indications (Dogs)	Dose (mg/kg)	Route	Interval (hr)	Duration (days)
Skin, pyoderma	22	PO	8	14–28*
Systemic, orthopedic infections	22	IV, IM, SC, PO	6–8	28*

*Treatment duration varies, usually 5–7 days beyond resolution of infection by culture testing.

ADDITIONAL DOSAGES. Respiratory infections, Table 88–8.

DISPENSING INFORMATION. Keep reconstituted oral suspension in refrigerator, discard unused portions after 2 weeks.

CHLORAMPHENICOL

CLASS. Acetamide.

ACTION. Bacterostatic; binds to 50s ribosomes of bacteria, inhibiting protein synthesis.

MORE INFORMATION. See FLORFENICOL, see elsewhere THIAMFENICOL. See Chapter 34, chloramphenicol; references: 34:117, 34:176.

PHARMACOKINETICS. GI absorption dependent on formulation. Crystalline salt is better, may cause salivation in cats but has good bioavailability with rapid absorption. Oral palmitate is better tolerated but gives poor systemic drug availability in anorectic cats (34:176). In dogs, drug availability with the palmitate is similar to tablets. The inactive palmitate is hydrolyzed in small intestine to release active absorbable drug. Sodium succinate ester can be given IV, SC, IM. Systemic availability is similar with each route, but IM injection is more painful. The succinate ester lacks antimicrobial activity but is hydrolyzed in liver, lung, and kidney to release active drug. It produces better bioavailability than chloramphenicol in aqueous suspensions or dissolved in organic solvents. Chloramphenicol is lipid soluble and distributed well to all tissues, including skeleton, prostate, CNS. Order of decreasing tissue concentrations is as follows: lymph node, spleen, pancreas, liver, kidney, lung, muscle, brain (34:176). Penetrates pleural, ascitic, and synovial fluids, saliva, milk, prostatic and amniotic fluids. Tissue concentrations often exceed those in plasma, but the drug is slower (3–4 hr) to penetrate the intact brain and CSF barriers. Compared with plasma, concentrations are 23% in aqueous and 77% in CSF (34:176). Concentrations are not altered appreciably by inflammation. Metabolized in liver by glucuronyl transferase; in dogs 90% of drug is metabolized and metabolites are excreted in urine. Only 5%–10% of a dose in adult dogs and 25% in cats and neonatal dogs is excreted unchanged in urine. Urine concentrations are 10–20 times blood concentrations and are therapeutic. Optimum activity at a urine pH of 7.5–8.0.

SPECTRUM. Gram positive: *Streptococcus, Staphylococcus.* **Gram negative:** *Salmonella, Shigella, Escherichia, Proteus, Bordetella.* **Anaerobes:** *Clostridium, Fusobacterium, Bacteroides.* Resistance can develop during use. **Others:** *Chlamydia, Rickettsia, Mycoplasma, Ehrlichia, Leptospira, Borrelia.* **Most effective:** anaerobic infections, rickettsial infections. **Ineffective:** *Mycobacterium, Pseudomonas, Enterobacter, Serratia, Klebsiella* may be resistant or develop it during treatment.

INDICATIONS. Cats: chronic rhinitis-sinusitis, pneumonia, pyothorax, periodontitis-gingivitis, bacterial enteritis, biliary infections, intra-abdominal sepsis, lower urinary infection, haemobartonellosis, bordetellosis, rickettsiosis, anaerobic infections (abscesses). Dogs: tetracycline-resistant *Ehrlichia canis* infections without myelosuppression; respiratory, urinary, and soft tissue infections.

CONTRAINDICATIONS. Pre-existing leukopenia or anemia; hepatic dysfunction requires reducing dose to lower risk of marrow suppression. Avoid in pregnancy, neonates, hepatic insufficiency, cats with renal failure. Avoid IV use in animals with cardiac failure because it depresses myocardium. Do not use in breeding animals because it may affect gonadal function. No reduction in dosage needed in dogs with mild renal insufficiency, but a 10% reduction is recommended in uremia as a result of protein catabolic effects of the drug.

ADVERSE REACTIONS. Protein synthesis inhibitor; theoretically, might delay wound healing or immunoglobulin synthesis. High plasma concentrations can be toxic for prenatal or neonatal animals owing to immature hepatic metabolism. Inhibits ferrochelatase, an enzyme in hemoglobin synthesis, resulting in reversible nonregenerative anemia. Reversible myelosuppression affecting the maturation of granulocytes occurs in dogs and cats. This should be differentiated from severe, often fatal irreversible idiosyncratic pancytopenia that occurs in some people (34:117). Dogs: with > 2–3 weeks of treatment at > 175 mg/kg/day may develop depression, anorexia; at > 225 mg/kg/day, myelosuppression, reticulocytopenia. No morphologic bone marrow effects are found in treated dogs. Erythropoietic response is suppressed at therapeutic dosages in dogs with pre-existing or concurrent blood loss when therapy commences. Regeneration occurs when therapy is discontinued. Cats: at 25–40 mg/kg/day for 3 weeks or 120 mg/kg/day for 1 week develop depression, dehydration, anorexia, weight loss, diarrhea, vomiting, myelotoxicity. Reversible erythroid maturation arrest, vacuolation of marrow elements, and pancytopenia occur.

INTERACTIONS. Avoid prescribing it with other drugs metabolized in the liver, especially to cats. Inhibits cytochrome P–450 activity and resultant hepatic biotransformation of drugs, which may potentiate by prolonging action of pentobarbital, phenobarbital, primidone, warfarin, salicylates, inhalation anesthetics, diphenylhydantoin, digoxin (34:68). Action of cyclophosphamide is inhibited because its metabolites are active. Effect on P-450 activity has even been noted with topical ophthalmic preparations. Does not alter the effects or duration of ketamine-xylazine anesthesia. Prolongs propofol anesthesia in dogs (34:93, 34:113). Decreases effectiveness of iron, B_{12} aminoglycosides, penicillins. Rifampin and phenobarbital decrease the effectiveness of chloramphenicol. Oral coadministration of calcium lactate, kaolin-pectin, aluminum hydroxide preparations may increase bioavailability. May cause a spurious positive test result for glucose using glucose oxidase strips.

Availability	Type	Sizes	Preparations (Company)
Human	Oral capsules	250 mg, 500 mg	*Chloromycetin* (Parke-Davis)*
	Oral liquid (palmitate)	50 mg/ml	*Chloromycetin* Palmitate (Parke-Davis)*
	Powder for injection (sodium succinate)	1-g, 10-g vials (100 mg/ml)	*Chloromycetin*
Veterinary	Oral tablets, film coated	100 mg, 250 mg, 500 mg, 1 g	*Amphicol* (Butler)*, generic (Phoenix)
	Capsules	100 mg, 250 mg, 500 mg	*Chloromycetin,* generic (many)*

*No longer available in USA.

INTERNATIONAL PREPARATIONS. *Aquamycetin, Biophenicol, Chemicetina, Chlorcol, Cloranfe, Dispaphenicol, Globenicol, Fenicol, Hortfenicol, Kemicetin, Septicol, Sificetina, Troymycetin.*

HANDLING. Oral palmitate suspension, tablets, capsules should be stored at room temperature away from light. Stable for several years at room temperature. The sodium succinate powder should be kept at controlled room temperatures. Once reconstituted, is stable for 1 mo at room temp or 6 mo if frozen.

ADMINISTRATION. Oral administration is generally satisfactory. Sodium succinate can be given IV, IM, SC, although pain or irritation may result at extravascular sites. SC or IM for fractious, unconscious animals or animals with GI disturbance; IV for high rapid levels in severe systemic infections. If no response to therapy in 3–5 days, reconsider diagnosis and treatment. Should recheck CBC for myelotoxicity at 1-wk and 2-wk intervals in cats and dogs, respectively.

DOSAGE

Indications	Dose	Route	Interval (hr)	Duration (days)
Dogs				
Urinary, rickettsial, localized soft tissue infections	25–50 mg/kg	PO	8	7
Systemic infection	50 mg/kg	IV, IM, SC, PO	6–8	3–5
Severe bacteremia, sepsis	50 mg/kg	IV, IM, SC	4–6	3
Cats				
Urinary, localized soft tissue infections	50 mg/cat	PO	12	14
Systemic infections	25–50 mg/kg	IV, IM, SC, PO	12	≤14
Bacteremia, sepsis	50 mg/cat	IV, IM, SC, PO	6–8	≤5

ADDITIONAL DOSAGES. Canine distemper, Table 3–5; ehrlichiosis, Table 28–4; Rocky Mountain spotted fever, Table 29–3; haemobartonellosis, Table 30–1; streptococcal infections, Table 35–2; enteric bacterial infections, Table 39–1; anaerobic infections, Table 41–10; Lyme borreliosis, Table 45–3; plague, Table 47–1; actinomycosis, Table 49–1; opportunistic mycobacteriosis, Table 56–5; feline abscesses, Table 52–2; musculoskeletal infections, Table 86–3; bacteremia, Table 87–7; respiratory disease, Table 88–8; oral infections, Table 89–4; colitis, Table 89–14; intra-abdominal infections, Table 89–15; hepatobiliary infections, Table 90–4; urinary infections, Table 91–8; CNS infections, Table 92–5; topical for ocular infections, Table 93–4.

DISPENSING INFORMATION. This drug is potentially toxic to people. Wear latex gloves when handling and administering to pets. Return animal every 2 weeks for hematologic testing. Can be administered with food. Tablets or capsules may be bitter if crushed. Shake suspensions well before use.

CIPROFLOXACIN HYDROCHLORIDE

CLASS. Fluoroquinolone.

ACTION. Bactericidal; interferes with DNA gyrase and synthesis of bacterial DNA.

MORE INFORMATION. See ENROFLOXACIN; Chapter 34, quinolones, Table 34–11.

PHARMACOKINETICS. See also ENROFLOXACIN. More variable and slower absorption than enrofloxacin. Well absorbed in dogs (70%) after PO administration. Food may delay rate but not degree of absorption. Approximately 40%–50% excreted unchanged in urine. Urinary metabolites have lower antibacterial activity. Wide tissue distribution. Concentrations in genital tissues of both sexes are high. Present in active form in saliva, nasal and bronchial secretions, sputum, skin blister fluid, lymph, peritoneal fluid, bile and prostatic secretions. Lower concentrations in lung, skin, fat, muscle, cartilage, bone. In people, concentrations in CSF are 40%–90% of serum with inflammation and less than 10% if uninflamed. Concentrations in aqueous humor are 4%–25% of serum, with low concentrations in vitreous..

SPECTRUM. See also ENROFLOXACIN. **Gram positive:** *Staphylococcus* (including methicillin-resistant strains), most *Streptococcus* are moderately susceptible. **Gram negative:** *Escherichia, Klebsiella, Enterobacter, Citrobacter, Salmonella, Campylobacter, Brucella, Pasteurella,* some *Pseudomonas* develop resistance. **Anaerobes:** most are resistant. **Others:** *Mycoplasma, Leptospira, Borrelia, Chlamydia, Mycobacterium tuberculosis,* some opportunistic mycobacteria, but not *Mycobacterium avium-intracellulare* complex. Increased activity and spectrum may occur in combined therapy with metronidazole, clindamycin, β-lactam drugs, or aminoglycosides. **More effective:** gram-negative bacteria. **Ineffective:** *Enterococcus, Actinomyces, Nocardia, Ehrlichia,* obligate anaerobes, *M. avium-intracellulare* complex.

INDICATIONS. See also ENROFLOXACIN. Complicated or chronic urinary tract infections or prostatitis caused by *Escherichia, Klebsiella, Enterobacter, Serratia, Proteus, Citrobacter, Pseudomonas, Staphylococcus.* Infectious diarrhea caused by pathogenic gram-negative bacteria such as enterotoxigenic *Escherichia, Campylobacter,* and *Salmonella.* Lower respiratory, skin, bone, and joint infections with very susceptible organisms. Gram-negative bacterial meningitis.

CONTRAINDICATIONS. See also ENROFLOXACIN. In reduced renal function, there is slight prolongation of ciprofloxacin elimination: reduce dose (once daily) in renal failure. Owing to arthropathy, should not be used in growing animals or in pregnant or lactating animals. Avoid in animals with previously documented adverse reaction.

ADVERSE REACTIONS. See also ENROFLOXACIN. Nausea, anorexia, vomiting, diarrhea are most frequent side effects. Malaise and inappetence occurs in cats. May cause CNS stimulation with tremors or seizures in predisposed animals. Permanent cartilage damage and lameness develop in growing animals. Dermal hypersensitivity reactions have occurred. High overdosages in dogs have resulted in nephrotoxicity from crystal deposition in kidneys (especially alkaline urine), cataracts, reduced spermatogenesis. These have not been seen with therapeutic dosages. Tendon ruptures have been observed in people.

INTERACTIONS. Concurrent use with theophylline results in elevated theophylline concentrations and increased risk of CNS stimulation.

Availability	Type	Sizes	Preparations (Company)
Human	Film coated oral tablets	250 mg, 500 mg, 750 mg	*Cipro* (Miles-Bayer)
	Parenteral (IV) solution	200 mg, 400 mg	*Cipro*

INTERNATIONAL PREPARATIONS. *Baycip, Belmacina, Catex, Ceprimax, Ciflox, Ciloxan, Ciprobay, Ciproxin, Cunesin, Flociprin, Quipro.*

HANDLING. Add parenteral solution of 0.9% NaCl or 5% dextrose. Stable for 14 days if refrigerated, but protect from light. Do not mix with clindamycin or clavulanate. Can be formulated for smaller tablet size by IDEXX at 1–888-RxIDEXX.

ADMINISTRATION. For IV, dilute in saline before administration and give slowly over 1 hr using large veins. Orally, food slows or reduces absorption of the drug. Preferred dosing is 2 hr after meal. Concurrent administration of antacids containing magnesium or aluminum hydroxide may reduce bioavailability to 90%. Sucralfate given within 2 hr of oral dosing similarly reduces absorption.

DOSAGE

Indications (Dogs)	Dose (mg/kg)	Route	Interval (hr)	Duration (days)
Urinary tract infections	5–8	PO	12	7–14
Skin, local soft tissue infections	7–11	PO	12	7–14
Bone and systemic infections, bacteremia and more resistant pathogens (e.g., *Enterobacter*)	10–15	PO	12	7–14

ADDITIONAL DOSAGES. Gram-negative bacterial infections, Table 37–2; musculoskeletal infections, Table 86–3; bacteremia and endocarditis, Table 87– 7.

DISPENSING INFORMATION. Administer at least 1 hr before or 2 hr after meals and do not give concurrently with antacids or sucralfate.

CLARITHROMYCIN

CLASS. Macrolide, methylerythromycin derivative.

ACTION. Bacteriostatic; inhibits bacterial RNA-dependent protein synthesis by binding to 50s subunit of ribosome.

MORE INFORMATION. See AZITHROMYCIN; Chapter 34, Macrolides.

PHARMACOKINETICS. Best absorbed macrolide with or without ingesta (55% bioavailable) because stable in gastric acid. Better absorption and tissue penetration than erythromycin with prolonged elimination half-life. Concentrated in and transported by phagocytes. High concentration reached in sputum, lung, tonsil, nasal sinus, stomach, uterus, ovary, cervix, prostate. Accumulates in pulmonary tissue. Penetrates and concentrates intracellularly in macrophages and neutrophils, facilitating killing of intracellular pathogens. Does not penetrate well into CNS. Metabolized in liver by hydroxylation and methylation, forming a very biologically active hydroxymetabolite and inactive demethylated compound. Metabolites are excreted in urine. From 20%–40% of dose may appear in urine as unchanged drug, depending on the formulation (tablets or powder, respectively).

SPECTRUM. See ERYTHROMYCIN for gram-positive and gram-negative aerobic bacteria. **Anaerobes:** *Bacteroides, Clostridium, Peptococcus,* and *Propionibacterium.* Best activity against gram-positive aerobes and anaerobes. **Others:** opportunistic mycobacteria, *M. avium-intracellulare complex (MAC), Borrelia, Bartonella, Toxoplasma, Chlamydia.* **More effective:** than erythromycin against *Streptococcus, Staphylococcus, Campylobacter, Helicobacter,* and obligate anaerobes.

INDICATIONS. Lower respiratory tract and skin infections, enteropathogenic bacterial infections, nasal sinusitis, *Toxoplasma* (combined with pyrimethamine), many cutaneous opportunistic mycobacterial infections, including those caused by *Mycobacterium avium-intracellulare* complex (recommend combining with other effective agents). Used in Lyme borreliosis and gastric helicobacteriosis. A substitute for erythromycin with less GI irritation, lower dose but higher cost.

CONTRAINDICATIONS. Previous erythromycin hypersensitivity. Reduce dose for renal or severe hepatic failure. Active urinary metabolite will not be produced with hepatic dysfunction. Avoid in pregnancy; has adverse effects on fetal development in experimental animals.

ADVERSE REACTIONS. Nausea, diarrhea, abdominal pain, cholestatic hepatitis, increased liver enzymes, thrombocytopenia, rare eosinophilia, allergic skin reactions. Should hepatic enzyme elevations occur, use lower dosage range. May be less likely than erythromycin to cause GI disturbances.

INTERACTIONS. See ERYTHROMYCIN; interferes with metabolism of drugs by cytochrome P–450 system. May inhibit benzodiazepine or digoxin metabolism.

Availability	Type	Sizes	Preparations (Company)
Human	Tablets	250 mg, 500 mg	*Biaxin* (Abbott), *Klacid* (many countries)
	Granules for oral suspension	125 mg/5 ml, 250 mg/5 ml	*Biaxin*

INTERNATIONAL PREPARATIONS. *Biclar, Cyllind, Klacid, Klaciped, Klariced, Macladin, Mavid, Veclam.*

HANDLING. Do not refrigerate suspension because it develops a bitter taste; keep at room temperature and use within 14 days.

ADMINISTRATION. Can be given with or without fasting, but food delays absorption.

DOSAGE

Indications	Dose (mg/kg)	Route	Interval (hr)	Duration (days)
Dogs	5–10	PO	12	prn
Cats	7.5	PO	12	prn

ADDITIONAL DOSAGES. Helicobacteriosis, Table 39–3; mycobacterial infections, Tables 50–4 and 50–5.

DISPENSING INFORMATION. Can be given with food. Shake suspension before administration. May cause diarrhea or vomiting.

CLINDAMYCIN

CLASS. Lincosamide; semisynthetic derivative of lincomycin.

ACTION. Bacteriostatic and antiprotozoal activity; binds to 50s subunit of bacterial and protozoal ribosome inhibiting protein synthesis. Potentiates opsonization and phagocytosis.

MORE INFORMATION. See LINCOMYCIN; Chapter 34, Lincosamides; references: 34:16, 34:57, 34:60, 71:12.

PHARMACOKINETICS. After oral administration, GI absorption approached 90%. For oral suspension, palmitate ester is hydrolyzed to active base while aqueous drops are readily absorbed. Absorption is delayed but not prevented by food. Better absorbed than lincomycin. Widely distributed to most tissues, including skin, muscle, bone, body fluids (pleural, peritoneal, synovial) to therapeutic levels. Active transport into phagocytic cells and abscess fluids, killing susceptible intracellular bacteria. Lowest levels reached are in intact CNS and CSF. Levels in inflamed meninges are 40% of blood concentration. Crosses placenta and enters milk. Hepatic metabolism to active and inactive moieties with excretion in bile, feces, urine. Prolonged enterohepatic circulation and excretion in stool for up to 2 weeks after last dose. It is predominantly (80%–90%) excreted in bile with 10%–20% renally excreted.

SPECTRUM. Gram positive: Aerobic cocci, including *Streptococcus* (not enterococci) and more susceptible *Staphylococcus, Nocardia,* and few *Corynebacterium.* **Gram negative:** *Campylobacter, Helicobacter.* **Anaerobes:** *Peptostreptococcus, Peptococcus, Actinomyces, Propionibacterium, Eubacterium, Clostridium* (except *C. difficile*), *Bacteroides, Fusobacterium.* **Others:** *Chlamydia;* protozoa *Toxoplasma, Neospora, Babesia, Pneumocystis.* **Ineffective:** most gram-negative aerobic bacteria, *Mycobacterium,* and *Mycoplasma.* Whenever resistance to lincomycin or erythromycin exists. Bacterial resistance may develop during treatment and usually also involves lincomycin.

INDICATIONS. For gram-positive aerobic and in anaerobic infections. Intra-abdominal or GI abscesses and infections (perforating ulcers, penetrating injuries, biliary infections, ischemic bowel, colitis, hepatic or biliary abscesses, soft tissue or subcutaneous abscesses, pelvic genital infections, or prostatitis caused by anaerobes, chronic sinusitis or otitis, bacterial pharyngitis, stomatitis, bite wounds, dental infections); for oral, dental, or upper respiratory tract procedures, pleuropulmonary infections (pyothorax, aspiration pneumonia, pleuritis, pulmonary abscesses). Skin and soft tissue infections (staphylococcal pyoderma); osteomyelitis; diskospondylitis; prophylaxis for head, neck, and open bowel surgery (for the latter, combine with aminoglycosides); endocarditis prophylaxis (after amoxicillin and erythromycin), streptococcal or staphylococcal septicemia. Very effective in treating anaerobic infections and could be preferred over chloramphenicol or metronidazole because of less toxicity. Usually combined with an aminoglycoside or quinolone to treat gram-negative aerobic bacterial infections. Toxoplasmosis and neosporosis: can be used in combination with pyrimethamine. Systemic toxoplasmosis in dogs and cats and enteroepithelial toxoplasmosis in cats. Pneumocystosis: combined with primaquine. Babesiosis: combined with quinine.

CONTRAINDICATIONS. Bacterial resistance to lincomycin. Reduce dose with hepatic dysfunction and biliary obstruction from any cause. Reduce dose with severe renal failure. Safety in reproductively active animals or pregnancy is uncertain.

ADVERSE REACTIONS. GI signs; generally less vomiting than with lincomycin, transient diarrhea when dose is reduced or temporarily discontinued. Pseudomembranous colitis, documented for other species, not a substantiated complication in dogs and cats. Local or systemic or dermal hypersensitivity reactions occur rarely. Local pain and sterile abscesses can form after IM and phlebitis after IV. Oral clindamycin may cause lip smacking and hypersalivation in some cats. Anorexia, vomiting, diarrhea owing to GI irritation can be overcome by parenteral rather than PO use and dosage reductions. May cause diarrhea in pups or kittens of dams receiving therapy. Can produce neuromuscular blockade. May cause leukopenia or increased serum hepatic enzyme activity. Cardiac arrhythmias may develop with bolus infusions of undiluted drug.

INTERACTIONS. Neuromuscular blockade compounded by other similar-acting agents such as aminoglycosides. Erythromycin and chloramphenicol interfere with the action of clindamycin in vivo. Do not use with macrolides.

Availability	Type	Sizes	Preparations (Company)
Human	Oral suspension (palmitate)	15 mg/ml	*Cleocin* (Pharmacia & Upjohn)
	Solution for injection (phosphate)	150 mg/ml	*Cleocin*
	Oral capsules	75 mg, 150 mg, 300 mg	*Cleocin*
Veterinary	Oral capsules	25 mg, 75 mg, 150 mg	*Antirobe* (Pharmacia & Upjohn)
	Oral solution (hydrochloride)	25 mg/ml	*Antirobe Aquadrops*

INTERNATIONAL PREPARATIONS. *Clindatech, Dalacin.*

HANDLING. Parenteral phosphate solution can be stored at room temperature, compatible with most isotonic IV solutions. Contains no preservatives, and if refrigerated, crystals will form that dissolve on rewarming. Oral hydrochloride is stable at room temperature for extended periods. Once reconstituted, palmitate stable for 2 weeks at room temperature but congeals if refrigerated. Parenteral solution of 300–900 mg diluted in 20 ml of 10% dextrose solution, is stable in frozen storage for 30 days. Parenteral solution is incompatible in infusions with aminophylline, calcium gluconate, ceftriaxone, barbiturates, ampicillin.

ADMINISTRATION. Oral preparations can be given with food, which does not modify the normal absorption of drug. For IV use, always dilute or administer parenteral solution in 0.9% sodium chloride, 5% dextrose, or lactated Ringer's. IV preparation can be added to solutions containing aminoglycosides (some), penicillins, cephalosporins, glucocorticoids, potassium chloride, sodium bicarbonate. Each dose can be given IV over 4–6 hr or slow IV bolus over 20-min period. Never give greater than 15 mg/min. Pain at IM or SC injection site. Manufacturer recommends a treatment interval of 5–28 days. Monitor hepatic, renal function, and hematologic test results during prolonged (≥ 30 day) therapy.

DOSAGE

Indications	Dose (mg/kg)	Route	Interval (hr)	Duration (days)
Dogs				
Staphylococcal pyoderma	11	PO	24	7–28
Wounds, abscesses, dental infections, stomatitis	5–11	PO	12	7–28
Neosporosis, toxoplasmosis	5–20	IV, IM, SC, PO	12	15
Neosporosis	13.5	PO	8	21
Osteomyelitis	11	PO	12	28
Systemic, bacteremia	3–10	IV, IM, SC, PO	8	prn
Cats				
Skin and soft tissue infections	11–24	PO, SC	24	7–28
Skin and soft tissue infections, stomatitis	5–11	PO, SC	12	7–28
Enteroepithelial toxoplasmosis	25–50	PO	24	7–14
Systemic toxoplasmosis	8–16	PO, SC	8	14–28
	12.5–25	PO, SC	12	14–28

ADDITIONAL DOSAGES. FIV stomatitis, Table 14–5; endotoxemia, Table 38–1; *Clostridium perfringens* diarrhea, Table 39–4; anaerobic infections; Table 41–10; tetanus, Table 43–2; actinomycosis, Table 49–1; feline abscesses, Table 52–2; hepatozoon, Table 74–2; babesiosis, Table 77–3; toxoplasmosis, Table 80–3; neosporosis, Table 80–7; pneumocystosis, Table 83–2; musculoskeletal infections, Table 86–3; oral infections, Table 89– 4; intra-abdominal infections, Table 89–15; hepatobiliary infections, Table 90–4; local use for ocular infections, Table 93–4.

DISPENSING INFORMATION. Shake oral suspension before each administration. Give liquid or capsules with small amount of food if vomiting occurs; otherwise give on an empty stomach. Cats may salivate when treated with PO preparations. Report any persistent or bloody vomiting or diarrhea to the veterinarian.

CLOFAZIMINE

CLASS. Iminophenazine dye.

ACTION. Antimycobacterial; binds preferentially to mycobacterial DNA. Some antiprotozoal and antifungal activity.

MORE INFORMATION. See Chapters 34 and 50; reference: 34:74.

PHARMACOKINETICS. Good absorption (45%–60%) from GI tract. Highly lipophilic, taken up in adipose and mononuclear phagocytes. Retained in tissues for long periods and can be excreted via bile into feces for months. Small amounts present in other body secretions.

SPECTRUM. *M. avium-intracellulare* complex, opportunistic rapid-growing mycobacteria. Weak activity against *Mycobacterium leprae*. Resistance rarely develops during treatment.

INDICATIONS. *M. avium-intracellulare* complex infections, leprosy, opportunistic mycobacteriosis. Combination therapy with other drugs (see Chapter 50) overcomes resistance and increases efficacy in treating mycobacteriosis. Combined with dapsone to treat leprosy. On a limited basis has been used to treat human leishmaniasis and topical mycoses. Has anti-inflammatory activity. Has some antileishmanial activity.

CONTRAINDICATIONS. During pregnancy can cause fetotoxicity and should be avoided in pre-existing gastrointestinal illness. Consider doxycycline or quinolones as alternatives.

ADVERSE REACTIONS. GI pain resulting from crystalline deposits of drug in viscera (nausea, vomiting, abdominal pain). Reduce or discontinue drug use if signs occur. Skin and body fluid discoloration (pink to brown) especially when exposed to sunlight. CNS signs, high serum hepatic transaminases.

INTERACTIONS. Interactions with dapsone are uncertain but combined therapy may be necessary.

Availability	Type	Sizes	Preparation (Company)
Human	Oral capsules	50 mg, 100 mg	*Lamprene* (Geigy)

INTERNATIONAL PREPARATIONS. *Lampren.*

HANDLING. Store at room temperature in moisture-proof containers. Capsules contain micronized drug in an oil-wax base, making it difficult to give partial amounts.

ADMINISTRATION. When given with food, absorption improved.

DOSAGE

Indications	Dose	Route	Interval (hr)	Duration (weeks)
Dogs	4–8 mg/kg	PO	24	4
Cats	8 mg/kg	PO	24	4
	50 mg/cat	PO	24	4

ADDITIONAL DOSAGES. Mycobacterial infections, Tables 50–4 and 50–5.

DISPENSING INFORMATION. Administer with meals. Medicine may turn animal's skin pink and its excretions a brownish-black color.

CLOTRIMAZOLE

CLASS. Imidazole-antifungal.

ACTION. Fungistatic; inhibits ergosterol formation in fungal cell wall.

MORE INFORMATION. See ENILCONAZOLE; Topical Antifungal Therapy, Chapter 57 and Tables 57–3, 58–4, 65–3, and reference 65:11.

PHARMACOKINETICS. Minimally (3%) not absorbed when used topically in mucosa and 0.5% through intact skin. Any absorbed is metabolized and excreted in bile with low concentrations of active drug and predominantly metabolites appearing in urine.

SPECTRUM. Dermatophytes, yeasts *(Candida, Malassezia),* and *Aspergillus.*

INDICATIONS. Dermatophytosis, yeast-induced otitis externa, nasal aspergillosis.

CONTRAINDICATIONS. Previous hypersensitivity, avoid ocular contact.

ADVERSE REACTIONS. Irritating, burning sensation, erythema, nasal discharge when used in nasal passages. Use of commercial preparations containing propylene glycol or isopropyl alcohol may cause severe airway obstruction. Clotrimazole may prolong barbiturate anesthesia.

Availability	Type	Sizes	Preparations (Company)
Human	Topical solution 1% (also cream, lotion)	10 ml, 30 ml	*Lotrimin* (Schering-Plough Animal Health), *Mycelex* (Miles)
	Vaginal tablets	100 mg, 500 mg	*Lotrimin*

INTERNATIONAL PREPARATIONS. *Antifungol, Candibene, Canesten, Trimysten.*

HANDLING. Flush for nasal aspergillosis: crush 1 g (two 500-mg tablets) of clotrimazole. Add to 100 ml of polyethylene glycol 400 (PEG–400) and stir on a hot plate until mixed. Keep suspension warm until used.

ADMINISTRATION. Intranasal: surgically place indwelling tubes in nasal passage or anesthetize animal and flush retrograde in nostrils. See procedure under ENILCONAZOLE and in Chapter 65. The 1% clotrimazole is sufficiently viscous to pass through the tubes yet remain in the passages. Two 60-ml dose syringes containing the drug are attached to tubes. Initially 30 ml of the solution is flushed into each cavity. Then the remainder is flushed slowly over 60 min while the animal remains anesthetized (see Figure 65–5). **Topical:** apply to dermatophyte lesions twice daily for 3 to 4 weeks.

DOSAGES. See Chapter 65 and Tables 65–3, 66–1, 69–1, 85–6, and 85–8 for topical usages and formulations.

CLOXACILLIN

CLASS. Isoxazolyl penicillin.

ACTION. Bactericidal; inhibits bacterial cell wall synthesis.

MORE INFORMATION. See DICLOXACILLIN, OXACILLIN; Chapter 34, Penicillins; Table 34–1.

PHARMACOKINETICS. Only partially absorbed (40%–50%) from the GI tract after PO administration, and food reduces this further. Distributed to most tissues and body fluids with the exception of CNS and CSF. Metabolized by the liver to active and inactive moieties, predominantly excreted in the urine and minor amounts in bile and feces.

SPECTRUM. *Staphyloccocus,* including β-lactamase producers, other gram-positive aerobic cocci, some gram-positive anaerobes.

INDICATIONS. Staphylococcal infections, especially pyoderma in dogs.

CONTRAINDICATIONS. Hypersensitivity, hepatotoxicity.

ADVERSE REACTIONS. See OXACILLIN.

INTERACTIONS. See OXACILLIN.

Availability	Type	Sizes	Preparations (Company)
Human	Oral capsules (as sodium)	250 mg, 500 mg	*Cloxapen* (SmithKline Beecham), *Tegopen* (Bristol), generic (various)
	Oral powder (as sodium)	125 mg/5 ml	*Tegopen*

INTERNATIONAL PREPARATIONS. *Alclox, Anaclosil, Bactopen, Cloxypen, Ekvacillin, Orbenin, Rivoclox.*

HANDLING. Store oral powder and capsules at room temperature. Reconstituted oral solution is stable for 14 days if refrigerated, 3 days at room temperature.

ADMINISTRATION. Give without food.

DOSAGE

Indications (Dogs and Cats)	Dose (mg/kg)	Route	Interval (hr)	Duration (days)
Localized soft tissue infections, staphylococcal pyoderma, diskospondylitis, osteomyelitis	10–15	PO	6	14–84
Systemic infection, bacteremia	20–40	PO	6–8	7–14

ADDITIONAL DOSAGES. Musculoskeletal infections, Table 86–3; CNS infections, Table 92–5.

DISPENSING INFORMATION. Give 1 hr before or 2 hr after feeding.

DAPSONE

CLASS. Sulfone.

ACTION. Antimycobacterial, antiprotozoal.

MORE INFORMATION. See Chapter 34, Antituberculous Drugs, and Chapter 50.

PHARMACOKINETICS. Complete absorption from GI tract after PO administration. Enters all body tissues and fluids, being retained in skin, muscle, liver, and kidney. Achieves steady state after 1 week. Metabolized in liver and undergoes enterohepatic circulation. Metabolites are excreted in urine for an extended period after drug is stopped.

SPECTRUM. *Mycobacterium leprae, M. lepraemurium, Leishmania, Pneumocystis.*

INDICATIONS. Leprosy, leishmaniasis, *Pneumocystis* pneumonia. Has been used to prevent systemic toxoplasmosis in immunosuppressed people.

APPROVED USES. Humans: leprosy and dermatitis herpetiformis.

CONTRAINDICATIONS. Previous hypersensitivity, anemia, pregnancy, lactation. Reduce dosage in renal failure.

ADVERSE REACTIONS. Dermatologic eruption, vomiting, diarrhea, anorexia, sulfone syndrome (dose-related hemolytic anemia, resulting from methemoglobinemia; especially with glucose-6-phosphate dehydrogenase deficiency), CNS signs, myelotoxicity, carcinogenic.

INTERACTIONS. Toxicity of dapsone and folate antagonists is increased when used in combination perhaps because of increased concentrations. Rifampin accelerates metabolism and removal of dapsone. Increased levels of both drugs occur when coadministered with trimethoprim. Dapsone should be combined with rifampin or clofazimine or another drug to treat mycobacterial infections and avoid resistance. It should be combined with pyrimethamine or trimethoprim to treat *Pneumocystis* pneumonia.

Availability	Type	Sizes	Preparation (Company)
Human	Oral tablets	25 mg, 100 mg	*Dapsone* (Jacobus)

INTERNATIONAL PREPARATIONS. *Aulosulfon, Disulone, Isoprodian, Maloprim.*

HANDLING. Tablets should be stored at room temperature away from light.

ADMINISTRATION. An oral suspension can be prepared by grinding tablets, putting in a sweet syrup, and adjusting pH to <5. Stable for 2 weeks if refrigerated. A proprietary liquid form is available (Jacobus) for investigational use.

DOSAGE

Indications (Mycobacteriosis)	Dose (mg/kg)	Route	Interval (hr)	Duration (days)
Dogs				
Initial	1.1	PO	6	Until remission
Maintenance	0.3	PO	8–12	After recovery
Cats	8.0	PO	24	6 weeks

ADDITIONAL DOSAGES. Opportunistic mycobacterial infections, Table 50–5.

DISPENSING INFORMATION. Avoid prolonged exposure of treated animals to sunlight because photosensitivity may develop.

DICLOXACILLIN

CLASS. Isoxazolyl penicillin.

ACTION. Bactericidal; inhibits bacterial cell wall synthesis.

MORE INFORMATION. See OXACILLIN, CLOXACILLIN; Chapter 34 and Table 34–1.

PHARMACOKINETICS. Partially absorbed (35%–70%) from GI tract after PO administration, which is reduced by ingesta. Well distributed to tissues and body fluids with exception of CNS and CSF.

SPECTRUM. *Staphylococcus,* including β-lactamase producers, other gram-positive aerobic cocci, some gram-positive anaerobes.

INDICATIONS. Staphylococcal infections, pyoderma.

CONTRAINDICATIONS. See OXACILLIN.

ADVERSE REACTIONS. See OXACILLIN.

INTERACTIONS. See OXACILLIN.

Availability	Type	Sizes	Preparations (Company)
Human	Oral capsules (as sodium)	125 mg, 250 mg, 500 mg	*Pathocil* (Wyeth), *Tegopen* (Bristol), generic (various)
	Oral powder for suspension (as sodium)	125 mg/5 ml	*Pathocil, Tegopen*

INTERNATIONAL PREPARATIONS. *Diclocil, Dicloxan, Diclocillin, Dynapen, Novapen.*

HANDLING. Store capsules and powder at controlled room temperature. Once reconstituted, oral solution is stable for 14 days when refrigerated, 7 days at room temperature.

ADMINISTRATION. Food interferes with absorption.

DOSAGE

Indications (Dogs and Cats)	Dose (mg/kg)	Route	Interval (hr)	Duration (days)
Localized soft tissue infections, staphylococcal pyoderma	10–25	PO	8	14–84
Problematic staphylococci, systemic infections, bacteremia	25–40	PO	8	7–14

DISPENSING INFORMATION. Give at least 1 hr before or 2 hr after feeding. Store oral suspension in refrigerator.

DIFLOXACIN

CLASS. Fluoroquinolone.

ACTION. Bactericidal, inhibits bacterial DNA gyrase.

MORE INFORMATION. See ENROFLOXACIN, MARBOFLOXACIN, ORBIFLOXACIN; Chapter 34; Table 34–11.

PHARMACOKINETICS. Bioavailability exceeds 80%. Active drug comprises 90% of plasma levels following oral or IV administration. Low plasma protein binding of 46% to 52%. Readily diffuses into tissues. Lipophilic with most (80%) elimination in biliary tract as glucuronide and only 5% excreted in urine. Undergoes enterohepatic circulation. Does not accumulate when a 24-hour interval of administration is used.

BODY FLUID/TISSUE DISTRIBUTION IN DOGS. After a single dose of 10 mg/kg PO (expressed as μg/ml or μg/g).

Body System	2 hours (n = 2)	6 hours (n = 1)	24 hours (n = 1)
Hematopoietic			
Whole Blood	2.3	1.1	0.6
Plasma	2.6	1.2	0.8
Bone	6.5	7.2	6.5
Lymph Node	3.1	2.5	1.7
Liver	10.7	7.8	4.6
Spleen	3.5	1.1	1.1
Urogenital			
Urine*	22.6	21.0	10.7
Kidney	5.0	2.8	1.5
Bladder Wall	3.0	1.8	1.7
Testes	3.1	1.6	0.8
Prostate	3.4	1.5	1.4
Gastrointestinal			
Stomach	66.7	8.5	9.9
Small intestine	18.3	38.7	16.4
Cardiopulmonary			
Lung	3.2	0.9	0.8
Heart	3.8	1.6	1.1
Other Tissues			
Muscle	4.1	1.2	1.1
Fat	0.7	0.8	0.8

*Based on percent of dose with urine output at 50 ml/kg/day.

SPECTRUM. **Gram positive:** *Staphylococcus.* **Gram negative:** *Escherichia, Pasteurella, Enterobacter, Pseudomonas, Proteus, Klebsiella.* **Anaerobes:** Not effective. **Others:** *Mycoplasma, Chlamydia, Rickettsia,* some opportunistic mycobacteria. **More Effective:** Anaerobic and facultative gram-negative organisms. **Ineffective:** *Enterococcus, Actinomyces, Nocardia, M. avium-intracellulare, Leptospira, Ehrlichia,* and obligate anaerobes.

INDICATIONS. Skin, soft tissue, and complicated or recurrent urinary infections. Alternative to aminoglycosides in presence of renal failure or when oral therapy is desired. See also ENROFLOXACIN.

APPROVED USES. Skin, soft tissue, and urinary infections in dogs.

CONTRAINDICATIONS. See ENROFLOXACIN.

ADVERSE REACTIONS. See ENROFLOXACIN.

INTERACTIONS. See ENROFLOXACIN.

Availability	Type	Sizes	Preparations (Company)
Veterinary (dogs)	Oral tablets (as hydrochloride)	11.4 mg; 45.4 mg; 136 mg	Dicural (Fort Dodge)

HANDLING. Store between 15°C and 30°C away from moisture.

ADMINISTRATION. See ENROFLOXACIN.

DOSAGE

Indications	Dose (mg/kg)	Route	Interval (hrs)	Duration (days)
Skin and soft tissue	5–10	PO	24	*

*Give for 2 to 3 days beyond resolution of clinical signs to a maximum of 30 days.

DISPENSING INFORMATION. See ENROFLOXACIN.

DIIODOHYDROXYQUIN

(See IODOQUINOL)

CLASS. 8-hydroxyquinoline.

ACTION. Antiprotozoal.

MORE INFORMATION. See IODOQUINOL.

DIMINAZENE ACETURATE

CLASS. Aromatic diamidine.

ACTION. See PENTAMIDINE.

MORE INFORMATION. See PENTAMIDINE, IMIDOCARB, AMICARBALIDE; Chapter 71 and Table 71–1; references: 71:8, 71:20, 71:26–29.

PHARMACOKINETICS. Not well absorbed orally. Rapid uptake after IV or IM administration, distributed extensively in tissues. Some hepatic metabolism with gradual urinary excretion of metabolites and active drug. Residues may persist for weeks in liver and kidneys, with lower amounts in GI tract, lungs, muscle, brain, fat, milk (71:27).

SPECTRUM. African *Trypanosoma, Babesia, Leishmania, Hepatozoon, Cytauxzoon;* some resistance may develop with repeated use.

INDICATIONS. African trypanosomiasis, babesiosis, cytauxzoonosis.

APPROVED USES. African trypanosomiasis in cattle.

CONTRAINDICATIONS. Pre-existing cardiomyopathy or heart failure.

ADVERSE REACTIONS. Less likely to produce acute anaphylaxis than other drugs in this class. Dosages up to 12 mg/kg are more effective in eliminating the organism but are more toxic. In general doses > 10 mg/kg should be avoided. Like other diamidines may produce CNS signs, including behavioral changes, nystagmus, ataxia, extensor rigidity, opisthotonus, sometimes death. Acute hemorrhagic gastroenteritis and cardiomyopathy have been reported. Delayed onset (1 week later) of CNS signs may relate to intracerebral killing of *Babesia*. Cats become anorectic, febrile, and depressed after initial treatment for cytauxzoon.

INTERACTIONS. For *T. congolense,* best response when combined with the experimental drug, difluoromethylornithine (DFMO), Hoechst Marion Roussel, Cincinnati, Ohio, (513)-948–7003 (71:26). Synergism against trypanosomes has also been observed with suramin. To prevent adverse reactions, antihistamines or nonsteroidal anti-inflammatory drugs (respectively, mepyramine maleate or piroxicam) have been used (71:29).

Availability	Type	Sizes	Preparations (Company)
Veterinary	Parenteral injection	Diluted to 70 mg/ml	Berenil (Bayer); not available in U.S.

INTERNATIONAL PREPARATIONS. *Azidine, Ganaseg, Ganasegur, Veriben.*

HANDLING. To ensure stability, should be kept refrigerated in sealed glass light-proof containers. At room temperature, solution is stable for at least 10–15 days. Lyophilized powder has an extended shelf-life for months at room temperature.

ADMINISTRATION. For *Babesia,* more effective treatment to eliminate resistant infections has been achieved by 3.5 mg/kg diminazene followed in 24 hr by 5 mg/kg imidocarb (71:28). Trypanosomes may disappear from the blood within 24 hr of treatment, but hematologic changes take at least 3 weeks to correct. CBC should be performed weekly. May have to repeat as needed if parasitemia recurs. Some suggest one or two additional daily treatments for resistant infections, but toxicity increases. Has been used topically to treat cutaneous leishmaniasis. Cats become more depressed, febrile, and anorectic after one injection presumably related to parasite death. A second injection is given after these signs subside.

DOSAGE

Indications	Dose (mg/kg)	Route	Interval (hr)	Duration (days)
Dogs				
African trypanosomiasis *(T. brucei brucei, T. congolense)*	7.0	IM	24	1
Babesiosis				
Babesia canis	3..5–5.0	IM, SC	24	1
Babesia gibsoni	7.5–10	IM, SC	24	1
Cats				
Cytauxzoonosis	2.0	IM, SC	96	*

*A second dose is given at an interval of 72–96 hr after the first injection or when adverse signs of the first injection subside.

ADDITIONAL DOSAGES. African trypanosomiasis, Table 72–1; hepatozoonosis, Table 74–2; cytauxzoonosis, Table 76–1, babesiosis, Table 77–3.

DOXYCYCLINE

CLASS. Tetracycline.

ACTION. Bacteriostatic; inhibits bacterial protein synthesis by binding 30s ribosomal unit.

MORE INFORMATION. MINOCYCLINE; TETRACYCLINE; Chapter 34; Table 34–7; references: 34:127, 34:138.

PHARMACOKINETICS. In presence of food, 93% absorption of PO dose; blood concentration after PO dose is equivalent to IV dose. More lipid soluble (five times) than tetracycline, allowing better GI absorption and good penetration into most tissues and body fluids, including difficult areas such as prostate, female reproductive tract, eye, CNS, lung, sputum, bile. Persists in respiratory and prostatic secretions. Crosses placenta to accumulate in fetal bone, teeth and enters milk. Penetrates well into nasal sinuses. Long half-life for a tetracycline, making twice-daily dosing feasible. Primary elimination into digestive tract by nonbiliary secretion as inactive compounds with up to 90% eliminated in feces. Has some biliary elimination with enterohepatic circulation. Approximately 20% appears in urine via glomerular filtration. Higher plasma protein binding in cats makes it less well distributed, and plasma concentrations are approximately twice those of dogs given the same dose (34:128).

SPECTRUM. **Gram positive:** few *Streptococcus*, few *Staphylococcus, Nocardia, Listeria, Bacillus.* **Gram negative:** *Bartonella, Brucella, Francisella, Pasteurella, Campylobacter, Helicobacter, Yersinia, Enterobacter, Klebsiella, Bordetella.* **Anaerobes:** *Clostridium, Fusobacterium, Actinomyces.* **Others:** *Haemobartonella, Chlamydia, Mycoplasma, Rickettsiae (Coxiella, Rickettsia, Ehrlichia),* Spirochetes *(Leptospira, Borrelia),* opportunistic rapid-growing mycobacteria, *M. avium-intracellulare* complex, *Entamoeba, Balantidium,* Coccidia, *Toxoplasma.* **More effective:** *Borrelia, Rickettsia, Leptospira.* **Ineffective:** *Proteus, Enterobacter, Klebsiella, Escherichia, Pseudomonas.* Gram-negative bacteria frequently develop resistance. Cross-resistance between other tetracyclines occurs.

INDICATIONS. Acute urinary infections, chronic prostatitis, respiratory tract infections, nasal and sinus infections, rickettsial diseases, borreliosis, chlamydial and mycoplasma infections, haemobartonellosis, tularemia, actinomycosis, nocardiosis, canine ehrlichiosis, borreliosis, Rocky Mountain spotted fever, leptospirosis, bartonellosis, intestinal amebiasis. Combined with aminoglycosides in treatment of brucellosis. Reduces severity of articular cartilage breakdown in various animal models of noninfectious arthritis (34:14), which questions the assumption that all doxycycline-responsive polyarthritis is infectious. In leptospirosis, has been used to clear the carrier state.

CONTRAINDICATIONS. Pregnancy, lactation, and young (< 6 mo of age before permanent tooth eruption; in pregnancy, can retard fetal skeletal development or be embryotoxic). Minimal dose adjustment needed with hepatic or renal failure. Unlike other tetracyclines, doxycycline does not accumulate in renal failure in dogs because it diffuses passively into the intestinal lumen (34:128). Therefore, it is the best tetracycline for use in an azotemic animal.

ADVERSE REACTIONS. Vomiting and GI irritation can be reduced by administering with food. Esophagitis and esophageal ulcers that form can be reduced by giving liquids after dosing and not giving to recumbent animals. May relate to formulation because capsules are more irritating than tablets or enteric coated preparations. The monohydrate salt is less acidic and ulcerogenic than the hydrochloride or hyclate formulations. Gastroenteritis can develop, especially in cats, but this drug is better tolerated than other tetracyclines in this species, causing less fever, anorexia, and vomiting compared with other tetracyclines. Because of more complete absorption, microfloral alterations and diarrhea are less frequent with other tetracyclines. Hypotension or vomiting may be observed with rapid IV infusion of doxycycline hyclate. Photosensitivity and skin eruptions may develop. Teeth and bone deposition and discoloration occur in young, but of all tetracyclines, doxycycline is least likely to have this effect. Diarrhea is less common than with tetracycline, presumably because of the better absorption and lower dosage needed with doxycycline. Hepatotoxicity can occur in dogs and cats after oral or parenteral therapy. Dramatic increases in serum alanine transaminase and alkaline phosphatase are noted. Thrombocytopenia, neutropenia, and eosinophilia have been observed in people, and neutropenia has been observed in dogs.

INTERACTIONS. GI absorption reduced by divalent and trivalent cations as found in iron preparations, aluminum hydroxide gels, sodium bicarbonate, bismuth subsalicylate, calcium, and magnesium salts. Having a high lipid solubility, it has less affinity for calcium binding as do other tetracyclines. Ingesta has relatively little effect on GI absorption. Half-life of anticonvulsants (phenobarbital, diphenylhydantoin) may be reduced, and these drugs reduce doxycycline serum concentrations. Rifampin may also increase clearance, lowering doxycycline efficacy. Interferes with activity of aminoglycosides, cephalosporins, penicillins. Renal failure can develop owing to calcium oxalate nephrolithiasis after methoxyflurane anesthesia.

Availability	Type	Sizes	Preparations (Company)
Human	Oral capsules or tablets (hyclate)	50 mg, 100 mg	*Doxychel* (Rachelle), *Vibramycin* (Pfizer), generic (various)
	Oral syrup (calcium)	50 mg/5 ml	*Vibramycin*
	Powder for oral suspension (monohydrate)	25 mg/5 ml	*Vibramycin*
	Powder for injection (hyclate)	100 mg, 200 mg	*Doxychel, Vibramycin* IV
Veterinary	Oral tablets	20 mg, 100 mg	*Ronaxan* (Rhone Merieux)
	Oral, gingival paste (for dogs)	Dispensing syringe	*Periodontal Disease Therapeutic* (Heska)

INTERNATIONAL PREPARATIONS. *Abadox, Biocyclin, Cyclidox, Diolan, Doxina, Doxydyn, Doxyhexal, Doxymycine, Dumoxin, Gewacyclin, Helvedoclyn, Rudocycline, Unacil.*

HANDLING. Parenteral hyclate solution is reconstituted with sterile water. Compatible when diluted to 1 mg/ml in 0.9% NaCl, 5% dextrose, Ringer's, and lactated Ringer's. Solutions of infusion fluids are generally stable for at least 12 hr at room temperature to 72 hr if refrigerated. Incompatible with solutions containing lidocaine, penicillin G, and piperacillin-tazobactam. Store tablets and capsules at room temperature in airtight light-proof containers. The PO suspension is stable at room temperature for 2 weeks.

ADMINISTRATION. This is the only tetracycline recommended for IV use, because it is less likely to cause thrombophlebitis or hepatic toxicity. For IV use, give as slow infusion over at least 1 hr in diluted form. Do not give IM or SC. Oral fluids, given at the time of medication, will reduce the effects of esophageal irritation and ulceration. Must avoid liquids containing polyvalent cations, which affect absorption. If gastric irritation occurs, give medication with food or milk, because the latter does not affect absorption of doxycycline as much as with other tetracyclines.

DOSAGE

Indications	Dose	Route	Interval (hr)	Duration (days)
Dogs				
General	3–5 mg/kg	PO	12	7–14
Soft tissue, urinary	4.4–11 mg/kg	PO, IV	12	7–14
Cats				
Haemobartonellosis	5–10 mg/kg	PO	24	7
Bartonellosis	50 mg/cat	PO	12	14–28
Systemic infection, bacteremia	5–11 mg/kg	PO, IV	12	prn

ADDITIONAL DOSAGES. Canine infectious tracheobronchitis, Table 6–1; salmon poisoning, Table 27–2; ehrlichiosis, Table 28–4; Rocky Mountain spotted fever, Table 29–3; Haemobartonellosis, Table 30–1; canine brucellosis, Table 40–2; leptospirosis, Table 44–4; Lyme borreliosis, Table 45–3; nocardiosis, Table 49–2; mycobacterial infections, Tables 50–4 and 50–5; feline abscesses, Table 52–2; feline bartonellosis, Table 54–3; hepatozoonosis, Table 74–2; babesiosis, Table 77–3; musculoskeletal infections, Tables 86–2 and 86–3; respiratory infections, Table 88–8; hepatobiliary disease, Table 90–4.

DISPENSING INFORMATION. May be given with food if necessary. Do not give with antacids, dairy products (less of a problem), iron supplements.

ENDOTOXIN ANTISERA

CLASS. Immunogloblin.

ACTION. Neutralizes gram-negative endotoxin.

MORE INFORMATION. Chapters 8, 38, and 100; references: 100:34, 100:114.

PHARMACOKINETICS. Enters systemic circulation at time of infusion.

SPECTRUM. *Salmonella typhimurium* antiserum of equine origin.

INDICATIONS. Canine or feline parvoviral diarrhea with signs of bacterial sepsis, gram-negative bacterial infections with endotoxemia.

APPROVED USES. Gram-negative endotoxemia.

CONTRAINDICATIONS. Younger than 8 weeks of age, use only once.

ADVERSE REACTIONS. Anaphylactic reactions likely after repeated administration. If anaphylactoid reaction occurs, administer epinephrine. A second administration is not indicated because the course of illness is limited.

INTERACTIONS. For adjunctive therapy, see Table 38–1.

INDICATIONS. Canine or feline endotoxemia or parvoviral infections with associated endotoxemia.

Availability	Type	Sizes	Preparations (Company)
Veterinary	Equine-origin antisera	50-ml bottles	*SEPTI-serum* (Imvac)

HANDLING. If refrigerated, 36-mo shelf-life. Use or dispose of entire contents once opened.

ADMINISTRATION. Warm solution to room (or preferably body) temperature before use. Given IV, diluted 1:1 with sterile isotonic saline or lactated Ringer's. Give only once over at least a 30-min period.

DOSAGE

Indications	Dose	Route	Interval (hr)	Duration (days)
Dogs and cats	4–8 mg/kg	IV	Once	1

ENILCONAZOLE

CLASS. Triazole.

ACTION. Antifungal. See KETOCONAZOLE.

MORE INFORMATION. See Chapters 57 and 65; Tables 57–1, 57–3; reference: 57:47.

PHARMACOKINETICS. Not absorbed from the GI tract after PO administration. Only used topically and not absorbed.

SPECTRUM. *Microsporum, Trichophyton, Aspergillus.*

INDICATIONS. Topical for dermatophytosis in dogs and for IN installation in dogs with nasal aspergillosis.

APPROVED USES. Dermatophytosis in dogs.

CONTRAINDICATIONS. Not recommended for use in cats owing to toxicity.

ADVERSE REACTIONS. Systemic reactions in cats. Oral ingestion during administration can cause salivation, inappetence, weight loss, increased hepatic enzymes. In conscious dogs with surgically implanted tubes, drooling, sneezing, head shaking may occur for 10–15 min with each flush.

Availability	Type	Size	Preparation (Company)
Veterinary	Topical solution (for ringworm in cattle, horses, and dogs)	100 mg/ml (10%)	Imaverol (Janssen); not licensed in U.S.

HANDLING. Concentrated solution diluted 1:50 with lukewarm water to produce 0.2% (2 mg/ml) emulsion. Do not discharge any into streams or untreated water supplies.

ADMINISTRATION. Dermatophytosis: remove crusts on diseased skin. Shave long-haired dogs. Apply diluted emulsion 3-day intervals for four treatments. **Aspergillosis surgical tube placement method:** under anesthesia, holes are drilled in the frontal sinuses and tubes inserted. Combine with turbinectomy initially or later if disease recurs. After anesthetic recovery, infuse 10 mg/kg of 10% solution, diluted 50:50 with sterile water, through tubes twice daily for 10 days. **Nonsurgical method:** see Chapter 65 for tube placement. Put dog under general anesthesia, take calculated diluted dose as just described, infuse equally into each nostril, and wait 30 min before anesthetic recovery. The nonsurgical method using enilconazole or clotrimazole has gained preference because of lower cost and noninvasive method.

DOSAGE

Indications	Dose	Route	Interval (hr)	Duration (days)
Dogs				
Nasal aspergillosis	10 mg/kg	Topically vial indwelling tubes	12	7–14

ADDITIONAL DOSAGES. Dermatophytosis, Table 58–4; aspergillosis, Table 65–3.

DISPENSING INFORMATION. For nasal flush with indwelling tubes, dilute dispensed solution volume for each dose 50:50 with provided water and infuse via syringe.

ENROFLOXACIN

CLASS. Fluoroquinolone.

ACTION. Bactericidal; inhibits bacterial DNA gyrase.

MORE INFORMATION. See CIPROFLOXACIN, DIFLOXACIN, MARBOFLOXACIN, ORBIFLOXACIN; Chapter 34; Table 34–11; references: 34:1, 34:3, 34:4.

PHARMACOKINETICS. Well absorbed from GI tract. Widely distributed in body tissues, including skeleton, CNS, CSF. Highest concentrations in liver, bile, kidney, genital tissues and secretions, urine (34:170). Penetrates and concentrates in macrophages, neutrophils. Carried to sites of inflammation and surrounding tissues and fluids. Concentrations in bone, lungs, prostate, kidneys are sufficient to affect aerobic and facultative gram-negative bacteria. High concentration in saliva, genital, nasal, bronchial secretions. Adequate concentrations in CNS and CSF are only reached at higher doses or with inflamed meninges. Ciprofloxacin, the major metabolite of enrofloxacin, achieves prostatic concentrations 30 times that in blood (34:3). Compared with ciprofloxacin, tissue enrofloxacin concentrations are often higher than in blood owing to less protein binding, high tissue penetration, extended serum half-life. Concentrations in skin exceed those in blood after several days of therapy and are suitable to treat dermal staphylococcal isolates (34:151). Predominate routine of excretion is renal with up to 50% unchanged. The remainder is metabolized to less active compounds and to active ciprofloxacin with biliary (fecal) and renal excretion (34:84). Distribution in the body: enrofloxacin penetrates into all canine and feline tissues and body fluids. Concentrations of drug equal to or greater than the minimal inhibitory concentration (MIC) for many pathogens (see following table) are reached in most tissues by 2 hr after dosing at 2.5 mg/kg and are maintained for 8–12 hr after dosing. Particularly high levels of enrofloxacin are found in urine. A summary of the body fluid–tissue drug levels at 2–12 hr after dosing at 2.5 mg/kg is given in Table (part 3).

BODY FLUID–TISSUE DISTRIBUTION OF ENROFLOXACIN (POSTTREATMENT) IN DOGS AND CATS FOR USE WITH MIC DATA FROM ISOLATED ORGANISMS (SINGLE ORAL DOSE = 2.5 mg/kg [1.13 mg/lb])*

	Canine (n = 2)		Feline (n = 4)	
Variable	**2 hr**	**8 hr**	**2 hr**	**12 hr**
Body Fluids (μg/ml)				
Bile	—	—	2.13	1.97
Cerebrospinal fluid	—	—	0.37	0.10
Urine	43.05	55.35	12.81	26.41
Eye fluids	0.53	0.66	0.45	0.65
Whole blood	1.01	0.36	—	—
Plasma	0.67	0.33	—	—
Serum	—	—	0.48	0.18
Tissues (μg/g) Hematopoietic System				
Liver	3.02	1.36	1.84	0.37
Spleen	1.45	0.85	1.33	0.52
Bone marrow	2.10	1.22	1.68	0.64
Lymph node	1.32	0.91	0.49	0.21
Urogenital System				
Kidney	1.87	0.99	1.43	0.37
Bladder wall	1.36	0.98	1.16	0.55
Testes	1.36	1.10	1.01	0.28
Prostate	1.36	2.20	1.88	0.55
Ovaries	—	—	0.78	0.56
Uterine wall	1.59	0.29	0.81	1.05
Gastrointestinal and Cardiopulmonary Systems				
Lung	1.34	0.82	0.91	0.33
Heart	1.88	0.78	0.84	0.32
Stomach	3.24	2.16	3.26	0.27
Small intestine	2.10	1.11	2.72	0.40
Large intestine	—	—	0.94	1.10

Variable	Canine (n = 2)		Feline (n = 4)	
	2 hr	8 hr	2 hr	12 hr
Other				
Fat	0.52	0.40	0.24	0.11
Skin	0.66	0.48	0.46	0.17
Muscle	1.62	0.77	0.53	0.29
Brain	0.25	0.24	0.22	0.12
Mammary Gland	0.45	0.21	0.36	0.30
Feces	1.65	9.97	0.37	4.18

*Data provided by product insert.

SPECTRUM. **Gram positive:** *Staphylococcus,* variable *Streptococcus.* **Gram negative:** *Brucella, Pasteurella, Escherichia, Aeromonas, Proteus, Shigella, Salmonella,* and other enteropathogens such as *Campylobacter, Yersinia,* and some *Pseudomonas.* **Anaerobes:** not effective. **Others:** *Mycoplasma, Chlamydia, Rickettsia, Haemobartonella,* some slow-growing, opportunistic mycobacteria (see Chapter 50). **More effective:** aerobic and facultative gram-negative organisms. **Ineffective:** *Enterococcus, Actinomyces, Nocardia, Mycobacterium avium-intracellulare* complex, *Leptospira, Ehrlichia,* and obligate anaerobes. Resistance can develop by chromosomal mutation, although plasmid-mediated resistance does not occur.

INDICATIONS. Complicated or recurrent urinary tract infections caused by more resistant gram-negative bacteria; prostatitis. Good alternative to aminoglycoside in presence of renal dysfunction. Respiratory infections from resistant gram-negative bacteria (often nosocomial). Osteomyelitis and joint infections because quinolones have good penetration and safety for long-term use in gram-negative infections. With staphylococcal osteomyelitis, additions of rifampin may assist. Complicated SC infections caused by *Staphylococcus,* gram negatives, or opportunistic mycobacteria. Always use in combination for treating brucellosis. For severe otitis externa caused by *Pseudomonas.* For enteropathogenic bacterial gastroenteritis (e.g., salmonellosis or campylobacteriosis; see Chapter 39) (34:135). GI infections caused by gram-negative bacteria, urinary tract infections, respiratory tract infections, infections of skin, eyes, and joints (34:135) and canine bacterial pyoderma (34:70, 34:119). Can be used topically (see Handling) for resistant gram-negative otitis externa to avoid aminoglycoside toxicity). Fluoroquinolones in combination have been shown to improve in vivo efficacy of some antifungal azoles.

CONTRAINDICATIONS. During rapid growth period, young animals should not receive the drug because of the potential of cartilaginous injury. Avoid in small- and medium-breed dogs (> 8 mo), large breeds (< 12 mo), and giant breeds (< 18 mo), and cats younger than 8 weeks. Some reduction in dosage is advised for marked renal failure, but hepatic elimination should compensate in minor renal dysfunction. Caution is advised with quinolones in pregnant animals, although side effects are not documented. Dosages of 15 mg/kg to males and to females of various stages of gestation and during lactation had no adverse effects. Animals being treated must always be adequately hydrated. Use cautiously in animals with seizure histories.

ADVERSE REACTIONS. Vomiting when IM solution is given IV. Intravascular hemolysis has been observed in some cats given parenteral solution IM or undiluted parenteral solution IV. Diarrhea and depression are occasionally seen in dogs (34:85), especially with higher dosages. Neurotoxicity or seizures at very high (supratherapeutic) IV dosages or with rapid IV infusion. In animals with seizures history, causes increase in the frequency and intensity of seizures in phenobarbital-treated dogs (34:170). Cats receiving 50 mg/kg have had neurologic signs, and some dogs receiving 10 mg/kg enrofloxacin have had seizures. Nonsteroidal anti-inflammatory drugs (e.g., fenbufen) may accentuate this problem. Occasional anorexia, vomiting, or diarrhea, especially with higher dosages. Cartilaginous damage to weight-bearing joints of immature growing dogs and cats. IM and SC injections are painful. Focal alopecia may occur over sites of SC injection. Efficacy in treating urinary tract infections can be enhanced by raising the urine pH with bicarbonate, but this may favor nephrotoxicity from renal tubular crystalluria. Because of the potential for renal dysfunction with overdosages, hydration should be maintained. Streptococcal superinfection with necrotizing fasciitis has been observed in dogs receiving prior treatment with enrofloxacin (see Chapter 35).

INTERACTIONS. Additive antibacterial effects with doxycycline, minocycline, or aminoglycosides for brucellosis. For leprosy or opportunistic mycobacteriosis, may be synergistic with dapsone or clofazimine. The coadministration of clindamycin or amoxicillin with quinolones results in increased serum bactericidal activity against gram-positive bacteria. Use of metronidazole and clindamycin do not affect pharmacokinetics of quinolones (34:9). Reduced GI absorption caused by preparations containing polyvalent cations (Al, Mg, Ca, Fe, Zn). Antacids containing these and sucralfate given within 24 hr can interfere with absorption (34:120). Concurrent cimetidine can delay quinolone elimination. May interfere with theophylline elimination, producing CNS signs. May potentiate effects of vitamin K antagonist rodenticides. The effectiveness of quinolones is reduced by protein-synthesis inhibitors such as chloramphenicol, rifampin, and erythromycin. Enrofloxacin and digoxin do not alter either drug's metabolism when coadministered to dogs (34:114).

Availability	Type	Sizes	Preparations (Company)
Veterinary	Tablets	5.7 mg, 22.7 mg, 68 mg	Baytril (Bayer)
	Parenteral solution for IM use	22.7 mg/ml	Baytril

HANDLING. Parenteral solution should be stored away from direct sunlight and never frozen. For topical otic preparation, take one 22.7-mg tablet and crush it with a mortar and pestle. Add powder to petrolatum and mix well with tongue depressor. Place mixture in syringe and administer in ear canals at least once daily.

ADMINISTRATION. Can give in combination with doxycycline, minocyclines, aminoglycosides, or rifampin to improve efficacy in certain disorders. Allow 4–6 hr between giving antacid, cation-containing preparations, or sucralfate and quinolones. Ingesta may delay absorption slightly, but may prevent vomiting that occasionally occurs. Preferably, administer on empty stomach. Always administer slowly IV, over at least 5 min, to avoid seizures. The manufacturer's suggested maximum duration of treatment is 10 days. An IV preparation is not available; however, some have given the IM solution IV. Dilute 1 part parenteral solution to 9 parts sterile water before IV infusion and give it over 10 min.

DOSAGE

Infection Indications/Site (Dogs and Cats)	Dose	Route	Interval (hr)	Duration (days)
Urinary infections (cats)	5.7 mg/cat	PO	12	7–14
Skin, urinary infections	2.5–5 mg/kg	PO	12	7–14
Skin, urinary, respiratory infections	5 mg/kg	PO	24	7–14
Skin infections (deep, refractory pyoderma)	10 mg/kg	PO	12–24	7–84
Prostate infections	5 mg/kg	PO	12	7–14
Haemobartonellosis	5 mg/kg	PO, IM	12	7–14
Systemic, orthopedic infections	5–11 mg/kg	PO, IM, IV, SC	12	10
Pseudomonas in tissues	11 mg/kg	PO, IM	12	7–14
Bacteremia, sepsis	11–15 mg/kg	PO, IM, IV, SC	8–12	prn

ADDITIONAL DOSAGES. Rocky Mountain spotted fever, Table 29–3; gram-negative infections, Table 37–2; endotoxemia, Table 38–1; enteric pathogenic bacteria, Table 39–1; leptospirosis, Table 44–4; mycobacteria, Tables 50–4 and 50–5; cytauxzoonosis, Table 76–1; canine pyoderma, Table 85–3; musculoskeletal infections, Table 86–3; bacteremia, endocarditis, Table 87–7; respiratory disease, Table 88–8; oral infections, Table 89–4; gastrointestinal infections, Table 89–11; intra-abdominal infections, Table 89–15; hepatobiliary infections, Table 90–4; urinary infections, Table 91–8.

DISPENSING INFORMATION. Give medication without feeding, unless vomiting occurs. Never give antacids or GI protectants within 2 hr of medication. Always be certain pet has plenty of fresh water to drink.

ERYTHROMYCIN

CLASS. Macrolide.

ACTION. Bacteriostatic; binds to 50s ribosomes of bacteria-inhibiting protein synthesis.

MORE INFORMATION. AZITHROMYCIN, CLARITHROMYCIN, ROXITHROMYCIN; Chapter 34, Macrolides; Table 34–8.

PHARMACOKINETICS. Several oral formulations exist. The degree of absorption from the GI tract depends on the formulation, gastric pH, presence of ingesta (see Table 34–8). Erythromycin is absorbed in the proximal small intestine and must withstand effects of gastric acid. Estolate and ethylsuccinate compounds resist degradation in the stomach and release free base for absorption in duodenum. Estolate is better absorbed than ethylsuccinate. Enteric-coated tablets required for free base and stearate formulations to prevent gastric acid inactivation. Unlike estolate and ethylsuccinate esters, absorption of the base and stearate are reduced by ingesta. Absorption of coated base tablets is less affected by food than stearate. Enteric-coated pellets are better absorbed than tablets. Well distributed to most body tissues, especially skin and respiratory tract, enters pleural and ascitic fluids, respiratory secretions but only the inflamed meninges. Enters the prostate and concentrates in leukocytes. Primarily eliminated by hepatic metabolism and biliary excretion. Does not achieve high enough levels in urine for likely therapeutic efficacy (4% of oral and 15% of parenteral dose). Bioavailability is lower by SC (40%) than IM (65%) routes.

SPECTRUM. **Gram positive:** *Staphylococcus, Streptococcus, Corynebacterium, Listeria, Erysipelothrix, Bacillus.* Predominantly for gram-positive infections. **Gram negative:** *Pasteurella, Campylobacter, Bordetella, Legionella.* Not for most gram-negative infections. Cross-resistance can occur with other macrolides and lincosamides. **Anaerobes:** *Fusobacterium, Clostridium* (limited activity). **Others:** *Chlamydia, Mycoplasma* (susceptibility varies), *Borrelia, Leptospira;* protozoa, e.g., amebae. **More effective:** *Campylobacter, Legionella, Mycoplasma.* **Ineffective:** most Enterobacteriaceae.

INDICATIONS. Gram-positive infections involving the GI tract, skin, respiratory tract, soft tissue infections as an alternative to β-lactams (e.g., penicillins, first-generation cephalosporins) when hypersensitivity exists. Campylobacteriosis.

CONTRAINDICATIONS. Previous hypersensitivity, pre-existing hepatic dysfunction, reduce dose in severe liver diseases, minimal dosage adjustment in renal failure.

ADVERSE REACTIONS. Vomiting—specific cholinergic effect. Abdominal discomfort or GI irritability—anorexia, vomiting, diarrhea. Can occur with parenteral preparations because of excretion in the bile. Thrombophlebitis with IV; pain on IM injection; rare ototoxicity; and hepatotoxicity (cholestatic hepatitis). The latter syndrome can be reduced in frequency of occurrence by shorter treatment regimens.

INTERACTIONS. Chloramphenicol and lincosamides (lincomycin, clindamycin) have similar action and should not be used in combination. Increases cyclosporin concentrations with resultant nephrotoxicity. Increases blood digoxin, methylprednisolone, theophylline concentrations, and other hepatic metabolized drugs as a result of cytochrome P-450 interactions.

Availability	Type	Sizes	Preparations (Company)
Human	Base oral tablets, enteric coated	250 mg, 333 mg, 500 mg	*E-mycin* (Pharmacia & Upjohn), *Ilotycin* (Dista)
	Estolate oral tablets	500 mg	*Ilosone* (Dista)
	Oral capsules, chewable tablets	125 mg, 250 mg	*Ilosone*
	Oral suspension	125 mg/5 ml, 250 mg/5 ml	*Ilosone*
	Stearate oral tablets, enteric coated	250 mg, 500 mg	*Erpar* (Parke-Davis), *Erythril* (E.R. Squibb), generic (various)
	Ethylsuccinate		
	Oral tablets	200 mg (125 mg base), 400 mg (250 mg base)	E.E.S generic (various), *E-Mycin E* (Pharmacia & Upjohn)
	Oral suspension or powder for suspension	100 mg/5 ml, 62.5 mg/5 ml, 200 mg/ 5 ml (125 mg/5 ml base), 400 (250 mg/5 ml base)	*Eryped* (Abbott), *Pediamycin* (Ross)
	Gluceptate IV solution	250 mg, 500 mg, 1 g	*Ilotycin Gluceptate* (Dista)
	Lactobionate IV infusion	500 mg, 1 g	*Erythrocin Lactobionate-IV* (Abbott)
Veterinary	Polyethylene injectable solution	100 mg/ml, 200 mg/ml	*Erythro* (Sanofi), *Erythromycin–200* (RXV)

INTERNATIONAL PREPARATIONS. *Abboticine, Aknemycin, Betamycin, Cusimicina, Doranol, Eboren, Erycinum, Erythromid, Erytran, Erytrocina, Meromycin, Primacine, Stiemycin.*

HANDLING. Lactobionate is stable at room temperature in dry form. Parenteral solutions are stable at room temperature Cold temperature may cause solidification, which can be reversed by immersion in warm water for 15–20 min. Once reconstituted the lactobionate is stable for 24 hr and 2 weeks, and the gluceptate for 24 hr and 1 week, at room and refrigerated temperatures, respectively. Erythromycin solutions are more unstable at acid pH (4.0–6.0). Oral suspensions (estolate, ethylsuccinate) should be refrigerated and generally have 14-day stability.

ADMINISTRATION. Given PO, administer on an empty stomach (base and stearate forms) unless GI upset occurs, then take with food. Estolate, ethylsuccinate, and enteric-coated forms can be taken with food. Capsules containing enteric-coated pellets *ERYC* (Parke-Davis) can be opened and sprinkled on food. Ethylsuccinate is nonirritating, tasteless, and suitable as a PO preparation for puppies and kittens. Dilute IV solutions given over 20–60 min. Give slowly IV by intermittent or continuous infusion using concentrations diluted to 1 to 5 mg/ml. IV route is preferred for very ill animals or those with GI signs. If given IM, must be deep into large muscles. IM preparations contain lidocaine. Should not be given SC or IP.

DOSAGE

Indications (Dogs and Cats)	Dose (mg/kg)	Route	Interval (hr)	Duration (days)
Localized, soft tissue infections	15–25	PO	12	7–10
Localized, soft tissue infeicitons	10–15	PO	8	7–10
Systemic, bacteremia infecions	22	PO, IV	8	prn

ADDITIONAL DOSAGES. Streptococcal infections, Table 35–2; *Rhodococcus* infection, Table 35–6; enteric bacterial infections, Table 39–1; actinomycosis, Table 49–1; nocardiosis, Table 49–2; canine pyoderma, Table 85–3; gastrointestinal infections, Table 89–11; local ocular treatment, Table 93–4.

DISPENSING INFORMATION. May cause GI irritation and resultant vomiting and diarrhea. If so, give first few doses with food to reduce irritation but then give to fasted animal.

ETHAMBUTOL

CLASS. Synthetic antimycobacterial.

ACTION. Inhibits intracellular metabolism of mycobacterial cells.

MORE INFORMATION. See Tuberculosis, Chapter 50; Table 50–4.

PHARMACOKINETICS. Readily absorbed from GI tract and 80% bioavailable, unaffected by food. Diffuses into tissues and fluids, including the CSF, with inflamed meninges. A lower percentage is metabolized by liver, and some is excreted in feces; most is excreted in urine as unchanged drug and metabolites.

SPECTRUM. *Mycobacterium tuberculosis, M. bovis, M. avium-intracellulare* complex.

INDICATIONS. Tuberculosis caused by *M. tuberculosis* or *M. bovis* in combination with other antimycobacterial drugs.

CONTRAINDICATIONS. Reduce dose by extending interval of dose administration in renal insufficiency. Has caused teratogenesis in laboratory animals during pregnancy.

ADVERSE REACTIONS. In people, reduced visual acuity from optic neuritis; anorexia, vomiting, abdominal pain, CNS signs, and thrombocytopenia.

INTERACTIONS. Often combined with isoniazid, rifampin, pyrazinamide, or aminoglycosides for tuberculosis. For *M. avium-intracellulare* complex infections, may be given in combination with fluoroquinolones, azithromycin or clarithromycin, aminoglycosides, rifampin, or clofazimine.

Availability	Type	Sizes	Preparation (Company)
Human	Oral tablets	100 mg, 400 mg	*Myambutol* (Lederle)

INTERNATIONAL PREPARATIONS. *Afimocil, Cidanbutol, Dexambutol, Etapiam, Servambutol.*

HANDLING. Keep in airtight containers at controlled room temperature, protected from moisture, heat, and light. Can mix with water and heat to 49°C for 10 min to dissolve and then put in suspension, which can be refrigerated for 1 week.

ADMINISTRATION. Aluminum-containing compounds reduce absorption. Administering with food reduces GI irritation. Use only in combination with other antimycobacterial drugs.

DOSAGE

Indications	Dose (mg/kg)	Route	Interval (hr)	Duration (mo)
Dogs	15	PO	24	3–6
	25	PO	72	3–6*

*Long-term suppressive therapy may be needed.

ADDITIONAL DOSAGES. Tuberculosis, Table 50–4.

DISPENSING INFORMATION. This medicine can be given with food.

FENBENDAZOLE

CLASS. Benzimidazole.

ACTION. Antihelminthic, antiprotozoal.

MORE INFORMATION. Chapter 71; Table 71–1; Reference: 71:2.

PHARMACOKINETICS. Minimal amount absorbed following oral administration, and any absorbed drug is rapidly metabolized. Administration with food, irrespective of fat content, increases its bioavailability. A majority of the drug is excreted unchanged in the feces, and minimal amounts (<1%) of the administered dose appear in the urine.

SPECTRUM. *Giardia;* in addition to approved uses, it is effective against various intestinal helminths and *Capillaria aerophila, Filaroides hirthi,* and *Paragonimus kellicotti.*

INDICATIONS. Helminths, *Giardia.*

APPROVED USES. For control of ascarids *(Toxocara canis, Toxascaris leonina),* hookworms *(Ancylostoma caninum, Uncinaria stenocephala),* whipworms *(Trichuris vulpis),* and tapeworms *(Taenia pisiformis)* in dogs.

CONTRAINDICATIONS. Unknown. Has been safe when administered to cats and pregnant animals.

ADVERSE REACTIONS. Unusual; vomiting occurs uncommonly when given with food. Other drugs of this class have been reported to cause hepatotoxicity. With large burdens of helminths, allergic reactions to dying tissue forms may be noted.

INTERACTIONS. Myelotoxicity was reported with coadministration of trimethoprim-sulfonamide in one dog. It was reversible after treatment was discontinued.

Availability	Type	Sizes	Preparations (company)
Dog	Oral granules 22.2%, packets or jar	1 g; 2 g; 4 g; 1-lb jar	Panacur (Hoechst Marion Roussel)
Horse	Oral granules 22.2%, packets	5.2 g	Panacur
	Paste 10%	25-g syringe	Panacur
Cattle and horse	Oral paste 10%	92-g syringe	Panacur
	Oral suspension 10%	1 liter	Panacur
Cattle	Oral paste 10%	290-g syringe	Panacur
	Oral suspension 10%	1 gallon	Panacur

HANDLING. Product should be stored away from moisture at a controlled (15–30°C) temperature.

ADMINISTRATION. For a dose of 50 mg/kg, use 1 g of packet granules for each 10 lb of body weight. Mix the correct amount of granules with a small amount of the usual diet. If dry food is fed, add water to facilitate mixing with the drug. To be effective, the drug must be administered for a minimum of 3 days. Treatment for more resistant protozoa or helminths continues for up to 14 days.

DOSAGE

Indications	Dose (mg/kg)	Route	Interval (hrs)	Duration (days)
Helminths, *Giardia*	50	PO	24	3

ADDITIONAL DOSAGES. Giardiasis, Table 78–2.

DISPENSING INFORMATION. Place amount indicated on canned pet food or moistened dry food. Make sure all the drug is taken by withholding other food until it is eaten.

FLORFENICOL

CLASS. Acetamide.

ACTION. Binds to 50s ribosome of bacteria-inhibiting protein synthesis.

MORE INFORMATION. See CHLORAMPHENICOL; Chapter 34.

PHARMACOKINETICS. Similar to chloramphenicol.

SPECTRUM. See CHLORAMPHENICOL.

INDICATIONS. See CHLORAMPHENICOL.

CONTRAINDICATIONS. Pregnancy.

ADVERSE REACTIONS. Chemical modification of this drug has alleviated the myelotoxic effect, although toxicity studies are not available for dogs and cats. Also not associated with human myelotoxicity. Can be locally irritating to animals when administered or to mucosae of sensitive people inadvertently contacting the drug.

INTERACTIONS. See CHLORAMPHENICOL.

INDICATIONS. Systemic bacterial or rickettsial infections when potential myelotoxicity in animals or people is to be avoided.

Availability	Type	Sizes	Preparation (Company)
Veterinary (cattle)	Parenteral solution 300 mg/ml	100, 250, and 500 ml	*Nuflor* (Schering-Plough Animal Health)

HANDLING. Can be stored between 2°C and 30°C, although refrigeration is not necessary. Color is pale yellow and does not affect patency.

ADMINISTRATION. Can be given IM or SC; the former may cause pain and irritation.

DOSAGE

Indications	Dose (mg/kg)	Route	Interval (hr)	Duration (days)
Dogs				
Systemic infections	25–50*	IM, SC	8	3–5
Cats				
Systemic infections	25–50*	IM, SC	12	3–5

*Extrapolated from dosages for chloramphenicol.

ADDITIONAL DOSAGES. Canine distemper, Table 3–5.

FLUCONAZOLE

CLASS. Bis-triazole.

ACTION. Antifungal; inhibits sterol and cytochrome P-450 synthesis.

MORE INFORMATION. See KETOCONAZOLE, ITRACONAZOLE; Chapter 57; Table 57–1; references: 57:7, 57:18, 57:22.

PHARMACOKINETICS. High bioavailability, > 90% systemic availability after IV or PO administration. GI absorption is unaffected by food intake or changes in gastric acidity caused by cimetidine or antacids containing magnesium or aluminum (57:50). In people, reaches effective tissue concentrations by 5–10 doses, which is 5–10 days with once-daily dosing or by 2 days if loading with twice the recommended dose is used the first day. Penetrates all body cavities and tissues, including eye and CNS. Sites having concentrations equal to or exceeding those in blood are skin, urine, skin blister fluids, nails, saliva, sputum, reproductive tissues. Penetration into CSF is 50%–90% of plasma levels independent of inflammation. Primarily eliminated (80%) by renal excretion of active drug (57:7, 57:22).

SPECTRUM. *Cryptococcus, Candida, Blastomyces, Histoplasma, Coccidioides;* variable against *Aspergillus*, dermatophytes.

INDICATIONS. Systemic fungal infections involving difficult-to-reach tissues (e.g., CNS). Blastomycosis, coccidioidomycosis, histoplasmosis, cryptococcosis, especially for cryptococcal infections of the brain, spinal cord, or eye. Nasal aspergillosis. Higher doses, if tolerated, may improve therapeutic efficacy.

APPROVED USES. Human: for treatment of esophageal candidiasis and maintenance therapy of cryptococcal meningitis and for treatment failures of candidiasis.

CONTRAINDICATIONS. Reduce dose in renal failure; avoid in pregnancy.

ADVERSE REACTIONS. See also KETOCONAZOLE. Can cause vomiting, diarrhea, abdominal discomfort. Dermal eruptions, hepatotoxicity (elevated transaminases, cholestasis, hepatitis, hepatic failure). Hepatotoxicity is much less frequent than with ketoconazole. Does not suppress adrenal or sex hormones like ketoconazole. Alopecia, dry skin and mucosae, and dizziness have been reported only in people.

INTERACTIONS. Cimetidine interferes with absorption. Fluconazole increases concentrations of thiazide diuretics, rifampin, cyclosporine, glipizide, antihistamines, diphenylhydantoin, and theophylline. Potentiates bleeding caused by anticoagulant rodenticides.

Availability	Type	Sizes	Preparations (Company)
Human	Oral tablets	50 mg, 100 mg, 150 mg, 200 mg	*Diflucan* (Pfizer)
	Powder for oral suspension	10 mg/ml, 40 mg/ml reconstituted	*Diflucan*
	Parenteral injection	2 mg/ml	*Diflucan*

INTERNATIONAL PREPARATIONS. *Biozolene, Elazor, Fungata, Lavisa, Loitin, Triflucan.*

HANDLING. Keep tablets at controlled room temperature in airtight containers. PO suspension: store powder at room temperature and dilute in distilled water; shake before using. Store reconstituted suspension between refrigerated and room temperature up to 2 weeks. Parenteral injection should be stored at room or refrigerator temperature. Do not add anything or freeze.

ADMINISTRATION. Give twice calculated daily dose for the first day of treatment. Give for 2–3 days if rapidly advancing or severe disseminated mycosis. IV solution should be given over 1–2 hr. Often treat neurologic or ocular cryptococcosis for at least 12 weeks or for 2 weeks after CSF examination shows resolution of inflammation and antigen test results on serum and CSF are negative. The best therapeutic response in CNS cryptococcosis of cats is with the 200 mg/cat/day dosages (57:7).

DOSAGE

Indications	Dose	Route	Interval (hr)	Duration (days)
Dogs				
Cryptococcosis, candidiasis	2.5–5 mg/kg	PO, IV	24	56–84
Meningitis	2.5–5.0 mg/kg	PO, IV	12	56–84
	5.0–10 mg/kg	PO, IV	24	56–84
Systemic mycoses	2.5–5.0 mg/kg	PO	24	8–12
Nasal aspergillosis	1.25–2.5 mg/kg	PO	12	56
Cats				
Nasal or dermal cryptococcosis	2.5–10 mg/kg	PO	12	*
	25 mg/cat	PO	12	*
	50 mg/cat	PO	24	*
CNS, cryptococcosis	50–100 mg/cat	PO	12	*
Systemic or CNS infection	50 mg/cat	PO	8	*
	150–200 mg/cat	PO	24	*

*Treatment should continue until antigen testing results of blood or CSF (with CNS disease) are negative.

ADDITIONAL DOSAGES. Blastomycosis, Table 59–1; histoplasmosis, Table 60–1; cryptococcosis, Table 61–4; coccidioidomycosis, Table 62–3; nasal aspergillosis, Table 65–3; candidiasis and trichosporonosis, Table 66–2; protothecosis, Table 69–1.

DISPENSING INFORMATION. This medication can be given with food.

FLUCYTOSINE

CLASS. Fluorinated pyrimidine.

ACTION. Antifungal; converted by specific enzyme in fungal cells to metabolites like 5-fluorouracil that interfere with fungal thymidylate synthase and resultant DNA and RNA synthesis.

MORE INFORMATION. See Chapter 57; Table 57–1.

PHARMACOKINETICS. Well absorbed from GI tract and widely distributed in tissues and body fluids, including joints, peritoneal fluid, and aqueous humor. CSF concentration is 70%–90% that in serum. Only 4% absorbed drug being metabolized, 80%–90% is excreted unchanged in urine.

SPECTRUM. *Candida, Cryptococcus.* Some effect against *Aspergillus.* Always used in combination with amphotericin B. Resistance may develop during treatment. **Ineffective:** filamentous fungi and dermatophytes.

INDICATIONS. Serious (disseminated) infections with *Candida* or *Cryptococcus* such as sepsis, endocarditis, meningitis.

APPROVED USES. In combination therapy for systemic yeast infections.

CONTRAINDICATIONS. Reduce dose or avoid in renal failure. Avoid with pre-existing myelosuppression, pregnancy, or in neonates.

ADVERSE REACTIONS. Myelosuppression (leukopenia, thrombocytopenia), teratogenic in laboratory animals. Renal failure, crystalluria, dermal eruptions, vomiting, diarrhea, abdominal pain, hepatotoxicity (cholestatic hepatitis—icterus and increased liver enzymes), CNS signs. Converted by GI flora to 5-fluorouracil, which can be toxic when absorbed producing myelosuppression or enterocolitis.

INTERACTIONS. Synergistic with amphotericin B, but renal toxicity of both drugs is enhanced.

Availability	Types	Sizes	Preparation (Company)
Human	Oral capsules	250 mg, 500 mg	*Ancobon* (Roche)

INTERNATIONAL PREPARATIONS. *Alcobon, Ancotil.*

HANDLING. Store capsules in airtight, light-proof containers at controlled room temperature.

ADMINISTRATION. Food may slow but not reduce drug absorption after PO administration. Repeatedly monitor hemogram, renal and hepatic test results every 2 weeks during treatment. Assess renal function at least twice a week if amphotericin B is also used.

DOSAGE

Indications (Dogs and Cats)	Dose (mg/kg)	Route	Interval (hr)	Duration (days)
Cryptococcosis, candidiasis*	25–50	PO	6	42
	50–65	PO	8	42
Cryptococcosis*	50	PO	6	42

*Must give in combination with a polyene or azole antifungal drug.

ADDITIONAL DOSAGES. Cryptococcosis, Table 61–4; CNS infections, Table 92–5.

DISPENSING INFORMATION. Monitor animal for any GI signs or bruising tendencies.

FOSCARNET SODIUM (PHOSPHONOFORMATE)

CLASS. Pyrophosphate analog.

ACTION. Antiviral; inhibits replication of all known herpesviruses. Inhibits virus-specific DNA and RNA polymerases and reverse transcriptases at concentrations that do not affect those in cells.

MORE INFORMATION. See Chapter 2; Table 2–1; references: 2:18, 2:23.

PHARMACOKINETICS. PO bioavailability 35% in cats, 10% in dogs. A derivative (thiofoscarnet) has higher PO bioavailability (2:22). IV route produces higher concentrations and is preferred for systemic therapy. At physiologic pH, it is ionized and has limited cellular penetration. Penetrates CSF (40% of blood concentration) with some accumulation in bone from where it is eliminated slowly. Drug undergoes little metabolism and is excreted mainly unchanged in urine. Clearance from plasma in young cats is quicker than in older cats (2:23).

SPECTRUM. DNA viruses and RNA viruses, including retroviruses. Most effective against herpesviruses.

INDICATIONS. Herpesvirus infections, retroviral infections. Acyclovir-resistant herpesvirus infections.

APPROVED USES. Human: cytomegalovirus retinitis in AIDS patients.

CONTRAINDICATIONS. Renal failure. Use caution in pregnant and lactating animals owing to potential for fetotoxicity and damage to bones and teeth of young animals.

ADVERSE REACTIONS. Nephrotoxicity; must monitor renal function during therapy. Renal dysfunction is evident in most people after 2 weeks of therapy. Maintenance of adequate hydration, diuresis, and discontinuation of the drug facilitate reversal of nephrotoxicity. Chelates divalent cations such as calcium, so that hypocalcemia, hyperphosphatemia or hypophosphatemia, hypomagnesemia, and hypokalemia may develop. Ulceration of the genital epithelium may occur with urine contamination. Anemia and granulocytopenia may develop. Young cats given high dosages develop widened growth plates, increased osteoid, mineralization failure.

INTERACTIONS. With concurrent pentamidine, may exacerbate hypocalcemia. Renal toxicity increased with concurrent use of amphotericin B or aminoglycosides. Cannot use with other nephrotoxic drugs such as ganciclovir because of additive effect.

Availability	Type	Sizes	Preparation (Company)
Human	Injectable solution	24 mg/ml in 500-ml and 250-ml bottles for IV infusion	*Foscavir* (Astra)

INTERNATIONAL PREPARATIONS. *Triapten, Virudin.*

HANDLING. Store at room temperature (15–30°C) and not frozen. Should use only if bottle and seal are intact.

ADMINISTRATION. Weakness or paresthesias may occur during infusion. Do not infuse as a bolus. This will increase the risk of toxicity. IV maximum rate of infusion of 1 mg/kg/min. Experimentally, has been given PO to dogs and cats (2:18, 2:23).

DOSAGE

Indications	Dose (mg/kg)	Route	Interval (hr)	Duration (days)
Dogs	20–30	IV, PO	8	prn
Cats: Retroviral infection	13.3	IV, PO	8	prn

DISPENSING INFORMATION. This drug can cause oral irrritation when given by mouth. Report any decrease in appetite or signs of oral bleeding to your veterinarian.

FURAZOLIDONE

CLASS. Nitrofuran.

ACTION. Antibacterial, antiprotozoal by unknown action; potentially interferes with carbohydrate metabolism of microorganism.

MORE INFORMATION. NITROFURANTOIN; Chapter 34, Nitrofurans; Table 34–9; Antiprotozoals, Chapter 71; Table 71–1.

PHARMACOKINETICS. Small amounts are absorbed from GI tract, the majority is not absorbed and is active in the intestinal lumen. Absorbed fraction may be responsible for most of adverse reactions. Rapid tissue and hepatic metabolism of any absorbed drug. Colored metabolites are excreted in urine and major amount in feces.

SPECTRUM. Gram positive: *Staphylococcus*. **Gram negative:** *Escherichia*, *Salmonella*, *Proteus*, *Aerobacter*, *Campylobacter*, and *Helicobacter*. **Protozoa:** *Giardia*, *Trichomonas*, Coccidia.

INDICATIONS. Bacterial or protozoal enteritis caused by susceptible pathogens. Gastric helicobacteriosis.

APPROVED USES. Humans: for bacterial and protozoal enteritis.

CONTRAINDICATIONS. Prior sensitivity. Avoid in pregnant and lactating animals and neonates.

ADVERSE REACTIONS. Vomiting, diarrhea, fever, dermatologic eruption, brown urine, hypoglycemia. Hemolysis in animals with glucose–6-phosphate dehydrogenase deficiency, or potentially in neonatal animals.

INTERACTIONS. Increased vasopressor effects of sympathomimetic drugs.

Availability	Type	Sizes	Preparation (Company)
Human	Oral liquid	50 mg/ 15 ml	*Furoxone* (Procter and Gamble)
	Oral tablets	100 mg	*Furoxone*

INTERNATIONAL PREPARATIONS. *Nifuran.*

HANDLING. Store in airtight, light-proof containers at controlled room temperature. If exposed to light, liquids will darken.

ADMINISTRATION. Oral suspension makes medication of cats convenient and dosing more accurate. Tablets can be crushed and added to corn syrup to improve palatability.

DOSAGE

Indications	Dose	Route	Interval (hr)	Duration (days)
Human				
Adult giardiasis	100 mg/person	PO	6	7
Child giardiasis	1.25 mg/kg	PO	6	7–10
Dogs				
Coccidiosis	8–20 mg/kg	PO	24	7
Entamebiasis	2.2 mg/kg	PO	8	7

Table continued on following page

Indications	Dose	Route	Interval (hr)	Duration (days)
Cats				
Coccidiosis	8–20 mg/kg	PO	24	7
Giardiasis	4 mg/kg	PO	12	5–10
Amebiasis	2.2 mg/kg	PO	8	7

ADDITIONAL DOSAGES. Giardiasis, Table 78–2; coccidiosis, Table 81–2.

DISPENSING INFORMATION. Reduce feeding of tyramine-containing foods to your pet such as aged cheese and smoked or pickled meat while administering drug. This drug may cause gastrointestinal side effects in your pet and brown discoloration of urine.

GANCICLOVIR (*Cytovene*; Syntex). See ACYCLOVIR and Chapter 2, Acyclovir.

GENTAMICIN

CLASS. Aminoglycoside.

ACTION. Bactericidal; inhibits bacterial protein synthesis by binding to the 30s ribosomal subunit.

MORE INFORMATION. AMIKACIN, KANAMYCIN, STREPTOMYCIN; Chapter 34, Aminoglycosides; Table 34–5; references 34:47, 34:48.

PHARMACOKINETICS. Poor absorption from the GI tract after PO administration. IM absorption (>90%) is more predictable and rapid than SC. Distribution restricted into extracellular fluids (see AMIKACIN). Therapeutic concentrations achieved in some tissues, including lung, bone, and heart; also distributes in limited extent to bile, synovial, peritoneal, abscess, pleural fluids. Low levels in CNS, CSF, or eyes even with inflammation. Must inject intrathecally to achieve adequate concentrations in CSF. Accumulation in kidneys and inner ear may be responsible for intoxication. Small amounts excreted in bile, most excreted in urine as unchanged drug. Can cross placental barrier, which can be risk for fetus.

SPECTRUM. Gram positive: *Corynebacterium*, some *Streptococcus*, *Staphylococcus*. **Gram negative:** *Escherichia*, *Pasteurella*, *Proteus*, some *Pseudomonas*, *Klebsiella*, *Serratia*, *Aerobacter*, *Citrobacter*, *Enterobacter*, *Salmonella*. No specific advantages over other aminoglycosides except possible synergy with penicillins against *Enterococcus*. **More effective:** gram-negative aerobes. **Ineffective:** obligate anaerobes, some resistance developing in strains of *Klebsiella*, *Escherichia*, and *Pseudomonas*.

INDICATIONS. Synergism with β-lactams is documented in vivo. Use in combination with β-lactams for high-risk animals requiring treatment or prophylaxis of established bacteremia or potential bacteremia during urologic, genital, digestive manipulations, or surgery. With clindamycin for surgery on open fractures; with metronidazole before digestive surgery; with quinolones before endoscopic or radiologic urinary tract procedures. Aminoglycosides are rarely recommended as single agents or for self-limiting infections when less toxic drugs are available. Genitourinary, respiratory, or skin and soft tissue infections caused by gram-negative bacilli; systemic infections (including bacteremia and endocarditis) caused by *Staphylococcus*; persistent fever in neutropenic animals. In serious infections caused by unknown organisms, usually combined with a penicillin or cephalosporin; combine with parenteral carbenicillin for serious infections caused by *Pseudomonas*. Can use in nebulization chambers (2.2 mg/kg) for aerosol treatment of bacterial pneumonia.

APPROVED USES. Many, human and veterinary.

CONTRAINDICATIONS. Avoid usage or greatly reduce dosage in renal failure; reduce dose in neonates. Can cause fetal intoxication during pregnancy. Nephrotoxicity is increased by dehydration, shock, renal failure, cardiac failure, hypotension, nonsteroidal anti-inflammatory (antiprostaglandin) drugs, metabolic acidosis, diuretics, calcium, or magnesium deficiencies. Should not be used in dogs that require hearing or balance for work or sport.

ADVERSE REACTIONS. See also Chapter 34, Aminoglycosides. Higher (> once daily) frequency and dosage is associated with nephrotoxicity and ototoxicity. Higher protein diets reduce nephrotoxicity in dogs (34:47). More ototoxic than amikacin in cats. Topical lavage of open wounds or body cavities with parenteral formulation (50 mg/ml) can lead to significant absorption and nephrotoxicity (34:100). Topical application of 3 mg/ml otic solution was not ototoxic in ear canals of dogs with intact or ruptured eardrums (34:153). Often added at 3 mg/ml in tris-EDTA lavage solutions for *Pseudomonas* (see Chapter 34, Table 34–12). Neuromuscular blockade can result after lavage of pleural or peritoneal cavities.

INTERACTIONS. Increased nephrotoxicity when administered with some older parenteral first-generation cephalosporins, amphotericin B, osmotic (mannitol) or loop (furosemide) diuretics, vancomycin, or anesthesia with methoxyflurane or enflurane. Can potentiate paralysis by neuromuscular blockers (*d*-tubocurarine, pancuronium, atracurium). Increased ototoxicity with concurrent use of furosemide and with reduced renal function. Effectiveness of gentamicin is reduced with concurrent use of penicillin, ampicillin, or carbenicillin.

Availability	Type	Sizes	Preparations (Company)
Human	Injectable solution (sulfate)	40 mg/ml, 10 mg/ml	*Garamycin, Garamycin* Pediatric (Schering-Plough Animal Health), generic (various)
	Intrathecal solution	2 mg/ml without preservatives	*Garamycin Intrathecal*
Veterinary	Injectable solution (sulfate)	50 mg/ml (dogs and cats) 100 mg/ml (equine)	*Gentocin* (Schering-Plough Animal Health) *Gentocin*

INTERNATIONAL PREPARATIONS. *Akomicin, Biogen, Cidomycin, Dispagent, Gentalline, Gentamen, Gentax, Genticol, Gentogram, Geomycine, Martigenta, Refobacin, Sulmycin.*

HANDLING. Store at controlled room temperature and never refrigerate or freeze. Never admix aminoglycosides and β-lactams owing to inactivation in vitro but can be coadministered separately. For IV dose, can be diluted in 5% dextrose or 0.9% saline for infusion, or give as IV bolus.

ADMINISTRATION. Can be administered IV or IM, but the former preferred for serious life-threatening bacteremia, animals in shock, those with reduced muscle mass, extensive skin lesions, or heart failure. Dosage frequency is greater but toxicity increased in these serious infections. Usually treat for a maximum of 7–10 days. Renal function must be monitored wherever possible. Monitor urine for fixed specific gravity, casts, albumin, glucose or blood. Increasing the interval of administration to at least 24 hr will reduce toxicity. If toxicosis is noted, the drug should be stopped immediately and fluid and osmotic diuresis instituted. Appearance of nephrotoxicity may be delayed for 1–3 weeks after dosage is discontinued. Intrathecal dose is 2–4 mg total dose/day. After lumbar or cisternal puncture, remove 1 ml/10 kg CSF volume. Dilute the gentamicin with an equal volume of sterile saline or aspirated CSF (if clear) before infusing over 3–5 min.

DOSAGE

Indications	Dose (mg/kg)	Route	Interval (hr)	Duration (days)
Dogs				
Localized, urinary infections	2.2*	IM, SC	12	7–10
Orthopedic infections	2	IV, IM, SC	8–12	<7†
Systemic infections	2.2	IV	6–8	<7†
Bacteremia, sepsis	2–4	IV, IM, SC	8–12	<7†
	6.6	IV, IM, SC	24	<7†
	8–12	IV, IM, SC	24	<7†
Cats‡				
Urinary, soft tissue infections	1–3	IV, IM, SC	8–12	<7†
Systemic, bacteremia	3	IV, IM, SC	8	<7†

*Recommended to give 4.4 mg/kg for first dose to help establish tissue levels.
†Renal function must be closely monitored by serum urea nitrogen and urinalysis.
‡Maximum amount for obese cat is 2.5 mg/kg per dose (34:182).

ADDITIONAL DOSAGES. Canine viral enteritis, Table 8–1; feline panleukopenia, Table 10–1; *Rhodococcus equi* infection, Table 35–6; gram-negative infections, Table 37–2; enteric bacterial infections, Table 39–1; canine brucellosis, Table 40–2; plague, Table 47–1; opportunistic mycobacterial infection, Table 50–5; dermatophilosis, Table 51–1; otitis externa, Table 85–6; musculoskeletal infections, Tables 86–2 and 86–3; bacteremia, Table 87–7; respiratory disease, Table 88–8; oral infections, Table 89–4; enteric infections, Table 89–11; intraabdominal infections, Table 89–15; hepatobiliary infections, Table 90–4; local ocular infections, Table 93–4.

DISPENSING INFORMATION. Must be given SC; therefore, not advised for home administration. Monitoring for renal toxicity is also needed.

GRANULOCYTE COLONY-STIMULATING OR HEMATOPOIETIC GROWTH FACTOR (FILGRASTIM)

CLASS. Cytokine.

ACTION. Stimulates myeloid progenitors in bone barrow.

MORE INFORMATION. Chapters 58 and 100; references: 100:48, 100:49, 100:125.

PHARMACOKINETICS. Human recombinant product, increases blood neutrophil counts in various animals. In dogs and cats, short-term increases in neutrophil counts are followed by neutropenia with continued use owing to development of neutralizing antibodies to this heterologous protein. Neutrophilia occurs by day 7 and reaches maximal levels from 10–14 days of treatment.

INDICATIONS. To stimulate production and function of neutrophils and monocytes. In dogs, for short-term use in treating neutropenia from whole body irradiation, parvovirus and *Ehrlichia* infections, myelosuppressive drugs. Potential uses in cats are leukopenias associated with feline panleukopenia virus, feline immunodeficiency virus, feline leukemia virus, myeloproliferative disease, lymphoid tumors, aplastic anemias. Best for short-term (≤21 days) use for treatment of neutropenia caused by infectious agents, chemotherapy, or total body irradiation. Neutropenia caused by toxins (e.g., cancer chemotherapeutics, estrogens, chloramphenicol, trimethoprim-sulfonamides) or infections (e.g., ehrlichiosis, parvoviral infections).

CONTRAINDICATIONS. Treatment for longer than 3 weeks.

ADVERSE REACTIONS. Bone discomfort or splenomegaly, allergic reactions. Persistent antibodies against endogenous canine or feline granulocyte colony-stimulating factor, resulting in rebound neutropenia.

INTERACTIONS. Artifactual increased serum lactic dehydrogenase and alkaline phosphatase from bone isoenzyme in people.

Availability	Type	Size	Preparation (Company)
Human	Solution for injection	300 μg/ml in 1-ml vial	*Neupogen* (Amgen)

HANDLING. Stock solution can be diluted with sterile physiologic buffered saline and bovine serum albumin. The final dilution is 100 μg/ml, which is stored at 4°C. The vial should not be frozen or exposed to sunlight. Incompatible in solution with amphotericin B, some cephalosporins, clindamycin, furosemide, methylprednisolone sodium succinate, metronidazole, and piperacillin.

ADMINISTRATION. Can be given SC or IV. Should give along with supportive care such as concurrent blood transfusions for concurrent anemia or thrombocytopenia or antibiotics for leukopenia. For IV use, may be further diluted to 5 to 15 μg/ml with addition of 5% dextrose. Albumin is added (12 mg/ml) to prevent absorption to plastics. Infusion rate IV should be over at least 15 min. Should not be given earlier than 24 hr after cytotoxic chemotherapy or 24 hr before. Bone pain can be alleviated by concurrent administration of nonsteroidal anti-inflammatory drugs. SC injection should be spaced out at different sites for each injection and may be more effective than IV use.

DOSAGE

Indications (Neutropenia)	Dose (μg/kg)	Route	Interval (hr)	Duration (days)
Dogs	10–100	SC	24	≤21
	5–20	SC	24	3
Cats	3–10	SC	12	≤21
	20–25	SC	24	3

ADDITIONAL DOSAGES. Feline immunodeficiency virus infection, Table 14–5.

DISPENSING INFORMATION. Animal should return for monitoring at least twice weekly with a complete blood count.

GRISEOFULVIN

CLASS. Antifungal antibiotic derived from *Penicillium* sp.

ACTION. Fungistatic; binds to keratin and inhibits fungal growth by disrupting mitosis.

MORE INFORMATION. See Chapter 57, Griseofulvin; Table 57–1; reference: 57:38.

PHARMACOKINETICS. Variable absorption can be increased by feeding a high fat content meal. Ultramicrocrystalline size (<1 μm) is better absorbed (>95%) than microsized (4 μm) preparation (30%–75%) lowering the equivalent dosage. Concentrated in dermis and appendages. Becomes incorporated in newly formed keratinized epithelium. Metabolized in liver to inactive compounds that are excreted.

SPECTRUM. *Microsporum, Trichophyton.* **Ineffective:** *Actinomyces, Nocardia, Aspergillus, Sporothrix, Blastomyces, Histoplasma, Cryptococcus, Coccidioides.*

INDICATIONS. "Ringworm," dermatophytosis of hair, nails, and skin. Should not be used in cases that are self-limiting or adequately confined for topical therapies.

APPROVED USES. Dermatophytosis in people and animals.

CONTRAINDICATIONS. Hepatic dysfunction, pregnancy, anemia, leukopenia, or feline retroviral infections, especially with leukopenias.

ADVERSE REACTIONS. Nausea, vomiting, diarrhea are most common. Systemic and dermal hypersensitivity (dermal edema and pruritus), hepatotoxicity. May be teratogenic and interferes with spermatogenesis. Myelotoxicity is idiosyncratic, uncommon, and independent of dosage, causing anemia, leukopenia, and/or thrombocytopenia. Neurotoxicity, usually associated with overdosage; ataxia and disorientation, cerebellar signs; may not resolve and may prove fatal (57:30).

INTERACTIONS. Interferes with porphyrin metabolism. Reduces effectiveness of barbiturates and warfarin rodenticides. Phenobarbital or other anticonvulsants may reduce griseofulvin's effectiveness.

Availability	Type	Sizes	Preparations (Company)
Human	Microsize: oral tablets	250 mg, 500 mg	*Fulvicin-U/F* (Schering-Plough Animal Health), *Grisactin* (Wyeth Ayerst)
	Oral capsules	125 mg, 250 mg	*Grisactin*
	Oral suspension	125 mg/5 ml	*Grifulvin V* (Ortho), *Grisactin*
	Ultramicrosize: tablets	125 mg, 165 mg, 250 mg, 330 mg	*Fulvicin P/G, Grisactin Ultra, Gris-PEG* (Allergan Herbert)
Veterinary	Microsize: oral tablets	250 mg, 500 mg	*Fulvicin-U/F*
		125 mg	*Grisovin* (Schering-Plough Animal Health)

INTERNATIONAL PREPARATIONS. *Biogrisin, Delmofulvina, Fulcin, Fulcine, Fungivin, Gricin, Griséfuline, Griseoderm, Griseomed, Griseostatin, Grisol, Grisovin, Grisovina, Lamoryl, Microcidal.*

HANDLING. Store at controlled room temperature in airtight containers. Protect suspension from light.

ADMINISTRATION. Therapy should continue until fungal cultures are negative or for at least 2 weeks after resolution of signs and for at least 5 mo for onychomycosis. Usually need 4–6 weeks of treatment because of drug incorporation into forming keratin. May combine with adjunctive topical therapy. Give tablet size most convenient by 1/4, 1/2, or whole-tablet increments. Give with a fatty meal or corn oil to enhance absorption and decrease GI irritation. Monitor CBC at least every 2 weeks during treatment.

DOSAGE. The dose recommended by the manufacturer of the microsize veterinary formulation (11–22 mg/kg/day) is much less than currently recommended for use in dogs and cats because it does not account for the more rapid clearance of the drug in dogs and cats.

Indications	Dose (mg/kg)	Route	Interval (hr)	Duration (days)
Dogs				
Dermatophytosis (microsized)	25	PO	12	42–56*
Dermatophytosis (ultramicrosized)	5–10	PO	24	42*
Cats				
Dermatophytosis (microsized)	25–50	PO	24	42–70
	12.5–25	PO	12	42–70
Dermatophytosis (ultramicrosized)	5–10	PO	24	42

*May have to treat longer for *Trichophyton* than for *Microsporum*.

ADDITONAL DOSAGES. Dermatophytosis, Table 58–5.

DISPENSING INFORMATION. Return for CBC weekly or biweekly. Duration of therapy at least 6 weeks for skin infections and 5 mo for onychomycotic lesions. May take up to 2.5 mo for mycologic cure of skin infection in many cases (57:38).

HETACILLIN

CLASS. Penicillin.

ACTION. Bactericidal; inhibits bacterial cell wall synthesis.

MORE INFORMATION. See also AMPICILLIN; Chapter 34, Aminopenicillins; Table 34–1.

PHARMACOKINETICS. Hydrolyzed in the stomach to ampicillin. See AMPICILLIN.

SPECTRUM, INDICATIONS, CONTRAINDICATIONS, ADVERSE REACTIONS, AND INTERACTIONS. See AMPICILLIN.

Availability	Type	Sizes	Preparation (Company)
Veterinary	Oral tablets (potassium)	50 mg, 100 mg, 200 mg	*Hetacin-K* (Fort Dodge)

INTERNATIONAL PREPARATIONS. *Etaciland.*

HANDLING AND ADMINISTRATION. See AMPICILLIN.

DOSAGE

Indications	Dose	Route	Interval (hr)	Duration (days)
Dogs				
Urinary tract	11–22 mg/kg	PO	12	7–14
Systemic infections, difficult organism	22–44 mg/kg	PO	12	14
	11–22 mg/kg	PO	8	14
Cats				
Urinary infections	50 mg/cat	PO	12	7–14
Systemic infections	10–20 mg/kg	PO	8	7–14

DISPENSING INFORMATION. Give 1 hr before or 2 hr after feeding.

IMIDOCARB DIPROPIONATE

CLASS. Aromatic diamidine.

ACTION. Antiprotozoal. Interferes with nucleic acid metabolism.

MORE INFORMATION. See DIMINAZENE, AMICARBALIDE, PHENAMIDINE, PENTAMIDINE; Chapter 71; Table 71–1; references: 71:16, 71:23, 71:28, 77:26a.

PHARMACOKINETICS. Slowly metabolized and excreted after IM injection. Persists for long periods in plasma and tissues and gradually eliminated. Protects dogs from infection for up to 5 weeks.

SPECTRUM. *Ehrlichia, Babesia.* Some variation in species and strain susceptibility. Not effective against *E. platys.* See Table 77–3 for efficacy against *Babesia* species.

INDICATIONS. Ehrlichiosis, babesiosis.

APPROVED USES. Babesiosis.

CONTRAINDICATIONS. Use of organophosphates or cholinesterase-inhibiting drugs may increase toxicity. Reduce dose or avoid use with pre-existing pulmonary impairment or renal or hepatic failure. Safety and efficacy have not been determined for puppies or for breeding, lactating, or pregnant dogs. Not recommended for IV use.

ADVERSE REACTIONS. Pain swelling or ulceration at injection site; periorbital edema, hypersalivation, nasal drip, shivering, lacrimation, diarrhea, vomiting, mental agitation, or depression. Posttreatment vomiting is one of the most consistent side effects. The less toxic dipropionate salt produces hypotension and signs similar to those of organophosphate intoxication when given IV (less with IM), but this reaction can be prevented by prior administration of atropine. Reversal with atropine is recommended. Occasional renal tubular necrosis develops. Dose range of 7–10 mg/kg has been tolerated by dogs but approached toxic levels. Doses of 10 mg/kg cause mild transient tachycardia, and higher dosages may cause premature ventricular tachycardia. Elevations of serum alanine transaminase and aspartate transaminase are observed proportional to dosages used as a result of hepatic necrosis. Hepatic vacuolization occurs at therapeutic IV dosage and consistent at overdosages of 20 mg/kg; massive fatal hepatic necrosis after very high (60 mg/kg) accidental overdosage (71:16). Oncogenesis at high dosages in rats. For adverse reaction reporting in the U.S., call 1-800-224-5318.

INTERACTIONS. For *Babesia,* synergistic with one injection of diminazene 24 hr later. Potentiates organophosphate toxicity as a result of inherent anticholinesterase activity. Should not be used simultaneously with exposure to cholinesterase-inhibiting substances.

Availability	Type	Sizes	Preparations (Company)
Veterinary	Parenteral solution	12% solution, multidose vial (120 mg/ml) in 10-ml sterile vials	*Forray–65* (Hoeschst Marion Roussel), *Imizol* (Schering-Plough Animal Health) AgriVet

INTERNATIONAL PREPARATIONS. *Carbesia.*

HANDLING. Store between 2°C and 25°C away from light.

ADMINISTRATION. Follow CBC up to 12–20 weeks to monitor response to therapy.

DOSAGE

Indications (Dogs)	Dose (mg/kg)	Route	Repeat Inoculation (days)
Ehrlichiosis	5.0	IM, SC	14–21
	5.0	IM	84
Babesiosis	5.0–6.6*	IM, SC	14
	7.5	IM, SC	None

*Higher dose from product insert, Schering-Plough.

ADDITIONAL DOSAGES. Ehrlichiosis, Table 29–4; hepatozoonosis, Table 74–2; cytauxzoonosis, Table 76–1; babesiosis, Table 77–3.

IMIPENEM-CILASTATIN SODIUM

CLASS. Imipenem is a β-lactam of the carbapenem group. It is used in a 1:1 ratio with cilastatin, an inhibitor of renal dehydropeptidase–1 that degrades cilastatin. Meropenem, a newer carbapenem, does not require cilastatin coadministration.

ACTION. Bactericidal; imipenem inhibits synthesis of bacterial cell wall peptidoglycan.

MORE INFORMATION. See Chapter 34; Table 34–1.

PHARMACOKINETICS. Poorly absorbed from GI tract, but good systemic availability (75% of IV) after IM administration. Imipenem degradation by renal tubular enzyme is inhibited by cilastatin, which increases urine concentration of active drug and reduces potential nephrotoxicity from metabolites. Most of the drug is renally excreted. Penetrates all tissues and fluid compartments, including aqueous humor. Concentrations in CSF with inflamed and normal meninges are lower than in other tissues and body fluids, with the lowest levels in CSF, vitreous, placenta, milk.

SPECTRUM. Very broad antibacterial activity. Resistant to most bacterial β-lactamases. **Gram positive:** *Staphylococcus,* some *Streptococcus,* including *S. viridans, Listeria, Nocardia,* some *Enterococcus* (not methicillin-resistant strains). **Gram negative:** most gram-negatives, *Escherichia, Klebsiella, Pseudomonas, Citrobacter, Enterobacter, Serratia.* Resistance to *Pseudomonas* can develop during use. **Anaerobes:** *Bacteroides, Fusobacterium, Peptostreptococcus.* **Others:** *Mycobacterium avium-intracellulare* complex. **More effective:** widest spectrum of any single antibacterial, little if any cross-resistance to penicillins or cephalosporins.

INDICATIONS. Bowel ruptures, skin infections, abscesses, cellulitis, wounds, endometritis, lower respiratory tract infections. Single, mixed, and resistant gram-negative bacterial infections. Intra-abdominal and genital infections caused by both gram-negative and anaerobic bacteria. May replace combined therapy with aminoglycoside or cephalosporin plus metronidazole or clindamycin. Good for lower respiratory tract infections, bacterial meningitis, bacteremia, sepsis caused by resistant organisms. IM route for less severe infections in soft tissue.

APPROVED USES. Serious and multiple-resistant bacterial infections when a single agent is needed.

CONTRAINDICATIONS. Severe or life-threatening infections, including bacterial sepsis, endocarditis, or shock. The dosage should be reduced in renal failure. Not determined whether safe for pregnant animals. Cross-hypersensitivity to penicillins.

ADVERSE REACTIONS. Allergic reactions to vehicle, treat as anaphylaxis with epinephrine, oxygen, airway management, glucocorticoids. IV preparation may produce phlebitis, pain, erythema at injection site. In people, systemic signs during infusion have been nausea, diarrhea, vomiting, fever, hypotension, seizures, dizziness, urticaria. All β-lactams can cause seizures if underlying brain disease or if overdosed related to body size and renal function. Laboratory alterations include increased bilirubin, hepatic transaminases, hyponatremia, azotemia, thrombocytosis or thrombocytopenia, eosinophilia. The IM product contains lidocaine hydrochloride, which is contraindicated with known hypersensitivity, with shock, or heart block.

INTERACTIONS. Antagonistic interaction may reduce effectiveness of this drug coadministered with other β-lactam drugs or chloramphenicol. Addition of aminoglycosides or trimethoprim-sulfonamide may be synergistic against certain organisms.

Availability	Type	Sizes	Preparations (Company)
Human	Powder for injection as 1:1 combination with cilastatin	250 mg, 500 mg, in vials and bottles for IV	*Primaxin* (Merck)
		500 mg and 750 mg for IM (suspension)	*Primaxin* I.M.

INTERNATIONAL PREPARATIONS. *Tenacid, Tienam, Tracix, Zienam.*

HANDLING. Store powder at refrigerated or controlled room temperature. For IV, dilute contents into at least 100 ml of appropriate infusion solution (0.9% NaCl, 5% dextrose, sodium bicarbonate, mannitol [2.5–10%], and KCl [0.15%]). Maintains potency for 4–10 hr at room temperature 24–48 hr if refrigerated; the longer time periods are with 0.9% NaCl diluent. Never freeze. Give by intermittent IV infusion over 20–60 min. Do not mix with other drugs. For IM, solutions reconstitute with 1% lidocaine (without epinephrine); should be used within 1 hr.

ADMINISTRATION. For IM, use a 21-gauge needle and deep injection. Aspirate before injection to avoid inadvertent IV administration.

DOSAGE

Indications (Dogs and Cats)	Dose (mg/kg)	Route	Interval (hr)	Duration (days)
Bacteremia/sepsis	2.0–7.5	IV, IM	8	3–5
Sepsis, more resistant organism	3.0–10	IV	6–8	3–5

ADDITIONAL DOSAGES. Gram-negative bacterial infections, Table 37–2; endotoxemia, Table 38–1; nocardiosis, Table 49–2; bacteremia and endocarditis, Table 87–7; respiratory infections, Table 88–8; intra-abdominal infections, Table 89–15.

INTERFERON-α (IFN-α)

CLASS. Cytokine produced by recombinant means to match human protein. The 2a and 2b forms differ in the sequence of two amino acids and purification.

ACTION. Acts on terminal stages of virus production by preventing assembly and budding of mature virions, also immunomodulating influences.

MORE INFORMATION. Chapters 2 and 100; Table 2–1; references: 100:27, 100:102b, 100:112; 100:124, 100:168a, 100:169; 100:175. Previously known as leucocytic or lymphoblastoid interferon.

PHARMACOKINETICS. Low-dose oral: (1–30 U) possibly stimulates oropharyngeal tonsils locally, not much absorbed systemically as destroyed by gastric acid. **High-dose parenteral:** SC (1.6 x 10^6 U/kg) resulted in plasma concentration measurable for 8 hr. Well absorbed after SC or IM injection. After IV injection, the drug is distributed primarily to liver and kidneys, with lesser amounts in thyroid, spleen, GI mucosae. Filtered at renal glomerulus, catabolized by kidneys, and excreted in urine. At lower concentrations (10^5 U/kg), the neutralizing antibody titers that develop to IFN- (see later) were proportionally lower.

SPECTRUM. Many viruses, immunostimulant.

INDICATIONS. Oral: adjunct to alleviate clinical manifestations of ill feline leukemia virus (FeLV)–infected cats suffering from immunosuppressive (not neoplastic) effects of FeLV. It may prolong cat's well-being and associated survival time. Stimulates appetite. Does *not* affect viremia but may have some effect on virus-induced myelosuppression. Use only in ill FeLV-positive cats. Can be tried in cats with feline immunodeficiency virus (FIV) or chronic upper respiratory tract disease or dogs with systemic mycotic infections as an adjunct to antifungal therapy. There has been subjective improvement in these situations but no controlled studies. **Parenteral:** may decrease retroviral viremia for limited periods. Use of recombinant human IFN parenterally can induce neutralizing antibody, which interferes with activity after several weeks. Cats receiving high doses (10^6 U/cat) for 21 days had neutralizing antibody titers develop and therapeutic refractoriness (2:32, 2:33). Cats receiving high dose (10^6 U/cat) had reduced lymphocyte blastogenesis compared with those receiving 10^4 or 10^2 U/kg, which had enhanced lymphocyte activity (2:30). Not routinely recommended for parenteral use in animals for these reasons. Low-dose oral is the preferred method of administration. Low doses (1–30 U/cat) given orally have been used in milder cases of noneffusive FIP, when it may help suppress disease progression (100:168a). High doses ($> 2 \times 10^4$ U/kg) given IM have been used as an immunomodulator in conjunction with glucocorticoids to treat effusive FIP (100:168a). **Intralesional:** for viral papillomatosis in people; might be tried for these lesions in dogs (Chapter 9) and cats (Chapter 21). **Topical:** used in conjunction with topical antiviral drugs in cats with chronic herpesvirus keratitis and conjunctivitis (2:21). See Chapter 93.

APPROVED USES. In people for various malignancies and viral diseases.

CONTRAINDICATIONS. Limited efficacy of high-dose parenteral human interferon in cats because of neutralizing antibodies (2:33). May become refractory 3–7 weeks after initiating treatment. PO, topical, or intralesional treatment does not induce this refractoriness.

ADVERSE REACTIONS. Parenteral: in cats, allergic reactions, fever, lethargy, myalgia, myelotoxicity; in people, also neurotoxicity, hepatotoxicity. **Oral, intralesional, topical:** none.

INTERACTIONS. Unknown.

Availability	Type	Sizes	Preparations (Company)
Human	Interferon-α_{2a}, solution or powder for injection	3, 6, or 36 $\times$ 10^6 U vials	*Roferon A* (Roche)
	Interferon-α_{2b}, powder for injection	3, 5, 10, 18, 25, or 50 $\times$ 10^6 U vials	*Intron A* (Schering-Plough Animal Health)
	Interferon-α_{n3} solution for injection	5 $\times$ 10^6 U vials	*Alferon N* (Purdue Frederick)

HANDLING. For 3-U/ml solution: make 1:100 dilution of commercial solution (3 x 10^6 U/ml) using sterile water giving 3 x 10^4 U/ml. Take 0.1 ml and add to 1 L of 0.9% NaCl containing 4 ml of 25% serum albumin (albumin is optional but adds stability at low concentrations). Package 3 U/ml solution in 15-ml aliquots in sterile injection vials and store frozen (−70°C desirable). Thaw vials as needed, then store refrigerated for administration. Discard unused portion 60 days after first using refrigerated solution. Discard unused 3 x 10^4 U/ml solution within 2 to 3 hr after making initial dilutions. **For 30-U/ml solution:** dilute entire contents of commercial solution (3 x 10^6 U/ml) into 1 L sterile IV fluid bag containing saline to give a solution of 3000 U/ml. This can be divided in 1- or 10-ml aliquots and frozen. The commercial solution or 3000-U/ml solution can be frozen for years without losing activity. The 3000-U/ml solution can be added to 1 ml/100 ml sterile saline or to a 10 ml/1 L IV fluid bag to produce either 100 or 1000 ml of 30-U/ml solution for administration (100:169).

ADMINISTRATION. Oral: for 3 U/ml solution, remove 0.3 ml (1 U) using sterile needle and 1.0-ml syringe. For 30 U/ml, remove 1-ml solution. Remove needle from hub and squirt dose into the oral cavity once each day of treatment. If syringes are reused, a short reusable rubber or plastic catheter segment may aid in keeping syringe from contacting oral mucosae to help preserve sterility of 15- or 30-ml refrigerated aliquots. **Parenteral:** not recommended because it stimulates antibody formation. **Intralesional:** into papillomas, inject 1 $\times$ 10^6 μ/0.1 ml into up to five warts three times/week until regression occurs.

DOSAGE

Indications	Dose	Units	Route	Interval (hr)	Duration (days)
Cat					
FeLV and appetite stimulation	1*	U/cat	PO	24	7†
	30	U/cat	PO	24	7‡
FIP exudative (wet)	2 $\times$ 10^4	U/kg	IM	24	14–21
FIP nonexudative (dry)	30	U/cat	PO	24	7‡
Dog					
Immunosuppression	1	U/5 kg	PO	24	7†

*Although daily doses of 30 U have been recommended (100:169), other studies with FeLV-infected cats have shown 1 U to be superior to 5 U (100:27).
†Treat alternate weeks or continuously (100:27).
‡Treat alternate weeks (100:169).

ADDITIONAL DOSAGES. FIP, Table 11–3; antiprotozoals, Table 71–1.

DISPENSING INFORMATION. Keep medication refrigerated and discard unused portions after 60 days. Use a short catheter on the end of the syringe to keep it from becoming contaminated with oral bacteria. This treatment will not reverse the FeLV-positive status of the cat but may improve appetite, general attitude, health.

INTERFERON-β_{1b} (IFN-β)

CLASS. Polypeptide cytokine from fibroblasts. Produced by recombinant DNA methods.

ACTION. Antiviral and immunoregulatory.

MORE INFORMATION. Previously known as fibroblast interferon. See Chapter 2, Antivirals, and Chapter 100, Immunotherapy.

PHARMACOKINETICS. Not detectable in blood or tissues after SC administration. Bioavailability is 50% with SC use. After IV use, reaches low levels in blood with rapid clearance.

INDICATIONS. In people for treatment of multiple sclerosis, also in immunosuppressed people with AIDS from HIV infection, myelogenous or metastatic neoplasia, some viral hepatitis. No immediate uses in dogs and cats but might be considered in similar disorders.

CONTRAINDICATIONS. Pregnancy, leukopenia, anemia.

ADVERSE REACTIONS. In people similar to IFN-α: myelosuppression, fever, chills, myalgia, photosensitivity, systemic allergic reactions, abortion.

INTERACTIONS. Decreased clearance of AZT given currently.

Availability	Type	Size	Preparation (Company)
Human	Powder for injection	0.3 mg (9.6 mIU) contains human albumin	*Betaseron* (Berlex)

HANDLING. Powder should be stored refrigerated. Inject sterile 0.9% NaCl into vial to dissolve drug. After reconstituting solution is 0.25 mg/ml. Only good for single use once reconstituted.

ADMINISTRATION. Injected SC.

DOSAGE

Indications	Dose	Route	Interval (hr)	Duration (years)
Human	0.25 mg (8 mIU)	SC	48	≤2

INTERFERON-γ_{1b} (IFN-γ)

CLASS. Polypeptide lymphokine with antiviral, immunomodulatory, and antiproliferative effects.

ACTION. Biologic response modifier, potent phagocyte-activating effects potentiate killing of intracellular organisms such as virulent *Staphylococcus, Toxoplasma, Leishmania, Listeria, Mycobacterium avium-intracellulare* complex.

MORE INFORMATION. Previously known as immune interferon. Chapter 100, Immunotherapy; references: 100:50.

PHARMACOKINETICS. Absorbed slowly after IM or SC administration. Rapid clearance after IV use. Slower elimination and high bioavailability (89%) makes SC use desirable.

SPECTRUM. Immunostimulating for defense against persistent intracellular organisms. Has been effective in experimental animal infections of toxoplasmosis, *Pneumocystis carinii* pneumonia, cryptosporidiosis (71:30). Some dose relationship; higher dosages were associated with improved efficacy.

INDICATIONS. Immunodeficiency caused by neutrophil phagocyte defects. Helps prevent infection.

CONTRAINDICATIONS. Pregnancy, leukopenia, thrombocytopenia.

ADVERSE REACTIONS. In people, CNS signs of mental depression and gait dysfunction, myelosuppression, abortion. Because these compounds are species specific, antibody might develop with chronic use in dogs and cats and limit effectiveness.

INTERACTIONS. May be synergistic with concurrent antimicrobial chemotherapy such as roxithromycin, trimethoprim-sulfonamide, sodium stilbogluconate.

Availability	Type	Size	Preparation (Company)
Human	Solution for injection	100 μg (3 × 10^6 U)/0.5 ml	*Actimmune* (Genentech)

HANDLING. No preservatives in vial; must be for single dose; keep refrigerated 2°C–8°C. Must be discarded if left unrefrigerated > 12 hr.

ADMINISTRATION. Drug is given SC. Liquid should be gently mixed but not shaken and should not be discolored or contain particulate matter.

DOSAGE

Indications (human)	Dose	Route	Interval	Duration (days)
Body surface > 0.5 m^2	50 μg/m^2	SC	3x weekly	prn
Body surface < 0.5 m^2	1.5 μg/kg	SC	3x weekly	prn

IODIDE (POTASSIUM AND SODIUM)

CLASS. Inorganic halogen.

ACTION. Antifungal but exact mechanism uncertain. May facilitate phagocytic killing of fungal cells.

MORE INFORMATION. Chapter 57; Table 57–4; Chapter 63.

PHARMACOKINETICS. Unknown.

SPECTRUM. *Sporothrix, Basidiobolus.*

INDICATIONS. Sporotrichosis, some treatment failures occur. Preferred for dogs owing to good clinical response and low toxicity. Has been effective in some cases of subcutaneous phycomycosis in people.

APPROVED USES. Antithyroidal agent, sporotrichosis, expectorant.

CONTRAINDICATIONS. Hyperthyroidism, iodide hypersensitivity, renal failure, dehydration, pregnancy.

ADVERSE REACTIONS. Cats often develop toxic signs of iodism, including vomiting, anorexia, muscle twitching, cardiomyopathy, heart failure, death. Enteric-coated tablets have caused bowel ulceration in people. Prolonged use has caused hypothyroidism, goiter, thyroid adenomas, and dermatitis in people.

INTERACTIONS. Concurrent use with other potassium-containing medications can cause hyperkalemia.

Availability	Type	Sizes	Preparations (Company)
Human KI	Oral solution	1 g KI/mL (300 ml/bottle)	*SSKI* (Upsher-Smith), generic (many)
	Oral syrup (black raspberry flavor)	325 mg/5 ml	*Pima* Syrup (Fleming)
Veterinary, NaI	Parenteral solution	200 mg/ml	Sodium Iodide (ProLabs, Vet Tek, Lextron, RXV)

HANDLING. Can produce saturated solution of KI in lieu of commercial preparations or 20% NaI solutions (200 mg/ml). Parenteral NaI solutions listed contain only water. If commercial KI or NaI solutions are used, they should not contain other ingredients intended as expectorants.

ADMINISTRATION. For accuracy, always aspirate dose in graduated 1-ml syringes. Always administer by placing drops directly on food to decrease GI irritation. Continue for at least 1 mo beyond clinical cure.

DOSAGE

Indications	Dose (mg/kg)	Route	Interval (hr)	Duration (days)
Dogs				
Sporotrichosis	40	PO	8	≥60
Cats				
Sporotrichosis	20	PO	12–24	≥60

ADDITIONAL DOSAGES. Drug therapy for sporotrichosis, Table 63–1.

DISPENSING INFORMATION. Administer by placing liquid on animal's food or give orally immediately after feeding. Report any loss of appetite or other signs to veterinarian.

IODOQUINOL

CLASS. 8-hydroxyquinoline; also called diiodohydroxyquin.

ACTION. Antibacterial, antifungal, and antiprotozoal.

MORE INFORMATION. See elsewhere, Clioquinol (Moebiquin, Vioform); Chapter 71; Table 71–1.

PHARMACOKINETICS. Poorly absorbed (8%) from GI tract, high concentration in intestinal lumen. Will only treat luminal and not systemic spread.

SPECTRUM. *Entamoeba*, *Balantidium*, yeasts. Acts strictly in the gut lumen.

INDICATIONS. Intraluminal treatment of intestinal amebiasis and balantidiasis. Topical antifungal.

APPROVED USES. Human amebiasis.

CONTRAINDICATIONS. Not effective with extraintestinal (hepatic) amebiasis. Do not use in animals with neurologic, renal, or liver impairment or pre-existing thyroid dysfunction.

ADVERSE REACTIONS. Dermatologic eruption, enlarged thyroids, vomiting, diarrhea; optic nerve or peripheral neuropathy after prolonged use at high dosages. Neurotoxicity found in dogs treated with 5 g of a 3% clioquinol topical preparation for 28 days. Causes discoloration of tongue, urine, feces. Oral use of this drug and Clioquinol is restricted because of neurotoxicity.

INTERACTIONS. Interferes with thyroid testing as a result of iodination.

Availability	Type	Sizes	Preparations (Company)
Human	Oral tablets	210 mg, 650 mg	*Yodoxin* (Glenwood)
	Oral powder	25 g	*Yodoxin*

INTERNATIONAL PREPARATIONS. Diodoquin, Direxiode, Floraquin, Sebaquin.

HANDLING. Insoluble in water and minimally in alcohol. For smaller doses, tablets must be crushed or powder placed on moist food.

ADMINISTRATION. Topical use of this drug as an antifungal has been toxic to dogs.

DOSAGE. Not recommended for use in small animals. Amebiasis is uncommon in dogs and cats.

IPRONIDAZOLE

CLASS. Nitroimidazole.

ACTION. See METRONIDAZOLE.

MORE INFORMATION. See METRONIDAZOLE, TINIDAZOLE.

SPECTRUM. *Giardia*, *Trichomonas*.

INDICATIONS. Used in veterinary medicine to treat blackhead in turkeys. For giardiasis, when added to drinking water in kennel dogs.

CONTRAINDICATIONS. Pregnancy.

ADVERSE REACTIONS. Not noted, although mutagenesis is possible.

INTERACTIONS. See METRONIDAZOLE.

Availability	Type	Sizes	Preparation (Company)
Veterinary	Available as feed/water additive for turkeys*	Unknown	*Ipropran* (Roche)

*Not available in the USA.

ADMINISTRATION. Mix desired amount in drinking water. Do not give other sources of water until dose is finished.

DOSAGE

Indication	Dose	Route	Interval (hr)	Duration (days)
Dogs	126–378 mg/L	In water	24	7–14

ISONIAZID (INH)

CLASS. Hydrazide: isonicotinic acid hydrazide.

ACTION. Interferes with nucleic acid and lipid biosynthesis in bacteria.

MORE INFORMATION. Chapter 34; Chapter 50; Table 50–2; reference: 34:171.

PHARMACOKINETICS. Rapid and completely absorbed after PO administration. All formulations are well absorbed. Inactivated in liver and 85% of unchanged drug and metabolites are excreted in urine. Portion metabolized by acetylation and excreted in urine; 50–70% excreted unchanged.

SPECTRUM. *Mycobacterium.*

INDICATIONS. *M. tuberculosis* or *M. bovis* infections.

APPROVED USES. Human mycobacteriosis.

CONTRAINDICATIONS. Reduce dose in hepatic dysfunction and in severe renal failure.

ADVERSE REACTIONS. Vomiting; hepatotoxicity—elevated enzymes, bilirubin, hepatic necrosis; peripheral neuropathy in people. Vitamin B_6 (pyridoxine) deficiency, which in dogs causes recurrent tonic clonic seizures followed by salivation, diarrhea, vomiting, incoordination, cardiac arrhythmias (34:171). To treat accidental overdosage, 50 mg/kg or more of pyridoxine hydrochloride at a gram-for-gram dose equal to the amount ingested as a 5%–10% total wt/vol IV infusion over 30–60 min. A bolus if in status epilepticus. Additional anticonvulsants diazepam and phenobarbital as needed.

INTERACTIONS. Reduces levels of ketoconazole. Increases levels of benzodiazepines, diphenylhydantoin, hepatotoxicity enhanced with halothane, rifampin. Glucocorticoids decrease its effectiveness.

Availability	Type	Sizes	Preparations (Company)
Human	Oral tablets	50 mg, 100 mg, 300 mg	*Laniazid* (Geigy), generics (various)
	Parenteral injection	100 mg/ml	*Nydrazid* (Apothecon)

INTERNATIONAL PREPARATIONS. *Cemidon, Dipasic, Inapsade, Isotamine, Isozid, Laniazid, Nicazide, Nicotibine, Nydrazid, Pyreazid, Rimifon, Tibinide.*

HANDLING. Store in airtight and light-proof containers. Incompatible with sugars. Sterilize solution by autoclaving.

ADMINISTRATION. A 10-mg/ml suspension can be prepared by using 12 100-mg tablets, distilled water to dissolve, and adding aqueous 50% sorbitol to bring the volume to 120 ml. This should be refrigerated and is stable for 3 weeks. Shake well before using. Always use in combination with other antimycobacterial drugs. Aluminum-containing compounds interfere with absorption. Administer on empty stomach.

DOSAGE

Indication (Dogs)	Dose	Route	Interval (hr)	Duration (days)
Tuberculosis	10 mg/kg	PO	24	prn

ADDITIONAL DOSAGES. Mycobacterial Infections, Table 50–4.

DISPENSING INFORMATION. Give for 3–6 mo after cytologic or culture data suggest cure. Usual treatment is at least 6 mo.

ITRACONAZOLE

CLASS. Synthetic triazole antifungal.

ACTION. Inhibits synthesis of fungal cell membrane. Greater potency and less toxicity than ketoconazole.

MORE INFORMATION. See KETOCONAZOLE, FLUCONAZOLE, CLOTRIMAZOLE; Chapter 57, Azoles; Table 57–1; references: 57:3a, 57:36.

PHARMACOKINETICS. PO bioavailability 40% with fasting but up to 99% when given with a high-fat meal such as canned food. Once absorbed, highly (>99%) protein bound to albumin. Capsules can be opened, and a fraction of the dose can be mixed in the food. Variable in some cats requiring higher doses (10 mg/kg) for better efficacy. Requires acid pH for absorption. Extensively distributed into lipophilic tissues: concentrations in liver, kidney, adrenals, lung, fat, skin at least twice that in blood. Does not penetrate well into CSF, saliva, aqueous humor. However, it has been used to treat animals with fungal meningitis and ophthalmitis. Therapeutic concentrations maintained longer in tissues than plasma. Requires 14–21 days to reach steady state (57:3a). Drug concentrations increase after several weeks of therapy. They are three to five times higher compared with single dosing after 2 weeks of treatment of dogs and 21 days in cats. Hepatotoxicity may be seen in 10% of dogs owing to inordinately high serum concentrations that develop. Primarily metabolized in liver with biliary and some urinary excretion of metabolites. Low activity in the urinary tract makes it unsuitable for treatment of urinary tract infections. Experimentally, oral dose of 5 mg/kg to cats is equivalent to 0.75–1 mg/kg IV or 1.25–1.5 mg/kg of oral solution because of the low bioavailability of oral capsules (57:3a). Oral solution is better absorbed and may be more efficacious on a milligram basis in cats.

SPECTRUM. *Blastomyces, Histoplasma, Cryptococcus, Coccidioides, Aspergillus.* **Variable activity:** *Trichophyton, Candida, Sporothrix, Acanthamoeba, Malassezia, Microsporum, Pythium.* Broader and more potent in vivo than ketoconazole. **Others:** *Acanthamoeba, Trypanosoma.*

INDICATIONS. Fungal: blastomycosis, histoplasmosis, aspergillosis, coccidioidomycosis, candidiasis, cryptococcosis, sporotrichosis, fungal keratitis, zygomycosis, chromomycosis, onychomycosis. Also effective in some cases of dermatophytosis when griseofulvin was not effective or has caused toxicity. Cutaneous and systemic sporotrichosis least toxic and most effective, although expensive. Nasal, disseminated, and meningeal cryptococcosis. Poor to variable efficacy in nasal and disseminated aspergillosis and no additive effect to that produced by topical enilconazole alone. **Protozoal:** Acanthamebiasis not involving the CNS, cutaneous leishmaniasis. No need to adjust dose in renal insufficiency, unlike fluconazole (57:20).

APPROVED USES. Human systemic fungal infections.

CONTRAINDICATIONS. Hepatic disease or insufficiency. Must reduce if used with hepatic disease or dysfunction. Teratogenic and embryotoxic effects have been seen at high dosages in lab animals, so should avoid in pregnancy.

ADVERSE REACTIONS. Vomiting, diarrhea, abdominal pain, inappetence, increased liver enzymes, peripheral edema, fever, hypertension, skin rash (57:14). Less hepatotoxic than ketoconazole and unlike ketoconazole, does not affect adrenal or reproductive steroid synthesis. Nausea, anorexia, vomiting, hepatic injury, increased serum alanine transaminase (ALT) are more common in cats; anorexia is associated with increased ALT and serum alkaline phosphatase. ALT decreases after drug is stopped for 1–2 weeks or until appetite returns or serum hepatic enzymes return toward reference levels; then treatment can be restarted at 50% dose or alternate days. Monitor serum hepatic enzyme activity every 2 weeks thereafter. Serious hepatotoxicity leads to icterus and death (57:14, 57:36). High doses can produce hypokalemia. Ulcerative dermatitis and hepatotoxicity occur more in dogs receiving higher (10 mg/kg) daily dosages. It subsides if dosage is stopped or reduced to 5 mg/kg once daily (see ITZ, Adverse Effects, Chapter 57).

INTERACTIONS. Do not coadminister with ketoconazole, cisapride, terfenadine; fatal cardiac arrhythmias may occur. Absorption decreased with concurrent antacids or any disease raising gastric pH. Prolongs effects and increases toxicity of benzodiazepines (midazolam), cyclosporine, glucocorticoids, antihistamines, quinidine, digoxin, vincristine, warfarin, sulfonylureas. H_2-receptor antagonists (cimetidine), diphenylhydantoin, itraconazole, rifampin decrease efficacy of itraconazole. For blood levels, send to Fungus Testing Laboratory, University of Texas Health Science Center, 7703 Floyd Curl Dr, San Antonio, TX 78284; (210) 567-4131.

AVAILABILITY. 100-mg capsules must be split or formulated for cats and small dogs before use. Expensive, which may limit use. PO solution available, and injectable solution under development. Oral solution has greater bioavailability in cats than capsules.

Availability	Type	Sizes	Preparations (Company)
Human	Oral capsules Oral solution	100 mg 100 mg/10 ml	*Sporanox* (Janssen) *Sporanox*

INTERNATIONAL PREPARATIONS. *Beltop.*

HANDLING. Before availability of the commercially available solution, liquid preparations were made from capsules based on the manufacturer's recommendation. **Oral syrup:** a small amount of oral suspension can be made from capsules for cats and small dogs. Six 100-mg capsules are placed into glass mortar. Add 1.25 ml of 95% ethyl alcohol USP and let it stand 3 min to soften. Grind into a paste and let dry. Add 4 ml of corn syrup and transfer to 15-ml bottle. Continue to add up to 15-ml to wash the mortar and transfer it to the bottle. The final concentration is 40 mg/ml. It is stable refrigerated for 35 days. Should be shaken well before using. **Oral liquid:** each capsule can be dissolved in 2 ml of 0.2 *N* HCl. After 15 min, 20 ml of cranberry juice (pH < 2) is added. The final concentration (mg/ml) is total number of capsules × 100 divided by the total ml of juice used. Stable for 14 days when refrigerated. **In butter:** see Dispensing Information.

ADMINISTRATION. Treatment of more resistant or "walled-off" systemic mycosis may require 10 mo or more. To achieve a higher steady state in rapidly advancing mycosis, consider initial higher loading dose followed by a lower maintenance level. For sporotrichosis in humans, treatment lasts 3–18 mo. Treatment for dermatophytosis is at least 1 week beyond clinical and mycologic cure (57:38). Coadminister with amphotericin B with rapidly progressive life-threatening infections. Increasing gastric acid secretion improves absorption. Administration with or immediately after a meal (especially with high fat) improves absorption. Monitor serum ALT monthly or cyclosporine, often increases in cats after 60 days. Anorexia or increased ALT is managed by reducing dosage. If toxicity develops at any dose, reinstitute dose at 50% after the adverse signs have abated. The capsules containing beads can be emptied and separated to smaller gelatin capsules or placed directly on food. For young kittens with dermatophytosis, can use 10 beads/day placed on food. Some concentration of itraconazole can be measured to ensure therapeutic level (≥ 2 μg/ml) is being acheived. Measured by Fungus Testing Laboratory, University of Texas, Health Science Center, 7703 Floyd Care Dr, San Antonio, TX 78284; (210) 567-4131.

DOSAGE

Indications	Dose	Route	Interval (hr)	Duration (days)
Dogs				
Systemic blastomycosis	5 mg/kg	PO	24	≥60*
Ocular or CNS blastomycosis	5 mg/kg	PO	12	≥60*
	10 mg/kg	PO	24	≥60*
Sporotrichosis	5–10 mg/kg	PO	12–24	†
Cats				
Dermatophytosis	10 mg/kg	PO	24	28–70‡
Histoplasmosis	5–10 mg/kg	PO	12	60–130 days§
Sporotrichosis	5 mg/kg	PO	12–24	†
Cryptococcosis (< 3.2 kg weight)	50 mg/cat	PO	24	To 8 weeks after clinical recovery
Cryptococcosis (≥ 3.2 kg weight)	100 mg/cat	PO	24	To 8 weeks after clinical recovery

*Continue therapy for at least 60 days after clinical recovery.
†Continue therapy for at least 30 days after clinical recovery.
‡Some clear in 4–8 weeks; others take 6–10 weeks.
§If relapse, may need a second course.

ADDITIONAL DOSAGES. Dermatophytosis, Table 58–5; blastomycosis, Table 59–1; histoplasmosis, Table 60–1; cryptococcosis, Table 61–4; coccidioidomycosis, Table 62–3; sporotrichosis, Table 63–1; nasal aspergillosis, Table 65–3; disseminated aspergillosis, Table 65–4; candidiasis and trichosporosis, Table 66–2; protothecosis, Table 69–1; fungal otitis, Table 85–6.

DISPENSING INFORMATION. Administer capsules with food to improve absorption and reduce gastrointestinal side effects. Owners should mix small beads within 100-mg capsule with ½ to 1 teaspoon of soft butter to a sausage shape on a plate, or aluminum foil, to be placed in freezer. This can be cut into appropriate amount for individual daily dosage. Most cats or dogs will readily eat this. Oral solution should be given without food, and dosage can be 25%–50% of that listed because of inherently better absoprtion. Recheck clinical signs and renal/hepatic tests at 2 weeks, monthly for 3 mo, and every 3 mo thereafter.

KANAMYCIN

CLASS. Aminoglycoside.

ACTION. Bactericidal; inhibits bacterial protein synthesis.

MORE INFORMATION. See GENTAMICIN; Chapter 34; Table 34–5.

PHARMACOKINETICS. See GENTAMICIN. For PO therapy, most of the dose is not absorbed and acts locally.

SPECTRUM. Gram positive: Some *Staphylococcus, Listeria.* **Gram negative:** *Escherichia, Proteus, Salmonella, Citrobacter.* Similar to gentamicin except poor against *Pseudomonas.* **Anaerobes**: ineffective. **Ineffective**: *Pseudomonas*, inconsistent against *Staphylococcus.*

INDICATIONS. Skin, soft tissue, and genitourinary infections caused by *Escherichia, Proteus, Enterobacter, Klebsiella, Serratia, Salmonella, Acinetobacter, Mycobacterium avium-intracellulare* complex infections.

CONTRAINDICATIONS. See GENTAMICIN; avoid or reduce dosage in renal failure.

ADVERSE REACTIONS. Ototoxicity and nephrotoxicity. See GENTAMICIN. Pain and muscle injury after repeated IM injection.

INTERACTIONS. See GENTAMICIN.

Availability	Type	Sizes	Preparations (Company)
Human	Solution for injection	250 mg/ml	*Kantrex* (Bristol-Myers Squibb); generic (various)
Veterinary	Solution for injection	50 mg/ml, 200 mg/ml	*Kantrim* (Fort Dodge)
		50 mg/ml	*Amiglyde-V* (Fort Dodge)
	Oral solution for enteric therapy (with bismuth and absorbent)	100 mg/5 ml	*Amforol* (Fort Dodge)
	Oral tablets for enteric therapy (with bismuth and absorbent)	100 mg	*Amforol*

INTERNATIONAL PREPARATIONS. *Kamycine, Kanamytrex, Kanescin, Kannasyn, Kemicina.*

HANDLING. Can be diluted in 0.9% NaCl or 5% dextrose.

ADMINISTRATION. For IV, do not mix with other antibacterials. Give as dilute solution over 1 hr. For IM, deep injection into large muscle. Can be given as aerosol by nebulization: add 250 mg to 3 ml 0.9% NaCl and put in nebulizer chamber. Repeat two to four times daily. Monitor for renal dysfunction and neurologic signs. Treat urinary infection until asymptomatic and culture results are negative. After 3 days of no response, re-evaluate treatment. Maximum treatment period is 10 days.

DOSAGE

Indications	Dose (mg/kg)	Route	Interval (hr)	Duration (days)*
Dogs				
Skin, soft tissue infection	10	SC, IM	12	7
Genitourinary infection	10	SC, IM	12	7–10
Systemic infection	5.0–7.5	SC	8	7
Enteric infection	5	PO	8	<5
Cats				
Soft tissue, systemic infection	5.5	IM, SC	12	<7

*Must closely monitor renal function during treatment.

ADDITIONAL DOSAGES. Plague, Table 47–1; opportunistic mycobacterial infections, Table 50–5; respiratory infections; Table 88–8.

KETOCONAZOLE

CLASS. Imidazole antifungal.

ACTION. Antifungal; impairs ergosterol synthesis in fungal cell wall.

MORE INFORMATION. See ITRACONAZOLE, FLUCONAZOLE; Chapter 57; Table 57–1.

PHARMACOKINETICS. Absorbed variably and usually incompletely from GI tract, acid environment in stomach and smaller amounts of food generally enhance absorption. High concentrations of drug reach the liver, kidney, pituitary, adrenals. Highly protein bound but reaches urine, saliva, milk, sweat, ceruminous secretions. CSF concentrations are minimal: dosages of 40 mg/kg/day are required for measurable amounts in CSF, although even then these levels are unpredictable. Metabolized by liver to inactive metabolites, with majority excreted in bile and feces. Very low (3%–4%) amounts reach the urine unmetabolized.

SPECTRUM. Fungi: *Blastomyces, Candida, Histoplasma, Paracoccidioides, Coccidioides, Trichophyton, Microsporum, Malassezia, Phialophora.* **Others:** *Leishmania.*

INDICATIONS. Localized or disseminated candidiasis, systemic mycoses: blastomycosis, histoplasmosis, coccidioidomycosis, paracoccidioidomycosis. In rapidly progressing systemic mycoses, treat with amphotericin B first or 1 week of high-dose itraconazole. High (often toxic) doses of ketoconazole required for CNS mycoses. For dermatophytes resistant to topical therapy; but griseofulvin or itraconazole are preferred for feline dermatophytosis. Not a first choice if CNS or ocular involvement. In more resistant canine nasal aspergillosis, may use ketoconazole combined with topical enilconazole or clotrimazole, but itraconazole or fluconazole preferred (57:47). Although ketoconazole is less expensive, toxicity and treatment failure rates are higher (57:46). For sporotrichosis, but more side effects and less effective than itraconazole. Has been used in treatment of leishmaniasis (see Chapter 73). High dosages have been used to suppress steroidogenesis in canine hyperadrenocorticism.

APPROVED USES. Antifungal for human use.

CONTRAINDICATIONS. Pregnancy or lactation; itraconazole or fluconazole a better choice for CNS, intraocular, or testicular infections. The slow response to therapy has made itraconazole preferred for animals with severe or rapidly progressing mycoses.

ADVERSE REACTIONS. Anorexia may be observed within the first 30 days of therapy in some animals. Fever, depression, vomiting, diarrhea, abdominal pain, weight loss, hepatocellular necrosis, thrombocytopenia, occasional nonregenerative anemia, teratogenic in pregnant and mutagenic in nursing animals. Fetal death causing abortion of mummified fetuses and stillbirths has been found in treated bitches. Hepatotoxicity is associated with increased hepatic enzymes, anorexia, vomiting, and/or icterus. Frequently, adverse effects of GI effects and hepatotoxicity necessitate dosage reduction. At clinical dosages (10–30 mg/kg/day), cats are more sensitive to the hepatotoxic effects than are dogs, although the tolerance is individualistic. One cat received 72 mg/kg/day for 10 mo without obvious signs of toxicity. Reduced production of cortisol and testosterone in dogs at 30 mg/kg/day. Only a transient reduction in testosterone in male cats. In people (and potentially in animals) decreased libido, gynecomastia, azoospermia, impotence in males, and suppressed reproductive cycling in females. Pruritus and alopecia when used at high dosages for extended periods in dogs and cats. Lightening of the haircoat owing to loss of guard hairs and more visible undercoat occurs after 3–4 mo of treatment. It resolves when the drug is discontinued or the dosage is reduced. Cats most consistently develop dry haircoats and weight loss from reduced appetite.

INTERACTIONS. Avoid rifampin and theophylline owing to their decreased activity. Effects of glucocorticoids enhanced owing to increased absorption and reduced clearance. Diphenylhydantoin, rifampin, barbiturates, cyclosporine alter its metabolism. Gastric alkalinizing agents (antacids, H_2 blockers, proton pump inhibitors) and achlorhydria decrease oral absorption. Increases activities of midazolam and diphenylhydantoin and activity and toxicity of cyclosporine.

Availability	Type	Size	Preparations (Company)
Human	Oral tablets, scored	200 mg	*Nizoral* (Janssen)

INTERNATIONAL PREPARATIONS. *Panfungal.*

HANDLING. To make suspension: dissolve or crush 200-mg tablet + 0.8 ml 1 *N* HCl + 3.1 ml water; gives 50 mg/ml concentration. Add this solution to syrup and 13 mg/ml methylcellulose or 2 g/100 ml DMSO (increases odor and dermal penetration) for topical applications. Stable for 6 mo if refrigerated. Shake well before using. Can be formulated for smaller dosage sizes by IDEXX at 1-888-RxIDEXX.

ADMINISTRATION. Monitor serum hepatic enzyme (alanine transaminase and alkaline phosphatase) activities, bilirubin, bile acids before and during treatment (at least monthly). Transient subclinical elevations in liver enzymes are tolerated and expected. With significant hepatotoxicity, temporarily discontinue or decrease dosage, go to alternate-day therapy or switch to alternative drugs. Do not give simultaneously with H_2 blockers, anticholinergics, antacids. Space 2 hr between. Treat dermatophyte infections at least 1 mo. Dividing daily dose and giving with small amounts of food help produce an acidic gastric environment favorable to absorption. Higher doses may be used during initial treatment. Once the disease is under control, the dosage can be reduced and therapy continued for months or years if relapse is anticipated.

DOSAGE

Indications	Dose	Route	Interval (hr)	Duration (days)
Dogs				
Nasal aspergillosis	10 mg/kg	PO	24	6 weeks*
	5 mg/kg	PO	12	2–18 weeks*
Systemic mycosis	10–20 mg/kg	PO	12	2–9 mo*
	15–30 mg/kg	PO	24	2–9 mo*
Sporotrichosis	15 mg/kg	PO	12	2–4 mo*
Cats				
Dermatomycosis	5–10 mg/kg	PO	24	4–9 mo*
Coccidioidomycosis	50 mg/cat	PO	24	9–12 mo*
	25–75 mg/cat	PO	12–48	9–12 mo*
Sporotrichosis	5–10 mg/kg	PO	12–24	2–4 mo*

*This is an expected range of time. Therapy should continue for at least 1 mo beyond last detection of dectable infection.

ADDITIONAL DOSAGES. Dermatophytosis, Table 58–5; cryptococcosis, Table 61–4; coccidioidomycosis, Table 62–3; sporotrichosis, Table 63–1; candidiasis and trichosporosis, Table 66–2; protothecosis, Table 69–1; protozoal infections, Table 71–1; oral infections, Table 89–4.

DISPENSING INFORMATION. Medication should be given on an empty stomach, but if vomiting occurs give with a small amount of food. Treating every other day may reduce side effects if they develop.

LACTOFERRIN

CLASS. Protein.

ACTION. Binds iron, reducing its availability for bacteria.

MORE INFORMATION. See Stomatitis, Chapter 89; reference: 14:173.

PHARMACOKINETICS. Used for its local effects in the oral cavity. Applied in oral cavity.

INDICATIONS. Stomatitis resulting from chronic calicivirus infections, dental disease, secondary to concurrent feline leukemia virus and feline immunodeficiency virus (FIV) infections.

CONTRAINDICATIONS. None.

ADVERSE REACTIONS. None.

INTERACTIONS. None.

AVAILABILITY. Must be purchased from chemical suppliers.

HANDLING. Powder is mixed in solution.

ADMINISTRATION. Drug is given by syringe into oral cavity to contact local mucosal surfaces.

DOSAGE

Indication	Dose	Route	Interval (hr)	Duration (days)
FIV	40 mg/kg	PO topically	24	14

ADDITIONAL DOSAGES. FIV Infection, Table 14–5.

DISPENSING INFORMATION. Take specified amount of liquid in syringe and squirt into cat's mouth. Do not mix with food.

LINCOMYCIN

CLASS. Lincosamide.

ACTION. Bacteriostatic, binds to 50s bacterial ribosomal subunit inhibiting protein synthesis.

MORE INFORMATION. See CLINDAMYCIN and LINCOMYCIN; Chapter 34.

PHARMACOKINETICS. Absorption from GI tract is incomplete and further impaired by food. IM or IV administration yields higher blood concentrations. Good tissue penetration except for meninges, where concentrations reach 40% of those in blood, even with meningitis. Concentrates in areas of low pH (e.g., abscesses). Metabolized in liver, unchanged drug and metabolites excreted in milk, bile, feces, urine. Most (77%) of PO dose given to a fasting animal is excreted in the bile, only 14% in urine. When given IM, 38% and 49% are excreted in bile and urine, respectively.

SPECTRUM. **Gram positive:** *Staphylococcus, Streptococcus, Nocardia, Corynebacterium, Erysipelothrix.* **Gram negative:** poor activity. **Anaerobes:** *Bacteroides, Propionibacterium, Fusobacterium, Peptostreptococcus, Peptococcus, Clostridium, Actinomyces.* **Others:** *Mycoplasma, Leptospira.* **More effective:** gram-positive aerobes, obligate anaerobes. Ineffective: most gram-negative aerobes, *Enterococcus, Mycobacterium.* Bacterial resistance may develop during treatment and usually also involves clindamycin.

INDICATIONS. Staphylococcal pyoderma in dogs. Infections caused by gram-positive bacteria involving upper respiratory tract, skin, wound infections, septicemia, abscesses in dogs and cats. Clindamycin is less toxic and better absorbed and may be preferred but is more costly.

APPROVED USES. Oral preparations for dogs and cats. Parenteral solution for dogs and swine.

CONTRAINDICATIONS. *Malassezia* or *Candida* infection or previous hypersensitivity to a lincosamide. Avoid or reduce dose with renal or hepatic dysfunction. In dogs, no problems with breeding performance, during gestation, or with neonates. May cause diarrhea in nursing puppies if dam is being medicated.

ADVERSE REACTIONS. Diarrhea, occasional vomiting (especially cats), anorexia, polydipsia, polyuria. Slight increases in blood hepatic enzyme activities may occur. IM injections cause local pain, and too-rapid IV infusion may cause hypotension and cardiopulmonary arrest.

INTERACTIONS. Reduces activity of coadministered erythromycin, enhanced activity of neuromuscular blockers.

Availability	Type	Sizes	Preparations (Company)
Veterinary	Oral tablets	100 mg, 200 mg, 500 mg	*Lincocin* (Pharmacia & Upjohn)
	Oral liquid (hydrochloride)	50 mg/ml	*Lincocin* Aquadrops
	Parenteral solution (licensed for swine)	100 mg/ml	*Lincocin* Sterile Solution

INTERNATIONAL PREPARATIONS. *Albiotic, Lincocine, Cillimicina, Cillimycin.*

HANDLING. Store at controlled room temperature (15°C–30°C). IV solution stable for at least 24 hr when mixed with IV fluids.

ADMINISTRATION. Ingesta and kaolin-pectin preparations reduce PO absorption. Can be given IM with slight pain or discomfort. For IV, dilute with 5% dextrose or 0.9% saline and give as slow (drip) infusion.

DOSAGE

Indications	Dose (mg/kg)	Route	Interval (hr)	Duration (days)
Dogs				
Skin, soft tissue infection	15.4	PO	8	21–42,* or 56†
	22	PO	12	21–42*, or 56†
Systemic infection	22	IM, SC, IV‡	24	≤12
	11	IM, SC	12	≤12
Bacteremia, sepsis	11–22	IV	8	≤12
Cats				
Skin and soft tissue infection	11	IM	12	≤12
	22	IM	24	≤12
Systemic infection	15	PO	8	≤12
	22	PO	12	≤12

*Superficial pyoderma.
†Deep, resistant pyoderma.
‡Must be diluted; see Administration.

ADDITIONAL DOSAGES. *Rhodococcus equi* infection, Table 35–6; canine pyoderma, Table 85–3; local ocular administration, Table 93–4.

DISPENSING INFORMATION. Give on empty stomach.

LUFENURON

CLASS. Chitin synthesis inhibitor.

ACTION. Interferes with formation of fungal cell wall and insect exoskeleton.

MORE INFORMATION. Coccidioidomycosis, Chapter 62.

PHARMACOKINETICS. Rapid and complete absorption from the GI tract after PO administration. Highly lipophilic, it enters the adipose, then redistributes back into the blood for approximately 30 days. Concentrates in the milk of lactating dams.

SPECTRUM. Fungi: *Coccidioides*, perhaps other systemic fungi, fleas.

INDICATIONS. Resistant systemic mycotic infections, alone or in combination with a polyene or azole antifungal drug.

APPROVED USES. Flea control for dogs and cats.

CONTRAINDICATIONS. None; appears safe in breeding animals.

ADVERSE REACTIONS. None at recommended concentrations. Anorexia at supratherapeutic doses.

INTERACTIONS. Appears safe in combination with other insecticides and does not alter cholinesterase activity.

Availability	Type	Sizes	Preparations (Company)
Veterinary	Oral tablets	Dogs: 45.0 mg, 90 mg, 204.9 mg, 409.8 mg	*Program* (Ciba-Geigy Animal Health)
	Oral liquid	Cats: Pouch containing liquid 135 mg; 270 mg	*Program*

HANDLING. Stored at room temperature (15°C–30°C). No special precautions for human contact.

ADMINISTRATION. Feeding enhances absorption. Suspension for cats is mixed in a palatable diet.

DOSAGE

Indications	Dose (mg/kg)	Route	Interval (hr)	Duration (days)
Systemic mycosis				
Dogs	5	PO	24	4
Cats	15	PO	24	4*

*Dose for cats is extrapolated and may have to be adjusted.

ADDITIONAL DOSAGES. Coccidioidomycosis, Table 62–3.

DISPENSING INFORMATION. Administer in conjunction with a full meal. Tablets or liquid can be placed in small amount of food to ensure it is eaten.

MARBOFLOXACIN

CLASS. Fluoroquinolone.

ACTION. Bactericidal; inhibits bacterial DNA gyrase.

MORE INFORMATION. See ENROFLOXACIN; Chapter 34; Table 34–11.

PHARMACOKINETICS. Well absorbed from GI tract. Widely distributed in tissues. Concentrations in muscle, liver, kidney, lung, skin are ≥ those in blood. Low protein binding occurs. Minimal metabolism (< 5% of dose). Renal excretion of 2/3 of dose with therapeutic levels in urine 2–5 days after 4-mg/kg dose. One third of the dose appears in feces.

SPECTRUM. Gram positive: *Staphylococcus*, some *Streptococcus*. **Gram negative:** *Escherichia, Klebsiella, Pseudomonas, Proteus, Salmonella, Serratia, Shigella, Citrobacter, Enterobacter, Brucella, Pasteurella*. Anaerobes: poor. Others: see ENROFLOXACIN.

More effective: gram-negative aerobes and facultative anaerobes. **Ineffective:** obligate anaerobes. See ENROFLOXACIN.

INDICATIONS. See ENROFLOXACIN.

APPROVED USES. Dog and cat, skin and urinary infections.

CONTRAINDICATIONS. Has been given at 6 mg/kg for 3 mo to growing dogs. Do not use in growing dogs (< 18 mo for large breeds) or growing cats (< 16 weeks).

ADVERSE REACTIONS. See ENROFLOXACIN.

INTERACTIONS. See ENROFLOXACIN.

Availability	Type	Sizes	Preparation (Company)
Veterinary	Oral tablets	5 mg, 20 mg, 80 mg	*Marbocyl* (Vetoquinol, Lure Cedex, France)

HANDLING. Store tablets in airtight, moisture-proof containers at room temperature.

ADMINISTRATION. See ENROFLOXACIN.

DOSAGE

Indications	Dose (mg/kg)	Route	Interval (hr)	Duration (days)
Dogs				
Urinary infections	2	PO	24	10–28
Skin, pyoderma	2	PO	24	49–126
Systemic infection	2–4	PO	12	<10
Cats				
Urinary, skin infection	2	PO	24	10–28

ADDITIONAL DOSAGES. Enteric bacterial infections, Table 39–1; otitis externa, Table 85–6.

DISPENSING INFORMATION. Can give medicine with food, especially if vomiting is noted.

MEGLUMINE ANTIMONATE

CLASS. Pentavalent antimonial, antiprotozoal.

ACTION. Antiprotozoal; interferes with energy metabolism of *Leishmania*.

MORE INFORMATION. See STIBOGLUCONATE; Chapter 71; Table 71–1; references: 71:10, 71:36, 73:51, 73:54.

PHARMACOKINETICS. Bioavailability in dogs is 92% after IM and SC injection because polar molecule has limited tissue distribution (71:36). High concentrations are reached in skin, spleen, liver in decreasing order. Rapidly eliminated by renal excretion. Liposomal-encapsulated formulations are being evaluated to reduce side effects (71:36a). These formulations have delayed uptake following SC compared with IM.

SPECTRUM. *Leishmania*. Resistance to drug may develop during treatment of infected dogs (71:10).

INDICATIONS. Leishmaniasis.

APPROVED USES. Humans for leishmaniasis; not available in U.S.

CONTRAINDICATIONS. Previous hypersensitivity, hepatic or renal insufficiency, cardiac arrhythmias, leukopenia.

ADVERSE REACTIONS. Pain, swelling, lameness with IM injection, SC preferred. Thrombophlebitis with IV use. See also STIBOGLUCONATE.

INTERACTIONS. May combine with allopurinol for increased efficacy.

Availability	Type	Size	Preparation (Company)
Veterinary	*N*-methylglucamine antimoniate	300 mg/ml as antimony in 5-ml ampules	*Glucantime* (Merial)

HANDLING. Store solution in sterile container at room temperature.

ADMINISTRATION. Continue medication until clinical signs or skin lesions have resolved. Give by slow IV, deep IM, or by SC or IP. For resistant cases, can give alternate dosing with Pentamidine *(Lomidine)*. Treatment involves 10–12 injections in succession if initiated early and 18–20 injections if chronic manifestations (dermatitis) are present. Injections are given 2–3 days apart.

DOSAGE

Indications (Dogs)	Dose	Route	Interval (hr)	Duration (days)
Leishmaniasis	100 mg/kg	SC	24	10*†
	200 mg/kg	SC, IV	48	20–40†
	5–10 ml	IV, IM, IP	48–72	‡
	10–20 ml	IV, IM, IP	48–72	‡
	20–30 ml	IV, IM, IP	48–72	‡

*Give for 10 days on and off for 1–8 months of treatment.
†More effective if combined with allopurinol, which is continued up to 8 months.
‡Package insert dosage regimen (treat for 10–12 injections if acute and 18–20 injections if chronic).

ADDITIONAL DOSAGES. Leishmaniasis, Table 73–4.

METHENAMINE MANDELATE (or HIPPURATE)

CLASS. Urinary antiseptic.

ACTION. Produces acid urine, which is bacteriostatic.

MORE INFORMATION. Chapter 34.

PHARMACOKINETICS. Readily absorbed from GI tract but 10%–30% destroyed by gastric acid unless enteric-coated tablets are used. Minimal blood or tissue levels but enters placenta and milk. Excreted (>90%) in urine within 24 hr. In acid urine, methenamine is hydrolyzed to ammonia and formaldehyde. The acid salts (mandelate and hippurate) help lower urine pH. Coadministration of acids (e.g., ascorbate) may help maintain low urine pH.

SPECTRUM. Gram positive: *Staphylococcus, Enterococcus.* **Gram negative:** *Escherichia.* **Ineffective:** in alkaline urine or against *Enterobacter* and other urea-splitting organisms (*Proteus, Pseudomonas*), which raise urine pH.

INDICATIONS. Chronic or recurrent urinary tract infections for long-term suppression/elimination of infection. Do not use in place of appropriate antimicrobial therapy to eliminate infection. Must eliminate infection by urea-splitting bacteria to allow methenamine to be effective. Only choice in predisposed animals in which anatomic causes cannot be eliminated.

APPROVED USES. Human: urinary infections.

CONTRAINDICATIONS. Pregnancy, lactation, renal or hepatic insufficiency (because of ammonia loading). Use of sulfonamides. Drug itself is not toxic in renal failure; organic acids it produces may be detrimental with mandelate; crystals may form in renal failure.

ADVERSE REACTIONS. Dysuria, bladder irritation, increased serum hepatic transaminases, vomiting, oral irritation.

INTERACTIONS. Urinary alkalinizing agents reduce effectiveness. Coadministration with sulfonamides may induce crystalluria and renal tubular damage in some species, but, because of unique sulfonamide metabolism, dogs are usually not affected. Drug combines with sulfonamides in urine, which results in mutual ineffectiveness of the drugs.

Availability	Type	Sizes	Preparations (Company)
Human	Oral tablets	1 g (as hippurate)	*Hiprex* (Marion Merrell Dow), *Urex* (3M Pharmaceuticals)
	Oral tablets	500 mg (as mandelate)	*Mandelamine* (Parke-Davis), Generic (various)
	Oral suspension	500 mg/5 ml (as mandelate)	Generic (various)

HANDLING. Store at room temperature and avoid contact with acids or metallic salts.

ADMINISTRATION. Offer animal free choice water. Give with meals to reduce GI irritation. Also available in combinations with other antimicrobials, pH reducers, urinary analgesics. Feeding diets that decrease urine pH are additive.

DOSAGE

Indication	Dose	Route	Interval (hr)	Duration (days)
Dogs	16.5 mg/kg	PO	24	prn*

*Therapy can be extended for months to suppress bacterial growth.

DISPENSING INFORMATION. Report any gastrointestinal signs to your veterinarian.

METRONIDAZOLE

CLASS. Nitroimidazole.

ACTION. Bactericidal, also antiprotozoal; penetrates cells by diffusion, metabolized in anaerobic organisms to intermediates that prevent DNA synthesis.

MORE INFORMATION. See TINIDAZOLE; Chapters 34 and 71; references: 34:108, 34:111, 71:7.

PHARMACOKINETICS. Virtually 100% GI absorption. Food delays systemic availability in people but not in dogs; also absorbed rectally. Good tissue penetration to all sites, including hard-to-reach areas such as brain, bone, placenta, fetal tissues, fluids (CSF, milk, saliva). Higher concentration in prostate than plasma of dog (34:111). Penetrates abscesses and pyothorax well. Metabolized in liver with predominantly active metabolites (60%–80%). Excreted mainly in urine and 10%–15% in feces. PO and IV routes give similar blood drug concentrations, but parenteral route is more expensive.

SPECTRUM. Anaerobic protozoa: *Trichomonas, Giardia, Entamoeba* (trophozoites), *Balantidium*. **Anaerobic bacteria:** *Bacteroides, Veillonella, Fusobacterium, Peptococcus,* most *Clostridium, Eubacterium,* few *Peptostreptococcus*. Alternative choices for anaerobic bacteria are chloramphenicol, clindamycin, cefoxitin. **Others:** *Helicobacter,* oral spirochetes, variable for *Campylobacter.* **More effective:** consistently good against *Bacteroides*. **Ineffective:** *Actinomyces,* yeasts, aerobic bacteria, and aerobic protozoa.

INDICATIONS. Recurrent or persistent anaerobic infections that fail to respond to penicillins, clindamycin, chloramphenicol. Anaerobic infections: intra-abdominal, anaerobic meningitis, intracranial abscesses, bacteremia, osteomyelitis, dermatitis, synovitis, soft tissue infections, chronic colitis, intestinal bacterial overgrowth (34:108), stomatitis, oral ulceration, tetanus, *Helicobacter*-associated gastritis, bacterial vaginitis, and prophylaxis (with aminoglycosides) for colorectal surgery. As antiprotozoal for trichomoniasis, giardiasis, amebiasis, balantidiasis.

APPROVED USES. Human: anaerobic infections and abscesses, gastric helicobacteriosis.

CONTRAINDICATIONS. Dose reduction (50%) with liver failure and some reduction with severe renal failure. Reduced dosage for neonates. Avoid in pregnancy because carcinogenic and mutagenic when laboratory rodents given chronic high doses.

ADVERSE REACTIONS. Profuse salivation, anorexia, weight loss with PO administration to cats. Can discolor urine reddish-brown. Vomiting, diarrhea, glossitis, stomatitis. Neurologic complications are seizures, encephalopathy, cerebellar dysfunction. Generalized ataxia and vertical positional nystagmus. *Never* exceed 30 mg/kg/day for dogs and cats. CNS toxicity in dogs has resulted with high (≥ 60 mg/kg/day) dosages, often after 7–10 days treatment. Cerebellar and vestibular nuclear injury (71:7). Degenerative changes in Purkinje's cells and associated cerebellar and vestibular axons. CNS signs may progress rapidly and develop after acute or chronic overdosage. Signs may take several days to months to resolve, but some dogs develop uncontrollable seizures, fatal encephalopathy, coma. CSF analysis may show increased protein concentration. Peripheral neuropathy with long-term use in people. Rarely pancreatitis, reversible mild leukopenia, thrombocytopenia. Long-term use may cause *Candida* overgrowth in GI tract.

INTERACTIONS. Barbiturates may alter metabolism, reducing metronidazole's therapeutic efficacy. Potentiates vitamin K antagonist rodenticides. Cimetidine may increase its concentration and enhance toxicity, whereas phenobarbital and diphenylhydantoin may decrease it. May interfere with measurement of serum triglycerides or some hepatic enzymes. In people, has been given in combination with tetracycline or amoxicillin and bismuth subsalicylate tablets to treat *Helicobacter*-associated gastritis and ulcers (see Chapter 39). Clarithromycin has been substituted for metronidazole when resistance is suspected. In some countries, metronidazole is available combined with spiramycin for treatment of mixed aerobic and anaerobic infections such as stomatitis, abscesses, genital and cutaneous infections. See SPIRAMYCIN.

Availability	Type	Sizes	Preparations (Company)
Human	Oral tablets	250 mg, 500 mg	*Flagyl* (Searle), generic (various)
	Powder for injection	500 mg (as HCl)	*Flagyl* IV
	Solution for injection	500 mg	*Flagyl* IV, *Metronidazole Redi-Infusion (Elkins-Sinn)*
Veterinary	Solution for injection	5 mg/ml	*Torgyl* (Merial)

INTERNATIONAL PREPARATIONS. *Abbonidazole, Acuzole, Anabact, Anaerobex, Anaeromet, Arilin, Ascacea, Bemetrazole, Clinazole, Elyzol, Metrazole, Metrogyl, Metrolyl, Metronide, Metrostat, Metrozol, Metryl, Narobic, Nidazol, Oecozol, Pharmaflex, Protostat, Rathimed, Rozex, Trichozole, Trikacide, Zagyl, Stomorgyl* (combined with *Spiramycin*).

HANDLING. Store tablets and powders in airtight, light-resistant containers. IV solution can be diluted with 0.9% NaCl or bacteriostatic water for injection, and further diluted in lactated Ringer's, 0.9% NaCl, or 5% dextrose. The pH is low (0.5–2), so before infusion add 5 mmol sodium bicarbonate for each 500 mg used to raise pH to 6–7. CO_2 bubbles may form during this, and the pressure needs an outlet. The neutralized solution should not be refrigerated, or precipitates may form. It must be used in 24 hr. If not neutralized, it is stable for 96 hr at room temperature. Should not contact aluminum (including needles), or solution may discolor to reddish-brown. Can be mixed in solutions with most aminoglycosides, cephalosporins, and penicillins. Protect from exposure to light. Refrigerated or concentrated (> 8 mg/ml) solutions will precipitate.

ADMINISTRATION. When possible, preferably give whole coated tablets to cats to reduce oral contact with bitter drug. Has a metallic taste that is distasteful to cats. Generic tablets can be crushed and powder placed in syrup gum, tragacanth, or melted butter to improve palatability. See administration of ITRACONAZOLE for details on mixing with butter. Can be formulated for smaller doses by IDEXX at 1–888-RxIDEXX. This drug is less palatable to cats than furazolidone for giardiasis, and there is risk of neurotoxicity at higher dosages (71:7). Can be given with food, and in dogs, absorption is enhanced.

DOSAGE

Indications	Dose	Route	Interval (hr)	Duration (days)
Dogs				
Giardiasis, trichomoniasis	30 mg/kg	PO	24	5–7
Stomatitis, colitis	10 mg/kg	PO	12	10
	20 mg/kg	PO	24	10
Stomatitis, soft tissue infection	7.5 mg/kg	PO	8	10
Systemic bacteremia, meningitis	10 mg/kg	PO, IV	8	14
Cats				
Giardiasis, trichomoniasis	10–25 mg/kg	PO	24	5
	8–10 mg/kg	PO	12	10
Anaerobic bacteremia or meningitis	10 mg/kg	PO, IV	8	prn
Soft tissue infection	7.5 mg/kg	PO	8–12	prn
Giardiasis	250 mg/cat	PO	24	5–7
	10 mg/kg	PO	24	5–7
	4 mg/kg	PO	12	5

ADDITIONAL DOSAGES. FIV infection, Table 14–5; endotoxemia, Table 38–1; enteric bacterial infections, Table 39–1; gastric helicobacteriosis, Table 39–3; *Clostridium perfringens* diarrhea, Table 39–4; anaerobic infections, Table 41–10; tetanus, Table 43–2; feline abscesses, Table 52–2; enteric protozoal infections, Table 78–2; bacteremia and endocarditis, Table 87–7; oral infections, Table 89–4; gastrointestinal infections, Table 89–11; colitis, Table 89–14; intra-abdominal infections, Table 89–15; hepatobiliary infections, Table 90–4; CNS infections, Table 92–5.

DISPENSING INFORMATION. Has an unpleasant metallic taste. May cause excessive salivation if tablets are bitten; do not crush or break. May darken urine color. May cause GI upset; take with food.

MINOCYCLINE

CLASS. Tetracycline.

ACTION. Bacteriostatic; inhibits protein synthesis by binding to 30s ribosomal unit.

MORE INFORMATION. DOXYCYCLINE, TETRACYCLINES; Chapter 34; Table 34–7.

PHARMACOKINETICS. More lipid soluble (10×) than tetracycline; 100% absorbed from GI tract. Penetrates well into most tissues, body fluids, difficult areas such as prostate, female reproductive tract, lung, bronchial secretions, saliva, bile, CSF, CNS. The only tetracycline that penetrates CNS with noninflamed meninges. Crosses the placenta to accumulate in fetal bones and teeth. Clears primarily by extensive hepatic metabolism and biliary elimination. Only small amount excreted in feces in unchanged form; active drug does not accumulate in liver failure. Minimal (4%–9%) urinary excretion; dose reduction not needed for renal failure.

SPECTRUM. See DOXYCYCLINE. **More effective:** than tetracycline against *Staphylococcus* and *Nocardia*. **Ineffective:** see DOXYCYCLINE.

INDICATIONS. Brucellosis (combined with other drugs), borreliosis, nosocomial infections against bacteria resistant to other drugs.

APPROVED USES. Human: bacterial infections of skin and respiratory and urinary tracts.

CONTRAINDICATIONS. Pregnancy, lactation, and young (< 6 mo). Dosage does not need reducing in renal failure because drug is excreted by biliary tract. However, drug does not accumulate in liver disease.

ADVERSE REACTIONS. Nausea, vomiting, yellow dental staining in young animals, increased hepatic enzyme activity, rare ototoxicity. Hypotension, shivering, dyspnea, cardiac arrhythmias, shock, and urticaria have developed in dogs given rapid IV doses that may have been caused by the drug vehicle. Certain vehicles such as propylene glycol in other IV tetracycline preparations may be responsible for acute systemic allergic reactions. In comparison, rapid IV infusions of doxycycline (5 mg/kg) has not produced systemic reactions. Vestibular side effects seen in people are related to a peculiar biotransformation of minocycline that does not occur in dogs and cats. Minocycline, at 10–20 mg/kg daily for 1 mo, decreased erythrocyte mass and increased blood alanine transaminase activity. Daily IV doses of 40 mg/kg produced increased urine calcium and Bromsulphalein retention, decreased food consumption, and weight loss. None of the effects were seen with similar PO dosages.

INTERACTIONS. GI absorption reduced by iron preparations, aluminum hydroxide gels, sodium bicarbonate, calcium, and magnesium salts.

Availability	Type	Sizes	Preparations (Company)
Human	Oral capsules	50 mg, 100 mg	*Minocin* (Lederle)
	Oral tablets	50 mg, 100 mg	*Minocin*
	Oral suspension	50 mg/5 ml	*Minocin*
	Powder for injection (IV)	100-mg vial	*Minocin*

INTERNATIONAL PREPARATIONS. *Aknosan, Aknoral, Dynacin, Klinotab, Mestacine, Minoclir, Minogal, Minomycin, Mynocine, Oracyclin.*

HANDLING. Reconstituted IV solution is stable at room temperature for 24 hr; activity declines to 92% after 1 week storage at room temperature and to 98% if refrigerated. Oral capsules should be stored at room temperature away from light. Oral suspension should be stored at room temperature but not frozen.

ADMINISTRATION. For IV, given diluted in 5% dextrose or 0.9% sodium chloride. Feeding does not affect absorption of oral preparations. Do not administer rapidly IV.

DOSAGE

Indications	Dose (mg/kg)	Route	Interval (hr)	Duration (days)
Dogs				
Soft tissue, urinary infections	5–12	PO, IV	12	7–14
Brucellosis (in combination)	12.5	PO	12	14–21
Cats				
Haemobartonellosis	6–11	PO	12	21

ADDITIONAL DOSAGES. Ehrlichiosis, Table 28–4; haemobartonellosis, Table 30–1; canine brucellosis, Table 40–2; actinomycosis, Table 49–1; nocardiosis, Table 49–2; musculoskeletal infections, Table 86–3.

DISPENSING INFORMATION. Can be given with food.

MYCOBACTERIAL CELL WALL EXTRACT

CLASS. Bacterial component.

ACTION. Immunostimulatory. Production of tumor necrosis factor and other cytokines.

MORE INFORMATION. Chapter 100 and Table 100– 21.

PHARMACOKINETICS. From nonpathogenic species and strain of mycobacteria, contains purified mycobacterial cell wall fractions with known immunostimulatory properties. Contains low-level analgesic and a green tracking solution to facilitate location of intra-tumor administration.

SPECTRUM. Stimulates activation of macrophages and thymic lymphocytes in tissue and blood cells. Increases interleukin–1 production.

INDICATIONS. Parenteral nonspecific immunostimulant, vaccine adjuvant, intralesional for antitumor therapy. Canine mammary tumors.

APPROVED USES. Adenocarcinomas in dog and sarcoids in horses.

CONTRAINDICATIONS. Previous allergic reactions to the drug. Pre-existing mycobacterial disease. Concurrent immunosuppression or glucocorticoid therapy.

ADVERSE REACTIONS. Fever, anorexia, systemic inflammatory reaction. Pain at the time of injection.

INTERACTIONS. Increased response of horses to herpesvirus vaccination when given IM, at the same time, but different site.

Availability	Type	Sizes	Preparations (Company)
Veterinary	Intratumoral (canine and equine)	10-ml vials	*Regressin-V* (Vetrepharm)
	IV (equine)	1.5-ml syringes	*Equimune I.V.* (Vetrepharm)

HANDLING. Store in a refrigerator (36°F–45°F [2°C–7°C]) but do not freeze. Mix the emulsion thoroughly until milky white in color immediately before use. May heat to 65°C to facilitate mixing.

ADMINISTRATION. Using a 20-gauge needle or smaller, mammary tumors are injected intralesionally and perilesionally under sedation or anesthesia once 2–4 weeks before surgery. Without surgery, repeat injections every 1–3 weeks for up to four treatments. Tumors that fail to respond after 4 treatments are considered refractory.

DOSAGE

Indications	Dose (ml)	Route	Interval (hr)	Duration (days)
Equine vaccine adjuvant	1.5	IM (deep)	24	1
Equine respiratory disease	1.5	IV	24	1

NEOMYCIN

CLASS. Aminoglycoside.

ACTION. Bactericidal, inhibits protein synthesis.

MORE INFORMATION. See GENTAMICIN; Aminoglycosides, Chapter 34; Tables 34–5, 34–6.

PHARMACOKINETICS. Poorly absorbed (<5%) from intact GI tract. Topical use for ulcerative lesions may allow increased uptake and potential toxicity. Majority of oral dose is excreted unchanged in feces. Any absorbed drug is excreted unchanged in urine.

SPECTRUM. See GENTAMICIN, less effective than gentamicin against many *Pseudomonas, Klebsiella, Escherichia.*

INDICATIONS. Not used parenterally because more toxic and less effective than other aminoglycosides. Commonly used orally for reduction of enteric flora or pathogens. Effect lasts for 48–72 hr after single dosing. Used orally for prophylaxis before intestinal or colonic surgery and to reduce bacterial ammonia production in hepatic insufficiency or coma.

APPROVED USES. Veterinary, farm animals.

CONTRAINDICATIONS. Pregnancy, because small absorbed amounts are fetotoxic; GI obstruction or ulcerative disease of GI tract suggested by hemoptysis, melena, or hematochezia.

ADVERSE REACTIONS. Diarrhea owing to microflora alterations, nephrotoxicity, ototoxicity, interference with intestinal bacterial vitamin K synthesis and fat malabsorption.

INTERACTIONS. Potentiates vitamin K deficiency and associated coagulopathy. Decreases absorption of digoxin, methotrexate, penicillin V, vitamin K.

Availability	Type	Sizes	Preparations (Company)
Human	Oral tablets (as sulfate)	500 mg	Generic (Biocraft)
	Oral solution (as sulfate)	125 mg/5 ml	*Mycifradin* (Pharmacia & Upjohn); Generic (various)
Veterinary	Oral liquid (as sulfate)	140 mg/ml	*Biosol* (Pharmacia & Upjohn)
	Oral solution (as sulfate)	50 mg/ml	*Biosol*
	Oral tablets (as sulfate)	100 mg	*Biosol* tablets

INTERNATIONAL PREPARATIONS. *Bykomycin, Francetin, Myciguent, Nebacetin, Neo-fradin, Neointestin.*

HANDLING. Store at room temperature in airtight and lightproof container.

ADMINISTRATION. PO: can give undiluted or diluted with water. Can be added to the sole source of drinking water to be consumed in 24 hr but must be made as fresh solution each day. Can also give by syringe or gavage. Not recommended for parenteral use.

DOSAGE

Indications (Dogs and Cats)	Dose	Route	Interval (hr)	Duration (days)
Bacterial enteritis, reducing GI flora, hepatic encephalopathy	10–15 mg/kg	PO	6–24	≤14

ADDITIONAL DOSAGES. Endotoxemia, Table 38–1; otitis externa (topical), Tables 85–6 and 85–8; local ocular use, Table 93–4.

DISPENSING INFORMATION. If animal shows persistent vomiting or bloody diarrhea, discontinue medication and notify veterinarian immediately.

NIFURTIMOX

CLASS. Nitrofuran derivative.

ACTION. Antiprotozoal; oxidative effects on trypanosomal enzymes, especially involving nucleic acid biosynthesis.

MORE INFORMATION. See Chapters 71, 72; Table 71–1.

PHARMACOKINETICS. Well absorbed from GI tract after PO administration, low plasma concentrations. Undergoes rapid biotransformation in liver to metabolites; little (≤0.5%) of active drug is excreted in urine.

SPECTRUM. *Trypanosoma cruzi.* African trypanosomiasis at higher dosages (second choice).

INDICATIONS. American trypanosomiasis. Some effect on African trypanosomiasis. Reduces severity of acute disease but ineffective in chronic phases; suppresses infection rather than cures. Pre-existing seizures or renal or hepatic disease. Alternative drug is benznidazole. Use of allopurinol has not been well studied in this disease.

CONTRAINDICATIONS. Despite toxicity, may be one of few effective drugs for this disease. Pre-existing seizures or renal or hepatic disease. Alternative drug is benznidazole.

ADVERSE REACTIONS. Frequent toxicity, including anorexia, vomiting, weight loss, CNS signs, polyneuritis, pulmonary infiltrates, skin eruptions, mitogenic (chromosomal aberrations). Hemolysis with glucose-6 phosphate dehydrogenase deficiency. In people, children tolerate the drug better than adults.

INTERACTIONS. Alcohol ingestion in people enhances adverse reactions.

Availability	Type	Size	Preparation (Company)
Human	Investigation drug for human use only in U.S. from CDC, (404) 639–3670; available in other countries	Oral tablets 120 mg	*Lampit* (Bayer)

HANDLING. Store at room temperature in airtight container.

ADMINISTRATION. Reduce dosage if GI disturbances occur.

DOSAGE

Indications (Human)	Dose (mg/kg)	Route	Interval (hr)	Duration (days)
Trypanosomiasis (*T. cruzi*)				
Adults	2–2.5	PO	6	90
Children	3–3.5	PO	6	90

ADDITIONAL DOSAGES. Trypanosomiasis, Table 72–1.

DISPENSING INFORMATION. Can be given with food but may cause gastrointestinal upsets. Food tends to reduce the gastrointestinal irritation.

NITROFURANTOIN

CLASS. Nitrofuran.

ACTION. Bactericidal or bacteriostatic; inhibits bacterial carbohydrate metabolism and cell wall formation.

MORE INFORMATION. See Nitrofurans, Chapter 34; Table 34–9.

PHARMACOKINETICS. Well absorbed (85–95%) from GI tract after PO administration. Bioavailability enhanced and irritation reduced by giving with food. The macrocrystalline formulation is less irritating to GI tract but more slowly absorbed. The microcrystals are absorbed faster, reaching higher and more rapid peak urinary bladder levels. Most of the drug is metabolized with 30%–50% excreted unchanged in urine. Concentrations in blood or tissues are too low to be effective but are sufficient to treat urinary tract infections.

SPECTRUM. **Gram positive:** *Staphylococcus, Streptococcus, Enterococcus.* **Gram negative:** *Escherichia*, some *Klebsiella*, some *Enterobacter, Salmonella.* **Ineffective:** *Proteus, Serratia, Pseudomonas, Acinetobacter.*

INDICATIONS. Urinary tract infections caused by susceptible organisms.

APPROVED USES. Human urinary tract infections.

CONTRAINDICATIONS. Reduce dosage in renal failure, oliguria, pregnancy, breeding males or females.

ADVERSE REACTIONS. Interstitial pneumonitis, hemolysis with glucose–6-phosphate dehydrogenase deficiency, cholestatic hepatitis, peripheral neuropathy. (The latter was noted in a dog by the author.) Vomiting is most common side effect in dogs and cats. May discolor urine to dark brown.

INTERACTIONS. Coadministered anticholinergics increase bioavailability while magnesium salts reduce absorption. May interfere with efficacy of fluoroquinolones.

Availability	Type	Sizes	Preparations (Company)
Human	Oral suspension	25 mg/ml	*Furadantin* (Proctor & Gamble)
	Oral capsules (microcrystalline)	25 mg, 50 mg, 100 mg	*Macrodantin* (Proctor & Gamble), generics (various) Nitrofurantoin generic (various)
	Oral capsules (regular)	50 mg, 100 mg	*Furadantin*

INTERNATIONAL PREPARATIONS. *Chemiofuran, Cistofuran, Cystit, Furabid, Furedan, Macrobid, Microdoïne, Nephronex, Novofuran, Phenurin, Urantoin, Urodid, Urolong.*

HANDLING. Store in airtight, light-proof containers at room temperature. May darken with light exposure. Avoid contact with most metals.

ADMINISTRATION. Bioavailability and GI tolerance is enhanced by giving with food. For long-term prophylaxis, give in evening to maintain nighttime levels in urine. Suspension can be mixed with milk to facilitate administration to animals.

DOSAGE

Indications (Dogs and Cats)	Dose (mg/kg)	Route	Interval (hr)	Duration (days)
Urinary infections				
Severe or difficult	4	PO	6	14–28
Routine	2.2–4.4	PO	8	7–14
Long-term prophylaxis	3–4	PO	24	≥90

ADDITIONAL DOSAGES. Urinary infections, Table 91–8.

DISPENSING INFORMATION. Give with food.

NORFLOXACIN

CLASS. Fluoroquinolone.

ACTION. Inhibits bacterial DNA gyrase.

MORE INFORMATION. See ENROFLOXACIN, MARBOFLOXACIN; Fluoroquinolones, Chapter 34; Table 34–11.

PHARMACOKINETICS. Lower bioavailability (30%–40%) than other quinolones after PO administration. Food reduces absorption. Hepatic metabolism to less active metabolites with biliary and urinary excretion. Penetrates well into genitourinary tract and its secretions.

SPECTRUM. Gram positive: *Staphylococcus.* **Gram negative:** *Escherichia, Proteus, Pseudomonas, Enterobacter.* Activity is lower than with ciprofloxacin and enrofloxacin. **Anerobes:** Minimal activity against obligate anaerobes. Resistance may develop when treating infections caused by *Klebsiella, Pseudomonas, Enterococcus.* **Others:** See ENROFLOXACIN. **More Effective:** aerobic or facultative anaerobic gram-negative bacteria. **Ineffective:** obligate anaerobes.

INDICATIONS. See ENROFLOXACIN.

CONTRAINDICATIONS. See ENROFLOXACIN.

ADVERSE REACTIONS. See ENROFLOXACIN. Interactions: See ENROFLOXACIN.

Availability	Type	Size	Preparation (Company)
Human	Oral tablets	400 mg	*Noroxin* (Merck)

HANDLING. Store in airtight, light-proof containers at room temperature.

ADMINISTRATION. Food can delay absorption but not considered to be critical.

DOSAGE

Indications (Dogs and Cats)	Dose (mg/kg)	Route	Interval (hr)	Duration (days)
Skin, urinary infections*	5–11	PO	12	14–21
Soft tissues, systemic† infections	11–22	PO	12	14–21
Bacteremia	22	PO, IM	12	prn

**Staphylococcus, Escherichia coli, Klebsiella, Serratia.*
†Pseudomonas, Enterobacter.

ADDITIONAL DOSAGES. Bacteremia and endocarditis, Table 87–7.

DISPENSING INFORMATION. Give medication on empty stomach. Do not give with dairy products or other antacids.

NOVOBIOCIN

CLASS. Coumarin antibiotic.

ACTION. Usually bacteriostatic; interferes with bacterial cell wall synthesis and nucleic acid synthesis.

MORE INFORMATION. See Novobiocin, Chapter 34.

PHARMACOKINETICS. Well absorbed from the GI tract, but food may reduce. High degree of serum protein binding so tissue and body fluid concentrations are low. Little penetration of CSF, even in meningitis. Predominantly excreted in bile and feces with little appearing in urine.

SPECTRUM. Gram positive: some *Streptococcus, Staphylococcus*, few *Enterococcus*. **Gram negative:** most resistant except *Proteus, Pasteurella*, and some *Pseudomonas*. **Anaerobes:** most resistant. **Ineffective:** most *Enterococcus*, and gram negatives.

INDICATIONS. Staphylococcal infections, upper respiratory tract infections in dogs, in combination with tetracycline with or without prednisolone.

CONTRAINDICATIONS. Hepatic insufficiency, biliary obstruction, myelosuppressive diseases.

ADVERSE REACTIONS. Allergic hypersensitivity, dermal eruptions, hepatic dysfunction, vomiting, diarrhea, bone marrow dyscrasia.

INTERACTIONS. May prolong excretion and increase blood concentrations of β-lactam and cephalosporin drugs. May inhibit excretion of bilirubin and Bromsulphalein. Often administered in combination with tetracycline or rifampin to prevent resistance.

Availability	Type	Sizes	Preparations (Company)
Human	Oral capsules	250 mg	*Albamycin* (Pharmacia & Upjohn)
	Oral syrup	125 mg/5 ml	*Albamycin*
Veterinary	Novobiocin (as sodium) and tetracycline (as HCl)	60 mg each or 180 mg each	*Albaplex* and *Albaplex–3X* (Pharmacia & Upjohn)
		also with prednisolone (1.5 or 4.5 mg)	*Delta Albaplex* and *Delta Albaplex–3X*

HANDLING. Store in airtight containers at room temperature.

ADMINISTRATION. Preferably give on empty stomach. If vomiting occurs, give with small amount of food. Available in combination with tetracycline, with or without prednisolone, for use in dogs. Tetracycline absorption in the combined preparations is more affected by ingesta than is novobiocin.

DOSAGE

Indications (Dogs)	Dose (mg/kg)	Route	Interval (hr)	Duration (days)
Respiratory infections	10	PO	8	5–7
	22*	PO	12	5–7

*Combined with tetracycline.

DISPENSING INFORMATION. Give at least 1 hr before or 2 hr after feeding. If vomiting occurs, consult veterinarian.

OFLOXACIN

CLASS. Fluoroquinolone.

ACTION. Bactericidal; inhibits bacterial enzyme DNA gyrase.

MORE INFORMATION. See ENROFLOXACIN; Chapter 34, Table 34–11.

PHARMACOKINETICS. Systemic availability after PO administration, bioavailability is 98% (the highest of the class). Maximum blood concentrations in 1–2 hr. Wide distribution in body tissues and fluids. Detected in blister fluid, genital tissues, lung. CSF concentrations are 40%–90% serum, if inflamed. Human aqueous humor concentration is 44%–88% serum. Minimal metabolism, primarily renally excreted.

SPECTRUM. Gram positive: *Staphylococcus*, some *Streptococcus*, poor activity against *Enterococcus*. **Gram negative:** *Enterobacter, Klebsiella, Pseudomonas, Proteus, Salmonella, Serratia, Yersinia, Campylobacter.* **Anaerobes:** poor activity. *Bacteroides* and *Clostridium* are inhibited in vitro.

INDICATIONS. Complicated urinary tract infections; also lower respiratory tract, skin, and soft tissue infections caused by susceptible gram-negative bacteria.

CONTRAINDICATIONS. Drug clearance reduced with renal failure so must use lower dosages. Avoid in pregnancy or lactation.

ADVERSE REACTIONS. Arthropathies in immature animals. High overdosages have not produced lenticular opacities or crystalluria, although these can occur with other drugs of this class. Nausea, vomiting, diarrhea may occur. All quinolones have potential to cause CNS hyperexcitability and seizures. Phototoxicity has been seen with use of some compounds in this class.

INTERACTIONS. Theophylline concentrations will increase when given concurrently. Should not give orally within 2–4 hr of receiving sucralfate or preparations containing polyvalent cations (Al, Ca, Mg, Fe, Zn).

Availability	Type	Sizes	Preparations (Company)
Human	Tablets	200 mg, 300 mg, 400 mg	*Floxin* (Ortho)
	IV solution	200 mg, 400 mg	*Floxin*

INTERNATIONAL PREPARATIONS. *Floxal, Surnox, Tarivid, Trafloxal.*

HANDLING. Store tablets in tightly closed containers below 30°C. Solution can be added to 0.9% NaCl, 5% dextrose, or solutions containing KCl.

ADMINISTRATION. Effect of food on absorption has not been well studied, but it may be better to avoid dosing with food.

DOSAGE

Indications (Dogs and Cats)	Dose (mg/kg)	Route	Interval (hr)	Duration (days)
Uncomplicated urinary infections	2.5	PO	12	7
Complicated urinary, genital infections	5–7.5	PO	12	10
Lower respiratory tract infections	7.5–10	PO	12	14

DISPENSING INFORMATION. Monitor animal for adequate water intake; avoid sucralfate and vitamins with iron and mineral supplements and antacids within 4 hr of administration.

ORBIFLOXACIN

CLASS. Fluoroquinolone.

ACTION. Bactericidal; inhibits bacterial DNA gyrase.

MORE INFORMATION. See ENROFLOXACIN, MARBOFLOXACIN; Chapter 34; Table 34–11.

PHARMACOKINETICS. Well absorbed orally (97% bioavailable) with peak plasma concentrations within 1 hr of administration. Plasma protein binding low (7%–14%). In dogs, after 3 hours of giving 5 mg/kg dose, tissue concentrations are 6.0 μg/ml in prostate and 4.1 μg/ml in lung. It is predominantly (50%) excreted unchanged in urine with concentrations of 100 μg/ml, between 0 and 6 hours after administration of 2.5 mg/kg.

SPECTRUM. Gram-negative and some gram-positive bacteria. Not effective against anaerobes. See ENROFLOXACIN.

INDICATIONS. Skin and soft tissue infections (wounds, abscesses, pyoderma) and urinary tract infections.

CONTRAINDICATIONS. Young growing animals, seizure-prone animals. Safety in pregnancy and breeding dogs has not been established.

ADVERSE REACTIONS. Can cause CNS stimulation and seizures in predisposed animals. Immature animals may develop arthropathy when treated. Avoid in rapid growth phase of 2–8 mo in small and medium breeds and up to 18 mo in giant breeds. See also ENROFLOXACIN.

INTERACTIONS. See also ENROFLOXACIN. Compounds such as sucralfate, antacids, and multivitamins that contain divalent and trivalent cations (iron, aluminum, calcium, magnesium or zinc) may interfere with absorption.

Availability	Type	Sizes	Preparation (Company)
Veterinary (dog and cat)	Oral tablets (scored)	5.7 mg (yellow), 22.7 mg (green), 68 mg (blue)	*Orbax* (Schering-Plough Animal Health)

HANDLING. Store tablets at controlled temperature between 2°C and 30°C.

ADMINISTRATION. For skin and soft tissue infections, give for 2–3 days beyond cessation of signs for a maximum of 30 days. Effect of feeding on dose has not been determined.

DOSAGE

Indications	Dose* (mg/kg)	Route	Interval (hr)	Duration (days)
Urinary infections	2.5–5.0	PO	24	10†
Soft tissue infections	5.0–7.5	PO	24	10†
Systemic infection, bacteremia	5.0	PO	12	prn

*Flexible dosage labeling.
†A maximum of 30 days has been evaluated in safety trials.

DISPENSING INFORMATION. Give medication without feeding, unless vomiting occurs. Never give antacids or GI protectants within 2 hr of medication.

ORMETROPRIM-SULFONAMIDE

CLASS. Diaminopyrimidine and sulfonamide.

ACTION. Combination is bactericidal, causes synergistic two-step inhibition of microbial folic acid synthesis. Antibacterial, antiprotozoal.

MORE INFORMATION. Similar to baquiloprim-sulfadimethoxine licensed in Europe. See TRIMETHOPRIM-SULFONAMIDE, BAQUILOPRIM-SULFONAMIDE; Chapter 34; Table 34–10; references: 34:104; 34:144.

PHARMACOKINETICS. Sulfadimethoxine and ormetoprim in a 5:1 ratio. Both have an extended blood half-life permitting once-a-day dosing. The sulfadimethoxine is highly protein bound, maintaining high and long-duration blood levels, is slowly excreted by dogs largely unchanged in the urine. Sulfadimethoxine has high solubility in the urine and kidney of dogs precluding precipitation and crystalluria. See also TRIMETHOPRIM-SULFONAMIDE.

SPECTRUM. Gram positive: *Staphylococcus, Nocardia.* **Gram negative:** *Proteus, Escherichia, Salmonella, Klebsiella, Brucella, Bordetella,* coccidiosis. **Anaerobes:** *Clostridium.* **Others:** Coccidia, *Pneumocystis, Neospora.* **Ineffective:** *Pseudomonas.* The combined drugs potentiate activity of each other.

INDICATIONS. Treatment of pyoderma, wounds, abscesses in dogs caused by susceptible strains of *Staphylococcus* and gram-negative organisms like *Escherichia.*

APPROVED USES. Skin and soft tissue infections caused by susceptible organisms in dogs.

CONTRAINDICATIONS. Pre-existing hepatic disease, blood dyscrasias, or known previous reaction to sulfonamide. Safety in breeding and pregnant animals is not established; should avoid.

ADVERSE REACTIONS. See also TRIMETHOPRIM-SULFONAMIDE. Keratoconjunctivitis, immune complex–mediated reaction (polyarthritis, urticaria, facial swelling, fever, hemolytic anemia, thrombocytopenia, leukopenia), hepatotoxicity, vomiting, anorexia, diarrhea, polydipsia, polyuria. Rare: generalized anaphylaxis. PO administration of this drug to dogs for 8 weeks at 27.5 mg/kg/day resulted in hypothyroidism (thyroid enlargement, follicular hyperplasia, reduced serum thyroid hormone), reflecting interference with thyroidal hormone synthesis (34:54). Very high doses in dogs cause CNS signs, depression, and seizures.

INTERACTIONS. Prolonged use can cause hypothyroidism.

Availability	Type	Sizes	Preparation (Company)
Veterinary	Oral tablet (sulfadimethoxine-ormetroprim in 5:1 ratio)	120 mg, 250 mg, 600 mg, 1200 mg	*Primor* (Pfizer Animal Health)

HANDLING. Keep tablets stored in airtight containers at room temperature.

ADMINISTRATION. Not recommended by manufacturer for treatment longer than 21 days; longer periods require careful monitoring. Treatment for infections such as pyoderma requires 3–9 weeks. Continue therapy for at least 2 days after remission of signs. Can be dosed once daily, even in bacterial skin disease (34:70). Although soluble in urine, adequate water should be provided at all times. Dehydration and acid urine favor crystal formation.

DOSAGE

Indications	Dose* (mg/kg)	Route	Interval (hr)	Duration (days)
Dogs				
Soft tissue, infection, coccidiosis	27.5	PO	24	21
Chronic pyoderma	27.5†	PO	24	21–63‡
Coccidiosis	66†	PO	24	23
Cats				
Coccidiosis	66	PO	24	≤23

*Dose includes combined sulfadimethoxime-ormetroprim in 5:1 ratio.
†Use twice this dose on the first day.
‡Not approved for longer than 21 days, but chronic skin disease often warrants longer treatment.

ADDITIONAL DOSAGES. Coccidiosis, Table 81–2; Canine pyoderma, Table 85–3; otitis externa, Table 85–6.

DISPENSING INFORMATION. Supply animal with unlimited water to drink; notify clinician of any signs of dry eyes, fever, GI upsets, skin eruptions, swelling, lameness, or worsening of clinical condition.

OXACILLIN

CLASS. Isoxazolyl penicillin.

ACTION. Bactericidal; inhibits bacterial cell wall synthesis.

MORE INFORMATION. Chapter 34; Table 34–1.

PHARMACOKINETICS. Bioavailability after PO administration is 60%–70%. One of few penicillins that has predominant hepatic inactivation and biliary excretion. Urinary excretion of unchanged drug is 30%–70% of that absorbed.

SPECTRUM. Gram positive: *Staphylococcus* (including β-lactamase producers), other gram-positive aerobic cocci, some gram-positive anaerobes.

INDICATIONS. Staphylococcal pyoderma, staphylococcal infections of the respiratory tract or soft tissues.

CONTRAINDICATIONS. Penicillin hypersensitivity.

ADVERSE REACTIONS. See PENICILLIN. Thrombophlebitis when given IV. Neutropenia in people when given IV for several weeks. Vomiting and diarrhea with oral formulations.

INTERACTIONS. Inactivates aminoglycosides when given in the same parenteral solution. Amikacin is most stable aminoglycoside in the presence of penicillins. Antagonism in activity with tetracyclines or chloramphenicol. Sulfonamides inhibit GI absorption of oxacillin.

Availability	Type	Sizes	Preparations (Company)
Human	Capsules	250 mg, 500 mg	*Bactocill* (SmithKline Beecham), *Prostaphlin* (Apothecon)
	Powder for oral solution	250 mg/5 ml	*Bactocill*
	Powder for injection	250 mg, 500 mg, 1 g, 2 g, 4 g, 10 g	*Bactocill*

INTERNATIONAL PREPARATIONS. *Bristopen, Penstapho, Stapenor.*

HANDLING. Reconstitute powder for injection with sterile NaCl or water. For IV, solution stable for 6 hr at room temperature at concentrations of 0.5–40 mg/ml. Compatible with 5% dextrose, Ringer's solution, and 0.9% NaCl. For IM, solution of 250 mg/1.5 ml stable for 3 days at room temperature, 7 days if refrigerated.

ADMINISTRATION. Infuse IV over at least 10 min. Food interferes with PO absorption.

DOSAGE

Indications (Dogs)	Dose (mg/kg)	Route	Interval (hr)	Duration (days)
Bacterial pyoderma	22	PO	8	14–21
Bacterial pyoderma	15–25	PO	12	14–21
Orthopedic infection	22	IV, IM, SC, PO	6–8	21–42

ADDITIONAL DOSAGES. Canine pyoderma, Table 85–3; musculoskeletal infections, Table 86–3; CNS infections, Table 92–5.

DISPENSING INFORMATION. Administer at least 1 hr before feeding or 2 hr after a meal.

OXYTETRACYCLINE

CLASS. Tetracycline.

ACTION. Bacteriostatic; interferes with bacterial protein synthesis. See TETRACYCLINE.

MORE INFORMATION. TETRACYCLINE; Tetracyclines, Chapter 34; Table 34–7.

PHARMACOKINETICS. See TETRACYCLINE.

SPECTRUM. See TETRACYCLINE.

INDICATIONS. See TETRACYCLINE.

APPROVED USES. Equine and food animal.

CONTRAINDICATIONS. See TETRACYCLINE.

ADVERSE REACTIONS. See TETRACYCLINE. Localized pain and allergic or anaphylactic reactions have occurred in dogs after parenteral use. This has been a particular problem with repeated doses of long-acting IM formulations.

INTERACTIONS. See TETRACYCLINE.

Availability	Type	Sizes	Preparations (Company)
Human	Capsules	250 mg (as HCl)	*Terramycin* (Pfizer)
	Solution for injection (IV)	500-mg vials	*Terramycin* IV
	Solution for injection (IM) with lidocaine	500 mg/ml, 125 mg/ml	*Terramycin* IM
Veterinary	Solution for injection	50 mg/ml, 100 mg/ml	*Oxytet* (Vedco), *Oxybiotic* 100 (Butler), *Intacycline* (Intervet), *Terramycin* (Pfizer), generic (various)
	Repositol solution for injection (licensed for cattle and pigs in U.S. dogs and cats in U.K.)	200 mg/ml	*Liquamycin* LA–200 (Pfizer)
		50 mg/ml, 100 mg/ml	*Engemycin* (Mycofarm)

INTERNATIONAL PREPARATIONS. *Aknin, Imperacin, Innolyre, Oxymycin, Terramycine.*

HANDLING. Store in airtight containers protected from light. Solutions are acidic and incompatible with alkaline solutions and many parenteral antimicrobials and other drugs.

ADMINISTRATION. No more than 1–2 ml should be injected at any one site when using IM route. IM route is painful and produces lower blood concentrations than by oral or IV route. Not recommended to use LA–200 by IV route. It is a long acting, less painful formulation developed for use in food-producing animals consisting of a vehicle containing a solvent, 2-pyrrolidone, with a povidone base. Administer PO to fasting animal. Do not give with dairy products or substances containing multivalent cations (Fe, Al, Mg, Ca, Bi).

DOSAGE

Indications	Dose (mg/kg)	Route	Interval	Duration (days)
Dogs				
Systemic infections	22	PO	8 hr	7–14
	20	IM (repositol)	7 days	7*
Cats				
Haemobartonellosis	10–25	PO, IV	8 hr	5–7

*May be repeated every 7 days.

ADDITIONAL DOSAGES. Salmon poisoning disease, Table 27–2; ehrlichiosis, Table 28–4; haemobartonellosis, Table 30–1; leptospirosis, Table 44–4; hepatozoonosis, Table 74–2; bacterial overgrowth, Table 89–11.

DISPENSING INFORMATION. Give PO on an empty stomach.

PAROMOMYCIN (AMINOSIDINE)

CLASS. Aminoglycoside.

ACTION. Antiprotozoal, antibacterial, anthelmintic.

MORE INFORMATION. See Chapter 34; Cryptosporidiosis, Chapter 82; Table 34–5; Table 71–1; reference: 71:4.

PHARMACOKINETICS. Minimal absorption from GI tract after PO administration. Most excreted unchanged in the feces.

SPECTRUM. Gram positive: poor. **Gram negative:** *Salmonella, Shigella.* **Protozoa:** *Cryptosporidium, Pentatrichomonas.* Other: some tapeworms. **Less effective:** *Giardia, Leishmania, Entamoeba.*

INDICATIONS. Cryptosporidiosis, amebiasis, hepatic insufficiency, to reduce enteric microflora production of NH_3. Second choice for *Entamoeba* and *Leishmania* (71:29a).

CONTRAINDICATIONS. Intestinal stasis or obstruction, GI ulceration. Not effective in extraintestinal infections (not absorbed when given PO).

ADVERSE REACTIONS. Nephrotoxicity or ototoxicity if absorbed from ulcerative bowel lesions or if given parenterally. Overgrowth of resistant bacterial or fungal enteric microflora. Oral use: self-limiting diarrhea, malabsorption at high doses. If given parenterally: ototoxicity, nephrotoxic, pancreatitis.

INTERACTIONS. See as for NEOMYCIN (oral).

Availability	Type	Sizes	Preparation (Company)
Human	Oral capsules	250 mg (as sulfate)	*Humatin* (Parke-Davis)

INTERNATIONAL PREPARATIONS. *Gabbroral, Humagel, Sinosid.*

HANDLING. Store in airtight containers.

ADMINISTRATION. Dosage levels appear to be important in therapeutic studies in experimental animals. For example, 100 mg/kg/day in dairy calves and immunosuppressed mice is effective, whereas 25 mg/kg/day and 50 mg/kg day is not. In piglets, 500 mg/kg/day is effective, whereas doses of 250 mg/kg/day and 125 mg/kg/day are less or not effective. Must be given parenterally for *Leishmania* infections.

DOSAGE

Indications (Dogs and Cats)	Dose (mg/kg)	Route	Interval (hr)	Duration (days)
Cryptosporidiosis	125–165	PO	12	5
Leishmania (dog)	10	SC	24	28

ADDITIONAL DOSAGES. Cryptosporidiosis, Table 82–1; *Pentatrichomonas,* Table 78–2.

DISPENSING INFORMATION. Give with meals. Observe pet for vomiting or diarrhea, dizziness, hearing loss.

PENICILLIN G

CLASS. Benzylpenicillin.

ACTION. Bactericidal, inhibits bacterial cell wall synthesis.

MORE INFORMATION. Penicillins; Chapter 34; Table 34–1.

PHARMACOKINETICS. PO: Unpredictable inactivation by gastric acid when given PO. **IV:** rapid high but transient blood levels. **IM:** procaine salt lasts 12–15 hr; benzathine lasts up to 4 weeks but produces very low concentrations. Diffuses readily into liver, lung, heart, skin, kidneys, bone, prostate, spleen, intestines, serosal fluids (synovial, peritoneal, ascitic), bile, urine, wound secretions. Penetration into CSF, brain, or ocular tissues poor unless inflammation present. Crosses placenta but does not enter milk. Excretion occurs unchanged in the urine.

SPECTRUM. Gram positive: *Staphylococcus, Streptococcus, Corynebacterium, Erysipelothrix, Bacillus, Listeria.* **Gram negative:** *Proteus, Salmonella, Enterobacter, Escherichia, Streptobacillus moniliformis, Pasteurella.* **Anaerobes:** *Clostridium, Peptococcus* sp, *Peptostreptococcus, Fusobacterium, Eubacterium, Actinomyces.* **Other:** *Borrelia, Leptospira.* **Ineffective:** *Enterococcus* (*Streptococcus faecalis*), β-lactamase-producing *Staphylococcus.*

INDICATIONS. PO administration requires higher doses because of gastric acid activation. Generally used parenterally. Penicillin V is an alternative for oral use. Use IV soluble form in presence of severe systemic infections or bacteremia. Recommended for actinomycosis, tetanus, rat bite fever, listeriosis, pasteurellosis, erysipelas, anthrax, streptococcosis, fusospirochetosis of oropharynx, some gram-negative bacteremias, leptospirosis (bacteremic phase), borreliosis.

CONTRAINDICATIONS. Use lower dosages in renal failure.

ADVERSE REACTIONS. IV: thrombophlebitis, convulsions, hyperkalemia with potassium salt. **IM:** peripheral nerve damage.

INTERACTIONS. Penicillins may inactivate aminoglycosides if mixed before administration.

Availability	Type	Sizes	Preparations (Company)
Human	Aqueous solutions (potassium or sodium)	2,000,000–20,000,000/U in powder for reconstitution	Generic (various)
	Oral tablets (as potassium)	200,000–800,000/U	Generic (various)
Veterinary	Procaine suspension for IM injection	300,000–500,000 U/ml	*Crystacillin* (Solvay); *Microcillin* (Anthony)
	Benzathine parenteral	300,000 U/ml	*Crystiben* (Solvay); *Flo-Cillin* (Fort Dodge)
	Procaine and benzathine combined equally	300,000–600,000 U/ml total	*Ambi-Pen* (Butler); *Crystiben* (Solvay); *Duo-Pen* (RX Vet, Vet Tek); *DuraPen* (Vedco)

HANDLING. Dry aqueous powder for injection stable in refrigerator. Dissolve in sterile water, 0.9% sodium chloride, or dextrose. Avoid alkaline dextrose solutions. After reconstitution, keep refrigerated, good for 1 week. Store procaine and benzathine preparations in refrigerator (not frozen). Before use, warm to room temperature and shake well.

ADMINISTRATION. Aqueous sodium or potassium solutions: given IM or by continuous IV infusion; give highest dose IV. For IM, use 100,000 U/ml concentration. For IV, determine daily fluid needs; add required aqueous penicillin and infuse over 24 hr. Local infusion (pleural, peritoneal) prepare as for IM, dilute in 1/4 to 1/2 volume compared with that of fluid aspirated from cavity. **Oral tablets:** administer 1 hr or more before feeding or at least 2 hr or more afterward. Dose for oral use is higher because of gastric acid degradation. **Procaine or benzathine:** administer by deep IM injection. Maximum volume at one site 10 ml.

DOSAGE

Indications	Dose (U/kg)*	Route	Interval (hr)	Duration (days)
Dogs				
Potassium				
Bacteremia, systemic infection	20,000–40,000	IV	4–6	prn
Orthopedic infection	20,000–40,000	IV	6	prn
Soft tissue infection	40,000–60,000	PO	8	prn
Procaine	20,000–40,000	IM, SC	12–24	prn
Benzathine	40,000	IM	120	prn
Cats				
Potassium				
Soft tissue, systemic infection	40,000	PO	6–8	prn
Procaine				
Soft tissue infection	20,000	IM, SC	12	prn
Orthopedic infection	20,000–40,000	IM	8	prn
Resistant organisms†	50,000–100,000	IM, SC	12	prn
Benzathine	50,000	IM	120	prn

*Na penicillin G for injection ≈ 1600 U/mg; procaine penicillin G ≈ 1000 U/mg; benzathine penicillin G ≈ 1200 U/mg.
†*Actinomyces*.

ADDITIONAL DOSAGES. Streptococcal infections, Table 35–2; anaerobic infections, Table 41–10; tetanus, Table 43–2; leptospirosis, Table 44–4; Lyme borreliosis, Table 45–3; actinomycosis, Table 49–1; feline abscesses, Table 52–2; musculoskeletal infections, Table 86–3; bacteremia and endocarditis, Table 87–7; hepatobiliary infections, Table 90–4; CNS infections, Table 92–5; local ocular infections, Table 93–4.

DISPENSING INFORMATION. Give all PO tablets at least 1 hr before, or 2 hrs after feeding.

PENICILLIN V POTASSIUM (PHENOXYMETHYLPENICILLIN)

CLASS. Penicillin.

ACTION. Bactericidal; inhibits bacterial cell wall synthesis.

MORE INFORMATION. PENICILLIN G.

PHARMACOKINETICS. Acid stable with absorption two to five times greater than penicillin G from GI tract after oral administration. For distribution in tissues and body fluids, see PENICILLIN G.

SPECTRUM. See PENICILLIN G. Same as for penicillin G except less active against *Salmonella, Escherichia, Proteus, Fusobacterium, Eubacterium*.

INDICATIONS. Preferred oral therapy when narrow-spectrum penicillin is indicated; borreliosis, streptococcal infections, staphylococcal infections.

CONTRAINDICATIONS. See PENICILLIN G.

ADVERSE REACTIONS. See PENICILLIN G.

INTERACTIONS. See PENICILLIN G.

Availability	Type	Sizes	Preparations (Company)
Human	Tablets (potassium)	125 mg, 250 mg, 500 mg	*Pen-Vee K* (Wyeth-Ayerst), *Beepen-VK* (SmithKline Beecham), various others
	Powder for oral suspension (potassium)	125 mg/5 ml, 250 mg/5 ml	

INTERNATIONAL PREPARATIONS. *Abbocillin-VK, Acipen-V, Apocillin, Arcasin, Calciopen, Cilicaine VK, Cliacil, Femepen, Oracilline, Penebene.*

HANDLING. Store products in airtight containers at room temperature. Oral suspension is stable for 2 wks if refrigerated.

ADMINISTRATION. Food interferes with absorption.

DOSAGE

Indications (Dogs and Cats)	Dose	Route	Interval (hr)	Duration (days)
Soft tissue infection	10 mg/kg	PO	8	7

*Equivalency ≈ 1600 U/mg.

ADDITIONAL DOSAGES. Streptococcal infections, Table 35–2 and 35–4; actinomycosis, Table 49–1; dermatophilosis, Table 51–1; feline abscesses, Table 52–2; musculoskeletal infections, Table 86–3.

DISPENSING INFORMATION. Give at least 1 hr before or 2 hr after feeding pet.

PENTAMIDINE ISETHIONATE

CLASS. Aromatic diamidine.

ACTION. Interferes with nuclear metabolism and inhibits the synthesis of DNA, RNA, proteins and phospholipids.

MORE INFORMATION. Chapter 71; Table 71–1; for inhalation therapy, reference: 71:14; for *Acanthamoeba*, reference: 71:32

PHARMACOKINETICS. Not absorbed from GI tract after PO administration. Must be given IV, topical (by inhalation), or IM (well absorbed). Lung tissue levels are lower after parenteral injection than by nebulization. One third excreted unchanged in urine within a few hours, but urinary excretion continues for weeks.

SPECTRUM. *Acanthamoeba, Pneumocystis, Leishmania, Babesia.* Less effective: for treatment of babesiosis, diminazene, imidocarb, or amicarbalide are preferred if available.

INDICATIONS. Invasive acanthamebiasis not involving the CNS. *Pneumocystis carinii* pneumonia by inhalation (nebulization). May add trimethoprim-sulfonamide plus pentamidine for some *Babesia* infections.

APPROVED USES. Humans: aerosolized drug for prophylaxis of *Pneumocystis* pneumonia.

CONTRAINDICATIONS. Renal failure: elimination is impaired but renal elimination is a minor factor in dogs.

ADVERSE REACTIONS. Systemic therapy (IV or IM): hypotension (vasodilation and reduced blood pressure); systemic anaphylaxis, nausea, salivation, vomiting, diarrhea; hypoglycemia (islet cell necrosis and hyperinsulinemia), then diabetes mellitus; myelosuppression; renal failure. Hypocalcemia and hypokalemia are frequent. To avoid allergic reactions, pretreatment with antihistamines just before administration is recommended. IM use causes pain or necrosis at the site of injection. **Inhalation therapy** is associated with lower toxicity. In dogs results in cilia loss, epithelial atrophy, submucosal hemorrhage in the nasal passages.

INTERACTIONS. Concomitant use of potentially nephrotoxic drugs should be avoided.

Availability	Type	Sizes	Preparations (Company)
Human	Powder for injection	300 mg/vial	*Pentam* (Lyphomed)
	Powder for aerosolization	300 mg/vial	*NebuPent* (Lyphomed)
Veterinary	Solution for injection	40 mg/ml in 20-ml vial	*Lomidine* (Merial)

INTERNATIONAL PREPARATIONS. *Pentacarinat; Pneumopent.*

HANDLING. Store powders away from light at controlled room temperature. For aerosolization reconstitute with sterile water (6 ml) to 50 mg/ml. For IM dissolve in 3 ml sterile water. For IV dissolve in 3–5 ml sterile water or 5% dextrose; can be further diluted into 50–250 ml of 5% dextrose. Do not dilute with any other solution or precipitate will form. Solution stable for 48 hr at room temperature.

ADMINISTRATION. Aerosol: fit mask over the dog's muzzle. **IV:** give over 60 min to reduce risk of hypotension. Should monitor for azotemia once or twice weekly. Do not give IV or SC. People administering drug in this manner should wear face masks and protective eyewear to prevent exposure to nebulized drug. **IM:** give deep injection in a large muscle or split dose at several sites. Use aseptic technique with a new needle at each site. In dogs, the IP route can be used by diluting product with 10 volumes physiologic saline and using long needles.

DOSAGE

Indications	Dose (mg/kg)	Route	Interval (hr)	Duration (days)
Human				
Acanthamebiasis	4.0	IV or IM	24	28 7 days every 4th wk
Pneumocystis prophylaxis	1.3	Aerosolized	24	
Leishmaniasis*	4.0	IM, IP	48	30 to 40
Babesiosis	4.0	IM	24	1

*Alternate with meglumine *(Glucantine)* if resistant to treatment.

ADDITIONAL DOSAGES. Babesiosis, Table 77–3; pneumocystosis, Table 83–2.

PHENAMIDINE ISETHIONATE

CLASS. Aromatic diamidine.

ACTION. Antiprotozoal.

MORE INFORMATION. See PENTAMIDINE as an alternative and closely related drug; Chapter 71; Table 71–1.

SPECTRUM. *Babesia.*

INDICATIONS. Second choice for babesiosis, other aromatic diamidines (e.g., imidocarb) are preferred for dogs and cats.

CONTRAINDICATIONS. See PENTAMIDINE.

ADVERSE REACTIONS. See PENTAMIDINE, antihistamine (oxomemazine) included to counter allergic reactions and irritation at the injection site.

INTERACTIONS. See PENTAMIDINE.

Availability	Type	Size	Preparation (Company)
Veterinary	Solution for injection	15 mg/ml in 10-ml ampules with 1 mg/ml oxomemazine	*Oxopirvedine* (Merial)

HANDLING. May be diluted in sterile 5% dextrose solution immediately before injection.

ADMINISTRATION. One 10-ml ampule can be given (SC preferred) for each 8.5 to 12.5 kg body weight. The dose can be given in one dose or divided in two doses given at a 24-hr interval.

DOSAGE

Indication (Dogs)	Dose (mg/kg)	Route	Interval (hr)	Duration (days)
Babesiosis *(B. gibsoni)*	7.5	IM, SC	24	2
	15.0	IM, SC	24	1

ADDITIONAL DOSAGES. Babesiosis, Table 77–3.

PIPERACILLIN SODIUM

CLASS. Semisynthetic penicillin.

ACTION. Bactericidal; inhibits bacterial cell wall synthesis.

MORE INFORMATION. Chapter 34, Penicillins; Table 34–1.

PHARMACOKINETICS. Not absorbed from the GI tract so administered parenterally. Penetrates blood-brain barrier. CSF-serum concentration ratio is 0.06 in noninflamed states and 0.3 in inflammation. Larger volume of distribution and more rapid clearance in pregnancy. Undergoes both biliary and renal excretion; can be used with renal compromise or biliary or hepatic dysfunction and to treat hepatobiliary infections. Majority (60%–80%) of dose is renally excreted.

SPECTRUM. Gram positive: *Enterococcus, Streptococcus,* non β-lactamase–producing *Staphylococcus.* **Gram negative:** *Escherichia, Proteus, Serratia, Klebsiella, Enterobacter, Citrobacter, Salmonella, Shigella, Pseudomonas* (synergistic with aminoglycosides), *Yersinia.* **Anaerobes:** *Actinomyces, Bacteroides, Clostridium, Eubacterium, Fusobacterium, Peptococcus, Peptostreptococcus.* **Others:** against *Pseudomonas,* use in combination with an aminoglycoside. Combine for treatment of bacteremia, endocarditis, osteomyelitis, pneumonia; use alone in treating of meningitis, urinary infection, invasive otitis. Combination with β-lactamase inhibitor, tazobactam, which increases spectrum to include resistant *Escherichia, Enterobacter, Pseudomonas, Enterococcus.* Useful combination to treat skin, soft tissue, respiratory, intra-abdominal, gynecologic infections.

INDICATIONS. Serious infections of abdomen, urinary, genital, lower respiratory tracts, skin, soft tissue, bone, joints, septicemia. Prophylaxis for intra-abdominal surgery. To treat suspected polymicrobial infections, singly, before isolation of causative organisms.

CONTRAINDICATIONS. Reduce dose in severe renal or hepatic failure.

ADVERSE REACTIONS. Local or systemic allergic reactions such as thrombophlebitis or anaphylaxis. Sudden endotoxin release when treating sepsis. Low toxicity characteristic of the penicillin group. Occasional diarrhea, azotemia, reversible neutropenia, thrombocytopenia, hemorrhagic manifestations.

INTERACTIONS. Prolongs action of some muscle relaxants.

Availability	Type	Sizes	Preparations (Company)
Human	Powder for injection	2 g, 3 g, 4 g, 40 g	*Pipracil* (Lederle)

INTERNATIONAL PREPARATIONS. *Avocin, Ivacin, Picillin, Pipcil, Piperacine, Pipérilline, Piperzam, Pipril.*

HANDLING. Stable in sterile water, 0.9% NaCl, 5% dextrose. Should not be refrigerated or frozen, stable for 24 hr at room temperature. **IV:** can also use Ringer's or lactated Ringer's or additives such as 40 mmol/L KCl; dissolve powder in at least 5 ml diluent, then add to desired infusion. **IM:** dilute to 2 g/5 ml, can use 0.5%–1.0% lidocaine without epinephrine. Do not mix with aminoglycosides or will cause inactivation.

ADMINISTRATION. IV for serious infections: given as a 20- to 30-min infusion every 4–6 hr. IV bolus over 3–5 min is shortest possible duration but risks phlebitis. For surgical prophylaxis, begin IV infusion 30 min before incision and continue no longer than 24 hr afterward. **IM:** limit to 2 g (5 ml) per site, use large muscle, avoid peripheral nerves.

DOSAGE

Indications (Dogs)	Dose	Route	Interval (hr)	Duration (days)
Skin infection, bacteremia	25–50 mg/kg	IV, IM	8–12	prn

ADDITIONAL DOSAGES. Bacteremia and endocarditis, Table 87–7; respiratory infection, Table 88–8.

PIPERACILLIN-TAZOBACTAM

CLASS. Semisynthetic + penicillin β-lactamase inhibitor in 8:1 ratio.

ACTION. Bactericidal; inhibits bacterial cell wall synthesis and β-lactamase activity.

MORE INFORMATION. See other β-lactam–β-lactamase inhibitor combinations such as AMPICILLIN-SULBACTAM, TICARCILLIN-CLAVULANATE, AMOXICILLIN-CLAVULANATE; Chapter 34; Tables 34–1 and 34–2.

PHARMACOKINETICS. Tazobactam does not affect pharmacokinetics of piperacillin. High, rapid onset of plasma concentration after IV infusion. Piperacillin is partially metabolized to an active metabolite, whereas tazobactam is metabolized to an inactive form. About 70% of piperacillin and 80% of tazobactam are excreted unchanged in urine, and there is some biliary excretion.

SPECTRUM. **Gram positive:** see PIPERACILLIN. **Gram negative:** See PIPERACILLIN. *Acinetobacter, Klebsiella.* **Anaerobes:** see PIPERACILLIN. **More effective:** piperacillin alone is active against most *Streptococcus,* some *Pseudomonas,* many Enterobacteriaceae. Adding tazobactam extends the spectrum to include *Staphylococcus,* more anaerobes, and additional gram-negative bacteria, including *Acinetobacter* and *Klebsiella.*

INDICATIONS. Lower respiratory tract, skin, soft tissue, intra-abdominal, gynecologic infections. Treatment of bacteremia or life-threatening infections in neutropenic or immunocompromised hosts. For piperacillin-resistant bacteria.

APPROVED USES. For humans with resistant intra-abdominal, cutaneous, and lower respiratory tract infections.

CONTRAINDICATIONS. Lower dosage advisable in renal impairment. Previous allergic reaction to penicillins, cephalosporins, or β-lactamase inhibitors.

ADVERSE REACTIONS. Vomiting, diarrhea, systemic allergies, leukopenia, elevated liver enzymes, hyperbilirubinemia.

INTERACTIONS. Not compatible in solution with lactated Ringer's, Ringer's, aminoglycosides but can infuse separately. False-positive urine glucose with copper reduction methods.

Availability	Type	Sizes	Preparation (Company)
Human	Powder for injection	2 g, 3 g, 4 g piperacillin with 0.25 g, 0.375 g, 0.5 g tazobactam, respectively	*Zosyn* (Lederle)

INTERNATIONAL PREPARATIONS. *Fluxapril, Tazobac, Tazobac, Tazocilline, Tazocin.*

HANDLING. Reconstitute powder in at least 5 ml, then place into IV fluid (0.9% NaCl, 5% dextrose). Compatible with 40 mmol of KCl added. Stability of stock solutions is 24 hr at room temperature or 48 hr if refrigerated.

ADMINISTRATION. IV: 30-min infusions every 6 hr, usually treat for 1 week in hospitalized animals.

DOSAGE

Indications (Dogs)	Dose (g/dog)	Route	Interval (hr)	Duration (days)
Bacterial sepsis	3.4	IV	6	7
	4.5	IV	8	7

ADDITIONAL DOSAGES. Intra-abdominal infections, Table 89–15.

PRIMAQUINE PHOSPHATE

CLASS. 8-aminoquinolone.

ACTION. Antiprotozoal; binds to protozoal DNA and alters mitochondria.

PHARMACOKINETICS. Rapid absorption after PO administration; highest concentrations in liver, brain, lungs, cardiac and skeletal muscle. Metabolizes to compounds with variable activity with small amount (<1%) excreted unchanged in urine.

SPECTRUM. *Hepatozoon, Babesia, Pneumocystis.*

INDICATIONS. Hepatozoonosis.

APPROVED USES. Human malaria. Being evaluated in combination with clindamycin for pneumocystosis.

CONTRAINDICATIONS. Concurrent hemolysis or bone marrow suppression. Concurrent quinacrine or other myelosuppressive drugs, leukopenia, other hemolytic drugs.

ADVERSE REACTIONS. Methemoglobinemia, hemolysis (with glucose-6-phosphate dehydrogenase), myelosuppression.

INTERACTIONS. Quinacrine increases toxicity.

Availability	Type	Size	Preparation (Company)
Human	Oral tablets	26.3 mg (15 mg active base)	*Primaquine phosphate* (Sanofi-Winthrop)

HANDLING. Store tablets in airtight container away from heat, light, and moisture.

ADMINISTRATION. Check CBC at least once weekly while being treated. May be given with food to avoid GI side effects.

DOSAGE

Indications	Dose	Route	Interval (hr)	Duration (days)
Dogs	0.3 (active base) mg/kg	PO	24	14

*Human dose, extrapolated.

ADDITIONAL DOSAGES. Hepatozoonosis, Table 74–2; babesiosis, Table 77–3; pneumocystosis, Table 83–2.

DISPENSING INFORMATION. Give drug with a small amount of food to reduce vomiting if it occurs.

PROPIONIBACTERIUM ACNES (CORYNEBACTERIUM PARVUM)

CLASS. Bacterial product, killed bacterial cells.

ACTION. Stimulates macrophage activation resulting in the release of various cytokines. Immunostimulant.

MORE INFORMATION. Chapter 100; references 100:9, 100:25.

SPECTRUM. Antiviral and immunostimulatory. Stimulates mononuclear phagocytes and interleukin (IL–1, IL–6, tumor necrosis factor).

INDICATIONS. Canine staphylococcal pyoderma, feline leukemia virus (FeLV) infection, feline herpesvirus infection. Aids in achieving clinical remission or improvement in pyoderma of dogs. May increase hematopoiesis in FeLV-positive cats but does not alter viremic status.

CONTRAINDICATIONS. Canine lymphoma or leukemia with CNS involvement.

ADVERSE REACTIONS. Fever, chills, lethargy involvement within 24 hr after administration. Localized pain and swelling if IV extravasation occurs.

INTERACTIONS. Not recommended for animals concurrently receiving glucocorticoids. Concurrent antibacterial therapy recommended.

Availability	Type	Sizes	Preparations (Company)
Veterinary*	Solution for injection		*ImmunoRegulin* (Immunovet, Vetoquinol)
	0.4 mg/ml (in ethanol)	5 ml vials	
	0.4 mg/ml (in ethanol)	5-ml and 50-ml vials	Equine product *EqStim* (Immunovet)

*Human products *Arthrokehlan "A"*, *Coparvax* (Immunovet)

HANDLING. Unopened vials are stored at room temperature. Keep refrigerated once opened.

ADMINISTRATION. IV or IP. Direct intralesional injection in tumors has also been done. No improvement after 12 weeks indicates that treatment is ineffective and should be discontinued. Some give one injection per month to maintain remission of pyoderma.

DOSAGE

Indications/ Body Weight	Dose (ml)	Route	Interval	Duration (weeks)
*Dogs, pyoderma**				
7 kg	0.250	IV	Twice weekly	2†
7–20 kg	0.50	IV	Twice weekly	2†
20–34 kg	1.00	IV	Twice weekly	2†
>34 kg	2.00	IV	Twice weekly	2†
Cats, antiviral				
5 lb	0.25	IV	Twice weekly	2†
10 lb	0.50	IV	Twice weekly	2‡

*Maximum dose in any dog is 2.0 ml.
†Once weekly thereafter until remission and once monthly after that to maintain clinical improvement.
‡Once weekly thereafter for 3 weeks and once monthly for 2 months for a total of nine injections. Some protocols for FeLV suggest follow-up with injections once weekly for 20 weeks or longer as needed.

PYRIMETHAMINE (and SULFONAMIDE)

CLASS. Folic acid inhibitor.

ACTION. Inhibits dihydrofolate reductase.

MORE INFORMATION. Toxoplasmosis and neosporosis, Chapter 71; Table 71–1.

PHARMACOKINETICS. After PO administration, well absorbed. Enters many tissues including CNS and CSF. Highly protein bound and suppressive effects of the drug may remain in the plasma for 1–2 weeks. Metabolized by the liver, and metabolites are excreted in urine.

SPECTRUM. Protozoa: *Toxoplasma gondii, Neospora caninum, Pneumocystis carinii.* **Ineffective:** bacteria (pyrimethamine).

INDICATIONS. Used for treatment of toxoplasmosis, neosporosis, pneumocystosis in combination with sulfonamides.

CONTRAINDICATIONS. Pregnancy because teratogenic. Folate deficiency or previous hypersensitivity. Reduced dose needed with hepatic but not with renal impairment.

ADVERSE REACTIONS. Vomiting, leukopenia, myelosuppression, fetal teratogenesis, myelodysplasia. Folate deficiency can be treated with folinic acid at 5–15 mg/day PO or parenterally.

INTERACTIONS. Use care in dosing with other folate inhibitors (trimethoprim or methotrexate) or other myelosuppressive drugs.

Availability	Type	Sizes	Preparations (Company)
Human	Oral tablets	25 mg	*Daraprim* (Burroughs Wellcome)
	Combined product	25 mg pyrimethamine; 500 mg sulfadoxine	*Fansidar* (Roche)

HANDLING. Tablets should be stored in airtight containers away from heat, direct light, and moisture. Formulation of smaller dosage sizes can be done by IDEXX at 1–888-RxI-DEXX.

ADMINISTRATION. If vomiting occurs, give with meals. Periodically check hemogram.

DOSAGE

Indications		Dose	Route	Interval (hr)	Duration (days)
Dogs					
Neosporosis	Pyrimethamine	1	PO	24	14
	plus				
	Sulfonamide	60	PO	24	13
	Pyrimethamine	1	PO	24	28
	plus				
	Trimethoprim-sulfonamide	15	PO	12	28
Cat					
Toxoplasmosis	Pyrimethamine	0.25–1	PO	24	14–28
	plus				
	Trimethoprim-sulfonamide	15	PO	12	14–28

ADDITIONAL DOSAGES. Hepatozoonosis, Table 74–2; toxoplasmosis, Table 80–3; neosporosis, Table 80–7.

DISPENSING INFORMATION. If gastrointestinal signs develop, they can be minimized by giving this drug with food.

QUINACRINE (MEPACRINE) HYDROCHLORIDE

CLASS. 9-aminocridine dye.

ACTION. Antiprotozoal.

MORE INFORMATION. Antiprotozoal Chemotherapy, Chapter 71; Table 71–1; Giardiasis, Chapter 78.

PHARMACOKINETICS. Readily absorbed from GI tract and widely distributed in tissues. Accumulates in liver with slow release up to 2 mo after a single dose. Crosses the placenta.

SPECTRUM. Protozoa: Coccidia, *Giardia*, *Leishmania*. **Others:** some tapeworms.

INDICATIONS. Giardiasis, alternative to nitroimidazoles, sometimes cutaneous leishmaniasis (except caused by *L. aethiopica*, *L. braziliensis*).

CONTRAINDICATIONS. Hepatic dysfunction, pregnancy.

ADVERSE REACTIONS. GI upsets, vomiting, diarrhea, CNS signs, fever, blood dyscrasias, dermatologic eruptions, yellow urine, skin, and sclera.

INTERACTIONS. Avoid use with other drugs that cause myelodyscrasias.

Availability	Type	Size	Preparation (Company)
Human	Oral tablets	100 mg	*Atabrine* HCl (Winthrop); not available in U.S. since 1992

HANDLING. More palatable if administered within gelatin capsules. Can add to liquids but is not stable in solution for more than 6 hrs so should be used immediately in this form. Solution for intralesional injections in leishmaniasis is prepared by grinding three 100-mg tablets in a mortar to a fine powder. A solution of 30 ml 0.9% NaCl is added. This is filtered through coarse filter paper and rinsed with 0.9% saline. The mixture is filtered through a 5-µm filter needle into a sterile empty vial. The final concentration is adjusted to 5%.

ADMINISTRATION. For intralesional injections in leishmaniasis, has been mixed as a 5% solution given at intervals of 3–5 days.

DOSAGE

Indications	Dose	Route	Interval (hr)	Duration (days)
Dogs				
Giardiasis	50–100 mg/dog	PO	12	3*
Cats				
Coccidiosis	10 mg/kg	PO	24	5

*Skip 3 days, then repeat again for one more course of therapy.

ADDITIONAL DOSAGES. Enteric protozoal infections, Table 78–2; coccidiosis, Table 81–2.

DISPENSING INFORMATION. Tablets can be crushed and placed in honey or ice cream to increase palatability by masking taste to animals that are difficult to medicate.

RIBAVIRIN

CLASS. Nucleoside (guanosine) analog.

ACTION. Antiviral; interferes with DNA and mRNA synthesis; weaker anticellular activity.

MORE INFORMATION. Chapter 2; references: 2:26–28.

PHARMACOKINETICS. Erythrocytes sequester large amounts of drug. Crosses blood-brain barrier, CSF concentration 50%–100% of blood levels.

SPECTRUM. Virostatic against DNA and RNA viruses, including herpes-, orthomyxo-, pox-, paramyxo-, influenza-, arena-, bunya-, and immunodeficiency viruses. Also feline infectious peritonitis virus (2:1, 2:29), canine parainfluenza virus, feline calicivirus. Has not been as effective against feline calicivirus in vivo as in vitro studies suggest.

INDICATIONS. Humans: aerosol therapy of infants with respiratory syncytial virus. IV or PO for adults with influenza A or acute viral hemorrhagic fever, for arthropod-borne encephalomyelitis. Not recommended for coronaviral infection in cats because of poor efficacy whether in aqueous or liposomal encapsulated form (2:28).

APPROVED USES. Humans for respiratory syncytial virus.

CONTRAINDICATIONS. Pre-existing anemia, leukopenia, thrombocytopenia, pregnancy.

ADVERSE REACTIONS. Toxic in cats when used alone at therapeutic dosages or higher (22 or 44 mg/kg) (2:27). Diarrhea, myelotoxicity (megakaryocytic hypoplasia, increased myeloid-erythroid ratio, anemia, leukopenia, thrombocytopenia), increased blood alanine transaminase, alkaline phosphatase, creatine kinase activities, enteritis, hepatocellular vacuolation or necrosis, fetotoxic, teratogenic, GI hemorrhage, and ulceration. Treated cats with calicivirus infection have had increased severity of illness, depressed bone marrow, weight loss, increased hepatic enzymes, icterus. Kittens treated for coronaviral infection had pronounced multifocal hemorrhages throughout body tissues (2:27). None of these abnormalities have been found in beagle dogs given 60 mg/kg of ribavirin for 2 weeks, although nonregenerative anemia develops in people and other animals given similar dosages.

INTERACTIONS. For cats, use at lower dosages in combination with interferon-α.

Availability	Type	Size	Preparation (Company)
Human	Powder for reconstitution for aerosol	6 g	*Virazole (ICN)*

HANDLING. Vials of powder are stored in a dry place at room temperature. Do not mix with any other drug. Solubilize drug with sterile water at final concentration of 20 mg/ml. Reconstituted drug is stable for 24 hr at 20–30°C.

ADMINISTRATION. Aerosol: dilute in reservoir and nebulize by a small particle aerosol generator. Deliver via face mask, ventilator, oxygen hood. Unfortunately, aerosols can leak and be inhaled by health care personnel. **IV:** relative toxicity and dose have been reduced by incorporation of the drug in liposomes but liposome-encapsulated drug was less effective than free ribavirin in treating coronavirus-infected cats (2:28).

DOSAGE

Indications (Cats)	Dose (mg/kg)	Route	Interval (hr)	Duration (days)
Systemic viral infections	11	PO, IM, IV	24	7
Children	2.5	PO	6	7

DISPENSING INFORMATION. Can be given orally by placing powder in gelatin capsules.

RIFAMPIN (RIFAMPICIN)

CLASS. Ansamycin.

ACTION. Binds to and inactivates bacterial DNA-dependent RNA polymerase while not affecting mammalian cells.

MORE INFORMATION. Similar to rifabutin *(Mycobutin, Ansatipine);* Chapter 34.

PHARMACOKINETICS. Rapid and almost complete absorption from GI tract. Food reduces rate and extent of absorption. High lipid solubility, penetrates most tissues, including CNS. Penetrates cells, including phagocytes, and organisms in extracellular cavitary spaces or caseous lesions, reaching therapeutic concentrations in abscessed tissues and discharges. Metabolized in liver and active metabolites excreted in urine (30%) and bile (70%), in the former as unchanged and metabolized drug.

SPECTRUM. Gram positive: staphylococci, *Rhodococcus.* **Gram negative:** *Bartonella, Brucella.* **Others:** *Neisseria, Haemophilus, Mycobacterium.* Antiviral (adenoviruses, poxviruses) and antichlamydial at very high doses. Some mycobacteria resistant to rifampin may be susceptible to rifabutin.

INDICATIONS. Resistance develops rapidly. Should always be combined with other drugs to improve efficacy and hinder resistance development. Chronic refractory pyoderma, bacterial abscesses, or granulomas. Resistant staphylococcal infections in difficult sites: osteomyelitis, endocarditis, CNS infections, infection of prosthetic implants. Rhodococcosis, granulomatous, mycobacterial infections, brucellosis, chlamydiosis. Can facilitate penetration of other antimicrobials, such as amphotericin B or flucytosine for fungal infections or isoniazid in tuberculosis. Facilitates metabolism and urinary excretion of bile acids, reducing pruritogenic substances.

APPROVED USES. Human mycobacteriosis and *Neisseria* meningitis.

CONTRAINDICATIONS. Reduce dosage in hepatic dysfunction or biliary obstruction. This drug induces its own accelerated metabolism and excretion. In pregnancy, can cause teratogenesis in laboratory animals.

ADVERSE REACTIONS. Hepatotoxicity: use lower dosages; vomiting, elevated liver enzymes, icterus, hemolytic anemia, thrombocytopenia. Urine, stool, saliva, tears may be discolored orange-red color by drug. CNS disturbances. Higher dosages (30–60 mg/kg PO daily) are more likely to be associated with side effects and should be avoided. Some cats have shown erythema, especially of the pinna, pruritus, dyspnea, and respiratory distress as a result of anaphylaxis, which may require dilute epinephrine and glucocorticoid administration. Pretreatment with antihistamines and reducing the dose has been beneficial in reducing this untoward reaction.

INTERACTIONS. Accelerates metabolism and may reduce effectiveness of drugs metabolized by microsomal enzymes: glucocorticoids, cardiac glycosides, sulfonylureas, benzodiazepines, chloramphenicol, doxycycline, digitoxin, ketoconazole, theophylline, barbiturates, verapamil. Hepatotoxicity increased when used with isoniazid or halothane. Inhibits assays for serum vitamin B_{12} and folate.

Availability	Type	Sizes	Preparations (Company)
Human	Oral capsules	150 mg, 300 mg	*Rifadin* (Marion Merrell Dow), *Rimactane* (Geigy)
	Powder for injection	600 mg	*Rifadin* IV

INTERNATIONAL PREPARATIONS. *Diabacil, Eremfat, Fenampicin, Fimizina, Rifa, Rifagen, Rifaldin, Rifapiam, Rifcin, Rifocina, Rifoldin, Rimactan, Rimycin.*

HANDLING. Store at room temperature in moisture and light-resistant containers. Powder for injection reconstituted with sterile water. Stability best in 5% dextrose. After reconstitution can store for 4 weeks at room temperature or refrigerated. To make PO suspension (10 mg/ml), mix contents of four 300-mg caps with simple syrup and bring to 120 ml with syrup. Keep refrigerated, stable for 4 weeks. May have to reformulate into smaller dosage capsules for cats by adding cornstarch and placing it in new capsules.

ADMINISTRATION. Food interferes with absorption; administer to fasted animal 1 hr before or 2 hr after meals. *Always give in combination* with at least one other drug when treating mycobacteria or other persistent intracellular infections.

DOSAGE

Indications	Dose (mg/kg)	Route	Interval (hr)	Duration (day)
Dogs				
Pyoderma	5–10	PO	24	prn
	5–10	PO	12	prn
	10–20	PO	24	prn
Systemic*	10	IV, IM	12–24	prn
Cats				
Bartonellosis, mycobacteriosis†	5–10	PO	24	14

*Maximum 8 mg/kg/day if hepatic function is impaired.
†Use in combination with doxycycline for bartonellosis, see Chapter 54, and for other antimycobacterial drugs, see Chapter 50.

ADDITIONAL DOSAGES. Actinomycosis, Table 49–1; mycobacterial infections, Tables 50–2 and 50–4; *Bartonella*, Table 54–3; CNS infections, Table 92–5.

DISPENSING INFORMATION. Give to fasting animal. May cause harmless reddish-orange discoloration of body excretions and secretions.

ROXITHROMYCIN

CLASS. Macrolide.

ACTION. Bacteriostatic, interferes with bacteria protein synthesis.

MORE INFORMATION. See ERYTHROMYCIN; reference: 34:88.

PHARMACOKINETICS. Rapidly absorbed from GI tract after PO administration, and 50% bioavailable. Acid stable in stomach, better absorbed than erythromycin. Feeding increases absorption in dogs. High concentration in pulmonary, prostatic, tonsillar, and pleural fluid. Does not enter saliva, milk, or CSF in absence of inflammation.

SPECTRUM. See ERYTHROMYCIN for bacteria; coccidia.

INDICATIONS. Respiratory, prostatic, urethral infections.

CONTRAINDICATIONS. Reduce dose in renal or hepatic dysfunction.

ADVERSE REACTIONS. See ERYTHROMYCIN.

INTERACTIONS. See ERYTHROMYCIN.

Availability	Type	Size	Preparation (Company)
Human	Oral capsules	150 mg	*Rulide* (Roussel-Uclaf)

INTERNATIONAL PREPARATIONS. *Assoral, Claramid, Macrosil, Rossitrol, Rotesan, Rotramin, Rulid, Surlid.*

DOSAGE

Indications (Dogs)	Dose	Route	Interval (hr)	Duration (days)
Soft tissue, respiratory, urinary infections	15 mg/kg	PO	24	prn

ADDITIONAL DOSAGES. Coccidiosis, Table 81–2.

DISPENSING INFORMATION. May be administered with food.

SPECTINOMYCIN

CLASS. Aminocyclitol related to aminoglycoside.

ACTION. Usually bacteriostatic; inhibits bacterial protein synthesis by acting on 30s ribosomal subunit.

MORE INFORMATION. Related to a new derivative trospectomycin, *Spexil* (Pharmacia & Upjohn).

PHARMACOKINETICS. Minor (<8%) absorption from GI tract. When given orally, used to reduce intestinal microflora or treat enteric pathogens. Rapid absorption after IM injection. Tissue concentrations are lower than in blood. Like aminoglycosides, does not enter CSF or ocular tissues and only slightly with inflammation. Majority (70%–80%) excreted in urine as active drug.

SPECTRUM. Gram positive: *Streptococcus*. Gram negative: *Proteus, Enterobacter, Salmonella, Escherichia, Klebsiella*. **Anaerobes:** little activity. **Others:** some *Mycoplasma*. **More effective:** most effective single agent for gram-negative bacteria in chemoprophylaxis of open bowel surgery. Used in people to treat gonorrhea. **Less effective:** *Chlamydia*, spirochetes, *Pseudomonas*.

INDICATIONS. Intra-abdominal infections or prophylaxis for abdominal surgery. If used orally, for bacterial gastroenteritis or to reduce enteric flora in cases of hepatic encephalopathy.

APPROVED USES. As single injection for penicillin-resistant human gonoccocal infections.

CONTRAINDICATIONS. Pre-existing renal failure, hypersensitivity to this drug.

ADVERSE REACTIONS. Pain or irritation at injection site; elevation in blood hepatic enzymes and urea with repeated doses. Less ototoxic and nephrotoxic than aminoglycosides. Cholestatic hepatitis in people. Can cause neuromuscular blockade, reversible with IV calcium.

INTERACTIONS. Effectiveness reduced when used with tetracycline or chloramphenicol. Can combine with lincomycin for increased efficacy against *Mycoplasma*.

Availability	Type	Sizes	Preparations (Company)
Human	Powder for injection	2 g (as HCl)	*Trobicin* (Pharmacia & Upjohn)
	Powder for oral suspension	2 mg/ml, 4 g/ml	
Veterinary	Solution for injection (poultry approval)	100 mg/ml	*Spectam* (Sanofi)

INTERNATIONAL PREPARATIONS. *Kempi, Stanilo, Trobicine.*

HANDLING. Store at room temperature. Mix powder well after diluting. Stable 4 weeks at room temperature, although it is recommended to use reconstituted drug within 24 hr.

ADMINISTRATION. Administer IM in large muscle.

DOSAGE

Indications (Dogs and Cats)	Dose	Route	Interval (hr)	Duration (days)
Prophylactic for bowel surgery, peritonitis	10 mg/kg	IM, SC	8–12	*

*Immediately before and during surgery.

SPIRAMYCIN

CLASS. Macrolide.

ACTION. Bacteriostatic; inhibits bacterial protein synthesis; binds to 50s ribosomal subunits.

MORE INFORMATION. See ERYTHROMYCIN, METRONIDAZOLE (interactions); Antiprotozoals, Chapter 71; Table 71–1.

PHARMACOKINETICS. Incompletely absorbed from GI tract, unaffected by food. Widely distributed except in CSF. Metabolized in liver to active metabolites with a majority excreted in the bile and 10% in urine. Enters milk. Persists in some tissues.

SPECTRUM. Anaerobic bacteria: *Campylobacter, Helicobacter.* Similar antibacterial spectrum as erythromycin but less active. **Others:** *Toxoplasma, Cryptosporidium.*

INDICATIONS. Toxoplasmosis, cryptosporidiosis. Combined with metronidazole for periodontitis and stomatitis.

CONTRAINDICATIONS. Pre-existing hepatic disease.

ADVERSE REACTIONS. Irritating after IM injection. Vomiting and diarrhea (similar to erythromycin), allergic reactions, cholestatic hepatitis. Cutaneous irritation to veterinarians exposed to the drug during preparation or administration.

Availability	Type	Sizes	Preparations (Company)
Human	Oral tablets	1 g	*Rovamycine* (Rhone-Pôulenc Rorer)
Veterinary	Oral tablets	46.9 mg* S, 25 mg M 234 mg S, 125 mg M 469 mg S, 250 mg M	*Stomorgyl* (Rhone-Merieux EC) (*Rodogyl* human drug counterpart containing S and M)

*46.9 mg spiramycin is 150,000 U.
S = spiramycin; M = metronidazole.

INTERNATIONAL PREPARATIONS. *Rovamycin, Rovamycina, Selectomycin.*

HANDLING. Store tablets at room temperature in containers away from light and moisture.

ADMINISTRATION. Can give tablets with a meal.

DOSAGE

Indications	Dose (mg/kg)	Route	Interval (hr)	Duration (days)
Human				
Pediatric toxoplasmosis	50–100	PO	24	21–28
Dogs and Cats				
Periodontal, oral infection	23.4 S 12.5 M	PO	24	5–10

S = spiramycin; M = metronidazole.

ADDITIONAL DOSAGES. Coccidiosis, Table 81–2; oral infections, Table 89–4.

DISPENSING INFORMATION. Do not break or crush tablets.

STAPHYLOCOCCAL PHAGE LYSATE

CLASS. Immunostimulant.

ACTION. Increases immune response against *Staphylococcus*. Stimulates production of interleukin-γ, interleukin-6, tumor necrosis factor, and γ-interferon.

MORE INFORMATION. Chapter 100; Table 100–21; references: 100:32, 100:82.

FORMULATION. Bacteriologically sterile preparation containing cell wall components of *S. aureus*, a bacteriophage, and some culture media, in solution. Each ml of solution contains 120–180 CFU of *S. aureus* before phage lysis.

INDICATIONS. Chronic or recurrent pyoderma in dogs caused by staphylococci.

CONTRAINDICATIONS. Previous severe hypersensitivity reaction to the product.

ADVERSE REACTIONS. Possible anaphylaxis. Rare fever, chills. Transient swelling, redness, and pruritus at site of inoculation.

Availability	Type	Sizes	Preparation (Company)
Veterinary	Solution for injection	1-ml ampules, 10-ml multidose vials	*Staphage Lysate* (Delmont Labs)

HANDLING. Store refrigerated (2°–8°C). Do not freeze. Use entire contents when vial is opened. No preservatives, so must be handled aseptically. Should not use if solution is cloudy.

ADMINISTRATION. Concomitant antibiotic therapy is recommended for the initial 4- to 6-week treatment period. Subcutaneous injection: to test for hypersensitivity, can perform intradermal skin test of 0.05 to 0.1 ml. Should precede initial use. Observe animal and inoculation site for 1 hr for immediate reactions and 48 hr for delayed reactions. Allergic reactions may require epinephrine administration.

DOSAGE

Indication	Dose (ml)	Route	Interval (hr)	Duration
Canine pyoderma	0.1–0.2	SC	3–7	*
	0.5	SC	Twice weekly	10–12 weeks†

*Increase dose in increments every 3–7 days until dose is 1.0 ml. Maximum dose in large dogs is 1.5 ml.
†Then 0.5–1.0 ml every 1–2 weeks. The interval may be lengthened to the longest interval that maintains control of the disease.

DISPENSING INFORMATION. Observe the injection site for pain, swelling, or discharge. Should this develop, the dosage can be reduced.

STAPHYLOCOCCAL PROTEIN A

CLASS. Bacterial extract, IgG binding reagent used for its affinity to purify mixtures of Ig.

ACTION. Immunostimulant; activates antibody synthesis, interferon induction, lymphocytes; binds immune complexes. Binds the Fc portion of antibodies (IgG class) by a nonimmune mechanism, without disturbing antigen binding. Reaction is generally not species specific.

MORE INFORMATION. See in Chapter 13, Antivirals and Immunotherapy; references: 100:102b; 100:102c.

PHARMACOKINETICS. Unknown.

INDICATIONS. Feline leukemia virus (FeLV) viremic cats with clinical signs caused by immunosuppression.

APPROVED USES. Reagent grade chemical for experimental purposes.

CONTRAINDICATIONS. Previous hypersensitivity to this compound or closely related compounds.

ADVERSE REACTIONS. Anaphylaxis, low-grade peritonitis.

INTERACTIONS. None.

Availability	Type	Size	Preparations (Company)
5 mg	Lyophilized powder (reagent grade)	3 ml volume diluted	Pharmacia Biotech

HANDLING. Powder (5 mg) is reconstituted according to manufacturer's recommendations using sterile technique. The resulting solution is filtered through a 0.3 μ filter and added to 500 ml of sterile saline to give 10 μg/ml. This is frozen in 5-ml aliquots, which can be frozen for several years. The solution should not be refrozen after thawing, and self-defrosting freezers with freeze-thaw cycles should be avoided.

ADMINISTRATION. Clip fur from abdominal wall, scrub to remove surface bacteria with detergents. Give injection IP.

DOSAGE

Indications	Dose	Route	Interval	Duration (weeks)
FeLV illness	10 μg/kg	IP	twice weekly	10*

*Then once a month for the life of the animal.

STIBOGLUCONATE (SODIUM)

CLASS. Pentavalent antimonial.

ACTION. Antiprotozoal: interferes with energy metabolism of *Leishmania* amastigotes.

MORE INFORMATION. See MEGLUMINE ANTIMONIATE; Chapter 71, Table 71–1.

PHARMACOKINETICS. Rapid systemic availability after parenteral administration, attains high serum concentrations, most of drug is excreted in urine within 24 hr. Some accumulation and with delayed excretion occurs after multiple doses.

SPECTRUM. *Leishmania.* Some increased resistance has been noted.

INDICATION. Leishmaniasis.

CONTRAINDICATIONS. Pre-existing cardiac arrhythmias or renal dysfunction.

ADVERSE REACTIONS. Musculoskeletal pain or injection, increased hepatic transaminases (usually reversible), pancreatitis, myocardial injury, hemolytic anemia, leukopenia, vomiting, diarrhea, cardiac arrhythmias, renal dysfunction, shock, sudden death. IV use can cause thrombophlebitis. In people, children tolerate the drug better than adults.

INTERACTIONS. Has been combined with paromomycin or pentamidine for resistant leishmaniasis.

Availability	Type	Size	Preparation (Company)
Human	Solution for parenteral injection. Not available in U.S. for animal use, only for humans through CDC, Atlanta, GA, (404) 639-3670; available in other countries	100 mg antimony/ml in 100 ml multidose vials	*Pentostam* (Glaxo Wellcome)

HANDLING. Protect from ultraviolet light. Can sterilize solutions by autoclaving.

ADMINISTRATION. Give IV or IM. If adverse reactions occur, can give on alternate days for longer periods. If given IV, should do it slowly (over 5 min) through a fine needle or catheter to avoid thrombophlebitis.

DOSAGE

Indications (Human)	Dose* (mg/kg)	Route	Interval (hr)	Duration (days)
Leishmaniasis (cutaneous)	10–20 antimony	IM	24	20
Leishmanasis (visceral)	20 antimony	IM, IV	24	20–28

*Doses are expressed as equivalent antimony.

ADDITIONAL DOSAGES. Leishmaniasis, Table 71–1.

STREPTOMYCIN

CLASS. Aminoglycoside.

ACTION. Bactericidal; interferes with bacterial protein synthesis.

MORE INFORMATION. See GENTAMICIN; Aminoglycosides, Chapter 34; Tables 34–5 and 34–6.

PHARMACOKINETICS. See GENTAMICIN.

SPECTRUM. Gram positive: some *Streptococcus.* **Gram negative:** *Escherichia,* some *Pasteurella, Salmonella, Yersinia, Francisella, Brucella.* Bacterial resistance is common with this aminoglycoside. **Others:** *Mycobacterium tuberculosis.*

INDICATIONS. Brucellosis, tularemia, plague, mycobacteriosis. Should always be used in combination.

CONTRAINDICATIONS. Avoid use in cats because of toxicity. Avoid with renal insufficiency, myasthenia gravis.

ADVERSE REACTIONS. Ototoxicity, neuromuscular blockade, renal damage.

INTERACTIONS. Ototoxicity and nephrotoxicity increased with concurrent diuretics (mannitol, furosemide), cephalosporins.

Availability	Type	Size	Preparations (Company)
Human	Injectable solution	400 mg/ml	*Streptomycin sulfate* (Pfizer); discontinued in U.S.; available only for human use by CDC. Presently for investigational use by veterinarians in U.S. by Roerig, Division of Pfizer; voice: 800-254-4445; Fax: 800-251-9445.

INTERNATIONAL PREPARATIONS. *Cidan Est, Novostrep, Solustrep, Streptocol, Strepto-Fatol.*

HANDLING. Stored at refrigerated 2°C–8°C temperatures. If diluted in fluid for IV use, stable for 24 hr.

ADMINISTRATION. IM use only. If insufficient muscle mass, may give dose in 100 ml of 0.9% NaCl or 5% dextrose and administer it over 30–60 min.

DOSAGE

Indication (Dogs)	Dose	Route	Interval (hr)	Duration (days)
Brucellosis	10–20 mg/kg	IM	12	7*

*Dose given for first and fourth week of treatment along with concurrent doxycycline (see Chapter 40 and Table 40–2).

ADDITIONAL DOSAGES. Canine brucellosis, Table 40–2; plague, Table 47–1; mycobacterial infections, Table 50–4; musculoskeletal infections, Table 86–3; local ocular treatment, Table 93–4.

SULFADIAZINE

CLASS. Sulfonamide.

ACTION. Bacteriostatic; inhibits bacterial folic acid synthesis.

MORE INFORMATION. TRIMETHOPRIM-SULFONAMIDE; Chapter 34, Sulfonamides; Table 34–10.

PHARMACOKINETICS. Rapid absorption after PO administration, 70%–100% absorbed, distributed through body tissues and fluids. Therapeutic levels achieved in eye, CNS, pleura, synovia. Enters placental and fetal tissues. Hepatic metabolism by acetylation. Pantothenic acid deficiency or "slow acetylating" animals may have increased risk of toxicity or accumulation of drug. Metabolites and active drug excreted in urine. Crystals are less soluble in acid urine and with restricted fluid intake.

SPECTRUM. Gram positive: *Streptococcus, Staphylococcus, Nocardia.* **Gram negative:** *Klebsiella, Proteus, Escherichia, Shigella, Salmonella.* **Anaerobes:** poor in vivo. **Others:** *Pneumocystis,* Coccidia, *Toxoplasma.*

INDICATIONS. Urinary tract infections, meningitis, nocardiosis, otitis media-interna, toxoplasmosis (with pyrimethamine).

CONTRAINDICATIONS. Hypersensitivity to sulfonamides, thiazide diuretics, or local anesthetics that have similar chemical structure. Avoid with blood dyscrasias, renal or hepatic insufficiency.

ADVERSE REACTIONS. High or overdoses can cause CNS signs or acute vomiting and abdominal pain. Hypersensitivity reactions (see TRIMETHOPRIM-SULFONAMIDE). GI irritation, dermatologic eruptions, polydipsia and polyuria, keratoconjunctivitis sicca. Resembles: goitrogens inhibiting T_4 production; diuretics causing polydipsia, polyuria; sulfonureas causing hypoglycemia.

INTERACTIONS. Chronic administration results in reduced thyroid hormone synthesis. It may increase warfarin activity, phentoin concentrations, thiopental activity, sulfonurea concentrations in treated animals. Increases toxicity of methotrexate, which also affects folate metabolism.

Availability	Type	Size	Preparation (Company)
Veterinary	Tablets	500 mg	Generic (various)

HANDLING. Store in airtight containers at room temperature.

ADMINISTRATION. Once daily suitable for urinary tract infections, but twice daily needed to maintain blood and tissue levels. Maintain hydration and adequate fluid therapy, especially in cats.

DOSAGE

Indications	Dose (mg/kg)	Route	Interval (hr)	Duration (days)
Dogs				
Soft tissue, urinary infections	30	PO	24	7–14
Cats				
Soft tissue, urinary infections	15	PO	12	7–14

ADDITIONAL DOSAGES. Nocardiosis, Table 49–2; hepatozoon (with trimethoprim), Table 74–2; see also TRIMETHOPRIM-SULFONAMIDE for combined use in other infections.

DISPENSING INFORMATION. Watch for vomiting, diarrhea, systemic illness, or reduced tear production.

SULFADIMETHOXINE

CLASS. Sulfonamide.

ACTION. Bacteriostatic; inhibits bacterial synthesis of folic acid from para-aminobenzoic acid. Antiprotozoal.

MORE INFORMATION. See SULFADIAZINE; the SULFONAMIDES; Chapter 34; Table 34–10.

PHARMACOKINETICS. See also SULFADIAZINE. Rapidly absorbed from GI tract. High plasma protein binding allows for sustained blood levels, prolonged excretion, longer dosing intervals. Diffuses especially into tissues that are less acid and in those having high leukocyte concentrations. In the dog, because the drug is excreted unchanged, the potential for drug-induced nephrotoxicity is low.

SPECTRUM. Gram positive: *Streptococcus, Staphylococcus.* **Gram negative:** *Klebsiella, Proteus, Escherichia, Shigella, Salmonella.* **Anaerobes:** poor in vivo. **Others:** coccidia, some activity against *Cryptosporidium.* **Ineffective:** viruses and *Rickettsia, Pseudomonas.*

INDICATIONS. Treatment of bacterial respiratory, enteric, genitourinary tract, soft tissue infections. Coccidiosis.

CONTRAINDICATIONS. Dehydration. See SULFADIAZINE.

ADVERSE REACTIONS. Few in dogs, diarrhea at higher than therapeutic dosages. IM injections are too painful to be practical.

INTERACTIONS. Reduced thyroid hormone synthesis with chronic (6 weeks) treatment. See SULFADIAZINE.

Availability	Type	Sizes	Preparations (Company)
Veterinary	Oral tablets (approved dogs and cats)	125 mg; 250 mg; 500 mg	*Albon* (Pfizer), *Bactrovet* (Schering-Plough)
	Liquid for injection (approved cats, dogs, horses, cows)	400 mg/ml	*Albon*
	Oral suspension (approved dogs, cats)	250 mg/5 ml	*Albon*
		125 mg/ml	*Bactrovet*

HANDLING. Store injectable liquid at room temperature. If crystals form, dissolve by warming slightly.

ADMINISTRATION. Parenteral liquid: IV or SC to obtain rapid blood levels or to treat anorectic, vomiting, fractious animal. IM route is very painful and should be avoided. PO suspension is custard flavored. Animals should maintain adequate water intake.

DOSAGE

Indications	Dose (mg/kg)	Route	Interval (hr)	Duration (days)
Dogs and Cats				
Systemic infections, coccidiosis	27.5*	IV, IM, PO	24	3–5
Cats				
Coccidiosis	50.0	PO	24	10
	27*	PO	24	prn†

*Give twice this dose the first day.
†Or 48 hr after signs resolve; usual course for coccidiosis may be 14–29 days.

ADDITIONAL DOSAGES. Coccidiosis, Table 81–2; pyoderma (with ormetroprim), Table 85–3. For combination therapy, see also TRIMETHOPRIM-SULFONAMIDE, ORMETROPRIM-SULFONAMIDE, and BAQUILOPRIM-SULFONAMIDE for treatment of other infections.

DISPENSING INFORMATION. Make sure animal has access to water at all times.

SULFASALAZINE (SALICYLAZOSULFAPYRIDINE)

CLASS. Sulfonamide.

ACTION. Inhibits bacterial folic acid synthesis combined to salicylic acid. The salicylate component is believed to be the active moiety, mainly anti-inflammatory.

MORE INFORMATION. See Chapter 34, Sulfonamides; Table 34–10.

PHARMACOKINETICS. After PO administration, one third of dose is absorbed from small intestine. The remaining two thirds pass to the colon, where it is hydrolyzed by resident microflora to 5-aminosalicylic acid and sulfapyridine; most of the latter is absorbed and metabolized. Within 3 days, 91% of drug and metabolites is recovered in the urine.

INDICATIONS. Inflammatory large bowel diseases of dogs and cats.

CONTRAINDICATIONS. Previous hypersensitivity to sulfonamides, intestinal, or urinary obstruction. Use caution in treating cats because of salicylate content.

ADVERSE REACTIONS. Anorexia, vomiting, hypersensitivity reactions. Use of enteric-coated tablet may alleviate GI side effects in cats. CNS signs (ataxia, depression), polydipsia, polyuria may inhibit thyroid hormone and produce thyroid enlargement (goiter). Orange-yellow discoloration of urine or skin, reduced spermatogenesis; keratoconjunctivitis sicca. Folate-deficiency anemia, especially in cats on long-term treatment. See TRIMETHOPRIM-SULFONAMIDE.

INTERACTIONS. Reduced thyroid hormone synthesis with chronic (5–6 weeks treatment).

Availability	Type	Sizes	Preparations (Company)
Human	Oral tablets ± enteric coating	500 mg	*Azulfidine* (Pharmacia & Upjohn), generic (various)
	Oral suspension	250 mg/5 ml	*Azulfidine*

INTERNATIONAL PREPARATIONS. *Colo-Pleon, Gastroprotetto, Salazopyrin, Salisulf, Sulazine, Sulfazine.*

HANDLING. Tablets should be stored at room temperature. Shake PO suspension before using and refrigerate after use; do not store longer than 14 days after reconstitution.

ADMINISTRATION. Give with food if causes vomiting. Subdividing the dose or using enteric-coated tablets helps avoid GI irritation.

DOSAGE

Indications	Dose (mg/kg)	Route	Interval (hr)	Duration (days)
Dogs				
Colitis	10–15*	PO	6–8	2–4†
Cats				
Inflammatory bowel disease	10–20	PO	12	14–42
	25‡	PO	24	14–42

*Maximum of 1 g daily.
†Then re-evaluate treatment response. After 4–5 weeks may reduce dose to 12 to 24 hr interval for 2–3 weeks before discontinuing.
‡Maximum of 250 mg total dose (1/2 tablet) can be given every 24 hr.

ADDITIONAL DOSAGES. Gastroenteric infections, Table 89–11; colitis, Table 89–14.

DISPENSING INFORMATION. See SULFADIAZINE; watch for reduced tear production.

TEICOPLANIN

CLASS. Glycopeptide.

ACTION. Bactericidal; binds to bacterial cell wall peptidoglycan.

MORE INFORMATION. See VANCOMYCIN; Chapter 34.

PHARMACOKINETICS. Not absorbed from GI tract. Usually given IV or IM and 90% bioavailable. After parenteral administration, enters liver, pancreas, bone, mucosal tissues, and peritoneal, biliary, and blister fluids. Poor entry into CNS or CSF with noninflamed meninges. Longer plasma half-life than vancomycin, can give once daily. Little metabolism, most renally excreted unchanged. Slow elimination phase.

SPECTRUM. Gram positive: Only against gram-positive aerobes and gram-positive obigate anaerobes; more activity and less resistance than with vancomycin.

INDICATIONS. β-lactam–resistant gram-positive infections as a result of *Staphylococcus, Streptococcus, Enterococcus, Listeria, Corynebacterium, Clostridium.* Should be combined with aminoglycoside to treat staphylococcal endocarditis, septicemia, endocarditis, skin, soft tissue, and lower respiratory infections, osteomyelitis. For catheter-induced infections; has also been impregnated on IV catheters for prophylaxis. Orally is not absorbed but is given to treat enterococcal and clostridial enterocolitis.

CONTRAINDICATIONS. Renal failure. Should monitor function during therapy.

ADVERSE REACTIONS. Injection site pain (IM) or phlebitis (IV), urticarial rash, eosinophilia, neutropenia, thrombocytopenia, vomiting, diarrhea.

INTERACTIONS. Synergistic with aminoglycosides, imipenem, and rifampin.

Availability	Type	Sizes	Preparation (Company)
Human	Powder for injection	200 mg, 400 mg	*Targocid* (Marion Merrell Dow)

INTERNATIONAL PREPARATIONS. *Targocid.*

HANDLING. Do not mix with other drugs in solution. See VANCOMYCIN.

ADMINISTRATION. Can give over 5-min period compared with 60-min duration required for vancomycin.

DOSAGE

Indications (Dogs)	Dose (mg/kg)	Route	Interval (hr)	Duration (days)
Skin, urinary, soft tissue infections	3	IV, IM	24	prn
Systemic infections	6	IV, IM	24	prn
Bacteremia with resistant organisms	12	IV, IM	24	prn

Often give twice the dose the first day.

TERBINAFINE

CLASS. Allylamine.

ACTION. Inhibits fungal sterol synthesis. Antifungal.

MORE INFORMATION. Reference 57:13.

PHARMACOKINETICS. In people, well absorbed (>70%) from the GI tract. Distributed in high concentrations in tissues, skin, sweat, sebum, nail bed, hair. Excreted into milk. A majority of the drug (70%) eliminated in the urine. Topical preparations are minimally (≤5%) absorbed.

SPECTRUM. Dermatophytes, some activity against *Sporothrix* and systemic fungi. In combination with itraconazole was successful in treatment of cellulitis caused by *Pythium insidiosum.*

INDICATIONS. Onychomycosis. Dermatophytosis. Reduced treatment time, improved cure rates, and lower relapse rate compared with griseofulvin.

CONTRAINDICATIONS. Reduce dosage in renal failure or hepatic dysfunction.

ADVERSE REACTIONS. GI disturbances, vomiting, abdominal pain, diarrhea. Hepatotoxicity, intrahepatic biliary stasis, increase hepatic enzyme activities, neutropenia, pancytopenia. In humans, loss of taste sensation.

INTERACTIONS. Cimetidine increases blood concentrations while rifampin decreases it.

Availability	Type	Sizes	Preparations (Company)
Human	Oral tablets (as hydrochloride)	125 mg; 250 mg	*Lamisil* (Sandoz)
	Topical cream (as hydrochloride)	1%	Not available in U.S.

INTERNATIONAL PREPARATION. *Daskil.*

HANDLING. Store tablets at room temperature in an airtight, light-proof container. May have to crush tablets and recompound the drug in gelatin capsules to achieve low dose needed.

ADMINISTRATION. Some increase in absorption is noted with administration of food. Must treat for extended periods in onychomycosis to become incorporated into nail surface.

DOSAGE

Indications (Dogs and Cats)	Dose* (mg/kg)	Route	Interval (hr)	Duration (days)
Onychomycosis	3–10	PO	24	42–84
Dermatophytosis	2–10	PO	24	28

*Extrapolated human dose. Tablets may have to be reformulated to achieve this dose level.

DISPENSING INFORMATION. This drug may cause GI upsets manifested by anorexia, vomiting, diarrhea.

TETRACYCLINE

CLASS. Tetracycline.

ACTION. Bacteriostatic; inhibits bacterial protein synthesis by binding to 30s ribosomal subunit. Has anti-inflammatory effects by suppression of leukocyte chemotaxis.

MORE INFORMATION. OXYTETRACYCLINE; Tetracyclines, Chapter 34; Antiprotozoals; Table 34–7; Chapter 71; Table 71–1.

PHARMACOKINETICS. 77%–80% absorption from GI tract (fasting). Unabsorbed drug appears in feces and may alter GI flora. Readily enters most body fluids and tissues. Crosses the placenta to accumulate in fetal bones and teeth. Reaches highest concentration in CSF than other tetracyclines except minocycline or doxycycline. Levels in the CNS and CSF may be therapeutic. Primarily (50%–70%) renal excretion by glomerular filtration. Highest concentrations reached in liver, kidney, urine.

SPECTRUM. Gram positive: *Streptococcus,* some *Staphylococcus, Bacillus.* **Gram negative:** *Escherichia, Pasteurella, Klebsiella, Enterobacter, Brucella, Bordetella, Aerobacter,* some *Salmonella.* **Anaerobes:** Clostridia, *Actinomyces.* **Others:** Rickettsiae *(Rickettsia, Ehrlichia, Haemobartonella), Chlamydia, Mycoplasma, Balantidium.* **Ineffective:** *Mycobacterium, Proteus, Pseudomonas.*

INDICATIONS. Tick-borne diseases (Rocky Mountain spotted fever [RMSF], ehrlichiosis, borreliosis), leptospirosis, oral spirochetosis, gram-negative bacterial gastroenteritis, yersiniosis, pasteurellosis, campylobacteriosis, brucellosis, chlamydiosis, intestinal amebiasis. Urinary tract infections caused by *Staphylococcus* and *Escherichia.* Intrapleural administration of tetracycline as a sclerosing agent to treat recurrent spontaneous pneumothorax and lymphatic leakage (34:89). Intense chest pain is an undesirable side effect of this therapy. Has been used for other uses as an anti-inflammatory agent for polyarthritis (see Chapter 34, Borreliosis) and for treatment of autoimmune skin disease (34:179a).

CONTRAINDICATIONS. Pregnancy, lactation, and young (<6 mo); renal or hepatic insufficiency. Reduce dose or avoid in renal failure.

ADVERSE REACTIONS. Fewer GI upsets than other tetracyclines. GI side effects are increased when coadministered with theophylline. Sometimes diarrhea from altered GI microflora. Yellow dental staining in young animals. Catabolic effect may exacerbate azotemia in renal failure. Esophagitis, anorexia, nausea, vomiting, occasional anaphylaxis, Fanconi-like syndrome if outdated drug given. Fever (≤41.1°C [106°F]) that resolves when treatment is discontinued. Cats very susceptible to these toxicities. Signs of GI irritation include depression, fever, anorexia, vomiting, diarrhea. Hepatotoxicity, hepatic necrosis, fever in cats (34:74). Nephrotoxicity has been associated with concurrent use of methoxyflurane anesthesia. Rapid IV injection may cause cardiac arrhythmias, presumably owing to chelation of calcium.

INTERACTIONS. GI absorption reduced by iron, bismuth, aluminum hydroxide, sodium bicarbonate, cimetidine, calcium, magnesium, kaolin and pectin, milk products. May interfere with penicillin activity when coadministered.

Availability	Type	Sizes	Preparations (Company)
Human	Oral suspension	125 mg/5 ml	*Achromycin-V* (Lederle); *Sumycin* (Squibb)
	Oral capsules, tablets	100 mg, 250 mg, 500 mg	*Achromycin*, generic (various), *Panmycin* (Pharmacia & Upjohn), *Sumycin*
	Powder for IV injection, also IM	100 mg, 250 mg, 500 mg vials	*Achromycin*
Veterinary	Oral liquid (chocolate-mint flavor)	100 mg/ml	*Panmycin* Aquadrops, *Actinomycin*, *Sumycin*, Tetra-Vet
	Oral capsules	250 mg	Generic (various)

INTERNATIONAL PREPARATIONS. *Acromicina, Austramycin, Hostacyclin, Latycin.*

HANDLING. Store capsules and tablets at room temperature in airtight, dry, light-resistant containers. PO suspension is stable at room temperature. Shake PO liquid well before administering. IV and IM products are stable at 12 and 24 hr, respectively, after reconstitution.

ADMINISTRATION. Administer to fasting animal. Do not mix with dairy products or substances containing multivalent cations (e.g., Fe, Al, Mg, Ca). Usually does not cause vomiting but can be given with a *small* amount of food if necessary.

DOSAGE

Indications	Dose	Route	Interval (hr)	Duration
Dogs				
Urinary infections	16 mg/kg	PO	8	7–14 days
Rickettsiosis, borreliosis	22 mg/kg	PO	8	14 days
Systemic bacteremia, brucellosis	22–50 mg/kg	PO	8	28 days
Cats				
Soft tissue infections	20 mg/kg	PO	8	21 days
Haemobartonellosis	10–25 mg/kg	PO	8–12	21 days
Bacteremia, systemic infections	7 mg/kg	IV, IM	12	prn

ADDITIONAL DOSAGES. Canine distemper, Table 3–5; salmon poisoning, Table 27–2; ehrlichiosis, Table 28–4; RMSF, Table 29–3; haemobartonellosis, Table 30–1; salmonellosis and other enteric bacterial infections, Table 39–1; helicobacteriosis (in combination), Table 39–3; *Clostridium perfringens* diarrhea, Table 39–4; brucellosis (in combination), Table 40–2; tetanus, Table 43–2; leptospirosis, Table 44–4; plague, Table 47–1; protothecosis, Table 69–1; hepatozoonosis (in combination), Table 74–2; enteric protozoa, Table 78–2; musculoskeletal infections, Tables 86–2 and 86–3; respiratory infections, Table 88–8; oral infections, Table 89–4; gastrointestinal infections; Table 89–11; hepatobiliary infections, Table 90–4; urinary tract infection, Table 91–8.

DISPENSING INFORMATION. Give on an empty stomach.

TICARCILLIN

CLASS. Carboxypenicillin.

ACTION. Bactericidal, inhibits bacterial cell wall synthesis.

MORE INFORMATION. See CARBENICILLIN; Penicillins, Chapter 34; Table 34–1.

PHARMACOKINETICS. Not absorbed after PO administration, so given parenterally. Reaches many extracellular fluids, soft tissues, and bone. Crosses blood-brain barrier, primarily with inflammation. CSF–serum ratio is 0.06:1 with noninflamed meninges and 0.4:1 with meningitis. Eliminated primarily by renal excretion.

SPECTRUM. **Gram positive:** *Staphylococcus* (non β-lactamase producers), some *Streptococcus,* some *Enterococcus.* **Gram negative:** *Escherichia, Proteus, Salmonella, Enterobacter, Pseudomonas, Citrobacter, Serratia.* **Anaerobes:** *Clostridium, Peptococcus, Peptostreptococcus, Bacteroides, Fusobacterium.* **More effective:** more potent than carbenicillin against *Pseudomonas.* Because of low toxicity, can cause large doses to have activity against some resistant strains of *Pseudomonas.*

INDICATIONS. Bone, joint infections, bacterial sepsis, skin, soft tissue infections, acute, chronic respiratory infections, genitourinary infections, intra-abdominal, pelvic infections. Infections of these areas involving *Pseudomonas* or anaerobes.

CONTRAINDICATIONS. Reduce dosage in renal failure.

ADVERSE REACTIONS. See CARBENICILLIN.

INTERACTIONS. Often combined with β-lactamase inhibitor, clavulanate (see TICARCILLIN-CLAVULANATE). May also use with aminoglycoside (administered separately) for additional activity against gram-negative aerobes and facultative anaerobes in severe infections.

Availability	Type	Sizes	Preparation (Company)
Human	Powder for injection	1 g, 3 g, 6 g, 20 g, 30 g	*Ticar* (SmithKline Beecham)

INTERNATIONAL PREPARATIONS: *Aerugipen, Tarcil, Ticarpen, Ticillin, Triacilline.*

HANDLING. Store powder at room temperature. **IM:** dilute with sterile water, 0.9% NaCl or 1% lidocaine solution. **IV:** dilute to 1 g/4 ml in 0.9% NaCl or 5% dextrose. Should refrigerate if not used within 1 hr because precipitation may occur. Stable for 24 hr at room temperature and 72 hr if refrigerated. Continuous drip required or intermittent pulse administration over 30 min to 2 hr. Never mix solutions with aminoglycosides because they become inactivated; however, they can be given separately at different sites.

ADMINISTRATION. Often given IV for bacterial sepsis, with an aminoglycoside.

DOSAGE

Indications	Dose (mg/kg)	Route	Interval (hr)	Duration (days)
Dogs				
Soft tissue, systemic infections	15–25	IV, IM, SC	6–8	prn
Septicemia	40–50	IV, IM	4–6	prn
Difficult, severe systemic infections	100	IV	6–8	prn
Cats (Pseudomonas)				
Soft tissue, systemic infections	15–24	IV, IM, SC	8	prn
Systemic, bacteremia	40–50	IV	6	prn

ADDITIONAL DOSAGES. Gram-negative bacterial infection, Table 37–2; otitis externa, topical, Table 85–6; bacteremia and endocarditis, Table 87–7; respiratory infections, Table 88–8; hepatobiliary infections, Table 90–4.

TICARCILLIN-CLAVULANATE

CLASS. Carboxypenicillin and β-lactamase inhibitor in 30:1 ratio.

ACTION. Bactericidal; ticarcillin interferes with bacterial cell wall synthesis; clavulanate inactivates plasmid-mediated β-lactamases; that cause resistance to penicillins and cephalosporins.

MORE INFORMATION. See TICARCILLIN; Penicillins, Chapter 34; Tables 34–1 and 34–2.

PHARMACOKINETICS. See also TICARCILLIN. Ticarcillin is not systemically available after PO administration. Parenteral dosages produces good concentration in tissues, bile, pleural and interstitial fluids; CSF in inflamed meninges. Mainly renal elimination, with 60–70% ticarcillin and 35%–45% clavulanate excreted unchanged in urine. Dogs excrete clavulanate more rapidly than ticarcillin.

SPECTRUM. Gram positive: *Staphylococcus, Streptococcus, Enterococcus.* **Gram-negative:** *Pseudomonas, Proteus, Enterobacter, Salmonella, Klebsiella, Escherichia, Citrobacter, Serratia, Acinetobacter, Pasteurella, Bordetella.* **Anaerobes:** *Bacteroides, Clostridium, Fusobacterium, Peptostreptococcus, Eubacterium, Peptococcus.*

INDICATIONS. Nosocomial pneumonia, severe skin, soft tissue infections; septicemia; bone, joint, urinary tract, intra-abdominal, gynecologic infections. Synergistic with aminoglycosides against some strains of *Pseudomonas.*

CONTRAINDICATIONS. Reduce dose in renal failure.

ADVERSE REACTIONS. Platelet dysfunction, hypersensitivity reactions, seizures, vomiting, diarrhea, myelotoxicity. Rarely hepatotoxicity in people.

INTERACTIONS. Synergistic with aminoglycoside for severe infections.

Availability	Type	Size	Preparation (Company)
Human	Powder for injection	3.1 g (3.0 g ticarcillin, 0.1 g clavulanate)	*Timentin* (SmithKline Beecham)

INTERNATIONAL PREPARATIONS. *Betabactyl, Claventin, Clavucar, Timenten.*

HANDLING. Concentrated reconstituted solution (200 mg/ml) stable up to 6 hr at room temperature or 72 hr if refrigerated. Can be diluted to 10–100 mg/ml with 5% dextrose, 0.9% NaCl, lactated Ringer's, and is stable for 24 hr at room temperature 7 days refrigerated, and 30 days frozen. For 5% dextrose solution, storage is only 7 days at frozen temperatures. Incompatible with bicarbonate in solution.

ADMINISTRATION. IV slowly over 30 min. Administer any concurrent aminoglycosides separately.

DOSAGE

Indications	Dose (mg/kg)	Route	Interval (hr)	Duration (days)
Dogs				
Bacteremia, *Pseudomonas* sepsis	40–50	IV	6–8	prn
Cats				
Bacteremia, *Pseudomonas* sepsis	40	IV, IM	6	prn

ADDITIONAL DOSAGES. Gram-negative bacterial infections, Table 37–2; respiratory disease, Table 88–8; intra-abdominal infections, Table 89–15.

TINIDAZOLE

CLASS. Nitroimidazole.

ACTION. Bactericidal, antibacterial, also antiprotozoal; see METRONIDAZOLE, IPRONIDAZOLE.

MORE INFORMATION. See METRONIDAZOLE; Chapter 34; Chapter 71; Table 71–1; references: 34:137, 34:138, 34:140, 34:141.

PHARMACOKINETICS. Almost complete absorption (≥90%) from GI tract. Widely distributed in tissues and body fluids. Therapeutic concentrations also in gingival crevice fluid. Metabolized in liver to active metabolites. Repeated administration at the pharmacologic dose does not lead to drug accumulation. Elimination half-life 8.4 hr in cats, 4.4 hr in dogs. Unchanged drug and metabolites are excreted in urine and to lesser extent in feces. In people, half-life of tinidazole is longer than metronidazole, but there is no difference in dogs (34:140).

SPECTRUM. See METRONIDAZOLE. **Anaerobes:** Excellent activity against *Porphyromonas* spp in canine gingival crevice and most obligate anaerobes including β-lactamase–producing *Bacteroides.* **Others:** anaerobic protozoa *Giardia, Entamoeba, Trichomonas.* **Ineffective:** aerobic and facultative anaerobic bacteria. **More effective:** anaerobic bacteria and anaerobic protozoa.

INDICATIONS. Gingivitis, oral ulceration, periodontitis, abscesses, anal sacculitis, chronic diarrhea of bacterial or protozoal (giardiasis, amebiasis, balantidiasis) association, osteomyelitis, peritonitis, pyothorax, pyometra, animal bite wounds. Invasive amebiasis. Used like metronidazole but has a longer duration of action. See also METRONIDAZOLE.

CONTRAINDICATIONS. No dosage modification in renal failure. Avoid in pregnant or lactating animals.

ADVERSE REACTIONS. Vomiting and diarrhea, cutaneous reactions, thrombophlebitis after IV use, stomatitis, glossitis, dry mucous membranes, neutropenia, neurologic signs (vestibular), metallic taste.

INTERACTIONS. See METRONIDAZOLE.

Availability	Type	Sizes	Preparation (Company)
Human	Oral tablets Parenteral solution	150 mg, 500 mg 5 mg/ml	*Fasigyn* (Pfizer, Europe)

INTERNATIONAL PREPARATIONS. *Fasigyne, Simplotan, Sorquetan, Tricolam, Trimonase.*

HANDLING. See METRONIDAZOLE.

ADMINISTRATION. Delayed or reduced absorption with food. Often given as a single daily PO dose with or after feeding. It can also be given IV.

DOSAGE

Indications	Dose (mg/kg)	Route	Interval (hr)	Duration (days)
Dogs				
Stomatitis, anaerobic bacterial infections	15–25	PO	12	7
Cats				
Stomatitis, anaerobic bacterial infections	15	PO	24	7

ADDITIONAL DOSAGES. Enteric protozoal infections (e.g., *Giardia*), Table 78–2.

DISPENSING INFORMATION. Drug can be given with or without food.

TOBRAMYCIN

CLASS. Aminoglycoside.

ACTION. Bactericidal; inhibits bacterial protein synthesis.

MORE INFORMATION. GENTAMICIN, Chapter 34, Aminoglycosides; Table 34–5.

PHARMACOKINETICS. See GENTAMICIN.

SPECTRUM. See GENTAMICIN. Similar to gentamicin but more active against *Pseudomonas.*

INDICATIONS. Classically used to treat severe infections caused by *Pseudomonas, Proteus, Klebsiella, Enterobacter,* and *Escherichia.*

CONTRAINDICATIONS. See GENTAMICIN. Reduce dose in renal failure.

ADVERSE REACTIONS. Ototoxicity and nephrotoxicity, see GENTAMICIN. May be more nephrotoxic to cats than gentamicin or amikacin.

INTERACTIONS. See GENTAMICIN.

Availability	Type	Sizes	Preparation (Company)
Human	Solution for injection	10 mg/ml, 40 mg/ml	*Nebcin* (Eli Lilly)

INTERNATIONAL PREPARATIONS. *Brulamycin, Gernebcin, Mytobrin, Nebcina, Obracin, Tobral, Tobralex, Tobramaxin, Tobrex.*

HANDLING. Do not mix with other drugs before infusion. Store at room temperature. Do not use if becomes discolored.

ADMINISTRATION. IM: inject deep into large muscle. **IV:** dilute in 0.9% NaCl or 5% dextrose; administer slowly over 30–60 min.

DOSAGE

Indications	Dose (mg/kg)	Route	Interval (hr)	Duration (days)
Dogs				
Soft tissue, systemic infections	1–1.7	IV	8	<7
Systemic infections	2	SC	8–12	<7
Persistent bacteremia	3–5	IV, IM, SC	8	<7
Cats				
Soft tissue, systemic infections	2	IV, IM, SC	12	<5
Persistent bacteremia	2	IV, IM, SC	8	<5

*There is evidence that administration of higher dosages less frequently may reduce the toxic potential of aminoglycosides without reducing efficacy, thus, the total daily dose calculated can be administered once every 24 hr.

ADDITIONAL DOSAGES. Otitis externa topical, Table 85–6; bacteremia or endocarditis, Table 87–7; respiratory infections, Table 88–8, local ocular treatment, Table 93–4.

TOLTRAZURIL

CLASS. Triazinon.

ACTION. Antiprotozoal.

MORE INFORMATION. Chapter 71; Table 71–1.

SPECTRUM. Coccidia, *Hepatozoon.*

Availability	Type	Sizes	Preparation (Company)
Veterinary	Oral solution 2.5%	100 ml, 1L bottle	*Baycox* (Bayer)

DOSAGE

Indication (Dogs)	Dose (mg/kg)	Route	Interval (hr)	Duration (days)
Coccidiosis	5–20	PO	24	1
	7	PO	24	2

ADDITIONAL DOSAGES. Hepatozoonosis, Table 74–2; toxoplasmosis, Table 80–3; coccidiosis, Table 81–2.

TRIMETHOPRIM-SULFONAMIDE

CLASS. Pyrimidine and sulfonamide in 1:5 ratio.

ACTION. Bactericidal, antiprotozoal; synergistic blockade of microbial synthesis of folinic acid.

MORE INFORMATION. See ormetroprim-sulfonamide above, and trimethoprim-sulfonamide, Chapter 34; Table 34–10.

PHARMACOKINETICS. Well absorbed orally, rapid and complete. Wide distribution in body tissues. Most (60%–80%) excreted in urine of dogs as unchanged drug. Small amount metabolized by liver and renally excreted. Acetylated metabolites do not accumulate in dogs, which reduces risk of nephrotoxicity compared with cats and people.

SPECTRUM. Gram positive: some *Staphylococcus* (coagulase negative). **Gram negative:** *Escherichia, Proteus, Klebsiella, Enterobacter, Bordetella, Salmonella, Pasteurella; Nocardia* and *Brucella* at high doses. **Anaerobes:** *Fusobacterium, Clostridium.* Despite in vitro efficacy, in vivo effectiveness against anaerobes is poor. **Others:** *Pneumocystis;* weak against *Toxoplasma* (pyrimethamine-sulfonamide better); enteric coccidia; *Cyclospora, Acanthamoeba.* **Ineffective:** many *Pseudomonas, Mycobacterium, Leptospira, Erysipelothrix,* many anaerobes, including *Bacteroides, Mycoplasma.*

INDICATIONS. Uncomplicated urinary tract infection as a result of susceptible bacteria. *Pneumocystis* pneumonia, acute and chronic prostatitis, antimicrobial prophylaxis for immunocompromised host; bacterial CNS infections/meningitis in dogs and cats. Long-term, low-dose therapy for chronic urinary infections. Microsporidiosis.

CONTRAINDICATIONS. Reduce dose with renal dysfunction. Pregnancy: teratogenic at high doses to laboratory animals but safe at therapeutic dosages in dogs. Dogs with reduced Schirmer Tear test values. Doberman pinschers have a decreased ability to detoxify sulfonamide hydroxylamine metabolites resulting in increased susceptibility to toxicity (34:29). Avoid use in dogs with congenital bleeding disorders because they increase the potential risk of hemorrhage should thrombocytopenia develop (34:34, 34:35). Avoid in animals with pre-existing hepatic parenchymal disease, anemia, or leukopenia.

ADVERSE REACTIONS

1. Dogs: keratoconjunctivitis sicca (KCS), dogs weighing less than 12 kg appear more at risk. KCS can develop within 1 week of treatment and up to 7 mo after discontinuation (34:7, 34:32).
2. Hepatotoxicity—cholestatic hepatitis: anorexia, depression, icterus, hepatic necrosis, especially with pre-existing hepatobiliary disease (34:133, 34:162).
3. Megaloblastic—folate acid deficiency anemia; more dramatic in cats after several weeks; large doses and longer treatment will affect dogs. Dietary supplement with folinic acid (Leukovorin) at 2.5 mg/kg/day can overcome the folate deficiency. Folic acid supplementation should not be used because its activation to folinic acid is blocked by trimethoprim. With folinic supplements, effectiveness against enterococci and some protozoa is reduced.
4. Immune-mediated polyarthritis, retinitis, glomerulitis, vasculitis, serum sickness, anemia, thrombocytopenia, urticaria, erythema multiforme, toxic epidermal necrolysis, facial swelling, conjunctivitis (34:157). For skin reactions see cutaneous drug eruption, next. Seems more common in large-breed dogs; Doberman pinschers have shown a predilection for immune-complex complications. Signs usually develop 1–3 weeks after first use of the drug or within 1 hr to 10 days after repeated usage. Signs begin to subside within 24–48 hr of withdrawal of the drug and commencement of glucocorticoid therapy.
5. Cutaneous drug eruption—erythema multiforme, erythroderma, exfoliative dermatitis, urticaria, toxic epidermal necrolysis, vesiculobullous disease, otitis externa, pemphigus, and pemphigoid-like disease (34:31, 34:99, 34:101). Large-breed dogs, particularly Doberman pinschers and golden and Labrador retrievers, have been most affected (34:49). Fewer cases of sulfamethoxazole-induced immune reactions exist and those that do are of the cutaneous drug eruption.
6. Renal failure—sulfonamide nephromicrolithiasis, polydipsia, and polyuria primarily seen in cats.
7. Salivation, diarrhea, and vomiting—especially in cats given crushed or broken tablets. Cats may show consistent vomiting after PO dosing, which may necessitate parenteral therapy. Parenteral therapy can cause local irritation.
8. Ataxia has been observed in dogs and cats given higher therapeutic dosages. Signs usually disappear within 24–48 hr after therapy is discontinued.
9. May interfere with thyroid hormone synthesis as do other sulfonamides (see ORMETROPRIM-SULFONAMIDE). Chronic (6 weeks dosing) to euthyroid dogs results in decreased serum T_3, T_4 (34:54).
10. Hyperkalemia—interferes with renal potassium excretion.

INTERACTIONS. Prolongs effects of anticoagulants, diphenylhydantoin, increased blood levels or activity of dapsone, sulfonylureas.

Availability	Type	Sizes	Preparations (Company)
Human	Trimethoprim-sulfamethoxazole (1:5 ratio) oral tablets	480 mg, 960 mg	*Bactrim* (Roche), *Cotrim* (Lemmon); *Septra* (Burroughs Wellcome), generic (various)
	Oral suspension	240 mg/5 ml	*Bactrim; Septra;* generic (various)
	IV solution	480 mg/5 ml	*Bactrim* IV, *Septra* V
Veterinary	Trimethoprim-sulfadiazine (1:5 ratio)		
	Oral tablets (approved for dogs)	30 mg, 120 mg, 480 mg, 960 mg	*Delvoprim* (Mycofarm, UK), *Di-Trim* (Syntex); *Duphatrim* (Solvay-Duphar), *Tribrissen* (Schering-Plough Animal Health)
	Oral suspension (approved for dogs)	60 mg	*Tribrissen* oral suspension

INTERNATONAL PREPARATIONS. *Abactrim, Antrima, Chemitrim, Comox, Coptin, Cotribene, Eusaprim, Fectrim, Isotrim, Polytrim, Resprim, Septrin, Sulfatrim, Sulfotrim, Trimatrim, Ultrasept.*

HANDLING. Store all products at room temperature in airtight containers. Cats should be given whole tablets or PO suspension to avoid hypersalivation. Crushing tablets or putting them on food has little influence on the absorptive process. Once-daily dosing should only be used for treatment of chronic urinary and skin infections, and prophylaxis for urinary infections. Twice-daily dosing is more effective in eliminating established infection.

ADMINISTRATION. Concurrent treatment with folinic and (2.5 mg/kg/day) will reduce the potential of megaloblastic anemia in cats. Hemogram should be done weekly for the first 2 weeks to check for myelotoxic effects. Hematologic studies should be performed at least once a month thereafter if treatment is extended. Always provide plenty of drinking water. Parenteral solutions are used to treat severe infections and for use in comatose or vomiting animals.

DOSAGE

Indications	Dose (mg/kg)	Route	Interval (hr)	Duration (days)
Dogs				
Urinary, pyoderma	30	PO	24	14
Urinary, pyoderma, soft tissue infection	15	PO	12	14
Chronic pyoderma, acanthamebiasis	30	PO	12	21–42
Systemic, bacteremia	30–45	PO	12	3–5
Cats				
Urinary infections	30	PO	24	7–14
Urinary, soft tissue infections	15	PO	12	7–14
Coccidiosis (weight ≥4 kg)	30–60	PO	24	6
(weight < 4 kg)	15–30	PO	24	6

ADDITIONAL DOSAGES. Canine infectious tracheobronchitis, Table 6–1; enteric bacterial infections, Table 39–1; plague, Table 47–1, opportunistic mycobacterial infections, Table 50–5; hepatozoonosis, Table 74–2; toxoplasmosis, Table 80–3; neosporosis, Table 80–7; coccidial infections, Table 81–2; pneumocystosis, Table 83–2; canine pyoderma, Table 85–3; bacteremia, endocarditis, Table 87–7; respiratory infections, Table 88–8; gastrointestinal infections, Table 89–11; hepatobiliary infections, Table 90–4; urinary infections, Table 91–8; CNS infections, Table 92–5.

DISPENSING INFORMATION. Watch for systemic signs such as fever, lameness, vomiting, yellowing of mucosae, or lack of tear production.

TRIMETREXATE GLUCURONATE

CLASS. Diaminoquinazoline.

ACTION. Bacteriostatic, antibacterial, and antiprotozoal; inhibitor of enzyme dihydrofolate reductase.

MORE INFORMATION. Reference: 71:37.

PHARMACOKINETICS. Not absorbed well orally, must be given by IV route. Metabolized by liver and excreted in bile. Metabolites and some (10% to 30%) unchanged drug excreted in urine.

SPECTRUM. *Pneumocystis, Toxoplasma.*

INDICATIONS. *Pneumocystis* pneumonia refractory or resistant to trimethoprim-sulfas or pentamidine. As an adjunct or second choice to clindamycin in treatment of toxoplasmosis.

APPROVED USES. Human: *Pneumocystis* pneumonia refractory or resistant to trimethoprim-sulfas or pentamidine.

CONTRAINDICATIONS. Previous sensitivity. Pregnancy.

ADVERSE REACTIONS. Dermatologic eruption, myelosuppression, stomatitis, increased hepatic serum transaminases, vomiting or diarrhea, folic acid deficiency anemia or leukopenia. Fetotoxic and teratogenic.

INTERACTIONS. Co-administer with folinic acid (leucovorin) to minimize mammalian cell toxicity.

Availability	Type	Size	Preparations (Company)
Human	Powder for injection	25 mg vials	*Neutrexin* (US Bioscience)

HANDLING. Store powder at controlled room temperatures away from light. Wear gloves while handling. Just before use, reconstitute by adding 2 ml of 5% dextrose or sterile water until powder is completely dissolved without opacity. Further dilute with 5% dextrose to 0.5–2 mg/ml. Solution stable for 24 hr at room temperature or refrigerated. Discard unused drug after 24 hr.

ADMINISTRATION. Must be given concurrently with folinic acid for 3 days after last dose of trimetrexate. Give IV separately from the folinic acid through a flushed IV catheter. Give over 60 min every 6 hr. IV catheters must be flushed with 10 ml of 5% dextrose before and after administering drug.

DOSAGE

Indications	Dose	Route	Interval (hr)	Duration (days)
Human Pneumocystosis or Toxoplasmosis				
Trimetrexate	45 mg/m^2	IV	24	21
with				
folinic acid	20 mg/m^2	IV	6	24
Dog				
Trimetrexate	10 mg/kg	IV	24	21

ADDITIONAL DOSAGES. Pneumocystosis, Table 83–2.

DISPENSING INFORMATION. Recheck hemogram and biochemical tests every 2 weeks.

TYLOSIN

CLASS. Macrolide.

ACTION. Bacteriostatic, antibacterial, similar to erythromycin.

MORE INFORMATION. Chapter 34; reference: 34:142.

PHARMACOKINETICS. Absorbed primarily in the small intestine. Excreted in urine and bile.

SPECTRUM. Gram positive: *Streptococcus, Staphylococcus, Chlamydia, Mycoplasma.* **Gram negative:** *Campylobacter, Helicobacter.*

INDICATIONS. Campylobacteriosis, helicobacteriosis, inflammatory bowel disease, chronic colitis, upper respiratory tract infections in cats owing to *Mycoplasma, Chlamydia.* Bacterial sensitivity often follows that of erythromycin.

APPROVED USES. Food-producing animals.

CONTRAINDICATIONS. Pre-existing cardiac arrhythmia, cardiomyopathy, myocarditis.

ADVERSE REACTIONS. Pain and irritation with IM injection. Inject no more than 1–2 ml/site. Nausea and vomiting with PO administration. Wide safety margin. High dosages (200–400 mg/kg/day, given for a 2-year period) tolerated by clinically healthy dogs with no apparent side effects. Dosages as low as 5 mg/kg have increased the tendency of dogs to develop ventricular tachycardia after experimental myocardial ischemia. Contact dermatitis has developed in some veterinarians who handled the drug.

INTERACTIONS. Erythromycin, chloramphenicol, lincomycin, clindamycin have similar action and should not be used together.

Availability	Type	Sizes	Preparations (Company)
Veterinary	Soluble powder astartrate Injection	100 g containers (~3 g/teaspoon) 50 mg/ml; 200 mg/ml	*Tylan* soluble (Elanco) *Tylan* injection (Elanco); generic (Fermenta, Lextron)

HANDLING. Should not mix injectable product with other drugs. Store in airtight containers. Unstable at low pH forming an inactive degradation product, desmycosin.

ADMINISTRATION. PO powder: measured amounts placed on food or in gelatin capsules, or diluted with water and given by gavage. Wear gloves when handling, especially when applying the powder to food. Powder can be mixed with dextrose or cornstarch in a 1:9 ratio to make it ~300 mg/teaspoon for more convenient dosing amounts in small animals.

DOSAGE

Indications (Dogs and Cats)	Dose (mg/kg)	Route	Interval (hr)	Duration (days)
Staphylococcal pyoderma	20	PO	12	15–35
	10	PO	12	17–35
Upper respiratory disease,	6.5–12.5	IM	12	prn
inflammatory bowel	5–10	PO	12	prn
Clostridium perfringens diarrhea	20–40	PO	12–24	5–7

ADDITIONAL DOSAGES. Enteric bacterial infections, Table 39–1; *Clostridium perfringens*, Table 39–4; gastrointestinal infections, Table 89–11; colitis, Table 89–14.

DISPENSING INFORMATION. Use gloves when administering capsules or placing on food.

VANCOMYCIN

CLASS. Glycopeptide.

ACTION. Bactericidal; interferes with peptidoglycan biosynthesis in cell walls of replicating gram-positive bacteria. Less effect on cytoplasmic RNA synthesis.

MORE INFORMATION. See also TEICOPLANIN. Chapter 34; references: 34:71, 34:183a.

PHARMACOKINETICS. Not well absorbed orally. Given PO for treatment of bacterial enterocolitis. For systemic infections it is given parenterally (IV) because IM is painful After IV injection, fair penetration into body tissues. Clinically useful concentrations in tissues such as heart, lung, kidney, bone, synovial and peritoneal fluids. Primarily eliminated by kidneys via glomerular filtration. Concentration in inflamed meninges may be too low for therapeutic effects so that intrathecal administration would be needed. Similar low concentrations in pleural and pericardial fluids and bile.

SPECTRUM. Gram positive: some *Staphylococcus*, most *Streptococcus*, some *Enterococcus*, *Corynebacterium*. Some resistance to *Enterococcus* and *Staphylococcus* occurs. Combination with aminoglycoside increases activity against these organisms. Those with low-level resistance are still susceptible to teicoplanin; however, some *Enterococcus* have high-level resistance, but development of resistance during treatment is unknown. **Anaerobes:** *Clostridium difficile*, other *Clostridium*, *Bacillus anthracis*, *Actinomyces*. **Others:** *Entamoeba*. **More effective:** Gram positive. **Ineffective:** most gram negative bacteria except *Neisseria*, *Mycobacterium*.

INDICATIONS. Bacterial cholangiohepatitis in cats (34:71). Prophylaxis or treatment of staphylococcal or streptococcal septicemia or endocarditis, for clostridial enterocolitis, and for resistant of gram-positive bacterial infections. Resistant *Enterococcus* urinary infections. Prophylaxis for orthopedic surgery combined with aminoglycoside. Orally used to treat *Clostridium difficile*–associated diarrhea in people, a rare condition in animals; enterococcal or clostridial enterocolitis is more likely in dogs and cats that might require vancomycin.

CONTRAINDICATIONS. Reduce dosage in renal failure.

ADVERSE REACTIONS. If too rapid IV inoculation, anaphylaxis-like or urticarial reaction may occur. Preadministered antihistamine (H_1 antagonists) prevents the problem. In toxicity studies, dogs receiving bolus IV infusion developed hypotension and bradycardia. Reversible neutropenia and thrombocytopenia. Nephrotoxicity (hematuria, proteinuria, urine casts, azotemia) is infrequent and rare. May cause auditory ototoxicity.

INTERACTIONS. Concurrent administration of an aminoglycoside and sometimes rifampin potentiates the activity of vancomycin. Use with aminoglycosides may potentiate nephrotoxicity.

Availability	Type	Sizes	Preparations (Company)
Human	Powder for injection	500 mg; 1 g; 5 g	*Vancocin* (Lilly); *Lyphocin* (Lyphomed)
	Oral solution and capsules *(Pulvules)*	125-mg, 250-mg capsules; 1-g, 10-g solution bottles	*Vancocin*

INTERNATIONAL PREPARATIONS. *Vancocine, Vancoled, Vancor.*

HANDLING. Incompatible in IV solutions with chloramphenicol, glucocorticoids, aminophylline, methicillin, barbiturates, sodium bicarbonate, heparin. Parenteral solutions stable for 14 days if refrigerated as concentrated stock solution. In infusion bottles is only stable for 24 hr at room temperature but 60 days if refrigerated. The oral solution is reconstituted with distilled water and is stable in refrigerator for 2 weeks.

ADMINISTRATION. IV slowly over 30–60 min in 5% dextrose or 0.9% saline or lactated Ringer's. Rate should be less than 15 mg/min. For CNS infections, 5 mg is placed in CSF by intrathecal injection to provide a concentration of about 25 μg/ml. Given orally, it is not absorbed and reaches high intraluminal concentrations for treatment of enteric bacterial infections.

DOSAGE

Indications (Dogs)	Dose (mg/kg)	Route	Interval (hr)	Duration (days)
C. difficle enterocolitis	10–20	PO	6	5–7
Skin, urinary, soft tissue infections	10–20	IV	12	7–10
Systemic infection, bacteremia	15	IV	6	10

ADDITIONAL DOSAGES. Hepatobiliary infections, Table 90–4; local treatment ocular infections, Table 93–4.

DISPENSING INFORMATION. The oral solution may be given with small amounts of food or both. Keep refrigerated.

ZIDOVUDINE

Formerly AZIDOTHYMIDINE, AZT.

CLASS. Nucleoside (thymidine) analog.

ACTION. Antiviral; inhibits viral reverse transcriptase. Prevents infection of new cells but virus replication may continue when existing cells are already infected.

MORE INFORMATION. Chapter 2; Table 2–1; references: 2:3, 2:7, 2:8.

PHARMACOKINETICS. Absorbed rapidly and completely from GI tract. Has a short half-life. Widely distributed and penetrates well into CNS and CSF, crosses placenta. Metabolized in liver to inactive metabolites, and rapidly excreted in urine.

SPECTRUM. Retroviruses, feline leukemia virus (FeLV), feline immunodeficiency virus (FIV), some herpesviruses. Some resistance by FIV strains has been noted in vitro (2:17). Some antibacterial activity against Enterobacteriaceae and synergistic with trimethoprim-sulfonamide.

INDICATIONS. Clinically affected cats with FIV. Has been used in combination with investigational drug PMEA (2:3). Reduces viral replication and delays onset of immunodeficiency when given prophylactically to FIV infected cats (2:10). Higher doses (30 mg/kg day) did not affect viremia in FeLV-infected cats but reduced FOCMA antibody titers (2:9). Does not cure retroviral infections but reduces the risk of opportunistic infections.

APPROVED USES. Human use: for clinically affected people with HIV infection.

CONTRAINDICATIONS. Dose must be reduced or dosage interval increased with hepatic insufficiency.

ADVERSE REACTIONS. Myelosuppression, megaloblastic anemia at high dosages (30 mg/kg/day) in cats (2:9, 2:20). Hematocrit of treated cats declines within 3 weeks of initiating treatment to 60% of baseline (2:32, 2:33). Effectiveness at 50 mg/kg/day was greatest in suppressing viral replication but most toxic in causing myelosuppression and anemia. At 5 mg/kg every 8 hr, was effectively reduced clinical signs of FIV infection and less toxic (2:6). Neutropenia is less frequent than anemia. In people fever, malaise, GI signs, myalgia, rash also reported.

INTERACTIONS. Additive effect on FeLV, FIV if given concurrently with PMEA. Delayed metabolism of drug if coadministered with sulfonamides, narcotics, nonsteroidal antiinflammatory drugs.

Availability	Type	Sizes	Preparations (Company)
Human	Oral capsules	100 mg	*Retrovir* (Glaxo Wellcome)
	Oral syrup	50 mg/5 ml	*Retrovir*
	Solution for injection	10 mg/ml	*Retrovir*

HANDLING. Store capsules and syrup away from moisture and light. Store vials at 15°–25°C away from light. Injection: remove calculated dose from vial and add to 5% dextrose. Should not add to biologic fluids (plasma or blood). Stable after reconstitution for 24 hr at room temperature, 48 hr if refrigerated.

ADMINISTRATION. Can begin with IV infusions over 1 hr, given every 4 hr. Switch from IV to PO when able to tolerate it. Doses 30 mg/kg/day are more effective in suppressing virus, but are more myelotoxic to cats.

DOSAGE

Indication (Cats)	Dose (mg/kg)	Route	Interval (hr)	Duration (days)
FIV	10	SC	12	21
	10–20*	PO	8	≤77
	5	PO	8	≥42

[a]At higher dosages, cats have more chance for myelotoxicity. These are various doses published in the references listed under More Information.

ADDITIONAL DOSAGES. FIV Infection, Table 14–5; FeLV, under Antivirals and Immunotherapy, Chapter 13.

Dispensing Information: Return once weekly for physical examination and blood count evaluation.

Index

Note: Page numbers in *italics* refer to illustrations; page numbers followed by t refer to tables.

ISBN 0-7216-2737-4